Sixth Edition

OH'S INTENSIVE CARE MANUAL

Edited by

Andrew D Bersten MB BS MD FANZCA FJFICM

Professor, Department of Critical Care Medicine, Flinders Medical Centre and School of Medicine, Flinders University, Adelaide, Australia

Neil Soni MB Chb MD FANZCA FRCA FJFICM

Consultant in Intensive Care and Anaesthesia, Director and Lead Clinician, Intensive Care Unit, Magill Department of Anaesthesia, Intensive Care and Pain Management
Honorary Senior Lecturer, Imperial College Medical School, Chelsea and Westminster Hospital, London, UK

BUTTERWORTH HEINEMANN

ELSEVIER

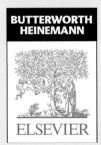

BUTTERWORTH
HEINEMANN
ELSEVIER

An imprint of Elsevier Limited

First published 1979
Second edition 1985
Third edition 1990
Fourth edition 1997
Fifth edition 2003
Sixth edition 2009
Reprinted 2009

ISBN 978-0-7020-3096-3

British Library Cataloguing in Publication Data
A catalogue record for this book is available from the British Library

Library of Congress Cataloging in Publication Data
A catalog record for this book is available from the Library of Congress

Notice
Medical knowledge is constantly changing. Standard safety precautions must be followed, but as new research and clinical experience broaden our knowledge, changes in treatment and drug therapy may become necessary or appropriate. Readers are advised to check the most current product information provided by the manufacturer of each drug to be administered to verify the recommended dose, the method and duration of administration, and contraindications. It is the responsibility of the practitioner, relying on experience and knowledge of the patient, to determine dosages and the best treatment for each individual patient. Neither the Publisher nor the authors assume any liability for any injury and/or damage to persons or property arising from this publication.

The Publisher

Printed in China
Last digit is the print number: 9 8 7 6 5 4 3 2

Contents

Contributors

Rinaldo Bellomo MB BS MD FRACP FCCP
Professor, Director of Intensive Care Research, Department of Intensive Care, Austin and Repatriation Medical Centre, Heidelberg, Victoria, Australia

Andrew D Bersten MB BS MD FANZCA FJFICM
Professor, Department of Critical Care Medicine, Flinders Medical Centre and School of Medicine, Flinders University, Adelaide, Australia

David Bihari FRCP FRACP FJFICM
Associate Professor, University of New South Wales, Lismore Base Hospital, Lismore, NSW, Australia

Stephen Brett MD FRCA
Consultant and Honorary Senior Lecturer in Intensive Care Medicine, Imperial College Healthcare NHS Trust, Department of Anaesthesia and Intensive Care, Hammersmith Hospital, London, UK

Craig Carr MB ChB MSc DA FRCA DICM
Head of Department of Intensive Care Medicine, The Royal Marsden Hospital, London, UK

Jeremy Cohen FRCA MRCP FJFICM
Staff Specialist, Department of Intensive Care, Royal Brisbane and Ipswich Hospitals, University of Queensland, Australia

Frances B Colreavy MBBch FFARCSI FJFICM
Department of Anaesthesia and Intensive Care, Mater Miseriocordiae, University Hospital, Dublin, Ireland

D J (Jamie) Cooper BMBS MD FRACP FJFICM
Professor of Medicine and Surgery, Monash University, Head Trauma Intensive Care, Alfred Hospital, Melbourne, Victoria, Australia

Lester A H Critchley BMedSci MBChB MD FFARCSI FHKAM
Department of Anaesthesia and Intensive Care, Prince of Wales Hospital, Shatin, Hong Kong, The People's Republic of China

Andrew R Davies MBBS FRACP FJFICM
Deputy Director of Intensive Care Unit, The Alfred Hospital, Melbourne, Victoria, Australia

Anthony Delaney MBBS MSc FACEM FJFICM
Senior Lecturer, Northern Clinical School, Faculty of Medicine, University of Sydney; Staff Specialist Intensive Care, Intensive Care Unit, Royal North Shore Hospital, St Leonards, NSW, Australia

Karl D Donovan MB FRACP FRCPI FJFICM
Specialist in Intensive Care, Intensive Care Unit, Royal Perth Hospital, Perth, WA, Australia

Graeme Duke MBBS FJFICM FANZCA
Critical Care Director, Critical Care Department, The Northern Hospital, Epping, Australia

Alan W Duncan MBBS FRCA FANZCA FJFICM
Director, Paediatric Intensive Care, Princess Margaret Hospital for Children, Perth, WA, Australia

Cyrus Edibam MBBS FFANZCA FJFICM
Senior Staff Specialist in Intensive Care, Department of Intensive Care Medicine, Royal Perth Hospital, Perth, WA, Australia

Evan Everest BSc ChB FRACP
Senior Consultant, Department of Critical Care Medicine, Flinders Medical Centre, Bedford Park, Adelaide, Australia

Patricia Figgis MBBS FRACP FJFICM
Staff Specialist, Department of Critical Care Medicine, Prince of Wales Hospital, Randwick, NSW, Australia

Simon Finfer MBBS FRCP FRCA FJFICM
Professor, Faculty of Medicine, University of Sydney; Senior Staff Specialist in Intensive Care, Intensive Care Unit, Royal North Shore Hospital, St Leonards, NSW, Australia

Malcolm McD Fisher AO MB CHB FJFICM FRCA MD
Clinical Professor, Anaesthesia and Medicine, University of Sydney; Senior Staff Specialist, Royal North Shore Hospital of Sydney, St Leonards, NSW, Australia

David Fraenkel BM BS FRACP
Princess Alexandria Hospital, Brisbane

Martyn A H French MB CRB MD FRCPath FRCP FRACP
Consultant Clinical Immunologist and Clinical Associate Professor in Pathology, Department of Clinical Immunology, Royal Perth Hospital, Perth, WA, Australia

Raffaele de Gaudio MD
Professor of Anaesthesiology and Intensive Care, Critical Care, University of Florence; Director of Anaesthesia and Intensive Care Unit, Ospedale di Careggi, Florence, Italy

Tony Gin MBChB BSc MD DipHSM FRCA FANZCA FHKAM
Professor, Department of Anaesthesia and Intensive Care, The Chinese University of Hong Kong, Prince of Wales Hospital, Shatin, Hong Kong, The People's Republic of China

David R Goldhill MA MBBS FRCA MD EDIC
Consultant, Anaesthesia and Intensive Care, The Royal National Orthopedics Hospital, Stanmore, UK

Charles D Gomersall N BSc FRCP FRCA EDIC FJFICM
Associate Professor, Department of Anaesthesia and Intensive Care, The Chinese University of Hong Kong, Shatin, Hong Kong, The People's Republic of China

Munita Grover BSc (Hons) MBBS FRCA
Specialist Registrar, Chelsea and Westminster Hospital, London, UK

Geoff A Gutteridge MBBS FANZCA FJFICM
Director of Intensive Care, Intensive Care Unit, Austin Hospital, Heidelberg, Victoria, Australia

Jonathan Handy BSc MBBS FRCA
Consultant Intensivist, Chelsea and Westminster Hospital; Honorary Senior Lecturer, Imperial College London, London, UK

Felicity Hawker MBBS FJFICM
Director, Intensive Care Unit, Cabrini Hospital, Malvern, Victoria, Australia

Michelle Hayes MD FRCA
Consultant in Anaesthesia and Intensive Care, Chelsea and Westminster Hospital, London, UK

Victoria Heaviside MB BS FRCA
Intensive Care Unit, Chelsea and Westminster Hospital

Peter V van Heerden MBBCh MMed (Anaes) PhD DA(SA) FFARCSI FANZCA FJFICM FCCP
Senior Intensive Care Specialist and Clinical Professor, Department of Intensive Care, Sir Charles Gardiner Hospital, Nedlands, Peryh, WA, Australia

Robert D Henning FRCA FJFICM DCH
Staff Specialist, Intensive Care Unit, Royal Children's Hospital, Parkside, Victoria, Australia

Bernard E F Hockings MB BS MD FRACP
Cardiologist and Clinical Associate, Professor of Medicine, University of Western Australia, Perth, WA, Australia

Andrew Holt MB BS FANZCA FFICANZCA
Critical Care Specialist, Department of Critical Care, Flinders Medical Centre, Bedford Park, Adelaide, Australia

Anwar Hussein BSc BMBCh DPhil FRCA
Consultant in Anaesthesia and Intensive Care Medicine, Epsom and St Helier University Hospitals NHS Trust, Epsom, Surrey, UK

James P Isbister MB BS BSc(Med) FRACP FRCPA
Clinical Professor of Medicine, Haematology and Transfusion Medicine, Sydney University; Clinical Professor of Medicine, Royal North Shore Hospital of Sydney, Sydney, NSW, Australia

Mandy Oade Jones PhD MSc MCSP SRP
Lecturer Physiotherapy, Brunel University, School of Health Science and Social Care, Uxbridge, Middlesex, UK

Gavin M Joynt MBBCh FFA(SA)(Crit Care) FHKCA(IC) FJFICM
Professor, Department of Anaesthesia and Intensive Care, The Chinese University of Hong Kong, Shatin, Hong Kong, The People's Republic of China

James A Judson MB ChB FFARACS FJFICM
Specialist Intensivist, Department of Critical Care Medicine, Auckland City Hospital, Auckland, New Zealand

Richard T Keays MB BS MD FRCP FRCA
Consultant Intensive Care Medicine, Magill Department of Anaesthetics, Chelsea and Westminster Hospital, London, UK

Warwick D Ngan Kee BHB MBChB MD FANZCA FHKCA FHKAM (Anesthesiology)
Professor, Director of Obstetric Anaesthesia, Department of Anaesthesia and Intensive Care, The Chinese University of Hong Kong; Department of Anaesthesia and Intensive Care, Prince of Wales Hospital, Shatin, Hong Kong, China

Angus M Kennedy MB BS MRCP MD
Consultant Neurologist, Chelsea and Westminster Hospital, London, UK

Geoff Knight FRACP FJFICM
Intensive Care Physician, PICU Princess Margaret Hospital for Children, Perth, WA, Australia

Richard Leonard BA MB BChir FRCP FRCA FANZCA FJFICM
Director, Intensive Care Unit, St Mary's Hospital, London, UK

Jeffrey Lipman MBBCh DA FFA(Crit Care) FJICM
Professor and Head, Anaesthesiology and Critical Care, University of Queensland; Director, Department of Intensive Care Medicine, Royal Brisbane and Women's Hospital, Brisbane, Queensland, Australia

David P Mackie MB ChB FRCA
Anesthesiologist/Intensivist, Red Cross Hospital, Beverwijk, The Netherlands

Neil T Matthews MB BS(NSW) FJFICM FANZCA
Senior Lecturer in Paediatrics, University of Adelaide; Director, Department of Paediatric Critical Care Medicine, Women's and Children's Hospital, Adelaide, Australia

Colin McArthur MBChB FANZCA FJFICM
Clinical Director, Department of Critical Care Medicine, Auckland City Hospital, Auckland, New Zealand

Angela McLuckie FRCA FJFICM
Consultant Intensivist and Clinical Lead for Critical Care, Guy's and St Thomas' NHS Foundation Trust, Department of Critical Care, London, UK

Fiona Herris Moffatt MSc BSc (Hons) MCSP SRP
Clinical Specialist Physiotherapist Critical Care Outreach Team, Nottingham University Hospital NHS Trust (Queen's Medical Centre), Ruddington, Nottingham, UK

Cliff J Morgan BM FRCA
Consultant in Critical Care and Anaesthesia, Department of Critical Care and Anaesthesia, Royal Brompton Hospital, London, UK

Thomas John Morgan MBBS FJFICM
Senior Specialist, Intensive Care Unit, Mater Adult Hospital, South Brisbane, Queensland, Australia

Peter T Morley MBBS FRACP FANZCA FJFICM
Clinical Associate Professor, School of Population Health, Faculty of Medicine, Dentistry and Health Sciences, The University of Western Australia, Clinical Associate Professor, Department of Medicine, Royal Melbourne & Western Hospitals, The University of Melbourne; Intensive Care Unit, Royal Melbourne Hospital, Victoria, Australia

Raymond G Morris PhD
Chief Medical Scientist, Associate Professor of Clinical Pharmacology, Department of Clinical Pharmacology, The Queen Elizabeth Hospital, Woodville, South Australia

Blair Munford BMedSc MBChB FANZCA
Senior Retrieval Specialist, NRMA CareFlight, Westmead Hospital, Westmead, Australia

John A Myburgh PhD FJFICM
Professor of Critical Care, University of New South Wales, Department of Intensive Care Medicine, St George Hospital, Sydney, Australia

Michael Mythen MD MBBS FRCA
Smiths Medical Professor of Anaesthesia and Crtitical Care, University College London, London, UK

Matthew T Naughton MD FRACP
Head, General Respiratory and Sleep Medicine, Department of Allergy, Immunology and Respiratory Medicine, Alfred Hospital, Melbourne, Victoria, Australia

Alistair D Nichol BA MB BCh BAO FRCARCSI
Senior Research Fellow, Australian New Zealand Intensive Care Research Center, Department of Epidemiology and Preventative Medicine, Monash University, Melbourne, Victoria, Australia

Helen Ingrid Opdam MBBS FJFICM FRACP
Intensive Care Specialist, Austin Hospital Intensive Care Unit, Victoria, Australia

Simon P G Padley MB BS BSc MRCP FRCR
Consultant Radiologist and Honorary Lecturer, Department of Radiology, Chelsea and Westminster Hospital, London, UK

Mark Palazzo MB ChB FRCA FRCP MD
Chief of Service Critical Care Medicine, Hammersmith Hospitals NHS Trust, London, UK

Marcus Peck MBBS MRCP FRCA
Specialist Registrar in Anaesthesia and Intensive Care Medicine, The National Hospital for Neurology and Neurosurgery, Queen Square, London, UK

Michael E Pelly MSc (Clin TropMed) FRCP DTM+H
Consultant Physician, Chelsea and Westminster Hospital, London, UK

David V Pilcher MBBS MRCP FRACP FJFICM
Consultant in Intensive Care, The Alfred Hospital, Melbourne, Victoria, Australia

Didier Pittet MD MS
Director, Infection Control Program, University of Geneva Hospital, Geneva, Switzerland

Brad Power MBBS FRACP FJFICM
Director of Intensive Care, Joondalup Health Campus, Joondalup, Sir Charles Gairdner Hospital, NedLands Perth, WA, Australia

Raymond F Raper MBBS BA MD FRACP FJFICM
Head, Intensive Care Unit, Royal North Shore Hospital, Sydney, NSW, Australia

Bernard Riley MBE BSc MBBS FRCA
Consultant, Adult Critical Care, Queen's Medical Centre, University Hospital, Nottingham, UK

John E Sanderson MA MD FRCP FACC
Professor of Clinical Cardiology, Department of Cardiovascular Medicine, The Medical School, University of Birmingham, Edgbaston, Birmingham, UK

Hugo Sax MD
Consultant Physician, Infection Control Program, University of Geneva Hospitals, Geneva, Switzerland

Frank A Shann MB BS MD FRACP FJFICM
Professor of Critical Care Medicine, Department of Paediatrics, University of Melbourne; Staff Specialist in Intensive Care, Royal Children's Hospital, Melbourne, Victoria, Australia

Ramachandran Sivakumar MD MRCP
Consultant Physician, Ipswich Hospital, Ipswich, UK

Elizabeth Sizer MBDS FRCA
Senior Trainee in Intensive Care of Anaesthetics, Institute of Liver Studies, King's College Hospital, London, UK

George A Skowronski MBBS(Hons) FRCP FRACP FJFICM
Conjoint Associate Professor, Anaesthetics, Intensive Care and Emergency Medicine, Faculty of Medicine, University of New South Wales; Senior Staff Specialist,

Department of Intensive Care, St George Hospital, Sydney, NSW, Australia

Anthony J Slater BMed SCMB BS FRACP FJFICM
Senior Staff Specialist, Department of Paediatric Critical Care Medicine, North Adelaide, Australia

Martin Smith MBBS FRCA
Consultant in Neuroanaesthesia and Neurocritical Care, The National Hospital for Neurology and Neurosurgery, University College London Hospitals, London, UK

Neil Soni MB ChB FANZCA FRCA MD FJFICM
Consultant in Intensive Care and Anaesthesia, Director and Lead Clinician, Intensive Care Unit, Magill Department of Anaesthesia, Intensive Care and Pain Management; Hon. Senior Lecturer, Imperial College Medical School, Chelsea and Westminster Hospital, London, UK

Stephen J Streat BSc MB ChB, FRACP
Intensivist, Department of Critical Care Medicine; Clinical Director, Organ Donation New Zealand; Honorary Clinical Associate Professor, Department of Surgery, Auckland City Hospital, New Zealand

David J Sturgess MBBS FRACGP
Intensive Care Fellow, Department of Intensive Care, The Wesley Hospital, Brisbane, Queensland, Australia

Joseph J Y Sung MD PhD FRCP FRACP FRCP(Edin) FRCP (Glas) FACG FHKAM FHKCP
Professor of Medicine, Department of Medicine and Therapeutics, The Chinese University of Hong Kong; Honorary Consultant, Prince of Wales Hospital, Shatin, Hong Kong, The People's Republic of China

Ian K S Tan MBBS MRCP (UK) FHKCA FHKCA (Int Care) FANZCA FJFICM
Consultant Intensivist, Director, Critical Care Services, Mount Elizabeth Hospital, Singapore

Chris Theaker RGN
Clinical Research Fellow, Intensive Care, Chelsea and Westminster Hospital, London, UK

James Tibballs MB BS BMedSci(Hons) MEd MBA MD MHlth & MedLaw FANZCA FJFICM FACTM
Associate Professor, Australian Venom Research Unit, Department of Pharmacology and Department of Paediatrics, The University of Melbourne; Associate Director, Paediatric Intensive Care Unit, Royal Children's Hospital, Melbourne, Victoria, Australia

David Treacher MA FRCP
Consultant in Intensive Care, and Clinical Physiology, St Thomas' Hospital, Guy's and St Thomas' NHS Foundation Trust, London, UK

David V Tuxen MB BS FRACP DipDHM MD FJFICM
Senior Intensivist, Intensive Care Office, The Alfred Hospital, Melbourne, Victoria, Australia

Richard N Upton BSc PhD
Principal Medical Scientist, Royal Adelaide Hospital, Adelaide, Australia

Balasubramanian Venkatesh MBBS MD(IntMed) FRCA FFARCSI MD(UK) FFICANZCA
Professor of Medicine, Princess Alexandra and Wesley Hospitals, University of Queensland, Brisbane, Australia; Department of Intensive Care, Princess Alexandra Hospital, Queensland, Australia

Adrian T J Wagstaff BSc(Hons) MBBS(Hons) MRCP FRCA
Clinical Research Fellow, Magill Department of Anaesthesia, Intensive Care and Pain Management, Imperial College London, London, UK

Carl S Waldmann MA MB BChir FRCA EDICM
Consultant in Intensive Care and Anaesthesia, Royal Berkshire Hospital, Reading, UK

John R Welch BSc(Hons) MSc RGN ENB 100
Nurse Consultant, Critical Care, Kingston Hospital, Kingston upon Thames, UK

Julia Wendon MBChB FRCP
Senior Lecturer and Consultant in Intensive Care, Institute of Liver Studies, King's College Hospital, London, UK

Steve Wesselingh BMBS PhD FRACP
Dean, Monash University, Melbourne, Australia

Ubbo F Wiersema MBBS FRACP FJFICM
Intensivist, Department of Intensive Care Medicine, Middlemore Hospital; Cardiothoracic and Vascular Intensive Care Unit, Auckland City Hospital, Auckland, New Zealand

Duncan LA Wyncoll MB BS FRCA EDIC DipICM(UK)
Consultant Intensivist Guy's and St Thomas' NHS Foundation Trust, London, UK

Steve M Yentis BSc MBBS FRCA MD MA
Consultant Anaesthetist, Department of Anaesthesia, Chelsea and Westminster Hospital, London, UK

Preface to the sixth edition

In the five years since the last edition there have been significant advances in most areas of intensive care medicine as the specialty has continued to evolve. This has included continued insights into both normal biology and disease, translation of this knowledge to the bedside, and results from large clinical trials directly relevant to clinical practice. Concurrently, health care professionals, patients and their relatives have unparalleled access to new knowledge through the internet. The original manual sought to provide useful and usable information at the bedside by distilling the immense amount of available information into a relevant and practical format. The burgeoning information highway that is the web does present a real challenge to a new edition of *Oh's Intensive Care Manual* but it also mandates this edition, which seeks to make that information more readily usable at the bedside. Well-known and well-respected clinicians have once again produced an edition that presents a current framework with the most up-to-date contextual references which we hope will be an important and practical contribution to the practice of intensive care medicine.

Many chapters have been extensively updated, and a number of new authors have faced the difficulty of summarising their field and choosing the key new references. While trying to prevent the manual from becoming any larger, we also felt the increasing importance and contribution of large clinical trials required a specific chapter. However, given the vast area of knowledge covered by the manual, there will be times when the reader wants further detail. The sixth edition will have been a success if it provides a clear framework for additional detail, and if it cites most of the key references. Indeed, this has been the successful format of previous editions that has made them so useful. More importantly, the sixth edition will have been worthwhile if it continues to make a positive contribution to the care of the critically ill.

ADB
NS

ACKNOWLEDGEMENTS

Since the fifth edition we have received a lot of feedback from readers. We are thankful for constructive comments received from medical students, residents, trainees, colleagues, nurses and other health professionals. Hopefully some of the issues have been addressed. Without the great efforts of the authors, their colleagues and mentors and publishers there would not be a sixth edition. We also thank our wives and children (Libby, Eleanor, David and Ben; Alison, Kate and Ben) for their unfailing and generous support.

ADB
NS

Part One

Organisational Aspects

1

Design and organisation of intensive care units

Felicity Hawker

An intensive care unit (ICU) is a specially staffed and equipped area of a hospital dedicated to the management of patients with life-threatening illnesses, injuries or complications. ICUs developed from the postoperative recovery rooms and respiratory units of the 1920s, 1930s and 1940s when it became clear that concentrating the sickest patients in one area was beneficial. Intermittent positive-pressure ventilation (IPPV) was pioneered in the treatment of respiratory failure in the 1948–1949 poliomyelitis epidemic and particularly in the 1952 Copenhagen poliomyelitis epidemic when IPPV was delivered using an endotracheal tube and a manual bag.[1] Subsequently mechanical ventilators were developed and became increasingly used for the treatment of thoracic surgery, general surgery, tetanus and 'crushed chests'.

The 1970s saw a heightened interest in intensive care medicine, with research into the pathophysiological processes, treatment regimens and outcomes of the critically ill and the founding of specialty journals, training programmes and qualifications dedicated to intensive care. Modern intensive care or critical care medicine is not limited to postoperative care or mechanical ventilation. It is a separate specialty and, although some period of training in an ICU is valuable to all specialties, it can no longer be regarded as 'part of' anaesthesia, medicine, surgery or any other discipline.

As outlined below, the ICU is not just a ward but a department with dedicated medical, nursing and allied health staff: it operates with defined policies and procedures and has its own quality improvement, continuing education and research programmes. Through its care of critically ill patients in the ICU and its outreach activities (see Chapter 2), the intensive care department provides an integrated service to the hospital, without which many programmes (e.g. cardiac surgery, trauma, transplantation) could not function.

CLASSIFICATION AND ROLE DELINEATION OF AN ICU

The delineation of roles of hospitals in a region or area is necessary to rationalise services and optimise the use of resources. Each ICU should similarly have its role in the region defined and should support the defined duties of its hospital. In general, small hospitals require ICUs that provide basic intensive care. Critically ill patients who need complex management and sophisticated investigative back-up should be managed in an ICU located in a large tertiary referral hospital. Three levels of adult ICUs are classified as follows by the Joint Faculty of Intensive Care Medicine (Australia and New Zealand).[2] The European Society of Intensive Care Medicine has a similar classification.[3] The American College of Critical Care Medicine also has a similar classification but uses a reversed-numbering system.[4] It should be noted that full-time directors and directors with qualifications in intensive care medicine are less common in the USA,[5] as are the requirement for a dedicated doctor for the ICU around the clock and referral to the attending ICU specialist for management.[6]

1. *Level I adult ICU*: a level I adult ICU has a role in small district hospitals. It provides resuscitation and short-term cardiorespiratory support of critically ill patients and monitors and prevents complications in 'at-risk' medical and surgical patients. It is capable of providing mechanical ventilatory support and simple invasive cardiovascular monitoring for a limited period. The medical director should be an intensive care specialist. Referral and transport policies are required.
2. *Level II adult ICU*: a level II adult ICU is located in larger general hospitals. It provides a high standard of general intensive care, including multisystem life support, in accordance with the role of its hospital (e.g. regional centre for acute medicine, general surgery, trauma). It has a medical officer on site and access to pharmacy, pathology and radiological facilities at all times, but may not have all forms of complex therapy and investigations (e.g. interventional radiology, cardiac surgical service). The medical director and at least one other consultant are intensive care specialists. Patients admitted are referred to the attending intensive care specialists for management. Referral and transport policies are required.

Table 1.1 UK classification of critical care beds

Level 0
Patients whose needs can be met through normal ward care in an acute hospital
Level I
Patients at risk of their condition deteriorating, or those recently relocated from higher levels of care whose needs can be met on an acute ward with additional advice and support from the critical care team
Level II
Patients requiring more detailed observation or intervention, including support for a single failing organ system or postoperative care, and those stepping down from higher levels of care
Level III
Patients requiring advanced respiratory support alone or basic respiratory support together with support of at least two organ systems. This level includes all complex patients requiring support for multiorgan failure (http://www.ics.ac.uk/icmprof/downloads/icsstandards-levelsofca.pdf)

3. *Level III adult ICU*: a level III adult ICU is located in a major tertiary referral hospital. It should provide all aspects of intensive care required by its referral role for indefinite periods. The unit is staffed by specialist intensivists with trainees, critical care nurses, allied health professionals and clerical and scientific staff. Complex investigations and imaging and support by specialists of all disciplines required by the referral role of the hospital are available at all times. All patients admitted to the unit must be referred to the attending intensive care specialist for management.

The classification of types of ICU must not be confused with the description of critical care beds throughout a hospital, as with the UK classification of critical care beds (Table 1.1).

TYPE AND SIZE OF AN ICU[2]

Within each of these classifications, an ICU may not be able to provide intensive care for all subspecialties, or may need to be more oriented towards a particular area of expertise (e.g. neurosurgery, cardiac surgery, burns or trauma). An institution may organise its intensive care beds into multiple units, under separate management by single-discipline specialists, for example, medical ICU, surgical ICU and burns ICU. Although this may be functional in some hospitals, Australasian experience has favoured the development of general multidisciplinary ICUs. Thus, with the exception of dialysis units, coronary care units (CCUs) and neonatal ICUs, critically ill patients are admitted to the hospital's multidisciplinary ICU and are managed by intensive care specialists (or paediatric intensivists in paediatric hospitals).

There are good economic and operational arguments for a multidisciplinary ICU as against separate, single-discipline ICUs. Duplication of equipment and services is avoided. Critically ill patients develop the same pathophysiological processes no matter whether they are classified as medical or surgical and they require the same approaches to support of vital organs. Doctors without intensive care training lack the experience and expertise to deal with the complexities of multiorgan failure.

The number of ICU beds in a hospital usually ranges from 1 to 4 per 100 total hospital beds. This depends on the role and type of ICU. Multidisciplinary ICUs require more beds than single-specialty ICUs, especially if high-dependency beds are integrated into the unit. ICUs with fewer than four beds are considered not to be cost-effective and are too small to provide adequate clinical experience for skills maintenance for medical and nursing staff. On the other hand, the emerging trend of ICUs having 26[7] or more beds creates major management problems. Although the evidence is scant, there is a suggestion that efficiency deteriorates once the number of critically ill patients per medical team exceeds 12.[8] Consequently two or more medical teams may need to work together in these 'mega-units'.

HIGH-DEPENDENCY UNIT (HDU)[9,10]

An HDU is a specially staffed and equipped area of a hospital that provides a level of care intermediate between intensive care and general ward care. Although HDUs may be located in or near specialty wards, increasingly they are located within or immediately adjacent to an ICU complex and are often staffed by the ICU personnel.

The HDU provides invasive monitoring and support for patients with or at risk of developing acute (or acute on chronic) single-organ failure, particularly where the predicted risk of clinical deterioration is high or unknown. It may act as a 'step-up' or 'step-down' unit between the level of care delivered on a general ward and intensive care, but does not normally accept patients requiring mechanical ventilation. Several older studies have shown benefits to outcome associated with the introduction of HDUs,[9] whereas a more recent study has questioned these findings.[11]

PAEDIATRIC ICU (PICU)[2]

A PICU is a separate area in the hospital capable of providing complex, multisystem life support for indefinite periods to infants and children less than 16 years of age. It is a tertiary referral centre for children needing intensive care and has extensive back-up laboratory and clinical services to support this tertiary role. Consultants in a PICU are paediatric intensive care specialists with expertise different from their adult intensive care colleagues. All patients admitted to the PICU are referred to the attending PICU specialists for management.

DESIGN OF AN ICU[1,3,12]

The ICU should be sited in close proximity to relevant acute areas, that is, operating rooms, emergency department, CCU, labour ward and acute wards, and to investigational departments (e.g. radiology department, cardiac catheterisation laboratory). Safe transport of critically ill patients to and from the ICU should be facilitated by sufficient numbers of lifts and these, with doors and corridors, should be spacious enough to allow easy passage of beds and equipment – vital points often ignored by 'planning experts'.

There should be a single entry and exit point, attended by the unit receptionist. Through traffic of goods or people to other hospital areas must never be allowed. An ICU should have areas and rooms for public reception, patient management and support services. The whole unit should be 2.5–3 times the area of the specific patient care areas.

PATIENT AREAS

Each patient bed area in an adult ICU requires a minimum floor space of 20 m^2 (215 ft^2), with single rooms being larger (at least 25 m^2), to accommodate patient, staff and equipment without overcrowding. The ratio of single-room beds to open-ward beds will depend on the role and type of the ICU, but with a recommended range of between 1:6 and 1:2. They should be equipped with an anteroom of 2.5 m^2. Single rooms are essential for isolation and, less importantly, privacy for conscious long-stay patients. The emergence of resistant bacterial strains in ICUs around the world has increased the need for isolation facilities in recent years. A non-splash hand wash basin with elbow- or foot-operated taps should be close to each bed and a hand disinfection facility at each bed.

Bedside service outlets should conform to local standards and requirements (including electrical safety and emergency supply, such as to the Australian Standard, Cardiac Protected Status AS3003).

Utilities per bed space as recommended for a level III ICU are:

- 4 oxygen
- 3 air
- 3 suction
- 16–20 power outlets
- a bedside light
- a telephone and data outlets

Adequate and appropriate lighting for clinical observation must be available. How the services are supplied (e.g. from floor column, wall-mounted, or ceiling-pendant) depends on individual preferences. There should be room to place or attach additional portable monitoring equipment and, as much as possible, equipment should be kept off the floor. Space for charts, syringes, sampling tubes, pillows, suction catheters and patient personal belongings should be available, often in a moveable bedside trolley.

All central staff and patient areas must have large clear windows. Lack of natural light and windowless ICUs give rise to patient disorientation and increased stress to all. Efforts should be made to reduce sound transmission and therefore noise levels, e.g. walls and ceilings should be constructed of materials with high sound-absorbing capability. Suitable and safe air quality should be maintained at all times. Air conditioning and heating should be provided with an emphasis on patient comfort.

Since critical care nursing is at the bedside, staffing of a central nurse station is less important than in a CCU. Nevertheless, the central station and other work areas should have adequate space for staff to work in comfort and situated so that patients can be seen. This central station usually houses a central monitor, satellite pharmacy and drug preparation area, satellite storage of sterile and non-sterile items, telephones, computers with internet connections, patient records, reference books and policy and procedure manuals. A dedicated computer for the picture archive and communication system (PACS) or a multidisplay X-ray viewer should be located within the patient care area.

STORAGE AND SUPPORTING SERVICES AREAS

Storage areas should take up a total floor space of about 25–30% of all the patient and central station areas. They should have separate access remote from the patient area for deliveries and be no farther than 30 m from the patient area. Frequently used items (e.g. intravenous fluids and giving sets, sheets and dressing trays) should be located closer to patients than infrequently used or non-patient items. There should be an area for storing emergency and transport equipment within the patient area with easy access to all beds.

Floor areas for supporting services should make up about 20–25% of the patient and central station areas. Utility rooms must be clean and separate, each with its own access. Disposal of soiled linen and waste must be catered for, including contaminated items from infectious patients, using one-way traffic schemes. Facilities for estimating blood gases, glucose, electrolytes, haemoglobin, lactate and sometimes clotting status are usually sufficient for the unit's laboratory. There should be a pneumatic tube or other system to transfer specimens to pathology. A good communication network of phones/intercoms is vital to locate and inform staff quickly. Adequate arrangements for offices, doctor-on-call rooms, staff lounge (with food/drinks facilities), wash rooms, education (seminar room) and a waiting room (see below) complete the unit.

RELATIVES AREA

Apart from a waiting room, levels II and III ICUs should have a separate room to interview and comfort distressed relatives. There should be facilities for tea/coffee making and a water dispenser and toilets should be located close by. Television and/or music should be provided.

STAFFING[2–5]

The level of staffing depends on the type of hospital and a tertiary hospital ICU requires a large team. Whatever the size of the team, it is crucial that there is free communication and collaboration among team members and a true multidisciplinary approach. Knaus *et al.* in a classic study[13] first showed a relationship between the degree of coordination in an ICU and the effectiveness of its care. Other studies have shown relationships between collaboration and teamwork and better outcomes for patients and staff.[14,15] Inadequate communication is the most frequent root cause of sentinel events.[16]

MEDICAL STAFF[17]

An intensive care department should have a medical director who is qualified in intensive care medicine and who coordinates the clinical, administrative and educational activities of the department. The duties of the director should involve patient care, supervision of trainees/other junior doctors, the drafting of diagnostic and therapeutic protocols, responsibility for the quality, safety and appropriateness of care provided and education, training and research. It is recommended that the director be full-time in the department.

The director should be supported by a group of other specialists trained in intensive care medicine who provide patient care and contribute to non-clinical activities. In an ICU of level II or III there must be at least one specialist exclusively rostered to the unit at all times. Specialists should have a significant or full-time commitment to the ICU ahead of clinical commitments elsewhere. There should be sufficient numbers to allow reasonable working hours, protected non-clinical time and leave of all types. The recent increase in ICU outreach activities (medical emergency team calls, outpatient review: see Chapter 2) has increased the workload of intensive care specialists as well as junior staff in many hospitals, resulting in the need to increase the size of the medical team.

There should also be at least one junior doctor with an appropriate level of experience rostered exclusively to level II and III units at all times. Junior medical staff in the ICU may be intensive care trainees, but should ideally also include trainees of other acute disciplines (e.g. anaesthesia, medicine and surgery). It is imperative that junior doctors are adequately supervised, with specialists being readily available at all times.

This physician staffing model has been used in Australia and New Zealand for many years, but has not been common in the USA. A systematic review[18] has shown that when there has been mandatory intensivist consultation (or closed ICU – see below) compared with no or elective intensivist consultation or open ICU, both ICU and hospital survival were improved and there was a reduced length of stay in ICU and in hospital.

NURSING STAFF

Critical care nursing is covered in Chapter 6. The bedside nurse conducts the majority of patient assessment, evaluation and care in an ICU. In ICUs supporting tertiary hospitals 1:1 nursing is required for all ventilated patients, whereas one nurse per two patients is appropriate for HDU patients. Some complex patients with multiple supports may require more than one nurse. When leave of all kinds is factored in, long-term 24-hour cover of a single bed requires a staff complement of six nurses. Nurse shortages have been shown to be associated with increased patient mortality and nurse burnout and adversely affect outcome and job satisfaction in the ICU.[19,20]

There should be a nurse manager who is appointed with authority and responsibility for the appropriateness of nursing care and who has extensive experience in intensive care nursing as well as managerial experience. In tertiary units the nurse manager should participate in teaching, continuing education and research. Ideally, all nurses working in an ICU should have training and certification in critical care nursing.

ALLIED HEALTH

Major ICUs must have 24-hour access to pathology and radiological services. Access to physiotherapists, dieticians, social workers and other therapists should also be available. A dedicated ward clinical pharmacist is invaluable and participation of a pharmacist on ward rounds has been associated with a reduction in adverse drug events.[21] Respiratory therapists are allied health personnel trained in and responsible for the equipment and clinical aspects of respiratory therapy, a concept well established in North America, but not the UK, continental Europe and Australasia. Technical support staff,[22] either as members of the ICU staff, or seconded from biomedical departments, are necessary to service, repair and develop equipment.

OTHER STAFF

Provision should be made for adequate secretarial support.[23] Transport and 'lifting' orderly teams will reduce physical stress and possible injuries to nurses and doctors. If no mechanical system is available to transport specimens to the laboratories (e.g. air-pressurised chutes), sufficient and reliable couriers must be provided to do this day and night. The cleaning personnel should be familiar with the ICU environment and infection control protocols. There should also be a point of contact for local interpreters, chaplains, priests or officials of all religions, when there is need for their services.

CLINICAL ACTIVITIES

OPERATIONAL POLICIES[2]

Clear-cut administrative policies are vital to the functioning of an ICU. An *open* ICU has unlimited access to multiple doctors who are free to admit and manage their patients. A *closed* ICU has admission, discharge and referral policies under the control of intensivists. Improved cost benefits are likely with a closed ICU and patient outcomes are better, especially if the intensivists have full clinical responsibilities.[18,24] Consequently ICUs today, especially levels II and III, should be *closed* under the charge of a medical specialist director. All patients admitted to the ICU are referred to the director and his/her specialist staff for management, although it is important for the ICU team to communicate regularly with the parent unit and to make referrals to specialised services when appropriate.

There must be clearly defined policies for admission, discharge, management and referral of patients. Lines of responsibilities must be delineated for all staff members and their job descriptions defined. The director must have final overall authority for all staff and their actions, although in other respects each group may be responsible to respective hospital heads, for example, director of nursing.

Policies for the care of patients should be formulated and standardised. They should be unambiguous, periodically reviewed and familiarised by all staff. Examples include infection control and isolation policies, policies for intra- and interfacility transport, end-of-life policies (e.g. do not resuscitate (DNR) procedure) and sedation and restraint protocols. It should be noted, however, that when protocols involve complex issues (such as weaning from mechanical ventilation) they may be less efficient than the judgement of experienced clinicians.[25] Clinical management protocols, e.g. for feeding and bowel care, can be laminated and placed in a folder at each bed or loaded on to the intranet.

EQUIPMENT

The type and quantity of equipment will vary with the type, size and function of the ICU and must be appropriate to the workload of the unit. There must be a regular programme in place for checking its safety. Protocols and in-service training for medical and nursing staff must be available for the use of all equipment, including steps to be taken in the event of malfunction. There should also be a system in place for regular maintenance and service. The intensive care budget should include provision to replace old or obsolete equipment at appropriate times. A system of stock control should be in place to ensure consumables are always in adequate supply. The ICU director should have a major role in the purchase of new equipment to ensure it is appropriate for the activities of the unit.

PATIENT CARE

ICU patient management should be multidisciplinary, with medical, nursing and other staff working together to provide the best care for each patient. The critical care nurse is the primary carer at the bedside and monitors, manages and supports the critically ill patient (see Chapter 6). The medical team consists of one or more registrars, residents or fellows who direct medical care with an intensive care specialist. The patient should be assessed by a formal ward round of the multidisciplinary team twice daily, usually at a time when the junior medical staff are handing over from one shift to the next. The nurse coordinating the floor and in larger units allied health staff such as pharmacists and dieticians also take part. Each patient should be assessed clinically (examination, observations and pathology, radiological and other investigation results), the medication chart reviewed, progress determined and a management plan developed for the immediate and longer term. The ward round is also an opportunity to assess compliance with checklists such as Fast Hug.[26] Clearly, unstable patients will require much more frequent assessment and intervention.

It is crucial that all observations, examination findings, investigations, medical orders, management plans (including treatment limitations) and important communications with other medical teams and patients' families are clearly documented in the appropriate chart or part of the medical record either electronically or in writing.

Wherever possible clinical management should be evidence-based and derived through consensus of the members of the ICU team, accepting, however, that evidence-based medicine has limitations when applied to intensive care medicine.[27]

CARE OF FAMILIES[28]

ICU care includes sensitive handling of relatives. It is important that there are early and repeated discussions with patients' families to reduce family stress and improve consistency in communication. Ideally one senior doctor should be identified as the ICU representative to liaise with a particular family. Discussions should be interactive and honest and an attempt made to predict the likely course, especially with respect to outcome, potential complications and the duration of intensive care management required. The time, date and discussion of each interview should be recorded. Cultural factors should be acknowledged and spiritual support available, especially before, during and after a death. Open visiting hours allow families maximum contact with their loved one and promote an atmosphere of openness and transparency.

Education and debriefing may be necessary for staff, especially in relation to difficult and/or unexpected deaths and grieving families.

OUTREACH

ICU outreach activities are described in Chapter 2.

NON-CLINICAL ACTIVITIES[2]

Non-clinical activities are very important in the ICU, as they enhance the safety, quality and currency of patient care. The Joint Faculty of Intensive Care Medicine recommends that full-time intensive care specialists should have as protected non-clinical time three half-day sessions per week.[29] Nursing and allied health staff should also seek protected time for these activities.

QUALITY IMPROVEMENT[30,31]

It is essential that senior medical and nursing staff promote a culture of quality improvement (QI) within the ICU, whatever its size and role. All ICUs should have demonstrable and documented formal audit and review of its processes and outcomes in a regular multidisciplinary forum. Staff who collect and process the data should have dedicated QI time.

Quality indicators can be considered under three headings:

1. *Structure.* Structural indicators assess whether the ICU functions according to its operational guidelines and conforms to the policies of training and specialist bodies (e.g. clinical work load and case mix, staffing establishment and levels of supervision).
2. *Clinical process.* Clinical process indicators assess the way care is delivered. Examples include whether deep-vein thrombosis prophylaxis is given, time to administration of antibiotics and glycaemic control.
3. *Outcome.* Examples of outcome measures include survival rate, quality of life of survivors and patient satisfaction.

The QI process involves *identification* of the indicator to be improved (e.g. high ventilator-associated pneumonia (VAP) rate), *development* of a method to improve it (e.g. checklist such as Fast Hug[26]), *implementation* of the method to improve it (e.g. requrement to tick off the checklist on the morning ward round), re-evaluation of the indicator (e.g. VAP rate) to ensure the intervention has improved the outcome and finally to *ensure sustainability* (e.g. print checklist on ICU chart).

Activities that assess processes include clinical audit (including morbidity and mortality meetings and delayed transfer out of ICU), compliance with protocols, guidelines and checklists and critical incident reporting.

Activities that assess outcomes are calculating risk-adjusted mortality using a scoring system such as the Acute Physiology and Chronic Health Evaluation II (APACHE II) and calculation of standardised mortality ratios (see Chapter 3), measurement of rates of adverse events such as central venous catheter-associated blood stream infection rate or serious adverse drug event rate and surveys (e.g. patient or relative satisfaction, bad backs from lifting in ICU nurses).

Risk management is a closely related field. In the ICU, risks can be identified from critical incident reports, morbidity and mortality reviews and complaints from staff, patients or family members. Using similar methodology to the QI process risks must be identified, assessed and analysed, managed and re-evaluated. A major patient safety incident should result in a root cause analysis.[32]

EDUCATION

All ICUs should have a documented orientation programme for new staff. There should be educational programmes for medical staff and a formal nursing education programme. Educational activities for intensive care trainees include lectures, tutorials, bedside teaching and trial examinations (written, clinical and viva). Apart from clinical reviews, meetings to review journals and new developments should be held regularly. Nurses are usually required to undergo annual assessment for advanced life support and sometimes other assessments (e.g. medication safety). Increasingly, simulation centres are used to teach and assess skills and teamwork in crisis scenarios.[33] A number of ICUs are also involved in undergraduate medical teaching. All staff should also participate in continuing education activities outside the hospital (e.g. local, national or international meetings).

RESEARCH

Level III ICUs should have an active research programme, preferably with dedicated research staff, but all units should attempt to undertake some research projects whether they be unit-based or contributions to multicentre trials.

THE FUTURE

In the USA critical care medicine is thought to account for 1–2% of the gross domestic product[34] and has become increasingly used and prominent in the delivery of health care. Although the total number of hospitals, hospital beds and inpatient days has decreased, there has been shown to be a large increase in the number of intensive care beds and bed days.[35] There is every reason to expect that other developed countries will follow this trend. As ICUs become larger and ICU staff become larger still (because of outreach activities: see Chapter 2) it is crucial that the basic principles outlined in this chapter are followed and that standards of ICU design, staffing and clinical and non-clinical activities are maintained.

REFERENCES

1. Trubuhovich R. On the very first, long-term, large-scale use of IPPV. Albert Bower and V Ray Bennett: Los Angeles, 1948–1949. *Crit Care Resusc* 2007; **9**: 91–100.
2. *Minimum Standards for Intensive Care Units.* Policy document IC-1. Melbourne: Joint Faculty of Intensive Care Medicine; 2003.
3. Ferdinande P and Members of the Task Force of the European Society of Intensive Care Medicine. *Intens Care Med* 1997; **23**: 226–32.
4. Haupt MT, Bekes CE, Brilli RJ *et al.* Guidelines on critical care services and personnel: recommendations based on a system of categorization of three levels of care. *Crit Care Med* 2003; **31**: 2677–83.
5. Brilli RJ, Spevetz A, Branson R *et al.* Critical care delivery in the intensive care unit: defining clinical roles and the best practice model. *Crit Care Med* 2001; **29**: 2007–19.
6. Angus DC, Shorr AF, White A *et al.* Critical care delivery in the United States: distribution of services and compliance with the Leapfrog recommendations. *Crit Care Med* 2006; **34**: 1016–24.
7. Martin J, Anderson T, Turton C *et al. Intensive Care Resources and Activity: Australia and New Zealand 2003–2005.* Melbourne: ANZICS; 2006.
8. Dara SI, Afessa B. Intensivist-to-bed ratio: association with outcomes in the medical ICU. *Chest* 2005; **128**: 567–72.
9. Boots R, Lipman J. High dependency units: issues to consider in their planning. *Anaesth Intens Care* 2002; **30**: 348–54.
10. *Minimum Standards for High Dependency Units Seeking Accreditation for Training in Intensive Care.* Policy document IC-13. Melbourne: Joint Faculty of Intensive Care Medicine; 2000.
11. Bellomo R, Goldsmith D, Uchino J *et al.* A before and after trial of the effect of a high-dependency unit on post-operative morbidity and mortality. *Crit Care Resusc* 2005; 7: 16–21.
12. Society of Critical Care Medicine. Guidelines for intensive care unit design. *Crit Care Med* 1995; **23**: 582–8.
13. Knaus WA, Draper EA, Wagner DP *et al.* An evaluation of outcome from intensive care in major medical centers. *Ann Intern Med* 1986; **104**: 410–18.
14. Baggs JG, Schmitt MH, Mushlin AI *et al.* Association between nurse–physician collaboration and patient outcomes in three intensive care units. *Crit Care Med* 1998; **27**: 1991–8.
15. Reader TW, Flin R, Mearns K *et al.* Interdisciplinary communication in the intensive care unit. *Br J Anaesth* 2007; **98**: 347–52.
16. Joint Commission on Accreditation of Health Care Organizations (JCAHO). *Statistics: Root Cause Statistics – Root Causes of Sentinel Events (All Categories).* Oakbrook Terrace, Ill: JCAHO, 2005.
17. *The Duties of an Intensive Care Specialist in Hospitals Accredited for Intensive Care Training.* Policy document IC-2. Melbourne: Joint Faculty of Intensive Care Medicine; 2000.
18. Pronovost PJ, Angus DC, Dorman T *et al.* Physician staffing patterns and clinical outcomes in critically ill patients. *JAMA* 2002; **288**: 2151–62.
19. Tarnow-Mordi W, Hau C, Warden A *et al.* Hospital mortality in relation to staff workload: a 4-year study in an adult intensive care unit. *Lancet* 2000; **356**: 185–9.
20. Ulrich BT, Lavandero R, Hart KA *et al.* Critical care nurses' work environments: a baseline status report. *Crit Care Nurse* 2006; **26**: 46–57.
21. Leape LL, Cullen DJ, Demspey Clapp M *et al.* Pharmacist participation in physician rounds and adverse drug events in the intensive care unit. *JAMA* 1999; **282**: 267–70.
22. Carter BG, Kiraly N, Hochmann N *et al.* ICU staffing: identification and survey of staff involved in providing technical services to Australian and New Zealand intensive care units. *Anaesth Intens Care* 2007; **35**: 259–65.
23. *Administrative Services to Intensive Care Units.* Policy document IC-7. Melbourne: Joint Faculty of Intensive Care Medicine; 2006.
24. Hanson CW, Deutschman CS, Anderson HL *et al.* Effects of an organised critical care service on outcomes and resource utilization: a cohort study. *Crit Care Med* 1999; **27**: 270–4.
25. Krishnan JA, Moore D, Robeson C *et al.* A prospective, controlled trial of a protocol-based strategy to discontinue mechanical ventilation. *Am J Respir Crit Care Med* 2004; **169**: 673–8.
26. Vincent JL. Give your patient a fast hug (at least) once a day. *Crit Care Med* 2005; **33**: 1225–9.
27. Vincent JL. Evidence-based medicine in the ICU: important advances and limitations. *Chest* 2004; **126**: 592–600.
28. Davidson JE, Powers K, Hedayat KM *et al.* Clinical practice guidelines for the support of the family in the patient-centered intensive care unit: American College of Critical Care Medicine Task Force 2004–2005. *Crit Care Med* 2007; **35**: 605–22.
29. Joint Faculty of Intensive Care Medicine. *Intensive Care Specialist Practice in Hospitals Recognised for Training in Intensive Care Medicine IC-2.* Available online at JFICM australia http://www.anzca.edu.au/jficm/resources/policy/IC-2-2005.pdf.
30. Curtis JR, Cook DJ, Wall RJ *et al.* Intensive care quality improvement: a 'how-to' guide for the interdisciplinary team. *Crit Care Med* 2006; **34**: 211–18.
31. *Quality Assurance.* Policy document IC-8. Melbourne: Joint Faculty of Intensive Care Medicine; 2000.

32. Batty L, Holland-Elliot K, Rosenfeld D. Investigation of eye splash and needlestick incidents from an HIV-positive donor on an intensive care unit using root cause analysis. *Occup Med* 2003; **53**: 147–50.
33. Hammond J. Simulation in critical care and trauma education and training. *Curr Opin Crit Care* 2004; **10**: 325–9.
34. Gipe BT. Financing critical care medicine in 2010. *N Horiz* 1999; 7: 184–97.
35. Halpern NA, Pastores S, Greenstein RJ. Critical care medicine in the United States 1985–2000: an analysis of bed numbers, use and costs. *Crit Care Med* 2004; **32**: 1249–59.

2

Outreach

David R Goldhill and John R Welch

CRITICAL CARE OUTREACH

A key innovation in critical care has been the development of dedicated outreach and medical emergency/rapid response services aiming 'to ensure equity of care for all critically ill patients irrespective of their location'.[1]

Outreach is multidisciplinary 'collaboration and partnership between critical care and other departments to ensure a continuum of care for patients and to enhance the skills and understanding of all staff in the delivery of critical care'.[2] Outreach services primarily focus on patients with potential or actual critical illness on general wards. They are not a substitute for insufficient critical care beds, poor ward facilities or inadequate staffing.

BACKGROUND

Many patients who require critical care are on a ward for part of their hospital admission. Comparison of outcomes of patients admitted to a critical care unit from the emergency department, operating theatre/recovery area and wards shows that the highest number of deaths is found in patients admitted from wards.[3] The longer patients are in hospital before admission to critical care, the higher their mortality.[4] Reports from many countries show that hospital patients frequently suffer adverse events and that these events can cause major morbidity or death.[5] Suboptimal treatment is common before admission to critical care and is associated with worse outcomes.[6] Crucially, the baseline characteristics of patients who receive suboptimal care are not significantly different from those who are well managed. Differences in mortality are attributable to differences in the quality of care rather than differences between patients themselves. Many factors are implicated, including lack of knowledge and failure to appreciate clinical urgency and to seek advice, compounded by poor organisation, breakdown in communication and inadequate supervision.

About one-quarter of all 'critical care deaths' occur *after* patients have been discharged back to wards from critical care. Patients discharged inappropriately early have an increased mortality.[7,8] There are also deaths among surgical patients who have returned to the ward following surgery without ever being admitted to critical care.

Nonetheless, these at-risk patients are in hospital, so they are accessible. If such patients can be identified early, prompt intervention may improve outcomes.

Even in well-resourced health care systems, critical care beds are a small proportion of all acute beds and have high rates of occupancy. Hospital lengths of stay have fallen and hospital admission criteria have been made more stringent in recent years. The result is that many ward patients have serious medical problems, although only the most unstable gain admission to a critical care unit. Therefore, many at-risk patients are cared for in inappropriate areas by staff unpractised in managing critical illness.

Changes in nursing education have reduced nurses' training time in acute and critical care areas, while such key tasks as measuring respiratory rate and blood pressure are delegated to untrained staff who may not understand the significance of abnormal values. Many hospitals use temporary staff who may not provide the stability and commitment essential for effective working. Medical education is also problematic. Recently qualified doctors are often unable to recognise or treat life-threatening problems and, because training is shorter and more specialised, consultants may also be less experienced in managing critical illness.

With shorter hospital stays and sicker patients, the system of care must be able to respond rapidly to changes in a patient's condition. For some patients, even daily medical review may not be enough.

OUTREACH SYSTEMS

Medical emergency teams (METs) were first introduced in Australia in 1990. METs expanded the role of the hospital cardiac arrest team to include the pre-arrest period, with call-out criteria generally based upon markedly deranged physiological values.[9] In the UK, critical care outreach (CCO) services became relatively widespread following negative publicity about shortages of critical care facilities and the national review of critical care services in 2000.[10] This led to some additional funding for critical care beds and outreach services. Other countries have also recognised the needs of critically ill patients outside designated critical care areas and have introduced their own systems to address these problems.

There are now many models and a variety of terms for outreach services.[11,12] Some organisations have enthusiastically embraced the concept whereas others have reservations. METs are usually physician-led, while CCO teams and rapid response teams (RRTs) are typically nurse-led but may include physiotherapists and other allied health professionals as well as doctors. Most teams respond to defined triggers, although some, particularly CCO services, also work proactively with known at-risk patients such as intensive care unit (ICU) discharges.

These systems have the following features in common:

- a mechanism for identifying ward patients who are, or have the potential to become, critically ill
- a trigger designed to initiate a response when certain criteria are fulfilled
- a prompt response from personnel with the required skills, experience and resources

The aim is to prevent unnecessary critical care admissions, to ensure timely transfer to critical care when needed, to facilitate safe discharge from critical care back to the ward, to share critical care skills and to improve standards of care throughout the hospital. There may also be a role in outpatient support for patients and their families after hospital discharge (Table 2.1).

Table 2.1 Functions of critical care outreach

- Identification of at-risk patients
- Support for ward staff caring for at-risk patients and those recovering from critical illness
- Referral protocols for obtaining timely, effective critical care treatments
- Immediate availability of expert critical care and resuscitation skills when required
- Facilitation of timely transfer to a critical care facility when needed
- Education for ward staff in recognition of fundamental signs of deterioration, and in understanding how to obtain appropriate help promptly
- Outpatient support to patients and their families following discharge from hospital
- Development of systems of coordinated, collaborative, continuous care of critically ill and recovering patients across the hospital and also in the community
- Audit and improvement of basic standards of acute and critical care – and of the outreach team itself – to minimise risk and optimise treatment of the critically ill throughout the hospital

Together, these elements comprise a system to deliver safe, quality care by proactive management of risk and timely treatment of critical illness

RECOGNISING CRITICAL ILLNESS

Critically ill patients are identified by review of the history, by examination and investigations. Higher risks are associated with extremes of age, with significant comorbidities or with serious presenting conditions. Outcome is often related to and can be predicted by abnormal physiology. Many studies show patients have abnormal physiology for hours and sometimes days before critical events such as cardiopulmonary arrest.[13–18] However, measuring and recording of vital signs on general wards are often inadequate.[19]

A physiologically based system for identifying critical illness should have certain attributes (Table 2.2).

For early recognition of hospital patients to be effective:

- Abnormal physiological values or biochemistry or other patient factors should enable identification
- There must be enough time to identify the patients – and to obtain expert assistance
- Early intervention should be beneficial

ABNORMAL PHYSIOLOGY AND ADVERSE OUTCOME

There is an association between abnormal physiology and adverse outcome. Critical care severity scoring systems such as Acute Physiology, Age and Chronic Health Evaluation II (APACHE II)[20] are based on this relationship. Patients who suffer cardiopulmonary arrest or who die in hospital generally have abnormal physiological values recorded in the preceding period, as do patients requiring transfer to the critical care unit.

It therefore follows that vital signs can predict many adverse events. These principles have been incorporated into a number of early-warning scoring (EWS) systems. The systems incorporate different combinations of physiological parameters, a range of approaches to scoring and various trigger thresholds. Examples of the variables included in a few of the scoring systems are given in Table 2.3.

In the UK these methods are often called track and trigger warning systems. They can be broadly summarised as single-parameter systems, multiple-parameter systems, aggregate weighted scoring systems or combinations (Table 2.4).[1]

In Australia, MET call-out criteria are usually based upon markedly deranged physiological values, although ward staff concern is also a trigger (Table 2.5).[21]

Table 2.2 Ideal attributes of an early-warning (track and trigger) scoring system

Timely	Measurable
Reliable	Reproducible
Inexpensive	Non-invasive
Repeatable	Safe
Accurate	Independent of disease state

Table 2.3 Variables used by different scoring systems to trigger referrals to a critical care service

Variable	Critical care service						
	METa[1]	METb[2]	METc[3]	PART[4]	CCLS[5]	EWS[6]	MEWS[7]
Airway	√		√				
Breathing							
Spo_2/blood gas		√	√	√	√		
Respiratory rate	√	√	√	√	√	√	√
Circulation							
Heart rate	√	√	√	√	√	√	√
Systolic blood pressure		√	√	√	√	√	√
Neurology	√	√	√	√	√	√	√
Renal		√		√			√
Temperature						√	√
Clinical concern	√	√	√	√			√

MET, medical emergency team; PART, patient at-risk team; CCLS, critical care liaison service; EWS, early-warning score; MEWS, modified early-warning score.
[1]Lee A, Bishop G, Hillman DM *et al*. The medical emergency team. *Anaesth Intens Care* 1995; **23**: 183–6.
[2]Bellomo R, Goldsmith D, Uchino S *et al*. A prospective before-and-after trial of a medical emergency team. *Med J Aust* 2003; **179**: 283–7.
[3]Buist MD, Moore GE, Bernard SA *et al*. Effects of a medical emergency team on reduction of incidence of and mortality from unexpected cardiac arrests in hospital: preliminary study. *Br Med J* 2002; **324**: 387–90.
[4]Goldhill DR, Worthington L, Mulcahy A *et al*. The patient-at-risk team: identifying and managing seriously ill ward patients. *Anaesthesia* 1999; **54**: 853–60.
[5]Hickey C, Allen MJ. A critical care liaison service. *Br J Anaesth* 1998; **81**: 650P.
[6]Morgan RJM, Williams F, Wright MM. An early warning score for detecting developing critical illness. *Clin Intens Care* 1997; **8**: 100.
[7]Stenhouse C, Coates S, Tivey M *et al*. Prospective evaluation of a modified Early Warning Score to aid earlier detection of patients developing critical illness on a surgical ward. *Br J Anaesth* 2000; **84**: 663–4P.
(Reproduced from Bright D, Walker W, Bion J. Clinical review: outreach – a strategy for improving the care of the acutely ill hospitalized patient. *Crit Care* 2004; **8**: 33–40.)

Table 2.4 Classification of track and trigger warning systems

Single-parameter systems
Tracking
Periodic observation of selected basic signs
Trigger
One or more extreme observational values
Multiple-parameter systems
Tracking
Periodic observation of selected basic vital signs
Trigger
Two or more extreme observational values
Aggregate weighted scoring systems
Tracking
Periodic observation of selected basic vital signs and the assignment of weighted scores to physiological values with calculation of a total score
Trigger
Achieving a previously agreed trigger threshold with the total score
Combination systems
Elements of single- or multiple-parameter systems in combination with aggregate weighted scoring

(Definitions taken from Department of Health/Modernisation Agency. *Critical Care Outreach 2003 – Progress in Developing Services: National Outreach Report*. London: Department of Health, 2003.)

Table 2.5 Medical emergency team call-out criteria

Airway	Respiratory distress Threatened airway
Breathing	Respiratory rate < 6 or > 30 breaths/min Spo_2 < 90% on oxygen Difficulty speaking
Circulation	Systolic blood pressure < 90 mmHg despite treatment Heart rate > 130 beats/min
Neurology	Unexplained decrease in consciousness Agitation or delirium Repeated or prolonged seizures
Other	Concern about patient Uncontrolled pain Failure to respond to treatment Unable to obtain prompt help

(Call-out criteria from Buist MD, Moore GE, Bernard SA *et al*. Effects of a medical emergency team on reduction of incidence of and mortality from unexpected cardiac arrests in hospital: preliminary study. *Br Med J* 2002; **324**: 387–90.)

Table 2.6 Early-warning score (EWS)

Variable	Score 3	2	1	0	1	2	3
Heart rate (beats/min)		≤ 40	41–50	51–100	101–110	111–130	≥ 130
Systolic blood pressure (mmHg)	< 70	71–80	81–100	101–199			≥ 200
Respiratory rate (breaths/min)		< 8		9–14	15–20	21–29	≥ 30
Temperature (°C)			≤ 35	35.1–36.5	36.6–37.4	≥ 37.5	
Central nervous system				A	V	P	U

This EWS is the one originally published by Morgan RJM, Williams F, Wright MM. An early warning score for detecting developing critical illness. *Clin Intens Care* 1997; **8**: 100.
A, alert; V, responds to voice; P, responds to pain; U, unresponsive.

The use of physiological values in the form of a multiple-parameter EWS to identify at-risk ward patients was first described by Morgan *et al.*[22] There are different formats but they follow a similar theme, awarding points for varying degrees of derangement of different physiological functions (Table 2.6). The higher the total score, the more the patient is 'at risk'.

To date, EWSs have been devised using clinical acumen and common sense. They have yet to be scientifically validated as predictors of preventable adverse outcomes. Crucially, the calculated score depends on the definition of normal physiological values and how much relative importance is attributed to the derangements of each measured parameter.

Physiologically based EWS systems are now widely used to identify at-risk patients. There is little concrete evidence about the most important parameters and the exact values that identify critical illness. It is possible that a combination of factors and analysis of changes over time may be the best way of identifying such patients.

MEASURING OUTCOME

The concept of outreach is based upon the premise that early detection and treatment of critical illness should improve patient outcomes. The quality of an outreach service may be evaluated against these and other measures, including indicators of effective processes (Table 2.7).

Table 2.7 Possible outcome and process measures

- Numbers of staff trained to recognize critical illness and respond appropriately
- Completeness of physiological values recording and other documentation
- Response times to triggers
- Appropriateness and timeliness of interventions
- Cardiopulmonary arrests, unexpected deaths and adverse events
- The interface with critical care departments, e.g. timeliness of patient transfer to critical care
- Numbers of admissions to critical care (and readmissions)
- Critical care and hospital mortality
- Critical care and hospital lengths of stay
- Patient and staff satisfaction

Outreach systems have certainly highlighted shortcomings in the care of ward patients and contributed to a change in attitude and more attention to at-risk patients. They have been instrumental in improving ward monitoring and charting and in disseminating critical care skills. There is much anecdotal evidence of benefit to individual patients. There is published evidence that outreach services improve the recognition of at-risk patients on wards and can reduce length of stay, cardiac arrest rates, unplanned admissions to critical care and morbidity and mortality of such patients.[21,23–26] However, there are as many reports that do not show significant effects. In fact there are as yet few good-quality studies, with just two randomised controlled trials.[26,27]

Positive studies include a UK randomised trial of phased introduction of a 24-hour outreach service to 16 wards in a general acute hospital.[26,28] The outreach team routinely followed up patients discharged from critical care to the wards and saw referrals generated by ward staff concern or use of an aggregate weighted scoring system. There was a statistically significant reduction in hospital mortality in wards where the service was operational. In contrast, a large prospective randomised trial of METs in Australia did not find improvements in cardiac arrests, unplanned admissions to critical care or unexpected deaths.[27] The study did reveal many shortcomings in the identification and care of critically ill patients. One possible conclusion is that for outreach to work there must be a whole-systems approach to early identification of at-risk patients and to obtaining an appropriate, timely and effective response.

It can be argued that outreach should not be necessary in a properly run and funded first-world health care system. Time will tell if outreach services are simply a stopgap solution to compensate for hospital system failings. Nonetheless, there is no doubt that there are significant numbers of patients on hospital wards with potential or actual critical illness whose care should and could be improved. Outreach systems are one method of addressing these issues.

SETTING UP AN OUTREACH SERVICE

Patients with potential or actual critical care illness may be found in almost every area of the acute hospital, so systems to identify and treat at-risk patients promptly and improve quality across an institution need to be planned at an organisational level. Involvement of managerial and clinical staff at all levels, particularly from the general wards, is essential. It is particularly important that there is agreement and clarity about how the outreach team interacts with the parent/primary medical team. The Institute for Healthcare Improvement has useful information on setting up a rapid response team.[29]

KEY STEPS IN PLANNING AN OUTREACH SERVICE

- Appoint senior clinical and managerial leads to develop the service.
- Institute organisational needs analysis, audit and evaluation, asking:
  - Which patients are at risk of critical illness and where are they located?
  - Where do cardiopulmonary arrests and unexpected deaths occur?
  - What is the source of unplanned admissions to ICU?
  - What is the pattern of adverse events where actual harm can be attributed to the process of care?
  - What are the other relevant clinical governance/risk management issues, e.g. complaints, or morbidity and mortality data?
- A point prevalence study can give snapshot views of the location of patients with physiological derangement.
- Review of unplanned ICU admissions can identify systems failings, including quality of patient management and appropriateness and timeliness of intensive care admission. Practice can be assessed against specific, measurable standards set locally or nationally/internationally.
- Such analyses should also highlight staff education and training needs.

Other factors to consider include:

- The patient case mix
- Existing skills of general ward staff
- Proposed hours of service
- Size of hospital – and likely demand
- Existing services such as pain teams, nutrition teams, tracheostomy specialist practitioners, respiratory specialists, renal specialists, night teams
- Training facilities for nursing, medical and other clinical staff
- Outreach service location and equipment needs, including information technology facilities
- Funding

THE OUTREACH TEAM

The composition and skills of the outreach team should be designed to meet the specific needs identified by individual organisations. At a minimum, a team should be capable of assessment, diagnosis, initiation of resuscitation and rapid triage of the patient to a higher level of care with authority to act. Such clinical skills as airway management techniques, venepuncture and cannulation are essential and so are skills in education and training, research and audit. A multiprofessional team is likely to be required in order for this range of skills to be available and also for the team to be able to communicate readily with the whole range of staff in the hospital.

A pragmatic, staged implementation could include:

1. Establishing an education programme in fundamental care of the critically ill for general ward staff so that all staff can recognise basic signs of deterioration and understand the necessity and means of obtaining timely help. Staff should update their skills annually
2. Introducing a physiological track and trigger warning system and defined referral/response protocols
3. Developing clinical bedside support – incrementally if necessary – increasing the number of clinical areas covered by the team and the hours of work. This might include follow-up of patients discharged from critical care and responding to patients identified through the track and trigger system or by referral from ward staff
4. It is essential that robust data are collected on the work of the service and that this information is used for audit and evaluation – and for feedback to ward managers and clinical staff. Successes should be highlighted and areas for improvement in practice identified. Data may include:
   - Numbers of referrals and patient follow-ups
   - Date and time of episode
   - Patient details, e.g. age, sex, date of hospital admission, location, emergency/elective admission, medical/surgical, resuscitation status
   - Trigger event, e.g. EWS, cardiac arrest call
   - Key problems identified
   - Interventions performed
   - Patient outcomes

REFERENCES

1. Department of Health and Modernisation Agency. *The National Outreach Report 2003.* London: Department of Health; 2003.

2. The Intensive Care Society. *Guidelines for the Introduction of Outreach Services.* London: Intensive Care Society; 2002.
3. Goldhill DR, Sumner A. Outcome of intensive care patients in a group of British intensive care units. *Crit Care Med* 1998; **26**: 1337–45.
4. Goldhill DR, McNarry AF, Hadjianastassiou VG *et al.* The longer patients are in hospital before intensive care admission the higher their mortality. *Intens Care Med* 2004; **30**: 1908–13.
5. Vincent C, Neale G, Woloshynowych M. Adverse events in British hospital: preliminary retrospective record review. *Br Med J* 2001; **322**: 517–19.
6. McQuillan P, Pilkington S, Allan A *et al.* Confidential inquiry into quality of care before admission to intensive care. *Br Med J* 1998; **316**: 1853–8.
7. Daly K, Beale R, Chang RW. Reduction in mortality after inappropriate early discharge from intensive care unit: logistic regression triage model. *Br Med J* 2001; **322**: 1274–6.
8. Goldfrad C, Rowan K. Consequences of discharges from intensive care at night. *Lancet* 2000; **355**: 1138–42.
9. Lee A, Bishop G, Hillman KM *et al.* The medical emergency team. *Anaesth Intens Care* 1995; **23**: 183–6.
10. Department of Health. *Comprehensive Critical Care. A Review of Adult Critical Care Services.* London: Department of Health, 2000.
11. DeVita MA, Bellomo R, Hillman K *et al.* Findings of the first consensus conference on medical emergency teams. *Crit Care Med* 2006; **34**: 2463–78.
12. Esmonde L, McDonnell A, Ball C *et al.* Investigating the effectiveness of critical care outreach services: a systematic review. *Intens Care Med* 2006; **32**: 1713–21.
13. Berlot G, Pangher A, Petrucci L *et al.* Anticipating events of in-hospital cardiac arrest. *Eur J Emerg Med* 2004; **11**: 24–8.
14. Buist MD, Jarmolowski E, Burton PR *et al.* Recognising clinical instability in hospital patients before cardiac arrest or unplanned admission to intensive care. A pilot study in a tertiary-care hospital. *Med J Aust* 1999; **171**: 22–5.
15. Harrison GA, Jacques TC, Kilborn G *et al.* The prevalence of recordings of the signs of critical conditions and emergency responses in hospital wards – the SOCCER study. *Resuscitation* 2005; **65**: 149–57.
16. Jacques T, Harrison GA, McLaws ML *et al.* Signs of critical conditions and emergency responses (SOCCER): a model for predicting adverse events in the inpatient setting. *Resuscitation* 2006: **69**: 175–83.
17. Kause J, Smith G, Prytherch D *et al.* A comparison of antecedents to cardiac arrests, deaths and emergency intensive care admissions in Australia and New Zealand, and the United Kingdom – the ACADEMIA study. *Resuscitation* 2004; **62**: 275–82.
18. Cullinane M, Findlay G, Hargraves C *et al.* An acute problem. London: National Confidential Enquiry into Patient Outcome and Death; 2005.
19. Audit Commission. Critical to Success. Audit Commission for Local Authorities and the London: National Health Service in England and Wales; 1999.
20. Knaus WA, Draper EA, Wagner DP *et al.* APACHE II: a severity of disease classification system. *Crit Care Med* 1985; **13**: 818–29.
21. Buist MD, Moore GE, Bernard SA *et al.* Effects of a medical emergency team on reduction of incidence of and mortality from unexpected cardiac arrests in hospital: preliminary study. *Br Med J* 2002; **324**: 387–90.
22. Morgan RJM, Williams F, Wright MM. An early warning score for detecting developing critical illness. *Clin Intens Care* 1997; **8**: 100.
23. Bellomo R, Goldsmith D, Uchino S *et al.* A prospective before-and-after trial of a medical emergency team. *Med J Aust* 2003; **179**: 283–7.
24. Bellomo R, Goldsmith D, Uchino S *et al.* Prospective controlled trial of effect of medical emergency team on postoperative morbidity and mortality rates. *Crit Care Med* 2004; **32**: 916–21.
25. Ball C, Kirkby M, Williams S. Effect of the critical care outreach team on patient survival to discharge from hospital and readmission to critical care: non-randomised population based study. *Br Med J* 2003; **327**: 1014–17.
26. Priestley G, Watson W, Rashidian A *et al.* Introducing critical care outreach: a ward-randomised trail of phased introduction in a general hospital. *Intens Care Med* 2004; **30**: 1398–404.
27. Hillman K, Chen J, Cretikos M *et al.* Introduction of the medical emergency team (MET) system: a cluster-randomised controlled trial. *Lancet* 2005; **365**: 2091–7.
28. Watson W, Mozley C, Cope J *et al.* Implementing a nurse-led critical care outreach service in an acute hospital. *J Clin Nurs* 2006; **15**: 105–10.
29. Institute for Healthcare Improvement. http://www.ihi.org/IHI/Topics/CriticalCare/IntensiveCare/Changes/EstablishaRapidResponseTeam.htm. Accessed 4 December 2006.

3

Severity of illness and likely outcome from critical illness

Mark Palazzo

At present scoring systems are not sufficiently accurate to make outcome predictions for individual patients.

Clinical assessment of severity of illness is an essential component of medical practice. It influences the need and speed for supportive and specific therapy. Initial acuity may also indicate likely prognosis when other factors such as comorbidity and organisational aspects of critical care delivery are considered. It is intuitive to consider whether patterns and severity of physiological disturbance can predict patient outcome from an episode of critical illness.

Perhaps the earliest reference to grading illness was in an Egyptian papyrus which classified head injury by severity.[1] More recently it has been the constellation of physiological disturbances for specific conditions which popularised an approach which linked physiological disturbance to outcome in the critically ill. Examples include the Ranson score for acute pancreatitis,[2] the Pugh modification of Child–Turcotte classification for patients undergoing portosystemic shunt surgery and now widely used for classification of end-stage liver disease,[3] Parsonnet scores for cardiac surgery[4] and the Glasgow Coma Score (GCS) for acute head injury.[5] The earliest attempts to quantify severity of illness in a general critically ill population was by Cullen *et al.*[6] who devised a therapeutic intervention score as a surrogate for illness. This was followed in 1981 with the introduction of the Acute Physiology, Age and Chronic Health Evaluation (APACHE) scoring system by Knaus *et al.*[7] Since then numerous scoring systems have been designed and tested in populations across the world.

The potential advantages of quantifying critical illness include:

- providing a common language for discussion
- provision of risk-adjusted expected mortality rates facilitating acuity comparisons for clinical trials
- estimates of prognosis
- providing a method by which critical care practice and processes can be examined

The least controversial use for scoring systems has been as a method for comparing patient groups in clinical trials. While this seems to have been widely accepted by the critical care community, there has been less enthusiasm to accept the same systems as comparators for between-unit and even between-country performances, unless of course your performance is good. Most clinicians agree that scoring systems have limited value for individual patient decision pathways, although recently an APACHE II score above 25 under appropriate circumstances has been included in the guidelines for the administration of recombinant human activated protein C for severe sepsis and septic shock. Much of the sceptical views among clinicians are based on studies which show poor prognostic performance from many of the models proposed.[8–14] The fundamental problem for these scores and prognostic models is poor calibration for the cohort of patients studied, often in countries with different health service infrastructures, to where the models were first developed. Other calibration issues arise either because there is poor adherence to the rules for scoring methodology by users, or patient outcomes improve following introduction of new techniques and treatments or models failed to include important prognostic variables. For example it has become clearer that prognosis is as much affected by local organisation, patient pathways, location prior to admission and preadmission state as it is by acute physiological disturbances.[15,16]

Score systems would be better calibrated if developed from a narrow number of countries with similar health services. However this limits their international usefulness for clinical studies. The latter can be improved by score systems developed from a wider international cohort; however when used for an individual country it can be expected to calibrate poorly. Simplified Acute Physiology Score 3 (SAPS 3: developed across the globe) has provided customisation formulae so that the risk-adjusted expected mortality can be related to the geographical location of the unit.[16]

Inevitably, as advances occur, risk-adjusted mortality predictions become outdated with some old models overestimating expected mortality[14,17] and others underestimating observed mortality.[18] The designers of the scoring systems have recognised the changing baselines

Table 3.1 Revision dates for the most common internationally recognized risk adjusted models for mortality prediction

Severity of illness model	Year	Timing of score	Cohort size	ICU units	ICU countries
SAPS	1984	First 24 hours	679	8	France
SAPS 2	1993	First 24 hours	13 152	137	Europe/USA
SAPS 3	2005	Admission	16 784	303	Europe, Australia, South and Central America
MPM I	1987	Admission	1997	1	USA
MPM II_0	1993	Admission	19 124		USA/Europe
APACHE I	1981	First 24 hours	805	2	USA
APACHE II	1985	First 24 hours	5815	13	USA
APACHE III	1991	First 24 hours	17 440	40	USA
APACHE IV	2006	First 24 hours	110 558	104	USA

ICU, intensive care unit; SAPS, Simplified Acute Physiology Score; MPM, Mortality Probability Model; APACHE, Acute Physiology, Age and Chronic Health Evaluation.

and review the models every few years, Table 3.1 outlines some characteristics of the upgraded systems.

FACTORS INDICATING RISK AND SEVERITY OF ILLNESS THAT MIGHT HELP PREDICT LIKELY OUTCOME

- Degree of physiological disturbance
- Primary pathological process causing the physiological disturbance
- Patient's physiological reserve specific, comorbid states and age
- Source of admission and mode of presentation
- Organ support prior to admission
- Unit organisation and processes

PHYSIOLOGICAL DISTURBANCE

An insult which potentially interferes with normal organ function is usually followed by increasing compensatory activity in order to retain vital organ activity. Most compensatory mechanisms are mediated through the endocrine and autonomic nervous system directed to maintain effective circulating volume, oxygenation and acid–base homeostasis to ensure normal mitochondrial function and vital organ function. Therefore hyperventilation, tachycardia, vasoconstriction and consequent oliguria – all signs of compensation – are hallmarks of early untreated critical illness. Once overwhelmed, the compensatory mechanisms lead to signs of decompensation such as hypotension, progressive coma, icterus and metabolic acidosis.

Most organs have limited ways in which they manifest their dysfunction in response to a systemic illness, for example the brain responds by becoming confused, developing seizures or progressive coma, while respiratory function is limited to hyperventilation, hypoventilation, wheezing or coughing with commensurate changes in blood gases. Therefore it is not surprising that most systemic pathophysiological processes result in common acute physiological disturbances. Consequently severity of illness can be assessed from a limited number of vital sign and biochemical observations. However it is not so clear what the magnitude of a response should be for a given insult. Therefore severity of illness for most conditions has been traditionally measured by the magnitude of physiological response rather than size of insult. The physiological response is further confounded by:

- Natural variability between patients
- Variable physiological reserve between patients
- Non-linear organ dysfunction in response to an insult, for example both the liver and kidney only manifest biochemical abnormality when a significant proportion of organ mass is malfunctioning
- Poor understanding of relative equivalence of degrees of malfunction between organs, e.g. what degree of jaundice is equivalent to a tachycardia 130 beats/min as an objective measure of severity of illness?
- Impact of organ support on physiological measurements, e.g. inotropes

Some scoring systems such as Mortality Probability Model (MPM II_0) and SAPS 3 estimate severity of illness on or near admission to intensive care in order to avoid the confounding effect of supportive therapy.

PRIMARY PATHOLOGICAL PROCESS

The primary pathology leading to intensive care admission has a significant influence on prognosis. Therefore, for a given degree of acute physiological disturbance, the most serious primary pathologies or underlying conditions are likely to have the worst predicted outcomes. For example, similar degrees of respiratory decompensation in an asthmatic and a patient with haematological malignancy are likely to lead to different outcomes. Furthermore the potential reversibility of a primary pathological process, whether spontaneous or through specific treatment, also greatly influences outcome, e.g. patients with diabetic ketoacidosis can be extremely unwell but insulin and volume therapy can rapidly reverse the physiological disturbance.

Both APACHE and the most recent SAPS systems include diagnostic categories with different weightings which improve the precision of estimated risk of hospital death calculations.

PHYSIOLOGICAL RESERVE, AGE AND COMORBIDITY

Physiological reserve is a surrogate term which broadly combines age and health status prior to critical illness. Age may be associated with diminishing physiological capacity but not in a predictable fashion.

- Chronological age alone is not a very strong influence on outcome.
- Biological age is a vague term usually used to imply physiological reserve below that expected for a patient's chronological age. Biological age greater than chronological age is common in patients who smoke heavily, abuse alcohol or who have insidious systemic diseases such as diabetes and hypertension; these patients typically have reduced reserve of one or more organs.

Chronic health states such as immunosuppression, cirrhosis, cancer and haematological malignancies all result in significant diminution of physiological reserve and may have an overwhelming influence on outcome. These conditions are commonly included in any assessment of critical illness.

SOURCE OF ADMISSION AND MODE OF PRESENTATION

Patients arriving in intensive care either come as an emergency or for a variety of reasons come following elective surgery. There are a very small number of patients who come to intensive care for elective medical reasons. By its very nature emergency admission implies that patients are likely to be unstable and that the acute physiological disturbances are in the process of being managed. Most scoring systems quantifying risk of death include an adjustment for emergency admission. It has become widely recognised that the source of admission also influences the likely outcome. This might in part be because it increases the likelihood of patients having resistant organisms, such as those admitted from a health care environment.

ORGAN SUPPORT PRIOR TO ADMISSION

Many patients may arrive in ICU already ventilated, and receiving inotropes. Assessment of severity of illness at this stage when some physiological abnormalities have been corrected would make a physiologically based assessment underscore. Therefore either the assessment has to be adjusted to a time when no organ support was provided or some allowance has to be made for the support in the assessment. The approach to this has been varied; for example, SAPS 3 makes an adjustment for patients on inotropes, whereas MPM II allows measurements for the hour on either side of admission to be included.

UNIT ORGANISATION AND PROCESSES

Soon after the introduction of APACHE II it was recognised that units with effective teams, nursing and medical leadership, good communications and run by dedicated intensive care specialists potentially had better outcomes than those without such characteristics.[19–21]

OTHER FACTORS

Some factors have not been included in risk-adjusted models for prediction of mortality; these include socioeconomic and genetic variables. However SAPS 3 has included a customisation adjustment to calibrate their model for patients in different parts of the world, possibly taking account of local factors and health care systems.

RISK-ADJUSTED EXPECTED OUTCOME AND ITS MEASUREMENT

Physiological disturbance, physiological reserve, pathological process and mode of presentation can be related to expected outcome by statistical methods. Common outcome measures for clinical trials are ICU mortality, or mortality at 28 days; however most models used for risk-adjusted mortality prediction are based on hospital mortality. Patient morbidity might also be considered nearly as important an endpoint as mortality, since many patients survive with serious functional impairment.[22,23] For socioeconomic reasons there would be a strong argument to consider 1-year survival and time to return to normal function or work as endpoints.[24,25] These latter measures however have been more closely related to chronic health status.

Hospital mortality is the most common outcome measure because it is frequent enough to act as a discriminator and is easy to define and document.

PRINCIPLES OF SCORING SYSTEM DESIGN

CHOICE OF INDEPENDENT PHYSIOLOGICAL VARIABLES AND THEIR TIMING

The designers of the original APACHE and SAPS systems chose variables which they felt would represent measures of acute illness. The chosen variables were based on expert opinion weighted equally on an arbitrary increasing linear scale, with the highest value given to the worst physiological value deviating from normal.[26,27] Premorbid conditions, age, emergency status and diagnostic details were also included in these early models and from these parameters a score and risk of hospital death probability could be calculated. Later upgrades to these systems, SAPS 2, APACHE III and the MPM,[28] used logistic regression analysis to determine the variables which should be included to explain the observed hospital mortality. Variables were no longer given equal importance but different weightings and a logistic regression equation were used to calculate a probability of hospital death. The more recent upgrades, APACHE IV and SAPS 3, have continued to use logistic regression techniques to identify variables that have an impact on hospital outcome.

The extent of physiological disturbance changes during critical illness. Scoring systems therefore needed to predetermine when the disturbance best reflected the severity of illness which additionally facilitated discrimination between likely survivors and non-survivors. Most systems are based on the worst physiological derangement for each parameter within the first 24 hours of ICU admission. However some systems, such as MPM II_0, are based on values obtained 1 hour either side of admission; this is designed to avoid the bias that treatment might introduce on acute physiology values.[29]

DEVELOPING A SCORING METHODOLOGY AND ITS VALIDATION

All the scoring systems have been based on a large database of critically ill patients, usually derived from at least one country and from several ICUs (Table 3.2). Typically, in the more recent upgrades of the common scoring systems, part of the database is used to develop a logistic regression equation with a dichotomous outcome – survival or death, while the rest of the database is used to test out the performance of the derived equation. The equation includes those variables which are statistically related to outcome. Each of these variables is given a weight within the equation. The regression equation can be tested, either against patients in the developmental dataset using special statistical techniques such as 'jack-knifing' and 'boot-strapping' or against a new set of patients – the validation dataset – who were in the original database but not in the developmental dataset. The aim of validation is to demonstrate that the derived model from the database can be used not only to measure severity of illness but also to provide hospital outcome predictions.

Table 3.2 Ability of scores to discriminate correctly between survivors and non-survivors when tested on similar casemixes. A value of 1 represents perfect prediction

Score	Area under ROC curve
APACHE II	0.85
APACHE III	0.90
SAPS 2	0.86
MPM II_0	0.82
MPM II_{24}	0.84
SAPS 3	0.84
APACHE IV	0.88

ROC, receiver operating characteristic; APACHE, Acute Physiology, Age and Chronic Health Evaluation; SAPS, Simplified Acute Physiology Score; MPM, Mortality Probability Model.

Once a satisfactory equation has been developed it can be used to calculate a probability of death for an individual patient. Similarly an overall probability of death can be calculated for a group of patients; however, this methodology can not indicate which of the patients in the cohort is going to die. These models are not powerful enough to provide sufficiently accurate discrimination.

In a perfect model the aim would be that:

- Overall predicted and observed outcomes should be the same.
- Individual patients observed to die or survive have been predicted.

The performance of a mortality prediction model used on a cohort of patients other than the developmental set is usually judged by two functions: first, its ability to predict which patients will survive and which will die (discrimination) and second, how well a model correctly predicts the overall observed mortality (calibration). The appendix shows some commonly calculated measures for a scoring system.

DISCRIMINATION

The discriminating power of a model can be determined by defining a series of threshold probabilities of death such as 50, 70, 80% above which a patient is expected to die if their calculated risk of death exceeds these threshold values and then comparing the expected number of deaths with what was observed in those patients at the various probability cut-off points. For example, the APACHE II system revealed a misclassification rate (patients predicted to die who survived and those predicted to survive who died) of 14.4, 15.2, 16.7 and 18.5% at 50, 70, 80 and 90% cut off points above which all patients with such predicted risks were expected to die. These figures indicate that the model predicted survivors and non-survivors best i.e., discriminated likely survivors from non-survivors when it was assumed that any patient with a risk of death greater than 50% would be a non-survivor.

A conventional approach to displaying discriminating ability is to plot sensitivity, true positive predictions on the *y*-axis against false-positive predictions (1 – specificity) on the *x*-axis for several predicted mortality cut-off points, and producing a receiver operator characteristic curve (ROC) (Figure 3.1).

The ROC area under the curve (AUC) summarises the paired true-positive and false-positive rates at different cut-off points (Figure 3.1) and provides a curve which defines the overall discriminating ability of the model. A perfect model would show no false positives and would therefore follow the *y*-axis and has an area of 1, a model which is non-discriminating would have an AUC 0.5, whereas models which are considered good would have AUC greater than 0.8. The AUC can therefore be used for comparing discriminating ability of severity of illness predictor models.

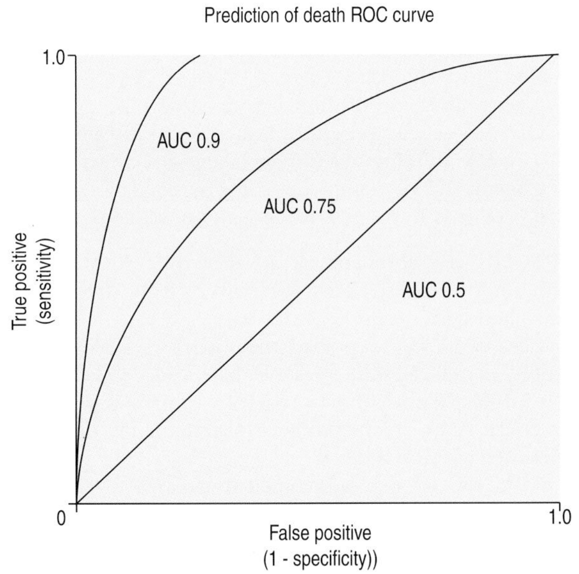

Figure 3.1 A receiver operator curve (ROC) plots true-positive against false-positive rates for a series of cut-off points for risk of death. For example, a risk of death cut-off point of 10% would predict that all patients with a risk greater than 10% will die and all those below will survive. This would be compared with the observed rates in those patients. The prediction would be expected to be frequently wrong and would reflect itself in the calculation of true-positive and false-positive rates. These calculations would represent one point on the ROC curve. The exercise is repeated at different cut-off points, such as 15, 20, 25, 30, from which a curve can be constructed. The resulting area under the curve (AUC) reflects the ability of the model to predict survival correctly. This is a measure of discriminatory power. The best models have values greater than 0.85.

CALIBRATION

A model with good calibration is one that for a given cohort predicts a similar percentage mortality as that observed. (Hosmer–Lemeshow goodness-of-fit C statistic compares the model with the patient group.)[30]

Observations with many models have revealed that, unless the casemix of the test patients is similar to that used to develop the model, the models may underperform due to poor calibration. This is particularly true when the testing is done for patients in different countries.[12,16,31,32]

COMMONLY USED SCORING SYSTEMS

GLASGOW COMA SCORE

Introduced in 1974 to quantify level of consciousness after the first 6 hours of head injury, it individually scores best eye opening, verbal and motor responsiveness, provides an overall scale between 3 (profound coma) and 15 (normal alert state). The Glasgow Coma Score (GCS) has been included in a number of general severity-of-illness scoring systems.

Its main characteristics are:

- Consistency between expert and non-expert observers and has been adopted worldwide.[33,34]
- Consistency has allowed head-injury management protocols to be based on the initial scale at presentation; decision-making is based on GCS trends.
- When combined with age it provides some assessment of prognosis.

The standard form of GCS is inapplicable to infants and children below the age of 5 years and has been modified to recognise that the expected normal verbal and motor responses must be related to the patient's age.[35]

THERAPEUTIC INTERVENTION SCORING SYSTEM (TISS)

Introduced in 1974 with the aims of estimating severity of illness, the burden of work for ICU staff and nursing resource allocation,[6] it requires the daily collection of 76 listed items, primarily interventions or treatments, although a cut-down version has been suggested – TISS 28.[36,37]

Its main characteristics are:

- good indicator of nursing and medical work
- poor measure of severity of illness
- successfully used as a method of accountancy through allocation of average costs per point

ACUTE PHYSIOLOGY AGE AND CHRONIC HEALTH EVALUATION (APACHE) SYSTEMS I–IV

In 1981 Knaus and colleagues described APACHE, a physiologically based classification system for measuring severity of illness in groups of critically ill patients. They suggested it could be used to control for casemix, compare outcomes, evaluate new therapies and study the utilisation of ICUs. APACHE II, a simplified version, was introduced in 1985[27] and, although superseded by APACHE III in 1991,[38] APACHE II has remained the most widely studied and extensive used severity-of-illness scoring system. APACHE IV was introduced in 2006 and, like APACHE, remains a proprietary system. Consequently, worldwide it is predominantly APACHE II rather than the later versions which is continued to be used for reporting severity of illness.

APACHE II was developed and validated on 5030 non-coronary artery bypass or burns patients admitted to ICUs in the USA.

It is the sum of three components:

1. an acute physiology score (APS)
2. a chronic health score based on defined premorbid states
3. a score based on the patient's age

The 12 variables of the APS and their relative weights were decided by expert opinion. These variables are collected in the first 24 hours after admission to intensive care and should represent the worst physiological values. The APACHE II score can be included in a logistic regression equation with a coefficient for one of 50 diagnostic categories representing the reason for admission and a factor for emergency surgery to provide a risk of death probability for an individual.

APACHE II functions best when the ICU patient cohort is similar to the original database used for its development and as expected, is less well calibrated when used for cohorts with limited diagnostic categories or in countries not represented in the developmental database. It has been noted that as critical care management and organisation improve, this older scoring system has tended to overestimate mortality predictions. Modifying old scoring systems does not readily correct the calibration problems, hence the need to develop upgraded systems from completely new databases.

MODIFICATIONS OF APACHE II

Bion *et al.*[39] and Chang *et al.*[40] separately were the first to explore the possibility of using APACHE II in a dynamic scoring system. The former used a modified APACHE II in the Sickness Score System, in which the day 1 score was compared with day 4 and risk of mortality was predicted. Chang *et al.*, on the other hand, used the product of daily APACHE II scores with a modified Organ Failure Score and calculated thresholds above which individual patient mortality could be predicted.[40]

APACHE III

APACHE III, based on a larger reference database, was introduced in 1991 and was designed:

- to improve prognostic estimates by re-evaluating the selection and weighting of physiological variables
- to examine how outcome is related to patient selection for ICU admission and its timing
- to clarify the distinction between using the APACHE scoring system to stratify by risk of mortality within particular patient groups and using it to make individual estimates of mortality

Characteristics of the new system

- The database is threefold larger (17 440 patients) from 40 US hospitals equally divided between developmental and validation groups.
- Exclusions included admission for less than 4 hours, age less than 16 years, burn injuries or patients admitted with chest pain.
- Coronary artery bypass patients were a separate group.
- Seventeen physiological variables and their weights were chosen through statistical analysis. There were 78 diagnostic categories.
- Treatment location immediately prior to ICU admission was included.
- A revised version of the GCS was used.
- Only those comorbidities which seem to affect the patient's immune status were taken into consideration
- Chronic disease and age contributed 15% to total mortality risk, the rest being acute physiology.

APACHE III represents an advance over APACHE II with improved discriminatory power (ROC 0.9 versus 0.85) and better calibration.[38]

Castella *et al.*[41] reported that, whereas APACHE II proved better calibrated results than SAPS and MPM I in a mixed-patient cohort of 14 745 from European and American ICUs, it failed to be as discriminating or as well calibrated as APACHE III.

APACHE III not only aimed to provide a calculated risk of death based on the worst first-day values but also if calculated on subsequent days gave an updated risk of death calculation. The coefficients for the regression equations are not in the public domain, and this has made independent assessment of the predictive aspect of the scoring system more difficult.

APACHE IV

It was the failure of customisation techniques with APACHE III to account for observations in subgroup analysis that indicated that a new model might be needed. Further the authors of APACHE IV revealed that when APACHE III in its modified form was applied to patients collected between 2002 and 2003, measures of calibration were poor.[17]

In 2006 there was consequently a further upgrade to the APACHE system based on a new database of 104

US ICUs in 45 hospitals. The selected hospitals had the APACHE III computerised data collection and analysis system already installed. The database, drawn from 131 618 admissions, analysed 110 558 patients, 60% of whom were randomly selected to make up the developmental dataset. The analysed patients excluded patients admitted for less than 4 hours, patients with burns, those < 16 years old and those who had received organ transplants other than kidney or liver. In addition patients in hospital for more than a year or who had no APS on the first day were excluded. Only first admissions were counted and those admitted from another ICU were excluded. The statistical and modelling techniques included cubic regression splines which allow a non-linear relationship between variable and outcome. This technique was applied to age, acute physiology and prior length of stay.

Variables included in APACHE IV

- Age
- Retained variables and weights of APACHE III and worst value collected on day 1
- Chronic health status
- 116 diagnostic categories for reason for admission
- Hospital length of stay and location prior to admission
- Emergency surgery status
- Ability to determine GCS
- Mechanical ventilation
- $Pa\text{O}_2/\text{Fi}\text{O}_2$ ratio
- Thrombolytic therapy for acute myocardial infarction

A different series of variables was used to develop a model for coronary artery bypass graft patients.

The AUC ROC (see Table 3.2) derived from the model used on a validation dataset was 0.88, indicating very good discrimination.

The APACHE IV mortality prediction model (Table 3.3) is in the public domain and can be found at www.criticaloutcomes.cerner.com.

The APACHE IV system has not been tested outside the USA and therefore may not be appropriately calibrated. Indeed, this may also be the case within the USA, given the selected units used for the database.[42]

Table 3.3 The relative contribution of predictor variables (%) for hospital mortality in APACHE IV

Acute physiology	65.5
Diagnosis	16.5
Age	9.4
Chronic health	5.0
Admission source and previous length of stay	2.9
Mechanical ventilation	0.6

APACHE, Acute Physiology, Age and Chronic Health Evaluation.

SIMPLIFIED ACUTE PHYSIOLOGY SCORE (SAPS 1–3)

The SAPS was originally based on data derived from French ICUs, based almost entirely on acute physiological variables.[26] The 14 physiological variables chosen were based on expert opinion and the points ascribed to deviation of these variables from normal were arbitrary. Initially the score was not related to an equation for predicting probability of death, although later this was possible. Unlike APACHE II, this system did not include a diagnostic category or chronic health status as part of the estimate of severity of illness.

In 1993 SAPS 2 was introduced and this was based on European and North American patients[43] The database contained 13 152 patients divided 65% and 35% between developmental and validation samples. Patients under 18 years, burns patients, coronary care and post cardiac surgery patients were excluded.

The weightings given to physiological derangements were derived from logistic regression analysis. This included 12 physiological variables and specific chronic health conditions such as the presence of acquired immunodeficiency syndrome (AIDS), haematological malignancies, cirrhosis and metastasis. Like SAPS, there was no requirement for inclusion of diagnostic groups to calculate probability of hospital mortality. The probability for hospital death could be readily calculated from a logistic regression equation based on APS and chronic health weightings. In the validation sample the area under the ROC curve was 0.86. It had equivalent calibration and discrimination to the APACHE III and MPM II systems. It is the most commonly used scoring system in Europe.

SAPS 3

SAPS 3 was introduced in 2005[15,16] and developed from a database of 16 784 patients from 303 ICUs from around the world, including South and Central America. The model used multilevel logistic regression equations based on 20 variables.

The variables were separated by the authors into those which were related to the period prior to admission, those concerning the admission itself and the acute physiological derangement (Table 3.4). These variables allow calculation of a SAPS 3 score which can be used to derive a risk of death from a logistic regression equation. Discrimination was good, with ROC AUC 0.848; however, the calibration varied depending on the geographical area tested. The best fits for the general SAPS 3 risk adjustment model were for northern European patients whereas the worst was for Central and South America, reflecting the number of patients used in the developmental dataset to derive the overall model. However the model can be customised with alternative equations to improve calibration for different regions of the world, and the authors suggest that customisation in future may allow within-country models.

Table 3.4 Factors considered in SAPS 3

Patient characteristics before admission	Circumstances surrounding admission	Acute physiological changes within 1 hour before and after admission
Age	Planned or unplanned	GCS
Comorbidities	Reason for admission (diagnostic group)	Bilirubin
Length of stay before ICU admission	Medical or surgical	Temperature
Hospital location before admission	Anatomical site of surgery	Creatinine
Vasoactive agents before admission	Acute infection at time of surgery	Leukocytes
		pH
		Systolic blood pressure
		Oxygenation and mechanical ventilation

SAPS, Simplified Acute Physiology Score; GCS, Glasgow Coma Score; ICU, intensive care unit.

The authors found that 50% of the explanatory power of the model for predicting hospital mortality was from patient characteristics prior to admission while circumstances surrounding admission and acute physiology parameters accounted for 22.5 and 27.5% respectively. Thus far experience with this model remains limited.

MORTALITY PREDICTION MODELS (MPM I AND II)

Introduced in 1985 to provide an evidence-based approach to constructing a scoring system,[44] the data were derived from a single US institution and included observations at the time of admission to ICU and within the first 24 hours. MPM I_0 was based on the absence or presence of some physiological and diagnostic features at the time of admission while a further prediction model, MPM I_{24}, was based on variables reflecting the effects of treatment at the end of the first ICU day. Unlike APACHE and SAPS systems, it does not calculate a score but computes the hospital risk of death from the presence or absence of factors in a logistic regression equation.

MPM II is based on the same dataset as SAPS 2.[28] The system is a series of four models which provide an outcome prediction estimate for ICU patients at admission and at 24, 48 and 72 hours. In common with the early APACHE and SAPS systems the models excluded burns, coronary care and cardiac surgery patients. The models were derived by using logistic regression techniques to choose and weight the variables, with the additional criterion that variables had to be 'clinically plausible'.

MPM II_0 and $MPMII_{24}$ have similar discriminatory power to SAPS 2, with ROC and AUC of 0.82 and 0.84 respectively.

In a comparison between MPM II, SAPS 2 and APACHE III and the earlier versions of these systems, all the newer systems performed better than their respective older versions. However no system stood out as being superior to the others.[41]

POSSUM

In 1991 Copeland *et al.* introduced a scoring system in the UK as a tool for adjusting for the risk of mortality and morbidity.[45] Physiological and Operative Severity Score for the enumeration of Mortality and Morbidity (POSSUM) includes 12 acute physiological parameters divided into four grades measured at the time of surgery and variables related to the severity of surgery (Table 3.5).

The POSSUM system was originally designed to predict risk of death by 30 days based on a logistic regression formula. However in 1996 Whiteley *et al.* noted that the POSSUM system overpredicted risk of death, particularly in those with very low risk (10%), by sixfold.[46] Whiteley

Table 3.5 Factors assessed for POSSUM risk of death

Acute physiological variables at time of surgery	Variables related to operative severity
Age Cardiac signs and chest X-ray findings Respiratory signs and chest X-ray findings Systolic blood pressure Pulse rate Glasgow Coma Score Urea Sodium Potassium Haemoglobin White cell count Electrocardiogram	Presence of malignancy Operative magnitude, e.g. minor, intermediate, major, major + Number of operations within 30 days Blood loss per operation Peritoneal contamination Timing of operation, e.g. elective, emergency < 2 hours or < 24 hours

POSSUM, Physiological and Operative Severity Score for the enumeration of Mortality and Morbidity.

et al. proposed that the POSSUM system was modified using the same parameters but a different logistic regression equation predicting risk of hospital mortality. This modification was named the Portsmouth-POSSUM (P-POSSUM) based on where it was developed. The P-POSSUM equation is more commonly used.

There have since been more modifications of the POSSUM logistic regression equation to obtain better calibration for other forms of surgery, e.g. vascular surgery (V-POSSUM), and Colon cancer resection (Cr-POSSUM).

POSSUM cannot be used for patients who do not have surgery and because the equation includes operative detail it cannot be used as a tool to make decisions as to whether surgery is undertaken. However it has become a very useful audit tool for surgeons who needed a risk adjustment tool for comparing their relative performances.

ORGAN FAILURE SCORES

These are simple prognostic values relating the number of failed organs and their duration to probability of mortality. The organ system failures (OSF) were defined for five organs in an all-or-nothing manner and the number of failures summed.[47] The outstanding observations were that:

- Single OSF lasting more than 1 day produced a hospital mortality rate of 40%.
- Two OSFs for more than 1 day (medical and surgical) increased rates to 60%.
- With three or more OSFs lasting more than 3 days, the mortality rate was 98%.
- Advanced chronologic age increased both the probability of developing OSF and the probability of death once OSF occurred.

Scores to take account of grades of dysfunction and supportive therapy have been proposed, including the multiple organ dysfunction score (MODS), which was based on specific descriptors in six organ systems (respiratory, renal, neurological, haematological, cardiovascular and hepatic). Progressive organ dysfunction was measured on a scale of 0–4; the intervals were statistically determined for each organ based on associated mortality. The summed score (maximum 24) on the first-day score was correlated with mortality in a graduated fashion.[48]

ICU mortality was approximately:

- 25% at 9–12 points
- 50% at 13–16 points
- 75% at 17–20 points
- 100% at levels of > 20 points

Good discrimination was seen, with areas under the ROC curve of 0.936 in the development set and 0.928 in the validation set.

SEQUENTIAL ORGAN FAILURE ASSESSMENT (SOFA)

This score was originally associated with sepsis, It takes into account six organs (brain, cardiovascular, coagulation, renal, hepatic, respiratory) and scores organ function from zero (normal) to 4 (extremely abnormal). Experts defined the parameter intervals.[49]

It was intended to provide the simplest daily description of organ dysfunction for use in clinical trials. It has the merit of including supportive therapy and, although increasing scores can be shown to be associated with increasing mortality, it was not designed for estimation of outcome probability. This simple method has become a popular method by which to track and describe patient changes in morbidity.

Logistic Organ, Dysfunction System (LODS) is an organ failure score that could be used for hospital outcome prediction.[50] Based on the patient cohort used to derive the SAPS 2 and MPM II systems, logistic regression was used on first-day data to propose an organ failure score. The LOD system identified 1–3 levels of organ dysfunction for six organ systems and between 1 and 5 LOD points were assigned to the levels of severity. The resulting LOD scores ranged from 0 to 22 points. Calibration and discrimination were good. LODS demonstrated that neurological, cardiovascular and renal dysfunction carried the most weight for predictive purposes followed by pulmonary and haematologic dysfunction, with hepatic dysfunction carrying the least weight. Unlike SOFA, the system takes into account the relative severity between organs and the degree of severity within an organ system by attributing different weights.

SCORES FOR INJURY AND TRAUMA

This is a relatively homogeneous group for assessment of severity of illness. There are two principal methods:

1. Injury Severity Score (ISS) scores the extent of anatomical injury.[51] Based on the Abbreviated Injury Scale (AIS), which assigns a code and a value from 1 (minor) to 6 (unsurvivable) to six body regions, and incorporates a modification for blunt and penetrating injury,[52] ISS is calculated from the sum of the squares of the highest AIS score in each of the three most severely injured body regions. (The square of values transformation results in a relatively linear relationship with mortality and other measures of severity.) The highest score is 5 (6 is fatal) in each body region and consequently the highest ISS is 75 (3×25).
2. Major trauma is defined as an ISS greater than 16 and this is associated with a greater than 10% risk of mortality. The ISS is a purely anatomical system that ignores physiological derangements or chronic health status.
3. Trauma Score (TS) is a physiologically based triage tool for use in the field, based on systolic blood pressure, capillary refill, respiratory rate and chest expansion and GCS. It could be used with anatomical and age data.[53]

The Revised Trauma Score (RTS)[54] is based on disturbances in three variables: (1) GCS; (2) systolic blood pressure; and (3) respiratory rate. Each is coded between 1 and 4. The physiological disturbance was further modified by use of a coefficient to indicate a relative weighting for that organ.

The ISS and RTS individually had flaws as indicators of outcome, but they were successfully combined by Boyd *et al.* to provide the Trauma Injury Severity Score (TRISS) methodology for outcome prediction. TRISS also included the presence of penetrating injury and age in its methodology.[51,54,55]

It uses coefficients derived from the data of 30 000 injured patients, from which it calculates an estimated probability of survival for individual trauma victims. It also provides a comparative measure of quality of care by trauma centres, using expected and observed outcomes.

A Severity Characterisation of Trauma (ASCOT) was introduced to rectify perceived problems with TRISS.[56] There are more details on injuries in the same body region, more age subdivisions and the use of emergency room acute physiology details rather than field values. ASCOT predicts survival better than TRISS, particularly for blunt injury. Reluctance to use ASCOT derives from increased complexity for only a modest gain in predictive value.

APPLICATION OF SCORING SYSTEMS

Standardised mortality ratio (SMR) is the comparison of predicted with observed mortality rates. This is used as surrogate evidence for good quality of care and a value of 1 is considered normal, above 1 worse than normal, below 1 better than normal but:

- standard deviations for SMR were not defined, therefore whether a unit significantly deviates from normal is unquantifiable
- SMR should be considered in the context of casemix and calibration[32]
- ideally samples should be very large and of a similar casemix as the original development database

The introduction of scoring systems has brought some standardisation and a new language that allows clinicians to describe the physiological disturbance of their casemix relatively accurately.

Such descriptions have led to numerous potential uses, including:

- stratification of patients for clinical trials
- comparison of predicted and observed outcomes
- relating resource allocation to severity of illness at presentation
- predicting length of stay for a cohort[57]

Decision-making for an individual patient based on the predictions of scoring systems is widely considered an inappropriate use because such systems are unable to discriminate patient outcome with certainty. The logistic regression equations only provide a probability for a dichotomous event, such as death or survival, and therefore they have no potential use as a guide to further treatment or limitation orders for an individual. When APACHE II was tested against an identical casemix to that from which it was derived and used as a predictor of outcome for individuals it at best had a misclassification rate of 15%.[27] The performance of these systems may be worse with different casemixes.[58–60]

Attempts to correct for this have included recalibrating the APACHE II system[61] and the use of neural networks. Neural networks use ongoing patient data input to modify predictor equations continually. This approach theoretically gets closer and closer to predicting outcome for a specific casemix but it never reaches certainty.

While scoring systems might facilitate recognition of hopelessly ill patients it is likely that patient management decisions will remain based on clinical judgement for the foreseeable future.

There are good reasons for not using severity score predictions to guide management but they can be used as a valid benchmark method for stratifying comparable patient groups for clinical studies. This stratification is best based on estimates of risk of death.

Unfortunately, unless there is a strict protocol for the collection of data across critical care units comparison of performance based on scoring systems can be very misleading particularly if further confounded by casemix differences which alter calibration. Clinical trials can control the quality of their data more easily than is achieved on a day-to-day basis in individual ICUs. Consequently comparison of risk of death and outcome between two patient groups might be more robust.

In order for between-ICU comparison to be representative of efficacy of care, some fundamental assumptions must be made:

- All pre ICU care is identical between hospitals and has no differential impact on ICU or hospital outcome.
- Patients in the different hospitals are drawn from the same population (casemix).
- The samples are large enough to obey the mathematical principles of logistic regression calculations.
- Data acquisition is both flawless with respect to the rules of the scoring system and consistent between units.

Although SMR may be misleading for between-unit comparisons as a measure of performance, it may remain a useful tool for within-ICU comparisons where it is assumed many of the confounding factors are the same. In such circumstances changes in ICU process or improvements prior to ICU admission while casemix remains the same may be revealed through improvements in SMR.

In the context of patient management scoring systems can be used as guidelines. A simple example is the use of a

GCS cut-off value below or equal to 8 for elective intubation and ventilation of a patient before transfer from the scene of injury. This has contributed to a reduction in secondary brain injury.

More controversial is the recent protocol for administration of recombinant human activated protein C, which suggests that it is only administered to patients with APACHE II scores > 25.[62]

REFERENCES

1. Breasted J. *The Edwin Smith Papyrus.* Chicago: University of Chicago; 1930.
2. Ranson JH, Rifkind KM, Turner JW. Prognostic signs and nonoperative peritoneal lavage in acute pancreatitis. *Surg Gynecol Obstet* 1976; **43**: 209–19.
3. Pugh RN, Murray-Lyon IM, Dawson JL *et al.* Transection of the oesophagus for bleeding oesophageal varices. *Br J Surg* 1973; **60**: 646–9.
4. Parsonnet V, Dean D, Bernstein AD. A method of uniform stratification of risk for evaluating the results of surgery in acquired adult heart disease. *Circulation* 1989; **79**: I3–12.
5. Jennett B, Teasdale G, Braakman R *et al.* Predicting outcome in individual patients after severe head injury. *Lancet* 1976; **1**: 1031–4.
6. Cullen DJ, Civetta JM, Briggs BA *et al.* Therapeutic intervention scoring system: a method for quantitative comparison of patient care. *Crit Care Med* 1974; **2**: 57–60.
7. Knaus WA, Zimmerman JE, Wagner DP *et al.* APACHE – acute physiology and chronic health evaluation: a physiologically based classification system. *Crit Care Med* 1981; **9**: 591–7.
8. Apolone G, Bertolini G, D'Amico R *et al.* The performance of SAPS II in a cohort of patients admitted to 99 Italian ICUs: results from GiViTI. Gruppo Italiano per la Valutazione degli interventi in Terapia Intensiva. *Intens Care Med* 1996; **22**: 1368–78.
9. Moreno R, Morais P. Outcome prediction in intensive care: results of a prospective, multicentre, Portuguese study. *Intens Care Med* 1997; **23**: 177–86.
10. Moreno R, Miranda DR, Fidler V *et al.* Evaluation of two outcome prediction models on an independent database. *Crit Care Med* 1998; **26**: 50–61.
11. Rowan KM, Kerr JH, Major E *et al.* Intensive Care Society's APACHE II study in Britain and Ireland – II: Outcome comparisons of intensive care units after adjustment for case mix by the American APACHE II method. *Br Med J* 1993; **307**: 977–81.
12. Bastos PG, Sun X, Wagner DP *et al.* Application of the APACHE III prognostic system in Brazilian intensive care units: a prospective multicenter study. *Intens Care Med* 1996; **22**: 564–70.
13. Zimmerman JE, Wagner DP, Draper EA *et al.* Evaluation of acute physiology and chronic health evaluation III predictions of hospital mortality in an independent database. *Crit Care Med* 1998; **26**: 1317–26.
14. Popovich MJ. If most intensive care units are graduating with honors, is it genuine quality or grade inflation? *Crit Care Med* 2002; **30**: 2145–6.
15. Metnitz PG, Moreno RP, Almeida E *et al.* SAPS 3 – from evaluation of the patient to evaluation of the intensive care unit. Part 1: Objectives, methods and cohort description. *Intens Care Med* 2005; **31**: 1336–44.
16. Moreno RP, Metnitz PG, Almeida E *et al.* SAPS 3 – from evaluation of the patient to evaluation of the intensive care unit. Part 2: Development of a prognostic model for hospital mortality at ICU admission. *Intens Care Med* 2005; **31**: 1345–55.
17. Zimmerman JE, Kramer AA, McNair DS *et al.* Acute Physiology and Chronic Health Evaluation (APACHE) IV: hospital mortality assessment for today's critically ill patients. *Crit Care Med* 2006; **34**: 1297–310.
18. Le Gall JR, Neumann A, Hemery F *et al.* Mortality prediction using SAPS II: an update for French intensive care units. *Crit Care* 2005; **9**: R645–52.
19. Zimmerman JE, Rousseau DM, Duffy J *et al.* Intensive care at two teaching hospitals: an organizational case study. *Am J Crit Care* 1994; **3**: 129–38.
20. Zimmerman JE, Shortell SM, Rousseau DM *et al.* Improving intensive care: observations based on organizational case studies in nine intensive care units: a prospective, multicenter study. *Crit Care Med* 1993; **1**: 443–51.
21. Knaus WA, Draper EA, Wagner DP *et al.* An evaluation of outcome from intensive care in major medical centers. *Ann Intern Med* 1986; **104**: 410–18.
22. Connors AF, Dawson NV, Thomas C *et al.* Outcomes following acute exacerbation of severe chronic obstructive lung disease. The SUPPORT investigators (Study to Understand Prognoses and Preferences for Outcomes and Risks of Treatments). *Am J Respir Crit Care Med* 1996; **154**: 959–67.
23. Hamel MB, Goldman L, Teno J *et al.* Identification of comatose patients at high risk for death or severe disability. SUPPORT Investigators. Understand Prognoses and Preferences for Outcomes and Risks of Treatments. *JAMA* 1995; **273**: 1842–8.
24. Ridley S, Plenderleith L. Survival after intensive care. Comparison with a matched normal population as an indicator of effectiveness. *Anaesthesia* 1994; **49**: 933–5.
25. Sage W, Rosenthal M, Silverman J. Is intensive care worth it? An assessment of input and outcome for the critically ill. *Crit Care Med* 1986; **14**: 777–82.
26. Le Gall JR, Loirat P, Alperovitch A *et al.* A simplified acute physiology score for ICU patients. *Crit Care Med* 1984; **12**: 975–7.
27. Knaus WA, Draper EA, Wagner DP *et al.* APACHE II: a severity of disease classification system. *Crit Care Med* 1985; **13**: 818–29.
28. Lemeshow S, Teres D, Klar J *et al.* Mortality Probability Models (MPM II) based on an international cohort of intensive care unit patients. *JAMA* 1993; **270**: 24–86.

29. Boyd O, Grounds M. Can standardized mortality ratio be used to compare quality of intensive care unit performance? *Crit Care Med* 1994; **22**: 1706–9.
30. Lemeshow S, Hosmer DW Jr. A review of goodness of fit statistics for use in the development of logistic regression models. *Am J Epidemiol* 1982; **115**: 92–106.
31. Vazquez Mata G, Rowan K, Zimmerman JE *et al.* International comparisons of intensive care: meeting the challenges of different worlds of intensive care. *Intens Care Med* 1996; **22**: 156–7.
32. Harrison DA, Brady AR, Parry GJ *et al.* Recalibration of risk prediction models in a large multicenter cohort of admissions to adult, general critical care units in the United Kingdom. *Crit Care Med* 2006; **34**: 1378–88.
33. Teasdale G, Jennett B. Assessment of coma and impaired consciousness. A practical scale. *Lancet* 1974; **2**: 81–4.
34. Teasdale G, Knill Jones R, van der Sande J. Observer variability in assessing impaired consciousness and coma. *J Neurol Neurosurg Psychiatry* 1978; **41**: 603–10.
35. Reilly PL, Simpson DA, Sprod R *et al.* Assessing the conscious level in infants and young children: a paediatric version of the Glasgow Coma Scale. *Childs Nerv Syst* 1988; **4**: 30–3.
36. Keene A, Cullen D. Therapeutic Intervention Scoring System: update 1983. *Crit Care Med* 1983; **11**: 1–3.
37. Miranda DR, de Rijk A, Schaufeli W. Simplified Therapeutic Intervention Scoring System: the TISS-28 items – results from a multicenter study. *Crit Care Med* 1996; **24**: 64–73.
38. Knaus WA, Wagner DP, Draper EA *et al.* The APACHE III prognostic system. Risk prediction of hospital mortality for critically ill hospitalized adults. *Chest* 1991; **100**: 1619–36.
39. Bion JF, Aitchison TC, Edlin SA *et al.* Sickness scoring and response to treatment as predictors of outcome from critical illness. *Intens Care Med* 1988; **14**: 167–72.
40. Chang RW, Jacobs S, Lee B. Predicting outcome among intensive care unit patients using computerised trend analysis of daily Apache II scores corrected for organ system failure. *Intens Care Med* 1988; **14**: 558–66.
41. Castella X, Artigas A, Bion J *et al.* A comparison of severity of illness scoring systems for intensive care unit patients: results of a multicenter, multinational study. The European/North American Severity Study Group. *Crit Care Med* 1995; **23**: 1327–35.
42. Afessa B. Benchmark for intensive care unit length of stay: one step forward, several more to go. *Crit Care Med* 2006; **34**: 2674–6.
43. Le Gall JR, Lemeshow S, Saulnier F. A new Simplified Acute Physiology Score (SAPS II) based on a European/North American multicenter study. *JAMA* 1993; **270**: 2957–63.
44. Lemeshow S, Teres D, Pastides H *et al.* A method for predicting survival and mortality of ICU patients using objectively derived weights. *Crit Care Med* 1985; **13**: 519–25.
45. Copeland GP, Jones D, Walters M. POSSUM: a scoring system for surgical audit. *Br J Surg* 1991; **78**: 355–60.
46. Whiteley MS, Prytherch DR, Higgins B *et al.* An evaluation of the POSSUM surgical scoring system. *Br J Surg* 1996; **83**: 812–15.
47. Knaus WA, Draper EA, Wagner DP *et al.* Prognosis in acute organ-system failure. *Ann Surg* 1985; **202**: 685–93.
48. Marshall JC, Cook DJ, Christou NV *et al.* Multiple organ dysfunction score: a reliable descriptor of a complex clinical outcome. *Crit Care Med* 1995; **23**: 1638–52.
49. Vincent JL, Moreno R, Takala J *et al.* The SOFA (Sepsis-related Organ Failure Assessment) score to describe organ dysfunction/failure. On behalf of the Working Group on Sepsis-Related Problems of the European Society of Intensive Care Medicine. *Intens Care Med* 1996; **22**: 707–10.
50. Le Gall JR, Klar J, Lemeshow S *et al.* The Logistic Organ Dysfunction system. A new way to assess organ dysfunction in the intensive care unit. ICU scoring group. *JAMA* 1996; **276**: 802–10.
51. Baker S, O'Neill B, Haddon Jr W *et al.* The injury severity score: a method for describing patients with multiple injuries and evaluating emergency care. *J Trauma* 1974; **14**: 187–96.
52. American Association for Advancement of Automotive Medicine. The Abbreviated Injury Scale, 1990 revision. Arlington Heights, IL: American Association for Advancement of Automotive Medicine; 1990.
53. Champion HR, Sacco WJ, Carnazzo AJ *et al.* Trauma score. *Crit Care Med* 1981; **9**: 672–6.
54. Champion HR, Sacco WJ, Copes WS *et al.* A revision of the Trauma Score. *J Trauma* 1989; **29**: 623–9.
55. Boyd CR, Tolson MA, Copes WS. Evaluating trauma care: the TRISS method. Trauma Score and the Injury Severity Score. *J Trauma* 1987; **27**: 370–8.
56. Champion HR, Copes WS, Sacco WJ *et al.* A new characterization of injury severity. *J Trauma* 1990; **30**: 539–45.
57. Zimmerman JE, Kramer AA, McNair DS *et al.* Intensive care unit length of stay: benchmarking based on Acute Physiology and Chronic Health Evaluation (APACHE) IV. *Crit Care Med* 2006; **34**: 2517–29.
58. Metnitz PG, Lang T, Vesely H *et al.* Ratios of observed to expected mortality are affected by differences in case mix and quality of care. *Intens Care Med* 2000; **26**: 1466–72.
59. Murphy Filkins R, Teres D, Lemeshow S *et al.* Effect of changing patient mix on the performance of an intensive care unit severity-of-illness model: how to distinguish a general from a specialty intensive care unit. *Crit Care Med* 1996; **24**: 1968–73.
60. Ridley S. Severity of illness scoring systems and performance appraisal. *Anaesthesia* 1998; **53**: 1185–94.
61. Rowan KM, Kerr JH, Major E *et al.* Intensive Care Society's Acute Physiology and Chronic Health Evaluation (APACHE II) study in Britain and Ireland: a prospective, multicenter, cohort study comparing two methods for predicting outcome for adult intensive care patients. *Crit Care Med* 1994; **22**: 1392–401.
62. Bernard GR, Vincent JL, Laterre PF *et al.* Efficacy and safety of recombinant human activated protein C for severe sepsis. *N Engl J Med* 2001; **344**: 699–709.

APPENDIX

Calculations of sensitivity and specificity for a prediction model for mortality

	Observed deaths	Observed survivors	Total
Predicted deaths	450	100	550
Predicted survivors	40	410	450
Total	490	510	1000

Sensitivity: the proportion of observed deaths that are predicted correctly (i.e. true positive).
Sensitivity = 450/(490) = 0.92.
Specificity: the proportion of survivors that are predicted to survive (i.e. true negative).
Specificity = 410/(510) = 0.80.
1 – specificity is proportion of survivors that were predicted to be dead (i.e. false positive).
Positive predictive value: observed deaths as a percentage of predicted deaths = 450/(550) = 0.82.
Negative predictive value: observed survivors as a percentage of those predicted to survive = 410/(450) = 0.91.
Misclassification rate is the proportion of patients wrongly predicted: (100 + 40)/1000 = 14%.
Correct classification rate is the proportion of patients correctly predicted = 450 + 410/1000 = 86%.
False-positive rate = 100% – positive predictive value = 18%.
False-negative value = 100% – negative predictive value = 9%.
Prevalence of death: 490/1000 = 49%.

4

Transport of the critically ill

Evan Everest and Blair Munford

All intensive care units (ICUs) are required to move critically ill patients for investigations or procedures that cannot be performed in the ICU. These patients have reduced or absent physiological reserves and even short trips can result in significant adverse events.[1,2] These events can be reduced by the use of trained personnel.[3,4]

In addition, ICU personnel are frequently involved in the stabilisation and transfer of critically ill patients into an ICU,[5] and some units may be involved in the transport of patients from the site of a prehospital incident, or between hospitals.[6,7] The interhospital transfer could be due to the increasing sophistication of critical care facilities in tertiary hospitals compared with district or rural hospitals, different subspecialty capabilities, local bed shortages[3] or, in certain health systems, for insurance or financial reasons. In some cases, the complexity of these interhospital transfers can be further complicated by the need for rapid transport, or the distances involved. All patient movement is associated with an increase in mortality or morbidity, but with an integrated approach using high-level clinical personnel who have the correct equipment and undertake sufficient planning, adverse events can be reduced.[3,4,6–8] Regular ambulances or untrained hospital staff should not be expected to manage ICU patients. Compared with specialist transport teams, standard ambulances with junior doctor escorts are associated with more cases of hypotension, acidosis and death.[9]

The hospital of the future has been described as the critical care hub of a dispersed network of facilities linked by information systems and critical care transport services.[10] Critical care transport should be part of a regional intensive care network and adhere to promulgated minimum standards for transport of the critically ill.[11,12]

INTERHOSPITAL TRANSPORT

The general principles of patient transport regarding equipment, patient monitoring and checking after movement are identical, whether intrahospital or interhospital. In interhospital transport the same problems are encountered but compounded by distance and the vehicular environment.

Patients are generally moved from the ICU for two reasons:

- diagnostic imaging that cannot be performed in the ICU, and
- for procedures, traditionally in the operating theatre, but increasingly for radiologically guided procedures including vascular embolisation, angioplasty, percutaneous drainage and stent insertion.

Moving an ICU patient is a high-risk procedure but with sufficient planning and preparation there should be little or no compromise to the patient's condition. Unfortunately, this is not always achieved, as there are often a number of distractions that will divert staff from monitoring the patient, or disconnection of infusions or ventilation. In up to 70% of ICU patient transports, adverse events occur, in which:

- one-third are equipment-related[13]
- acute deterioration of $Pa\text{O}_2/Fi\text{O}_2$ ratio is common
- ventilator-associated pneumonia is significantly increased[14,15]

However management is changed in 40–50% of patients, thus justifying the risk. Sufficient notification will allow the assembly of equipment, monitoring and sufficient staff who are trained and familiar with the equipment and the patient. The more complex the patient, the more capable the team required. In unstable patients the minimum team should consist of a suitably trained doctor (e.g. one capable of reintubating a ventilated patient and able to manage any changes occurring in the patient's condition), the patient's nurse and two assistants to move the bed and help to lift the patient. For more stable, less complicated patients the patient's nurse and assistants may be sufficient.

COMPUTED TOMOGRAPHY SCANNING

The most common diagnostic investigation necessitating transport is computed tomography (CT). On most occasions very little planning and preparation is required for what is almost a routine procedure. The exceptions are patients with head injuries, the administration of nasogastric contrast and the increased aspiration risk in patients with decreased gastric motility. Repeated CT scanning of head-injury patients is common. In those patients with decreased cerebral compliance, movement and changes in body position or $Paco_2$ can result in marked changes in intracranial pressure (ICP). Prior to transport, $Etco_2$ should be measured on the transport monitor while the patient remains connected to the ICU ventilator. ICP changes caused by ventilator-induced variations in $Paco_2$ when switching to the transport ventilator can be reduced by adjusting the minute volume to maintain a stable $Etco_2$. Adequate sedation will also decrease movement-induced rises in ICP. Ideally, the ICP should be measured on the transport monitor but this is often not possible. Whether a staff member remains in the scanner room or views the patient and monitor from outside depends on patient stability. Radiation exposure is small and is not considered a risk, and depends on where personnel stand in relation to the scanner's 'doughnut', from where the radiation is emitted.

MAGNETIC RESONANCE IMAGING SCANNING

The hazards to a patient in magnetic resonance imaging (MRI) are greater due to limitations in the proximity of infusion pumps, ventilators and monitors to the magnet, and at times on catheters and pacemakers inserted in the patient. The need for the MRI should be balanced against the information likely to be gained. The three main problems with transport equipment are:

1. metal objects becoming projectiles when in close proximity to the magnet
2. equipment interfering with the MRI
3. the MRI causing failures in transport equipment

MRI units vary in policy, from prohibiting any equipment in the room to having minimal equipment that is placed as far away from the magnet as possible. The ability of ventilators and infusion pumps to function in the MRI scan room must have been tested prior to any patient being scanned, as some modern transport ventilators have failed in the MRI. Ideally, the equipment should be left outside the room with extensions added to the infusion and ventilator tubing, but this increases the risk of disconnection. There is one reported case of the external part of a pulmonary artery catheter burning through during an MRI scan,[16] probably caused by the development of radiofrequency eddy currents. Thermodilution pulmonary artery catheters are probably safe, but although patients with internal defibrillators and permanent pacemakers have been scanned with no consequence, deaths have been reported. Prior discussion with individual MRI units on how ICU patients can be scanned is required.

INTERHOSPITAL TRANSPORT

ORGANISATIONAL ASPECTS

Provision of critical care transport services needs to be a part of regional ICU services. The staffing of critical care transport teams will depend on the workload, with around 300 per year being the threshold for a specific transport roster, depending on transport duration and regulations affecting duty times. Other factors include regional demographics, resources and geography. A team from within that unit, or from another ICU, or an emergency department, or a stand-alone transport service may provide transport of patients to a particular ICU. The merits of each system have been summarised.[17] Whatever arrangement is chosen, staff should not be conscripts but selected from those interested in critical care transport, and should be appropriately trained. Use of junior inexperienced staff is associated with increases in preventable mortality and morbidity.[18,19] Rostering of teams needs to be appropriate for the workload and take into account the potential for significant overtime hours when urgent requests occur near shift changeovers. If personnel are also allocated to other clinical duties, they need to be readily relieved when required. Equipment should be prechecked and the team should have a practised routine to enable prompt departure.

A coordination centre should be used in systems involving multiple requests and transport teams.

PERSONNEL

The aim of the transport team is at least to maintain but preferably to enhance the level of care. This requires transport teams to have diagnostic and procedural skills to provide the full complement of care for the full range of patients transported. Ideally, the personnel caring for the patient in transit should be equivalent to the 'front-line' clinical team at the destination, implying a physician-based team, although transport of well-stabilised patients by non-physician teams has been reported.[20]

The transport team should be a minimum of two people. For multiple patients a formula of $n + 1$ personnel for n critical patients has been suggested.[21] Multidisciplinary teams of physicians, nurse and/or ambulance officers offer advantages of a wider range of skills and training than a team from any single profession. In certain circumstances, other specialised staff may need to be taken, for example a surgeon or obstetrician.[6] It is preferable and safer to add a specialist to the standard team because of the latter's familiarity with the practicalities of the transport environment. Other desirable attributes in staff include: good teamwork and communication skills; adaptability; reasonable body habitus and physical condition; and no significant visual or auditory impairment or susceptibility to motion sickness. Travel sickness medications such as hyoscine (scopolamine) are of limited value, needing to be taken up to 4 hours pretransport and possibly causing significant side-effects.[22]

Training should encompass:

- principles and practicalities of clinical care in transport
- vehicle familiarisation
- relevant communication, safety and emergency procedures

Staff should have:

- appropriate personal protective equipment
- light-weight fireproof overalls or other clothing
- uniforms for prehospital responses, which should be of high visibility and bear identification

PATIENT SELECTION

The best utilisation of a critical care transport system is when it is activated for appropriate patients, which will depend on the levels of care available within the ambulance services. The need for critical care transport may be identified by:

- a diagnosis with the potential to deteriorate
- the requirement for physiological monitoring and acute interventions
- the continuation of treatment already instituted during transport

Both receiving hospitals and ambulance services need to be alert to possible cases where critical care transport is indicated, but not identified by the referring team. A mechanism that is highly sensitive and specific at identifying patients unsuitable for standard ambulance transport is required. Triage mechanisms and tables to aid in patient selection have been described.[23,24]

COMMUNICATIONS

A systematic approach is necessary to ensure a smooth response when the need for transport of a critically ill patient is identified. A single toll-free telephone number with conference call capability is the ideal. Facsimile and teleradiology capabilities may also be of value. The one call for assistance should result in the provision of clinical advice if required, the dispatch of a transport team, and finding a bed in an appropriate hospital. Concise, simple clinical advice appropriate for the capabilities of the referring hospital by either the receiving hospital or the transport service is paramount. No matter how fast the transport team's response, without some interim care the patient with major airway, breathing or circulatory compromise will not survive.[6,7] Ongoing advice, including stabilisation and preparation of the patient for transport, may be required prior to the arrival of the transport team. The provision to referring hospitals of a checklist for patient management and preparation for transport may assist.

The transport team should communicate with the receiving hospital, especially where changes in the patient's condition change the time of arrival, posttransport management or destination within the hospital or to another centre. Cellular telephones have revolutionised communication in transit, but their use may not be possible in all circumstances. Radio communication between ground and air ambulances and relevant hospitals is a preferred back-up.

EQUIPMENT

GENERAL CONSIDERATIONS

Minimum standards for supplies, equipment and monitoring for critical care transport have been developed.[10,17] Equipment selection is a compromise between providing for every conceivable scenario and being mobile. The aim should be to have a core set of equipment plus optional items for specific scenarios plus some back-up redundancy for vital supplies and equipment such as oxygen, airway devices and basic circulatory monitoring. A suggested equipment schedule is given in Table 4.1. Meticulous checking of equipment after each use and on a regular basis is essential.

Table 4.1 Suggested equipment schedule for interhospital critical care transport

Respiratory equipment
Intubation kit
Endotracheal tubes and connectors – adult and paediatric sizes
Introducers, bougies, Magill forceps
Laryngoscopes, blades, spare globes and batteries
Ancillaries: cuff syringe and manometer, clip forceps, 'gooseneck' tubing, heat moisture exchanger/filter(s), securing ties, lubricant
Alternative airways:
Simple: Guedel and nasopharyngeal
Supraglottic: laryngeal masks and/or Combitube
Infraglottic: cricothyrotomy kit and tubes
Oxygen masks (including high-Fio_2 type), tubing, nebulisers
Suction equipment:
Main suction system – usually vehicle-mounted
Spare (portable) suction – hand, O_2 or battery-powered
Suction tubing, handles, catheters and spare reservoir
Self-inflating hand ventilator, with masks and positive end-expiratory pressure (PEEP) valve
Portable ventilator with disconnect and overpressure alarms
Ventilator circuit and spares
Spirometer and cuff manometer
Capnometer/capnograph.
Pleural drainage equipment:
Intercostal catheters and cannulae
Surgical insertion kit and sutures (see below)
Heimlich-type valves and drainage bags
Main oxygen system (usually vehicle-mounted) of adequate capacity with flowmeters and standard wall outlets
Portable/reserve oxygen system with flowmeter and standard outlet
Circulatory equipment
Defibrillator/monitor/external pacemaker, with leads, electrodes and pads
Intravenous fluid administration equipment:
Range of fluids: isotonic crystalloid, dextrose, colloids
High-flow and metered-flow giving sets
Intravenous cannulae in range of sizes: peripheral and central/long lines

Continued

Table 4.1 Suggested equipment schedule for interhospital critical care transport—*Continued*

- Intravenous extension sets, three-way taps and needle-free injection system
- Syringes, needles and drawing-up cannulae
- Skin preparation wipes, intravenous dressings and BandAids
- Pressure infusion bags (for arterial line also)

Blood pressure-monitoring equipment:
- Arterial cannulae with arterial tubing and transducers
- Invasive and non-invasive (automated) blood pressure monitors
- Aneroid (non-mercury) sphygmomanometer and range of cuffs (preferably also compatible with non-invasive arterial blood pressure)

Pulse oximeter, with finger and multisite probes
Syringe/infusion pumps (minimum 2) and appropriate tubing

Miscellanous equipment

Urinary catheters and drainage/measurement bag
Gastric tubes and drainage bag
Minor surgical kit (for intercostal catheter, central venous lines, cricothyrotomy, etc.):
- Sterile instruments: scalpels, scissors, forceps, needle holders
- Suture material and needles
- Antiseptics, skin preparation packs and dressings
- Sterile gloves (various sizes); drapes ± gowns

Cervical collars, spinal immobilisation kit, splints
Pneumatic antishock garment (military antishock trousers (MAST) suit)
Thermometer (non-mercury) and/or temperature probe/monitor
Reflective (space) blanket and thermal insulation drapes
Bandages, tapes, heavy-duty scissors (shears)
Gloves and eye protection
Sharps and contaminated waste receptacles
Pen and folder for paperwork
Torch ± head light
Drug/additive labels and marker pen
Nasal decongestant (for barotitis prophylaxis)

Pharmacological agents

Central nervous system drugs:
- Narcotics ± non-narcotic analgesics
- Anxiolytics/sedatives
- Major tranquillisers
- Anticonvulsants
- Intravenous hypnotics/anaesthetic agents
- Antiemetics
- Local anaesthetics

Cardiovascular drugs:
- Antiarrhythmics
- Anticholinergics
- Inotropes/vasoconstrictors
- Nitrates
- α- and β-blockers; other hypotensives

Electrolytes and renal agents:
- Sodium bicarbonate
- Calcium (chloride)
- Magnesium
- Antibiotics
- Oxytocics
- Potassium
- Loop diuretics
- Osmotic diuretics

Endocrine and metabolic agents:
- Glucose (concentrate) ± glucagon
- Insulin
- Steroids

Other agents:
- Neuromuscular blockers: depolarising and non-depolarising
- Anticholinesterases (neuromuscular block reversal)
- Narcotic and benzodiazepine antagonists
- Bronchodilators
- Antihistamines
- H_2-blockers/proton pump inhibitors
- Anticoagulants
  - Thrombolytics
- Vitamin K
- Tocolytics

Diluents (saline and sterile water)

Additional/optional equipment

Transvenous temporary pacing kit and pacemaker
Blood (usually O negative) and/or blood products
Additonal infusion pumps and associated intravenous sets
Obstetrics kit
Additional paediatric equipment (depending on capability of basic kit)
Antivenene (polyvalent or specific)
Specific drugs or antagonists

Transport monitors, infusion pumps and ventilators must work outside the transport vehicle. This requires equipment to be battery-powered and readily portable. Although newer monitors and other devices have rechargeable batteries with improved endurance, problems can still occur. The equipment-checking process includes different charging regimes. Nickel cadmium (NiCad) batteries need to be fully discharged before recharging to decrease memory effect, which reduces endurance, whereas sealed lead–acid or lithium batteries perform best when continually charged between uses.[25]

Internal batteries should not be relied upon unless transport duration is less than half the estimated battery life. For longer trips, a supplementary power source from either an external battery pack or the transport vehicle should be available to reduce battery use or even charge the batteries. An external supply combined with a wiring harness to run and recharge internal batteries on all devices is preferable. Spare batteries are not ideal, as many devices are not amenable to rapid 'on-the-job' battery swaps without interruption of monitoring and therapy.

Portability can be addressed in two ways. Equipment can be vehicle-mounted but readily detachable to accompany the patient, either as individual devices or more conveniently as a modular unit.[26] Alternatively, a mobile intensive care module can be incorporated into the stretcher, either in the base[27] or as a 'stretcher bridge' straddling the patient.[28] Such designs are now widely used and allow the patient and equipment to be assembled into one unit at the referral point; this reduces loading and unloading time, ventilator and other device disconnections, and the risk of leaving equipment behind. Minor disadvantages include the increase in weight (25–30 kg), with corresponding reduction in maximum patient weight, and slight top-heaviness of the stretcher/patient combination.

MONITORING

Clinical observation by experienced personnel remains the mainstay of monitoring,[10] but some clinical assessments such as auscultation are impossible during transit. Hence monitoring by appropriate equipment should be at the same level or a higher level than what the patient receives in the stationary setting. Referring institutions should not allow patients to be transported by teams with inferior monitoring capability. Compact transport monitors offering electrocardiogram (ECG), Sp_{O_2}, non-invasive and multichannel invasive pressures, capnography and temperature monitoring have largely superseded older techniques, such as systolic pressure estimation by palpation and mean arterial pressure monitoring via an aneroid interface and gauge. These older techniques can still be used for backup, as can defibrillators for ECG, while small hand-held pulse oximeters and Et_{CO_2} detector are also available. Non-invasive blood pressure and pulse oximetry devices are susceptible to artefact[29,30] and the use of invasive arterial monitoring or shielding pulse oximetry probes may be required. Mercury-containing devices are unsuitable, especially in aircraft. For longer transports, or patients with major biochemical or respiratory disturbances, compact biochemical and blood gas analysers may be valuable.[31]

VENTILATION AND RESPIRATORY SUPPORT

A mechanical ventilator should be used on all ventilated patients during transport. Manual ventilation occupies one team member fully and cannot reliably deliver constant tidal volumes and stable Et_{CO_2}.[32] Transport ventilators are a compromise between portability and features.

The characteristics of an ideal transport ventilator are outlined in Table 4.2. No currently available transport ventilator meets all of these, and different models are optimised for different scenarios, so selection of a transport ventilator should take into account likely clinical and operational requirements. Back-up manual ventilation equipment must be available. In some cases of severe respiratory disease, a standard ICU ventilator may be needed. This may require medical air and AC power, although newer hybrid ICU/transport ventilators can provide enhanced ventilation capability without supply of these.[33] Similar requirements will apply to transport of patients on extracorporeal membrane oxygenation.

The provision of continuous positive airways pressure (CPAP) in transport remains problematic. 'Clapperboard'-type systems are economical on gas consumption, but being gravity-driven perform poorly during movement. Conventional CPAP systems have extremely high gas consumption, rendering them impractical except for short road transports. Electronically triggered CPAP is a feature of some newer transport ventilators; however, though they have been successfully used on occasions, poor performance with mask CPAP has been reported,[34] and some patients may need to be converted to synchronised intermittent mandatory ventilation or intermittent positive-pressure ventilation (IPPV) for transport.

Table 4.2 Features of an ideal transport ventilator

- Small, light, robust and cheap
- Not dependent on external power source
- Easy to use and clean, with foolproof assembly
- Economical on gas consumption
- Suitable for patients from neonates to large adults
- Fi_{O_2} continuously variable from ambient air to 100% oxygen
- Able to deliver positive end-expiratory pressure, continuous positive airways pressure, synchronised intermittent mandatory ventilation and pressure support
- Variable inspiratory-to-expiratory ratios
- Flow or pressure generator modes
- Integrated monitoring and alarm functions with audio and visual signals
- Altitude compensated

Maintenance of humidification of inspired gases is important during transport. In most cases, heat and moisture exchangers should provide adequate protection for intubated patients.[35] In special circumstances, for example, in neonates and cystic fibrosis patients, it may be necessary to use active humidification.

A suction system and preferably a reserve are needed during all phases of transport. These may be Venturi systems, electrical-powered pumps or manual aspirators. Oxygen Venturi systems are lighter than electrical systems and outperform manual aspirators, but have high oxygen consumption, > 40 l/min.[36]

INFUSIONS

Critically ill patients often have multiple drug infusions which need to be continued during transport. A reduction in pumps may be obtained by combining sedation infusions or by suspending some infusions for transport and giving them as intermittent boluses.

During the referral process it is important to ascertain the number of infusions running to ensure sufficient pumps are taken. Modern light-weight syringe drivers are preferable for most infusions but a volumetric pump is superior if an infusion of large volumes of fluid is required. Older 'drop-counting'-type infusion pumps are susceptible to disruption by movement and ambient pressure change and should not be used. Infusion pressure bags should also be available to maintain intravenous flow rates, as only minimal elevation of fluid bags is possible in most transport vehicles.

MISCELLANEOUS EQUIPMENT

Transcutaneous pacing is adequate in an emergency, or during very short transports, but in other circumstances elective transvenous pacing should be instituted. Equipment to institute or maintain other specialised therapy en route should be carried if required. In some situations, such as with an intra-aortic balloon pump, the equipment may be bulky and can influence the selection of the transport vehicle.[37]

Heimlich or similar one-way flap valves for pleural drainage are essential, as underwater seal drainage systems are not suitable for transport, owing to the likelihood of tipping and/or syphoning. Equipment to maintain nasogastric, urinary and wound drainage is also required.

MODE OF TRANSPORT

Three types of transport vehicle are commonly employed: road, aeroplane (fixed-wing), and helicopter (rotary-wing). Basic requirements for critical care transport vehicles are listed in Table 4.3. Ideally, dedicated vehicles for all transport modes should be used, but the workload may not justify this and often vehicles that can be readily converted for mobile ICU use are seconded as required. The mode of transport depends on distances involved between referring and receiving hospitals and transport team locations; it also depends on the urgency of the case, which is often influenced by the clinical capability of the referring centre. Guidelines for vehicle utilisation should be developed but should have some flexibility for special circumstances, e.g. workload, traffic congestion, weather. Features and limitations of different modes of transport are summarised in Table 4.4.

ROAD TRANSPORT

The ground ambulance remains the most commonly used critical care vehicle. With patients for whom time is not critical and level of care in transit is more important than speed, road transport over considerable distances is feasible and may be safer in some patient groups.[38]

Table 4.3 Essential features of transport vehicles

- Readily available
- Adequate operational safety
- Capable of carrying at least one stretcher and mobile intensive care equipment set
- Safe seating for full medical team, including at head and side of patient
- Adequate space and patient access for observation and procedures
- Equipped with adequate supply of oxygen/other gases for duration of transport
- Fitted with medical power supply of appropriate voltage and current capacity
- Appropriate speed, coupled with comfortable ride, without undue exposure to accelerations in any axis
- Acceptable noise and vibration levels
- Adequate cabin lighting, ventilation and climate control
- Fitted with overhead intravenous hooks, and sharps/biohazard waste receptacles
- Straightforward embarcation and disembarcation of patient and team
- Fitted with appropriate radios and mobile telephone

FIXED-WING TRANSPORT

Conventional aircraft are the most suitable for long-range transport. Their faster speed is offset by the secondary ambulance transport at both ends. Advantages over helicopters include pressurised cabins (in most models), decreased cabin noise compared with helicopters and the ability to fly in icing conditions.

ROTARY-WING TRANSPORT

Helicopters remain the most controversial, high-profile and expensive vehicles which require significant internal adaptations by clinical teams to enable them to perform patient care. Smaller helicopters are relatively or totally unsuitable as air ambulances. Appropriate helicopters are versatile vehicles, with the ability to perform transport both inside and beyond their 50–30-km optimum range 'doughnut'. Maximum value is obtained with a high workload, ensuring efficient clinical team utilisation, and between hospitals with on-site helipads to avoid secondary transport.

SAFETY AND TRAINING

Transport by any mode involves risk to staff and patients, and also imposes limitations on the delivery of care. In the aeromedical environment unfamiliar personnel perform clinical tasks poorly,[39] so teams must be appropriately trained and equipped to function effectively and safely in each mode of transport. They need to be familiar with use of the various transport vehicles' oxygen, suction, medical power, communications systems, and other equipment and stores. A senior member of their own professional group should train and accompany new personnel for several missions. Other specialist staff added to a team should receive a thorough safety brief and work under the direction of regular transport team members. Aeromedical crew training should encompass safety equipment, crash response, emergency egress and survival. Safety should be a foremost consideration in any transport. Activities that compromise road and air safety such as hazardous driving or flying below safe minima are not acceptable, and clinical teams must avoid attempting to coerce drivers or pilots to take risks. This has been recognised as a contributor to air ambulance accidents.[40]

ALTITUDE AND TRANSPORT PHYSIOLOGY

All transport modes result in increased noise, vibration, turbulence and accelerations in various or all axes (see Table 4.4). Personnel need to be aware of altitude-related complications that can occur with air transport. Increasing altitude results in decreasing oxygen partial pressure in accordance with Dalton's law; while gas volumes increase or where volume change is restricted, relative increases in pressure occur in accordance with Boyle's law (Table 4.5). Good introductory[41,42] and more detailed[43,44] aviation physiology texts are available.

Table 4.4 Properties of transport vehicles

	Road	Helicopter	Fixed wing
Launch time	3–5 min	5–10 min (more if IFR)	30–60 min
Speed	10–120 km/h dependent on roads and traffic	120–150 knots (220–290 km/h), straight line	140–180 knots (piston) 230–270 knots (turboprop) 375–460 knots (jet)
Secondary transport	Not applicable	Sometimes	Inevitable
Effective range	0–100 km (longer if required)	50–300 km (longer or shorter in special cases)	200–2000 km
Noise	Low, except at high speed	Moderate to high (headsets required)	Low to moderate (cruise). Higher on take-off/landing
Vibrations	Variable with speed and road surface	Moderate in most phases (varies with rotor type)	Low in cruise, moderate or high on take-off/landing
Accelerations	Variable and sometimes unpredictable in all axes	Minimal and usually vertical only	Significant (fore/aft) on take-off and landing
Special features	Base vehicles readily available	Versatility; point-to-point capability	Cabin pressurisation and all-weather capability (most)
Acquisition cost	Lowest	High (US$ 1–4.5 million new) depending on capabilities	Moderate (piston) to very high (jet)
Operating costs (per km)	Intermediate	Intermediate to high	Low to intermediate

IFR, international flight rules.

OXYGENATION AND HYPOXIA

Critical patients who are already dependent on an increased FiO_2 will be compromised by reduction in atmospheric pressure. Further oxygen supplementation will be required to maintain arterial PaO_2. Only in special or unexpected circumstances, for example, alpine helicopter operations or cabin decompression, would hypoxia be expected to affect the medical crew; however, they should be aware of the risk and be alert to symptoms. The manifestations of hypoxia are well described elsewhere.[37–40]

GAS EXPANSION

Expansion of trapped gases can manifest in: (1) physiological air spaces; (2) pathological air spaces; and (3) air-containing equipment.

The first category includes the middle ear, nasal sinuses and the gastrointestinal tract. These manifestations can affect crew as well as patients; consequently staff with upper respiratory tract infections or gastrointestinal disturbances should not fly.

The second category includes pneumothoraces, emphysematous lung cysts or bullae, intraocular or intracranial air from open injuries, bowel obstruction or rupture and gas emboli. Such patients should be transported at the lowest possible cabin or ambient altitude, with close monitoring and extreme care, especially on the ascent phase. The effect of trapped gas expansion can be reduced with denitrogenation by breathing 100% O_2 before and during flight.

Air-containing equipment includes: endotracheal and tracheostomy tube cuffs; Sengstaken–Blakemore tubes; pulmonary artery catheter balloons; air splints, pneumatic antishock garments (military antishock trousers (MAST) suit); and pleural, gastric and some wound drainage bags. Endotracheal cuff pressures need to be adjusted during flight, or filled with water. Increases in tidal volume in pneumatically controlled ventilators can occur with altitude, necessitating setting changes.[45]

CABIN PRESSURISATION

Most fixed-wing air ambulances have pressurised cabins, which decreases hypoxia and gas expansion. The pressurisation creates a cabin pressure equivalent to flying at a lower altitude, hence the term 'cabin altitude'. The maximum pressure differential that can be generated depends on the aircraft model. Most turboprop air ambulances can provide around 350 mmHg (46.7 kPa) differential, or cabin altitude of 1000 m (3000 ft) while flying at 6500 m (20 000 ft). Once maximum differential has been achieved, lower cabin altitude can only be provided by lower flight, which may be relatively or absolutely contraindicated – for example, a slower more turbulent flight or beneath lowest safe altitude, respectively. The medical team should not request a lower cabin altitude than what

Table 4.5 Changes with altitude

Altitude (ft)	Pressure (mmHg)	Alveolar Po_2		Gas space expansion	Standard temperature (8°C)	Notes
		(on air)	(100% O_2)			
Sea level	760	103	663	–	15	158°C is 'reference' average temperature – actual obviously varies
1000 (304.8 m)	733	98	636	13.6%	13	Minimum altitude above ground level for helicopter transports
2000 (609.6 m)	706	94	609	18%	11	Likely altitude for most (VFR) helicopter flights over sea-level terrain
3000 (914.4 m)	681	89	584	112%	9	Likely range of cabin altitude for standard flights in most turboprop air ambulance craft (e.g. Raytheon–Beech King Air series)
4000 (1219.2 m)	656	85	559	116%	7	
7000 (2133.6 m)	586	73	489	129%	1	Standard cabin altitude for airliners and most jet air ambulances (e.g. Lear 35)
10 000 (3048 m)	523	61	426	145%	25	Likely ceiling of helicopter operations and hypoxic threshold in normal individuals
15 000 (4572 m)	429	45	332	177	214.5	Threshold for hypoxic decompensation in non-acclimatised individuals
20 000 (6096 m)	349	34	252	1117	224.5	Likely upper range of cruise altitude for turboprop aircraft. Decompression at these altitudes causes rapid loss of consciousness and death without O_2
25 000 (7620 m)	282	30	185	1170	234	
40 000 (12 192 m)	141	10	61	1439	256	Cruise ceiling for airliners and jets. Limit for survivable decompression, even with 100% O_2 for flight crew

VFR, visual flight rules.

is required, with the final decision resting with the pilot. Failure of cabin pressurisation is rare, but if sudden can have dramatic consequences, and teams should be aware of procedures to follow.

OTHER CONSIDERATIONS

Temperature falls by 2°C for every 300 m (1000 ft) altitude increase. Water partial pressure also falls and is not corrected by cabin pressurisation. Respiratory and other exposed mucosa can become dehydrated and could eventually lead to systemic hypovolaemia. All intubated patients should have at least passive humidification. On prolonged journeys, staff may also be affected. Staff rostered for air transport should refrain from compressed-gas diving for at least 24 hours prior to the shift.[46]

PATIENT PREPARATION FOR TRANSPORT

The preparation phase for transport will depend on the patient's diagnosis and condition. If possible, the patient should be stable; efforts, which may include surgery, should be undertaken to obtain stability. The exception would be a patient requiring time-critical intervention at the receiving hospital. These transports are riskier, but are likely to be less futile than attempting to stabilise an inevitably deteriorating patient. Prior to any transport all patients must have a secure airway, either self-maintained or intubated and ventilated, and intravenous access. Any external bleeding should be controlled. Urgent investigations (e.g. X-rays, arterial blood gases) should be obtained where indicated, and possible in the time available. The patient should be secured on the stretcher and connected to ventilators and monitoring commensurate to the degree of stability and time constraints. Infusions should be rationalised and sedation may need to be increased during the trip.

Intercostal drains, if present or placed, should be connected to Heimlich-type valves. If parenteral nutrition is discontinued, an appropriate dextrose infusion should be substituted, with interval blood glucose estimation.

Appropriate documentation, including a referral letter, results of investigations and hospital and ambulance observations, needs to accompany the patient. The team should ensure that any relevant legal requirements have

Table 4.6 Suggested predeparture checklists

A. Before leaving hospital	
Patient identity and next of kin	Recorded
Consent for transport	Obtained and documented
Paperwork and X-rays	Collected
Drugs for transport	Present and sufficient
Emergency drugs/equipment	Available
Medical equipment	Collected and repacked
Monitors, ventilator and infusions	Connected and on
Tubes, lines, drains and catheters	Secured
Altitude request (if applicable)	Passed to pilot
Receiving unit	Contacted and updated
B. In-vehicle and predeparture	
Stretcher and patient restraints	Secured and checked
Oxygen supply	On and sufficient
Monitors, ventilator and infusions	Working and secure
Emergency drugs/equipment	Stowed and accessible
Other medical packs	Stowed
Intravenous fluids	Hung and running
Intravenous injection port	Accessible
Medical power	On and connected
Communications	Checked as applicable
Seatbelts	On and checked
Staff/patient headsets	On/checked (if applicable)

been complied with and, where possible, consent for transport obtained.[47] The final step prior to transport should be a series of checks, as listed in Table 4.6.

PATIENT CARE DURING TRANSPORT

If the patient is adequately prepared this phase should be uneventful. Special vigilance should be employed in the initial stages of movement, as this is the most likely time for either physiological decompensation or technical problems such as disconnections to occur. Once in the transport vehicle, a further set of checks is advisable (see Table 4.6). Therapy, monitoring and documentation should continue during transport. Transported patients are vulnerable to hypothermia, especially if intubated and/or paralysed and/or receiving multiple infusions.[2,48] Active heating in transit may be possible using the vehicle heating, while passive heat conservation should be practised during loading and unloading. Transport crews should be restrained during transport. If a critical event occurs necessitating the crew leaving their seats, the driver or pilot should be informed.

Death in transport should be a rare occurrence.[6,7] If it does occur, distance and the expectations and location of relatives should be taken into account in making the decision whether or not to continue transport to the destination. Carriage of relatives remains a controversial issue. For conscious patients, especially children, the presence of family members may have a beneficial effect. For unconscious patients it is less clear and needs to be balanced against space constraints in the mobile ICU vehicle, and the potential reaction of relatives in case of a critical event. Transport services should have policies in place both for carriage of relatives and for death in transit.

QUALITY ASSURANCE IN EDUCATION AND RESEARCH

Critical care transport is a recent development where accepted standards and guidelines are still evolving.[49] This means there is still considerable likelihood of problems, errors and critical incidents, with corresponding scope for research and quality improvement. This requires good clinical and operational data collection and patient outcomes. The process should be sensitive to the existence of system errors as well as individual patient, equipment or staff incidents. Preliminary results from the use of a critical incident monitoring system have been reported.[13] Users of the service must be informed of recommendations and system changes resulting from this process. Innovation and research by staff involved in this area should be encouraged.

SPECIAL TRANSPORT SITUATIONS

PERINATAL TRANSPORT

This encompasses both in utero and extrauterine transport of the neonate. Specialised neonatal teams normally perform neonatal transport.[50] Alternatively, part or all of the regular transport team may accompany specialist neonatal personnel. Neonatal transport stretchers are bulky and heavy, and require a vehicular power output of up to 250 W for the incubator and active humidifier as well as monitors, ventilator and infusion pumps. They also require a supply of medical air to allow precise regulation of FiO_2.[51] Transport of the pregnant patient carries the risk of precipitating labour, and in rare cases, delivery in transit.[52] This is suboptimal, especially where the baby is premature or otherwise at risk. Where labour cannot be suppressed, consideration should be given to delivery at the referring hospital, with subsequent neonatal and maternal transport.

TRANSPORT OF DIVING-INJURY PATIENTS

Patients with decompression sickness or arterial gas embolus require expeditious transport to a recompression facility. This must be balanced against the risk of even small decreases in ambient pressure; even a 10-m (30-ft) increase in altitude can exacerbate pathogenesis.[42] Divers with other problems such as marine animal envenomation or other medical conditions will still have increased total body nitrogen stores and can be at risk of developing evolved gas disorders during air transport. The use of transportable hyperbaric chambers has been reported[53] but their use severely compromises speed of response, and therapy possible in transit. Transport at or very near sea-level cabin pressure on 100% oxygen is the usual procedure.

INTERNATIONAL AND LONG-DISTANCE TRANSPORTS

International transport of critically ill patients is becoming increasingly common. There are often complex medical, social and economic factors for returning patients to their own medical system. These must be balanced against the immigration, visa and logistic requirements, and medical problems of ultralong-distance transport.[54] A physician-based team is less likely to have problems relating to drug carriage and status compared with a paramedical team. Logistic problems include carriage of sufficient supplies, and clinical staff to work shifts for prolonged transports. Pressure may be exerted to utilise cheaper regular passenger transport services instead of much more expensive air ambulances. Most international airlines will accept a stable seated patient, but there is considerable variation among airlines willing to carry stretcher patients and associated equipment. Such transports require considerable planning to arrange stretcher fitment and sufficient supplies of oxygen and electric power. A separate oxygen system for critical care transports is required as the aircraft's emergency oxygen system is not permitted for patient care and the oxygen systems for in-flight use by passengers with medical conditions can only deliver up to 4 l/min.[50] Airline engineering clearance of medical equipment is often required. Aircraft power needs to be negotiated or sufficient batteries carried. An air ambulance may be indicated for cases that are urgent, infective or require low cabin altitude, whereas stable post myocardial patients can be safely transported in commercial aircraft with appropriate escorts.[55]

CRITICAL CARE SCENE RESPONSES

Critical care teams offer a wide range of measures to complement standard prehospital providers, especially for major trauma, including: sedative/relaxant-assisted intubation; cricothyrotomy; tube thoracostomy; intravenous cutdown or central line insertion; and blood administration, as well as triage to an appropriate hospital.[56] These teams are only useful for trapped patients in the urban setting,[57] but combined with helicopter transport can improve outcomes in rural patients with blunt trauma.[56,58,59] In these situations the team should include an experienced prehospital provider. With appropriate activation the team may reach the patient at the scene or supplement management at the local hospital.

Critical care teams may also be of value in disaster situations.[60] Disaster medicine involves a change in emphasis to performing a small number of basic life-saving procedures on a large number of patients. Personnel with transport/prehospital experience are likely to be better trained and equipped to work at disaster scenes than traditional hospital disaster teams.[61] The order of priority remains the same as traditional critical care transport: triage, treatment and then transport.

REFERENCES

1. Braman S, Dunn S, Amico CA *et al.* Applications of intrahospital transport in critically ill patients. *Ann Intern Med* 1987; **107**: 469–73.
2. Ridley S, Carter R. The effects of secondary transport on critically ill patients. *Anaesthesia* 1989; **44**: 822–7.
3. Duke GJ, Green JV. Outcome of critically ill patients undergoing interhospital transfer. *Med J Aust* 2001; **174**: 122–5.
4. Edge WE, Kantar RK, Weigle CG *et al.* Reduction of morbidity in interhospital transport by specialised paediatric staff. *Crit Care Med* 1994; **22**: 186–91.
5. Hourihan F, Bishop G, Hillman KM *et al.* The medical emergency team: a new strategy to identify and intervene in high risk patients. *Clin Int Care* 1995; **6**: 269–72.
6. Gilligan JE, Griggs WM, Jelly MT *et al.* Mobile intensive care services in rural South Australia. *Med J Aust* 1999; **171**: 617–20.
7. Havill JH, Hyde PR, Forrest C. Transport of the critically ill: example of an integrated model. *NZ Med J* 1995; **108**: 378–80.
8. Flabouris A. Patient referral and transportation to a regional tertiary ICU: patient demographics, severity of illness and outcome comparison with non-transported patients. *Anaesth Intens Care* 1999; **27**: 385–90.
9. Bellingan G, Olivier T, Batson S *et al.* Comparison of a specialist retrieval team with current United Kingdom practice for the transport of critically ill patients. *Intens Care Med* 2000; **26**: 740–4.
10. Goldsmith JC. The US health care system in the year 2000. *JAMA* 1986; **256**: 3371–5.
11. Joint Faculty of Intensive Care, Australian and New Zealand College of Anaesthetists, and Australasian College of Emergency Medicine. Policy document IC10. *Minimum Standards for Transport of Critically Ill Patients*, 2003. Available online at: www.anzca.edu.au/jficm/resources/policy/ic10_2003.
12. Commission on Accreditation of Medical Transport Systems. *Accreditation Standards.* Anderson, SC: CAMTS; 1997.
13. Waydhas C. Intrahospital transport of critically ill patients. *Crit Care* 1999; **3**: R83–9.
14. Predictors of respiratory function deterioration after transfer of critically ill patients. *Intens Care Med* 1998; **24**: 1157–62.
15. Kollef MH, Von Harz B, Prentice D *et al.* Patient transport from intensive care increases the risk of developing ventilator-associated pneumonia. *Chest* 1997; **112**: 765–73.
16. ECRI. A new MRI complication. *Health Devices Alert 1988.* ECRI.
17. Flabouris A, Seppelt I. Optimal interhospital transport systems for the critically ill. In: Vincent JL (ed.) *2001 Yearbook of Intensive Care and Emergency Medicine.* Berlin: Springer-Verlag; 2001: 647–60.
18. Deane SA, Gaudry PL, Woods WPD *et al.* Interhospital transfer in the management of acute trauma. *Aust NZ J Surg* 1990; **60**: 441–6.
19. Gentleman D, Jennett B. Hazards of interhospital transfer of comatose head injured patients. *Lancet* 1981; **2**: 853–5.
20. Beyer AJ IIIrd, Land G, Zaritsky A. Non-physician transport of intubated paediatric patients: a system evaluation. *Crit Care Med* 1992; **20**: 961–6.

21. International Society of Aeromedical Services Australasian chapter. *Aeromedical Standards.* Arncliffe, Sydney: ISAS Australasia; 1993.
22. Benson AJ. Motion sickness. In: Ernsting J, King PF (eds) *Aviation Medicine.* Oxford: Butterworth-Heinemann; 1988: 318–38.
23. Lee A, Lum ME, Beehan SJ *et al.* Interhospital transfers: decision making analysis in critical care areas. *Crit Care Med* 1996; **24**: 618–23.
24. New South Wales Health Department/Ambulance Service. *Guidelines for Retrieval of the Critically Ill.* Sydney: NSW Health Department; 1995.
25. Gates Energy Products Technical Marketing Staff. *Rechargeable Batteries Applications Handbook.* Stoneham, MA: Butterworth-Heinemann; 1992.
26. Noy-Man Y, Papa MZ, Margaliot SZ. Portable air mobile life support unit. *Aviat Space Environ Med* 1985; **56**: 598–600.
27. Grant-Thompson JC. The Mobile Intensive-care Rescue Facility (MIRF): a close look at the intensive care aeromedical evacuation capability. *US Army Med Dept J* 1997; Sept–Oct: 23–6.
28. Wishaw KJ, Munford BJ, Roby HP. The Care Flight stretcher bridge: a compact mobile intensive care module. *Anaesth Intens Care* 1990; **18**: 234–8.
29. Rutten AJ, Isley AH, Skowronski GA *et al.* A comparative study of mean arterial blood pressure using automatic oscillometers, arterial cannulation, and auscultation. *Anaesth Intens Care* 1986; **14**: 58–65.
30. Lawless ST. Crying wolf: false alarms in a paediatric intensive care unit. *Crit Care Med* 1994; **22**: 981–5.
31. Hankins DG, Herr DM, Santrach PJ *et al.* Utilisation of a portable clinical analyser in air rescue. In: *ADAC/International Society of Aeromedical Services AIRMED 96 Congress Report.* Munich: Wolfsfellner Medizin Verlag; 1997: 109–11.
32. Erler CJ, Rutherford WF, Rodman G *et al.* Inadequate respiratory support in head injury patients. *Air Med J* 1993; **12**: 223–6.
33. Wong LS, McGuire NM. Laboratory assessment of the Bird T–Bird VS ventilator performance using a model lung. *Br J Anaesth* 2000; **84**: 811–17.
34. Porges KJ, Kelly SL. A comparison of the imposed work of breathing in continuous positive pressure ventilation mode between three different ventilators. *Emerg Med* 1999; **1**: 111–17.
35. Hedley RM, Allt-Graham J. Heat and moisture exchangers and breathing filters; a review. *Br J Anaesth* 1994; **73**: 227–36.
36. Russell WJ. Venturi suction. In: *Equipment for Anaesthesia and Intensive Care*, 2nd edn. Adelaide, SA: WJ Russell; 1997: 27–9.
37. Mertlich G, Quaal SJ. Air transport of the patient requiring intra-aortic balloon pumping. *Crit Care Nursing Clin North Am* 1989; **1**: 443–58.
38. Schneider NS, Borok Z, Heller M *et al.* Critical cardiac transport: air versus ground. *Am J Emerg Med* 1988; **6**: 449–52.
39. Harris BH. Performance of aeromedical crew members: training or experience? *Am J Emerg Med* 1986; **4**: 409–13.
40. *National Transportation Safety Board (US) Safety Study: Commercial Emergency Medical Services Helicopter Operations.* SS/88/01. USA: NTSB; 1988.
41. Blumen IJ, Callejas S. Transport and physiology: a reference for air medical personnel. In: Blumen IJ, Lemkin DL (eds) *Principles and Direction of Air Medical Transport.* Salt Lake City, UT: Air Medical Physician Association; 2003: 357–77.
42. Martin TE, Rodenberg HD. The physiological effects of altitude. In: Martin TE, Rodenberg HD (eds) *Aeromedical Transportation: A Clinical Guide.* Aldershot, UK: Avebury Aviation; 1996: 37–54.
43. De Hart RL (ed.) *Fundamentals of Aerospace Medicine.* Philadelphia: Lea & Febiger; 1985.
44. Ernsting J, King PF (eds) *Aviation Medicine.* Oxford: Butterworth-Heinemann; 1988.
45. Thomas G, Brimacombe J. Function of the Drager Oxylog ventilator at high altitude. *Anaesth Intens Care* 1994; **22**: 276–80.
46. Edmonds C, Lowry C, Pennefather J (eds) *Diving and Subaquatic Medicine*, 3rd edn. Oxford, UK: Butterworth-Heinemann; 1992: , 434–6.
47. Dunn JD. Legal aspects of transfers. *Problems Crit Care* 1990; **4**: 447–8.
48. Fiege A, Rutherford WF, Nelson DR. Factors influencing patient thermoregulation in flight. *Air Med J* 1996; **15**: 18–23.
49. Robinson KJ, Kamin R. Quality improvement for transport programs. In: *Principles and Direction of Air Medical Transport.* Salt Lake City, UT: Air Medical Physician Association; 2003: 148–56.
50. American Academy of Pediatrics Task Force on Interhospital Transport. *Guidelines for Air and Ground Transport of Neonatal and Pediatric Patients.* Elk Grove, IL: American Academy of Pediatrics; 1993.
51. James AG. Neonatal resuscitation, stabilisation and emergency neonatal transportation. *Intens Care World* 1995; **11**: 53–7.
52. Low RB, Martin D, Brown C. Emergency air transport of pregnant patients: the national experience. *Am J Emerg Med* 1988; **6**: 41–8.
53. Gilligan JE, Gorman DF, Millar I. Use of an airborne recompression chamber and transfer under pressure to a major hyperbaric facility. In: Shields TG (ed.) *Proceedings of the XIV Meeting of the European Undersea Biomedical Society.* Aberdeen, UK: European Undersea Biomedical Society; 1988; abstract (paper no. 5).
54. Munford BJ, Roby HP, Xavier X. Considerations in international air medical transport. In: *Principles and Direction of Air Medical Transport.* Salt Lake City, UT: Air Medical Physician Association; 2003: 59–75.
55. Essebag V, Lutchmedial S, Churchill-Smith M. Safety of long distance aeromedical transport of the cardiac patient: a retrospective study. *Aviat Space Environ Med* 2001; **72**: 182–7.

56. Garner A, Rashford S, Lee A *et al.* Addition of physicians to paramedic helicopter services decreases blunt trauma mortality. *Aust NZ J Surg* 1999; **69**: 697–700.
57. Hanrahan BJ, Munford BJ. Air medical scene response to the entrapped trauma patient. In: *AIRMED 96. ADAC/International Society of Aeromedical Services Congress Report.* Munich: Wolfsfellner Medizin Verlag; 1997: 375–80.
58. Baxt WG, Moody P. The impact of a physician as part of the aeromedical prehospital team in patients with blunt trauma. *JAMA* 1987; **257**: 3246–50.
59. Schmidt U, Scott BF, Nerlich ML *et al.* On-scene helicopter transport of patients with multiple injuries – comparison of a German and American system. *J Trauma* 1992; **33**: 548–55.
60. Nocera A, Dalton AM. Disaster alert! The role of physician staffed helicopter emergency medical services. *Med J Aust* 1994; **161**: 689–92.
61. Garner A, Nocera A. Should New South Wales hospital disaster teams be sent to major incident sites? *Aust NZ J Surg* 1999; **69**: 702–7.

5

Physiotherapy in intensive care

Fiona H Moffat and Mandy O Jones

Historically, physiotherapy in the intensive care unit (ICU) was confined to the treatment of respiratory problems performed routinely on all patients. Evidence-based practice has demonstrated that there is no longer a place for routine physiotherapy treatment in ICU.[1] Physiotherapeutic intervention is based on clinical reasoning following the identification of physiotherapy-amenable problems, which are elucidated from a thorough systematic assessment.

There is still some debate about the precise role of the physiotherapist within ICU, which may vary,[2] but the main features include:

- optimisation of cardiopulmonary function
- assistance in the weaning process utilising ventilatory support and oxygen therapy
- instigation of an early rehabilitation/mobilisation programme to assist in preventing the consequences of enforced immobility
- advice on positioning to protect joints and to minimise potential muscle, soft-tissue shortening and nerve damage
- optimisation of body position to effect muscle tone in the brain-injured patient
- optimisation of voluntary movement to promote functional independence and improve exercise tolerance
- management of presenting musculoskeletal pathology
- advice and education of family and carers
- liaison with medical and nursing staff on the continuation and monitoring of ongoing physiotherapy devised care plans

CARDIOPULMONARY PHYSIOTHERAPY

TREATMENT MODALITIES TO OPTIMISE CARDIOPULMONARY FUNCTION

Patients who are critically ill may present with impaired cardiopulmonary physiology secondary to both the underlying pathology and the therapeutic interventions employed to treat them. In their approach to any individual patient, physiotherapists may use specific treatment techniques targeted at improving ventilation/perfusion (V/Q) disturbances, increasing lung volumes, reducing the work of breathing and removing pulmonary secretions. Physiotherapy treatment modalities may differ depending on the presence of an endotracheal tube, although patient participation with treatment is encouraged and promoted at the earliest point during intubation. Each intervention is rarely used in isolation, but as part of an effective treatment plan. Some physiotherapeutic techniques may have short-lived beneficial effects on pulmonary function, and some have no clear evidence to validate their effectiveness (Table 5.1).

MANUAL HYPERINFLATION

In this technique a self-inflating circuit is used to deliver a volume of gas 50% greater than tidal volume (V_T) via an endotracheal or tracheostomy tube. An augmented V_T may recruit atelectatic lung secondary to reduced airflow resistance and enhanced interdependence via the collateral channels of ventilation.[3] Bronchial secretions may be mobilised by the increased expiratory flow rate and/or stimulation of a cough.[4] However, ventilator hyperinflation, the delivery of an augmented V_T via the ventilator, has been shown to be as effective in the removal of secretions and maintenance of static lung compliance as conventional manual hyperinflation (MHI).[5] This may also avoid cardiopulmonary instability associated with ventilator disconnection and loss of positive end-expiratory pressure (PEEP). In an emergency situation an Ambu-bag and facemask can be used to perform MHI in the self-ventilating patient. However, an alternative technique such as intermittent postitive-pressure breathing (IPPB) should be considered when an augmented V_T is required during a therapeutic intervention (Table 5.2).

RECRUITMENT MANOEUVRES

Recruitment manoeuvres may be employed to reverse hypoxaemia in patients with acute lung injury (ALI)/acute respiratory distress syndrome (ARDS). A recruitment manoeuvre involves a transient increase in transpulmonary

Table 5.1 Treatment modalities to optimise cardiopulmonary function

Invasively ventilated patients	Non-invasive/self-ventilating patients
Manual hyperinflation (MHI)	Active cycle of breathing technique (ACBT)
Suction	Manual techniques
Manual techniques	Positioning
Positioning	Intermittent positive-pressure breathing (IPPB)
Mobilization/ rehabilitation	Continuous positive airways pressure (CPAP)
	Non-invasive ventilation (NIV)
	Nasopharyngeal/oral suction
	Positive expiratory pressure (PEP) mask, flutter valve
	Mobilization/rehabilitation

Table 5.2 Potential advantages and complications of manual hyperinflation

Potential advantages
Reversal of acute lobar atelectasis[3]
Alveolar recruitment via channels of collateral ventilation[3]
Improvement in arterial oxygenation
Mobilisation of secretions and contents of aspiration[5]
Improved static lung compliance[5]
Effectiveness may be increased when combined with appropriate positioning and manual techniques[1]
Potential complications
Absolute contraindications include undrained pneumothorax and unexplained haemoptysis
Cardiovascular and haemodynamic instability[6]
Loss of PEEP, inducing hypoxia and potential lung damage. This can be minimised by incorporating a PEEP valve into the circuit of a 'PEEP-dependent' patient
Risk of volutrauma, barotrauma and pneumothorax,[7] which can be reduced by including a manometer in the circuit
Risk of increased intracranial pressure
Increased patient stress and anxiety

PEEP, positive end-expiratory pressure.

pressure in an attempt to reinflate and maintain atelectatic lung units.[8] No standard approach exists; however, common options include: the application of incremental levels of continuous positive airways pressure (CPAP) with no tidal excursion; incremental increases in PEEP with additional V_T; and the application of intermittent larger 'sigh' breaths. In randomised studies, although recruitment manoeuvres may transiently improve oxygenation, there is as yet no proven outcome benefit.[9]

SUCTION

Suction is used to clear secretions from central airways when a cough reflex is impaired or absent. A suction catheter is passed via an endotracheal or tracheostomy tube or via a nasal/oral airway to the carina, and this may stimulate a cough in a non-paralysed patient (Table 5.3). The catheter is pulled back 1 cm before suction is applied on withdrawal. The suction catheter diameter should not be greater than 50% of the diameter of the airway through which it is inserted as large negative pressure can be generated intrathoracically without air entrainment. The use of suction following effective MHI optimises removal of secretions.[10] Instillation of normal saline prior to suctioning remains controversial; however, it may stimulate a cough, maximising secretion mobilisation and clearance.

Table 5.3 Potential advantages and complications of suction

Potential advantages
Stimulation of a cough when reflex is impaired by mechanical stimulation of the larynx, trachea or large bronchi
Removal of secretions from central airways when cough is ineffective or absent
Potential complications
Tracheal suction is an invasive procedure and should only be undertaken when there is a clear indication
Absolute contraindications to suctioning are unexplained haemoptysis, severe coagulopathies, severe bronchospasm, laryngeal stridor, base-of-skull fracture and a compromised cardiovascular system
Hypoxaemia can be induced secondary to suctioning. This can be limited by pre- and postoxygenation
Cardiac arrhythmias may be more common in the presence of hypoxia
Tracheal stimulation may produce increased sympathetic nervous system activity or a vasovagal reflex producing cardiac arrhythmias and hypotension

MANUAL TECHNIQUES

CHEST SHAKING AND VIBRATIONS

Shaking and vibrations are oscillatory movements of large and small amplitude performed during expiration, and are thought to increase expiratory flow rate, aiding mucociliary clearance.[11] These techniques are believed to be more effective when performed at high lung volumes.

CHEST WALL COMPRESSION

Compression of the chest wall can be used to augment an expiratory manoeuvre such as a 'huff' (see section on active cycle of breathing technique (ACBT), below) or a cough by providing tactile stimulation, or wound support.

CHEST CLAPPING/PERCUSSION

Chest clapping is a rhythmical percussion applied over specific areas of the chest. It may mobilise secretions secondary to the transmission of mechanical oscillations through the chest wall. However, there is little evidence to support this claim.

NEUROPHYSIOLOGICAL FACILITATION (NPF) OF RESPIRATION

NPF of respiration is a set of techniques designed for the treatment of the neurologically impaired adult. Manual externally applied stimuli to the thorax, abdomen and mouth can be used to stimulate increased V_T, a cough reflex, augmented contraction of the abdominal muscles or an increased conscious level.[12,13]

POSITIONING

A simple change of position can have a profound effect on cardiopulmonary physiology[14,15] (Table 5.4). As such, positioning is commonly utilised to achieve several different goals: drainage of secretions using gravity-assisted positioning (GAP), reduction of the work of breathing/breathlessness or to optimise V/Q matching.

GRAVITY-ASSISTED POSITIONING

GAP facilitates the removal of excess bronchial secretions by positioning a specific bronchopulmonary segment perpendicular to gravity (Table 5.5). This technique is not used in isolation but in conjunction with augmented V_T, via the ventilator, MHI or ACBT in a spontaneously breathing patient. An individual position exists for each bronchopulmonary segment based on the anatomy of the bronchial tree;[16] however, these may need modification in the ICU setting.

REDUCTION OF THE WORK OF BREATHING

A reduction in the work of breathing/breathlessness can be achieved by putting a patient in a position that optimises the length–tension relationship of the diaphragm, promotes relaxation of the shoulder girdle and upper chest and facilitates the use of breathing control.[17] This approach to positioning is particularly effective when used in conjunction with non-invasive ventilation (NIV). Adequately supported high side-lying is a useful position to promote relaxation of the breathless patient. In addition, it can discourage the overuse of accessory muscles of respiration, which may reduce energy expenditure. Some patients prefer forward lean-sitting with their arms placed in front of them on a high table. In this position the length–tension relationship of the diaphragm is optimised secondary to forward displacement of the abdominal contents.

Table 5.4 Potential advantages and complications of mobilisation[14]

Potential advantages	
Positioning supine to upright	**Mobilisation**
↑ Lung volumes	↑ Ventilation
↑ Lung compliance	↑ V/Q matching
↓ Airway closure	↑ Recruitment of lung units
↑ Pa_{O_2}	↑ Surfactant production/ distribution
↓ Work of breathing	↑ Mobilisation of secretions
↑ Mobilisation of secretions	↑ Cardiopulmonary fitness and exercise capacity
Potential complications	
Cardiovascular/neurological/ haematological instability	
Increased oxygen/ventilatory requirement	

(Adapted from Dean E: The effects of positioning and mobilization on oxygen transport. In: Pryor JA, Webber BA (eds) *Physiotherapy for Respiratory and Cardiac Problems,* 2nd edn. Edinburgh: Churchill Livingstone; 1998: 125.)

Table 5.5 Potential advantages and complications of gravity-assisted positioning (GAP)

Potential advantages
Maximises removal of excess bronchial secretions when combined with active cycle of breathing technique
Allows accurate treatment of specific bronchopulmonary segments
Self-treatment can be included in a home programme on discharge
Potential complications
Positions need modification when used in the presence of cardiovascular/neurological instability, haemoptysis or gastric reflux

VENTILATION/PERFUSION

Appropriate positioning of a patient can maximise V/Q.[18] In the self-ventilating adult, V/Q matching increases from non-dependent to dependent areas of lung.[19] However, in adults receiving positive-pressure ventilation lung mechanics are altered, producing V/Q inequality. In this situation non-dependent areas of lung are preferentially ventilated while dependent regions are optimally perfused; as such, a regular change of position is recommended.

In an extreme form prone positioning has been used to improve refractory hypoxaemia in patients with ALI/ARDS. The mechanisms behind these improvements are complex, but likely centre around a combination of a redistribution of some pulmonary perfusion together with a more homogeneous distribution of ventilation, leading to improved V/Q matching. Although prone positioning improves oxygenation in 70% of patients with ALI/ARDS, its role in improving outcome remains controversial.[20]

ACTIVE CYCLE OF BREATHING TECHNIQUE

The ACBT is a cycle of breathing exercises used to remove excess bronchial secretions (Table 5.6). The cycle can be adapted for each patient according to existing

Table 5.6 Potential advantages and complications of active cycle of breathing technique (ACBT)

Potential advantages
Mobilises and clears excess bronchial secretions[21,22]
Improves lung function[23]
Minimises the work of breathing
Individual components of the cycle can be utilised/emphasised to target specific problems
Can be used in combination with other manual techniques, gravity-assisted positioning, *V/Q* matching, positioning to reduce breathlessness and during activities such as walking
Self-treatment can be included in a home programme
Potential complications
Without adequate periods of breathing control, bronchospasm and desaturation can occur
Poor technique can lead to ineffective treatment and unnecessary energy expenditure

underlying pathology and presenting clinical signs. It consists of:

- breathing control × 4–6 breaths
  - normal tidal breathing using the lower chest
  - minimising the use of accessory muscles of respiration
  - promoting relaxation
- lowering thoracic expansion × 4–6 breaths
  - with/without an inspiratory hold
- forced expiration technique
  - expiration with an open glottis ('huff'), combined with breathing control

Although mainly used in the self-ventilating patient, alert, cooperative, ventilated patients can participate with this technique. The ACBT can be delivered via MHI in sedated and ventilated patients requiring mobilisation of secretions and airway clearance.

MECHANICAL ADJUNCTS

INTERMITTENT POSITIVE-PRESSURE BREATHING

IPPB is a patient-triggered, pressure-cycled mechanical device mainly used in self-ventilating patients to increase ventilation, mobilise bronchial secretions and re-expand lung tissue by augmenting V_T[24] (Table 5.7). Positive airway pressure is maintained throughout inspiration. Expiration is passive. IPPB requires constant adjustment of pressure and flow rates and careful patient monitoring to maintain effectiveness and cooperation. Effectiveness is increased when used in conjunction with positioning, ACBT and manual techniques[24] (Table 5.8).

CONTINUOUS POSITIVE AIRWAYS PRESSURE

CPAP maintains a positive airway pressure throughout inspiration and expiration. It is used in both intubated and self-ventilating patients to increase/normalise functional residual capacity (FRC) via recruitment of atelectatic lung. Clinically increased FRC is associated with improved lung compliance, improved oxygenation and a reduced work of breathing.[24] Effectiveness is increased when used in conjunction with appropriate positioning. The self-ventilating patient must be able to generate an adequate V_T as this volume is not augmented with CPAP (see Table 5.7).

Table 5.7 Site and action of intermittent positive-pressure breathing (IPPB), continuous positive airways pressure (CPAP) and non-invasive ventilation (NIV)

	IPPB	CPAP	NIV
Lung volume affected	↑ V_T	↑ FRC	↑ V_T and FRC
Action	Assists removal of excess bronchial secretions	Reverses atelectasis	Ventilatory support

FRC, functional residual capacity.

Table 5.8 Potential advantages and complications of intermittent positive-pressure breathing (IPPB), continuous positive airways pressure (CPAP) and non-invasive ventilation (NIV)

Potential advantages
Improves lung volumes
Improves gaseous exchange
Decreases the work of breathing
IPPB and NIV can mobilise excess bronchial secretions by improving V_T
IPPB and NIV can improve lung and chest wall compliance
CPAP reduces left ventricular afterload by reducing the transmural pressure gradient
Patients can be mobilised while on CPAP and some modes of NIV. Alteration of ventilator settings might be indicated to maximise patient potential/exercise tolerance during treatment
Settings can be adjusted to augment physiotherapy intervention, e.g. increased inspiratory positive airway pressure to assist removal of secretions
Potential complications
Absolute contraindications include severe bronchospasm, undrained pneumothorax, pneumomediastinum, unexplained haemoptysis and facial fractures. Use with care in pre-existing bullous lung disease
Haemodynamic/neurological instability
Risk of decreased urine output with CPAP and NIV
Risk of carbon dioxide retention with CPAP
Risk of aspiration

IPAP, Inspiratory positive airway pressure.

NON-INVASIVE VENTILATION

In recent years there has been an expansion in the role of NIV in the ICU. This includes the prevention of invasive ventilation in patients with chronic obstructive pulmonary disease,[25] pulmonary oedema and immunocompromise; early weaning from mechanical ventilation; and potentially the prevention of reintubation in those who suffer extubation failure. In addition, V_T may be augmented during physiotherapy treatment to remove secretions, or when mobilising the patient (see Table 5.7). Improved oxygenation may be achieved using NIV when the patient is positioning to optimise V/Q (see Table 5.8).

TREATMENT ADJUNCTS AND TECHNIQUES

Positive expiratory pressure mask and flutter devices are specialised mucociliary clearance devices used by some patients with chronic lung disease. These devices are rarely introduced in the ICU setting.

Table 5.10 Deconditioning and the respiratory system[31–33]

Respiratory system
Adverse effects on:
Functional residual capacity
Compliance (lung and chest wall)
Resistance
Closing volume
Respiratory muscle function – impaired strength and endurance, reduced performance of ventilatory pump, ↑ days of mechanical ventilation, complex weaning issues
Concept of ventilator-induced diaphragmatic dysfunction proposed (atrophy, fibre remodelling, oxidative stress and structural injury). Time-dependent reduction in force-generating capacity, secondary to disuse and passive shortening
Respiratory muscle weakness may be limited by judicious choice of ventilation mode. Role of inspiratory muscle training unclear

CRITICAL CARE REHABILITATION

The effects of deconditioning on the cardiovascular (Table 5.9), respiratory (Table 5.10) and neuromusculoskeletal system (Table 5.11) are well documented.[26–28] This phenomenon occurs as a result of restricted physical activity, and reduces the ability to perform work. The effects of deconditioning can occur with even relatively short periods of immobility, and are significantly influenced by age, premorbid condition, nature of the illness/injury and pharmacological factors. The consequences of deconditioning are significant in terms of patient outcome, length of hospital stay, duration of rehabilitation and subsequent ability to function independently in the community.[29] The psychological impact of deconditioning should not be underestimated. Inability to function at a 'normal' level of activity may result in depression and reduced self-efficacy.

Table 5.9 Deconditioning and the cardiovascular system[26,28,30]

Cardiovascular system
↓ Stroke volume – ventricular remodelling and reduced preload (see ↓ Plasma volume)
↑ Heart rate (resting and exercising): ↓ vagal tone, ↑ sympathetic catecholamine secretion and ↑ cardiac β-receptor activity
↓ Cardiac output and systemic oxygen delivery
↓ $\dot{V}O_{2max}$: magnitude highly correlated to duration, static exercise effective in preventing some decrease. Related to changes centrally (cardiac output) and peripherally (oxygen delivery and utilisation)
↓ Plasma volume: secondary to fluid shift and altered renin–angiotensin–aldosterone activity. Contributes to ↓ orthostatic tolerance
Orthostatic intolerance develops more rapidly in the elderly or those with cardiovascular pathology. Often slow to resolve
Increased blood viscosity and vascular stasis: predisposition to thromboembolism
Altered cardiovascular reflexes: proposed attenuated baroreflex-mediated sympathoexcitation and enhanced cardiopulmonary receptor-mediated sympathoinhibition. Contributes to orthostatic intolerance
Altered arterial/venous vascular function

An increasing volume of research suggests that the deleterious consequences of immobility may be in part attenuated by selected rehabilitation interventions.[38,39] The physiotherapist possessing expertise in rehabilitation and exercise physiology should direct the multiprofessional team in evaluating individual patients, devising a therapeutic strategy and referring to other specialties (e.g. speech and language therapy, occupational therapy) as required. Considerations must include:

- current physiological reserve
- extent of physiological impairment (associated with deconditioning and coexisting pathology, e.g. sepsis, multiorgan failure, neurological insult, inotrope dependence)
- nutritional status
- premorbid physiological reserve
- premorbid functional ability
- extent of patient participation
- external limitations (e.g. surgical instructions, traction, sedation, paralysing agents)
- risk assessment for moving and handling
- selection of appropriate/validated outcome measures

Traditionally, exercise rehabilitation has progressed linearly from activity in bed, then sitting, and finally to standing/walking. The model demonstrated in Figure 5.1 represents a three-stage functional rehabilitation programme. It is supported by evidence that suggests that a multimodal training regime is required to maintain/restore both

Table 5.11 Deconditioning and the neuromusculoskeletal system[26,34–37]

Neuromusculoskeletal system
Muscle atrophy – protein degradation (loss of contractile protein, increased non-contractile tissue, e.g. collagen) and cytokine activity. Reduction in strength, especially lower-limb antigravity muscles (i.e. those involved with transferring and ambulation). Inactivity amplifies the catabolic response of skeletal muscle to cortisol, therefore there is more marked atrophy following trauma or illness. Particularly significant in patient groups with low relative muscle mass, e.g. the elderly. Nutritional countermeasures should be considered and carefully titrated to meet demands best
↓ Muscle endurance (cf. Table 5.10) – reduced muscle blood flow/red cell volume/capillarisation/oxidative enzymes and biochemical changes. Generally longer to rehabilitate compared to reduction in muscle strength
Muscle shortening or changes in peri-/intra-articular connective tissue (including chest wall and thoracic spine) → contractures, ↓ joint range of motion, pain. Positioning and stretching maintain range and delay invasion of non-contractile protein
Decreased bone mineral density (particularly trabecular bone) – may be attenuated by standing or resistance exercise. Rate of recovery tends to lag behind that of muscle strength. Increased risk of fracture on remobilisation, especially in elderly
Microvascular and biochemical changes in peripheral nerves impair neuromuscular function. Adversely affects maximal voluntary contraction, and balance/proprioceptive activity
Critical illness neuropathy and myopathy frequently develop in patients hospitalised in an ICU for > 1 week. Risk factors include sepsis, SIRS and severe MOF. Associated with higher mortality rate, prolonged ventilation and rehabilitation, disability and reduced quality of life

ICU, intensive care unit; SIRS, systemic inflammatory response syndrome; MOF, multiorgan failure.

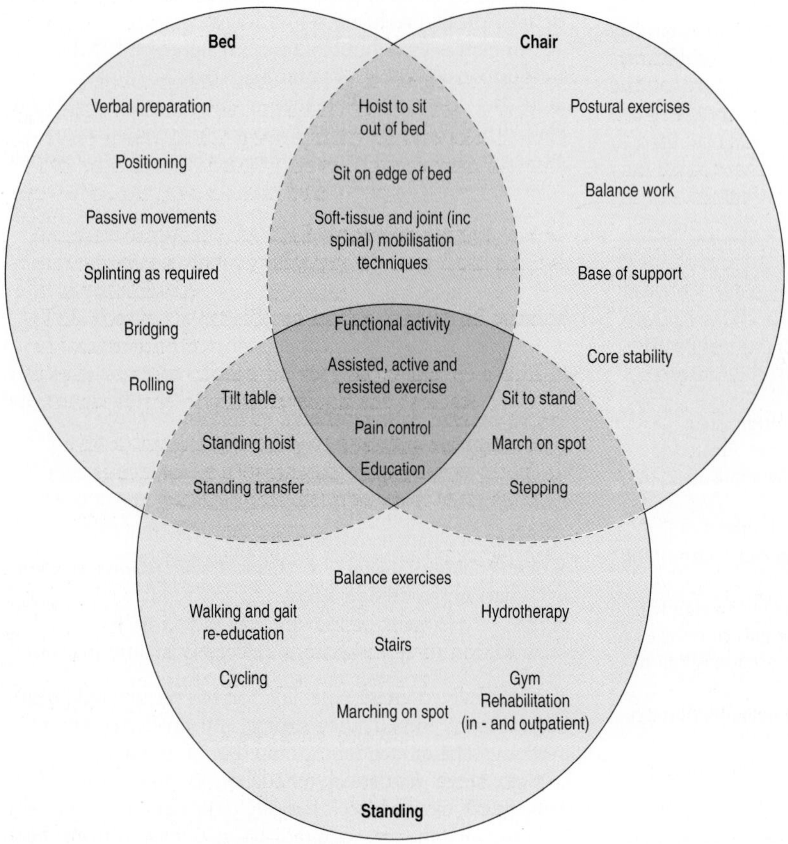

Figure 5.1 Schemata representing three-stage functional rehabilitation programme.[41]

physiological and psychological performance after a period of immobility and illness.[39] The use of interlinking circles is intended to reflect the non-linear pattern of exercise progression more commonly utilised in patients with critical illness, e.g. patients may be able to stand using a tilt-table before they are able to tolerate sitting out of bed. The central shaded area represents the core components that should be addressed at every stage in the patient's recovery. The areas bordered by the broken lines represent the progression or regression from one stage to the next. During all stages, the patient's cardiopulmonary response must be closely monitored, and exercise titrated accordingly. Modifications (e.g. temporarily increasing the FiO_2 and/or level of ventilatory assistance) during exercise and in the early postexercise period may be necessary. Such modifications are commonly required as increasing physical activity invariably coincides with weaning from ventilatory support – both significant challenges to the physiological reserve.

The wealth of evidence regarding deconditioning should play a central role in planning treatment, both preventive and rehabilitative. For example, those muscle groups known to be most adversely affected by disuse should be the first to be targeted with a gradual, progressive regime. During the remobilisation period, the multiprofessional team must be particularly mindful of those elements with delayed recovery, e.g. orthostatic tolerance and bone mass (predisposition to falls and fractures) and muscle endurance (diminished exercise tolerance).

It has been suggested that, in order to improve long-term outcomes for survivors of ICU (e.g. late mortality, ongoing morbidity, neurocognitive defects, functional disability, quality of life, economic burden), critical illness and its management should be viewed on a continuum and not merely the time spent in a critical care facility.[29] Consequently, rehabilitation must also reflect this change in focus, continuing into the community, outpatient or follow-up clinic setting.[40]

In recent years the concept of 'prehabilitation' has been introduced. Some have argued the case for exercise training prior to planned ICU admissions in order to ameliorate functional capacity. It is proposed that this would enable an individual to withstand better the stressor of inactivity and decrease the duration of dependency post critical care discharge.[26]

PATIENT PROBLEMS AFTER ICU DISCHARGE

A prolonged stay in ICU can be debilitating mentally and physically and can affect recovery after discharge (Table 5.12). In order to optimise a fast and effective recovery, a patient's care plan should be multidisciplinary in origin with ongoing appropriate rehabilitation following discharge from the ICU and indeed hospital.

PHYSIOTHERAPY ROLE EXPANSION

The nature of the critical care environment offers diverse opportunities for role expansion. The lead physiotherapist for the service must possess specialist cardiopulmonary and rehabilitative skills, as well as an expert knowledge of exercise physiology in health and disease. Furthermore, as a member of a dynamic multiprofessional team, it may be appropriate to extend diagnostic or clinical skills beyond the remit of conventional physiotherapy, e.g. developing weaning strategies, advanced tracheostomy management, bronchoscopy, prescription, arterial blood gas sampling and managing NIV services.

As an educator, the clinician must ensure that all professionals who provide physiotherapy input are competent in their assessment, clinical reasoning and skill execution. A commitment to audit and research is essential in order to ensure evidence-based service provision, clinical governance and best possible patient outcome.

PHYSIOTHERAPY AND CRITICAL CARE OUTREACH TEAMS

The development of specialist physiotherapist posts within critical care outreach teams (CCOTs) constitutes a prime example of role expansion. Following the publication of *Comprehensive Critical Care*[42] CCOT services were developed to meet the actual or potential needs of patients through critical care provision 'without walls':

- Avert critical care admission where possible
- Facilitate timely critical care admission when appropriate

Table 5.12 Psychological, cardiopulmonary and functional problems often encountered after discharge from the intensive care unit

Psychological	Cardiopulmonary	Functional
Depression	Compromised cardiopulmonary system	Back pain
Fear	Difficulty clearing retained secretions (trache tube, mini-trach in situ)	Shoulder pain
Anxiety		Muscle atrophy/decreased strength
Confusion	Decreased lung volumes	Inability to carry out activities of daily living independently
Disorientation	Oxygen dependence	
Flashbacks		Limited mobility
Lack of motivation		Poor exercise tolerance
Functional dependence		Poor gait pattern

- Empower all health care staff by disseminating ward-based critical care skills
- Optimise patient management and make best use of critical care resources via effective clinical decision-making

The introduction of CCOT has been associated with a varied approach to team configuration; however it has been suggested that those following a multiprofessional model are most likely to affect clinical and organisational improvements.[43] Consequently, many teams have elected to employ a designated specialist physiotherapist who can bring physiotherapeutic expertise to the service whilst also developing generic outreach practitioner skills (e.g. advanced tracheostomy management, cannulation, venopuncture, prescription via patient group directions, arterial blood gas sampling, drug administration, advanced life support, management of central/peripheral lines, 12-lead electrocardiogram interpretation, ordering/interpreting blood results and chest X-rays).

SUMMARY

The physiotherapist has an important and varied role within the ICU/high-dependency unit setting working as part of the multidisciplinary team to optimise cardiopulmonary function and functional ability. The physiotherapist is often uniquely placed to follow and treat a patient from the acute stages at ICU admission, through the rehabilitation process to subsequent discharge from hospital and, if necessary, treatment can be continued in the outpatient setting.

There is no longer a place for routine physiotherapy treatment. Regular systematic assessment will identify physiotherapy-amenable problems that contribute to a multidisciplinary care plan. Implementation of any physiotherapy treatment should always utilise continuous analytical reassessment.

ACKNOWLEDGEMENT

The authors wish to acknowledge the contributions made by Eleanor Douglas, Bronwen Jenkinson and Ann Alderson.

REFERENCES

1. Stiller K. Physiotherapy in intensive care. Towards an evidence-based practice. *Chest* 2000; **118**: 1801–13.
2. Norrenberg M, Vincent JL. Intensive care medicine. A profile of European intensive care unit physiotherapists. *Eur Soc Intens Care Med* 2000; 7: 988–94.
3. Denehy L. The use of manual hyperinflation in airway clearance. *Eur Respir J* 1999; **14**: 958–65.
4. Hodgson C, Denehy L. Ntoumenopoulos G. *et al.* An investigation of the early effects of manual lung hyperinflation in critically ill patients. *Anaesth Intens Care* 2000; **28**: 255–61.
5. Berney S, Denehy L. A comparison of the effects of manual and ventilator hyperinflation on static lung compliance and sputum production in intubated and ventilated intensive care patients. *Physiother Res Int* 2001; 7: 100–8.
6. Singer M, Vermaat J, Hall G *et al.* Haemodynamic effects of manual hyperinflation in critically ill mechanically ventilated patients. *Chest* 1994; **106**: 1182–7.
7. Clarke RCN, Kelly BE, Convery PN *et al.* Ventilatory characteristics in mechanically ventilated patients during manual hyperventilation for chest physiotherapy. *Anaesthesia* 1999; **54**: 936–40.
8. Lapinsky SE, Sangeeta M. Bench-to-bedside review: recruitment and recruiting maneuvers. *Crit Care* 2005; **9**: 60–5.
9. Brower RG, Lanken PN, MacIntyre NR *et al.* Higher versus lower positive end-expiratory pressures in patients with the acute respiratory distress syndrome NIH/NHLBI ARDSNET. *N Engl J Med* 2004; **351**: 327–36.
10. Choi JS, Jones AY. Effects of manual hyperinflation and suctioning on respiratory mechanics in mechanically ventilated patients with ventilator acquired pneumonia. *Aust J Physiother* 2005; **51**: 25–30.
11. McCarren B, Alison JA, Herbert RD. Vibration and its effect on the respiratory system. *Aust J Physiother* 2006; **52**: 39–43.
12. Bethune D. Neurophysiological facilitation of respiration in the unconscious adult patient. *Physiother Canada* 1975; **27**: 241–5.
13. Chang AT, Boots RJ, Brown MG *et al.* Ventilatory changes following head up tilt and standing in healthy subjects. *Eur J Appl Physiol* 2005; **95**: 409–17.
14. Dean E. The effects of positioning and mobilization on oxygen transport. In: Pryor JA, Webber BA (eds) *Physiotherapy for Respiratory and Cardiac Problems*, 2nd edn. Edinburgh: Churchill Livingstone; 1998: 125.
15. Jones AY, Dean E. Body position change and its effect on haemodynamic and metabolic status. *Heart Lung* 2004; **33**: 281–90.
16. Thoracic Society. The nomenclature of bronchopulmonary anatomy. *Thorax* 1950; **5**: 222–8.
17. Dean E. Effects of position on pulmonary function. *Phys Ther* 1985; **65**: 613–18.
18. Fink JB. Positioning versus postural drainage. *Respir Care* 2002; **47**: 769–77.
19. West JB. *Respiratory Physiology*, 5th edn. Baltimore: Williams & Wilkins; 1995: 51–69.
20. Gattinoni L, Tognoni G, Pesenti A *et al.* Effect of prone positioning on the survival of patients with acute respiratory failure. *N Engl J Med* 2001; **345**: 568–73.
21. Webber BA, Pryor JA. Physiotherapy techniques. In: Pryor JA, Webber BA (eds) *Physiotherapy for Respiratory and Cardiac Problems*, 2nd edn. Edinburgh: Churchill Livingstone; 1998: 137–209.
22. Pryor JA, Webber BA, Hodson ME *et al.* Evaluation of the forced expiration technique as an adjunct to postural drainage in treatment of cystic fibrosis. *Br Med J* 1979; **2**: 417–18.

23. Webber BA, Hofmeyr JL, Morgan MDL *et al.* Effects of postural drainage, incorporating forced expiratory technique on pulmonary function in cystic fibrosis. *Br J Dis Chest* 1986; **80**: 353–9.
24. Denehy L, Berney S. The use of positive pressure devices by physiotherapists. *Eur Respir J* 2001; **17**: 821–9.
25. British Thoracic Society guidelines. Noninvasive ventilation in acute respiratory failure. *Thorax* 2002; **57**: 192.
26. Topp R, Ditmyer M, King K *et al.* The effect of bed rest and potential of prehabilitation on patients in the intensive care unit. *AACN Clin Issues* 2002; **13**: 263–76.
27. Convertino VA, Bloomfield SA, Greenleaf JE. An overview of the issues: physiological effects of bed rest and restricted physical activity. *Med Sci Sports Exerc* 1997; **29**: 187–90.
28. Convertino VA. Cardiovascular consequences of bed rest: effect on maximal oxygen uptake. *Med Sci Sports Exerc* 1997; **29**: 191–6.
29. Angus DC, Carlet J. Surviving intensive care: a report from the 2002 Brussels roundtable. *Intens Care Med* 2003; **29**: 368–77.
30. Mueller PJ, Cunningham JT, Patel KP *et al.* Proposed role of the paraventricular nucleus in cardiovascular deconditioning. *Acta Physiol Scand* 2003; **177**: 27–35.
31. Jubran A. Critical illness and mechanical ventilation: effects on the diaphragm. *Respir Care* 2006; **51**: 1054–61.
32. Chang AT, Boots RJ, Brown MG *et al.* Reduced inspiratory muscle endurance following successful weaning from prolonged mechanical ventilation. *Chest* 2005; **128**: 553–9.
33. Gayan-Ramirez G, Decramer M. Effects of mechanical ventilation on diaphragm function and biology. *Eur Respir J* 2002; **20**: 1579–86.
34. Bloomfield S. Changes in musculoskeletal structure and function with prolonged bed rest. *Med Sci Sports Exerc* 1997; **2**: 197–206.
35. Kawakami Y, Akima H, Kubo K *et al.* Changes in muscle size, architecture, and neural activation after 20 days of bed rest with and without resistance exercise. *Eur J Appl Physiol* 2001; **84**: 7–12.
36. Latronico N, Peli E, Botteri M. Critical illness myopathy and neuropathy. *Curr Opin Crit Care* 2005; **11**: 126–32.
37. Paddon-Jones D. Interplay of stress and physical inactivity on muscle loss: Nutritional countermeasures. *J Nutr* 2006; **136**: 2123–6.
38. Vernikos J, Ludwig DA, Ertl AC *et al.* Effect of standing or walking on physiological changes induced by head down bed rest: implications for spaceflight. *Aviat Space Environ Med* 1996; **67**: 1069–79.
39. Greenleaf JE. Intensive exercise training during bed rest attenuates deconditioning. *Med Sci Sports Exerc* 1997; **29**: 207–15.
40. Elliott D, McKinley S, Alison JA *et al.* Study protocol: home-based physical rehabilitation for survivors of a critical illness. *Crit Care* 2006; **10**: R90.
41. Douglas E. The Nottingham Critical Care Rehabilitation Model, University of Nottingham Division of Physiotherapy. Personal communication, 2006.
42. Department of Health. *Comprehensive Critical Care: A Review of Adult Critical Care Services.* London: Department of Health; 2002.
43. Wood D. Designing an outreach service. In: Cutler L, Robson W (eds) *Critical Care Outreach.* Chichester: John Wiley; 2006: 13–30.

6

Critical care nursing

John R Welch and Chris Theaker

NATURE AND FUNCTION OF CRITICAL CARE NURSING

Nurses are the one round-the-clock constant for critically ill patients and their families, acting as the 'glue' that holds the critical care service together. Nurses ensure safety and provide continuity and fine-tuning, coordinating and communicating all the elements of treatment and care needed by the patient.

Skilled critical care nurses provide:

- continuous, close monitoring of the patient and attached apparatus
- dynamic analysis and synthesis of complex data
- anticipation of complications
- decision-making, execution and evaluation of interventions to minimise adverse effects
- enhancement of the speed and quality of recovery
- emotional support of the patient and family, including support through the process of death[1]

Nursing in critical care is influenced by both the essential nature of nursing and the specific characteristics of the field. Fundamental concerns for all nurses are said to take in:

- the concept of holism
- an appreciation of the whole range of influences on all areas of life
- the pursuit of health rather than treatment of illness[2]

There is inevitably an emphasis on technology in the intensive care unit (ICU), and nurses must be technically competent. However, treatments should be administered with an understanding of the essential human elements of care. ICU patients report that such care is often missing: one described his experience as 'rooted in the minute analysis of charts and the balancing of chemicals, not so much in the warmth of human contact'.[3]

Patients are not usually able to control what happens to them during the first phases of critical illness, but seek to reassert their autonomy as they begin to recover, e.g. when weaning from ventilation or with the transition to lower levels of care. Critical care nurses can enable patients to have a say in the management of these processes while still ensuring safe progression through different stages of treatment. Studies highlight the value of connecting with patients both psychologically and physically,[4] and that patient-centred care and emotional support can be lost when the nursing resource is reduced.[5] Fundamental care (e.g. personal cleansing, protection of tissue integrity, prevention of infection) is also generally undertaken or supervised by nurses. Other important functions (e.g. chest physiotherapy, mobilisation, delivery of nutrition) may be managed by other specialists, but it is nurses who integrate these treatments into a complete package of care.

A SYSTEMATIC APPROACH TO CARE

Nursing the critically ill patient is highly complex. It is vital to structure the patient review in order to clarify and prioritise patient needs, so that the whole range of patient function – and dysfunction – is addressed. In acute situations, assessment in turn of the fundamental A–B–C–D–E aspects of physiology is a useful method:

A. *Airway*: establishment and maintenance of airway patency (usually with the use of artificial devices), removal of pulmonary secretions, etc.
B. *Breathing*: adequacy of oxygenation and ventilation, optimising patient position, etc.
C. *Circulation*: circulatory volume and pressures; perfusion of brain, heart, lungs, kidneys, gut and other organs; control of bleeding, haematology, etc.
D. *Disability*: consciousness/reduced consciousness, and the factors that affect it; systemic and localised neurology.
E. *Exposure*: hands-on, head to toe, front and back examination, and everything else (!); wounds and drains; electrolytes and biochemistry, renal function.

Appropriate treatment strategies can be prioritised using this schema, which has the additional benefit that it will be familiar to colleagues trained in advanced life support and similar systems.

Further detail may then be gained from review of:

F. *fluid* and electrolyte balance, fluid input, urine output
G. *gastrointestinal* tract function: nutritional needs; elimination
H. *history* and *holistic* overview of the patient
I. *infection* and infection control; microbiology
L. *lines* – utility and risks
M. *medications*
N. *nursing* and interdisciplinary teamwork: ensuring resources are sufficient for the patient's severity of illness and the physical demands of care
P. *psychology* – pain and comfort, rest and sleep; managing the dying process
R. *relatives* – communication of the plan of care and prognosis in the short, medium and longer term (after Hillman *et al.*[6])

More sophisticated models can be used to frame a wider impression of the patient and to reflect a particular philosophy or approach to nursing. For example, the Roy model[7] expresses a view of nursing as a vehicle for enabling adaptive adjustments to any dysfunction. The model prompts analysis of both immediate and other contributing influences in a systematic consideration of oxygenation, nutrition, elimination, activity and rest, protective mechanisms, sensory function, fluid, electrolyte and acid–base balance, neurological and endocrine function, as well as the patient's self-concept, role-mastery and psychosocial interdependence.[7] Such an approach has a commendable breadth of vision, but may be too complex for the novice. Articulation of patient problems may be aided by the use of validated nursing diagnoses, as developed in North America. This system provides definitions and recommended nursing responses for many problems, and specifies appropriate outcome measures. What is most important is that any system used gives unambiguous definitions of patient problems and a clear statement of specific, measurable therapeutic goals.

NURSING AND PATIENT SAFETY

Inadequate nurse staffing is linked to increases in adverse events, patient morbidity and mortality. Significant numbers of patients suffer serious harm caused by errors in clinical practice, but nurses prevent many more incidents by intercepting and mitigating errors made by other professionals.[8] Direct observation and patient care remain key to patient safety:[9] it has been calculated that at least seven nurses need to be employed for each patient if a nursing presence is required continually 24 hours a day.[1] No particular system of critical care nursing has been shown to be definitively superior to others,[9] but ensuring appropriate nursing numbers, skills and experience to meet patient need is a gold standard of care[10] (see Staffing the critical care unit, below).

EVOLVING ROLES OF CRITICAL CARE NURSES

Critical care nurses' range of practice has evolved rapidly with progress in technology and with changes in the working of interdisciplinary team colleagues. The benefits of developing new skills must be balanced against ensuring the maintenance of fundamental patient care.[11] There remains a large variation in the array of tasks undertaken by nurses in critical care, with invasive procedures and drug prescriptions still usually performed by doctors. However, from 2006 qualified nurse (and pharmacist) prescribers in the UK have been enabled – in theory at least – to prescribe licensed medicines for the whole range of medical conditions. Nurse prescribing is not as yet a widespread phenomenon in critical care, but may become a routine part of practice in the future.

Critical care nurses also have a large and developing role in decision-making regarding the ongoing adjustment, titration and troubleshooting of such key treatments as ventilation, fluid and inotrope administration, and renal replacement therapy. The use of less invasive techniques (e.g. transoesophageal Doppler ultrasonography for cardiac output estimation) means that it is possible for nurses to institute relatively sophisticated monitoring and administer appropriate therapies for restoration of homeostasis. There is evidence that nurses can achieve good outcomes in these areas, especially with the use of clinical guidelines and protocols; for example, by reducing the time to wean respiratory support.[12] This indicates that further development of protocols, guidelines, care pathways and the like can be used to enhance the nursing contribution to critical care.

NEW NURSING ROLES IN CRITICAL CARE

Medical and nursing staffing in the ICU is an ongoing problem in many countries. This has led to the development of various new ways of working to deliver both fundamental and more sophisticated modes of care.[13] New nursing roles include those that essentially substitute for medical roles, as well as those that retain a nursing focus and aim to fill gaps in health care with nursing practice rather than medical care. For example, the UK has designated a relatively small number of nurse consultant posts in all areas of health care, with the largest proportion in critical care, particularly in outreach roles. These are advanced practitioners focusing primarily on clinical practice but also required to demonstrate professional leadership and consultancy, development of appropriate education and training, macrolevel practice and service development, research and evaluation.[14]

Other sorts of non-nursing staff are increasingly being used to deliver what has been seen as basic nursing care (e.g. oral and ocular care, recording of vital signs), in order to support trained nurses and enable them to concentrate on more advanced practices.[15] Nursing shortages may make such developments inevitable in some areas, but it is imperative that nurses continue to ensure best outcomes for patients with proper arrangements for training, support and working systems.

CRITICAL CARE NURSING BEYOND THE ICU: CRITICAL CARE OUTREACH

Around the world, general wards are required to manage an increasing throughput of patients who are, on average, older than before, with more complex, chronic diseases, and more acute and critical illness. Review of admissions to ICU from general wards shows that many patients experience substandard care before transfer.[16] Various factors are implicated, including lack of knowledge and failure to appreciate clinical urgency and to seek advice, compounded by poor organisation, breakdown in communication and inadequate supervision.

These issues are problems for the whole interdisciplinary team, but the nursing contribution is significant. It is nurses who record or supervise the recording of vital signs, suggesting that there is often poor understanding of the seriousness of such indicators, or failures to communicate effectively with medical staff, or difficulty in ensuring that appropriate treatment is prescribed and administered. Nurse-led outreach teams can support ward staff caring for at-risk and deteriorating patients, and facilitate transfer to intensive care when appropriate[17] (see Chapter 2). They can also support the care of patients on wards after discharge from ICU, and after discharge from the hospital (see Chapter 8). Potential problems with these approaches include a loss of specialist critical care staff from the ICU, and being sure that outreach teams have the necessary skills to manage high-risk patients in less well-equipped areas, particularly when there are limitations placed on nurses prescribing and administering treatments.

NURSING IN THE INTERDISCIPLINARY TEAM

Effective critical care is based on interdisciplinary teamwork, with:

- 'clear individual roles
- members who share knowledge, skills, best practice and learning
- systems that enable shared clinical governance, individual and team accountability, risk analysis and management'.[18]

QUALITY OF CARE

Robust systems of audit are the foundation of quality care. Various measures have been suggested as indicators of the effectiveness of nursing structures, processes and outcomes, e.g. pressure ulcer prevalence, nosocomial infection rates and patient satisfaction. Although nurses should take responsibility for the care that they deliver, there are few, if any, nursing activities that can be considered entirely separately from other variables that influence patient outcomes. Furthermore, there are few, if any, medical interventions that are unaffected by nursing care. Rather, quality care depends on a collective interdisciplinary commitment to continuous improvement.[19] This interdependence of different critical care personnel was illustrated in a multicentre investigation where interaction and communication between team members were more significant predictors of patient mortality than the therapies used or the status of the institution.[20]

CRITICAL CARE NURSING MANAGEMENT

The critical care nurse manager role is crucial to the performance of the service. The responsibilities and challenges of the nurse manager vary across different national systems and hospitals, but the most important concern for the manager is probably the problem of attracting and retaining a flexible, developing and consistently effective nursing team that works well with other health care professionals to meet patient needs within a limited budget.

STAFFING THE CRITICAL CARE UNIT[1]

The starting point for calculations of staffing requirements is an understanding of patient needs – and the knowledge and skills that will be required to meet those needs – with an awareness that there will be unpredictable variations over time.

- Patient need has many components, including:
  - the severity and complexity of the acute illness and chronic disease
  - other physical characteristics, e.g. mobility, body weight, skin integrity, continence
  - consciousness and cognition (alert, oriented, cooperative or confused, agitated, at risk of self-harm)
  - mood and emotionality (e.g. anxiety, depression, motivation)
  - the frequency and complexity of observation/monitoring and intervention required
  - the needs of relatives
- The staff resource includes members of the clinical team and a whole range of ancillary staff, and support services. Collectively, these personnel must be adequate to meet patient needs. This requires evaluation of:
  - nursing numbers and skill-mix
  - interdisciplinary team skill-mix, and consideration of variations in the continuous availability of team members (e.g. doctors, respiratory/physiotherapists, equipment technicians)

- The context of care is also significant:
  - The physical environment, e.g. the ease with which patients can be observed, whether in groups or in separate rooms
  - Workload variations – peaks, troughs and overall activity in the department, e.g. admissions, discharges, transfers

OTHER RESPONSIBILITIES

The manager is also typically responsible for:

- the coordinated operational management of the area
- the quality of nursing care
- management of nursing pay and non-pay budget
- personnel management

There are dynamic political, social and economic forces bearing on the organisational objectives and resources of the hospital and the ICU. The nurse manager needs to have an understanding of these factors and how they influence the practical delivery of patient care and the maintenance of a healthy environment for individual and team development. The manager must be able to communicate the key issues to the whole team in the form of an agreed strategy and a clear, regularly updated operational plan for the department. This should enable a shared understanding of exactly what needs to be done in practice, and where each team member fits into the plan. Externally, the manager represents the service and ensures that other disciplines and the organisation are informed about critical care issues.

Teams perform most effectively when individuals believe that they are working toward some common and worthwhile goals. A key role of the manager is to provide such coherence not just within the unit but also by integrating the views of all users of the service, including patients and their families, into the departmental plan. The principles of shared governance can be usefully applied in this perspective, whereby staff collectively review and learn from existing practices in order to develop and improve patient care within the unit. This has to be in the context of:

- the strategic agendas of the unit and the hospital
- the development of the service
- financial issues, budgets and budgetary restraints
- an appreciation of day-to-day working issues

Not surprisingly, the complexity and range of requirements may be too much for one person, so that different individuals are employed to take responsibility for particular aspects of management.

STRESS MANAGEMENT AND MOTIVATION

The ICU can be extremely stressful, demanding considerable cognitive, affective and psychomotor effort. Supervisory arrangements and feedback mechanisms should be in place to alleviate such demands, and enable prompt recognition of staff who are having difficulties at work. Regular individual performance reviews and formulation of development plans provide positive assurance and encouragement and can identify individuals' personal requirements, such as educational needs. They also provide an opportunity to identify poor practice that can then be rectified in a constructive manner. Study of human resource practices in acute hospitals has found a strong association between the quantity and quality of staff appraisal and patient mortality.[21] Organisations that emphasise training and team-working also have better outcomes.[21] Developing nurses' critical thinking and decision-making skills is important for effective working. The nurse manager should provide a system that facilitates such training.

Occupational psychology suggests that providing staff at all levels with opportunities to feel that they can influence and perhaps change the working environment tends to decrease stress and increase motivation. Flexibility to work in different ways at different times, while still meeting the overall demands of the department, is important. It is the manager's job to balance and meet the needs of staff, patients and the organisation. One method is to give staff choice regarding rostering, so that a nurse may opt to work with particular patients for a period in order to practise particular skills, and to promote continuity and coordination of care. This can have real benefits for patients and their families too.

NURSE EDUCATION

Critical care nurses generally enjoy well-established educational programmes, although there is variability in the content and quality of such training. Nurses usually wish to gain formal academic credentials, and there is a role for study of relevant philosophy, nursing theory and research methods. However, there is a fundamental requirement for learning that focuses on clinical practice issues and problem-solving that benefits patients.[22] It is also clear that there should be more widespread deployment of critical care nursing skills. These imperatives drive a need to produce unambiguous statements about the standards necessary for proper nursing assessment and nursing management of critically ill patients.

Summarised examples of competencies for critical care nurses might include the following:[23]

- Safe, effective, appropriate nursing management of patient requiring invasive ventilation, using:
  - a range of suitable ventilatory modes
  - pulmonary recruitment manoeuvres (e.g. prone positioning)
  - strategies for weaning
  - consideration of patient comfort (sedation, etc.)
- Safe, effective, appropriate nursing management of patient suffering from cardiovascular instability, including:
  - acute coronary syndromes
  - cardiac dysrhythmias

Table 6.1 Assessment of critical care nurses' performance

Rating	Definition	Observed behaviour	Prompts
Novice	Limited skill and/or knowledge, inconsistent practice, variable interpersonal skill. Limited understanding of wider context, inflexible rule-governed behaviour	Lacks coordination and confidence. Potential for omissions or inaccuracies. Unable to demonstrate accurate and safe performance despite repeated attempts	Requires frequent directive prompts, supervision and advice
Advanced beginner	Some skill and knowledge, generally consistent practice and interpersonal skill; variable ethical thought. Some appreciation of situational influences	Coordinated and confident in fundamental tasks. Easily distracted or unable to integrate other aspects of patient care	Requires occasional directive prompts and some supervision
Competent	Consistent safe, accurate and effective practice, interpersonal skill and ethical thought. Conscious and deliberate planning with consideration of immediate context	Skillful, confident and coordinated patient-focused practice, with evident integration of other aspects of care. Prioritisation of workload	Self-directing without supervision
Proficient	Consistent safe, accurate and effective practice, higher-level interpersonal skill and ethical reasoning. Conscious and deliberate planning with consideration of longer-term goals. Adapts care in response to changing situations	Skilled and accomplished practice, proactive and flexible approach to care. Problem-solving and decision-making through reflection. Role model	Capable of supporting and demonstrating skills to others

(After Benner P. *From Novice to Expert: Excellence and Power in Clinical Nursing Practice.* Menlo Park: Addison-Wesley; 1984.)

  - haemodynamic instability secondary to other factors
  - circulatory failure
  - periarrest situations
  - cardiopulmonary arrest
- Safe and effective management of prerenal failure, intrinsic renal failure and postrenal failure, with appropriate nursing care, including:
  - fluid and drug therapies
  - urinary drainage devices
  - renal replacement techniques (in the appropriate setting)

These statements outline the types of competencies that might be required by nurses, and can be used to structure indepth descriptors of the skills, applied knowledge and attitudes needed to achieve specific patient outcomes. Clear detailing of specific skills is essential, but there also needs to be consideration of how individual actions are integrated into holistic care, and the role of independent clinical judgement. Appraisal of performance requires suitable assessors to observe and question the nurse in practice, but this places great demands on hard-pressed clinical areas. It may be that increasingly sophisticated simulators can be used to test performance away from the practice setting.

Various frameworks to identify different levels of performance have been developed, e.g. based on Benner's hierarchy[4] (Table 6.1). These can be used to mark progression to particular standards in core skills.

CRITICAL CARE NURSING RESEARCH

Critical care services treat small numbers of patients at high cost. Critical care has great physical and psychological impact, but often uses somewhat untested methods. Patient outcomes are influenced by different organisational approaches, staff characteristics, varied working practices and treatment methods, as well as differences between patients themselves. Therefore, a range of quantitative and qualitative investigative procedures is needed to gain a comprehensive understanding of the issues and to develop best practice. The approach chosen depends on the nature of the research question, and also the objectives of the researcher and the resources available.

REVIEWING RESEARCH

The methods used to appraise research depend partly on the type of work under review. The following questions may be used to structure a critique:

- Justification for the research: are the background and rationale of the study clearly established?
- Scientific content: is there a specific question/hypothesis?
- Originality: is it a new idea, or re-examining an old problem differently or better?
- Methodology and study design: are the methods appropriate and are they likely to produce an answer to the question? For example:
  - comparisons of different treatments generally require quantitative measurements of particular end-points, e.g. the dose of a drug needed to achieve a target physiological variable, or the time taken to wean from ventilation
  - understanding how an individual thinks or feels usually involves analysis of qualitative material, e.g. data from interviews with patients and families to obtain their views of the service[24]

- Is the research method described in a way that can be readily understood, and replicated?
- Are the relevant results shown? Are data given that provide details of the individuals under investigation (e.g. demographics) and details of how representative these might be of a larger population?
- Is the analysis appropriate and is the power of the study adequate? (This is usually determined by the numbers involved and the size of the difference being examined.)
- Interpretation and discussion: are the conclusions and comments reasonable in the light of the results? Do the conclusions follow from the analysis?
- Are any references to background literature reasonably comprehensive and appropriate?
- What can be taken from the study, that is, what value does the study have in terms of supporting or developing clinical practice?
- What is the overall impression of the work? Is it credible? Is the presentation clear and informative?
- If evaluating a paper, has the work undergone proper peer review?

UNDERTAKING A RESEARCH PROJECT

STAGE 1: IDENTIFY AND CLARIFY THE TOPIC TO BE EXAMINED

Research in clinical settings is most valued when it is relevant to practice. The researcher is more likely to gain support for investigation of high-risk and high-cost processes. Current political priorities in health care may also be significant. Many everyday methods and treatments warrant examination too, particularly when there are significant variations in practice. The researcher should determine how the topic of interest might be described in a measurable way, and formulate the investigation as a question, with some consideration of how answers can be obtained.

STAGE 2: GATHER RELEVANT BACKGROUND INFORMATION

It is important to collect information that enables an understanding of the issues under investigation, and helps justify performing the study. Hospital libraries are useful, not least because there may be staff who can give advice about the project. Indexes for journals and books are in print and computer-based formats, with databases and texts also available through the internet. A good starting point is Google Scholar (http://scholar.google.com/). This uses a broad approach to locating articles in searches across many disciplines and sources. More specific medical/nursing websites include:

- PubMed, a service from the US National Library of Medicine (http://www.nlm.nih.gov/), with access to the MEDLINE (Medical Literature, Analysis, and Retrieval System Online) biomedical database
- the Cumulative Index to Nursing and Allied Health (CINAHL) at http://www.cinahl.com
- the Cochrane Collaboration of systematic reviews of health care interventions (http://www.cochrane.org)
- EMBASE (http://www.embase.com/) is particularly good for pharmacological information

The most important piece of advice when conducting a search is not to enter the first word that comes to mind into the database or search engine, but to start by formulating a question and then break it down into its component parts. Training in searching databases is recommended.

The researcher must also evaluate the quality of the information gathered. Different types of research are traditionally considered to have different weights, e.g. results obtained from randomised controlled trials are considered to be high-grade evidence, whereas observational studies are deemed less useful.[25] This hierarchy is not always applicable and may devalue some sorts of valuable work, but it does emphasise the need to examine critically the credibility of research.

STAGE 3: DESIGN A METHOD THAT:

- will provide data that will answer the question
- is adequate to answer the question (e.g. studies that use statistics require consideration of the numbers of data items needed to demonstrate differences between different groups or categories)
- is feasible to do in practice
- is ethical

STAGE 4: COLLECT THE DATA

This is usually relatively simple provided that the data items to be collected are clearly defined at the planning stage of the study. A common pitfall is to collect vast amounts of unnecessary data and lose the focus of the original question. Data should be collected in a manageable format, often using some type of database.

STAGE 5: ORGANISE THE DATA

By this stage, a large amount of material may have been gathered from primary and secondary sources. It is important that:

- a system of categorisation and analysis is used that meets the objectives of the investigation
- the analysis addresses the original question
- appropriate statistical methods are used (specialist expertise or advice may be required)

STAGE 6: PRESENT AND EXPLAIN THE DATA

Prsentation can take many forms, but it is always necessary to set out the question asked, to describe the research method so that it is clear what was done, to illustrate the results and their analysis and to present the key findings and conclusions. The conclusions should follow from the analysis, without inappropriate extrapolations. Any applications to clinical practice should be highlighted. The report must be presented succinctly and in a constructive manner, but with any shortcomings or

Table 6.2 Issues for consideration in the review of research proposals

Particular to the patient/research subject	Particular to study design/integrity
• The possibility of risk of harm • The degree of inconvenience to the patient/research subject (or associated persons, e.g. patients' relatives) • The duration of the study period (for the patient/subject) • Whether the individual patient or research subject may obtain a direct or indirect benefit from participating • The characteristics of the population to be studied • Inclusion and exclusion criteria, and the rationale for inclusion and exclusion • Whether any of the patients/research subjects are enrolled into other research projects that could influence the new study	• The credentials of the researchers • Whether the researchers are subject to any conflicts of interest • The benefits of the research balanced against its detriments • What is needed to fund and resource the study • Whether there is an effective mechanism for managing adverse events • Whether there is an effective mechanism for terminating the study • The frequency of occurrence of the phenomenon to be studied • The duration of the study • The feasibility of recruiting sufficient patients or research subjects to meet statistical power requirements • Where, when and how patients or research subjects are to be recruited, and who will be doing the recruiting • How long the patient or research subject will be given to decide whether or not to take part • What happens if the patient agrees to take part but subsequently wishes to withdraw • How data will be collected, scrutinised, stored – and subsequently disposed of – in order to protect patient confidentiality • Whether the research is analysing an established procedure or a novel method

problems in the study discussed. The goal is that the reader can understand the methodology and how the results were interpreted, while acknowledging any limitations of the work.

The main point of research is to share what has been learnt: the researcher should think about how the work may be made available to as large an audience as is possible or appropriate.

STAGE 7: EVALUATE THE PROJECT

The final phase is reflective. Conducting research is a process that can always be improved. Constructive feedback from colleagues is an effective way of determining the value of a study. The researcher should review what has been learnt from the process as well as from the results of the study, and consider how the work might be further developed in the future.

RESEARCH ETHICS

The practitioner must always consider the ethical issues associated with conducting research: in many countries it is a criminal offence to undertake medical research without ethical approval. The researcher generally needs to submit a detailed application document for approval to an ethics committee. There are local differences in the process of obtaining ethical approval for research on humans, but most systems incorporate the principles of the Declaration of Helsinki (see the World Medical Association website at http://www.wma.net/e/policy/b3.htm).

One important area is the question of how informed consent will be obtained from patients. Even if patients are awake it does not necessarily mean that they have the capacity to provide informed consent. Some countries adopt the practice of obtaining consent from a patient's next of kin in an effort to circumvent this issue, but this is in fact obtaining 'assent' rather than 'consent'. In the European Union, this approach is only legal when the research is a clinical trial for medicinal products.

An ethics committee is usually made up of professional and lay members attached to hospitals or universities. The committee looks beyond the stated necessity and significance of the proposed research to evaluate a range of matters particular to the patients who may be involved, and to aspects of the study design. Some of these issues are summarised in Table 6.2.

REFERENCES

1. Royal College of Nursing. *Guidelines for Nurse Staffing in Critical Care.* London: Royal College of Nursing; 2003.
2. Chinn P, Kramer M. *Integrated Knowledge Development in Nursing.* St Louis, MO: Mosby; 2003.
3. Watt B. Patient: *The True Story of a Rare Illness.* London: Penguin; 1996.
4. Benner P. *From Novice to Expert: Excellence and Power in Clinical Nursing Practice.* Menlo Park: Addison-Wesley; 1984.

5. Ball C, McElligot M. Realising the potential of critical care nurses: an exploratory study of the factors that affect and comprise the nursing contribution to the recovery of critically ill patients. *Intens Crit Care Nurs* 2003; **19**: 226–38.
6. Hillman K, Bishop G, Flabouris A. Patient examination in the intensive care unit. *Yearbook of Intensive Care and Emergency Medicine 2002*. Berlin: Springer-Verlag; 2002.
7. Roy C, Andrews H. *The Roy Adaptation Model*. Englewood Cliffs, NJ: Prentice-Hall; 1999.
8. Rothschild J, Hurley A, Landrigan C *et al.* Recovery from medical errors: the critical care nursing safety net. *Jt Comm J Qual Patient Safe* 2006; **32**: 63–72.
9. Coombs M, Lattimer V. Safety, effectiveness and costs of different models of organising care for critically ill patients: literature review. *Int J Nurs Stud* 2007; **44**: 115–29.
10. American Association of Critical-Care Nurses. *AACN Standards for Establishing and Sustaining Healthy Work Environments*. Aliso Viejo, CA: American Association of Critical Care-Nurses; 2005.
11. Mullally S. Improving the quality of clinical practice. *Nurs Ethics* 2000; 7: 531–2.
12. Kollef M, Shiparo S, Silver P *et al.* A randomized, controlled trial of protocol directed versus physician directed weaning from mechanical ventilation. *Crit Care Med* 1997; **25**: 567–74.
13. Scholes J, Furlong S, Vaughan B. New roles in practice: charting three typologies of role innovation. *Nurs Crit Care* 1999; **4**: 268–75.
14. NHS Executive. *Health Service Circular 1999/217. Nurse, Midwife and Health Visitor Consultants*. Leeds: NHS Executive; 1999.
15. Hind M, Jackson D, Andrews C *et al.* Health care support workers in the critical care setting. *Nurs Crit Care* 2000; **5**: 31–9.
16. Cullinane M, Findlay G, Hargraves C *et al. An Acute Problem? A Report of the National Confidential Enquiry into Patient Outcome and Death*. London: NCEPOD; 2005.
17. Watson W, Mozley C, Cope J *et al.* Implementing a nurse-led critical care outreach service in an acute hospital. *J Clin Nurs* 2006; **15**: 105–10.
18. Department of Health-Emergency Care Team. *Quality Critical Care: Beyond 'Comprehensive Critical Care': A Report by the Critical Care Stakeholder Forum*. London: Department of Health-Emergency Care Team; 2005.
19. Curtis J, Cook D, Wall R *et al.* Intensive care unit quality improvement: a 'how-to' guide for the interdisciplinary team. *Crit Care Med* 2006; **34**: 211–18.
20. Tarnow-Mordi W, Hau C, Warden A *et al.* Hospital mortality in relation to staff workload: a 4-year study in an adult intensive care unit. *Lancet* 2000; **356**: 185–9.
21. West M, Borrill C, Dawson J *et al.* The link between the management of employees and patient mortality in acute hospitals. *Int J Hum Resource Manage* 2002; **13**: 1299–310.
22. Wigens L, Westwood S. Issues surrounding educational preparation for intensive care nursing in the 21st century. *Intens Crit Care Nurs* 2000; **16**: 221–7.
23. SW London Critical Care Nursing Curriculum Planning Group. *Critical Care Competencies*. London: Kingston University and St George's Hospital Medical School Faculty of Healthcare Sciences; 2002.
24. Wilcock P, Brown G, Bateson J *et al.* Using patient stories to inspire quality improvement within the NHS Modernization Agency collaborative programmes. *J Clin Nurs* 2003; **12**: 422–30.
25. Concato J, Shah N, Horwitz R. Randomized, controlled trials, observational studies, and the hierarchy of research designs. *N Engl J Med* 2000; **342**: 1887–92.

FURTHER READING

Gerrish K, Lacey A (eds) *The Research Process in Nursing*, 5th edn. Oxford: Blackwell; 2006.
Wedderburn Tate C. *Leadership in Nursing*. Edinburgh: Churchill Livingstone; 1999.

7

Ethics in intensive care

Raymond F Raper and Malcolm McD Fisher

DEFINITION

Ethics is the study of how one ought to behave. In contrast, the law defines how one must behave to avoid punishment. Ethics is concerned with differentiating right from wrong behaviour. For most people, a sense of ethics is innate. Medical ethics particularly relates to the relationships between health care practitioners and patients and is not limited to doctors even if it is particularly applicable to doctors. Ethical conflict almost always involves a clash of values and appropriate resolution depends on recognition of the conflicting interests and values.

ETHICAL FRAMEWORK

Medical ethics are usually discussed in the context of principles. These principles inform ethical behaviour and can be summarised as:

1. *Autonomy*: the principle of individual self-determination in respect of medical care.
2. *Beneficence*: the principle of 'doing good', an obligation always to act in the best interests of patients with respect to saving lives, curing illness and alleviating pain and suffering.
3. *Non-maleficence*: the principle of doing no harm.
4. *Fidelity*: faithfulness to duties and obligations, a principle underlying confidentiality, telling the truth, keeping up with medical knowledge (i.e. continuing professional development) and not neglecting patient care.
5. *Social justice*: the principle of equitable access of all citizens to medical care according to medical need.
6. *Utility*: the principle of doing most good for the most number of people; that is, achieving maximum benefits for society without wasting health resources.

Utility is a consequentialist concept, where the right or wrong of an action is determined by the outcome rather than by an a priori principle. The 'correct' action may thus vary with the particular circumstances. This is sometimes seen as an entirely different framework from the rights or principles-based system. The utility principle is more applicable to systems development in medical practice and may create conflict with individual patient responsibility. It is important that intensivists participate in the public debate that determines how much of society's goods are to be allocated to medicine and how much of the health budget is to be allocated to intensive care without, at the same time, surrendering responsibility for the interests of individual patients. Moving between these public and private spheres of functioning can be challenging but is essential to good medical practice.

Ethical conflict is most often encountered where there is a clash of values. Rationing, for instance, involves a clash between the values of individual rights and collective rights. Euthanasia usually involves a clash between the values of sanctity of life and autonomy. Resolution of ethical conflict depends on recognition of the values that are in dispute and of the principles that are operative. Absolutist terms such as 'futility' tend to mask the values-in-clash and are thus unhelpful in resolution of ethical conflict. Consideration of the various interests involved is also helpful in foregrounding the real issues behind an ethical conflict.

ICU ETHICAL PROBLEMS

END-OF-LIFE MANAGEMENT

During its relatively brief history, intensive care has seen a dramatic increase in both capacity and capability. Practice has become codified and at least partly standardised and intensive care is more generally accessible. Greater emphasis on individual rights has seen an increased demand for medical resources in general and this has flowed on to intensive care. The great challenge for intensive care lies in the reality that prolonged life support is often quite easily achieved without there being either inevitable recovery or intractable demise. Of the sickest patients in the intensive care unit (ICU), only a proportion ultimately recovers and can be returned to a reasonable quality of life. Even this would not be a problem if it were possible to predict survival with any degree of certainty and a great deal of effort has been expended in an attempt to achieve this. Unfortunately, this has met with only limited success and consideration of the appropriateness of ongoing intensive care is necessarily conducted against a background of prognostic uncertainty.[1]

In consequence of this, death in ICU usually involves some limitation or withholding of life-sustaining treatment.[2,3] This has now been well documented in many studies from around the world and the driving factors are now reasonably well understood.[2–9] The ethical principles underpinning this practice are those described above. Intensive care is inevitably burdensome and requires a commensurate benefit to conform to beneficence and non-maleficence. While life itself has a value, this is considerably offset if it is brief, painful and non-interactive. As death becomes increasingly imminent, its deferment at any cost becomes less appropriate. Considerations of justice should rarely intrude at the bedside. However, prolongation of life by artificial means in a patient with little or no chance of survival may challenge the rights of survivable patients to limited intensive care resources.[10] Where resources are publicly owned, offering to one patient treatment that cannot be made available to all patients in similar circumstances is fundamentally unethical. The collective has the ethical right to regulate access to even beneficial therapy provided it does so in a non-discriminatory fashion. The intensive care specialist does not have a right unilaterally to apply or withhold resources against the will of the collective. Unfortunately, the will of the collective is rarely known.

End-of-life management in the intensive care setting has been subjected to a considerable research endeavour over the past several years.[2,4,11–13] Insights that can be gleaned from published studies include:

- Patients not infrequently die in some discomfort in ICU receiving unwanted therapy.
- Considerable dissatisfaction has been reported by both patients and families with management at the end of life.
- Patient wishes with respect to end-of-life treatment are commonly unknown.
- Patients and families may be quite ignorant of the nature and prognosis of end-of-life initiatives such as cardiopulmonary resuscitation.[14]
- Active interventions including obligatory, outside consultations have not been particularly effective in improving the quality of end-of-life management.
- There is a good deal of practice variability across countries and communities with respect to attitudes to death, dying and the withholding and withdrawing of active treatment.[2,8]
- The reported variability in practice relates to attitudes of doctors and nurses, decision-making processes and to actual practices once a treatment-limiting decision has been made.
- Although some form of treatment limitation is common, withdrawal of treatment is not practised and is even illegal in some communities while active foreshortening and active euthanasia are reported in others.
- There remains some confusion concerning the distinction between active foreshortening of life and administration of drugs that both relieve unwanted symptoms and shorten the dying process. The nature and doses of agents used actively to shorten life are not necessarily different from those used to relieve symptoms without the intention of accelerating death and the time to death may also not be affected.[2]
- Most patients and families report a preference for some form of collaboration in end-of-life decision-making.[15–17]

PRACTICAL CONSIDERATIONS

- Decisions to limit treatment in ICU depend on a careful consideration of the burdens and benefits of treatment.
- Prognostication in ICU practice is imperfect so that decision-making is based on probability rather than certainty.
- Decision-making is usually an evolving process, commonly involving several discussions of therapeutic possibilities, quality of life and patient preferences.[9,11]
- Competent patients should always be involved in discussions and inclusion of family members should be encouraged and fostered.
- Given the common desire for collaborative decision-making, seeking patient preferences and consensus in a proposed management plan is more appropriate than either surrendering decision-making responsibility to patients or surrogates or systematically excluding patients and/or carers.
- The important role of nurses and allied health practitioners in the management of critically ill patients warrants respect by inclusion in discussions. Failure to do so has resulted in nurses inappropriately taking unilateral, surreptitious action justified as patient advocacy. Legal action for unlawful termination of life has also resulted.

ADVANCE DIRECTIVES AND POWER OF ATTORNEY

Patients may formally signal their preferences for end-of-life care in a written document or may nominate a surrogate decision-maker in the event of future incompetence. The legal standing of such documents is highly variable. Nevertheless, as expressions of self-determination they have considerable ethical validity and warrant respect. Unfortunately, advance directives are often insufficiently specific and it is not always possible to be sure that decisions included in such documents were fully informed and rational. Given the frequent reticence of patients to consider end-of-life matters,[14] advance directives are unlikely to become widely pervasive.

EUTHANASIA

This term is strictly applicable only to situations of active termination of life with the knowledge of and usually at the request of a patient suffering a terminal and/or debilitating, incurable illness. Physician-assisted suicide is a variation of this practice. This is a subject of considerable debate and is now legal in a small number of jurisdictions though likely practised surreptitiously in many more. Ethicists, largely on consequentialist grounds, maintain no distinction between this and the terminal withdrawal or withholding of treatment[18] (sometimes inappropriately termed 'passive euthanasia'). For intensive care practice, however, the distinction seems obvious and essential. The distinction is most often argued on the basis of intent. Although there may well be a difference in intent between active euthanasia and withdrawal of treatment, relief of pain and suffering may be at the heart of both activities. Even if this is the case, active euthanasia is certainly a disproportionate means to the end. Treatment limitation is arguably an essential component of intensive care practice while euthanasia is not and there is usually a clear and obvious difference in the acts themselves. While it may be true that in some instances there is no moral distinction between euthanasia and withdrawal of treatment, this does not mean that there is never such a distinction.

TREATMENT WITHDRAWAL

- Once a decision has been made to withdraw or withhold treatment, the decision, the participants, the rationale and the details of the treatment limitation should be clearly documented in the patient records. Surreptitious treatment limitation is difficult to justify and potentially hazardous.
- There is no moral hierarchy of treatments but ventilator withdrawal is more obviously terminal than, say, withdrawal of renal replacement therapy or antibiotics.
- Although treatment may sometimes be withdrawn or withheld in ICU, care must never be withdrawn. An alternative, palliative management plan focusing on symptom relief and patient dignity should be instituted and documented.
- From a practical perspective, progressive treatment withdrawal enables progressive management of any resultant discomfort. It also helps foster an appreciation that death is a consequence of disease or organ system failure rather than of the withdrawal of treatment.
- Symptom relief with especially sedatives and narcotics may sometimes appear to hasten death. This is often justified on the 'double effect' principle, as the acceleration of death, though foreseen, was not intended. More importantly, however, this should be seen simply as a trade-off of two aims where the relief of unwanted symptoms assumes a higher priority than avoidance of the foreshortening of life. Certainly, it is difficult to justify unnecessary pain and suffering at the end of life on ethical grounds. Finally clinical experience suggests that, rather than shortening life, narcotics and sedatives commonly prolong the dying process by reducing cardiovascular stress.

CONSENT

Informed consent lies at the heart of the doctor–patient relationship and has both ethical and legal implications. Consent relates both to treatment (especially to invasive procedures) and to participation in research. General principles relating to consent can be listed:

- Patient consent is a fundamental tenet of medical practice. Routine or minor procedures may be included in the general consent to treatment.
- Consent may be waived in an emergency for treatment that is immediately necessary to save life or avoid significant physical deterioration. This applies whether or not the patient is technically competent.
- Valid consent is dependent on the provision of adequate information, including benefits and risks, and must be voluntary and free from coercion.
- Written consent provides evidence of the consent process, but consent itself need not be in writing, unless specifically required by a local authority.
- Competent patients are entitled to refuse consent to treatment even when doing so may result in harm or death.
- Surrogate consent for more elective procedures relies for ethical justification on the principle of autonomy. Patients' interests must be paramount. Legal requirements relating to surrogate consent are highly variable and 'surrogate' is often formally defined and limited by local statute.
- Autonomy also provides the ethical justification for advance directives, the legal status of which is also highly variable.
- An enduring power of attorney generally applies to financial affairs rather than to consent to treatment. Again, the ethical basis relates to self-determination.
- Competent minors may or may not have a legal right to consent but age does not affect ethical considerations independently of insight and understanding. Even incompetent minors have some entitlement to confidentiality and all are entitled to protection from harm, even if that harm devolves from parental or guardian decisions based on well-meaning conviction or prejudice.
- Consent is especially required to involve a patient in research, where the importance of full disclosure is even greater. Medical research imposes some particular ethical issues, to be discussed below.
- Consent is also required for teaching purposes, such as video recording and photographing patients and teaching practical procedures.
- There may be a legal requirement for consent for testing for diseases such as human immunodeficiency virus (HIV)/acquired immunodeficiency syndrome (AIDS) and hepatitis. These diseases are not especially unique from an ethical perspective, however, and patients' rights to privacy are not absolute.

Because intensive care patients are often unable to provide formal consent and because critical illness itself may negate the preconditions for consent, this issue is commonly neglected. Consent to 'routine' or everyday procedures in critically ill patients is often presumed or rather subsumed under the general consent to treatment. Near-universal consent is possible, however.[19] The precise role for consent in the intensive care context has not been fully defined but deviations from the general requirement for consent require some justification. The legal requirement for consent varies with different interpretations and jurisdictions. If taken to extreme, such as enabling surrogate refusal for 'routine' procedures such as central venous access, consent-related autonomy may become incompatible with the beneficence and non-maleficence principles and may largely become untenable.

RATIONING AND SOCIETAL ROLE

Intensive care is, by nature, expensive. This creates a tension and a potential ethical conflict for intensive care practitioners. It is essential to find a balance between responsibilities to individual patients and to those of the collective. In theory, this is achieved by removing all rationing decisions from the bedside. Established norms rather than temporal availability or personal influence should determine access to ICU. Treatment is withheld or withdrawn not because there is a 'more deserving' patient at the door but because it would always be withheld or withdrawn under the particular clinical circumstances. Wide variations in access to medical care for similar patients across a single society cannot be ethically justified. More challenging is the definition of society. If a sufficiently broad perspective is adopted, most intensive care is difficult to justify. The ethically responsible intensive care practitioner will both advocate for individual patients and participate in the mostly unstructured social debate that determines what proportion of community resources is expended on medicine and on intensive care in particular.

PROFESSIONALISM

Medical practitioners occupy a unique and, usually, a privileged position in society. With this come a number of responsibilities. These are generally well covered in codes of conduct issued from time to time by professional societies and institutions of learning. The oldest and perhaps best known is the hippocratic oath. Professional, ethical responsibilities may be sorely tested where the well-being of the practitioner is at risk from medical practice, as with infectious disease epidemics and acts of terrorism. Resolution of this potential conflict has not been satisfactorily determined to date.

Among the ethical responsibilities of medical practitioners are:

- Maintenance of professional standards by continuing education and professional development
- Maintenance of appropriate professional relationships with patients
- Appropriate documentation of medical interactions
- Participation in quality and safety initiatives and practices
- Respect for patient and staff confidentiality
- Respect for the tenets of the law

INDUSTRY AND CONFLICT OF INTEREST

Relationships among doctors and the medical technology and pharmaceutical companies are complex.[20] Doctors and industry are somewhat interdependent. Medical advances do not occur in a vacuum and the invention, assessment, development and marketing of new drugs and technologies necessitate close relationships among doctors and industry. While doctors are entitled to fair consideration for their skills and effort, the relationships must be overt and openly scrutinised if conflicts of interests are not to occur. The nature of the rewards offered by companies for medical involvement in product development is diverse but includes both direct and indirect payments. The economic justification for all these payments depends on their effects on subsequent product marketing. The propriety of travel and related support is questionable unless it is directly and attributably related to openly contracted services. Involvement of companies with vested interests in pseudoeducational initiatives and even guideline development may be little more than covert marketing.[21] Some open labelled research initiatives with large, practitioner reward programmes are similarly worrisome. Initiatives designed to limit these conflicts of interest include open disclosure of all financial relationships and voluntary and involuntary codes of conduct on both sides of the relationship. Financial inducements can be easily concealed, however, and specific financial relationships can be obscured by their volume and pervasiveness. Although this potential for ethical conflict exists in many other commercial relationships, the nature of medicine and the associated expenditure of, often, public funds dictate that this is not an entirely private consideration.

RESEARCH

Critically ill patients can rarely consent themselves to participation in research projects and yet they are able to benefit from the results of earlier studies with similarly problematic consent issues. Locating surrogate decision-makers within a timeframe appropriate for some types of research can also be impossible. This has been recognised and enacted in a consent waiver for even randomised clinical trials. The potential ethical conflict in this situation lies in the use of a patient as an instrument to achieve another's end without express consent. There is a potential 'slippery slope' in valuing the rights of the collective over those of the individual and yet the individual can be seen to have an interest in the resolution of some of these important clinical questions. The conduct of such research must be carefully scrutinised by outside agents and careful consideration must be given to the balance between risk and benefit. A potentially greater benefit might help justify a potentially greater risk even if the benefit might not be directly applicable to the subject. Studies of, for example, disease mechanisms involving little or no potential direct patient benefit would need to involve no material risk. In general, the principles of consent detailed above are applicable. When a waiver is applied, patients and/or surrogates should be afforded an opportunity to withdraw from study at the earliest opportunity.

RESOLVING ETHICAL CONFLICT

Ethical conflict most commonly arises where there is a clash of values or interests. Resolution is often difficult because of entrenched positions and convictions. The innate sense of right and wrong lends itself to strong convictions in a way not seen in other human activities. The fundamental basis of resolution is discussion, enabling exposure of the values or interests that are in conflict. This may require a third party or mediator. Absolutist convictions such as 'sanctity of life' and absolutist terminology such as 'futility' impede conflict resolution and have to be unravelled.

There are several useful guidelines informing practice, particularly in relation to end-of-life decision-making. Individual practitioners should be aware of these and adapt them to local circumstances. Institution-based guidelines that conform to more overarching documents are probably most useful. Most learned colleges and professional societies now promulgate such practice guidelines in various forms.

Ethics committees have an important role in establishing frameworks for ethical practice. There is some evidence that formal ethics consultations improve end-of-life management but the principles utilised are those of open discussion and full disclosure that should inform normal bedside communication. Committees should normally have no individual decision-making role.

Recourse to legal processes may be essential but should be infrequent as the legal system does not cope well with the complexity of medical decision-making and is generally slow and ponderous. Practice should conform to legal norms, however, so long as these are not unethical.

REFERENCES

1. Logan RL, Scott PJ. Uncertainty in clinical practice: implications for quality and costs of health care. *Lancet* 1996; **347**: 595–8.
2. Sprung CL, Cohen SL, Sjokvist P *et al.* End-of-life practices in European intensive care units. The Ethicus study. *JAMA* 2003; **290**: 790–7.
3. Prendergast TJ, Luce JM. Increasing incidence of withholding and withdrawing of life support from the critically ill. *Am J Respir Crit Care Med* 1997; **155**: 15–20.
4. Cook D, Rocker G, Marshall J *et al.* Level of care study investigators and the Canadian critical care trials group. Withdrawal of mechanical ventilation in anticipation of death in the intensive care unit. *N Engl J Med* 2003; **349**: 1123–32.
5. Hamel MB, Teno JM, Goldman L *et al.* Patient age and decisions to withhold life-sustaining treatments from seriously ill, hospitalized adults. SUPPORT investigators. Study to Understand Prognoses and Preferences for outcomes and Risks of Treatment. *Ann Intern Med* 1999; **130**: 116–25.
6. Phillips RS, Hamel MB, Teno JM *et al.* Patient race and decisions to withhold or withdraw life-sustaining treatments for seriously ill hospitalized adults. SUPPORT investigators. Study to Understand Prognoses and Preferences for Outcomes and Risks of Treatments. *Am J Med* 2000; **108**: 14–9.
7. Kolleff M. Private attending physician status and the withdrawal of life-sustaining interventions in a medical intensive care unit population. *Crit Care Med* 1996; **24**: 968–75.
8. Fisher M. An international perspective on dying in the ICU. In: Curtis JR, Rubenfeld GD (eds) *Managing Death in the ICU.* New York: Oxford University Press; 2001: 273–88.
9. Fisher MM, Raper RF. Withdrawing and withholding treatment in intensive care. *Med J Aust* 1990; **153**: 217–29.
10. Fisher M, Raper RF. Delay in stopping treatment can become unreasonable and unfair. *Br Med J* 2000; **320**: 1268–9.
11. Faber-Lagendorf K, Bartels DM. Process of foregoing life-sustaining treatment in a university hospital: an empirical study. *Crit Care Med* 1996; **24**: 968–75.
12. The SUPPORT investigators. A controlled trial to improve care for seriously ill, hospitalized patients. The Study to Understand Prognoses and references for Outcomes and Risks of Treatment (SUPPORT). *JAMA* 1995; **274**: 1591–8.
13. Angus DC, Barnato AE, Linde-Zwirble WT *et al.* Use of intensive care at the end of life in the United States: an epidemiologic study. *Crit Care Med* 2004; **32**: 638–43.
14. Heyland DK, Frank C, Groll D *et al.* Understanding cardiopulmonary resuscitation decision making: perspectives of seriously ill hospitalised patients and family members. *Chest* 2006; **103**: 419–28.
15. Heyland DK, Rocker GM, O'Callaghan CJ *et al.* Dying in the ICU: perspectives of family members. *Chest* 2003; **124**: 392–7.
16. Ferrand E, Robert R, Ingrand P *et al.* Withholding and withdrawal of life support in intensive-care units in France: a prospective survey. French LATAREA group. *Lancet* 2001; **357**: 9–14.
17. Sjokvist P, Nilstun T, Svantesson M *et al.* Withdrawal of life support-who should decide? *Intens Care* 1999; **25**: 949–54.

18. Rachels J. Active and passive euthanasia. *N Engl J Med* 1975; **292**: 78–80.
19. Davis N, Pohlman A, Gehlbach B *et al.* Improving the process of informed consent in the critically ill. *JAMA* 2003; **289**: 1963–8.
20. Gale EAM. Between two cultures: the expert clinician and the pharmaceutical industry. *Clin Med* 2003; **3**: 538–41.
21. Eichacker PQ, Natanson C, Danner RL. Surviving sepsis – practice guidelines, Marketing campaigns, and Eli Lilly. *N Engl J Med* 2006; **355**: 1640–2.

8

Common problems after ICU

Carl S Waldmann

Until recently, an intensive care unit (ICU) stay was deemed successful if a patient survived to go to the ward. No consideration was taken of the patient dying on the ward or soon after leaving hospital or indeed if the patient went home with an appalling quality of life.

Mortality figures for patients leaving our own ICU recently are shown in Figure 8.1.

A Kings Fund report[1] in 1989 concluded that it was necessary to look at the morbidity following critical illness as well as mortality: 'There is more to life than measuring death'.

Publications such as that of the Audit Commission (*Critical to Success*)[2] and that of the National Expert Group[3] (*Comprehensive Critical Care*) have supported the development of follow-up for patients following a stay in intensive care. In 2007, the National Institute for Clinical Excellence (NICE) began to take an interest in the rehabilitation of critically ill patients and it is hoped will make recommendations to facilitate the introduction of follow-up programmes in all hospitals looking after critically ill patients.

In Reading, a follow-up programme has been ongoing since 1993. Until recently the rehabilitation of patients after a critical illness has fallen between too many stools. Following multiorgan dysfunction, it is difficult to categorise a patient to an individual specialty such as cardiac, respiratory or the stroke rehabilitation teams. Family doctors often have difficulty taking on the complexity of these patients, with the result that they are denied vital advice and assistance and lack an advocate with 'teeth' to ensure timely help.

SETTING UP A FOLLOW-UP SERVICE

Funding such a follow-up programme has posed local problems in many trusts. The service in Reading was initially approved and funded by local then regional audit committees.

The service is staffed by a follow-up sister who spends most of her time in this role helped by a staff nurse and an ICU consultant for the clinics held as a formal outpatient clinic 2/3 times monthly.

Patients who were in ICU for more than 4 days are seen in clinic at 2 months, 6 months and 1 year after discharge and, occasionally, we see patients who have been in ICU for a shorter time period and we also see referrals from other hospitals where follow-up isn't happening. It is important to identify clerical and IT support, and to achieve good collaboration with other hospital departments and general practitioners (GPs) to ensure patients do not make unnecessary journeys to the hospital, by trying to coordinate their visits and ensuring that transport is organised where necessary. Very often, patients will voluntarily come from long distances if they had initially been admitted from other geographical locations – out-of-area transfers.

The logistics of running the service include arranging specific tests that may be required for the visit, such as pulmonary function tests, swabs for methicillin-resistant *Staphylococcus aureus* (MRSA), blood/urine for creatinine clearance. There may be special tests such as magnetic resonance imaging (MRI)[4] for patients who had a tracheostomy during their stay in ICU.

The service in Reading costs £30 000 annually which, in the context of the bigger picture (£4.5 million budget for our ICU), is a small price to pay (Figure 8.2). An unexpected bonus is that the clinic is often seen by the patients as a convenient place to make donations to the ICU.

SPECIFIC PROBLEMS POST-ICU

The range of problems seen after intensive care is vast and ranges from nightmares and sleep disturbance through to ill-fitting clothes. Many of the problems are very specific to the individual but there are also recurrent themes. Flashbacks are common, as are taste loss, poor appetite, nail and hair disorders and sexual dysfunction.

There are several quality-of-life tools used in follow-up studies (Table 8.1). Objective measurements may be inappropriate because they look at aspects such as return to work: often, patients in their 50s may not return to work after a traumatic episode, including ICU, and subjective measures would be more applicable, such as Perceived Quality Of Life (PQOL).

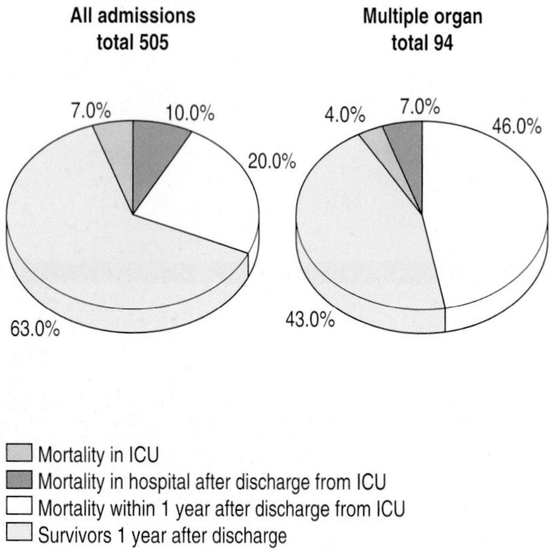

Figure 8.1 Mortality rates for leaving the intensive care unit (ICU).

Follow-up clinic

Nursing	£18 000
Medical	£6 000
Administration	£4 000
Laboratory tests and X-rays	£2 000
Total	**£30 000**

Figure 8.2 Costs of running a service.

Table 8.1 Quality-of-life tool examples

Objective	
QALY	Quality of Life tool[5]
Subjective	
HAD	Hospital Anxiety and Depression[6]
PQOL	Perceived Quality of Life[7]
EuroQol	'European' tool[8]
SF 36	36-item short-form survey[9]

TRACHEOSTOMY

Since percutaneous techniques performed by intensivists started to replace surgical tracheostomy in 1991, we have seen an increasing number of patients tracheostomised earlier in their ICU stay.

The long-term sequelae have been assessed by lung function tests, nasoendoscopy and MRI screening (Figure 8.3). There are minor cosmetic problems, such as

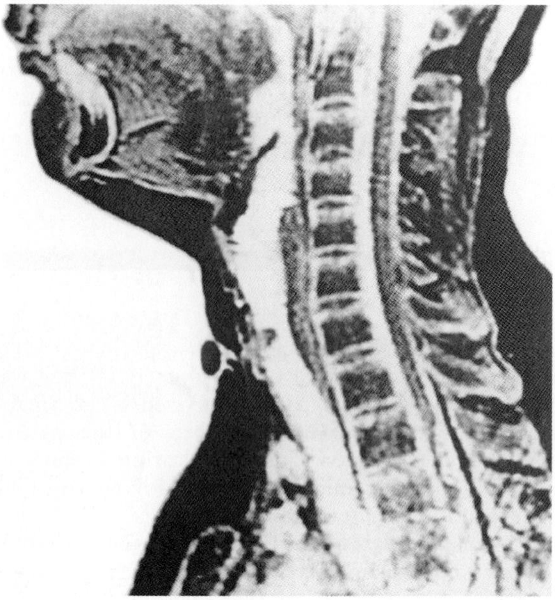

Figure 8.3 Assessment of long-term sequelae.

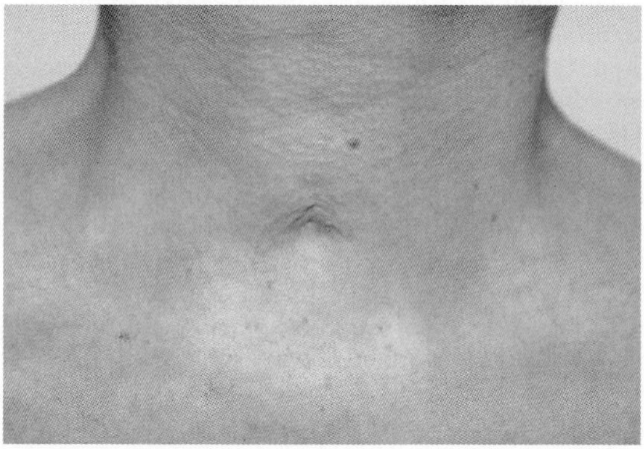

Figure 8.4 Tethering.

tethering (Figure 8.4). Tethering is easily dealt with in ear, nose and throat outpatients under local anaesthetic.

More difficult to manage is tracheal stenosis, defined as a 15% reduction in tracheal diameter. However, there have only been two cases to date. These were seen in the first series of 30 cases.[4]

MOBILITY

Even in the absence of trauma, patients can expect to need 9 months to 1 year to regain full mobility. This is usually due to a mixture of joint pain, stiffness and muscle weakness. In one study,[10] the duration of ICU stay was associated with mobility problems probably associated with loss of muscle mass. If questioned, patients will often

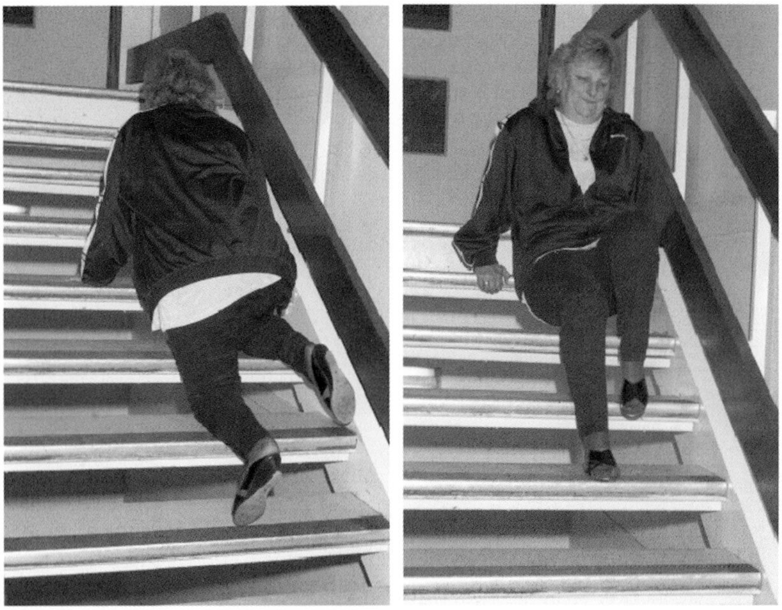

Figure 8.5 Climbing and descending stairs.

report climbing stairs on all fours and descending on their bottoms (Figure 8.5). Muscle wasting can present as a severe localised problem.

This may be associated with critical illness polyneuropathy (CIP),[11] which not only prolongs ventilatory weaning but frequently both complicates and delays rehabilitation. Muscle relaxants have been implicated in the development of CIP[12] but have not been shown to be statistically significant in terms of delayed weaning of intermittent positive-pressure ventilation and duration of stay in ICU.[13]

Until now, there have been no specific rehabilitation programmes for patients recovering from critical illness, although rehabilitation programmes for heart attack, stroke and respiratory disease are well established. A three-centre study has shown that a self-help physiotherapy guided rehabilitation exercise programme will speed up physical recovery after intensive care.[14]

It is important for a member of the team to try and spend time with patients at their homes to assess their special needs and liaise with the GPs, district nurses, community physiotherapists and occupational therapists.

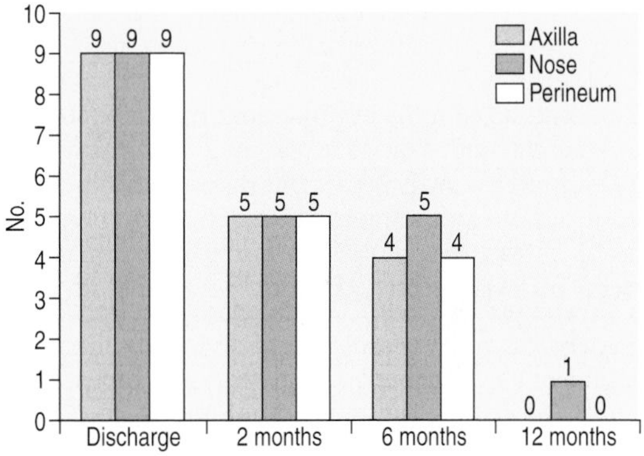

Figure 8.6 Colonisation with methicillin-resistant *Staphylococcus aureus* (MRSA).

Colonisation with MRSA often persists for up to 9 months or longer (Figure 8.6). It is common to hear that patients are being treated as 'lepers' by their own family.

SKIN

Patients complain of a variety of non-specific disorders, including hair loss and nail ridging. Severe pruritus used to be common and not amenable to treatment and was traced back to the use of high-molecular-weight starch solutions in ICU. Described in 2000,[15] in 85 cardiac surgical patients, pruritus was absent in the 26 patients who did not receive starch, but there was a 22% incidence in the 59 patients who did receive starch. This is now supposedly less of a problem with the newer starches.

SEXUAL DYSFUNCTION

Any patients who estimate their sex-life activity to be less active than before ICU admission are deemed to have sexual dysfunction.

In a group of 57 patients,[16] there was a 39% incidence of sexual dysfunction, although in 4 patients, sex life had improved. Sexual dysfunction improves with time, from a frequency of about 26% at 2 months post-ICU down to 16% at 1 year.[17] Sexual dysfunction is often thought to be a psychological problem but, interestingly, following severe burns, it has been reported that there is no correlation between the incidence of posttraumatic stress syndrome and sexual dysfunction.[18] Nevertheless, withdrawing sexual intimacy because of fear of failure can damage relationships. Often sexual dysfunction may go untreated because people are too embarrassed to mention the problem when they have recovered from a life-threatening illness.

Sexual dysfunction affects both men and women. In men it usually manifests itself as impotence or inability to maintain an erection sufficient for satisfactory sexual activity. For management guidelines for erectile dysfunction, see Ralph and McNicholas.[19]

In investigating sexual dysfunction, it is important to eliminate causes such as the use of drugs e.g. L-dopa and H_2-blockers and certain types of surgery (aortic aneurysm) or trauma/radiotherapy to the pelvic region. The patients may be diabetic.

Treatments available include intracavernous or transureteral alprostadil or oral Viagra. Patients with cardiovascular dysfunction have to be carefully assessed before being given Viagra. Non-pharmacological therapies include the use of vacuum devices and inflatable penile prostheses.

In females, sexual dysfunction may occur due to surgery or trauma to the pelvis. More commonly, there is a reduction in desire. Various lubricating gels can be used. As yet, the role of Viagra for women has to be determined. In 127 patients asked to fill in a questionnaire while attending the clinic, the incidence of sexual dysfunction was 45%.[20] There was no link with gender but there was a close association with posttraumatic stress disorder (PTSD).

OTHER PHYSICAL PROBLEMS

A variety of other problems have been seen during follow-up:

- Visual acuity – particularly in patients who have been profoundly hypotensive, visual problems may occur. Occasionally ischaemic changes may be seen on fundoscopy (Figure 8.7a), which may be amenable to laser therapy (Figure 8.7b).
- Facial scarring, where the tape securing the endotracheal tube has been too tight. This scarring can be the whole thickness of the cheek.
- Unneccessary medication. Frequently medication started in ICU as a temporary measure may have been continued (e.g. amiodarone started for sepsis-related arrhythmias).

PSYCHOLOGICAL PROBLEMS

Most patients admitted to ICU have no warning of their admission (emergency admission) and these are the patients who are very much at risk of psychological sequelae post-ICU.

The majority of patients do not have a structured memory of their ICU stay. Those who do may have upsetting memories which may be relatively innocuous, such as being thirsty and hearing a can of Coke being opened, or of a far more profound nature.

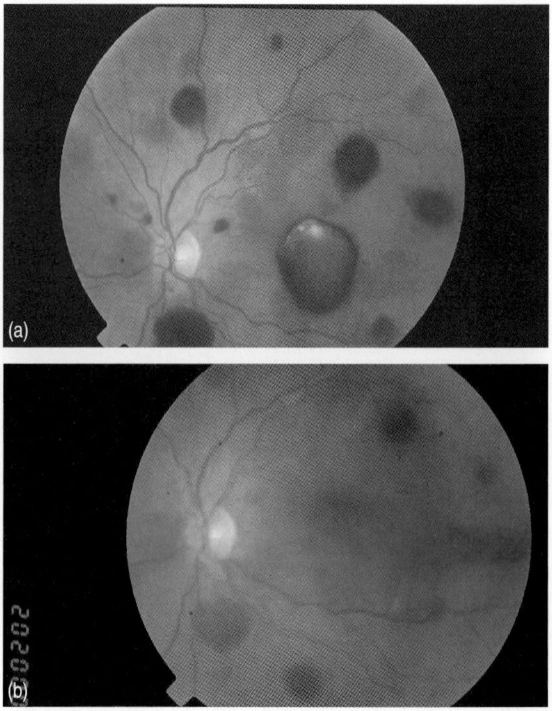

Figure 8.7 (a, b) Ischaemic changes in fundoscopy.

The story of 'torture' experiences is not unusual when you talk to an ex-ICU patient. The psychological impact of the experience may be formidable and may be resented by the patient. The memory of hearing that a patient is about to be 'bagged' was interpreted as being put into a body bag rather than a physiotherapy manoeuvre and the use of a tape measure was interpreted as being measured for a coffin and not as part of the cardiac output measurements. Previous studies demonstrate a high incidence of anxiety, depression and posttraumatic stress.[21] It is common for patients to have memories of being trapped, of being unable to move easily, of being unable to see what is happening and of feeling intensely vulnerable. The anxiety of impending death is also reported.

Below is a typical nightmare of one of our patients:

> *I was in a tunnel knee-deep in mud. It was pitch black, but I could see light at the end. I felt a cold chill on my neck as if someone was breathing down my neck. I thought it was the grim reaper, I knew I had to get to the light.*

There may be several reasons for these experiences (Table 8.2). There is a common belief that, when on ICU, it is better that a patient does not remember anything. However, it is increasingly realised that false memories or delusions during an ICU stay can have a

Table 8.2 Psychological problems

Illness
Sedation technique
Withdrawal
No communication aids
Lack of clear night/day
Continuous noise of alarms
Sleep disturbance – lack of rapid-eye-movement sleep

significant impact on psychological recovery after ICU[22] and factual memories of ICU may reduce anxiety.[23]

It now seems likely that delusional memories of ICU and nightmares are associated with PTSD.

PTSD is a normal reaction to severe stress and is similar to a grief reaction to bereavement. It occurs in about 1% of the population and increases to 10% in victims of road traffic accidents and 65% in prisoners of war. About 15% of patients have the typical disorder post-ICU. In those with adult respiratory distress syndrome, the incidence increases to 27.5%.

PTSD is the development of characteristic symptoms after being subjected to a traumatic event. PTSD can be triggered by any memory or mention of something to do with the traumatic event and is characterised by intrusive recollections, avoidance behaviour and hyperarousal symptoms.[24]

Chronic fatigue syndrome (CFS), previously known as myalgic encephalitis (ME), is thought to describe the condition of many patients post-ICU who have had a period of prolonged inactivity. CFS is diagnosed by the presence of fatigue at 6 months post-ICU with impairment of daily living, social and leisure pursuits and with no medically significant cause of the fatigue. There is no doubt that a graded exercise programme is of benefit to aid physical recovery in such ICU patients.[14] Drugs such as fluoxetime (Prozac) do not seem to benefit such patients, even though there is a great temptation to use antidepressants in these patients.[25]

Various strategies to deal with the psychological sequelae of ICU stay have been tried.

DURING ICU STAY

- There is no doubt that continuous intravenous sedation has been identified as an independent predictor of a longer duration of mechanical ventilation, ICU stay and total hospital stay.[26] Kreiss *et al.*[27] demonstrated that, in 128 adults, ICU stay was reduced from an average of 7.3 to 4.9 days by the daily interruption of the sedative regime. This regime may have had an impact by reducing PTSD as the patients are more likely to have some recollection of their ICU stay, thus helping them to understand the reasons for the need for their prolonged rehabilitation period. Concerns have been raised as to the type of sedative agent used in ICU. It is well known that etomidate may cause an excess in mortality in trauma patients in ICU[28] and propofol may do the same in head-injured patients at doses greater than 5 mg/kg per h.[29] The decision to use benzodiazepines such as midazolam increasingly may be associated with dependence. This has been studied; 21 out of 148 ICU patients were discharged home on oral benzodiazepine, of whom 10 were still taking them at 6 months post-discharge having not been on them pre-ICU.[30] Lorazepam has been promoted as the benzodiazepine of choice for sedation in ICU[31] and is preferred by a task force in the USA for adult patients in ICU.[32]
- Encouraging the use of communication aids, involving speech therapists particularly in patients with tracheostomies[33] and training more nurses to lip-read can be invaluable.
- When building or modifying ICUs, remember that windows and 24-hour clocks visible to patients may help re-establish circadian rhythms and the use of curtains to ensure patient dignity should not be forgotten. There has been some interest in appropriate colours that should be used in ICU décor, avoiding colours that cause alarm in the animal kingdom, such as red, yellow and black.
- Use of aromatherapy and massage whilst patients receive their ICU does seem to reduce stress levels and encourages contact between the patient and relatives, reducing the feeling of isolation.[34]

POST-ICU DISCHARGE

Visiting patients on the ward post ICU discharge and giving them an information booklet helps to prepare them better for the long rehabilitation process ahead.

As well as three ICU follow-up clinic appointments in the year after their discharge, patients with PTSD are encouraged to visit the ICU and, with the help of a diary, reconstruct the lost period of time in the patient's life. We are considering the use of photos of patients whilst they are on ICU to help them understand how ill they actually were.

CONCLUSION

It is important to assess patient satisfaction or dissatisfaction with their follow-up. This may be audited by questionnaire during their third visit to the follow-up clinic at 1 year post ICU discharge.[35]

The findings have been reassuring. The response rate was 87 out of 88 patients and all but one of the 87 patients found benefit from the clinic, particularly because questions could be answered (often their GP could not help). Other findings are as follows:

- 28% benefited from referral to other specialists
- 26% had PTSD counseling
- 25% felt they derived some benefit from returning to the ICU and having a diary written for them
- 48% felt they were helping the staff of the ICU

The comments were very useful, e.g.:

- 'You helped me retrace the time lost whilst under sedation'
- 'It was frightening leaving ICU to go back to the ward. My wife slept next to me in the ward on a mattress on the floor'

There is no end to the surprises and unexpected problems that arise in patients after intensive care. It is not unusual to see patients who were initially deemed inappropriate for surgery and ICU who have done well and who on questioning have an excellent quality of life. It is only by the ICU specialists undertaking to follow up patients that we can assess the appropriateness of our decision-making and treatments.

In the UK follow-up clinics were recommended by the Audit Commission in 1999 (*Criticial to Success*)[2] and in the *Comprehensive Critical Care* document in 2000[3], yet only a small number of hospitals have been able to fund such a service. Griffiths *et al.*[36] demonstrated that clinics are not widely established and show marked heterogeneity. Of those established, only two-thirds are funded and most do not have a prenegotiated access to other outpatient services. It is hoped that NICE will support their growth and that the National Outreach Forum will support the idea that follow-up will be one of the quality indicators of a hospital's resolve to set up a comprehensive service for patients who have been critically ill. Meanwhile there is an exponential increase in literature related to outcome following critical illness as health economists and intensivists try and make some sense out of the cost-effectiveness of intensive care.[37–40] Further studies are under way. The DiPEx study seeks to obtain a variety of patient and relative experiences of critical care (www.dipex.org). I-CANUK is a website that is being set up to provide a forum and voice for those involved in patient care following intensive care discharge and to support research into potential therapies following critical illness. The results of the PraCTICaL (Pragmatic Randomised Controlled Trial of Intensive Care Follow-up clinics in improving longer-term outcomes trial from critical illness) should be available by the end of 2008.

REFERENCES

1. Kings Fund. Intensive care in the United Kingdom; a report from the Kings Fund Panel. *Anaesthesia* 1989; **44**: 428–30.
2. Audit Commission. *Critical to Success. The Place of Efficient and Effective Critical Care Services within the Acute Hospital.* London: Audit Commission; 1999.
3. National Expert Group. *Comprehensive Critical Care. A Review of Adult Critical Care Services.* London: Department of Health; 2000.
4. Bernau F, Waldmann CS, Meanock C *et al.* Long-term follow-up of percutaneous tracheostomy using ßow-loop and MRI scanning. *Intens Care Med* 1996; **22**: S295.
5. Harris J. Qualifying the value of life. *J Med Ethics* 1987; **13**: 117–73.
6. Zigmond AS, Snaith RP. The hospital anxiety and depression scale. *Acta Psychiatry Scand* 1983; **67**: 361–70.
7. Patrick DL, Davis M, Southerland LI *et al.* Quality of life following intensive care. *J Gen Int Med* 1988; **3**: 218–23.
8. Williams A. The Euro Qol – a new facility for the measurement of health related quality of life. *Health Policy II* 1990; **16**: 199–208.
9. Ware JE, Sherbourne CD. The MOS 36-item short-form health survey (SF-36): I. Conceptual framework and item selection. *Med Care* 1992; **30**: 473–81.
10. Jones C, Griffiths RD. Identifying post intensive care patients who may need physical rehabilitation. *Clin Intens Care* 2000; **11**: 35–8.
11. Leijten FSS, de Weerd AW. Critical illness polyneuropathy. A review of literature, definition and pathophysiology. *Clin Neurol Neurosurg* 1994; **96**: 10–19.
12. Barohn RJ, Jackson CE, Rogers SJ *et al.* Prolonged paralysis due to non-depolarising neuromuscular blocking agents and corticosteroids. *Muscle Nerve* 1994; **17**: 647–54.
13. Zifko UA, Zipko HT, Bolton CF. Clinical and electrophysiological finding in critical illness polyneuropathy. *J Neurol Sci* 1998; **159**: 186–93.
14. Jones C, Skirrow P, Griffith RD. Rehabilitation after critical illness, a randomised controlled trial. *Crit Care Med* 2003; **31**: 2456–61.
15. Morgan PW, Berridge JC. Giving long-persistent starch as volume replacement can cause pruritis after cardiac surgery. *Br J Anaesth* 2000; **85**: 676–99.
16. Quinlan J, Gager M, Fawcett D *et al.* Sexual dysfunction after intensive care. *Br J Anaesth* 2001; **87**: 348.
17. Quinlan J, Waldmann CS, Fawcett D. Sexual dysfunction after intensive care. *Br J Anaesth* 1998; **81**: 809–10.
18. De Rios MD, Norac A, Achauer BH. Sexual dysfunction and the patient with burns. *Burn Care Rehabil* 1997; **18**: 37–42.
19. Ralph D, McNicholas T. UK management guidelines for erectile dysfunction. *Br Med J* 2000; **321**: 499–503.
20. Griffiths J, Gager M, Alder N *et al.* A self-report based study of the incidence and associations of sexual dysfunction in the survivors of intensive care treatment. *Intens Care Med* 2006; **32**: 445–51.
21. Koshy G, Wilkinson A, Harmsworth A *et al.* Intensive care unit follow-up program at a district general hospital. *Intens Care Med* 1997; **23**: S160.
22. Griffiths RD, Jones C, McMillan I. Where is the harm in not knowing? Care after intensive care. *Clin Intens Care* 1996; **7**: 144–5.
23. Jones C, Griffiths RD, Humphries G. Factual memories of intensive care may reduce anxiety post-ICU. *Br J Anaesth* 2000; **82**: 793.

24. Horowitz MJ. *Stress response syndromes – a review of post-traumatic stress and adjustment disorders.* In: Wilson JP, Raphael B (eds) *International Handbook of Traumatic Stress Syndromes.* New York: Plenum Press; 1993: 49–60.
25. Jones C, Skirrow P, Griffiths RD *et al.* The characteristics of patients given antidepressants while recovering from critical illness. *Br J Anaesth* 2000; **84**: 666.
26. Kollef MH, Levy NT, Ahrens TS *et al.* The use of continuous IV sedation is associated with prolongation of mechanical ventilation. *Chest* 1998; **114**: 541–8.
27. Kreiss JP, Pohlman AS, O'Connor MF *et al.* Daily interruption of sedative infusions in critically ill patients undergoing mechanical ventilation. *N Engl J Med* 2000; **342**: 1471–7.
28. Ledingham IM, WattI. Influence of sedation in multiple trauma patients. *Lancet* 1983; **8336**: 1270.
29. Cremer OL, Moons GM, Bouman EAC *et al.* Long-term propofol infusion and cardiac failure in adult head-injured patients. *Lancet* 2001; **357**: 117–18.
30. Conway DH, Eddleston J, Turner S. Prevalence of oral sedation dependency following intensive care. *Intens Care Med* 1999; **25** (suppl. 1): S169.
31. Meagher DJ. Delirium: optimising management. *Br Med J* 2001; **322**: 144–9.
32. Shapiro BA, Warren J, Egol AB *et al.* Practice parameters for intravenous analgesia and sedation in the intensive care unit: an executive summary. *Crit Care Med* 1995; **23**: 1596–600.
33. Etchels MC. Personal communication. ICU talk. Available online at: www.computing.dundee.ac.uk/projects/icutalk.
34. Waldmann CS, Tseng P, Meulman P *et al.* Aromatherapy in the intensive care unit. *Care Crit Ill* 1993; **9**: 170–4.
35. Hames KC, Gager M, Waldmann CS. Patient satisfaction with specialist ICU follow-up. *Br J Anaesth* 2001; **87**: 372.
36. Griffiths JA, Barber VS, Cuthbertson BH *et al.* A national survey of intensive care follow up clinics. *Anaesthesia* 2006; **61**: 950–5.
37. Griffiths RD, Jones C. *Intensive Care Aftercare.* Oxford: Butterworth-Heinemann; 2002.
38. Angus DC, Carlet J. *Surviving Intensive Care.* Update in Intensive Care and Emergency Medicine 39. Berlin: Springer-Verlag; 2003.
39. Wu A, Gao F. Long term outcomes in survivors of critical illness. *Anaesthesia* 2004; **59**: 1049–52.
40. Herridge MS, Cheung A, Tansey C *et al.* One year outcomes in survivors of the acute respiratory distress syndrome. *N Engl J Med* 2003; **348**: 683–93.

9

Clinical information systems

David Fraenkel

Clinical record-keeping requires an integrated system to manage the information, including its acquisition during clinical care, and archiving and availability for future clinical, business and research uses.

The term 'clinical information systems' (CIS) refers to computerised systems for managing the clinical record, often within specialised areas of a hospital, such as intensive care, emergency medicine, operating theatres or cardiology. CIS for intensive care units (ICUs) have been developing since the late 1980s; however, their implementation has been limited by cost, functionality and clinician acceptance.[1–8]

The electronic medical record (EMR) and electronic health care records (EHR) embrace respective hospital and community-wide electronic systems for managing patient records which may be integrated with the more specialised CIS. Over the next decade we can expect to see EHR implementation throughout the health systems of the more developed nations. The driving incentive is community concern for safety and quality in health care and the EHR is the single most powerful measure to produce a safer, more effective and efficient health care system.[8–12]

In the UK the National Health Service (NHS) has embarked on an ambitious National Programme for Information Technology (NPfIT) featuring a national summary care record (SCR) or 'spine' to hold limited essential information on each consenting patient. Additional features include picture archiving and communication systems (PACS), more detailed data held on integrated local computer systems, electronic prescribing and computerised physician order entry (CPOE).[13,14]

The US government has placed a high priority on electronic health records, although progress will be uneven due to the fragmented nature of its health system. The Veterans Health Administration (VHA) has a system-wide EHR (VistA) that is closely integrated with its quality monitoring and enhancement programme and is delivering tangible results.[15–17] Similarly, the Partners HealthCare System at the Brigham and Women's Hospital and Massachusetts General Hospital has demonstrated real improvements in health care with cost and quality benefit outcomes.[18–21]

The coordination of effort in Europe will be similarly challenging, although the need is recognised by the European Commission. In Australia, the HealthConnect strategy is largely focused on broadband connections for primary health care providers and establishing data dictionaries and standards with limited strategies or funding for actual implementation of EHRs.[22]

FUNCTIONS AND ADVANTAGES OF CIS

CIS seek to deliver several key benefits (Table 9.1).[23] These include the automation of repetitive manual tasks, improved accuracy through reductions in human error, attributable records simultaneously available from multiple points of care and integration with other bedside equipment and information systems. The built-in error checking and knowledge-based systems should also provide a safer and higher-quality clinical process. The CIS electronically capture the data and make this information potentially available to a multitude of systems. This obviates the need for repetitive manual data entry or transcription, while making the data accessible for a range of purposes which may include clinical, business and research reporting.

The ICU is already a technology-rich environment, where bedside devices process and provide data elements in electronic format. Similarly, many clinical measurements are available on monitors, ventilators and pumps. Traditionally, these electronically derived values are transcribed on to observation charts and paper-based clinical records, as are repetitive clinical observations and arithmetic calculations which are often performed manually or with the aid of a calculator. The voluminous observation charts present a challenge for both storage and access, and transcription errors and arithmetic errors are prolific in these paper systems.

The CIS automates the process of electronic data collection from monitors, ventilators, infusion pumps, dialysis/filtration equipment, cardiac assist devices and other bedside devices and provides a real-time spreadsheet with arithmetic accuracy. Incorporation of clinical documentation and progress notes provides a legible and attributable record of events.

The patient record can then be accessed from geographically distant workstations in the ICU, the hospital,

Table 9.1 Clinical information systems (CIS) benefits

1. Recording of bedside observations
   (a) Automation of physiological data collection
   (b) Reduction in transcription and arithmetic errors
   (c) Downloading from bedside therapeutic devices (e.g. pumps, ventilators)
2. Clinical documentation
   (a) Legible and attributable clinical record
   (b) Structures and cues encourage comprehensive documentation
   (c) Electronic record of drug prescription and administration
   (d) Attributable record simultaneously available from multiple points of care
3. Access to additional clinical information at the bedside
   (a) Pathology results
   (b) Digitised medical imaging and reports
   (c) Digital clinical photographs
   (d) Other hospital systems (e.g. admission/discharge/transfer (ADT), CIS)
4. Bedside decision support systems
   (a) Passive
      (i) Improved and accessible clinical record
      (ii) Online clinical policies and procedures
      (iii) Online knowledge bases
      (iv) Online literature searches
   (b) Active
      (i) Investigative and therapeutic management algorithms
      (ii) Clinical pathways
      (iii) Drug allergy and interaction alerts
      (iv) Drug dosing and monitoring support
      (v) Antibiotic selection and prescribing
      (vi) Ventilation and haemodynamic management systems
5. Medicolegal archiving
   (a) Audit trail for all changes during episode of care
   (b) No ability to change once archived
   (c) Secure long-term storage and ensured availability
6. Clinical database
   (a) Long-term accessible storage of relevant clinical data
   (b) Industry-standard database format
   (c) Efficient and flexible query and reporting solutions
   (d) Scheduled and ad hoc reports
   (e) Clinical, research and management requirements

and even from other more remote sites. As long as the system is running, the record is easy to locate and always available.

A major contribution of CIS to clinical safety and quality is through the provision of an electronic prescribing and administration record for drugs and fluids. Errors in prescription and administration are a leading cause of adverse events with associated morbidity.[18,24] CIS provide both legibility and varying levels of decision support which may include defining usual dosages and administration routes, suggesting dose modification in the setting of organ failures, or preventing prescribing in cases of known allergy or likely drug interaction.[25]

ARCHITECTURE AND COMPONENTS OF CIS

BASIC CIS ARCHITECTURE

All CIS share certain basic components consisting of workstations, a network and central servers (Figure 9.1). The user interface is presented at the workstation, which is usually at each bedside but may also be in nearby central and administrative areas, such as the nurses' station, or more distant in the offices of clinical or administrative staff. Workstations commonly consist of relatively standard personal computer (PC) hardware being desk-, pendant or trolley-mounted, but may include laptops or personal digital assistants (PDAs) with wireless systems where technical challenges related to speed and reliabiltiy of data transmission can be overcome.

Most CIS allow other applications, such as PACS, word processing or e-mail, to be run on the same PC, but this is potentially a rich source of system conflicts and requires careful administration.

Workstations are linked to each other and a centralised set of servers through a network of communication cables. Hubs, switches and routers control network traffic. A dedicated network, either actual or virtual, enhances system performance but it is important to ensure built-in redundancy in network loops and power sources to minimise potential interruptions from physical disruption or component failure.

The configuration of computer servers varies widely but it is common to have 'paired' or 'mirrored' servers, which duplicate their partner's function. This provides protection from hardware failure, minimising system down time, and provides some degree of data protection. Servers have a finite capacity to process data from multiple workstations and other peripheral connections, and so larger systems may require multiple server pairs.

CIS usually require a separate workstation or server to manage the interfaces with other systems. These include hospital demographics (ADT systems for admission/discharge/transfer), pathology laboratory, pharmacy, radiology and hospital finance. Interfacing requires a software platform known as an interface engine. Additional software identifies the relevant data and directs and processes these data to the correct field in the appropriate format. Due to the huge variety of current and legacy systems, this process almost always requires custom-written code and programming, representing one of the major risks and expenses of systems integration.[13]

Bedside monitoring systems usually include a central station or server that can be linked with the CIS servers to transfer their downloaded information back to the bedside. Transferring data from other bedside devices is usually achieved by a cable connection from the device to a bedside concentrator in the patient bay. The connection requires an electronic decoder, specific to the

Figure 9.1 Clinical information systems architecture. LAN, local area network; WAN, wide area network; ADT, admission/discharge/transfer; CVHD, continuous venovenous haemodialysis.

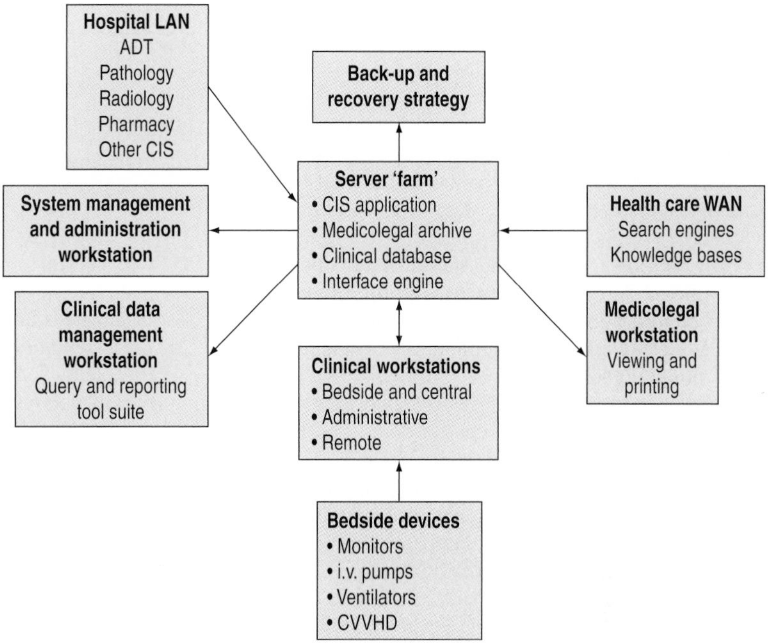

manufacturer and model of the device. The concentrator must then communicate with the central servers via a subsidiary server that provides the software translator to complete the interface. A selection of established interfaces to commonly utilised equipment exists but often additional customised interfaces must be written.

MEDICOLEGAL STORAGE

Electronic data capture does not necessarily result in long-term electronic data storage. Many CIS sites have continued to require the printing-out of all reports from the patient episode to store in the paper-based hospital medical record. Modern servers have extensive storage capacity but this can be rapidly consumed by the equally enormous amount of data being collected from every patient. Some server pairs can only hold 2–3 months of data before data begin to be purged or overwritten. Although hard-disk memory is ever-increasing and more affordable, additional strategies such as more efficient databases or offline storage formats may be needed. When the choice of storage solution is made, it is equally important to be aware that the format of data storage is determined by the anticipated use of the data and to ensure that future software upgrades do not render the stored data unreadable.

Data archiving for medicolegal purposes requires that the clinical information be readily accessible and preferably presented in exactly the same format as it was recorded and reviewed by the clinicians during the episode of patient care. Any changes to the clinical record during the patient episode must be clearly displayed and attributable – this is known as an audit trail or change history. An audit trail is a standard feature of most CIS and actually offers improved accountability over paper-based systems. It may be desirable to make it impossible to alter the record after the patient episode, which requires specialised storage formats or strict access restrictions to the data archive.

Once the record is stored, by whatever method, it must be protected from accidental loss. This usually requires a carefully engineered and documented management plan with regular scheduled back-ups, off-site storage of duplicates and robust recovery strategies. When these requirements are fulfilled, the electronic medicolegal archive can readily exceed the performance of a paper-based record through its assured availability and authenticity.

CLINICAL DATABASE STORAGE

A major objective of CIS is to provide a comprehensive clinical database which will accumulate data in real time that can be stored and queried for a wide range of reports for a variety of purposes. The relevant data need to be held in an accessible and readily searchable database that will allow a variety of sophisticated reports to be prepared on both a scheduled and ad hoc basis. These requirements are quite different from those of medicolegal storage and usually require a separate form of data storage, commonly known as a clinical database, data repository, data warehouse or data management solution.

It may be desirable to adopt a significantly different database structure from the core CIS database which may have been designed with prospective user configurability in mind, rather than allowing easy location of data fields in a structure designed for rapidly processing queries. The design of the clinical database is a compromise between saving effectively the large amount of data collected while maintaining speed and ease of use in running queries. Even when the vendor has utilised an industry-standard database application, such as Oracle or SQL, in the core CIS application, designing and running queries may still present a challenging specialist task because of the complexity of the table structure or the huge amount of aggregated data.

The clinical data management solutions currently offered are quite diverse. One solution simply provides an industry-standard data transfer protocol (e.g. 'ODBC driver') as a means of accessing the data. The local circumstances of each hospital then dictate customised queries or secondary database designs for local use. Alternatively, an industry-standard query tool is used to generate reports from the core CIS database, but the number of queries that can be designed and preconfigured in this fashion is often limited, particularly as the user configurations of the CIS vary widely. There is inevitably a compromise between standardisation and flexibility. Data fields must be standardised in the configuration of the CIS to allow standard queries to be performed. Some CIS solutions offer a proprietary subsidiary database containing selected clinical data with a wider range of reports preconfigured into the query tool.

EVALUATION AND IMPLEMENTATION OF CIS

Clinicians frequently underestimate the managerial requirements, human resource demands and opportunity costs of CIS implementation.[11] The process should be viewed as a major project requiring advanced planning and management skills (Table 9.2). The project team must be multidisciplinary, consult widely and consider workplace flows and processes, or else a suboptimal result is guaranteed, as has been demonstrated in the literature.[26,27] The CIS will impact on medical, nursing, allied health, managerial and technical staff within the ICU, together with those from other clinical disciplines. Involvement of hospital information management and medical records staff is strongly recommended. Extensive documentation and continued scheduled reviews are required throughout the process.

Business case development to secure funding is less problematic than previously and assisted by the quality benefits of CIS implementation.[11,21] The most basic system can be expected to cost in the order of AUD $25 000–50 000 per bed, while more advanced systems may be two to three times that cost. Annual recurrent costs are significant and usually exceed 20% of the capital cost of the system.

The CIS industry is subject to the same vagaries as other parts of the IT industry, including high turnover of personnel and frequent inability to deliver on promised functionality and timelines. CIS selection is best conducted as a formal tender process, and the evaluation of submissions is a complex task (Table 9.3). Availability and expense of on-site support during and following implementation are also critical factors.

Implementation planning should be detailed and requires a full-time project officer on site. A standard implementation needs 4–6 months prior to the 'go live' date with hospital-wide consultation, issue management and carefully scheduled staff training. It is desirable to have as many as possible of the interfaces and bedside devices linked to the CIS at the implementation date. This will maximise perceived benefits early and thereby encourage acceptance of the system. It should be implemented through the whole ICU as partial implementations are rarely successful.

Post-implementation review is essential to progress outstanding issues, which are usually prolific, and help establish

Table 9.2 Clinical information systems (CIS) implementation

1. Professional project management
   - (a) Structured multidisciplinary team
     - (i) Sponsor, director, manager, representatives
     - (ii) Medical, nursing, allied health, managerial
   - (b) Comprehensive documentation
   - (c) Consultative approach
     - (i) Medical records department
     - (ii) IT/IM department
     - (iii) Hospital and business managers
2. Project framework
   - (a) Needs analysis
   - (b) Definition of scope
   - (c) Management of expectation and scope creep
3. Tender evaluation (see Table 9.3)
4. Implementation process
   - (a) Implementation plan and schedule
   - (b) Training
   - (c) Installation
   - (d) Schedule of payments
   - (e) Quality monitoring of process
5. Postimplementation review
   - (a) Actual outcomes of plan
   - (b) Unresolved issues
   - (c) Process improvement
6. System management plan
   - (a) Identification of system components
   - (b) Departmental and individual roles and responsibilities
   - (c) Identification of vendor responsibilities
   - (d) Back-up schedules and recovery plans
7. Support contracts
   - (a) Scope and level of support
   - (b) Pricing
8. Future issues
   - (a) Ongoing management of 'special projects'
   - (b) Continued development and innovation
   - (c) System upgrades
   - (d) Scheduled hardware replacement
   - (e) System obsolescence and replacement

Table 9.3 Clinical information systems (CIS) evaluation

1. Vendor characteristics
   (a) Monitoring of software experience
   (b) Niche specialty products, cf. health care-wide
   (c) Development base by specialty and geography
2. Preliminary evaluation
   (a) Evaluate tender documents
   (b) Product demonstration
   (c) Prepared and impromptu scenario testing of product
   (d) Ensure all required components identified, e.g. database, interfaces, etc.
   (e) Comparative levels of best fit for needs and specifications
3. Site visits to installed customer base
   (a) Reference sites and 'sites like us'
   (b) Demonstrations with vendor
   (c) Candid visits without vendor
   (d) Observe functionality
   (e) Examine interfaces
   (f) Explore support issues
4. Interfaces
   (a) Identify requirements
   (b) Assess vendor capabilities
   (c) Inspect working interfaces
   (d) Customisation scope and cost
5. Technical issues
   (a) Industry-standard hardware and software
   (b) Local acceptability
   (c) Integration with existing systems
   (d) Upgrade paths
   (e) Network specifications
   (f) Network costs and management
6. Support issues
   (a) Location and availability
   (b) Product support specialists
   (c) Technical engineers
   (d) Level of risk-sharing
   (e) Whole-of-life costing

the arrangements for the support and continued development of the system. A system management plan identifies the responsibility centres for management of the CIS components and clarifies requirements and expectations. A permanent on-site system management position is required for system maintenance, progressing outstanding issues and managing future upgrades and developments.

BENEFITS OF CIS: THE STATE OF THE ART

Basic CIS requirements are fulfilled by the majority of systems currently available:

- Charting, including tabulation of bedside observations and measurements such as fluid balance. The flow sheets are usually more than adequately flexible and configurable to meet local requirements.
- Bedside device interfaces. New devices may not have the necessary decoders and software. The expense of developing new interfaces can be considerable when calculated on a per-bed basis.
- Clinical progress notes. These are adequate but the free text may not be 'searchable', and structured text may be only marginally better.
- Keyboard skills are increasingly widespread but may still be an issue with some clinicians.
- Drug and fluid prescription and administration are good but not always incorporated in some systems, necessitating a separate system.

Decision support systems have previously been disappointing but their further development offers substantial benefits.[25,28] A legible and available record of previous and ongoing care does offer an improved level of decision support, albeit one that the general community would already expect and see as mandatory. Passive decision support with access to knowledge-based systems through CIS and hospital intranets, as well as resources such as pharmacopoeia, literature search engines and online texts and journals, is widely available. It is intuitive that these resources would improve the quality of clinical outcomes; but there is little evidence to support this.

Active decision support has not been generally available, including the flagging of drug allergies and interactions and the integration of relevant information, such as baseline renal function, recent urine output, last measured creatinine and required dose of aminoglycoside. Decision support systems to recommend antimicrobial prescribing, ventilatory therapy or haemodynamic measurement have been developed in dedicated centres of excellence, but are also not generally available nor necessarily able to be migrated successfully across boundaries of international practice. The provision of prompts has been shown to be effective for routine prophylaxis and care processes, supported by clinical pathways and guidelines.[19,29] Increasing emphasis on decision support from safety and quality initiatives may be expected to accelerate developments.

CPOE is exemplified in electronic prescribing, but its benefits extend to other areas such as pathology and radiology orders and results viewing. There is good evidence that a reduction in ordering occurs through reduced duplication and timeliness and access to results.[25,28] The availability of CPOE (computerised physician order entry) varies with the level of systems integration and compatibility with other legacy and proprietary computer systems. Standardised communications protocols (e.g. HL-7) are helpful but only provide similarities of electronic language. High-level interfaces require continued maintenance and development and therefore expenditure. Other solutions include seamless and simultaneous operation in multiple systems (Clinical Context Object Workgroup) or placing all data in a single repository for access by multiple applications.[13]

Clinical databases remain a significant challenge, whether at a local departmental, hospital, regional or national level.

Although many products are purported to include data management and query solutions, those that are available 'off the shelf' may be quite rudimentary and their development may require additional expenditure and a major commitment from the clinical staff. Part of the problem is the need for clinicians to define prospectively what is expected of the system. This requires exhaustive definition of the questions that the system should be able to answer and therefore also specification of the detailed nature of the data and queries that will be required.

Accurate analysis of diagnoses and procedures requires that key information is entered correctly and consistently and that reliable and high-quality data capture is achieved. Data entry should be 'once-only', simple and robust, and should be easily performed as the clinical scenario unfolds. There is very limited agreement and standardisation between clinicians with respect to mandatory data fields, diagnostic criteria and classifications. Standardised reports are therefore difficult to develop in different clinical environments, let alone regions or countries. The eventual adoption of common international standards and classifications (e.g. SNOMED for diagnoses, National Library of Medicines for pharmaceuticals) would greatly facilitate solution design and querying. Other issues, including the speed of data access in huge data repositories, the development of unique patient/episode identifiers and privacy considerations, are still significant.

FUTURE DEVELOPMENTS

Over the next decade the EHR will provide the most significant and comprehensive improvement in the delivery of health care in developed nations. Central clinical repositories will probably initially hold sentinel data for consenting patients such as identifiers, past and present diagnoses, medications and allergies. More detailed data will be held in peripheral repositories where the challenge is ensuring appropriate accessibility and/or systems integration. The use of CIS with active decision support and computerised order entry will be an integral part of delivering and monitoring improved patient care. Despite requiring huge levels of investment, these developments are happening now and should include clinical involvement and leadership to realise and maximise their benefits.

REFERENCES

1. Teich JM, Glaser JP, Beckley RF *et al.* The Brigham integrated computing system (BICS): advanced clinical systems in an academic hospital environment. *Int J Med Inform* 1999; **54**: 197–208.
2. de Keizer NF, Stoutenbeek CP, Hanneman LA *et al.* An evaluation of patient data management systems in Dutch intensive care. *Intens Care Med* 1998; **24**: 167–71.
3. Harrison JP, Palacio C. The role of clinical information systems in health care quality improvement. *Health Care Manage (Frederick)* 2006; **25**: 206–12.
4. Metnitz PG, Lenz K. Patient data management systems in intensive care – the situation in Europe. *Intens Care Med* 1995; **21**: 703–15.
5. Urschitz M, Lorenz S, Unterasinger L *et al.* Three years experience with a patient data management system at a neonatal intensive care unit. *J Clin Monit Comput* 1998; **14**: 119–25.
6. Fraenkel DJ. Clinical information systems in intensive care. *Crit Care Resusc* 1999; **1**: 179.
7. Ash JS, Bates DW. Factors and forces affecting EHR system adoption: report of a 2004 ACMI discussion. *J Am Med Inform Assoc* 2005; **12**: 8–12.
8. Bates DW, Gawande AA. Improving safety with information technology. *N Engl J Med* 2003; **348**: 2526–34.
9. Bates DW, Cohen M, Leape LL *et al.* Reducing the frequency of errors in medicine using information technology. *J Am Med Inform Assoc* 2001; **8**: 299–308.
10. Leape LL, Berwick DM. Five years after To Err Is Human: what have we learned? *JAMA* 2005; **293**: 2384–90.
11. Frisse ME. Comments on return on investment (ROI) as it applies to clinical systems. *J Am Med Inform Assoc* 2006; **13**: 365–7.
12. The Leapfrog Group Fact Sheet. Available online at http://www.leapfroggroup.org/about_us/leapfrog-factsheet. Accessed 7 November 2006.
13. Tackley R. Integrating anaesthesia and intensive care into the national care record. *Br J Anaesth* 2006; **97**: 69–76.
14. National Health Service. NHS Connecting for Health. Available online at: http://www.connectingforhealth.nhs.uk/. Accessed 7 November 2006.
15. Asch SM, McGlynn EA, Hogan MM *et al.* Comparison of quality of care for patients in the Veterans Health Administration and patients in a national sample. *Ann Intern Med* 2004; **141**: 938–45.
16. Hynes DM, Perrin RA, Rappaport S *et al.* Informatics resources to support health care quality improvement in the Veterans Health Administration. *J Am Med Inform Assoc* 2004; **11**: 344–50.
17. United States Department of Veterans Affairs. VA VISTA Innovations Award. Available online at: http://www.innovations.va.gov/innovations/. Accessed 7 November 2006.
18. Bates DW, Leape LL, Cullen DJ *et al.* Effect of computerized physician order entry and a team intervention on prevention of serious medication errors. *JAMA* 1998; **280**: 1311–16.
19. Kucher N, Koo S, Quiroz R *et al.* Electronic alerts to prevent venous thromboembolism among hospitalized patients. *N Engl J Med* 2005; **352**: 969–77.
20. Wang SJ, Middleton B, Prosser LA *et al.* A cost–benefit analysis of electronic medical records in primary care. *Am J Med* 2003; **114**: 397–403.
21. Kaushal R, Jha AK, Franz C *et al.* Return on investment for a computerized physician order entry system. *J Am Med Inform Assoc* 2006; **13**: 261–6.

22. Health Connect. Available online at: http://www.health.gov.au/internet/hconnect/publishing.nsf/Content/home. Accessed 7 November 2006.
23. Fraenkel DJ, Cowie M, Daley P. Quality benefits of an intensive care clinical information system. *Crit Care Med* 2003; **31**: 120–5.
24. Brennan TA, Leape LL, Laird NM *et al.* Incidence of adverse events and negligence in hospitalized patients. Results of the Harvard Medical Practice study I. *N Engl J Med* 1991; **24**: 370–6.
25. Teich JM, Osheroff JA, Pifer EA *et al.* Clinical decision support in electronic prescribing: recommendations and an action plan: report of the joint clinical decision support workgroup. *J Am Med Inform Assoc* 2005; **12**: 365–76.
26. Han YY, Carcillo JA, Venkataraman ST *et al.* Unexpected increased mortality after implementation of a commercially sold computerized physician order entry system. *Pediatrics* 2005; **116**: 1506–12.
27. Sittig DF, Ash JS, Zhang J *et al.* Lessons from 'Unexpected increased mortality after implementation of a commercially sold computerized physician order entry system.' *Pediatrics* 2006; **118**: 797–801.
28. Garg AX, Adhikari NK, McDonald H *et al.* Effects of computerized clinical decision support systems on practitioner performance and patient outcomes: a systematic review. *JAMA* 2005; **293**: 1223–38.
29. Evans RS, Pestotnik SL, Classen DC *et al.* A computer-assisted management program for antibiotics and other antiinfective agents. *N Engl J Med* 1998; **338**: 232–8.

10

Clinical trials in critical care

Simon Finfer and Anthony Delaney

> *Evidence based medicine is the conscientious, explicit, and judicious use of current best evidence in making decisions about the care of individual patients. The practice of evidence based medicine means integrating individual clinical expertise with the best available external clinical evidence from systematic research.*[1]

The most reliable evidence, and thus the best evidence for guiding clinical practice in critical care, will generally come from adequately powered and properly conducted randomised clinical trials (RCTs). It is commonly the case, however, that there are no individual RCTs that adequately address a particular question, and so clinicians may have to assess the ability of other studies such as cohort studies, case-control studies and systematic reviews to supplement their clinical expertise. It is important that clinicians are familiar with the underlying principles and potential sources of bias in each of these study designs, so that they can incorporate evidence from reliable trials into their clinical practice and treat with appropriate caution those studies whose design makes it possible that they will produce unreliable results.

RANDOMISED CLINICAL TRIALS

The result of any clinical trial may be due to three factors:

1. a true treatment effect;
2. the effects of bias or confounding; or
3. the play of chance.

RCTs, when properly designed, conducted and analysed, offer the optimal conditions to minimise bias and confounding, and to define the role that chance may have played in the results. As such, they represent the best study design to delineate true treatment effects under most circumstances. However, it is imperative that RCTs are designed, conducted, analysed and reported correctly. Studies that have not adhered to the principles outlined below still may produce results that do not reflect a true estimate of treatment effects.

THE QUESTION TO BE ADDRESSED

Every trial should seek to answer a focused clinical question that can be clearly articulated at the outset. For example, 'we sought to assess the influence of different volume replacement fluids on outcomes of intensive care patients' is better expressed as the focused clinical question 'we sought to address the hypothesis that when 4 percent albumin is compared with 0.9 percent sodium chloride (normal saline) for intravascular-fluid resuscitation in adult patients in the ICU, there is no difference in the rate of death from any cause at 28 days'.[2] The focused clinical question defines the interventions to be compared, the population of patients to be studied and the primary outcome to be considered. This approach can be formalised using the PICO system. PICO stands for patient, intervention, comparison and outcome. In the example above:

- Patient – adult intensive care unit (ICU) patient
- Intervention – albumin
- Comparison – saline
- Outcome – 28-day all-cause mortality

The question that a trial is designed to address will vary somewhat depending on the stage of development of the proposed treatment. After development and testing in animal models, the testing of pharmaceutical agents in humans is generally conducted in three phases. Sometimes a fourth phase is added:

1. Phase I trial – testing in healthy volunteers
2. Phase II trial – first testing in population of patients with disease to be modified. Usually small trials focused on establishing safety and evidence of efficacy using surrogate outcome measures. Phase II trials provide an estimate of treatment effect and baseline outcomes which can be used to calculate the sample size for phase III trials
3. Phase III – large-scale trial in patients that is powered to determine the effect of the treatment on the primary outcome of interest.
4. Phase IV – postmarketing open label trials to confirm efficacy and safety profile once the agent is introduced into routine clinical practice

Trials may be designed to answer two quite different questions about the same treatment and the design will be quite different depending on the questions to be answered. An *efficacy trial* seeks to determine whether a treatment will work under optimal conditions whereas an *effectiveness trial* seeks to determine the effects of the intervention when applied in normal clinical practice. For a detailed comparison of the features of efficacy and effectiveness trials, please see Hebert *et al.*[3]

POPULATION AND SAMPLE SIZE

The population to be studied will be defined by the study question. Efficacy trials may have a very narrowly defined population, with strict eligibility criteria and many exclusion criteria, whereas effectiveness trials are likely to have more broad inclusion criteria and few exclusion criteria. In any case the population included in the study should be well described. This will allow readers to assess the scientific merit of the study. It also allows clinicians to judge whether the results of the study could apply to their patients, to assess the generalisability of the results. Trials that look only at a very narrowly defined population may also face difficulties in recruiting sufficient participants to reach a definitive conclusion.

How large do trials need to be to reach a definitive conclusion? In a parallel-group trial the number of patients required to answer a question depends on four factors:

1. The percentage of patients expected to have the outcome in the control group – the control group outcome rate
2. The expected change (usually reduction) that may result from the treatment being tested – the treatment effect
3. The level of probability to be accepted to indicate that the difference did not occur by chance, i.e. the probability level at which a treatment effect will be deemed to be real – significance level or α (alpha)
4. The desired percentage chance of detecting a clinically important treatment effect if one truly exists (power)

It is clear that many published trials addressing issues of importance in intensive care medicine are too small to detect clinically important treatment effects;[4] fortunately this is now changing.[2,5] This has almost certainly given rise to a significant number of false-negative results (type II errors). Type II errors result in potentially beneficial treatments being discarded. In order to avoid these errors, clinical trials have to include a surprisingly large numbers of participants. Examples of sample size calculations based on different baseline incidences, different treatment effects and different power are given in Table 10.1.

RANDOMISATION AND ALLOCATION CONCEALMENT

Two components of the randomisation procedure are critically important. The first is the generation of a truly random allocation sequence; modern computer programs make this relatively straightforward. The second is the concealment of this allocation sequence from the investigators, so that the investigators and participants are unaware of the treatment allocation (group) prior to each participant entering the study.

There are a number of benefits of using a random process to determine treatment allocation. Firstly, it eliminates the possibility of bias in treatment assignment (selection bias). In order for this to be ensured, both a truly random sequence of allocation must be produced and this sequence must not be known to the investigators prior to each participant entering the trial. Secondly, it reduces the chance that the trial results are affected by confounding. It is important that, prior to the intervention in a RCT being delivered, both groups have an equal chance of developing the outcome of interest. A clinical characteristic (such as advanced age, gender or disease severity, as measured by Acute Physiology, Age and Chronic Health Evaluation (APACHE) or Sequential Organ Failure Assessment (SOFA) scores) that is associated with the outcome is known as a confounding factor. Randomisation of a sufficient number

Table 10.1 Examples of sample size calculations

Control group outcome rate (%)	Treatment group outcome rate (%)	ARR	Power (β)	Total sample size
50	30	20	80	206
50	30	20	90	268
30	15	15	90	348
30	20	10	90	824
30	25	5	90	3428
15	10	5	90	1914
15	12	3	90	5582
10	8	2	80	6626
10	8	2	90	8802

ARR, absolute risk reduction.
All calculations performed with STATA 8.2, assuming a two-sided $\alpha = 0.05$.

of participants ensures that both known and unknown confounding factors (for example, genetic polymorphisms) are evenly distributed between the two treatment groups. The play of chance may result in uneven distribution of known confounding factors between the groups and this is particularly likely in trials with fewer than 200 participants.[6] The third benefit of randomisation is that it allows the use of probability theory to quantify the role that chance could have played when differences are found between groups.[7] Finally, randomisation with allocation concealment facilitates blinding, another important component in the minimisation of bias in clinical trials.[8]

The generation of the allocation sequence must be truly random. There are a number of approaches to generating a truly random allocation sequence, most commonly using a computer-generated sequence of random numbers. More complicated processes where randomisation is performed in blocks or is stratified to ensure that patients from each hospital in a multicentre trial or those with certain baseline characteristics are equally distributed between treatment groups can also be used. Allocation methods based upon predictable sequences, such as those based on medical record numbers or days of the week do not constitute true randomisation and should be avoided. These methods allow researchers to predict to which group participants will be allocated prior to them entering the trial; this introduces the possibility of selection bias.

Whatever method is used to produce a random allocation sequence, it is important that allocation concealment is maintained. Methods to ensure the concealment of allocation may be as simple as using sealed opaque envelopes,[9] or as complex as the centralised automated telephone-based or web-based systems commonly used in large multicentre trials. Appropriate attention to this aspect of a clinical trial is essential as trials with poor allocation concealment produce estimates of treatment effects that may be exaggerated by up to 40%.[10]

THE INTERVENTIONS

The intervention being evaluated in any clinical trial should be described in sufficient detail that clinicians could implement the therapy if they so desired, or researchers could replicate the study to confirm the results. This may be a simple task if the intervention is a single drug given once at the beginning of an illness, or may be complex if the intervention being tested is the introduction of a process of care, such as the introduction of a medical emergency team.[11] There are two additional areas with regard to the interventions delivered in clinical trials that require some thought by those conducting the trial and by clinicians evaluating the results, namely blinding and the control of concomitant interventions.

BLINDING

Blinding, also known as masking, is the practice of keeping trial participants (and, in the case of critically ill patients, their relatives or other legal surrogate decision-makers), care-givers, data collectors, those adjudicating outcomes and sometimes those analysing the data and writing the study reports unaware of which treatment is being given to individual participants. Blinding serves to reduce bias by preventing clinicians from consciously or unconsciously treating patients differently on the basis of their treatment assignment within the trial. It prevents data collectors from introducing bias when recording parameters that require a subjective assessment, for example pain scores and sedation scores or the Glasgow Coma Score. Although many ICU trials cannot be blinded, for example, trials of intensive insulin therapy cannot blind treating staff who are responsible for monitoring blood glucose and adjusting insulin infusion rates, the successful blinding of the Saline versus Albumin Fluid Evaluation (SAFE) trial demonstrated the possibility of blinding even large complex trials if investigators are sufficiently committed and innovative.[2] Blinded outcome assessment is also necessary when the chosen outcome measure requires a subjective judgement. In such cases the outcome measure is said to be subject to the potential for ascertainment bias. For example, a blinded outcome assessment committee should adjudicate the diagnosis of ventilator-associated pneumonia (VAP) and blinded assessors should be used when assessing functional neurological recovery using the extended Glasgow Outcome Scale; both the diagnosis of VAP and assessment of the Glasgow Outcome Scale require a degree of subjective assessment and are therefore said to be prone to ascertainment bias.

It has been traditional to describe trials as single-blinded, double-blinded or even triple-blinded. However these terms can be interpreted by clinicians to mean different things, and the terminology may be confusing.[12] We recommend that reports of RCTs include a description of who was blinded and how this was achieved, rather than a simple statement that the trial was ‘single-blind’ or ‘double-blind’.[13] Blinding is an important safeguard against bias in RCTs, and although not thought to be as essential as maintenance of allocation concealment, empirical studies have shown that unblinded studies may produce results that are biased by as much as 17%.[10]

CONCOMITANT TREATMENTS

Concomitant treatments are all treatments that are administered to patients during the course of a trial other than the study treatment. With the exception of the study treatment, patients assigned to the different treatment groups should be treated equally. When one group is treated in a way that is dependent on the treatment assignment, but not directly related to the treatment, there is the possibility that this third factor will influence the outcome. An example might be a trial of pulmonary artery catheters (PACs), compared to management without a PAC. If the group assigned to receive management based on the data from a PAC received an additional daily chest X-ray to confirm the position of the PAC, they could conceivably have other important complications noted earlier, such as pneumonia, pulmonary oedema or pneumothoraces, and this may affect outcome in a fashion unrelated to the data available from the PAC. Maintaining balance in concomitant treatments is facilitated by blinding. When trials cannot be blinded, use of concomitant treatments that may alter outcome should be recorded and reported, so that the potential impact of different concomitant treatments can be assessed.

OUTCOME MEASUREMENT

All clinical trials should be designed to detect a difference in a single outcome. In general there are two types of outcome: clinically meaningful outcomes and surrogate outcomes.

A *clinically meaningful outcome* is a measure of how patients feel, function or survive.[14] Clinically meaningful outcomes are the most credible end-points for clinical trials that seek to change clinical practice. Phase III trials should always use clinically meaningful outcomes as the primary outcome. Examples of clinically meaningful outcomes include mortality and measures of health-related quality of life. In contrast, a *surrogate outcome* is a substitute for a clinically meaningful outcome; a reasonable surrogate outcome would be expected to predict clinical benefits based upon epidemiologic, therapeutic, pathophysiologic or other scientific evidence.[14] Examples of surrogate end-points would include cytokine levels in sepsis trials, changes in oxygenation in ventilation trials or blood pressure and urine output in a fluid resuscitation trial.

Unless a surrogate outcome has been validated, it is unwise to rely on changes in surrogate outcomes to guide clinical practice. For example, it seemed intuitively sensible that after myocardial infarction the suppression of ventricular premature beats (a surrogate outcome) which were known to be linked to mortality (the clinically meaningful outcome) would be beneficial. Unfortunately the Cardiac Arrhythmia Suppression Trial (CAST) trial found increased mortality in participants assigned to receive antiarrhythmic therapy.[15] The process for determining whether a surrogate outcome is a reliable indicator of clinically meaningful outcomes has been described.[16]

ANALYSIS

Even when trials are well designed and conducted, inappropriate statistical analyses may result in uncertain or erroneous conclusions. A detailed discussion of the statistical analysis of large-scale trials is well beyond the scope of this chapter but certain guiding principles can be articulated:

- All trials should adhere to a predetermined statistical analysis plan; otherwise the temptation to perform multiple analyses and only report those that support the preconceived ideas of the investigators may prove irresistible. A predetermined analysis plan protects the investigators from such temptation and allows readers to give appropriate weighting to the results.
- The convention of accepting a *P*-value of <0.05 to indicate statistical significance is based on assessment of a single outcome. Assessing multiple outcomes increases the likelihood of finding a *P*-value of <0.05 purely due to the play of chance. Each trial should have a single predefined primary outcome measure. If more than one primary outcome measure is used then the *P*-value used to indicate statistical significance should be reduced. The simplest method is to perform a Bonferoni correction which divides 0.05 by the number of outcomes examined to determine the new level of statistical significance. Thus, for two outcomes the *P*-value must be below 0.025, and for three it must be below 0.017. The *P*-value may also have to be further reduced if the trial employs interim analyses.

Clinicians should pay close attention to the analysis to make certain that a true intention-to-treat analysis is presented, and that any subgroup analysis is viewed with an appropriate amount of caution.

INTENTION-TO-TREAT ANALYSIS

Trials should be analysed using the intention-to-treat principle. This means that all participants are analysed in the group to which they were randomised regardless of whether they received all or any of the treatment to which they were assigned. To some readers the intention-to-treat principle may appear intuitively incorrect; it is reasonable to ask why patients who did not receive the intended treatment should be included in the analysis. Use of intention-to-treat analysis prevents bias arising from the selective exclusion of patients – attrition bias. In an appropriately sized trial, loss of patients at random should occur equally in both groups and inclusion of those patients will not alter the result. If loss of patients is occurring as a non-random event (for example, because of protocol violations or intolerance of the treatment in one arm of the trial) then the trial result will be different if the lost patients are excluded. Consider a trial of a 5-day course of N^G-monomethyl L-arginine (L-NMMA) for the treatment of patients with septic shock. In the trial a number of patients who receive L-NMMA die in the first 24–48 hours and are excluded from the analysis as they have received only a little of the study treatment. A trial report based on the remaining patients who completed the treatment protocol (per-protocol analysis) will not give a true estimate of the effect of using L-NMMA in clinical practice. Although this is an extreme example, once patients are included in a trial their outcome should always be accounted for in the study report.

SUBGROUP ANALYSIS

Particular difficulties arise from the selection, analysis and reporting of subgroups. Subgroups should be predefined and kept to the minimum number possible. When many subgroups are examined, the likelihood of finding a subgroup where the treatment effect is different from that seen in the overall population increases. A well-known example of this was the analysis of the treatment effect of aspirin in patients with myocardial infarction in the large second International Study of Infarct Survival (ISIS-2) trial. Overall the trial indicated that aspirin reduced the relative risk of death at 1 month by 23%. To illustrate the unreliability of subgroup analyses, the participants were divided into subgroups according to their astrological birth signs; the analysis showed that patients born under Libra or Gemini did not benefit from treatment with aspirin.[17] Although it is easy to identify this as a chance subgroup finding, this may be much harder when the choice of the subgroup appears rational and a theoretical explanation for the findings can be advanced. For example, in the Gruppo Italiano per lo Studio della Streptochinasi nell'infarto miocardico (GISSI) trial, subgroup analysis suggested that fibrinolytic therapy did not reduce mortality in patients who had suffered a previous myocardial infarct.[18] Although this finding appears biologically plausible, subsequent trials have shown quite clearly that fibrinolytic therapy is just as effective in patients with prior infarction as in those without.[19]

Separation of patients into subgroups should be on the basis of characteristics that are apparent at the time of randomisation. Selection of subgroups using features identified after randomisation risks introducing bias as the patients have already been subjected to the different study treatments and the subgroup analysis will therefore not be comparing like with like.

TESTS OF INTERACTION VERSUS WITHIN-SUBGROUP COMPARISONS

Even when subgroups are selected appropriately many readers will be tempted to draw inappropriate conclusions from the results. As the trial will have been designed and powered to examine the effect of the treatment on the primary outcome in the whole study population, the best assessment of the treatment effect in any subgroup will be the effect seen in the trial as a whole. When analysing a subgroup result, the investigators should seek to answer the following question: is the treatment effect in the subgroup different from the treatment effect seen in the remaining participants? This is a test of interaction or of heterogeneity. Often the investigators err and perform within-subgroup comparisons which instead answer the question: what was the effect of treatment A versus treatment B in this subgroup? Within-subgroup comparisons are more likely to lead to unreliable results.

For example, the SAFE study identified patients with severe sepsis at baseline as an a priori subgroup. In the overall population studied the relative risk of death for those assigned albumin versus those assigned saline was 0.99 (95% confidence interval (CI) 0.91–1.09). In those with severe sepsis at baseline, the relative risk was 0.87 (95% CI 0.74–1.02, $P = 0.09$); the mortality rate for patients assigned albumin was 30.7% (185 deaths in 603 patients) versus 35.3% (217 deaths in 615 patients) for patients assigned saline. Despite this result, the most likely estimate for the treatment effect in the subgroup is the effect seen in the trial as a whole, namely a relative risk (RR) of 0.99. The investigators reported the test of common RR (a test of heterogeneity) which asked whether the RR in the subgroup of patients with severe sepsis (RR 0.87, 95% CI 0.74–1.02) was different from that in those without severe sepsis (RR 1.05, 95% CI 0.94–1.17); the *P*-value for this comparison was 0.06. This means that the probability that the difference in RR (0.87 versus 1.05) arose by chance is 0.06; a *P*-value of this order suggests that it would be reasonable to conduct an appropriately powered trial of albumin versus saline in patients with severe sepsis.

REPORTING

The reporting of RCTs has been greatly improved by the work of the Consolidated Standards of Reporting Trials (CONSORT) group.[13,20] The CONSORT statement provides a framework and checklist (Table 10.2) which can be followed by investigators and authors to provide a standardised high-quality report.[20] An increasing number of journals require authors to follow the CONSORT recommendations when reporting the results of an RCT. The group also recommends the publication of a structured diagram which documents the flow of patients through four stages of the trial: enrolment, allocation, follow-up and analysis (Figure 10.1). It is likely that the use of the CONSORT statement to guide the reporting of RCTs does lead to improvements, at least in the quality of reporting of RCTs.[21]

Trials may report results using a number of values that, taken together, will give readers a full understanding of the trial results. These may include a *P*-value, CI and number needed to treat (or harm).

- Probabilities – the *P*-value represents the probability that a difference has arisen by chance. In very large trials, small and clinically insignificant differences may give rise to *P*-values of less than 0.05. Conversely, a moderately sized trial may report a clinically important difference with a *P*-value that is close to or greater than 0.05. *P*-value should not be viewed in isolation but assessed in combination with other measures such as CI and the number needed to treat (or harm).
- CI give an indication of the precision of the result. Whenever a trial reports a difference it is reporting a difference found in a finite sample of the population of interest. If the same trial is repeated it is highly likely a slightly or very different result will be reported. If the

Table 10.2 The CONSORT checklist

	Item number	Descriptor	Reported on page number
Title and abstract	1	How participants were allocated to interventions (e.g. 'random allocation', 'randomised', or 'randomly assigned')	
Introduction			
Background	2	Scientified background and explanation of rationale	
Methods			
Participants	3	Eligibility criteria for participants and the settings and locations where the data were collected	
Interventions	4	Precise details of the interventions intended for each group and how and when they were actually administered	
Objectives	5	Specific objectives and hypotheses	
Outcomes	6	Clearly defined primary and secondary outcome measures and, when applicable, any methods used to enhance the quality of measurements (e.g. multiple observations, training of assessors, etc.)	
Sample size	7	How sample size was determined and, when applicable, explanation of any interim analyses and stopping rules	
Randomisation			
Sequence generation	8	Method used to generate the random allocation sequence, including details of any restriction (e.g. blocking, stratification)	
Allocation concealment	9	Method used to implement the random allocation sequence (e.g. numbered containers or central telephone), clarifying whether the sequence was concealed until interventions were assigned	
Implementation	10	Who generated the allocation sequence, who enrolled participants, and who assigned participants to their groups	
Blinding (masking)	11	Whether or not participants, those administering the interventions, and those assessing the outcomes were aware of group assignment. If not, how the success of masking was assessed	
Statistical methods	12	Statistical methods used to compare groups for primary outcomes(s); methods for additional analyses, such as subgroup analyses and adjusted analyses	
Results			
Participant flow	13	Flow of participants through each stage (a diagram is strongly recommended). Specifically, for each group, report the numbers of participants randomly assigned, receiving intended treatment, completing the study protocol, and analysed for the primary outcome. Describe protocol deviations from study as planned, together with reasons	
Recruitment	14	Dates defining the periods of recruitment and follow-up	
Baseline data	15	Baseline demographic and clinical characteristics of each group	
Numbers analysed	16	Number of participants (denominator) in each group included in each analysis and whether the analysis was by 'intention to treat'. State the results in absolute numbers when feasible (e.g. 10/20, not 50%)	
Outcomes and estimation	17	For each primary and secondary outcome, a summary of results for each group, and the estimated effect size and its precision (e.g. 95% CI)	
Ancillary analyses	18	Address multiplicity by reporting any other analyses performed, including subgroup analyses and adjusted analyses, indicating those prespecified and those exploratory	
Adverse events	19	All important adverse events or side-effects in each intervention group	
Discussion			
Interpretation	20	Interpretation of the results, taking into account study hypotheses, sources of potential bias or imprecision and the dangers associated with multiplicity of analyses and outcomes	
Generalisability	21	Generalisability (external validity) of the trial findings	
Overall evidence	22	General interpretation of the results in the context of current evidence	

(Reproduced from Moher D, Schulz KF, Altman DG. The CONSORT statement: revised recommendations for improving the quality of reports of parallel-group randomised trials. *Lancet* 2001; **357**: 1191–4.)

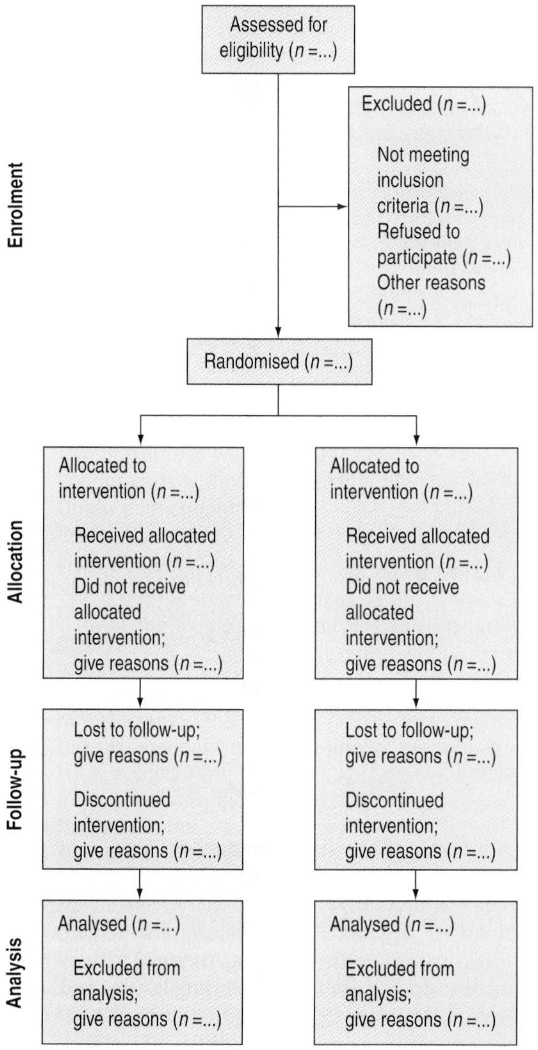

Figure 10.1 Flow diagram of the progress through the phases of a randomised trial. (Reproduced from Moher D, Schulz KF, Altman DG. The CONSORT statement: revised recommendations for improving the quality of reports of parallel-group randomised trials. *Lancet* 2001; **357**: 1191–4.)

trial is reporting relatively small number of patients with the outcome of interest (small number of events) then the difference between the results may be large; if the trial reports a large number of events then it is likely the two results will be quite close to each other. CIs give a range of values within which it is likely the 'true' result lies – they give an indication of the precision of the result. The most commonly quoted are the 95% CIs; these are the limits within which we would expect 95% of study results to lie if the study was repeated an infinite number of times. They are often interpreted to mean that we can be 95% confident that the 'true' result lies within these limits.

- Number needed to treat (or harm) – a useful concept for clinicians is the number needed to treat (or harm). This is the reciprocal of the absolute difference in outcomes arising from two treatments. For example, in the ISIS-2 trial, patients randomised to intravenous streptokinase had an absolute reduction in mortality of 2.8%. Thus the number needed to treat to prevent one death is 100/2.8 or 35.7 patients. As the trial was very large with a large number of events (17187 participants and 1820 deaths), this relatively small absolute reduction in mortality (2.8%) yielded a *P*-value of less than 0.000 001. The same calculation can be performed to calculate the number needed to harm. For example, in the Corticosteroid Randomisation After Significant Head injury (CRASH) trial, patients with traumatic brain injury treated with high-dose steroids had a 3.4% increase in the absolute risk of death. The number needed to harm is calculated as 100/3.4, or one extra death for every 29.4 patients treated with high-dose corticosteroids. Again, as this was a large trial (10 008 participants and 1945 deaths), the *P*-value is small ($P = 0.00001$).

ETHICAL ISSUES SPECIFIC TO CLINICAL TRIALS IN CRITICAL CARE

The ethical principles guiding the conduct of research in human subjects are outlined in the *International Ethical Guidelines for Biomedical Research Involving Human Subjects*.[22] In addition country-specific guidelines are provided by various national bodies. The ethical principles of integrity, respect for persons, beneficence and justice should be considered whenever research is conducted and an appropriately convened human research ethics committee or equivalent should assess all research to ensure adherence to these principles. As the potential participants in critical care research are particularly vulnerable due to the nature of their clinical conditions and the limitations to communication that exist, special consideration needs to be given to a number of areas, including informed consent.

INFORMED CONSENT

That all mentally competent participants in clinical research should give informed consent prior to entering a study is an important ethical principle. This is rarely possible for people suffering critical illness, where the disease process (e.g. traumatic brain injury, encephalitis, severe hypoxaemia) or the required treatment (e.g. intubation, use of sedative medications) may make it impossible to obtain informed consent. Even awake, alert patients may not be able to give fully informed consent when they are facing stressful and potentially life-threatening situations.[23] This applies equally to surrogate decision-makers. However, the treatment of critically ill patients can only be improved through the conduct of research and in many jurisdictions this has been recognised by making special provisions for consent in emergency research, including research in the critically ill. In some circumstances, it may be ethical to allow a waiver of consent for research involving treatments that must be given in a time-dependent fashion (e.g. in the setting of cardiac arrest). A waiver of consent may well improve recruitment into clinical trials; it is unclear if this approach is universally acceptable. Another approach has been to allow delayed consent, where patients are included in the study and consent from the patient or the relevant surrogate decision-maker is sought as soon as practical. Neither approach is without problems.[24]

CRITICAL APPRAISAL

Clinicians reading reports of RCTs should use a structured framework to assess the methodological quality of the trial and the adequacy of the trial report. They should also address the magnitude and precision of reported treatment effects and ask themselves whether the results of the trial can be applied to their own clinical practice. There are a number of resources available to assist clinicians in this task, notably the *Users' Guides to Evidence-Based Practice*, originally published in the *Journal of the American Medical Association*, and the *Critical Appraisal Skills* programme from Oxford, UK, both of which are freely available on the internet.[25,26] These resources provide a structured framework which allows any reader to perform a systematic critical appraisal of almost any piece of medical literature. A checklist is provided for the appraisal of RCTs (Table 10.3).

Table 10.3 Critical appraisal checklist for randomised controlled trials

I. Are the results of the study valid?

Primary guides

1. Was the assignment of patients to treatments randomised?
2. Were all patients who entered the trial properly accounted for and attributed at its conclusion?
3. Was follow-up complete?
4. Were patients analysed in the groups to which they were randomised?

Secondary guides

1. Were patients, health workers and study personnel 'blind' to treatment?
2. Were the groups similar at the start of the trial?
3. Aside from the experimental intervention, were the groups treated equally?

II. What were the results?

1. How large was the treatment effect?
2. How precise was the estimate of the treatment effect?

III. Will the results help me in caring for my patients?

1. Can the results be applied to my patient care?
2. Were all clinically important outcomes considered?
3. Are the likely treatment benefits worth the potential harms and costs?

(Reproduced from Centre for Health Evidence. Users' guides to evidence-based practice, 2007. Avilable online at: http://www.cche.net/usersguides/main.asp.)

OBSERVATIONAL STUDIES

Although RCTs are the optimal study design for deciding whether or not a treatment 'works', not all research questions can be addressed with this type of study. When the disease is rare, the outcome is rare or the treatment may be associated with harm, other study designs may be more appropriate. In these circumstances a cohort study or case-control study may be used to explore potential associations between exposure to a treatment and the occurrence of outcomes.

DESCRIPTIVE STUDIES

Case reports, case series and cross-sectional studies are all examples of descriptive studies. These types of studies may be important in the initial identification of new diseases such as human immunodeficiency virus (HIV)/acquired immunodeficiency syndrome (AIDS)[27–30] and severe acute respiratory syndrome (SARS).[31] The purpose of these studies will be to describe the 'who, when, where, what and why' of the condition, and so further the understanding of the epidemiology of the disease. It is important that clear and standardised definitions of cases are utilised, so that the information gathered can be used by clinicians and researchers to identify similar cases. While there are some famous examples where data from simple observational studies have been used to solve particular problems,[32] in general only very limited inferences can be drawn from descriptive data. In particular, it is dangerous to draw conclusions about 'cause and effect' using data from descriptive studies alone.[33]

ANALYTICAL OBSERVATIONAL STUDIES

There are two main types of analytical observational studies: case-control studies and cohort studies.

Case-control studies are performed by identifying patients with a particular condition (the 'cases'), and a group of people who do not have the condition (the 'controls'). The researchers then look back in time to ascertain the exposure of the members of each group to the variables of interest.[34] A case-control design may be appropriate when the disease has a long latency period and is rare. *Cohort studies* are performed by identifying a group of people who have been exposed to a certain risk factor and a group of people who are similar in most respects apart from their exposure to the risk factor. Both groups are then followed to ascertain whether they develop the outcome of interest. Cohort studies may be the appropriate design to determine the effects of a rare exposure, and have the advantage of being able to detect multiple outcomes that are associated with the same exposure.[35]

Both types of observational study are prone to bias. In particular, although it is possible to correct for known confounding factors using multivariate statistical techniques, it is not possible to control for unknown or unmeasured confounding factors. There are a number of other biases that may distort the results of observational studies; these include selection bias, information bias and differential loss to follow-up.[35,36] Critical appraisal guides for observational studies are available to help readers assess the validity of these studies.[37] These limitations and inherent biases mean that observational studies may not always provide reliable evidence to guide clinical practice, although it has been argued that this is not always the case.[38,39]

SYSTEMATIC REVIEWS AND META-ANALYSIS

Systematic reviews have been proposed as a solution to the problem of the ever expanding medical literature.[40] A systematic review utilises specific methods to identify and critically appraise all the RCTs that address a particular clinical question, and, if appropriate, statistically combine the results of the primary RCTs in order to arrive at an overall estimate of the effect of the treatment. By systematically assembling all RCTs that address one specific topic, a methodologically sound systematic review can provide a valuable overview for the busy clinician. Systematic reviews play an important role in providing an objective appraisal of all available evidence and may reduce the possibility that treatments with moderate effects will be discarded due to false-negative results from small or underpowered studies.[41] The use of meta-analysis could have resulted in the earlier introduction of life-saving therapies such as thrombolysis.[42] By using systematic methods, meta-analyses can provide more accurate and unbiased overviews, drawing conclusions that are often at odds with those of 'experts' and narrative reviews.[43,44]

In spite of these advantages and benefits there are still problems with interpretation of meta-analyses. Like all clinical trials, they need to be performed with attention to methodological detail. There are guidelines for performing and reporting systematic reviews.[45,46] It is clear that in the critical care literature these guidelines are not always followed.[47] Clinicians should critically appraise the reports of all systematic reviews and meta-analyses regardless of the source of the review, using an appropriate guide.[48,49] Problems with interpretation can arise when the results of a meta-analysis are at odds with the results of large RCTs which address the same issue;[50,51] this is not uncommon and clinicians will have to compare the methodological quality of meta-analysis and the RCTs included in the meta-analysis to the validity of the large RCT in order to decide which provides the most reliable evidence.[2,52]

REFERENCES

1. Sackett DL, Rosenberg WM, Gray JA *et al.* Evidence based medicine: what it is and what it isn't. *Br Med J* 1996; **312**: 71–2.
2. The SAFE Study Investigators. A comparison of albumin and saline for fluid resuscitation in the intensive care unit. *N Engl J Med* 2004; **350**: 2247–56.
3. Hebert PC, Cook DJ, Wells G *et al.* The design of randomized clinical trials in critically ill patients. *Chest* 2002; **121**: 1290–300.
4. Roberts I, Schierhout G, Alderson P. Absence of evidence for the effectiveness of five interventions routinely used in the intensive care management of severe head injury: a systematic review. *J Neurol Neurosurg Psychiatry* 1998; **65**: 729–33.
5. Edwards P, Arango M, Balica L *et al.* Final results of MRC CRASH, a randomised placebo-controlled trial of intravenous corticosteroid in adults with head injury – outcomes at 6 months. *Lancet* 2005; **365**: 1957–9.
6. Lachin JM. Properties of simple randomization in clinical trials. *Control Clin Trials* 1988; **9**: 312–26.
7. Schulz KF, Grimes DA. Generation of allocation sequences in randomised trials: chance, not choice. *Lancet* 2002; **359**: 515–19.
8. Armitage P. The role of randomization in clinical trials. *Stat Med* 1982; **1**: 345–52.
9. Doig GS, Simpson F. Randomization and allocation concealment: a practical guide for researchers. *J Crit Care* 2005; **20**: 18–91; discussion 191–3.
10. Schulz KF, Chalmers I, Hayes RJ *et al.* Empirical evidence of bias. Dimensions of methodological quality associated with estimates of treatment effects in controlled trials. *JAMA* 1995; **273**: 408–12.
11. Hillman K, Chen J, Cretikos M *et al.* Introduction of the medical emergency team (MET) system: a cluster-randomised controlled trial. *Lancet* 2005; **365**: 2091–7.
12. Montori VM, Bhandari M, Devereaux PJ *et al.* In the dark: the reporting of blinding status in randomized controlled trials. *J Clin Epidemiol* 2002; **55**: 787–90.
13. Altman DG, Schulz KF, Moher D *et al.* The revised CONSORT statement for reporting randomized trials: explanation and elaboration. *Ann Intern Med* 2001; **134**: 66–94.
14. De Gruttola VG, Clax P, DeMets DL *et al.* Considerations in the evaluation of surrogate endpoints in clinical trials. Summary of a National Institutes of Health workshop. *Control Clin Trials* 2001; **22**: 485–502.
15. Echt DS, Liebson PR, Mitchell LB *et al.* Mortality and morbidity in patients receiving encainide, flecainide, or placebo. The Cardiac Arrhythmia Suppression Trial. *N Engl J Med* 1991; **324**: 781–8.
16. Bucher HC, Guyatt GH, Cook DJ *et al.* Users' guides to the medical literature: XIX. Applying clinical trial results. A. How to use an article measuring the effect of an intervention on surrogate end points. Evidence-Based Medicine Working Group. *JAMA* 1999; **282**: 771–8.

17. ISIS-2 (Second International Study of Infarct Survival) Collaborative Group. Randomised trial of intravenous streptokinase, oral aspirin, both, or neither among 17 187 cases of suspected acute myocardial infarction: ISIS-2. *Lancet* 1988; **2**: 349–60.
18. Gruppo Italiano per lo Studio della Streptochinasi nell'Infarto Miocardico (GISSI). Effectiveness of intravenous thrombolytic treatment in acute myocardial infarction. *Lancet* 1986; **1**: 397–402.
19. Fibrinolytic Therapy Trialists' (FTT) Collaborative Group. Indications for fibrinolytic therapy in suspected acute myocardial infarction: collaborative overview of early mortality and major morbidity results from all randomised trials of more than 1000 patients. *Lancet* 1994; **343**: 311–22.
20. Moher D, Schulz KF, Altman DG. The CONSORT statement: revised recommendations for improving the quality of reports of parallel-group randomised trials. *Lancet* 2001; **357**: 1191–4.
21. Plint AC, Moher D, Morrison A *et al.* Does the CONSORT checklist improve the quality of reports of randomised controlled trials? A systematic review. *Med J Aust* 2006; **185**: 263–7.
22. Council for International Organizations of Medical Sciences. *International ethical guidelines for biomedical research involving human subjects*, 2002. Available online at: http://www.cioms.ch/frame_guidelines_-nov_2002.htm.
23. Wilets I, Schears RM, Gligorov N. Communicating with subjects: special challenges for resuscitation research. *Acad Emerg Med* 2005; **12**: 1060–3.
24. Harvey SE, Elbourne D, Ashcroft J *et al.* Informed consent in clinical trials in critical care: experience from the PAC-Man Study. *Intens Care Med* 2006; **32**: 2020–5.
25. Centre for Health Evidence. Users' guides to evidence-based practice, 2007. Avilable online at: http://www.cche.net/usersguides/main.asp.
26. Learning and Development, Public Health Resource Unit. *Critical Appraisal Skills Programme and Evidence-Based Practice.* Oxford: Public Health Resouce Unit; 2005.
27. Masur H, Michelis MA, Greene JB *et al.* An outbreak of community-acquired *Pneumocystis carinii* pneumonia: initial manifestation of cellular immune dysfunction. *N Engl J Med* 1981; **305**: 1431–8.
28. Gottlieb MS, Schroff R, Schanker HM *et al. Pneumocystis carinii* pneumonia and mucosal candidiasis in previously healthy homosexual men: evidence of a new acquired cellular immunodeficiency. *N Engl J Med* 1981; **305**: 1425–31.
29. Durack DT. Opportunistic infections and Kaposi's sarcoma in homosexual men. *N Engl J Med* 1981; **305**: 1465–7.
30. Siegal FP, Lopez C, Hammer GS *et al.* Severe acquired immunodeficiency in male homosexuals, manifested by chronic perianal ulcerative herpes simplex lesions. *N Engl J Med* 1981; **305**: 1439–44.
31. Zhong NS, Zheng BJ, Li YM *et al.* Epidemiology and cause of severe acute respiratory syndrome (SARS) in Guangdong, People's Republic of China, in February, 2003. *Lancet* 2003; **362**: 1353–8.
32. 150th anniversary of John Snow and the pump handle. *MMWR Morb Mortal Wkly Rep* 2004; **53**: 783.
33. Grimes DA, Schulz KF. Descriptive studies: what they can and cannot do. *Lancet* 2002; **359**: 145–9.
34. Schulz KF, Grimes DA. Case-control studies: research in reverse. *Lancet* 2002; **359**: 431–4.
35. Grimes DA, Schulz KF. Cohort studies: marching towards outcomes. *Lancet* 2002; **359**: 341–5.
36. MacMahon S, Collins R. Reliable assessment of the effects of treatment on mortality and major morbidity, II: observational studies. *Lancet* 2001; **357**: 455–62.
37. Levine M, Walter S, Lee H *et al.* Users' guides to the medical literature. IV. How to use an article about harm. Evidence-Based Medicine Working Group. *JAMA* 1994; **271**: 1615–9.
38. Benson K, Hartz AJ. A comparison of observational studies and randomized, controlled trials. *N Engl J Med* 2000; **342**: 1878–86.
39. Concato J, Shah N, Horwitz RI. Randomized, controlled trials, observational studies, and the hierarchy of research designs. *N Engl J Med* 2000; **342**: 1887–92.
40. Cook DJ, Meade MO, Fink MP. How to keep up with the critical care literature and avoid being buried alive. *Crit Care Med* 1996; **24**: 1757–68.
41. Egger M, Smith GD. Meta-analysis. Potentials and promise. *Br Med J* 1997; **315**: 1371–4.
42. Lau J, Antman EM, Jimenez-Silva J *et al.* Cumulative meta-analysis of therapeutic trials for myocardial infarction. *N Engl J Med* 1992; **327**: 248–54.
43. Antman EM, Lau J, Kupelnick B *et al.* A comparison of results of meta-analyses of randomized control trials and recommendations of clinical experts. Treatments for myocardial infarction. *JAMA* 1992; **268**: 240–8.
44. Mulrow CD. The medical review article: state of the science. *Ann Intern Med* 1987; **106**: 485–8.
45. Higgins JPT, Green S (eds). *Cochrane Handbook for Systematic Reviews of Interventions* version 5.0.0 (updated February 2008). The Cochrane Collaboration 2008. Available from www.cochrane-handbook.org.
46. Moher D, Cook DJ, Eastwood S *et al.* Improving the quality of reports of meta-analyses of randomised controlled trials: the QUOROM statement. Quality of Reporting of Meta-analyses. *Lancet* 1999; **354**: 1896–900.
47. Delaney A, Bagshaw SM, Ferland A *et al.* A systematic evaluation of the quality of meta-analyses in the critical care literature. *Crit Care* 2005; **9**: R5–82.
48. Delaney A, Bagshaw SM, Ferland A *et al.* The quality of reports of critical care meta-analyses in the Cochrane Database of Systematic Reviews: an independent appraisal. *Crit Care Med* 2007; **35**: 589–94.

49. Oxman AD, Cook DJ, Guyatt GH. Users' guides to the medical literature. VI. How to use an overview. Evidence-Based Medicine Working Group. *JAMA* 1994; **272**: 1367–71.

50. LeLorier J, Gregoire G, Benhaddad A *et al.* Discrepancies between meta-analyses and subsequent large randomized, controlled trials. *N Engl J Med* 1997; **337**: 536–42.

51. Villar J, Carroli G, Belizan JM. Predictive ability of meta-analyses of randomised controlled trials. *Lancet* 1995; **345**: 772–6.

52. Cochrane Injuries Group Albumin Reviewers. Human albumin administration in critically ill patients: systematic review of randomised controlled trials. *Br Med J* 1998; **317**: 235–40.

Part Two

Shock

11

Shock – an overview

Angela McLuckie

DEFINITION

Shock is a clinical state, with characteristic symptoms and signs, which occurs when an imbalance between oxygen supply and demand results in the development of tissue hypoxia. Although changes in systemic perfusion are always present in shock, oxygen delivery to the tissues is not invariably reduced, and indeed may be increased in shock due to severe sepsis.[1]

CLASSIFICATION

Physiologically, tissue hypoxia may be considered as hypoxic (low Pao_2), anaemic (low haemoglobin level or increased levels of carboxy- or met-haemoglobin), stagnant (low cardiac output) or histotoxic (e.g. cyanide poisoning). Clinically, it is more common to subdivide shock into cardiogenic, obstructive, hypovolaemic or septic. Infrequently it may be neurogenic or anaphylactic in origin (Table 11.1).

Most often, cardiogenic shock is the result of myocardial disease, e.g. infarction, myocarditis. However, valvular abnormalities, e.g. mitral regurgitation due to papillary muscle rupture, and mechanical problems, e.g. ischaemic ventriculoseptal defect, may also be implicated. The term 'obstructive shock' is applied to situations where pump failure is due to extrinsic cardiac obstruction rather than primary myocardial pathology, with the two most common causes being pulmonary embolus and cardiac tamponade.

Hypovolaemic shock is usually the result of uncontrolled haemorrhage, but may be due to excessive fluid loss from the gastrointestinal and urinary tracts, and even the skin in severe burns. Any type of infection – bacterial, fungal or viral – can be complicated by the development of shock. The clinical findings, perhaps with the exception of the cutaneous manifestations of meningococcal disease, are not specific to the type of organism involved, and it is not generally possible to determine the nature of the infecting organism from clinical examination alone.[2]

In practice, there is often considerable overlap between the different types of shock and it is not unusual, for example, to find both hypovolaemia and myocardial dysfunction in patients with predominantly septic shock. Even in cardiogenic shock, some improvement in cardiac function may be achieved with a careful volume challenge if the patient has been overaggressively diuresed.

PATHOPHYSIOLOGY

Oxygen delivery to the tissues (Do_2) is reduced in hypovolaemic, obstructive and cardiogenic shock. Several factors contribute to this, including low cardiac output, anaemia and hypoxaemia. In hypovolaemic shock, the diminished cardiac output is secondary to a reduction in myocardial preload. In obstructive shock venous return to the left ventricle is also reduced, whilst in cardiogenic shock impaired contractility predominates.

During the initial stages of hypovolaemic and cardiogenic shock, as oxygen delivery begins to fall, the tissues are able to maintain their oxygen uptake (Vo_2) at a normal level (170 ml/min per m^2) by extracting more oxygen from each unit of blood (supply-independent Vo_2). However, once oxygen delivery falls below a critical value of 330 ml/min per m^2, this compensatory mechanism is insufficient and oxygen uptake begins to decline (supply-dependent Vo_2). This phase is associated with the accumulation of an 'oxygen debt', and its severity may be gauged by the degree to which blood lactate is elevated (Figure 11.1).

In septic shock, microbial components or their toxins are recognised by soluble cell-bound receptors, e.g. the lipopolysaccharide of Gram-negative bacteria binds to CD14 and Toll-like receptor 4 (TLR4), whilst the peptidoglycan of Gram-positive bacteria binds to TLR2. This process stimulates the release of proinflammatory (tumor necrosis factor-α (TNF-α), interleukin-1 (IL-1), IL-6) and anti-inflammatory (IL-10, IL-1ra, TNF receptors) cytokines, generation of complement, activation of coagulation and platelet aggregation. There is also increased synthesis of arachidonic acid metabolites, reactive oxygen species and nitric oxide.[3] The combined effect of these changes is to produce vasodilatation, increased cardiac output despite impaired contractility and reduced intravascular volume secondary to increased capillary permeability.

Do_2 in septic shock is supranormal, mainly as a result of the elevated cardiac output. Vo_2 is also raised, due to an increase in tissue metabolic activity. At levels of Do_2 above the normal critical threshold, although Vo_2 is increased, it appears to be inadequate and a lactic acidosis

Table 11.1 Classification of shock

Physiological	Clinical
Hypoxic	Cardiogenic
Anaemic	Obstructive
Stagnant	Hypovolaemic
Histotoxic	Septic
	Neurogenic
	Anaphylactic

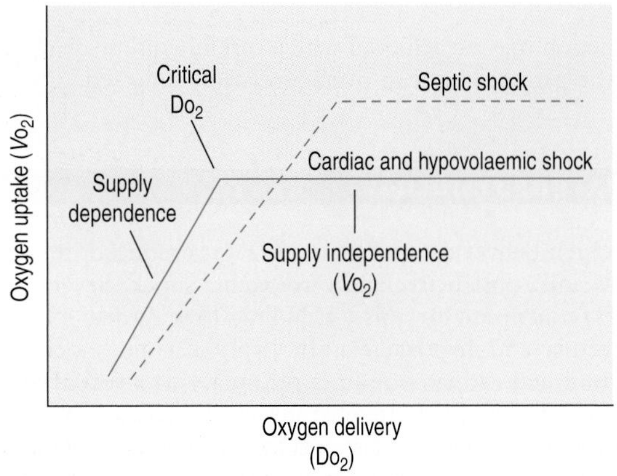

Figure 11.1 Relationship between oxygen uptake (Vo_2) and oxygen delivery (Do_2) in cardiogenic, hypovolaemic and septic shock.

develops. Supply dependency is thus observed over a wider range of oxygen delivery values than usual. This may be explained by abnormalities in perfusion at a microcirculatory level, resulting in locally reduced Do_2 despite a supranormal global value. Alternatively, sepsis-induced mitochondrial dysfunction may prevent oxygen utilisation at a cellular level.

In all forms of shock, anaerobic cellular metabolism leads to depletion of adenosine triphosphate and failure of the cell membrane sodium–potassium pump. Cell swelling occurs due to the influx of sodium and water. Anaerobic metabolism also leads to a worsening lactic acidosis. Mitochondrial calcium loss further impairs the efficiency of oxidation and phosphorylation, and may interfere with other organ-specific functions such as myocardial contractility.

If untreated, or suboptimally treated, shock will eventually progress via multiple-organ dysfunction to frank failure.

CLINICAL PRESENTATION

The clinical picture observed with the different types of shock can be divided into two categories, depending upon whether cardiac index is reduced (hypodynamic shock) or increased (hyperdynamic shock).

Hypovolaemic, obstructive and cardiogenic shock are usually associated with a low cardiac index; however blood pressure may be normal due to compensatory sympathetic and neurohormonal responses. Classically, the patient is confused, pale, tachycardic, tachypnoeic, poorly perfused and oliguric. The combination of extreme respiratory difficulty and inspiratory crepitations on auscultation of the chest should alert the physician to the possibility of pulmonary oedema due to left ventricular failure, which occurs frequently in cardiogenic shock. Clinically, estimation of central venous pressure (CVP) may help to differentiate between hypovolaemic and cardiogenic shock, since it is invariably low in the former and often raised in the latter. However, in obstructive shock the CVP is also raised.

In contrast septic shock is usually hyperdynamic, unless the patient is also significantly hypovolaemic. By definition, the patient must have a proven source of infection, be hypotensive (or requiring vasopressors to maintain a systolic blood pressure of 90 mmHg), exhibit two or more signs of systemic inflammation (tachycardia, tachypnoea, hypo-/hyperthermia, leukocytosis/leukopenia) and have dysfunction of at least one end-organ.[4] As with other forms of shock, the patient is often confused, tachycardic, tachypnoeic and oliguric. However, in contrast to hypovolaemic, obstructive and cardiogenic shock, peripheral pulses are bounding and the extremities are warm to touch. In meningococcal septicaemia a characteristic purpuric rash may be visible.

INVESTIGATIONS

LABORATORY, RADIOLOGICAL AND NON-INVASIVE CARDIAC INVESTIGATIONS

Investigations should be tailored to the history and clinical findings. In most cases, a few simple blood tests (full blood count, clotting, electrolytes, urea and creatinine, arterial blood gas, lactate, troponin and blood cultures), in conjunction with an electrocardiogram and chest X-ray, will be sufficient to confirm the nature of the shock.

In cardiogenic and obstructive shock echocardiography is invaluable, since it provides an objective measure of ventricular function, can identify and quantify abnormalities of regional wall motion and valvular function, and excludes cardiac tamponade or massive pulmonary embolus. Where the history and preliminary findings raise the suspicion of pulmonary embolus, alternative confirmatory tests include spiral computed tomography (CT), which is readily available in most hospitals, and pulmonary angiography.[5]

Hypovolaemic shock, due to concealed haemorrhage, may require further invasive and radiological investigations such as diagnostic peritoneal lavage, abdominal ultrasound, or CT scanning. When hypovolaemia is due to excessive gastrointestinal or renal losses, electrolyte disturbances can be severe, and urea and creatinine are often markedly elevated. Haemoconcentration may also be noted. Further investigations will depend upon the likely pathology, but may include supine and erect abdominal X-rays in bowel obstruction, abdominal ultrasound in acute cholecystitis and serum amylase and abdominal CT scan in pancreatitis.

Septic shock can lead to a rise or fall in the white cell count, the latter being associated with a particularly poor prognosis. Best practice dictates that blood and other relevant cultures are taken prior to initiating antibiotic therapy wherever possible, and in certain cases measurement of C-reactive protein and procalcitonin may be of value.[6,7] Disseminated intravascular coagulation, diagnosed by the combination of prolonged clotting, thrombocytopenia and reduced fibrinogen, is often present. When measured, antithrombin III, protein C and protein S levels are commonly low.

Blood lactate is elevated in all forms of shock, and indicates the presence of tissue hypoxia. The degree to which it is elevated corresponds to the severity of the shock, and it is frequently used as a guide to the effectiveness of therapeutic interventions.[8] Furthermore, lactate, base excess or a combination of the two can be used to predict outcome in patients admitted to the intensive care unit (ICU).[9]

INVASIVE HAEMODYNAMIC MEASUREMENTS

Whilst the therapeutic efficacy of the pulmonary artery catheter (PAC) remains controversial,[10] the measurements obtained from it are undoubtedly extremely useful in differentiating between the four major types of shock (Table 11.2).

Pulmonary artery catheterisation is rarely required to aid in the diagnosis of uncomplicated hypovolaemic shock. The clinical picture and presence of a low CVP are usually sufficient. However, the additional information obtained from a PAC may be invaluable in differentiating cardiogenic shock due to acute myocardial infarction (pulmonary artery occlusion pressure (PAOP) elevated, CVP normal or elevated, pulmonary artery pressure (PAP) normal), from pulmonary embolus (PAOP normal, CVP and PAP elevated) and cardiac tamponade (PAOP and CVP identical and elevated). It may also be helpful in cases of septic shock that are not clinically hyperdynamic, particularly in relation to optimising fluid, inotrope and vasopressor therapy. Alternatively, optimisation of cardiac preload and index in all forms of shock may be guided by measurement of stroke volume variation and cardiac index using lithium dilution (LiDCO) or intrathoracic blood volume index, extravascular lung water, stroke volume variation and cardiac index by transpulmonary thermodilution (PiCCO).[11–13]

PRINCIPLES OF MANAGEMENT

Management may be considered in terms of general measures that are applicable to all shocked patients, and specific measures that are appropriate in shock of a particular aetiology. Irrespective of the type of shock, it should be treated as a medical emergency. Resuscitation and investigation must therefore proceed in parallel and not in series.

GENERAL MEASURES

OXYGEN THERAPY AND MECHANICAL VENTILATION

All shocked patients should be given high-flow oxygen via a facemask, with the aim of improving arterial oxygen saturation and oxygen delivery to the tissues. Tachypnoea is common, and work of breathing is greatly increased, particularly in those cases with either cardiogenic or non-cardiogenic pulmonary oedema. Mechanical ventilation has much to commend it in this situation, since it will reduce oxygen consumption by the respiratory muscles at a time when their oxygen supply is compromised. Intubation at an early stage will also facilitate the insertion of invasive haemodynamic monitoring devices, which are invariably required to monitor and deliver fluid and inotropic therapy, but may be difficult to insert safely in a confused, agitated patient.

FLUID THERAPY

Optimising cardiac preload and restoring circulating volume are fundamental aspects of correcting tissue hypoxia in patients with shock. In cases of hypovolaemic and septic shock several litres of fluid are usually needed to achieve this, but occasionally even some patients with cardiogenic shock may benefit from a judicious volume challenge. In patients with severe sepsis, aggressive volume replacement within 6 hours of presentation in conjunction

Table 11.2 Values obtained from the pulmonary artery catheter in the four major types of shock

	Septic shock	Cardiogenic shock	Hypovolaemic shock	Obstructive shock
Cardiac index	↑	↓	↓	↓
Pulmonary artery occlusion pressure (PAOP)	Normal or ↓	↑	↓	Normal or ↑
Central venous pressure (CVP)	Normal or ↓	Normal or ↑	↓	↑
Systemic vascular resistance (SVR)	↓	↑	↑	↑
Oxygen delivery ($D\text{O}_2$)	↑	↓	↓	↓

with targeting a central venous oxygen saturation > 70% ($S_{cv}O_2$ > 70) and haemoglobin level > 10 g/dl can reduce hospital mortality by up to 16%.[14]

CVP is often used as a surrogate for myocardial preload in uncomplicated hypovolaemic shock. However, in patients with ischaemic heart disease PAOP is usually preferred. Intrathoracic blood volume, an alternative measure of cardiac preload, offers theoretical advantages over both CVP and PAOP, particularly in mechanically ventilated patients, and is obtained using either double (COLD) or single (PiCCO) indicator dilution.[12,13] More recently, stroke volume variation (SVV) with respiration has been shown to be the best predictor of volume responsiveness, and has the advantage of being relatively easy to obtain through analysis of the arterial waveform trace.[15] When SVV is 9.5% or greater a 100 ml volume load will increase stroke volume by at least 5%.[16] It is less useful in patients with atrial fibrillation or frequent ventricular ectopics, where wide fluctuations in baseline stroke volume are present.

Logically, the fluid used to correct any deficit should reflect the type of fluid lost, and patients who have significant bleeding will clearly require blood. In intensive care patients without acute coronary syndromes, it appears safe to aim for a haemoglobin level of 7–9 g/dl once the acute resuscitation phase has passed. Indeed, targeting this level is associated with a lower mortality than 10–12 g/dl.[17] At present, the use of blood substitutes such as diasprin cross-linked haemoglobin is not recommended in haemorrhagic shock, as they are linked to a higher death rate.[18]

Given that blood is usually supplied in the form of red cell concentrates, the clinician must decide whether to combine it with a crystalloid, human albumin or a synthetic colloid in order to restore circulating volume. The same dilemma, over whether to use a crystalloid or a colloid during resuscitation, also arises in patients with septic shock. One property in favour of colloids is that they restore circulating volume more efficiently than crystalloids, since approximately 1.5 times as much crystalloid must be infused to achieve the same haemodynamic end-point.[19] It is therefore common to begin resuscitation with a colloid to restore intravascular volume, and to continue with crystalloid to correct interstitial and intracellular losses. A recent, large placebo-controlled trial of normal saline versus 4% albumin for resuscitation in ICU may challenge this practice, however, since no differences in mortality or morbidity could be demonstrated between the groups, and crystalloids are undoubtedly much cheaper to use.[19]

In addition, several papers have raised concerns regarding the safety of colloids. A systematic review of randomised studies comparing the use of crystalloids and colloids in the resuscitation of critically ill patients concluded that the use of colloid was associated with a 4% increase in mortality.[20] The specific issue of renal failure was highlighted in a randomised controlled study comparing the use of the synthetic colloid hydroxyethyl starch (MMW-HES 200 kDa, 0.6–0.66 substitution) with 3% gelatine in patients with sepsis and septic shock. In this study the incidence of renal failure was significantly higher in the HES group.[21] The use of high-molecular-weight hydroxyethylstarch (HMW-HES 450 kDa, 0.5 substitution) has also been associated with abnormal clotting and increased bleeding.[22]

A number of recent publications have focused on the use of hypertonic crystalloids, such as 7.5% sodium chloride alone or in conjunction with dextran 70, for initial resuscitation. While most of the large studies have failed to show a clear survival benefit in the general trauma population, hypertonic solutions may be useful in certain subgroups, such as those with severe head injuries, in whom the administration of large volumes of isotonic crystalloid may worsen cerebral oedema.[23,24] Most studies also show that the use of hypertonic solutions is associated with a reduction in fluid and blood transfusion requirements.[25]

INOTROPIC SUPPORT

Inotropic support is rarely required in hypovolaemic shock, except when it is severe and surgical control of bleeding is delayed. In most instances, fluid replacement alone is sufficient to restore cardiac output and blood pressure. Although fluid therapy is also important in patients with septic shock, it is rarely helpful in those with cardiogenic shock, and in both septic and cardiogenic shock vasoactive drugs are often required to improve tissue perfusion and reverse tissue hypoxia.

In cardiogenic shock cardiac output and blood pressure are characteristically low, and systemic vascular resistance increased. Ideally an inodilator, e.g. dobutamine or milrinone, should be selected, provided that blood pressure is not unduly compromised. When hypotension is a prominent feature, the use of an inoconstrictor, e.g. epinephrine or dopamine, or a pure constrictor in combination with an inodilator, e.g. norepinephrine and dobutamine, is often preferred. A number of adverse side-effects are to be expected with epinephrine, including hyperglycaemia, hypokalaemia and hyperlactataemia.[26,27] Consequently, use of epinephrine should be taken into account when interpreting blood lactate measurements. Levosimendan, a new inotropic agent that exerts its effect by binding to troponin C and increasing myocyte sensitivity to calcium, is being used increasingly in the setting of acute heart failure.[28] It has the advantage of not increasing myocardial oxygen consumption when compared to dobutamine, and is particularly useful in cases where an element of load-induced right ventricular failure exists since it also reduces pulmonary artery resistance.[29,30]

Septic shock classically results in a high cardiac output and low blood pressure due to excessive peripheral vasodilatation. This so-called peripheral circulatory failure is mediated via increased production of nitric oxide due to stimulation of inducible nitric oxide synthase in vascular smooth muscle and endothelium. Once cardiac preload is optimised, use of a pure vasoconstrictor, e.g. norepinephrine, is recommended. If cardiac output is reduced, it is often helpful to combine norepinephrine with dobutamine or milrinone. Theoretically, the inoconstrictor dopamine could also be used in this situation, if it were not for a number of problematic side effects. These include adverse effects on pituitary function (reduced prolactin, growth hormone and TRH), T-cell function, gut mucosal perfusion and renal medullary oxygen consumption.[31,32]

DIURETICS

The use of 'low-dose' or 'renal-dose' dopamine, to prevent renal failure in shocked patients, does not reduce the number of patients who subsequently require renal replacement therapy, and, given the concern about possible adverse effects of dopamine, should be abandoned.[33,34] If a natriuresis is desired, this can usually be achieved with furosemide, given by intermittent bolus (10–80 mg) or continuous infusion (3–10 mg/h). Care should be taken to ensure that the patient is adequately volume-resuscitated before a diuretic is given, so that hypovolaemia is not exacerbated by an inappropriate diuresis.

SPECIFIC MEASURES

HYPOVOLAEMIC SHOCK

Surgical, radiological or endoscopic intervention may be required in haemorrhagic shock, and should be undertaken in a timely fashion. In most situations fluid resuscitation precedes definitive intervention, but in some trauma patients outcome may be improved if fluid resuscitation is delayed until bleeding is controlled.[35] Hypovolaemic shock due to other intrabdominal pathologies, e.g. perforation/obstruction, may also warrant surgery. In these cases, measures taken to improve the condition of the patient preoperatively, such as correcting hypovolaemia, hypoxia and anaemia, and increasing oxygen $D\text{O}_2$, can reduce perioperative mortality substantially.[36,37]

SEPTIC SHOCK

Source control

Infected fluid collections should be drained, either radiologically or surgically. Surgical intervention may also be required for other sources of sepsis, for example bowel perforation.

Antibiotics

It is vital to select an appropriate antibiotic(s) and to ensure that the dosing regimen is optimal. This latter task is often the more difficult, especially when re-dosing depends upon monitoring of drug levels. Any delay in obtaining a level can expose the patient to a significant period of suboptimal antibiotic therapy. In order to reduce this problem, antibiotics whose efficacy does not depend upon peak levels, e.g. vancomycin, may be given by continuous infusion (0.5–2 g/day, depending on renal function) with a random level taken once daily.[38] In the absence of culture results, initial antibiotic therapy is designed to cover a broad range of likely pathogens. However, once culture results are available, antibiotic cover should be narrowed and directed at the identified organism(s).

Steroids

Large doses of steroid (30–120 mg/kg of methylprednisolone) given within 24 hours of the onset of shock result in haemodynamic improvement but not lower mortality, a finding that may be explained by the increased incidence of secondary infection associated with their use.[39,40] More recently, administration of lower doses of steroid (300 mg/day hydrocortisone), particularly to those patients with a 'flat' Short Synacthen Test (SST), became common practice following a study demonstrating a beneficial effect on both haemodynamics and mortality.[41] However, the merits of this practice are now being re-evaluated following publication of a large randomized, double-blind, placebo controlled trial (CORTICUS) that failed to demonstrate a mortality benefit from steroids (300 mg hydrocortisone/day), irrespective of the SST result. Worryingly even low doses of steroid appear to be associated with more episodes of superinfection, including new sepsis and septic shock.[42] At present it would seem prudent to reserve steroid therapy for patients who are poorly responsive to adequate fluid therapy and vasopressor support, and to limit the dose to < 300 mg of hydrocortisone/day.

L-NMMA

The results of phase I and II trials of N^{G}-monomethyl-L-arginine hydrochloride (L-NMMA), a non-selective nitric oxide synthase inhibitor, in septic shock appeared promising. When infused at a maximum rate of 20 mg/kg per h for 8 hours, there was a 60–80% reduction in the amount of norepinephrine required to maintain a mean arterial pressure of 70 mmHg or greater.[43] Unfortunately, the subsequent phase III study demonstrated an increased mortality in the L-NMMA group. This was largely due to L-NMMA-induced increases in both systemic and pulmonary vascular resistances that resulted in cardiac failure.[44] Further investigations in this area are likely to focus on the development of a selective inducible nitric oxide synthase inhibitor.

Vasopressin

Vasopressin secretion from the posterior pituitary is an important homeostatic mechanism for restoring blood pressure in various forms of shock. In septic shock vasopressin levels may be inappropriately low, due to either impaired secretion or depletion.[45,46] In cases of septic shock with refractory hypotension despite high doses of catecholamines, the addition of an intravenous infusion of vasopressin (0.04 U/min) can increase mean arterial pressure, systemic vascular resistance and urine output.[47] A recent large, double-blind trial (VASST) comparing vasopressin (0.01–0.03 U/min) and norepinephrine (5–15 μg/min), in addition to open-label vasopressors in patients with septic shock requiring more than 5 μg norepinephrine, failed to show a difference in

28 day mortality. Reassuringly, given previous concerns regarding the potential of vasopressin to cause tissue ischaemia, there was no significant difference in the incidence of serious adverse events between the two groups.[48]

Activated protein C

Activated protein C is an endogenous protein capable of promoting fibrinolysis and inhibiting thrombosis and inflammation. In sepsis, the conversion of protein C from an inactive to active form, which is stimulated by thrombin bound to thrombomodulin, is impaired due to downregulation of thrombomodulin by inflammatory cytokines. In patients with severe sepsis, infusing activated protein C (24 μg/kg per h) for up to 96 hours reduces absolute risk of death by 6%.[49] Hospital survival is increased from 65.1% to 70.3%.[50] Administering the drug in this fashion does however result in an increased risk of serious bleeding, and its effect on mortality has not been studied in patients who are at increased risk of bleeding, including those who have had recent surgery or trauma.

It is of no benefit in patients with a low risk of death, such as those with single-organ failure or an Acute Physiology, Age and Chronic Health Evaluation (APACHE) score less than 25. Indeed, it is contraindicated in this group of patients, since its use is associated with an increased incidence of serious bleeding complications.[51]

High-volume haemofiltration

Haemofiltration is frequently used to manage severe metabolic acidosis, as well as renal failure itself, in patients with septic shock. Numerous studies have demonstrated that haemodynamic status often improves following commencement of haemofiltration, and it is postulated that this is due to cytokine removal in the ultrafiltrate and by adsorption on to the filter.[52,53] In patients with sepsis, there is some evidence to suggest that using a higher 'dose' of haemofiltration, e.g. 45 ml/kg per h, may improve outcome.[54] However, a rigorous, randomised, controlled study of high-volume haemofiltration in septic patients has not been undertaken to date.

CARDIOGENIC SHOCK

PERCUTANEOUS CORONARY INTERVENTION (PCI), THROMBOLYSIS, CORONARY ARTERY BYPASS GRAFTING

For the treatment of myocardial infarction with ST-segment elevation, PCI is superior to thrombolysis in terms of short-term mortality, non-fatal reinfarction, stroke and a composite of all three.[55] This benefit is maintained, even when patients have to be transferred to a specialist centre to undergo PCI, provided that the transfer takes 2 hours or less.[56] Coronary artery bypass grafting may be undertaken in a small number of patients who are not suitable for PCI. Thrombolysis alone does not reduce the mortality of cardiogenic shock complicating acute myocardial infarction (55% at 30 days).[57]

INTRA-AORTIC BALLOON PUMP

The intra-aortic balloon pump provides a useful bridge to surgery in cases of cardiogenic shock due to papillary muscle rupture and ischaemic ventricular septal defect. Its use as a supportive therapy, in conjunction with other aggressive invasive treatments, in the wider population of patients with acute myocardial infarction is also associated with a reduction in 1-year mortality.[58]

OBSTRUCTIVE SHOCK

PULMONARY EMBOLUS

Even patients without hypotension or shock may benefit from thrombolysis, if they have evidence of pulmonary hypertension or right ventricular dysfunction. Those who receive heparin alone are more likely to require an escalation in their therapy (catecholamine infusion, secondary thrombolysis, intubation, cardiopulmonary resuscitation or embolectomy).[59]

CARDIAC TAMPONADE

Surgical or percutaneous drainage of pericardial fluid should be undertaken immediately for pericardial tamponade. Whenever possible percutaneous drainage should be guided by echocardiography.

OUTCOME

Outcome in shock depends upon a multitude of factors, including aetiology, severity of illness at presentation, response to therapy and comorbidity. In general terms, the mortality associated with hypovoalemic shock is considerably lower than that for either cardiogenic or septic shock, provided that the source of bleeding can be controlled. Even in good centres, where patients receive aggressive therapy, mortality from septic shock is approximately 30–50%, and often higher for cardiogenic shock.[60]

REFERENCES

1. Vincent JL, Van der Linden P. Septic shock: particular type of acute circulatory failure. *Crit Care Med* 1990; **18**: S70–4.
2. Wiles JB, Cerra FB, Siegel JH *et al.* The systemic septic response: does the organism matter? *Crit Care Med* 1990; **8**: 55–60.
3. Vincent JL, De Backer D. Pathophysiology of septic shock. *Adv Sepsis* 2001; **1**: 87–92.
4. Members of the American College of Chest Physicians/Society of Critical Care Medicine Consensus Conference Committee. ACCP/SCCM Consensus Conference: Definitions for sepsis and organ failure and guidelines for the use of innovative therapies in sepsis. *Crit Care Med* 1992; **20**: 864–74.
5. Pruszczyk P, Torbicki A, Pacho R *et al.* Non-invasive diagnosis of suspected severe pulmonary embolism: transoesophageal echocardiography vs spiral CT. *Chest* 1997; **112**: 722–8.

6. Povoa P, Almeida E, Moreira P *et al.* C-reactive protein as an indicator of sepsis. *Intens Care Med* 1998; **24**: 1052–6.
7. Assicot M, Gendrel D, Carsin H *et al.* High serum procalcitonin concentrations in patients with sepsis and infection. *Lancet* 1993; **341**: 515–8.
8. Bakker J. Lactate: may I have your votes please?. *Intens Care Med* 2001; **27**: 6–11.
9. Smith I, Kumar P, Molloy S *et al.* Base excess and lactate as prognostic indicators for patients admitted to intensive care. *Intens Care Med* 2001; **27**: 74–83.
10. Connors AF, Speroff T, Dawson NV *et al.* The effectiveness of right heart catheterisation in the initial care of critically ill patients. *JAMA* 1996; **276**: 889–97.
11. Linton R, Band D, O'Brien T *et al.* Lithium dilution cardiac output measurement: a comparison with thermodilution. *Crit Care Med* 1997; **25**: 1796–800.
12. Lichtwarck-Aschoff M, Zeravik J, Pfeiffer UJ. Intrathoracic blood volume accurately reflects circulatory volume status in critically ill patients with mechanical ventilation. *Intens Care Med* 1992; **18**: 142–7.
13. Sakka SG, Ruhl CC, Pfeiffer UJ *et al.* Assessment of cardiac preload and extravascular lung water by single transpulmonary thermodilution. *Intens Care Med* 2000; **26**: 180–7.
14. Rivers E, Nguyen B, Havstad S. Early goal-directed therapy in the treatment of severe sepsis and septic shock. *N Engl J Med* 2001; **345**: 1368–77.
15. Hofer CK, Muller SM, Furrer L *et al.* Stroke volume and pulse pressure variation for prediction of fluid responsiveness in patients undergoing off-pump coronary artery bypass grafting. *Chest* 2005; **128**: 848–54.
16. Berkenstadt H, Margalit N, Hadani M *et al.* Stroke volume variation as a predictor of fluid responsiveness in patients undergoing brain surgery. *Anaesth Analg* 2001; **92**: 984–9.
17. Hebert PC, Wells G, Blajchman MA *et al.* A multicentre, randomised, controlled clinical trial of transfusion requirements in critical care. *N Engl J Med* 1999; **340**: 409–17.
18. Sloan EP, Koenigsbers M, Gens D *et al.* Diasprin cross-linked haemoglobin (DCLHb) in the treatment of severe traumatic haemorrhagic shock. A randomised controlled efficacy trial. *JAMA* 1999; **282**: 1857–64.
19. The SAFE Study Investigators. A comparison of albumin and saline for fluid resuscitation in the intensive care unit. *N Engl J Med* 2004; **350**: 2247–56.
20. Schierhout G, Roberts I. Fluid resuscitation with colloid or crystalloid solutions in critically ill patients: a systematic review of randomised trails. *Br Med J* 1998; **316**: 961–4.
21. Schortgen F, Lacherade J-C, Bruneel F *et al.* Effects of hydroxyethylstarch and gelatin on renal function in severe sepsis: a multicentre randomised study. *Lancet* 2001; **357**: 911–6.
22. Boldt J, Knothe C, Zickmann B *et al.* Influence of different intravascular volume therapies on platelet function in patients undergoing cardiopulmonary bypass. *Anaesth Analg* 1993; **76**: 1185–90.
23. Vassar MJ, Perry CA, Gannaway WL *et al.* 7.5% sodium chiloride/dextran for resuscitation of trauma patients undergoing helicopter transport. *Arch Surg* 1991; **126**: 1065–72.
24. Vassar MJ, Fischer R, O'Brien P *et al.* A multicentre trial for resuscitation of injured patients with 7.5% sodium chloride. The effect of added dextran 70. The multicentre group for the study of hypertonic saline in trauma patients. *Arch Surg* 1993; **128**: 1003–11.
25. Younes RN, Aun F, Accioly CQ *et al.* Hypertonic solutions in the treatment of hypovolaemic shock: a prospective randomised study in patients admitted to the emergency room. *Surgery* 1992; **111**: 380–5.
26. Day NPJ, Phu NH, Bethel DP *et al.* The effects of dopamine and adrenaline infusions on acid–base balance and systemic haemodynamics in severe infection. *Lancet* 1996; **348**: 219–23.
27. Totaro RJ, Raper RF. Epinephrine-induced lactic acidosis following cardiopulmonary bypass. *Crit Care Med* 1997; **25**: 1693–9.
28. Huang L, Weil MH, Tang W *et al.* Comparison between dobutamine and levosimendan for management of post resuscitation myocardial dysfunction. *Crit Care Med* 2005; **33**: 487–91.
29. Morelli A, Teboul J-L, Maggiore SM *et al.* Effects of levosimendan on right ventricular afterload in patients with acute respiratory distress syndrome: a pilot study. *Crit Care Med* 2006; **34**: 2287–93.
30. Kerbaul F, Rondelet B, Demester J-P *et al.* Effects of levosimenden versus dobutamine on pressure load-induced right ventricular failure. *Crit Care Med* 2006; **34**: 2814–9.
31. Van den Berge G, De Zegher F. Anterior pituitary function during critical illness and dopamine treatment. *Crit Care Med* 1996; **24**: 1580–90.
32. Pawlik W, Mailman D, Shanbour L *et al.* Dopamine effects on the intestinal circulation. *Am Heart J* 1976; **75**: 325–31.
33. ANZICS clinical trials group. Low-dose dopamine in patients with early renal dysfunction: a placebo-controlled randomised trial. *Lancet* 2000; **356**: 2139–43.
34. Kellum JA, Decker JM. Use of dopamine in acute renal failure. *Crit Care Med* 2001; **29**: 1526–31.
35. Bickell WH, Wall MJ, Pepe PE *et al.* Immediate versus delayed fluid resuscitation for hypotensive patients with penetrating truncal injuries. *N Engl J Med* 1994; **331**: 1105–9.
36. Shoemaker WC, Appel PL, Kram HB *et al.* Prospective trail of supranormal values of survivors as therapeutic goals in high-risk surgical patients. *Chest* 1988; **94**: 1176–86.
37. Boyd O, Grounds RM, Bennett ED. A randomised clinical trial of the effect of deliberate perioperative increase of oxygen delivery on mortality in high-risk surgical patients. *JAMA* 1993; **270**: 2699–707.
38. James JK, Palmer SM, Levine DP *et al.* Comparison of conventional dosing versus continuous-infusion vancomycin therapy for patients with suspected or

documented Gram-positive infections. *Antimicrob Agents Chemother* 1996; **40**: 696–700.
39. Sprung CL, Caralis PV, Marcial EH. The effects of high-dose corticosteroids in patients with septic shock. A prospective, controlled study. *N Engl J Med* 1984; **311**: 1137–43.
40. Bone RC, Fisher CJ, Clemmer TP. A controlled clinical trial of high-dose methylprednisolone in the treatment of severe sepsis and septic shock. *N Engl J Med* 1987; **317**: 653–8.
41. Bollaert P-E, Charpentier C, Levy B *et al.* Reversal of late septic shock with supraphysiological doses of hydrocortisone. *Crit Care Med* 1998; **26**: 645–50.
42. Sprung CL, Annane D, Keh D *et al.* Hydrocortisone therapy for patients with septic shock. *N Engl J Med* 2008; **358**: 111–24.
43. Grover R, Zaccardelli D, Colice G *et al.* An open-label dose escalation study of the nitric oxide synthase inhibitor, *N*-methy-L-arginine hydrochloride (546C88), in patients with septic shock. *Crit Care Med* 1999; **27**: 913–22.
44. Grover R, Lopez A, Lorente J *et al.* Multicentre, randomised, placebo-controlled, double blind study of nitric oxide synthase inhibitor 546C88: effect on survival in patients with septic shock. *Crit Care Med* 1999; **27** (Suppl. 1): A33.
45. Sharshar T, Blanchard A, Palliard M *et al.* Circulating vasopressin levels in septic shock. *Crit Care Med* 2001; **31**: 1752–8.
46. Mutlu GM, Factor P. Role of vasopressin in the management of septic shock. *Intens Care Med* 2004; **30**: 1276–91.
47. Tsuneyoshi T, Yamada H, Hakihana Y *et al.* Haemodynamic and metabolic effects of low-dose vasopressin infusions in vasodilatory septic shock. *Crit Care Med* 2001; **29** 487: 93.
48. Russell JA, Walley KR, Singer J *et al.* Vasopressin versus norpinephrine infusion in patients with septic shock. *N Engl J Med* 2008; **358**: 877–87.
49. Bernard GR, Vincent JL, Laterre P-F *et al.* Efficacy and safety of recombinant human activated protein C for severe sepsis. *N Engl J Med* 2001; **344**: 699–709.
50. Angus DC, Laterre P-F, Helterbrand J *et al.* The effect of drotregogin alfa (activated) on long-term survival after severe sepsis. *Crit Care Med* 2004; **32**: 2199–206.
51. Abraham E, Laterre P-F, Garg R *et al.* Drotrecogin alfa (activated) for adults with severe sepsis and a low risk of death. *N Engl J Med* 2005; **353**: 1332–41.
52. Heering P, Morgera S, Schmitz FJ *et al.* Cytokine removal and cardiovascular haemodynamics in septic patients with continuous venovenous haemofiltration. *Intens Care Med* 1997; **23**: 288–96.
53. Honore PM, Jamez J, Wauthier M *et al.* Prospective evaluation of short-term, high-volume isovolaemic haemofiltration on the haemodynamic course and outcome in patients with intractable circulatory failure resulting from septic shock. *Crit Care Med* 2000; **28**: 3581–7.
54. Ronco C, Bellomo R, Homel P. Effects of different doses in continuous veno-venous haemofiltration on outcomes of acute renal failure: a prospective randomised trial. *Lancet* 2000; **355**: 26–30.
55. Keeley EC, Boura JA, Grines CL. Primary angioplasty versus intravenous thrombolytic therapy for acute myocardial infarction: a quantative review of 23 randomised trials. *Lancet* 2003; **361**: 13–20.
56. Andersen HR, Nielsen TT, Rasmussen K *et al.* A comparison of coronary angioplasty with fibrinolytic therapy in acute myocardial infarction. *N Engl J Med* 2003; **349**: 733–42.
57. Holmes DR, Bates ER, Kleinman NS *et al.* Contemporary reperfusion therapy for cardiogenic shock: the GUSTO-I trial experience. *J Am Coll Cardiol* 1995; **26**: 668–74.
58. Holmes DR, Califf RM, Van de Werf F *et al.* Difference in countries' use of resources and clinical outcome for patients with cardiogenic shock after myocardial infarction: results from the GUSTO trial. *Lancet* 1997; **349**: 75–8.
59. Konstantinides S, Geibel A, Heusel G *et al.* Heparin plus alteplase compared with heparin alone in patients with submassive pulmonary embolus. *N Engl J Med* 2002; **347**: 1143–50.
60. Brun-Buisson C, Doyon F, Carlet J *et al.* Incidence, risk factors, and outcome of severe sepsis and septic shock in adults. *JAMA* 1995; **274**: 968–74.

12

Haemodynamic monitoring

David J Sturgess and Thomas John Morgan

Haemodynamics is the study of blood flow. Haemodynamic monitoring therefore refers to the monitoring of blood flow through the cardiovascular system. In the intensive care unit (ICU), haemodynamic monitoring is used to detect cardiovascular insufficiency, differentiate contributing factors and guide therapy.

There has been debate over the risks and benefits of invasive haemodynamic monitoring in critically ill patients. Because there are scant data to show that invasive monitoring leads to improved survival, there has been a steady trend toward less invasive monitoring in the ICU. Regular clinical assessment remains an important component of haemodynamic monitoring, and any acquired physiological data must be interpreted in the clinical context. Importantly, monitoring must be combined with effective therapy in order to demonstrate an impact on outcome.[1]

As an aid to understanding haemodynamics, several circulatory models have been proposed, each with limitations. The standard model consists of a non-pulsatile pump and a hydraulic circuit with discrete sites of flow resistance. Heart rate and stroke volume determine cardiac output. The concepts of preload, contractility and afterload (Frank–Starling mechanism) are incorporated as determinants of stroke volume. In practice, quantification of these parameters is difficult, both clinically and in the laboratory. The model itself is simplistic, and does not allow for the pulsatile interaction of the cardiac pump with the elastance of the arterial tree. More complex models based on electrical circuits have been devised, but are still unable to quantify afterload and contractility precisely.

At the bedside the clinician must work with inexact surrogates of preload, contractility and afterload, measured or derived from arterial blood pressure (systemic or pulmonary), volume or pressure indices of cardiac filling, cardiac output and various markers of tissue well-being. In this chapter we focus on all these measurements except for those of tissue well-being, which are discussed elsewhere.

ARTERIAL BLOOD PRESSURE

The systemic pulse wave propagates from the aortic valve at 6–10 m/s. During its passage into the peripheral vasculature there is a progressive increase in systolic (SBP) and reduction in diastolic blood pressures (DBP), as standing and reflected waves become incorporated into the waveform, a process known as distal pulse amplification. Consequently, systemic arterial pressure measurements vary according to the site of measurement.

Mean arterial pressure (MAP) is arguably a more relevant index to monitor than either SBP or DBP for three reasons:

1. MAP is least dependent on measurement site or technique (invasive versus non-invasive).
2. MAP is least altered by measurement damping.
3. MAP determines tissue blood flow via autoregulation (apart from the left ventricle, which autoregulates from DBP).

In the absence of sophisticated waveform analysis, arterial pressure is poorly correlated with cardiac output. Hence clinical estimation of cardiac output from arterial pressure and heart rate is unreliable until extreme hypotension occurs.[2]

NON-INVASIVE ARTERIAL BLOOD PRESSURE (NIBP) MEASUREMENT

In ICU, most standard NIBP instruments are automated intermittent oscillometric devices. Finger plethysmography and arterial tonometry can monitor both arterial pressure and waveforms continuously, but there are concerns regarding their accuracy.

Oscillometric NIBP is often used to check the reliability of invasive measurements, or can be used alone when beat-to-beat monitoring is not required. Contraindications to NIBP are relative, and influence the site of cuff placement. For instance, it is preferable to avoid extremities with severe peripheral vascular disease, venous cannulation, arteriovenous fistula or previous lymph node clearance (for example, radical mastectomy).

To make an oscillometric blood pressure measurement, a pneumatic cuff is inflated around a limb until all oscillations in cuff pressure are extinguished. The occluding pressure is then lowered stepwise, so that oscillations reappear over a discrete interval. Proprietary algorithms compute MAP, SBP and DBP from the alterations in oscillatory amplitude during deflation.

Oscillometry overestimates low pressures and underestimates high pressures, but for the normotensive range the 95% confidence limits are ± 15 mmHg (2 kPa). Dysrhythmias increase the error. Cuff width should be 40% of the mid-circumference of the limb. Narrower cuffs overestimate and wider cuffs underestimate blood pressures.

Complications are unusual. Repeated cuff inflations can cause skin ulceration, oedema and bruising, more so when the consciousness is impaired by illness and sedation. Ulnar nerve injury is also possible, especially with low cuff placement.

INVASIVE BLOOD PRESSURE MEASUREMENT[3]

Invasive blood pressure measurement is desirable in the presence of haemodynamic instability, end-organ disease requiring beat-to-beat blood pressure monitoring, during therapeutic manipulation of the cardiovascular system or if non-invasive methods fail. Cannulation of a systemic artery allows continuous monitoring of the arterial pressure waveform, heart rate and blood pressure, and also facilitates frequent arterial blood gas analysis. Relative contraindications include coagulopathy and vascular abnormality or disease.

The radial artery is the most common site for cannulation. Nothing larger than a 20-gauge cannula is advisable, and either a modified Seldinger technique or direct cannulation can be used. Once inserted, the cannula is usually infused with normal or heparinised saline at 3 ml/h, with a snap flush rate of 30–60 ml/h. Although it appears not to prolong patency, the use of heparinised saline (2–4 units/ml) might improve accuracy.[4] It should be avoided if heparin-induced thrombocytopenia syndrome is suspected.

The axillary, brachial, femoral, posterior tibial and dorsalis pedis arteries can all be used without apparently raising the complication profile (Table 12.1). In severe circulatory compromise, gaining peripheral arterial access may be difficult and time-consuming. Rapid femoral cannulation by the Seldinger percutaneous technique usually remains feasible, with the added advantage that femoral arterial monitoring more accurately reflects aortic pressure in low-output states.

Cannulae are usually removed or resited between days 5 and 7, or earlier if a complication is suspected. Distal perfusion should be checked at least 8-hourly, and the cannula removed if there is persistent blanching, coolness with sluggish capillary refill, loss of pulses or evidence of raised muscle compartment pressures. Complications associated with arterial cannulation are presented in Table 12.1.

PHYSICAL PROPERTIES OF CLINICAL PRESSURE MEASUREMENT SYSTEMS[5,6]

In the standard set-up, the arterial cannula is connected to a linearly responsive pressure transducer via fluid-filled non-compliant tubing < 1 m in length. Modern disposable transducers are precalibrated using electrical signals, and are not normally calibrated further against known pressures. The system is zeroed to the level of the phlebostatic axis, normally the mid-axillary line at the fourth intercostal space. Subsequent lowering of the transducer relative to this axis will cause pressure overestimation, while raising it will cause underestimation.

The *natural resonant frequency* of the system should ideally exceed 30 Hz (> 10 harmonics) for heart rates up to 180 beats/min (3 Hz) to prevent distortion of the biological signal by sine-wave system oscillations. *Damping* refers to any property of an oscillatory system that reduces the amplitude of oscillations. Factors that increase oscillation in the system, such as increased tubing length, diameter or compliance, cause underdamping. Overdamping tends to smooth the waveform, causing underestimation of SBP and overestimation of DBP, while MAP tends to be preserved. Contributing factors include clots, air bubbles and loose connections. Damping can be assessed clinically by the fast-flush test (Table 12.2).[7]

Upstream resistance or turbulence can result in a flow-dependent pressure reduction at the cannula site that differs from damping in that the MAP, SBP and DBP are all reduced. This is described as *attenuation* and is often observed in 'positional' arterial lines.

ADDITIONAL INFORMATION FROM THE ARTERIAL WAVEFORM

Measurement systems used in ICU do not precisely quantify the rate of arterial pressure rise and fall. Nevertheless, the wide pulse pressure of aortic regurgitation and the slowed upstroke of severe aortic stenosis may be detected. Pulsus paradoxus can readily be quantified in the spontaneously breathing patient. Systolic time intervals can provide an indication of ventricular contractility.

The systemic arterial pressure waveform can also assist in the prediction of fluid responsiveness (see Functional haemodynamic monitoring, below).

Estimation of stroke volume and cardiac output[8]

Estimation of stroke volume by analysis of the arterial pressure waveform, in particular various properties of the pulse pressure (pressure above diastolic) component, has been studied for many years. Pulse contour analysis calculates stroke volume from the area under the systolic portion of the arterial pressure waveform. After individual calibration, these monitors can determine stroke volume beat-to-beat. Cardiac output, derived by multiplying stroke volume by heart rate, appears to offer reliable continuous cardiac output monitoring, even during haemodynamic instability.[9] However, accuracy in the presence of arrhythmia has not been validated.

Transpulmonary indicator dilution (discussed below) is the usual method of calibration. Pulse contour devices that use thermodilution or lithium ion calibration are commercially available.[10] Comparisons with pulmonary artery catheter (PAC) cardiac output measurements have shown good agreement, with mean bias values ≤ 0.1 l/min and precision (SD of bias) of the order of 0.6 l/min.

Table 12.1 Complications of arterial cannulation, with suggested preventive and treatment options[61]

Complication	Prevention	Treatment
Vascular thrombosis (ranges from 7 to 30% following radial artery cannulation). Risk factors for digital ischaemia include: shock, sepsis, embolus of air or clot, hyperlipoproteinaemia, vasculitis, female sex, prothrombotic states, accidental intra-arterial injection of drugs	Risks reduced by smaller catheter, larger artery, decreased duration of cannulation, avoiding traumatic insertion and multiple attempts. Allen's test (including modifications such as Doppler, plethysmography and digital blood pressure) is probably unhelpful	Remove cannula. Arterial thrombosis is usually self-limiting. Severe ischaemic damage estimated at $< 0.01\%$. Anticoagulation and/or vascular surgery/ intervention may be necessary
Distal embolisation	Diligent catheter care and observation	As for thrombosis
Proximal embolisation of clot or air (can result in stroke)	Diligent catheter care and observation. Exclude air from pressurised system. Avoid axillary, subclavian or carotid access	Tailored to sequelae
Vascular spasm	Smaller catheter, larger artery. Avoid traumatic insertion and multiple attempts	Remove cannula. Resite if necessary
Skin necrosis at catheter site	Diligent catheter care and observation	Surgical debridement and skin grafting may be necessary
Line disconnection and bleeding/ exsanguination	Minimise connections. Diligent catheter care and observation	Control bleeding. Transfusion may be necessary
Accidental drug injection	Clearly label arterial line near ports	Leave cannula in situ to facilitate treatment if required. Depends on drug injected. May require papaverine or procaine, analgesia, sympathetic block of limb and anticoagulation
Infection – local or systemic	Diligent catheter care and observation	Remove cannula and send tip for culture. Resite if necessary. Immobilise and elevate affected upper limb. Start empiric antibiotics if sepsis or septic shock is present
Damage to nearby structures such as nerves, directly or due to haematoma (e.g. compartment syndrome or carpal tunnel syndrome). Arteriovenous fistula. Femoral approach can be associated with bowel damage	Careful insertion technique. Seek assistance from experienced operator	Tailored to sequelae. Haematomas can develop into pseudoaneurysms requiring surgery

Table 12.2 Fast-flush test to assess dynamic response (damping) of the blood pressure-monitoring system

Make a paper record of transducer output
Snap the valve of the continuous flush system. This produces a square wave on the output trace
Repeat the process at least twice
Resonant frequency is the distance between successive peaks divided by the paper speed in millimetres per second
Damping is satisfactory (critical damping) if each snap test has two to three oscillation waves, with each wave one-third or less the size of the preceding wave

Disadvantages of such techniques can include:

- calibration against another method, such as thermodilution
- recalibration every few hours is advisable to allow for changes in systemic vascular resistance. This is especially important if there is haemodynamic instability or during the administration of vasoactive drugs
- alterations in abdominal pressure or changes in body position, particularly in the obese, can alter aortic compliance, necessitating recalibration
- dependence on arterial site. Clinical validation studies usually document femoral cannulation
- aortic aneurysms and significant aortic regurgitation are both difficult to model and invalidate the technique

Recently developed proprietary algorithms continuously measure stroke volume and cardiac output without requiring calibration against another method.[11] Additional clinical validation is awaited.

CENTRAL VENOUS CATHETERISATION (CVC)

CVC is indicated for monitoring of central venous pressure (CVP) and administration of certain drugs and parenteral nutrition. Modified catheters are also available which continuously monitor central venous oxygen saturation ($S_{cv}O_2$). Contraindications to CVC are relative and reflect potential complications of the procedure (Table 12.3). These should be considered in selecting the site for catheter insertion. Particular attention should be paid to the coagulation profile and factors which affect coagulation such as thrombolysis and activated protein C therapy.

Traditionally, puncture of the central vein is performed by passing a needle along the anticipated line of the vein

Table 12.3 Complications of central venous catheterisation, with preventive and treatment options[62]

Complication	Prevention	Treatment
Intravascular loss of guidewire	Ensure guidewire is always secured. Avoid retracting guidewire into insertion needle. Seek assistance from experienced operator	Interventional radiology or surgery may be required for retrieval
Air embolism	Proper patient positioning, including Trendelenburg (head-down tilt) for jugular or subclavian insertion. Consider alternative insertion sites. Ensure connections are tight	Left lateral Trendelenburg position. Administer 100% oxygen and ventilatory support. If catheter in place, tighten all connections and attempt to aspirate air. Basic/advanced life support if necessary
Dysrhythmias and conduction defects such as right bundle branch block	Continuous electrocardiographic monitoring during insertion. Correct placement of catheter tip	Withdraw or remove guidewire or catheter
Damage to nearby structures: Pneumothorax/haemothorax/chylothorax/hydrothorax, particularly with approaches to subclavian vein. Nerve injury such as phrenic, recurrent laryngeal, Horner's syndrome. Arterial puncture – including injury to carotid, subclavian, aorta or pulmonary artery. Haematoma, pseudoaneurysm, arteriovenous fistula can result. Stroke may result from carotid artery injury. Tracheal injury. Femoral approach can be associated with bowel damage	Identify risk factors such as previous surgery, skeletal deformity or scarring at site of insertion. Seek assistance from experienced operator. Select insertion site depending on impact of potential complications. Consider ultrasound guidance. Scheduled, routine replacement of catheter increases risk of mechanical complications	Tailored to sequelae
Line disconnection and bleeding	Minimise connections. Proper catheter care and observation	Control bleeding. Transfusion may be necessary
Infection – local or systemic (including endocarditis)	Aseptic insertion technique. Lower risk with subclavian compared to internal jugular or femoral insertion. Antimicrobial-impregnated catheters. Disinfect catheter hubs. Routine scheduled resiting appears not to reduce systemic infection rates. Remove catheter when no longer required	Remove catheter; resite if necessary. Culture blood and catheter tip. Start empiric antibiotics if sepsis or septic shock is present
Superior vena caval erosion can result in haemothorax or cardiac tamponade	Remove catheter when no longer required	Early detection and surgical intervention
Thrombosis	Remove catheter when no longer required. Subclavian insertion lower risk than internal jugular or femoral	Anticoagulation, vascular or endovascular intervention may be required

with reference to surface anatomical landmarks (landmark method). Catheterisation is usually achieved via the subclavian, internal jugular or external jugular veins into the superior vena cava.[12] The median cubital and basilic veins are used less commonly. Access to the subclavian vein is usually via the infraclavicular approach, but the supraclavicular approach is safe and reliable in experienced hands.

The use of ultrasound has been advocated to optimise the success rate of CVC insertion and minimise complications.[13] Two-dimensional imaging can be used to localise the vein and define anatomy prior to placement of a CVC by standard landmark techniques. Ultrasound can also provide real-time, two-dimensional guidance during CVC insertion. Alternatively, audio-guided Doppler ultrasound can aid localisation of the vein and differentiate it from its companion artery during CVC insertion.

In 2002, the UK National Institute for Clinical Excellence issued guidelines recommending the use of ultrasound for elective catheterisation of the internal jugular vein, and consideration of ultrasound guidance in most clinical situations.[14] These recommendations for ultrasound-guided internal jugular catheterisation are supported by meta-analysis.[15] However, there are limited data supporting its use for subclavian and femoral veins.

The right tracheobronchial angle and carina are common radiological markers of insertion depth. In an attempt to reduce further the incidence of venous erosion (which is rare but potentially catastrophic), some practitioners place the catheter tip lower in superior vena cava or even in the upper right atrium, ensuring that the catheter is parallel to the long axis of the vein so that the tip does not abut the vein or heart wall end-on.[16]

Femoral venous catheterisation with radiological positioning of the tip close to the right atrium produces pressure measurements in good agreement with the subclavian CVP.[17]

CENTRAL VENOUS PRESSURE

Jugular venous pressure, CVP and right atrial pressure (RAP) are often used interchangeably. However, in situations associated with increased central venous resistance, such as central vein sclerosis, these pressures may not be the same.

The normal CVP in the spontaneously breathing supine patient is 0–5 mmHg, while 10 mmHg is generally accepted as the upper limit during mechanical ventilation. In health there is a good correlation between CVP and pulmonary artery occlusion pressures (PAOP), but this is lost in many types of critical illness such as pulmonary hypertension, pulmonary embolism, right ventricular infarction, left ventricular hypertrophy and myocardial ischaemia. The relationship between CVP and right ventricular end-diastolic volume (RVEDV: preload) is altered in critical illness by changes in right ventricular diastolic compliance and juxtacardiac pressures.[18]

Except at extreme values, static measures of CVP do not differentiate patients likely to respond to fluid therapy from non-responders. However, dynamic changes in CVP either in response to volume loading or related to respiration can assist in evaluating volume status.[19] For instance, a steep increase in CVP following volume challenge suggests the heart is functioning on the plateau portion of the Frank–Starling curve. Severe hypotension with a low or normal CVP is unlikely to be due to acute pulmonary embolism, cardiac tamponade or tension pneumothorax.

Although fluid manometry is sufficient to measure the CVP, the frequency response is low and waveform analysis impossible (Table 12.4). Therefore, an electrical transducer system is normally used.

In a trend toward less invasive monitoring, peripheral venous pressure and non-invasive estimates of CVP have demonstrated potential as alternatives to direct CVP measurement.[20,21]

$S_{cv}O_2$

A recent prospective randomised study of patients with severe sepsis and septic shock demonstrated a survival advantage with the use of this monitoring technique and an emergency department treatment protocol (early goal-directed therapy).[22] $S_{cv}O_2$ has been proposed as a marker of tissue hypoxia (see Chapter 14). It is mentioned here as an example of the scant data relating haemodynamic monitoring to improved survival.

Table 12.4 Analysis of central venous pressure waveform

Condition	Pressure changes	Waveform changes
Tricuspid regurgitation	Increased RA pressure	Prominent v-wave, x descent obliterated, y descent steep
Right ventricular infarction	RA and RV pressure elevated. RAP does not fall and may rise in inspiration	Prominent x and y descents
Constrictive pericarditis	RA, RV diastolic, PA diastolic and occlusion pressures elevated and equalised. RAP may rise in inspiration	Prominent x and y descents
Pericardial tamponade	RA, RV diastolic, PA diastolic and occlusion pressures elevated and equalised. RAP usually falls in inspiration	y descent damped or absent

RA, right atrial; RV, right ventricular; RAP, right atrial pressure; PA, pulmonary artery.

PULMONARY ARTERY CATHETER

Right-heart catheterisation using a flow-directed balloon-tipped catheter was introduced by Swan and Ganz in 1970.[23] The ability to monitor sophisticated haemodynamic and gas exchange variables at the bedside appealed to clinicians, and the PAC was rapidly accepted into routine critical care.

In 1996 a non-randomised cohort study of PAC use in American teaching hospitals appeared to show that, in any of nine major disease categories, PAC in the first 24 hours increased 30-day mortality (odds ratio 1.24, 95% confidence interval (CI) 1.03–1.49), mean length of stay and mean cost per hospital stay.[24] A simultaneous editorial called for a moratorium on PAC use, and for a prospective multicentre trial.[25]

A subsequent Cochrane database systematic review of PAC monitoring in adult ICU patients incorporated data from two recent multicentre trials and 10 other studies.[26] The pooled mortality odds ratio for studies of general ICU patients was 1.05 (95% CI 0.87–1.26) and for studies of high-risk surgery patients was 0.99 (95% CI 0.73–1.24). PAC monitoring had no impact on ICU or hospital length of stay (where reported). A recent multicentre trial incorporating protocolised haemodynamic management of patients with acute lung injury compared PAC-guided with CVC-guided therapy.[27] There were no significant differences in 60-day mortality or organ function between groups. Overall, these data suggest that PAC monitoring in critically ill patients is not associated with increased mortality or with survival benefit.

On the other hand, recent data suggest a differential association between PAC use and mortality dependent upon severity of illness. Logistic regression analyses of data from a tertiary-care university teaching hospital[28] and from the National Trauma Data Bank (American College of Surgeons)[29] suggest that PAC use may be associated with survival benefit in the most severely ill/injured patients.

Overall, the PAC still finds application as a haemodynamic monitoring tool in the ICU and the operating room. However, its role is under increasing scrutiny, and continues to decline in favour of less invasive alternatives. It could be argued that future PAC use should be guided by studies to determine optimal management protocols and appropriate patient groups.[26]

Traditional indications for PAC monitoring have been to:

- characterise haemodynamic perturbation (e.g. distributive, cardiogenic, obstructive and hypovolaemic shock or combinations)
- differentiate cardiogenic from non-cardiogenic pulmonary oedema
- guide use of vasoactive drugs, fluids (including renal replacement therapy) and diuretics, especially when haemodynamic disturbances are coupled with increased lung water, right ventricular or left ventricular dysfunction, pulmonary hypertension and organ dysfunction

Contraindications for insertion reflect those for CVC. If known in advance, atypical cardiac or vascular anatomy, either congenital or secondary to trauma or surgery, should also be considered. Less invasive monitoring might provide the data that are sought. Also, PAC monitoring does not exclude simultaneous recourse to other monitoring techniques.

CATHETER INSERTION[30]

A 7.5–9 F 15-cm introducer sheath is first inserted by the Seldinger technique. The subclavian and internal jugular veins are most commonly used. Access is feasible with the 110-cm catheter via the median cubital, basilic and femoral veins. The external jugular veins can also be used, although difficulty may be encountered passing the introducer both into the vein and then subsequently below the clavicle into the subclavian vein.

Balloon volume is 1.5 ml. The balloon should be tested prior to insertion into the sheath. Deflation should always occur passively to minimise the risk of balloon damage. Before passage through the heart the balloon should be inflated to assist flow guidance and protect against myocardial injury and dysrhythmias. Inflation should not be forced, and should not alter the waveform prior to wedging. The right atrium is reached at 15–20 cm from the internal jugular vein, 10–15 cm from the subclavian vein, 30–40 cm from the femoral vein and 40 and 50 cm respectively from the right and left basilic veins. The right ventricle and pulmonary artery (PA) are then entered at additional 10-cm intervals, with a further 10 cm to PA occlusion.[31] Waveforms seen as the catheter floats to the wedged position are shown in Figure 12.1.

MEASURED VARIABLES

The PAC remains unique in its ability to measure right ventricular and pulmonary arterial pressures directly at the bedside. In acute respiratory distress syndrome (ARDS), where pulmonary hypertension and increased right ventricular afterload are linked to excess mortality,[32] a PAC can assist in the titration of afterload-reducing therapies such as inhaled prostacyclin or nitric oxide.

In this context echocardiography might be considered as a less invasive alternative, since it provides a qualitative assessment of right ventricular loading[33] and can estimate PA pressures via Doppler techniques.[34] However, these are largely confined to intermittent 'snapshot' assessments, and can be challenging in mechanically ventilated patients.

Normal pressures are given in Table 12.5.

PULMONARY ARTERY OCCLUSION PRESSURE

Measurements of PAOP should be performed by slow injection of air into the balloon while watching the PA waveform. Overwedging can lead to falsely high occlusion pressures or pulmonary arterial rupture. Less than 1.5 ml air may be required. Deflation after PAOP measurement should re-establish the normal pulmonary

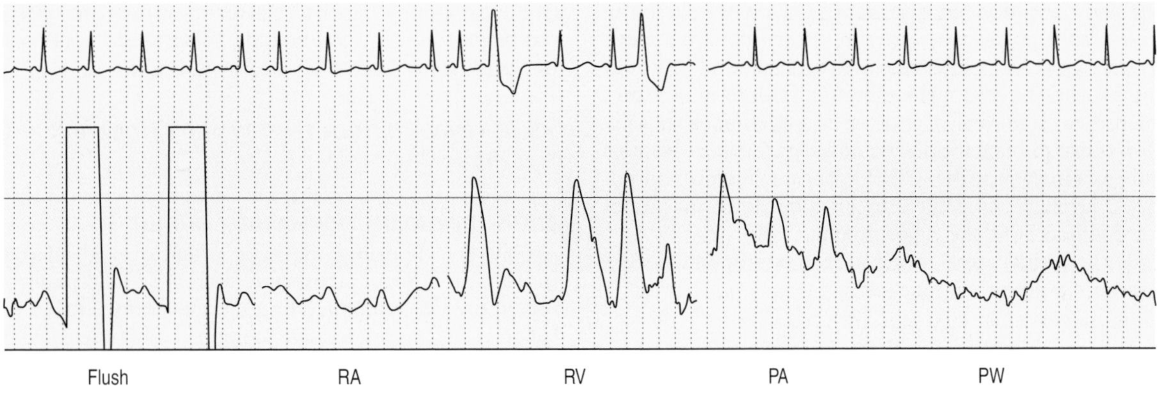

Figure 12.1 Pressure tracings and electrocardiogram (ECG) trace obtained on insertion of a pulmonary artery catheter. The snap flush test confirms an appropriate frequency response and degree of damping. RA, right atrial trace; RV, right ventricular trace (note simultaneous premature ventricular contractions during RV passage of the catheter); PA, pulmonary artery trace (note dichrotic notch and elevated diastolic pressure); PW, pulmonary wedge trace (note respiratory variation). (Reproduced with permission from Leatherman JW, Marini JJ. Pulmonary artery catheterization: interpretation of pressure recordings. In: Tobin MJ (ed.) *Principles and Practice of Intensive Care Monitoring.* New York: McGraw Hill; 1998: 822.)

Table 12.5 Measured and derived variables from pulmonary artery catheter

Site	mmHg	kPa
Right atrium: mean	−1–7	0.13–0.93
Right ventricle: systolic	15–25	2.0–3.3
Right ventricle: diastolic	0–8	0–1.1
Pulmonary artery: systolic	15–25	2.0–3.3
Pulmonary artery: diastolic	8–15	1.1–2.0
Pulmonary artery: mean	10–20	1.3–2.6
Pulmonary artery occlusion pressure	6–15	0.8–2.0

arterial waveform. If not, distal migration has occurred and the catheter should be withdrawn until the waveform is re-established.

PAOP should be measured during end-expiration and ideally in end-diastole, using the electrocardiogram (ECG) P-wave as a marker. PAOP has been termed the back-pressure to pulmonary blood flow,[35] and is also a key determinant of pulmonary capillary pressure (see below) and hence extravascular lung water. When the catheter wedges in a branch of the PA it creates a static column of blood which equilibrates with downstream pressure at the site where it rejoins the flowing pulmonary venous system (the j point). Here the blood is very near the left atrium. PAOP therefore closely approximates left atrial pressure (LAP), which approximates left ventricular end-diastolic pressure (LVEDP). The validity of PAOP as a surrogate of preload depends on a number of assumptions (Figure 12.2). These assumptions are often incorrect in critically ill patients and the use of PAOP to reflect preload has been questioned.[36]

Zone 3 or not?[37]

The catheter tip usually floats to a level at or below the left atrium. To maintain a column of fluid between the

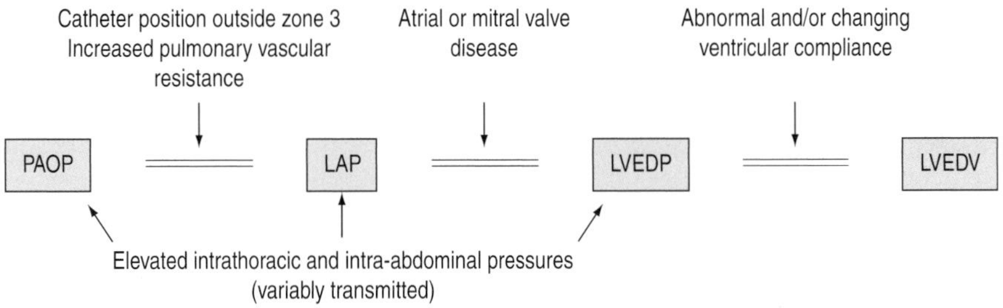

Figure 12.2 Factors affecting the accuracy of pulmonary artery occlusion pressure (PAOP) as a measure of preload in critically ill patients. Clinically, left ventricular end-diastolic volume (LVEDV) is usually accepted as a surrogate of preload. LAP, left atrial pressure; LVEDP, left ventricular end-diastolic pressure.

pressure transducer and the LAP, the tip should be in West's zone 3 (alveolar pressure < pulmonary venous pressure). Factors which increase the likelihood of wedging in zones 1 and 2 include high intrathoracic pressures when there is normal or increased lung compliance (e.g. obstructive pulmonary disease and high intrinsic positive end-expiratory pressure (PEEP)) and low cardiac output states. Here, rotating the relevant lung down maximises the likelihood of zone 3 positioning.

At the bedside, tests which suggest appropriate zone 3 catheter tip positioning include:

- tip of the catheter at or below the left atrium on lateral supine chest radiograph
- clearly delineated atrial waveforms
- respiratory variation of PAOP is ≤ 50% static airway pressure (peak – plateau)
- PAOP alters by < 50% of PEEP alterations

Waveform analysis

As with CVP, analysis of the PAOP waveform may give some indication of cardiac pathology. Constrictive pericarditis and pericardial tamponade show the same abnormalities (but less clearly) as in the CVP trace. Mitral regurgitation may cause a large v-wave, which may be confused with the PA waveform. The two can be distinguished by examining the timing of the waves relative to the T-wave of the ECG. The peak of the PA systolic wave occurs before and the v-wave occurs after the T-wave. Large v-waves may also be associated with mitral stenosis, congestive heart failure or ventricular septal defect.

Potential substitutes for PAOP

Measurement of PAOP requires wedging, which is associated with a number of risks (Table 12.6). The normal PA diastolic pressure (PADP) to PAOP gradient is < 5 mmHg, so that PADP may normally be used as a close approximation for PAOP. However, tachycardia (> 120 beats/min) and conditions that increase pulmonary vascular resistance (such as ARDS, chronic obstructive pulmonary disease and pulmonary embolism) variably increase this gradient, invalidating direct substitution of PADP for PAOP. The relationship between PADP and PAOP tends to be stable over hours. Once this is determined, PADP can be used to track PAOP in the short term without repeated wedge manoeuvres.

Echocardiographic (non-invasive) estimation of PAOP has recently been described in critically ill patients.[38]

PULMONARY CAPILLARY HYDROSTATIC PRESSURE (P_{cap})[39]

P_{cap} tends to force fluid out of the pulmonary capillaries into the interstitium, and when elevated can contribute to the development of pulmonary oedema. In critical illness such as ARDS and sepsis, variability in the distribution of the precapillary and postcapillary resistance alters the relationship between P_{cap} and PAOP. Because of this, a normal PAOP may substantially underestimate the tendency for fluid leakage from the pulmonary capillaries. Although it can be challenging, measurement of P_{cap} can be performed at the bedside by analysis of a pressure transient after an acute PA occlusion (Figure 12.3).

MIXED VENOUS OXYGEN TENSION AND SATURATION

See Chapter 14.

BOLUS THERMODILUTION CARDIAC OUTPUT

A bolus injection into the right atrium of cold injectate (usually 5% dextrose) transiently decreases blood temperature in the PA (monitored by a thermistor proximal to the balloon). The mean decrease in temperature (calculated by integrating temperature over time) is inversely proportional to the cardiac output, which can be determined by a modification of the Stewart–Hamilton equation:

$$Q = \frac{V \times (Tb - Ti)K1 \times K2}{Tb(t)dt}$$

where Q = cardiac output; V = volume injected; Tb = blood temperature; Ti = injectate temperature; $K1$ and $K2$ = corrections for specific heat and density of injectate and for blood and dead space volumes; and $Tb(t)dt$ = change in blood temperature as a function of time.

This is an indicator dilution method, using temperature change instead of indocyanine green dye, radioisotopes or chemicals such as sodium thiocyanate and hypertonic saline. Advantages are:

- The indicator is non-toxic.
- It does not recirculate. Repeat measurements are limited only by volume constraints and the time to regain temperature stability between injections.
- The method shows good agreement with the Fick and indocyanine green methods. However, there is considerable variability. A clinically significant change in cardiac output cannot be diagnosed with certainty unless there is a difference of approximately 15% between the mean of three cardiac output determinations and the previous mean.[40]

Too much or too little injectate will respectively underestimate and overestimate cardiac output. Cold injectate (preferably 0–4°C, but up to 12°C is usually accepted) improves the signal-to-noise ratio, but causes a brief decrease in heart rate, reducing cardiac output while it is being measured. Room temperature injectate introduces a small decrement in bias and precision, but has acceptable accuracy. However, the accuracy using room temperature injectate is further degraded at extremes of cardiac index, high ambient temperatures (and thus injectate temperature) or in patient hypothermia.[29]

Respiration causes fluctuations in cardiac output and PA temperature. Reproducibility is improved by taking measurements in expiration, though this may not reflect cardiac output throughout the respiratory cycle. Timing can be difficult and in practice an average of three evenly spaced measurements is taken. Causes of inaccurate measurements are listed in Table 12.7.

Table 12.6 Complications encountered with the pulmonary artery catheter (PAC) with proposed measures for prevention and treatment[63]

Complications	Prevention	Treatment
During insertion		
Damage to adjacent structures	As for central venous cannulation	As for central venous cannulation
Perforation of pulmonary artery	Ensure balloon inflated throughout insertion. Continuously monitor pulmonary artery waveform. Avoid distal PAC tip position	As for pulmonary artery rupture below
Air embolism	Raise venous pressure prior to insertion. Always occlude open ends during insertion. Use sheaths with pneumatic valve. Periodically check and tighten all connections. Remove air from fluid bag and tubing. Dress site with occlusive dressing after removal	Left lateral Trendelenburg position. Administer 100% oxygen and ventilatory support. If PAC in place, tighten all connections and attempt to aspirate air from right atrium or right ventricle. Basic/advanced life support if necessary
Dysrhythmia	Keep balloon inflated during passage from RA to PA. Minimise insertion time	For sustained ventricular tachycardia, remove PAC from right ventricle. For ventricular fibrillation, remove PAC and defibrillate
Right bundle branch block/complete heart block	Avoid PAC insertion in patients with left bundle branch block (LBBB) if possible. Insert PAC with pacing electrodes in patients with LBBB	Use pacing equipment as required
Catheter knotting/kinking	Minimise insertion time. Do not advance catheter against resistance. Check for waveform change from RA to RV or RV to PA after advancing 15 cm; if not, withdraw catheter	Check chest X-ray. Pull knot back then remove the sheath and catheter. If no sheath used, a cut-down to vein under local anaesthesia may be required. Exploration by a vascular surgeon is indicated if unsuccessful (5% of occasions)
Valve damage	Ensure balloon is inflated during forward passage through the heart and deflated prior to any retraction	Cardiothoracic consultation
During maintenance		
Dysrhythmia (37%)	Remove PAC when no longer required	See above
Thrombosis	As for central venous cannulation	As for central venous cannulation
Pulmonary artery rupture (0.2%)	Risk factors include pulmonary hypertension, anticoagulation and in situ duration $>$ 3 days. Maintain high level of suspicion. Avoid distal PAC tip position. Minimise wedge procedures. Continuously monitor pulmonary artery waveform – withdraw PAC if spontaneous wedging occurs, inflate with only enough air to change PA to PAOP waveform. Withdraw PAC if PAOP obtained with $<$ 1.25 ml air	Check PAC position on chest X-ray, deflate and pull back. If applicable, stop anticoagulation therapy. Lateral position, affected side down. Selective bronchial intubation. PEEP. Surgical repair
Pulmonary infarction	As for pulmonary artery rupture	Check PAC position on chest X-ray, deflate and pull back. Observe
Infection – including endocarditis	As for central venous cannulation	As for central venous cannulation
Air embolism	High suspicion of balloon rupture. Avoid repeating failed attempts to inflate	See above

RA, right atrial; PA, pulmonary artery; RV, right ventricular; PEEP, positive end-expiratory pressure; PAOP, pulmonary artery occlusion pressure.

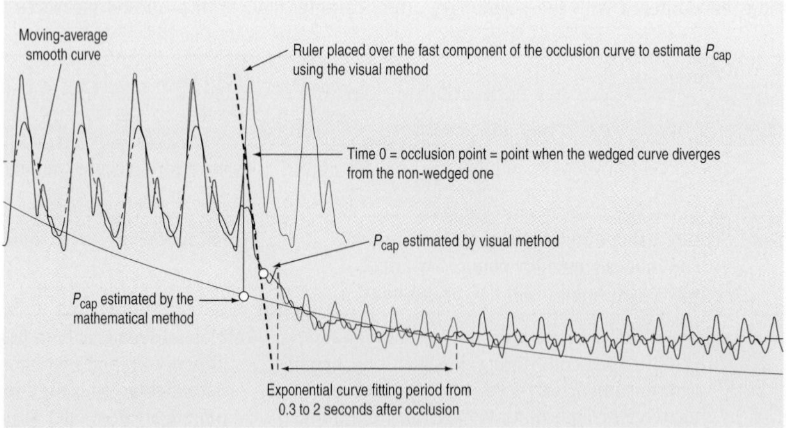

Figure 12.3 Capillary pressure (P_{cap}) has been estimated from the pulmonary artery pressure decay following occlusion with balloon inflation. For better visualisation the occlusion trace is superimposed on a non-occluded trace, both recorded during an expiratory hold during mechanical ventilation. An additional trace using 20 data point moving average smoothing of the original trace (collected at 100 Hz) is superimposed on the curves. This further facilitates the visual estimation of the capillary pressure by defining more exactly the point of divergence of the occluded and non-occluded curves. In addition, an exponential curve has been fitted on the curve 0.3–2 s after occlusion. This fitted curve has then been extrapolated to the time of occlusion to provide the capillary pressure. (Reproduced from Takala J. Pulmonary capillary pressure. *Intens Care Med* 2003; **29**: 890–3, Figure 1, with kind permission of Springer Science and Business Media.)

Table 12.7 Causes of inaccurate bolus thermodilution cardiac output measurements

Catheter malposition
Wedge position
Thermistor impinging on vessel wall
Abnormal respiratory pattern
Intracardiac shunts
Tricuspid regurgitation (common in mechanically ventilated patients)
Cardiac dysrhythmias
Incorrect recording of injectate temperature (minimised by siting thermistor on injection port)
Rapid intravenous infusions, especially if administered via the introducer sheath
Injectate port close to or within introducer sheath
Abnormal haematocrit values (affecting *K*2 value)
Extremes of cardiac output (room temperature injectate)
Poor technique
Slow injection (> 4 s)
Incorrect injectate volume

SEMICONTINUOUS THERMODILUTION CARDIAC OUTPUT[41]

This method uses the same principles as bolus thermodilution, but allows semicontinuous measurement by employing a thermal filament wrapped around the right ventricular segment of the catheter. This transmits low-power pulses of heat. 'On–off' heat pulses in pseudorandom binary code are delivered in cycles. The downstream thermistor detects the heat pulses, which are then cross-correlated with the input sequence and power (to allow differentiation of thermal signal from noise).

The method shows good experimental agreement with the Fick and bolus thermodilution methods, with bias and precision in the ranges of −0.08 to +0.35 and 0.5–1.2 l/min respectively.

Drawbacks of the technique are:

- inaccuracy during thermal disequilibrium,[42] such as rapid infusions of cool fluids or after cardiac bypass
- delay in detecting sudden changes in cardiac output[42]
- magnetic resonance imaging is contraindicated (it can melt the thermal filament)
- electrocautery can interfere with measurements

DERIVED VARIABLES

A number of variables can be derived from the measurements obtained with a standard PAC (Table 12.8).

VOLUMETRIC PAC[43]

A recently available PAC incorporating a rapid-response thermistor allows semicontinuous assessment of cardiac output, right ventricular ejection fraction (RVEF) and RVEDV. This algorithm supersedes RVEDV based on bolus thermodilution. The new algorithm uses the slaved electrocardiograph signal and generates a relaxation waveform, which resembles the bolus thermodilution washout decay curve. The waveform is generated by accumulating the temperature change for each on- and each off-segment of the input signal. Calculation of RVEF is based on estimation of the exponential decay time constant (t) of this curve and heart rate (HR):

$$\text{RVEF} = 1 - \exp(-60/[t \times \text{HR}])$$

Table 12.8 Derived haemodynamic variables

Parameter	Abbreviation	Formula	Normal range	Units
Mean arterial pressure	MAP	DBP + 0.33 × (SBP − DBP)	70–105	mmHg
Mean pulmonary artery pressure	MPAP	PADP + 0.33 × (PASP − PADP)	9–16	mmHg
Mean right ventricular pressure	MRVP	CVP + 0.33 × (PASP − CVP)		mmHg
LV coronary perfusion pressure	LVCPP	DBP − PAOP		mmHg
RV coronary perfusion pressure	RVCPP	MAP − MRVP		mmHg
Cardiac index	CI	CO/BSA	2.8 – 4.2	l/min per m^2
Stroke volume index	SVI	CI/HR	35 – 70	ml/beat per m^2
Systemic vascular resistance index	SVRI	(MAP − CVP)/CI × 79.92	1760 – 2600	dyn s/cm^5 per m^2
Pulmonary vascular resistance index	PVRI	(PAP − PAOP)/CI × 79.92	44 – 225	dyn s/cm^5 per m^2
Left ventricular stroke work index	LVSWI	SVI × MAP × 0.0144	44 – 68	g m/m^2 per beat
Right ventricular stroke work index	RVSWI	SVI × PAP × 0.0144	4 – 8	g m/m^2 per beat
Body surface area	BSA	Weight $(kg)^{0.425}$ × height $(cm)^{0.725}$ × 0.007184		m^2

DBP, diastolic blood pressure; SBP, systolic blood pressure; PADP, pulmonary artery diastolic pressure; PASP, pulmonary artery systolic pressure; CVP, central venous pressure; LV, left ventricular; PAOP, pulmonary artery occlusion pressure; RV, right ventricular; CO, cardiac output; HR, heart rate.

RVEDV is calculated from cardiac output (CO) and RVEF as follows:

$$RVEDV = (CO/HR)/RVEF$$

The correlation between thermodilution RVEDV and thermodilution cardiac output is not fully explained by mathematical coupling of these variables.[44] Thermodilution techniques appear to overestimate RVEDV and underestimate RVEF.[45] However, right ventricular geometry is complex and there are limited options for bedside volumetric evaluation.

COMPLICATIONS OF PAC

These are listed in Table 12.6. A catheter may not actually be knotted, despite a chest X-ray appearance to suggest this. If knotting is suspected, other catheters should be removed in reverse order to which they were inserted, and the chest X-ray repeated.

TRANSPULMONARY INDICATOR DILUTION

With this technique, thermal and other indicators injected into a central vein are detected in a systemic artery. Because the indicators pass through all chambers of the heart as well as the entire pulmonary circulation, information additional to cardiac output can be gained. In particular, central blood volumes and indices of extravascular lung water can be quantified (Figure 12.4).

TRANSPULMONARY THERMODILUTION[8,46]

A fibreoptic thermistor is positioned in the femoral artery at the tip of a modified 4F arterial catheter. Cardiac output is measured by administering a central venous bolus of cold injectate, constructing an arterial thermodilution curve and applying the Stewart–Hamilton equation. The axillary artery can also be used, but placing the sensor in more peripheral arteries such as the radial causes overestimation of cardiac output. Curves are longer and flatter than PAC curves due to thermal equilibration with intrathoracic blood and extravascular lung water, but are unaffected by the respiratory phase of injection. Measurements are in good agreement with pulmonary thermodilution and direct Fick methods. There is a positive bias of about 5%, perhaps because of indicator loss, or because transpulmonary measurements are less affected by the transient decrease in heart rate induced by cold thermodilution.

USE OF A SECOND INDICATOR

Combining thermal dilution with simultaneous dye dilution is the basis of the double-indicator technique. Indocyanine green is used because it is non-toxic and highly

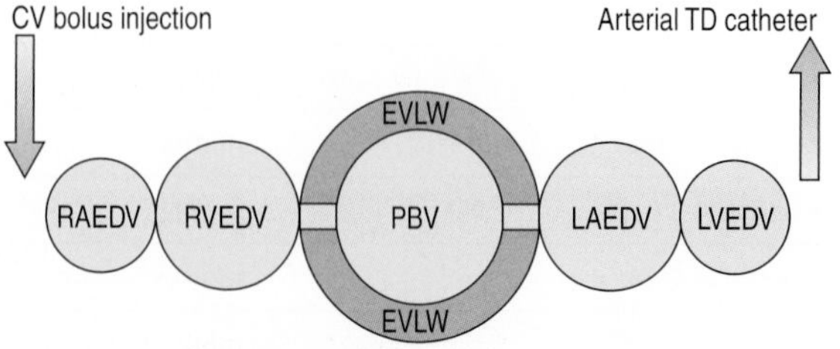

Figure 12.4 Diagrammatic representation of the mixing chambers of the cardiopulmonary system. CV, central venous; EVLW, extravascular lung water; LAEDV, left atrial end-diastolic volume; LVEDV, left ventricular end-diastolic volume; PBV, pulmonary blood volume; RAEDV, right atrial end-diastolic volume; RVEDV, right ventricular end-diastolic volume; TD, thermodilution. ITTV is the whole volume between the points of injection and detection, including the EVLW. Pulmonary thermal volume (PTV) is the sum of PBV + EVLW. ITBV is the sum of RAEDV + RVEDV + PBV + LAEDV + LVEDV. EVLW = ITTV – ITBV. GEDV is the sum of RAEDV + RVEDV + LAEDV + LVEDV. (Reproduced from Hudson ERGN, Beale RF. Lung water and blood volume measurements in the critically ill. *Curr Opin Crit Care* 2000; **6**: 222–6.)

albumin-bound, remaining confined to the intravascular space on its initial circulation. Rapid-response measurements can now be achieved using an in vivo fibreoptic sensor at the catheter tip.

Calculations

The equilibration volumes for each indicator between injection and detection points are calculated as the product of the transpulmonary thermodilution cardiac output (CO_{TPTD}) and the mean transit time (MTT), where MTT is first determined from a semilogarithmic transformation of the indicator dilution curve. Hence:

$$CO_{TPTD} \times MTT_{dye} = \text{intrathoracic blood volume (ITBV)}$$
$$CO_{TPTD} \times MIT_{thermal} = \text{intrathoracic thermal volume (ITTV)}$$
$$ITTV - ITBV = \text{extravascular lung water (EVLW)}$$

Indocyanine green concentrations after complete mixing can then be used to calculate the circulating blood volume and the subsequent concentration decay can serve as a liver function test.

ITBV

Unlike CVP and PAOP, ITBV is a volumetric preload index. Interpretation is thus independent of alterations in juxtacardiac pressures or myocardial compliance, and should be superior to conventional pressure indices. There is experimental and clinical evidence that this is so.[47]

EVLW[48]

EVLW is a marker of the severity of illness. Following EVLW as a therapeutic end-point may reduce positive fluid balances and ventilator and ICU days. EVLW also appears to offer prognostic information in sepsis and acute lung injury.

EXTENDED APPLICATION OF TRANSPULMONARY THERMODILUTION (SINGLE INDICATOR)[8,46]

This approach retains the advantages of the double indicator method, while being much easier and less expensive, and thermodilution-derived EVLW* and ITBV* show good agreement with the double-indicator method. (Note: asterisks differentiate parameters derived from the single-indicator method (EVLW* and ITBV*) from the identically named/labelled double-indicator parameters.) However, errors in volume measurement may occur in the presence of large aortic aneurysms, intracardiac shunts, pulmonary embolism or acute changes in chamber size (such as recent pulmonary lobectomy or pneumonectomy).

The pulmonary thermal volume (PTV; Figure 12.4) can be determined from the product of cardiac output and the 'exponential downslope time' (DST) on the semilogarithmic thermodilution curve. This relationship assumes that the majority of temperature decay occurs in the largest mixing chamber (PTV). This allows calculation of the global end-diastolic volume (GEDV), which is said to represent the volume of blood in all chambers of the heart at end-diastole. Hence:

$$ITTV - PTV = GEDV$$

ITBV* can be derived as a linear function of GEDV:

$$ITBV^* = 1.25 \times GEDV - 28.4\ \text{ml}$$

Like ITBV, GEDV has been shown to be a more reliable measure of cardiac preload than conventional pressure-based surrogates.[49] Interpretation of measurements should account for the lack of differentiation between left and right cardiac volumes. For example, the clinical context and supplemental data may be important in differentiating acute cor pulmonale from left ventricular failure. Both these conditions could result in elevated ITBV/GEDV but require different therapy. Also low ITBV/GEDV does not mandate fluid challenge. For instance, low ITBV/GEDV in the setting of restrictive or constrictive pathology might not represent inadequate intravascular volume. These conditions may be associated with high CVP despite low ITBV/GEDV.

A device is available which employs transpulmonary thermodilution both to measure EVLW* and the preload indices ITBV* and GEDV, and to calibrate continuous cardiac output measurements by the pulse contour technique. The method is suitable for small children, in whom PAC is not feasible.

LITHIUM DILUTION CARDIAC OUTPUT[50]

Lithium can also serve as a transpulmonary indicator. The small doses of lithium required are non-toxic and easily measured with an ion-selective electrode. Following injection, there is no significant first-pass loss from the circulation. Blood is sampled from an arterial line via a three-way tap. A peristaltic pump limits sampling to 4 ml/min. After passing through the sensor, blood is discarded.

The main advantage over thermodilution is that more peripheral arteries such as the radial can be used without loss of accuracy. Also, injection can be performed peripherally if central venous access is unavailable. The technique shows good agreement with bolus thermodilution (PAC). It is able to measure cardiac output safely and accurately in adult and paediatric populations.

Limitations include:

- It cannot be used in patients receiving lithium therapy (background lithium concentration contributes to overestimation of cardiac output).
- Electrode drift can occur in the presence of high peak doses of muscle relaxants.
- Abnormal shunts can result in erroneous cardiac output measurements (true for all indicator dilution methods).
- Ex vivo analysis requires disposal of sampled blood.

PULSED-DYE DENSITOMETRY[51]

Pulsed-dye densitometry allows intermittent cardiac output measurement based on transpulmonary dye dilution, with transcutaneous signal detection adapted from pulse oximetry. After central venous injection of indocyanine green, the concentration is estimated in the arterial blood by optical absorbance measurements. Using the Stewart–Hamilton formula, the cardiac output can be calculated from the resultant dye dilution curve.

Poor peripheral circulation, vasoconstriction, interstitial oedema, movement artefact and ambient light influences impair peripheral signal detection. This technique still has significant limitations.

ULTRASOUND

Two approaches are available to measure stroke volume (and thereby, cardiac output) using sound waves. The first involves the use of echocardiography to measure systolic and diastolic left ventricular volumes. Stroke volume is calculated as the difference between these two volumes. Access to expensive echocardiographic equipment and trained personnel limits the usefulness of this technique for haemodynamic monitoring. The second method uses Doppler techniques to measure stroke volume (Figure 12.5).[52] This approach is less dependent on image quality and shows better agreement with thermodilution.[53] Although ultrasonic measurements tend to be operator-dependent, Doppler measurement of aortic blood flow demonstrates good reproducibility (intraobserver, interobserver and day-to-day variability 3.2 ± 2.9%, 5.4 ± 3.4% and 3.3 ± 3.1%, respectively).[54]

The Doppler principle states that the frequency of reflected sound is altered by a moving target, such as red blood cells. Continuous and pulsed-wave Doppler are the main techniques employed to measure flow. Physical principles for the two techniques are similar. Pulsed-wave Doppler allows the site (depth) of sampling to be specified; the target sample is usually central laminar flow. With continuous-wave Doppler, a piezoelectric crystal transmits the ultrasound beam while another measures the frequency of

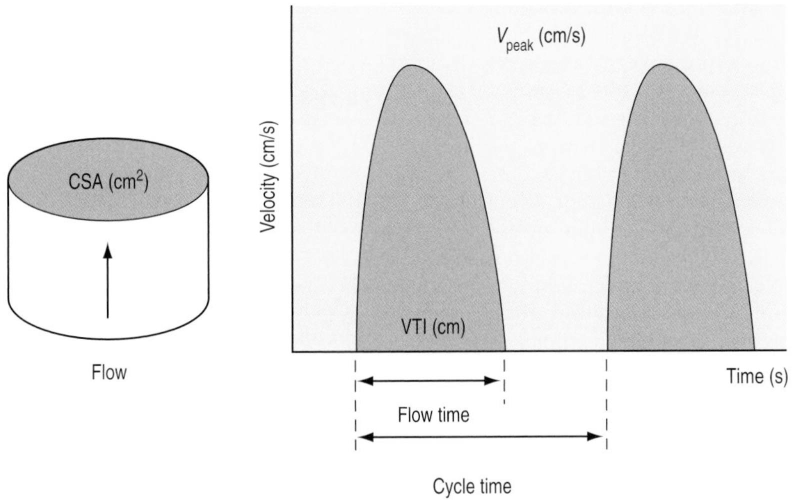

Figure 12.5 Doppler stroke volume calculation. The cross-sectional area (CSA) of flow is calculated as a circle from echocardiographic measurements or nomogram-based estimations. Velocity–time integral (VTI) is the integral of Doppler velocity with regard to time. Stroke volume (SV) is calculated as the product of CSA and VTI (ml/s in this example). Cardiac output is calculated from the product and SV and heart rate. Peak velocity of flow (V_{peak}) is also indicated.

reflected waves. The velocities of all the red blood cells moving along the path of the ultrasound beam are recorded. As a result, a continuous-wave Doppler recording consists of a full spectral envelope with the outer border corresponding to the fastest-moving blood cells. The flow velocity (V) of red cells can be determined from the Doppler shift in the frequency of reflected waves.

$$V = (2F_0 \times \cos\theta)^{-1} \times C\Delta F$$

where C is the speed of ultrasound in tissue (1540 m/s), ΔF is the frequency shift, F_0 is the emitted ultrasound frequency, and θ is the angle of incidence. The most accurate results are obtained when the ultrasound beam is parallel to flow ($\theta = 0°$, $\cos\theta = 1$; $\theta = 180°$, $\cos\theta = -1$). However, angles up to 20° still yield acceptable results ($\theta = 20°$, $\cos\theta = 0.94$).

In addition to measuring stroke volume, Doppler assessment of aortic blood flow can provide additional haemodynamic information. For instance, the duration of the aortic velocity signal corrected for heart rate (corrected flow time: FT_c) is inversely related to the systemic vascular resistance; hence, it is a marker of left ventricular afterload. A decrease in left ventricular preload can be associated with an increase in afterload (low FT_c). Other causes include excessive vasopressor doses, heart failure and hypothermia (all produce a low FT_c).[55] The peak velocity of aortic blood flow (V_{peak}) has been proposed as an index of contractility. Also, respiratory variation in V_{peak} (ΔV_{peak}) has been described as a predictor of increased cardiac output in response to fluid challenge.[56]

OESOPHAGEAL DOPPLER MONITORING[8,57]

Oesophageal Doppler measures blood flow velocity in the descending aorta with a Doppler probe (usually 4-MHz continuous wave or 5-MHz pulsed wave depending upon device) incorporated in the tip of a flexible probe. The probe is positioned in the oesophagus about 30–40 cm from the teeth. At this point, the aorta runs parallel to the oesophagus and the systolic cross-sectional area varies least. The probe is rotated to obtain a characteristic aortic signal. The aortic cross-sectional area is either determined from nomograms of age, weight and height, or calculated from a measured diameter (M-mode ultrasound). Calibration against other cardiac output methods is also possible.

Oesophageal Doppler appears to offer a useful alternative to thermodilution techniques for monitoring cardiac output and its variation. Moreover, randomised studies using the technique to guide fluid titration have demonstrated benefit in high-risk surgical patients. Lower complication rates and shorter hospital stay have been demonstrated after cardiac and abdominal surgery and after femur fracture fixation.

ADVANTAGES

- Only a short period of training is required. Nurses at the bedside can follow volume challenge protocols guided by Doppler indices.
- The probes (6 mm in diameter) are minimally invasive, and can be inserted nasally or orally.
- Contraindications are few. They include severe agitation, pharyngo-oesophageal pathology, aortic balloon counterpulsation, aortic dissection or severe aortic coarctation.[43]
- Insertion is simple, allowing reduced time to data acquisition and treatment.
- Probes are relatively stable once placed. If displaced they can be repositioned quickly, and can be left in place for days in a sedated, ventilated patient.

DISADVANTAGES

- Assumptions that descending aortic flow is 70% of total cardiac output and that nomograms accurately determine aortic cross-section can be incorrect. This limits usefulness when there is aortic pathology or compression, or abnormal upper-/lower-body blood flow distributions.
- Flow in the aorta is not always laminar. Conditions such as tachycardia, anaemia and aortic valve disease can cause turbulent aortic blood flow and alter velocity measurements.
- Assumptions that the aorta is cylindrical with a fixed systolic cross-section are not always valid. The cross-sectional area of the aorta is actually dynamic and is dependent on the pulse pressure and aortic compliance. This may be particularly relevant in children, where aortic cross-section fluctuates in systole.
- Finding and maintaining optimal probe positioning is important for consistency in trend measurements.
- The probe may be poorly tolerated in non-sedated patients. Oral insertion is usually reserved for intubated patients receiving sedation. Trends toward minimal sedation and shorter duration of endotracheal intubation might decrease the practicality of this technique in many patients.

TRANSCUTANEOUS DOPPLER MONITORING

In the past, stroke volume and cardiac output have been measured with varying success by placing Doppler probes externally at the cardiac apex and suprasternal notch. Recently, an external continuous-wave Doppler monitoring device capable of measuring transpulmonary (parasternal) and transaortic (suprasternal) cardiac output has become available. Flow diameters are estimated by a proprietary algorithm based upon the linear association between height and cardiovascular dimensions.[58] This allows measurement of stroke volume without two-dimensional echocardiographic measurements of valve diameters, which can be technically difficult.[52] If diameters are known, this information can be entered into the device.

Like oesophageal Doppler, this method appears to offer a clinically useful alternative to thermodilution techniques for monitoring cardiac output and its variation.[59] The technique can be used in all age groups and can be comfortably performed in non-sedated patients.

PARTIAL REBREATHING OF CO_2[8,10,51]

The Fick principle is an extension of the law of conservation of mass and states that the amount of a substance taken up by an organ (or the whole body) per unit time is the product of the arteriovenous concentration difference by the blood flow to the organ (or body). Historically it has been used to determine cardiac output by analysing oxygen uptake from the lungs (direct Fick method). This method requires PA catheterisation to sample mixed venous blood. Traditionally, it has been considered the 'gold standard', but in most ICU patients the stringent preconditions for accuracy are not met. Further error is introduced by the elevated oxygen consumption of inflamed lungs. Use is therefore mainly confined to cardiac laboratories.

The Fick principle can be applied to indicators other than oxygen. The indirect Fick method employs CO_2 as an alternative. The indirect Fick method can be represented mathematically by the formula:

$$\text{Cardiac output} = V\text{CO}_2/(\text{CvCO}_2 - \text{CaCO}_2)$$

where $V\text{CO}_2$ is whole-body CO_2 elimination, and CaCO_2 and CvCO_2 are the CO_2 contents of arterial and mixed venous blood respectively.

A partial rebreathing technique can be used to eliminate the need to measure CvCO_2 directly. The rebreathing values are obtained by introducing an additional 150 ml of dead space into the ventilator circuit (disposable rebreathing loop) and taking measurements once a new equilibrium has been established. Cardiac output can be measured at 3-minute intervals. Assuming that the CvCO_2 concentration does not change significantly throughout the rebreathing period, the terms associated with CvCO_2 cancel each other out and are not needed to calculate cardiac output.

The CO_2 concentration and airflow during a breathing cycle are measured by a mainstream infrared and airflow sensor. $V\text{CO}_2$ is obtained by multiplying airflow by CO_2 concentration. CaCO_2 is derived from end-tidal CO_2 (etCO_2) and the slope of the CO_2 dissociation curve (S). This is represented mathematically as:

$$\text{Cardiac output} = \Delta V\text{CO}_2/(S \times \Delta\text{etCO}_2)$$

Partial CO_2 rebreathing really measures non-shunted pulmonary capillary blood flow rather than total cardiac output. Therefore a correction for venous admixture is added based on FiO_2 and SaO_2 (measured by pulse oximetry).

PROBLEMS WITH THE PARTIAL REBREATHING OF CO_2 METHOD

- It is unsuitable for non-intubated patients (who have variable tidal volumes and leakage around facemasks).
- Changes in mechanical ventilator settings that alter dead space or ventilation/perfusion relationships may result in an artefactual change in cardiac output measurements. The accuracy of the technique also appears to be challenged by spontaneous mechanically assisted ventilation.
- etCO_2 may not accurately reflect change in pulmonary end-capillary and $P\text{aCO}_2$, especially in chronic lung disease.
- $V\text{CO}_2$ may not reach steady state in the time available (especially in chronic lung disease).
- The value of S varies with haemoglobin concentration and $P\text{CO}_2$.
- Venous admixture cannot be calculated reliably from FiO_2 and SaO_2 when there is significant V/Q scatter (e.g. in chronic lung disease).
- Overall there is a lack of validation in chronic lung disease.

THORACIC ELECTRICAL BIOIMPEDANCE[8,10]

An alternating electrical current (high-frequency, very low magnitude) is passed through the thorax. Current is kept constant and fluctuations in electrical impedance are measured. Six electrodes are usually attached (two in the upper thorax/neck region and four in the lower thorax). These electrodes detect changes in bioimpedance and monitor cardiac electrical signals. The technique is very sensitive to any alteration in position or contact of the electrodes to the patient.

The change in aortic blood flow due to myocardial contraction (stroke volume) is measured from the changes in thoracic bioimpedance through the cardiac cycle. Other factors that contribute to a change in overall thoracic bioimpedance include changes in tissue fluid volume and changes in venous and pulmonary blood volume induced by respiration. Respiratory artefact is eliminated by averaging values over several cardiac cycles using the R-R interval as a synchronising signal.

Measuring whole-body rather than truncal impedance by placing electrodes on wrists and ankles also appears successful.

Inaccuracies can arise from numerous sources. These include motion artefact, electrical interference, dysrhythmias (including frequent premature atrial contractions and atrial fibrillation) and acute change in tissue water content (such as pulmonary oedema, pleural effusions or expansion of interstitial fluid). Despite these limitations, it is clinically appealing due to its non-invasive nature. Recent studies of second-generation technology have shown improved reliability of this technique.

FUNCTIONAL HAEMODYNAMIC MONITORING

The recently coined term, *functional haemodynamic monitoring*, implies a therapeutic application, independent of diagnosis.[60] It has been posed in response to the

Table 12.9 Variables described as indices of cardiac preload or fluid responsiveness in critically ill patients

Static	Dynamic
Intracardiac pressures	**Spontaneous respiratory effort**
Central venous pressure (CVP)/right atrial pressure (RAP)	Inspiratory decrease in right atrial pressure (ΔRAP)
Pulmonary artery occlusion pressure (PAOP)	
	Mandatory mechanical ventilation
Cardiovascular volumes	Systolic pressure variation (SPV)
Thermodilution right ventricular end-diastolic volume (RVEDV)	Decrease in systolic pressure (Δdown)
Echocardiographic RVEDV	Pulse pressure variation (PPV)
Echocardiographic left ventricular end-diastolic area (LVEDA)/volume (LVEDV)	Pulse contour analysis stroke volume variation (SVV)
Transpulmonary thermodilution global end-diastolic volume (GEDV)	Respiratory variation in peak aortic blood velocity (ΔV_{peak})
Transpulmonary thermodilution intrathoracic blood volume (ITBV)	Respiratory change in the pre-ejection period (ΔPEP)
	Respiratory systolic variation test (RSVT)
Doppler	
Duration of the aortic velocity signal corrected for heart rate (FT_c)	**Passive leg raising**
	Change in aortic blood flow
	Change in pulse pressure

Variables have been divided into static and dynamic categories. Static variables are estimates of ventricular preload at a point in time, usually end-expiration. Dynamic variables are characterised by measurement of variation in haemodynamic measurements in response to changes in cardiac loading conditions.[47,49,56,64–69]

observation that, although stated in physiological terms, haemodynamic questions must be practical and concrete in order to address clinical problems. Arguably the most relevant functional haemodynamic question is: 'Will stroke volume (or consequently cardiac output) increase with volume loading?' This question can help guide the resuscitation of haemodynamically unstable patients and defines the clinical usefulness of predicting fluid responsiveness. This is an area of increasing research and clinical interest beyond the scope of this chapter. For reference, variables that have been described as indices of preload or predictors of fluid responsiveness in critically ill patients are presented in Table 12.9.

REFERENCES

1. Bellomo R, Uchino S. Cardiovascular monitoring tools: use and misuse. *Curr Opin Crit Care* 2003; **9**: 225–9.
2. Wo CC, Shoemaker WC, Appel PL *et al.* Unreliability of blood pressure and heart rate to evaluate cardiac output in emergency resuscitation and critical illness. *Crit Care Med* 1993; **21**: 218–23.
3. Cousins TR, O'Donnell JM. Arterial cannulation: a critical review. *AANA J* 2004; **72**: 267–71.
4. Whitta RK, Hall KF, Bennetts TM *et al.* Comparison of normal or heparinised saline flushing on function of arterial lines. *Crit Care Resusc* 2006; **8**: 205–8.
5. Bentley MW, Lee CM. The frequency response of direct pressure measurement systems. *Australas Phys Eng Sci Med* 1988; **11**: 150–5.
6. Ercole A. Attenuation in invasive blood pressure measurement systems. *Br J Anaesth* 2006; **96**: 560–2.
7. Gardner RM. Direct blood pressure measurement – dynamic response requirements. *Anesthesiology* 1981; **54**: 227–36.
8. Chaney JC, Derdak S. Minimally invasive hemodynamic monitoring for the intensivist: current and emerging technology. *Crit Care Med* 2002; **30**: 2338–45.
9. Godje O, Hoke K, Goetz AE *et al.* Reliability of a new algorithm for continuous cardiac output determination by pulse-contour analysis during hemodynamic instability. *Crit Care Med* 2002; **30**: 52–8.
10. Parmley CL, Pousman RM. Noninvasive cardiac output monitoring. *Curr Opin Anaesthesiol* 2002; **15**: 675–80.
11. Manecke GR. Edwards FloTrac sensor and Vigileo monitor: easy, accurate, reliable cardiac output assessment using the arterial pulse wave. *Exp Rev Med Devices* 2005; **2**: 523–7.
12. Venus B, Satish P. Vascular cannulation. In: Civetta JM, Taylor RW, Kirby RR (eds) *Critical Care*. Philadelphia: Lippincott-Raven; 1997: 521–44.
13. Tan PL, Gibson M. Central venous catheters: the role of radiology. *Clin Radiol* 2006; **61**: 13–22.
14. National Institute for Clinical Excellence. *Guidance on the Use of Ultrasound Locating Devices for Placing Central Venous Catheters*. Technology Appraisal Guidance no. 49. London: National Institute for Clinical Excellence; 2002.
15. Keenan SP. Use of ultrasound to place central lines. *J Crit Care* 2002; **17**: 126–37.
16. Fletcher SJ, Bodenham AR. Safe placement of central venous catheters: where should the tip of the catheter lie? *Br J Anaesth* 2000; **85**: 188–91.
17. Joynt GM, Gomersall CD, Buckley TA *et al.* Comparison of intrathoracic and intra-abdominal measurements of central venous pressure. *Lancet* 1996; **347**: 1155–7.
18. Sturgess DJ, Marwick TH, Venkatesh B. Diastolic (dys)function in sepsis. In: Vincent JL (ed.) *Yearbook*

of Intensive Care and Emergency Medicine. Berlin: Springer-Verlag; 2007: 444–54.
19. Magder S. How to use central venous pressure measurements. *Curr Opin Crit Care* 2005; **11**: 264–70.
20. Desjardins R, Denault AY, Belisle S *et al.* Can peripheral venous pressure be interchangeable with central venous pressure in patients undergoing cardiac surgery? *Intens Care Med* 2004; **30**: 627–32.
21. Ward KR, Tiba MH, Barbee RW *et al.* A new noninvasive method to determine central venous pressure. *Resuscitation* 2006; **70**: 238–46.
22. Rivers E, Nguyen B, Havstad S *et al.* Early goal-directed therapy in the treatment of severe sepsis and septic shock. *N Engl J Med* 2001; **345**: 1368–77.
23. Swan HJ, Ganz W, Forrester J *et al.* Catheterization of the heart in man with use of a flow-directed balloon-tipped catheter. *N Engl J Med* 1970; **283**: 447–51.
24. Connors AF Jr, Speroff T, Dawson NV *et al.* The effectiveness of right heart catheterization in the initial care of critically ill patients. SUPPORT investigators. *JAMA* 1996; **276**: 889–97.
25. Dalen JE, Bone RC. Is it time to pull the pulmonary artery catheter? *JAMA* 1996; **276**: 916–18.
26. Harvey S, Young D, Brampton W *et al.* Pulmonary artery catheters for adult patients in intensive care. *Cochrane Database Syst Rev* 2006; **3**: CD003408.
27. Wheeler AP, Bernard GR, Thompson BT *et al.* Pulmonary-artery versus central venous catheter to guide treatment of acute lung injury. *N Engl J Med* 2006; **354**: 2213–24.
28. Chittock DR, Dhingra VK, Ronco JJ *et al.* Severity of illness and risk of death associated with pulmonary artery catheter use. *Crit Care Med* 2004; **32**: 911–15.
29. Friese RS, Shafi S, Gentilello LM. Pulmonary artery catheter use is associated with reduced mortality in severely injured patients: a National Trauma Data Bank analysis of 53 312 patients. *Crit Care Med* 2006; **34**: 1597–601.
30. Preas II HL, Suffredini AF. Pulmonary artery catheterization: insertion and quality control. In: Tobin MJ (ed.) *Principles and Practice of Intensive Care Monitoring*. New York: McGraw Hill; 1998: 773–95.
31. Worthley LIG. Vascular cannulation and haemodynamic pressure. In: Worthley LIG (ed.) *Synopsis of Intensive Care Medicine*. Edinburgh: Churchill Livingstone; 1994: 83–95.
32. Leeman M. Pulmonary hypertension in acute respiratory distress syndrome. *Monaldi Arch Chest Dis* 1999; **54**: 146–9.
33. McLean AS, Huang SJ. Intensive care echocardiography. In: Vincent JL (ed.) *Yearbook of Intensive Care and Emergency Medicine*. Berlin: Springer-Verlag; 2006: 131–41.
34. Ristow B, Ali S, Ren X *et al.* Elevated pulmonary artery pressure by Doppler echocardiography predicts hospitalization for heart failure and mortality in ambulatory stable coronary artery disease: the Heart and Soul Study. *J Am Coll Cardiol* 2007; **49**: 43–9.
35. Pinsky MR. Hemodynamic profile interpretration. In: Tobin MJ (ed.) *Principles and Practice of Intensive Care Monitoring*. New York: McGraw Hill; 1998: 871–88.
36. Calvin JE, Driedger AA, Sibbald WJ. Does the pulmonary capillary wedge pressure predict left ventricular preload in critically ill patients? *Crit Care Med* 1981; **9**: 437–43.
37. Summerhill EM, Baram M. Principles of pulmonary artery catheterization in the critically ill. *Lung* 2005; **183**: 209–19.
38. Bouhemad B, Nicolas-Robin A, Benois A *et al.* Echocardiographic Doppler assessment of pulmonary capillary wedge pressure in surgical patients with postoperative circulatory shock and acute lung injury. *Anesthesiology* 2003; **98**: 1091–100.
39. Ganter BG, Jakob SM, Takala J. Pulmonary capillary pressure. A review. *Minerva Anestesiol* 2006; **72**: 21–36.
40. Stetz CW, Miller RG, Kelly GE *et al.* Reliability of the thermodilution method in the determination of cardiac output in clinical practice. *Am Rev Respir Dis* 1982; **126**: 1001–14.
41. Bennett JA. Equipment review: Edwards vigilance continuous cardiac output monitor. *Am J Anesthesiol* 1995; **22**: 269–72.
42. Haller M, Zollner C, Briegel J *et al.* Evaluation of a new continuous thermodilution cardiac output monitor in critically ill patients: a prospective criterion standard study. *Crit Care Med* 1995; **23**: 860–6.
43. Wiesenack C, Fiegl C, Keyser A *et al.* Continuously assessed right ventricular end-diastolic volume as a marker of cardiac preload and fluid responsiveness in mechanically ventilated cardiac surgical patients. *Crit Care* 2005; **9**: R22–233.
44. Nelson LD, Safcsak K, Cheatham ML *et al.* Mathematical coupling does not explain the relationship between right ventricular end-diastolic volume and cardiac output. *Crit Care Med* 2001; **29**: 940–3.
45. Globits S, Pacher R, Frank H *et al.* Comparative assessment of right ventricular volumes and ejection fraction by thermodilution and magnetic resonance imaging in dilated cardiomyopathy. *Cardiology* 1995; **86**: 67–72.
46. Hudson ERGN, Beale RF. Lung water and blood volume measurements in the critically ill. *Curr Opin Crit Care* 2000; **6**: 222–6.
47. Reuter DA, Felbinger TW, Schmidt C *et al.* Stroke volume variations for assessment of cardiac responsiveness to volume loading in mechanically ventilated patients after cardiac surgery. *Intens Care Med* 2002; **28**: 392–8.
48. Kuzkov VV, Kirov MY, Sovershaev MA *et al.* Extravascular lung water determined with single transpulmonary thermodilution correlates with the severity of sepsis-induced acute lung injury. *Crit Care Med* 2006; **34**: 1647–53.
49. Hofer CK, Furrer L, Matter-Ensner S *et al.* Volumetric preload measurement by thermodilution: a comparison with transoesophageal echocardiography. *Br J Anaesth* 2005; **94**: 748–55.
50. Jonas MM, Tanser SJ. Lithium dilution measurement of cardiac output and arterial pulse waveform analysis:

an indicator dilution calibrated beat-by-beat system for continuous estimation of cardiac output. *Curr Opin Crit Care* 2002; **8**: 257–61.
51. Hofer CK, Zollinger A. Less invasive cardiac output monitoring: characteristics and limitations. In: Vincent JL (ed.) *Yearbook of Intensive Care and Emergency Medicine*. Berlin: Springer-Verlag; 2006: 162–75.
52. Quinones MA, Otto CM, Stoddard M *et al.* Recommendations for quantification of Doppler echocardiography: a report from the Doppler Quantification Task Force of the Nomenclature and Standards Committee of the American Society of Echocardiography. *J Am Soc Echocardiogr* 2002; **15**: 167–84.
53. McLean AS, Needham A, Stewart D *et al.* Estimation of cardiac output by noninvasive echocardiographic techniques in the critically ill subject. *Anaesth Intens Care* 1997; **25**: 250–4.
54. Gardin JM, Dabestani A, Matin K *et al.* Reproducibility of Doppler aortic blood flow measurements: studies on intraobserver, interobserver and day-to-day variability in normal subjects. *Am J Cardiol* 1984; **54**: 1092–8.
55. Singer M. The FTc is not an accurate marker of left ventricular preload. *Intens Care Med* 2006; **32**: 1089.
56. Feissel M, Michard F, Mangin I *et al.* Respiratory changes in aortic blood velocity as an indicator of fluid responsiveness in ventilated patients with septic shock. *Chest* 2001; **119**: 867–73.
57. Cholley BP, Payen D. Noninvasive techniques for measurements of cardiac output. *Curr Opin Crit Care* 2005; **11**: 424–9.
58. Nidorf SM, Picard MH, Triulzi MO *et al.* New perspectives in the assessment of cardiac chamber dimensions during development and adulthood. *J Am Coll Cardiol* 1992; **19**: 983–8.
59. Tan HL, Pinder M, Parsons R *et al.* Clinical evaluation of USCOM ultrasonic cardiac output monitor in cardiac surgical patients in intensive care unit. *Br J Anaesth* 2005; **94**: 287–91.
60. Pinsky MR. Functional hemodynamic monitoring. *Intens Care Med* 2002; **28**: 386–8.
61. Durbin CG Jr. Radial arterial lines and sticks: what are the risks? *Respir Care* 2001; **46**: 229–31.
62. McGee DC, Gould MK. Preventing complications of central venous catheterization. *N Engl J Med* 2003; **348**: 1123–33.
63. Complications encountered with the PAC. 2006. Available online at www.pacep.org. Accessed November 2006.
64. Bendjelid K, Romand JA. Fluid responsiveness in mechanically ventilated patients: a review of indices used in intensive care. *Intens Care Med* 2003; **29**: 352–60.
65. Monnet X, Rienzo M, Osman D *et al.* Esophageal Doppler monitoring predicts fluid responsiveness in critically ill ventilated patients. *Intens Care Med* 2005; **31**: 1195–201.
66. Perel A, Minkovich L, Preisman S *et al.* Assessing fluid-responsiveness by a standardized ventilatory maneuver: the respiratory systolic variation test. *Anesth Analg* 2005; **100**: 942–5.
67. Monnet X, Rienzo M, Osman D *et al.* Passive leg raising predicts fluid responsiveness in the critically ill. *Crit Care Med* 2006; **34**: 1402–7.
68. Bendjelid K, Suter PM, Romand JA. The respiratory change in preejection period: a new method to predict fluid responsiveness. *J Appl Physiol* 2004; **96**: 337–42.
69. Magder S, Georgiadis G, Cheong T. Respiratory variations in right atrial pressure predict the response to fluid challenge. *J Crit Care* 1992; **7**: 76–85.

13

Multiple organ dysfunction syndrome

Patricia Figgis and David Bihari

The incidence of multiple organ dysfunction syndrome (MODS) is increasing and accounts for up to one-half of deaths in intensive care. Some 50 years ago, multiple organ failure did not exist as a clinical entity. Patients could not be kept alive long enough for the sequential disturbances in the function of distant organs to occur. In the 1960s, acute respiratory failure characterised by bilateral infiltrates on chest radiograph, now termed acute respiratory distress syndrome (ARDS), was described following a variety of non-pulmonary insults. Finally, in 1973, the first description of multiple organ failure appeared in the surgical literature, describing the course of three patients who subsequently died following surgery for ruptured aortic aneurysm.[1]

Critical illness is often associated with a downward spiral through a systemic inflammatory response syndrome (SIRS) towards frank organ failure and death. Since organ failure is not an all-or-nothing phenomenon, and because dysfunction usually precedes and may progress to gross organ failure, the old term 'multiple organ failure' was deemed unsatisfactory. The American College of Chest Physicians/Society of Critical Care Medicine (ACCP/SCCM) consensus conference in 1992 proposed that the term 'dysfunction' identifies a phenomenon in which organ function is not capable of maintaining homeostasis (Table 13.1).[2] However, it should be remembered that it is only a descriptive definition and does not provide any insight into the aetiology or pathogenesis of MODS. In fact, it is not clear whether MODS is a single pathological process with variable clinical expression, or a limited phenotypic expression of a large number of pathological processes. As yet no therapeutic interventions specifically directed at MODS have significantly altered outcome.

AETIOLOGY

Uncontrolled infection was classically thought to be the main precedent leading to SIRS and subsequently to MODS. In an Australian epidemiological study, infection was not identified in 912 of a total of 1803 SIRS episodes.[4] Therefore it is thought that a substantial proportion of cases of MODS are not initiated by infection. Table 13.2 lists many of the causes of MODS, but is not exhaustive. It must be noted that any number of these causes may in fact act as a secondary insult precipitating MODS. The common features of non-infective aetiologies of MODS are ischaemia, hypoxia, cytokine release, mechanical injury or any combination of these. Thus MODS may occur after all forms of shock and compartment syndromes. Other important causes include trauma, major surgery, burns, pancreatitis, hepatic failure, pulmonary aspiration syndromes and mechanical ventilation.[5] Less commonly, cardiopulmonary bypass, blood product and cytokine infusions, and some drug reactions have been associated with MODS.[6]

PATHOPHYSIOLOGY

INFLAMMATION

The current explanation for the development of SIRS and MODS is local inflammation with activation of the innate immune system and subsequent unbridled systemic inflammation.[7] There is a spectrum of clinical sequelae, ranging from the mildest SIRS that just meets the definition, through organ dysfunction that resolves within a few days, to overwhelming SIRS and MODS. The balance between the inflammatory and regulatory arms of the host response may in part explain these varied responses.

Inflammation involves the activation of circulating immune cells (in particular natural killer (NK), T and B cells and macrophages), the endothelium, and multiple mediator cascades balanced by an anti-inflammatory system. Following injury, proinflammatory mediators are released locally to combat foreign antigens and promote wound healing. Concurrently, anti-inflammatory mediators are released to downregulate this process. If the regulatory mechanisms are unable to contain the response, then inflammatory mediators enter the systemic circulation, additional leukocytes are recruited and activated, and a whole-body response ensues. Homeostasis may be lost and so-called 'immunological dissonance' occurs, when the host's inflammatory or anti-inflammatory response to injury (or both) is excessive or inadequate (Figure 13.1).[8] Thus, MODS is not necessarily due to the primary insult, but more likely to be related to an

Table 13.1 Definition of systemic inflammatory response syndrome (SIRS) and multiple organ dysfunction syndrome (MODS)[3]

Systemic inflammatory response syndrome
The systemic inflammatory response to a variety of severe clinical insults is manifest by two or more of the following conditions:
Temperature >38°C or <36°C
Heart rate >90 beats/min
Respiratory rate >20 breaths/min or Pa_{CO_2} <32 mmHg (or ventilator dependence)
White blood cell count >12 000 cells/mm^3, <4000 cells/mm^3 or >10% band forms
Multiple organ dysfunction syndrome
The presence of altered function involving at least two or more organ systems in an acutely ill patient such that homeostasis cannot be maintained without intervention

Table 13.2 Causes of multiple organ dysfunction syndrome (MODS)

Infectious agents	Non-infectious insults	Mechanism
Bacteria	Mechanical ventilation	Ischaemia
Viruses	Aspiration	Hypoxia
Fungi	Surgery	Cytokine release
Protozoa	Burns	
	Reperfusion syndromes	
	Visceral ischaemia	
	Pancreatitis	
	Hepatic failure	
	Cardiopulmonary bypass	
	Massive transfusion	
	Transfusion reactions	
	Hyperthermia	
	Malignancy	

uncontrolled, aggressive systemic response of the host to that primary insult. Without intervention, SIRS may lead to MODS and death.

MOLECULAR MECHANISMS

In sepsis, activated cell/antigen products interact with a member of the Toll-like receptor family to signal gene expression of inflammatory mediators. Toll-like receptors are evolutionarily-conserved receptors expressed by monocytes and macrophages, which recognise whole subsets of pathogens, and represent the phylogenetically ancient innate immune system. Toll-like receptors mediate cell signalling through the same intracellular transcription pathways as cytokines themselves, most notably nuclear factor κB (NF-κB).[10] Non-infective causes of MODS seem to have this final common pathway, resulting in mediator release. For example, in ventilator-associated lung injury, the signalling cascade converting the physical stimulus into mediator release operates via NF-κB, but the upstream events remain unclear.[11] Large numbers of mediators are involved in inflammation, with chemotactic factors attracting, adhesion molecules focusing, and cytotoxic agents assisting this process. They include cytokines, leukotrienes, prostaglandins, platelet factors and the coagulation and complement systems.

Cytokines are the main mediators of inflammation, with several actions, including directing the cellular response, inducing enzyme production such as inducible nitric oxide synthase (iNOS) and altering adhesion molecules. Their actions are pleiotropic, acting on multiple target cells in different ways depending on timing and local tissue concentration. Several cytokines have been implicated in the development of SIRS and MODS, including tumour necrosis factor (TNF)-α, and interleukins (IL) 1β, 6, and 8. Cytokine and NF-κB concentrations appear to be linked to morbidity and mortality.[12,13] In response to proinflammatory mediators, there is endogenous production of anti-inflammatory cytokines such as IL-4, IL-10 and IL-13.

However, it seems that the prevailing internal milieu is likely to be more important than any absolute levels of one mediator or another. Patients at increased risk of SIRS and MODS, such as the elderly and those with pre-existing illnesses, seem to have abnormal cytokine levels.[14] The ability of a cell to synthesise pro- or anti-inflammatory mediators is influenced by many factors, both genetic and environmental in origin, but also by its previous state of activation. It may be that an initial insult, insufficient to cause MODS, nevertheless pre-primes a susceptible individual such that a subsequent or secondary insult generates a response that overwhelms homeostasis.

If a relative excess or deficiency of mediator expression can upset inflammatory homeostasis, then it is not surprising to find a strong genetic correlation. Families characterised by low TNF-α production have a 10-fold increased risk of fatal outcome in meningococcal disease, whereas high IL-10 production increases the risk 20-fold.[15] TNF-α and IL-10 receptor antagonist polymorphisms are associated with greater susceptibility and worse outcomes to severe sepsis.[16] Unfortunately genetic determinants are likely to be more complicated than simple quantitative expression of one mediator or another.

TISSUE INJURY

The final common pathway leading to MODS is often tissue hypoxia. Many factors can compromise oxygen

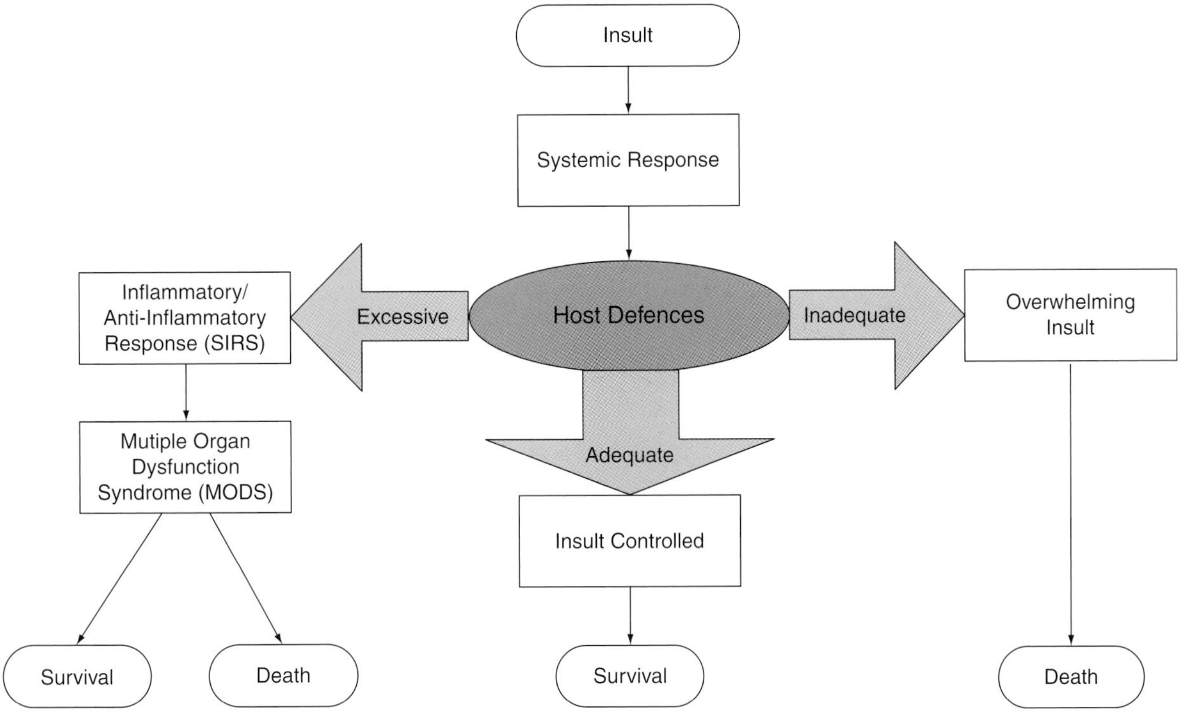

Figure 13.1 Varied host response to injury. (Adapted from Johnson D, Mayers I. Multiple organ dysfunction syndrome: a narrative review. *Can J Anaesth* 2001; **48**: 502–9, with permission).

delivery to tissues. Among these factors are arterial hypoxaemia due to acute lung injury, and reduced cardiac output from reduced left ventricular preload and/or impaired ventricular performance. Over and above oxygen delivery abnormalities, evidence is rapidly building that microcirculatory and mitochondrial dysfunction with an abnormal distribution of blood flow and defective oxygen utilisation ('tissue dysoxia') is central to the pathogenesis of MODS. Indiscriminate injury by mediators of inflammation leads to deranged endothelial function with altered vascular relaxation and abnormal modulation of coagulation, and mitochondrial and cellular damage. This is compounded by an ongoing initial or subsequent insult. Unchecked, cellular dysfunction leads to loss of ion gradients, leakage of lysosomal enzymes, proteolysis and cell death. If enough tissue injury occurs, organ dysfunction and ultimately failure ensue.

ENDOTHELIAL DYSFUNCTION

The endothelium is activated by the engagement of antigen, for example lipopolysaccharides from bacterial cell walls, with Toll-like receptors or inflammatory mediators with various receptors. At any stage other environmental factors such as hypoxia, hypoperfusion, increased temperature, acidosis and glycaemic perturbations may also affect endothelial function. The interaction of these extracellular factors with their receptors activates downstream signalling pathways, influencing transcription factors and altering cellular function and/or gene expression. Cell surface adhesion molecules are upregulated, leading to increased leukocyte rolling, adhesion and transmigration, with cytokine-mediated positive feedback and cellular recruitment enhancing this process.[17,18] Upregulation of iNOS leads to excessive amounts of NO production.

In addition, inappropriate intravascular coagulation is an important cause of tissue injury. Activation and amplification of the tissue factor pathway, and possibly downregulation of anticoagulatory pathways, lead to the generation of thrombin and hence fibrin formation. Coagulation may result in focal areas of ischaemia, and concurrent depletion of counterregulatory networks. The mechanisms that regulate inflammation, coagulation and the various cell types are intimately linked and cannot be thought of as discrete entities. A schematic diagram of the processes involved in endothelial dysfunction is shown in Figure 13.2.

It can therefore be seen that following endothelial cell activation, abnormal blood flow distribution may occur as a result of a combination of:

- NO-mediated extensive vasodilatation and increased endothelial cell permeability

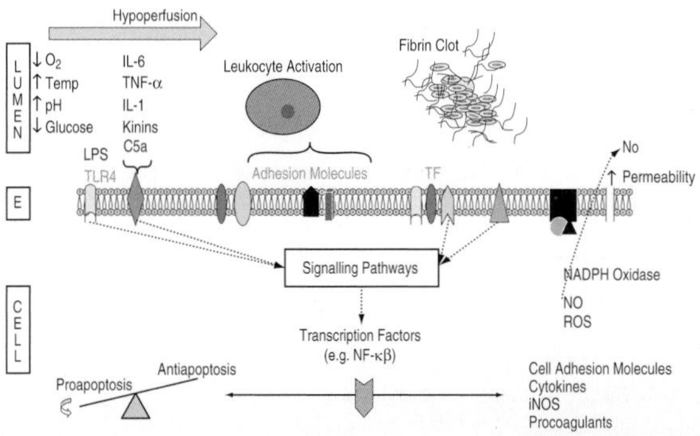

Figure 13.2 Mechanisms of endothelial dysfunction. The temporal sequence of events is depicted from left to right. E, endothelium; LPS, lipopolysaccharide; TLR, Toll-like receptor; IL, interleukin; TNF, tumour necrosis factor; C5a, complement factor 5a; NF-κB, nuclear factor κB; TF, tissue factor; NO, nitric oxide; ROS, reactive oxygen species; NADPH, nicotinamide adenine dinucleotide phosphate; iNOS, inducible nitric oxide synthase. (Adapted from Aird WC. The role of the endothelium in severe sepsis and multiple organ dysfunction syndrome. *Blood* 2003; **101**: 3765–77, with permission.)

- functional shunting
- obstruction of flow by microthrombi, platelet or leukocyte aggregates, abnormal red cell deformability, and possibly endothelial cell oedema
- hypoperfusion secondary to reduced cardiac output from various causes such as a reduction in cardiac preload (actual or relative hypovolaemia or a decrease in effective blood volume), myocardial depression (mediated by NO, IL-1β and TNF-α), and reduced lusitropy (mediated by NO)[19]

Relatively new non-invasive techniques such as orthogonal polarisation (Figure 13.3) have demonstrated these abnormalities in microcirculatory blood flow distribution in septic states compared with normal controls. As a consequence of the derecruitment of capillaries, the increased diffusion distances will in turn contribute to the development of hypoxia.

APOPTOSIS

Changes in the dynamics and regulation of apoptosis in critical illness contribute to organ dysfunction. Apoptosis is the fundamental physiological process by which cells activate an endogenous programme that leads to controlled death and clearance of cells without evoking an inflammatory response. In contrast, necrosis is uncontrolled cellular death with release of intracellular contents and subsequent inflammation. Alterations in the control of apoptosis are caused by changes in the expression of proapoptotic and antiapoptotic genes. Excessive apoptosis has been particularly implicated in gastrointestinal, liver, kidney and cardiac dysfunction. Interestingly, the apoptosis of lymphocytes is delayed, which could lead to prolonged injurious function.[20,21]

MITOCHONDRIAL DYSFUNCTION

Normally more than 85% of oxygen extracted by tissues is used in the mitochondrial respiratory chain to produce adenosine triphosphate (ATP), the main intracellular energy source. It is widely accepted that oxygen consumption, and hence extraction, is reduced in many disease states leading to MODS. This decrease in oxygen consumption may be out of proportion to any reduction in oxygen delivery caused by microcirculatory dysfunction. Abnormal mitochondrial respiration with markedly reduced ATP production has been implicated in some cases.[22] The strong inherited component to the heterogeneity seen in MODS outcome may be influenced by the natural genetic variation in mitochondrial DNA.[23]

Several mutually compatible mechanisms have been postulated to account for this tissue dysoxia (previously confused with 'cytopathic hypoxia'). There is diminished delivery of pyruvic acid to the tricarboxylic acid (TCA) cycle by inhibition of pyruvate dehydrogenase leading to increased lactate production. NO and reactive oxygen species (ROS) have been demonstrated to inhibit the mitochondrial respiratory chain significantly. ROS can also induce DNA damage, which activates poly (ADP-ribose) polymerase-1 (PARP-1), consuming NAD^+/NADH for repair as a consequence. Since NADH is the main reducing equivalent in oxidative phosphorylation, energy production is compromised. Animal studies suggest that tissue dysoxia occurs after the disease process is well established, which suggests that early intervention may prevent the evolution of MODS.[24,25]

In addition to energy production, mitochondria are critical for other aspects of cellular function, such as modulating calcium levels and the biosynthesis of haem and sulphur centres. Thus, mitochondrial dysfunction causes cell damage by a combination of reduced energy production, abnormal calcium homeostasis and oxidative stress through release of ROS. Furthermore, mitochondrial damage can contribute to deranged apoptosis by releasing proapoptotic factors into the cytoplasm.

The mechanisms of tissue injury described above are not mutually exclusive, but the result of interactions between multiple predisposing patient factors, a series of physiologic insults and an endogenous response effected via multiple cell types and hundreds of biochemical mediators. Figure 13.4 attempts to simplify and illustrate the pathogenesis and mechanisms of tissue injury.

CLINICAL FEATURES

As SIRS progresses, an often unpredictable but nonetheless sequential pattern of organ dysfunction ensues. Once two or more organs are involved, the term 'MODS' can

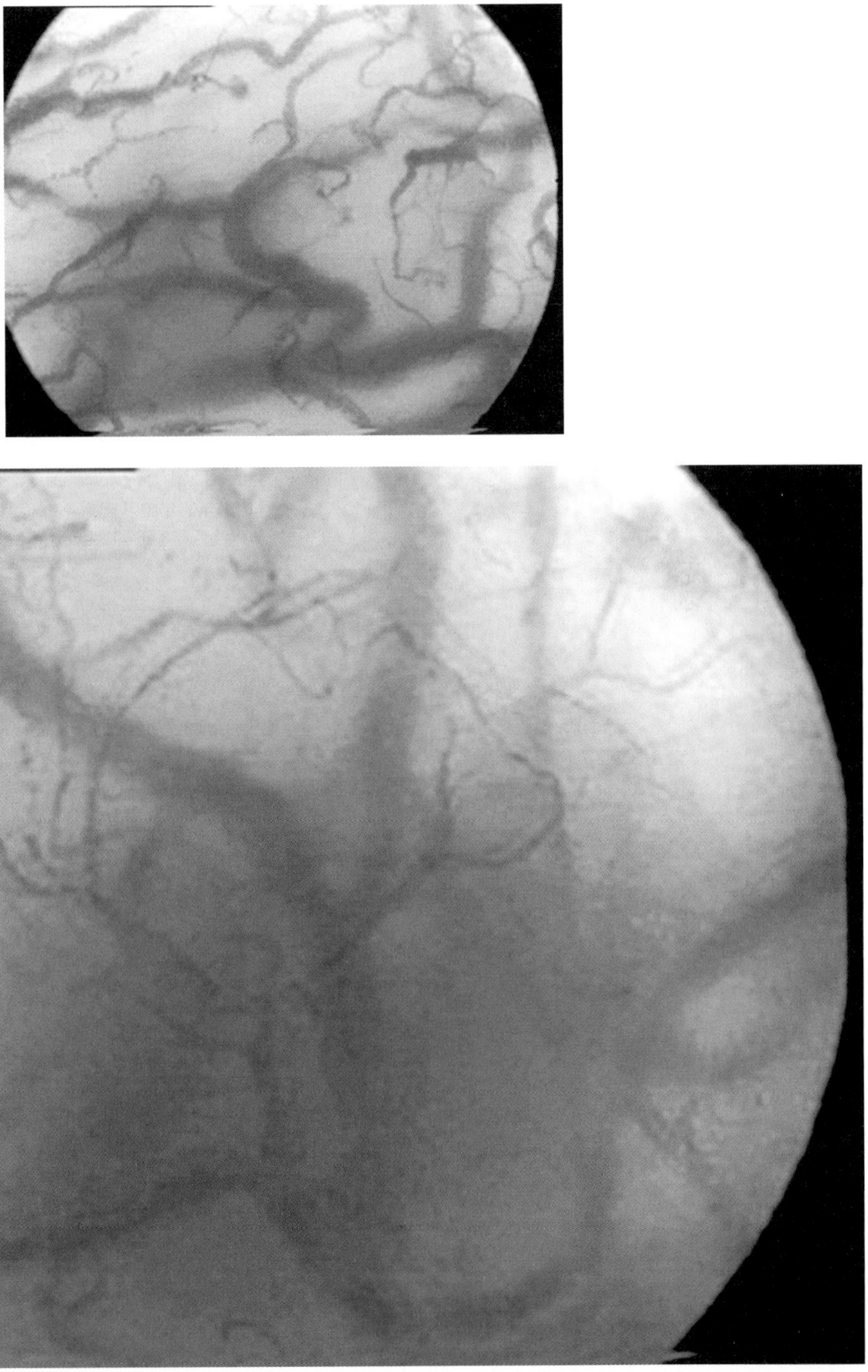

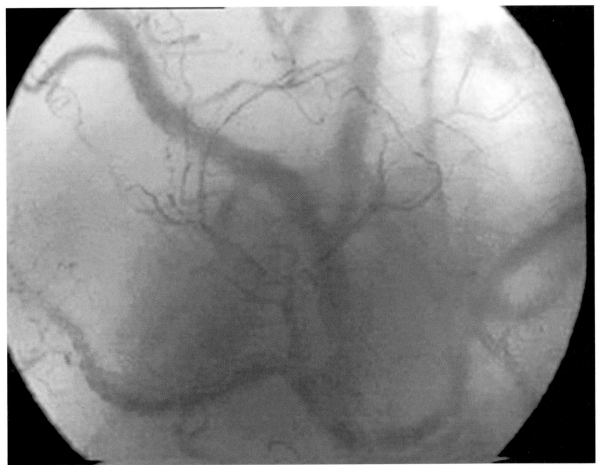

Figure 13.3 Orthogonal polarisation images of the sublingual mucosa in a normal (top) and a septic (bottom) patient. Note, firstly, paucity of smaller blood vessels in the septic sublingual mucosa with increased diffusion distances between blood vessels and, secondly, that the remaining blood vessels are of smaller calibre. (Courtesy of Cytometrics.)

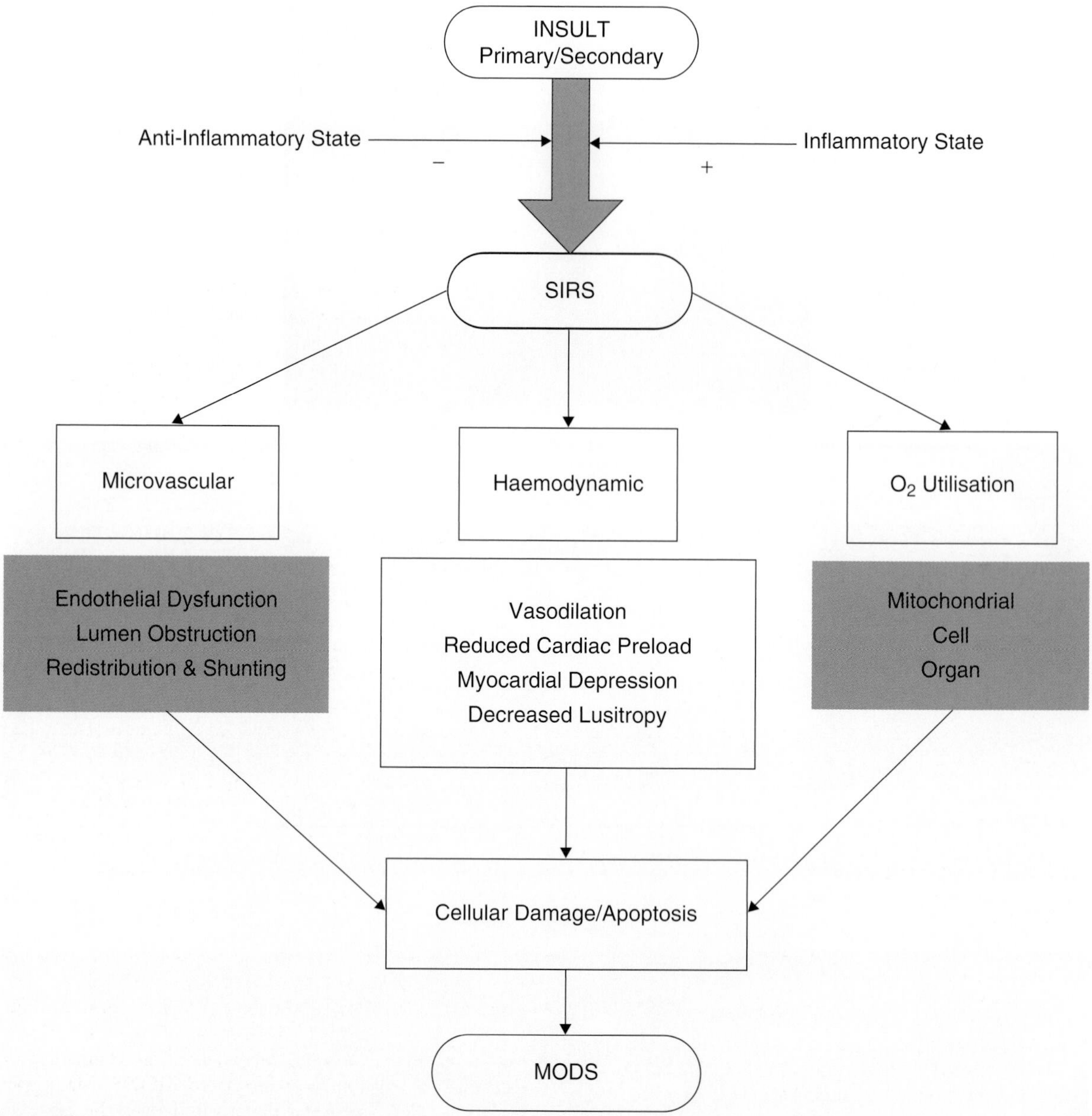

Figure 13.4 Summary of mechanisms of tissue injury. SIRS, systemic inflammatory response syndrome; MODS, multiple organ dysfunction syndrome. (Adapted from Johnson D, Mayers I. Multiple organ dysfunction syndrome: a narrative review. *Can J Anaesth* 2001; **48**: 502–9, with permission.)

be used. Table 13.3 lists the commoner organ systems affected and their associated clinical features.

Encephalopathy is very common and correlates with mortality in sepsis.[26] As many as 30% of patients have evidence of myocardial dysfunction (reduced ejection fraction) and ARDS complicates 60% of cases of septic shock.[3,27] There is a close relationship between increased intestinal permeability on intensive care unit (ICU) admission and the subsequent development of MODS.[28] Increased intestinal permeability may lead to the translocation of endotoxin, bacteria and other mediators. It can therefore be seen that many of these physiological changes can also act as secondary insults in the development of MODS.

Table 13.3 Commonly affected organs, with associated clinical features

Organ system	Associated clinical features	Physiological and biochemical changes
Neurological	Decreased level of consciousness/encephalopathy (confusion, agitation and/or drowsiness)	Abnormal EEG suggestive of metabolic encephalopathy
Cardiovascular	SBP $<$ 90 mmHg or a reduction of $>$40 mmHg from baseline Tachycardia $>$90 beats/min, dysrhythmia Oedema formation	Reduced systemic vascular resistance Myocardial depression and reduced lusitropy Increased capillary permeability
Respiratory	Tachypnoea $>$20 breaths/min Desaturation Central and peripheral cyanosis Requirement for mechanical ventilation	$Pa\text{CO}_2 < 32$ mmHg Hypoxaemia (reduced $Pa\text{O}_2/Fi\text{O}_2$ ratio) Increased work of breathing Increased lung water
Renal	Urinary output $<$ 0.5 ml/kg per h despite adequate fluid resuscitation	Increasing urea and creatinine
Gastrointestinal	Abdominal discomfort and distension Large nasogastric aspirates Failure to absorb enteral nutrition Haemorrhage	Increased intestinal permeability Splanchnic ischaemia Ileus Acalculous cholecystitis Pancreatitis Stress ulceration
Hepatic	Jaundice Encephalopathy	Increasing bilirubin Increasing lactate Hyperglycaemia (increased gluconeogenesis, impaired clearance) Hypoglycaemia (failing gluconeogenesis)
Haematological	Haemorrhage, petechial rash Peripheral cyanosis	White blood cell count $>$ 12 000 cells/mm^3, $<$ 4000 cells/mm^3 or $>$ 10% band forms DIC with coagulopathy and platelets reduced by 50% over 3 days, or $<$ 80 000 cells/mm^3 Anaemia

EEG, electroencephalogram; SBP, systolic blood pressure; DIC, disseminated intravascular coagulation.

MANAGEMENT

The cornerstones of the management of patients with SIRS and impending MODS are firstly, the prevention of secondary insults such as nosocomial infection; secondly, early identification of dysfunctional organs with regular clinical assessment and appropriate monitoring, and thirdly, the timely treatment of both primary and secondary insults. Good supportive care, including recognition of the requirement and instigation as necessary of fluid resuscitation, vasopressors/inotropes, mechanical ventilation (with lung protective strategies) and renal replacement therapies, reduce mortality from MODS. In addition, infection control, avoiding oversedation, pressure area care, nursing the patient head-up, early enteral nutrition, and stress ulcer and deep-vein thrombosis thromboprophylaxis are all paramount in reducing secondary insults.

A sobering consequence of high-quality clinical trials performed in the ICU over the past decade has been the realisation that making a normal or supranormal physiologic state the therapeutic target in a critically ill patient whose homeostasis is profoundly disrupted may be detrimental rather than beneficial and that many interventions carry the potential cost of inadvertent harm. The majority of research has been conducted in MODS of septic origin and it is unclear whether the results can be extrapolated to non-sepsis-mediated MODS. Many specific therapies have been investigated over the last two decades and have appeared to be promising. Although some of these so-called 'innovative' therapies have found their way into algorithms such as the 'Surviving Sepsis' guidelines, there remains much controversy regarding their benefits. Thus, at present, there is insufficient evidence to warrant graded recommendations for directed therapeutic interventions in MODS.

INNOVATIVE THERAPIES

GLYCAEMIC CONTROL

Hyperglycaemia has been reported to impair the immune system, increase endothelial cell apoptosis and cause mitochondrial dysfunction.[29] Moreover, insulin promotes endothelial cell survival.[30] Hence it may be that tight glucose control could have a protective effect on the endothelium.

In a single-centre study, an absolute mortality risk reduction of 3.4% from MODS and sepsis has been demonstrated in critically ill surgical intensive care patients treated with intensive insulin therapy (aiming for a blood glucose in the range of 4.1–6.1 mmol/l).[31]

LOW-DOSE GLUCOCORTICOIDS

There has been renewed interest in the therapeutic role of 'replacement doses' of steroids in SIRS and MODS, with some evidence suggesting improved survival in patients with septic shock.[32] Specifically, steroids inhibit NF-κB and the induction of iNOS by cytokines. Hence the mechanisms by which physiological, and perhaps beneficial, doses of corticosteroids are thought to act include:

- anti-inflammatory via a decreased transcription of proinflammatory cytokines and iNOS
- treatment of relative adrenocortical insufficiency
- restoration of catecholamine receptor sensitivity

MANIPULATION OF THE COAGULATION CASCADE

A 28-day absolute reduction in the risk of death of 6.1% ($P = 0.005$) has been reported with the administration of human recombinant activated protein C (APC) to patients with severe sepsis and evidence of organ dysfunction (PROWESS study group).[33] APC has several potentially beneficial effects:

- potent inhibition of factors Va and VIIIa (and a lesser effect on unactivated forms)
- promotion of fibrinolysis by indirectly inducing plasmin activity, and thus clot lysis
- complex anti-inflammatory effects
- possible inhibition of endothelial cell apoptosis

However, there is a small but significant increased risk of serious bleeding complications. Certain patient groups, notably those with low Acute Physiology and Chronic Health Evaluation (APACHE) II scores (less than 25) and children appear not to benefit from such treatment.[34,35] A confirmatory study in patients with APACHE II scores greater than 25 is planned by the original PROWESS investigators.[33]

Other research into the modulation of the coagulation system has proven disappointing. In contrast to the initial promising preclinical data on antithrombin III, a phase III trial failed to show any benefit, although a recent subgroup analysis of the trial hinted at improved survival in those who also received heparin.[36,37] Furthermore, treatment with recombinant tissue factor pathway inhibitor had no effect on all-cause mortality in patients with severe sepsis and high international normalised ratio (INR). Moreover, there was an increased risk of bleeding, irrespective of baseline INR.[38]

NUTRITION

Studies in ARDS and sepsis patients have suggested that ω-3 fatty acid administration may reduce the release of proinflammatory mediators with decreased cytokine production, NF-κB inhibition and macrophage-mediated systemic dysfunction.[39,40] Whilst some studies suggest a reduction in the severity of MODS in humans, conclusive clinical data are lacking. This raises the interesting possibility that not only may nutritional factors influence the course of MODS, but an individual may be susceptible to developing the syndrome in the first instance.

BLOOD PURIFICATION

High-volume haemofiltration (2–6 l/hour) with highly permeable biocompatible membranes has been postulated to remove large quantities of mediators either by filtration or by membrane absorption. While improved cardiovascular parameters have been observed, this may also be due to control of hyperthermia, correction of fluid overload, metabolic acidosis and electrolyte abnormalities.[41]

IMMUNE MODULATION

Extensive investigation has been undertaken with drugs targeted at manipulating the immune system. Not surprisingly, attempts to block or replace single mediators have failed to improve the outcome of SIRS and MODS. The therapeutic challenge in attempting to modulate the anti-inflammatory and proinflammatory responses is that the numbers of mediators are numerous, they are intimately interrelated and interdependent, their expression varies during the course of a particular illness and between patients, and laboratory measurement may not represent in vivo action.

NITRIC OXIDE INHIBITORS

Indiscriminate NOS inhibition with N^G-monomethyl-L-arginine hydrochloride (L-NMMA), whilst improving vasomotor tone, also leads to significantly increased myocardial and renal complications and mortality. Selective NOS inhibitors may have a role in the treatment of MODS in the future.[42]

OUTCOMES

The mortality from MODS is related to the number and duration of organ systems in failure,[43] and remains the leading cause of death in non-coronary ICUs.[44] A simple count of organs affected and the duration of dysfunction will stratify mortality in broad ranges, for example 60–98% depending on age, with three organs affected for more than 1 week.[45] Although the incidence and overall outcome of MODS did not seem to change very much in the 1980s, an analysis of the APACHE II and III databases suggests that patients with three or more organ systems in failure did indeed have a better outcome in the later APACHE III database.[46] Since the results of research into specific interventions have on the whole been disappointing, any improvement in outcome must be related to better (or earlier) resuscitation and supportive therapies. Survival rates do seem to be improving in this very sick population of patients, but whether MODS can be prevented by any new specific therapy remains to be seen.

MODS may serve as a useful outcome measure of disease severity for risk adjustment and outcome markers in critical care. The advantage of using MODS is that it may be a less biased measure of the original insult and subsequent care provided. One specific instrument designed to assess organ failure is the Sequential Organ Function Assessment (SOFA) score (see Appendix 8). Using the worst values for six commonly measured parameters ($Pa\text{O}_2/Fi\text{O}_2$ ratio, platelet count, bilirubin, blood pressure, Glasgow Coma Score and urine output or creatinine), a score is assigned on admission to intensive care and repeated every 48 hours until discharge. The advantage of the SOFA score is in its ability to describe the epidemiology of critical illness both at the time of admission and during ICU care. There is a positive association between total SOFA score on admission and ICU mortality before 7 days, but not after. Interestingly, ICU mortality after 7 days is associated with high SOFA scores on day 6 after adjusting for admission score. Thus, illness on admission becomes less important, and the course during the ICU stay becomes more relevant, with the presence or development of cardiovascular dysfunction having the strongest independent effect on the probability of death compared with other organ system dysfunctions.[47]

Although mortality is an important outcome measure in ICU, permanent restrictions in daily activities as measured by quality of life (QOL) scores are often also relevant to both the individual and society. MODS has been shown in a prospective observational study using the QOL score RAND-36 to have a statistically significant negative effect on vitality and emotional role limitations. Some 47.2% of all patients were unable to return to work and/or experienced severe limitations in their daily activities and 3.8% were unable to live at home 1 year after hospital discharge.[48] Similarly diminished QOL scores have been found in post cardiac surgery and acute lung injury patients.[49,50] However, patients with acute renal dysfunction appear to have a less marked deterioration in their QOL.

REFERENCES

1. Tilney NL, Bailey GL, Morgan AP. Sequential system failure after rupture of abdominal aortic aneurysms: an unsolved problem in postoperative care. *Ann Surg* 1973; **178**: 117–22.
2. American College of Chest Physicians/Society of Critical Care Medicine Consensus Conference. Definitions for sepsis and organ failure and guidelines for the use of innovative therapies in sepsis. *Crit Care Med* 1992; **20**: 864–74.
3. Parrillo JE, Parker MM, Natanson C *et al.* Septic shock in humans. Advances in the understanding of pathogenesis, cardiovascular dysfunction, and therapy. *Ann Intern Med* 1990; **113**: 227–42.
4. Finfer S, Bellomo R, Lipman J *et al.* Adult-population incidence of severe sepsis in Australian and New Zealand intensive care units. *Intens Care Med* 2004; **30**: 589–96.
5. Evans TW, Smithies M. ABC of intensive care: organ dysfunction. *Br Med J* 1999; **318**: 1606–9.
6. Suntharalingam G, Perry MR, Ward S *et al.* Cytokine storm in a phase 1 trial of the anti-CD28 monoclonal antibody TGN1412. *N Engl J Med* 2006; **355**: 1018–28.
7. Singer M, De Santis V, Vitale D *et al.* Multiorgan failure is an adaptive, endocrine-mediated, metabolic response to overwhelming systemic inflammation. *Lancet* 2004; **364**: 545–8.
8. Bone RC. Immunologic dissonance: a continuing evolution in our understanding of the systemic inflammatory response syndrome (SIRS) and the multiple organ dysfunction syndrome (MODS). *Ann Intern Med* 1996; **125**: 680–7.
9. Johnson D, Mayers I. Multiple organ dysfunction syndrome: a narrative review. *Can J Anaesth* 2001; **48**: 502–9.
10. Glauser MP. Pathophysiologic basis of sepsis: considerations for future strategies of intervention. *Crit Care Med* 2000; **28**: S–8.
11. Held HD, Boettcher S, Hamann L *et al.* Ventilation-induced chemokine and cytokine release is associated with activation of nuclear factor-kappaB and is blocked by steroids. *Am J Respir Crit Care Med* 2001; **163**: 711–16.
12. Pinsky MR, Vincent JL, Deviere J *et al.* Serum cytokine levels in human septic shock. Relation to multiple-system organ failure and mortality. *Chest* 1993; **103**: 565–75.
13. Paterson RL, Galley HF, Dhillon JK *et al.* Increased nuclear factor kappa B activation in critically ill patients who die. *Crit Care Med* 2000; **28**: 1047–51.
14. Bone RC. Toward a theory regarding the pathogenesis of the systemic inflammatory response syndrome: what we do and do not know about cytokine regulation. *Crit Care Med* 1996; **24**: 163–72.
15. Westendorp RG, Langermans JA, Huizinga TW *et al.* Genetic influence on cytokine production and fatal meningococcal disease. *Lancet* 1997; **349**: 170–3.
16. Freeman BD, Buchman TG. Gene in a haystack: tumor necrosis factor polymorphisms and outcome in sepsis. *Crit Care Med* 2000; **28**: 3090–1.
17. Vallet B. Bench-to-bedside review: endothelial cell dysfunction in severe sepsis: a role in organ dysfunction? *Crit Care* 2003; 7: 130–8.

18. Aird WC. The role of the endothelium in severe sepsis and multiple organ dysfunction syndrome. *Blood* 2003; **101**: 3765–77.
19. Drexler H. Nitric oxide synthases in the failing human heart: a doubled-edged sword? *Circulation* 1999; **99**: 2972–5.
20. Mahidhara R, Billiar TR. Apoptosis in sepsis. *Crit Care Med* 2000; **28**: N1–13.
21. Marshall JC. Inflammation, coagulopathy, and the pathogenesis of multiple organ dysfunction syndrome. *Crit Care Med* 2001; **29**: S99–106.
22. Brealey D, Brand M, Hargreaves I *et al.* Association between mitochondrial dysfunction and severity and outcome of septic shock. *Lancet* 2002; **360**: 219–23.
23. Baudouin SV, Saunders D, Tiangyou W *et al.* Mitochondrial DNA and survival after sepsis: a prospective study. *Lancet* 2005; **366**: 2118–21.
24. Fink MP. Bench-to-bedside review: cytopathic hypoxia. *Crit Care* 2002; **6**: 491–9.
25. Fink MP. Cytopathic hypoxia. Mitochondrial dysfunction as mechanism contributing to organ dysfunction in sepsis. *Crit Care Clin* 2001; **17**: 21–237.
26. Eidelman LA, Putterman D, Putterman C *et al.* The spectrum of septic encephalopathy. Definitions, etiologies, and mortalities. *JAMA* 1996; **275**: 470–3.
27. Kollef MH, Schuster DP. The acute respiratory distress syndrome. *N Engl J Med* 1995; **332**: 27–37.
28. Doig CJ, Sutherland LR, Sandham JD *et al.* Increased intestinal permeability is associated with the development of multiple organ dysfunction syndrome in critically ill ICU patients. *Am J Respir Crit Care Med* 1998; **158**: 444–51.
29. Baumgartner-Parzer SM, Wagner L, Pettermann M *et al.* High-glucose-triggered apoptosis in cultured endothelial cells. *Diabetes* 1995; **44**: 1323–7.
30. Hermann C, Assmus B, Urbich C *et al.* Insulin-mediated stimulation of protein kinase Akt: a potent survival signaling cascade for endothelial cells. *Arterioscler Thromb Vasc Biol* 2000; **20**: 402–9.
31. van den Berghe G, Wouters P, Weekers F *et al.* Intensive insulin therapy in the critically ill patients. *N Engl J Med* 2001; **345**: 1359–67.
32. Annane D, Sebille V, Charpentier C *et al.* Effect of treatment with low doses of hydrocortisone and fludrocortisone on mortality in patients with septic shock. *JAMA* 2002; **288**: 862–71.
33. Bernard GR, Vincent JL, Laterre PF *et al.* Efficacy and safety of recombinant human activated protein C for severe sepsis. *N Engl J Med* 2001; **344**: 699–709.
34. Abraham E, Laterre PF, Garg R *et al.* Drotrecogin alfa (activated) for adults with severe sepsis and a low risk of death. *N Engl J Med* 2005; **353**: 1332–41.
35. Nadel S, Goldstein B, Williams MD *et al.* Drotrecogin alfa (activated) in children with severe sepsis: a multicentre phase III randomised controlled trial. *Lancet* 2007; **369**: 836–43.
36. Warren BL, Eid A, Singer P *et al.* Caring for the critically ill patient. High-dose antithrombin III in severe sepsis: a randomized controlled trial. *JAMA* 2001; **286**: 1869–78.
37. Wiedermann CJ, Hoffmann JN, Juers M *et al.* High-dose antithrombin III in the treatment of severe sepsis in patients with a high risk of death: efficacy and safety. *Crit Care Med* 2006; **34**: 285–92.
38. Abraham E, Reinhart K, Opal S *et al.* Efficacy and safety of tifacogin (recombinant tissue factor pathway inhibitor) in severe sepsis: a randomized controlled trial. *JAMA* 2003; **290**: 238–47.
39. Mayer K, Fegbeutel C, Hattar K *et al.* Omega-3 vs. omega-6 lipid emulsions exert differential influence on neutrophils in septic shock patients: impact on plasma fatty acids and lipid mediator generation. *Intens Care Med* 2003; **29**: 1472–81.
40. Pacht ER, DeMichele SJ, Nelson JL *et al.* Enteral nutrition with eicosapentaenoic acid, gamma-linolenic acid, and antioxidants reduces alveolar inflammatory mediators and protein influx in patients with acute respiratory distress syndrome. *Crit Care Med* 2003; **31**: 491–500.
41. Heering P, Morgera S, Schmitz FJ *et al.* Cytokine removal and cardiovascular hemodynamics in septic patients with continuous venovenous hemofiltration. *Intens Care Med* 1997; **23**: 288–96.
42. Watson D, Grover R, Anzueto A *et al.* Cardiovascular effects of the nitric oxide synthase inhibitor N_G-methyl-L-arginine hydrochloride (546C88) in patients with septic shock: results of a randomized, double-blind, placebo-controlled multicenter study (study no. 144-002). *Crit Care Med* 2004; **32**: 1–20.
43. Knaus WA, Draper EA, Wagner DP *et al.* Prognosis in acute organ-system failure. *Ann Surg* 1985; **202**: 685–93.
44. Marshall JC, Cook DJ, Christou NV *et al.* Multiple organ dysfunction score: a reliable descriptor of a complex clinical outcome. *Crit Care Med* 1995; **23**: 1638–52.
45. Barriere SL, Lowry SF. An overview of mortality risk prediction in sepsis. *Crit Care Med* 1995; **23**: 376–93.
46. Zimmerman JE, Knaus WA, Wagner DP *et al.* A comparison of risks and outcomes for patients with organ system failure: 1982–1990. *Crit Care Med* 1996; **24**: 1633–41.
47. Nfor TK, Walsh TS, Prescott RJ. The impact of organ failures and their relationship with outcome in intensive care: analysis of a prospective multicentre database of adult admissions. *Anaesthesia* 2006; **61**: 731–78.
48. Pettila V, Kaarlola A, Makelainen A. Health-related quality of life of multiple organ dysfunction patients one year after intensive care. *Intens Care Med* 2000; **26**: 1473–9.
49. Nielsen D, Sellgren J, Ricksten SE. Quality of life after cardiac surgery complicated by multiple organ failure. *Crit Care Med* 1997; **25**: 52–7.
50. Weinert CR, Gross CR, Kangas JR *et al.* Health-related quality of life after acute lung injury. *Am J Respir Crit Care Med* 1997; **156**: 1120–8.

14

Monitoring oxygenation

Thomas John Morgan and Balasubramanian Venkatesh

THE ROLES OF OXYGEN IN AEROBIC ORGANISMS

Oxygen has several vital physiological roles:

1. *Bioenergetics.* Aerobic mitochondrial respiration accounts for 90% of oxygen consumption, generating adenosine triphosphate (ATP) by oxidative phosphorylation. Mitochondrial electron transfer oxidase systems provide the fundamental machinery, in particular the cytochrome oxidase of complex IV. Oxygen acts as terminal electron acceptor, combining with two protons to produce water.[1]
2. *Biosynthetics.* Oxygen transferase systems incorporate oxygen into substrates, such as prostanoids, catecholamines and some neurotransmitters.
3. *Biodegradation and detoxification reactions.* These mixed-function oxidase reactions require oxygen and a co-substrate (e.g. NADPH). The cytochrome P-450 hydroxylases are examples.
4. *Generation of reactive oxygen species.* These are essential antimicrobial defences deployed by neutrophils and macrophages.[2]

TISSUE HYPOXIA

As tissue Po_2 falls, the biosynthetic and biodegradation systems are the first to succumb. Cell signalling by reactive oxygen species, released at mitochondrial complex III, activates hypoxia-inducible factor-1, a transcription factor upregulating genes important in hypoxic cell survival.[3] Oxidative phosphorylation starts to fail at an intracellular Po_2 of 0.1–1 mmHg, equivalent to an extracellular Po_2 of around 5 mmHg. At this point oxygen-limited cytochrome turnover causes progressive ATP depletion, a process which has been termed 'dysoxia'.[4] Stopgap production continues by anaerobic glycolysis, but without correction of dysoxia there is progressive lactic acidosis and eventual cell death by apoptosis and necrosis. On reoxygenation, further release of reactive oxygen species causes oxidant stress, often overshadowing the hypoxic insult.[2]

CATEGORIES OF HYPOXIA

Classically, hypoxia has been categorised under three headings:[1]

1. stagnant hypoxia, where the primary abnormality is reduced tissue blood flow
2. hypoxaemic hypoxia, where the primary abnormality is a low arterial oxygen tension
3. anaemic hypoxia, where the primary abnormality is a low haemoglobin concentration

However in critical illness, tissue oxygenation can be disordered with a normal or even high tissue Po_2:

1. cytopathic hypoxia, defined as abnormal cellular oxygen utilisation despite adequate oxygen delivery[5]
2. oxygen toxicity, defined as abnormal cell function due to high oxygen tensions[6]

THE OXYGEN CASCADE

In unicellular organisms, oxygen reaches the mitochondria across a short diffusion path with a steep partial pressure gradient. In multicellular animals the much longer diffusion path traverses a series of small partial pressure reductions known as the oxygen cascade. As a result, oxygen arrives at intracellular organelles at tensions above the anaerobic threshold.

Important steps in the oxygen cascade include:

1. inspired gas
2. alveolar gas
3. arterial blood
4. microcirculation
5. interstitium
6. mitochondria and other intracellular organelles

The cascade can be jeopardised at any step, with downstream oxygen deprivation of mitochondria and other intracellular organelles. In this chapter we will consider how oxygenation can be monitored at strategic points along the cascade.

INSPIRED GAS

Monitoring the fraction of inspired oxygen (FiO_2) is necessary to prevent both hypoxaemia and the adverse effects of excess oxygen. The inspired oxygen tension (PiO_2) of humidified gas is determined by the FiO_2, the barometric pressure (BP) and the saturated vapour pressure of water (47 mmHg).

$$PiO_2 = FiO_2 \times (BP - 47) \qquad \textit{Equation 14.1}$$

Gas supply pressures are monitored continuously. Ventilators incorporate input pressure alarms and oxygen analysers within the inspiratory module to identify oxygen source failure. Direct measurement of circuit oxygen concentration can be performed.

TRANSFER OF INSPIRED GAS TO ALVEOLI

Communication between oxygen delivery system and pulmonary alveoli is open if:

1. There are no signs of upper-airway obstruction (Chapter 25).
2. Expired tidal and minute volumes and airway pressures for the ventilated patient are within correctly set alarm limits (Chapter 27).
3. There is an appropriate end-tidal CO_2 waveform (Chapter 34).

ALVEOLAR GAS

In a patient receiving 100% oxygen, alveolar PO_2 in individual lung units can range from < 40 mmHg to > 600 mmHg. Consequently, end-tidal PO_2 monitoring is of no value.

DISTRIBUTION OF ALVEOLAR VENTILATION

Clinicians routinely track chest movement, auscultate air entry and examine plain chest radiographs. Although computed tomography scanning can reveal occult overdistension,[7] it has logistical disadvantages and is a significant radiation hazard. Electrical impedance tomography is under development as an alternative, and shows promise.[8] Simple and non-invasive, it tracks lung volume changes in real time, with potential to optimise alveolar ventilation distribution while limiting overdistension.[9]

MATCHING OF VENTILATION AND PERFUSION

For efficient gas exchange, the majority of lung units must have well-matched alveolar ventilation and perfusion (V/Q ratios close to 1). Even in health there is a spread to lower and higher V/Q ratios, all clustered around unity. When lungs are diseased, V/Q scatter is much greater, with variable representation across the full spectrum from zero to infinity. Such complexity resists simple bedside quantification. The best method is the multiple inert gas technique (MIGET). MIGET generates a lung model with 50 compartments spanning the full range of V/Q ratios, by measuring the retention and elimination of six inert gases of varying solubility.[10,11] Because MIGET is impractical at the bedside, simpler non-invasive modelling of shunt and V/Q mismatch is under evaluation, using FiO_2 as a forcing function while tracking haemoglobin oxygen saturation.[12] Predictive capacity[13] and ease of application[14] are encouraging.

THE IDEAL ALVEOLUS AND THE THREE-COMPARTMENT LUNG MODEL

Meanwhile the simplest model of all, a three-compartment model devised in the mid 20th century, is still in use. No manipulations such as FiO_2 switching or inert gas infusions are needed. However, the trade-off is that the model is overly simplistic, with poor predictive capacity in many respiratory disorders. The three compartments are:

1. the ideal compartment, consisting of alveoli with perfectly matched perfusion and ventilation ($V/Q = 1$)
2. the venous admixture or shunt compartment, containing perfused non-ventilated alveoli ($V/Q = 0$)
3. the alveolar dead space compartment, made up of ventilated non-perfused alveoli. ($V/Q = \infty$)

The alveolar PO_2 in the ideal compartment (PAO_2) is calculated from the alveolar gas:

$$PAO_2 = PiO_2 - (1 - FiO_2 \times (1 - R)) \times PaCO_2/R \qquad \textit{Equation 14.2}$$

where R is the respiratory exchange ratio, either measured by indirect calorimetry or assumed to be 0.8. PiO_2 is calculated as in Equation 14.1. $PaCO_2$ is arterial PCO_2.

Most clinicians use the following approximation:

$$PAO_2 = PiO_2 - PaCO_2/0.8$$

It is important to remember that PAO_2 is not a physiological reality. It is an artificial construct. Other parameters based on the three-compartment lung model, such as the A-a gradient and venous admixture (see below) must be regarded in the same light.

TRANSFER FROM ALVEOLI TO ARTERIAL BLOOD (PULMONARY OXYGEN TRANSFER)

The MIGET technique has identified V/Q mismatch and intrapulmonary right-to-left shunt as the two main causes of reduced pulmonary oxygen transfer in critical illness.[15] Intrapulmonary shunt predominates in the acute respiratory distress syndrome (ARDS), in lobar pneumonia and after cardiopulmonary bypass, whereas V/Q mismatch without shunt is more prominent in chronic lung disease.[16]

BEDSIDE INDICES OF PULMONARY OXYGEN TRANSFER

These are either tension-based or content-based.

TENSION-BASED INDICES

A-a gradient

The A-a gradient is calculated as $PAO_2 - PaO_2$, where PAO_2 is the 'ideal' compartment alveolar PO_2 determined from the alveolar gas equation (Equation 14.2). Hypoxaemia can then be classified under two headings:

Normal A-a gradient

1. Alveolar hypoventilation (elevated $PACO_2$)
2. Low PIO_2 ($FIO_2 < 0.21$, or barometric pressure < 760 mmHg)

Raised A-a gradient

1. diffusion defect (rare)
2. V/Q mismatch
3. right-to-left shunt (intrapulmonary or cardiac)
4. increased oxygen extraction ($CaO_2 - CvO_2$)

Although the A-a gradient forms part of the Acute Physiology, Age and Chronic Health Evaluation (APACHE 2) score, several drawbacks reduce its clinical usefulness. They include:

1. Normal values which vary with FIO_2 and age. The normal A-a gradient breathing air is 7 mmHg in young adults and 14 mmHg in the elderly. On 100% oxygen, these values become 31 and 56 mmHg respectively.
2. An exaggerated FIO_2 dependence in intrapulmonary shunt[17] (Figure 14.1) and even more so in V/Q mismatch (Figure 14.2).

PaO_2/FIO_2 *ratio*

The PaO_2/FIO_2 ratio is used to define acute lung injury and ARDS,[18] and is an input variable in the Simplified Acute Physiology Score (SAPS II)[19] and lung injury scoring systems.[20] At sea level its normal value is ≥ 500 mmHg. In acute lung injury, $PaO_2/FIO_2 < 300$ mmHg, whilst in ARDS the ratio is < 200 mmHg.

Its only advantage is simplicity. There are several major disadvantages:

1. Barometric pressure alters the normal PaO_2/FIO_2 ratio. A ratio of 380 mmHg is unremarkable at 1600 metres elevation for a young adult breathing air, but not at sea level.
2. Unlike the A-a gradient, the PaO_2/FIO_2 ratio cannot distinguish hypoxaemia due to alveolar hypoventilation from other causes.
3. The ratio is markedly FIO_2-dependent, both in right-to-left shunt (the predominant ARDS abnormality)

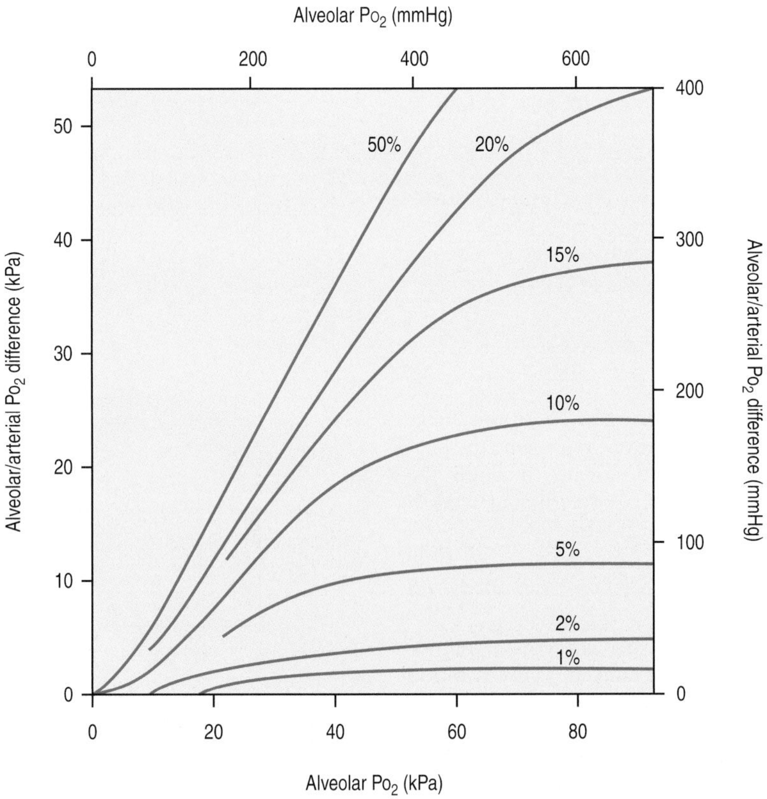

Figure 14.1 Effect of varying FIO_2 (PAO_2) on A-a gradient with different degrees of intrapulmonary shunt. (Reproduced from Nunn JF. Oxygen. In: Nunn JF (ed.) *Applied Respiratory Physiology*, 4th edn. Oxford, UK: Butterworth-Heinemann; 1993: 264, with permission.)

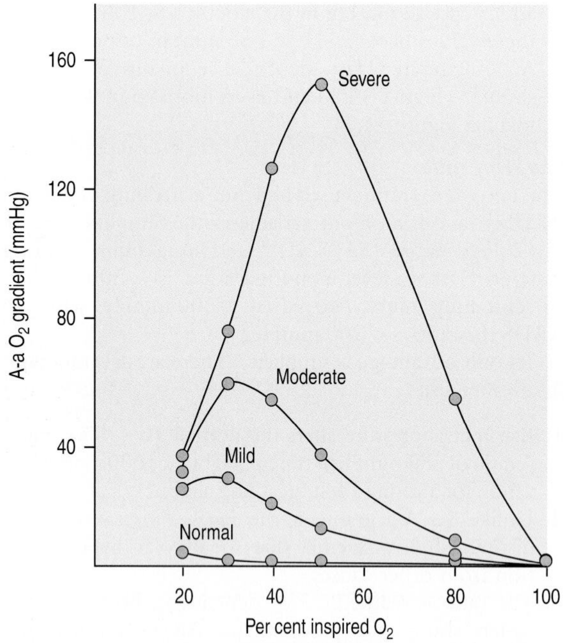

Figure 14.2 Effect of varying F_{IO_2} on A-a gradient with mild, moderate and severe *V/Q* mismatch. No allowance is made for absorption atelectasis or alterations in hypoxic pulmonary vasoconstriction. (Reproduced from D'Alonzo GE, Dantzker DR. Respiratory failure, mechanisms of abnormal gas exchange, and oxygen delivery. *Med Clin North Am* 1983; **67**: 557–71, with permission.)

and in lungs with a wide *V/Q* scatter (chronic obstructive pulmonary disease).[17,21]

4. The ratio is also highly dependent on $Ca_{O_2} - Cv_{O_2}$,[17] which tends to fluctuate markedly in sepsis.

CONTENT-BASED INDICES

Venous admixture (Q_s/Q_t)

Venous admixture, another construct based on the three-compartment lung model (see above), represents the proportion of mixed venous blood flowing through the shunt ($V/Q = 0$) compartment. It is determined according to the formula:

$$\frac{Q_s}{Q_T} = \frac{Cc'O_2 - Ca_{O_2}}{Cc'O_2 - Cv_{O_2}} \qquad \textit{Equation 14.3}$$

$Cc'O_2$, Ca_{O_2} and Cv_{O_2} are the oxygen contents of pulmonary end-capillary, arterial and mixed venous blood respectively. Ca_{O_2} and Cv_{O_2} are calculated using data from arterial and mixed venous blood gas analysis and CO oximetry (see Table 14.4, below). $Cc'O_2$ is derived differently, since pulmonary end-capillary blood cannot be sampled. $P_{C}^{1}O_2$ is assumed to equal PA_{O_2} as derived from the alveolar gas equation (Equation 14.2). $S_{C}^{1}O_2$ (normally close to 1) can then be computed from an algorithm for the HbO_2 dissociation curve.[22]

Advantages of venous admixture

1. unaffected by barometric pressure
2. unaffected by alveolar hypoventilation
3. provided intrapulmonary right-to-left shunt is the dominant pathology (e.g. ARDS), venous admixture is stable across the entire F_{IO_2} range, despite variations in $Ca_{O_2} - Cv_{O_2}$.[23]

Disadvantages of venous admixture

1. Sampling mixed venous blood requires a pulmonary arterial (PA) catheter.
2. In *V/Q* mismatch without right-to-left shunt, venous admixture varies markedly with F_{IO_2} and virtually disappears at $F_{IO_2} > 0.5$ (Figure 14.3). Venous admixture is thus of little use in conditions where the dominant gas exchange abnormality is not intrapulmonary right-to-left shunt, such as chronic obstructive pulmonary disease.

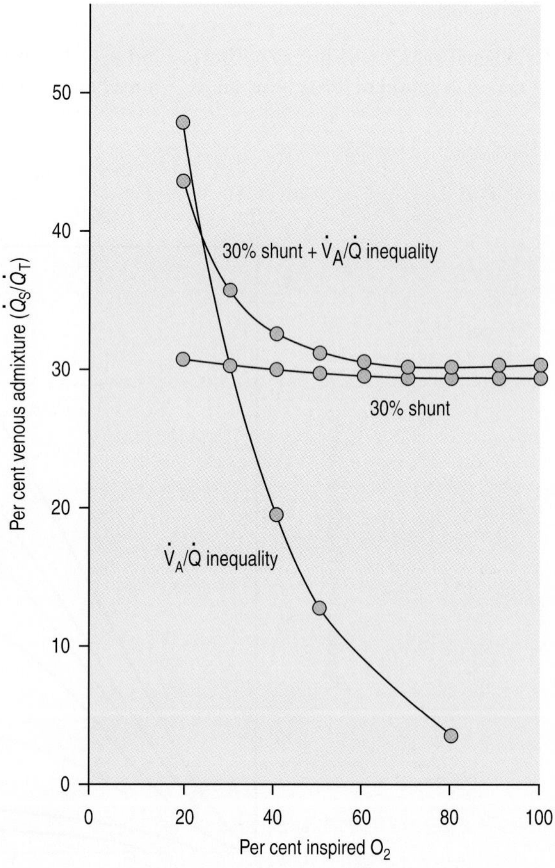

Figure 14.3 Effect of varying F_{IO_2} on venous admixture in various combinations of *V/Q* mismatch and shunt. No allowance has been made for absorption atelectasis or alterations in hypoxic pulmonary vasoconstriction. (Reproduced from D'Alonzo GE, Dantzker DR. Respiratory failure, mechanisms of abnormal gas exchange, and oxygen delivery. *Med Clin North Am* 1983; **67**: 557–71, with permission.)

When determined at $F_{IO_2} = 1$, venous admixture is an accurate measure of right-to-left shunt. However, exposure to 100% oxygen causes absorption atelectasis of unstable low *V/Q* units and increases intrapulmonary shunt.

Estimated shunt fraction

If a fixed $Ca_{O_2} - Cv_{O_2}$ can be assigned, no PA catheter is necessary. However, in critical illness $Ca_{O_2} - Cv_{O_2}$ can range from 1.3 to 7.4 ml/dl. The inaccuracy from assigning a fixed value is such that even the direction of change of estimated shunt can be wrong.[23]

Non-invasive estimates of V/Q mismatch and shunt

Simpler lung models using varying F_{IO_2} as a forcing function are under evaluation, as discussed above.[12–14]

ARTERIAL BLOOD

Indices of arterial oxygenation are Pa_{O_2} and Sa_{O_2}. They are linked by the HbO_2 dissociation curve (Figure 14.4).

Clinically significant hypoxaemia is defined as $Pa_{O_2} <$ 60 mmHg or $Sa_{O_2} < 0.9$. These values normally lie near the descending portion of the HbO_2 dissociation curve, so that a further drop in Pa_{O_2} leads to a marked fall in Sa_{O_2} and thus Ca_{O_2}.

BLOOD GAS ANALYSIS AND CO-OXIMETRY

Arterial blood is collected in a purpose-designed syringe containing lyophilised heparin to a final concentration of 20–50 U/mL. Pa_{O_2} measurements are made by a Clark electrode, and Sa_{O_2} by CO-oximetry. The Clark electrode works on polarographic principles, and CO-oximeters compute the concentrations of each of the four main haemoglobin species (HbO_2, Hb, COHb, MetHb) from light absorbances of haemolysed blood over several wavelengths. Sa_{O_2} is functional saturation, determined from concentrations of HbO_2 and Hb (see Table 14.4, below). Interference to CO-oximetry arises from substances with competing absorbance spectra, such as bilirubin, HbF, lipid emulsions and intravenous dyes. Newer multi-wavelength techniques reduce or eliminate this interference. Sa_{O_2} should always be measured rather than calculated.

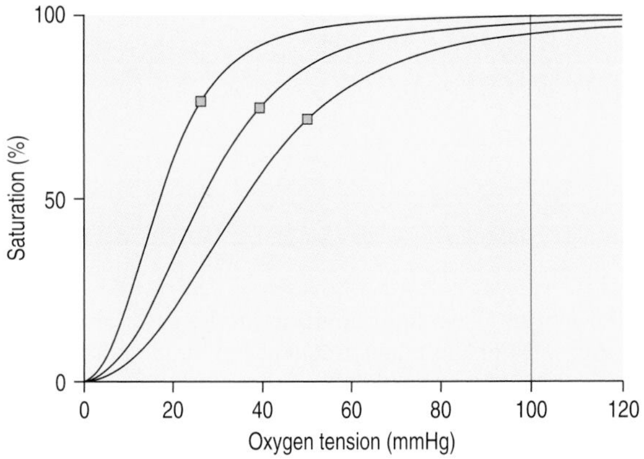

Figure 14.4 Three HbO_2 dissociation curves: normal (P50 = 26.7 mmHg), left-shifted (P50 = 17 mmHg) and right-shifted (P50 = 36 mmHg). The vertical line represents the normal oxygen loading tension (P_{O_2} = 100 mmHg). The filled squares represent an oxygen extraction of 5 ml/dl blood, assuming a haemoglobin concentration of 150 g/l. (Reproduced from Morgan TJ. The HbO_2 dissociation curve in critical illness. *Crit Care Resusc* 1999; **1**: 93–100, with permission.)

ERRORS (TABLE 14.1)

Temperature correction

All measurements are made at 37°C. Temperature-corrected values can be calculated if the core temperature of the patient is entered into the device software. Most clinicians interpret blood gas data at 37°C, except when evaluating the A-a gradient.

CONTINUOUS INTRA-ARTERIAL BLOOD GAS MONITORING (TABLE 14.2)[24]

Multiparameter fibreoptic sensors can be placed in the arterial stream. Fibreoptic sensors are called 'optodes', and those measuring P_{O_2} normally operate by fluorescence quenching. They require calibration with precision gases or solutions before use. Typical sensors are 0.5 mm in diameter, and can be inserted through 20-G arterial cannulae. The 90% in vitro response time to a change in P_{O_2} is 78 seconds. P_{O_2} drift in vivo is 0.03 mmHg/hour. Recalibration in vivo can be performed against conventional blood gas analysis. Accuracy on in vitro and animal testing is good.

Clinical trials evaluating the accuracy of these monitoring systems have revealed varying degrees of bias and imprecision. Trials demonstrating an improved outcome when therapeutic decisions are based on data from these devices are lacking. These factors, combined with the costs of these devices, have limited their bedside application.

Some problems encountered with intra-arterial sensors, particularly artefact due to flow and position, have prompted the development of extracorporeal monitors placed in line but ex vivo. These devices do not provide continuous real-time data. When a measurement is desired, a sample is drawn into the externally located cassette, and then returned. Results are available in 2 minutes. In preterm neonates this method has allowed significant reductions in red cell transfusions.[25]

TRANSCUTANEOUS P_{O_2} AND P_{CO_2} MONITORING

Continuous non-invasive assessment of blood gas tensions is possible with transcutaneous P_{O_2} and P_{CO_2} monitoring. Available systems incorporate P_{O_2} and P_{CO_2} electrodes with integral thermistors and servo-controlled heaters. P_{O_2} measurement utilises the principle of the Clark electrode, while the P_{CO_2} device is a pH-sensitive glass electrode. To achieve good correlation with arterial values, the skin is warmed to a temperature of 42–44°C.

Table 14.1 Preanalytic and analytic errors in Po_2 measurement

Preanalytic	Analytic
Oxygen diffusing into or out of air bubbles, according to the tension gradient	Interanalyser variability. There is 7–8% measurement variation on the same sample
Contamination with flush solution. Discard volume should be 2–3 times the internal volume of cannula and tubing	Inadequate anticoagulation, allowing protein deposition on the electrodes
Pseudohypoxaemia. Oxygen consumption in vitro from extreme leukocytosis	Non-linearity at high Po_2 (> 150 mmHg)
Artifactual Pao_2 elevations. With polypropylene syringes stored on ice, the semipermeable plastic allows oxygen ingress, facilitated by the cold-induced increase in oxygen solubility	Maintenance of electrode temperature within narrow limits (37 ± 0.1°C) is critical. Po_2 changes by 7% for every degree Celsius temperature change Interference by nitrous oxide and halothane is minimal, provided the polarizing voltage of the electrode does not exceed 600 mV Quality control materials such as aqueous, perfluorocarbon and bovine haemoglobin solutions are used for convenience, but tonometry is the primary reference method Arterial blood gas tensions fluctuate breath to breath Intermittent analysis is a snapshot

Table 14.2 Continuous intra-arterial Pao_2 monitoring – advantages and disadvantages

Advantages	Disadvantages
Eliminates preanalytic errors of intermittent blood gas analysis	The 'wall' effect – a sudden decrease in measured Pao_2 due to contact with the arterial wall, with averaging of arterial and wall oxygen tensions. The problem is reduced in larger arteries such as the femoral artery
More sensitive than pulse oximetry to changes in arterial oxygenation when $Pao_2 > 70$ mmHg (the flat part of the Hbo_2 dissociation curve).	The 'flush' effect. Unless the sensor is inserted a sufficient distance beyond the cannula tip, measured Pao_2 can be altered by contamination with the continuous flush solution
Free from the sources of error of pulse oximetry (see Table 14.3)	Damping of the arterial waveform
Near real-time Pao_2 allows prompt tracking of responses to changed ventilator settings	Large footprint of the free-standing monitor
Reduced exposure of personnel to potentially infected blood	
Reduced blood loss for diagnostic purposes	

Transcutaneous monitors generate reliable Pco_2 values in adequately perfused patients, but Po_2 measurements are more for trend analysis. Skin warming necessitates frequent site changes to prevent burns, and there is a need for regular recalibration. Monitoring in haemodynamically unstable patients is not recommended. The monitors have a role in the prevention of neonatal hyperoxia, a problem not reliably detected by pulse oximetry.[26]

PULSE OXIMETRY[27,28]

Pulse oximetry determines Spo_2 from the absorbance of light at wavelengths 660 nm (red) and 940 nm (infrared) by tissue capillary beds such as fingers, earlobes and the nasal septum. Two light-emitting diodes cycle on and off at multiples of the mains frequency. A single photodiode detects the transmitted light, and a third interval allows correction for background ambient light. The emergent signal is pulsatile due to arterial volume fluctuations. Subtraction of the background signal (tissue, capillary blood and venous blood) isolates the arterial component.

For both wavelengths, absorbance (A) is determined as follows:

$$A = \log_{10}(I_0/I)$$

where I_0 = incident light intensity, and I = emergent light intensity. For a given chromophore, A is proportional to its concentration (Beer's law) and to the path length (Lambert's law). From the pulsatile (AC) and background (DC) absorbance signals at both wavelengths, a ratio (R) is derived:

$$R = (AC_{660}/DC_{660})/(AC_{940}/DC_{940})$$

Spo_2 is then computed from R, using software 'look-up' tables of empirically derived relationships between R-values and either Sao_2 or fractional saturation ($FHbO_2$) measured in the arterial blood of volunteers breathing hypoxic gas mixtures.

Spo_2 is usually displayed as a percentage. Only two wavelengths are used, forcing the assumption that HbO_2 and Hb are the only haemoglobin species in the light path. This is always incorrect, but the error is trivial with normal dyshaemoglobin concentrations. Some manufacturers calibrate R against $FHbO_2$ rather than Sao_2 (functional saturation). Because volunteers generating the data have normal dyshaemoglobin concentrations, differences between the two calibrations are small.

SPEED OF RESPONSE

Spo_2 is averaged over 3–6 seconds, and updated every 0.5–1 second. With forehead probes a sudden reduction in Fio_2 produces a response within 10–15 seconds, whereas with finger probes and peripheral vasoconstriction the delay can exceed 1 minute.

ACCURACY

In the 90–97% saturation range, Spo_2 has a mean absolute bias of $< 1\%$, and a precision (standard deviaition of bias) of $< 3\%$. At $Sao_2 < 80\%$ there is significant imprecision and a tendency towards negative bias. This is because very low Sao_2 values are unsafe in volunteers, necessitating extrapolation from Spo_2/R relationships at higher saturations.

ERROR

Causes of error are set out in Table 14.3. A falsely high Spo_2 is of greatest concern.

Unlike CO-oximetry, pulse oximetry is not subject to interference from bilirubin, lipid emulsions and HbF.

Dyshaemoglobins and pulse oximetry

Pulse oximeters cannot distinguish COHb from HbO_2. When [COHb] is elevated, Spo_2 tends to overestimate Sao_2. Spo_2 can thus provide false reassurance when hypoxaemia is combined with a high [COHb], for example after an inhalational burn injury.

MetHb has more complex effects, since it absorbs both wavelengths. At normal saturations, increased [MetHb] causes underestimation of Sao_2, but at very low oxygen tensions overestimation is possible. At [MetHb] $\geq 35\%$, the R-value becomes unity, which translates to $Spo_2 = 85\%$.

IMPORTANCE OF PULSE OXIMETRY

Pulse oximeters generate accurate real-time information without calibration, within moments of sensor placement. Their use is mandatory in patient transport, and in high-acuity areas such as operating rooms, recovery rooms and intensive care units. They are also useful screening tools. On the down side, pulse oximeters are the most common source of false alarms in intensive care. They are also

Table 14.3 Causes of error in Spo_2 readings

Factor	Comment
Carboxyhaemoglobin	Measured as Hbo_2 – Spo_2 may be falsely high – see text
Methaemoglobin	Absorbs both wavelengths – see text
Low saturations	Progressive inaccuracy below 70–80%, usually falsely low Spo_2
Prominent venous signal	Dependent limb, tricuspid regurgitation (venous pulsations) – falsely low Spo_2
Non-pulsatile flow	Cardiopulmonary bypass – poor signal
Vasoconstriction, limb ischaemia, shock states	Low pulsatile signal
Motion artefact	Tremor, voluntary movement – falsely low Spo_2
Ambient light	Strong sunlight, fluorescent and xenon lamps, flickering light– falsely low Spo_2
Anaemia	No effect
Dyes	Methylene blue, indocyanine green, indigo carmine – falsely low Spo_2
Black skin pigmentation	Variable precision and bias. May require separate calibration
Nail polish	Especially blue. Falsely low Spo_2. Acrylic nails do not interfere
Optical shunting	Due to inadequate probe contact – falsely low Spo_2
Radiofrequency interference	Reported with magnetic resonance imaging scanners – falsely high Spo_2

insensitive to changes in arterial oxygenation at higher Pao_2 values (> 70–100 mmHg).

MONITORING HAEMOGLOBIN–OXYGEN AFFINITY

Haemoglobin–oxygen affinity is the relationship between the oxygen tension of blood and its oxygen content, described by the sigmoid-shaped HbO_2 dissociation curve (see Figure 14.4). The P50 is the oxygen tension at $So_2 = 0.5$. The normal value in humans is 26.7 mmHg. Factors which decrease haemoglobin–oxygen affinity increase the P50. They include acidaemia (the Bohr effect), hypercapnia, high levels of erythrocytic 2,3-diphosphoglycerate (2,3-DPG) and fever, whereas P50 is decreased (increased affinity) by alkalaemia, hypocapnia, low 2,3-DPG levels, hypothermia, COHb, MetHb and FHb.

In the intensive care unit, it is possible to calculate accurate P50 values from a single measurement of blood gases and Sao_2 up to $Sao_2 = 0.97$.[29] However the impact of haemoglobin–oxygen affinity on tissue oxygenation in critical illness appears to be small,[30] making routine monitoring unnecessary.

OXYGEN DYNAMICS

Common indices of oxygen dynamics are set out in Table 14.4.

Do_2/Vo_2 RELATIONSHIPS

More than 30 years ago an association was reported between hyperdynamic oxygen flow patterns and survival after high-risk non-cardiac surgery.[31] This led to the hypothesis that an induced perioperative hyperdynamic state is protective, subsequently supported by single-unit studies,[32–35] but not by larger multicentre studies.[36,37] Much of any benefit may be due to fluid loading, or even increased care and attention. Typical therapeutic goals have been cardiac index (CI) > 4.5 l/min per m^2, Do_2I > 600 ml/min per m^2, Vo_2I > 170 ml/min per m^2. More recently more emphasis has been placed on the Do_2I target, since supranormal Vo_2I values are much harder to achieve. It is now also clear that in sepsis, aggressive pursuit of hyperdynamic goals is counterproductive.[38]

MEASURING Do_2I

Although Do_2I determinations require accurate measurements of CI and Cao_2, a PA catheter is not essential (see Chapter 12). Normal ranges can be quoted (Table 14.4), but oxygen demand in critical illness is so variable that isolated Do_2I measurements are difficult to interpret.

MEASURING Vo_2I

The two methods of measuring Vo_2I are the reverse Fick method (Table 14.4) and indirect calorimetry.

Table 14.4 Oxygen dynamics – measured and derived indices

Parameter	Abbreviation	Formula	Normal range	Units
Functional haemoglobin concentration	$[Hb_{funct}]$	$[HbO_2] + [Hb]$	12.0–18.0	g/dl
Arterial oxygen tension	Pao_2	Measured	95 ± 5	mmHg
Mixed venous oxygen tension	$P\bar{v}o_2$	Measured	40 ± 5	mmHg
Functional saturation	So_2	$[HbO_2]/([HbO_2] + [Hb])$		
Fractional saturation	$FHbO_2$	$[HbO_2]/([HbO_2] + [Hb] + [COHb] + [MetHb])$		
Arterial functional saturation	Sao_2		0.97 ± 0.02	
Mixed venous functional saturation	$S\bar{v}o_2$		0.75 ± 0.05	
Blood oxygen content	CO_2	$1.39 \times [Hb_{funct}] \times So_2 + 0.0031 \times Po_2$		ml/dl
Arterial oxygen content	Cao_2		16–22	ml/dl
Mixed venous oxygen content	$C\bar{v}o_2$		12–17	ml/dl
Cardiac index	CI	CO/BSA	2.5–4.2	$l/min/m^2$
Oxygen delivery index	Do_2I	$CI \times Cao_2 \times 10$	460–650	ml/min per m^2
Oxygen consumption index	Vo_2I	$CI \times (Cao_2 - C\bar{v}o_2) \times 10$	96–170	ml/min per m^2
Oxygen extraction ratio	O_2ER	$(Cao_2 - C\bar{v}o_2)/Cao_2$ or Vo_2/Do_2	0.23–0.32	

HbO_2, oxyhaemoglobin; Hb, reduced haemoglobin; COHb, carboxyhaemoglobin; MetHb, methaemoglobin; BSA, body surface area.

Reverse Fick method

The reverse Fick method requires a PA catheter, and has large random errors, ranging from 17% overestimation to 13% underestimation. Changes cannot be detected reliably unless they exceed 20%. The error is increased by lung inflammation, when up to 20% of $\dot{V}O_2I$ can arise from the lungs alone.

Indirect calorimetry

Indirect calorimetry has better accuracy. $\dot{V}O_2I$ is determined from the volumes and oxygen concentrations of inspired and expired gas. However, high FiO_2 settings introduce error. Newer devices retain their accuracy up to $FiO_2 = 0.8$, with relative errors of $< 5\%$.[39]

MIXED VENOUS BLOOD

Mixed venous sampling is by gentle aspiration of blood from the distal port of an unwedged PA catheter. This ensures complete admixture of blood from superior and inferior venae cavae and coronary sinus. Mixed venous O_2 and CO_2 tensions and content are flow-weighted averages of the venous effluents of multiple tissues. The integrating process can conceal pockets of hypoxia and hypercapnia.

MIXED VENOUS PO_2 ($P\bar{v}O_2$)

Venous gas tensions reflect postcapillary and tissue gas tensions. At a $P\bar{v}O_2$ of 26 mmHg, the average intracellular PO_2 has fallen from 11 to 0.8 mmHg.[40] A $P\bar{v}O_2$ below this value is highly suggestive of intracellular hypoxia. However, a normal or high $P\bar{v}O_2$ does not exclude regional tissue hypoxia, whether cytopathic hypoxia[5] or hypoxia due to tissue shunting.[41]

MIXED VENOUS OXYGEN SATURATION ($S\bar{v}O_2$)

$S\bar{v}O_2$ is measured either intermittently by CO-oximetry on mixed venous samples or continuously by fibreoptic reflectance oximetry using a modified PA catheter. $S\bar{v}O_2$ measurements have a number of potential uses:

1. To calculate $C\bar{v}O_2$ (Table 14.4). $C\bar{v}O_2$ can then be used to determine Q_s/Q_t, $\dot{V}O_2I$ by the reverse Fick method, the oxygen extraction ratio (Table 14.4) and cardiac output by the Fick method.
2. As an indirect index of tissue hypoxia. A $S\bar{v}O_2$ value of 0.5 corresponds to the theoretical critical $P\bar{v}O_2$ of 26 mmHg. Values between 0.7 and 0.8 represent a desirable balance between global oxygen supply and demand (Table 14.4), with lactic acidosis appearing between 0.3 and 0.5.[42] Values exceeding 0.8 can be seen in high-flow states such as sepsis, hyperthyroidism and severe liver disease.

$S\bar{v}O_2$ as a therapeutic target (> 0.7) failed to improve survival in a multicentre trial.[43] Only two-thirds of the treatment group achieved the $S\bar{v}O_2$ target. Like $P\bar{v}O_2$, $S\bar{v}O_2$ is insensitive to cytopathic hypoxia and tissue shunting. In chronic heart failure, low values can be surprisingly well tolerated.

CENTRAL VENOUS SATURATION ($SCvO_2$)[43–45]

As with $S\bar{v}O_2$, $ScvO_2$ can be measured either continuously using a central venous catheter modified for reflectance oximetry, or by intermittent sampling and CO-oximetry. $ScvO_2$ is normally 2–3% lower than $S\bar{v}O_2$. However, in shock this difference can be reversed. Trends in $S\bar{v}O_2$ and $ScvO_2$ in response to management usually run in parallel.

In an influential single-centre study of the early hypodynamic phase of severe sepsis and septic shock, resuscitation guided by a $ScvO_2$ target of > 0.7, as well as by central venous pressure and mean arterial pressure values, appeared to reduce 28-day and 60-day mortality, and duration of hospitalization.[45] It remains to be seen whether this success can be replicated in larger trials, and if so whether intermittent sampling is of equivalent benefit. Nevertheless, $ScvO_2$ currently has equal billing with $S\bar{v}O_2$ in the management guidelines of the Surviving Sepsis Campaign.[46]

VENOARTERIAL PCO_2 GRADIENT (ΔPCO_2)

ΔPCO_2 (normally about 6 mmHg) is markedly increased during cardiac arrest and in experimental low-output states, but lacks sensitivity and specificity as a global index of tissue hypoxia. A sudden increase in the respiratory quotient ($\dot{V}CO_2/\dot{V}O_2$), or in the venoarterial CO_2 tension difference/arteriovenous O_2 content difference[47] may be more reliable markers of the onset of anaerobic metabolism.

PLASMA LACTATE AND REDOX INDICES

See Chapter 15.

REGIONAL OXYGENATION INDICES

REGIONAL PCO_2[48]

Regional PCO_2 reflects the balance between arterial blood CO_2 content, tissue blood flow and tissue CO_2 production. The CO_2 gap, which is regional $PCO_2 - PaCO_2$, was devised to correct regional PCO_2 for varying arterial CO_2 content. As tissue blood flow falls, reduced CO_2 clearance causes the CO_2 gap to increase. With the onset of anaerobic metabolism, tissue CO_2 production steadily decreases, although worsening regional metabolic acidosis generates some CO_2 by proton titration of tissue and capillary HCO_3^-. A rising CO_2 gap merely signals falling tissue blood flow. It cannot identify the onset of anaerobic metabolism.

GASTRIC TONOMETRY[49]

The impetus to develop regional gastric capnometry was the knowledge that splanchnic hypoperfusion occurs early in circulatory shock, tends to persist as 'covert shock', and is manifested by intramucosal hypercapnia and acidosis. A gastric tonometer was therefore developed as a modified nasogastric tube with a silicone balloon 11.4 cm from the tip. Gastric mucosal CO_2 equilibrates with luminal CO_2, which equilibrates with (and is measured in) fluid filling the balloon. Early on, this fluid was saline. Subsequently air was found to have more rapid equilibration characteristics, and automated cycling of air through an infrared CO_2 analyser was far more efficient than measuring saline $P\text{CO}_2$ intermittently and applying time-based correction factors.

The original concept involved calculation of intramucosal pH (pH_i) via the Henderson–Hasselbalch equation, using gastric luminal $P\text{CO}_2$ and arterial $[HCO_3^-]$. Intramucosal acidosis was defined as pHi < 7.3, and taken to indicate inadequate splanchnic perfusion. Changing the monitoring end-point from pH_i to the mucosal–arterial CO_2 gap (normally 8–10 mmHg) removed the most fundamental flaw – the use of arterial $[HCO_3^-]$ as a surrogate for mucosal $[HCO_3^-]$. Automated air tonometry combined with simultaneous end-tidal CO_2 measurement allows the regular calculation of a gastric to end-tidal CO_2 gap, a parameter linked to outcome in high-risk surgery.[50]

Even with these improvements, the technique has not found widespread application, and is unlikely to do so for several reasons:

1. the need for a nasogastric tube
2. signal degradation by luminal contents, including feeds and blood. Feeds must be stopped 2 hours prior to measurements, jeopardising nutritional support
3. inability to identify a clear hypoxic threshold. Empiric recommendations have been to target a CO_2 gap < 25 mmHg
4. a need to suppress gastric acidity to prevent luminal CO_2 generation by HCl titration of duodenal bicarbonate
5. a lack of convincing evidence that tonometry-guided therapy improves outcome[51]

SUBLINGUAL CAPNOMETRY[49,50]

Sublingual capnometry measures the interstitial CO_2 tension under the tongue, as its name suggests, using either electrode or optode technologies. Although the tongue vasculature is not part of the splanchnic circulation, it responds similarly to circulatory disturbances. It has the added advantage of accessibility with minimal invasion. Optode sensors in particular provide rapid-response $P\text{CO}_2$ signals. It is also possible to perform simultaneous inspections of the microcirculation using orthogonal polarisation spectral imaging.

At this stage, all that can be said is that sublingual $P\text{CO}_2$ seems to correlate with the severity of haemodynamic disturbances and with gastric mucosal $P\text{CO}_2$, and that in a limited number of shocked patients the sublingual CO_2 gap was correlated with survival. It remains to be seen whether the technique can be used to guide therapy.

CEREBROVENOUS OXYGEN SATURATION MONITORING

See Chapter 67.

DIRECT TISSUE $P\text{O}_2$ MEASUREMENT

In patients this is largely impractical. Measurements have been recorded primarily in animal models in the brain, subcutaneous tissue, muscle and renal beds under a variety of perfusion insults.[52] Tensions are commonly around 30–45 mmHg, but can range from < 10 mmHg in the renal medulla to > 70 mmHg in subcutaneous tissue.

OTHER REGIONAL TECHNIQUES

Orthogonal polarisation spectroscopy (OPS) allows real-time in vivo imaging of microcirculatory blood flow.[42] Tissue beds visualised in intensive care have included the sublingual, rectal, oral and ileal (via stoma) microcirculations. OPS can be combined with near-infrared spectroscopy to monitor deeper regional mitochondrial redox status, and with reflectance spectrophotometry for measurement of superficial microcirculatory oxygen saturation. Combinations of this type provide uniquely integrated information on oxygen transport distribution during sepsis and septic shock.

Other techniques showing promise include in vivo magnetic resonance imaging[53] and optical spectroscopy.[54]

REFERENCES

1. Schumacker PT. Cell metabolism and tissue hypoxia. In: Albert RK, Slutsky A, Ranieri M *et al.* (eds) *Clinical Critical Care Medicine.* Philadelphia: Mosby Elsevier; 2006: 41–50.
2. Bayir H. Reactive oxygen species. *Crit Care Med* 2005; **33** (Suppl.): S49–501.
3. Schumacker PT. Hypoxia-inducible factor-1 (HIF-1). *Crit Care Med* 2005; **33** (Suppl.): S423–5.
4. Connett RJ, Honig CR, Gayeski TE *et al.* Defining hypoxia: a systems view of $\dot{V}O_2$, glycolysis, energetics, and intracellular $P\text{O}_2$. *J Appl Physiol* 1990; **68**: 833–42.
5. Fink MP. Bench to bedside review: cytopathic hypoxia. *Crit Care* 2002; **6**: 491–9.
6. Deby-Dupont G, Deby C, Lamy M. Oxygen therapy in intensive care patients: a vital poison? In: Vincent J-L (ed.) *Yearbook of Intensive Care and Emergency Medicine.* Berlin: Springer-Verlag; 1999: 417–32.
7. Terragni PP, Rosboch G, Tealdi A *et al.* Tidal hyperinflation during low tidal volume ventilation in acute respiratory distress syndrome. *Am J Respir Crit Care Med* 2007; **175**: 160–6.
8. Dunlop S, Hough J, Riedel T *et al.* Electrical impedance tomography in extremely prematurely born infants and during high frequency oscillatory ventilation analyzed in the frequency domain. *Physiol Meas* 2006; **27**: 1151–65.
9. Wolf GK, Arnold JH. Noninvasive assessment of lung volume: respiratory inductance plethysmography and

electrical impedance tomography. *Crit Care Med* 2005; **33** (Suppl.): S163–9.
10. West JB. Ventilation–perfusion relationships. *Am Rev Respir Dis* 1977; **116**: 919–43.
11. Yu G, Yang K, Baker AB *et al.* The effect of bi-level positive airway pressure mechanical ventilation on gas exchange during general anaesthesia. *Br J Anaesth* 2006; **96**: 522–32.
12. Kjaergaard S, Rees S, Malczynski J *et al.* Non-invasive estimation of shunt and ventilation–perfusion mismatch. *Intens Care Med* 2003; **29**: 727–34.
13. Rees SE, Kjaergaard S, Andreassen S *et al.* Reproduction of MIGET retention and excretion data using a simple mathematical model of gas exchange in lung damage caused by oleic acid infusion. *J Appl Physiol* 2006; **101**: 826–32.
14. Kjaergaard S, Rees SE, Gronlund J *et al.* Hypoxaemia after cardiac surgery: clinical application of a model of pulmonary gas exchange. *Eur J Anaesthesiol* 2004; **21**: 296–301.
15. D'Alonzo GE, Dantzker DR. Respiratory failure, mechanisms of abnormal gas exchange, and oxygen delivery. *Med Clin North Am* 1983; **67**: 557–71.
16. Rodriguez-Roisin R, Roca J. Mechanisms of hypoxaemia. *Intens Care Med* 2005; **31**: 1017–9.
17. Nirmalan M, Willard T, Columb MO *et al.* Effect of changes in arterial-mixed venous oxygen content difference ($C(a\text{-}v)O_2$) on indices of pulmonary oxygen transfer in a model ARDS lung. *Br J Anaesth* 2001; **86**: 477–85.
18. Bernard GR, Artigas A, Brigham KL *et al.* Report of the American–European consensus conference on ARDS: definitions, mechanisms, relevant outcomes and clinical trial coordination. *Intens Care Med* 1994; **20**: 225–32.
19. Le Gall J-R, Lemeshow S, Saulnier F. A new simplified acute physiology score (SAPS II) based on a European/North American multicentre study. *JAMA* 1993; **270**: 2957–63.
20. Murray JF, Mathay MA, Luce JM *et al.* An expanded definition of the adult respiratory distress syndrome. *Am Rev Respir Dis* 1988; **138**: 720–3.
21. Whiteley JP, Gavaghan DJ, Hahn CE. Variation of venous admixture, SF6 shunt, PaO_2, and the PaO_2/FiO_2 ratio with FiO_2. *Br J Anaesth* 2002; **88**: 771–8.
22. Siggaard-Andersen O, Siggaard-Andersen M. The oxygen status algorithm: a computer program for calculating and displaying pH and blood gas data. *Scand J Clin Lab Invest* 1990; **50** (Suppl. 203): 29–45.
23. Nirmalan M, Willard T, Khan A *et al.* Changes in arterial–mixed venous oxygen content difference (CaO_2–$C\bar{v}O_2$) and the effect on shunt calculations in critically ill patients. *Br J Anaesth* 1998; **80**: 829–31.
24. Venkatesh B, Hendry S-P. Continuous intra-arterial blood gas monitoring. *Intens Care Med* 1996; **22**: 818–28.
25. Widness JA, Madan A, Grindeanu LA *et al.* Reduction in red blood cell transfusions among preterm infants: results of a randomized trial with an in-line blood gas and chemistry monitor. *Pediatrics* 2005; **115**: 1299–306.
26. Rudiger M, Topfer K, Hammer H *et al.* A survey of transcutaneous blood gas monitoring among European neonatal intensive care units. *BMC Pediatr* 2005; **5**: 30.
27. Jubran A. Pulse oximetry. In: Tobin MJ (ed.) *Principles and Practice of Intensive Care Monitoring*. New York: McGraw Hill; 1998: 261–87.
28. McMorrow RCN, Mythen MG. Pulse oximetry. *Curr Opin Crit Care* 2006; **12**: 269–71.
29. Morgan TJ, Koch D, Morris D *et al.* Red cell 2,3-diphosphoglycerate concentrations are reduced in critical illness without net effect on in vivo P50. *Anaesth Intens Care* 2001; **29**: 479–83.
30. Gutierrez G. The unpretentious role of 2,3-diphosphoglycerate in critical illness. *Crit Care Med* 2005; **33**: 2423–4.
31. Shoemaker WC, Montgomery ES, Kaplan E *et al.* Physiologic patterns in surviving and nonsurviving shock patients. *Arch Surg* 1973; **106**: 630–6.
32. Boyd O, Grounds M, Bennett D. A randomized clinical trial of the effect of deliberate perioperative increase of oxygen delivery on mortality in high-risk surgical patients. *JAMA* 1993; **270**: 2699–707.
33. Wilson J, Woods I, Fawcett J *et al.* Reducing the risk of major elective surgery: randomised controlled trial of preoperative optimisation of oxygen delivery. *Br Med J* 1999; **318**: 1099–103.
34. Lobo SM, Salgoda PF, Castillo VGT *et al.* Effects of maximizing oxygen delivery on morbidity and mortality in high-risk surgical patients. *Crit Care Med* 2000; **28**: 3396–404.
35. Pearse R, Dawson D, Fawcett J *et al.* Early goal-directed therapy after major surgery reduces complications and duration of hospital stay. A randomised, controlled trial. *Crit Care* 2005; **9**: 687–93.
36. Takala J, Meier-Hellmann A, Eddleston J *et al.* Effect of dopexamine on outcome after major abdominal surgery: a prospective, randomized, controlled multicenter study. European Multicenter Study Group on Dopexamine in Major Abdominal Surgery. *Crit Care Med* 2000; **28**: 3417–23.
37. Sandham JD, Hull RD, Brant RF *et al.* Canadian Critical Care Clinical Trials Group. A randomized, controlled trial of the use of pulmonary-artery catheters in high-risk surgical patients. *N Engl J Med* 2003; **348**: 5–14.
38. Gattinoni L, Brazzi L, Pelosi P. Does cardiovascular optimization reduce mortality? In: Vincent J-L (ed.) *Yearbook of Intensive Care and Emergency Medicine*. Berlin: Springer-Verlag; 1996: 308–18.
39. Walsh TS, Monaco F. Gas exchange measurement in the ICU. In: Vincent J-L (ed.) *Yearbook of Intensive Care and Emergency Medicine*. Berlin: Springer-Verlag; 2005: 632–43.
40. Siggaard-Andersen O, Fogh-Andersen N, Gøthgen IH *et al.* Oxygen status of arterial and mixed venous blood. *Crit Care Med* 1995; **23**: 1284–93.
41. Elbers PW, Ince C. Bench-to-bedside review: mechanisms of critical illness – classifying microcirculatory flow abnormalities in distributive shock. *Crit Care* 2006; **10**: 221.

42. Marx G, Reinhart K. Venous oximetry. *Curr Opin Crit Care* 2006; **12**: 263–8.
43. Gattinoni L, Brazzi L, Pelosi P *et al.* A trial of goal-orientated hemodynamic therapy in critically ill patients. *N Engl J Med* 1995; **333**: 1025–32.
44. Rivers E, Nguyen B, Havstad S *et al.* Early goal-directed therapy in the treatment of severe sepsis and septic shock. *N Engl J Med* 2001; **345**: 1368–77.
45. Pearse R, Dawson D, Fawcett J *et al.* Changes in central venous saturation after major surgery, and association with outcome. *Crit Care* 2005; **9**: R694–9.
46. Dellinger RP, Carlet JM, Masur H, *et al.* Surviving Sepsis Campaign guidelines for management of severe sepsis and septic shock. *Crit Care Med* 2004; **32**: 858–73.
47. Mekontso-Dessap A, Castelain V, Anguel N *et al.* Combination of venoarterial $P\text{CO}_2$ difference with arteriovenous O_2 content difference to detect anaerobic metabolism in patients. *Intens Care Med* 2002; **28**: 272–7.
48. Marik PE. Regional carbon dioxide monitoring to assess the adequacy of tissue perfusion. *Curr Opin Crit Care* 2005; **11**: 245–51.
49. Creteur J. Gastric and sublingual capnometry. *Curr Opin Crit Care* 2006; **12**: 272–7.
50. Lebuffe G, Vallet B, Takala J *et al.* A European, multicenter, observational study to assess the value of gastric-to-end tidal $P\text{CO}_2$ difference in predicting postoperative complications. *Anesth Analg* 2004; **99**: 166–72.
51. Miami Trauma Clinical Trials Group. Splanchnic hypoperfusion-directed therapies in trauma: a prospective, randomized trial. *Am Surg* 2005; **71**: 252–60.
52. Venkatesh B, Morgan TJ. Monitoring tissue gas tensions in critical illness. In: Vincent J-L (ed.) *Yearbook of Intensive Care and Emergency Medicine.* Berlin: Springer-Verlag; 2001: 251–65.
53. Zaharchuk G, Busse RF, Rosenthal G *et al.* Noninvasive oxygen partial pressure measurement of human body fluids in vivo using magnetic resonance imaging. *Acad Radiol* 2006; **13**: 1016–24.
54. Mayevsky A, Rogatsky G. Mitochondrial function in vivo evaluated by NADH fluorescence: From animal models to human studies. *Am J Physiol Cell Physiol* 2007; **292**: C615–40.

15

Lactic acidosis

D J (Jamie) Cooper and Alistair D Nichol

Lactic acidosis is defined by convention as the combination of an increased blood lactate concentration (> 5 mmol/l) and acidaemia (arterial blood pH of < 7.35).[1,2] However hyperlactaemia occurs whenever the blood lactate concentration is above the normal range (< 2 mmol/l). Lactic acidosis may be masked by coincident metabolic or respiratory alkalosis. Critically ill patients with lactic acidosis usually have a high mortality[3] and blood lactate concentrations > 8 mmol/l predict fatality.[4] A prospective study reported 83% mortality in patients with blood lactate concentrations of 10 mmol/l.[1] In each individual patient, however, prognosis is completely dependent on the underlying condition, with the initial degree of lactic acidosis being a clinically useful indicator of shock severity, and serial assessment allowing evaluation of response to therapy. Recently, blood lactate concentration has been identified as one marker of the degree of shock triggering treatment in septic patients who may benefit from early goal-directed therapy.[5] It is important to remember that, in healthy athletes, severe lactic acidosis during exercise is a normal, self-limited observation.

PATHOPHYSIOLOGY

There is a continuous cycle of lactate production and metabolism. Lactate is produced at about 0.8 mmol/kg per h, while simultaneous metabolism in liver, kidneys, skeletal muscle, brain and red blood cells ensures that blood lactate concentrations are normally low (< 1 mmol/l). Lactic acidosis occurs when lactate production exceeds metabolic capacity, or when metabolic capacity is decreased by organ dysfunction. The liver has a key role in lactate homeostasis and many patients who develop lactic acidosis have decreased metabolic capacity due to liver disease.[6]

Formation and metabolism of lactate in cells are catalysed by lactate dehydrogenase (LDH):

$$\text{Pyruvate} + \text{NADH} + \text{H}^+ \xleftrightarrow{\text{LDH}} \text{Lactate} + \text{NAD}^+$$

Lactate formation is in part dependent upon pyruvate concentrations and pyruvate is sourced from glycolysis (85%) and proteolysis (15%). Glucose is derived from absorption, glycogen and gluconeogenesis. Rate of glycolysis is controlled by three unidirectional enzymes and the activity of one of these enzymes is increased by increasing intracellular pH. Acidosis therefore decreases (and alkalosis increases) glycolysis and pyruvate, and consequently lactate production. In oxygen excess, pyruvate is oxidised and lactate does not accumulate. Anaerobic metabolism however, causes lactate accumulation and an increased lactate/pyruvate ratio. The blood lactate/pyruvate ratio is however a poor indicator of mitochondrial concentrations, and is not of clinical use.

In critically ill patients, lactic acidosis is often due to shock. In cardiogenic and hypovolaemic shock, hypoperfusion and tissue hypoxia increase lactic acid production while decreased hepatic perfusion decreases lactic acid metabolism. In septic shock, lactic acidosis is multifactorial. Contributors include global hypoperfusion, microvascular disruption causing regional hypoperfusion and impaired cellular oxygen utilisation by mitochondria.

CLASSIFICATION (TYPES A AND B)

The Cohen and Woods classification of lactic acidosis[7] defines two subgroups depending on the presence (type A) or absence (type B) of tissue hypoxia (Table 15.1). Type A lactic acidosis due to tissue hypoxia is common in critically ill patients. Type B (no tissue hypoxia) is much less common. Some patients with type B lactic acidosis have increased lactate generation (some malignancies and toxins impair oxygen utilisation by cells, despite adequate oxygen delivery), and other patients have decreased lactate clearance (liver disease). Patients with liver disease have greater hyperlactaemia during states of increased lactate production than those with normal liver function.[6]

COMBINED ABNORMALITIES (TYPES A AND B)

In clinical practice, separation of types A and B lactic acidosis is usually not helpful, because many critically ill patients have combined abnormalities. Increased lactate formation from tissue hypoxia and decreased lactate clearance often occur together. In patients with cancer, anaerobic glycolysis may be increased while hepatic lactate metabolism is impaired by tumour replacement. Diabetic patients may present with shock, but in non-insulin-dependent diabetes there may also be a defect in pyruvate

Table 15.1 Classification of lactic acidosis

Type A	Shock Very severe hypoxaemia Very severe anaemia Carbon monoxide poisoning
Type B1 (underlying disease)	Sepsis Liver failure Thiamine deficiency Malignancy Phaeochromocytoma Diabetes
Type B2 (drug or toxin)	Epinephrine Salbutamol Propofol Nucleoside analogue reverse transcriptase inhibitor Ethanol Methanol Paracetamol Nitroprusside Salicylates Ethylene (and propylene) glycol Biguanides Fructose Sorbitol Xylitol Cyanide Isoniazid
Type B3 (rare inborn errors of metabolism)	Glucose-6-phosphatase deficiency Fructose-1,6 diphosphatase deficiency Pyruvate carboxylase deficiency Deficiency of enzymes of oxidative phosphorylation

oxidation, and in diabetic ketoacidosis ketones may also inhibit hepatic lactate uptake. Thiamine and biotin are essential cofactors for pyruvate dehydrogenase activity and for conversion of pyruvate to oxaloacetate. Malnutrition (beri-beri) and inadequate parenteral nutrition have therefore been associated with lactic acidosis due to deficiencies of these cofactors. In these cases, pyruvate accumulation increases lactate production. In alcoholics, ethanol oxidation increases the conversion of pyruvate to lactate and inhibits other pathways of pyruvate metabolism. Phenformin therapy is associated with lactic acidosis for several reasons: phenformin increases glycolysis in peripheral tissues, inhibits pyruvate oxidation, increases splanchnic lactate production and decreases hepatic lactate clearance. Phenformin was therefore used to induce lactic acidosis in older animal models until it was recognised that phenformin is also a potent cardiac depressant. These studies reporting the effects of lactic acidosis on cardiac function were flawed. Both endogenous and infused catecholamines cause hepatic vasoconstriction and impair hepatic lactate clearance, and epinephrine also increases hepatic glycogenolysis to lactate.[8] Importantly, acidosis also stimulates adrenal catecholamine release, which may mask other cardiac effects of acidosis.

SEPSIS

There has been much recent debate[9] whether the hyperlactaemia of sepsis results from net increased cellular production[10] or reduced net clearance.[11] However the potential for sepsis to derange lactate metabolism is clear. Both impaired regional microvascular and mitochondrial dysfunction have been implicated in the pathogenesis of lactic acidosis during sepsis. Excess catecholamines may impair hepatic lactate extraction (by reducing regional hepatic blood flow) and increase lactate production (increased glycogenolysis). At the same time lactate clearance is decreased because pyruvate dehydrogenase activity is reduced in both skeletal muscle and liver. Mitochondrial pyruvate oxidation is impaired.

Tissue hypoxia may not be a major mechanism for regional lactate production during sepsis: hyperlactaemia is thought to be linked to the severity of the septic cellular inflammatory response and hypermetabolic state.[9,12] Net lactate production from the hepatosplanchnic bed is uncommon in septic patients[13] and nuclear magnetic resonance spectroscopy suggests that hyperlactaemia may occur without tissue hypoxia.[14]

LUNG INJURY

The lung is a primary source of lactate production in patients with acute lung injury, with pulmonary release of lactate being directly related to the severity of lung injury,[15,16] supporting the view that the primary contributors are the tissues with the most inflammation or injury. The increased lactate production by the injured lung is not only secondary to anaerobic metabolism in the hypoxic regions of the lung but also may be due to altered glucose metabolism and a direct effect of cytokines on pulmonary cells.[16]

Recent laboratory data suggest that both metabolic and respiratory acidosis protect the lung against injury whereas correction of acidosis compounded the injury.[17,18] The two ventilator trials[19,20] which demonstrated a positive impact on mortality in acute respiratory distress syndrome (ARDS) by limiting tidal volume and airway pressures differed widely on how they regarded the resultant hypercapnic acidosis. While Amato *et al.*[19] allowed elevation of the $Pa\text{CO}_2$ (permissive hypercapnia) and resultant acidosis, the ARDSnet group[20] in contrast aggressively corrected the hypercapnic acidosis by increasing the respiratory rate and allowing administration of sodium bicarbonate. There is growing evidence that not only may hypercapnic acidosis be beneficial in lung injury,[17,21] but the ARDSnet interventions aimed at correcting the acidosis may also be deleterious.[18,22] These findings have not only promoted a greater tolerance of acidosis in ARDS but also increased reluctance to buffer the acidosis exogenously towards 'normal' values.

ASTHMA

Lactic acidosis also often occurs in patients with acute severe asthma.[23] Fatiguing respiratory muscles have been implicated, but severe lactic acidosis also occurs in sedated, paralysed mechanically ventilated patients who have no endogenous respiratory muscle activity.[24] β-agonists, including salbutamol and epinephrine cause lactic acidosis by increasing gluconeogenesis, glycogenolysis, lipolysis and cyclic adenosine monophospate (AMP) activity. Clinical experience suggests that infusions of β-agonists are the primary cause of lactic acidosis in patients with asthma because decreasing intravenous salbutamol infusions to less than 10 mcg/min is usually associated with resolution of the acidosis. In asthma, lactic acidosis does not have specific prognostic implications.

CARDIAC SURGICAL PATIENTS

Hyperlactaemia during cardiopulmonary bypass is relatively frequent and is associated with an increased postoperative morbidity.[25] Recent work has suggested that this 'on-pump' hyperlactaemia is secondary to inadequate peripheral oxygen delivery (DO_2) which creates a condition similar to cardiogenic shock, leading to both direct lactate formation by dysoxic tissues and also to catecholamine release, insulin resistance and hyperglycemia-induced lactate production.

The use of epinephrine after cardiopulmonary bypass precipitates lactic acidosis in some patients.[26] This phenomenon is probably β-agonist-mediated, is associated with increased whole-body blood flow and resolves after substitution of norepinephrine. However there is emerging evidence that the severity of lactic acidosis following cardiac surgery is related to certain genetic polymorphisms in tumour necrosis factor and interleukin-10 genes.[27] Similar to asthma, lactic acidosis associated with the administration of epinephrine in this setting does not have the adverse implications of lactic acidosis associated with shock.

MESENTERIC ISCHAEMIA

The diagnosis of mesenteric ischaemia can be challenging to make in the critically ill due to a lack of clinical and diagnostic signs, difficulty transferring unstable patients for diagnostic imaging and concern about the deleterious effects of inappropriately administrating contrast agents. Animal models have shown that lactate increases within 1 hour of induced intestinal ischaemia. In addition, elevated lactate at the time of diagnosis of mesenteric ischaemia is a predictor of mortality.[28] However, although plasma lactate is a very sensitive marker (100%) for detecting acute mesenteric ischaemia, the low specificity of this marker (42%) is a particular problem in the critically ill, who frequently have many plausible alternate diagnoses.

D-lactate is the isomer of lactate that is produced by intestinal bacterial and not by humans. Experimental work suggests that ischaemic bowel allows the translocation of D-lactate into the systemic circulation; as D-lactate is not eliminated by the liver, plasma levels may be more specific markers of mesenteric ischaemia.[29] However, many issues need to be clarified, including the effect of antibiotic therapy on the intestinal bacteria, before D-lactate could be considered as a bedside diagnostic test.[30]

It is necessary to have a high index of suspicion for mesenteric ischaemia in a deteriorating patient with an elevated lactate in the absence of a convincing alternative diagnosis, as identification of mesenteric ischaemia is frequently made first at laparotomy in the critically ill.

CLINICAL PRESENTATION

Patients present with clinical signs appropriate to their primary disorder. Their lactic acidosis is usually only evident after laboratory testing. In critically ill patients with shock, however, the severity of lactic acidosis can be a valuable monitor of the efficacy of resuscitation. Repeated measures of arterial blood gases and blood lactate concentrations are required. In hypovolaemic shock, resolving lactic acidosis along with the clinical signs of improving perfusion is one of several indicators of successful resuscitation. Conversely, failure of lactic acidosis to resolve in hypovolaemic shock suggests inadequate resuscitation or another undetected or unresolved clinical problem. In patients with severe lactic acidosis[1] a blood lactate concentration of 5 mmol/l indicated a mortality approaching 80% and survival was best in patients whose hyperlactaemia resolved. In septic shock there are many contributors to lactic acidosis, so the time course of acidosis resolution in this setting is a less reliable indicator of the adequacy of shock resuscitation.

Lactic acidosis may also occur in critically ill patients in the absence of shock. Examples include hypermetabolic states where accelerated aerobic glycolysis may contribute (trauma, burns, sepsis), conditions with increased muscle activity (seizures) and during exogenous lactate administration (lactate buffered haemofiltration fluid). In many of these patients (for example, patients with seizures) very high blood lactate concentrations have no prognostic implications because the acidosis is rapidly cleared.

CARDIAC DYSFUNCTION – ASSOCIATION, CAUSE OR RESULT OF LACTIC ACIDOSIS

Cardiac dysfunction is common in shocked patients with lactic acidosis and it has often been assumed that therapies for lactic acidosis would improve cardiac function. However, cardiac dysfunction in these patients is very likely due to other factors, with cytokines (tumour necrosis factor-α, interleukins) being the major cause in septic shock, and with lactic acidosis a consequence or association rather than a cause of cardiac dysfunction. In lactic acidosis, some clinicians recommend normalisation of arterial pH based on two assumptions: (1) that acidosis causes cardiac dysfunction; and (2) that patients are better with 'normal' laboratory values.[31] Both of these assumptions are incorrect in most critically ill patients. First, early research in isolated muscle, isolated heart preparations, animal models and clinical case reports supported the view that acidosis decreased cardiac function and decreased the haemodynamic response to catecholamines. However later large animal studies in which preload, afterload and heart rate were carefully controlled found only marginal effects of lactic acidosis on contractility.[2,32] Also, laboratory reports of deceased cardiac function during acidosis studied an arterial pH much lower (pH 6.6–6.9) than that usually observed in critically ill patients.[33] Increasing experience with permissive hypercapnia in ARDS and asthma has supported the view that patients with respiratory acidosis have fewer complications and better outcomes when normal values are not targeted. The major haemodynamic effect of acute hypercapnic acidosis in ARDS and asthma was increased cardiac output and vasodilatation, not cardiac depression.[34] Therefore, targeting normal values in lactic acidosis is also unlikely in itself to be beneficial, and may be harmful.

MANAGEMENT

GENERAL

In critically ill patients, lactic acidosis is often an indicator of major patient pathology. Therefore the main focus is to identify and treat the cause rapidly. A clinical examination and search for occult sepsis, inadequate resuscitation, localised ischaemia or cardiovascular failure are urgently required. In each case, after diagnosis and initial management, lactic acidosis may then be used as an ongoing monitor of disease progression or resolution. pH correction with sodium bicarbonate has the disadvantage of removing this useful clinical monitor.

TREAT THE PRIMARY DISORDER

Specific therapies and supports must be directed at each underlying cause. In hypovolaemic and cardiogenic shock, restoration of an adequate global oxygen delivery is required. Vasoconstrictors may worsen tissue perfusion and should only follow adequate intravascular volume and appropriate cardiac supports. In septic shock, antibiotics appropriate to cover all likely sources of infection are a priority, and in patients with possible ischaemic gut, surgery may be required for both diagnosis and therapy. Postsurgical gastrointestinal leaks may sometimes be difficult to diagnose, may not be detectable on computed tomography and require early laparotomy. In status epilepticus, lactic acidosis is a result of muscle activity and rapid use of effective anticonvulsants is indicated. In diabetic ketoacidosis, insulin, appropriate fluid and treatment of precipitants enable resolution of all metabolic abnormalities, including associated lactic acidosis. In thiamine deficiency, highlighted during a nationwide American shortage of multivitamins for patients receiving total parenteral nutrition,[35] high-dose intravenous thiamine corrected both the vasodilated shock and associated lactic acidosis. In acute severe asthma, lactic acidosis is commonly a result of high-dose intravenous β-agonist therapy, and salbutamol dose reduction usually resolves the problem. In vasodilated patients after cardiopulmonary bypass, lactic acidosis may also be related to β-agonist therapy[26] and resolves after substitution of intravenous epinephrine with norepinephrine. In these cases, lactic acidosis is not related to decreased tissue perfusion and adverse effects upon prognosis have not been noted. Patients with human immunodeficiency virus (HIV) receiving nucleoside analogue reverse transcriptase inhibitor (NRTI) therapy have a high incidence of hyperlactaemia (8.3%) which can progress to a rapidly fatal metabolic lactic acidosis syndrome. These patients with NRTI-induced mitochondrial dysfunction require withdrawal of the therapy (if lactate > 5 mmol/l) and close monitoring.[36] In symptomatic patients an elevated lactate level is associated with mortality .

HYPERVENTILATION

Hyperventilation is a normal compensatory response to metabolic acidosis in conscious patients. Therefore in mechanically ventilated patients with lactic acidosis, most clinicians will use some hyperventilation to correct acidaemia partially. Clearly in patients with pulmonary pathology, hyperventilation may be difficult or inappropriate, and in some patients hyperventilation increases intrathoracic pressure, decreases venous return, decreases cardiac output and exacerbates the cause of lactic acidosis.

BICARBONATE

Bicarbonate therapy for lactic acidosis is controversial.[2,31,37] Correction of acidosis with bicarbonate might reverse depressed cardiac performance, but there is no evidence in critically ill patients that lactic acidosis depresses cardiac function, and more recent laboratory studies also report minimal depression in large animals.[32,38] Further, not all studies have demonstrated a rise in pH after the administration of bicarbonate.[39] Importantly, two randomised studies of bicarbonate therapy in critically ill patients with lactic acidosis and shock found no improvement in cardiac function or any other beneficial effects of pH correction.[33,40] One reason for these findings is that sodium bicarbonate has adverse effects, including acute hypercapnia and ionised hypocalcaemia,[33] which outweigh potential benefits in patients. Hypercapnia may increase intracellular acidosis (CO_2 crosses cell membranes rapidly), and hypocalcaemia decreases myocardial contractility.[41] Other side-effects of bicarbonate occur because bicarbonate is a hypertonic solution and include acute intravascular volume overload and cardiac depression. In addition, bicarbonate increases lactate production by increasing the activity of the rate-limiting enzyme phosphofructokinase, shifts the haemoglobin–oxygen dissociation curve, increases oxygen affinity of haemoglobin and thereby decreases oxygen delivery to tissues. Adverse effects of bicarbonate in patients can be reduced by using slow infusions in preference to rapid boluses, and by correcting side-effects, by increasing minute volume in ventilated patients and by correcting ionised hypocalcaemia.

Mechanical ventilation limits the ability to excrete the CO_2 evolved from bicarbonate administration with the potential to attenuate the resultant increase in pH. In support of this, two prospective randomised controlled trials conducted in mechanically ventilated patients with lactic acidosis demonstrated that bicarbonate administration resulted in minimal improvements in pH.[33,40] Furthermore, in the presence of severely limited ventilation such as a lung protection strategy, bicarbonate may lower arterial pH.[42] The ARDSnet group supported administration of bicarbonate to limit the pH effects of hypercapnia,[20] but emerging experimental work suggests that buffering of hypercapnic acidosis may be detrimental,[18] and may not therefore be advisable during protective ventilator strategies.

Importantly, however, despite decades of debate, bicarbonate has never been shown to be beneficial in any clinical trial and its use in patients with lactic acidosis is not now recommended, regardless of the degree of acidaemia.[2]

There are two subgroups of patients with lactic acidosis in whom bicarbonate may be considered. Patients with pulmonary hypertension and right heart failure (e.g. lung transplant recipients) may have pulmonary vasoconstriction which is exacerbated by acidosis. In these patients, although there are other useful therapies, including inhaled nitric oxide, partial pH correction may improve right heart function. Secondly, patients with significant ischaemic heart disease and lactic acidosis may be at increased risk of major arrhythmias, because severe acidosis lowers the myocardial threshold for arrhythmias. In both of these subgroups, slow bicarbonate infusions to keep the arterial pH above 7.15 can currently be justified.

ALTERNATIVE THERAPIES

CARBICARB

Carbicarb is an equimolar combination of sodium carbonate and sodium bicarbonate which generates less carbon dioxide than bicarbonate and may therefore have fewer adverse effects. Carbicarb more consistently increases intracellular pH, has inconsistent effects on haemodynamics, like bicarbonate does not address the underlying cause of lactic acidosis, and is not in clinical usage.

DICHLOROACETATE

Dichloroacetate (DCA) works by stimulating the phosphate dehydrogenase complex, the rate-limiting enzyme which regulates entry of pyruvate into the tricarboxylic acid cycle. DCA increases arterial pH and decreases lactate concentrations[43] but nevertheless, a large multicentre randomised clinical trial in patients with lactic acidosis found no benefit for either haemodynamics or patient outcome.[44] This study is really the best evidence currently available to support the view that correction of lactic acidosis in critically ill patients without improving the underlying primary disorder has no overall effect on patient outcome. DCA is not available commercially.

TRIS/THAM

Tris-hydroxymethyl aminomethane (THAM) is a commercially available weak alkali which is rarely used as a clinical therapy because of concerns about side-effects which include hyperkalaemia, hypoglycaemia, extravasation-related necrosis and neonatal hepatic necrosis. In acute lung injury, THAM has been demonstrated to be an effective buffer in ventilated patients, as it is not associated with an increased CO_2 load and is capable of ameliorating some of the haemodynamic effects of hypercapnia.[42,45] However, it is unclear whether buffering of hypercapnic acidosis in acute lung injury patients is of any benefit.

DIALYSIS/HAEMOFILTRATION

Peritoneal dialysis has been reported to be effective at removing lactate, but bicarbonate-buffered haemofiltration is ineffective, contributing to less than 3% of lactate clearance.[46] Indeed, haemofiltration was so ineffective that it has been noted that lactate concentrations remain a useful clinical marker of disease progression in patients on bicarbonate-buffered haemofiltration.

However, in lactate-intolerant patients (i.e. those with shock-induced lactic acidosis and/or liver disease), the use of lactate-based dialysis fluid may overload the patient's metabolic capacity for lactate, particularly if high-volume haemofiltration is employed.[47] In these patients bicarbonate-based dialysis should be chosen.

REFERENCES

1. Stacpoole PW, Wright EC, Baumgartner TG *et al.* Natural history and course of acquired lactic acidosis in adults. DCA-Lactic Acidosis Study Group. *Am J Med* 1994; **97**: 47–54.
2. Forsythe SM, Schmidt GA. Sodium bicarbonate for the treatment of lactic acidosis. *Chest* 2000; **117**: 260–7.
3. Gunnerson KJ, Saul M, He S *et al.* Lactate versus non-lactate metabolic acidosis: a retrospective outcome evaluation of critically ill patients. *Crit Care* 2006; **10**: R22.
4. Broder G, Weil MH. Excess lactate: an index of reversibility of shock in human patients. *Science* 1964; **143**: 1457–9.
5. Rivers E, Nguyen B, Havstad S *et al.* Early goal-directed therapy in the treatment of severe sepsis and septic shock. *N Engl J Med* 2001; **345**: 1368–77.
6. Berry MN. The liver and lactic acidosis. *Proc R Soc Med* 1967; **60**: 1260–2.
7. Cohen RD, Woods HF. Lactic acidosis revisited. *Diabetes* 1983; **32**: 181–91.
8. Stacpoole PW. Lactic acidosis. *Endocrinol Metab Clin North Am* 1993; **22**: 221–45.

9. Gutierrez G, Wulf ME. Lactic acidosis in sepsis: another commentary. *Crit Care Med* 2005; **33**: 2420–2.
10. Chiolero RL, Revelly JP, Leverve X *et al.* Effects of cardiogenic shock on lactate and glucose metabolism after heart surgery. *Crit Care Med* 2000; **28**: 3784–91.
11. Levraut J, Ciebiera JP, Chave S *et al.* Mild hyperlactatemia in stable septic patients is due to impaired lactate clearance rather than overproduction. *Am J Respir Crit Care Med* 1998; **157**: 1021–6.
12. Mizock BA. The hepatosplanchnic area and hyperlactatemia: a tale of two lactates. *Crit Care Med* 2001; **29**: 447–9.
13. De Backer D, Creteur J, Silva E *et al.* The hepatosplanchnic area is not a common source of lactate in patients with severe sepsis. *Crit Care Med* 2001; **29**: 256–61.
14. Hotchkiss RS, Karl IE. Reevaluation of the role of cellular hypoxia and bioenergetic failure in sepsis. *JAMA* 1992; **267**: 1503–10.
15. Kellum JA, Kramer DJ, Lee K *et al.* Release of lactate by the lung in acute lung injury. *Chest* 1997; **111**: 1301–5.
16. Iscra F, Gullo A, Biolo G. Bench-to-bedside review: lactate and the lung. *Crit Care* 2002; **6**: 327–9.
17. Laffey JG, Honan D, Hopkins N *et al.* Hypercapnic acidosis attenuates endotoxin-induced acute lung injury. *Am J Respir Crit Care Med* 2004; **169**: 46–56.
18. Laffey JG, Engelberts D, Kavanagh BP. Buffering hypercapnic acidosis worsens acute lung injury. *Am J Respir Crit Care Med* 2000; **161**: 141–6.
19. Amato MB, Barbas CS, Medeiros DM *et al.* Effect of a protective-ventilation strategy on mortality in the acute respiratory distress syndrome. *N Engl J Med* 1998; **338**: 347–54.
20. Ventilation with lower tidal volumes as compared with traditional tidal volumes for acute lung injury and the acute respiratory distress syndrome. The Acute Respiratory Distress Syndrome Network. *N Engl J Med* 2000; **342**: 1301–8.
21. Kregenow DA, Rubenfeld GD, Hudson LD *et al.* Hypercapnic acidosis and mortality in acute lung injury. *Crit Care Med* 2006; **34**: 1–7.
22. Conrad SA, Zhang S, Arnold TC *et al.* Protective effects of low respiratory frequency in experimental ventilator-associated lung injury. *Crit Care Med* 2005; **33**: 835–40.
23. Mountain RD, Heffner JE, Brackett NC Jr *et al.* Acid–base disturbances in acute asthma. *Chest* 1990; **98**: 651–5.
24. Manthous CA. Lactic acidosis in status asthmaticus: three cases and review of the literature. *Chest* 2001; **119**: 1599–602.
25. Demers P, Elkouri S, Martineau R *et al.* Outcome with high blood lactate levels during cardiopulmonary bypass in adult cardiac operation. *Ann Thorac Surg* 2000; **70**: 2082–6.
26. Totaro RJ, Raper RF. Epinephrine-induced lactic acidosis following cardiopulmonary bypass. *Crit Care Med* 1997; **25**: 1693–9.
27. Ryan T, Balding J, McGovern EM *et al.* Lactic acidosis after cardiac surgery is associated with polymorphisms in tumor necrosis factor and interleukin 10 genes. *Ann Thorac Surg* 2002; **73**: 1905–9; discussion 1910–11.
28. Newman TS, Magnuson TH, Ahrendt SA *et al.* The changing face of mesenteric infarction. *Am Surg* 1998; **64**: 611–6.
29. Murray MJ, Gonze MD, Nowak LR *et al.* Serum D(−)-lactate levels as an aid to diagnosing acute intestinal ischemia. *Am J Surg* 1994; **167**: 575–8.
30. van der Voort PH. Diagnostic and scientific dilemma: the ischemic bowel. *Crit Care Med* 2006; **34**: 1561–2.
31. Narins RG, Cohen JJ. Bicarbonate therapy for organic acidosis: the case for its continued use. *Ann Intern Med* 1987; **106**: 615–8.
32. Cooper DJ, Herbertson MJ, Werner HA *et al.* Bicarbonate does not increase left ventricular contractility during L-lactic acidemia in pigs. *Am Rev Respir Dis* 1993; **148**: 317–22.
33. Cooper DJ, Walley KR, Wiggs BR *et al.* Bicarbonate does not improve hemodynamics in critically ill patients who have lactic acidosis. A prospective, controlled clinical study. *Ann Intern Med* 1990; **112**: 492–8.
34. Thorens JB, Jolliet P, Ritz M *et al.* Effects of rapid permissive hypercapnia on hemodynamics, gas exchange, and oxygen transport and consumption during mechanical ventilation for the acute respiratory distress syndrome. *Intens Care Med* 1996; **22**: 182–91.
35. Centers for Disease Control. Lactic acidosis traced to thiamine deficiency related to nationwide shortage of multivitamins for total parental nutrition. United States; 1997. *MMWR Mortal Morbid Weekly Rep* 1997; **46**: 523–8.
36. Claessens YE, Chiche JD, Mira JP *et al.* Bench-to-bedside review: severe lactic acidosis in HIV patients treated with nucleoside analogue reverse transcriptase inhibitors. *Crit Care* 2003; 7: 226–32.
37. Stacpoole PW. Lactic acidosis: the case against bicarbonate therapy. *Ann Intern Med* 1986; **105**: 276–9.
38. Walley K, Cooper DJ, Baile E *et al.* Bicarbonate does not improve left ventiricular contractility during resuscitation from hypovolemic shock in pigs. *J Crit Care* 1992; 7: 14–21.
39. Graf H, Leach W, Arieff AI. Metabolic effects of sodium bicarbonate in hypoxic lactic acidosis in dogs. *Am J Physiol* 1985; **249**: F630–5.
40. Mathieu D, Neviere R, Billard V *et al.* Effects of bicarbonate therapy on hemodynamics and tissue oxygenation in patients with lactic acidosis: a prospective, controlled clinical study. *Crit Care Med* 1991; **19**: 1352–6.
41. Lang RM, Fellner SK, Neumann A *et al.* Left ventricular contractility varies directly with blood ionized calcium. *Ann Intern Med* 1988; **108**: 524–9.
42. Kallet RH, Jasmer RM, Luce JM *et al.* The treatment of acidosis in acute lung injury with *tris*-hydroxymethyl aminomethane (THAM). *Am J Respir Crit Care Med* 2000; **161**: 1149–3.

43. Stacpoole PW, Harman EM, Curry SH *et al.* Treatment of lactic acidosis with dichloroacetate. *N Engl J Med* 1983; **309**: 390–6.
44. Stacpoole PW, Wright EC, Baumgartner TG *et al.* A controlled clinical trial of dichloroacetate for treatment of lactic acidosis in adults. The Dichloroacetate-Lactic Acidosis Study Group. *N Engl J Med* 1992; **327**: 1564–9.
45. Weber T, Tschernich H, Sitzwohl C *et al.* Tromethamine buffer modifies the depressant effect of permissive hypercapnia on myocardial contractility in patients with acute respiratory distress syndrome. *Am J Respir Crit Care Med* 2000; **162**: 1361–5.
46. Benjamin E. Continuous venovenous hemofiltration with dialysis and lactate clearance in critically ill patients. *Crit Care Med* 1997; **25**: 4–5.
47. Naka T, Bellomo R. Bench-to-bedside review: treating acid–base abnormalities in the intensive care unit – the role of renal replacement therapy. *Crit Care* 2004; **8**: 108–14.

Part Three

Acute Coronary Care

16

Acute cardiac syndromes, investigations and interventions

Brad Power

Cardiovascular disease (CVD) accounts for 35–40%[1] of deaths in western industrialised society, with coronary artery disease (CAD) being responsible for about half of these. In patients over age 40, acute myocardial infarction (MI) is the cause of approximately 20% of all deaths. Up to 80–90% of these deaths occur outside hospital. Of patients admitted to hospital, mortality is 8–9%,[1] much higher in at-risk groups. Lowering in-hospital mortality from CAD requires us to identify rapidly patients who are at risk and to implement evidence-based treatment regimens.

MYOCARDIAL INFARCTION

MI is necrosis of myocardial cells due to ischaemic injury. Diagnosis is usually made on the basis of clinical suspicion, although tests such as electrocardiography (ECG) and biomarkers, echocardiography or autopsy findings are required to confirm the diagnosis.

Acute MI can occur in association with or result from a number of different pathological and epidemiological mechanisms:[2]

- a primary coronary artery event such as plaque erosion and/or rupture, fissuring or dissection
- a problem of oxygen supply demand such as coronary spasm, coronary embolism, vasculitis, drug abuse, arrhythmia, anaemia or hypotension
- sudden cardiac death where death precludes determination of causation
- percutaneous coronary intervention (PCI)
- coronary artery bypass grafting (CABG)

Each mechanism may have a different long-term prognosis despite similar biomarker and ECG changes. Such classifications may be clinically important when interpreting the results of clinical trials.[2]

ACUTE CORONARY SYNDROMES (ACS)

ACS represent the largest group of patients developing MI. They describe the spectrum of patients who present with chest discomfort or other symptoms caused by acute myocardial ischaemia (Figure 16.1). ACS can be further divided into acute MI and unstable angina (USA). Both are invariably caused by recent thrombus formation on pre-existing coronary artery plaque leading to impaired myocardial oxygen supply. In this sense they differ from stable angina, which is usually precipitated by increased myocardial oxygen demand with severe background coronary artery narrowing. Both represent medical emergencies and are one of the most frequent causes of hospital and coronary care unit (CCU) admission.

AETIOLOGY AND RISK FACTORS

Atheroma deposits in the walls of coronary arteries provide the substrate for the development of ACS. Major risk factors for the development of coronary artery atheroma are seen in Figure 16.2. Up to 90% of the adult population possess at least one risk factor for the development of atheroma and CAD.

Cessation of smoking, lowering plasma cholesterol (diet and medications) and adoption of a more active lifestyle can all help prevent the development of CAD. Treatment of hypertensive patients produces a large and early reduction in stroke incidence (35–40%) and mortality, and a significant fall in MI (20–25%).[3] Modification of risk factors is one of the most important means of decreasing the prevalence and mortality from CVD.

PATHOPHYSIOLOGY

Formation of thrombus upon disrupted, fissured or eroded atheromatous plaque is the usual precipitant of an ACS.[4] Atherosclerotic plaque formation is probably initiated by injury to the vessel wall that may commence even as early as childhood. Highly activated macrophages are attracted to the site of injury and differentiate into tissue macrophages. Macrophages incorporate blood stream lipids into the connective tissue fibres of the plaque, forming a thrombogenic soft lipid core. Plaque development is slow, but is rapidly accelerated in people with risk factors.

Acute coronary syndrome (ACS). A spectrum of clinical conditions characterized by acute chest pain or myocardial ischaemia. Pain is of recent origin or is more frequent, severe or prolonged than known angina, is more difficult to control with medication or occurs at rest or with minimal exertion. ACS includes myocardial infarction with ST-segment Elevation (STEMI), myocardial infarction in the absence of ST-Segment Elevation (NSTEMI) and unstable angina. An initial clinical subdivision of ACS is made on the presence or absence of ECG ST-segment Elevation

STEMI. Patients presenting with ST-segment Elevation ACS will invariably display initial or subsequent troponin elevation, although the extent of myocardial infarction and complications may be significantly moderated by intervention

NSTEACS. Patients who present without ST-segment Elevation, may later (after testing of biomarkers) be determined to have:

a. NSTEMI. Cardiac biomarkers elevated indicating myocardial infarction
b. Unstable Angina. No evidence of cardiac biomarker elevation

Figure 16.1 Classification of acute coronary syndromes.

Modifiable	Non modifiable
By lifestyle	Increasing age
Smoking	Male sex
Obesity	Family history (Genetic) an immediate relative having CAD, male <55 years, female <65 years
Physical inactivity	
By pharmacotherapy or lifestyle	
Hypertension	
Lipid disorders (elevated LDL, low HDL, elevated plasma TGs)	
Diabetes and insulin resistance	
Hyperhomocysteinaemia	
Other factors: Increased plasma viscosity, chronic inflammation	

LDL, low-density lipoprotein; HDL, high-density Lipoprotein; TG, Trigylceride.

Figure 16.2 Risk factors for the development of atherosclerosis and coronary artery disease (CAD).

'Vulnerable plaque' is often rich in lipid and covered by a thin fibrin cap. The cause of plaque rupture or fissuring is unknown but exposes thrombogenic lipid and collagen, which are potent activators of platelets. Development of thrombus upon this eroded plaque results from: (1) platelet adherence and activation; and (2) coagulation pathway activation.

Although many pathways initiate platelet activation, the final common pathway of thrombus formation is via activation of the glycoprotein (GP) IIb/IIIa receptor, the platelet surface membrane receptor for fibrinogen. Activated GP IIb/IIIa receptors cross-link fibrinogen between activated platelets, promoting the formation of platelet thrombi. Platelets aggregate to form 'white thrombus'; however this thrombus is seldom totally occluding. Activation of coagulation pathways by exposed lipid and fibrin, as well as by the now activated platelets, leads ultimately to thrombin activation and the laying-down of fibrin clot. Red cells are enmeshed in this so-called 'red thrombus' complex, which surrounds the 'white thrombus'. Sudden artery occlusion by thrombus may thus complicate even only moderate-sized plaque; 70% of ACS patients may have a < 50% stenotic lesion and in only 14% is the underlying stenosis > 70% of the lumen diameter (Figure 16.3).

These processes have immediate relevance to treatment:

- Antiplatelet agents prevent platelet adherence and heaping, which limits and even reverses the development of 'white thrombus'. These agents may target the adenosine diphosphate receptor (e.g. ticlopidine and clopidogrel) or may inhibit cyclooxygenase (e.g. aspirin). Although aspirin has been the major antiplatelet agent and blocks synthesis of thromboxane A_2, it fails to block platelet activation by thrombin, adenosine diphosphate and collagen.
- Fibrinolytic agents lyse 'red thrombus' but are not active against 'white thrombus'.
- Antithrombin agents (e.g. heparins) may limit thrombin activation. Current thrombolytic agents lyse fibrin and red cell thrombus, but paradoxically may increase surface thrombin activation.

Totally occluding thrombus causes myocardial necrosis unless there is good collateral flow or the thrombus is rapidly cleared. Occlusion is often accompanied by ST-segment elevation on the ECG. If thrombus is largely 'white thrombus', with minimal or non-occlusive red thrombus, ST-segment elevation is far less likely. Non-occlusive thrombus may be asymptomatic, may cause USA or may cause MI, especially if spasm or distal embolisation of thrombus occurs. Although non-occlusive thrombus is less likely to be associated with early or sudden death, it is indicative of unstable plaque

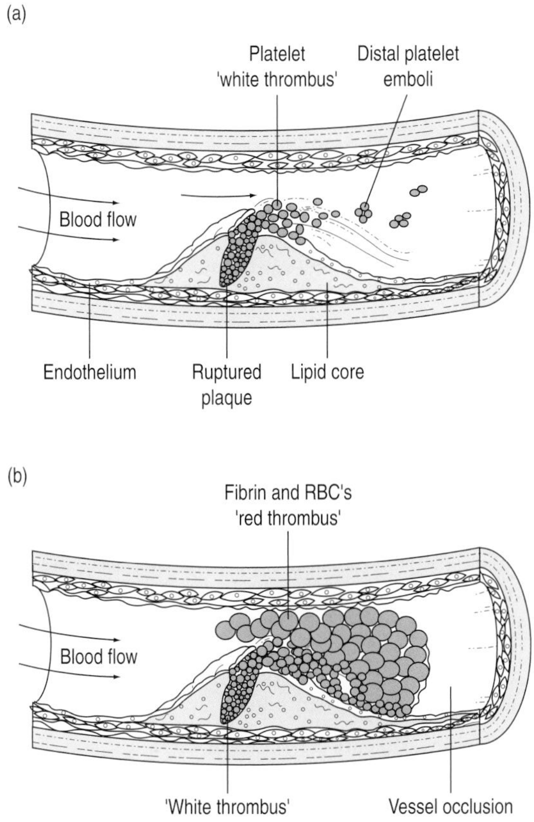

Figure 16.3 (a) Plaque rupture exposes thrombogenic lipid. 'White thrombus' is formed by adherent activated platelets. Coronary artery narrowing, distal platelet embolisation or arterial spasm can cause ischaemic myocardial pain and possible myocardial necrosis. This lesion is unstable and may lead to thrombin activation. 'White thrombus' is not removed by thrombolytic therapy. (b) Thrombin activation leads to a mesh of fibrin and red blood cells (RBCs) or 'red thrombus'. Arterial occlusion may result and, in arteries without adequate collateral circulation, myocardial necrosis follows. Complete arterial occlusion is suggested by ST-segment elevation on the electrocardiogram. Prompt reperfusion with thrombolytic therapy or with invasive coronary procedures may prevent extensive myocardial necrosis.

and is strongly associated with reinfarction and death in following months.

Ischaemia results in cellular disruption, loss of function, thinning and softening of the affected myocardium, and subsequently fibrosis and ventricular remodelling.

Infarct size determines:

- left ventricular (LV) systolic function impairment
- stroke volume decrease
- ventricular filling pressure rise (leads to pulmonary congestion and hypotension that may impair coronary perfusion pressures and exacerbate the myocardial ischaemia)
- LV diastolic dysfunction

Initially, infarcted muscle is softened, leading to an increase in ventricular compliance, but as fibrosis takes place compliance is decreased. With time, there is often expansion of the infarcted segment and compensatory hypertrophy of unaffected myocardial cells (i.e. ventricular remodelling). This can commence early after infarction, affecting overall ventricular function and prognosis.

CLINICAL PRESENTATION

The diagnosis of myocardial ischaemia is usually made (suspected) on the basis of clinical history and ECG.[2]

HISTORY

Patients with myocardial ischaemia can present with chest pain or pressure, syncope, palpitations, dyspnoea or sudden death. Prodromal symptoms of USA occur in the days preceding infarction in 20–60% of patients.

Typically, the pain of acute MI:

- is severe, constant and restrosternal, spreading across the chest
- lasts for more than 20 min and is without a clear precipitant
- may radiate to the throat and jaw, down the ulnar aspect of both arms and to the interscapular area

Sweating, nausea, pallor, dyspnoea and anxiety are common.

The pain of USA may be similar but milder in nature. Features that may suggest it to be ischaemic are:

- waxing and waning characteristics
- reproducibility upon minimal exertion or with emotion
- association with autonomic symptoms

The pain may sometimes be atypical:

- epigastric (leading to possible misdiagnosis)
- confined to the jaw, arms, wrists or interscapular region
- burning or a 'pressure-like' sensation
- sharp or stabbing in nature
- reproduced by chest pressure

These features do not necessarily exclude infarction.[5] Differential diagnosis includes:

- aortic dissection
- pericarditis

Atypical or silent presentations are common: 20–60% of non-fatal infarctions are unrecognised at onset.[4] This presentation is more common in patients who are elderly, diabetic, have hypertension, who smoke or take non-steroidal anti-inflammatory agents.

The assessment of clinical symptoms alone is insufficient for risk stratification and severity of pain does not usually correlate with the extent of infarction.

PHYSICAL EXAMINATION

Examination of patients with USA is often unremarkable. With more severe infarction and extensive myocardial injury, signs of autonomic activation (pallor, sweating, agitation, clamminess) as well as heart failure and even shock may be apparent. Pericardial friction rubs occur frequently after MI but are usually transient.

LV failure is associated with a higher mortality. Signs include gallop rhythm, tachycardia, tachypnoea and basal crackles. A fourth heart sound is often heard, but a third heart sound usually indicates a large infarction with extensive muscle damage. A systolic murmur may be present and may be transient or persistent. These murmurs can have prognostic significance and usually result from mitral regurgitation, due to either papillary muscle dysfunction or LV dilatation.

Cardiogenic shock, hypotension, oliguria and other features of low cardiac output are associated with particularly poor outcome. Shock may be present without hypotension[6] and may develop many hours after onset of symptoms. Right ventricle (RV) infarction results in hypotension and marked elevation of the jugular venous pressure (also seen with major LV dysfunction, usually in association with marked pulmonary venous congestion).

Conditions with similar presentations that do not benefit from thrombolysis are:

- pericarditis (auscultate for pericardial rub)
- aortic dissection (arterial pulses are compared; review chest X-ray if concerned)

INVESTIGATIONS

The presence of MI should also be qualified by:[2]

- anatomical location and size
- causation (e.g. ACS, post-CABG, post-PCI, in association with sudden death)
- time from occurrence (acute, early, late)

Technological advances allow accurate detection of very small infarcts (myocardial necrosis < 1.0 g)[7] that would not have been detected in earlier eras.

ELECTROCARDIOGRAPHY

Acute and complete occlusion of a coronary artery usually leads to serial ECG changes in leads subtending the area of ischaemia, where the:

- number of leads involved broadly reflects the extent of myocardium involved
- height of initial ST-segment elevation is modestly correlated with the degree of ischaemia
- acute resolution of ST-segment elevation correlates well with reperfusion[8]

Identification of classical acute and early changes where ST-segment elevation MI (STEMI) is present identifies patients in whom reperfusion therapy may interrupt, prevent or minimise myocardial necrosis (Figure 16.4). These are:

- *hyperacute* (0–20 min): tall, peaking T-waves and progressive upward coving and elevation of ST-segments
- *acute* (minutes to hours): persisting ST-segment elevation, gradual loss of R-wave in the infarcted area. ST-segments begin to fall and there is progressive inversion of T-waves
- *early* (hours to days): loss of R-wave and development of pathological Q-waves in area of ischaemia. Return of ST-segments to baseline. Persistence of T-wave inversion
- *indeterminate* (days to weeks): pathological Q-waves with persisting T-wave inversion. ST-segments normalise (unless there is aneurysm)
- *old* (weeks to months): persisting deep Q-waves with normalised ST-segments and T-waves

Other causes of acute ST-segment elevation and T-wave changes that should *not* receive thrombolytic therapy are:

- normal variant
- metabolic disturbance, particularly hyperkalaemia
- drug toxicity, pericarditis
- LV hypertrophy
- LV aneurysm
- Wolff–Parkinson–White syndrome and Brugada syndrome
- apical ballooning syndrome (Takotsubo syndrome or 'broken-heart' syndrome)

The Takotsubo syndrome is characterised by precordial ST-segment elevation, apical ballooning on echocardiography but normal vessels on angiography. It may follow the onset of recent severe stress and may cause up to 1–2% of STEMI.[9] It has been recognised in critical illness.[10]

Patients with ACS but without significant ST-segment elevation (generically, non-ST-segment elevation ACS

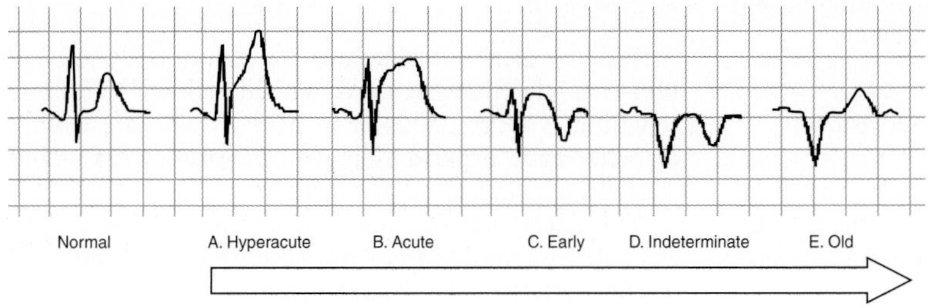

Figure 16.4 Total acute coronary occlusion leads to serial electrocardiogram changes. The evolution is variable and may be interrupted or altered by successful reperfusion. ST-segment elevation is an early and relatively specific indicator of the need for thrombolysis in patients with acute coronary syndrome.

(NSTEACS), until further subdivided by biomarker studies) may still be at high risk of infarction and death. They likely have active, non-occluding thrombus or, if it is occluding, then some collateral flow is present. ECGs in these patients may be normal or display:

- ST-segment depression
- ST-segment elevation (insufficient to meet thrombolysis criteria)
- T-wave inversion or 'normalisation' of previous inverted T-waves

A normal ECG does not exclude MI. Despite the absence of ST-segment elevation, a small percentage of patients progressively lose R-wave height and develop evidence of Q-waves and a small number progress to cardiogenic shock.

LOCALISATION OF INFARCTION

The left anterior descending (LAD) coronary artery supplies the anterior two-thirds of the interventricular septum (septal perforators), the anterior and lateral wall of the LV (diagonal branches) and sometimes part of the RV. The left circumflex artery supplies the LV lateral (anterolateral marginal branches) and posterior walls, and occasionally its inferior aspect (posterior LV arteries: 15% of patients) and the posterior septum. The right coronary artery (RCA) supplies the RV wall, and usually the posterior septum and inferior (diaphragmatic) wall of the left ventricle (posterior LV arteries; 85% of people). The RCA is 'dominant' (as opposed to the circumflex) if it gives rise to the posterior descending coronary artery (PDA) (Figure 16.5).

It is usual to use the ECG in initial clinical assessments to localise the area of myocardial ischaemia. The pattern of lead involvement may thus assist with localisation of the MI (Figure 16.6).[8,11,12] There is a reasonable correlation between the site of infarction as defined by the ECG and the occluded coronary artery and the infarcted region of myocardium (Figure 16.7). However, ECG localisation may differ from angiographic, echocardiographic and autopsy findings, especially where there is collateral circulation or previous CABG. Anterior wall infarctions usually result from occlusion of the LAD; inferior, true posterior and RV infarctions result from occlusion of the RCA or circumflex arteries.

Common ECG patterns of infarction are shown in Figure 16.6. Approximately 40–50% of patients present with anterior infarction and 50% with inferior infarction. Anterior wall infarctions may be extensive or localised (septal, anterior, lateral) whereas inferior infarctions may similarly involve extension to the lateral, posterior or RV myocardium. Of clinical importance:

- 8% of patients with MI will only display ST-elevation in posterior leads V_7–V_8 (true posterior) or in right precordial leads V_3R–V_6R (RV).[4,11]
- True posterior infarction involves 'mirror' changes in leads V_1 and V_2 and is important to diagnose because the amount of threatened myocardium is similar to that of inferior infarction.
- RV infarction is usually concurrent with inferior wall infarction and very rare in isolation. A V_4R lead (V_4 lead in an equivalent position on the right anterior chest wall) is sensitive and specific for RV infarction.[11,12]

The resting ECG does not have sufficient predictive value to stratify patients with NSTEACS reliably into those with infarction (NSTEMI) and those without (USA).

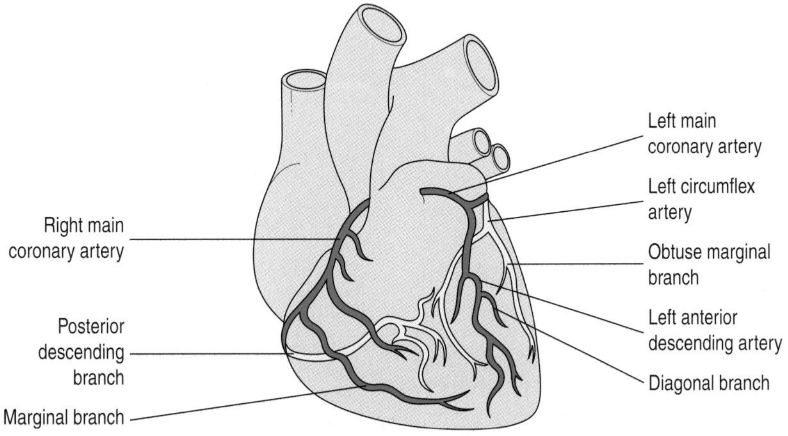

Figure 16.5 Coronary artery anatomy. Left anterior descending artery (LAD) supplies anterior two-thirds of the interventricular septum (septal perforators), anterior and lateral wall of the left ventricular (LV: diagonal branches) and sometimes part of the right ventricle (RV). Circumflex (Cx) supplies the LV lateral (anterolateral marginal branches) and posterior walls, and occasionally its inferior aspect (posterior LV arteries: 15% of patients) and the posterior septum. The right coronary artery (RCA) supplies the RV wall, and usually the posterior septum and inferior (diaphragmatic) wall of the LV (posterior LV arteries; 85% of people). The RCA is 'dominant' (as opposed to the circumflex) if it gives rise to the posterior descending coronary artery (PDA) and the posterior left ventricular arteries.

Localization	Leads (predominant)	Anatomy
ANTERIOR WALL		
'Extensive' anterior (anterior-lateral)	V_1–V_6, I, aVL	Proximal LAD occlusion
Septal	V_1–V_3(V_4)	Septal perforators of LAD
Anterior (localised or true)	V_4–V_6 (I, aVL, V_2)	Diagonal (supplies anterior LV wall). Occasionally marginal branches of Cx
Lateral (apical)	V_5, V_6 I, aVL	Distal LAD or circumflex
INFERIOR WALL		
Inferior (localized)	II, III, aVF	RCA or posterolateral branch of Cx
Inferior (extended)	II, III, aVF plus	
Infero-lateral	I, aVL, V_5, V_6	RCA or dominant Cx
Infero-posterior*	V_1–V_2	Posterior descending branch or RCA or posterolateral branch of Cx
Right ventricular	V_1, V_3R, V_4R (additional right chest leads helpful)	Proximal RCA occlusion

Figure 16.6 Electrocardiogram patterns of myocardial injury. RCA, right coronary artery; LAD, left anterior descending coronary artery; Cx, circumflex coronary artery. *Initial ST-segment depression and T-wave inversion in V_1–V_2, subsequent evolution to tall R-waves in V_1–V_2 and loss of R-wave in V_6. The correlation of electrocardiogram localisation with culprit artery (determined at angiography) and echocardiographic or autopsy localisation is variable.

Up to 18% of patients with MI show no changes on the initial ECG and up to 20% of patients with NSTEACS have normal or minimal CAD.[11,12] Cardiac biomarkers are necessary to confirm myocardial cellular injury and meet diagnostic criteria for MI.

CARDIAC BIOCHEMICAL MARKERS

- The increasing sensitivity and specificity of cardiac troponins (cTN) has made them the gold standard for the confirmation of myocardial necrosis. Elevated levels should be taken as evidence of myocardial injury and, in the correct setting, as confirmation of MI.[2,7]
- Troponin measurements have generally replaced creatinine kinase (CK) as the biomarker used to identify the presence of myocardial necrosis.

The typical rise and fall of cardiac markers after infarction are shown in Figure 16.8.

Two (cTnT, cTnI) of the three isoforms of the cTn complex are exclusively expressed in cardiac myocytes (specific). Troponin levels allow early and sensitive detection of myocardial necrosis.

TROPONINS

- These are more sensitive indicators than CK and its CK-MB isomer. Up to 20–40% of patients with ACS but normal CK-MB may have elevated cTn levels.
- There is a strong correlation between troponin level, intracoronary thrombus and amount of threatened or ischaemic myocardium.
- Identify patients who will derive benefit from therapies such as low-molecular-weight heparins (LMWHs), glycoprotein inhibitors (GPIs) and early PCI.

The increased sensitivity of troponins compared to CK means that a third of patients previously considered to have USA are now recognised or redefined as having evidence of myocardial necrosis. Troponins also have better specificity than CK, similar to that of its isomer CK-MB. They do not differentiate the cause of the myocardial injury (e.g. ischaemia, myocarditis, trauma), however, and thus clinical context must always be considered.[2] Troponins are more persistent in the serum (up to 7–10 days) and thus may be useful in diagnosis when presentation is delayed. Whilst CK-MB has traditionally been thought to be a better predictor of reinfarction, a rise in troponin of > 20% some 3–6 hours after onset of suspected reinfarction is also significant.[2]

Troponins should be checked in all patients with ACS and aggressive therapies should be targeted at patients with elevated levels.[5]

TROPONINS IN CRITICAL ILLNESS

Cardiac-specific troponins are frequently elevated in critical illness, including but not confined to sepsis, pulmonary embolus and renal insufficiency.[13] It is likely that they are

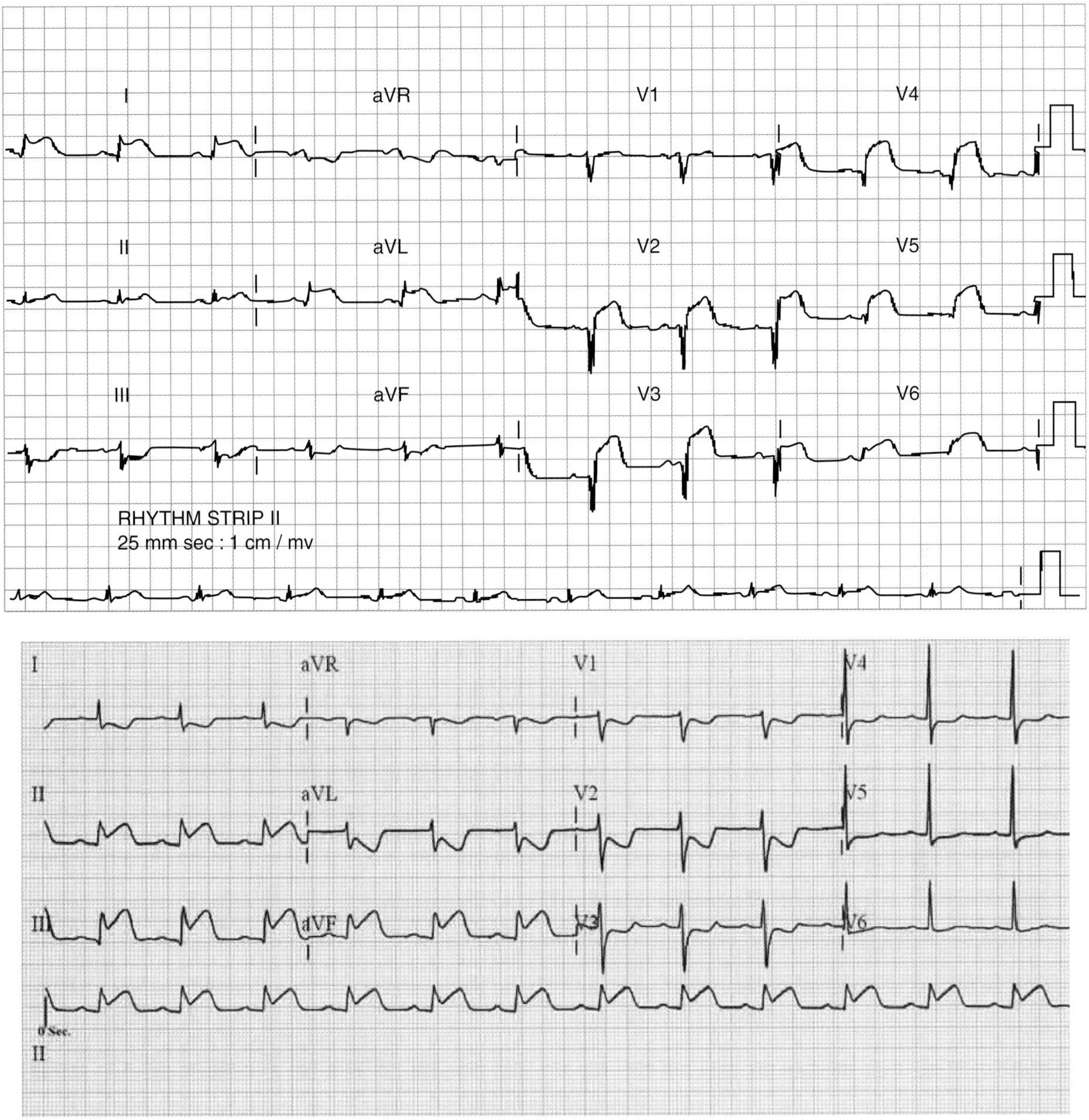

Figure 16.7 Acute Inferior myocardial infarction (ST-segment elevation in the inferior leads II, III and aVF) with reciprocal ST depression in leads I, aVL, V1 and V2. The addition of right sided (V4R) and posterior leads would help identify the presence of RV and posterior infarction. Reciprocal ST segment depression in leads remote from the site of infarction is a highly sensitive indicator of myocardial infarction. It may be seen in 70% of inferior and 30% of anterior infarctions.

of cardiac origin and are indicative of myocardial injury. Their elevation does correspond with adverse outcomes. Most will not be due to 'unstable plaque', however, and the role of standard NSTEMI therapies is uncertain. Clinical context is necessary to decide those likely to have significant underlying CAD that may require acute or subsequent investigation.[2]

Please also see the latest information at the end of the chapter.

ECHOCARDIOGRAPHY

Two-dimensional transthoracic echocardiography with colour Doppler has good clinical utility as a non-invasive investigation during admission for an ACS. Its primary role is in assessing the degree of regional and global LV dysfunction.

Echocardiography detects regional wall motion abnormalities, which can help confirm or exclude the diagnosis

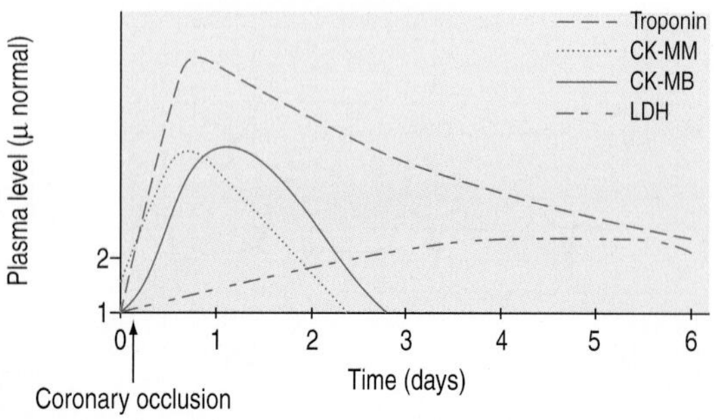

Figure 16.8 Serum biochemical marker changes after acute myocardial infarction. The sensitivity and specificity of cardiac troponins makes them useful for the early diagnosis of MI. Their delayed fall may allow diagnosis where presentation is late. CK or CK-MB are useful if re-infarction with secondary biomarker rise is queried.

of MI in the small percentage of cases where diagnosis is uncertain (e.g. left bundle branch block (LBBB) or old infarction with atypical presentations). Regional wall motion abnormality and loss of wall thickening with contraction are often present in these cases if due to ischaemia, while their absence suggests that ischaemia is not acute. It is useful for excluding differential diagnoses (e.g. aortic dissection or pericardial effusions), again in a small percentage of patients.[2]

Echocardiography is subsequently useful to:

- assess infarct size, especially if thrombolysis has interfered with biomarker measurement
- diagnose RV infarction and infarct extension
- assist management by bedside assessment of LV function
- diagnose specific complications, for example, mitral regurgitation, pericardial effusion, mural thrombus and myocardial rupture, including ventricular septal defect

Transoesophageal echocardiography may have an increasing role in the therapy of cardiogenic shock, giving some guide to volume therapy.

Dynamic or graded intravenous (IV) dobutamine stress echocardiography (2–10 days after MI) can assess myocardial viability and distinguish non-viable myocardium from stunned myocardium. Superiority to standard exercise testing has not been proven.

RADIONUCLIDE STUDIES

Radionuclide angiography has little practical role in the emergency-room diagnosis of ACS. Dynamic or functional radionuclide studies (thallium-201 or technetium-99m-sestamibi myocardial perfusion imaging studies) are useful in postinfarction risk stratification and are able to detect 'threatened myocardium'. They are useful in the later risk assessment of patients who have presented with USA or NSTEMI and where the clinical significance of lesions noted on angiography is uncertain.

STRESS TESTING

Stress testing may be useful in risk stratification and diagnosis of stable angina. Following infarction, the following may be of use:

- submaximal stress testing (to a heart rate of 120 beats/min), predischarge, upon patients with an uncomplicated course
- maximal symptom-limited stress test 3–6 weeks postinfarction

CORONARY ANGIOGRAPHY AND LEFT VENTRICULOGRAPHY

Coronary angiography is the gold standard for the diagnosis (and often treatment) of CAD; however the timing and need for this are determined by clinical risk. In the appropriate clinical setting, coronary angiography will usually identify a 'culprit artery' subtending an area of regional wall motion abnormality and additionally may allow definitive treatment of this abnormality. These indications are discussed later.

RISK STRATIFICATION OF ACUTE CORONARY SYNDROME (FIGURE 16.9)

An immediate goal is to identify patients with STEMI, who will then benefit from reperfusion therapy. This is almost always done on the basis of the presenting ECG.

STEMI

STEMI (including new, presumed new LBBB) with persistent pain is the most lethal form of ACS and is usually due to complete occlusion of a coronary artery (> 90% of patients).[5] It is an indication for reperfusion therapy. Such therapy may be successful and significantly reduce the size of the potential infarction, although some rise in troponin is usually inevitable. Patients who develop ST-segment elevation after admission should also then be stratified to this group.

NSTEACS

Patients have ischaemic chest pain but have 'non-specific' ECG changes (normal, ST-segment depression or minimal elevation, T-wave inversion). After serial biomarker testing, these patients will later prove to have either USA pectoris if troponins remain normal or NSTEMI (elevated troponin).

The therapy of NSTEMI aligns more clinically with that of USA than with that of STEMI. These two conditions, both forms of NSTEACS, represent a spectrum of disease and require common treatments directed at platelet inactivation and 'plaque stabilisation'. The term 'NSTEACS' recognises that they are clinically indistinguishable at presentation. The more severe the ischaemia,

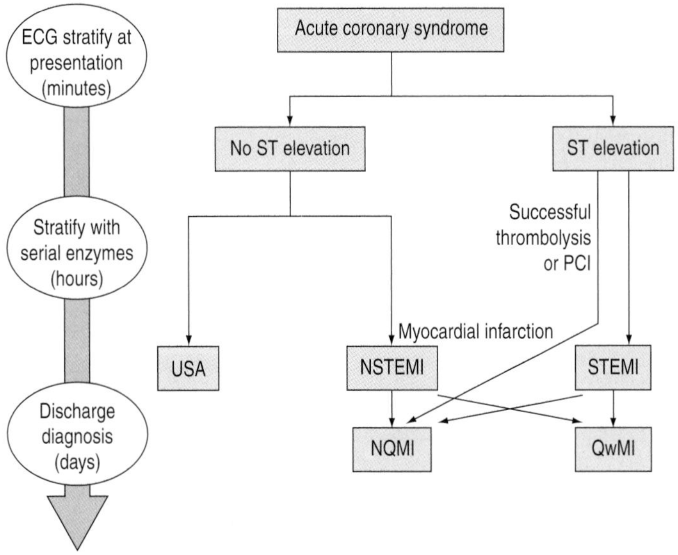

Figure 16.9 Immediate stratification of acute coronary syndrome (ACS) into those with and without ST-segment elevation identifies patients requiring reperfusion therapy. Early and serial biomarker results in non-ST-segment elevation acute coronary syndrome (NSTEACS) identify patients with unstable angina (normal levels) and those with NSTEMI (elevated levels). Discharge electrocardiogram identifies patients who have sustained Q-wave myocardial infarction (QwMI) and non-Q-wave myocardial infarction (NQwMI). Successful reperfusion therapy may avert or limit the extent of Q-wave development. USA, unstable angina; PCI, percutaneous coronary intervention.

the higher the need for more aggressive anticoagulation and invasive procedures. Early diagnostic classification using both ECG and troponins allows early risk stratification and evidence-based therapy. Only 35–75% of patients have evidence of coronary thrombus formation and thrombolytic therapy is not beneficial in this group. Indeed, it is associated with worse outcomes.[5,14]

Figure 16.10 displays the incidence of major coronary events over the following 12 months in patients presenting with and without ST-segment elevation. ST-segment depression has lesser early mortality but a similar or higher mortality at 6 months and at 10 years than those presenting with ST-segment elevation.[15,16] Features that correlate with risk are:

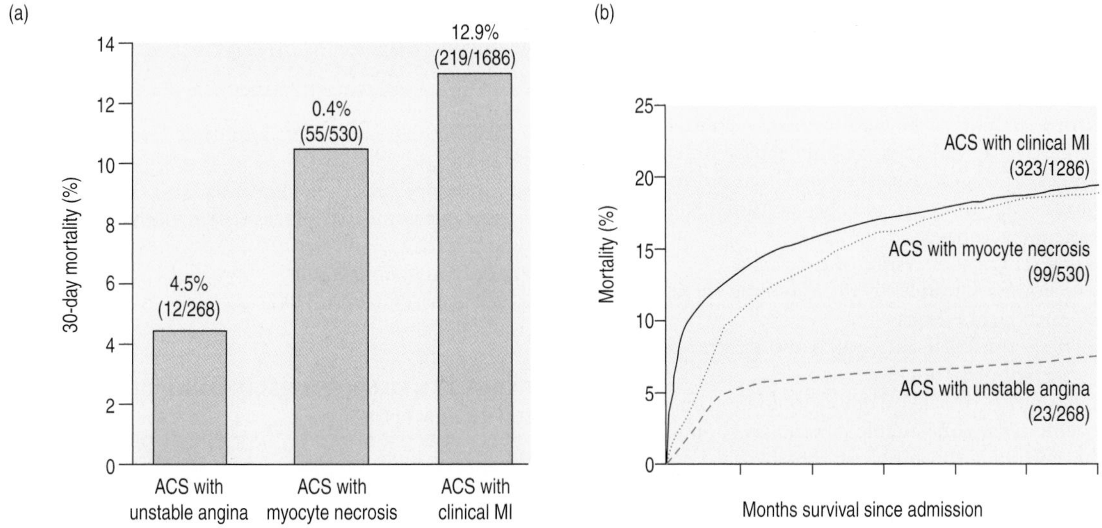

Figure 16.10 (a) Thirty-day mortality according to British Cardiac Society category. (b) Kaplan–Meier survival area curves for events from admission to 6 months. ACS, acute coronary syndrome. (Reproduced from Das R, Kilcullen N, Morrell C *et al.* The British Cardiac Society Working Group definition of myocardial infarction: implications for practice. *Heart* 2006; **92**: 21–6 with permission.)

- refractory angina with ischaemic ECG changes
- ischaemia associated with haemodynamic instability or arrhythmia
- recurrent ST-segment change with elevated cTn levels

Q-wave MI (QwMI) or non-Q-wave MI (NqwMI) are older terms used to describe MI. The 10-year mortality of NqwMI (70%) is 10% higher than that of QwMI.[16]

IMMEDIATE MANAGEMENT OF ACUTE CORONARY SYNDROMES

PREHOSPITAL CARE

- 50% of deaths from MI occur within the first hour of symptom onset. These deaths are usually due to ventricular fibrillation (VF). Treatment is defibrillation.

Review of trials comparing prehospital to in-hospital thrombolysis suggests a 17% decrease (95% confidence interval, 2–29%) in 30-day mortality.[17]

IMMEDIATE HOSPITAL CARE

1. Cardiac monitoring
2. Oxygen via facemask (6–8 l/min)
3. ECG (12-lead) should be taken within 5 min of arrival
4. Aspirin at 160–325 mg should be chewed and swallowed on arrival. IV aspirin can be given if necessary. Clopidogrel can be given if there is aspirin sensitivity or high risk[4]
5. Sublingual nitroglycerine (GTN) may have beneficial effects. Side-effects include hypotensive reactions and a hypotensive bradycardic response (the Bezold–Jarisch reflex)
6. Venous access is usually established
7. Pain relief should be provided. Pain produces catecholamines which increase ischaemia. GTN, reassurance and small incremental boluses (1–2 mg) of morphine, repeated until pain is relieved, can be given
8. Thrombolytic therapy should be considered for all those patients with ST-segment elevation or presumed new LBBB (STEMI) who have no major contraindication (Figure 16.11) and arrive within clinical timeframes
9. Emergent angioplasty (or rapid transfer to a centre capable of this) should be considered for these patients who have:
   - presented to a centre of excellence
   - a contraindication to thrombolytic therapy
   - cardiogenic shock
   - high risk with anticipated moderate response to thrombolytic therapy
10. β-adrenergic blockers (oral) should be commenced in haemodynamically stable patients as soon as possible (usually after thrombolytic therapy has been given[18] or before PCI)[5,19]
11. Pulmonary oedema if present is treated with upright posture, IV furosemide (40 mg furosemide) IV, GTN or IV nitrates and if severe, with continuous positive airway pressure ventilation
12. Prophylactic antiarrhythmics are *not* administered

Reperfusion therapy. Presentation ≤ 12 hours with ACS, unrelieved by GTN and:
• ST segment elevation in 2 or more contiguous leads > 2 mm in chest leads ($V_2 - V_6$) OR > 1 mm in limb leads (I, aVL, II, III, aVF) **OR**
• New-onset LBBB (include presumed new-onset) **OR**
• Posterior infarction (Dominant R wave and ST depression ≥ 2 mm in $V_1 - V_2$) **OR**
• Presentation 12 – 24 hours after onset of ACS with continuing pain and evidence of evolving infarction

Figure 16.11 Typical indications for reperfusion therapy in acute myocardial infarction.

ACUTE MANAGEMENT OF STEMI (FIGURE 16.12)

REPERFUSION THERAPY

Prompt initiation of reperfusion therapy (mechanical or pharmacologic) is the 'gold standard' for STEMI therapy and is far superior to placebo.

Reperfusion therapy should be considered for all patients presenting within 12 h of onset of STEMI.[5,20]

Indications and contraindications are given in Figures 16.11 and 16.13. Restoration of patency reduces infarct size, preserves LV function, reduces mortality and prolongs survival.

Strategies to achieve reperfusion can include:

1. fibrinolytic (thrombolytic) therapy
2. PCI, e.g. angioplasty with or without stent insertion
3. urgent CABG

Factors that influence treatment choice and outcome are:[5]

- skill and expertise of admitting hospital (availability of PCI)
- time since onset of symptoms
- age and comorbid illness (particularly risk of bleeding and stroke)
- haemodynamic status
- previous PCI or CABG

PERCUTANEOUS TRANSLUMINAL CORONARY INTERVENTION

When delivered in centres of excellence (door to balloon time < 90 min), primary PCI is superior to thrombolytic therapy, with reduced short-term mortality (5.3% versus 7.4%), nonfatal reinfarction (2.5% versus 6.8%) and stroke (1.0 versus 2.0%).

The survival benefit of primary PCI compared with thrombolytic therapy is of the order of 20 lives per

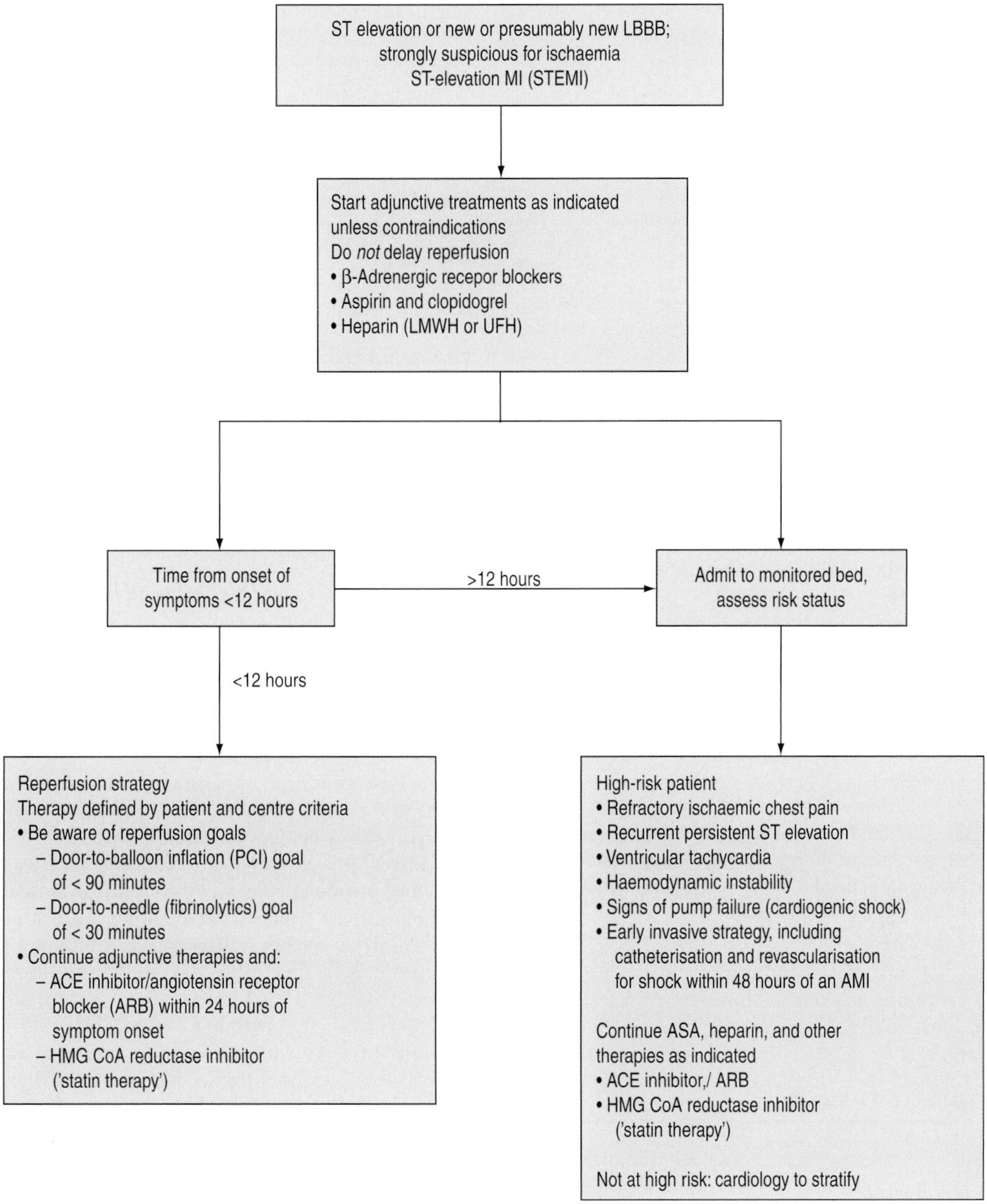

Figure 16.12 Management of ACS with ST-segment Elevation (STEMI). Aspirin, β-blockers and heparin (except if streptokinase used) should be given to all patients without contraindications. Immediate reperfusion with thrombolysis (available in all centres) should be commenced. Immediate PCI is preferred in centres of excellence, where there are contraindications to thrombolysis or where risk favours expedient transfer for such therapy. Glycoprotein IIb/IIIa receptor blockers may reduce complications during PCI.

1000 patients treated. These benefits are not uniform and are significantly influenced by its better outcomes in high-risk patients.

Urgent PCI in STEMI should be strongly considered in patients with:

- presentation to cardiological centres of excellence
- contraindications to thrombolysis
- high risk but with predicted small or moderate benefit from thrombolytic therapy (e.g. elderly, diabetic and with presentation beyond 3 h)
- cardiogenic shock even up to 12–36 h after infarction[21] (see Chapter 20)
- failed thrombolysis
- previous CABG

Absolute contraindications

- Previous haemorrhagic stroke
- Other stroke or cerebrovascular accident ≤ 6 months
- Intracranial neoplasm
- Active internal bleeding ≤ 2 weeks (menses excluded)
- Aortic dissection, known or suspected

Relative contraindications (advisory following clinical consideration)

- Severe uncontrolled hypertension on presentation (≥ 180/110 mmHg)
- Oral anticoagulation therapy (INR > 2.5); known bleeding diathesis
- Recent major trauma, surgery (≤ 4 weeks) including head trauma
- Pregnancy
- Traumatic CPR
- Active peptic ulcer disease
- Previous allergic reaction to drug to be used
- Recent streptokinase or anistreplase (≤ 5 days). Use different agent (risk of allergy, antibodies may reduce effectiveness)
- History of prior CVA or intracerebral pathology not covered in contraindications
- History of chronic hypertension

Specialist opinion should be sought urgently where doubt exists. Patients with contraindications may still benefit from urgent coronary angioplasty.

Figure 16.13 Contraindications and cautions for fibrinolytic use in myocardial infarction (advisory following clinical consideration). INR, international normalised ratio; CPR, cardiopulmonary resuscitation; CVA, cerebrovascular accident.

Very few patients have contraindications to PCI,[17] although caution is needed in those at risk of contrast-associated renal failure.

THROMBOLYTIC THERAPY

- Thrombolytic therapy (versus placebo) of patients with ST-elevation and/or new LBBB results in a significant mortality reduction (10.9% versus 13.4%; relative risk reduction 19%), a reduction of approximately 20 deaths per 1000 patients treated.[5,14]
- Outcomes are critically dependent upon time from symptom onset to administration of therapy. A goal is 'door to needle time' of less than 30 min. Delay is associated with excess mortality.

Thrombolysis within 6 h of symptom onset saves 30 lives per 1000 patients treated; within 7–12 h, the rate is 20 lives per 1000 patients treated, but there is no overall benefit for therapy beyond this time. Up to 40 lives per 1000 could be saved (relative risk reduction 50%) if treatment was given in the first hour.[22] Benefit is still present at 20-year follow-up.[23] Largest benefits are seen in anterior infarction (3.7% absolute mortality reduction), less in inferior (0.8% reduction).[5,14,24]

Age has a major impact upon survival following STEMI. Compared with controls thrombolysis reduces mortality at age < 55 years (3.4% versus 4.6%,), age 55–64 years (7.2% versus 8.9%, 18 lives per 1000 patients treated), age 65–75 years (11.1% versus 12.7%, 27 lives per 1000 patients treated) and age > 75 years (24.3% versus 25.3%, 10 lives per 1000). Thus, although the relative reduction in elderly patients is small (4%), the absolute reduction in mortality is still significant.[14]

THROMBOLYTIC AGENTS (FIBRINOLYTIC AGENTS)

Commonly licensed thrombolytic agents are streptokinase, tissue plasminogen activator (t-PA), alteplase (rt-PA), reteplase and tenecteplase. These drugs promote the conversion of plasminogen to plasmin, which then lyses fibrin thrombi. The fibrinolytic agents approved for therapy of STEMI differ in a number of ways, including fibrin specificity.

- Streptokinase is a first-generation fibrinolytic drug and is considered non-specific. It converts plasminogen to plasmin with a marked fall in circulating fibrinogen and other factors, resulting in a systemic lytic state. Streptokinase has a prolonged thrombolytic effect and concomitant IV heparin increases bleeding and rate of cerebral haemorrhage.[5,24,25] It is antigenic (beware previous exposure or recent streptococcal infection) and can result in hypotension and bradycardia, most evident in patients with inferior MI.
- t-PA, a non-antigenic, more fibrin-selective, shorter-acting proteolytic enzyme produced by vascular endothelium, was used as the basis for second-generation fibrinolytic agents (alteplase, recombinant t-PA or rt-PA). By acting more directly at the fibrin surface, and with less degradation of circulating fibrinogen, t-PA is associated with less systemic bleeding. An initial bolus of t-PA with subsequent infusion (accelerated regimen) produces higher patency rates than streptokinase. It has generally been used as the benchmark or control arm in trials.
- Third-generation fibrinolytic agents (reteplase, tenecteplase) are bioengineered products of t-PA with longer half-lives. These agents have gained popularity because they appear to have similar efficacy and side-effect profiles but are simpler to administer.

Major and minor contraindications are shown in Figure 16.13.

SIDE-EFFECTS AND CHOICE OF AGENT

Although newer-generation fibrin-specific agents that are available as a bolus (reteplase/tenecteplase) are generally the fibrinolytics of choice, streptokinase may still be a cost-effective treatment in many.

More efficient (fibrin-specific) thrombolytic agents improved upon the initial results of streptokinase. In

Global Utilization of Streptokinase and Tissue Plasminogen Activator to Treat Occluded Arteries (GUSTO-1), accelerated rt-PA regimens were shown to reduce mortality compared to streptokinase (6.3% versus 7.3%, relative rate 14% reduction), but at the price of a small excess of haemorrhagic strokes.[26,27] This represented an extra 10 lives saved per 1000 patients.

The tPA congeners reteplase and tenecteplase have very short initial half-lives, allowing convenient bolus dose administration. Trials of these agents against 'accelerated rt-PA' demonstrated equivalence.[28] Accordingly these agents have come into frequent use because of their ease of administration. Tenecteplase can be given as a single agent, making it useful for prehospital and emergency hospital use.

Aggressive thrombolysis regimens are associated with lower all-cause mortality rates despite higher rates of cerebral haemorrhage[5] that are fatal in 40–60% of cases.[25] Of concern with these regimens is that the number of non-fatal strokes (severe disability occurs in 50%) can be problematic in high-risk groups. Accelerated t-PA regimens may result in 5 disabled stroke survivors per 1000 patients treated; streptokinase with subcutaneous heparin may result in 3 per 1000 patients treated.[25] Age, recent stroke and hypertension on arrival significantly increase the risk of both lethal and non-lethal stroke. Since these patients were often excluded from trials, specialist input is required on a case-by-case basis to ascertain whether a less aggressive fibrinolytic agent (streptokinase) may be of use.[26] Alternatively, strong consideration is given to PCI when thrombolysis is likely to be associated with a high incidence of lethal or non-lethal stroke.

Failure to adjust the dose of fibrinolytic correctly to body weight may be associated with increased mortality and intracerebral haemorrhage.[17]

PRIMARY PCI VERSUS THROMBOLYTIC THERAPY

Despite the advantages of PCI over thrombolysis, many patients present to centres that do not offer primary PCI. Given the advantage of PCI over thrombolysis, the possible benefit of transfer to such a centre needs to be considered. Transfer, however, involves an inherent delay and, if this is prolonged, then the advantage of more reliable revascularisation may be rapidly removed by the death of myocardium occurring as a result of the delay.[17,29] Studies of groups of patients suggest that this advantage for groups may be lost if the transfer adds an additional 60–110 min to the process. This may represent an erosion of PCI's mortality advantage of 0.29–0.40% for every 10-min delay. Well-developed systems need to be in place to minimise transport delays.

The significance of transfer for an individual patient will vary significantly. The incremental effect of delay is most marked in patients who present early. The current results from thrombolytic therapy in patients presenting early (< 3 h) are very good as fresh clots seem more likely to be lysed. However transfer may be advisable in patients at high risk of bleeding or where presentation is late and where, despite thrombolysis, baseline or predicted mortality is high.

INVASIVE STRATEGY (PCI) IS CLEARLY SUPERIOR TO THROMBOLYSIS IF

- There are contraindications to thrombolytic therapy
- There is cardiogenic shock
- Angiography is needed to determine diagnosis and where an occluding lesion is found

INVASIVE STRATEGY (PCI) IS GENERALLY PREFERRED (CONSIDER TRANSFER) IF

- Skilled PCI lab is available with surgical back-up:[17]
  - Medical contact-to-balloon or door-to-balloon is < 90 min
  - (Door-to-balloon) – (door-to-needle) is < 1 hour and specialist centre
- High risk from STEMI:
  - Age > 75 years
  - Extensive anterior infarction with late presentation
  - High risk of bleeding
  - Previous MI or CABG
  - Killip class is ≥ 3
- Late presentation:[17]
  - Symptom onset was > 3 hours ago

FIBRINOLYSIS GENERALLY PREFERRED IF:[17]

- Early presentation (3 hours from symptom onset and delay to invasive strategy)
- Invasive strategy is not an option:
  - Catheterisation lab occupied or not available
  - Vascular access difficulties
  - Lack of access to skilled PCI lab
- Delay to invasive strategy:
  - Prolonged transport
  - (Door-to-balloon) – (door-to-needle) is > 1 hour and specialist centre
  - Medical contact-to-balloon or door-to-balloon is > 90 minutes

There is increasing evidence that, in the presence of failed thrombolysis where predicted mortality is high, rescue PCI confers survival benefit.[18] Trials of 'facilitated PCI' where pharmacological therapy is routinely followed immediately by PCI are controversial and current evidence favours worse outcomes with this routine approach.[17,18]

ADJUNCTIVE THERAPY USED WITH THROMBOLYSIS AND REPERFUSION (FIGURE 16.14)

- Improvement in adjunctive or supportive reperfusion therapies has been the major driver of improved outcomes from reperfusion strategies, contributing more than the development of newer antifibrinolytics.
- Compliance with guidelines for administration of these therapies is likely to improve outcomes significantly.

Acute intervention	Patients (*n*)	RCTs (*n*)
Intravenous thrombolytics	58 600	9
Aspirin	18 773	9
Anticoagulant	4 075	7
β-blocker	28 970	29
Nitrates	81 908	22
ACE inhibitors	100 963	15
Magnesium	60 366	2
Prophylactic lidocaine	12 385	21
Calcium antagonists	6 420	16

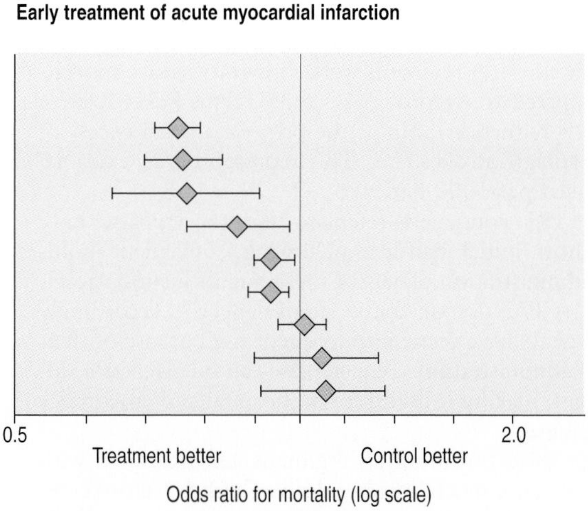

Figure 16.14 Effect of acute (early) interventions upon mortality following acute myocardial infarction. Results are from meta-analyses. Urgent percutaneous coronary intervention (not shown) has not been compared to placebo and offers superior results to thrombolysis for patients who present to centres of excellence. RCT, randomised controlled trial; ACE, angiotensin-converting enzyme.

Adjunctive therapy is necessary after thrombolysis due to the following:

- About 50% of patients fail to obtain or sustain coronary artery patency.
- The underlying artery remains unstable, evidenced by:
  - angiographic reocclusion in 30%
  - recurrence of ischaemia in 20%
- Current plasminogen activators (thrombolytics) destroy fibrin strands of 'red thrombus'. They have little effect on underlying exposed thrombin and indeed may be prothrombotic, requiring concomitant antithrombin (e.g. heparin) or anticoagulant therapy.
- Antiplatelet therapies are needed to 'pacify' underlying platelet-rich 'white thrombus' and plaque.

The major complication of adjunctive therapy is generally an increase in bleeding.

ASPIRIN AND CLOPIDOGREL

All patients undergoing reperfusion therapy for STEMI (PCI or fibrinolysis) should be given aspirin and clopidogrel unless contraindicated.[18]

Aspirin is one of the most significant and cost-effective treatments for STEMI. Given acutely in the second International Study of Infarct Survival (ISIS-2) it reduced mortality by 23% and gave a nearly 50% reduction in reinfarction and stroke. Streptokinase also reduced mortality (by 25%), while the combination had an additive effect and reduced mortality by 42%.[24,30] Treatment for a mean duration of 1 month resulted in approximately 25 fewer deaths and 10–15 fewer episodes of non-fatal reinfarction and non-fatal stroke for every 1000 patients treated.[30] It does not appear to increase bleeding and benefit is still present after 10 years.

Clopidogrel confers significant additional benefit. Given in conjunction with thrombolytics and aspirin, it reduces the risk of early vessel reocclusion without a significant rise in bleeding.[29,31] Patients who undergo PCI and have a stent inserted also benefit if they have received clopidogrel. Benefit is less evident in patients who undergo PCI but do not have a stent placed, and bleeding is problematic.

GLYCOPROTEIN IIB/IIIA INHIBITORS

It is reasonable to use abciximab with primary PCI, but GPIs offer little benefit in patients treated with thrombolytics (full or half-dose).

In theory, GPIs override the platelet activation caused by plasminogen activators, improving patency rates and allowing better reperfusion of small vessels beyond the occluding thrombus. In the setting of PCI, they are proven to be a most important adjunct to the procedure if a stent is placed or lesion dilated. Trials of GPIs in combination with full-dose thrombolytics found increased bleeding. These trials were done with half-dose thrombolytics. Results were again disappointing, with increased bleeding (especially in the elderly) but no survival benefit. In STEMI patients who have not received reperfusion therapy, GPIs do not appear to confer benefit.[29,31,32]

UNFRACTIONATED HEPARIN (UFH, STANDARD) AND LOW-MOLECULAR-WEIGHT HEPARIN

Antithrombin therapy is generally given in combination with PCI or with fibrin-specific fibrinolytic agents. The net benefit-to-risk ratio of using thrombin inhibitors in MI is not clear, however.

Prior to the use of fibrinolytics and aspirin, a limited number of small trials suggested that UFH reduced mortality (from 13.1% to 9.2%, 20–25% relative rate reduction). With the introduction of fibrinolytics and aspirin, UFH administration was continued. It was usually administered for 24–48 h after the fibrin-specific agents alteplase, reteplase or tenecteplase, reflecting the basis on which the drugs were trialled and licensed. Heparins do not lyse clot, but may decrease rethrombosis.

Despite UFH use, few trials (1239 patients) examined whether it added survival benefit to patients already treated with both thrombolytics and aspirin. At most the effect of UFH seems to be small (perhaps 5 lives saved per 1000 patients treated) and increased bleeding can be problematic.[24,33]

LMWHs are produced by chemical or enzymatic depolymerisation of UFH. Their theoretical advantages include:

- predictable pharmacokinetic profiles and anticoagulant response
- enhanced anti-Xa activity and less affected by platelet factors
- weight-adjusted dosing does not require activated partial thromboplastin time monitoring
- convenient to administer and do not require an IV line, although acquisition costs are higher than for UFH
- lower incidence of thrombocytopenia, skin necrosis, hypersensitivity reactions and catheter-related infections

Comparison of UFH and LMWH has often proven difficult because of large variations in duration of therapy. LMWH is probably superior[17,33–35] to UFH, resulting in lower rates of reinfarction, although the bleeding can be problematic in high-risk patients and caution should be used in this group.[17]

Meta-analysis[34] of LMWH versus placebo has suggested that, across the whole ACS spectrum, adjunctive antithrombin therapy with enoxaparin is associated with significantly superior efficacy. Among STEMI[34] patients, approximately 21 death or MI events were prevented for every 1000 patients treated with enoxaparin, at the cost of an increase of 4 non-fatal major bleeds.

Despite the increasing use of LMWHs, UFH may still be used where bleeding risk is high or where urgent PCI is anticipated.

The pentasaccharide factor Xa inhibitor fondaparinux has recently demonstrated a moderate reduction in mortality and reinfarction over 'usual care' (placebo or UFH). These benefits were seen without an increase in bleeding.[36] Like LMWH it has the advantage of ease of administration and absence of need for monitoring but is associated with fewer bleeding complications. Benefits were present in patients at higher risk and not undergoing PCI. End-catheter thrombus was problematic in patients undergoing PCI, suggesting the need for UFH if this therapy is subsequently required. Some benefit was seen in patients who did not receive reperfusion therapy.[36]

β-BLOCKERS

Haemodynamically stable patients should commence oral β-blockers within 24 h of the onset of symptoms unless contraindicated (pulmonary oedema, asthma, hypotension, bradycardia, advanced atrioventricular block).

Significant benefit from IV β-blockers was seen in the prethrombolysis era, but benefits appear small or absent in the postthrombolysis era.[18] More recent studies have suggested that the use of IV β-blockers is associated with a decrease in reinfarction and VF but with an increase in cardiogenic shock, producing no overall benefit. IV therapy may be useful in patients with hypertension or tachycardia (although it is wise to assess LV function, perhaps with echocardiography). IV β-blockers given to patients receiving PCI produce an early absolute mortality reduction of 1.7%: the benefit is confined to patients not on β-blockers at time of admission.[19]

OTHER THERAPIES

Although nitrates may have had a small benefit in prethrombolysis days, there is little evidence of outcome benefit in the postthrombolysis era and indeed complicating hypotension may be harmful. Glucose–insulin–potassium therapies have not been shown to provide benefit under trial conditions.[37]

COMPLICATIONS OF MYOCARDIAL INFARCTION (FIGURE 16.15)

ARRHYTHMIAS

Rhythm disturbance occurs in nearly all patients following acute MI and is most likely within the first few hours of onset and during reperfusion. There has been a decline in the incidence of VF from approximately 4.5% of admissions to 1% of admissions with MI. This decrease probably reflects the effect of thrombolytic therapies and better maintenance of electrolytes.

- Correct hypoxia, hypovolaemia or acid–base disturbances.
- Maintain serum potassium in the normal range (4.0–5.0 mmol/l).
- Maintain the serum magnesium level.

Prophylactic lidocaine tends to increase mortality and is thus reserved for the treatment of life-threatening ventricular arrhythmias. Prophylactic or routine IV magnesium (< 4 h) was of benefit in the Second Leicester Intravenous Magnesium Intervention Trial (LIMIT II) study but not in the larger ISIS-4 study, and is not of proven benefit.[5]

FAILED THROMBOLYSIS (RESCUE PCI)

A number of patients with STEMI will fail to show resolution of ST-segment elevation with fibrinolysis, suggesting failed reperfusion. Whether this should be treated with further fibrinolysis or PCI, or whether no

Diagnosis	CVP	PAOP	CO	Other findings on PAC	Echocardiography
Mechanical complications					
Free wall rupture	↑	↑	↓↓	Usually tamponade physiology: RA mean, RV and PA end-diastolic, and PAOP pressures are high and within 5mmHg	Pericardial effusion with tamponade and RV diastolic collapse; may visualise pseudoaneurysm
Acute ventricular septal defect	↑	↑	↓↓	Left-to-right shunt with O_2 step-up at RV level; V waves may be seen in PAOP tracing	Visualisation of left-to-right shunting with colour Doppler; can sometimes visualise defect as well
Acute mitral regurgitation	↑↑	↑↑	↓↓	V waves in PAOP tracing	Regurgitant jet apparent on colour Doppler; can diagnose papillary muscle rupture with flail leaflet
RV infarction	↑↑	↓ or normal	↓↓		RV dysfunction
Pump failure (cardiogenic shock)	↑↑	↑↑	↓↓		Decreased overall LV performance; regional wall motion abnormalities; dyskinetic or aneurysmal segments

CVP, central venous pressure; PAOP, pulmonary artery occlusion pressure; CO, cardiac output; PAC, pulmonary artery catheterisation; RV, right ventricular; RA, right atrial; PA, pulmonary artery

Figure 16.15 Mechanical complications of myocardial infarction. CVP, central venous pressure; PAOP, pulmonary artery occlusion pressure; CO, cardiac output; PAC, pulmonary artery catheterisation; RV, right ventricular; RA, right atrial; PA, pulmonary artery.

intervention should be undertaken, has been uncertain. Meta-analysis of a small number of trials suggests that further thrombolysis is not associated with survival or reinfarction benefit and indeed may be harmful. Rescue PCI, compared to conservative management, conferred no survival benefit but was associated with significant reductions in heart failure, requiring 9 patients to be treated to achieve this benefit. Treatment was associated with an increased risk of bleeding and possibly stroke. Consideration for rescue PCI should probably be considered on a case-by-case basis; most benefit is likely to be achieved in shocked or haemodynamically unstable patients.

CARDIAC FAILURE

LV dysfunction with the clinical signs of failure occurs in up to 30–40% of patients. It usually develops when the abnormally contracting segment exceeds 30% of the LV circumference: cardiogenic shock or death results when it exceeds 40%. It is more common in the setting of previous infarction, and is associated with a poor short- and long-term prognosis. With large MI there is progressive thinning of the affected myocardium, with stretching and dilatation of the ventricle, and sometimes frank aneurysm formation.

Angiotensin-converting enzyme (ACE) inhibitors appear to limit dilatation, preserve LV function and improve prognosis. Benefits are maximal in those with poor LV function. ACE inhibitors are thus recommended for all patients with significant LV dysfunction and are usually started early following MI. Captopril has a short half-life and may be started at very small doses in ICU patients (6.25 mg t.d.s.) if the systolic blood pressure is > 100 mmHg (13.3 kPa). Lower starting doses may be considered (e.g. 1–3 mg t.d.s.) in hypotensive but otherwise stable patients. The dose is titrated upwards and a longer-acting agent may be substituted prior to discharge.

RV failure secondary to RV infarction[38] should be distinguished from RV failure secondary to LV failure and should be considered in any patient with inferior MI. It is associated with significantly increased mortality. These patients have a markedly elevated jugular venous pressure with little or no pulmonary congestion. Treatment principles are different to those for LV dysfunction. Patients with RV infarction often respond to volume loading and it is important to maintain RV preload. The latter is guided by clinical response and echocardiography. Pulmonary flotation catheters, seeking to maintain an optimal LV filling pressure at around 16–18 mmHg (2.1–2.4 kPa), are now used less often. Diuretic therapy, afterload reduction and unrecognised hypovolaemia may aggravate hypotension and renal insufficiency in these patients.

CARDIOGENIC SHOCK (SEE FIGURE 16.15)

Mortality from cardiogenic shock remains very high (55–70%)[39] and is the major cause of hospital mortality from STEMI. Patients with cardiogenic shock may have 'stunned' myocardium that is capable of improvement with revascularisation and initial intensive medical support. Patients presenting with cardiogenic shock are treated with acute interventional revascularisation (PCI or CABG) in preference to thrombolysis and medical management: the benefits are still present beyond 5 years (survival 32.8% versus 19.6%).[21]

POSTINFARCTION ANGINA AND REINFARCTION

Postinfarction angina unresponsive to medical therapy or with significant ECG changes is an indication for aggressive anti-ischaemic therapy and early PCI. Reinfarction in the 10 days following MI occurs in up to 5–10%; it can be treated with further thrombolysis or angioplasty. Where streptokinase has previously been given, t-PA is preferred because of the possible presence of antibodies that may neutralise activity or cause anaphylaxis.

MITRAL REGURGITATION

Transient mitral valve dysfunction is common after MI. More severe, rupture of a papillary muscle and severe mitral regurgitation occur in about 4% of patients. A decrescendo systolic murmur may be present rather than the typical pansystolic murmur of chronic regurgitation. Posterior leaflet rupture is most common as it receives its blood supply from the dominant coronary artery (usually the RCA), whereas the anterior leaflet has a dual blood supply.

It can complicate even relatively small MI and the diagnosis should be considered if heart failure is disproportionate to the infarct size, even if a murmur cannot be heard. Surgery is usually required; pharmacological and mechanical afterload reduction often provides a bridge.

CARDIAC RUPTURE[20]

Rupture of the interventricular septum occurs in about 1–2% of cases of MI, usually in large infarctions (60% of cases). Anterior and inferior infarctions are equally represented.

- It is often heralded by a new long systolic murmur which initially may be soft or absent and the patient may not be haemodynamically compromised. Diagnosis is best confirmed by echocardiography.
- Almost always there is progressive clinical deterioration (untreated mortality of 54% at 1 week and 92% at 1 year). Surgical repair is considered as soon as the diagnosis is made; intra-aortic balloon counterpulsation often provides a bridge to surgery.

Free wall rupture occurs in 1–3% of all hospitalised patients with MI and often occurs very early. Acute rupture of the LV free wall is usually catastrophic, resulting in pulseless electrical activity and death. Subacute rupture (leaking blood is contained by pericardium forming a false aneurysm) is less common and may mimic reinfarction. It requires urgent surgery.

SYSTEMIC EMBOLI

Embolic (ischaemic) stroke occurs in approximately 1% of patients during their hospital admission and in 2% by 12 months.[40] Most of these cases occur following extensive anterior MI.[41]

- 30–40% of anterior Q-wave MIs may be complicated by mural thrombus (echocardiography). Embolisation is most frequent with large or protruding emboli and is uncommon following inferior infarction.
- 5–10% of these may undergo embolisation, usually within the first 10 days.

MANAGEMENT

- The patient is usually put on anticoagulant therapy for ≥ 3 months (initial heparin, then warfarin) if mural thrombus is proven or if extensive anterior regional wall motion abnormality suggests high risk.
- Extensive anterior-wall motion abnormality is best proven by echocardiography. Clinicians should have a high index of suspicion in the presence of large anterior infarction.
- Patients with poor LV function remain at long-term risk of embolic stroke.[41]

POST-MI INJURY SYNDROME (DRESSLER'S SYNDROME) AND PERICARDITIS

Pericarditis is a common early complication of extensive anterior and inferior infarction.

- Pericardial rub may be heard in 10–15% of patients with anterior MI, less often with inferior infarction.
- It occurs 24–72 hours after infarction and may mimic ischaemia.
- It is best treated with high-dose aspirin or non-steroidal anti-inflammatory medications.

Dressler's syndrome is now uncommon (< 1–3%) but is thought to be an immunopathic response to myocardial necrosis. It is characterised by fever, elevated erythrocyte sedimentation rate, a pericardial rub, pleuropericardial pain and arthralgia, and may occur some weeks after MI.

MANAGEMENT OF UNSTABLE ANGINA AND NSTEMI (NSTEACS) (FIGURE 16.16)

NSTEACS result from the development of non-occluding thrombus upon unstable plaque. Superimposed vasospasm and microembolisation may aggravate myocardial ischaemia. Therapies are directed at 'white thrombus' and plaque stabilisation, and at reduction of myocardial oxygen demand.

General principles of treatment are:

- immediate relief of ischaemic symptoms
- immediate introduction of antiplatelet therapy, usually in conjunction with an antithrombin agent, to stabilise plaque and prevent complete artery occlusion
- determination of benefits of early invasive versus medical therapy

Thrombolytic agents are generally contraindicated in the treatment of NSTEACS; their routine administration is associated with poorer outcome.[14,42]

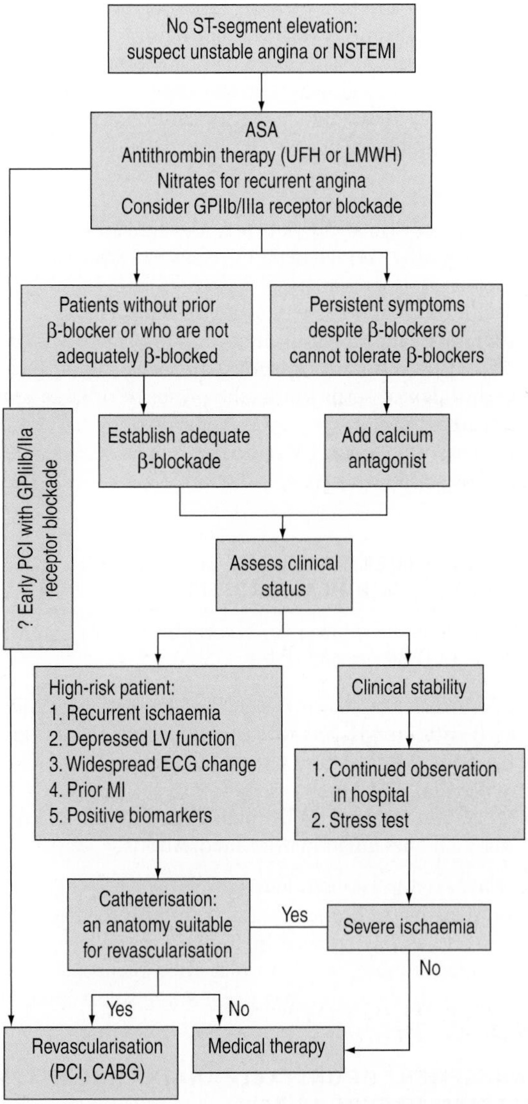

Figure 16.16 Management of acute coronary syndrome without ST-segment elevation. Aspirin, heparin and beta-blockers are administered to all without contraindications; nitrates are given for symptom control. Patients at intermediary or high risk may have best outcomes following early percutaneous coronary intervention with intravenous glycoprotein IIb/IIIa receptor blockade. Patients who stabilise may be treated medically followed by stress testing to screen for inducible myocardial ischaemia. ASA, acetylsalicylic acid; UFH, unfractionated heparin; LMWH, low-molecular-weight heparin; GP, glycoprotein; PCI, percutaneous coronary intervention; LV, left ventricle; ECG, electrocardiogram; MI, myocardial infarction; CABG, coronary artery bypass grafting. (Modified from Ryan TJ, Antman EM, Brooks NH *et al.* 1999 update: ACC/AHA guidelines for the management of patients with acute myocardial infarction. A report of the American College of Cardiology/American Heart Association Task Force on Practice Guidelines (Committee on Management of Acute Myocardial Infarction). *J Am Coll Cardiol* 1999; **34**: 890–911.)

EARLY INVASIVE VERSUS MEDICAL THERAPY IN NSTEACS

While medical therapy is introduced to all patients, keen observation should be continued for signs of instability which suggest that an invasive approach is appropriate. Prior to the introduction of potent antiplatelet inhibitors as ‘upstream therapy’ and coronary stents, early invasive therapy was associated with minimal benefit or with adverse outcome despite its theoretical attractiveness.[43] The development of better adjunctive agents (principally GPI blockers) has led to more recent studies suggesting that early invasive strategies are associated with reduced rates of MI and death.[44] The benefits of PCI are dependent upon the baseline risk to the patient. Emergent PCI is demonstrated to offer clinical benefit to patients with high-risk features such as elevated troponins, recurrent chest pain and recurrent ECG changes.[43]

ANTI-ISCHAEMIC AGENTS

1. *β-blockers* assist symptom control. ß-blockers, administered orally, should be started in the absence of contraindications. Caution is suggested in the early use of IV β-blockers, which should be targeted to specific indications and should be avoided with haemodynamic instability and heart failure.[4] IV therapy may be warranted for high-risk patients (e.g. with ongoing pain and hypertension) without contraindication to therapy. In these patients, metoprolol at 5 mg IV is commonly given incrementally every 5 min until symptoms are relieved, side-effects are experienced or a dose of 15 mg is reached. Ideally medication is titrated to attain a heart rate of 55–60 beats/min.
2. *Nitrates.* Sublingual nitroglycerine 300–600 μg is usually given in two doses at least some minutes apart (monitoring blood pressure) to relieve ischaemic pain. Patients with ongoing pain may receive IV nitrates. Evidence of improved outcome is lacking. Hypotension is a contraindication.
3. *Calcium channel blockers* may provide symptom relief when there are problems with β-blockers and nitrates. They may have a neutral or negative effect on mortality and progression to MI. Nifedipine without concomitant beta-blocker may increase mortality.[5] As sole agent, only those agents that reduce heart rate should be used (e.g. diltiazem or verapamil).[20]

ANTIPLATELET THERAPIES

1. *Aspirin* (acetylsalicylic acid) decreases ‘death or non-fatal MI’ in patients with NSTEACS by approximately 50%.[30,45]
2. *Clopidogrel* (in combination with aspirin) was demonstrated in the Clopidogrel in Unstable angina to prevent Recurrent Events (CURE) study to produce a

20% reduction in adverse events (compared to aspirin alone) when commenced early and continued in patients with NSTEMI. Reduction was mainly in MI. Significant early in-hospital benefit was seen.[46] Clopidogrel is preferred to ticlopidine, its older thienopyridine relative. (Clopidogrel is generally used in conjunction with aspirin in NSTEACS regardless of whether a conservative or invasive approach is planned. Its introduction or continuation should be reviewed if CABG is immediately imminent.[29,31])

3. *GP IIb/IIIa receptor blockers* reduce the 30-day risk of non-fatal MI by 38%[47,48] in NSTEMI patients undergoing PCI. Benefit seems to be confined to high-risk patients (elevated troponins) undergoing PCI. Pretreatment with tirofiban may be useful in this group.[29,31,49] They have not been shown to be beneficial in the routine management of 'medically treated' patients (GUSTO-IV-ACS).[50]

ANTITHROMBINS AND ANTICOAGULANTS

Heparins significantly reduce the composite of 'MI or death' in NSTEACS patients receiving aspirin, although the endpoint of mortality alone has not been significant. The same is true of LMWHs.

Meta-analyses that compared regimens of LMWHs to regimens of UFH found a minimal or less significant reduction in the composite of 'death, MI and need for urgent revascularisation' in favour of LMWHs than found when compared in STEMI patients.[33–35,51] However, despite higher acquisition costs, their simplicity, lack of need for monitoring and acceptable safety profile perhaps favour their administration.

Fondaparinux compared to enoxaparin in NSTEACS had similar early efficacy but appeared to do so with fewer bleeding complications. At later follow-up, fondaparinux was associated with lower mortality and cerebrovascular accidents; most of the benefit seemed to accrue from its lesser bleeding rate.[52] Substitution of fondaparinux for enoxaparin might save 6 lives per 1000 patients treated and might result in 19 less bleeds. There is concern that fondaparinux is not sufficient to prevent stent occlusion and concomitant UFH use is recommended in patients undergoing PCI.

ONGOING AND DISCHARGE CARE OF ACS (SECONDARY PREVENTION) (FIGURE 16.17)

A number of therapies have been studied in the long-term (secondary) treatment of ACS, both STEMI and NSTEACS:

1. *Aspirin* (75–160 mg/day) should be continued unless there are strong contraindications. In the first 2 years after MI, aspirin therapy results in an absolute decrease of approximately 36 vascular events (vascular death or non-fatal MI or stroke) for every 1000 patients treated.[30]
2. *Clopidogrel* is generally continued throughout the hospital stay in both STEMI[18] and NSTEMI. In patients who have undergone PCI, continued treatment after discharge is beneficial, although the duration of that treatment is unknown and dependent upon the nature of the stent placed. Given in conjunction with aspirin, clopidogrel is proven to be of benefit when administered long-term to patients at high risk of future cardiovascular events (the CURE study),[46] although it is associated with an increased risk of bleeding. Clopidogrel is also a useful treatment in patients with aspirin resistance.
3. *β-blockers* significantly reduce the incidence of sudden and non-sudden cardiac death in survivors of MI. Benefit is prolonged and is most marked in high-risk patients, for example those with extensive anterior infarction. Given at the time of MI and continued orally, β-blockers have an early and significant effect on mortality, which is apparent at 7 days, although therapy is not appropriate in patients with

Late interventions	Patients; *n*.	RCT's; *n*.
Anticoagulant	4975	12
Cardiac rehabilitation	5022	23
Beta-blockers	24 298	26
Cholesterol reduction	10 775	8
Antiplatelet agents	18 411	10
ACE inhibitors*	5984	3
Calcium antagonists	13 114	6
Class 1 antiarrhythm	6300	18
Amiodarone	1557	9

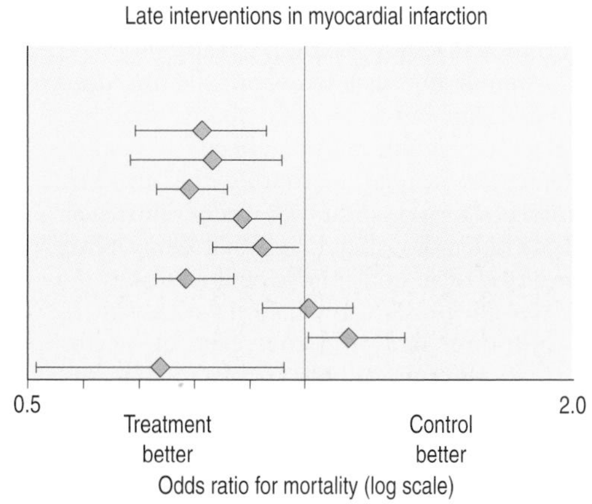

Figure 16.17 Late intervention in acute myocardial infarction.

contraindications.[18] Long-term administration after MI is also associated with survival and reinfarction benefit.[53,54]

4. *ACE inhibitors* are recommended in the treatment of all patients recovering from MI.[55] They significantly reduce mortality in high-risk patients or with symptomatic failure when commenced during recovery from MI. Patients with anterior MI and ejection fraction < 40% maintained on long-term ACE inhibitor therapy may experience a 20% relative reduction in mortality[56,57] and a significant reduction in the incidence of LV failure. Benefit is still seen at 4 years post-treatment.[56] Very early introduction of ACE inhibitors (within 36 h of infarction) may also reduce mortality. In patients intolerant of ACE inhibitors an ACE receptor blocker may be used.[55]

   The aldosterone antagonist eplerenone reduces mortality in asymptomatic patients with low EF post-MI and already receiving β-blockers and ACE inhibitors (see Chapter 20).
5. *Lipid-lowering agents.* Statins should be commenced in hospital for all patients with ACS. Benefit is maximal in patients with elevated cholesterol and other factors, but benefit is present at all cholesterol levels. Lowering elevated cholesterol concentrations following MI results in a decrease in mortality and reinfarction.[58] Although data are conflicting, benefit may be evident within 30 days and therapy should be commenced as early as possible. It is thought that statins reduce hypercholesterolaemia and inflammation, stabilising the lipid core, and early introduction may be beneficial.
6. *Other anti-ischaemia agents*:
   - Routine use of calcium channel blockers does not improve outcome and certain agents have been suggested to cause harm. They may be of symptomatic use in patients intolerant of β-blockers or where a concomitant antihypertensive effect is needed.[5,20]
   - Carvedilol may be of benefit in patients with ACS.
7. *Antiarrhythmic therapy* is not routinely continued. In the Cardiac Arrhythmia Suppression Trial (CAST), prolonged flecainide therapy was used to suppress ventricular ectopy. Despite doing so, mortality was increased.[59] Amiodarone in low doses (200 mg/day) may reduce mortality, but results of definitive trials are awaited and it has significant side-effects. It cannot currently be recommended as routine therapy. For patients with actual or who are at high risk of ventricular arrhythmia, consideration may be given to long-term amiodarone or use of an implantable defibrillator.
8. *Warfarin* given alone or in combination with aspirin is associated with lower rates of a composite of 'death, reinfarction and thromboembolic stroke'. Concerns about bleeding (especially in the elderly) probably still see its clinical application restricted. Warfarin is useful for patients with proven myocardial thrombus, a large area of regional wall motion abnormality or a generalised thrombotic tendency.[5]
9. *Lifestyle advice* is most important and all patients should cease smoking and receive advice on exercise and diet. Diabetes should be tightly controlled.

MYOCARDIAL INFARCTION IN THE INTENSIVE CARE UNIT

Myocardial ischaemia is a common problem in the ICU. It also commonly complicates perioperative care of major surgery, with mortality of up to 15–25%. Diagnostic criteria are uncertain but a system has been proposed by Devereaux *et al.*[60] There are few randomised controlled trials to guide therapy of postoperative infarction, or infarction complicating the care of the critically ill. Many patients with such presentations were excluded from trials of ACS therapy.

The pathophysiology of postoperative infarction and infarction in ICU patients is probably different to that of ACS.[61] Studies suggest that, in the presence of severe ischaemia, left main disease and triple-vessel disease are common and that ischaemia is secondary to oxygen supply-and-demand problems rather than thrombosis. However, data on this are conflicting.[61] The absence of thrombosis as an underlying pathological mechanism in many suggests that standard aggressive 'antithrombus' therapies will have different risk–benefit profiles, and that harm is exacerbated by the often high bleeding risk of these patients.

The patient with significant ST-segment elevation and haemodynamic instability in the ICU presents a difficult problem. Where underlying coronary artery is considered likely, an invasive approach is usually necessary. Thrombolysis is usually precluded by bleeding risk and by uncertainty regarding the causative process. Angiography will allow diagnosis and intervention if necessary; however, the use of adjunctive therapy (short- and intermediate-term) may be associated with significant bleeding. Reversible factors such as hypoxia, severe anaemia, anxiety and tachycardia must all be controlled where possible. Hypotension may limit the ability to administer β-blockers and control tachycardia.

Echocardiography may be useful in confirming regional wall motion abnormality and in confirming the amount of myocardium at risk. Of interest is the Takotsubo syndrome, where anterior ST-segment elevation and apical ballooning on echocardiography, often in association with elevated troponins, may occur in the presence of normal coronary arteries.[9,10]

BLEEDING COMPLICATIONS POSTREPERFUSION THERAPY

The increased use of aggressive fibrinolytic regimens and of adjunctive reperfusion agents has led to troublesome bleeding in some patients. Some knowledge of reversal of these agents is necessary.[62]

1. *GPIIb/IIIa blockers.* Abciximab, a chimeric monoclonal antibody, has a short half-life, but antiplatelet activity is still prolonged at 24–48 h. Fortunately transfused platelets are not affected and will assist with bleeding reversal. The newer agents tirofiban and eptifibitide have very short half-lives and antiplatelet action returns to normal 4–8 h after discontinuation. During this period, however, antiplatelet action is profound. It is suggested that administration of fresh frozen plasma (8 units) and platelets (2 units) is likely necessary to reverse antiplatelet action.[62]
2. *Clopidogrel.* It is recommended that clopidogrel be ceased at least 5 days before elective CABG, but this is not always possible in emergent surgery or in unstable cases. Major bleeding rates may approach 10% in these cases. Pharmacology suggests that platelet transfusions are necessary to moderate this but dose is unknown.
3. *LMWHs.* Reversal of LMWHs with protamine is variable and incomplete, even with doses of 100 mg. Protamine may reverse up to 60% of LMWH action. It is suggested that doses of protamine should equal doses of enoxaparin administered on a milligram-per-milligram scale.
4. *Fibrinolytic agents.* In the setting of life-threatening bleeding, large doses of cryoprecipitate (10–20 units) may be required to replete fibrinogen (target > 1 g/l) and coagulation factors (especially factor VIII). Fresh frozen plasma may supplement factor V and VIII levels. Platelet transfusions at high dose may replace platelets and supplement factor V levels. ε-Aminocaproic acid at a dose of 5 g (0.1 g/kg) over 30–60 min followed by continuous infusion (0.5–1.0 g/h) may assist with bleeding control.[62]

OUTCOME OF MYOCARDIAL INFARCTION

The in-hospital mortality from acute MI has been steadily decreasing over the past three decades from 15% to 30% in the 1970s to approximately 10% in 1980 and now to around 8–9% in the new millennium.[1] Despite improved mortality, 60% of all deaths occur within the first hour (usually from VF), and usually before reaching a medical facility.[1] Modern management of acute MI has undoubtedly contributed to decreased mortality. Further significant reductions in mortality must come from management strategies within the first hours of the onset of symptoms.

The major in-hospital changes are likely to come from:[63]

- better hospital organisation to increase access to PCI
- increased use of adjuvant therapies and discharge medications
- increased rates of thrombolysis or PCI in eligible patients

The latter cannot be underestimated. In one study, the in-hospital mortality was 5.7% for those who received thrombolysis but 14.8% for those who were eligible for but did not receive such therapy (9.3% versus 18% in eligible women who did not receive therapy, 10.5% versus 19% in eligible elderly). Up to 24% of eligible patients do not receive reperfusion therapy.[63]

NEW INFORMATION

The conclusions can be summarised.

- Cardiac troponin level is frequently increased in hospitalized patients in the absence of an ACS
- it portends poor short- and long-term outcomes
- Most of these patients have an alternative explanation for cardiac troponin increase
- Cardiac diagnostic procedures are frequently unhelpful in excluding a non-ACS-related troponin increase

Essentially Troponin I level had poor accuracy in discriminating patients with and wihout ACS. Alternative diagnoses included; sepsis, acute left heart failure, cerebrovascular events and a wide range of other conditions.

REFERENCES

1. Rosamond W, Flegal K, Furie K *et al.* Heart disease and stroke statistics – 2008 update. A report from the American Heart Association Statistics Committee and Stroke Statistics Subcommittee. *Circulation* 2008; **117**: e25–146.
2. Thygesen K, Alpert JS, White HD. Universal definition of myocardial infarction. *J Am Coll Cardiol* 2007; **50**: 2173–95.
3. Chobanian AV, Bakris GL, Black HR *et al.* The seventh report of the Joint National Committee on Prevention, Detection, Evaluation, and Treatment of High Blood Pressure: the JNC 7 report. *JAMA* 2003; **289**: 2560–72.
4. Anderson JL, Adams CD, Antman EM *et al.* ACC/AHA guidelines for the management of patients with unstable angina/non-ST-elevation myocardial infarction: a report of the American College of Cardiology/American Heart Association Task Force on Practice Guidelines (Committee to Revise the 2002 Guidelines for the Management of Patients with unstable angina/Non-ST-Elevation Myocardial Infarction). *J Am Coll Cardiol* 2007; **50**: e1–157.
5. Antman EM, Anbe DT, Armstrong PW *et al.* ACC/AHA guidelines for the management of patients with ST-elevation myocardial infarction: a report of the American College of Cardiology/American Heart Association Task Force on Practice Guidelines (Committee to Revise the 1999 Guidelines for the Management of Patients with Acute Myocardial Infarction). *Circulation* 2004; **110**: e82–292.
6. Menon V, Slater JN, White HD *et al.* Acute myocardial infarction complicated by systemic hypoperfusion without hypotension: report of the SHOCK trial registry. *Am J Med* 2000; **108**: 374–80.
7. Alpert JS, Thygesen K, Antman E *et al.* Myocardial infarction redefined – a consensus document of the Joint European Society of Cardiology/American College of Cardiology Committee for the redefinition of myocardial infarction. *J Am Coll Cardiol* 2000; **36**: 959–69.
8. Zimetbaum PJ, Josephson ME. Use of the electrocardiogram in acute myocardial infarction. *N Engl J Med* 2003; **348**: 933–40.

9. Prasad A. Apical ballooning syndrome: an important differential diagnosis of acute myocardial infarction. *Circulation* 2007; **115**: e56–9.
10. Tsuchihashi K, Ueshima K, Uchida T *et al.* Transient left ventricular apical ballooning without coronary artery stenosis: a novel heart syndrome mimicking acute myocardial infarction. *J Am Coll Cardiol* 2001; **38**: 11–18.
11. Sgarbossa EB, Birnbaum Y, Parrillo JE. Electrocardiographic diagnosis of acute myocardial infarction: current concepts for the clinician. *Am Heart J* 2001; **141**: 507–17.
12. Owens CG, Adgey AA. Electrocardiographic diagnosis of non-ST-segment elevation acute coronary syndromes: current concepts for the physician. *J Electrocardiol* 2006; **39**: 271.
13. Fromm RE Jr. Cardiac troponins in the intensive care unit: common causes of increased levels and interpretation. *Crit Care Med* 2007; **35**: 1–5.
14. Appleby P, Baigent C, Collins R *et al.* Indications for fibrinolytic therapy in suspected acute myocardial infarction: collaborative overview of early mortality and major morbidity results from all randomised trials of more than 1000 patients. *Lancet* 1994; **343**: 311.
15. Das R, Kilcullen N, Morrell C *et al.* The British Cardiac Society Working Group definition of myocardial infarction: implications for practice. *Heart* 2006; **92**: 21–6.
16. Herlitz J, Karlson BW, Sjolin M *et al.* Ten year mortality in subsets of patients with an acute coronary syndrome. *Heart* 2001; **86**: 391–6.
17. Boden EB, Eagle K, Granger CB. Reperfusion strategies in acute ST-segment elevation myocardial infarction. *J Am Coll Cardiol* 2007; **50**: 917–29.
18. Antman EM, Hand M, Armstrong PW *et al.* 2007 focused update on the ACC/AHA 2004 guidelines for the management of patients with ST-elevation myocardial infarction (a report of the American College of Cardiology/American Heart Association Task Force on Practice Guidelines). *J Am Coll Cardiol* 2008; **51**: 210–47.
19. Halkin A, Grines CL, Cox DA *et al.* Impact of intravenous beta-blockade before primary angioplasty on survival in patients undergoing mechanical reperfusion therapy for acute myocardial infarction. *J Am Coll Cardiol* 2004; **43**: 1780–7.
20. Van de Werf F, Ardissino D, Betriu A *et al.* Management of acute myocardial infarction in patients presenting with ST-segment elevation. The Task Force on the Management of Acute Myocardial Infarction of the European Society of Cardiology. *Eur Heart J* 2003; **24**: 28–66.
21. Hochman JS, Sleeper LA, Webb JG *et al.* Early revascularization and long-term survival in cardiogenic shock complicating acute myocardial infarction. *JAMA* 2006; **295**: 2511–5.
22. Boersma E, Maas ACP, Decker JW *et al.* Early thrombolytic treatment in acute myocardial infarction: reappraisal of the golden hour. *Lancet* 1996; **348**: 771.
23. van Domburg RT, Sonnenschein K, Nieuwlaat R *et al.* Sustained benefit 20 years after reperfusion therapy in acute myocardial infarction. *J Am Coll Cardiol* 2005; **46**: 15–20.
24. Collins R, Peto R, Baigent C *et al.* Aspirin, heparin, and fibrinolytic therapy in suspected acute myocardial infarction. *N Engl J Med* 1997; **336**: 847–60.
25. Gore JM, Granger CB, Simoons ML *et al.* Stroke after thrombolysis. Mortality and functional outcomes in the GUSTO-I trial. Global use of strategies to open occluded coronary arteries. *Circulation* 1995; **92**: 2811–8.
26. Walley T, Dundar Y, Hill R *et al.* Superiority and equivalence in thrombolytic drugs: an interpretation. *Q J Med* 2003; **96**: 155–60.
27. The GUSTO Investigators. An international randomized trial comparing four thrombolytic strategies for acute myocardial infarction. *N Engl J Med* 1993; **329**: 673–82.
28. Sinnaeve P, Alexander J, Belmans A *et al.* One-year follow-up of the ASSENT-2 trial: a double-blind, randomized comparison of single-bolus tenecteplase and front-loaded alteplase in 16,949 patients with ST-elevation acute myocardial infarction. *Am Heart J* 2003; **146**: 27–32.
29. Ting HH, Yang EH, Rihal CS. Narrative review: reperfusion strategies for ST-segment elevation myocardial infarction. *Ann Intern Med* 2006; **145**: 610–17.
30. Awtry EH, Loscalzo J. Aspirin. *Circulation* 2000; **101**: 1206–18.
31. Clappers N, Brouwer MA, Verheugt FW. Antiplatelet treatment for coronary heart disease. *Heart* 2007; **93**: 258–65.
32. De Luca G, Suryapranata H, Stone GW *et al.* Abciximab as adjunctive therapy to reperfusion in acute ST-segment elevation myocardial infarction: a meta-analysis of randomized trials. *JAMA* 2005; **293**: 1759–65.
33. Eikelboom JW, Quinlan DJ, Mehta SR *et al.* Unfractionated and low-molecular-weight heparin as adjuncts to thrombolysis in aspirin-treated patients with ST-elevation acute myocardial infarction: a meta-analysis of the randomized trials. *Circulation* 2005; **112**: 3855–67.
34. Murphy SA, Gibson CM, Morrow DA *et al.* Efficacy and safety of the low-molecular weight heparin enoxaparin compared with unfractionated heparin across the acute coronary syndrome spectrum: a meta-analysis. *Eur Heart J* 2007; **28**: 2077–86.
35. Yusuf S, Mehta SR, Xie C *et al.* Effects of reviparin, a low-molecular-weight heparin, on mortality, reinfarction, and strokes in patients with acute myocardial infarction presenting with ST-segment elevation. *JAMA* 2005; **293**: 427–35.
36. Yusuf S, Mehta SR, Chrolavicius S *et al.* Effects of fondaparinux on mortality and reinfarction in patients with acute ST-segment elevation myocardial infarction: the OASIS-6 randomized trial. *JAMA* 2006; **295**: 1519–30.
37. Mehta SR, Yusuf S, Diaz R *et al.* Effect of glucose-insulin-potassium infusion on mortality in patients with acute ST-segment elevation myocardial infarction: the CREATE-ECLA randomized controlled trial. *JAMA* 2005; **293**: 437–46.

38. O'Rourke RA, Dell'italia LJ. Diagnosis and management of right ventricular myocardial infarction. *Curr Probl Cardiol* 2004; **29**: 6–47.
39. Dauerman HL, Goldberg RJ, Malinski M *et al.* Outcomes and early revascularization for patients > or = 65 years of age with cardiogenic shock. *Am J Cardiol* 2001; **87**: 844–8.
40. Witt BJ, Ballman KV, Brown RD Jr *et al.* The incidence of stroke after myocardial infarction: a meta-analysis. *Am J Med* 2006; **119**: e1–9.
41. Cairns JA, Theroux P, Lewis HD Jr *et al.* Antithrombotic agents in coronary artery disease. *Chest* 2001; **119** (Suppl.): 228S–52S.
42. Antman EM, Anbe DT, Armstrong RW *et al.* ACC/AHA guidelines for the management of patients with ST-elevation myocardial infarction – executive summary: a report of the American College of Cardiology/American Heart Association Task Force on Practice Guidelines (Writing Committee to Revise the 1999 Guidelines for the Management of Patients with Acute Myocardial Infarction). *Circulation* 2004; **110**: 588–636.
43. Cannon CP, Weintraub WS, Demopoulos LA *et al.* Comparison of early invasive and conservative strategies in patients with unstable coronary syndromes treated with the glycoprotein IIb/IIIa inhibitor tirofiban. *N Engl J Med* 2001; **344**: 1879–87.
44. Bavry AA, Kumbhani DJ, Rassi AN *et al.* Benefit of early invasive therapy in acute coronary syndromes: a meta-analysis of contemporary randomized clinical trials. *J Am Coll Cardiol* 2006; **48**: 1319–25.
45. Antiplatelet Trialists Collaboration. Collaborative overview of randomised trials of antiplatelet therapy – I: Prevention of death, myocardial infarction, and stroke by prolonged antiplatelet therapy in various categories of patients. *Br Med J* 1994; **308**: 81–106.
46. The Clopidogrel in Unstable angina to prevent Recurrent Events (CURE) Investigators trial. I. Effects of clopidogrel in addition to aspirin in patients with acute coronary syndromes without ST-segment elevation. *N Engl J Med* 2001; **345**: 494–502.
47. Topol EJ, Moliterno DJ, Herrmann HC *et al.* Comparison of two platelet glycoprotein IIb/IIIa inhibitors, tirofiban and abciximab, for the prevention of ischemic events with percutaneous coronary revascularization. *N Engl J Med* 2001; **344**: 1888–94.
48. Topol EJ. A contemporary assessment of low-molecular-weight heparin for the treatment of acute coronary syndromes: factoring in new trials and meta-analysis data. *Am Heart J* 2005; **149** (Suppl. 1): S100–106.
49. Kastrati A, Mehilli J, Neumann FJ *et al.* Abciximab in patients with acute coronary syndromes undergoing percutaneous coronary intervention after clopidogrel pretreatment: the ISAR-REACT 2 randomized trial. *JAMA* 2006; **295**: 1531–8.
50. Simoons ML. Effect of glycoprotein IIb/IIIa receptor blocker abciximab on outcome in patients with acute coronary syndromes without early coronary revascularisation: the GUSTO IV-ACS randomised trial. *Lancet* 2001; **357**: 1915–24.
51. Eikelboom JW, Anand SS, Malmberg K *et al.* Unfractionated heparin and low-molecular-weight heparin in acute coronary syndrome without ST elevation: a meta-analysis. *Lancet* 2000; **355**: 1936.
52. Yusuf S, Mehta SR, Chrolevicius S *et al.* Comparison of fondaparinux and enoxaparin in acute coronary syndromes. *N Engl J Med* 2006; **354**: 1464–76.
53. Hennekens CH, Albert CM, Godfried SL *et al.* Adjunctive drug therapy of acute myocardial infarction – evidence from clinical trials. *N Engl J Med* 1996; **335**: 1660–8.
54. Gheorghiade M, Goldstein S. Beta-blockers in the post-myocardial infarction patient. *Circulation* 2002; **106**: 394–8.
55. Hunt SA. ACC/AHA 2005 Guideline update for the diagnosis and management of chronic heart failure in the adult: a report of the American College of Cardiology/American Heart Association Task Force on Practice Guidelines (Writing Committee to Update the 2001 Guidelines for the Evaluation and Management of Heart Failure). *J Am Coll Cardiol* 2005; **46**: e1–82.
56. Flather MD, Yusuf S, Kober L *et al.* Long-term ACE-inhibitor therapy in patients with heart failure or left-ventricular dysfunction: a systematic overview of data from individual patients. *Lancet* 2000; **355**: 1575.
57. Latini R, Tognoni G, Maggioni AP *et al.* Clinical effects of early angiotensin-converting enzyme inhibitor treatment for acute myocardial infarction are similar in the presence and absence of aspirin: systematic overview of individual data from 96 712 randomized patients. *J Am Coll Cardiol* 2000; **35**: 1801–7.
58. Cannon CP, Braunwald E, McCabe CH *et al.* Intensive versus moderate lipid lowering with statins after acute coronary syndromes. *N Engl J Med* 2004; **350**: 1495–504.
59. Pratt CM, Moye LA. The Cardiac Arrhythmia Suppression Trial: background, interim results and implications. *Am J Cardiol* 1990; **65**: 20B–9B.
60. Devereaux PJ, Goldman L, Yusuf S *et al.* Surveillance and prevention of major perioperative ischemic cardiac events in patients undergoing noncardiac surgery: a review. *CMAJ* 2005; **173**: 779–88.
61. Devereaux PJ, Goldman L, Cook DJ *et al.* Perioperative cardiac events in patients undergoing noncardiac surgery: a review of the magnitude of the problem, the pathophysiology of the events and methods to estimate and communicate risk. *CMAJ* 2005; **173**: 627–34.
62. Schroeder WS, Gandhi PJ. Emergency management of hemorrhagic complications in the era of glycoprotein IIb/IIIa receptor antagonists, clopidogrel, low molecular weight heparin, and third-generation fibrinolytic agents. *Curr Cardiol Rep* 2003; **5**: 310–17.
63. Gibson CM. NRMI and current treatment patterns for ST-elevation myocardial infarction. *Am Heart J* 2004; **148** (Suppl. 1): 29–33.

17

Adult cardiopulmonary resuscitation

Peter T Morley

The incidence and outcomes of cardiac arrests appeared not to have changed dramatically over a number of decades. However, a number of recent advances offer significant promise in our attempts to increase neurologically intact survival.

PREVALENCE AND OUTCOMES OF CARDIAC ARRESTS

Approximately 75% of deaths from cardiac arrests occur in the pre-hospital setting.[1] Cardiac arrests in the community occur at approximately 50–150/100 000 person-years.[2–4] This incidence (and the outcome) is dramatically affected by the definition of the denominator (e.g. all cardiac arrests (89/100 000 person-years) versus those with a presumed cardiac cause and where resuscitation was attempted (31/100 000 person-years)[3]).

In-hospital cardiac arrests occur at approximately 1–5/1000 admissions,[5,6] with a similar denominator effect (as the majority of in-hospital cardiac deaths are expected and occur without attempts at resuscitation[7]).

The majority of cardiac arrests in both pre- and in-hospital settings appear to be of cardiac origin, but the underlying causes, comorbidities and presenting rhythms vary significantly between studies.[4,6,8,9]

Outcomes of cardiac arrests are variable depending on the origin of the report, and are also critically dependent on the denominator.[2,3,10] The best outcomes from a cardiac arrest (near 100%) occur in the electrophysiology laboratory (where ventricular fibrillation [VF] is often deliberately induced). The outcomes from in-hospital cardiac arrest are surprisingly good (hospital discharge as high as 42%) despite significant comorbidities, and are probably related to their early detection and the early arrival of the advanced life support (ALS) team.[6]

INTERNATIONAL REVIEW PROCESS

Since the formation of the International Liaison Committee on Resuscitation in 1992, a cooperative international evaluation of the resuscitation science has resulted in the publication of international guidelines in 2000[11] and an international consensus on resuscitation science in 2005.[12] The published guidelines of the major resuscitation councils throughout the world (including the American Heart Association,[13] the Australian Resuscitation Council (www.resus.org.au) and the European Resuscitation Council[14]) are based on this document. The process for the 2005 consensus on resuscitation science involved the review of 276 topics by 281 international contributors, with the completion of 403 worksheets[15] (completed worksheets available at www.c2005.org). This science review process continues to be refined and a new consensus on resuscitation science document is planned for publication in 2010.

IMPORTANCE OF CHAIN OF SURVIVAL

The term 'chain of survival' has been used to define the important links in the chain for the resuscitation process.[10] The key links, which apply to both in- and out-of-hospital cardiac arrests, are: early recognition and the summoning of help, early basic life support (BLS), early access to defibrillation and early ALS, including postresuscitation care.[10]

RECENT CHANGES TO GUIDELINES

As a result of the science review published in 2005,[12] a number of important changes have been made to the guidelines for both basic and ALS.

In summary, the BLS changes include:

- commencing cardiopulmonary resuscitation (CPR) where there are no signs of life (unconscious/unresponsive, not breathing normally and not moving)
- two initial breaths instead of five
- a uniform compression-to-ventilation ratio of 30:2 for infants, children and adults (regardless of the number of rescuers)[16]

The ALS changes include:

- refocusing on the provision of good CPR (including minimising the interruptions to CPR)
- minimising the potential harm associated with ventilation
- maximising the likelihood of successful defibrillation (using a single-shock strategy and appropriate energy levels)[17]

These changes are discussed in more detail in the sections that follow.

BASIC LIFE SUPPORT

The general flow of BLS management is provided in the Australian Resuscitation Council BLS flowchart (www.resus.org.au; Figure 17.1).

COMMENCEMENT OF CPR

The use of a pulse check as a means of determining the need for external cardiac compressions was downplayed in the 2000 guidelines, largely as a result of the review of a number of papers suggesting that even experienced providers may have difficulty in accurately assessing the presence or absence of a pulse.[18] This was again confirmed in the current guidelines, where it has been recommended that CPR be commenced if the victim has no signs of life (unconscious/unresponsive, not breathing normally and not moving).[16] An appropriately trained ALS provider can check for a central pulse (e.g. carotid) for up to 10 seconds during this period of assessment for signs of life.

EXTERNAL CARDIAC COMPRESSION

SITE OF COMPRESSION

The desired compression point for CPR in adults is over the lower half of the sternum. Compressions that are provided higher than this become less effective, and compressions lower than this are also less effective and have an increased risk of damage to intra-abdominal organs. Previous techniques that were widely taught to find this compression point may have introduced delays in commencing and recommencing chest compressions.

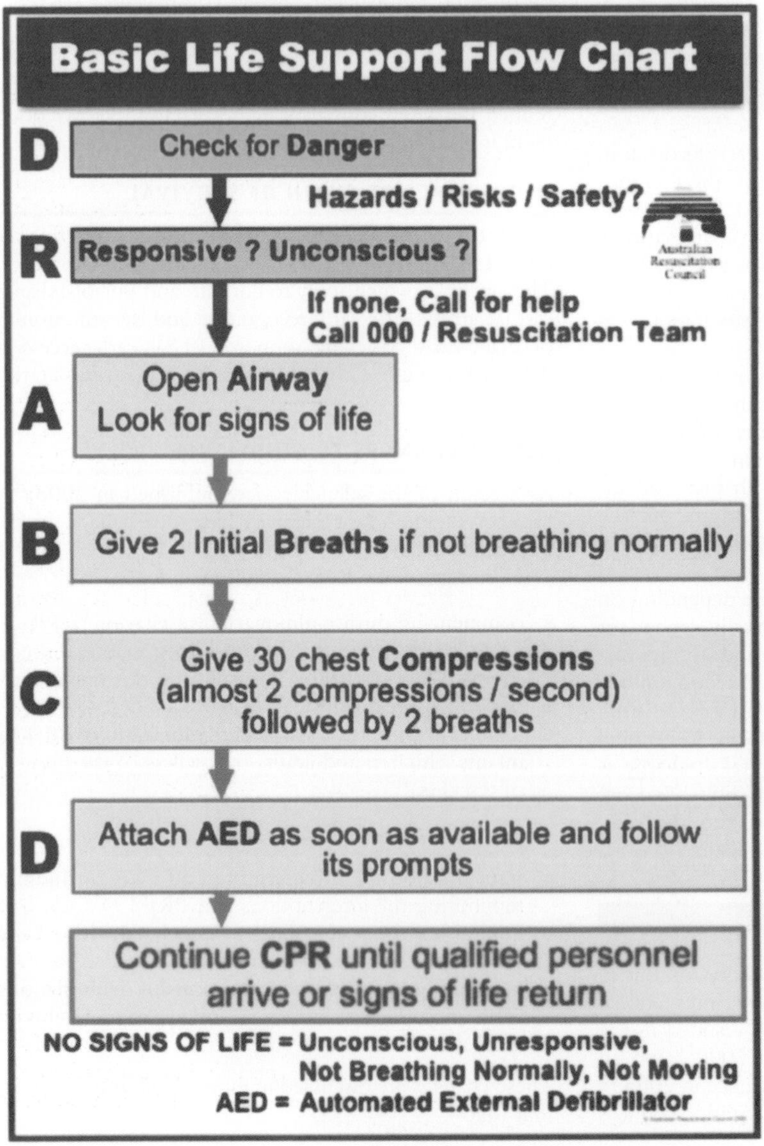

Figure 17.1 Basic life support flowchart. (Reproduced from the Australian Resuscitation Council (www.resus.org.au), with permission.)

To minimise pauses between ventilations and compressions, it is reasonable for laypeople and health care professionals to be taught to position the heel of their dominant hand in the centre of the chest of an adult victim (with the non-dominant hand on top).[2]

RATE OF COMPRESSION

The optimal rate of cardiac compression during cardiac arrest in adults has not yet been determined.[2] In a recent human study,[19] lower rates (e.g. < 80/min) were associated with worse outcomes and higher rates (> 120/min) with more fatigue and no benefits. It is recommended that chest compressions should be performed at a rate of approximately 100 compressions/minute.

DEPTH OF COMPRESSION

The ideal depth of compression is unknown. Compression depth is usually inadequate when it is measured in either manikin studies or actual cardiac arrests, and increasing depth of compression appears to be associated with higher defibrillation success.[20] It is currently recommended that, when performing chest compressions in adults, the chest should be compressed by at least 4–5 cm (or approximately one-third of its depth).

MINIMISE INTERRUPTIONS TO COMPRESSIONS

Interruptions in chest compressions ('hands-off time') are common, often prolonged, and are associated with a decrease in coronary perfusion pressure and a deceased likelihood of defibrillation success.[20–22] These adverse effects commence within 10 seconds, but appear to be at least partially reversible with the recommencement of chest compressions.[23] It is recommended that CPR (initial breaths, then chest compressions) be commenced as soon as the victim is confirmed to have no signs of life. Pauses in compressions for rhythm recognition or specific interventions (such as ventilations, defibrillation or intubation) should be minimised.

COMPRESSION–VENTILATION RATIO

The minute ventilation requirements during cardiac arrest are less than that in the non-arrested state, so the respiratory rate can be decreased. To increase the number of compressions given per minute, minimise interruptions to chest compressions and simplify instruction for teaching and skills retention, a single compression-to-ventilation ratio of 30:2 is recommended for adult BLS before the airway is secured (irrespective of the number of rescuers).[2] The tidal breath should be delivered within 1 second, and the desired tidal volume to be delivered is one that results in a visible chest rise.[2]

MONITORING THE QUALITY OF CPR

A number of different techniques are available to monitor the quality of CPR, some of which are more applicable to ALS. Simple monitoring techniques include observation of the rate, depth and positioning of chest compressions, the rate and depth of ventilation and palpation of central pulses. Additional monitoring techniques that can be used include end-tidal carbon dioxide (Table 17.1), mechanical devices (e.g. for monitoring the depth of compressions) and new monitor/defibrillators (e.g. for monitoring the depth and rate of compressions and ventilation). Feedback from these devices can improve the quality of CPR and should result in improved outcomes.[24]

Table 17.1 Utility of end-tidal carbon dioxide ($ETCO_2$) monitoring during cardiac arrest[24]

Cardiovascular (absolute value of $ETCO_2$)
Falls immediately at the onset of cardiac arrest
Increases immediately with chest compressions
Provides a linear correlation with cardiac index
Allows early detection of return of spontaneous circulation (sudden increase)
Respiratory ($ETCO_2$ waveform)
Allows assessment of endotracheal tube placement
Allows assessment of expiratory flow limitation
Prognosis (absolute value of $ETCO_2$)
Predicts successful resuscitation

'COMPRESSION-ONLY' CPR

Increasing anxiety about the performance of mouth-to-mouth ventilation has required the consideration of an alternative approach to traditional bystander CPR. A number of animal studies have suggested that ventilation may not be necessary during the initial phase of resuscitation from an arrest of a cardiac cause (e.g. where VF was electrically induced).[2] Recent research in human out-of-hospital cardiac arrests suggests that outcomes are not worse and may actually be better if ventilation is not initially attempted,[25,26] although no studies have compared 'compression-only' CPR with the BLS protocols that are currently recommended. It is recommended that if rescuers are unable, not trained, or unwilling to perform mouth-to-mouth ventilation (rescue breathing) then they should perform 'compression-only' CPR.

DEFIBRILLATION

Defibrillation is no longer only the domain of ALS. BLS providers are now often taught how to use an automated external defibrillator (AED). ALS providers can use defibrillators in automated or manual modes. Defibrillation remains the definitive treatment for VF, and it requires an appropriate combination of defibrillator waveform and energy level. Recent research has emphasised the importance of the timing of defibrillation in relation to other interventions.

EARLY DEFIBRILLATION VERSUS CPR BEFORE DEFIBRILLATION

The timing of defibrillation with regard to other interventions appears crucial. The traditional approach to the treatment of a shockable rhythm during cardiac arrest has been to perform defibrillation as soon as possible. In the scenario of recent-onset VF, this still holds, and the best outcomes are associated with defibrillation within 3 minutes (e.g. in electrophysiology labs or coronary care units). However, in situations where the VF has persisted for more than a few minutes, an initial period of CPR may actually improve the likelihood of shock success, and result in better outcomes.[23,27,28]

WAVEFORM FOR DEFIBRILLATION

No specific defibrillator waveform (either monophasic or biphasic) is consistently associated with a greater incidence of return of spontaneous circulation (ROSC) or increased hospital discharge rates from cardiac arrest due to VF.[29] Defibrillation with biphasic waveforms (either truncated exponential or rectilinear), using equal or lower energy levels, appears at least as effective for termination of VF as monophasic waveforms.[30,31]

ENERGY LEVELS

Recommendations for energy levels to be used for defibrillation vary according to the type of defibrillator (and the specific waveform) that the rescuers are using. Previous recommendations regarding energy levels were based on studies using monophasic waveforms that demonstrated increased heart block with higher energy levels. Current recommendations are based on maximising the likelihood of the success of each shock. The recommended energy level for defibrillation in adults where monophasic defibrillators are used is 360 J for all shocks. When using biphasic waveforms, the energy level should be set at 200 J for all shocks, unless there are relevant clinical data for the specific defibrillator that suggest that an alternative energy level provides adequate shock success (e.g. > 90%). There is no consistent evidence (e.g. survival benefit) to suggest that an escalation of energy levels is required for subsequent shocks.[29,32]

SINGLE-SHOCK TECHNIQUE

The use of a single-shock strategy for defibrillation is now recommended (i.e. deliver a single shock and then immediately commence CPR, rather than deliver up to three shocks in a sequence). This strategy has been proposed to decrease the interruptions to chest compressions which occur as a result of the repeated assessment of rhythm and signs of life that were inherent in the stacked-shock approach.[29] This protocol would be of particular benefit in scenarios where there is a significant time required for rhythm recognition and recharging of the defibrillator (i.e. > 10 seconds), such as with AEDs. The benefits of this strategy are clearly dependent on the quality of CPR, as the next shock will be delayed for at least 2 minutes while CPR is performed.

The Australian Resuscitation Council does however recommend the retention of a stacked-shock strategy (up to three shocks as necessary) in a specific circumstance: for the first defibrillation attempt in a witnessed arrest, where a manual defibrillator is immediately available, and the time required for rhythm recognition and charging of the defibrillator is short (e.g. < 10 seconds), resulting in delivery of the (up to) three shocks within 30 seconds. All subsequent shocks should be given using a single-shock strategy (see www.resus.org.au).

ADVANCED LIFE SUPPORT

The role of ALS is clearly established in the management of cardiac arrests. Interestingly, in itself, the provision of ALS (apart from defibrillation) has not been clearly demonstrated to be associated with improved outcomes. A number of these techniques are listed below; some of these are only available in the in-hospital setting.

ADVANCED LIFE SUPPORT FLOWCHART

The recommended sequence of treatment to be followed is designated on the ALS flowchart of the Australian Resuscitation Council (www.resus.org.au; Figure 17.2). This is designed to be used as an aide-mémoire and a teaching tool.

PRECORDIAL THUMP

The provision of a precordial thump in a witnessed and monitored arrest due to a shockable rhythm may be of value if a defibrillator is not immediately available.[29] However the technique is not without risks, and should not delay defibrillation.

CHEST COMPRESSIONS

The provision of good BLS is an essential part of the ALS management of both shockable and non-shockable rhythms. Interruptions to chest compressions for definitive procedures or interventions should be kept as brief as possible. Chest compressions should be continued up until defibrillation, and should be commenced again immediately following defibrillation (without checking the rhythm) and continued for at least 2 minutes unless signs of life return. Even if defibrillation has successfully reverted the rhythm into one that could generate a pulse, in the vast majority of cases this is not initially associated with an output.[33] Immediate compressions in these situations avoid the detrimental effects of prolonged interruptions in compressions, maintain the coronary perfusion pressure and are not associated with an increased risk of refibrillation.[34] After each 2 minutes of CPR (or if signs

Figure 17.2 Advanced life support flowchart. (Reproduced from the Australian Resuscitation Council (www.resus.org.au), with permission.)

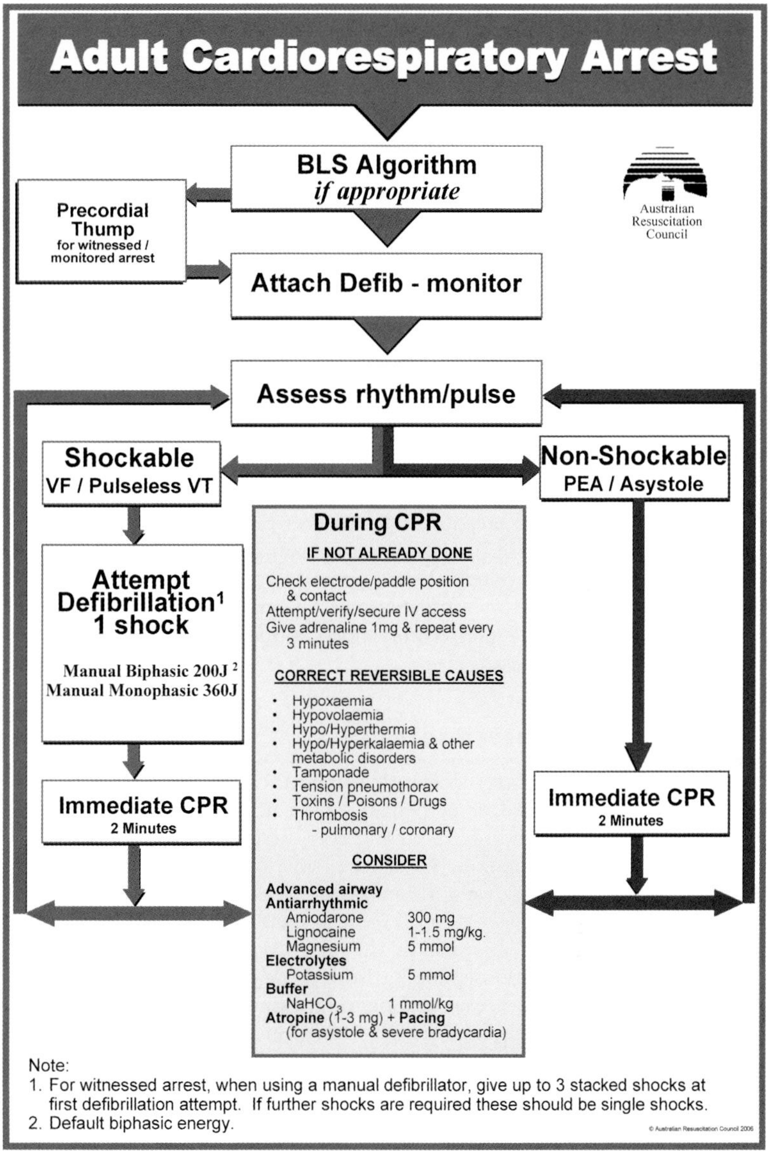

of life return), the underlying rhythm should be checked, and if a rhythm compatible with a return of spontaneous circulation is observed at this stage, then the pulse should also be checked.

AIRWAY MANAGEMENT DURING CPR

There are no data to support the routine use of any specific approach to airway management during cardiac arrest.[35] Despite this, endotracheal intubation remains the gold standard for airway maintenance and airway protection in CPR. If the victim is unconscious and has no gag reflex, and a trained operator is available, endotracheal intubation should be performed at the first appropriate opportunity, and the patient ventilated with 100% oxygen. The endotracheal tube provides optimal isolation and patency of the airway, allows suctioning of the airway and also provides access for the delivery of some drugs (e.g. adrenaline (epinephrine), lidocaine and atropine). However, attempts at endotracheal intubation should not interrupt cardiac compressions for more than 20 seconds. The routine use of an endotracheal tube during cardiac arrest management has not been shown to improve outcomes, and without adequate training and experience the incidence of complications, such as unrecognised oesophageal intubation, is unacceptably high. Alternatives to the endotracheal tube that have been studied during CPR include the bag-valve mask and other advanced airway devices such as the laryngeal mask airway and oesophageal–tracheal combitube.[35] The training and experience of the resuscitation team members and availability of such devices will determine the appropriate choice for airway adjunct.

VENTILATION DURING CPR

The minute ventilation requirements during cardiac arrest are less than those required in the non-arrested state. Hyperventilation during cardiac arrest is associated with increased intrathoracic pressure, decreased coronary and cerebral perfusion and, at least in animals, a decreased rate of return of spontaneous circulation.[36] A compression-to-ventilation ratio of 30:2 is recommended before the airway is secured, and after the airway is secured the recommended ventilation rate is 8–10/min.[2] One way to provide this, and to minimise interruptions to compressions, is to use a compression-to-ventilation ratio of 15:1 once the airway is secured (www.resus.com.au). If there is a concern about potential gas trapping, a period of disconnection from the ventilation circuit may be beneficial.[35] The tidal volume recommended is one that results in a visible chest rise.[2]

IDENTIFICATION OF REVERSIBLE CAUSES

Irrespective of the initial or subsequent rhythms, cardiac arrests can be precipitated or perpetuated by a number of conditions, which, if not detected and corrected, may prevent successful resuscitation. These 'reversible causes' are categorised in the ALS algorithm as the '4Hs and 4Ts' (www.resus.org.au; see Figure 17.2). A number of techniques are available to assist in the diagnosis and exclusion of these conditions (ranging from a good history, through careful clinical examination to investigations and interventions).[24] Echocardiography can potentially diagnose (or help exclude) a number of cardiac and non-cardiac reversible causes (Table 17.2). Transoesophageal echocardiography requires a more skilled technician, but useful information can be obtained after minimal training with the transthoracic approach.[24]

Table 17.2 Potentially useful diagnoses detectable by echocardiography[24]

Hypovolaemia*
Tamponade* (pericardial)
Tension pneumothorax*
Thrombosis – pulmonary* (thromboembolism)
Thrombosis – coronary* (regional or global wall motion abnormalities, including lack of cardiac motion)
Pacemaker capture
Unexpected ventricular fibrillation
Acute valvular insufficiency (e.g. papillary muscle rupture)
Ventricular rupture
Aortic dissection
Massive pleural effusion

*Reversible causes listed in the '4Hs and 4Ts' (www.resus.org.au).

DRUGS DURING CPR

Although various drugs are recommended for use during the management of cardiac arrests, there are no placebo-controlled studies that show that the routine use of any drugs at any stage during human cardiac arrest increase survival to hospital discharge.[35]

VASOPRESSORS

The putative beneficial effects of vasopressors during cardiac arrest are to increase the perfusion pressure to heart and brain. No vasopressor has been shown to improve long-term survival when compared with placebo for the management of cardiac arrests,[35] but despite this lack of confirmatory evidence, it is reasonable to continue to use a vasopressor routinely in the management of cardiac arrests. There are insufficient data to support any particular drug or combination of drugs.[35] Adrenaline remains the vasopressor of choice during the management of cardiac arrest (1 mg every 3 min). Vasopressin is an alternative drug, but studies have been unable to demonstrate any consistent benefit.[35,37]

ANTIARRHYTHMICS

No antiarrhythmic drug has been shown to improve long-term survival when compared with placebo for the management of cardiac arrests.[35] However, administration of amiodarone (300 mg or 5 mg/kg) for shock-refractory VF has been associated with an increased survival to hospital when compared with either placebo[38] or lidocaine.[39] Either amiodarone or lidocaine (but not both) should be considered in those patients still in VF after repeated attempts at defibrillation (including attempted defibrillation after the administration of adrenaline) have failed.

OTHER DRUGS

Other drugs that are listed in the ALS flowchart to be considered during cardiac arrest include electrolytes (such as magnesium or potassium), atropine and sodium bicarbonate (www.resus.org.au; see Figure 17.2). Additional specific drugs may be indicated depending on the specific circumstances of the arrest (see summary in Table 17.3).[40–42]

ADJUNCTS TO CPR

Many technologies and techniques have been evaluated as adjuncts to CPR in an attempt to improve survival in the management of cardiac arrests, but none have

Table 17.3 Cardiac arrest medications in specific circumstances[40–42]

Medication	Potential indications
Adrenaline (epinephrine)	Beta-blocker/calcium channel blocker toxicity
Atropine	Cholinergic/cardiac glycoside toxicity
Benzodiazepines	Sympathomimetic toxicity
Calcium	Hypocalcaemia, hypermagnesaemia, hyperkalaemia, beta-blocker/ calcium channel blocker toxicity
Digoxin-specific antibodies	Cardiac glycoside toxicity
Flumazenil	Benzodiazepine toxicity
Glucagon	Beta-blocker/calcium channel blocker toxicity
Magnesium	Hypomagnesaemia, hypokalaemia, hypercalcaemia, tricyclic antidepressant/cardiac glycoside toxicity, torsade de pointes
Naloxone	Opioid toxicity
Potassium	Hypokalaemia
Pyridoxine	Isoniazid toxicity
Sodium bicarbonate	Hyperkalaemia, tricyclic antidepressant/sodium channel blocker toxicity

been consistently associated with improved outcomes.[35] Active-compression decompression (ACD) CPR is the most widely evaluated technique, but it has not been associated with improved long-term survival.[35] An automated version of ACD CPR has been developed (LUCAS) and is currently being evaluated. A modification of vest CPR (the load-distributing band) has had recent conflicting results.[43,44] The impedance threshold valve appears promising (especially in combination with ACD CPR), and there has also been a resurgence of interest in extracorporeal techniques. At this stage there is insufficient supportive evidence to recommend the routine use of any of these adjunctive techniques.[35]

POSTRESUSCITATION CARE

The missing link in research in resuscitation has for a long time been the period of care after the return of spontaneous circulation. Survival after cardiac arrest is largely dependent on the patient's comorbidities and the initial hypoxic insults to the heart and brain. However it can also be influenced by subsequent complications (including secondary insults and the ensuing systemic inflammatory response).

INDUCED HYPOTHERMIA

Induced hypothermia has been used for postcardiac arrest management since the late 1950s, but it was brought to the attention of the wider medical community with the publication of two randomised controlled trials in 2002.[45,46] Both of these trials, in unconscious but haemodynamically stable survivors of out-of-hospital cardiac arrests due to VF, demonstrated improved neurologically intact survival with a 12–24-hour period of induced hypothermia (32–34°C).

Mild hypothermia is associated with a number of potential beneficial effects in the postarrest patient, but also a number of potential adverse effects (Table 17.4).[47] During hypothermia, the sedation and/or paralysis that may be needed to prevent the adverse effects of shivering may in turn mask seizure activity. Several techniques are available to cool patients, ranging from cold intravenous fluids through to commercial devices,[45–47] and these continue to be evaluated.

It is recommended that unconscious but haemodynamically stable survivors of out-of-hospital cardiac arrests due to VF should be cooled to 32–34°C for 12–24 hours. A period of induced hypothermia should also be considered for cardiac arrests due to other rhythms, as well as in-hospital arrests.[35,48]

OTHER FACTORS IN POSTRESUSCITATION CARE

Clearly other factors are important in the postarrest period, but studies are limited.[35] It is likely that hyperventilation and the resultant cerebral vasoconstriction are potentially harmful. Tight blood glucose control may be beneficial but its use remains controversial. Maintenance of cerebral perfusion, adequate oxygenation, treatment of seizures and good supportive care are likely to be beneficial. Norwegian investigators were able to double their survival to hospital discharge (with a favourable neurological outcome) for out-of-hospital cardiac arrests by introducing a standardised postresuscitation protocol. This protocol focused on vital organ function, including the use of therapeutic hypothermia, percutaneous coronary interventions (PCI) and the control of haemodynamics (mean arterial pressure (MAP) > 65 mmHg), blood glucose (5–8 mmol/l), ventilation (normocapnia) and seizures.[49]

BLOOD PRESSURE CONTROL

There are limited human data to guide hemodynamic management after cardiac arrest. Reported successful blood pressure goals have varied from a period of relative

Table 17.4 Potential risks and benefits of induced hypothermia after cardiac arrest[47]

Potential neurological benefits
Decreased cerebral oxygen consumption (6–7%/°C)
Decreased excitatory amino acids (especially glutamate)
Decreased free radical formation/oxidative stress
Decreased neuron-specific enolase
Decreased cerebral lactate
Decreased cerebral oedema
Decreased intracranial pressure
Decreased cell-destructive enzymes
Decreased expression of intercellular adhesion molecule-1 (ICAM-1)
Decreased neutrophil migration to ischaemic tissue
Downregulates ongoing inflammatory response
Anticonvulsant effects
Better redistribution of blood to ischaemic areas
Increased neurotrophic factors
Potential risks
Cardiovascular
Bradycardia
Vasoconstriction
Arrhythmias (uncommon at 33°C)
Haematological
Decreased numbers/function of white blood cells
Decreased numbers/function of platelets
Prolonged clotting times
Gastrointestinal
Decreased gut motility
Hyperglycaemia
Renal
Renal dysfunction
Diuresis
Metabolic
Hypokalaemia
Hypophosphataemia
Musculoskeletal
Shivering (with associated lactic acidosis)*

*Sedation and/or paralysis to control shivering may mask ongoing seizure activity.

hypertension (MAP 90–100 mmHg[45]) to more standard goals (MAP > 65–70 mmHg[49]). It is recommended to aim for a blood pressure equal to the patient's usual blood pressure or a systolic pressure greater than 100 mmHg.

GLUCOSE CONTROL

Tight blood glucose control (to normoglycaemia) in one study involving critically ill surgical patients improved survival,[50] but this has not been replicated in subsequent studies.[51] There is a large amount of circumstantial evidence to suggest that hyperglycaemia should be avoided but the optimal target for control is unknown.

PERCUTANEOUS CORONARY INTERVENTION

Thrombolysis and PCI are the mainstay of management after acute coronary syndromes. PCI has been used successfully when indicated in the early period after recovery of spontaneous circulation, and should be considered as part of routine postarrest care.[49,52]

MEDICAL EMERGENCY TEAMS (MET)

It has long been recognised that in-hospital cardiac arrests are usually preceded by some deterioration in physiological criteria.[7,53] A number of different mechanisms have been proposed to respond to these early signs.[35] The most common of these are variations of an MET (usually involving a multidisciplinary response to a single abnormality[5]) and early-warning systems (a response to an accumulated score). Commonly used criteria to initiate a MET call include:

- a threatened airway
- a respiratory rate (< 5 or > 36 breaths per minute)
- a pulse rate (< 40 or > 140 beats/min)
- a systolic blood pressure (< 90 mmHg)
- a fall in Glasgow Coma Score of 2 points
- prolonged seizures[5,7]

OUTCOMES

Promising data from studies using historical controls (or before-and-after methodology) suggested that the introduction of an MET response resulted in a number of benefits, including reductions in hospital deaths and cardiac arrest rates, and improved outcomes following cardiac arrest.[35] A large prospective cluster randomised study was performed in an attempt to confirm these benefits,[5] but it was unable to demonstrate any statistically significant improvement in outcomes (see Chapter 2).

PRE-MET

Recent observations have confirmed that minor derangements in vital signs predict adverse clinical outcomes.[54,55] Many of these derangements occur at a level that would not elicit either an MET call or an early-warning system response,[55] therefore ward-based systems are required to respond to these factors.

PROGNOSTICATION

It is impossible to predict accurately the degree of neurological recovery during or immediately after a cardiac arrest.[35,56] Relying on the neurologic examination during cardiac arrest to predict outcome is not recommended and should not be used as it has insufficient negative predictive value.[35] After cessation of sedation (and/or induced hypothermia), the probability of awakening decreases with each day of coma. Clinical examination (absence of pupillary response or motor response to pain on day 3), somatosensory evoked potentials and electro-encephalography offer the best prognostic estimates[35,56] (www.resus.org.au).

SUMMARY

Improved outcomes after cardiac arrest are now anticipated to occur as a result of a number of advances in management and the ongoing science evaluation process. Improvements within each link of the chain of survival are anticipated. These include: earlier recognition and activation of the emergency response (including MET and pre-MET); good BLS (maximising quality of and minimising interruptions to chest compressions); optimised defibrillation (with an appropriate sequence of CPR, and using optimal energy levels for the waveform used); and early and appropriate ALS with more focus on the period of postresuscitation care.

REFERENCES

1. 2005 American Heart Association Guidelines for Cardiopulmonary Resuscitation and Emergency Cardiovascular Care. Part 3: Overview of CPR. *Circulation* 2005; **112** (Suppl.): IV12–18.
2. 2005 International Consensus on Cardiopulmonary Resuscitation and Emergency Cardiovascular Care Science with Treatment Recommendations. Part 2: Adult basic life support. *Resuscitation* 2005; **67**: 187–201.
3. Finn JC, Jacobs IG, Holman CD *et al.* Outcomes of out-of-hospital cardiac arrest patients in Perth, Western Australia, 1996–1999. *Resuscitation* 2001; **51**: 247–55.
4. Jennings PA, Cameron P, Walker T *et al.* Out-of-hospital cardiac arrest in Victoria: rural and urban outcomes. *Med J Aust* 2006; **185**: 135–9.
5. Hillman K, Chen J, Cretikos M *et al.* Introduction of the medical emergency team (MET) system: a cluster-randomised controlled trial. *Lancet* 2005; **365**: 2091–7.
6. Sandroni C, Nolan J, Cavallaro F *et al.* In-hospital cardiac arrest: incidence, prognosis and possible measures to improve survival. *Intens Care Med* 2007; **33**: 237–45.
7. Kause J, Smith G, Prytherch D *et al.* A comparison of antecedents to cardiac arrests, deaths and emergency intensive care admissions in Australia and New Zealand, and the United Kingdom – the ACADEMIA study. *Resuscitation* 2004; **62**: 275–82.
8. Peberdy MA, Kaye W, Ornato JP *et al.* Cardiopulmonary resuscitation of adults in the hospital: a report of 14 720 cardiac arrests from the National Registry of Cardiopulmonary Resuscitation. *Resuscitation* 2003; **58**: 297–308.
9. Cohn AC, Wilson WM, Yan B *et al.* Analysis of clinical outcomes following in-hospital adult cardiac arrest. *Intern Med J* 2004; **34**: 398–402.
10. Perkins GD, Soar J. In hospital cardiac arrest: missing links in the chain of survival. *Resuscitation* 2005; **66**: 253–5.
11. American Heart Association in collaboration with the International Liaison Committee on Resuscitation (ILCOR). Guidelines 2000 for cardiopulmonary resuscitation and emergency cardiovascular care. *Circulation* 2000; **102** (suppl. I): I:13–403.
12. Proceedings of the 2005 International Consensus on Cardiopulmonary Resuscitation and Emergency Cardiovascular Care Science with Treatment Recommendations. *Resuscitation* 2005; **67**: 157–341.
13. 2005 American Heart Association Guidelines for Cardiopulmonary Resuscitation and Emergency Cardiovascular Care. *Circulation* 2005; **112** (Suppl.): IV1–203.
14. European Resuscitation Council guidelines for resuscitation 2005. *Resuscitation* 2005; **67** (Suppl. 1): S1–189.
15. Morley PT, Zaritsky A. The evidence evaluation process for the 2005 International Consensus Conference on cardiopulmonary resuscitation and emergency cardiovascular care science with treatment recommendations. *Resuscitation* 2005; **67**: 167–70.
16. Jacobs IG, Morley PT. The Australian Resuscitation Council: new guidelines for 2006. *Crit Care Resusc* 2006; **8**: 87–8.
17. Morley PT, Walker T. Australian Resuscitation Council: adult advanced life support (ALS) guidelines 2006. *Crit Care Resusc* 2006; **8**: 129–31.
18. Cummins RO, Hazinski MF. Guidelines based on fear of type II (false-negative) errors. Why we dropped the pulse check for lay rescuers. *Resuscitation* 2000; **46**: 439–42.
19. Abella BS, Sandbo N, Vassilatos P *et al.* Chest compression rates during cardiopulmonary resuscitation are suboptimal: a prospective study during in-hospital cardiac arrest. *Circulation* 2005; **111**: 428–34.
20. Edelson DP, Abella BS, Kramer-Johansen J *et al.* Effects of compression depth and pre-shock pauses predict defibrillation failure during cardiac arrest. *Resuscitation* 2006; **71**: 137–45.
21. Eftestol T, Sunde K, Steen PA. Effects of interrupting precordial compressions on the calculated probability of defibrillation success during out-of-hospital cardiac arrest. *Circulation* 2002; **105**: 2270–3.
22. Ewy GA. Cardiac arrest – guideline changes urgently needed. *Lancet* 2007; **369**: 882–4.
23. Eftestol T, Wik L, Sunde K *et al.* Effects of cardiopulmonary resuscitation on predictors of ventricular fibrillation defibrillation success during out-of-hospital cardiac arrest. *Circulation* 2004; **110**: 10–15.
24. Morley PT. Monitoring the quality of CPR. *Curr Opin Crit Care* 2007; **13**: 261–7.
25. Kellum MJ, Kennedy KW, Ewy GA. Cardiocerebral resuscitation improves survival of patients with out-of-hospital cardiac arrest. *Am J Med* 2006; **119**: 335–40.
26. Cardiopulmonary resuscitation by bystanders with chest compression only (SOS-KANTO): an observational study. *Lancet* 2007; **369**: 920–6.

27. Cobb LA, Fahrenbruch CE, Walsh TR *et al.* Influence of cardiopulmonary resuscitation prior to defibrillation in patients with out-of-hospital ventricular fibrillation. *JAMA* 1999; **281**: 1182–8.
28. Wik L, Hansen TB, Fylling F *et al.* Delaying defibrillation to give basic cardiopulmonary resuscitation to patients with out-of-hospital ventricular fibrillation: a randomized trial. *JAMA* 2003; **289**: 1389–95.
29. 2005 International Consensus on Cardiopulmonary Resuscitation and Emergency Cardiovascular Care Science with Treatment Recommendations. Part 3: defibrillation. *Resuscitation* 2005; **67**: 203–11.
30. Morrison LJ, Dorian P, Long J *et al.* Out-of-hospital cardiac arrest rectilinear biphasic to monophasic damped sine defibrillation waveforms with advanced life support intervention trial (ORBIT). *Resuscitation* 2005; **66**: 149–57.
31. Kudenchuk PJ, Cobb LA, Copass MK *et al.* Transthoracic incremental monophasic versus biphasic defibrillation by emergency responders (TIMBER): a randomized comparison of monophasic with biphasic waveform ascending energy defibrillation for the resuscitation of out-of-hospital cardiac arrest due to ventricular fibrillation. *Circulation* 2006; **114**: 2010–8.
32. Stiell IG, Walker RG, Nesbitt LP *et al.* BIPHASIC trial: a randomized comparison of fixed lower versus escalating higher energy levels for defibrillation in out-of-hospital cardiac arrest. *Circulation* 2007; **115**: 1511–7.
33. Rea TD, Shah S, Kudenchuk PJ *et al.* Automated external defibrillators: to what extent does the algorithm delay CPR? *Ann Emerg Med* 2005; **46**: 132–41.
34. Hess EP, White RD. Ventricular fibrillation is not provoked by chest compression during post-shock organized rhythms in out-of-hospital cardiac arrest. *Resuscitation* 2005; **66**: 7–11.
35. 2005 International Consensus on Cardiopulmonary Resuscitation and Emergency Cardiovascular Care Science with Treatment Recommendations. Part 4: advanced life support. *Resuscitation* 2005; **67**: 213–47.
36. Aufderheide TP. The problem with and benefit of ventilations: should our approach be the same in cardiac and respiratory arrest? *Curr Opin Crit Care* 2006; **12**: 207–12.
37. Aung K, Htay T. Vasopressin for cardiac arrest: a systematic review and meta-analysis. *Arch Intern Med* 2005; **165**: 17–24.
38. Kudenchuk PJ, Cobb LA, Copass MK *et al.* Amiodarone for resuscitation after out-of-hospital cardiac arrest due to ventricular fibrillation. *N Engl J Med* 1999; **341**: 871–8.
39. Dorian P, Cass D, Schwartz B *et al.* Amiodarone as compared with lidocaine for shock-resistant ventricular fibrillation. *N Engl J Med* 2002; **346**: 884–90.
40. 2005 American Heart Association Guidelines for Cardiopulmonary Resuscitation and Emergency Cardiovascular Care. Part 7.4: monitoring and medications. *Circulation* 2005; **112** (Suppl.): IV78–83.
41. 2005 American Heart Association Guidelines for Cardiopulmonary Resuscitation and Emergency Cardiovascular Care. Part 10.1: life-threatening electrolyte abnormalities. *Circulation* 2005; **112** (Suppl.): IV121–5.
42. 2005 American Heart Association Guidelines for Cardiopulmonary Resuscitation and Emergency Cardiovascular Care. Part 10.2: toxicology in ECC. *Circulation* 2005; **112** (Suppl.): IV126–32.
43. Ong ME, Ornato JP, Edwards DP *et al.* Use of an automated, load-distributing band chest compression device for out-of-hospital cardiac arrest resuscitation. *JAMA* 2006; **295**: 2629–37.
44. Hallstrom A, Rea TD, Sayre MR *et al.* Manual chest compression vs use of an automated chest compression device during resuscitation following out-of-hospital cardiac arrest: a randomized trial. *JAMA* 2006; **295**: 2620–8.
45. Bernard SA, Gray TW, Buist MD *et al.* Treatment of comatose survivors of out-of-hospital cardiac arrest with induced hypothermia. *N Engl J Med* 2002; **346**: 557–63.
46. Mild therapeutic hypothermia to improve the neurologic outcome after cardiac arrest. *N Engl J Med* 2002; **346**: 549–56.
47. Bernard SA, Buist M. Induced hypothermia in critical care medicine: a review. *Crit Care Med* 2003; **31**: 2041–51.
48. Nolan JP, Morley PT, Vanden Hoek TL *et al.* Therapeutic hypothermia after cardiac arrest: an advisory statement by the advanced life support task force of the International Liaison Committee on Resuscitation. *Circulation* 2003; **108**: 118–21.
49. Sunde K, Pytte M, Jacobsen D *et al.* Implementation of a standardised treatment protocol for post resuscitation care after out-of-hospital cardiac arrest. *Resuscitation* 2007; **73**: 29–39.
50. Van den Berghe G, Wouters P, Weekers F *et al.* Intensive insulin therapy in the critically ill patients. *N Engl J Med* 2001; **345**: 1359–67.
51. Van den Berghe G, Wilmer A, Hermans G *et al.* Intensive insulin therapy in the medical ICU. *N Engl J Med* 2006; **354**: 449–61.
52. Spaulding CM, Joly LM, Rosenberg A *et al.* Immediate coronary angiography in survivors of out-of-hospital cardiac arrest. *N Engl J Med* 1997; **336**: 1629–33.
53. Jacques T, Harrison GA, McLaws ML *et al.* Signs of critical conditions and emergency responses (SOCCER): a model for predicting adverse events in the inpatient setting. *Resuscitation* 2006; **69**: 175–83.
54. Buist M, Bernard S, Nguyen TV *et al.* Association between clinically abnormal observations and subsequent in-hospital mortality: a prospective study. *Resuscitation* 2004; **62**: 137–41.
55. Harrison GA, Jacques T, McLaws ML *et al.* Combinations of early signs of critical illness predict in-hospital death-the SOCCER study (signs of critical conditions and emergency responses). *Resuscitation* 2006; **71**: 327–34.
56. Zandbergen EG, de Haan RJ, Stoutenbeek CP *et al.* Systematic review of early prediction of poor outcome in anoxic-ischaemic coma. *Lancet* 1998; **352**: 1808–12.

18

Management of cardiac arrhythmias

Andrew Holt

CARDIAC ELECTROPHYSIOLOGY

The electrophysiological properties of cardiac cells are important in understanding cardiac arrhythmias and their management. Cardiac cells undergo cyclical depolarisation and repolarisation to form an action potential. The shape and duration of each action potential are determined by the activity of ion channel protein complexes on the myocyte surface. These highly selective ion channels determine the rate of ion flux which in turn determines the magnitude and rate of change of myocyte membrane potential. Many of these ion channels are the molecular targets for antiarrhythmic drugs.

Ion channel function can be affected by:

- genetic mutations of channel proteins
- changes in functional expression of channel protein genes
- acute ischaemia
- autonomic tone
- myocardial scarring
- electrolyte concentration

The spectrum of cardiac action potentials varies from *fast-response* cells – conducting and contractile myocytes (Figure 18.1a) – to *slow-response* cells of pacemaker myocytes – sinoatrial (SA) and atrioventricular (AV) nodes (Figure 18.1b). Fast myocytes lose their characteristic action potential and behave more like slow myocytes when ischaemic. The action potential is divided into five phases, as follows.

PHASE 0

In fast myocytes (Figure 18.1a) rapid depolarisation occurs due to activation of voltage-dependent Na^+ channels. Activation is initiated in an all-or-none response once the threshold is reached. The Na^+ channels are inactivated as membrane potential rises to +30 mV and remain inactivated until repolarisation occurs. Rapidity of depolarisation determines speed of conduction. In slow-response myocytes depolarisation does not involve Na^+ channels and the slower rate of depolarisation is due to a slow inward Ca^{2+} current via L- and T-type voltage-dependent Ca^{2+} channels.

PHASE 1

Early rapid incomplete repolarisation to approximately 0 mV occurs due to activation of transient outward current from I_{TO1} and I_{TO2} K^+ channels. Slow myocytes do not exhibit phase 1 or 2 characteristics (Figure 18.1b).

PHASE 2

The prolonged plateau repolarisation of fast myocytes is a consequence of low membrane conductance to all ions. The decreasing inward Ca^{2+} current of L- and T-type Ca^{2+} channels is initially balanced and then overcome by the outward K^+ current of the delayed rectifiers or the I_k family of K^+ channels. During this phase the rise in $[Ca^{2+}]_i$ is the trigger to release sarcoplasmic reticulum stores of Ca^{2+} and initiate the contractile process.

PHASE 3

Relatively rapid repolarisation occurs as outward K^+ current of the delayed rectifiers increases. The I_{kr} K^+ channel, one of the I_k delayed rectifiers, is the common mechanism whereby antiarrhythmic drugs prolong the action potential and refractoriness.

PHASE 4

This is a stable electrical state in fast non-pacemaker myocytes. In slow pacemaker myocytes the resting membrane potential (RMP) slowly depolarises until the action potential threshold is reached (Figure 18.1b). This inward or pacemaker current is due to I_f K^+ channels.

Fast-response and slow-response myocytes also have important differences in properties of refractoriness. In fast myocytes, Na^+ channels are progressively reactivated during phase 3 repolarisation as the membrane potential becomes more negative. When an extra stimulus occurs during phase 3, the magnitude of the resulting inward Na^+ current and likelihood of impulse propagation depend on the number of reactivated Na^+ channels. Refractoriness is therefore determined by the voltage-dependent recovery of Na^+ channels. The absolute refractory period (Figure 18.1) is that minimum time needed for recovery

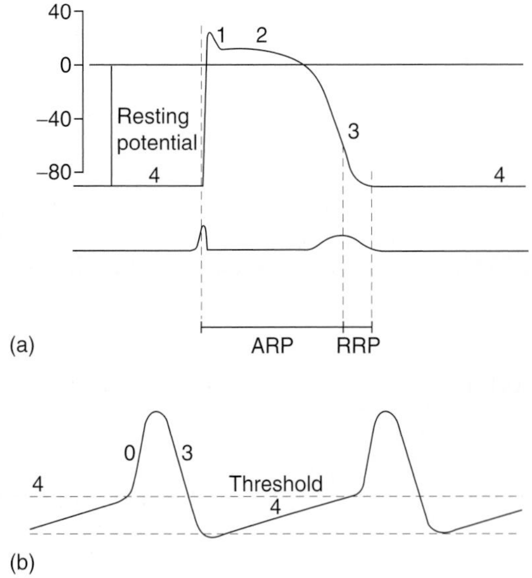

Figure 18.1 (a) Action potential in a fast-response, non-pacemaker myocyte: phases 0–4, resting membrane potential −80 mV, absolute refractory period (ARP) and relative refractory period (RRP). (b) Action potential in a slow-response, pacemaker myocyte. The upward slope of phase 4, on reaching threshold potential, results in an action potential.

of sufficient Na^+ channels for a stimulus to result in impulse propagation. However, once propagation in fast myocytes occurs, conduction velocity is normal. In contrast, slow-response or Ca^{2+} channel-dependent myocytes exhibit time-dependent refractoriness. Even after full repolarisation further time is needed before all Ca^{2+} channels are reactivated. Stimuli during this period produce reduced Ca^{2+} current and the propagation velocity of any resulting impulse is reduced. The conduction velocity independence of premature action potentials with fast-response myocytes is lost in the setting of Na^+ channel-blocking drugs or ischaemia because they behave increasingly like slow-response myocytes with resulting slowed impulse conduction.

GENETIC BASIS TO ARRHYTHMIA[1]

In the absence of structural abnormalities of the heart, primary electrical disease is associated with mutations in ion channel genes. The long-QT syndrome (LQTS), short-QT syndrome, Brugada syndrome (idiopathic ventricular fibrillation (VF)) and catecholaminergic polymorphic ventricular tachycardia (VT: causes of sudden cardiac death (SCD) in the young) are examples of primary electrical disease where genetic mutations encoding for ion channel proteins have been characterised. The ion channel basis of congenital LQTS has been verified with the discovery of disease-causing mutations in the *KCNQ1*, *KCNH2* and *SCN5A* genes that encode for the cardiac delayed rectifier K^+ (I_{Ks}, I_{Kr}) and sodium (I_{Na}) channels respectively. Single-gene mutations can also give rise to more than one distinct syndrome with mutation of the *SCN5A* gene producing both LQTS and Brugada syndromes. This phenotype complexity is presumably the result of interactions between gene expression and environmental factors or the effect of other modifier genes.

Genetic mutations can result in increased or decreased ion channel function. Mutations to the gene *KCNQ1* encoding for I_{Ks} K^+ channel can result in:

- reduced function, impaired repolarisation and LQTS type 1
- increased function, accelerated repolarisation and short-QT syndrome, which is also associated with SCD

Inheritable forms of structural ventricular disease are associated with atrial arrhythmias and SCD. Examples include hypertrophic and dilated cardiomyopathies and arrhythmogenic right ventricular dysplasia which are linked to mutations in sarcomeric, cytoskeletal and intercellular junction proteins, respectively.

The risk of cardiac arrhythmias and SCD in the setting of acquired structural heart disease such as ischaemic heart disease is in part genetically determined. Studies demonstrate an increased risk of SCD in patients who have a parental history of cardiac arrest.

MOLECULAR BASIS TO ARRHYTHMIA[1]

Structural and electrical remodelling in response to myocardial injury, altered haemodynamic loads and changes in neurohumoral signalling lead to alterations in:

- ion channel function
- intracellular calcium handling
- intercellular communication
- composition of intercellular matrix

All of these factors lead to heterogeneous slowing of conduction velocity and prolonged refractoriness.

Tachycardic remodelling of the atrium is associated with:

- reduced functional expression of L-type Ca^{2+} channels, intracellular Ca^{2+} overload and shortening action potential duration

Heart failure is associated with:

- downregulation of each of the major repolarising K^+ currents, prolonging repolarisation and resulting insusceptiblity to early afterdepolarisation (EADs). As these changes are heterogeneous they also create the substrate for re-entrant arrhythmias
- reduced Na^+ channel density decreasing conduction velocity

- increased expression of Na^+-Ca^{2+} exchanger protein, leading to intracellular Ca^{2+} overload and predisposition to delayed afterdepolarisation (DAD)-mediated arrhythmia

Intercellular ion channels or connexins at gap junctions are decreased and redistributed from the intercalated disc to lateral cell borders, slowing conduction velocity and uncoupling myocytes.

Myocardial infarction scar produces:

- heterogeneous action potential duration with zones of healing myocytes with shortened action potential and surrounding hypertrophic myocytes with prolonged action potentials
- potential anatomical circuits due to fibrous tissue separating myocyte bundles

ARRHYTHMOGENIC MECHANISMS[2–4]

Many factors in isolation or combination give rise to the substrate of arrhythmogenesis (Figure 18.2). Arrhythmia may arise from abnormalities of impulse generation or conduction. Table 18.1 demonstrates the relationship between mechanism and type of arrhythmia, and desired antiarrhythmic effect.

ABNORMAL IMPULSE GENERATION (TABLE 18.2)

ENHANCED NORMAL AUTOMATICITY

Automaticity is the property of spontaneous impulse generation by cardiac fibres. This results from spontaneous depolarisation during phase 4, due to an inward current carried by K^+ in SA node or subsidiary pacemaker myocytes.

ABNORMAL AUTOMATICITY

Abnormal automaticity is the mechanism by which spontaneous impulses are generated in fibres that are partially depolarised by a pathological process. This less negative RMP is associated with inactivation of the normal ionic currents of phase 4 depolarisation and the pacemaker potential results from inward Na^+ and Ca^{2+} currents and is not readily susceptible to overdrive suppression from normal pacemaker activity. Due to their less negative membrane potentials, these abnormal automatic fibres inactivate the phase 0 fast inward Na^+ current, resulting in an impaired rate of impulse conduction (as well as contractility) which further contributes to arrhythmia. In this setting, Ca^{2+} carries the major inward current on depolarisation in these fibres.

TRIGGERED ACTIVITY

Abnormal impulse generation from triggered activity originates from oscillations in the membrane potential that are initiated or triggered by a preceding action potential. There are two types of oscillations, EAD and DAD. EAD occurs during phase 2 or 3 of the action potential, whereas DAD occurs after the termination of depolarisation. The signal-averaged electrocardiograph (ECG) can detect after-depolarisations.

1. EAD appear as subthreshold humps during the plateau or depolarisation phases. On reaching threshold, single or multiple action potentials can be induced. Plateau EAD are caused by an increased inward Ca^{2+} current (at this level of membrane potential, fast inward Na^+ channels are inactivated) and produce slow rising and propagating action potentials. Phase 3 EAD are caused by a reduction in outward K^+ currents and produce relatively rapidly rising and propagating action potentials. EAD amplitude and likelihood of triggered arrhythmia increase as driving rate decreases and action potential is prolonged.

Figure 18.2 Factors that combine to form the substrate of arrhythmogenesis.

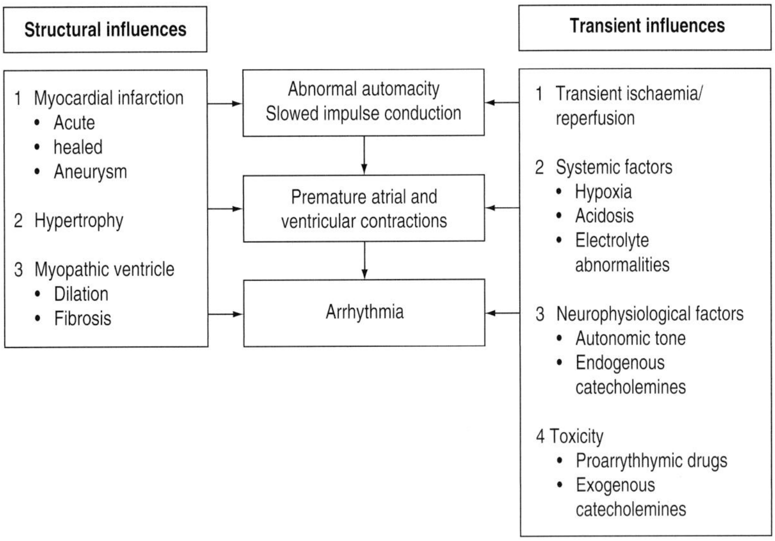

Table 18.1 Classification of mechanisms of arrhythmia and desired antiarrhythmic drug action

Mechanism of arrhythmia	Arrhythmia	Antiarrhythmic effect	Representative drugs
Automaticity-enhanced			
Normal	Inappropriate sinus tachycardia Unifocal atrial tachycardia	Decrease phase 4 depolarisation	β-blocker Sodium channel blockers
Abnormal	Unifocal atrial tachycardia Accelerated idioventricular rhythms VT post myocardial infarction	Hyperpolarise or decrease phase 4 depolarisation	Calcium or sodium channel blockers M_2 agonists
Triggered activity			
Early afterdepolarisation (EAD)	Torsade de pointes Digitalis-induced arrhythmias Some VT	Shorten action potential or suppress EAD	Increase heart rate with β-agonists or vagolytic agents, calcium channel blockers, β-blockers or magnesium
Delayed afterdepolarisation (DAD)		Decrease calcium overload or suppress DAD	Calcium or sodium channel blockers, β-blockers, adenosine
Re-entry: sodium channel-dependent			
Long excitable gap	Afl type 1 Circus movement tachycardia in Wolff–Parkinson–White syndrome (WPW) Monomorphic VT	Depress conduction and excitability Prolong refractory period	Sodium channel blockers Potassium channel blockers
Short excitable gap	Afl type 2 Atrial fibrillation Circus movement tachycardia in WPW Polymorphic and monomorphic VT Bundle branch re-entry Ventricular fibrillation		
Re-entry: calcium channel-dependent			
	Atrioventricular nodal re-entrant tachycardia Circus movement tachycardia in WPW VT	Depress conduction and excitability	Calcium channel blockers

VT, ventricular tachycardia.
(Modified with permission from Task Force of the Working Group on Arrhythmias of the European Society of Cardiology. The Sicilian gambit: a new approach to the classification of antiarrhythmic drugs based on their actions on arrhythmogenic mechanisms. *Circulation* 1991; **84**: 1831–51.)

Tachyarrhythmias induced by EAD are more likely to occur on the background of a bradycardia.

2. DAD are produced by Na^+-Ca^{2+} exchanger current-induced oscillations in inward calcium current. These oscillations are caused by $[Ca^{2+}]_i$ overload saturating sarcoplasmic reticulum sequestration mechanisms, thereby leading to Ca^{2+}-induced Ca^{2+} release. Unlike EAD, DAD depend on previous rapid rhythm for their initiation.

ABNORMAL IMPULSE CONDUCTION[5]

Abnormal impulse conduction may cause an arrhythmia by the phenomena of re-entry. Re-entry describes the re-excitation of an area or entire heart by a circulating impulse. Although the classic 'bifurcating Purkinje fibre' model of Schmitt and Erlanger has given way to a much more complex picture, the essential electrophysiological requirements for re-entrant excitation remain. Requirements for re-entry are (Figure 18.3):

- conduction block in one limb of the circuit
- slowed conduction in the other limb
- the impulse returns back along the limb initially blocked to re-enter and re-excite the pathway proximal to the block and complete the re-entry pathway

When these properties are present, the chance of a circulating impulse producing re-entrant excitation depends on pathway geometry, the electrical properties and length of the depressed area and conduction velocity within each

Table 18.2 Causes of abnormal impulse generation

Enhanced normal automaticity	Adrenergic stimulation
Abnormal automaticity	Ischaemia
Early afterdepolarisations	Hypoxia
	Hypercapnia
	Catecholamines
	Class IA antiarrhythmic drugs
	Class III antiarrhythmic drugs
	Other drugs that prolong repolarisation
Delayed afterdepolarisations	Digoxin toxicity
	Increased intracellular Na^+
	Decreased extracellular K^+
	Increased intracellular Ca^{2+}
	Intracellular Ca^{2+} overload
	Myocardial infarction
	Reperfusion after ischaemia

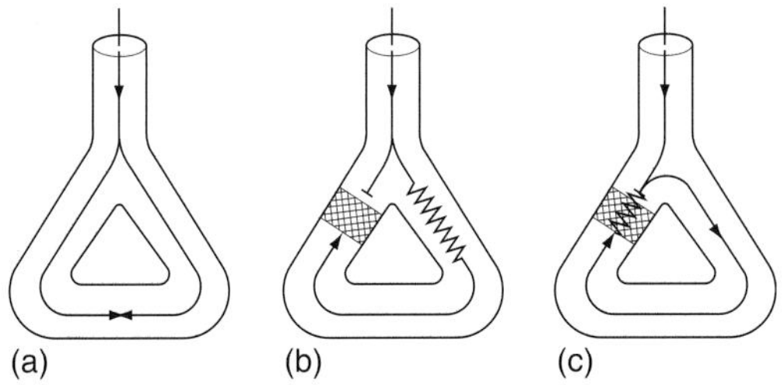

Figure 18.3 Re-entrant excitation. (a) Normal cardiac impulse conduction results in the impulse being extinguished. (b) Conduction down one limb is blocked by segment of refractory tissue (excitable gap). (c) The impulse is conducted back up the limb and arrives at the excitable gap which has recovered from refractoriness and retrograde conduction is complete. If geometry and electrical properties are favourable, the excitable gap circulates around the re-entry loop and arrhythmia is initiated.

component. The segment of the re-entry pathway that is initially refractory and therefore blocks conduction down one limb and recovers in time to conduct the return impulse is termed the 'excitable gap'. Therefore, the generation and subsequent maintenance of a circuit depend on this excitable gap of non-refractory tissue circulating between the advancing depolarising wave front and the repolarising tail. The resulting re-entrant impulse can be self-terminating, causing ectopic beats, or lead to atrial or ventricular tachyarrhythmias.

Risk of re-entry can be further modelled and quantified. Cardiac wavelength (λ) is the physical distance an electrical impulse travels in one refractory period. λ equals conduction velocity × refractory period (or action potential duration). Re-entry is critically dependent on the λ being shorter than the potential reentrant pathway. If λ exceeds the path length then the advancing impulse encroaches on the refractory tail and re-entry is terminated. Reducing λ (decreasing conduction velocity or refractory period) promotes re-entry circuits.

Re-entry may be terminated by:

- increasing conduction velocity: the excitable gap is abolished by the wave front arriving too early and meeting refractory tissue
- increasing refractory period: the excitable gap is lost
- slowing conduction: a unidirectional block can be converted into a complete block

Ordered re-entry occurs along anatomical pathways which are 'macroscopic' loops (macro-re-entry), as in Wolff–Parkinson–White (WPW) syndrome. Functional circuits can be created following myocardial infarction, resulting in VT. 'Microscopic' loops (micro-re-entry) occur at the level of single fibres where antegrade and retrograde impulse propagation occurs in parallel fibres. Random re-entry refers to the generation of a circulating impulse, not from a fixed circuit but from constantly changing electrophysiologically distinct fibres or pathways created by the circulating impulse, resulting in atrial fibrillation (AF) or VF.

The cellular properties that lead to impaired conduction include:

- inactivation of the phase 0 fast Na^+ channels, which reduces both the magnitude and rate of propagation of any resultant action potential
- intercellular uncoupling, which increases resistance to action potential propagation and slows conduction. Intercellular coupling is reduced by ischaemia, $[Ca^{2+}]_i$ overload, acidosis and reduced expression of intercellular ion channel connexin proteins in diseases such as chronic heart failure

ELECTROPHYSIOLOGICAL EFFECTS OF ISCHAEMIA

Both hypoxia and acidosis are implicated in the production of a less negative RMP in ischaemia. A rise in extracellular K^+ results from impairment of the adenosine triphosphate (ATP)-dependent K^+ inward channels. As $[K^+]_o/[K^+]_i$ is the major determinant of the RMP, intracellular K^+ loss results in a less negative RMP.

The consequences of this are:

- abnormal automaticity
- inactivation of the fast inward Na^+ channels, which slows the conduction velocity

ELECTROLYTE ABNORMALITIES AND ARRHYTHMIA[6]

POTASSIUM

Hyper- and hypokalaemia both cause arrhythmia mediated by the resultant changes in RMP (Table 18.3). In ischaemia, hyperkalaemia at the local tissue level caused by a

Table 18.3 Arrhythmogenic effects of potassium disturbance

	Arrhythmogenic effects	Electrocardiogram changes	Arrhythmia
Hyperkalaemia	Less negative RMP	Peaked T-waves	Sinus node suppression
	Inactivation of fast Na^+ channels	Widening of P-wave and QRS complex	Atrioventricular block
	Slowed conduction velocity		Ventricular fibrillation
Hypokalaemia	Prolongation of rapid repolarisation	U-waves	Atrial and ventricular ectopy
	Hyperpolarisation of RMP	ST-segment and T-wave changes	Atrial and ventricular ectopy tachyarrhythmias
	Increased pacemaker activity in Purkinje and ventricular fibres		

RMP, resting membrane potential.

pathological extracellular shift of K^+ is the major factor contributing to ventricular arrhythmia in this setting. In hypokalaemia, the dispersion of pacemaker activity and the effect on repolarisation are similar to the electrophysiological effects of cardiac glycosides and β-adrenergic agonists, and it is not surprising that a combination of these factors is associated with an increased incidence of arrhythmia. The increased risk of death in hypertensive patients treated with thiazide diuretics has been attributed to hypokalaemic (and possibly hypomagnesaemic)-induced arrhythmia (Multiple Risk Factor Intervention Trial). Thiazide-induced hypokalaemic ventricular ectopy is worsened by exercise.[7] Hypokalaemia is associated with VF and VT following acute myocardial infarction (AMI). The increased incidence of VF/VT with a serum K^+ less than 3.5 mmol/l is clearly established and the probability of VT increases as the serum K^+ decreases. During AMI the incidence of VF/VT was 15% at 4.5 mmol/l, 38% at 3.5 mmol/l, 55% at 3.0 mmol/l and 67% at 2.5 mmol/l.[8]

MAGNESIUM

The antiarrhythmic properties of Mg^{2+} are clearly established but a causal relationship between hypomagnesaemia and arrhythmia is largely circumstantial. Decreased extracellular Mg^{2+} by itself has little effect on the electrophysiological properties of myocytes or the ECG. Hypomagnesaemia has been implicated in the genesis of VT/VF in patients with hypertension and heart failure receiving thiazide or loop diuretics, acute alcohol intoxication or withdrawal and possibly with AMI. The product of K^+ and Mg^{2+} is the best predictor of arrhythmia in hypertensive patients taking thiazide diuretics.[9]

AUTONOMIC NERVOUS SYSTEM AND VENTRICULAR ARRHYTHMIA[10]

The autonomic nervous system, particularly vagal tone, has a significant effect on the occurrence of post myocardial infarction VF, as seen by the following:

- High vagal tone is associated with better outcome and less susceptibility to exercise-induced VF with new ischaemia in animal models.
- Post myocardial infarction exercise training results in an increased vagal tone, which inhibits induced VF.
- Implantable electrical vagal stimulation and muscarinic agents, including edrophonium, are protective.
- The protection is not heart rate-related as the protection remains even when atrial pacing is used to maintain the heart rate.
- The administration of atropine increases the likelihood of developing VF.

Vagal tone can be measured by variability in the heart rate (RR interval) or blood pressure rise induced by the pressor agent phenylephrine. Heart rate variability is considered a measure of tonic vagal activity whereas the phenylephrine method is considered a measure of magnitude of the vagal reflex in response to stimulus. A reduced vagal tone has been found postinfarction in humans, which returns to normal over a 3–6-month period. There is no relationship between vagal tone and ejection fraction and the origin of reduced vagal tone postinfarction appears to be due to afferent stimulation in response to necrotic tissue and impaired cardiac contractile geometry. This reduced vagal tone has also been shown to be predictive of mortality and inductility of arrhythmia at electrophysiological study (EPS).

PROARRHYTHMIC EFFECTS OF ANTIARRHYTHMIC DRUGS[11,12]

Concomitant proarrhythmia with the use of antiarrhythmic drugs is increasingly recognised. The 'quinidine syncope' due to VF and polymorphic VT at therapeutic concentrations was also seen with disopyramide. The Cardiac Arrhythmia Suppression Trial (CAST) clearly defined the magnitude of this deleterious side-effect in drugs that were previously perceived to be of benefit.[13] This study, which involved flecainide, encainide and moricizine (a class IA drug), was terminated early because of adverse outcome in the flecainide and encainide groups (relative risk of arrhythmic death or non-fatal cardiac arrest of 3.6, 95% confidence interval (CI) 1.7–8.5). Proarrhythmia is reported between 5.9% and 15.8% depending on agent, clinical setting and definition of proarrhythmia, and now considered ubiquitous with all antiarrhythmic drugs.

Proarrhythmia has been defined as an increase in frequency of ventricular ectopic beat (VEB) or aggravation of the target arrhythmia on Holter monitor or exercise test. Manifestations of proarrhythmia not only include VEB, monomorphic and polymorphic VT and VF, but also bradyarrhythmias and Afl with 1:1 AV conduction. Most proarrhythmic events occur soon after starting the drug, but late arrhythmias are also a significant problem.

Proarrhythmia appears to be correlated with the degree of drug-induced QT prolongation or characteristics of sodium channel blockade. Sodium channel blocking agents with a long time constant for recovery of the sodium channel blockade cause more pronounced blockade, even at slow heart rates, slow conduction to a greater extent and are mostly proarrhythmic. Agents with a short time constant of sodium channel blockade, where sodium channel blockade is more pronounced at fast heart rates (e.g. class IB: lidocaine and mexiletine) are less proarrhythmic than drugs with long time constants (e.g. class IC: flecainide and propafenone). Class III drugs and quinidine proarrhythmia correlate with degree of QT prolongation.

The mechanism of drug proarrhythmia is probably via both slowing of conduction and abnormal automaticity. Paradoxically slowing conduction, which may block a re-entry circuit, may also create the very substrate needed for re-entry, unidirectional block and an excitable gap. The existence of a re-entrant circuit requires the circulating wave front of the impulse not to catch up with the refractory tissue behind the tail. Re-entry is more likely to occur with a shorter refractory period and reduced conduction velocity (Figure 18.4).[11]

Increasing conduction velocity is an ideal antiarrhythmic property but there are no antiarrhythmic drugs that accelerate conduction. However antiarrhythmic drugs readily slow conduction and the degree of conduction slowing and therefore proarrhythmic tendency correlates with the potency of antiarrhythmic properties.

Prolonging the refractory period is also an ideal antiarrhythmic property, which increases the likelihood of abolishing any excitable gap by ensuring the wave front of a re-entrant circuit meets refractory tissue. The potency of class IA and III antiarrhythmic agents is dependent on the prolongation of the refractory period. This property is also protective against proarrhythmia due to re-entry mechanism. The effect of class IB agents on shortening the refractory period will contribute to proarrhythmia by this mechanism in this class.

Surface mapping of the heart has been used to quantify proarrhythmic effect. The scale of potency of proarrhythmia has been found to be:

flecainide > propafenone > quinidine > disopyramide > procainamide > mexiletine > lidocaine > sotalol[11]

Amiodarone was not included in this study but presumably its proarrhythmic potential is similar to other class III agents and less than the class I agents.

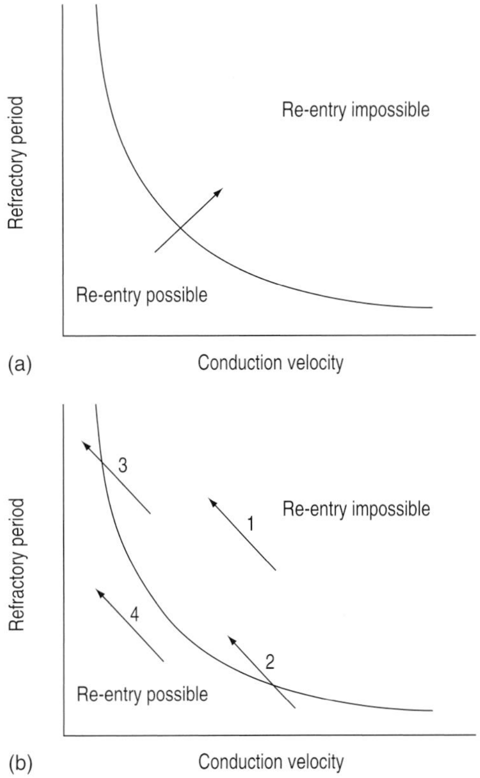

Figure 18.4 (a) Graph of refractory period of an excitable gap versus its conduction velocity around a theoretical re-entrant circuit. When conduction velocity is high enough so that refractory period of excitable gap exceeds circuit time, re-entry is impossible. Arrow demonstrates the action of an 'ideal' antiarrhythmic drug, which prolongs refractory period and increases conduction velocity. (b) With antiarrhythmic drugs that increase refractory period and slow conduction, the net effect of an antiarrhythmic drug may have no effect on proarrhythmia (arrows 1 and 4), decrease proarrhythmia (arrow 2) or increase proarrhythmia (arrow 3) depending on properties of a potential re-entrant circuit. (Adapted from Schwartz PJ, La Rovere MT, Vanoli E. Autonomic nervous system and sudden cardiac death. *Circulation* 1992; **85** (suppl. 1): 77–91 with permission.)

Antiarrhythmic drugs are effective at suppressing abnormal automaticity, with the exception of triggered automaticity due to EAD. Class IA, class III and many non-antiarrhythmic drugs can produce proarrhythmia via EAD. These drugs increase not only the frequency of EAD, but also the likelihood of them leading to triggered tachyarrhythmias. Slowing repolarisation, which leads to QT prolongation and slower heart rate, is central to this increased frequency and sensitivity to EAD. EAD manifests as prominent and bizarre T-U waves on the ECG and, if triggered activity results, VEB and ventricular tachyarrhythmias may occur. Torsade de pointes is the classical resulting arrhythmia, although less classical

Table 18.4 Factors facilitating antiarrhythmic drug proarrhythmia

Toxic blood levels due to excessive dose or reduced clearance from old age, heart failure, renal disease or hepatic disease
Severe left ventricular dysfunction. Ejection fraction less than 35%
Pre-existing arrhythmia or arrhythmia substrate
Digoxin therapy
Hypokalaemia or hypomagnesaemia
Bradycardia
Combinations of antiarrhythmic drugs and concomitant drugs with similar toxicity

(Adapted from Campbell TJ. Proarrhythmic actions of antiarrhythmic drugs: a review. *Aust NZ J Med* 1990; **20**: 275–82, with permission.)

polymorphic VT and VF result. Risk of proarrhythmia via this mechanism correlates with the degree of QT prolongation.

All antiarrhythmic drugs are capable of producing bradyarrhythmias via decreasing normal automaticity and slowing conduction. Digoxin can be proarrhythmic via the production of triggered activity due to DAD.

Antiarrhythmic drug proarrhythmia is facilitated by several factors, which are frequently found in patients on antiarrhythmic drugs or with heart disease (Table 18.4).

MANAGEMENT OF THE PATIENT WITH A CARDIAC ARRHYTHMIA

HISTORY AND PHYSICAL EXAMINATION

A careful history is important. Specific questions should confirm or exclude palpitations, syncope, chest pain, shortness of breath, ischaemic heart disease (especially previous myocardial infarction), congestive cardiac failure, valvular heart disease, thyrotoxicosis and diuretic therapy without adequate potassium supplements. A family history is helpful for arrhythmias associated with inherited disorders (e.g. LQTS and hypertrophic obstructive cardiomyopathy). The physical examination looks for underlying structural heart disease and signs to assist diagnosis, and assesses haemodynamic consequences of the arrhythmia.

VAGAL MANOEUVRES

Vagal manoeuvres may be undertaken during examination. These reflexly increase vagal tone, thereby prolonging AV node conduction and refractoriness. The effect may be:

- transient slowing of sinus tachycardia as SA nodal discharge rate is slowed
- termination of AV nodal re-entry tachycardia (AVNRT) and AV re-entry tachycardias (AVRT)
- unmasking (but not reversion) of atrial tachycardia, flutter (Figure 18.5) and fibrillation.

VT is not affected. Carotid sinus massage is most commonly used. Valsalva manoeuvre or iced water to the face may be useful. Eyeball pressure should be avoided as eye damage may result. Carotid sinus massage is performed with the patient supine, with head extended and turned away from the side to be massaged. After auscultation to exclude carotid bruits, the carotid bifurcation is gently palpated by placing two fingers anterior to the sternocleidomastoid muscle, just below the angle of the jaw. Massage is applied one side at a time, and never both sides simultaneously. It is contraindicated in those with known or suspected cerebrovascular disease.

INVESTIGATIONS

A 12-lead ECG should be recorded with a longer rhythm strip (usually lead II or V_1). If P-waves are not visible, atrial activity may be recorded using an oesophageal electrode or pacing lead, or via a central venous catheter or the right atrial injectate port of a pulmonary artery catheter, using 20% saline and a bedside monitor.[14]

Holter monitoring requires prolonged (usually 24–72 h), non-invasive, ambulatory ECG monitoring, sometimes combined with exercise testing.

EPS, which involves invasive electrophysiological testing with programmed electrical stimulation, attempts to reproduce the spontaneously occurring arrhythmia.[15,16] EPS is not clearly superior to Holter monitoring in evaluating drug treatment for ventricular arrhythmias.

Other investigative techniques being studied include signal-averaged ECG, heart rate variability and electrical alternans measurement.[10,17]

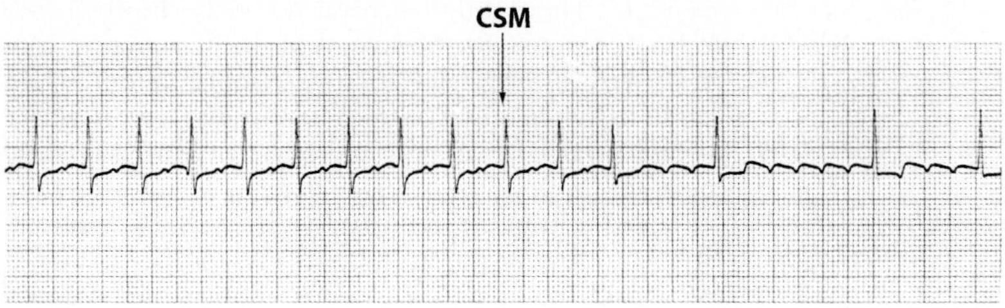

Figure 18.5 Atrial flutter with 2:1 atrioventricular (AV) block. Carotid sinus massage (CSM) increases AV block to 4:1 then 6:1.

MANAGEMENT OF SPECIFIC ARRHYTHMIAS

Treatment has two aspects: acute termination of the arrhythmia and long-term prophylaxis. The decision whether to treat depends on the rhythm diagnosis, haemodynamic consequences, aetiology of the arrhythmia and the prognosis (e.g. risks of sudden death or long-term complications).

ECTOPIC BEATS

These are premature impulses originating from the atria, AV junction or ventricles. The coupling interval (time between the ectopic and the preceding beat) is shorter than the cycle duration of the dominant rhythm.

PREMATURE VENTRICULAR ECTOPIC BEATS

These are also known as ventricular premature beats and ventricular premature complexes. The ventricle is not normally activated via the rapidly conducting bundle branches, and a wide QRS complex results from slow ventricular conduction.

ECG

There is no preceding P-wave.

- Premature complexes occur before the next expected QRS
- QRS is wide (> 120 ms)
- T-wave of opposite polarity to the QRS (Figure 18.6)
- VEB is not conducted retrogradely to the SA node.
- SA node is therefore not reset, and there is temporary AV dissociation with a full compensatory pause; the interval between the normal QRS complexes on either side of the VEB will usually be twice that of the dominant sinus rhythm.

Occasionally VEB may not produce any pause, and are said to be interpolated (see Figure 18.6). Interpolated VEB occur when the background sinus rhythm is slow. The retrograde conduction into the AV node renders it partially refractory to the next impulse and its conduction through the AV node is slowed and the PR interval is prolonged. A VEB following each sinus beat is ventricular bigeminy (Figure 18.7). Ventricular trigeminy refers to recurring sequences of a VEB followed by two sinus beats. Two VEB in succession are a couplet (Figure 18.8), and three, a triplet.

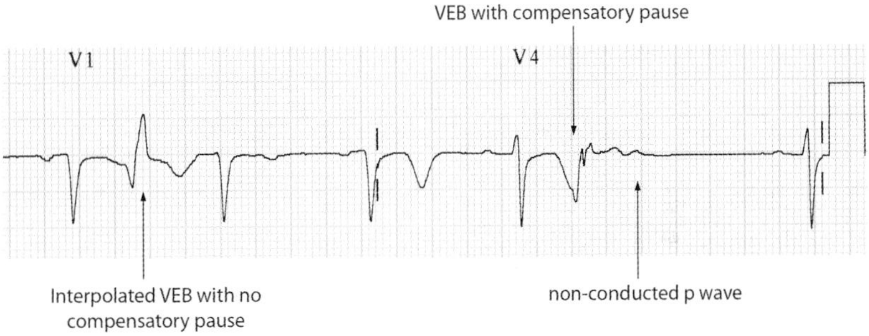

Figure 18.6 Sinus rhythm with an interpolated ventricular ectopic beat (VEB) without a compensatory pause and a VEB with a following non-conducted P-wave, resulting in a compensatory pause.

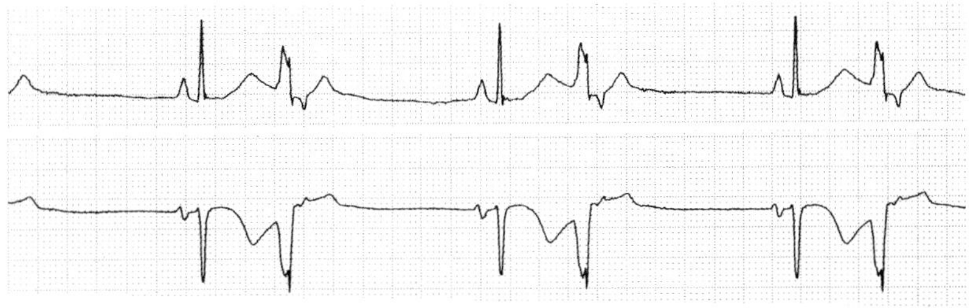

Figure 18.7 Sinus rhythm with ventricular bigeminy.

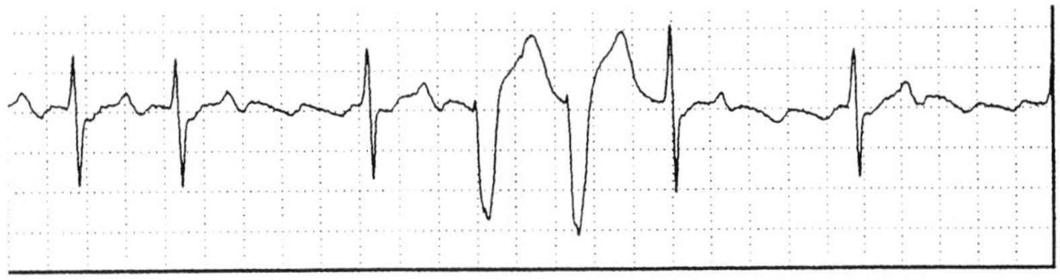

Figure 18.8 Atrial fibrillation with a ventricular couplet.

CLINICAL

Even when frequent, complex, or in short runs of non-sustained VT, VEB are not associated with risk of sudden death in asymptomatic healthy adults.[18] However, there is increased risk of cardiovascular death with:

- exercise-induced VEB: risk of death 2.53 (95% CI 1.65–3.88)[19]
- AMI and VEB. Frequent and complex VEB often precede VF or sustained VT and are a marker of risk of subsequent SCD

Apart from ischaemic heart disease, VEB may be associated with cardiomyopathy, valvular disease, myocarditis and non-cardiac precipitating factors (e.g. electrolyte and acid–base disturbances, hypoxia and drugs such as digoxin).

TREATMENT

Drug treatment of VEB is rarely indicated and may be dangerous.

- Correct potassium and magnesium.
- Severely symptomatic patients with frequent complex VEB may benefit from judicious β-blockade.
- The underlying cause of VEB is often more clinically relevant than the arrhythmia. Following myocardial infarction, β-adrenergic blockers, which are indicated for long-term benefit, will also likely suppress VEB.
- Prophylactic lidocaine following AMI will increase total mortality and has been abandoned.[20,21]
- Attempts at long-term VEB suppression with class IC agents (flecainide and encainide), even if successful, increase mortality.[13]

SUPRAVENTRICULAR TACHYCARDIAS[22,23] (TABLE 18.5)

Supraventricular tachycardias (SVT) are any tachycardias that require atrial or AV nodal tissue for their initiation and maintenance.

- SVT are usually conducted rapidly through the bundle branches so that QRS complexes are narrow.
- All narrow-complex tachycardias are SVT and wide-complex tachycardias are usually ventricular.
- However, SVT may be wide-complex in the setting of bundle branch block (BBB) and pre-excitation.

A clinically useful classification divides SVT into AV node-dependent and AV node-independent.

Distinguishing between AV node-dependent and independent SVTs can be difficult. Vagal manoeuvres or drugs that prolong AV nodal refractoriness (e.g. adenosine) may assist in diagnosis:

- Temporary AV block with unchanged atrial rate indicates AV node independence.
- Slowing or reversion of the tachycardia diagnoses AV dependence.

Table 18.5 Classification of supraventricular tachycardias

Atrioventricular (AV) node-dependent
AV nodal re-entry tachycardia: re-entry within the AV node
AV re-entry tachycardia: re-entry includes accessory pathway between atria and ventricles
Accelerated idionodal rhythm: increased automaticity of AV nodea
AV node-independent
Atrial flutter: re-entry confined to atria
Atrial fibrillation: multiple re-entry circuits confined to atria
Unifocal atrial tachycardia: usually due to increased automaticity
Multifocal atrial tachycardia: increased automaticity or triggered activity
Others: sinus node re-entry tachycardia

AV NODE-DEPENDENT SVT

In these SVT, sometimes referred to as junctional tachycardias, the re-entry circuit or ectopic focus involves the AV node or junction. Blocking the AV node with drugs such as adenosine or vagal manoeuvres will terminate these SVT.

AV NODE-INDEPENDENT SVT

Also referred to as atrial tachycardias, the atrial tissue only is required for the initiation and maintenance of the tachycardia. Blocking the AV node will not terminate these SVT; it will merely slow ventricular rate.

AV NODAL RE-ENTRY TACHYCARDIA (AVNRT) (FIGURE 18.9)

Re-entry tachycardia is confined to the AV node. Antegrade conduction to the ventricles usually occurs over the slow pathway and retrograde conduction over the fast pathway.

ECG

There is regular narrow-complex tachycardia (140–220 beats/min) with abrupt onset and termination. P-waves are not usually observed as they are buried in the QRS complexes (Figure 18.10).

CLINICAL

AVNRT is a common arrhythmia that is not usually associated with structural heart disease. The major symptom is palpitations.

TREATMENT

Vagal manoeuvres slow conduction through the AV node and may 'break' the tachycardia. If carotid sinus massage fails, adenosine is the drug of choice and nearly all AVNRT will revert with adenosine.[24,25] Verapamil has been used in the past, but causes hypotension, which may be prolonged if cardiac function is depressed or patients are receiving β-adrenergic blockers. Sotalol,

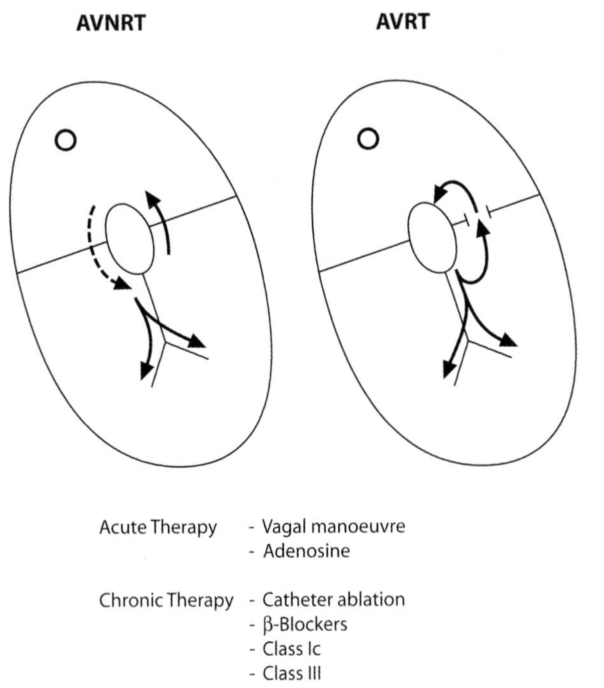

Figure 18.9 Arteriovenous nodal re-entry tachycardia (AVNRT) has both pathways in the AV node. The conduction occurs over the slow pathway and retrogradely over the fast pathway. AV re-entry tachycardia (AVRT) involves antegrade conduction through the AV node and retrograde conduction through an accessory pathway.

amiodarone and flecainide may also be effective but are rarely used. Rapid atrial pacing will usually terminate AVNRT but is rarely needed.

Cardioversion is occasionally necessary when drugs are ineffective or when severe haemodynamic instability is present.

PREVENTION

Troublesome recurring episodes of AVNRT can be cured by radiofrequency ablation, using a transvenous catheter to interrupt the re-entrant circuit permanently.[26]

AV RE-ENTRY TACHYCARDIA (SEE FIGURE 18.9)

The re-entry pathway consists of the AV node and an accessory pathway, which bypasses the AV node. The accessory pathway may be evident during sinus rhythm, with the ECG showing pre-excitation: short PR interval, delta wave and widening of the QRS (see WPW, below, under pre-excitation syndrome). However, in 25% of cases, the accessory pathway conducts only retrogradely from ventricle to atria and the ECG pre-excitation will be concealed in sinus rhythm. Orthodromic AVRT, with antegrade nodal and retrograde accessory pathway circuit, is the most common regular SVT in patients with accessory pathway.

ECG

The ECG is similar to AVNRT. The length of the re-entry circuit is however greater, and the accessory AV pathway is some distance from the AV node. It therefore takes longer for the impulse to be conducted backwards to the atria, and so the retrograde P-wave usually occurs after the QRS, sometimes at some distance, and is inverted in leads II, III and aVF (Figure 18.11 and 18.12).

CLINICAL

AVRT is similar to AVNRT, although antegrade conduction over the accessory pathway may be very rapid with WPW, if AF occurs.

TREATMENT[24,25]

Acute treatment is identical to AVNRT, but verapamil should be avoided in WPW syndrome, as it may block the AV node, facilitating very rapid conduction to the ventricles via the accessory pathway.[27]

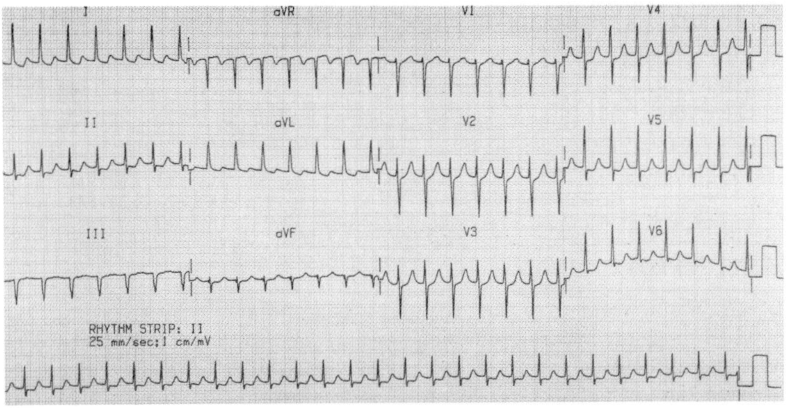

Figure 18.10 Arteriovenous nodal re-entry tachycardia (AVNRT). Narrow QRS tachycardia at 160 beats/min. P-waves are not apparent and are buried in the QRS complex.

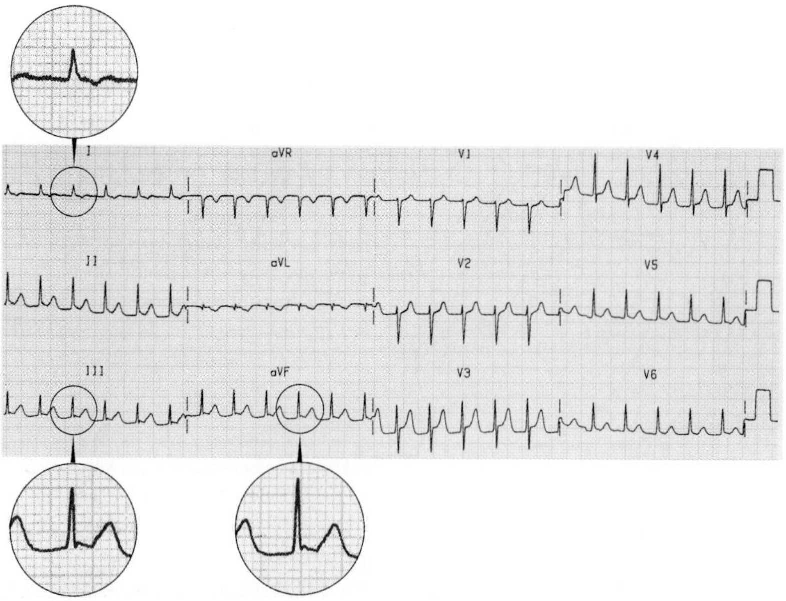

Figure 18.11 Arteriovenous re-entry tachycardia (AVRT). Narrow QRS tachycardia at 135 beats/min. Inverted P-wave in leads I, II, III and aVF just following the QRS complex.

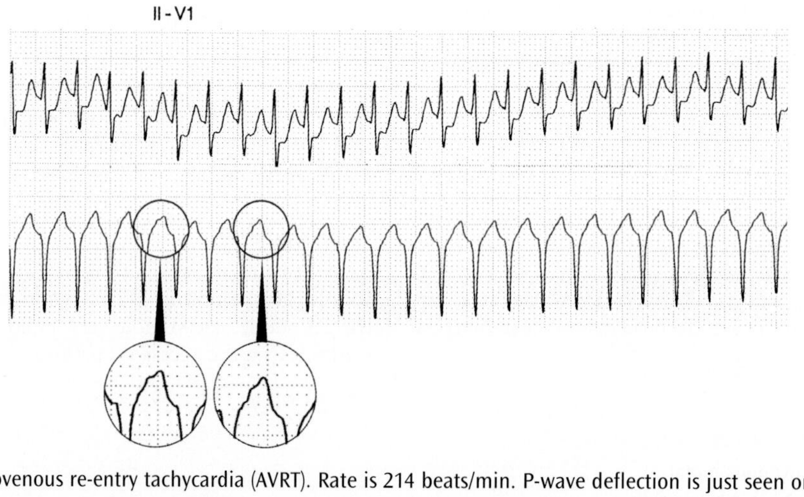

Figure 18.12 Arteriovenous re-entry tachycardia (AVRT). Rate is 214 beats/min. P-wave deflection is just seen on the upslope of the T-wave in lead V_1.

PREVENTION

Drugs such as sotalol and flecainide may prevent recurrence of the tachycardia. Radiofrequency ablation of the accessory pathway is usually curative.[26]

ACCELERATED IDIONODAL RHYTHM

Increased automaticity of the AV junction (above the inherent discharge rate of 40–60 beats/min) is the usual cause of this arrhythmia. The often-used term 'non-paroxysmal AV junctional tachycardia' is cumbersome and misleading: junctional rate is commonly 60–100 beats/min, not strictly a tachycardia. AV dissociation is often present, but there may be synchronisation of the two pacemakers – so-called isorhythmic dissociation.

ECG

There are narrow complexes on the ECG at a regular rate (60–130 beats/min) (Figure 18.13), often with independent atrial activity. With isorhythmic dissociation, P-wave is either fixed relative to the QRS complex (usually just after) or oscillates to and fro across the QRS in a rhythmical manner.

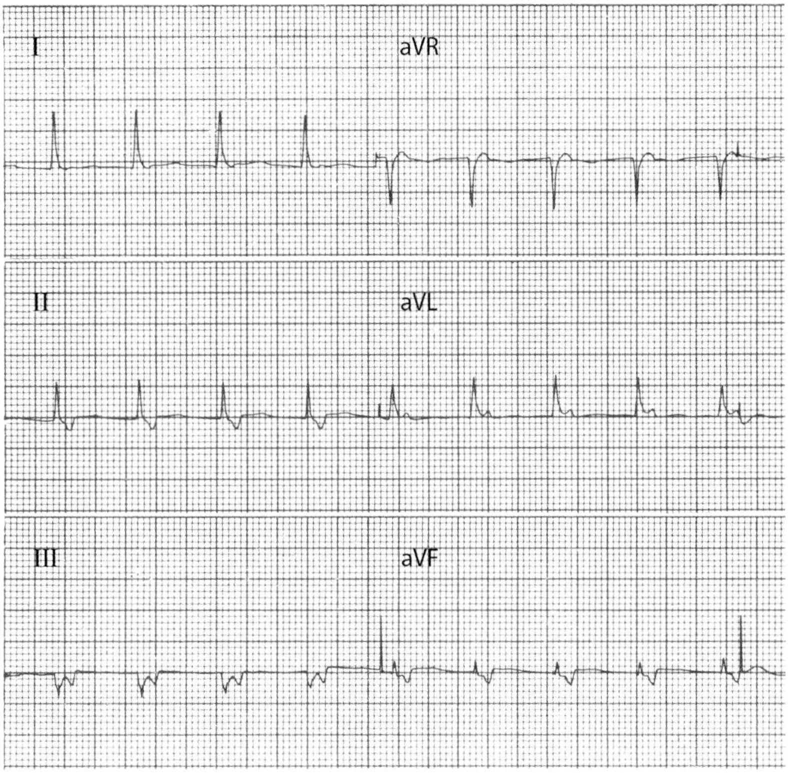

Figure 18.13 Accelerated idionodal rhythm: 105 beats/min. Inverted P-wave is immediately following the QRS complex in leads II, III and aVF.

CLINICAL

It may be observed in normal persons, but is often associated with structural heart disease, especially following inferior myocardial infarction. Digoxin intoxication is another important cause.

TREATMENT

In most cases, the rhythm is transient and well tolerated, and no treatment is required. Treatment is otherwise directed towards the underlying cause.

UNIFOCAL ATRIAL TACHYCARDIA

This is sometimes called ectopic atrial tachycardia to distinguish it from the atrial tachycardias (referring collectively to unifocal atrial tachycardia, Afl and AF). However, it is inappropriate to call atrial tachycardia paroxysmal atrial tachycardia. Paroxysmal, by definition, indicates an abrupt onset and termination, which applies less commonly to unifocal atrial tachycardia. Vagal manoeuvres will not terminate this arrhythmia, but AV block may be induced, or increased if already present.

ECG

P-wave morphology is abnormal but monomorphic. Atrial rate is often 130–160 beats/min, and may occasionally exceed 200 beats/min. Atrial rate distinguishes unifocal atrial tachycardia from atrial flutter (Afl), with Afl greater than 250 beats/min. The QRS complexes will usually be narrow (Figure 18.14). AV block is common (Figure 18.15).

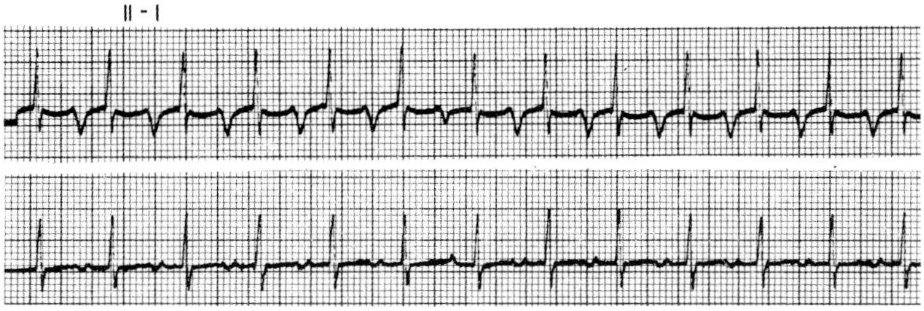

Figure 18.14 Unifocal atrial tachycardia with 1:1 arteriovenous conduction; rate is 140 beats/min. Large, inverted P-waves are seen in lead II.

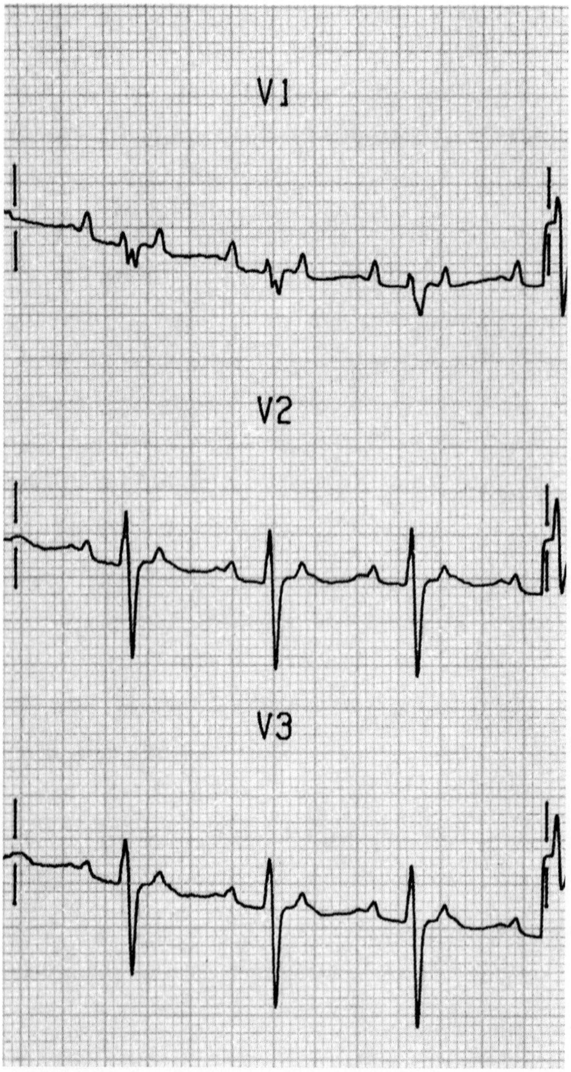

Figure 18.15 Unifocal atrial tachycardia with 2:1 arteriovenous conduction. Atrial rate is 170 beats/min.

CLINICAL

Digitalis intoxication is the most common cause, especially when AV block is present. Other causes include myocardial infarction, chronic lung disease and metabolic disturbances.

TREATMENT[25]

If applicable, digitalis is stopped and the toxicity treated. Otherwise digoxin may be used to control the ventricular rate. β-Adrenergic blockers or amiodarone are alternatives. Rapid atrial pacing may be ineffective if the arrhythmia is due to increased automaticity, although it may increase AV block, thereby slowing ventricular rate. Synchronised DC shock may be necessary, but is avoided if digitalis intoxication is suspected.

MULTIFOCAL ATRIAL TACHYCARDIA[28]

Multifocal atrial tachycardia (MAT) is defined as an atrial rhythm, with a rate greater than 100 beats/min, with organised, discrete non-sinus P-waves having at least three different forms in the same ECG trace. The baseline between P-waves is isoelectric, and the PP, PR and RR intervals are irregular. This is an uncommon arrhythmia, also known as chaotic or mixed atrial tachycardia.

ECG

There are irregular atrial rates, usually 100–130 beats/min, with varying P-wave morphology (at least three different P-wave morphologies and varying PR interval) and some degree of AV block (Figure 18.16). Most P-waves are conducted to the ventricles, usually with narrow QRS complexes.

CLINICAL

MAT is often misdiagnosed and inappropriately treated as AF. This rhythm occurs most commonly in critically ill elderly patients with chronic lung disease and often cor pulmonale, and is associated with a very high mortality from underlying disease. Theophylline has been implicated as a precipitating cause, and rarely digoxin.

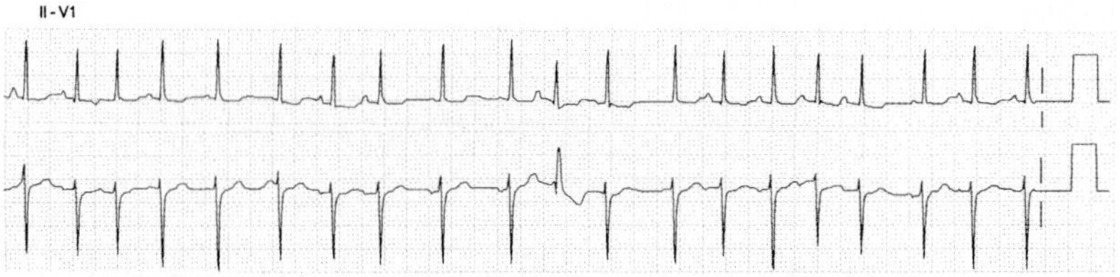

Figure 18.16 Multifocal atrial tachycardia with the rate about 130 beats/min. There is varying P-wave morphology and PR intervals. Note the wide complex preceded by a P-wave. The aberrant intraventricular conduction is related to the long–short cycle length sequence.

TREATMENT

Treatment should correct the underlying cause (e.g. treatment of cardiorespiratory failure, electrolyte and acid–base abnormalities and theophylline toxicity). Spontaneous reversion is common, and few patients require antiarrhythmic therapy. Magnesium is the drug of choice for acute control.[29] β-Blockers are probably more effective than diltiazem, but because of the common association of MAT with obstructive lung disease have limited utility.[30] Digoxin and cardioversion are ineffective, which highlights the need to differentiate MAT from AF. Longer-term control is best achieved with diltiazem in patients with good left ventricular (LV) function and amiodarone in those without.

ATRIAL FLUTTER[31]

Atrial rate during classical Afl is 250–350 beats/min, and in most cases, close to 300 beats/min. Afl is due to a single re-entry circuit lying within the right atrium and the wave of depolarisation in most patients is anticlockwise. If the right atrium is significantly enlarged the rate may be considerably slower. Studies in patients who had recently undergone cardiac surgery subdivided Afl into type I and II on the basis of rate and typical responses to atrial pacing.

Type I flutter was slower – rate 240–320 beats/min – and was readily entrained with overdrive pacing. Type II flutter was faster than type I, with rates of 340–430 beats/min. Type II flutter could not be entrained or terminated by pacing. Type II is thought to arise from a circus pathway with a very short excitable gap.

ECG

Afl waves (characteristic sawtooth appearance with no isoelectric baseline) are best seen in V_1 (Figure 18.17) or aVF, but leads II and III may also be useful. The flutter waves are usually negative in aVF. Rapid QRS waves may obscure typical flutter waves, and vagal manoeuvres may unmask them (see Figure 18.5). AV conduction block (usually 2:1) is usually present, so that alternate flutter waves are conducted to the ventricles, with a ventricular rate close to 150 beats/min. Frequently flutter waves are not obvious and a ventricular rate of 150 beats/min leads to the presumption of Afl (Figure 18.18). Type II Afl results in greater atrial and ventricular rates (Figure 18.19). Treatment with drugs that affect AV node conduction may lead to higher degrees of AV block (Figure 18.20) and/or variable AV block with irregular QRS duration. Rarely, Afl with 1:1 conduction occurs. This is usually associated with sympathetic overactivity or class I antiarrhythmic drugs (which slow atrial discharge rate to 200 beats/min, thereby allowing each atrial impulse to be conducted) (Figure 18.21). QRS complexes are usually narrow, as conduction through the bundle branches is normal.

CLINICAL

AFL is less common than AF. It may occur in ischaemic heart disease, cardiomyopathy, rheumatic heart disease and thyrotoxicosis, and after cardiac surgery.

TREATMENT[25]

No drug will reliably terminate Afl, although ibutillide and dofetilide have been shown to be most likely to result in

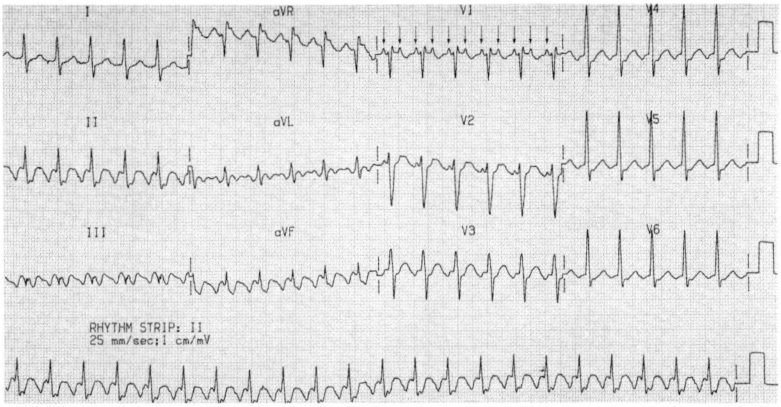

Figure 18.17 Atrial flutter with 2:1 arteriovenous conduction. Atrial rate is 270 beats/min (arrows V_1) and ventricular 135 beats/min. Characteristic 'sawtooth' inverted flutter waves are evident in leads II, III and aVF.

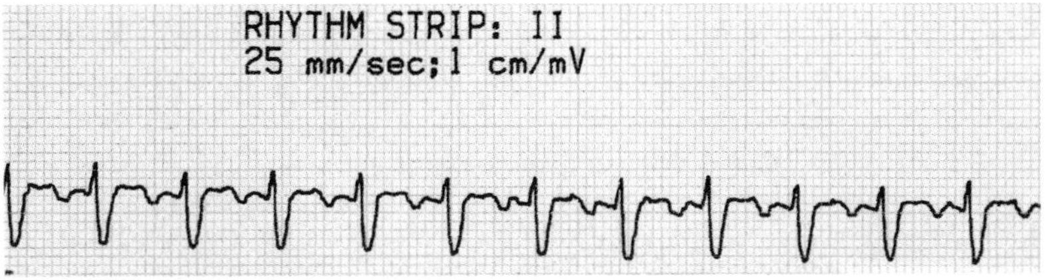

Figure 18.18 Atrial flutter with 2:1 arteriovenous (AV) conduction. Inverted flutter waves are difficult to differentiate from T-waves. Rate of 144 beats/min confirms atrial flutter with 2:1 AV conduction.

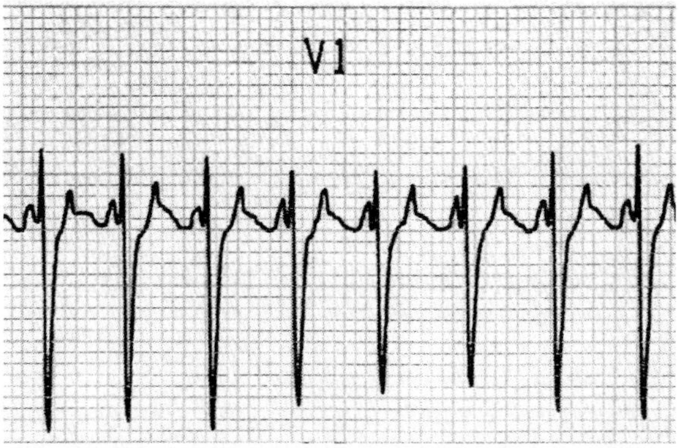

Figure 18.19 Atrial flutter with 2:1 arteriovenous conduction. Type II atrial flutter is confirmed by the rapid atrial rate of 380 beats/min.

pharmacological reversion. Attempts at slowing ventricular rate by drugs that will increase the degree of AV block are worthwhile in the first instance. Drugs such as digoxin, diltiazem, β-adrenergic blockers, sotalol and amiodarone may be tried; the choice depends on LV function. Flecainide and procainamide may occasionally be effective at terminating Afl. However, class IA and IC drugs may lead to 1:1 AV conduction. Class I drugs should probably be avoided unless ventricular response has been slowed with calcium channel or β-adrenergic blocking drugs.

Synchronised DC cardioversion, often with low energies (25–50 J), is a reliable treatment option. Rapid atrial pacing faster than the flutter rate will terminate classical or type I Afl in most patients.

Anticoagulation guidelines are the same as that for AF, although there are less supporting data.

PREVENTION

Prevention is difficult. Drugs used include sotalol and amiodarone at low doses. Class IC agents (e.g. flecainide) may be used in patients without significant structural heart disease. Increasingly recurrent or refractory Afl may be cured by radiofrequency ablation to create a linear lesion between the inferior tricuspid annulus and the eustachian ridge at the anterior margin of the inferior vena cava to interrupt the re-entry circuit.[26]

ATRIAL FIBRILLATION[32]

AF is the most common arrhythmia requiring treatment and/or hospital admission. The incidence increases with age: 5% of individuals over 70 years have this arrhythmia. There is also an age-independent increase in frequency due to increase in obesity and obstructive sleep apnoea. LV dyfunction increases risk of AF (4.5-fold in men and 5.9 in women) with atrial stretch and fibrosis causing electrical and atrial ionic channel remodelling.

AF is common in:

- congestive cardiac failure (40%)
- coronary artery bypass grafting (25–50%)
- critically ill patients (15%)

Idiopathic or lone AF (i.e. with no structural heart disease or precipitating factor) in someone aged under 60 years has an excellent prognosis; however, AF developing after cardiac surgery, for instance, is associated with increased stroke, life-threatening arrhythmias and longer hospital stays.

ECG

Atrial activity is chaotic with rapid (350–600 beats/min) and irregular depolarisations varying in amplitude and

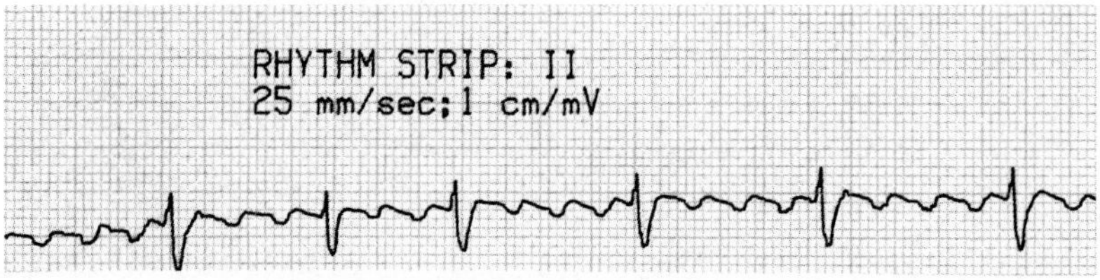

Figure 18.20 Atrial flutter varying between 3:1 and 4:1 arteriovenous (AV) conduction due to drug effect slowing AV node conduction.

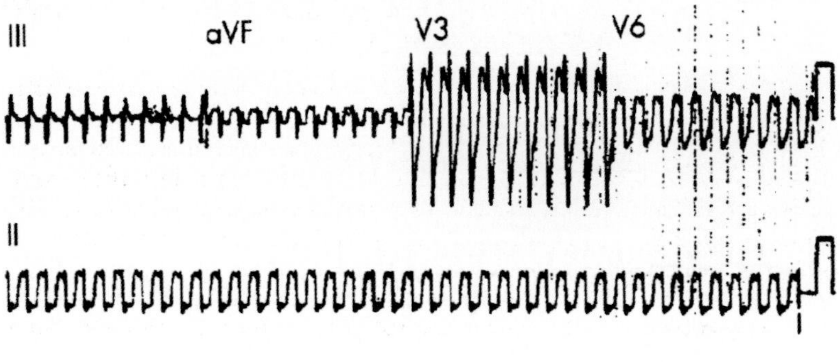

Figure 18.21 Atrial flutter with 1:1 conduction with a rate of 240 beats/min. Up-sloping of ST segment is easily mistaken as part of the QRS complex, giving the appearance of a broad QRS tachycardia in some leads. Lead III shows true narrow width of QRS complex.

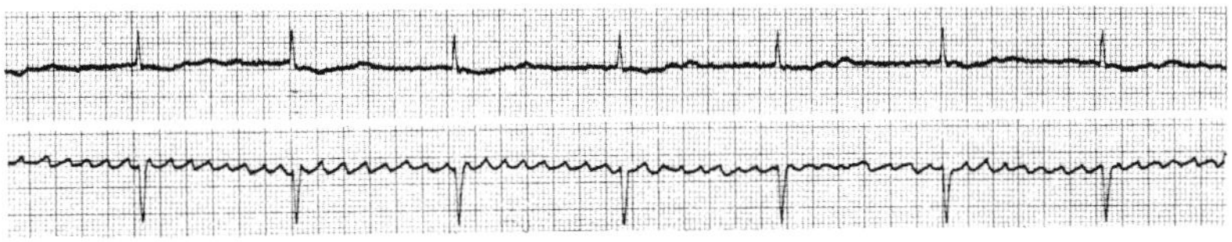
Figure 18.22 Atrial fibrillation. Irregular fibrillation waves with varying amplitude and morphology.

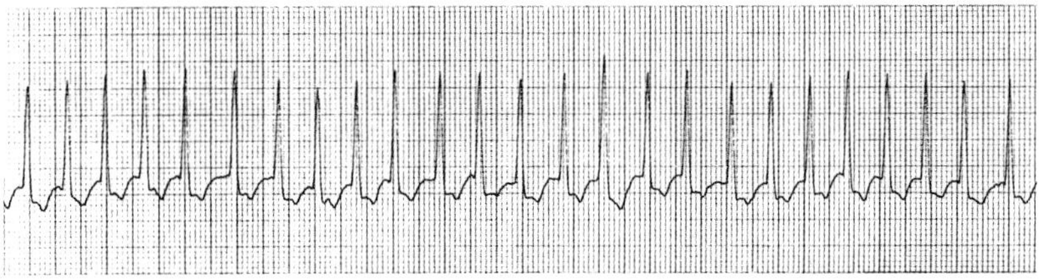
Figure 18.23 Atrial fibrillation with rapid ventricular rate. Ventricular irregularity and fibrillation waves are less evident when the rate is rapid.

morphology (fibrillation waves). Ventricular response is irregularly irregular (Figure 18.22). Most atrial impulses are not conducted to the ventricles, resulting in an untreated ventricular rate of 100–180 beats/min. QRS complexes will usually be narrow. When the ventricular rate is very rapid or very slow, ventricular irregularity may be missed (Figure 18.23).

CLINICAL

AF is more common in patients with underlying heart disease (particularly those with a dilated left atrium) and abnormal atrial electrophysiology. Causes include ischaemic and valvular heart disease, pericarditis, hypertension, cardiac failure, thyrotoxicosis and alcohol abuse. AF may also occur after cardiac surgery and thoracotomy. AF can be chronic, or intermittent with paroxysmal attacks. Chronic AF has a poorer prognosis.

AF is associated with:

- adverse haemodynamic effects. Rapid ventricular rate and loss of atrial systole may increase pulmonary capillary wedge pressure, while stroke volume and cardiac output decline
- systemic embolism and stroke
- tachycardiomyopathy. Reversible global cardiomyopathy secondary to rapid heart rate. Assessing LV function with echocardiogram before and after AV node ablation for AF refractory to medical therapy suggests that 10% of patients with AF have AF-induced tachycardiomyopathy[33]

TREATMENT[25,34,35]

The goals of treatment include ventricular rate control, anticoagulation where appropriate and conversion to sinus rhythm. There is increasing evidence available on the 'rate versus rhythm' control debate. Results from several recent major studies have challenged the previous belief that achievement of sinus rhythm is important in the long term (Table 18.6). When comparing control of ventricular rate versus reversion to sinus rhythm no clear survival benefit is apparent. However composite end-points of death, stroke and recurrent hospilisation favour rate control only.[36–39]

The possible reasons why rhythm control has not been shown to be superior include:

- Trials have included predominantly elderly high-risk patients.
- Sinus rhythm is difficult to achieve (39–63%).
- Rate control strategies can result in sinus rhythm in up to 35% of patients.
- Underlying heart disease that initiates the AF persists.
- There may be antiarrhythmic drug side-effects.
- Anticoagulation is still required even if rhythm control is successful.

However rhythm control (if possible) appears superior in patients with LV dysfunction, with both amiodarone and dofetilide reducing mortality when sinus rhythm is achieved.[40,41] The paucity of data in younger patients (less than 60 years) favours initial attempts at rhythm control, particularly in those with structurally normal hearts, in the hope that progressive atrial electrical and anatomical remodelling is prevented.

RECENT ONSET OR PAROXYSMAL AF

VENTRICULAR RATE CONTROL

The urgency of ventricular rate control depends on the clinical situation and spontaneous reversion of AF is common. Treatment may not be necessary, and a reasonable strategy is based on clinical status:

- Haemodynamically unstable with rapid ventricular rate requires immediate synchronised DC shock (in addition to drug therapy) to control rate urgently.
- Haemodynamically stable, symptomatic with depressed LV function: semiurgent synchronised DC shock or drug therapy, digoxin or amiodarone to control ventricular rate.
- Haemodynamically stable, symptomatic, normal LV function: control of ventricular response with

Table 18.6 Atrial fibrillation rate versus rhythm control debate

Study	Number	Follow-up (months)	Age (years)	Amiodarone use (%)	Sinus rhythm (%)	Warfarin (%)	Thromboembolism (%)	Mortality (%)
AFFIRM[36]		42						
Rate control	2027		70 ± 9	10	35	85	6	21
Rhythm control	2033		70 ± 9	70	63	70	7.5	24
RACE[37]		27						
Rate control	256		68 ± 9	–	10	96	5.5	17
Rhythm control	266		68 ± 9	–	39	86	7.9	13
STAF[38]		22						
Rate control	100		65 ± 9	0	0	–	0.6	5
Rhythm control	100		66 ± 9	0	–	–	3.1	2.5
PIAF[39]		12						
Rate control	125		61 ± 9	0	10	100	–	1.6
Rhythm control	125		60 ± 10	100	56	100	–	1.6

AFFIRM, Atrial Fibrillation Follow-up Investigation of Rhythm Management; RACE, Rate Control versus Electrical Cardioversion of persistent atrial fibrillation; STAF, Strategies of Treatment of Atrial Fibrillation; PIAF, Pharmacological Intervention in Atrial Fibrillation.

β-adrenergic blockers, diltiazem, digoxin (poor control with exertion and settings with increased sympathetic tone), magnesium (short-term), amiodarone or sotalol.

- Haemodynamically stable, with no structural heart disease and minimal or no symptoms: no immediate treatment is an option. Most cases will revert spontaneously within 24 h. Single-dose flecainide for paroxymal AF has been recommended (contra-indicated in patients with structural heart disease).[42]

Ideal rate control can be defined as a resting heart rate of 80 beats/min, peak rate of 110 beats/min with 6-minute walk and an average of 100 beats/min.

CONVERSION TO SINUS RHYTHM

Antiarrhythmic drugs or DC shock cardioversion can be used. The likelihood of short- and long-term success depends on the clinical situation. Conversion to sinus rhythm is more important in young patients and those with heart failure. Maintenance of sinus rhythm is problematic: sinus rhythm at 1 year is 60% with amiodarone and 40% with sotalol, and associated with significant drug cardiac and extracardiac toxicities. The risk of stroke and need for antithrombotic therapy due to frequent AF recurrences, which may be asymptomatic, remain. Achieving sinus rhythm (especially greater than 60 years) is less important than previously thought.[36]

DC SHOCK CARDIOVERSION

DC shock cardioversion is indicated either before 24–48 h or after appropriate anticoagulation protocol. Combining DC shock with antiarrhythmic drugs to promote maintenance of sinus rhythm is favoured, especially if risk factors for relapse exist. Cardioversion is less likely to be successful if:

- AF has been present for over 1 year
- left atrial size is greater than 45 mm
- untreated conditions are present, e.g. thyrotoxicosis, valvular heart disease and heart failure

Critically ill patients who are septic, postoperative or on drugs such as catecholamines are likely to relapse.

ANTICOAGULATION AND CARDIOVERSION[43,44]

Loss of atrial contraction with AF is associated with stasis of blood flow and formation of blood clots in the left atrium, particularly the atrial appendage. Reversion to sinus rhythm and return of more effective atrial contraction may cause expulsion of any atrial clots and systemic emboli. Once AF has been present for more than 48 h – some authors stipulate 24 h – the risk of systemic emboli is significant and anticoagulation is required prior to DC shock cardioversion. The current recommended period of anticoagulation prior to DC shock cardioversion is 3 weeks. This 3-week period can be shortened to 1 day for heparin and 5 days for warfarin if the left atrium can be demonstrated free of clot using transoesophageal echocardiography. With this accelerated approach heparin dose should be titrated to an activated partial thromboplastin time 2–3 times control or warfarin to produce an international normalised ratio (INR) of 2.0–3.0. In many clinical situations such as recent surgery or other bleeding risks, anticoagulation is contraindicated and elective cardioversion should be delayed until recommended anticoagulation cover is safe. Following successful cardioversion to sinus rhythm the risk of systemic embolism continues as the propensity to form atrial clot remains due to atrial contractile stunning and anticoagulation should be continued for 4–6 weeks.

ANTIARRHYTHMIC DRUGS

The drugs used for ventricular rate control – digoxin, diltiazem and β-adrenergic blockers – are unlikely to result in pharmacological cardioversion.

Antiarrhythmic drugs that may cardiovert are unfortunately relatively ineffective and may possibly be dangerous. They are more effective at retaining sinus rhythm. About 50% will remain in sinus rhythm 1 year after cardioversion with drugs and 25% without drugs.

Quinidine is more effective than placebo, but increases mortality through proarrhythmia (generally class IA and IC antiarrhythmic drugs are contraindicated). Ibutilide and dofetilide are newer antiarrhythmic drugs with particular success at pharmacological cardioversion. Pretreatment with ibutilide increased DC shock cardioversion from 72% for placebo to 100%. In placebo failures, crossover to ibutilide resulted in a 100% success rate with subsequent cardioversion. Ibutilide also resulted in reduction in DC shock energy required from 228 ± 93 J to 166 ± 80 J. However, ibutilide was associated with a 3% incidence of sustained polymorphous VT.[45] Dofetilide appears to cardiovert AF and Afl pharmacologically in about a third of patients (intravenous (IV) better than oral, recent onset better than prolonged and Afl may be more responsive than AF). Dofetilide is far superior to placebo and sotalol, with similar recurrence rates to amiodarone.[46]

Other drugs currently used to promote onset of sinus rhythm and prevent AF relapse include amiodarone, sotalol, procainamide, flecainide and propafenone. Amiodarone was found to be superior in preventing AF recurrence with a recurrence rate of 35% compared to a recurrence rate of 63% for sotalol and propafenone.[47]

The factors dictating choice are:

- degree of LV depression: amiodarone has the least and flecainide the greatest
- risk of proarrhythmia: worse with flecainide and propafenone
- long term side-effect profile: amiodarone is the worst

When using amiodarone for prevention of AF recurrence there was an 18% incidence of adverse effects versus 11% for sotalol and propafenone.[47]

ATRIAL FIBRILLATION ABLATION THERAPY

Ablation techniques for AF have been continuously refined since the original Maze III surgical procedure which involved numerous atrial incisions to form a maze-like pattern of scarring, blocking propagation of arrhythmia. The ultility of this procedure was limited because it was surgical, with longer bypass times, postoperative bleeding and impaired atrial contractility. The magnitude of this original procedure was based on the belief that the entire atrium was involved in the initiation and maintenance of the fibrillatory conduction. This may be true for long-standing AF but paroxysmal AF appears to originate primarily at the junction of the left atrium and pulmonary veins. AF in 94% of patients is initiated by rapid discharges from one or more foci at or near the pulmonary vein orifices.[48] Atrial tissue in this area has heterogeneous electrophysiological properties and there is also clustering of vagal inputs, which creates substrate for rapid discharges that initiate microre-entrant circuits or 'rotors'. These high-frquency periodic rotors send spiral wave fronts of activation into surrounding atria. Localised ablation of a single dominant foci and rotor is inadequate as there are usually multiple foci.

There is renewed interest in surgical AF ablation therapy in conjunction with cardiac surgery. Complications have been reduced with energy (cryotherapy, radiofrequency) rather than incisions and the extent of lesions reduced. The minimum lesion set is now considered to be encirclement of pulmonary veins, linear lesion from the inferior pulmonary vein to mitral annulus and from the coronary sinus to the inferior vena cava.

Left atrial catheter (transatrial septum) AF ablation isolating all four pulmonary veins using radiofrquency is being heralded as the possible AF cure. Results are improving as all pulmonary veins are now isolated and the encircling lesion is clear of the pulmonary vein antrum (reducing pulmonary vein stenosis). Success rates of 81% (75–88%) free of AF and off drugs are reported. Success appears long-term as recurrence occurs early. A further 10–20% may become responsive to antiarrhythmic drugs which were previously ineffective. Repeating the procedure can increase success to > 90% with failure only in patients found to have extensive atrial scarring (predicting and excluding patients with this extensive atrial scarring is a major future challenge). Although not yet the universal cure the results are two- to threefold better than antiarrhythmic drugs alone.

Complication rates are also falling associated with:

- intracardiac echocardiography ensuring safer transeptal puncture and positioning of isolating lesions clear of the pulmonary vein antra
- higher levels of procedural anticoagulation
- strict limitations on radiofrequency energy output

Transient ischaemic attacks, strokes, tamponade/perforation and symptomatic pulmonary vein stenosis are all well below 1% respectively. Proarrhythmia resulting from re-entrant tachycardias from incomplete ablative lesions is more common. Some are advocating ablation as first-line treatment whereas most are selecting younger patients (less than 70 years) with paroxysmal AF for whom antiarrhythmic therapy has failed, left atrial diameter is less than 5 cm and ejection fraction is greater than 40%.[26] Head-to-head studies comparing ablation and antiarrhythmic drugs are appearing with suggested survival benefit, improved quality of life, reduced adverse effects and cost-effectiveness after approximately 3 years with catheter AF ablation therapy.[49,50]

CHRONIC ATRIAL FIBRILLATION

Although most patients undergo at least one attempt at cardioversion to sinus rhythm, many are left in chronic AF, particularly those with dilated atria, poor LV function and valvular heart disease. In this setting, treatment aims at ventricular rate control and prevention of embolic stroke.

VENTRICULAR RATE CONTROL

Digoxin is often the drug of choice, particularly in patients with poor LV function. It is often ineffective at controlling ventricular rate during exercise and physiological stress. Judicious addition of a small dose of a β-adrenergic blocker may improve digoxin control. Amiodarone is particularly useful in patients with poor LV function. Higher-dose β-adrenergic blocker, diltiazem, sotalol or flecainide can be used in patients with good LV function. Rarely, His-bundle ablation with permanent cardiac pacing may be required for severe cases refractory to drug therapy.

ANTICOAGULATION FOR CHRONIC ATRIAL FIBRILLATION

Consider for all patients, especially those with risk factors (Table 18.7).

Table 18.7 Prognostic factors for ischaemic stroke and systemic embolism in patients with atrial fibrillation

High	Previous stroke, transient ischaemic attack, systemic embolism
	Mitral stenosis
	Prosthetic heart valve
Moderate	Age > 75 years
	Left atrial size > 45 mm
	Hypertension
	Congestive cardiac failure
	Diabetes mellitus
	Left ventricular ejection fraction < 35%
Low	Female
	Age 65–74 years
	Coronary artery disease
	Thyrotoxicosis

VALVULAR ATRIAL FIBRILLATION

A seventeen-fold increased risk of embolic stroke with rheumatic mitral valve disease requires warfarin (INR 2–3). With prosthetic valves there is a similar target range of INR, though the exact level is dependent on type of valve.

NON-VALVULAR ATRIAL FIBRILLATION

The risk of stroke is determined by $CHADS_2$ score (assign 1 point for congestive heart failure, hypertension, age = 75 years and diabetes mellitus, and 2 points for stroke/TIA)[51] (Tables 18.8 and 18.9).

The treatment options are discussed below.

WARFARIN

Adjusted-dose warfarin reduces relative risk of stroke by 62%. The absolute risk reduction is 2.8% per year for primary and 8.4% per year for secondary prevention, although intracranial haemorrhage occurs (0.3% per year). Low-dose warfarin (INR 1.5–2.0) is less effective than an INR of 2.0–3.0 but has fewer haemorrhagic complications. Embolic stroke rate doubles as INR falls from 2.0 to 1.7, and is markedly higher at an INR of 1.3 compared to 2.0.[43,52]

Table 18.8 $CHADS_2$ score stroke risk stratification in non-valvular atrial fibrillation

Prognostic factor	Relative risk*	$CHADS_2$ score
Congestive heart failure (ejection fraction < 35%)	1.4	1
History of hypertension	1.6	1
Age 75 years	1.4	1
Diabetes mellitus	1.7	1
Stroke or transient ischaemic attack in past	2.5	2

*Relative risk without any antithrombotic treatment compared to atrial fibrillation patients without these prognostic factors.
$CHADS_2$, congestive heart failure, hypertension, age = 75 years and diabetes mellitus, and 2 points for stroke/transient ischaemic attack.

Table 18.9 The adjusted annual stroke rate in non-valvular atrial fibrillation without any antithrombotic treatment

$CHADS_2$ score	Adjusted stroke rate	
	%/year	95% CI
0	1.9	1.2–3.0
1	2.8	2.0–3.8
2	4.0	3.1–5.1
3	5.9	4.6–7.3
4	8.5	6.3–11.1
5	12.5	8.2–17.5
6	18.2	10.5–27.4

$CHADS_2$, congestive heart failure, hypertension, age = 75 years and diabetes mellitus, and 2 points for stroke/transient ischaemic attack; CI, confidence interval.

ASPIRIN

Aspirin has reduced efficacy when compared with warfarin, with a 22% relative risk reduction and an absolute risk reduction of 1.5% and 2.5% per year for primary and secondary prevention. Warfarin compared with aspirin for AF will prevent 23 strokes and result in nine additional major bleeds per 1000 patients per year.

CLOPIDOGRIL PLUS ASPIRIN

Although warfarin is better under ideal circumstances, poor INR control will readily erode this benefit.

WARFARIN COMBINED WITH ANTIPLATELET THERAPY

There is no benefit over warfarin alone.

Recommendations for anticoagulation in patients with atrial fibrillation

Non-valvular AF

- $CHADS_2$ score = 0: aspirin
- $CHADS_2$ score = 1: either aspirin or warfarin
- $CHADS_2$ score = 2: warfarin

Valvular AF

- Warfarin

Risk of haemorrhage is reduced by keeping INR = 3, systolic blood pressure < 135 mmHg and avoiding antiplatelet drugs.

Temporary cessation of anticoagulation for AF with surgery is a common problem. Valvular AF requires heparin or enoxiparin until surgery and recommencement of heparin/enoxiparin, then warfarin as soon as safely possible. Non-valvular $CHADS_2$ score = 1 can have anticoagulation withheld with minimal risk. Non-valvular $CHADS_2$ score = 2 is increasingly managed as valvular AF.

Angioplasty and stenting of coronary arteries require aspirin and clopidogrel to maintain stent patency. Stenting in patients already on warfarin for AF is a common problem.

Recommendations for AF patients requiring coronary artery stenting

- Non-valvular $CHADS_2$ score = 1: cease warfarin as aspirin and clopidorel are started
- Valvular AF and non-valvular with $CHADS_2$ score = 2: add aspirin and clopidogrel to continued warfarin treatment

PRE-EXCITATION SYNDROME

Pre-excitation syndromes have an additional or accessory AV pathway. The term 'WPW syndrome' is usually applied when tachyarrhythmias are present.

ECG

During sinus rhythm, an atrial impulse will reach the ventricles via both the AV node and the accessory AV pathway. The latter conducts the atrial impulse to the ventricles before the AV node, resulting in ventricular pre-excitation and a short PR interval. On reaching the ventricles, the pre-excitation impulse is not conducted via the specialised conducting system. Hence, early ventricular activation will be slowed, resulting in a slurred upstroke of the QRS complex, the so-called delta (δ) wave (Figure 18.24). The abnormal ventricular activation also gives rise to secondary S-T segment and T-wave abnormalities. δ-wave polarity in a 12-lead ECG may help localise the anatomical position of the accessory pathway. Type A WPW is characterised by upright QRS deflections in the right precordial leads (tall R-waves in V_1 and V_2) (Figure 18.25). In type A WPW the accessory pathway is usually situated on the left with pre-excitation of the left ventricle. Type B WPW has a dominantly negative QRS complex in V_1 and the accessory pathway tends to be on the right with pre-excitation of the right ventricle (Figure 18.26).

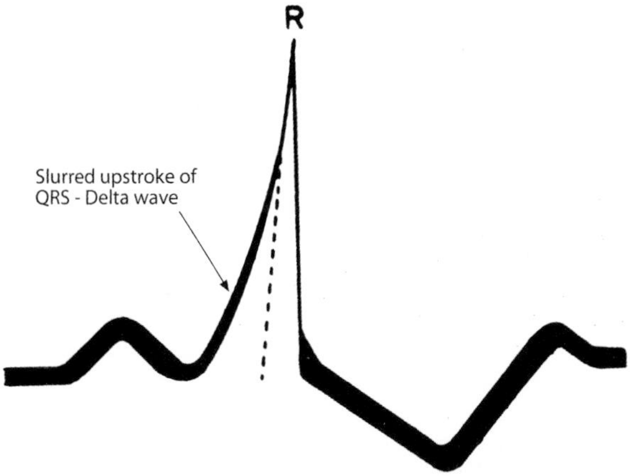

Figure 18.24 Ventricular pre-excitation via accessory pathway giving rise to a slurred upstroke and widened QRS complex.

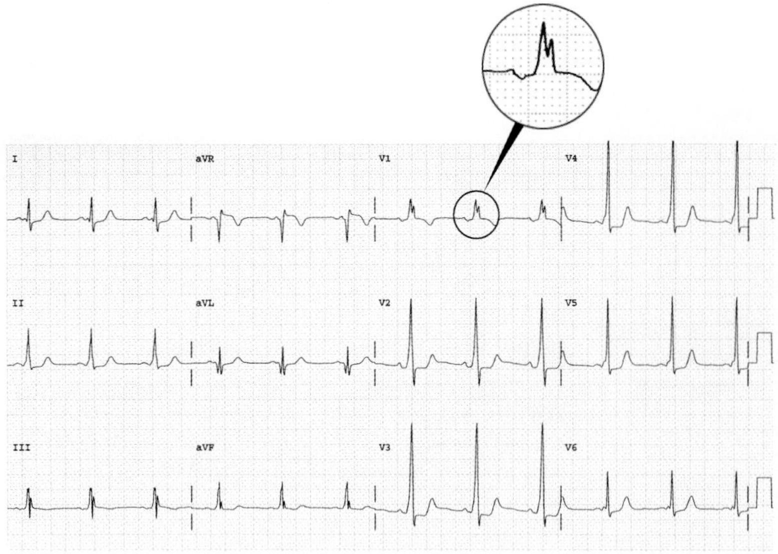

Figure 18.25 Type A Wolff–Parkinson–White syndrome with positive R-waves in the right precordial leads, short PR interval and δ-wave giving rise to a wide QRS complex.

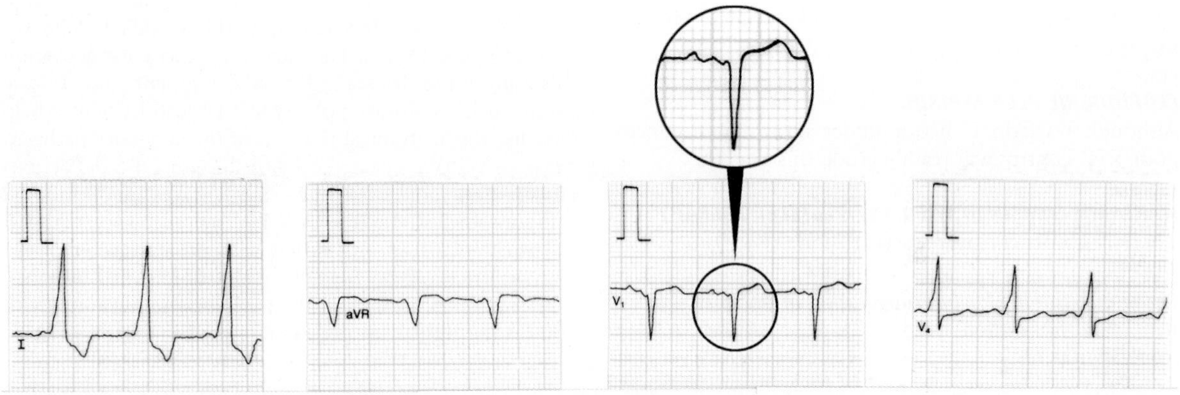

Figure 18.26 Type B Wolff–Parkinson–White syndrome with a negative QRS deflection in V_1.

CLINICAL

AVRT or AF can occur with WPW. During AVRT, the re-entry impulse usually travels down the AV node and back up the accessory pathway. Ventricular activation is via the normal conducting pathways and the QRS will be narrow. Occasionally, the re-entry impulse may pass in the opposite direction (down the accessory pathway and up the AV node), resulting in a wide QRS-complex tachycardia due to abnormal slow ventricular activation. Treatment is the same as for AVRT (i.e. IV adenosine). AF is uncommon in WPW, but may be life-threatening. Most impulses are conducted via the accessory pathway, leading to wide QRS complexes. The ECG of WPW with AF usually shows rapid, irregular QRS complexes with variable QRS width (Figure 18.27). Ventricular response is very rapid, leading to hypotension or cardiogenic shock. This arrhythmia may degenerate to VF.

TREATMENT[25]

Treatment usually involves synchronised DC shock. Antiarrhythmic drugs may be used when patients are haemodynamically stable and the ventricular rate is not excessively rapid.

- Drugs that prolong the refractory period of the accessory pathway are useful (e.g. sotalol, amiodarone, flecainide and procainamide).
- Drugs that shorten the refractory period (e.g. digoxin) are contraindicated as they may accelerate ventricular rate.
- Verapamil and lidocaine may increase the ventricular rate during AF, and are also best avoided.[26]
- β-Adrenergic blockers have no effect on the refractory period of the accessory pathway.

Long-term management by radiofrequency ablation of the accessory pathway is effective in selected patients.[25]

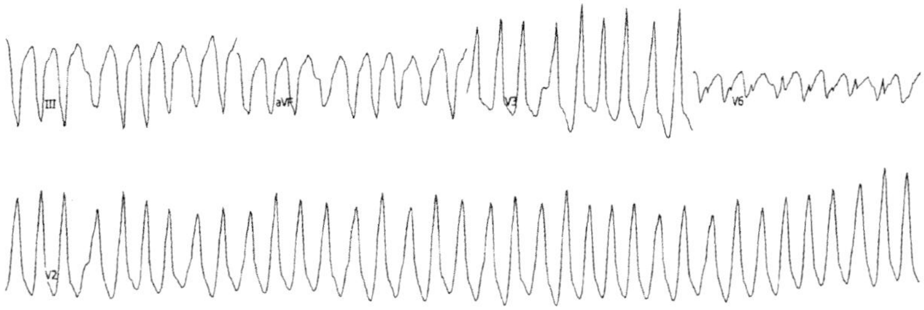

Figure 18.27 Wolff–Parkinson–White syndrome with atrial fibrillation. Rapid rate and irregularity of the broad QRS complexes help to distinguish from ventricular tachycardia.

VENTRICULAR TACHYCARDIA

VT is defined as three or more VEB at a rate greater than 130 beats/min, and may exceed 300 beats/min. VT lasting over 30 s is considered to be sustained. Non-sustained VT may not cause symptoms, but is associated with increased mortality in certain patients (e.g. after myocardial infarction). VT may be monomorphic (i.e. same QRS morphology) (Figure 18.28) or polymorphic (varying QRS morphology).

MONOMORPHIC VENTRICULAR TACHYCARDIA

This is the most common form of VT. It is commonly associated with previous myocardial infarction, and often causes symptoms (e.g. palpitations, shortness of breath, chest pain or syncope). It may result in cardiac arrest, due to the tachycardia itself or degeneration into VF. The most common mechanism is re-entry secondary to inhomogeneous activation of the myocardium and slow conduction through scar tissue from a previous myocardial infarction. AV dissociation (i.e. independent atrial and ventricular activity) (Figure 18.29) is present in about 75% of instances, whereas retrograde ventricle to atrial conduction occurs in about 25%. AV dissociation is virtually diagnostic for VT during a wide-complex tachycardia, but ECG recognition of independent (and slower) atrial activity can be difficult (Figure 18.30). VT is the most common cause of a wide-complex tachycardia (QRS > 120 ms) and any such tachycardia should be considered VT until proven otherwise. Mistakes in diagnosis are common: SVT with aberrant conduction is often mistaken for VT. Inappropriate treatment based on incorrect diagnosis can have disastrous consequences.

ECG

Older criteria (e.g. QRS > 140 ms and extreme electrical axis changes) are unhelpful in rhythm diagnosis.[53] ECG criteria initially proposed by Wellens and revised by Brugada *et al.* permit accurate diagnosis in four sequential steps (Figure 18.31).[54–56]

The sensitivity of these four consecutive steps was 0.987, with a specificity of 0.965.

- Step 1: is an RS complex present in any precordial lead? (QR, QRS, QS, monophasic R and rSR are not considered RS complexes.) If not (Figure 18.32), the diagnosis is VT.
- Step 2: if an RS is present, then measure the duration of the R-to-S nadir (lowest part of the S-wave). If this duration is > 100 ms in any V lead (Figure 18.33), the rhythm is VT.

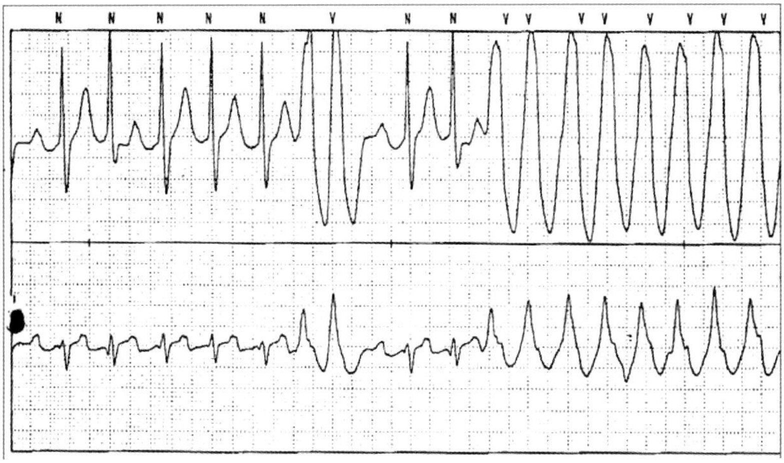

Figure 18.28 Monomorphic ventricular tachycardia preceded by a ventricular couplet.

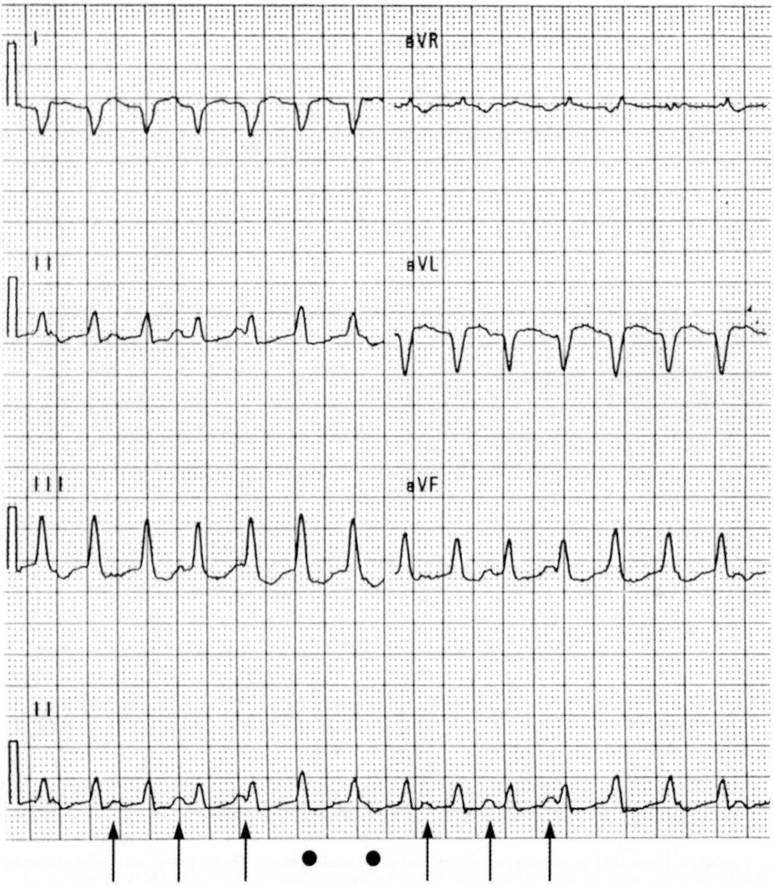

Figure 18.29 Ventricular tachycardia with obvious arteriovenous dissociation and independent P-waves are highlighted with arrows in lead II.

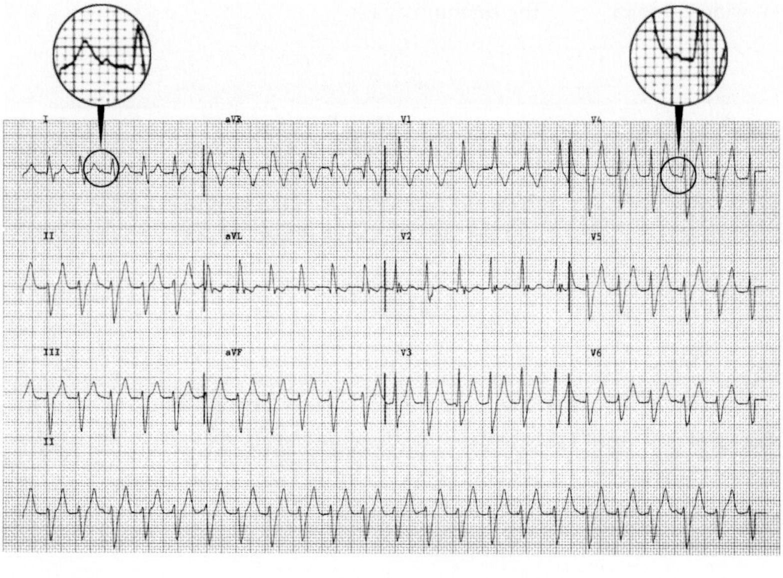

Figure 18.30 Ventricular tachycardia. Independent atrial activity can be difficult to see. Dissociated P-waves can just be seen in leads I and V_5.

Sequential ECG Criteria of Brugada for Diagnosis of Ventricular Tachycardia

1. Absent RS complex in all V leads → VT
2. R to S nadir >100msec in any V lead → VT
3. Atrio-ventricular dissociation → VT
4. Typical/Classical BBB pattern → No → VT

↓

Yes

↓

SVT

Figure 18.31 Algorithm proposed by Brugada *et al.*[54] to diagnose ventricular tachycardia in the setting of a broad QRS-complex tachycardia.

- Step 3: if RS < 100 ms, then AV dissociation is searched for (more QRS complexes than P-waves (see Figures 18.29 and 18.30)). Indirect evidence of AV dissociation such as capture or fusion beats may be present. Capture beats occur when atrial sinus impulses reach the AV node when it is no longer refractory from retrograde conduction of ventricular discharges: the AV node and ventricle are then 'captured' by the sinus impulse. The resultant QRS will occur earlier than the next expected VT complex and the QRS morphology will be that of the 'normal' underlying complexes for that patient. Similarly, a sinus impulse can penetrate the AV and 'fuse' with an already depolarising ventricle from the ectopic focus initiating the VT. The resulting QRS morphology of a fusion beat will be variable and depend on the relative contribution of the supraventricular and ventricular impulses to ventricular activation. Even a single capture or fusion beat confirms AV dissociation and VT (Figure 18.34).

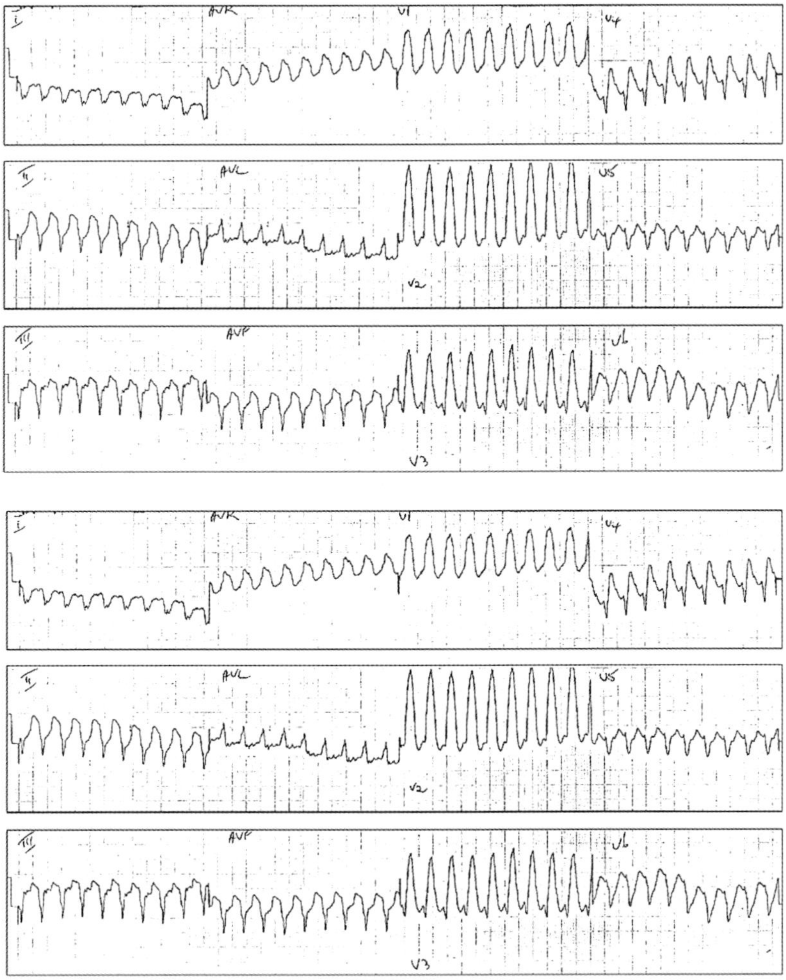

Figure 18.32 (a, b) Ventricular tachycardia. Broad QRS-complex tachycardia with absence of RS complex in all precordial leads.

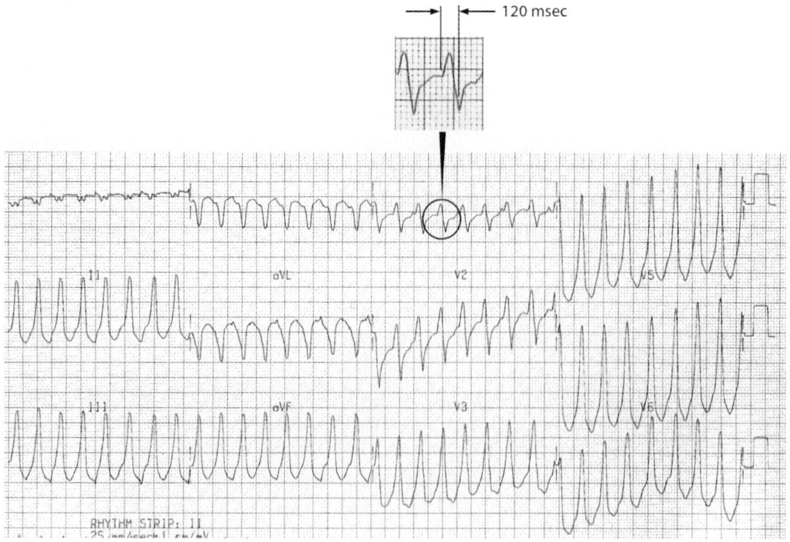

Figure 18.33 Ventricular tachycardia. Time duration of R to the nadir of the negative S-wave is 120 ms. Note also independent P-waves in lead V_1.

- Step 4: If AV dissociation is not present, then decide whether the wide QRS has a right or left BBB pattern. If the BBB is typical in both V_1 and V_6 leads, the rhythm is supraventricular in origin (see the section on BBB, below). If there are any atypical features, the rhythm is considered to be VT (see Figures 18.38 and 18.39, below).

Termination of a wide-complex tachycardia by IV adenosine strongly suggests the arrhythmia as SVT. However, adenosine in this setting has the risk of destabilising VT when blood pressure is barely compensated by vasodilatation or acceleration of accessory pathway conduction, and is not recommended by International Liaison Committee on Resuscitation (ILCOR) as a diagnostic strategy in wide-complex tachycardia.[25] Demonstration of AV dissociation by intracardiac ECG from a central venous catheter or a transvenous pacing lead signifies VT.

CLINICAL

The major cause of VT is significant coronary artery disease. Other causes include cardiomyopathy, myocarditis and valvular heart disease. Symptoms will depend on the ventricular rate, duration of tachycardia and underlying cardiac function. There are not necessarily any haemodynamic differences between VT and SVT with aberrant conduction but haemodynamic instability mandates management as for VT.

TREATMENT[25,57]

DC shock is indicated if a patient is haemodynamically unstable. Antiarrhythmic drug trial is indicated in haemodynamically stable VT.

- Amiodarone may terminate VT: there is less negative inotropy action but delayed effect.
- Sotalol and procainamide are more effective than lidocaine but are associated with significant myocardial depression.
- Although traditionally indicated, there are now doubts about the efficacy of lidocaine.

If drugs are ineffective, synchronised DC shock is indicated. Rapid right ventricular pacing may also be effective.

Long-term prevention of VT and sudden death is difficult. Sotalol guided by Holter ECG or electrophysiological testing, and empirical (i.e. non-guided) amiodarone are superior to other drugs in preventing arrhythmia recurrences. Empirical β-adrenergic blockers also have a role. Implantable defibrillators can recognise and automatically terminate VT by rapid ventricular pacing or, if this fails, by internal DC cardioversion, which may be life-saving.

POLYMORPHIC VENTRICULAR TACHYCARDIA AND TORSADE DE POINTES

This arrhythmia has QRS complexes at 200 beats/min or greater, which change in amplitude and axis so that they appear to twist around the baseline (Figure 18.35). Torsade de pointes usually has prolonged QT during sinus rhythm, and U-waves are often present (see section on long-QT syndrome, below). However, polymorphic VT may be associated with a normal QT interval in settings such as myocardial ischaemia, infarction or post cardiac surgery.

TREATMENT

Polymorphic VT associated with a normal QT interval during sinus rhythm (e.g. following AMI) should be treated in the same way as monomorphic VT. (See section on treatment of long-QT and polymorphic VT, below.)

ACCELERATED IDIOVENTRICULAR RHYTHM (AIVR)

This is often inappropriately called slow VT. Increased automaticity is probably the mechanism responsible for this relatively benign arrhythmia.

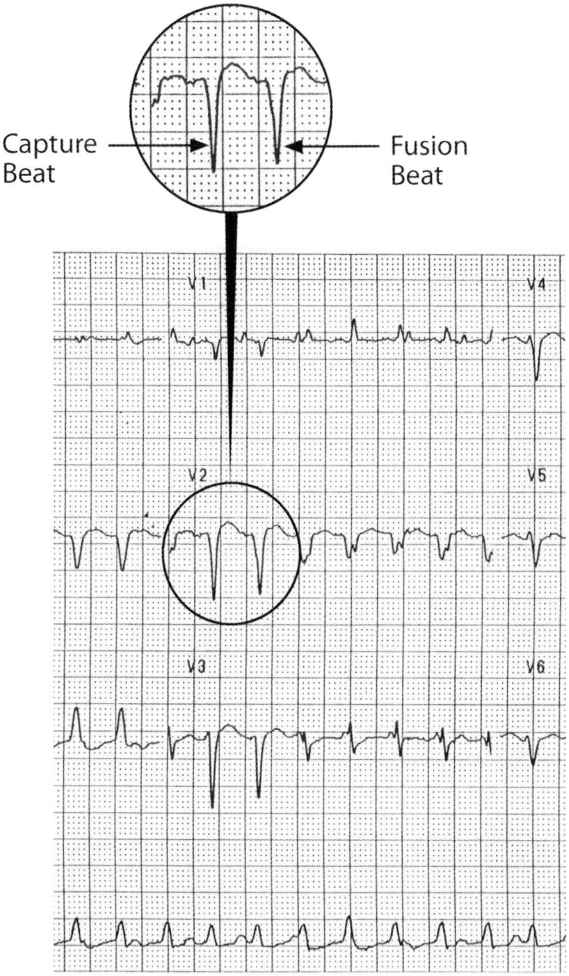

Figure 18.34 Ventricular tachycardia with a highlighted premature capture beat followed by a fusion beat showing transitional QRS morphology between the underlying normal QRS and VT complex. Note also independent P-waves.

ECG

There is a wide QRS with a rate of 60–110 beats/min (Figure 18.36). Sinus rate is often only slightly slower than the arrhythmia, so the dominant rhythm may be intermittent AIVR and sinus rhythm. Fusion beats are therefore common.

CLINICAL

The rhythm is commonly encountered in inferior myocardial infarction. AIVR may be misdiagnosed as VT. Occasionally, AIVR causes haemodynamic deterioration, usually due to loss of atrial systole. Increasing the atrial rate with either atropine or atrial pacing may then be necessary.

VENTRICULAR FIBRILLATION

VF always causes haemodynamic collapse, loss of consciousness and death if not immediately treated. Of patients resuscitated from VF, 20–30% have sustained an AMI, and 75% have coronary artery disease. VF (and VT) unassociated with AMI is likely to be recurrent; 50% die within 3 years.

ECG

The ECG shows irregular waves of varying morphology and amplitude (Figure 18.37).

CLINICAL

VF is usually associated with ischaemic heart disease, although other causes include cardiomyopathy, antiarrhythmic drugs, severe hypoxia and non-synchronised DC cardioversion.

TREATMENT[57]

Give an immediate non-synchronised DC shock at 200 J, and if ineffective, repeated at 200–360 and 360 J (or biphasic equivalent). Time should not be wasted with basic life support if immediate defibrillation can be delivered.

Figure 18.35 Torsade de pointes preceded by multifocal ventricular ectopic beats.

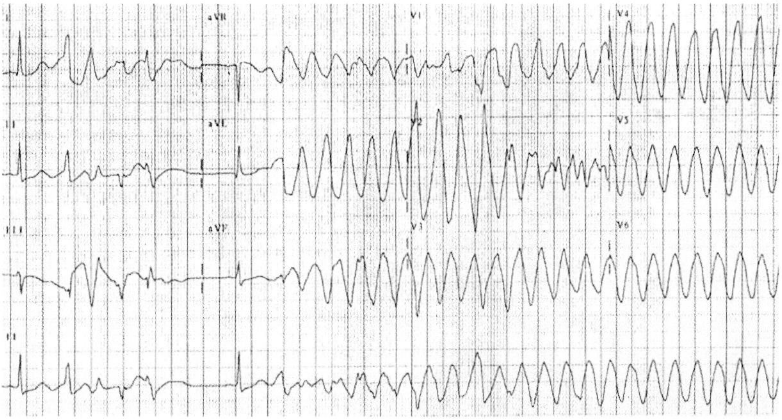

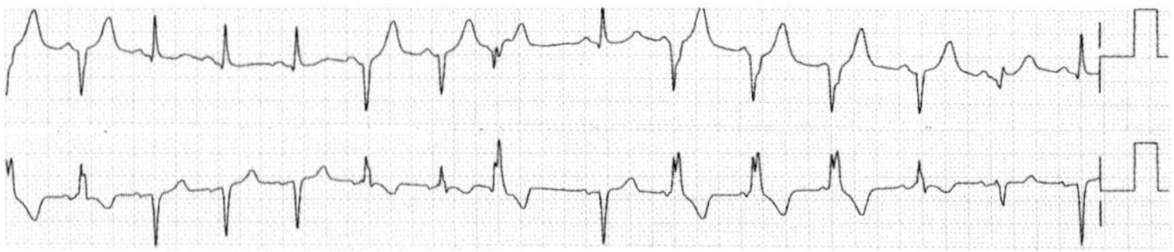

Figure 18.36 Sinus rhythm with short runs of accelerated idioventricular rhythm. Note frequent fusion beats as sinus rate is similar to the accelerated idioventricular rate.

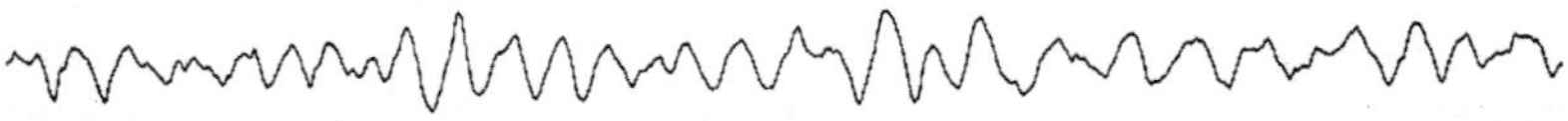

Figure 18.37 Ventricular fibrillation with waves of varying morphology and amplitude.

If DC shock sequence fails, basic and advanced life support aiming to maximise coronary blood flow with chest compressions and vasopressors is crucial to cardiac success. Until recently, any role of antiarrhythmic drugs in DC shock-resistant VF has been traditional rather than proven. Recommendations have varied from lidocaine and bretyllium to amiodarone. The ILCOR currently recommends consideration of a range of antiarrhythmic drugs, including amiodarone, lidocaine, magnesium and procainamide. Recent studies indicate amiodarone as the drug of choice for DC shock-resistant VF. Amiodarone (300 mg) was superior to lidocaine and, in another study, 5 mg/kg followed by 2.5 mg/kg if required was superior to lidocaine. There is an incidence of bradycardia and hypotension but no difference in adverse effect profile between lidocaine and this sizeable amiodarone dose.[58,59] After return of circulation, appropriate antiarrhythmic therapy is less clear but the role of lidocaine continues to disappear. Precipitating factors should be sought and treated (for long-term management issues, see the section on sudden cardiac death, below).

RIGHT BUNDLE BRANCH BLOCK (FIGURE 18.38)

In right BBB (RBBB) the normal rapid coordinated depolarisation of the right ventricle is lost due to conduction block in the right branch of the bundle of His. There is normal rapid depolarisation of the septum and the initial deflection of the QRS is not altered. The activation of the free wall of the left ventricle is also normal. However the final activation of the free wall of the right ventricle is slow and anomalous, leading to a broad QRS.

ECG

The ECG shows wide QRS (> 120 ms) and the QRS morphology in the right ventricular leads V_1 and V_2 is often M-shaped. This results in two R-waves, with the smaller of the R-waves being designated 'r' and the larger 'R'. The classical pattern is the M-shaped rSR in V_1 or V_2 and a broad S-wave in LV leads, especially I and V_6. In V_1 the R-wave is greater in amplitude than the R-wave. In V_6 the R-wave is greater than any S-wave present. Partial RBBB is identical, except the QRS duration is 110–120 ms.

CLINICAL

RBBB may be a normal variant, but may occur with massive pulmonary embolism, right ventricular hypertrophy, ischaemic heart disease and congenital heart disease (note that myocardial infarction can be diagnosed in the presence of RBBB).

LEFT BUNDLE BRANCH BLOCK (FIGURE 18.39)

In left BBB (LBBB), there is delayed and anomalous activation of the interventricular septum from right to left (i.e. in the opposite direction to normal) and the free wall of the left ventricle.

ECG

There is a wide QRS (> 120 ms) and in V_1 the characteristic morphology shows an rS or QS. In V_6 there are primary and secondary R-waves (RR′), often resulting in M-shaped or plateau morphology. Q-waves are never seen in LV leads (V_4–V_6) (note that myocardial infarction cannot usually be diagnosed in the presence of LBBB). Partial LBBB is similar, except that the QRS duration is 110–120 ms.

CLINICAL

LBBB is often associated with heart disease such as coronary artery disease, cardiomyopathy or LV hypertrophy. LBBB makes diagnosis of myocardial infarction difficult and the development of a new LBBB fulfils ECG criteria of acute infarction.

HEMIBLOCKS

The left branch of the bundle of His divides into the left anterosuperior division supplying the anterior superior lateral wall of the left ventricle and the posteroinferior division supplying the posterior inferior diaphragmatic surface of the left ventricle. Although block can occur in either division it is more common in the anterosuperior division, as it is more vulnerable to disease processes due to its longer course and thinner dimension. The anterosuperior division runs close to the aortic valve and tends to be involved in degenerative processes affecting this valve.

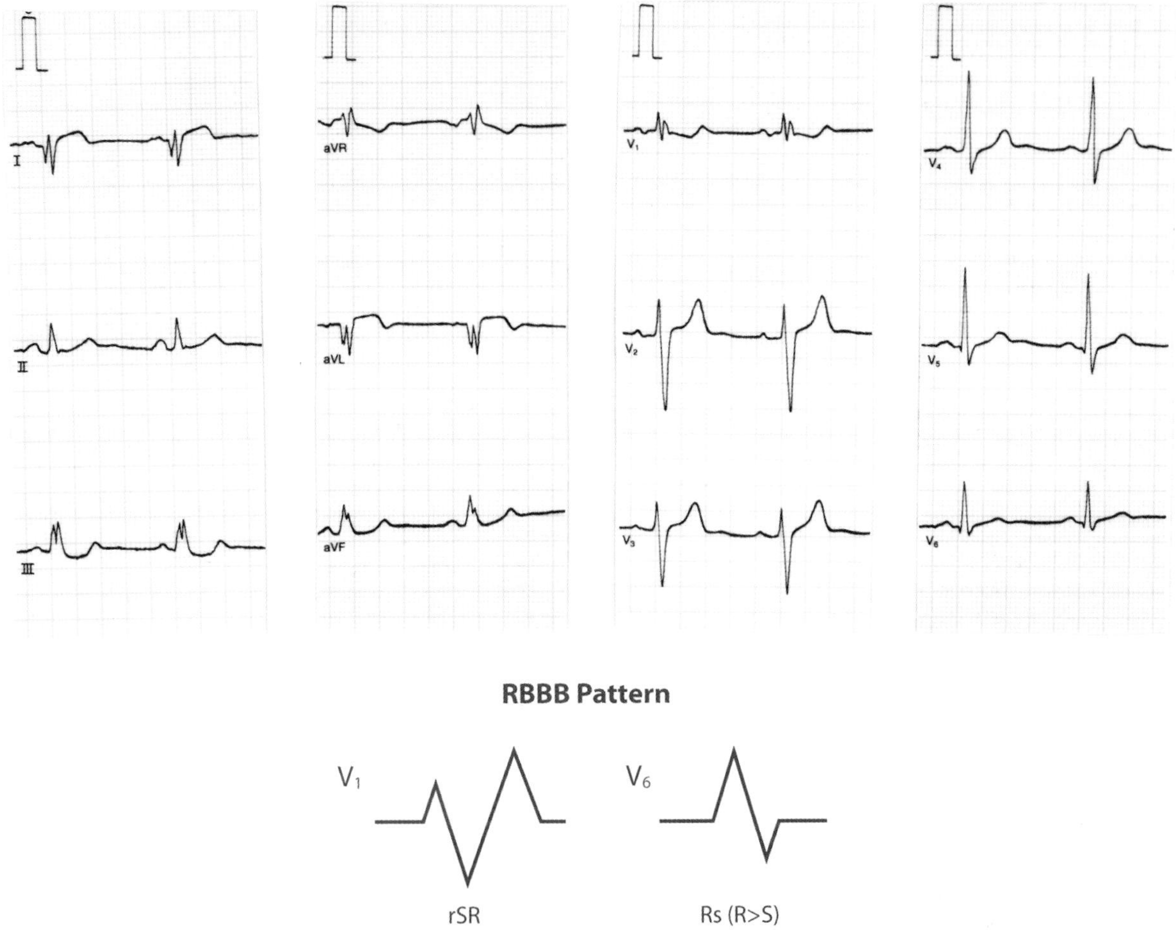

Figure 18.38 Right bundle branch block (RBBB) with characteristic M-shaped rSR complex in lead V_1 and Rs complex in V_6.

The posteroinferior division is shorter and thicker and, unlike the anterosuperior division, has a double blood supply.

LEFT ANTERIOR HEMIBLOCK

There is left-axis deviation (usually lead I predominantly positive, leads II and III predominantly negative) with initial R-wave in inferior leads (II, III, aVF).

LEFT POSTERIOR HEMIBLOCK

There is usually right-axis deviation (lead I predominantly negative and lead III predominantly positive). Other causes of right-axis deviation (e.g. right ventricular hypertrophy) need to be excluded.

CLINICAL

RBBB with either left anterior hemiblock (Figure 18.40) or left posterior hemiblock indicates an extensive conduction defect and a poor prognosis (high risk of complete heart block), especially in AMI.

HYPERKALAEMIA

A high serum K^+ can produce ECG changes (Figure 18.41). Early changes consist of tall peaked T-waves with reduced P-wave amplitude. Progressive widening of the QRS may be confused with BBB. Cardiac arrest may eventually occur.

ATRIOVENTRICULAR BLOCK[57]

AV block is a delay or failure of impulse conduction from the atria to the ventricles. AV block is classified according to whether conduction of atrial impulses is delayed (first-degree), blocked intermittently (second-degree) or blocked completely (third-degree).

FIRST-DEGREE AV BLOCK

ECG

PR interval (measured from the onset of the P-wave to the onset of the QRS) exceeds 200 ms (Figure 18.42).

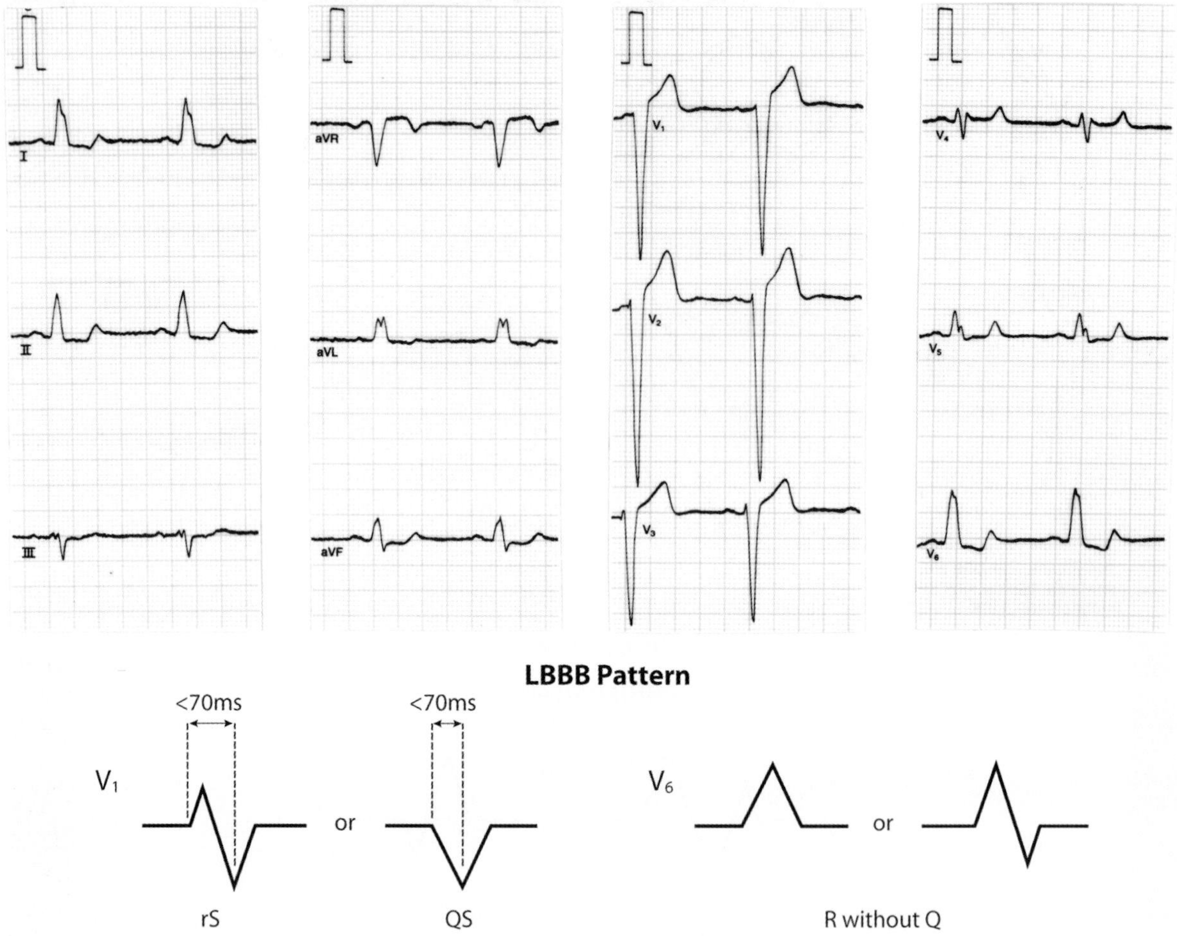

Figure 18.39 Left bundle branch block (LBBB).

Each P-wave is followed by a QRS. PR intervals may be prolonged to such a degree that the P-wave is buried in the previous T-wave or even QRS.

CLINICAL

First-degree AV block is commonly associated with increased vagal tone, and occasionally with drugs (especially digoxin), ischaemic heart disease (particularly inferior myocardial infarction) and rheumatic fever. It usually causes no symptoms and requires no treatment. If associated with digoxin, the drug should be ceased or the dose decreased.

SECOND-DEGREE AV BLOCK

Second-degree AV block is characterised by intermittent failure of AV conduction and is classified into Mobitz types I and II. Second-degree AV block can occur in SVTs; however the conduction block is a physiological 'protective' mechanism in the setting of rapid atrial impulses.

MOBITZ TYPE I (WENCKEBACH)

Delay in AV conduction increases with each atrial impulse until an atrial impulse fails to conduct. This is usually a repetitive pattern which may or may not begin with first-degree AV block. The level of AV block in type 1 is usually in the AV node itself and can be physiological (increased vagal tone) as well as pathological.

ECG

There is progressive lengthening of the PR interval over successive cardiac cycles, culminating in a non-conducted P-wave, resulting in a missed beat (Figure 18.43). Type 1 is common in fit healthy people in the presence of high levels of resting vagal tone (Figure 18.44).

CLINICAL

The condition is generally benign and does not carry the adverse likelihood of progression to complete AV block, although it may occur with inferior infarction. Treatment is rarely necessary.

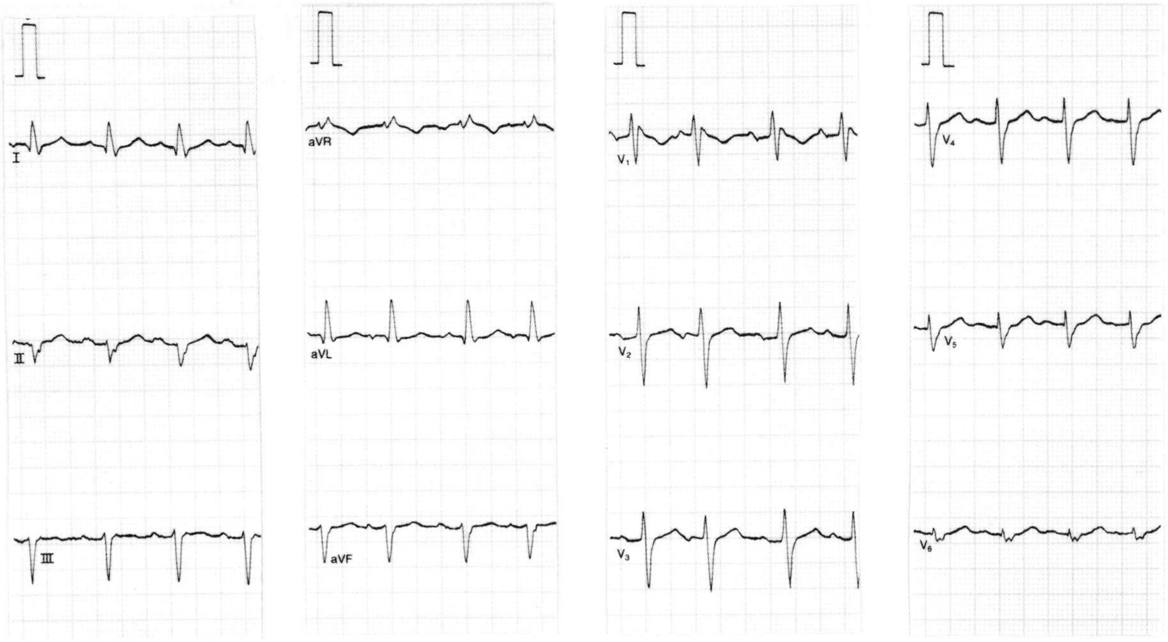

Figure 18.40 Right bundle branch block with left anterior hemiblock. There is left-axis deviation (mean frontal axis of −75 °) and small R-waves in II, III and aVF.

Figure 18.41 Sinus rhythm with peaked 'tent-shaped' T-waves in a patient with a serum potassium of 7.6 mmol/l.

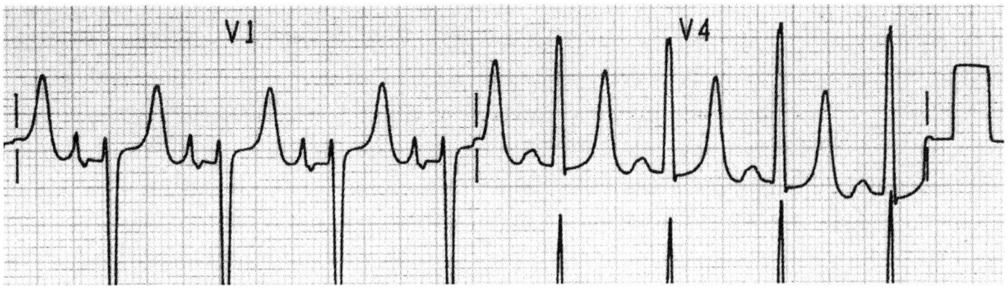

MOBITZ TYPE II

There is intermittent failure of conduction of atrial impulses to the ventricles without preceding increases in the PR interval. The ratio of conducted to non-conducted atrial impulses varies, e.g. every second or fourth atrial impulse may be conducted (i.e. 2:1 or 4:1 second-degree AV block). The lesion causing type ?? is usually situated in the bundle of His and is always pathological.

ECG

PR interval remains constant prior to the blocked P-wave. There is always a constant P-QRS-wave ratio: the P-waves are two (Figure 18.45), three (rare) or four times more frequent than QRS-waves.

CLINICAL

It is likely to be associated with structural heart disease. Slower symptomatic ventricular rates may require pacing. The AV block may be intermittent or persistent. The adverse prognosis relates to the frquency of progression to complete AV block.

THIRD-DEGREE (COMPLETE) AV BLOCK

This rhythm occurs when no atrial impulses are conducted to the ventricles; atrial and ventricular contraction are dissociated. The SA node usually continues to depolarise the atria, whereas ventricular activation depends on a standby escape pacemaker located below the block. The escape pacemaker may be close to the His bundle (narrow QRS, stable pacemaker usually 40–60 beats/min) (Figure 18.46), or more distal in ventricular tissue (wide QRS, relatively unstable pacemaker with a rate of 20–40 beats/min) (Figure 18.47). If no ectopic escape pacemaker emerges, ventricular asystole will occur, resulting in a Stokes–Adams attack, or death if the episode is prolonged. Torsade de pointes may also occur associated with the bradycardia.

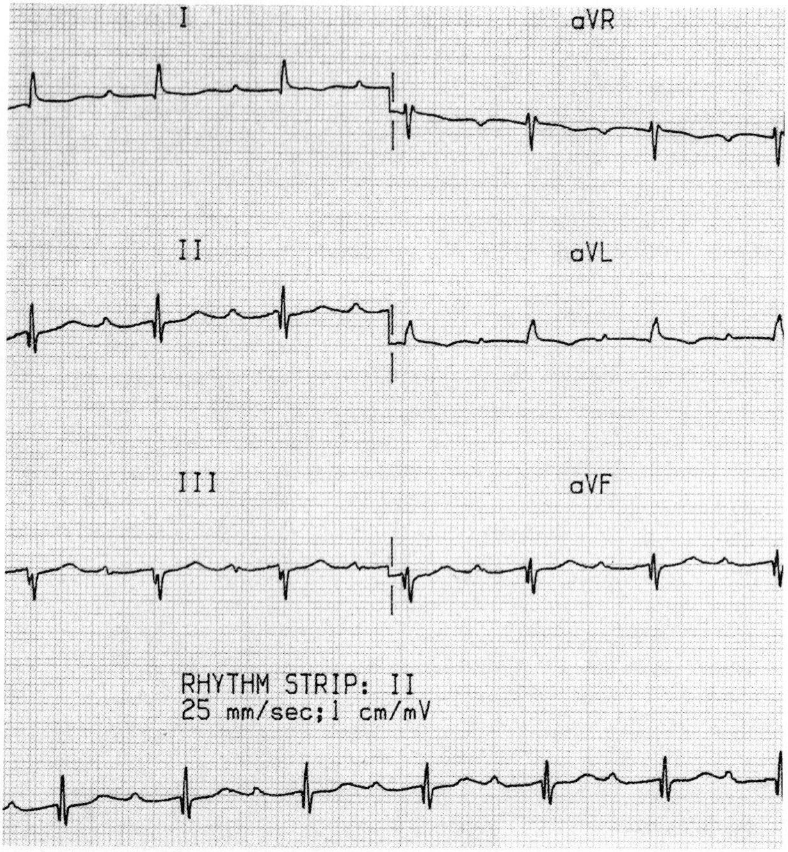

Figure 18.42 Sinus rhythm with first-degree AV block. The PR interval is 360 ms. Note inferior-wall myocardial infarction with Q-waves in II, III and aVF.

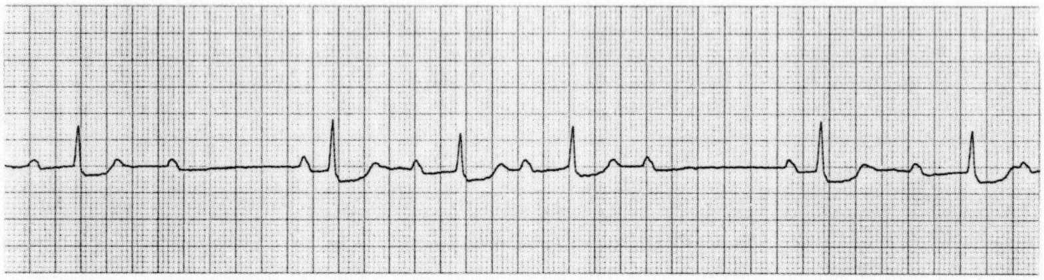

Figure 18.43 Mobitz type I (Wenckebach) second-degree arteriovenous block. Progressive lengthening of PR interval results in the failure of the second and sixth P-wave to be conducted.

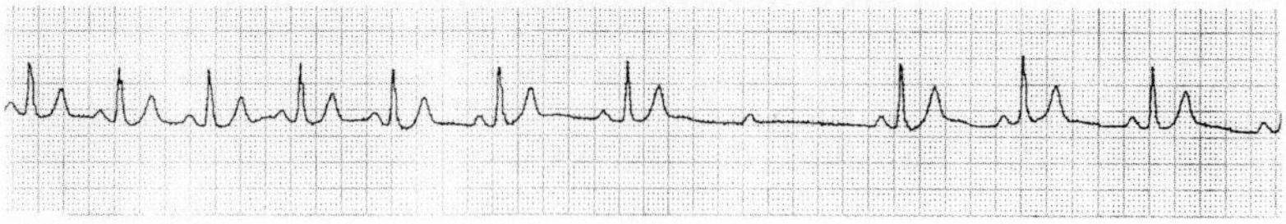

Figure 18.44 Intermittent type I second-degree arteriovenous block in a healthy male with obvious background sinus arrhythmia. Constant PR interval of 0.14 s suddenly increases to 0.22 s and next P-wave is not conducted.

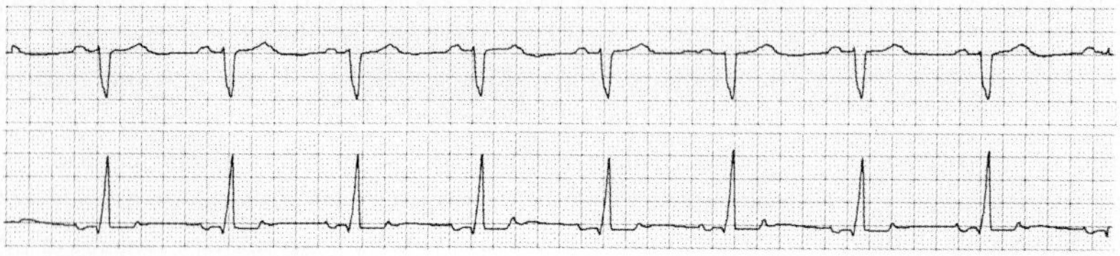

Figure 18.45 Mobitz type II second-degree arteriovenous (AV) block. Persistent 2:1 AV block with the atrial rate at 108 beats/min and the ventricular rate 54 beats/min.

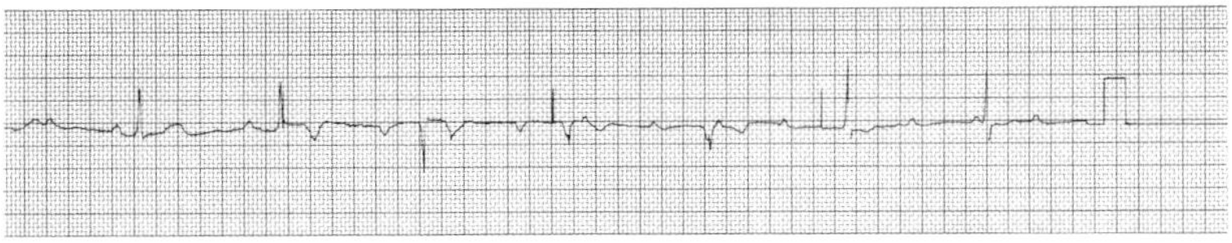

Figure 18.46 Leads I, aVR, V_1 and V_4 showing third-degree arteriovenous block. Complete dissociation of atrial activity at a rate of 107 beats/min and the ventricular rate at 46 beats/min. The escape rhythm is junctional (high up in the bundle of His) with a narrow QRS morphology.

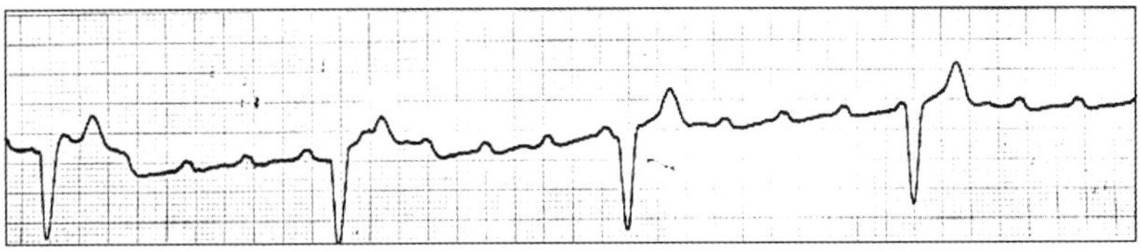

Figure 18.47 Third-degree arteriovenous block with an atrial rhythm at 135 beats/min and a broad distal ventricular escape rhythm which is unstable at a rate of 30 beats/min.

ECG

The ECG shows normal regular P-waves completely dissociated from QRS complexes. The QRS rate is always significantly slower than the P-wave rate and may be very slow at times.

CLINICAL

Idiopathic fibrosis of the conduction system is the most common cause. Other causes include myocardial infarction, valvular heart disease, cardiac surgery and a congenital form of complete heart block. Cardiac pacing is usually required to increase heart rate and cardiac output. Congenital forms often have a relatively fast escape ventricular rate, and patients may remain asymptomatic for many years.

SICK-SINUS SYNDROME

This consists of a number of sinus node abnormalities, including inappropriate sinus bradycardia, SA blocks or sinus arrest. When sinus bradycardia or SA block occurs, junctional escape rhythms are common. There may also be abnormalities of AV conduction. Paroxysms of AF or Afl may alternate with episodes of bradycardia (bradycardia–tachycardia syndrome) (Figure 18.48).

CLINICAL

The bradycardias associated with sick-sinus syndrome (SSS) may result in syncope or near-syncope. SSS is often not associated with structural heart disease, but may occur with ischaemic and congenital heart disease.

TREATMENT

Cardiac pacing is usually required to control bradycardia symptoms. Atropine and low-dose isoprenaline may be useful prior to pacing, in the haemodynamically compromised patient. Bradycardia–tachycardia syndrome may require both pacing (for the bradycardia) and antiarrhythmic drugs (for the tachycardia). Anticoagulation needs to be considered if episodes of AF occur.

CRITICALLY ILL PATIENTS AND ARRHYTHMIA[60]

In the general population or critically ill patients, excluding acute coronary syndromes and cardiac surgical patients, arrhythmia is common. The documented incidence is as high as 78%; however, the incidence of arrhythmia that requires treatment is much lower, at 15–30%. SVT are by far the most common arrhythmia that requires treatment.

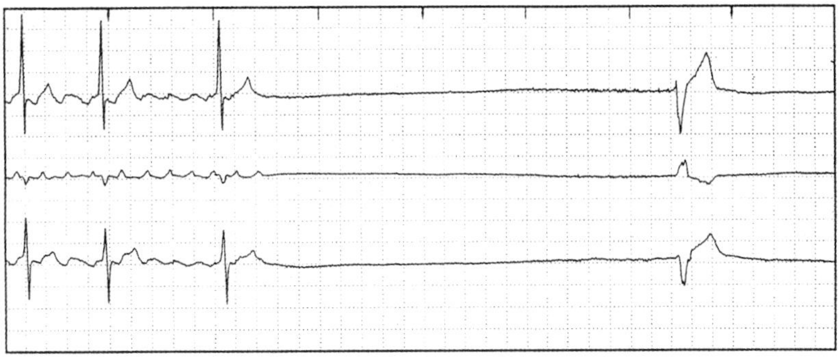

Figure 18.48 Characteristic findings in sick-sinus syndrome. Episodic atrial tachycardias (atrial flutter with variable block in this instance) with periods of sinus arrest and very slow ventricular escape rhythm upon spontaneous termination. CSM, carotid sinus massage.

AF, Afl and unifocal atrial tachycardias are the most frequent, in descending order. These SVTs are rarely the cause of admission but develop early in the admission, the majority by day 2. In critically ill patients, SVTs often result in:

- adverse myocardial oxygen supply–demand balance
- compromised blood pressure, cardiac output and systemic oxygen delivery
- impaired end-organ function such as oliguria and worsening gas exchange

The development of SVT in a critically ill patient is associated with a significant increase in mortality, especially in patients with sepsis and respiratory failure. Incidence of SVT is increased with:

- elderly patients
- evidence or past history of heart disease
- haemodynamic features of diastolic failure with elevated pulmonary artery occlusion pressure
- catecholamine infusion

The actual dose of the catecholamine infusion does not appear to be important and, although electrolyte disturbances are common in critically ill patients, low plasma potassium and magnesium levels do not appear to be important predictors of SVT development. The incidence of SVT, particularly AF, is so high in elderly patients with heart disease on a catecholamine infusion that consideration of prophylactic strategies is worthwhile.

TREATMENT OF SUPRAVENTRICULAR TACHYCARDIA IN CRITICALLY ILL PATIENTS

Continuing arrhythmogenic and chronotropic factors make rate control difficult.

- Digoxin often results in poor rate control due to persisting endogenous and exogenous sympathomimetic tone. The inotropic and vasopressor effects of acute digitalisation are beneficial. Digoxin (10 μg/kg) has been shown to provide superior circulatory support to dopamine at 8 μg/kg per min in septic patients.[61]
- Irrespective of plasma levels, magnesium has been shown to be effective at rate control; however, hypotension due to vasodilatation can be seen.
- Amiodarone is particularly effective and has allowed reliable acute rate control over a period of days in critically ill patients with circulatory shock requiring catecholamine infusions.[62] It can cause hypotension if patients are rapidly loaded. In another study, magnesium was at least as effective as amiodarone in rate control and time to reversion to sinus rhythm.[63]
- Other agents, such as diltiazem, sotalol and procainamide, are associated with prohibitive myocardial depression and hypotension.

Urgent cardioversion is indicated in unstable patients. The likelihood of remaining in sinus rhythm in the setting of high endogenous and exogenous sympathomimetic tone is low without concomitant use of an antiarrhythmic drug. Cardioversion is best reserved for hastening onset of sinus rhythm once a drug like amiodarone has controlled rate. Cardioversion should at least be attempted within 24–48 h of onset in the hope that embolic and anticoagulation issues are avoided.

MYOCARDIAL INFARCTION AND ARRHYTHMIA[21]

Arrhythmia is common following AMI. While early arrhythmia contributes significantly to mortality, treatment is largely expectant and secondary to re-establishing coronary blood flow, minimising infarct size and treating ongoing ischaemia and heart failure. Late ventricular arrhythmia is particularly challenging, as selecting patients at risk is difficult and treatment options are limited.

MANAGEMENT OF ACUTE MYOCARDIAL INFARCTION AND ARRHYTHMIA CONTROL

Modern management of AMI, although targeted to prevent or reduce infarct size, has also been very effective in reducing arrhythmia incidence and sequelae. Numerous studies have documented transient ventricular arrhythmias at the time of reperfusion resulting from thrombolysis and acute angioplasty. However, the most common arrhythmias seen in this setting are VEB, AIVRs and non-sustained VT, rather than VF or sustained VT.

Meta-analysis of thrombolytic trials has shown no increase in early VF following thrombolytic therapy in the first 24 h. The likelihood of developing VF at any time during a hospital episode is reduced following thrombolytic therapy but the risk of developing VT is increased. The mechanism of reperfusion arrhythmia is believed to be related to intracellular calcium overload and the resulting triggered activity in the form of DAD. Dipyridamole, which inhibits the cellular uptake of adenosine, has been shown to be effective in preventing and treating reperfusion ventricular arrhythmia.

Prior to the introduction of thrombolytic therapy, β-adrenergic receptor blockers significantly reduced the incidence of early VEB and VF. However, following routine use of thrombolytic therapy, the benefit of β-blockers relates to a reduction in postinfarction ischaemia and subsequent infarction.

The early work demonstrating survival benefit of magnesium was initially thought to be due to the prevention of arrhythmia.[64] However, the Leicester Intravenous Magnesium Intervention Trial (LIMIT-2) found the improved survival not to be related to a reduction in arrhythmia.[65] Subsequent studies in the thrombolytic era have failed to show any benefit at all with magnesium, although debate regarding optimal time of administration persists. Magnesium may have a role in patients in whom β-adrenergic blockers or thrombolytic therapy are contraindicated.

ELECTROLYTE CONCENTRATIONS AND ARRHYTHMIA FOLLOWING ACUTE MYOCARDIAL INFARCTION

Serum potassium following AMI is negatively correlated with the incidence of VEB and VT, with the probability of VT falling until serum potassium exceeds 4.5 mmol/l.[8] There is no evidence that magnesium levels in this setting have any effect on ventricular arrhythmia. Nonetheless, ILCOR recommendations not only include the maintenance of serum potassium greater than 4.0 mmol/l, but also serum magnesium levels greater than 1.0 mmol/l.

BRADYARRHYTHMIAS POST ACUTE MYOCARDIAL INFARCTION

One-third of patients with AMI develop sinus bradycardia because of increased vagal tone. In inferior infarcts due to occlusion of the right coronary artery, bradyarrhythmia is due to ischaemia of the SA and AV nodes. Reperfusion of the right coronary artery can also lead to sinus bradycardia and heart block that is due to accumulation of adenosine in nodal tissue. Bradycardia in this setting is resistant to atropine.

Second- or third-degree AV block occurs in approximately 20% of AMI patients. High-degree AV block occurs early when present, with 42% presenting with AV block and most, 66%, developing in the first 24 h. Similar to all post-AMI arrhythmias, thrombolytic therapy has reduced the incidence down to 12%. When present, high-degree AV block is associated with an increased mortality. However, high-degree AV block is not an independent predictor, rather a marker of extensive infarction and LV dysfunction.

Treatment is only indicated for sinus bradycardia associated with symptoms, hypotension or signs of poor cardiac output. Most often, first- and second-degree block also do not need treatment. Mobitz type I second-degree block may require treatment and atropine is indicated. However, in Mobitz type II, atropine usually has no effect on infranodal block and may precipitate third-degree block by increasing sinus rate and enhancing block. Atropine may improve heart rate with AV block occurring at the AV node, as demonstrated by a narrow QRS complex, by improving AV conduction or accelerating escape rhythm. Atropine is not indicated for infranodal third-degree block, which is diagnosed by the presence of a new wide QRS complex. When required, atropine is administered, 0.5–1.0 mg every 3 min until signs or symptoms are resolved, up to a maximum of 0.03–0.04 mg/kg. If atropine is not indicated or effective, cardiac pacing is required (Table 18.10). Transcutaneous pacing is indicated for initial management as a bridge until a transvenous temporary pacing wire can be inserted safely and with appropriate sterile technique. With the ready availability of transcutaneous pacing, IV catecholamines for bradyarrhythmias are to be avoided in the setting of AMI.

Table 18.10 Indications for pacing following myocardial infarction

Haemodynamically unstable bradycardia (< 50 beats/min)
Mobitz type II second-degree atrioventricular block
Third-degree heart block
Bilateral bundle branch block
Left anterior fascicular block
New left bundle branch block
Bundle branch block and first-degree atrioventricular block

ATRIAL FIBRILLATION POST ACUTE MYOCARDIAL INFARCTION

New-onset AF occurs in 10–15% of AMI. The incidence increases with age, large infarcts, LV hypertrophy and congestive cardiac failure. It is also related to atrial infarction with occlusion of the right coronary artery proximal to the sinus node branch or circumflex proximal to the left atrial circumflex branch. Later in the course of myocardial infarction, AF is related to postinfarct pericarditis.

Thrombolytic therapy has reduced the incidence of AF. In the setting of AMI, AF is usually self-limiting and requires no treatment. If rapid ventricular rates are associated with further ischaemic symptoms or haemodynamic compromise, cardioversion is indicated. β-Blockers, which are indicated in the treatment of AMI anyway, are the initial treatment of choice. Digoxin is not indicated in the setting of acute ischaemia as the likelihood of triggered activity associated with intracellular calcium overload is increased. AF following AMI is associated with an increase in mortality. Systemic emboli following AMI are three times more likely with AF and 50% occur in the first 24 h of onset of AF. For this reason, sustained AF is an indication for anticoagulation prior to the normal 48-h period following AMI.

VENTRICULAR ARRHYTHMIA POST ACUTE MYOCARDIAL INFARCTION[20,66,67]

VF/VT is the leading cause of mortality following AMI. Fifty per cent of patients dying from AMI do so pre-hospital due to VF/VT. Pre-hospital mortality is being reduced by improved community education, wider application of basic life support and availability of an automated external defibrillator (AED). Following admission to hospital, LV failure is the most common cause of death.

The major risk period for VF is the first 4 h following onset of symptoms, with 4–18% of patients having VF in this period. Once admitted to hospital, 5% develop VF, mostly in this first 4-h period. VF in this early 4-h period is termed 'primary VF'. VF later in the course of an AMI, usually associated with LV failure or cardiogenic shock, is called 'secondary VF'.

Thrombolytic therapy has reduced VF incidence. The Gruppo Italiano per lo Studio della Streptochinasi nell'infarto miocardico (GISSI) study[66] found an incidence of primary VF of 3.6% and secondary VF of 0.6%. The overall incidence of ventricular arrhythmia in the Global

Utilization of Streptokinase and Tissue plasminogen activator to treat Occluded arteries (GUSTO-1) report was VF, 4.1%, VT, 3.5% and both, 2.7%.

Primary VF increases in-hospital mortality and complications but not long-term mortality. Complex ventricular arrhythmias, defined as multiform VEB, couplets and non-sustained VT, occur in 35–40% of patients during hospital stay. They occur equally with Q-wave and non Q-wave infarction. Complex ventricular arrhythmia is a risk factor for subsequent VF/VT and SCD, particularly in non-Q-wave infarction. Polymorphous VT is less common after AMI and does not appear to be related to QT prolongation or electrolyte disturbances in the reported cases.

Lidocaine reduces primary VF by 33% but mortality is increased by a similar amount such that there is no net benefit and the third International Study of Infarct Survival (ISIS-3) reported an overall trend to increased mortality.[68] Being more selective as to which patients receive lidocaine has not been possible, as only 50% of patients who develop VF have 'warning' ventricular arrhythmia. In the 'thrombolytic and β-blocker' era of treatment of AMI, the use of prophylactic lidocaine, or any other antiarrhythmic drug, to prevent VF will have even less benefit. There are no conclusive data to support the use of lidocaine to prevent recurrent VF in those patients who have already suffered an episode of VF. Despite this, a short period of 6–24 h of lidocaine has been advocated.

Patients who survive a late or secondary episode of VF/VT following myocardial infarction require full evaluation for preventive strategies, as do survivors of SCD. All survivors of a myocardial infarction are at an increased risk for SCD but accurate prediction is not feasible. Risk factors that have been shown to be associated with increased risk of a subsequent episode of VF/VT after myocardial infarction include:

- age
- Holter monitoring and demonstration of non-sustained VT, couplets and frequent VEB (i.e. >10 beats/min)
- impaired LV function (i.e. ejection fraction less than 30–40%)
- signal-average ECG and detection of delayed after-potentials. In patients presenting with SCD after myocardial infarction, 68–87% have an abnormal signal-average ECG. However the positive predictive value is poor, at 15–25%
- demonstrated inducibility of VT postinfarction is associated with increased risk of SCD. However, the positive predictive value is again poor, at 20–30%

Combinations of these risk factors have been evaluated to predict risk after infarction. The combination of delayed potentials on signal-average ECG, LV ejection fraction of less than 40% and non-sustained VT on Holter monitor has been shown to be associated with up to 50% risk of SCD. Currently, there is no agreement on which patients require primary preventive strategies for VF/VT following myocardial infarction.

Using frequent VEB to identify patients at risk following myocardial infarction has been extensively used. There have been 54 randomised trials reported involving more than 20 000 patients using 11 different class I agents.

Class I agents showed no overall benefit on all-cause mortality and class IC agents have excess mortality despite arrhythmia suppression.[13]

Class II antiarrhythmics, β-blockers, have an established and broadening role, with recent evidence showing significant benefit.[69]

Class III agents lack a consistent class effect. Sotalol (Survival with oral D-sotalol: SWORD) was found to increase all-cause mortality and arrhythmia deaths.[70] Amiodarone (Canadian Amiodarone Myocardial Infarction Arrhythmia Trial: CAMIAT) reduces all-cause mortality in patients with frequent VEB post myocardial infarction[71] but another study (European Myocardial Infarction Amiodarone Trial: EMIAT) evaluated amiodarone in patients with ejection fraction less than 40% and found no effect on all-cause mortality but a 35% reduction in arrhythmia deaths.[72] Subsequent analysis of combined CAMIAT and EMIAT data has emphasised the importance of β-blockers. The combination of amiodarone and β-blockers in these post-infarct patients was better than either drug alone.[73]

CARDIOTHORACIC SURGERY AND ARRHYTHMIA

SVT AFTER CARDIOTHORACIC SURGERY[74]

AF predominates, with Afl and unifocal atrial tachyarrhythmia also commonly occurring after coronary artery bypass grafting, with an incidence of 11–40% and in over 50% following valvular surgery. In addition to mechanisms found in non-surgical patients, pericardial inflammation or effusion, increased catecholamine production and postoperative autonomic changes are implicated. Major risk factors include:

- previous history of AF
- increasing age
- postoperative withdrawal of β-blocker therapy

Extent of coronary artery disease, postoperative ischaemia, duration of aortic cross-clamping or cardiopulmonary bypass and method of myocardial protection do not influence incidence. SVT post cardiothoracic surgery is not a benign event, with the major consequence being thromboembolic complications. Stroke occurs following coronary artery bypass grafting in 1–6% of patients and postoperative atrial tachyarrhythmias increase the incidence threefold. Other adverse effects include:

- haemodynamic instability
- prolonged inotropic support
- need for intra-aortic balloon pump
- reoperation for bleeding
- longer and more expensive critical care unit and hospital episodes

PREVENTION OF SUPRAVENTRICULAR TACHYCARDIA[75,76]

Preoperative β-blocker treatment should be continued postoperatively. β-Blockers consistently reduce SVT across many studies with differing agents.

Amiodarone prophylaxis after elective cardiac surgery reduced postoperative AF from 53% to 25%. Diltiazem has also been shown to be effective at SVT prevention and there was associated improvement in haemodynamic variables and rates of myocardial ischaemia. Verapamil is not effective. Esmolol was found to be more effective than diltiazem. Sotalol is also effective but problematic bradycardia and hypotension are greater.[77] Atorvastatin is also effective.[78]

There is no relation between SVT incidence and serum magnesium levels and there are conflicting data relating to the efficacy of prophylactic magnesium. Digoxin has no role in prevention.

TREATMENT OF SUPRAVENTRICULAR TACHYCARDIA

Treatment is aimed at control of ventricular rate, prevention of thromboembolism and cardioversion.

Digoxin, atenolol, diltiazem and magnesium are appropriate choices to control rate.

In persisting AF, the timing of electrical cardioversion is debatable. Early electrical cardioversion, inside 24–48 h, avoids the need for anticoagulation but is associated with a significant recurrence rate as postoperative arrhythmogenic factors remain. In persistent or recurrent AF, sotalol and amiodarone, depending on myocardial function, are suitable antiarrhythmic drugs and should be continued for 6–12 weeks following cardioversion.

Timing of safe anticoagulation following cardiac surgery is also debatable. Many advocate delaying anticoagulation till 72 h postsurgery, which may be greater than 24–48 h after onset of SVT. Most cardiac surgical patients receive aspirin and low-dose heparin in the early postoperative period, which is likely to reduce risk. However, it is worth noting that, in other AF settings, 325 mg of aspirin decreased thromboembolic but 75 mg did not.

VENTRICULAR ARRHYTHMIA FOLLOWING CARDIAC SURGERY

Ventricular arrhythmia requiring treatment, DC shock or drug therapy is common following cardiac surgery and occurs in 23% of patients.[79] Arrhythmias requiring DC shock occur in the first 36 h and are associated with:

- advanced age
- failure to use an internal mammary artery conduit (which is likely to reflect preoperative assessment of high risk)
- SVT

The incidence was not related to previous myocardial infarction, ejection fraction of less than 50%, prolonged operative time, perioperative myocardial infarction or reduced number of vessels bypassed. In patients undergoing coronary artery bypass, grafting patients at high risk for sudden death, LV ejection fraction less than 36% and abnormalities on signal-averaged ECG had a 6.3% incidence of sustained VT and 4.3% VF.

VEB are common early on return from surgery, with frequent or complex ectopy associated with adrenergic effects of emerging from anaesthesia and hypokalaemia. The threshold to treat these arrhythmia varies with clinicians. Potassium must be regularly checked and maintained above 4 mmol/l.

If there is accompanying emergent hypertension, in addition to the antiarrhythmic action, the vasodilating properties of magnesium provide an ideal profile at this stage. Patients with VT/VF reverting with DC shock who are haemodynamically stable should have prophylactic antiarrhythmic cover until adrenergic stimulation associated with awakening and weaning from mechanical ventilation is past. Lidocaine has been the agent of choice, but magnesium, amiodarone and sotalol are all more effective. Maintaining antiarrhythmic levels of magnesium may not be conducive to weaning from ventilation. Extrapolating from post myocardial infarct data would support the conversion to β-blockers if there were no contraindications.

A smaller proportion of patients develop malignant VF/VT, most often in association with poor LV function and a postoperative low-cardiac-output state requiring catecholamine infusions. In this setting, ventricular arrhythmia is common, often initiated by short-coupling polymorphous VT (normal QT_c), due to ongoing ischaemia or reperfusion of ischaemic heart.

- High-dose amiodarone may work best in combination with antiarrhythmic levels of magnesium (1.8–2.0 mmol/l) or lidocaine.
- Many of these patients need an intra-aortic balloon pump to defend coronary artery perfusion pressure not only because of the likely poor LV function and low-output state, but also to minimise the adverse affects of antiarrhythmic drugs and recurrent DC shocks.
- Pacing may be required to counteract bradyarrhythmia associated with escalating doses of antiarrhythmic drugs. Pacing at faster rates (90–110 beats/min, which may not be ideal from a cardiac-output point of view) may be protective against recurrent episodes by promoting homogeneity of depolarisation and suppression of abnormal automaticity. The presence of epicardial or transvenous pacing wires also enables bedside-programmed stimulation and overdrive pacing for termination of recurrent VT, which has fewer deleterious effects than recurrent DC shocks.

LONG-QT SYNDROME[80]

The traditional criteria of prolonged QT is corrected heart rate (QT_c, Bazett's formula, QT divided by the square root of the RR interval) and a QT_c greater than 0.44 s. This should also be adjusted for age and gender. The causes of LQTS can be divided into acquired and idiopathic (Table 18.11). Common to all causes is a prolongation of repolarisation which creates the substrate for random re-entry, giving rise to polymorphous VT (classically of the torsade de pointes type), particularly under conditions of acute adrenergic arousal.

Action potential prolongation results from either enhancing depolarisation (Na channel, I_{Na}) or reducing repolarisation current (delayed rectifier K currents, I_{Kr} and I_{Ks}).

There is less capacity to respond to additional stresses that impair repolarisation such as hypokalaemia, hypomagnesaemia and drugs with class III action.

Prolonged action potential in LQTS prediposes to arrhythmia in two ways:

1. Extended plateau phase of action potential results in susceptibilty to EAD-initiated arrhythmia.
2. Heterogeneity of prolonged action potential creates spatial dispersion of repolarisation, leading to regions of refractory block and substrate for re-entrant arrhythmia. This mechanism appears important in pharmacological LQTS.

Table 18.11 Causes of long-QT syndrome

Acquired
Drugs
Class IA antiarrhythmic drugs
Quinidine, procainamide
Class III antiarrhythmic drugs
Amiodarone, sotalol
Tricyclic antidepressants
Macrolide antibiotics
Phenothiazines
Antihistamines
Cisapride
Myocardial ischaemia/infarction
Hypokalaemia
Cardiomyopathy
Acute myocarditis
Mitral valve prolapse
Acute cerebral injury
Hypothermia
Idiopathic
Familial: 90%
Linked to a DNA marker on the short arm of chromosome 11
Autosomal-dominant in most cases
Some cases linked to congenital deafness and autosomal-recessive
Sporadic: 10%
Non-familial – related to new gene mutation

IDIOPATHIC LQTS[81]

Idiopathic LQTS is characterised by genetic heterogeneity with mutations in seven gene loci (*LQT1–7*), described below.

LQT1 involves mutation of gene *KCNQ1* encoding for I_{Ks} K^+ channel, resulting in impaired K^+ repolarising current. This accounts for approximately 50% of idiopathic LQTS, with an incidence of SCD of 0.30%/year, and has an inheritance pattern of both autosomal-dominant and recessive.

LQT2 involves gene *KCNH2* encoding for I_{Kr} K^+ channel, again resulting in impaired K^+ repolarising current. This accounts for 30–40%, has an incidence of SCD of 0.60%/year and the inheritance pattern is autosomal dominant.

LQT3 involves gene *SCN5A* encoding for I_{Na} Na^+ channel, resulting in increased Na^+ depolarising current. It accounts for 5–10%, has an incidence of SCD of 0.56%/year and the inheritance pattern is autosomal dominant.

The other described genetic mutations leading to LQTS are rare.

CLINICAL FEATURES[82]

Prevalence is estimated to be 1 in 3000–5000.

Thirty per cent of patients with idiopathic LQTS present with unexplained syncope or aborted sudden death (which is often not the first episode). The majority (60%) are identified when family members are screened after syncope or cardiac arrest in a family member. Ten per cent are detected on routine evaluation of ECG. The majority of episodes of syncope or sudden death (60%) are precipitated by emotions, physical activity or auditory stimuli causing acute adrenergic arousal. The degree of QT_c prolongation is not predictive of syncope or sudden death.

MANAGEMENT

The first line of management of polymorphous VT with shock is DC shock, with magnesium being the anti-arrhythmic of choice.[83]

- Unresponsive rhythms or recurrence despite magnesium require pharmacological intervention (isoprenaline or adrenaline (epinephrine) depending on blood pressure) or electrical pacing.
- Factors associated with acquired LQTS need to be identified and eliminated.

Strategies for prevention of recurrence in idiopathic LQTS depend on the presentation. Patients who present with or have a history of syncope or aborted sudden death have a high risk of recurrence (5% per year). β-Blockers are the first line of treatment with the goal of reducing the exercise heart rate to less than 130 beats/min. Symptomatic bradycardia following adequate β-blockade requires a permanent pacemaker. Patients with recurrence despite these measures and those with an early malignant course need stellate sympathetic ganglionectomy. In 5% of these high-risk patients triple therapy fails and an implantable defibrillator is required. Asymptomatic patients with incidental LQTS (< 0.5% per year) and asymptomatic family members (0.5% per year) have a very low risk of syncope or sudden death. It is also very rare for the first episode to be fatal in these two groups so prophylactic measures are generally not required and close follow-up is sufficient.

Class IA, IC and III drugs may increase QT interval and should be avoided in polymorphous VT and torsade de pointes.

SUDDEN CARDIAC DEATH[84]

Arrhythmic causes of SCD can be divided into three categories:

1. primary VT or VF (most common)
2. primary SVT with a very rapid ventricular rate. This is usually associated with the development of AF or flutter in the presence of an accessory AV connection (but can occasionally be due to enhanced conduction over the normal AV conduction system)
3. bradycardia or asystole. Usually the result of an inadequate escape pacemaker mechanism associated with either a high-degree AV block or severe sinus node dysfunction. In addition, some patients with sinus node dysfunction have paroxysmal supraventricular arrhythmia (tachycardia–bradycardia syndrome) that on termination results in an exaggerated overdrive suppression of both the sinus node and escape pacemakers such that the prolonged pause evolves into asystole or VF

The causes of these arrhythmia can be divided into three general categories:

1. ischaemic heart disease. AMI or old myocardial infarction scar
2. non-ischaemic heart disease – cardiomyopathy, valvular heart disease, congenital heart disease, ventricular hypertrophy and cardiac trauma
3. no apparent structural heart disease – primary electrical disease, electrolyte abnormalities, prolonged QT syndromes and drugs

Contributing factors are often multifactorial, particularly the combination of structural heart disease, proarrhythmic drugs and electrolyte abnormalities.

EVALUATION OF A SURVIVOR OF SCD

Primary prevention of SCD has been disappointing due to difficulties in selecting patients at risk. Regardless of the aetiology of the SCD, the reported recurrence rate is high, at least 30–40% at 1 year. Therefore, in-hospital assessment is critical to establish the underlying cause and to guide therapy.

CORONARY ARTERY DISEASE AND SUDDEN CARDIAC DEATH

Extensive atherosclerotic coronary artery disease is the most common pathological finding in survivors and non-survivors of SCD. Fewer than 30% have evidence of a recent AMI. A larger proportion (up to 50%) has evidence of coronary artery thrombosis or plaque fissuring and rupture. In those patients not having an AMI, the majority (75%) have coronary artery stenosis (> 50% of lumen), and 60% have three-vessel disease. Approximately 50% have evidence of an old myocardial infarction. The fact that the typical pathological background for SCD is severe epicardial coronary artery disease, with or without an old myocardial infarction and evidence of a new ischaemic syndrome, underlines the central role that coronary artery disease plays in SCD.

INVESTIGATIONS[15–17]

- chest X-ray: cardiac size, presence of pulmonary oedema
- 12-lead ECG: acute ischaemia, previous infarction, ventricular aneurysm or LV hypertrophy. Abnormalities of rate, rhythm, conduction or sinus node dysfunction. PR interval, QRS complex duration or QT interval. Changes of electrolyte abnormalities
- plasma electrolytes: potassium, magnesium and calcium. Potassium levels may be difficult to interpret after a period of resuscitation
- cardiac enzymes: serial troponin, creatinine phosphokinase with myocardial band fractionation and lactate dehydrogenase to establish the presence of a recent AMI
- plasma blood levels of drugs that affect cardiac rhythm or conduction: while proarrhythmic effects of drugs are more likely at high levels, it should be emphasised that proarrhythmia can occur at normal or low plasma drug levels
- toxicology screen: substance abuse or drug overdose (cocaine, psychotropic drugs), particularly in patients without overt structural heart disease
- 24-h Holter monitor ECG: quantitative analysis of frequency of arrhythmia and to detect silent myocardial ischaemia
- assessment of LV function: LV ejection fraction. Gated pool scan gives a better estimate of global LV systolic function, but echocardiogram will give added diagnostic information such as valvular disease and myocardial hypertrophy. Both studies will detect segmental wall motion abnormalities
- exercise tolerance test: standard exercise ECG or thallium-201 scans. Echocardiogram immediately following exercise may be as informative
- signal-average ECG: averages between 100 and 400 heart beats, for identification of low-amplitude electrical signals, such as afterdepolarisations. These are

found in the terminal portion of the QRS complex and cannot be seen on the 12-lead ECG. Associated with an increased risk of spontaneous and inducible ventricular arrhythmia
- cardiac catheterisation and coronary angiogram: to quantify the degree of coronary artery disease.
- EPS: virtually always indicated to document and characterise ventricular tachyarrhythmia. The initial baseline EPS should be performed in the absence of any antiarrhythmic drugs. Inducibility of sustained ventricular arrhythmias at EPS is associated with worse outlook, with a 5-year risk of SCD of 32% versus 24% in those without inducible arrhythmia, and is an indication for an implantable defibrillator. The inducibility of VT/VF is less common in survivors of SCD (44%) than patients who present with recurrent sustained VT. In patients with sustained monomorphic haemodynamically stable VT, EPS mapping techniques are used to determine the possibility of surgical or catheter ablation. EPS is also important in other causes of SCD other than VT/VF. Patients with ventricular pre-excitation (WPW syndrome) require localisation of the accessory pathway. Propensity to develop complete heart block can be assessed by a His-bundle ECG.

PREVENTION OF RECURRENT VENTRICULAR ARRHYTHMIA IN SURVIVORS OF SUDDEN CARDIAC DEATH

MYOCARDIAL REVASCULARISATION AND SUDDEN CARDIAC DEATH

The Coronary Artery Surgery Study (CASS) registry looked at 13 476 patients with significant operable coronary artery disease and showed an incidence of SCD of 5.2% in the medical arm compared to 1.8% in those assigned to surgery.[85] The precise mechanism of the benefit of surgery in primary prevention is unclear but is probably associated with prevention of ischaemia rather than arrhythmia control. In summary, the near-universal practice of surgical coronary revascularisation in SCD survivors with critical stenoses is based upon this primary prevention data (and the central role that ischaemia and infarction are known to play in arrhythmia substrate) rather than data demonstrating arrhythmia control.

ANTIARRHYTHMIC DRUGS AND SUDDEN CARDIAC DEATH[13,70–73]

The CAST study has clearly demonstrated the poor results of antiarrhythmic drug therapy alone in the prevention of arrhythmic SCD. Data from studies in survivors of SCD using amiodarone are conflicting, but generally poor, even with EPS confirmation of lack of inducibility. Certainly patients with an ejection fraction less than 30% do poorly on amiodarone alone. The primary role of antiarrhythmic drugs in the secondary prevention of SCD has all but disappeared, but amiodarone may be indicated if there is demonstrable suppression of inducible VT at EPS and the patient has an ejection fraction greater than 30–40%.

SURGICAL AND CATHETER ABLATION TECHNIQUES AND SUDDEN CARDIAC DEATH[26]

As most sustained ventricular arrhythmias arise from a scar within the myocardium, surgical attempts were made to excise these areas completely. Catheter ablation techniques for VT are suitable for the minority of patients with haemodynamically stable VT who can withstand prolonged mapping procedures. Currently, the success rates for ablative techniques are such that a significant number still need additional preventive therapies.

IMPLANTABLE CARDIOVERTER DEFIBRILLATORS AND SUDDEN CARDIAC DEATH

The reduction in SCD and overall cardiac mortality with implantable cardioverter defibrillators (ICDs) has been so spectacular and the results of previous therapies so poor that ICDs were initially introduced with little randomised controlled data. More recently controlled studies have shown:

- reduction in 3-year mortality by 31% compared to antiarrhythmic drug therapy in SCD survivors[86]
- reduced risk of death in patients with poor LV function following myocardial infarction[87]
- improved survival in patients with hypertrophic cardiomyopathy[88]

However, no survival benefit was shown in high-risk patients following coronary artery bypass surgery.

Representative data from several studies are shown in Table 18.12. The benefit of ICD on survival persists for at least 8 years. Current indications are expanding, but the benefit is clear in the following groups of survivors of SCD and patients with documented VT/VF outside the early postinfarct phase:

- non-inducible VT/VF at EPS
- inducible VT/VF resistant to treatment
- VT/VF in patients with LV ejection fractions less than or equal to 30% regardless of results of EPS-directed drug therapy

Table 18.12 Mortality data for the various treatment regimens for sudden cardiac death

	Sudden death (%)	Total mortality (%)
Implantable cardioverter defibrillator	3.5	13.6
Empirical amiodarone	12.0	34.0
Electrophysiological study-directed drug treatment	14.0	24.0
Surgery	3.7	37.0

Further developments currently taking place include:

- transvenous catheter placement and subcutaneous patch avoiding the need for thoracotomy
- dual-chamber sensing to improve discrimination between SVT and VT that can be difficult on rate criteria alone, particularly in patients with intraventricular conduction delay
- technological advances reducing size, cost and increasing battery life

Although one of the proposed advantages of ICD is the avoidance of antiarrhythmic drug side-effects, particularly the myocardial depressant effects, current practice usually combines ICD with low-dose amiodarone. This enables improved arrhythmia control by reducing atrial tachyarrhythmia and slowing VT rate, and prolonging battery life by reducing the frequency of arrhythmia. The role of ICD in the management algorithms of SCD is shown in Figure 18.49 and 18.50. Given the current lack of available ICD, some advocate restriction to patients less than 75 years. With wider availability of ICD, fewer patients will be managed on drug-only strategies in the future.

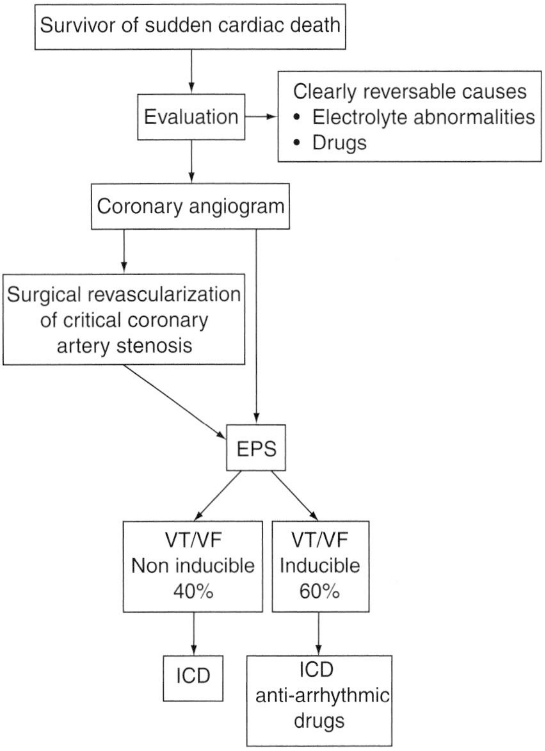

Figure 18.49 Management algorithm of a survivor of sudden cardiac death. This algorithm does not include the option of an antiarrhythmic drug alone in patients with intact left ventricular function who initially have inducible ventricular tachycardia/fibrillation (VT/VF) that is subsequently found to be suppressible on a drug with electrophysiological studies (EPS). ICD, implantable cardioverter defibrillator.

CLASSIFICATION OF ANTIARRHYTHMIC DRUGS

The time-honoured physiologically based classification of antiarrhythmic drugs is the Vaughan-Williams classification (Table 18.13), which has been modified over the years. This classification is a hybrid, with classes I and IV representing ion channel blockers, class II representing a receptor blocker and class III representing a change in an electrophysiological variable. The prolongation of repolarisation, the defining effect of

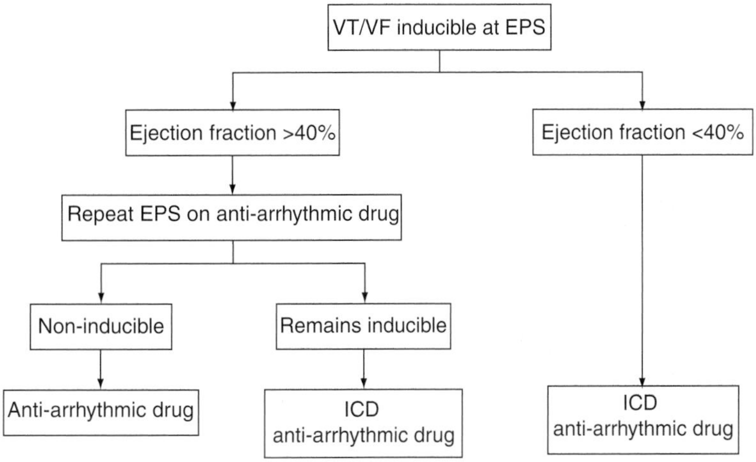

Figure 18.50 Patients found to have inducible ventricular tachycardia (VT) or fibrillation (VF) at electrophysiological studies (EPS), with an ejection fraction > 40% and subsequent drug suppression of their VT/VF, can be managed on antiarrhythmic drugs alone.

Table 18.13 Vaughan-Williams classification of antiarrhythmic drugs

	Mechanism of action	Effect on action potential	Indicative drugs
Class I	Sodium channel blockade	Depresses rate of rise of phase 0	
Class IA		Prolongs repolarisation	Procainamide Disopyramide Quinidine
Class IB		Shortens repolarisation	Lidocaine Mexiletine Phenytoin
Class IC		Minimal effect on repolarisation	Flecainide Encainide Propafenone
Class II	β-Adrenergic receptor blockers		Propranolol Atenolol Metoprolol Esmolol
Class III	Potassium channel blockers	Prolong repolarisation	Amiodarone Sotalol Ibutitide Bretylium
Class IV	Calcium channel blockers		Verapamil Diltiazem

class III agents, can be produced by a block of any one of several K^+ ionic channels (the delayed rectifier potassium current IKr responsible for phase 3 repolarisation is the ionic channel target of most class III agents) or from modification of Na^+ or Ca^+ channel function. This classification is also incomplete and does not include cholinergic agonists, digitalis, magnesium and adenosine. For this reason, an alternative classification has been advocated based upon molecular targets for drug action that include ion channels, receptors and pumps/carriers (Table 18.14).[2]

ANTIARRHYTHMIC DRUGS[68]

DIGOXIN

Digoxin is a muscurinic subtype 2 receptor (M_2) agonist and a highly potent Na^+,K^+-ATPase pump-blocking agent. Digoxin exerts its antiarrhythmic activity predominantly at the AV node where at lower doses conduction is slowed by the M_2 vagotonic effect. This effect is easily reversed by enhanced sympathetic tone in the setting of exercise, critical illness and postoperative state. At higher concentrations, digoxin has a direct effect on AV node conduction by the Na^+,K^+-ATPase pump blockade and is more resistant to sympathomimetic effects. The decrease in $[K^+]_i$ and increase in $[Na^+]_i$ results in hyperpolarisation, shortening of atrial action potential and an increase in AV nodal refractoriness. There is also increased availability of intracellular Na^+ for the Na^+-Ca^{2+} exchanger, increasing $[Ca^{2+}]_i$ which results in the positive inotropic effects of digoxin, making it an ideal agent in the setting of LV dysfunction. However, the positive inotropic effects of Na^+,K^+-ATPase blockade are deleterious in the setting of myocardial ischaemia and other causes of diastolic dysfunction. Digoxin also has weak vasopressor properties when administered as a slow bolus.[61] The major ECG effects of digoxin are PR prolongation and a non-specific alteration in ventricular repolarisation with characteristic reverse-tick S-T segments.

INDICATIONS AND DOSE

- AF: slowing of ventricular rate only
- loading dose: 15 μg/kg IV, typically administered over 30–60 min, but can be given faster
- maintenance dose depends on renal function

PLASMA LEVELS

Oral bioavailabiliy can be reduced, especially if intestinal microflora-altering antibiotics are coadministered. Therapeutic levels are 0.5–2.0 ng/ml. Plasma levels must be measured during the postdistribution phase some 6–8 h after dose. The elimination half-life is 36 h with normal renal function. Difference between therapeutic and toxic levels can be reduced by hypokalaemia, hypomagnesaemia, hypercalcaemia, hypoxia, cardiac surgery and myocardial ischaemia. Many drugs increase digoxin plasma levels by competing with the renal P-glycoprotein-mediated transport, or by reducing renal blood flow or function.

CONTRAINDICATIONS

Relative contraindications include myocardial ischaemia/infarction, diastolic heart failure due to hypertrophy and ischaemia, renal failure and hyperkalaemia, planned DC

Table 18.14 Actions of antiarrhythmic drugs on membrane channels, receptors and ionic pumps in the heart

Drug	Channels			Receptors						Pumps
	Na^+			Ca^{2+}	K^+	α	β	M_2	P	Na^+,K^+ ATPase
	Fast	Med	Slow							
Lidocaine	+									
Mexiletine	+									
Phenytoin	+									
Procainamide		+++			++					
Disopyramide		+++			++			+		
Quinidine		+++			++	+		+		
Propafenone		+++					++			
Flecainide			+++		+					
Encainide			+++							
Bretylium					+++	+/–	+/–			
Sotalol					+++		+++			
Amiodarone	+			+	+++	++	++			
Ibutilide					+++					
Dofetilide					+++					
Verapamil	+			+++		++				
Diltiazem				++						
Propranolol	+						+++			
Metoprolol							+++			
Esmolol							+++			
Atropine								+++		
Adenosine									A	
Digoxin								A		+++
Magnesium				+						A

Sodium channel blockers are subdivided into drugs with fast, medium and slow time constant for recovery from block. Receptors α, β-adrenoreceptors, muscarinic subtype 2 (M_2) and A_1 purinergic (P). Relative blocking potency: low +, moderate ++, high +++. Partial agonist/antagonist: +/–. Agonist: A.
(Modified with permission from Task Force of the Working Group on Arrhythmias of the European Society of Cardiology. The Sicilian gambit: a new approach to the classification of antiarrhythmic drugs based on their actions on arrhythmogenic mechanisms. *Circulation* 1991; **84**: 1831–51.)

shock cardioversion and tachycardia–bradycardia syndromes. Coadministration with other drugs that effect AV nodal conduction, typically β-adrenergic and calcium channel blockers, requires caution.

ADVERSE EFFECTS

The same increase in $[Ca]_i$ responsible for the positive inotropic effects of digoxin also forms the basis for toxicity arrhythmia. The increased inward calcium current is responsible for DAD-initiated arrhythmia. Digoxin toxicity can cause virtually any arrhythmia:

- DAD-related tachycardias with impairment of sinus node or AV nodal function
- unifocal atrial tachycardia with AV block is 'classic'
- ventricular bigeminy and various degrees of AV block occur

With advanced toxicity severe hyperkalaemia due to poisoning of Na^+,K^+-ATPase results. Profound bradycardia, which may be unresponsive to pacing, develops.

Any serious toxicity arrhythmia should be treated with antidigoxin Fab fragments. Magnesium is the drug of choice for digoxin-toxic tachyarrhythmias. Digoxin, particularly if at toxic levels, increases risk of VF precipitated by DC shock. Digoxin toxicity is associated with nausea, disturbances in cognitive function and blurred or yellow vision.

β-ADRENERGIC BLOCKERS

β-Adrenergic blocking or class II antiarrhythmic drugs have differing properties such as relative cardioselectivity (atenolol, metoprolol), non-cardioselectivity (propranolol), intrinsic sympathomimetic activity (pindolol), lipid solubility and central activity (metoprolol, propranolol) and membrane-depressant effects (propranolol). The antiarrhythmic properties appear to be a class effect and no agent has been shown to be superior. There are data to suggest that the survival benefit of β-adrenergic blockers post myocardial infarction may relate to some extent to the central modulation of autonomic tone of the more lipid-soluble agents. The direct membrane-stabilising or 'quinidine-like' effect of propranolol requires doses far greater than those used clinically and is of negligible clinical significance. β-Adrenergic blockers competitively inhibit catecholamine binding at the β-adrenergic receptor sites, which reduces the phase 4 slope of the action potential of pacemaker cells, prolongs their refractoriness and slows conduction in the AV node. Refractoriness and conduction in the His–Purkinje system are unchanged. β-Adrenergic blockers are most effective in arrhythmia associated with increased cardiac adrenergic stimulation (postoperative states, sepsis, thyrotoxicosis, phaeochromocytoma, exercise or emotion).

INDICATIONS

Supraventricular tachycardias

β-Adrenergic blockers may terminate SVT when the AV node is an intrinsic part of the re-entry circuit (AVNRT and AVRT); adenosine is more effective. AF and Afl do not revert with β-adrenergic blockers but the ventricular rate will be slowed. β-adrenergic blockers are effective at preventing SVT following cardiac surgery. Studies involving propranolol and atenolol have produced the best results. β-Adrenergic blockers are effective in MAT, but, as this arrhythmia is most often seen in patients with severe chronic airflow limitation and cor pulmonale, their utility is limited.[30]

Ventricular arrhythmias

β-Adrenergic blockers are ineffective for the emergency treatment of sustained VT. Empiric prophylactic administration of β-adrenergic blockers appears to be as effective in ventricular arrhythmia prevention as electrophysiologically guided drug methods. However ventricular arrhythmia most often occurs in the setting of poor LV dysfunction and β-adrenergic blockers are either poorly tolerated or contraindicated.

Myocardial infarction

Survival in patients with AMI treated with thrombolytics is probably improved by early IV β-adrenergic blockade. There may be other benefits such as decreased incidence of VF and relief of chest pain. Long-term β-adrenergic blockade reduces mortality following myocardial infarction, the benefit being greatest in those at highest risk for sudden death. However, suppression of ventricular ectopy is not a requisite for benefit. Drugs with intrinsic sympathomimetic activity have not been shown to improve survival after AMI.

ATENOLOL

Atenolol does not have significant central action due to poor lipid solubility and is eliminated predominantly by the kidneys with an elimination half-life of 7–9 h. Care is required in patients with poor or deteriorating renal function.

- loading dose IV: 5 mg every 10 min, maximum 10 mg
- loading dose oral: 50–100 mg
- maintenance dose oral: 50–200 mg/day
- ISIS-1 post-MI regime: 5 mg IV over 5 min, repeated 10 min later if heart rate exceeds 60 beats/min. If heart rate exceeds 40 beats/min 10 min later, oral 50 mg atenolol and continue at 100 mg daily
- SVT prophylaxis following cardiac surgery: 5 mg IV within 3 h of surgery, repeated 24 h later, followed by oral 50 mg daily for 6 days

METOPROLOL

Metoprolol is lipid-soluble and has significant central action. It is eliminated by the liver with an elimination half-life of 3–4 h.

- loading dose IV: 1–2 mg/min, maximum dose of 15–20 mg
- loading dose oral: 100–200 mg
- maintenance dose oral: 50–100 mg/12-hourly

PROPRANOLOL

Propranolol has been one of the most studied β-adrenergic blockers for SVT prophylaxis following cardiac surgery.

- dose: 10 mg orally 6-hourly starting the morning after surgery

ESMOLOL

Esmolol is an ultrashort-acting cardioselective β-adrenergic blocker, which is especially useful for rapid control of ventricular rate in AF or Afl. Esmolol has also been shown to prevent postoperative SVT. The distribution half-life is 2 min and the elimination half-life is 9 min. Esmolol is rapidly metabolised by hydrolysis of the ester linkage, chiefly by the esterases in the cytosol of red blood cells and not by plasma cholinesterases or red cell membrane acetyl-cholinesterase.

- loading dose IV: 500 μg/kg over 1 min
- maintenance dose IV: 50 μg/kg per min for 4 min. If satisfactory rate control is not achieved, the loading dose should be repeated and the maintenance dose increased to 100 μg/kg per min. If control is still not achieved after a further 4 min, then the procedure is repeated with 50 μg/kg per min increments in the maintenance infusion until 300 μg/kg per min is reached. Further increases in infusion rate are unlikely to be successful.

CONTRAINDICATIONS

Reversible airways disease and poor LV function are two common relative contraindications, which limit the utility of β-adrenergic blockers in patients with cardiac disease. β-Adrenergic blockers may also be poorly tolerated in diabetics and patients with severe peripheral vascular disease.

ADVERSE EFFECTS

β-Adrenergic blockers, particularly those that are centrally acting, are often poorly tolerated in the long term. These effects include fatigue, hypotension, bradycardia, dry mouth, dizziness, headache and cold extremities.

CALCIUM CHANNEL BLOCKERS

Calcium channel blockers or class IV antiarrhythmic drugs block the slow calcium channels in cardiac tissue. Verapamil and diltiazem have similar electrophysiological properties. The dihydropyridine group of calcium channel blockers, which include nifedipine, does not have any significant electrophysiological properties. Calcium channel blockers depress the slope of diastolic depolarisation in the SA node cells, the rate of rise of the phase 0 and action potential amplitude in the SA and AV nodal cells. They also slow conduction and prolong the refractory period of the AV node, which results in their main antiarrhythmic actions. Refractoriness of atrial, ventricular and accessory pathway tissue is unchanged. The sinus rate does not usually change significantly because calcium channel blockers induce peripheral vasodilatation, which causes reflex sympathetic stimulation of SA node. Verapamil particularity has marked negative inotropic actions and hypotension is often seen; however, cardiac index is generally maintained because of afterload reduction. Diltiazem has less negative inotropic effect than verapamil.

INDICATIONS

- SVT: calcium channel blockers are effective if the AV node is an integral part of the arrhythmia circuit. Verapamil has been superseded by adenosine for the first line of treatment for these with AVNRT and AVRT.
- AF and Afl: slow ventricular response in AF and Afl, but termination of the arrhythmia is uncommon. Verapamil may prolong episodes of AF through a proarrhythmic effect.
- MAT[30]: calcium channel blockers are effective.
- SVT following cardiac surgery: diltiazem has been shown not only to reduce, but also to decrease incidence of ventricular arrhythmia and postoperative ischaemia.
- AF associated with the WPW syndrome: calcium channel blockers may increase the ventricular response and should be avoided if this is suspected.[27]

In general, calcium channel blockers should not be given to patients with a wide-complex tachycardia not only because of the risk of accelerating accessory pathway conduction, but also because their myocardial depressant effects can result in cardiovascular collapse in the setting of VT and pre-existing myocardial dysfunction.

VERAPAMIL

Verapamil is cleared by the liver with an elimination half-life of 3–8 h. Therapeutic plasma concentration is 0.1–0.15 mg/l. With the availability of adenosine and the better tolerance of diltiazem, the use of verapamil has fallen substantially.

- loading dose IV: 1 mg/min to a maximum of 10–15 mg or 0.15 mg/kg
- maintenance dose IV: 5 mg/kg per min
- maintenance dose oral: 80–120 mg 6–8-hourly

DILTIAZEM

Diltiazem is cleared by the liver with an elimination half-life of 3.5 h. There is reduced oral absorption and extensive first-pass hepatic metabolism: only 40% of oral dose is available compared with IV.

- loading dose IV: 0.25 mg/kg, followed by 0.35 mg/kg if required
- maintenance dose IV: 5–15 mg per h
- maintenance dose oral: 60–120 mg 6–8-hourly
- SVT prophylaxis following cardiac surgery: 0.1 mg/kg per hour, starting at onset of bypass and continuing for 24 h. The dose can be titrated up for blood pressure control

MAGNESIUM

Magnesium is an emerging antiarrhythmic agent with a range of indications; however, as an antiarrhythmic agent, magnesium has largely defied classification. Magnesium has many reported electrophysiological effects, including blocking voltage-dependent L-type Ca^{2+} channels. Magnesium is a necessary cofactor for the membrane enzyme Na^+/K^+-ATPase that provides energy for the membrane Na/K channels.[89] The consequences of magnesium deficiency are as follows:

- Intracellular potassium falls and intracellular sodium rises, leading to a reduction in RMP.
- Intracellular sodium is elevated, increasing the availability of sodium for the Na/Ca counter transport mechanism.
- The resulting elevation in intracellular calcium predisposes to DAD-triggered activity.

Magnesium administration reduces the availability of intracellular Na^+ and therefore this Ca^{2+} inward current. The dependency of normal membrane potassium gradients on magnesium is demonstrated by the inability to correct intracellular potassium deficiency with the administration of potassium in the setting of hypomagnesaemia. The antiarrhythmic properties of supranormal levels of magnesium associated with pharmacological doses of magnesium appear to be largely due to augmentation of this physiological role of magnesium. Therefore, magnesium may be best classified as a Na/K pump agonist.

Magnesium in pharmacological doses decreases RMP, resulting in a reduction in automaticity. However, once depolarisation occurs, the maximum rate of depolarisation and action potential amplitude is increased, thereby improving conduction. Action potential duration is increased, thereby increasing absolute refractory period and reducing relative refractory period. The net result is a reduction in the vulnerable period and more synchronous conduction. All of these electrophysiological effects are augmented in the setting of increased extracellular potassium. It is not surprising that the utility of magnesium appears greatest in the setting of ischaemia where loss of potassium from the cell is a major consequence.

A secondary effect is the reduction in the availability of intracellular sodium to contribute to inward calcium flux, producing triggered activity. Magnesium has also been shown to elevate VF and ectopy threshold.[90]

INDICATIONS

- acute rate control of AF, and has been shown to be as effective as amiodarone[63]
- prevent postoperative SVT following cardiac surgery with varying efficacy
- acute control of MAT
- ventricular arrhythmia associated with triggered activity, such as torsade de pointes and digoxin toxicity[83]
- drug-induced polymorphous VT, particularly that caused by class I agents, can also be terminated with magnesium
- appears very effective at controlling transient ventricular arrhythmia in the setting of ischaemia such as post-infarct and cardiac surgery

DOSE

- AF rate and MAT control: 0.15 mmol/kg as slow IV push. Subsequent dose recommendation has varied from 60 mmol to 0.1 mmol/kg per h for 24 h. Magnesium levels following 0.1 mmol/kg per h were 1.92 ± 0.49 mmol/l at 24 h
- SVT prophylaxis following cardiac surgery: 20–25 mmol per day for 4 days
- transient ventricular arrhythmia: 10 mmol as a slow IV push, repeated if required
- LIMIT-2 post myocardial infarction dose: 8 mmol bolus over 5 min, followed by 65 mmol over 24 h. Mean plasma level 1.55 (SD 0.44) mmol/l[65]

PLASMA LEVELS

Observational data would suggest that plasma levels of magnesium required for potent antiarrhythmic action are at least 1.8 mmol/l.

ADVERSE EFFECTS

- When administered too rapidly, magnesium can cause hypotension by excessive peripheral vasodilatation; this is associated with an unpleasant hot-flush sensation.
- Prolonged administration or excessive dosing can produce plasma levels associated with skeletal muscle weakness, which can be clinically significant in acute-on-chronic respiratory failure.
- Excessive action can be seen if magnesium is used in the setting of hyperkalaemia, resulting in brady-arrhythmia and heart block.

PROCAINAMIDE

Procainamide is a class IA antiarrhythmic drug with potent Na^+ channel-blocking activity and intermediate K^+ channel-blocking activity. The Na^+ channel-blocking action has an intermediate time constant of recovery. Procainamide has similar electrophysiological and ECG effects to quinidine but lacks vagolytic and α-adrenergic blocking activity:

- decreases automaticity
- increases refractory period
- slows conduction

Procainamide is metabolised to *N*-acetyl procainamide. *N*-acetyl procainamide lacks Na^+ channel-blocking activity, but is equipotent in K^+ channel blockade and prolongation of action potential. The increasing effect of greater refractoriness and QT prolongation with chronic procainamide therapy relates to increased contribution of *N*-acetyl procainamide.

CLINICAL USE

Procainamide is used to treat both atrial and ventricular arrhythmias.

- IV procainamide is more effective than lidocaine for terminating VT.
- Procainamide controls ventricular rate in AF and Afl.
- It is effective for conversion of AVNRT, AVRT and possibly AF and Afl.
- It controls rapid ventricular rate due to accessory pathway conduction in pre-excitation syndromes and for wide-complex tachycardias that cannot be distinguished as being SVT or VT.

The need to infuse slowly to avoid hypotension is the major barrier to wider use in life-threatening arrhythmia. Maintenance therapy with procainamide is not widely used due to its side-effect profile.

- loading dose IV: 6–17 mg/kg at 20 mg/min until there is arrhythmia control, hypotension ensues or QRS duration increases by more than 50%. Up to 50 mg/min has been used in urgent situations
- maintenance dose IV: 1–4 mg/min
- plasma levels: *N*-acetyl procainamide has a longer duration of action
- adverse effects: as with quinidine, the ventricular response may be accelerated if given for SVT. QT-interval prolongation and torsade de pointes may also occur

A reversible lupus-like syndrome develops in 20–30% of patients receiving procainamide long-term. Other side-effects include gastrointestinal disturbances (less common than with quinidine), central nervous system manifestations and cardiac depression.

LIDOCAINE

Lidocaine, long considered an important antiarrhythmic drug for ventricular tachyarrhythmia, is now relegated to lower-choice options or missing from most treatment algorithms. Na^+ channel-blocking effect is increased in myocardial ischaemia and is unproven outside acute ischaemia settings. It has no effect on SA node automaticity, but it depresses automaticity in other pacemaker tissues. Normally, lidocaine has little or no effect on conduction. The ECG shows no changes in sinus rate, PR interval, QRS width or QT interval with lidocaine.

CLINICAL USE

Lidocaine has reducing importance.

- It is ineffective against SVT.
- Amiodarone has taken over as the antiarrhythmic of choice for DC shock-resistant VF.[58,59]
- Lidocaine increases the current required for defibrillation, increases the likelihood of post DC shock asystole and therefore is detrimental during an episode of VF.
- Prophylaxis to prevent VF in AMI can no longer be recommended.

Extensive first-pass hepatic metabolism precludes oral use of lidocaine; IV dose should be reduced by 30–50% in severe liver disease or heart failure. The distribution half-life is about 8 min, and the elimination half-life is 1.5 h in normal patients (but may be increased > 10h in severe heart failure or shock). An initial bolus of IV lidocaine 1.5–2.0 mg/kg over 1–2 min, followed by an infusion of 4 mg/min for 1 h, then 2 mg/min for 2 h, and thereafter 1–2 mg/min, is recommended. Increasing the maintenance infusion rate without an additional bolus requires about 6 h (four elimination half-lives) to reach a steady state. If the initial bolus is ineffective, another bolus of 1 mg/kg may be given after 5 min. Another dosage regimen is 1.5–2.0 mg/kg initially, and 0.8 mg/kg at 8-min intervals for three doses (i.e. three distribution half-lives), and thereafter 1–2 mg/min by infusion. The half-life of lidocaine increases after 24–48 h as the drug in effect inhibits its own hepatic metabolism and dose reduction is required.

ADVERSE EFFECTS

Central nervous system toxicity with high plasma concentrations are the most common adverse effects (e.g. dizziness, paraesthesia, confusion, and coma and convulsions). Uncommonly, AV block or cardiac depression may occur. Cimetidine reduces lidocaine clearance, potentially causing toxic drug concentrations.

FLECAINIDE

Flecainide exhibits rate-dependent Na^+ channel blockade with slow time constant of recovery, with marked slowing of conduction in all cardiac tissue, and little prolongation of refractoriness.

CLINICAL USE

- may revert AVNRT and AVRT, although adenosine and verapamil are more widely used
- useful in SVT, including AF and possibly Afl, particularly in the setting of accessory pathway syndromes
- flecainide has been given in life-threatening VT

Flecainide can be administered IV or orally. If flecainide is deemed necessary for prophylaxis of ventricular arrhythmias, therapy should start with ECG monitoring. In CAST, suppression of VEBs after myocardial infarction with flecainide was associated with increased mortality.[13]

- dose: IV loading 2 mg/kg at 10 mg/min
- oral maintenance: 100–200 mg 12-hourly

ADVERSE EFFECTS

- Depression of cardiac contractility. Flecainide is usually contraindicated in patients with abnormal LV function as it can worsen or precipitate heart failure.
- Conduction block. Avoid in high-degree AV block unless a pacemaker is in situ.
- Flecainide increases pacing capture threshold.
- Proarrhythmic events are common, especially in patients with depressed LV function, and may be life-threatening.
- Torsade de pointes may occur, even in patients without structural heart disease.
- Incessant VT may be induced, unresponsive to any therapy, including cardioversion.
- Although flecainide depresses intracardiac conduction, a paradoxical increase in ventricular rate may occur with Afl or fibrillation.
- Central nervous system effects include visual disturbances, dizziness and nausea.

PROPAFENONE

Propafenone has a similar electrophysiological, haemodynamic and side-effect profile to flecainide and encainide. In addition, propafenone has non-selective β-blocking properties. Similar to flecainide, propafenone could be considered in both ventricular and SVT arrhythmia in the setting of normal LV function. Use of long-term propafenone should probably be limited because of its class IC profile, even though it was not included in the CAST study.

- dose: IV 2 mg/kg at 10 mg/min

AMIODARONE

Amiodarone is a potent antiarrhythmic agent with a complex electrophysiological and pharmacological profile. The appealing broad spectrum and haemodynamic stability of amiodarone have resulted in it emerging as the most frequently used antiarrhythmic in critically ill patients. In this setting short-term use predominates and the formidable side-effect profile is much less significant. Amiodarone:

- prolongs action potential duration
- increases the refractoriness of all cardiac tissue
- has Na^+ channel blockade (class I), antiadrenergic (class II), calcium channel blockade (class IV) and antifibrillatory effects. The Na^+ channel blockade of amiodarone has a fast time constant for recovery
- QT prolongation reflects a global prolongation of repolarisation and is closely associated with its antiarrhythmic effects

When given IV, amiodarone has little immediate class III effect: the major action is on the AV node, causing a delay in intranodal conduction and a prolongation of refractoriness. This probably explains why IV amiodarone controls the ventricular rate in recent-onset AF, but is less effective for termination of this arrhythmia. Administration IV causes some cardiac depression, the magnitude depending on rate of administration and pre-existing LV function. Cardiac index is often unchanged because of its vasodilator properties.

CLINICAL USE

It is effective in suppressing both supraventricular and ventricular tachyarrhythmias.

SUPRAVENTRICULAR TACHYCARDIA

Amiodarone is effective in terminating and suppressing recurrences of AVNRT and AVRT tachycardias, although adenosine (for acute reversion) or verapamil (acute termination and long-term prophylaxis) is superior. Amiodarone IV is less effective in reverting Afl or AF, but the ventricular rate will slow. Administration over a longer time span (days to weeks) may be more effective in reverting recent-onset AF. In preventing recurrence of AF after reversion, amiodarone is comparable in efficacy to quinidine and flecainide but superior to sotalol and propafenone.[47]

DOSE

- Lower doses than that required for ventricular arrhythmia are usually sufficient.
- AVNRT and AVRT reversion AF and Afl rate control: 3–5 mg/kg IV over 10–60 min depending on blood pressure and myocardial function, followed by 0.35–0.5 mg/kg per h. Poor rate control can be improved with additional 1–2 mg/kg boluses.
- Postoperative AF prophylaxis: 200 mg orally 8-hourly for 5 days, followed by daily until hospital discharge.
- Long-term SVT control or AF rate control: 100–200 mg/day orally will usually suffice.

VENTRICULAR TACHYARRHYTHMIAS

Amiodarone IV may be effective in treating life-threatening ventricular tachyarrhythmias refractory to other drugs, especially in myocardial infarction and poor LV function. Amiodarone's efficacy in DC shock-resistant VF further confirms a prominent role in this setting.[58,59] Long-term oral amiodarone is useful is controlling symptomatic VT and VF, especially when other conventional antiarrhythmics have failed. The absence of negative inotropic effect is useful in those with severely depressed LV function, but its many adverse effects limit widespread use. The Cardiac Arrest in Seattle, Conventional versus Amiodarone Drug Evaluation (CASCADE) study demonstrated that empirical amiodarone treatment was superior to guided (non-invasive Holter or EPS) class I drugs in survivors of VF unassociated with AMI. Amiodarone prevented arrhythmia recurrence and decreased the incidence of sudden death. Amiodarone, presumably because it is better tolerated in patients with poor LV function and having less proarrhythmia, can be considered as first-line drug to prevent life-threatening ventricular tachyarrhythmias.[71–73] The rate of arrhythmia control is often slower with ventricular arrhythmia and may take several days to achieve. This delay appears to be independent of dose. The pharmacodynamic basis for this relates to the fact that much of the class III or K^+ channel-blocking activity is due to the amiodarone metabolite, desethylamiodarone, whereas the predominant actions of acute administration of amiodarone are due to its class I and class II activity. The full potency of the class III activity requires several days, at least, for the effects of desethylamiodarone to appear.

DOSE

- haemodynamic stable VT: 5–7 mg/kg over 30–60 min, followed by 0.5–0.6 mg/kg per h
- DC shock-resistant VF: 5 mg/kg, followed by 2.5 mg/kg if required[59]
- long-term prevention of ventricular arrhythmia: oral loading with 1200 mg/day for 1–2 weeks, reducing to 400–600 mg/day and then 100–400 mg/day after 2–3 months. The dose should probably not be reduced below 400 mg/day with life-threatening ventricular arrhythmia

MYOCARDIAL INFARCTION

Data are limited at present, but amiodarone may improve long-term survival in patients after myocardial infarction.

PHARMACOKINETICS

Oral bioavailabiliy of amiodarone is variable at 40–70% with a delayed onset of action (days to weeks); however loading doses reduce this interval. Initial IV dose recommendations were 5–7 mg/kg over 30 min, followed by 50 mg/h. The kinetics of amiodarone have been modelled to four compartments when given acutely. Following a slow IV bolus over 15 min, amiodarone is rapidly distributed to the active compartment ($t_{1/2}a$ = 4.2 min), with demonstrable prolongation of QTc and antiarrhythmic effect within 2–5 min. Subsequently, amiodarone is progressively redistributed to 'deeper' compartments ($t_{1/2}b$ = 36.6 min, $t_{1/2}g$ = 4.5 h and $t_{1/2}d$ = 33.6 h).[91] This is in contrast to the very prolonged terminal half-life – greater than 50 days – after long-term treatment. This redistribution of amiodarone explains why repeated boluses are often required in the first 24–48 h of treatment. Transient loading-dose hypotension due to myocardial depression or vasodilatation is dose-, rate- and patient-dependent. A loading dose of 5 mg/kg over 20 min resulted in significant further myocardial depression and a fall in cardiac index, whereas in patients without evidence of heart failure, 5 mg/kg over 1 min resulted in hypotension due to systemic vasodilatation and an increase in cardiac index.[92,93]

MONITORING

Plasma amiodarone concentrations have poor correlation with arrhythmia control, and therapeutic levels, 1.0–2.5 mg/l, have the greatest utility for avoidance of adverse effects in long-term treatment.

ADVERSE EFFECTS

Adverse effects will occur in the majority of patients if they receive amiodarone for long enough. Most are reversible when the drug is discontinued. Adverse effects include:

- dermatological: photosensitivity, bluish/grey skin discoloration (slate-blue skin)
- eye: corneal microdeposits (almost 100%) with little or no clinical significance
- gastrointestinal disturbances
- hypo- and hyperthyroidism
- liver dysfunction: asymptomatic increases in liver enzymes are common, and do not require amiodarone cessation unless enzymes are 2–3 times normal; hepatitis is rare
- neuropathy, myopathy and cerebellar abnormalities
- pulmonary toxicity: unexpected acute respiratory distress syndrome has been reported in patients on amiodarone undergoing procedures such as uncomplicated cardiopulmonary bypass surgery and pulmonary angiography. These observations suggest that amiodarone may predispose the lung to acute injury. Pulmonary toxicity is the most serious adverse effect, with a reported incidence of 10% at 3 years. Amiodarone pulmonary toxicity has been reported in one case after 13 days and 11.2 g cumulative dose and 11.2 g over 2 weeks in another. Patients on long-term amiodarone need regular respiratory function testing and an increase in diffusion limitation of carbon monoxide 15% above baseline requires dose modification or cessation. The severe syndrome of shortness of breath, cough and fever with pulmonary crepitations and widespread pulmonary infiltrates on chest X-ray has a mortality of 10%. Immediate discontinuation is necessary. Use of steroids is controversial

Amiodarone interacts with other drugs, potentiating warfarin, digoxin and other antiarrhythmic agents. When administered concurrently, doses of these drugs should be reduced accordingly. On the positive side, long-term amiodarone is unlikely to precipitate or worsen heart failure and proarrhythmias are uncommon.

SOTALOL

Sotalol prolongs action potential duration, thereby prolonging the effective refractory period in the atria, ventricles, AV node and accessory AV pathways. It is also a potent non-cardioselective β-adrenergic blocker (class II). Sotalol also has antifibrillatory actions which are superior to those of conventional β-blockers. It can worsen heart failure in patients with depressed LV function. The negative inotropic β-blocking effect is slightly offset by a weak positive inotropic effect due to prolongation of the action potential (resulting in more time for calcium influx into contracting myocardial cells).

CLINICAL USE

Higher doses of sotalol are required to prolong cardiac repolarisation than to cause β-blockade. Sotalol may be administered IV or orally, and is excreted by the kidneys (elimination half-life 15 h); IV dose is 0.5–1.5 mg/kg over 5–20 min. Oral therapy is initiated at 80 mg 12-hourly and increased to 160 mg 12-hourly, although doses of 320 mg 12-hourly have been administered.

SUPRAVENTRICULAR TACHYCARDIA

- effective in AVNRT and AVRT, although adenosine and verapamil are superior. Long-term sotalol will prevent recurrences of these arrhythmias
- probably ineffective for reversion of AF/Afl, but is effective in preventing recurrence of AF after cardioversion. If AF recurs, heart rate is likely to be well controlled with sotalol
- prevents postoperative SVT

VENTRICULAR ARRHYTHMIAS

Sotalol is superior to lidocaine to terminate sustained VT, and should be considered a first-line drug in patients without heart failure. Oral sotalol is more effective than class I drugs for the long-term prevention of VT or VF. Guided (Holter or EPS) sotalol and empirical amiodarone are first-line drugs to prevent recurrences of VT and VF over the long term; however, the worse outcome with sotalol in SWORD has significantly reduced the role of sotalol in this setting.[70]

ADVERSE EFFECTS

Side-effects of sotalol are mainly due to β-blockade (e.g. bronchospasm, heart failure or AV conduction problems) and prolongation of QT proarrhythmia (e.g. torsade de pointes, similar 2% incidence as quinidine, which may occur early during drug titration or later during long-term treatment).

IBUTILIDE

Ibutilide is an I_{Kr} K^+ channel blocker, which prolongs action potential and increases the refractory period. This agent, with class III effect, is recommended for acute pharmacological conversion of AF and Afl, or as an adjunct to improve success of DC shock cardioversion. The success rate for ibutilide alone is higher for Afl (50–70%) than that with AF (30–50%) and, as expected, efficacy is greatest in short-term AF/Afl without structural heart disease. The major role of ibutilide appears to be cardioversion pretreatment to facilitate reversion to sinus rhythm from AF.[45] Ibutilide has minimal effect on blood pressure and heart rate and the major adverse effect is proarrhythmia, with torsade de pointes occurring in 3–6% of patients. For this reason, patients should be monitored for at least 6 h after administration. Ibutilide has a short duration of action and other antiarrhythmic drugs are required to maintain sinus rhythm.

DOSE

For patients weighing more than 60 kg, 1 mg over 10 min, which can be repeated 10 min later if unsuccessful. In patients weighing less than 60 kg, 0.01 mg/kg is given as initial dose.

DOFETILIDE

Dofetilide is one of the latest class III I_{Kr} K^+ channel blockers being investigated in the hope of finding an antiarrhythmic drug for long-term use with amiodarone's efficacy but without its side-effect profile. Dofetilide's emerging role is again in pharmacological cardioversion of AF and Afl (superior to sotalol, similar to amiodarone but inferior to ibutilide) in about 30% of patients. Prevention of recurrence is similar to amiodarone and long-term oral therapy is not associated with increased mortality in post-MI and heart failure patients. It also appears safe in patients with LV dysfunction. Early (first 3 days) proarrhythmia (3.3% of patients developed torsade de pointes) also necessitates monitoring with commencement of therapy.[40,46,94,95]

DOSE

Recommended dose is 500 mg orally 12-hourly. Dose requires adjustment for renal function and QT-interval monitoring (QT_c interval > 500 ms necessitates cessation) for a minimum of 3 days.

ADENOSINE

Adenosine stimulates specific A_1 receptors present on the surface of cardiac cells, thereby influencing adenosine-sensitive K^+ channel cyclic adenosine monophosphate production. It slows the sinus rate and prolongs AV node conduction, usually causing transient high-degree AV block. The half-life of adenosine is usually less than 2 min as it is taken up by red blood cells and deaminated in the plasma. This ultrashort half-life is a major advantage over other antiarrhythmic drugs. The effects of adenosine, both antiarrhythmic and haemodynamic, can be antagonised by methylxanthines, especially theophylline and caffeine. Dipyridamole, an adenosine uptake blocker, potentiates the effect of adenosine. Adenosine effects are prolonged in patients on carbamazepine and in denervated transplanted hearts.

CLINICAL USE

- AVNRT and AVRT tachycardias: the drug of choice. Expected reversion rates exceed 90%.[24] The AV nodal-blocking actions of adenosine may unmask atrial activity (e.g. flutter waves in Afl).
- Diagnosis of a wide-complex tachycardia may be assisted by the use of adenosine.
- SVT with intraventricular conduction block will terminate with adenosine, whereas few VTs will revert. Whether adenosine should be used routinely to discriminate between VT and SVT with aberrancy in haemodynamically stable wide-complex tachycardia is unclear. Potential for haemodynamic collapse in VT is real and ILCOR advises against.

Adenosine will not revert AF. Ventricular rate may transiently increase AF associated with the WPW syndrome.

Adenosine is given as a rapid bolus through a large peripheral or central vein followed by a saline flush, at intervals less than 60 s. The usual dose is 6 mg, followed by 12 mg if response is ineffective. Another 18 mg can be given if the last dose was well tolerated.

ADVERSE EFFECTS

Most patients experience transient side-effects such as flushing, shortness of breath and chest discomfort. Adenosine should not be given to asthmatic patients as bronchospasm may result.

DIRECT CURRENT CARDIOVERSION[96]

DC cardioversion/defibrillation is an important treatment option in tachyarrhythmias. In addition to its emergency role in cardiac arrest from VF or VT, urgent DC cardioversion is indicated in haemodynamically unstable VT and sustained SVT that precipitate angina, heart failure or hypotension. More elective DC cardioversion is indicated in haemodynamically stable VT following a trial of antiarrhythmic drug therapy. Cardioversion is most commonly used in AF/Afl once potential precipitants have been eliminated and, again, usually after antiarrhythmic drug treatment to prevent further episodes. Digoxin toxicity is a relative contraindication to DC cardioversion, which should also be used with care in patients on digoxin.

MECHANISM OF ACTION

The exact mechanism of action is unknown. DC shocks need to produce a current density that depolarises a critical mass of myocardium, thereby leaving insufficient myocardium to maintain the re-entrant tachycardia and prevent reinitiation. For VF and AF, the critical mass involves the entire ventricles or atria, whereas for the more organised tachyarrhythmias, VT and Afl, which involve specific re-entrant circuits, regional depolarisation in the path of their circulating wave fronts is all that is required. DC shocks also prolong the refractoriness of myocardium and this effect will contribute to the arrhythmia termination and prevention of immediate recurrence.

ELECTRICAL ENERGY

Even though the goal is to achieve a certain current through the entire heart, atria or a region depending on the arrhythmia, DC shocks are prescribed as energy measured in joules (J) or watt-seconds. Obviously it would make more sense to be able to deliver a set current. This would prevent delivering inappropriately low currents in patients with high impedance and excessive current flow causing myocardial damage in patients with low impedance. Clinical studies to determine current doses are under way for defibrillation and cardioversion. The optimal current for VF using monophasic damped sinusoidal (MDS) waveform for cardioversion waveform appears to be 30–40 A. Current dosage for biphasic waveform is not available.

CURRENT WAVEFORM

Modern defibrillators deliver a current, the magnitude of which depends on the prescribed energy and thoracic impedance. This current can be delivered in a number of different waveforms.

MDS defibrillators deliver current that is in a single direction or polarity. They can be further characterised by the rate at which the current pulse returns to zero. MDS waveforms return to zero gradually, whereas truncated exponential waveform return instantaneously. Recent evidence suggests that biphasic waveform for cardioversion (BTE) provide equal efficacy at lower electrical energies. A sequence of two current pulses is generated; the polarity of the second is in the direction opposite to the first. Biphasic waveforms with lower shock energies are associated with fewer ST-segment changes and less postresuscitation myocardial dysfunction and have an ILCOR class IIa recommendation.

THORACIC IMPEDANCE

The magnitude of current flow is dependent on the resistance to current flow or thoracic impedance. The average adult thoracic impedance is 70–80 Ω. Factors which determine thoracic impedance include:

- energy selection
- electrode size
- electrode composition
- paddle-to-skin coupling
- distance between electrodes
- number of previous shocks
- time interval between previous and present shock
- pressure on electrodes
- phase of ventilation
- patient's body build
- recent sternotomy

Conductive gel reduces impedance, while hair trapping air between skin and paddle and self-adhesive monitor/defibrillator electrode pads may increase it. There is no clear relationship between body size and energy requirements but compensation for patient-to-patient differences in impedance can be achieved by changes in duration and voltage of shocks, or by a process called burping, which involves releasing the residual membrane charge.

PADDLE POSITION AND SIZE

ILCOR recommends standard placement of sternum paddle just to the right of the upper sternal border below the clavicle and the apex paddle to the left of the nipple, with the centre of the paddle in the mid-axillary line. Permanent pacemakers and ICD must be avoided as shock may cause malfunction or block current going to the heart. Inevitably, some current passes down the pacemaker lead and it is necessary to check pacing threshold postshock. Other alternative paddle placements can enable avoidance of pacemakers and ICD or perhaps improve current direction. Using self-adhesive electrodes, the sternum electrode can be placed posterior to the heart on the right infrascapular region and the apex on the left precordium. The use of right parasternal and left posterior infrascapula has been advocated for AF because this configuration provides an optimal vector of current delivery to the atria. Large electrodes or paddles have less impedance; however, excessively large electrodes may result in less transmyocardial current flow. The minimum recommended electrode size is 50 cm^2, with the sum of both electrodes exceeding 150 cm^2.

SYNCHRONISED CARDIOVERSION

With cardioversion of atrial tachyarrhythmias and VT, when time permits, synchronisation of DC shock with the R-wave of the QRS complex is required to reduce the possibility of inducing VF by delivering the shock during the relatively refractory portion of the T-wave of the cardiac cycle. Synchronisation in VT may be difficult and misleading because of the wide complex or polymorphous nature. Synchronisation should not delay DC shock in pulseless VT or VT associated with unconsciousness, hypotension or severe pulmonary oedema.

DIRECT CURRENT SHOCK DOSAGE

Recommendations for energy doses are changing, as biphasic waveform generators become more widely available. Where studied, BTE shocks have been consistently as effective as higher-energy MDS shocks. Recommended doses are always a balance between that energy likely to generate a critical current flow and an energy not likely to cause functional and morphological damage. Electrical energies greater than 400 J have been reported to cause myocardial necrosis.

- VF and pulseless VT: escalating MDS shocks, starting at 200 J, then 200–300 J and, finally, 360 J. Evidence for sequential escalation of the energy dose is not strong and repeated shocks at the same energy result in increasing current delivery as impedance falls. Repeated non-escalating lower-energy BTE shocks, in the range of 150–175 J, are as effective as escalating MDS recommendations.
- VT: energy dose for cardioversion of VT depends on morphology and rate. For monomorphic VT, synchronised 100 J MDS is the starting energy. For polymorphic VT, synchronised if possible, 200 J MDS is the starting energy and for both stepwise increases if the first shock fails.
- AF: initial energy is synchronised 100–200 J MDS and stepwise increases if first shock fails. Despite obvious concerns for myocardial injury, megadose energy at 720 J has been used with success in large patients with AF refractory to 360 J, without evidence of myocardial injury. Constant-current, rectilinear biphasic waveforms appear to be more effective in cardioverting AF. This biphasic waveform at the low energy of 120 J was superior to 200 J MDS.
- Afl, AVNRT and AVRT: these atrial tachyarrhythmias require least energy and the initial recommended energy is synchronised 50–100 J MDS.

SEDATION

A separate doctor expert in managing the airway must perform sedation for cardioversion. The dose of the sedating agent is titrated on the basis of patient factors and type of arrhythmia. Patients with poor myocardial function not only need reduced dose, but also onset time is slower because of low cardiac output. Sensitive tachyarrhythmias such as Afl require only low doses, whereas AF is likely to need higher and repeated doses as higher energy and repeated shocks may be necessary. Cardioversions should be performed with standard resuscitation equipment available and preoxygenation is crucial.

DIGOXIN AND CARDIOVERSION

Digoxin toxicity results in a significant reduction in the threshold for inducing ventricular arrhythmia with DC shock. If digoxin toxicity is a possibility, then reconsideration of the need for cardioversion or at least careful titration of energy is required. Clinical experience would suggest the latter procedure of starting with 10 J MDS, and a stepwise increase thereafter increases safety of DC shock in this setting.

ANTICOAGULATION FOR CARDIOVERSION[96]

Cardioversion of AF and, to a lesser extent, Afl is associated with catastrophic thromboembolism, especially stroke. Early studies suggested an incidence of up to 6.3% without anticoagulation. It is accepted that the propensity of clots to form in the left atrium after 48 h in AF and for these to be dislodged when sinus rhythm is restored is so high that anticoagulation is indicated prior to cardioversion in AF.

Anticoagulation for 3–4 weeks before cardioversion reduced the risk of embolism by 80%. The risk of thromboembolism following cardioversion continues for a period:

- Echocardiographic findings suggestive of atrial thrombi formation occur in up to 35% of patients postcardioversion.
- Left atrial appendage emptying velocities often decrease despite the development of coordinated electrical activity after cardioversion, presumably because of stunning of mechanical function.

Prolonged AF greater than 48 h requires anticoagulation for 3 weeks prior to cardioversion and warfarin therapy for at least another 4 weeks depending on risk of recurrence of AF.

Transoesophageal echocardiography, which allows detection of thrombi in the left atrial appendage with much greater accuracy, has been found to be a safe means of expediting cardioversion. Anticoagulation with heparin for 1 day or warfarin for 5 days prior to demonstrating the left atrium to be free of thrombi by transoesophageal echocardiography, then 4 weeks of warfarin following cardioversion, was as effective in preventing emboli as the conventional longer anticoagulation regime. However, there was a significant reduction in major haemorrhagic events in the transoesophageal echocardiography-guided, shorter lead-in anticoagulation strategy.

REFERENCES

1. Shah M, Akar FG, Tomaselli GF. Molecular basis of arrhythmias. *Circulation* 2005; **112**: 2517–29.
2. Task Force of the Working Group on Arrhythmias of the European Society of Cardiology. The Sicilian gambit: a new approach to the classification of antiarrhythmic drugs based on their actions on arrhythmogenic mechanisms. *Circulation* 1991; **84**: 1831–51.
3. Hoffman BF, Rosen MR. Cellular mechanisms for cardiac arrhythmias. *Circ Res* 1981; **49**: 1–15.
4. Binah O, Rosen MR. Mechanisms of ventricular arrhythmias. *Circulation* 1992; **85** (suppl. 1): 25–31.
5. Wit AL, Cranefield PF. Reentrant excitation as a cause of cardiac arrhythmias. *Am J Physiol* 1978; **235**: H1–17.
6. Gettes LS. Electrolyte abnormalities underlying lethal and ventricular arrhythmias. *Circulation* 1992; **85** (suppl. 1): 70–6.

7. Hollifield JW. Thiazide treatment of hypertension: effects of thiazide diuretics on serum potassium, magnesium and ventricular ectopy. *Am J Med* 1986; **80**: 8–12.
8. Nordrehaug JE, Johannessen K-A, von der Lippe G. Serum potassium concentration as a risk factor of ventricular arrhythmias early in acute myocardial infarction. *Circulation* 1985; **71**: 645–9.
9. Hollifield JW. Thiazide treatment of systemic hypertension: effects on serum magnesium and ventricular ectopic activity. *Am J Cardiol* 1989; **63**: G22–5.
10. Schwartz PJ, La Rovere MT, Vanoli E. Autonomic nervous system and sudden cardiac death. *Circulation* 1992; **85** (suppl. 1): 77–91.
11. Campbell TJ. Proarrhythmic actions of antiarrhythmic drugs: a review. *Aust NZ J Med* 1990; **20**: 275–82.
12. Dhein S, Muller A, Gerwin R *et al.* Comparative study on the proarrhythmic effects of some antiarrhythmic agents. *Circulation* 1993; **87**: 617–30.
13. The Cardiac Arrhythmia Suppression Trial (CAST) Investigators. Preliminary report: effect of encainide and flecainide on mortality in a randomized trial of arrhythmia suppression after myocardial infarction. *N Engl J Med* 1989; **321**: 227–33.
14. Donovan KD, Power BM, Hockings BE *et al.* Usefulness of atrial electrograms recorded via central venous catheters in the diagnosis of complex cardiac arrhythmias. *Crit Care Med* 1993; **21**: 532–7.
15. Mason JW. A comparison of electrophysiologic testing with Holter monitoring to predict antiarrhythmic drug efficacy for ventricular tachyarrhythmias. *N Engl J Med* 1993; **329**: 445–51.
16. Buxton AE, Lee KL, DiCarlo L *et al.* Electrophysiologic testing to identify patients with coronary artery disease who are at risk of sudden death. *N Engl J Med* 2000; **342**: 1937–45.
17. Gilman JK, Jalal S, Naccarelli GV. Predicting and preventing sudden cardiac death from cardiac causes. *Circulation* 1994; **90**: 1083–92.
18. Kennedy HL, Whitlock JA, Sprauguе MK *et al.* Long-term follow up of asymptomatic healthy subjects with frequent and complex ventricular ectopy. *N Engl J Med* 1985; **312**: 193–7.
19. Jouven X, Zuriek M, Desnos M *et al.* Long-term outcome in asymptomatic men with exercise-induced premature ventricular depolarisations. *N Engl J Med* 2000; **343**: 826–33.
20. Teo KK, Yusuf S, Furberg CD. Effects of prophylactic antiarrhythmic drug therapy in acute myocardial infarction: an overview of results from randomized controlled trials. *JAMA* 1993; **270**: 1589–95.
21. The American Heart Association in Collaboration with the International Liasion Committee on Resuscitation (ILCOR). Guidelines 2000 for cardiopulmonary resuscitation and emergency cardiovascular care. *Circulation* 2000; **102** (suppl. I): I172–203.
22. Ganz LI, Friedman PL. Supraventricular tachycardia. *N Engl J Med* 1995; **322**: 162–73.
23. Chauhan VS, Krahn AD, Klein GJ *et al.* Supraventricular tachycardia. *Med Clin North Am* 2001; **85**: 193–223.
24. Camm AJ, Garratt CJ. Adenosine and supraventricular tachycardia. *N Engl J Med* 1991; **325**: 1621–9.
25. The American Heart Association in Collaboration with the International Liasion Committee on Resuscitation (ILCOR). Guidelines 2000 for cardiopulmonary resuscitation and emergency cardiovascular care. *Circulation* 2000; **102** (suppl. I): I158–65.
26. Cappato R, Calkins H, Chen SA *et al.* Worldwide survey on the methods, efficacy and safety of catheter ablation for human atrial fibrillation. *Circulation* 2005; **111**: 1100–5.
27. Garratt C, Antoniou A, Ward D *et al.* Misuse of verapamil in pre-existent atrial fibrillation. *Lancet* 1989; **1**: 367–9.
28. Scher DL, Arsura EL. Multifocal atrial tachycardia: mechanisms, clinical correlates and treatment. *Am Heart J* 1989; **118**: 574–80.
29. McCord JK, Borzak S, Davis T *et al.* Usefulness of intravenous magnesium for multifocal atrial tachycardia in patients with chronic obstructive pulmonary disease. *Am J Cardiol* 1998; **81**: 91–3.
30. Arsura E, Lefkin AS, Scher DL *et al.* A randomized double-blind placebo-controlled study of verapamil and metoprolol in treatment of multifocal atrial tachycardia. *Am J Med* 1988; **85**: 519–24.
31. Olshansky B, Wilber DJ, Hariman RJ. Atrial flutter – update on the mechanism and treatment. *Pace* 1992; **15**: 2308–35.
32. Falk RH. Medical progress: atrial fibrillation. *N Engl J Med* 2001; **344**: 1067–78.
33. Ozcon C, Jahangir A, Frudman PA *et al.* Significant effects of atrioventricular node ablation and pacemaker implantation on left ventricular function and long-term survival in patients with atrial fibrillation and left ventricular dysfunction. *Am J Cardiol* 2003; **92**; 33–7.
34. Prichett ELC. Management of atrial fibrillation. *N Engl J Med* 1992; **326**: 1264–71.
35. Prystowski EN, Benson DW, Fuster V *et al.* Management of patients with atrial fibrillation. A statement for healthcare professionals. From the subcommittee on electrocardiography and electrophysiology: American Heart Association. *Circulation* 1996; **93**: 1262–77.
36. Atrial Fibrillation Follow-up Investigation of Rhythm Management (AFFIRM) Investigations. A comparison of rate control and rhythm control in patients with atrial fibrillation. *N Engl J Med* 2002; **347**: 1825–33.
37. Rienstra M, Van Veldhiusen DJ, Crijns HJ *et al.* Enhanced cardiovascular morbidity and mortality during rhythm control treatment in persistent atrial fibrillation in hypertensives: data of the RACE study. *Eur Heart J* 2007; **6**: 741–51.
38. Carlsson J, Miketic S, Windeler J *et al.* Randomized trial of rate-control in persistent atrial fibrillation: the Strategies of Treatment of Atrial Fibrillation (STAF) study. *J Am Coll Cardiol* 2003; **41**: 1690–6.
39. Holmloser S, Kuick K, Lilienthal J. Rhythm or rate control in atrial fibrillation: Pharmacological Intervention in Atrial Fibrillation (PIAF): a randomized trial. *Lancet* 2000; **356**: 1789–94.

40. Predersen OD, Brendorp B, Elnung H *et al.* Does conversion and prevention of atrial fibrillation enhance survival in patients with left ventricular dysfunction? Evidence from the Danish Investigations of Arrhythmia and Mortality On Dofetilide (DIAMOND) study. *Card Electrophysiol Rev* 2003; 7: 220–4.
41. Deedwandia PC, Singh B, Ellenbogen K *et al.* Spontaneous conversion and maintenance of sinus rhythm by amiodarone in patients with heart failure and atrial fibrillation: observations from the Veterans Affairs Congestive Heart Failure Survival Trial of Antiarrhythmic Therapy (CHF-STAT). *Circulation* 1998; **98**: 2574–9.
42. Fuster V, Ryden LE, Cannom DS *et al.* ACC/AHA/ESC 2006 Guidelines for the management of patients with atrial fibrillation: a report of the American College of Cardiology/American Heart Association Task Force on Practice Guidelines and the European Society of Cardiology Committee for Practice Guidelines. *Circulation* 2006; **114**: e257–354.
43. Hylek EM, Skates SJ, Sheehan MA *et al.* An analysis of the lowest effective intensity of prophylactic anticoagulation for patients with non-rheumatic atrial fibrillation. *N Engl J Med* 1996; **335**: 540–6.
44. Klein AL, Grimm RA, Murray RD *et al.* Assessment of cardioversion using transesophageal echocardiography investigators. Use of transesophageal echocardiography to guide cardioversion in patients with atrial fibrillation. *N Engl J Med* 2001; **344**: 1411–20.
45. Oral H, Souza JJ, Michaud GF *et al.* Facilitating transthoracic cardioversion of atrial fibrillation with Ibutilide pre-treatment. *N Engl J Med* 1999; **340**: 1849–54.
46. McCellan KJ, Markham A. Dofetilide: a review of its use in atrial fibrillation and atrial flutter. *Drugs* 1999; **58**: 1043–59.
47. Roy D, Talajie M, Dorian P *et al.* The Canadian Trial of Atrial Fibrillation Investigators. Amiodarone to prevent recurrence of atrial fibrillation. *N Engl J Med* 2000; **342**: 913–20.
48. Haissaguerre M, Jais P, Shah DC *et al.* Spontaneous initiation of atrial fibrillation by ectopic beat originating in the pulmonary veins. *N Engl J Med* 1998; **339**: 659–66.
49. Verma A, Natale A. Why atrial fibrillation ablation should be considered first-line therapy for some patients. *Circulation* 2005; **112**: 1214–22.
50. Pappone C, Rosamo S, Augello G *et al.* Mortality, morbidity and quality of life after circumferential pulmonary vein ablation for atrial fibrillation: outcomes from a controlled non randomized long-term study. *J Am Coll Cardiol* 2003; **42**: 185–97.
51. Gage BF, Waterman AD, Shannon W *et al.* Validation of clinical classification schemes for predicting stroke: results from the National Registry of Atrial Fibrillation. *JAMA* 2001; **285**: 2864–70.
52. Hart RG, Benavente O, McBride R *et al.* Antithrombotic therapy to prevent stroke in patients with atrial fibrillation: a meta-analysis. *Ann Intern Med* 1999; **131**: 492–501.
53. Wellens HJJ, Bar FWHM, Lie KL. The value of the electrocardiogram in the differential diagnosis of a tachycardia with a wide QRS complex. *Am J Med* 1978; **64**: 27–33.
54. Brugada P, Brugada J, Mont L *et al.* A new approach to the differential diagnosis of a regular tachycardia with a wide QRS complex. *Circulation* 1991; **83**: 1649–59.
55. Antunes E, Brugada J, Steurer G *et al.* The differential diagnosis of a regular tachycardia with a wide QRS complex on the 12-lead ECG: ventricular tachycardia, supraventricular tachycardia with aberrant intraventricular conduction, and supraventricular tachycardia with anterograde conduction over an accessory pathway. *Pacing Clin Electrophysiol* 1994; **17**: 1515–24.
56. Griffith MJ, Garratt CJ, Mounsey P *et al.* Ventricular tachycardia as a default diagnosis in broad complex tachycardia. *Lancet* 1994; **343**: 386–8.
57. The American Heart Association in Collaboration with the International Liasion Committee on Resuscitation (ILCOR). Guidelines 2000 for cardiopulmonary resuscitation and emergency cardiovascular care. *Circulation* 2000; **102** (suppl. I): I142–157.
58. Kudenchuk PJ, Cobb LA, Copass MK *et al.* Amiodarone for resuscitation after out-of-hospital cardiac arrest due to ventricular fibrillation. *N Engl J Med* 1999; **341**: 871–8.
59. Dorian P, Cass D, Schwartz B *et al.* Amiodarone as compared with lidocaine for shock-resistant ventricular fibrillation. *N Engl J Med* 2000; **346**: 884–90.
60. Artucio H, Pereira M. Cardiac arrhythmias in critically ill patients: epidemiologic study. *Crit Care Med* 1990; **18**: 1383–8.
61. Nasraway SA, Rackow EC, Astiz ME *et al.* Inotropic response to digoxin and dopamine in patients with severe sepsis, cardiac failure and systemic hypoperfusion. *Chest* 1989; **95**: 612–15.
62. Holt AW. Hemodynamic responses to amiodarone in critically ill patients receiving catecholamine infusions. *Crit Care Med* 1989; **17**: 1270–6.
63. Moran JL, Gallagher J, Peake SL *et al.* Parenteral magnesium sulfate versus amiodarone in the therapy of atrial tachyarrhythmias: a prospective, randomized study. *Crit Care Med* 1995; **23**: 1816–24.
64. Horner SM. Efficacy of intravenous magnesium in acute myocardial infarction in reducing arrhythmias and mortality: meta-analysis of magnesium in acute myocardial infarction. *Circulation* 1992; **86**: 774–9.
65. Woods KL, Fletcher S, Roffe C *et al.* Intravenous magnesium sulphate in suspected acute myocardial infarction: results of the second Leicester Intravenous Magnesium Intervention Trial (LIMIT-2). *Lancet* 1992; **339**: 1553–8.
66. Maggioni AP, Zuanetti G, Franzosi MG *et al.* Prevalence and prognostic significance of ventricular arrhythmias after acute myocardial infarction in the thrombolytic era: GISSI-2 results. *Circulation* 1993; **87**: 312–22.
67. Solomon SD, Ridker PM, Antman EM. Ventricular arrhythmias in trials of thrombolytic therapy for acute myocardial infarction: a meta-analysis. *Circulation* 1993; **88**: 2575–81.
68. The American Heart Association in Collaboration with the International Liasion Committee on Resuscitation (ILCOR). Guidelines 2000 for cardiopulmonary resuscitation and emergency cardiovascular care. *Circulation* 2000; **102** (suppl. I): I112–128.

69. Radford MJ, Krumholz HM. Beta-blockers after myocardial infarction – for few patients, or many? *N Engl J Med* 1998; **339**: 551–3.
70. Waldo AL, Camm AJ, de Ruyter H *et al.* Effect of D-sotalol on mortality in patients with left ventricular dysfunction after recent or remote myocardial infarction. The SWORD investigators. Survival with oral D-sotalol. *Lancet* 1996; **348**: 7–12.
71. Cairns JA, Connolly SJ, Roberts R *et al.* Randomized trial of outcome after myocardial infarction in patients with frequent or repetitive ventricular premature depolarizations: CAMIAT. Canadian Amiodarone Myocardial Infarction Arrhythmia Trial investigators. *Lancet* 1997; **349**: 675–82.
72. Julian DG, Camm AJ, Frangin G *et al.* Randomized trial of effect of amiodarone on mortality in patients with left-ventricular dysfunction after recent myocardial infarction: EMIAT. European Myocardial Infarction Amiodarone Trial investigators. *Lancet* 1997; **349**: 667–74.
73. Boutitie F, Boissel JP, Connolly SJ *et al.* Amiodarone interaction with beta-blockers: analysis of merged EMIAT (European Myocardial Infarction Amiodarone Trial) and CAMIAT (Canadian Amiodarone Myocardial Infarction Arrhythmia Trial) databases. The EMIAT and CAMIAT investigators. *Circulation* 1999; **99**: 2268–75.
74. Ommen SR, Odell JA, Stanton MS. Atrial arrhythmias after cardiothoracic surgery. *N Engl J Med* 1997; **336**: 1429–34.
75. Andrews TC, Reimold SC, Berlin JA *et al.* Prevention of supraventricular arrhythmias after coronary artery bypass surgery: a meta-analysis of randomized control trials. *Circulation* 1991; **84** (suppl. III): III236–44.
76. Kowey PR, Taylor JE, Rials SJ *et al.* Meta-analysis of the effectiveness of prophylactic drug therapy in preventing supraventricular arrhythmia early after coronary artery bypass grafting. *Am J Cardiol* 1992; **69**: 963–5.
77. Burgess DC, Kilborn MJ, Keech AC. Interventions for prevention of post-operative atrial fibrillation and its complications after cardiac surgery: a meta-analysis. *Eur Heart J* 2006; **27**: 2846–57.
78. Patti G, Chello M, Candura D *et al.* Randomized trial of atorvastatin for reduction of post operative atrial fibrillation in patients undergoing cardiac surgery: results of the ARMYDA-3 (Atorvastatin for Reduction of MYocardial Dysrhythmia After cardiac surgery) study. *Circulation* 2006; **114**: 1455–61.
79. Ferraris VA, Ferraris SP, Gilliam HS *et al.* Predictors of postoperative ventricular dysrrhythmias: a multivariate study. *J Cardiovasc Surg (Torino)* 1991; **32**: 12–20.
80. Moss AJ. Prolonged QT syndromes. *JAMA* 1986; **256**: 2985–7.
81. Moss AJ, Schwartz PJ, Crampton RS *et al.* The long QT syndrome: prospective longitudinal study of 328 families. *Circulation* 1991; **84**: 1136–44.
82. Moss AJ, Robinson J. Clinical features of the idiopathic long QT syndrome. *Circulation* 1992; **85** (suppl. 1): 140–4.
83. Tzivoni D, Bonai S, Schuger C *et al.* Treatment of torsade de pointes with magnesium sulphate. *Circulation* 1988; 77: 392–7.
84. Huikuri HV, Castellanos A, Myerburg RJ. Medical progress: sudden death due to cardiac arrhythmias. *N Engl J Med* 2001; **345**: 1473–82.
85. Holmes DR, Davis KB, Mock MB *et al.* The effect of medical and surgical treatment on subsequent cardiac death in patients with coronary artery disease: a report from the Coronary Artery Surgery Study. *Circulation* 1986; **73**: 1254–63.
86. The Antiarrhythmics Versus Implantable Defibrillators (AVID) investigators. A comparison of antiarrhythmic-drug therapy with implantable defibrillators in patients resuscitated from near fatal ventricular arrhythmias. *N Engl J Med* 1997; **337**: 1576–84.
87. Moss AJ, Zareba W, Hall WJ *et al.* Multicenter Automatic Implantable Defibrillator Trial II Investigators. Prophylactic implantation of a defibrillator in patients with myocardial infarction and reduced ejection fraction. *N Engl J Med* 2002; **346**: 877–83.
88. Maron BJ, Shen W-K, Link MS *et al.* Efficacy of implantable cardioverter-defibrillators for prevention of sudden death in patients with hypertrophic cardiomyopathy. *N Engl J Med* 2000; **342**: 365–73.
89. Watanabe Y, Dreifus L. Electrophysiological effects of magnesium and its interactions with potassium. *Cardiovasc Res* 1972; **6**: 79–88.
90. Ghani MF, Rabah M. Effects of magnesium chloride on electrical stability of the heart. *Am Heart J* 1977; **94**: 600–2.
91. Mostow ND, Rakita L, Vrobel TR *et al.* Amiodarone: intravenous loading for rapid suppression of complex ventricular arrhythmias. *J Am Coll Cardiol* 1984; **4**: 97–104.
92. Schwartz A, Shen E, Morady F *et al.* Hemodynamic effects of intravenous amiodarone in patients with depressed left ventricular function and recurrent ventricular tachycardia. *Am Heart J* 1983; **106**: 848–55.
93. Cote P, Bourassa MG, Delaye J *et al.* Effects of amiodarone on cardiac and coronary hemodynamics and on myocardial metabolism in patients with coronary artery disease. *Circulation* 1954; **67**: 1347–55.
94. Torp-Pedersen C, Moller M, Bloch-Thomsen PE *et al.* Dofetilide in patients with congestive heart failure and left ventricular dysfunction. *N Engl J Med* 1999; **341**: 857–65.
95. Roukoz H, Saliba W. Dofetilide: a new class III antiarrhythmic agent. *Exp Rev Cardiovasc Ther* 2007; **5**: 9–19.
96. The American Heart Association in Collaboration with the International Liasion Committee on Resuscitation (ILCOR). Guidelines 200 or cardiopulmonary resuscitation and emergency cardiovascular care. *Circulation* 2000; **102** (suppl. I): I112–28.

19

Cardiac pacing and implantable cardioverter/defibrillators

Karl D Donovan and Bernard E F Hockings

Cardiac pacing has rapidly evolved since its introduction by Zoll in 1952.[1] The technological knowledge gained in pacing has assisted in the even more rapidly advancing field of implantable cardioverter/defibrillators (ICDs). Although implantation and follow-up of permanent pacemakers and ICDs are in the domain of appropriately trained cardiologists, intensive care physicians should be familiar with such devices as a significant number of critically ill patients will have them in situ. It is also essential, when urgent pacing is required, that the intensivist is skilled in all aspects of temporary pacing, including lead insertion and testing.

Cardiac pacing repetitively delivers very low electrical energies to the heart, thus initiating and maintaining cardiac rhythm. Pacing may be temporary, with an external pulse generator, or permanent, with an implanted pulse generator. It is usually associated with the treatment of bradycardia, but rapid atrial or ventricular pacing can be used to terminate certain supraventricular tachycardias (SVTs) and ventricular tachycardias (VTs).

More recently, the indications for cardiac pacing have expanded beyond symptomatic bradycardia and include conditions such as hypertrophic obstructive cardiomyopathy (HOCM), congestive cardiac failure (cardiac resynchronisation therapy: CRT) and prevention of atrial fibrillation (AF).

CARDIAC PACING IN BRADYARRHYTHMIAS[2,3]

ELECTRODES

UNIPOLAR (FIGURE 19.1)

The pacing lead has only one conducting wire and electrode. Electric current returns to the pacemaker via the body fluids. A unipolar lead is rarely used for temporary pacing, as a skin electrode is also needed for the return current pathway, which may cause muscle twitching. Unipolar systems are sometimes used for permanent pacing. Oversensing of electromagnetic interference (EMI) or skeletal muscle potentials may be a significant problem.

BIPOLAR (FIGURE 19.2)

A bipolar lead has two conducting wires surrounded by a layer of insulation. Electric current travels down one wire to an electrode (usually the distal), passes through cardiac tissue to cause depolarisation, and returns to the pacemaker via the second electrode. Inappropriate sensing of EMI or myopotentials is uncommon. Bipolar pacing is the method of choice for temporary pacing. If one limb fails, a bipolar system can be converted to a unipolar system (see Figure 19.1) by connecting the other limb to one pacemaker pole (usually positive). The other pole (usually negative) is connected to an electrocardiogram (ECG) skin electrode to complete a unipolar pacing circuit.

PACING SITES

TRANSVENOUS ENDOCARDIAL PLACEMENT

The pacing lead is passed via a vein to the endocardial surface of the right atrium (RA), or most commonly, the right ventricle (RV). Rarely, the left atrium (LA) may be paced via the coronary sinus.

EPICARDIAL PLACEMENT

This is mainly used in conjunction with cardiac surgery, where the electrodes are attached directly to the epicardial surface of the atrium and/or ventricle.

TRANSCUTANEOUS EXTERNAL PACING

Transcutaneous pacing patches have high impedance, resulting in better current density and less pain and discomfort. Adequate, adjustable current outputs (50–150 mA) are delivered. Some patients will experience significant pain and may need analgesics. Although transcutaneous pacing can be initiated quickly by personnel unskilled in transvenous pacing, it is only a temporising measure until the latter can be instituted. Reliable transcutaneous pacing has rendered prophylactic temporary transvenous pacing obsolete.

Other pacing modalities such as the transoesophageal route are rarely used. A pacing Swan–Ganz catheter is

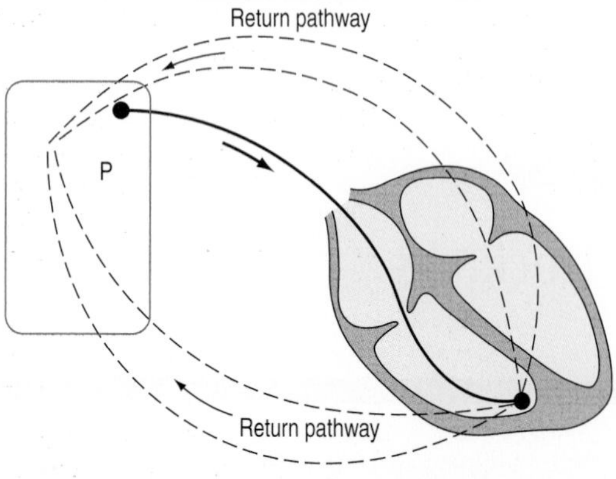

Figure 19.1 Unipolar pacing lead. P, pacemaker.

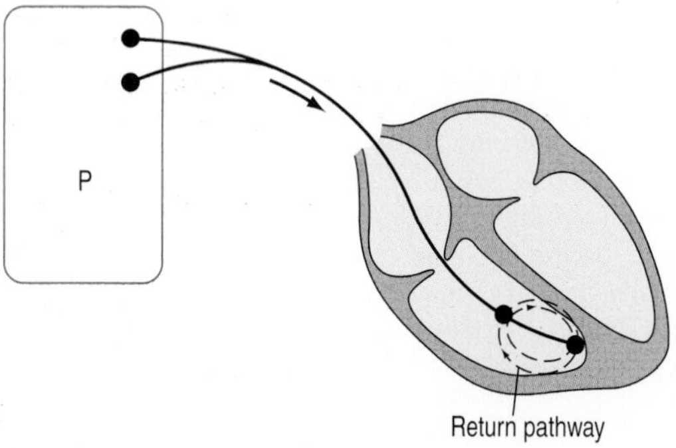

Figure 19.2 Bipolar pacing lead. P, pacemaker.

unstable and should not be relied upon in pacemaker-dependent patients.

PACING LEADS

TEMPORARY PACING

Ventricular pacing

(5–6 FG). Leads are relatively stiff but still flexible enough to be manipulated under fluoroscopic control to the correct position in the RV. Balloon-tipped leads which, in theory, float into a stable position in the RV are occasionally used in some units when fluoroscopy is not available.

Atrial pacing

Atrial leads have a preformed J-tip to hook into the RA appendage, as this usually ensures pacing lead stability with a low pacing threshold and good sensing capacity.

PERMANENT PACING

Leads for permanent pacing commonly use passive fixation with protrusions close to the tips to ensure wedging or entanglement of the electrode in the trabeculations of the RV. Alternatively, active fixation with myocardial penetration by an extendable screw at the electrode tip is used. Steroid eluting leads may reduce pacing stimulation thresholds. Pacing lead insulation problems remain a limiting factor in pacing lead longevity.

PACEMAKER MODES

The North American Society of Pacing and Electrophysiology (NASPE) and the British Pacing and Electrophysiology Group (BPEG) developed the NBG code[4] for pacing. It is a generic code used to identify modes of pacing (Table 19.1). The code was updated in 2002 to include multisite pacing therapy (position V).[5]

Table 19.1 The North American and British Group (NBG) pacemaker code

Position I	Position II	Position III	Position IV	Position V
Chamber(s) paced	Chamber(s) sensed	Response to sensing	Rate modulation	Multisite pacing
0 = none	0 = none	0 = none	0 = none	0 = none
A = atrium	A = atrium	T = triggered	R = rate modulation	A = atrium
V = ventricle	V = ventricle	I = inhibited		V = ventricle
D = dual	D = dual	D = dual		D = dual
(A + V)	(A + V)	(T + I)		(A + V)
Manufacturer's designation only:				
S = single	S = single			
(A or V)	(A or V)			

Note: Positions I–III are used exclusively for antibradycardia function.
(Reproduced from Bernstein AD, Daubert JC, Fletcher RD *et al.* Pacing. *Clin Electrophysiol* 2002; **25:** 260.)

- **Position I**: refers to the chamber(s) paced: A = atrium; V = ventricle; and D = dual chambers, i.e. both A and V.
- **Position II**: refers to chamber(s) in which sensing occurs: A = atrium; V = ventricle; and D = dual chambers, i.e. both A and V.
- **Position III**: refers to the pacemaker's response to a sensed event. This may be:
  - (a) I (inhibition) – a pacemaker's discharge is inhibited (switched off) by a sensed signal, for example, VVI, where ventricular pacing is inhibited by spontaneous ventricular activity.
  - (b) T (triggering) – a pacemaker's discharge is triggered by a sensed signal.
  - (c) D (dual) – both T and I responses can occur. This designation is reserved for dual-chamber systems. A depolarisation sensed in the atrium inhibits the atrial output but triggers ventricular pacing. There is, however, a delay (the AV interval) between the sensed atrial depolarisation and the triggered ventricular pacing which mimics the normal P-R interval. If a spontaneous ventricular depolarisation is sensed, ventricular pacing is inhibited.
- **Position IV**: refers to *R* or rate modulation. An *R* indicates that the pacemaker incorporates a sensor to vary the pacemaker independently of intrinsic cardiac activity. A sensor,[6] in effect an artificial sinoatrial (SA) node, increases or decreases the heart rate according to the body's metabolic needs. Two different sensors are widely used:
  1. Activity sensors with vibration detectors (accelerometer or piezoelectric crystal) have the disadvantage that they may respond to non-physiological stimuli, for example, pacing rate increase may occur when the patient is using an electrical drill. On occasions this response can be used to good effect, for example, an inappropriate bradycardia in a shocked patient with a rate-adaptive (activity sensor) permanent pacemaker can usually be speeded up by tapping the skin over the unit.
  2. Minute ventilation sensors (respiratory rate times tidal volume, which is estimated by measuring impedance differences between the pacing electrode and the pacemaker unit) rely on minute volume changes to alter the pacing rate. This sensor may occasionally inappropriately accelerate the pacing rate, for example, in a mechanically ventilated patient requiring a large minute volume. Changing the 'upper rate' limit of the pacemaker or switching the rate-adaptive function 'off' will usually solve the problem.

  Other sensors, such as ventricular paced Q-T interval systems, have also been successfully used in clinical practice. Recently, rate-adaptive systems with dual sensors, where one sensor cross-checks the other and only responds if both sensors are receiving consistent data, have become available.

  All modern permanent pacemakers are programmable, i.e. multiple pacing parameters, such as current output, rate and mode, can be changed by an external device (programmer).
- **Position V:** is now used to indicate whether multisite pacing is present: O = none of the cardiac chambers; A = one or both atria; V = one or both ventricles; or D = any combination of atria and ventricles, e.g. the code for a patient with dual-chamber, rate-adaptive pacing (DDDR) and biventricular pacing is DDDRV.

SPECIFIC PACING MODES

The three-position code (Figure 19.3) is adequate to describe emergency temporary pacing and most forms of permanent pacing in the intensive care unit (ICU) (Table 19.2).

SINGLE-CHAMBER PACING

1. AOO and VOO (asynchronous atrial and ventricular) pacing. There is no ability to sense cardiac activity (Figure 19.4). Such pacing is virtually obsolete, except in some pacing emergencies (see later).
2. AAI (atrial demand) pacing. This is indicated for sinus bradycardia provided AV conduction is intact (to maintain AV synchrony).
3. VVI (ventricular demand) pacing (Figure 19.5). This is the most commonly used mode and the mode of choice in life-threatening bradyarrhythmias. Spontaneous cardiac rhythm is sensed, and there is minimal danger of pacemaker-induced ventricular tachyarrhythmia (Figure 19.6). AV synchrony is, however, lost and there is no 'speed-up for need'.

DUAL-CHAMBER PACING

Two sets of electrodes are required (atrial and ventricular).

DVI (AV SEQUENTIAL) PACING

Atria and ventricles are paced in sequence (Figure 19.7). After a stimulus is delivered to the atrium, there is a delay and an impulse is then delivered after atrial stimulation, to the ventricles. If AV conduction is successful, the ventricular output of the pacemaker is inhibited; otherwise the ventricle is paced. The advantage of this mode is that the atria and ventricles usually contract in sequence. To maintain AV synchrony in the absence of atrial sensing, the pacemaker discharge rate must be greater than the spontaneous atrial rate; asynchronous atrial pacing can precipitate AF. Self-inhibition ('cross-talk') can occasionally occur, that is, inappropriate detection of the atrial pacing stimulus by the ventricular channel. If there is no escape rhythm, asystole may result. DVI pacing is indicated when there is impaired AV conduction with an atrial bradycardia. It is of no value when atrial tachyarrhythmias are present.

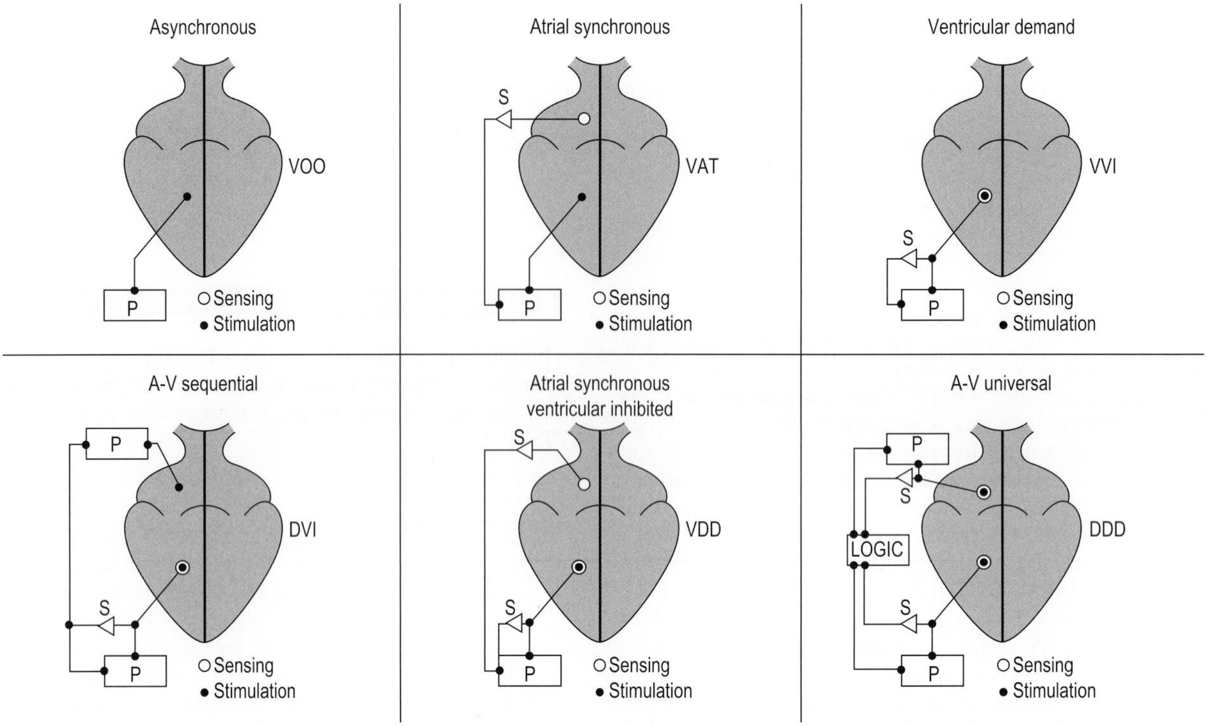

Figure 19.3 Examples of pacemaker modes and their three-position (letter) codes. P, pacemaker; S, sensing.

Table 19.2 Examples of pacemaker modes

Code		Common description	Comment
VOO	Paces the ventricle, no sensing	Fixed-rate, asynchronous	Obsolete – except for pacemaker testing and 'emergency' pacing
VVI	Paces the ventricle, senses ventricular activity, ventricular activity inhibits the pacemaker	Ventricular demand	Most commonly used in life-threatening bradycardia
AAI	Paces the atrium, senses atrial activity, atrial activity inhibits the pacemaker	Atrial demand	Indicated in sinus bradycardia with intact AV conduction
VAT	Paces the ventricle, senses atrial activity, atrial activity triggers ventricular pacing	Atrial synchronised, P-wave triggered	Obsolete – replaced by VDD and DDD
DVI	Paces both atrium and ventricle, senses only ventricular activity, ventricular activity inhibits atrial and ventricular pacing	AV sequential	Commonly used dual-chamber pacing mode in ICU
VDD	Paces the ventricle only, senses atrial and ventricular activity	Atrial synchronous, ventricular inhibited DDD	May be useful when normal sinus rhythm is present with a high-degree AV block
DDD	Paces and senses both atrium and ventricle: atrial activity triggers ventricular pacing	DDD	Often ideal but more complicated
DDI	Paces and senses both atrium and ventricle. Atrial activity not tracked; thus atrial tachyarrhythmias do not trigger rapid atrial pacing	AV sequential, non-P synchronous	Useful for sinus bradycardia with AV block and intermittent atrial tachyarrhythmias

AV, atrioventricular; ICU, intensive care unit.

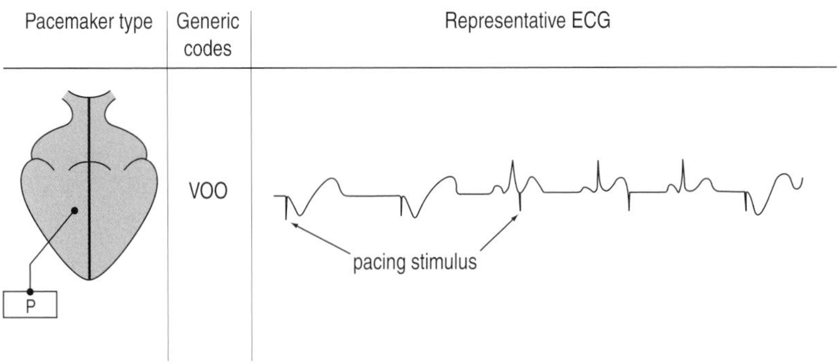

Figure 19.4 Fixed-rate ventricular pacing VOO. P, pacemaker.

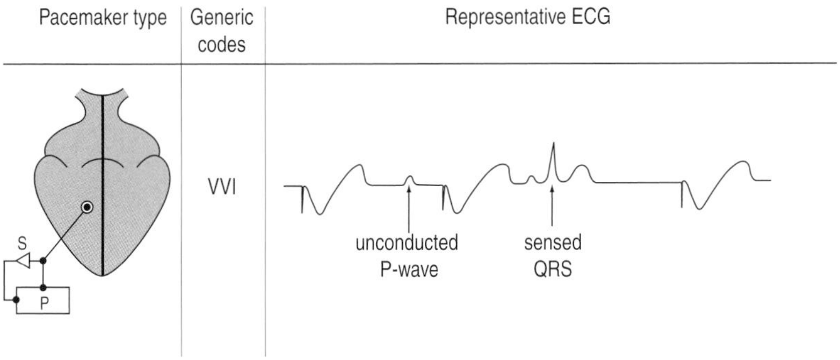

Figure 19.5 Ventricular demand pacing VVI. P, pacemaker; S, sensing.

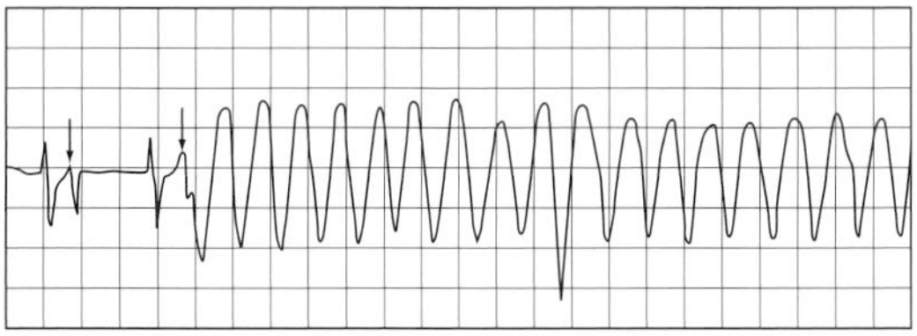

Figure 19.6 Non-sensing of QRS (see first two beats). Pacing spikes (arrows) fall on the T-wave with subsequent pacemaker-induced ventricular tachycardia.

VDD (ATRIAL SYNCHRONOUS VENTRICULAR INHIBITED) PACING

This mode paces only the ventricle. Sensing takes place in both atrium and ventricle. A sensed P-wave triggers ventricular pacing. VDD pacing is used in some permanent pacemaker systems as a single-lead system capable of pacing the ventricle in response to atrial sensing (from an electrode situated in the intra-atrial part of the lead) with ventricular electrodes at the apex of the RV.

DDD PACING

There is pacing and sensing in both chambers (Figure 19.8). An atrial impulse will trigger a ventricular output and simultaneously inhibit an atrial output. If the impulse is conducted normally to the ventricle, the ventricular output is then inhibited, as with the DVI mode. Upper rate-limiters prevent the pacemaker from following excessive atrial activity with paced ventricular responses. DDD pacemaker function depends on the underlying cardiac rhythm:

1. atrial bradycardia with intact AV conduction – atrial pacing
2. normal sinus rhythm with high-degree AV block – tracking of P-waves with synchronised ventricular pacing
3. sinus bradycardia with AV block – pacing the atria and ventricles sequentially
4. normal sinus rhythm and AV conduction – inhibition of both atrial and ventricular pacing

Self-inhibition can be prevented by introducing a ventricular blanking (refractory) period coinciding with the atrial pacing stimulus. With DDD and VDD pacing, re-entry pacemaker-mediated 'endless-loop' tachycardias are possible.[7] These are commonly initiated by a ventricular premature beat (Figure 19.9) conducted retrogradely to the atria, where it is sensed and ventricular pacing is triggered with an endless loop: the circuit's anterograde limb is the pacemaker, and the retrograde limb is via the AV

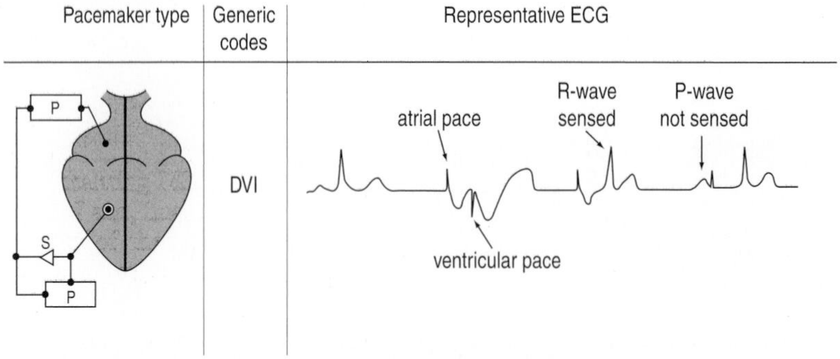

Figure 19.7 Atrioventricular sequential demand pacing DVI. P, pacemaker; S, sensing.

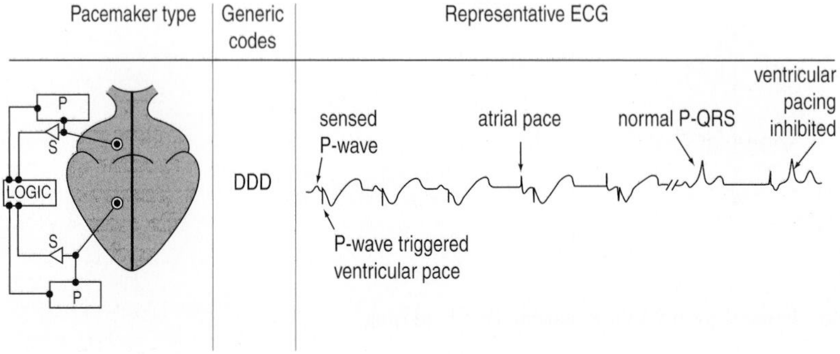

Figure 19.8 DDD pacing. P, pacing; S, sensing.

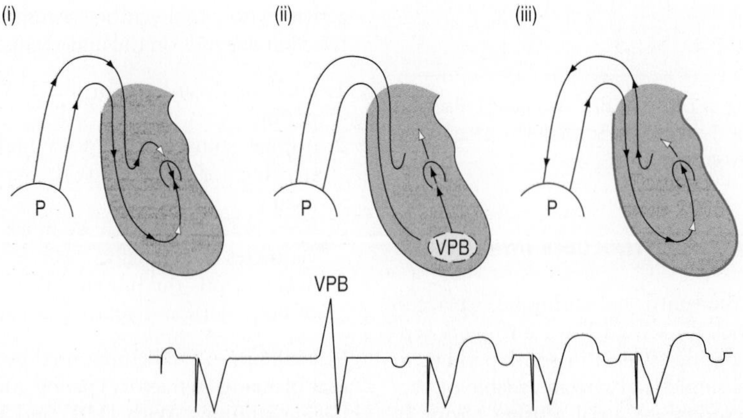

Figure 19.9 Pacemaker-mediated 'endless-loop' tachycardia: (i) under normal conditions (first beat) there is no conduction from the ventricles to the atria because of ventriculoatrial block or because the atrial and ventricular impulses collide and extinguish each other in the atrioventricular node; (ii) if a ventricular premature beat (VPB) is conducted retrogradely to the atria (second beat), inducing an inverted 'p'-wave, this may be sensed by the pacemaker (P) which then triggers a ventricular paced beat (third beat); (iii) if the paced ventricular beat is then retrogradely conducted from the ventricle to the atria and sensed, an 'endless loop' may occur (beats 4, 5); that is, pace ventricle VA conduction 'p' wave (sensed) ventricular pace, and so forth.

node. Conversion to asynchronous (non-sensing) mode or DDI or increasing the postventricular atrial refractory period (PVARP) will prevent endless-loop tachycardia.

DDI PACING (AV SEQUENTIAL, NON-P-WAVE SYNCHRONOUS)

Sensing occurs in both atria and ventricle, but sensed atrial events do not trigger ventricular pacing. This mode prevents endless-loop tachycardias or tracking of SVTs. It is also useful in patients with SA node dysfunction and episodes of atrial tachyarrhythmias, although DDD (R) with mode switching (ability to change to DDI, DDIR, DVI or DVIR with the onset of an atrial tachyarrhythmia) is preferable. During atrial tachyarrhythmias, the DDI pacemaker will simply pace the ventricle at its back-up rate and not track the tachycardia.

HAEMODYNAMICS OF CARDIAC PACING

In the normal heart, cardiac output increases three- to fourfold during exercise, due mainly to increased heart rate and increases in stroke volume. Atrioventricular synchrony – the normal activation sequence of the heart in which the atria contract first and then, after an appropriate delay, the ventricles contract – contributes only about 20% of cardiac output.[8] Thus the ability of pacemakers to increase heart rate is paramount, although AV synchrony may on occasions be vital (e.g. in low-cardiac-output states). Many permanent pacemakers are rate-adaptive. When temporary pacing is used, the arbitrary back-up rate of 70–80 beats/min may need to be increased if oxygen delivery is inadequate. For life-threatening bradyarrhythmias, increasing heart rate with VVI mode pacing is the treatment of choice. Permanent VVIR pacing (most commonly using an activity or respiration sensor) will allow heart rate modulation. However, in the ICU, adaptive rate changes may not occur. For example, no activity will be sensed in a patient with septic shock, even when the cardiac output is low.

During VVI and VVIR pacing the atria and ventricles beat independently and AV synchrony is lost. Occasionally this can have deleterious effects and cause a 'pacemaker syndrome'.[9] The pacemaker syndrome is, however, a complex of clinical signs and symptoms associated with loss of AV synchrony. A fall in blood pressure coinciding with the onset of ventricular pacing is consistent with the pacemaker syndrome. It was initially recognised with VVI pacing but can occur with any pacing mode if there is AV dissociation, and can be compared to the effects in patients with complete heart block and AV dissociation. The atria contract against closed AV valves with significant regurgitation of blood into the pulmonary and systemic circulation. Blood pressure, stroke volume and cardiac output may fall. The pacemaker syndrome can be eliminated by restoring AV synchrony.

Emergency and long-term haemodynamic effects of DDD or AAI pacing are generally superior to VVI pacing. In studies of patients with permanent pacing, there is a consistent lower mortality with DDD or AAI pacing compared to VVI pacing, and a significantly lower incidence of AF.[2] DDD and/or DVI pacing requires two pacing leads, one each in the RA and RV. Under appropriate conditions AAI and DVI pacing provide AV synchrony but not rate adaptation. DDD pacing will usually ensure AV synchrony and heart rate responsiveness, provided the SA node is normal.

Dual-chamber pacemakers require the AV interval to be set as close as possible to the normal P-R interval (140–200 ms). Traditionally, the pacing AV interval is arbitrarily set at about 150–200 ms. If interatrial conduction time (between the RA and LA) is significantly prolonged, the LV may contract before or at the same time as the LA, causing DDD pacemaker syndrome[10] with decreased stroke volume and cardiac output (due to LA contraction against a closed mitral valve). Hence, if there is evidence of inadequate cardiac output or impaired oxygen delivery, the AV interval may need to be increased appropriately, or optimised using thermodilution cardiac output or echocardiographic techniques at various AV intervals.

INDICATIONS FOR CARDIAC PACING IN BRADYARRHYTHMIAS

TEMPORARY PACING

Cardiac pacing is indicated for any sustained symptomatic bradycardia that does not promptly respond to medical treatment. Pacing may also be indicated if a bradycardia predisposes to malignant ventricular arrhythmias. The decision to pace is based on bradycardia associated with haemodynamic deterioration, and not on the specific rhythm disturbance. For example, pacing is indicated in a patient with AF and a ventricular response of 50/min associated with a blood pressure of 70/40 mmHg (9.3/5.3 kPa), cardiac failure and oliguria. Pacing is not indicated in an asymptomatic normotensive patient with an inferior infarction, complete heart block and a ventricular rate of 45/min.

Temporary pacing is indicated for the treatment of heart block or sinus bradycardia after cardiac surgery. In high-risk patients, for example, aortic or mitral valve replacement, prophylactic epicardial electrodes are often attached during surgery. DDD (dual-chamber) epicardial pacing has been shown to increase cardiac output at any given heart rate compared to VVI (single-chamber) pacing.[11] Temporary perioperative cardiac pacing strategies to increase stroke volume and cardiac output include optimisation of AV delay and occasionally multisite pacing.[12] Temporary pacing may be required for bradycardia during cardiac catheterisation and percutaneous transluminal coronary angioplasty. Asymptomatic patients with bifascicular block do not require prophylactic pacing prior to general anaesthesia, although transcutaneous pacing should be readily available. Patients with second- or

Table 19.3 Complete atrioventricular (AV) block in acute myocardial infarction

Feature	Inferior	Anterior
Onset	Slow (usually via Mobitz 1)	Sudden (usually via Mobitz II)
QRS complex	Narrow	Wide
Ventricular rate	>45 beats/min	<45 beats/min (often 20–30 beats/min)
Escape pacemaker	Stable	Unstable
Drug response (e.g. atropine)	Yes	No
Haemodynamic effects	No (usually)	Yes
Permanent pacing	No (usually)	Yes (if high-degree AV block persists)
Prognosis	Good	Very poor

third-degree AV block should be paced prior to general anaesthesia and surgery.

Caution should be exercised in patients with acute myocardial infarction as many patients will have received thrombolytic agents; central venous cannulation should be avoided, although if necessary the femoral vein can be used. Prognosis is related to infarct size rather than the degree of AV block. Transcutaneous pacing obviates the need for prophylactic temporary transvenous pacing leads in high-risk patients. Pacing is sometimes required for patients with anterior or inferior myocardial infarction (Table 19.3).

PERMANENT PACING

Guidelines for permanent pacing have been published.[13]

1. *Class I.* Indicated. For example, chronic symptomatic second- or third-degree AV block, SA node dysfunction with documented symptomatic bradycardia and recurrent syncope associated with hypersensitive carotid sinus.
2. *Class II–IIa.* Good supportive evidence. For example, asymptomatic complete AV block with average ventricular rate >40/min in an awake patient. *IIb.* Weak supportive evidence. For example, first-degree heart block (>0.3 seconds) in patients with depressed left ventricular function and symptoms of left ventricular failure.
3. *Class III.* Pacing is not indicated. For example, in asymptomatic first-degree heart block or reversible AV block secondary to drug toxicity.

OTHER INDICATIONS

There are also non-bradycardia indications for pacing for haemodynamic improvement. Evolving indications include the following:[2,3]

1. *HOCM.* Pacing is usually reserved for symptomatic patients with a high gradient in the left ventricular outflow tract (LVOT). DDD pacing with a short AV interval causes RV apical activation with altered septal activation, thereby decreasing both the LVOT gradient and systolic anterior motion (SAM) of the mitral valve. The results of trials to date have been mixed and it is unclear whether pacing is a preferred treatment option for HOCM. Currently, it is a class IIb indication (weak supportive evidence).
2. *Heart failure.* A significant number of patients with dilated cardiomyopathy have an intraventricular conduction disturbance, usually left bundle branch block (LBBB) with significant ventricular dyssynchronisation and associated paradoxical septal motion and mitral regurgitation. CRT refers to re-establishing synchronous contraction between the left ventricular free wall and the ventricular septum, resulting in improvements in LV performance. Generally, CRT has been used to describe biventricular or multisite ventricular pacing. CRT improves the symptoms of heart failure and improves survival in specific patient groups. In the most recent American College of Cardiology/American Heart Association Task Force on Practice Guidelines[13] for pacing, biventricular pacing is included as a class IIa indication in medically refractory symptomatic New York Heart Association class III/IV patients with idiopathic dilated or ischaemic cardiomyopathy, prolonged QRS (>130 ms), left ventricular end-diastolic diameter >55 mm and left ventricular ejection fraction <0.35. The underlying rhythm should be sinus or AF with a ventricular response slow enough to allow continuous biventricular stimulation and capture. The chronic use of CRT via a permanently implantable biventricular pacemaker (the LV lead is usually passed via a tributary of the coronary sinus to the epicardial surface of the LV) is gaining widespread acceptance for treatment of heart failure. Biventricular pacing is usually reserved for permanent pacing. Temporary biventricular pacing with a temporary transvenous pacemaker lead passed to a coronary vein via the coronary sinus has been used successfully in cardiogenic shock and high-degree AV block.[14] More recently, permanent devices combining CRT and implantable defibrillators have been developed.
3. *AF prevention.* Atrial pacing may be effective in preventing episodes of paroxysmal AF. Most trials have been performed in patients requiring permanent pacing for bradycardia who also incidentally have episodes of paroxysmal AF. Synchronous dual-site pacing of either RA and LA or two different RA sites may be superior to single-site atrial pacing by virtue of

decreasing dispersion of refractoriness.[15] Single-site RA pacing (back-up rate slightly faster than intrinsic sinus rhythm, usually 80–110 beats/min) decreases the incidence of AF after cardiac surgery.[16,17] Dual-site, RA and LA, or two-site RA are more complicated but may be superior to single-site RA pacing for AF prevention.[18,19]

ELECTROMAGNETIC INTERFERENCE

Any signal that can be sensed by the pacemaker, or ICD, constitutes EMI and can cause pacing problems such as failure to pace (inappropriate sensing), asynchronous pacing ('safety pacing' when excess 'noise' is detected), pacemaker reprogramming and occasionally damage to the pacemaker (DC shock, diathermy) or the heart itself. The most important source of potentially harmful electromagnetic radiation in hospitals is magnetic resonance imaging (MRI). MRI is generally considered to be contraindicated in patients with a pacemaker or ICD. Recently, several studies have demonstrated the potential for MRI to be performed in pacemaker or ICD patients.[20] The risks presented by MRI must be outweighed by the diagnostic benefit of this powerful imaging modality on a case-by-case assessment.

In critically ill patients, potential EMI sources include DC shocks, diathermy and possibly mobile telephones. In general, mobile telephones, especially analogue systems, are reasonably safe. Digital telephones have a greater theoretical risk for EMI and it is recommended that telephones do not come into close contact with the pacemaker, for example the mobile telephone should not be rested on the skin over the implanted device. If there is any doubt the pacemaker (or ICD) should be checked and reprogrammed.

CARDIOVERSION/DEFIBRILLATION IN PATIENTS WITH A PERMANENT PACEMAKER (OR ICD)

Place paddles in the anterior–posterior position, at least 10 cm from the unit. Make sure a suitable programmer is available and check the pacemaker (or ICD) afterwards. In patients with a temporary transvenous pacemaker, keep the external unit and the leads well away from the paddles.

DIATHERMY

Bipolar diathermy should be used whenever possible. When diathermy is used in pacemaker-dependent patients, it may be safer to change the mode to asynchronous pacing. This can be achieved in permanent pacemakers by reprogramming the pacemaker: close liaison with the patient's cardiologist is very important. In an emergency (e.g. asystole in a patient whose pacemaker is inhibited by diathermy), placing a magnet over the permanent pacemaker will usually result in a fixed-rate mode. Modern pacemakers may not be magnet-responsive, but they are also less likely to be affected by diathermy. Patients with temporary transvenous pacing can be switched to VOO or DOO mode. ICD devices should be switched off before diathermy is used. In contradistinction to pacemakers, placing a magnet over the ICD will deactivate the unit, although pacing functions will not be altered. After surgery the pacemaker or ICD should be tested and reprogrammed appropriately.

TECHNIQUE OF TEMPORARY TRANSVENOUS PACING

VENTRICULAR PACING

A sterile technique is mandatory. In emergencies, transcutaneous pacing (VVI) is used first while transvenous VVI pacing is being prepared. A bipolar lead introduced under fluoroscopic control is most commonly used.

Percutaneous insertion via the right internal jugular vein probably offers least complications with ease of manipulation and stability of the lead. The infraclavicular (subclavian vein) approach allows more freedom for patient arm movement. Antecubital veins are associated with lead instability and thrombophlebitis. The femoral vein is best avoided except in patients who have received thrombolytic agents, because of problems with sterility and increased risk of deep-vein thrombosis. The pacing lead is introduced using the Seldinger technique and manipulated under fluoroscopic control to the apex of the RV (Figure 19.10). After the lead has been manipulated to a satisfactory position, a chest X-ray should be

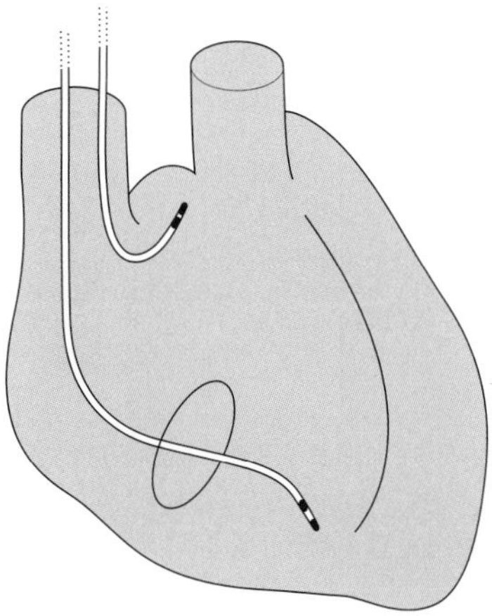

Figure 19.10 Characteristic appearance of temporary transvenous pacing leads ideally positioned in (a) the right atrium (right atrial appendage) and (b) apex of right ventricle.

obtained to exclude pneumothorax and to confirm adequate lead positioning. The lead should be sutured to the skin at two different sites: one where the lead exits the skin, and a second to a loop formed with the lead. Occasionally, transvenous RV pacing may not be feasible, owing to the presence of a prosthetic tricuspid valve or a congenital anomaly.

ATRIAL PACING

Insertion of the atrial J-lead is similar to that of the ventricular lead. Correct positioning requires experience. The right atrial appendage is anterior and medial, and the tip is advanced anteriorly and to the patient's left, after passing from the superior vena cava to the RA (see Figure 19.10). The correct position can be confirmed by a lateral chest X-ray or fluoroscopy.

DUAL-CHAMBER PACING

Modern external pacemakers are available (Figure 19.11) which will pace in all modes. These units are small, easy to use and can fit into a small pouch suitable for mobile patients.

TESTING THE PACING LEADS

Pacing threshold and sensing should be tested adequately using the external pacemaker.

Pacing threshold

The lead is attached to the external pulse generator with the distal electrode connected to the negative pacemaker terminal. The cardiac chamber is then paced at 5–10 beats/min faster than patient heart rate, while the pulse generator's output is slowly decreased until consistent capture outside the myocardial refractory period is lost. Threshold testing is always performed at an identical pulse duration, usually 0.5–1.0 ms. Ideally, ventricular pacing threshold should be 1.0 mA and the atrial threshold 2.0 mA. Pacemaker output is usually set at 2–3 times pacing threshold and always > 3 mA to allow a reasonable safety margin. After acute myocardial infarction the amplitude must not be set higher than necessary, as inadvertent pacing during the vulnerable period of the cardiac cycle may result in VT or ventricular fibrillation (VF).

Sensing

A pacemaker senses the potential difference between the two pacing electrodes. The amplitude of the ventricular signal is commonly 5–15 mV and the atrial signal 2–5 mV. Modern external pacemakers can sense signals as small as 0.8 mV for the ventricle, and 0.4 mV for atrial depolarisation. Before testing the sensitivity, pacing output is set at zero, thereby avoiding potentially dangerous competition between the pacemaker and the spontaneous cardiac rhythm. Pacing rate is then set lower than the spontaneous rate of the tested cardiac chamber, and the pacemaker sensitivity is decreased until there is competition between paced and spontaneous cardiac rhythms. The pacemaker sensitivity is then set at twice that value. This involves reducing the numerical sensitivity value (e.g. changing sensitivity from 2.0 to 1.0 mV will double the sensitivity). Testing pacemaker sensing should not be attempted in pacemaker-dependent patients.

Assessment of sensing is important, particularly in inferior infarction with RV involvement, when the intracardiac ventricular signal may be very small and not sensed. This resultant competition between pacemaker and spontaneous cardiac rhythm can initiate VT (see Figure 19.6) or VF.

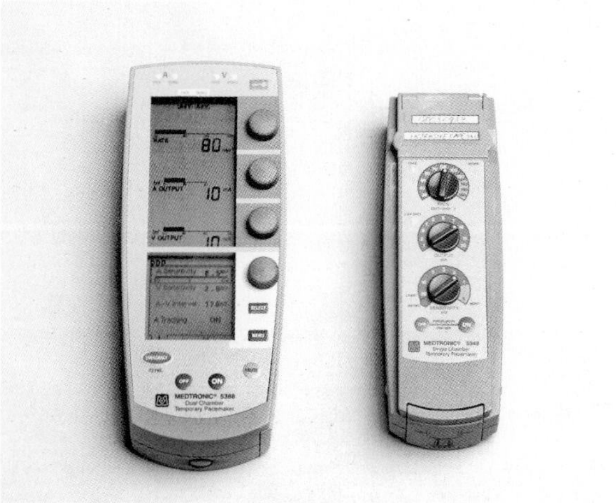

Figure 19.11 External pacemakers. Medtronic, Inc. (i) Model 5388 (dual-chamber); (ii) model 5348 (single-chamber). Both are capable of rapid pacing for certain tachycardias (see text).

COMPLICATIONS OF TEMPORARY PACING[21]

Temporary transvenous pacemaker insertions should have a low complication rate. There are, however, problems when inexperienced and/or inadequately trained operators insert the pacing lead. Several studies from the UK report complications in a third to a half of all cases.[22,23] Temporary pacing involves two components: (1) obtaining central venous access; and (2) intracardiac placement of the pacing lead. Complications include:

- those associated with central venous line insertion, such as pneumothorax, haemothorax, arterial puncture, AV fistula. Perforation of the RV can occur, but rarely results in cardiac tamponade
- undersensing, with pacemaker-induced arrhythmias; oversensing, with pacemaker inhibition and loss of pacing stimuli; and failure to capture, usually due to device defects, unstable lead position, increasing pacing threshold and occasionally RV perforation

- extracardiac stimulation, usually diaphragmatic (may be associated with RV perforation) and local muscle stimulation can also occur
- thrombus formation and infection occasionally

FAILURE TO PACE

A life-threatening situation may arise if the pacemaker suddenly fails. The following is an ordered approach to such an emergency:

1. Make sure the pacemaker is switched on and connected to the pacing lead(s).
2. The pacemaker output should be increased to its maximum setting (usually 20 mA or 10 V).
3. Asynchronous DOO/VOO mode(s) is selected to prevent oversensing.
4. Connect the pacemaker directly to the pacing lead, as occasionally the connecting wires may be faulty.
5. Give consideration to replacing the pacemaker unit or the batteries.
6. External transcutaneous pacing should be immediately available and commenced while a new pacing system is being inserted.
7. Cardiopulmonary resuscitation and positive chronotropic drugs such as atropine, isoprenaline or adrenaline (epinephrine) should be available.

PACEMAKER PROGRAMMING

An external programmer emits signals capable of changing ('programming') various pacing parameters (Table 19.4). Virtually all modern permanent pacemakers are capable of programming rate, voltage, output, pulse width, sensitivity, mode and AV interval. Programmability is also helpful in assessing various pacemaker problems. The pacemaker format best suited to a particular patient's needs may change with time, and programmability enables optimal pacemaker function to be achieved, i.e. 'prescribed'. Pacing changes may be indicated under certain circumstances, for example, decreased pacing rate in a patient with angina or acute myocardial infarction to reduce myocardial oxygen consumption, or increased rate in a patient with haemorrhagic shock.

Table 19.4 Multiprogrammable permanent dual-chamber pacemakers

Parameter	Adjustment	Comments
Rate	Increase	Increase cardiac output
	Decrease	Reduce myocardial oxygen consumption To assess underlying cardiac rhythm
Output	Increase	Increasing output may result in successful pacing when there is failure to capture
	Decrease	Increases battery life
Sensitivity	Increase	Reducing numerical value increases sensing ability May cause oversensing occasionally
	Decrease	Increasing numerical value decreases sensing ability Useful in oversensing, e.g. T-wave sensing
Mode	DDD to DDI	To prevent endless-loop tachycardias and to prevent tracking of episodic atrial tachyarrhythmias Mode switching can be automated and programmed either 'on' or 'off'
Atrioventricular interval (AVI)	Increase/ decrease	To optimise stroke volume and cardiac output AVI can be rate-adaptive, i.e. AVI shortens as the heart rate increases
Refractory period (atrial/ ventricular)	Increase	To minimise oversensing, e.g. to prevent ventricular sensing in AAI pacing
	Decrease	To optimise sensing under certain circumstances
Hysteresis		To preserve AV synchrony by delaying the onset of VVI pacing until the spontaneous heart rate is significantly less than the back-up ventricular pacing rate
Polarity	Unipolar mode	To improve sensing. Occasionally to allow pacing to continue when fracture of the other conducting wire occurs
	Bipolar mode	To prevent oversensing, e.g. muscle potentials

CARDIAC PACING IN TACHYARRHYTHMIAS

Certain tachyarrhythmias may be treated safely and effectively by rapid pacing and/or premature electrical stimulation. These include:

- AV nodal re-entry tachycardia (AVNRT)
- AV re-entry tachycardia (AVRT)
- atrial flutter
- unifocal atrial tachycardia
- ventricular tachycardia

AVNRT and AVRT rarely require rapid atrial pacing as treatment with drugs such as adenosine or verapamil is usually successful. Atrial flutter, however, is often resistant to drug therapy, and rapid atrial pacing will usually convert it to sinus rhythm. When unifocal atrial tachycardia is associated with an atrial re-entry circuit, rapid atrial pacing will often revert this arrhythmia; conversely, when due to automatic focus discharging at a rapid rate, the arrhythmia is usually incessant and will respond only intermittently, if at all, to atrial pacing. Occasionally, dual-chamber pacing with a short AV interval can be used to prevent drug-resistant AVNRT or AVRT. Rapid continuous atrial pacing can be used to slow ventricular rate during resistant SVTs associated with a rapid ventricular response, by inducing AF and a high degree of AV block. Sustained VT is responsive to rapid ventricular pacing, but this should not be used for very rapid ventricular rates (e.g. >300/min), or when severe haemodynamic compromise is present, as immediate DC cardioversion is indicated. Rapid cardiac pacing may at times have advantages over DC cardioversion (Table 19.5) and drug therapy (Table 19.6), but is of no value in sinus tachycardia, AF and VF (Table 19.7).

Table 19.5 Pacing versus cardioversion for the treatment of tachyarrhythmias

- Pacing may assist in rhythm diagnosis
- Pacing may be used (cautiously) in digitalis intoxication
- Pacing does not require a general anaesthetic
- Pacing avoids complications of DC shock, especially myocardial depression
- Repeated reversions are easier with pacing
- Standby pacing is immediately available if bradycardia or asystole occurs after electrical reversion

Table 19.6 Pacing versus drug therapy for the treatment of tachyarrhythmias

- Pacing may aid in arrhythmia diagnosis
- Pacing avoids drug-induced cardiac depression and other drug side-effects
- Pacing can be used when drug therapy has failed
- Termination of the tachycardia with pacing is often immediate
- Standby pacing is immediately available

Table 19.7 Indications for rapid cardiac pacing in suitable arrhythmias

- Failure of drug therapy
- Recurrent arrhythmias
- Contraindication for cardioversion (e.g. digitalis intoxication)
- Aid to arrhythmia diagnosis (e.g. wide-complex tachycardia to differentiate ventricular tachycardia from supraventricular tachycardia)

TORSADE DES POINTES

Only re-entrant monomorphic VT can be reverted with rapid ventricular pacing. In the acquired long QT syndrome the polymorphic tachycardia of torsade des pointes is invariably preceded/precipitated by pauses or bradycardia. Torsade des pointes can usually be prevented by pacing the atrium or the ventricle at 90–110 beats/min.

SUPRAVENTRICULAR TACHYARRHYTHMIAS

The pacing lead is manipulated to a suitable position in the RA. Atrial pacing is started at a slow rate (e.g. 60–80/min) and slowly increased to about 10–20% faster than the spontaneous atrial rate. Inadvertent ventricular pacing, especially at rapid rates, must be avoided. The atrium is paced for about 30 seconds and the pacemaker is then switched off. Normal sinus rhythm should ensue (Figure 19.12). If not, the pacing lead is manipulated to a different position and/or a faster pacing rate is tried. A more prolonged pacing period may be effective. If sinus rhythm still does not result, AF is deliberately precipitated by rapid atrial pacing at 400–800/min. This is an unstable rhythm which usually reverts spontaneously to normal sinus rhythm. AF persists occasionally, but the ventricular rate is usually slower and more responsive to drug therapy than with SVT.

VENTRICULAR TACHYCARDIA

Useful techniques to pace VT include the following:

1. Ventricular burst pacing (similar to rapid atrial pacing) is simple and effective. The ventricle is paced at a rate about 120% of the spontaneous VT rate for 5–10 beats. Normal sinus rhythm should ensue (Figure 19.13). Potential complications include entrainment (Figure 19.14), that is, speeding up of VT, and occasionally precipitation of VF. Trained personnel, a defibrillator and resuscitation facilities must be available.
2. Underdrive ventricular pacing at rates less than that of the tachycardia may occasionally be successful.
3. Overdrive atrial pacing may be useful if there is 1:1 AV conduction and the ventricular rate is relatively slow (e.g. 120–180/min).

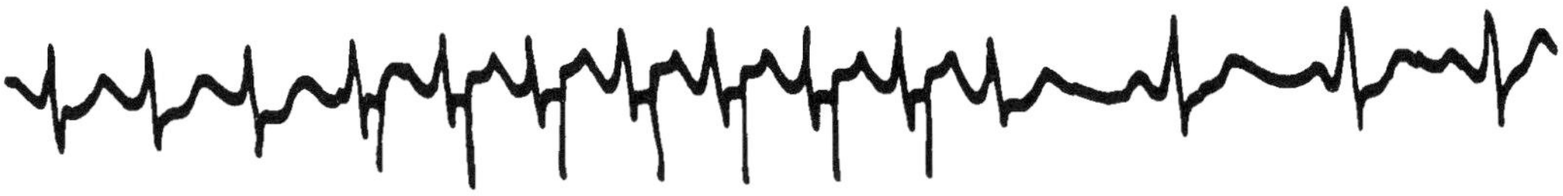

Figure 19.12 Narrow-complex tachycardia. Rapid atrial pacing with atrial capture results in sinus rhythm on cessation of pacing.

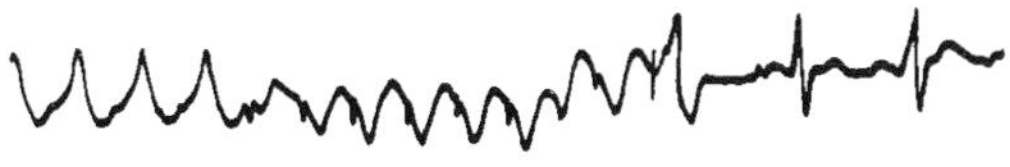

Figure 19.13 Wide-complex tachycardia. Ventricular burst pacing with ventricular capture results in normal sinus rhythm on cessation of pacing.

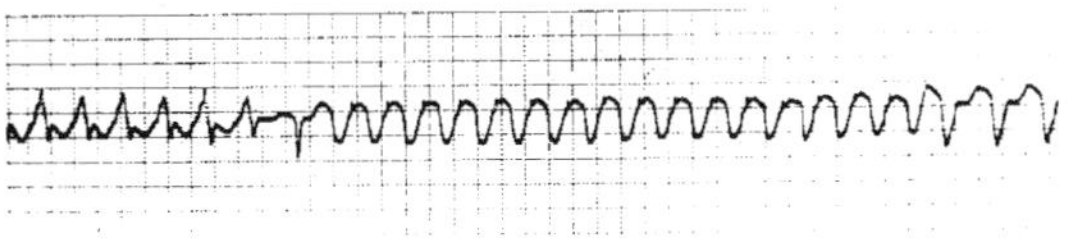

Figure 19.14 Example of entrainment. Wide-complex tachycardia is followed by ventricular burst pacing. When pacing is discontinued, a wide-complex tachycardia of opposite polarity is precipitated.

IMPLANTABLE CARDIOVERTER/DEFIBRILLATOR[2]

This is an implantable device which can recognise and automatically terminate VT and VF. Guidelines[13] have been published for ICD implantation; nevertheless, this is a rapidly evolving field with many trials in progress. ICDs are of proven survival benefit (class I) in patients who have had a cardiac arrest due to VF or VT, not due to transient or reversible cause. In other clinical situations ICD implantation may be a reasonable approach, for example, syncope with inducible VT at electrophysiology study which is poorly tolerated haemodynamically, and antiarrhythmic drugs are ineffective and/or contraindicated. A trial[24] in over 1200 patients with recent myocardial infarction (> 1 month) and low LV ejection fraction (30%) has demonstrated a decrease in mortality when prophylactic ICD implantation was compared to conventional treatment. ICDs are standard therapy to prevent sudden cardiac death in such high-risk patients.

Virtually all ICD systems are implanted transvenously and include antitachycardia pacing and back-up ventricular bradycardia pacing, dual-chamber pacing with rate-adaptive options. Single- or dual-chamber ICDs may be implanted. One trial[25] suggests that single-chamber ICDs may be superior to dual-chamber ICDs in patients who do not have an associated bradycardia. Current devices continuously monitor the patient's heart rate and deliver therapy when the heart rate exceeds a predetermined limit. There is a graded response which is programmable:

1. 'slow' VT (e.g. ventricular rate 160–180/min) – antitachycardia pacing, that is, pacing at a rate faster than the intrinsic rate. If this is unsuccessful, antitachycardia pacing might be attempted at a faster rate; or
2. DC shock(s) (synchronised during VT, asynchronous during VF), initially at low energies. If unsuccessful, then high-energy shocks are delivered. All shocks are biphasic as these are more efficient and require lower energies than monophasic waveforms
3. pacing back-up (single- or dual-chamber) is usually available if there is a significant bradycardia after cardioversion/defibrillation

COMPLICATIONS

Occasionally, multiple ICD discharges occur. This is a true clinical emergency. Shocks may be appropriate or inappropriate. Frequent malignant ventricular arrhythmias may result in multiple appropriate discharges. If DC shocks are unsuccessful, the device may need to be reprogrammed to deliver higher-energy shocks; conversely, if the multiple shocks are successful in defibrillating the patient during an arrhythmia 'storm', then the ICD device should probably be inactivated and external transthoracic defibrillation and antiarrhythmic drug therapy should be given as required. This will save battery power and allow the patient's ICD system to be tested later. If inappropriate ICD shocks arise, the ICD device should be switched off at once. The most common reason for inappropriate shocks is AF or some other SVT. Reprogramming the device may solve the problem. Occasionally sensing of EMI may cause ICD discharge. Avoidance of EMI source and/or reprogramming may be necessary. Nerve stimulators have been sensed by an ICD.

REFERENCES

1. Zoll PM. Resuscitation of the heart in ventricular standstill by external electric stimulation. *N Engl J Med* 1952; **247**: 768–71.
2. Hayes DL, Zipes DP. Cardiac pacemakers and cardioverter-defibrillators. In: Zipes DP, Libby P, Bonow RO *et al.* (eds). *Braunwald's Heart Disease: A Textbook of Cardiovascular Medicine*, 7th edn. Philadelphia: Elsevier Saunders; 2005: 767–802.

3. Trohman RG, Kim MH, Pinski SL. Cardiac pacing: the state of the art. *Lancet* 2004; **364**: 1701–19.
4. Bernstein AD, Camm AJ, Fletcher RD *et al.* The NASPE/BPEG generic pacemaker code for antibradyarrhythmic and adaptive rate pacing and antitachyarrhythmic devices. *Pace* 1987; **10**: 794–9.
5. Bernstein AD, Daubert JC, Fletcher RD *et al.* North American Society of Pacing and Electrophysiology/ British Pacing and Electrophysiology Group: the revised NASPE/BPEG generic code for antibradycardia, adaptive-rate, and multisite pacing. *Pacing Clin Electrophysiol* 2002; **25**: 260–4.
6. Leung S-K, Lau C-P. Developments in sensor-driven pacing. *Cardiol Clin* 2000; **18**: 113–55.
7. Furman S, Fisher JD. Endless-loop tachycardia in an AV universal (DDD) pacemaker. *Pace* 1982; **5**: 486–9.
8. Donovan KD, Dobb GJ, Lee KY. The haemodynamic importance of maintaining atrioventricular synchrony during cardiac pacing in critically ill patients. *Crit Care Med* 1991; **19**: 320–6.
9. Johnson AD, Laiken SL, Engler RL. Hemodynamic compromise associated with ventriculoatrial conduction following transvenous pacemaker placement. *Am J Med* 1978; **65**: 75–81.
10. Pierantozzi A, Bocconcelli P, Sgarbi E. DDD pacemaker syndrome and atrial conduction time. *Pace* 1994; **17**: 374–6.
11. Baller D, Hoeft A, Korb H *et al.* Basic physiological studies on cardiac pacing with special reference to the optimal mode and rate after cardiac surgery. *Thorac Cardiovasc Surg* 1981; **29**: 168–73.
12. Spotnitz HM. Optimizing temporary perioperative cardiac pacing. *J Thorac Cardiovasc Surg* 2005; **129**: 5–8.
13. Gregoratos G, Abrams, J, Epstein ET *et al.* ACC/ AHA/NASPE 2002 guideline update for implantation of cardiac pacemakers and antiarrhythmia devices. Summary article: a report of the American College of Cardiology/American Heart Association Task Force on Practice Guidelines (ACC/AHA/NASPE commmittee to update the 1998 pacemaker guidelines). *Circulation* 2002; **106**: 2145–61.
14. Guo H, Hahn D, Olshansky B. Temporary biventricular pacing in a patient with subacute myocardial infarction, cardiogenic shock, and third-degree atrioventricular block. *Heart Rhythm* 2005; **2**: 112.
15. Bryce M, Spielman SR, Greenspan AM *et al.* Evolving indications for permanent pacemakers. *Ann Intern Med* 2001; **134**: 1130–41.
16. Greenberg MD, Katz NM, Iuliano S *et al.* Atrial pacing for the prevention of atrial fibrillation after cardiovascular surgery. *J Am Coll Cardiol* 2000; **35**: 1416–22.
17. Blommaert D, Gonzalez M, Muccumbitsi J *et al.* Effective prevention of atrial fibrillation by continuous atrial overdrive pacing after coronary artery bypass surgery. *J Am Coll Cardiol* 2000; **35**: 1411–5.
18. Levy T, Fotopoulos G, Walker S *et al.* Randomized controlled study investigating the effect of biatrial pacing in prevention of atrial fibrillation after coronary artery bypass grafting. *Circulation* 2000; **102**: 1382–7.
19. Daubert JC, Mabo P. Atrial pacing for the prevention of postoperative atrial fibrillation: how and where to pace? *J Am Coll Cardiol* 2000; **35**: 1423–7.
20. Faris OP, Mitchell S. Magnetic resonance imaging of pacemaker and implantable cardioverter-defibrillator patients. *Circulation* 2006; **114**: 1232–3.
21. Donovan KD, Lee KY. Indications for and complications of temporary transvenous cardiac pacing. *Anaesth Intens Care* 1985; **13**: 63–70.
22. Betts TR. Regional survey of temporary transvenous pacing procedures and complications. *Postgrad Med J* 2003; **79**: 463–5.
23. Murphy JJ. Problems with temporary cardiac pacing. *Br Med J* 2001; **323**: 527.
24. Moss AJ, Zareba W, Hall WJ *et al.* Prophylactic implantation of a defibrillator in patients with myocardial infarction and reduced ejection fraction. *N Engl J Med* 2002; **346**: 877–83.
25. Wilkoff BL, Cook JR, Epstein AE *et al.* Dual-chamber pacing or ventricular backup pacing in patients with an implantable defibrillator: the Dual chamber and VVI Implantable Defibrillator (DAVID) trial. *JAMA* 2002; **288**: 3115–23.

20

Acute heart failure

David Treacher

The pattern of heart failure seen in the community, outpatients clinics and specialist cardiac wards is dominated by the acute coronary syndromes and chronic heart failure, predominantly caused by ischaemic heart disease and hypertension.[1,2] Heart failure is the commonest cause of hospital admission in people over 65 years of age and it has been estimated that in North America and Europe over 15 million patients have heart failure and 1.5 million new cases are diagnosed each year.[3] Patients present with chest pain, shortness of breath, fatigue and oedema and will usually have single-organ failure. Management focuses on reducing cardiac work to relieve symptoms and prevent further myocardial damage.[4,5]

Patients either admitted with or who develop acute heart failure on the intensive care unit (ICU) frequently have overt or occult underlying coronary artery disease, but will usually have significant other organ dysfunction. Management in this setting focuses on both improving global and regional oxygen delivery and maintaining perfusion pressure, often with the use of drugs that stimulate rather than rest the myocardium.[6–8] The resolution of this apparent paradox requires that for each patient management should attempt to achieve the frequently difficult balance between the best interests of the myocardium and the circulatory requirements of the other vital organs. The critical care physician should target the minimum necessary oxygen delivery and arterial pressure to maintain other organ function at maximum cardiac efficiency (e.g. ensuring adequate fluid resuscitation before starting beta-agonists) so that cardiac work and the risk of myocardial ischaemia and necrosis from exuberant beta-agonist use are minimised and the cardiologist should consider the wider circulation and other organ requirements when instituting strategies to protect the myocardium.

DIAGNOSIS OF ACUTE HEART FAILURE

The diagnosis of acute heart failure in critically ill patients can be more difficult than is commonly recognised. Although the underlying pathology in most patients with acute heart failure on intensive care will be coronary artery disease, other diagnoses must be considered (Table 20.1).

It is also important to reassess critically the patient referred with a diagnosis of acute heart failure to decide whether this is indeed the primary problem. The history, examination and initial investigations with routine blood tests, electrocardiogram (ECG) and chest X-ray may be compatible with this diagnosis but many such patients are elderly with multiple comorbidities and deciding whether the patient is suffering from a primary myocardial pathology as opposed to a pulmonary problem or indeed systemic sepsis[9] can be difficult. Equally, patients believed to have a primary respiratory problem may fail to wean from ventilatory support because of a failure to realise that they have left ventricular failure with a high left atrial pressure and incipient pulmonary oedema, causing a reduction in pulmonary compliance, an increased work of breathing and respiratory distress when ventilatory support is withdrawn.

Further investigations that can help to confirm or refute an initial diagnosis of acute heart failure are echocardiography and the measurement of recently available biomarkers such as troponin and brain natriuretic peptide.

ECHOCARDIOGRAPHY (SEE CHAPTER 23)

Echocardiography is an extremely valuable investigation in the management of the critically ill patient with acute heart failure[10] and the modern critical care physician should at least be able to perform a basic examination. It will frequently establish the underlying cardiac pathology and can be used to monitor the response to treatment. It will:

1. identify pericardial effusions and determine whether ventricular filling is impaired (tamponade) and whether drainage is indicated. However, ultimately tamponade is a clinical diagnosis based on the full haemodynamic picture in the context of pericardial fluid demonstrated on the echocardiogram. Many of the diagnostic features related to alterations with respiration are affected by positive-pressure ventilation and drainage may be appropriate even if such classic echocardiographic criteria are not present. Even small effusions may cause tamponade since it is the rate of accumulation of fluid rather than the amount of fluid that determines the degree of cardiac compromise
2. identify obstruction to cardiac filling from other intrathoracic space-occupying lesions that increase

Table 20.1 Causes of acute heart failure on the intensive care unit

Coronary artery disease
Infection – systemic sepsis,[9] myocarditis
Mechanical – endocarditis, pulmonary emboli, valve problems, septal defects, tamponade, high intrathoracic pressure with inadequate preload
Drugs – beta-blockers, calcium antagonists, cytotoxic therapy
Hypoxaemia
Metabolic – acidaemia, thiamine deficiency, hypocalcaemia, hypophosphataemia
Myocardial contusion – blunt thoracic trauma
Myocardial infiltration – tumour, sarcoidosis, amyloidosis
Vasculitis – rare

intrathoracic pressure, particularly in ventilated patients (pleural effusion, alveolar gas trapping in asthma)
3. assess adequacy of *volume* preload of left ventricle, particularly in the context of raised preload *pressures* and monitor response to fluid challenge
4. identify primary valvular heart disease (critical aortic stenosis, acute mitral regurgitation from papillary muscle rupture, acute endocarditis) when urgent surgery is indicated and distinguish this from functional valvular regurgitation due to primary ventricular disease for which surgery could be lethal
5. identify septal defects, regional wall motion abnormalities and aneurysmal dilatation from recent or previous myocardial infarction
6. identify the presence of intracardiac thrombus or clot
7. identify increased end-systolic and diastolic dimensions, indicating ventricular contractile failure. However the use of ejection fraction as an index of ventricular dysfunction can be misleading, especially in patients on inotropic drugs
8. identify diastolic dysfunction when high-pressure preload measurements fail to reflect true volume preload and extra fluid volume may be indicated
9. identify pulmonary hypertension associated with tricuspid regurgitation when an estimate of pulmonary artery (PA) pressure can be made

The images obtained with transthoracic echocardiography (TTE) may be poor in ventilated patients but the experienced operator can achieve considerable improvement using microbubble contrast techniques.[11]

Transoesophageal echo (TOE) gives excellent views of the aorta (dissections), the atria and left heart valves and is indicated if transthoracic views are very difficult to obtain or if better resolution is required. Right heart structures and the left ventricle are less well imaged.

MEASUREMENT OF TROPONIN AND BRAIN NATRIURETIC PEPTIDE

Myocardial injury and the development of acute heart failure are common but frequently unrecognised complications of critical illness occurring not only in patients with an overt acute coronary syndrome but also in other conditions such as sepsis and major pulmonary embolism (PE).[12] Relying on blood tests alone to establish a diagnosis or to plan management is inadvisable but, when interpreted in conjunction with the wider clinical picture, brain-type natriuretic peptide (BNP) and cardiac troponin are two tests that are becoming routinely available and appear to be sensitive markers of myocardial stress and necrosis and to have significant prognostic significance.

BRAIN-TYPE NATRIURETIC PEPTIDE

BNP was first isolated from porcine brain but the major source is the ventricular myocardium. The main stimulus for synthesis and release is myocardial wall stress. As a triage tool in the emergency department it is able to discriminate patients with heart failure from those with pulmonary or other non-cardiac causes for acute dyspnoea and has been shown to reduce rates of ICU admission, length of hospital stay and cost.[13] Several studies have demonstrated that, below a cut-off of 100 pg/ml, BNP has a sensitivity of almost 90% and a specificity approaching 80% as a test for excluding heart failure.[14] It is now included in both the European and UK National Institute for Clinical Excellence guidelines for the management of heart failure[15,16] and BNP has also been shown to be a marker of myocardial dysfunction and prognosis in severe sepsis.[17]

CARDIAC TROPONIN I AND T (cTnI, cTnT)

Troponin is part of the thin filament of the myocyte contractile apparatus and has three subunits: (1) I, which binds actin to inhibit actin-myosin contraction; (2) T, which binds tropomyosin to facilitate contraction; and (3) C, which binds calcium ions. The cardiac isoforms cTnI and cTnT are specific to the heart and can be measured in the blood after myocyte necrosis with 50% release by 4 hours, peaking at 12–24 hours and remaining elevated for up to 10 days. It is far more sensitive than the traditional cardiac enzyme tests such as creatine kinase and indeed it has substantially changed the diagnosis and management of acute myocardial infarction, as reflected in the new guidelines issued by the European Society of Cardiology[15] and American College of Cardiologists. Troponin may be released in conditions other than acute coronary ischaemia[18] such as sepsis and after chemotherapy and in the absence of evidence of myocardial necrosis as in acute heart failure or major PE, where it is believed that the acute ventricular dilatation causes increased membrane permeability. Raised troponin levels are also associated with increased morbidity and mortality in surgical ICU patients.[19]

In combination with BNP, cTnI is valuable in screening for massive PE: in massive and submassive PE both are raised and further investigation with computed tomography pulmonary angiogram (CTPA) is indicated but in minor PE both will be negative.

Raised levels of either of these markers, but particularly BNP indicating early myocardial stress, may have an important role in alerting the clinician to impending myocardial failure and the need to review the use of drugs that stimulate the myocardium and to consider the introduction of a beta-blocker, particularly in the context of tachycardia.

It should be remembered that, for critically ill patients with acute heart failure not resulting from primary myocardial infarction, if the precipitating cause is successfully treated without significant myocardial necrosis occurring, the acute heart failure will resolve, cardiac function will return to its premorbid state and the prognosis will be improved.

The remainder of this chapter addresses the assessment and principles of management of ventricular function in patients admitted to the ICU with acute heart failure. This inevitably involves reference to circulatory failure and the state of the peripheral circulation but the more detailed aspects of oxygen delivery and control of the regional and microcirculation are considered elsewhere[20] (see Chapters 11 and 12), as are the acute coronary syndromes[2] (see Chapter 16) and chronic heart failure.[1]

CIRCULATORY FAILURE OR 'SHOCK'

The principal function of the heart is the generation of the energy necessary to perfuse the lungs with venous blood and to propel the oxygenated arterial blood through the systemic circulation at a rate and pressure that ensure that the fluctuating metabolic requirements of the various organs are met at rest and during exercise. This should be performed at maximum efficiency so that the work performed is not at the cost of unnecessarily high myocardial energy expenditure and the risk of myocardial ischaemia is minimised.

Failure to maintain an adequate oxygen supply to the tissues with the consequent development of anaerobic cellular metabolism defines circulatory failure or 'shock', a term that benefits from brevity but little else since it implies neither cause nor prognosis, but its use is now widespread and inescapable. Table 20.2 classifies circulatory 'shock'.

In considering these causes of circulatory failure, several points require emphasis:

1. Acute heart failure resulting in cardiogenic shock is not a pathological diagnosis but a collective term that embraces all causes of myocardial failure. Treatment must focus on the underlying diagnosis.
2. Patients admitted to ICU may have acute heart failure either as the primary reason for admission, e.g. severe myocardial infarction, or develop it as part of multiple organ failure triggered by an extracardiac cause, frequently the delayed or ineffective treatment of severe sepsis.
3. Pre-existing cardiac disease, usually ischaemic heart disease, is an important factor in determining the physiological response to critical illness. Several studies investigating the effect of manipulating oxygen delivery have demonstrated the poor prognosis associated with the inability of the heart to achieve a hyperdynamic response to critical illness either spontaneously or with volume loading and inotropic support.[7,8,21] Preoperative assessment with exercise testing is probably appropriate for all patients undergoing major surgery as a means of identifying those with poor physiological reserve so that the true risk of surgery can be identified and perioperative management planned accordingly.
4. Although hypotension is often considered to be the cardinal sign of circulatory failure, other global features (persistent tachycardia, confusion, tachypnoea, impaired peripheral perfusion, progressive metabolic acidaemia) occur earlier since the body has powerful homeostatic mechanisms that maintain pressure at the expense of flow.
5. The heart must provide its own blood supply and, if coronary blood flow does not match myocardial oxygen requirements, coronary ischaemia develops and cardiac and global circulatory failure may ensue.[22]
6. The primary problem in hypovolaemic, cardiogenic and obstructive shock is a progressive decline in cardiac output (CO) and global oxygen delivery, which, if not corrected, leads to secondary failure of the peripheral circulation and progressive organ dysfunction. In septic, anaphylactic and neurogenic shock, however, the primary problem is the loss of control of the peripheral circulation resulting in systemic hypotension and disordered distribution of blood flow, although CO and global oxygen delivery are usually increased.[23]
7. Although a primary cause for the circulatory failure may be identified, other causes may contribute to the

Table 20.2 Major categories of circulatory failure or 'shock'

Cardiogenic	Myocardial infarction, myocarditis, vasculitis, valve dysfunction (e.g. critical aortic stenosis, mitral regurgitation, acute endocarditis), post cardiac bypass surgery, drug overdose (β-blockers, calcium antagonists)
Hypovolaemic	Haemorrhage, burns, gastrointestinal fluid loss
Obstructive	Pulmonary embolus, cardiac tamponade, tension pneumothorax
Anaphylactic	Drugs, blood transfusion, insect sting
Septic	Bacterial infection, non-infective inflammatory conditions, e.g. pancreatitis, burns, trauma
Neurogenic	Intracranial haemorrhage, brainstem compression, spinal cord injury

evolution of the final pathology. For example, in septic shock the initial and major derangement is peripheral: it is characterised by microcirculatory chaos triggered by cytokine release, white-cell activation, disruption of the coagulation cascade resulting in microthrombi that occlude the microvasculature and endothelial disruption resulting in interstitial oedema. This same process occurs in the coronary microvasculature impairing myocyte function.[24] There is also widespread loss of fluid from the intravascular to the extravascular space, resulting in hypovolaemia. The primary peripheral circulatory failure may therefore be compounded by both cardiogenic and hypovolaemic shock.

8. 'Early' and 'late' shock are terms that reflect the association between the duration and severity of the circulatory derangement and prognosis. Early intervention in circulatory shock has a major impact on survival.[25] If treatment is delayed until organ failure is established, the underlying pathological processes are frequently irreversible.
9. Although not a true 'mixed' venous sample, the oxygen saturation of blood taken from an internal jugular ($S_{ij}O_2$) or subclavian cannula has been shown to be valuable in assessing whether global oxygen delivery (DO_2) is adequate for global tissue oxygen consumption. A value $< 70\%$ should prompt consideration of whether a fluid challenge or other strategy to increase DO_2 is indicated. A value $> 70\%$ is not necessarily reassuring in patients with established hyperdynamic shock as this may reflect an inability of the tissues to extract and utilise oxygen.

ASSESSMENT OF VENTRICULAR FUNCTION

Making the considerable assumption that the circulation can be analysed as a constant-flow, fixed-compliance system, six key measurements traditionally define ventricular performance:

- Right and left atrial pressures (RAP, LAP or ventricular preload)
- Mean systemic and pulmonary arterial pressures (MAP, PAP or ventricular afterload)
- Heart rate (HR)
- CO (Q_t)

Table 20.3 illustrates typical values in normal subjects and in the common causes of circulatory failure with calculation of the associated vascular resistances and oxygen delivery. The values quoted are merely examples that indicate the pattern of circulatory derangement produced by these pathologies: pre-existing cardiopulmonary disease and the severity of the condition will affect the precise figures obtained in individual cases and the response to vasoactive therapy.

Stroke volume (SV) is calculated from CO and heart rate:

$$SV = Q_t/HR$$

Three factors determine stroke volume: (1) preload; (2) afterload; and (3) myocardial contractility.

VENTRICULAR PRELOAD

Ventricular preload, traditionally assessed from the atrial filling pressures, determines the end-diastolic ventricular volume, which, according to Starling's law of the heart and depending on ventricular contractility, dictates the stroke work generated by each ventricle at the next cardiac contraction. The resulting stroke volume depends on the resistance or afterload that confronts the ventricle.[26]

On the general ward the jugular venous pressure (JVP) is measured from the sternal angle but in ICU vascular pressures are measured from the mid-axillary line in the fifth intercostal space. From this reference point, in the supine position, the normal RAP is between 4 and 8 mmHg and the LAP, or wedge pressure, is between 8 and 12 mmHg. Relative changes in either the contractility of the two ventricles or the respective vascular resistances will change the relationship between the atrial pressures, which must then be independently assessed.[27]

The predominant factor determining preload is venous return, which depends on the intravascular volume and venous tone, which is controlled by the autonomic nervous system, circulating catecholamine levels and local factors, particularly PO_2, PCO_2 and pH.

The systemic venous bed is the major intravascular capacitance or reservoir of the circulation with a compliance that can vary from 30 to over 300 ml/mmHg and which provides a buffer against the effects of intravascular volume loss. It also explains the response observed in major haemorrhage and subsequent transfusion. As volume is lost, venous tone increases, preventing the large falls in atrial filling pressures and CO that would otherwise occur. If the equivalent volume is returned over the subsequent few hours the RAP gradually returns to normal as the intravascular volume is restored and the reflex increase in sympathetic tone abates. However, rapid reinfusion of the same volume does not allow sufficient time for the venous and arteriolar tone to fall and may result in the LAP rising to a level that precipitates pulmonary oedema, although the intravascular volume has only been returned to the prehaemorrhage level and left ventricular function is normal (Figure 20.1).

If the preload is low and either blood pressure or CO is inadequate, the priority is volume loading to restore intravascular volume and venous return.

Raised preload pressures reflect: (1) high intravascular volume; (2) impaired myocardial contractility; or (3) increased afterload.

Preload may be reduced by:

- removing volume from the circulation (diuretics, venesection, haemofiltration) or increasing the capacity of the vascular bed with venodilator therapy (e.g. glyceryl trinitrate, morphine[28])
- improving contractility
- reducing afterload[29]

Table 20.3 Measurements in a normal 75-kg adult and in various conditions causing circulatory 'shock'

	RAP (mmHg)	LAP (mmHg)	PAP (mmHg)	MAP (mmHg)	HR (per min)	Cardiac output (l/min)	SVR*	PVR*	Stroke work (g.m)		Venous compliance (ml/mmHg)	CaO_2 (l/100 ml)	DO_2 (ml/min)
									LV	RV			
Normal	5	10	15	90	70	5.0	17	1.0	78	10	300	20	1000
Major haemorrhage	0	3	10	80	100	3.2	25	2.2	34	4.4	40	16	510
Left ventricular failure	7	19	23	90	100	3.6	23	1.1	35	8	80	18	650
Cardiac tamponade	14	16	19	65	110	2.3	22	1.3	14	1.4	50	20	460
Major PE	10	6	35	70	110	2.6	23	11.0	21	8	40	16	420
Exacerbation of COAD	10	9	35	80	100	6.5	11	4.0	63	22	150	13	850
Septic shock:													
(i) pre-volume	2	7	17	49	130	4.2	11	2.4	18	7	350	15	630
(ii) post-volume	10	14	25	68	120	8.0	7	1.4	49	14	200	14	1120

Typical circulatory measurements in a normal adult and in various cardiorespiratory conditions that may cause shock. The severity of the condition and pre-existing cardiorespiratory disease will affect the precise figures obtained in individual cases.

Pressures referenced to zero at mid-axillary line in supine patient. Subtract vertical distance from mid-axilla to sternal angle (approximately 5–7 mmHg) if sternal angle used as reference point.

LV, Left ventricle; RV, right ventricle; CaO_2, arterial oxygen content; DO_2, global oxygen delivery; PAP/MAP, mean pulmonary artery/arterial pressure; SVR*/PVR*, systemic/pulmonary vascular resistance $\times$ 80 to give SI units: $dyn{\cdot}s{\cdot}cm^{-5}$.

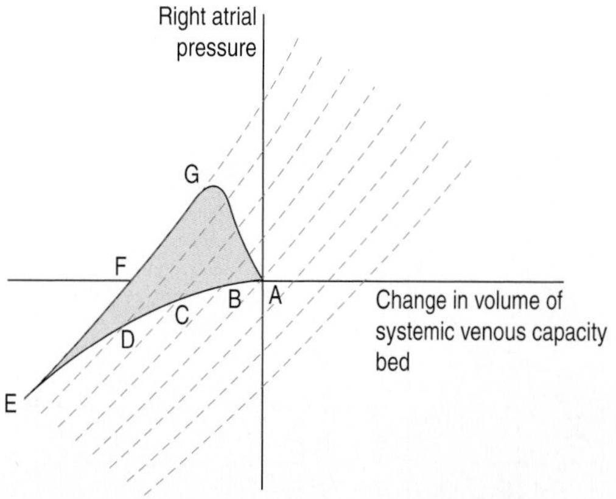

Figure 20.1 Venous compliance curves. Each dotted line represents a line of constant venous compliance ranging from low compliance (increased tone) on the left to increased compliance (reduced tone) on the right. Line ABCDE shows the effect of progressive haemorrhage with the reduction in venous compliance limiting the fall in atrial pressure. Line EFGA shows the effect of rapid reinfusion of the same volume that was removed but at a rate that does not allow the sympathetically mediated increase in venous tone to abate. Each dotted line represents a line of constant venous compliance ranging from minimum on the left to diminished venous tone on the right.

In assessing preload, end-diastolic *volume* rather than pressure is relevant and when interpreting atrial *pressures* as measures of preload, two points must be considered:

1. Intravascular pressure (P_v) measurements are misleading if the intrathoracic pressure (P_t) is raised, since the true distending pressure that determines ventricular end-diastolic volume is the transmural pressure ($P_v - P_t$). This is particularly relevant if there is significant alveolar gas trapping generating intrinsic or auto positive end-expiratory pressure (PEEP), as in asthma, and positive-pressure ventilation with high PEEP levels and an inverse inspiratory-to-expiratory time ratio.[30,31]
2. When the ventricle is dilated and poorly compliant, the end-diastolic pressure–volume relationship is not necessarily linear and *pressure* will not necessarily reflect the adequacy of *volume* preload.

Alternative methods of assessing ventricular preload are discussed later in this chapter under "Assessment of intravascular volume status" and in Chapter 12.

VENTRICULAR AFTERLOAD

The vascular resistance against which each ventricle works is calculated, by analogy with Ohm's law, as the pressure gradient across the vascular bed divided by the CO (Table 20.4).

Circulatory management requires a clear understanding of this relationship between pressure, flow and resistance. If ventricular work is constant, increased vascular resistances produce higher pressures but with a lower CO. A systemic dilator such as sodium nitroprusside will reduce systemic resistance and blood pressure and increase CO. Although such manipulation is attractive in increasing CO for the same cardiac work, it is important to maintain a blood pressure that ensures appropriate distribution of blood flow and a diastolic pressure sufficient to maintain coronary artery perfusion, particularly in patients with known ischaemic heart disease or pre-existing hypertension.

The effects of some of the commonly used vasoactive agents are shown in Table 20.5 and considered in more detail later (see Chapters 79 and 80).

Table 20.4 Calculation of ventricular afterload and stroke work

Systemic vascular resistance (SVR)	$= [(\text{MAP} - \text{RAP})/Q_t] \times 80$ dyn.s.cm^{-5}
	$= [(90 - 5)/5] \times 80 = 1360$ dyn.s.cm^{-5}
SVRI	$=$ SVR $\times$ BSA $= 1360 \times 1.65 = 2244$ dyn.s.cm^{-9}
Pulmonary vascular resistance (PVR)	$= [(\text{PAP} - \text{LAP})/Q_t \times 80$ dyn.s.cm^{-5}
	$= [(15 - 5)/5] \times 80 = 160$ dyn.s.cm^{-5}
PVRI	$=$ PVR $\times$ BSA $= 160 \times 1.65 = 264$ dyn.s.cm^{-9}
Stroke volume (SV)	$= Q_t/\text{HR} = 72$ ml
Stroke volume index (SVI)	$= 72/1.65 = 44$ ml/m^2
Ventricular stroke work (VSV)	$=$ SV $\times$ (afterload $-$ preload)
LVSW	$=$ SV $\times$ (MAP $-$ LAP) $\times$ 0.0136 g.m
	$= 72 \times (90 - 10) \times 0.0136 = 78$ g.m
LVSWI	$= 78/1.65 = 47$ g.m
RVSW	$=$ SV $\times$ (PAP $-$ RAP) $\times$ 0.0136 g.m
	$= 72 \times (15 - 5) \times 0.0136 = 10$ g.m
RVSWI	$= 10/1.65 = 6$ g.m

MAP, mean arterial pressure; PAP, mean pulmonary artery pressure.
Pressures are measured in mmHg, cardiac output (Q_t) in l/min.
Values for resistance, stroke work are frequently indexed by dividing by the patient's body surface area (BSA) derived from height and weight.
In calculating ventricular stroke work, 0.0136 converts from ml.mmHg to SI units of g.m.
Example calculations assume a normal 75-kg individual with BSA 1.65 m^2.

Table 20.5 Circulatory effects of commonly used vasoactive drug infusions

Drug	Receptors	Cardiac contractility	Heart rate	Blood pressure	Cardiac output	Splanchnic blood flow	SVR	PVR
Dopamine								
(<5 μg/kg per min)	DA1, β1, α	+	0/+	0/+	+	0/+	0/+	0/+
(>5 μg/kg per min)	β1, α, DA1, β2	++	+	+	++	0	+	+
Epinephrine	β1, α, β2	++	+	++	+++	−	+	+
Norepinephrine	α, β1	0/+	0	++	−	− −	++	++
Isoprenaline	β1, β2	+	++	+/0	+	0/+	−	−
Dobutamine	β1, β2, α	+	+	+/0/−	++	0	−	−
Dopexamine	β2, DA1, DA2	+	+	0	+	+	−	−
Glyceryl trinitrate	via NO	0	+	−	+	+	−	−
Nitroprusside	via NO	0	+	− −	+	+	− −	−
Milrinone	PDE	+	+	−	++	0/+	− −	−
Nitric oxide (inhaled)	via NO	0	0	0	0/+	0	0	− −
Prostacyclin		0	+	− −	+	+	−	− −

+, increases; 0, no change; −, decreases.
These effects are guidelines only. The response will depend on the circulatory state of the patient when the drug is started and the differential effects on α, β, dopamine (DA1, DA2), phosphodiesterase (PDE) receptors and nitric oxide/cGMP with increasing dose.

VENTRICULAR CONTRACTILITY AND EFFICIENCY

The work that the ventricle performs under given loading conditions defines contractility.

For each ventricle it may be expressed mathematically as the gradient and intercept of the relationship between atrial filling pressure and stroke work (Figure 20.2). The resulting stroke volume varies with the resistance of the vascular bed into which the ventricle is ejecting. Although the right ventricle generates a much smaller stroke work, the afterload (pulmonary vascular resistance) against which it ejects is correspondingly lower since the right and left ventricular stroke volumes must necessarily be the same over time.

The work generated by each ventricle with each heart beat is the ventricular stroke work and is calculated as shown in Table 20.4.

Consideration of ventricular work is important since optimum circulatory management requires that the necessary pressures and flows to maintain satisfactory organ perfusion and oxygen delivery are achieved at maximum cardiac efficiency, i.e. for the minimum ventricular work to avoid myocardial ischaemia.

Left ventricular efficiency is the ratio of work output to energy input and may be less than 20% in patients with acute heart failure, with over 80% of energy lost as heat. A technique, based on thermodynamic principles and requiring only measurement of temperature and oxygen content difference across the left ventricular capillary bed, is simpler, clinically applicable and more accurate than earlier methods.[32] It will allow selection of therapies based on both global circulatory and myocardial metabolic considerations.

If circulatory failure is due to impaired myocardial contractility, as defined by a 'flattened' stroke work/filling pressure equation (see Figure 20.2), the atrial pressures will often already be raised. Provided such pressures reflect volume preload, further increases are not helpful since the ventricle becomes increasingly distended with high wall tension, as predicted by Laplace's law:

$$\text{Wall tension} = (\text{intraventricular pressure} \times \text{radius}) \div (\text{wall thickness} \times 2)$$

This increase in wall tension compromises myocardial blood supply, particularly epicardial to endocardial blood flow, resulting in endocardial ischaemia, further impairment of ventricular contractility and the risk of pulmonary oedema developing.

The remaining therapeutic options are:

- *Reduce afterload* using an arteriolar dilator (nitrates, α-blocker, phosphodiesterase inhibitor, angiotensin-converting enzyme (ACE) inhibitor), although this strategy is frequently limited by the resulting fall in systemic pressure.[33]
- *Increase myocardial contractility*, either by removing negatively inotropic influences (acidaemia, hyperkalaemia, drugs, e.g. β-blockers) or by using a positive inotrope, which may be defined as an agent that increases the gradient of the stroke work to filling pressure relationship, resulting in a larger stroke volume for the same pre- and afterload pressures. When considering

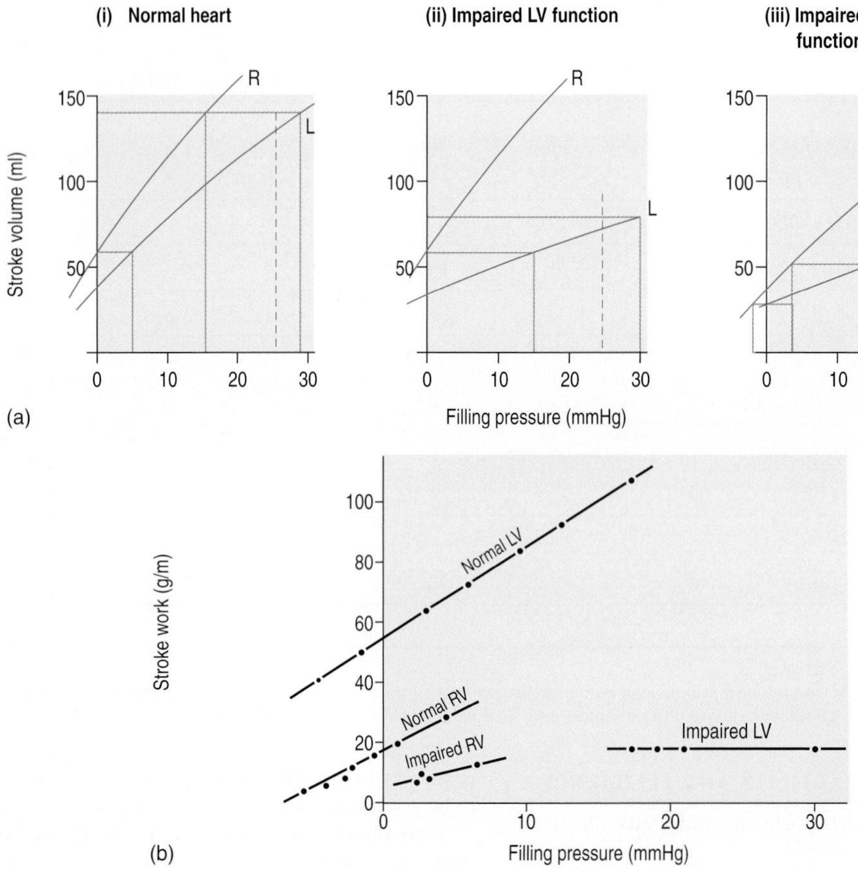

Figure 20.2 Ventricular function curves. (a) Relationship between stroke volume (ml) and atrial filling pressure for left (L) and right (R) ventricles in patients with normal and impaired ventricular function. (b) Relationship between stroke work (g.m) and atrial filling pressure (in mmHg) for the left (L) and right (R) ventricles for a normal subject and a patient with severe left and right ventricular failure.

the use of an inotropic agent (Table 20.5), the adverse effects of vasoactive agents on ventricular efficiency, metabolic rate and regional distribution of flow should be considered.[34]

HEART RATE AND RHYTHM

In cardiac failure the stroke volume is usually constant for rates up to 100/min and thereafter falls as restriction of diastolic filling time limits end-diastolic volume. Increasing the heart rate from 70 to 90/min will increase CO by almost 30%. Achieving this with a chronotrope such as the β_1-agonist isoproterenol increases myocardial work and oxygen consumption and also ventricular irritability. In patients with ischaemic heart disease and particularly after a recent myocardial infarction, atrial or atrioventricular sequential pacing (which maintains coordinated atrial contraction in heart block) improves haemodynamics without stimulating myocardial metabolism and increasing myocardial irritability.[35]

Heart rates above 110 beats/min, particularly with an irregular rhythm, should be controlled by either drugs or DC cardioversion after ensuring that plasma potassium and magnesium levels have been corrected. If the rhythm is supraventricular and unstable with intermittent periods of sinus rhythm, pharmacological control is indicated using either digoxin or amiodarone. Digoxin is appropriate for atrial fibrillation and has a temporary positive inotropic effect.[36] However amiodarone is suitable for all supraventricular rhythms and is more likely to restore sinus rhythm. A meta-analysis showed that, used prophylactically, it reduced the rate of arrhythmic episodes and sudden death in patients with recent myocardial infarction or congestive cardiac failure.[37] It is however a negative inotrope and this can be significant in the patient with severe heart failure.

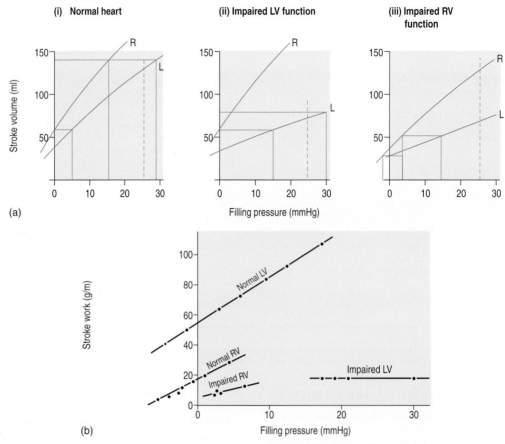

A fixed rate of 150/min suggests atrial flutter and should prompt careful inspection of the ECG and a trial of adenosine. A persistent sinus tachycardia unexplained by fever may be due to hypovolaemia, pain or anxiety.

ASSESSMENT OF MYOCARDIAL FUNCTION

Of the six key circulatory variables that define ventricular function, three (RAP, MAP and HR) can be assessed clinically and are routinely monitored in ICU patients. However additional monitoring, traditionally using the PA catheter, is required to *measure* the other variables (LAP, PAP and Q_t) and answer the questions:

1. Is further intravascular volume indicated?
2. Is CO too low and compromising global oxygen delivery?
3. Is dilator, constrictor or inotropic therapy appropriate?

It is certainly not always necessary to use invasive monitoring.[38] Initial management can be based on clinical assessment of intravascular volume and CO. The discipline of committing to an estimate of these key variables ensures that both the analysis of the circulation and the approach to treatment are logical. Further monitoring should be instituted if the initial management does not produce clinical improvement. Alternative, less invasive methods are available for assessing CO such as transoesophageal Doppler,[39] lithium dilution,[40] continuous CO by pulse contour analysis (PiCCO) and echocardiography[10] – techniques which can also provide data on the volume rather than pressure preload of the left ventricle. Table 20.6 lists some features of the techniques available for measuring CO and whether they provide information on left ventricular preload. Further details of circulatory monitoring and these other techniques are described in the section on haemodynamic monitoring (see Chapter 12). A recent International Consensus Conference produced guidelines for the haemodynamic monitoring and management of patients with shock.[41]

KEY POINTS WHEN ASSESSING CARDIAC FUNCTION

- Pressure is no guarantee of flow
- Trends and changes are more important than a single observation
- Dynamic tests (fluid challenge, pulse pressure variation with respiration) are more revealing than static tests (RAP, central venous pressure)
- Monitoring devices may be complex with many potential sources of error, e.g. 'blocked' catheters, failure to re-level the transducer after a change in the patient's position. Readings should always be interpreted with care and in conjunction with clinical assessment
- Invasive monitoring has its own hazards (infection, trauma, immobility) and should be removed if no longer required

PULMONARY ARTERY CATHETERISATION

This remains *one of* the most widely used methods for measurement of left atrial and PA pressures and assessment of CO using the thermodilution technique.[42] Although generally viewed as the 'gold standard' for determining CO, the error is at least 10%, even with fastidious attention to technical detail.

Inflation of the balloon at the end of the catheter provides a PA occlusion or wedge pressure, which reflects left atrial pressure provided there are no significant

Table 20.6 Comparison of methods for assessing cardiac output

Method	Invasion/risk	Ventricular preload assessed	Complexity	Measurement error	Cost
Indicator dilution					
Thermodilution (using PA catheter)	+++	From 'wedge' pressure	++	+	++
Fick	+++	No	+++	+	++
Indocyanine green	+++	No	++	+	++
Lithium	++	Yes	+	+	+
Respired gas					
Modified Fick	+	No	++	++	+
Inert gas rebreathing	+	Yes	+++	++	+
Doppler (transoesophageal)	+	Yes	++	++	+++
Echocardiography	0	Yes	++	+++	+
Impedance cardiography	0	No	++	++	+
Pulse contour analysis	+	Yes (ITBV)	+	++	+
Clinical assessment	0	Yes	+	++	0

Table 20.7 Indications for pulmonary arterial catheterisation in patients with heart failure

Failure to improve with initial circulatory management and uncertainty about adequacy of cardiac output and relationship between atrial filling pressures
Assessment of left ventricular preload when the relationship between right and left atrial pressures is uncertain due to recent myocardial infarction, valvular abnormalities or high pulmonary vascular resistance. A low wedge pressure indicates that further volume is indicated but a high value does not necessarily exclude the need for further volume
Measurement of cardiac output by thermodilution to direct appropriate choice of vasoactive drug and to manipulate therapy, particularly when high doses are being used
Need to monitor pulmonary arterial pressures and assess right ventricular function

pulmonary vascular bed abnormalities, as occur in chronic obstructive airways disease and long-standing mitral valve disease. Despite obtaining a good-quality wedge tracing, the measurement must be interpreted with caution since increased intrathoracic pressure and diastolic dysfunction make this pressure measurement an unreliable index of true left ventricular volume preload.

The focus on 'goal-directed therapy' led to the widespread use of PA catheters, but their indiscriminate use was challenged by a multicentre case-controlled study which suggested that patients managed with a PA catheter had a poorer outcome than those managed without such intervention.[43] This study probably reflected the enthusiasm for inappropriate goal-directed therapy prevalent at that time, poor training in the use of the catheter and an inability of clinicians to respond appropriately to the data obtained.[44]

Table 20.7 lists the indications for PA catheterisation in heart failure. Other aspects of haemodynamic monitoring are discussed in Chapter 12.

ASSESSMENT OF INTRAVASCULAR VOLUME STATUS

CLINICAL

This is conventionally based on measurement of the right atrial filling pressure and the assumption that a normal relationship exists between the atrial filling pressures, which is not necessarily valid in the critically ill patient, particularly in cardiogenic shock.[27] Although values < 12 mmHg suggest hypovolaemia, higher levels are more difficult to interpret, particularly in the ventilated patient. The RAP should therefore be interpreted carefully and in light of other clinical evidence. However such static tests for assessing the intravascular volume are less valuable than dynamic tests, such as the fluid challenge and the effect of positive-pressure ventilation, which assess the circulatory response to an intervention.

Intravascular volume depletion is suggested if hypotension is precipitated by sedation, analgesia and postural change. In the patient receiving positive-pressure ventilation respiratory fluctuation in the arterial pressure tracing also suggests relative hypovolaemia. This is confirmed if brief disconnection from the ventilator causes the blood pressure to rise and venous pressure to fall: the measurement off the ventilator more accurately reflects the ventricular end-diastolic *transmural* pressure. This manoeuvre is relatively contraindicated in patients with acute respiratory distress syndrome since loss of positive end-expiratory pressure may cause widespread alveolar collapse.

FLUID CHALLENGE

If hypovolaemia is suspected, 200 ml of colloid should be administered and the impact on blood pressure, flow and preload observed. In the volume-depleted patient blood pressure and flow will increase with only a small, transient increase in filling pressure. While pulmonary gas exchange remains satisfactory there is less anxiety about giving further colloid. Sufficient volume will have been given when either the target pressures are achieved and the evidence of poor peripheral perfusion and organ dysfunction has resolved, or when there is a sustained rise in filling pressures to a level above which there is a risk of pulmonary oedema developing.

Deciding on the appropriate fluid volume to give in sepsis can be difficult and frequently represents a balance between giving sufficient volume to prevent the use of excessive doses of constricting inotropes and giving excessive amounts with consequent tissue oedema and deterioration in pulmonary gas exchange.

If there is concern about administering even 200 ml of fluid, a reversible fluid challenge can be given in sedated patients by elevating the legs to 60° from the horizontal for 2 minutes.

VALSALVA MANOEUVRE

The effect of changes in intrathoracic pressure can be used to assess intrathoracic blood volume and provide an estimate of true left ventricular preload. Figure 20.3 shows the classic Valsalva response in a normal subject and in a patient with a high intrathoracic blood volume. If a normal-type trace is observed on the monitor, further volume is indicated, whereas a square-wave response indicates an adequate left ventricular volume preload.[45] This response can be quantified by calculating the ratio of the pulse pressure during phase 2 of the manoeuvre to the baseline value. This correlates with measurements of PA wedge pressure[46] and can be applied at the bedside in sedated, ventilated patients.[47] However, if the patient is breathing spontaneously, this test is difficult both to perform and to interpret.

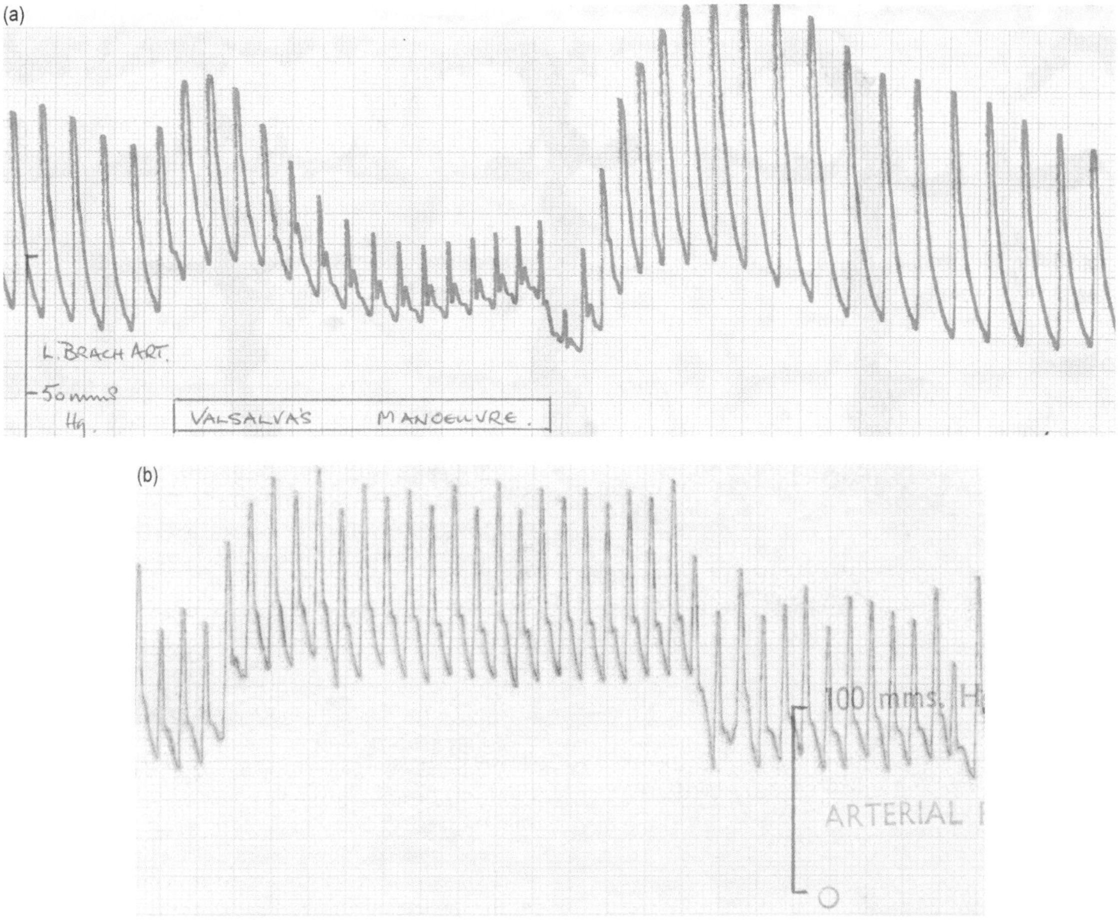

Figure 20.3 Valsalva traces. (a) Normal pulse pressure response to Valsalva's manoeuvre. (b) Square-wave pulse pressure response to Valsalva's manoeuvre.

ECHOCARDIOGRAPHY

Echocardiography is useful in identifying inadequate volume preload and the need for further fluid resuscitation, particularly when the preload pressures are high, as may occur with diastolic dysfunction. Performing serial studies to assess the response to therapy (fluid challenge, starting vasoactive therapy, changing ventilator settings) can be particularly valuable.

MANAGEMENT OF CARDIAC FUNCTION IN THE CRITICALLY ILL

Circulatory management should be regularly reviewed in the critically ill patient. Following initial assessment and with knowledge of the primary diagnosis, the need for extra monitoring should be decided, provisional targets should be set for fluid balance, ventricular preload, mean and diastolic arterial pressures and a management plan agreed on how to achieve these goals. Generally a MAP > 65 mmHg with diastolic pressure > 50 mmHg is acceptable but adequate cerebral, coronary, splanchnic and renal perfusion may require higher pressures, particularly in the elderly patient with pre-existing hypertension or widespread atheroma.

CORRECTION OF METABOLIC FACTORS

The following metabolic factors should be promptly corrected:

- hypoxaemia: $Po_2 < 8$ kPa
- acidaemia: pH < 7.20
- hyperkalaemia: $K^+ > 5.5$ mmol/l
- hypomagnesaemia: $Mg^{2+} < 0.9$ mmol/l
- hypocalcaemia: ionised $Ca^{2+} < 1.0$ mmol/l
- hypophosphataemia: $PO_4^- < 0.8$ mmol/l
- anaemia: Hb < 9 g%
- thiamine deficiency (malnutrition, excess alcohol, diuretic or digoxin treatment)

Metabolic acidaemia with pH < 7.20 or base deficit > 10 mmol/l should be corrected since myocardial contractility increases linearly with rising pH to values > 7.40. The suggestion that sodium bicarbonate should not be used as it produces a damaging paradoxical intracellular acidosis is misleading since the experiments demonstrating this effect were performed in vitro using non-physiological solutions, within a closed system that allowed no correction for any rise in carbon dioxide concentration and in which the sodium bicarbonate was given by bolus rather than by slow infusion.[48] The case for using bicarbonate to correct a metabolic acidaemia in the clinical setting has been recognised[49] and is supported by studies looking at the use of bicarbonate rather than lactate as the buffer solution in haemofiltration.[50] Figure 20.4 shows the effect of correcting a severe metabolic acidaemia on CO by changing from lactate to bicarbonate haemofiltration.

Although a prospective randomised study demonstrated an improved survival for critically patients if haemoglobin concentration was maintained at 7–9 g% rather than at 10–12 g%, this did not apply to the elderly and those with coronary artery disease, in whom the haemoglobin level should be maintained > 9 g%.[51]

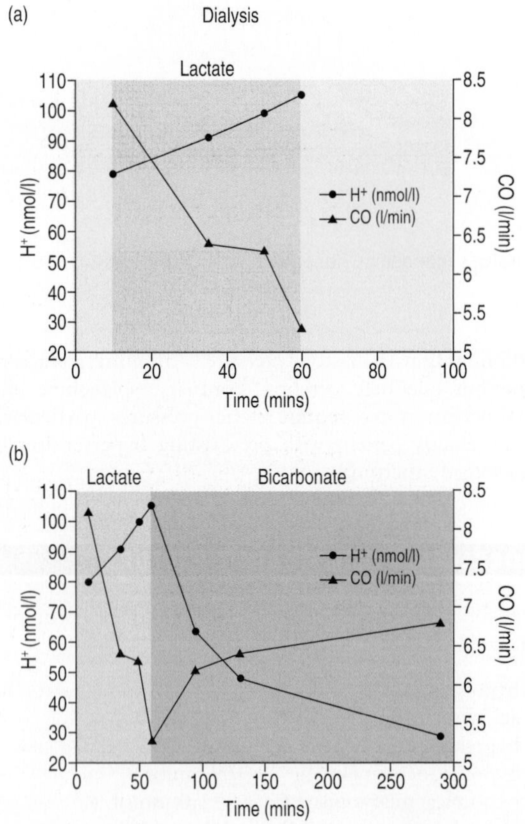

Figure 20.4 Effect of dialysis: (a) rising hydrogen ions and falling CO with lactate buffer dialysis; (b) change to bicarbonate buffer – there is falling hydrogen ion concentration and a rising cardiac output.

Patients with poor dietary thiamine intake, chronic alcohol abuse and those on chronic furosemide or digoxin therapy are at risk of thiamine deficiency, resulting in impaired myocardial function. Oral thiamine (200 mg/day) improves left ventricular function in these patients.[52]

SELECTION OF APPROPRIATE VASOACTIVE AGENTS (SEE CHAPTER 82)

The choice of vasoactive agent when treating acute heart failure represents a balance between the global circulatory requirements and those of a stressed myocardium. The properties of commonly used agents are shown in Table 20.5.

The impact of these drugs in individual patients will be influenced by the baseline state of the circulation, i.e. if either intensely constricted or dilated, the same drug will potentially produce different effects on pressure, flow and its distribution. The initial choice of vasoactive agent will depend on the mean arterial pressure (MAP), CO and derived systemic vascular resistance (SVR). For example:

- CO and MAP are both low with a high SVR: an inotropic and dilating (inodilator) effect is required and dobutamine would be appropriate. If CO rises but MAP falls, as may happen with dobutamine, and a more powerful inotropic effect is required, a combination of adrenaline (epinephrine) and glyceryl trinitrate is appropriate. However, increasing doses of adrenaline risk myocardial ischaemia with ventricular irritability and splanchnic ischaemia and the development of lactic acidosis.[53]
- MAP and SVR are low with high CO – this is frequently seen in sepsis: arteriolar constriction with noradrenaline (norepinephrine) is indicated after adequate volume resuscitation.
- MAP is at or above target but CO is low with raised SVR: a dilating agent (nitrate, e.g. glyceryl trinitrate) or an inodilator is appropriate.

When pulmonary vascular resistance and RAP are acutely raised, a pulmonary vasodilator to offload the right ventricle and maintain CO is required: a nitrate or β-agonist would be appropriate but hypotension may result from arteriolar dilatation and hypoxaemia can develop due to increased ventilation–perfusion mismatch.

Dopamine has been widely used in the erroneous belief that it selectively improves renal blood flow. However, if the patient has been fully volume-resuscitated and a modest inotropic effect with only a small increase in SVR and a natriuretic effect are required, then a low-dose dopamine infusion (< 4 μmol/kg per min) is appropriate.[54]

Dopexamine is used to improve splanchnic blood flow but, despite reported benefits when used with volume loading in perioperative patients,[55] there is little evidence of outcome benefit in established shock.

Patients with chronic heart failure and those receiving long-term β-agonist infusion often develop tolerance with reduced catecholamine receptor responsiveness, resulting in less effect in raising intracellular cyclic adenosine monophosphate (cAMP) levels and increasing myocardial contractility. Phosphodiesterase inhibitors (enoximone, milrinone) offer an alternative strategy. Milrinone competitively inhibits the phosphodiesterase III isoenzyme, responsible for the breakdown of cAMP, thereby increasing intracellular cAMP levels and improving myocardial contractility independent of β-receptor stimulation. There is also improvement in ventricular diastolic relaxation. However, these agents are powerful vasodilators and hypotension frequently limits their use or requires a noradrenaline infusion. The dose should be reduced in renal failure.

Levosimendan is an intracellular calcium sensitiser and bypasses the receptors through which other inotropic agents act. Administered as an infusion over 3 days, it has a long-lasting metabolite which results in any improvement in myocardial contractility being sustained for several weeks.[56] It has mainly been used in chronic heart failure and its role in severe acute heart failure and cardiogenic shock following acute myocardial infarction is uncertain but promising. As a potassium channel blocker, it dilates smooth muscle and may cause hypotension. In the patient with severe heart failure already on inotropic drugs, treatment should start with a low-dose infusion (0.05 μg/kg per min) and no loading dose should be given. If tachycardia develops or persists it is theoretically logical to consider addition of a beta-blocker but it is advisable to start with a small dose of a short-acting drug such as metoprolol or esmolol.

BETA-BLOCKADE

The use of β-blockers in patients with heart failure remains controversial. Large studies have demonstrated their benefit early after acute myocardial infarction[4,57] and atenolol given intravenously perioperatively produces a survival benefit for up to 2 years after non-cardiac surgery in patients deemed to be at high risk of coronary artery disease.[58] This evidence would appear to conflict with an increasing number of studies of perioperative optimisation that show benefit from increasing oxygen delivery with volume loading and the use of β-agonists.[55] The explanation may be that in surgical patients the majority of the benefit derives from achieving adequate volume resuscitation and the additional use of a β-agonist is beneficial if the CO and oxygen delivery remain inadequate and the heart rate is less than 100/min, whereas the subset of patients with underlying coronary artery disease and a persisting tachycardia after fluid resuscitation may benefit from β-blockade rather than β-stimulation.

MECHANICAL SUPPORT FOR THE HEART

Continuous positive airway pressure (CPAP) by facemask[59] and invasive positive-pressure ventilation are the most common forms of mechanical support provided in heart failure. The benefits result from improved oxygenation and reducing or eliminating the work of breathing, which may account for up to 30% of oxygen consumption.[60] This reduction in oxygen consumption reduces left ventricular workload and alleviates myocardial ischaemia. When instituting mechanical ventilation the clinician must be prepared to give volume and even adrenaline as the sedation and other anaesthetic agents given for intubation will reduce endogenous levels of catecholamines, producing arteriolar and venular dilatation and potentially catastrophic hypotension.

The intra-aortic counterpulsation balloon pump (IABP) is physiologically attractive since it both improves coronary and peripheral circulatory perfusion and decreases cardiac work. This results in a more efficient cardiac performance and improved myocardial oxygenation.[61]

Left ventricular assist devices (LVAD) can temporarily take over myocardial function but are only indicated if all other treatment options have been explored and improvement in myocardial function can be anticipated.[62] There are significant problems with bleeding, infection, thromboembolism and stroke. Both IABP and LVAD should be viewed as 'bridges to recovery' after cardiac surgery or recent myocardial infarction or when there is a realistic prospect of cardiac transplantation.

CARDIOGENIC SHOCK AFTER ACUTE MYOCARDIAL INFARCTION

In patients admitted to intensive care with cardiogenic shock resulting from an acute myocardial infarction, some additional points should be noted:

- The effects of management on myocardial oxygenation must be considered as well as global circulatory targets.
- Although the patient may be ventilated on ICU, therapies demonstrated to improve myocardial salvage must not be overlooked or delayed. Thrombolysis may be contraindicated but the benefits of aspirin alone are significant if given in the early hours after infarction; if necessary the aspirin can be given rectally. β-blockers[57] and an ACE inhibitor[63] should be started as soon as possible but bradycardia, heart block, hypotension and impairment of renal function may cause delay. A trial of a short-acting beta-blocker, either a low-dose esmolol infusion or a small dose of metoprolol may be appropriate, particularly if there is a tachycardia, since studies have suggested that the benefit from beta-blockers may be even greater in patients with heart failure.[57] Patients with left ventricular dysfunction and heart failure should also be started on an aldosterone receptor antagonist therapy, such as spironolactone or eplerenone[64] which reduce BNP levels and cardiac morbidity and mortality. Urgent coronary angiography to allow angioplasty and stenting should be considered and the early use of an intra-aortic balloon pump[65] is preferable to escalating doses of inotropic drugs.

- In patients admitted following an arrest witnessed out of hospital, therapeutic hypothermia (cooling to 32–34°C) has been shown to be beneficial but, if planned, this should not prevent other interventions such as primary angioplasty being performed if appropriate. It must also be realised that monitoring the patient is more complex in the hypothermic patient since paralysis is often necessary to prevent shivering, most of the techniques for CO measurement are invalidated and both bedside assessment of the circulation and interpretation of acid–base and lactate data are difficult.
- It is important to recognise:
  - right ventricular infarction (ST elevation in lead V_4R) since further monitoring may be necessary to ensure appropriate volume loading and to direct therapy to offload the right ventricle[66]
  - the development of either a ventricular septal defect or mitral regurgitation from papillary rupture since insertion of an intra-aortic balloon pump and urgent surgery may be indicated[67]

REFERENCES

1. Packer M. Pathophysiology and treatment of chronic heart failure. *Lancet* 1992; **340**: 88–95.
2. Simoons ML, Boersma E, van der Zwaan C *et al.* The challenge of acute coronary syndromes. *Lancet* 1999; **353** (suppl. II): 1–4.
3. Redfield MM. Heart failure – an epidemic of uncertain proportions. *N Engl J Med* 2002; **347**: 1442–4.
4. Yusuf S, Peto R, Lewis J *et al.* Sleight P. Beta-blockade during and after myocardial infarction: an overview of the randomised trials. *Prog Cardiovasc Dis* 1985; **27**: 335–71.
5. MERIT-HF Study Group. Effect of metoprolol CR/XL in chronic heart failure: metoprolol CR/XL randomised intervention trial in congestive heart failure (MERIT-HF). *Lancet* 1999; **353**: 2001–7.
6. Shoemaker WC, Appel PL, Kram HB *et al.* Prospective trial of supranormal values of survivors as therapeutic goals in high-risk surgical patients. *Chest* 1988; **94**: 1176–87.
7. Hayes MA, Timmins AC, Yau EH *et al.* Elevation of systemic oxygen delivery in the treatment of critically ill patients. *N Engl J Med* 1994; **330**: 1717–22.
8. Gattinoni L, Brazzi L, Pelosi P *et al.* A trial of goal-orientated haemodynamic therapy in critically ill patients. *N Engl J Med* 1995; **333**: 1025–32.
9. Turner A, Tsamitros M, Bellomo R. Myocardial cell injury in septic shock. *Crit Care Med* 1999; **27**: 1775–80.
10. Price S, Nicol E, Gibson DG *et al.* Echocardiography in the critically ill: current and potential roles. *Intens Care Med* 2006; **32**: 48–59.
11. Gmaurer G. Contrast echocardiography: clinical utility. *Echocardiography* 2000; **17**: 5–9.
12. Guest TM, Ramanathan AV, Tuteur AV *et al.* Myocardial injury in critically ill patients: a frequently unrecognized complication. *JAMA* 1995; **273**: 1945–9.
13. Mueller C, Scholer A, Laule-Kilian K *et al.* Use of B-type natriuretic peptide in the evaluation and management of acute dyspnea. *N Engl J Med* 2004; **350**: 647–54.
14. McCullough PA, Nowak RM, McCord J *et al.* B-type natriuretic peptide and clinical judgement in emergency diagnosis of heart failure: analysis from Breathing Not Properly (BNP) multinational study. *Circulation* 2002; **106**: 416–22.
15. Niemenen MS, Bohn M, Drexler H *et al.* New practice guidelines of the European Society of Cardiology: management of acute heart failure. *Eur Heart J* 2005; **26**: 384–416.
16. NICE guidelines for the management of chronic heart failure in adults in primary and secondary care 2003. Available online at: htpp://www.nice.org.uk.
17. Charpentier J, Luyt CE, Fulla Y *et al.* Brain natriuretic peptide: a marker of myocardial dysfunction and prognosis during severe sepsis. *Crit Care Med* 2004; **32**: 660–5.
18. Arlati S, Brenna S, Prencipe L *et al.* Myocardial necrosis in ICU patients with acute non-cardiac disease: a prospective study. *Intens Care Med* 2000; **26**: 31–7.
19. Relos RP, Hasinof IK, Beilman GJ. Moderately elevated serum troponin concentrations are associated with increased morbidity and mortality rates in surgical intensive care unit patients *Crit Care Med* 2003; **31**: 2598–603.
20. Leach RM, Treacher DF. Oxygen delivery and consumption in the critically ill. *Thorax* 2002; **57**: 170–7.
21. Shoemaker WC, Appel PL, Waxman K *et al.* Clinical trial of survivors' cardiorespiratory patterns as therapeutic goals in critically ill postoperative patients. *Crit Care Med* 1982; **10**: 398–403.
22. Corday E, Williams JH, DeVera LB *et al.* Effect of systemic blood pressure and vasopressor drugs on coronary blood flow and the electrocardiogram. *Am J Cardiol* 1959; **3**: 626.
23. Parillo JE. Pathogenetic mechanisms in septic shock. *N Engl J Med* 1993; **328**: 1471–7.
24. Kumar A, Thota V, Dee L *et al.* Tumour necrosis factor-α and interleukin 1β are responsible for in vitro myocardial cell depression induced by human septic shock serum. *J Exp Med* 1996; **183**: 949–58.
25. Rivers E, Bguyen B, Havstad S *et al.* Early goal directed therapy in the treatment of severe sepsis and septic shock. *N Engl J Med* 2001; **345**: 1368.
26. Sarnov SJ, Bergland E. Ventricular function 1. Starling's law of the heart studied by means of simultaneous right and left ventricular function curves. *Circulation* 1954; **9**: 706.
27. Bradley RD, Jenkins BS, Branthwaite MA. The influence of atrial pressure on cardiac performance following myocardial infarction complicated by shock. *Circulation* 1970; **42**: 827–37.
28. Vismara LA, Leamon DM, Zelis R. The effects of morphine on venous tone in patients with acute pulmonary oedema. *Circulation* 1976; **54**: 335–7.
29. Ross JJ. Afterload mismatch and preload reserve: a conceptual framework for the analysis of ventricular function. *Prog Cardiovasc Dis* 1976; **18**: 255–64.

30. Cournand A, Motley HL, Werko L *et al.* Physiological studies of the effects of intermittent positive pressure breathing on cardiac output in man. *Am J Physiol* 1948; **152**: 162.
31. Buda AJ, Pinsky MR, Ingels NB *et al.* Effect of intrathoracic pressure on left ventricular performance. *N Engl J Med* 1979; **301**: 453–9.
32. Stewart JT, Simpson IA. Left ventricular energetics: heat production by the human heart. *Cardiovasc Res* 1993; **27**: 1024–32.
33. Francis GS. Vasodilators in the intensive care unit. *Am Heart J* 1991; **121**: 1875–8.
34. Mueller H, Ayers SM, Gianelli S *et al.* Effect of isoproterenol, L-norepinephrine and intra-aortic counterpulsation on haemodynamics and myocardial metabolism in shock following acute myocardial infarction. *Circulation* 1972; **45**: 335.
35. Chamberlain DA, Leinbach RC, Vassaux CE *et al.* Sequential atrioventricular pacing in heart block complicating acute myocardial infarction. *N Engl J Med* 1970; **282**: 577–82.
36. Smith TW. Digoxin in heart failure. *N Engl J Med* 1993; **329**: 51–3.
37. Amiodarone Trials Meta-Analysis Investigators. Effect of prophylactic amiodarone on mortality after acute myocardial infarction and in congestive heart failure: meta-analysis of individual data from 6500 patients in randomised trials. *Lancet* 1997; **350**: 1417–24.
38. Goodwin J. The importance of clinical skills. *Br Med J* 1995; **310**: 1281–2.
39. Singer M, Clarke J, Bennett ED. Continuous haemodynamic monitoring by oesophageal Doppler. *Crit Care Med* 1989; **17**: 447–52.
40. Linton RAF, Band DM, O'Brien T *et al.* Lithium dilution cardiac output measurement: a comparison with thermodilution. *Crit Care Med* 1997; **25**: 1796–800.
41. Antonelli M, Levy M, Andrews PJD *et al.* Haemodynamic monitoring in shock and implications for management. International Consensus Conference, Paris, France, April 2006. *Intens Care Med* 2007; **33**: 575–90.
42. Steingrub JS, Celori G, Vickers-Lahti M *et al.* Therapeutic impact of pulmonary artery catheterisation in a medical/surgical ICU. *Chest* 1991; **99**: 1451–5.
43. Connors AF, Speroff T, Dawson NV *et al.* The effectiveness of right heart catheterisation in the initial care of critically ill patients. *JAMA* 1996; **276**: 889–97.
44. Iberti TJ, Fischer EP, Leibowitz AB *et al.* A multicentre study of physicians' knowledge of the pulmonary artery catheter. *JAMA* 1990; **264**: 2928–32.
45. Sharpey-Schafer EP. Effects of Valsalva's manoeuvre on the normal and failing circulation. *Br Med J* 1955; **1**: 693–5.
46. McIntyre KM, Vita JA, Lambrew CT *et al.* A noninvasive method of predicting pulmonary capillary wedge pressure. *N Engl J Med* 1992; **327**: 1715–20.
47. Marik PE. The systolic blood pressure variation as an indicator of pulmonary capillary wedge pressure in ventilated patients. *Anaesth Intens Care* 1993; **21**: 405–8.
48. Ritter JM, Doctor H, Benjamin M. Paradoxical effect of bicarbonate on cytoplasmic pH. *Lancet* 1990; **335**: 1243–6.
49. Narius RG, Cohen JJ. Bicarbonate therapy for organic acidosis: the case for its use. *Ann Intern Med* 1987; **106**: 615–18.
50. Hilton PJ, Taylor J, Formi LG *et al.* Bicarbonate-based haemofiltration in the management of acute renal failure with lactic acidosis. *Q J Med* 1998; **91**: 279–83.
51. Hebert PC, Wells G, Blajchman MA *et al.* A multicenter, randomized, controlled clinical trial of transfusion requirements in critical care. *N Engl J Med* 1999; **340**: 409–17.
52. Leslie D, Gheorghiade M. Is there a role for thiamine supplementation in the management of heart failure? *Am Heart J* 1996; **131**: 1248–50.
53. Day NPJ, Phu NH, Bethell DP *et al.* The effects of dopamine and adrenaline infusions on acid–base balance and systemic haemodynamics in severe infection. *Lancet* 1996; **348**: 219–23.
54. Australian and New Zealand Intensive Care Society (ANZICS) Clinical Trials Group. Low-dose dopamine in patients with early renal dysfunction: a placebo-controlled randomised trial. *Lancet* 2000; **356**: 2139–43.
55. Wilson J, Woods I, Fawcett J *et al.* Reducing the risk of major elective surgery: randomized, controlled trial of preoperative optimisation of oxygen delivery. *Br Med J* 1999; **318**: 1099–103.
56. Hasenfuss G, Pieske B, Castell M *et al.* Influence of the novel inotropic agent levosimendan on isometric tension and calcium coupling in failing human myocardium. *Circulation* 1998; **98**: 2141–7.
57. Gottlieb SS, McCarter RJ, Vogel RA *et al.* Effect of beta blockade on mortality among high risk and low risk patients after myocardial infarction. *N Engl J Med* 1998; **339**: 489–97.
58. Mangano DT, Layug EL, Wallace A *et al.* Effect of atenolol on mortality and cardiovascular morbidity after noncardiac surgery. *N Engl J Med* 1996; **335**: 1713–20.
59. Bersten AD, Holt AW, Vedig AE *et al.* Treatment of severe cardiogenic pulmonary oedema with continuous positive airway pressure delivered by facemask. *N Engl J Med* 1991; **325**: 1825–30.
60. Aubier M, Trippenbach T, Roussos C. Respiratory muscle fatigue during cardiogenic shock. *J Appl Physiol Respir Environ Ex Physiol* 1981; **51**: 499–508.
61. Nanas JN, Moulopouloss D. Counterpulsation: historical background, technical improvements, hemodynamic and metabolic effects. *Cardiology* 1994; **84**: 156–67.
62. Westaby S, Katsumata T, Houel R *et al.* Jarvik 2000 heart: potential for bridge to myocyte recovery. *Circulation* 1998; **98**: 1568–74.
63. Pfeffer MA, Braunwald E, Moye LA *et al.* Effect of captopril on mortality and morbidity in patients with left ventricular dysfunction after myocardial infarction. Results of the survival and ventricular enlargement trial. *N Engl J Med* 1992; **327**: 669–77.

64. Pitt B, Remme W, Zannard F *et al.* Epleronone, a selective aldosterone blocker in patients with left ventricular dysfunction after myocardial infarction. *N Engl J Med* 2003; **348**: 1309–21.
65. Mueller HS. Role of intra-aortic counterpulsation in cardiogenic shock and acute myocardial infarction. *Cardiology* 1994; **84**: 168–74.
66. Kohn JN, Guiha NH, Broder MI *et al.* Right ventricular infarction: clinical and haemodynamic features. *Am J Cardiol* 1974; **33**: 209–14.
67. Hasdai D, Topol EJ, Califf RM *et al.* Cardiogenic shock complicating acute coronary syndromes. *Lancet* 2000; **356**: 749–56.

21

Valvular and congenital heart disease

John E Sanderson

VALVULAR HEART DISEASE

Valvular heart disease is still a common cause for symptoms and disability worldwide. In most economically developed countries the main cause is no longer rheumatic heart disease: congenital valve abnormalities such as mitral valve prolapse and bicuspid aortic valves, degenerative valve disease or infective endocarditis are more common causes.[1] However, in many parts of the world, rheumatic fever and rheumatic heart disease are still major health problems, especially in the young.[2,3] Diseases of heart valves produce stenosis, incompetence or both.

RHEUMATIC FEVER

This acute febrile illness is due to a cross-reaction following a group A β-haemolytic streptococci pharyngitis, which causes inflammatory lesions involving the joints, heart and subcutaneous tissues. It presents with polyarthritis, carditis, subcutaneous nodules, rash (erythema marginatum) and chorea. Carditis consists of:

- murmurs (most commonly mitral, aortic regurgitation or the mid diastolic Carey–Coombs murmur)
- pericarditis
- cardiomegaly
- congestive heart failure[4]

Chronic rheumatic heart disease occurs in about 40% of those with apical and basal diastolic murmurs, and 70% with heart failure or pericarditis during the acute attacks. It is still common in the Middle East, India, Africa and South America, and causes 20–40% of all cardiovascular disease in the Third World.[2] It is now rare in North America, western Europe, Australasia and parts of Asia.

MITRAL STENOSIS

Rheumatic fever is the main cause of mitral stenosis; rarer causes are:

- left atrial myxoma
- ball-valve thrombus
- calcification of the annulus
- systemic lupus erythematosus

Scarring or fibrosis of the valves, especially at the edges and sometimes involving the subvalvular apparatus, causes narrowing and hence increased left atrial pressure, pulmonary venous hypertension and pulmonary arterial hypertension. Thus the lungs and right ventricle suffer the most burden. Main symptoms are breathlessness on exertion, recurrent bronchitis, fatigue, palpitations due to paroxysmal atrial fibrillation (AF), haemoptysis and stroke. The onset of AF is usually associated with marked symptomatic deterioration and significantly increases the risk for left atrial thrombus formation and embolism.

Classic signs of mitral stenosis are:

- mitral facies (peripheral cyanosis on the cheeks)
- a small-volume pulse which may be irregular (AF is common)
- right ventricular hypertrophy
- a tapping apex due to a palpable first heart sound
- a loud first heart sound, and an opening snap with a rumbling diastolic murmur

The first clue to the diagnosis is often the loud first heart sound, which should prompt a careful search for the diastolic rumble which may be soft, low-pitched and localised to the apex. An opening snap is present if the valve is not calcified and this occurs 0.04–0.10 s after S_2.

An electrocardiogram (ECG) shows a broad P-wave in lead 2 due to left atrial hypertrophy. Chest X-ray shows an enlarged left atrium and appendage, prominent upper-lobe pulmonary veins, but heart size is usually within normal limits. The diagnosis can readily be confirmed by echocardiography, which allows assessment of the valve anatomy, and estimation of valve area and gradient. Severe stenosis is considered to be present if the valve area is $< 1\ cm^2$ (Figure 21.1).

Treatment is the use of β-blockers to slow the heart rate and increase diastolic filling time diuretics, and digoxin is given if the patient is in AF. Anticoagulation is essential if there is significant mitral stenosis and AF. Mitral balloon valvuloplasty has been shown to be very successful therapy with excellent long-term outcome, and compares well with surgical treatment.[5] The main contraindications to balloon valvuloplasty are significant mitral regurgitation and heavy calcification when mutual valve replacement should be done.

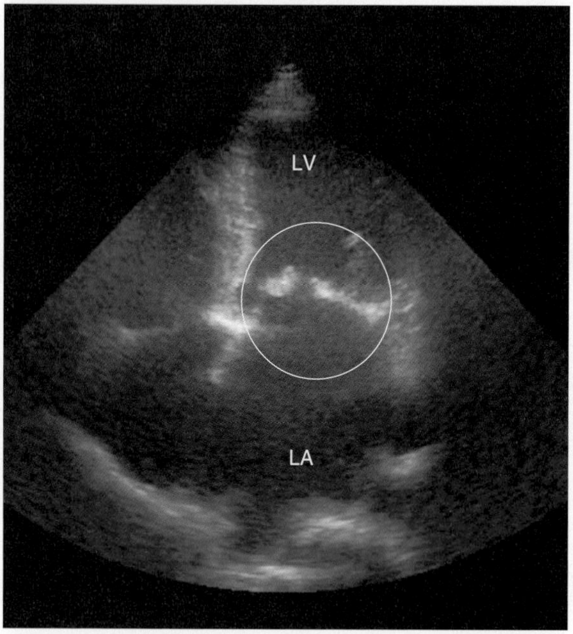

Figure 21.1 Mitral stenosis. Thickened and calcified anterior and posterior mitral valve leaflets with reduced opening. LV, left ventricle; LA, left atrium.

MITRAL REGURGITATION

There is a considerable difference between acute and chronic mitral regurgitation (Table 21.1). In chronic mitral regurgitation, there is time for the left ventricle and left atrium to adapt to the increasing regurgitation, leading to their gradual enlargement. In acute mitral regurgitation, the sudden pressure overload of the left atrium and pulmonary veins leads to severe pulmonary oedema. The treatment for acute mitral regurgitation is urgent surgery. The management of chronic mitral regurgitation is more difficult. Initially, medical therapy can be helpful, but the probability of postoperative death or persistent severe heart failure after valve replacement increases abruptly when the left ventricular (LV) end-systolic diameter exceeds 45 mm on echocardiography, or ejection fraction falls below 60%.[6] In patients without mitral stenosis, mitral valve repair is preferable to replacement, and evidence suggests that preservation of the chordae improves postoperative LV function.[7]

MITRAL VALVE PROLAPSE[8]

This is a common condition affecting 5% of the adult population – more women than men. It has a number of synonyms, such as Barlow and click–murmur syndrome. It is due to myxomatous degeneration of the valve, with redundancy of the leaflets, which may affect both the anterior and posterior valves. At the end of diastole, the valve closes normally, but as LV pressure rises during systole, a portion of the valve leaflet prolapses in the left atrium, with associated regurgitation. It is usually mild, but can progress and become more severe, and, rarely, the chordae may rupture to produce severe acute regurgitation.

Mitral valve prolapse is usually asymptomatic, but a wide variety of symptoms have been associated, including odd chest pains, palpitations and fatigue. On examination, typical findings are a mid-systolic click and a late systolic murmur, which are separated from the first heart sound, but usually reaching the second heart sound. The murmur may have a crescendo/decrescendo quality. It is usually louder with the Valsalva manoeuvre and on standing. As the prolapse worsens with age the murmur becomes more pansystolic. Echocardiography is diagnostic, and can accurately assess the degree of severity of mitral valve prolapse (Figure 21.2). In most patients, mitral prolapse is a benign condition with a good prognosis. It poses a risk for infective endocarditis, which then leads to a substantial risk of death and need for mitral valve surgery.[9] There is a very small increased incidence of embolic neurological ischaemic events.

AORTIC STENOSIS

The commonest cause of aortic stenosis is degeneration of a bicuspid aortic valve. Valve stenosis leads to increased LV systolic pressure, LV hypertrophy and reduced LV compliance. The increased LV work may induce subendocardial ischaemia, arrhythmias and sudden death.

The main symptoms are angina, syncope and breathlessness. Typical findings on examination are a slowly rising small-volume pulse, evidence of LV hypertrophy without an enlarged heart, and a harsh ejection systolic murmur radiating into the neck. If the valve is calcified, there is no click and the A_2 is soft.

An ECG confirms LV hypertrophy. The chest X-ray may show:

- a normal heart size
- a poststenotic dilatation in the ascending aorta
- presence of calcification

Echocardiography is diagnostic, and allows the measurement of the aortic valve area, gradient and the degree of aortic incompetence (Figure 21.3).

Medical treatment is not effective. Valve replacement should be performed as soon as the patient is symptomatic, if asymptomatic with LV systolic dysfunction, or if the jet velocity is > 4 m/s in patients undergoing coronary artery bypass surgery.[10]

AORTIC REGURGITATION

Like mitral regurgitation, the features of chronic and acute aortic regurgitation are different. Chronic aortic regurgitation has a number of causes, including:

- rheumatic, connective tissue disorders (e.g. ankylosing spondylitis, Reiter's syndrome and rheumatoid disease)
- syphilitic aortitis
- cystic medial necrosis (Marfan's syndrome)
- aortic root dilatation due to hypertension
- a congenital bicuspid aortic valve
- endocarditis, which can produce aortic regurgitation in a normal valve

The leak from the aorta increases LV volume, causing LV dilatation and LV hypertrophy. Initially, this is well tolerated but eventually LV function declines.

Main symptoms are fatigue and dyspnoea. Typical findings on examination are a large-volume, bounding, wide pulse pressure which is collapsing in nature. Other classical physical signs include Corrigan's (visible carotid pulsation) and nail bed capillary pulsation (Quincke sign), which all reflect the rapid run-off. The heart is usually enlarged with a displaced apex, and there is a high-pitched early diastolic blowing murmur which radiates from the left sternal edge to the apex. There may be a mid-diastolic murmur (Austin Flint) due to the regurgitant aortic jet hitting the anterior mitral valve leaflet.

An ECG shows LV hypertrophy, usually with a strain pattern. A chest X-ray shows an enlarged heart with a dilated aorta. Echocardiography is diagnostic and can demonstrate the degree of aortic regurgitation, LV size and function.

The decision to undertake aortic valve replacement in patients with pure aortic regurgitation is difficult. Many patients can survive despite enlarged left ventricles. In general, patients should be advised to have an operation before LV end-systolic dimension exceeds 55 mm or ejection fraction < 60%. Medical therapy with vasodilators such as nefedipine or angiotensin-converting enzyme inhibitors may delay the need for valve replacement.[6,11] However, surgery should not be delayed for too long, otherwise irreversible LV dysfunction ensues.

Acute aortic regurgitation is a severe disease with a high mortality, usually due to endocarditis (*Staphylococcus* or *Pneumococcus*).[12] There is acute LV diastolic pressure and volume overload, which leads to severe pulmonary oedema without LV dilatation. It can be difficult to diagnose

Table 21.1 Mitral regurgitation

	Chronic	Acute
Causes	Mitral valve prolapse Rheumatic heart disease LV dilatation (IHD, cardiomyopathies, etc.) Prosthetic valves	Ruptured chordae Ruptured papillary muscle Perforation of leaflet Prosthetic valves
Physiology	LV volume overload LV dilatation and hypertrophy Increased LA size (mean pressure normal initially because of increased compliance)	Sudden pressure overload of LA and pulmonary veins No change in LV dimension LA may be normal size
Symptoms	Asymptomatic initially Fatigue Dyspnoea	Severe dyspnoea
Examination	Pansystolic apical murmur radiating to axilla/lower sternal edge Third heart sound	Harsh pansystolic murmur radiating to axilla and back Third heart sound
Electrocardiogram	LV hypertrophy LA hypertrophy	No change (or acute MI)
Chest X-ray	Increased-size LV Increased-size LA	Normal LV and LA dimension Pulmonary oedema
Echocardiography	Diagnostic	Diagnostic
Treatment	Vasodilators and ACE inhibitors (reduce afterload) Diuretics and digitalis Surgery if symptoms and LV size increase (before LV end-systolic diameter > 4.5 cm or LV ejection fraction < 60%)	Preload and afterload reduction and prepare for urgent surgery

MI, myocardial infarction; LV, left ventricle/ventricular; IHD, ischaemic heart disease; IE, infective endocarditis; LA, left atrium/atrial; ACE, angiotensin-converting enzyme.

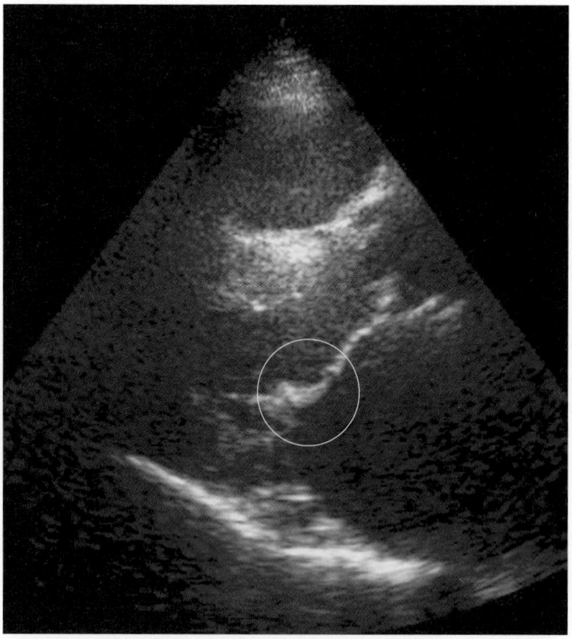

Figure 21.2 Mitral valve prolapse with bowing of the anterior mitral valve leaflet with enlargement of the left atrium but normal left ventricle size.

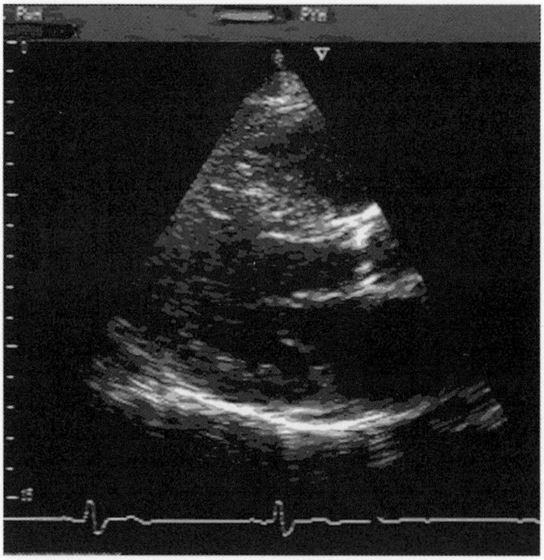

Figure 21.3 Aortic stenosis. A calcified thickened valve with reduced opening and the presence of left ventricular hypertrophy.

clinically, because the early diastolic murmur is very short and soft. An echocardiogram, however, is completely diagnostic, and can demonstrate severe aortic regurgitation, and, more importantly, early closure of the mitral valve. The treatment is urgent surgery without delay.

TRICUSPID REGURGITATION

Tricuspid regurgitation is usually secondary to right ventricular (RV) dilatation/hypertrophy because of pulmonary hypertension. However, increasingly, infective endocarditis (usually *Staphylococcus*) in drug addicts is a common cause.[13] The diagnosis is made by the presence of large V-waves in the jugular venous pressure, pansystolic murmur at the left sternal edge and echocardiography. Surgery may be necessary if the degree of valvular regurgitation is severe.

INFECTIVE ENDOCARDITIS

This is one of the most important diagnoses not to miss because untreated it is lethal.[14,15] A delay in diagnosis considerably lowers the probability of survival. The old adage that 'fever + murmur = endocarditis' until proven otherwise remains true. In fact any unexplained illness in a patient with a murmur should raise the question of infective endocarditis. The pattern of infective endocarditis is changing; it may be acquired in the community but increasingly in hospitals particularly as a result of procedures involving vascular catheterization, especially in elderly patients. Prior invasive procedures are more common than dental procedures as a cause. Consequently *Staphylococcus aureus* is now more common than *Streptococcus viridans* or enterococci in blood cultures. Infective endocarditis may also affect native valves that were previously thought to be normal and increasingly is a problem associated with intravenous drug abuse.

Clinical features of chronic endocarditis may be misleading. The symptoms are vague ill health, weight loss, malaise with night sweats and mild fever, and many patients are assumed to have influenza. In more chronic cases, there may be nail and conjunctival splinter haemorrhages, clubbing, splenomegaly and anaemia. Regurgitant murmurs (aortic, mitral or tricuspid) are usually present, and heart failure is a bad prognostic sign. Emboli may occur, causing strokes. Cerebral mycotic aneurysms are frequently lethal due to late rupture, which may occur many months after succesful treatment of infective endocarditis (see Appendix).

NATIVE VALVE ENDOCARDITIS (NVE)

Most community-acquired NVE is now more likely to be caused by *Staphylococcus aureus* and by coagulase-negative staphylococci than by the classical oral viridans streptococci. Enterococci are a less common cause but their incidence is increasing. In staphylococcal infective endocarditis the skin lesion may be quite trivial. Some strains of staphylococci are particularly virulent and can attack a previously normal valve, whereas streptococci and enterococci seem to infect only previously abnormal valves. Hospital-acquired NVE is almost always caused by staphylococci but occasionally coagulase-negative staphylococci and often *S. epidermidis* may be responsible. Increasingly, more cases of methicillin-resistant *S. aureus* (MRSA) endocarditis are being seen, usually from intravascular access site infections.

PROSTHETIC VALVE ENDOCARDITIS (PVE)

The risk of infection is always present. Preventive measures are extremely important in these patients as prosthetic PVE is a cardiological disaster. Even in the best centres, mortality remains high and reoperation is often necessary. The distinction between early infective endocarditis (theatre infection) and late infective endocarditis (community-acquired) is artificial as bacteria acquired in the theatre (such as *S. epidermidis*) may present many months or even longer after surgery. Since the infection involves the sewing ring, vegetations may not be present but more commonly paraprosthetic leaks or abscesses are found: these usually require transoesophageal echocardiography, cardiac magnetic resonance imaging (MRI) or computed tomography (CT) scanning to visualise.

INTRAVENOUS DRUG ABUSE

Infection usually affects the tricuspid valve and the condition is frequently misdiagnosed as pneumonia. Vegetations from the tricuspid valve embolise into the lung, causing patchy infarction with infection. Paradoxical embolism may occur into the systemic circulation through a patent formen ovale or atrial septal defect, helped by a high right atrial pressure secondary to the tricuspid regurgitation. Infected vegetations can cause cerebral, splenic or peripheral infarction. The tricuspid murmur may be very soft and the degree of tricuspid regurgitation may not be severe. The diagnosis therefore is not always obvious and will always need to be considered in any intravenous drug addict with a fever.

DIAGNOSIS OF INFECTIVE ENDOCARDITIS

The most important investigation remains the blood culture (three sets) before antibiotics are given. Although echocardiography is extremely useful in infective endocarditis, there is a misconception that endocarditis can be diagnosed or excluded by echocardiography. This is not true. Vegetations may be small and not visualised, and large vegetations may be old and sterile. It is not necessary to delay taking blood cultures while waiting for a spike of temperature. It is probably also not necessary to take samples from different sites. Levels of C-reactive protein will usually be elevated in infective endocarditis. The peripheral white cell count is often very high in those infections caused by *Staphylococcus* but may be normal in those caused by less virulent organisms. Occasionally, patients have so-called blood culture-negative infective endocarditis despite convincing clinical and echocardiographic evidence. In these cases, it is important to look specifically for other organisms such as fastidious bacteria and fungi (or suspect previous antibiotic therapy). Q fever due to *Coxiella burnetii* is common in certain areas such as Canada and parts of the USA and it can be caught from household cats. Diagnosis can be difficult as the illness is often indolent and fever may be absent. Serology is necessary to make the diagnosis, although *C. burnetii* antibodies cross-react with *Bartonella* species. Often the diagnosis is only made by histology of a replaced valve.

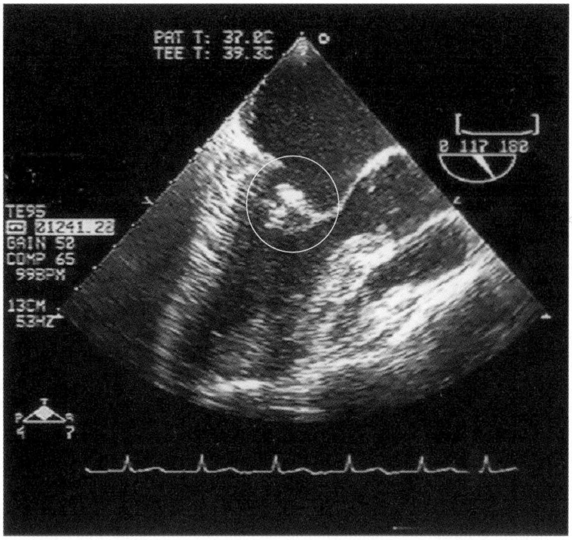

Figure 21.4 A large vegetation can be seen on the anterior mitral valve leaflet during transoesophageal echocardiography.

Echocardiography may show vegetations if they are > 3 mm and will give useful information on the degree of regurgitation, any intramyocardial spread (abscess formation) and LV function. Transoesophageal echocardiography is much more useful than transthoracic, particularly for mitral valve endocarditis or PVE and the detection of an abscess (Figure 21.4).[16]

TREATMENT

In acute endocarditis treatment should not be delayed while awaiting the results of blood cultures, although this may be acceptable in the patient who has been unwell for weeks or months. There are a number of guidelines for antibiotic treatment which can be consulted[17] (for current antibiotic treatment, see Tables 21.2, 21.3 and 21.4). The duration of treatment is traditionally 6 weeks. However, shorter courses with oral therapy have been successfully used for sensitive *Streptococcus* infections. Treatment of *C. burnetii* requires treatment for 18 months to 3 years with multiple antibiotics. Current recommendations for prophylaxis can be found in appendix.

PERSISTENT FEVER

A number of possibilities need to be considered, including infection elsewhere either in the heart or outside, such as an infection of a central line which should be removed and sent for culture. Abscesses, paravalvular or intracardiac, are an important cause of persistent or recurrent fever and require surgery. It is nearly always impossible to eradicate an abscess by medical therapy only, and it is generally better to undertake surgery earlier than later. In some patients who appear to be well controlled, an abscess may be detected by transoesophageal

Table 21.2 Antibiotic treatment for infective endocarditis caused by penicillin-susceptible (MIC < 0.1 mg/l) or penicillin relatively resistant (0.1 < MIC ≤ 0.5 mg/l) streptococcal endocarditis

	No allergy to penicillin		Allergy to penicillin		Duration
	Drug	Dosage	Drug	Dosage	
Penicillin-susceptible streptococci (MIC < 0.1 mg/l)					
Non-complicated native valve IE	Penicillin G or amoxicillin or ceftriaxone ± gentamicin*	200–300 000 U/kg per day 100 mg/kg per day 2 g/day 3–5 mg/kg per day	Vancomycin or teicoplanin ± gentamicin*	30 mg/kg per day 6–10 mg/kg per day 3–5 mg/kg per day	2 weeks combination or 4 weeks β-lactam
Complicated and/or prosthetic valve IE	Penicillin G or amoxicillin + gentamicin*	200–300 000 U/kg per day 100 mg/kg per day 3–5 mg/kg per day	Vancomycin or teicoplanin ± gentamicin*	30 mg/kg per day 6–10 mg/kg per day 3–5 mg/kg per day	2 weeks combination + 2–4 weeks β-lactam
Penicillin-relatively resistant streptococci G† (0.1< MIC ≤ 0.5 mg/l)					
Non-complicated native valve IE	Penicillin G or amoxicillin + gentamicin*	300–400 000 U/kg per day 200 mg/kg per day 3–5 mg/kg per day	Vancomycin or teicoplanin + gentamicin*	30 mg/kg per day 6–10 mg/kg per day 3–5 mg/kg per day	2 weeks combination + 2 weeks β-lactam
Complicated and/or prosthetic valve IE	Penicillin G or amoxicillin + gentamicin*	300–400 000 U/kg per day 200 mg/kg per day 3–5 mg/kg per day	Vancomycin or teicoplanin + gentamicin*	30 mg/kg per day 6–10 mg/kg per day 3–5 mg/kg per day	2 weeks combination + 2–4 weeks β-lactam

IE, infective endocarditis; MBC, minimal bactericidal concentration; MIC, minimal inhibitory concentration.
*Other choice: netilmicin (5–6 mg/kg per day); for both drugs, once-daily administration.
†Including tolerant streptococci (MBC/MIC >32), for which amoxicillin is to be preferred to penicillin.
Hoen B. Epidemiology and antibiotic treatment of infective endocarditis: an update. *Heart* 2006; **92**: 1694–700.

echocardiography, but after stopping the antibiotics the infection will recur (Figure 21.5). Extracardiac infection may be due to a myocotic aneurysm which can cause fever or metastatic infection. Myocotic aneurysms of the brain can be a particular problem and may lead to rupture many months or even years later.

ROLE OF SURGERY

If the patient is not recovering or the fever is not under control, then surgery should always be considered. Major indications are haemodynamic deterioration with increasing aortic or mitral regurgitation and an abscess. Staphylococcal endocarditis in particular may cause rapid destruction of the valve and require urgent surgery. Infections by fungi nearly always require surgery, as does infective endocarditis due to Q fever. The question of surgery to prevent embolism in a patient with a large vegetation is sometimes difficult. Vegetations > 10 mm in diameter are associated with an increased risk of embolism but it has not been shown that this is a necessary indication for surgery. If there is existing severe regurgitation then the decision to operate is easier. In general, if a large vegetation is seen then it is best to operate early, as after antibiotic therapy there is a lower risk of embolism. It is a general principle that surgery should be considered early and it is not necessary to wait for antibiotic treatment to take effect. Late surgery will always be more difficult with increasing complexity of the operation, difficulty in suturing the new valve because of destruction of the valve ring, and increased complications such as renal failure.

CONGENITAL HEART DISEASE IN ADULTS

The number of adults with congenital heart disease is steadily increasing, and includes not only patients with congenital heart disease who have survived into adulthood, but an increasing number of patients who have had cardiac surgery. The commonest congenital conditions found in adults are ostium secondum atrial septal defects, pulmonary valve stenosis, patent ductus arteriosus, uncomplicated congenitally corrected transposition of the great arteries, small panmembranous ventricular septal defects and Fallot's tetralogy.

OSTIUM SECUNDUM ATRIAL SEPTAL DEFECT

This is the commonest congenital cardiac abnormality in adults. It is often unrecognised because symptoms may be absent and the physical signs are subtle. Older patients may develop atrial fibrillation and cardiac failure. Paradoxical emboli through the defect are rare.

Table 21.3 Antibiotic treatment for enterococcal, nutritionally variant and penicillin-resistant (MIC > 0.5 mg/l) streptococcal endocarditis

Condition	No allergy to penicillin		Allergy to penicillin		Duration
	Drug	Dosage	Drug	Dosage	
Enterococcal strain susceptible to penicillin, aminoglycosides and vancomycin	Amoxicillin or penicillin G + gentamicin*	200 mg/kg per day 300–400 000 U/kg per day 3 mg/kg per day	Vancomycin or teicoplanin + gentamicin*	30 mg/kg per day 6–10 mg/kg per day 3 mg/kg per day	4–6 weeks†
Enterococcal strain susceptible to penicillin, streptomycin, and vancomycin and resistant to gentamicin	Amoxicillin or penicillin G + streptomycin‡	200 mg/kg per day 300–400 000 U/kg per day 15 mg/kg per day	Vancomycin or teicoplanin + streptomycin‡	30 mg/kg per day 6–10 mg/kg per day 15 mg/kg per day	4–6 weeks†
Enterococcal strain resistant to penicillin (intrinsic resistance), susceptible to gentamicin and vancomycin	Vancomycin or teicoplanin + gentamicin*	30 mg/kg per day 6–10 mg/kg per day 3 mg/kg per day	Vancomycin or teicoplanin + gentamicin*	30 mg/kg per day 6–10 mg/kg per day 3 mg/kg per day	6 weeks
Enterococcal strain resistant to penicillin (β-lactam-producing), susceptible to gentamicin and vancomycin	Co-amoxiclav + gentamicin*	175 mg/kg per day amoxicillin 3 mg/kg per day	Vancomycin or teicoplanin + gentamicin*	30 mg/kg per day 6–10 mg/kg per day 3 mg/kg per day	6 weeks
Streptococcal and enterococcal strains with high-level resistance to all aminoglycosides	Amoxicillin	> 200 mg/kg per day	Vancomycin	30 mg/kg per day	≥ 8 weeks
Enterococcus faecalis resistant to penicillin, aminoglycosides and vancomycin	Amoxicillin + ceftriaxone or imipenem	200 mg/kg per day 2 g/day 2 g/day	–	–	≥ 8 weeks
E. faecium resistant to penicillin, aminoglycosides and vancomycin	Linezolid or quinupristin-dalfopristin	1200 mg/day 22.5 mg/kg per day	Linezolid or quinupristin-dalfopristin	1200 mg/day 22.5 mg/kg per day	≥ 8 weeks

*Two or three daily doses.
†Duration of aminoglycoside administration could be shortened to 2–3 weeks; the total duration of treatment should be 6 weeks when vancomycin or teicoplanin is used.
‡Two daily doses.
Hoen B. Epidemiology and antibiotic treatment of infective endocarditis: an update. *Heart* 2006; **92**: 1694–700.

Examination typically shows a pulmonary ejection systolic murmur with a wide and fixed second heart sound.

ECG usually shows a right bundle branch block (and a left axis deviation with a primum defect). Chest X-ray will show pulmonary plethora.

Echocardiography, especially transoesophageal echocardiography, can demonstrate the defect and give an estimate of the pulmonary artery pressure. There is an increased risk of developing Eisenmenger's syndrome but no risk of endocarditis. Many patients can live to a good age but overall life expectancy is not normal. Closure is by surgery or more usually now an occluder introduced percutaneously is usually recommended if the size of the shunt is > 1.5:1.0. Patent foramen ovale can now also be closed percutaneously. This is often done if there is evidence of paradoxical emboli.[18]

PATENT DUCTUS ARTERIOSUS

This congenital abnormality is often asymptomatic and survival is usual. At the age of about 20, the risk of infective endocarditis increases, and at the age of about 30, patients with sizeable left-to-right shunts will begin to develop cardiac failure. Patients with significant shunts should have

Table 21.4 Antibiotic treatment for staphylococcal infective endocarditis (IE)

	No allergy to penicillin		Allergy to penicillin		Duration
	Drug	Dosage	Drug	Dosage	
Native valve IE					
Oxa-S strain	Oxacillin†	150–200 mg/kg per day	Vancomycin§	30 mg/kg per day	4–6 weeks (5 days combination)
	+ gentamicin‡	3 mg/kg per day	or cefamandole**	75–100 mg/kg per day	
			+ gentamicin‡	3 mg/kg per day	
Oxa-R strain	Vancomycin§	30 mg/kg per day	Vancomycin§	30 mg/kg per day	4–6 weeks (5 days combination)
	± gentamicin‡	3 mg/kg per day	± gentamicin‡	3 mg/kg per day	
Prosthetic valve IE*					
Oxa-S strain	Oxacillin†	150–200 mg/kg per day	Vancomycin§	30 mg/kg per day	≥ 6 weeks combination (aminoglycoside no longer than 15 days)
	+ gentamicin‡	3 mg/kg per day	+ gentamicin‡	3 mg/kg per day	
	+ rifampicin	20–30 mg/kg per day	+ rifampicin	20–30 mg/kg per day	
Oxa-R, genta-S strain	Vancomycin§	30 mg/kg per day	Vancomycin§	30 mg/kg per day	≥ 6 weeks combination (aminoglycoside no longer than 15 days)
	+ rifampicin	20–30 mg/kg per day	+ rifampicin	20–30 mg/kg per day	
	+ gentamicin‡	3 mg/kg per day	+ gentamicin‡	3 mg/kg per day	
Oxa-R, genta-R strain	Vancomycin§	30 mg/kg per day	Vancomycin§	30 mg/kg per day	≥ 6 weeks combination
	+ rifampicin¶	20–30 mg/kg per day	+ rifampicin¶	20–30 mg/kg per day	
	+ other antistaphylococccal drug, if available		+ other antistaphylococccal drug, if available		

oxa, oxacillin; R, resistant; S, susceptible.
*Valve replacement should be considered, inasmuch as IE develops early after valve implantation.
†Other choices: cloxacillin 100–150 mg/kg per day; cefamandole 75–100 mg/kg per day.
‡Other choice: netilmicin (5–6 mg/kg per day).
§Other choice: teicoplanin, target serum trough concentrations 25–30 mg/l.
¶If strain resistant to rifampicin, combine vancomycin with one or two other antistaphylococcal drugs, according to susceptibility pattern.
**The use of a cephalosporin is not recommended in patients with a history of anaphylactic reaction to penicillin.
Hoen B. Epidemiology and antibiotic treatment of infective endocarditis: an update. *Heart* 2006; **92**: 1694–700.

the patent ductus arteriosus closed by surgery or, increasingly, by transcatheter using an umbrella device.[19]

VENTRICULAR SEPTAL DEFECTS

These are very common at birth but are seldom found in adults. The occasional adult will survive with a persistent small perimembranous ventricular septal defect which is not haemodynamically significant but a risk for endocarditis.

FALLOT'S TETRALOGY

This is the cyanotic malformation most frequently associated with survival to adulthood. In these patients, the pulmonary stenosis is usually sufficient to prevent excessive pulmonary blood flow, but not so severe as to cause

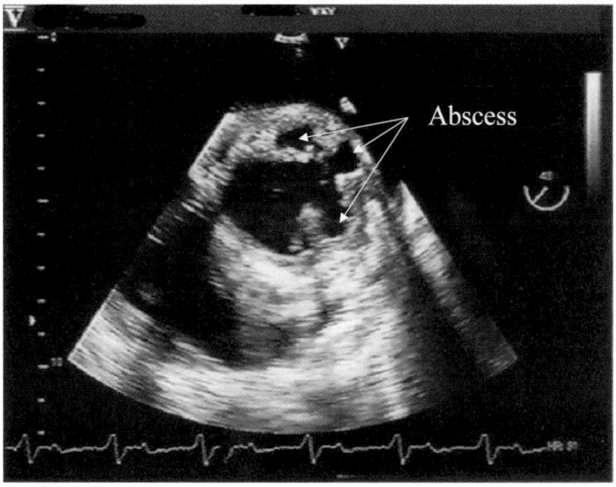

Figure 21.5 Abscess cavities seen in the aortic root during transoesophageal echocardiography.

large degrees of shunting from the right to the left ventricle. An increasing number of patients who have had complete repair are surviving into adulthood, and overall outcome is excellent.[20] The 30-year actuarial survival rate is 90% of the expected, and late health status is very good. However, in some RV fibrosis and damage may lead to ventricular arrhythmias and sudden death. Also there is an increased risk of conduction defects (heart block).

NON-CARDIAC SURGERY

CYANOTIC CONGENITAL HEART DISEASE

These patients have an increased risk of acute cholecystitis caused by calcium bilirubinate stones, and cholecystectomy is a procedure to be anticipated. Blood taken for phlebotomy can be stored for transfusion later. Oxygen inhalation appears to be desirable. Care must be taken with all intravenous lines, infusions and drugs, so that air is not introduced because of the risk of systemic embolism. If patients with Fallot's tetralogy have a sudden fall in blood pressure because of a fall in systemic resistance, intense cyanosis and occasionally death may occur. Conversely, a sudden rise in systemic resistance may severely depress systemic blood flow. Prophylaxis is required for infective endocarditis. Cyanotic patients with elevated fixed pulmonary vascular resistance (Eisenmenger's syndrome) are not able to respond rapidly to haemodynamic changes. In these patients, a sudden fall or rise in systemic vascular resistance can be very dangerous.

OSTIUM SECUNDUM ATRIAL SEPTAL DEFECT

In asymptomatic adults with this malformation and with normal pulmonary artery pressure, there is little risk during non-cardiac surgery. However, a rise in peripheral vascular resistance will increase left-to-right shunting; with hypotension, right-to-left shunting may occur. Systemic paradoxical emboli from leg veins can occur and early mobilisation is recommended.

CONGENITAL COMPLETE HEART BLOCK

If the QRS is narrow and the subsidiary pacemaker is reliable with a reasonable ventricular rate, then temporary RV pacing is not required. However, all vagotonic stimuli should be minimised. If the QRS complex is wide and there is a relatively slow ventricular response, a temporary pacemaker should be inserted preoperatively.

REFERENCES

1. Soler-Soler J, Galve E. Worldwide perspective of valve disease. *Heart* 2000; **83**: 721–5.
2. Sanderson JE, Woo KS. Rheumatic fever and rheumatic heart disease – declining but not gone. *Int J Cardiol* 1994; **43**: 231–2.
3. Eisenberg MJ. Rheumatic heart disease in the developing world: prevalence, prevention, and control. *Eur Heart J* 1993; **14**: 122–8.
4. Barlow JB. Aspects of active rheumatic carditis. *Aust NZ J Med* 1992; **22**: 592–600.
5. Reyes VP, Raju BS, Wynne J *et al.* Percutaneous balloon valvuloplasty compared with open surgical commissurotomy for mitral stenosis. *N Engl J Med* 1994; **331**: 961–7.
6. Bonow Ro *et al.* ACC/AHA 2006 Guidelines for the management of patients with valvular heart disease: Executive Summary. In a report of the American College of Cardiology/American Heart Association Task Force on Practice Guidelines. *J Am Coll Cardiol* 2006; **48**: 598–675.
7. Enriquez-Sarano M, Schaff HV, Orszulak TA *et al.* Valve repair improves the outcome of surgery for mitral regurgitation: a mutivariate analysis. *Circulation* 1995; **91**: 1022–8.
8. Pellerin D, Brecker S, Veyrat C. Degenerative mitral valve disease with emphasis on mitral valve prolapse. *Heart* 2002; **88**: 20–28.
9. Frary W, Devereux RB, Kramer-Fox R *et al.* Clinical and health-care cost consequences of infective endocarditis in mitral valve prolapse. *Am J Cardiol* 1994; **73**: 263–7.
10. Otto C. Valvular aortic stenosis: disease severity and timing of intervention. *J Am Coll Cardiol* 2006; **47**: 2141–51.
11. Scognamiglio R, Rahimtoola SH, Fasoli G *et al.* Nifedipine in asymptomatic patients with severe aortic regurgitation and normal left ventricular function. *N Engl J Med* 1994; **331**: 689–94.
12. Benolti JR. Acute aortic insufficiency. In: Dalen JE, Alpert JS (eds) *Valvular Heart Disease*, 2nd edn. Boston: Little, Brown; 1987: 319–52.
13. Robbins MJ, Sveiro R, Fishman WH *et al.* Right-sided valvular endocarditis: etiology, diagnosis and approach to therapy. *Am Heart J* 1986; **109**: 558–66.
14. Moreillon P, Que YA. Infective endocarditis. *Lancet* 2004; **363**: 39–49.

15. Li JS, Sexton DJ, Mick N *et al.* Proposed modifications to the Duke criteria for the diagnosis of infective endocarditis. *Clin Infect Dis* 2000; **30**: 633–8.
16. Rinaldi CA, Hall RJ. Echocardiography in endocarditis. In: Izzart MB, Sanderson JE, Sutton MG (eds) *Echocardiography in Adult Cardiac Surgery.* Oxford: ISIS Medical Media; 1999: 155–6.
17. Hoen B. Epidemiology and antibiotic treatment of infective endocarditis: an update. *Heart* 2006; **92**: 1694–700.
18. Meier B. Closure of patent foramen ovale: technique, pitfalls, complications and follow-up. *Heart* 2005; **91**: 444–8.
19. Schenek MH, O'Laughlin MP, Rokey R *et al.* Transcatheter occlusion of patent ductus arteriosus in adults. *Am J Cardiol* 1993; **72**: 591–5.
20. Murphy JG, Gersh BJ, Mair DD *et al.* Long-term outcome in patients undergoing surgical repair of tetralogy of Fallot. *N Engl J Med* 1993; **329**: 593–9.

APPENDIX

NICE GUIDANCE

Antimicrobial prophylaxis against infective endocarditis in adults and children undergoing interventional procedures (March 2008)

Antibacterial prophylaxis and chlorhexidine mouthwash are not recommended for the prevention of endocarditis in patients undergoing dental procedures.

Antibacterial prophylaxis is not recommended for the prevention of endocarditis in patients undergoing procedures of the:

- upper and lower respiratory tract (including ear, nose, and throat procedures and bronchoscopy);
- genito-urinary tract (including urological, gynaecological, and obstetric procedures);
- upper and lower gastro-intestinal tract.

Whilst these procedures can cause bacteraemia, there is no clear association with the development of infective endocarditis. Prophylaxis may expose patients to the adverse effects of antimicrobials when the evidence of benefit has not been proven.

Any infection in patients at risk of endocarditis[1] should be investigated promptly and treated appropriately to reduce the risk of endocarditis.

If patients at risk of endocarditis[1] are undergoing a gastro-intestinal or genito-urinary tract procedure at a site where infection is suspected, they should receive appropriate antibacterial therapy that includes cover against organisms that cause endocarditis.

Patients at risk of endocarditis[1] should be:

- advised to maintain good oral hygiene;
- told how to recognise signs of infective endocarditis, and advised when to seek expert advice.

From BNF: http://www.bnf.org/bnf/bnf/55/102053.htm

22

Intensive care after cardiac surgery

Raymond F Raper

Coronary artery bypass surgery is one of the most frequently undertaken surgical procedures. Because of the prevalence of cardiac disease, cardiac surgery has significant health and economic implications. Intensive care may account for up to 40% of the total hospital costs for these patients and much of the short-term morbidity and mortality is based on perioperative events.

The overall mortality of cardiac surgery is low (approximately 3%). However, this ranges from less than 1% for elective coronary artery bypass grafting to in excess of 30% for more complicated surgery in patients with significant myocardial dysfunction and associated disorders. Usually, intensive care post-cardiac surgery involves a short period of recovery before discharge to the ward but, for a small percentage of patients, at least potentially remediable complications may require the complete intensive care armamentarium, with a highly significant impact on the intensive care unit (ICU) and hospital budgets and resources.

ORGANISATION

The convergence of large numbers of patients with very similar problems in the cardiac ICU provides an ideal environment for the standardisation of care based on protocols and clinical pathways. One of the traps of postoperative cardiac care is that the sameness of the patients tends to obscure their particularity. Individual patient assessment must carefully address the multisystemic manifestations of cardiovascular and degenerative diseases.

Cardiac surgery involves a continuum of care from presentation to postdischarge management and rehabilitation. The intensive care specialist must be involved in this continuum, not functioning in isolation from surgeons, anaesthetists, cardiologists and family practitioners.

The postoperative stage is largely set by the preoperative and operative phases of management. A component of postoperative management is active participation both in principle and in particular in patient selection and preparation as well as in the conduct of anaesthesia and surgery. Relevant aspects include suitability and preparation for surgery, advanced care planning and more technical issues such as temperature management, invasive monitoring, haemodynamic management and transport. Movement from the operating theatre to the ICU and later to the ward will only appear seamless if the management systems have been well coordinated in advance.

CARDIOVASCULAR MANAGEMENT

The first step in the intensive care management of the newly arrived patient who has undergone cardiac surgery involves a simple transfer of ventilation, monitoring and drug administration from transport to ICU systems. This should be structured to minimise disruption.

- Confirm integrity and position of endotracheal and gastric tubes and intravascular catheters.
- Re-establish mechanical ventilation of both lungs.
- Undertake chest radiography; to assess lung expansion, pleural integrity and catheter placement.
- Perform early 12-lead electrocardiography to exclude or identify acute ischaemia.

Management is conveniently dictated by standardised protocols, which should cover investigations, fluid and electrolyte management, vasoactive and other drug administration and mechanical ventilation. Standardisation is probably more important than the particulars of the protocol, which might vary considerably among institutions. Optimal cardiovascular management requires a sound knowledge of normal and abnormal cardiovascular physiology. It also requires an understanding of the haemodynamic changes usually seen in the postoperative patient (Figure 22.1).[1]

MONITORING

Electrocardiography and continuous invasive blood pressure and central venous pressure monitoring are standard. Flotation pulmonary artery (PA) catheterisation has become somewhat controversial. It is now reasonably well established that PA catheterisation is safe but may not alter outcomes.[2]

- Surgery can be safely undertaken at least in low-risk patients without PA catheterisation.[3]
- Collateral evidence supports PA catheter use in more complicated cases.

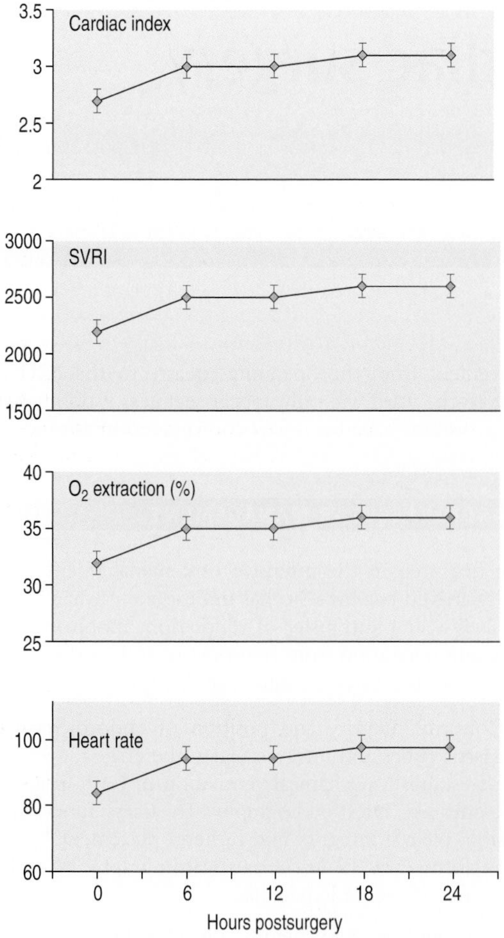

Figure 22.1 Haemodynamic changes following cardiac surgery. Systemic vascular resistance index (SVRI).

- It is essential that the known limitations and complications of PA catheters are considered in usage and interpretation.[4]

Cardiac output measurement by pulse contour analysis and a variety of ultrasound techniques is becoming more commonplace. A precise role for these techniques is not established, especially in the postsurgical patient, where Doppler-enabling windows may be difficult to obtain. Pulse contour analysis is invalidated by intra-aortic counterpulsation. Nevertheless, these techniques and continuous mixed venous saturation monitoring are attractive and very useful in individual patients.

Transoesophageal echocardiography is now almost routine in the operating theatre, at least for more complicated patients. The technique is less suitable for monitoring in the ICU but is helpful in the diagnosis and management of cardiovascular instability in postoperative patients.

FLUID AND ELECTROLYTE MANAGEMENT

Despite generous intraoperative fluid administration, effective hypovolaemia is common in the early postoperative period, especially as warming with associated vasodilatation occurs.

RESUSCITATION FLUID

- Use of isotonic fluid is essential.
- No benefit for any particular resuscitation fluid has been established. The suggestion that albumin may not be safe has been essentially dispelled.[5]
- Larger volumes of crystalloid than colloid solutions are required.

Polyuria is frequently observed in the early postoperative period, possibly related to hypothermia, haemodilution and the after-effects of non-pulsatile cardiopulmonary bypass on stretch and baroreceptors. This usually settles within the first 6 hours but often necessitates considerable volume replacement in the meantime.

POTASSIUM AND MAGNESIUM HOMEOSTASIS

Hypomagnesaemia and hypokalaemia are frequent in the early postoperative stage. These are exacerbated by polyuria. Late hyperkalaemia is also quite common, especially in patients with renal impairment or prior angiotensin-converting enzyme (ACE) inhibitor administration. Treatment for hyperkalaemia is rarely required in the absence of significant renal impairment. Especially in patients with atrial or ventricular ectopy or tachydysrhythmias, potassium and magnesium levels must be maintained in the high normal range.

Calcium homeostasis is generally not threatened by cardiopulmonary bypass. Massive transfusion, however, frequently causes hypocalcaemia. Ionised calcium levels are now easily monitored by ward-based blood gas machines.

HYPOTENSION

Hypotension is both a consequence and a cause of myocardial dysfunction. The major causes include:

- hypovolaemia
- vasodilation
- pericardial tamponade
- heart failure

Other causes of low cardiac output state (Table 22.1) should be considered and excluded. Whatever the cause, hypotension frequently causes myocardial ischaemia and consequent heart failure, especially if it occurs in the first 12–24 hours postoperatively. Angiography during this time almost always shows a significant reduction in the calibre of native coronary arteries, indicating increased coronary resistance and, presumably, altered coronary vasodilator reserve. Treatment of hypotension is urgent if a spiral of ischaemia and heart failure is to be averted.

Table 22.1 Low cardiac output

Preload
• Hypovolaemia, including haemorrhage
• Tamponade, pericardial constriction
• Left ventricular diastolic dysfunction
• Hypertrophy
• Ischaemia
• Oedema
• Cardiomyopathy
• Pulmonary hypertension
• Right ventricular failure
Afterload
• Excessive vasoconstriction
• Aortic stenosis
• Functional left ventricular obstruction
• Obstructive cardiomyopathy
• Systolic anterior motion of the mitral valve
Myocardial function
• Mechanical (ventricular septal defect, valve pathology)
• Cardiomyopathy
• Ischaemia, postischaemic stunning
• Metabolic, electrolyte abnormalities, pharmacolgical depression

MANAGEMENT

Successful management of hypotension depends on:

- rapid diagnostic assessment
- diagnosis-specific intervention

Context is very helpful. Early hypotension in patients with well-preserved ventricular function and no obvious ischaemia usually responds well to fluid administration. Patients with poor ventricular function and increasing inotrope requirement are likely to have a more sinister pathophysiology.

Vasoconstrictors may be useful in breaking the cycle of hypotension–ischaemia–hypotension but must be used cautiously in patients with impaired ventricular function, and especially in patients with major vascular or aortic pathology, for whom a hypertensive overshoot may be catastrophic.

HYPERTENSION

Complications associated with hypertension include:

- bleeding
- heart failure
- vascular (especially aortic) injury
- myocardial ischaemia

Significant postoperative hypertension is more common in patients having a history of hypertension and with cessation of β-blockade, but is reasonably common in the early postoperative period. Both absolute pressure and *dp/dt* are important factors in vascular injury. Vascular resistance declines over the first few hours (see Figure 22.1), so that therapy during this period is best undertaken with agents with a short duration of action. Nitroglycerine is theoretically more appropriate than nitroprusside because of the possibility of coronary steal with the latter agent.[6] In practice, this is almost never apparent and nitroprusside appears to be more effective. Simple measures such as the provision of adequate analgesia and sedation should also be considered.

The target blood pressure varies with the indication. Excessive reduction of blood pressure risks reducing myocardial oxygen supply more than demand. Under most circumstances, a mean arterial pressure between 90 and 100 mmHg (12.0 and 13.5 kPa) seems optimal.[7] Much lower target pressures may be applicable for the management of heart failure or in the presence of a vulnerable aorta, such as occurs with aortic trauma, dissection or aneurysm. Reduction of *dp/dt* with beta-blockade is more important than absolute blood pressure control in the management of aortic dissection.

LOW CARDIAC OUTPUT

The aetiology of a low cardiac output following heart surgery is diverse (see Table 22.1). The most common causes include:

- intravascular volume depletion
- systolic heart failure
- pericardial tamponade

Transient, reversible myocardial depression may follow an episode of acute ischaemia (preoperative or intraoperative) and is especially problematic where intraoperative myocardial protection has been difficult or suboptimal. Recognition of a low-output state in the absence of invasive monitoring may be difficult. Many of the usual signs of low output are also consequences of anaesthesia and surgery. Tachycardia may be obscured by drugs, hypothermia and heart disease, and even lactic acidosis may be an unreliable marker in this patient group.[1]

In the early postoperative period, a relatively low cardiac output may not warrant intervention, providing tissue oxygen delivery is adequate. Since beta-blockade is beneficial in the postoperative cardiac patient, beta-agonists should not be used unquestioningly. Nevertheless, optimisation of cardiac function does confer some benefit[8] and intervention is clearly required when tissue oxygen delivery is inadequate.

Low cardiac output is associated with increased gastrointestinal, renal and neurological complications.

MANAGEMENT OPTIONS

1. Establish the diagnosis, including aetiology. Distinguishing tamponade from heart failure may require

cardiac imaging with transthoracic or transoesophageal echocardiography. This should be the first recourse when uncertainty remains following conventional haemodynamic assessment. Tamponade may not be detectable using transthoracic echocardiography in the early phase after surgery.[9] The principal role of echocardiography is thus the investigation of possible alternate diagnoses.

2. Correct all easily reversible factors, including hypovolaemia, tamponade, acute myocardial ischaemia, electrolyte abnormalities and dysrhythmias.
3. Vasodilators are helpful in the presence of hypertension and ventricular dilatation. Postsurgical vasodilation after the first 4–8 hours often obviates any ongoing role for these agents.
4. Use of inotropic agents. Because of the associated vasodilatation, ino-constricting agents are frequently required, alone or in combination. Useful agents include:
   - dobutamine, an essentially pure β_1-agonist with inotropic, lusotropic and some chronotropic effects
   - noradrenaline (norepinephrine), metaraminol, vasopressin and high-dose dopamine which, being predominantly vasoconstrictors, are hazardous in the presence of hypovolaemia and should probably not be used alone in the presence of a low cardiac output
   - adrenaline (epinephrine), the metabolic effects of which (especially lactic acidosis) make usage in cardiac surgical patients problematic.[10] Adrenaline is, nevertheless, a potent ino-constrictor and recent studies suggest that it is as effective and as safe as noradrenaline, in the general patient population at least
   - milrinone, which has a long duration of action and potent vasodilating properties. These make milrinone relatively difficult to introduce and to wean. It is, however, a very effective inotropic agent, especially in patients with beta-receptor downregulation
   - levosimendan, a novel calcium-sensitising agent, has a promising role both perioeratively and as rescue therapy for postsurgery heart failure[11]
5. Intra-aortic balloon counterpulsation (IABC; see below).
6. Ventricular assist devices (VAD) are expensive and technically far more demanding than IABC. They are effective in resting the heart while supporting organ and tissue oxygen delivery. Indications for implantation have not been well established but include intractable heart failure, and failure to wean from cardiopulmonary bypass in spite of full cardiovascular support. A combination of haemodynamic and cardiac support-level criteria seems most useful and early utilisation offers improved outcomes.[12,13] Usage is relatively infrequent so that management expertise is difficult to acquire. Some centres thus prefer to re-establish or continue cardiopulmonary bypass as short-term, biventricular support. Most published VAD data relate to non-surgical patients in whom the role of heart assist devices is increasingly established as both 'bridge to transplant' and as 'destination therapy'.
7. Delayed sternal closure has an established role in improving outcome after cardiac surgery.[14] Cardiac output is increased and inotropic requirement reduced. Subsequent sternal closure has an acceptably low complication rate. The sternum may be left open following an initial attempt at closure or reopened with later deterioration. Sternal retraction may be required.
8. Mechanical ventilation is generally continued throughout the period of low output. This reduces cardiac workload by removing the work of breathing. Positive intrathoracic pressure reduces left ventricular afterload, which is beneficial to the dilated left ventricle. Positive pressure may be detrimental, however, in the presence of diastolic ventricular dysfunction or hypovolaemia, where the reduction in venous return may further reduce ventricular preload.

INTRA-AORTIC BALLOON COUNTERPULSATION

IABC has an established role in support of cardiac surgery. Its two actions are: (1) augmentation of diastolic coronary perfusion pressure; and (2) left ventricular afterload reduction. This is achieved by balloon inflation (30–50 ml capacity) within the aorta during diastole and rapid deflation of the balloon immediately before aortic valve opening. The catheter is usually inserted using a Seldinger technique, but can be placed by femoral artery cutdown or directly into the descending thoracic aorta. Timing of inflation and deflation is critical to optimal function. This is best achieved using the pressure waveform and a 1:2 ratio (Figure 22.2).

Inflation is timed to coincide with the dicrotic notch. Deflation is timed to occur as late as possible in diastole,

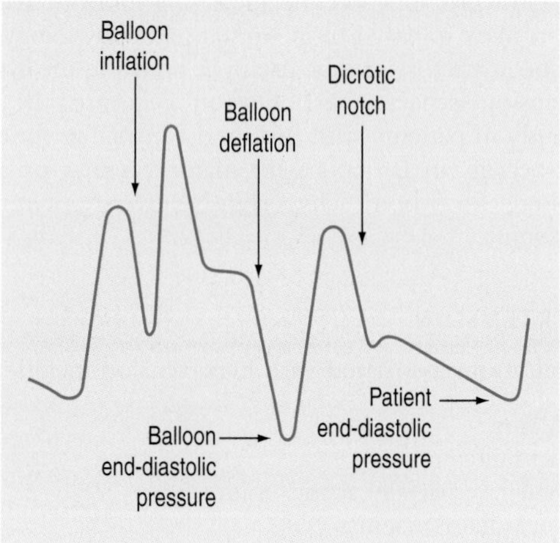

Figure 22.2 Intra-aortic balloon counterpulsation pressure waveform.

Table 22.2 Indications for intra-aortic balloon counterpulsation

Prophylactic
- Cardiac surgery
  - Two of: left main >70%, left ventricular ejection fraction <0.4, unstable angina, reoperation
- Non-cardiac procedures
  - Severe left ventricular impairment, unstable angina
- Failure to wean from cardiopulmonary bypass
- Cardiogenic shock
  - *Reversible* myocardial depression
  - Support for reperfusion, revascularisation
  - Bridge to transport

ensuring that the IABC end-diastolic pressure is lower than the patient's end-diastolic pressure. IABC increases cardiac index and coronary perfusion and reduces left ventricular filling pressure, myocardial lactate production and oxygen extraction percentage.

Indications for IABC are summarised in Table 22.2.

IABC improves:

- mortality in high-risk cardiac surgery[15,16]
- clinical outcomes when used in support of infarct-related, non-surgical coronary reperfusion[17]

IABC is not helpful in the management of cardiogenic shock from irremediable causes except as a bridge to transplant. Complications are:

- limb ischaemia (6–16%)
- vascular trauma, dissection
- infection (cutdown>percutaneous)
- balloon rupture
- bleeding
- thrombocytopenia
- malposition, vascular obstruction
- malfunction, failure to unwrap

Limb ischaemia is the most frequent complication and optimal management requires early recognition based on routine, systematic observation.

ISCHAEMIA

Postoperative myocardial ischaemia predicts a more complicated course.[18] Recognition is enhanced by automated multilead ST analysis with confirmatory electrocardiography, although diagnosis may be difficult in the presence of preoperative electrocardiographic abnormalities.

Ischaemia may be due to graft failure. Remedial options include coronary angiography and/or reoperation. Angiography offers the potential for tailored reoperation or non-operative intervention. Management decisions may be influenced by surgical factors such as the availability of further conduit and the state of the native arteries. Thus close liaison among ICU personnel, cardiologists and surgeons is essential.

DIASTOLIC DYSFUNCTION

Ventricular hypertrophy is the commonest cause of diastolic dysfunction, and is exacerbated by poor myocardial protection during surgical procedures. Myocardial ischaemia, right ventricular (RV) dilatation and pericardial abnormalities (including tamponade) can also reduce left ventricular volume in spite of elevated filling pressures.[19] Recognition and management can be very difficult.

Diagnosis generally requires:

- demonstration of small ventricular volumes (using echocardiography or other techniques)
- the presence of increased pressures

MANAGEMENT

- Treatable causes should be addressed.
- Blood volume must be maintained, with blood transfusion where necessary.
- Maintenance of sinus rhythm is helpful, if not essential.
- Atrial pacing at an enhanced heart rate is often beneficial since the stroke volume is fixed and the diastolic filling time is foreshortened.
- β-agonists and milrinone improve diastolic relaxation and hence ventricular compliance.

DYSRHYTHMIAS

Ventricular and supraventricular dysrhythmias are common. Prevention and treatment of electrolyte abnormalities may be prophylactic. New occurrence of complex ventricular dysrhythmias should stimulate a search for causal ischaemia and graft malfunction.

- Ventricular fibrillation and pulseless ventricular tachycardia require rapid defibrillation, preferably before external cardiac massage, which may cause mechanical injury poststernotomy. If haemodynamic stability cannot be rapidly restored, open cardiac massage should be instituted.
- Facilities for atrioventricular pacing are essential as transient heart block is common.

ATRIAL FIBRILLATION (AF)

AF is the most common complication of cardiac surgery.[20,21] Its incidence varies from 10 to 40% in patients undergoing coronary artery surgery and up to 50% with some valvular procedures. Predisposing factors include a history of AF, valvular heart disease (especially mitral valve pathology), increasing age and prolonged P-wave duration. AF can be effectively treated and its recurrence prevented with intraoperative radiofrequency ablation and left atrial reduction during cardiac surgery.[22] AF is probably less frequently observed following 'off-pump' surgery, and is most frequently encountered around the second and third postoperative days, but may occur weeks after surgery and hospital discharge.

AF is a potentially serious complication. Apart from discomfort, it may provoke or complicate haemodynamic instability. The major complication of AF, however, is stroke, with an increased risk of approximately threefold. Based on echocardiography, there is the potential for embolic stroke within 3 days of onset of AF.

AF is also associated with:

- increase in inotrope usage
- increased use of IABC
- increased reoperation for bleeding
- prolonged ICU and hospital stay
- increased costs

Several strategies are beneficial in preventing AF:[23]

- β-blockade
- amiodarone
- sotolol
- diltiazem
- atrial pacing
- dexamethasone

Treatment should be tempered with an understanding that spontaneous reversion to sinus rhythm is frequent. A treatment strategy is summarised in Table 22.3.

- Beta-blockade is best established.
- Digitalis is not more effective than placebo at reverting AF and may not be helpful in ventricular rate control in the presence of catecholamine stimulation.
- Anticoagulation should be considered where AF persists for longer than 48 hours and in all cases where elective cardioversion is undertaken.
- Early cardioversion tends to be ineffective and potentially harmful and should only be undertaken to correct severe haemodynamic compromise.

Table 22.3 Management of atrial fibrillation (AF)

Rate control
• β-blockade
• Calcium channel blockers
• Amiodarone
• Sotolol
• Digitalis
Cardioversion
• Ibuletide
• Amiodarone
• Magnesium
• Electrical cardioversion
Anticoagulation
• Always for elective cardioversion
• Consider if atrial fibrillation persists beyond 48 hours

RIGHT VENTRICULAR DYSFUNCTION

RV failure following cardiac surgery is reasonably common. Aetiological factors include:

- direct RV ischaemia or infarction
- poor myocardial protection
- anteriorly placed RV
- bypass-related pulmonary hypertension

Management involves:

- volume resuscitation
- maintenance of RV perfusion pressure with vasoconstrictors
- IABC as required
- inotrope administration
- RV afterload reduction

Useful afterload-reducing agents include nitric oxide,[24] prostaglandins and sildenafil.[25] Conventional vasodilators tend to produce excessive systemic vasodilatation. Occasionally, RV balloon counterpulsation or an RV assist device may be required. Delayed sternal closure has an established role.

EMERGENCY REOPERATION

Emergency re-sternotomy is indicated as part of resuscitation when haemodynamic stability cannot be rapidly re-established with conventional means.[26,27] Advantages compared to closed-chest resuscitation include:

- establishment of the cause of instability
- correction of the cause (e.g. tamponade, kinked graft)
- more effective cardiac massage
- direct establishment of atrial and ventricular pacing

Re-sternotomy also enables the re-establishment of cardiopulmonary bypass and regrafting or correction of mechanical abnormalities as required. Infectious complications of emergency re-sternotomy are probably increased but the incidence is not prohibitive.

RESPIRATORY MANAGEMENT

Postoperative mechanical ventilation remains routine in cardiac surgical patients. Immediate extubation appears to offer little patient benefit[28] but may be expedient. Neither is routine ventilation beyond 12 hours essential.[29] Extubation can be safely undertaken with simple protocols. Reintubation is rarely required, but is more likely in older patients with pre-existing lung and vascular disease and impaired ventricular function. Reoperative surgery and bleeding requiring massive transfusion also increase the likelihood of early extubation failure.[30]

Hypoxia is very common in the early postoperative period. It is mostly attributable to atelectasis and responds well to simple measures such as positive end-expiratory pressure (PEEP), prolonged inspiration and simple recruitment manoeuvres. Atelectasis is a consequence of cardiopulmonary bypass and intraoperative ventilation with high inspired oxygen and without PEEP. Long-term sequelae are rare. Incentive spirometry and chest physiotherapy are commonly utilised in the postoperative period, without good supportive evidence. Early mobilisation appears most beneficial. Adequate analgesia facilitates physiotherapy and mobilisation. Local analgesic initiatives may be helpful[31] whereas some non-steroidal agents may increase the risk of complications.[32]

More sinister causes of hypoxia include severe heart failure and hypoxaemic respiratory failure (acute respiratory distress syndrome: ARDS). The aetiology of ARDS is diverse, but includes shock, massive blood product administration and cardiopulmonary bypass itself. Management is not particular to this group of patients. Occasionally, profound hypoxia accompanies minor atelectasis with moderate pulmonary hypertension. Patent foramen ovale (which is seen in 10–15% of the normal population) with right-to-left intracardiac shunt is the likely mechanism.

Pulmonary embolism is an uncommon complication of cardiac surgery, probably due to bypass-induced platelet dysfunction, routine postoperative antiplatelet therapy and thromboprophylaxis.[33] 'Off-pump' surgery may be associated with an increase in this complication and so may warrant a more aggressive prophylactic regimen.[34]

POSTOPERATIVE COMPLICATIONS

HAEMORRHAGE

Excessive postoperative bleeding is a major cause of increased morbidity and mortality. Mechanisms are complex and include preoperative anticoagulation, thrombolysis and antiplatelet therapy as well as activation of haemostatic mechanisms, including fibrinolysis. 'Off-pump' surgery may be associated with excessive bleeding because of administration of anticoagulant and antiplatelet therapy out of fear of early graft closure.

Most studies of pharmacological strategies to minimise postoperative blood loss have involved preoperative or intraoperative intervention. Extrapolation to the postoperative phase is intuitive rather than established. Aprotinin and the lysine analogues aminocaproic acid and tranexamic acid reduce bleeding and exposure to blood and blood products. Aprotinin has been associated with an increased risk of serious end-organ damage.[35] Desmopressin is probably less effective and has been associated with an increased risk of myocardial infarction.[36]

Effective postoperative measures include reversal of residual heparin (including 'heparin rebound') and correction of coagulopathy with blood products. Application of PEEP has been shown to be effective in some studies, but not others. Retransfusion of shed blood reduces autologous transfusion requirements without apparent side-effects. Controlled tamponade with discontinuation of drain suction and even clamping of drains has also been reported.[37] Finally, at least in reasonably stable patients, reduction of the transfusion threshold to at least 80 g/l reduces exposure to autologous blood transfusion[38] without adverse consequences.

RENAL FAILURE

Depending on definition and patient groups, acute renal failure is observed in 1–5% of patients undergoing cardiac surgery. Risk factors include increasing age, heart failure, prolonged bypass, diabetes, pre-existing renal impairment and postoperative shock.[39] Surgery without cardiopulmonary bypass may be relatively protective.[40] Morbidity, mortality and costs are significantly increased. Effective preventive strategies beyond careful haemodynamic management and minimisation of associated nephrotoxic insults have not been established. Nevertheless, attention to urine output in the presence of known risk factors appears warranted.

SHIVERING

Shivering is frequent following cardiac surgery. Mechanisms are complex and not entirely related to core temperature. Shivering causes a significant increase in metabolic rate and hence cardiac workload. This is especially important in the patient with impaired cardiac function and limited reserve. Effective preventive agents include dexamethasone, clonidine, high-dose morphine and external warming. Pethidine effectively reduces the duration of shivering. Short-term neuromuscular blockade is occasionally required.

STERNAL INFECTION

Deep sternal wound infection is uncommon (0.5–2.5%). Associated morbidity and mortality are significant. Risk factors have been variously reported but consistently include diabetes, obesity and use of internal mammary arteries, especially if bilateral. Other contributing factors include prolonged surgery, chronic lung disease, male sex, low postoperative cardiac output, blood transfusion, sternal reopening and dialysis. Rigid control of blood sugar levels in diabetics[41] and preoperative nasal and oropharyngeal decontamination[42] may help prevent infection.

NEUROLOGICAL COMPLICATIONS

Neurological complications of cardiac surgery include neuropsychiatric deterioration as a consequence of cardiopulmonary bypass, delirium and a range of peripheral neuropathies, the most frequent of which is a unilateral phrenic nerve palsy. Paraplegia is a recognised complication of thoracic aortic surgery.

The most devastating neurological complication is cerebral infarction. The incidence varies with patient selection, but ranges from 1 to 5%. The pathophysiology is mostly embolic. Risk factors include carotid artery stenosis, hypertension, AF, aortic atheroma, impaired ventricular function and peripheral vascular disease.[43] 'Off-pump' surgery is almost certainly protective and other operative techniques may also reduce the incidence.

GASTROINTESTINAL COMPLICATIONS

Peptic ulcer disease, pancreatitis, cholecystitis, gut ischaemia, ileus and hepatic dysfunction are uncommon (<1%) after cardiac surgery. Morbidity, however, is quite high. Risk factors include increased age, more complicated surgery and postoperative shock. The incidence of gastrointestinal complications may be reduced with 'off-pump' surgery.[44]

LONG-TERM CONSIDERATIONS

Patients surviving cardiac surgery have a continuing risk of disease progression. It is important that effective secondary prevention strategies be considered or recommenced in the postoperative period. Initiatives with proven long term benefit in patients with ischaemic heart disease include anti-platelet therapy, beta blockade, ACE inhibitors, lipid-lowering statins and exercise. Treatment for hypertension, diabetes and other intercurrent disorders should also be reinstituted.

A small percentage of patients require long-term ICU management for a variety of complications. Excellent long-term survival and quality of life are possible in this group of patients, especially if the prolonged ICU stay results from pulmonary complications rather than severe heart failure or neurological dysfunction.[45]

NON-CARDIAC SURGERY

Non-cardiac surgery poses a significant risk to the patient with cardiac disease.[46,47] Postoperative cardiac complications result in significantly increased immediate and late mortality. Simple preoperative assessment enables risk stratification which might lead to deferment or cancellation of non-essential surgery. Indications for specific investigations and treatments are probably not different in the preoperative patient. However, this might be the first time that a cardiac assessment has been undertaken and hence significant cardiac pathology identified. Risk factors are summarised in Table 22.4. Cumulative factors are more than additive. Patients undergoing vascular procedures have a high risk of associated coronary artery disease and should be carefully assessed preoperatively. Perioperative risk can be modified by anaesthetic technique and by optimal medical (or surgical) management of heart disease, which might include myocardial revascularisation.[46]

Table 22.4 Risk factors for cardiac patients undergoing non-cardiac surgery

- High-risk surgery (abdominal, thoracic, major vascular)
- History of ischaemic heart disease
- History of congestive heart failure
- History of cerebrovascular disease
- Treatment with insulin
- Renal impairment

High risk: three or more factors.

The principles of postoperative management are the same as those outlined for the cardiac surgical patient. The period of risk for cardiac complications extends for some days after surgery and close monitoring to identify and manage events during this time is desirable in high-risk patients. The immediate perioperative period poses risks associated with anaesthesia, bleeding, fluid and electrolyte imbalance, haemodynamic instability and temperature abnormalities. These can be effectively managed. Early reinstitution of protective treatment (aspirin, beta-blockers, ACE inhibition, statins, antihypertensive therapy) may protect against later complications.

REFERENCES

1. Raper RF, Cameron G, Walker D *et al.* Type B lactic acidosis following cardiopulmonary bypass. *Crit Care Med* 1997; **25**: 46–51.
2. Shah MR, Hasselbad V, Stevenson LW *et al.* Impact of the pulmonary artery catheter in critically ill patients. Maeta-analysis of randomized clinical trials. *JAMA* 2005; **294**: 1664–70.
3. Leibowitz AB, Beilin T. Pulmonary artery catheters and outcome in the perioperative period. *N Horiz* 1997; **5**: 214–22.
4. Taylor RW. Controversies in pulmonary artery catheterization. *N Horiz* 1997; **5**: 173–296.
5. Finfer S, Bellomo R, Boyce N *et al.* A comparison of albumin and saline for fluid resuscitation in the intensive care unit. *N Engl J Med* 2004; **350**: 2247–56.
6. Fremes C, Weisel RD, Mickle DAG *et al.* A comparison of nitroglycerine and nitroprusside: 1. Treatment of postoperative hypertension. *Ann Thorac Surg* 1985; **39**: 53–60.
7. Fremes C, Weisel RD, Baird RJ *et al.* Effects of postoperative hypertension and its treatment. *J Thorac Cardiovasc Surg* 1983; **86**: 47–56.
8. Polonen P, Ruokonen E, Hippelainen M *et al.* A prospective randomized study of goal-oriented haemodynamic therapy in cardiac surgical patients. *Anesth Analg* 2000; **90**: 1052–9.
9. Price S, Prout J, Gibson DG *et al.* 'Tamponade' following cardiac surgery: terminology and echocardiography may both mislead. *Eur J Cardiothporacic Surg* 2004; **26**: 1156–60.

10. Totaro RJ, Raper RF. Epinephrine-induced lactic acidosis following cardiopulmonary bypass. *Crit Care Med* 1997; **25**: 1693–9.
11. Raja SG, Raven BS. Levosimendan in cardiac surgery: curent best available evidence. *Ann Thorac Surg* 2006; **81**: 1536–46.
12. Morales DLS, Mehmet CO. Mechanical circulatory assist devices in critical care management. *N Horiz* 1999; **7**: 489–503.
13. Samuels LE, Kaufman MS, Thomas MP *et al.* Pharmacological criteria for ventricular assist device insertion following postcardiotomy shock: experience with the Abiomed BVS system. *J Card Surg* 1999; **14**: 288–93.
14. Furnary AP, Magovern JA, Simpson KA *et al.* Prolonged open sternotomy and delayed sternal closure after cardiac operations. *Ann Thorac Surg* 1992; **54**: 233–9.
15. Dietl CA, Berkheimer MD, Woods EL *et al.* Efficacy and cost effectiveness of preoperative IABP in patients with ejection fraction of 0.25 or less. *Ann Thorac Surg* 1996; **62**: 401–9.
16. Christenson JT, Simonet F, Badel P *et al.* Optimal timing of preoperative intraaortic balloon support in high-risk coronary patients. *Ann Thorac Surg* 1999; **68**: 934–9.
17. Ohman EM, George BS, White CJ *et al.* Coronary heart disease/myocardial infarction/peripheral vascular disease: use of aortic counterpulsation to improve sustained coronary artery patency during acute myocardial infarction: results of a randomised trial. *Circulation* 1994; **90**: 792–9.
18. Yazigi A, Richa F, Gebara S *et al.* Prognostic importance of automated ST-segment monitoring after coronary artery bypass graft surgery. *Acta Anaesth Scand* 1998; **42**: 532–5.
19. Raper RF, Sibbald WJ. Misled by the wedge? The Swan Ganz catheter and left ventricular preload. *Chest* 1986; **89**: 427–34.
20. Bharucha DB, Kowey PR. Management and prevention of atrial fibrillation after cardiovascular surgery. *Am J Cardiol* 2000; **85**: 24D–4D.
21. Ommen SR, Odell JA, Stanton MS. Current concepts: atrial arrhythmias after cardiothoracic surgery. *N Engl J Med* 1997; **336**: 1429–34.
22. Scherer M, Therapidis P, Miskovic A *et al.* Left atrial size reduction improves the sinus rhythm conversion rate after radiofrequency ablation for continuous atrial fibrillation in patients undergoing concomitant cardiac surgery. *Thorac Cardiovasc Surg* 2006; **54**: 34–8.
23. Crystal E, Garfinkle MS, Connolly SS *et al.* Interventions for preventing post-operative atrial fibrillation in patients undergoing heart surgery. *Cochrane Database Systenaic Rev* 2004; **4**: CD003611.
24. Argenziano M, Choudhri AF, Moazami N *et al.* Randomized, double-blind trial of inhaled nitric oxide in LVAD recipients with pulmonary hypertension. *Ann Thorac Surg* 1998; **65**: 340–5.
25. Trachte AL, Lobato EB, Urdaneta F *et al.* Oral sildenafil reduces pulmonary hypertension after cardiac surgery. *Ann Thorac Surg* 2005; **79**: 194–7.
26. Birdi I, Chaudhuri N, Lenthall K *et al.* Emergency reinstitution of cardiopulmonary bypass following cardiac surgery: outcome justifies the cost. *Eur J Cardiothorac Surg* 2000; **17**: 743–6.
27. Raman J, Saldanha RF, Branch J *et al.* Open cardiac compression in the postoperative cardiac intensive care unit. *Anaesth Intens Care* 1989; **17**: 129–35.
28. Montes FR, Sanchez SI, Giraldo JC *et al.* The lack of benefit of tracheal extubation in the operating room after coronary artery bypass surgery. *Anesth Analg* 2000; **91**: 776–80.
29. Hickey RF, Cason BA. Timing of tracheal extubation in adult cardiac surgery patients. *J Cardiac Surg* 1995; **10**: 340–8.
30. Rady MY, Ryan T. Perioperative predictors of extubation failure and the effect on clinical outcome after cardiac surgery. *Crit Care Med* 1999; **27**: 340–7.
31. McDonald SB, Jacobshn E, Kopacz DJ *et al.* Parasternal block and local anaesthetic infiltration with levobupivocaine after cardiac surgery with desflurane: the efect on postoperative pain, pulmonary function, and tracheal extubation times. *Anesth Analg* 2005; **100**: 25–32.
32. Nussmeier NA, Whelton AA, Brown MT *et al.* Complications of the COX-2 inhibitors parecoxib and valdecoxib after cardiac surgery. *N Engl J Med* 2005; **352**: 1133–5.
33. Shammas NW. Pulmonary embolus after coronary artery bypass surgery: a review of the literature. *Clin Cardiol* 2000; **23**: 637–44.
34. Mariani MA, Gu J, Boonstra PW *et al.* Procoagulant activity after off-pump coronary operation: is the current antocoagulation adequate? *Ann Thorac Surg* 1999; **67**: 1370–5.
35. Mangano DT, Tudor IC, Dietzel C. The risk associated with aprotinin in cardiac surgery. *N Engl J Med* 2006; **354**: 353–65.
36. Levi M, Cromheecke ME, deJonge E *et al.* Pharmacological strategies to decrease excessive blood loss in cardiac surgery: a meta-analysis of clinically relevant endpoints. *Lancet* 1999; **354**: 1940–7.
37. Aravot DJ, Barak J, Vidne BA. Induction of controlled tamponade in the management of massive unexplained postcardiotomy bleeding. Case report and review of the literature. *J Cardiovasc Surg* 1986; **27**: 613–17.
38. Bracey AW, Radovancevic P, Riggs SA *et al.* Lowering the haemoglobin threshold for transfusion in coronary artery bypass procedures: effect on patient outcome. *Transfusion* 1999; **39**: 1070–7.
39. Mangano CM, Diamondstone LS, Ramsay J *et al.* Renal dysfunction after myocardial revascularization: risk factors, adverse outcomes, and hospital resource utilization. *Ann Intern Med* 1998; **128**: 194–203.
40. Ascione R, Lloyd CT, Underwood MJ *et al.* On-pump versus off-pump coronary revascularization: evaluation of renal function. *Ann Thorac Surg* 2000; **68**: 493–8.
41. Furnary AP, Zerr KJ, Grunkemeier GL *et al.* Continuous intravenous insulin infusion reduces the incidence of deep sternal wound infection in diabetic patients

after cardiac surgical procedures. *Ann Thorac Surg* 1999; **67**: 352–60.
42. Segers P, Speekenbrink RGH, Ubbink DT *et al.* Prevention of nosocomial infection in cardiac surgery by decontamination of the nasopharynx and oropharynx with chlorhexidine gluconate. A randomized controlled trial. *JAMA* 2006; **296**: 2460–6.
43. Das SK, Brow TD, Pepper J. Continuing controversy in the management of concomitant coronary and carotid disease: an overview. *Int J Cardiol* 2000; **74**: 47–65.
44. Raja SG, Haider Z, Ahmad M. Predictors of gastrointestinal complications after conventional and beating heart coronary surgery. *Surgeon* 2003; **1**: 221–8.
45. Wahl GW, Swinburne AJ, Fedullo AJ *et al.* Long-term outcome when major complications follow coronary artery bypass graft surgery. *Chest* 1996; **110**: 1394–8.
46. Eagle KA, Charanjit S, Mickel MC *et al.* Cardiac risk of noncardiac surgery: influence of coronary disease and type of surgery in 3368 operations. *Circulation* 1997; **96**: 1882–7.
47. Lee TH, Marcantonio ER, Mangione CM *et al.* Derivation and prospective validation of a simple index for prediction of cardiac risk of major noncardiac surgery. *Circulation* 1999; **100**: 1043–9.

23

Echocardiography in intensive care

Karl D Donovan and Frances B Colreavy

Echocardiography refers to a group of interrelated ultrasound applications used to examine the heart and great vessels. The reflected and processed sonic waves are displayed on a monitor and the images can be stored on videotape or disk. Echocardiography includes: (1) two-dimensional (2-D) anatomical imaging; (2) M-mode echocardiography, usually obtained with 2-D guidance; and (3) Doppler techniques. Echocardiography is a safe non-invasive technique which is integral to clinical cardiology. More recently, echocardiography has evolved into a powerful diagnostic and management tool in critically ill patients, especially in cardiovascular emergencies of uncertain cause.[1,2]

Cardiologists, although highly skilled in echocardiography, may not appreciate the complex pathophysiology of critically ill patients in intensive care, and they have time commitments elsewhere. Echocardiography is operator-dependent; optimal image acquisition requires both technical knowledge of the machine's capabilities as well as a degree of manual dexterity. As a general rule, echocardiography is not an efficient technique for monitoring haemodynamic indices over the medium term (hours–days) in the intensive care unit (ICU). Echocardiography can help determine whether and when continuous haemodynamic monitoring should be commenced.[3] Repetitive trend measurements, such as stroke volume, cardiac output and pulmonary artery wedge pressure, are more suited to the pulmonary artery catheter. Moreover, intensive care staff are skilled and experienced in its use. Echocardiography technicians are not present in ICU, especially out of hours; intensivists must be able to act as their own sonographers as well as interpreting and reporting on the echographic images obtained. It is important that intensivists acquire all requisite skills so that echocardiography becomes more widely available.

PRINCIPLES AND TECHNICAL CONSIDERATIONS[4]

Echocardiography uses the reflection of sound waves at tissue boundaries to construct a 2-D image of cardiac structures. The human ear hears only sound waves with a frequency between 20 Hz and 20 kHz; higher frequencies are referred to as ultrasound. Echocardiography uses sound in the frequency 1–10 MHz. A piezo electrical crystal generates and receives the ultrasound waves.

2-D ECHOCARDIOGRAPHY

2-D echocardiography is the cornerstone of cardiac ultrasound as Doppler and M-mode are usually performed with reference to the 2-D image. Each 2-D image is defined by the position of the transducer (acoustic window) and image plane which is determined by the axis of the heart and not the spine (Table 23.1).

M-MODE ECHOCARDIOGRAPHY

Rapidly repeated transmit and receive cycles allow production of images with good resolution. M-mode echocardiography complements 2-D echocardiography. The beam is not scanned but stays in a fixed position, allowing the display of structures along the beam as a function of time. The rapid sampling rate makes identification of thin moving structures, such as valve leaflets, relatively easy. The cursor is usually directed through a 2-D image, giving a one-dimensional slice or 'icepick' view. Distance (depth) is on the vertical and time is on the horizontal axis (Figure 23.1).

DOPPLER ECHOCARDIOGRAPHY[4,5]

Doppler echocardiography is vital for obtaining haemodynamic information and is an integral part of every echocardiographic study.

The *Doppler effect* is based on changes in sound frequency that occur when a sound source moves towards or away from an observer. One classic example is that of an ambulance siren; as it comes toward a listener, the sound frequency increases (higher pitch) and after the ambulance moves away from the observer the sound frequency decreases (lower pitch).

The *Doppler shift* is the difference between frequencies that are transmitted and received by a transducer after striking red blood cells.

The *Doppler equation* is the mathematical relationship between the Doppler shift and the velocity of red blood cells that produce it.

$$V = C \times \Delta f / 2f_t \times \cos\theta$$

where V = velocity of blood flow, C = speed of sound in soft tissue (1540 m/s), Δf = Doppler (frequency) shift:

Table 23.1 Some standard views in transthoracic and transoesophageal echocardiography

Acoustic window	Image plane
Transthoracic	
Parasternal	Long axis
	Short axis
Apical	Four-chamber
	Two-chamber
	Long axis
Subcostal	Multiple
Transoesophageal*	
Transgastric	e.g. Short axis
	Long axis
Deep transgastric	e.g. Long axis/five-chamber
Lower transoesophageal	e.g. Four-chamber
	Two-chamber
	Long axis
Upper transoesophageal	e.g. Short axis of aortic valve
	Long axis of aortic valve
	Right ventricular inflow–outflow

*Multiple image planes from 0° to 180°.

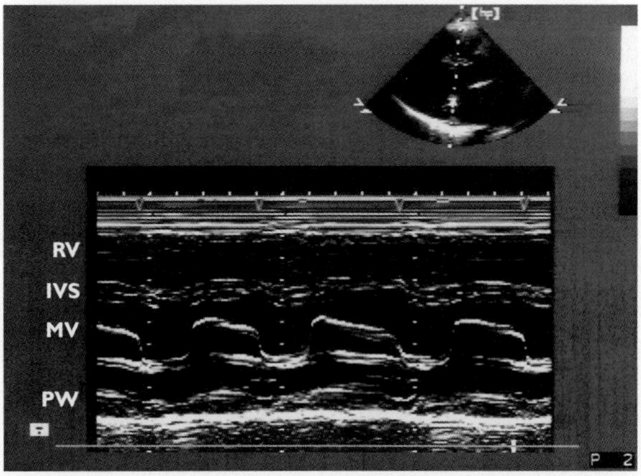

Figure 23.1 M-mode echocardiogram guided by M-mode cursor on the two-dimensional (2-D) image (see top). The transducer is anterior with the cursor directed through the right ventricle (RV), intraventricular septum (IVS), mitral valve (MV) and posterior wall (PW) of the left ventricle. The mitral valve leaflets are thickened and there is reduced diastolic slope of the anterior leaflet and the posterior leaflet moves anteriorly during diastole due to commissural fusion.

difference in frequency between received (f_r) and transmitted (f_t) ultrasound and θ = angle between ultrasound beam and direction of blood flow (Figure 23.2). Echocardiographic machines contain computers that automatically calculate the Doppler shift which is then entered into the Doppler equation. Blood flow velocity (m/s) is calculated and displayed on the monitor.

It is very important that the ultrasound beam is parallel or nearly parallel with the direction of blood flow. If

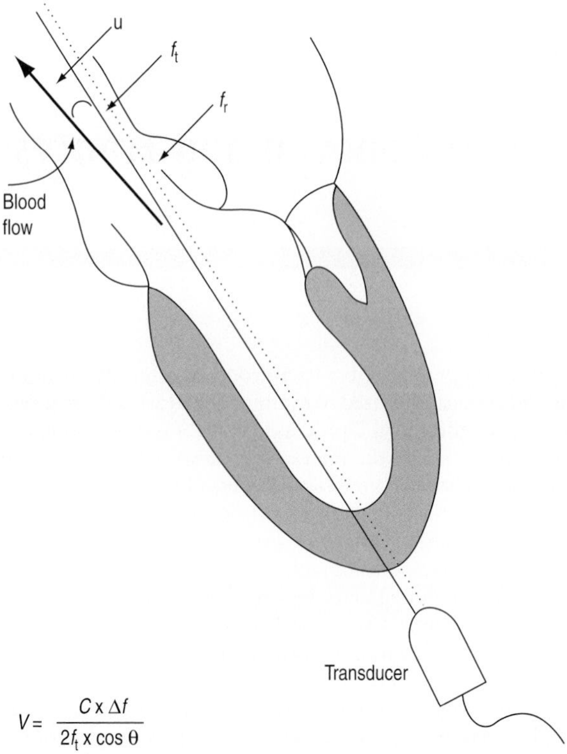

$$V = \frac{C \times \Delta f}{2f_t \times \cos\theta}$$

Figure 23.2 The Doppler equation.

θ equals 0 then cosign θ equals 1; however, if $\theta > 20°$ then the velocity of blood flow will be significantly underestimated. Doppler data are processed and a spectral display plots instantaneous blood velocities over time. Blood flow velocity can be expressed as peak velocity or mean velocity throughout a cardiac cycle (velocity–time integral: VTI) (Figure 23.3).

The most common uses of Doppler are pulsed-wave (PW), continuous-wave (CW) and colour-flow Doppler (CFD).

PULSED-WAVE DOPPLER

PW Doppler is usually performed with a duplex transducer (2-D and Doppler): a single ultrasound transducer transmits and receives ultrasound signals. Blood flow velocities of a small volume of blood, the sample volume, are obtained at a specific depth so it is useful for velocity measurements at specific sites such as the left ventricular outflow tract (LVOT). Due to technical limitations the maximum measurable velocity is usually < 2 m/s.

CONTINUOUS-WAVE DOPPLER

The transducer consists of two crystals: one continuously transmits and the other continuously receives ultrasound waves. It can measure high-velocity blood flow, such as occurs in aortic stenosis. Unlike PW Doppler, CW

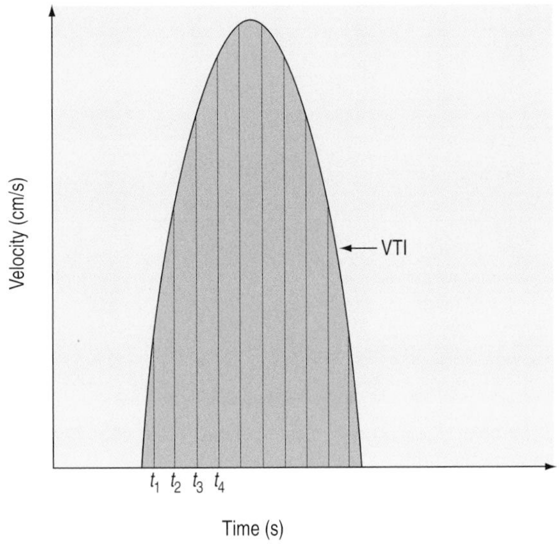

Figure 23.3 Velocity–time integral (VTI: cm/s) = area under the velocity curve: sum of velocities (cm/s) during the ejection time (s); t_1 = time one, t_2 = time two, etc.

Doppler measures all the frequency shifts along the beam path and it is not possible to estimate the velocity at a specific site (range ambiguity).

Blood flow velocities measured by either PW or CW Doppler can be converted to pressure gradients using the simplified Bernoulli equation, $\Delta P = 4V^2$ (where ΔP is the instantaneous pressure gradient and V is the instantaneous velocity), to provide estimates of pressure.

COLOUR-FLOW DOPPLER

This is based on PW Doppler principles. Multiple sample volumes are recorded with blood flow velocities encoded in colour (flow towards the probe is coloured red, away blue) and superimposed on 2-D images. Thus, CFD information displayed includes: (1) direction of blood flow; (2) timing of CFD signals; (3) a crude estimation of blood flow velocity; and (4) laminar flow can be differentiated from turbulent flow.

THREE-DIMENSIONAL

Three-dimensional (3-D) echocardiography is an evolving technique. Current equipment provides 'real-time' 3-D images (Figure 23.4a). The acquisition of a complete volume data set typically requires four sequential cardiac cycles. This 3-D data set must then be viewed and analysed. The full 3-D volume can then be 'cropped' so that the interior is exposed (Figure 23.4b). The 3-D volume set can be 'opened' in any imaging plane, providing both long- and short-axis views of cardiac structures. The 3-D volumetric probe can also be used for simultaneous acquisition of true real-time biplane (Figure 23.5a) and triplane (Figure 23.5b) images.

SAFETY

Ultrasound at the power levels used clinically to image cardiac structures has no known adverse biologic effects. Transoesophageal echocardiography (TOE) in trained, experienced hands is a well-developed and safe procedure. Nevertheless, TOE is semi-invasive and serious complications and even deaths have occurred. TOE is contraindicated in the presence of oesophageal stricture or neoplasm. Caution should be exercised in other situations such as previous oesophageal surgery or total gastrectomy. TOE should be deferred in patients with any symptoms of dysphagia until the cause has been found. Oesophageal varices, severe coagulopathy and significant cervical spine abnormalities are relative contraindications to TOE. Routine antibiotic prophylaxis does not appear to be necessary before TOE in intensive care patients.

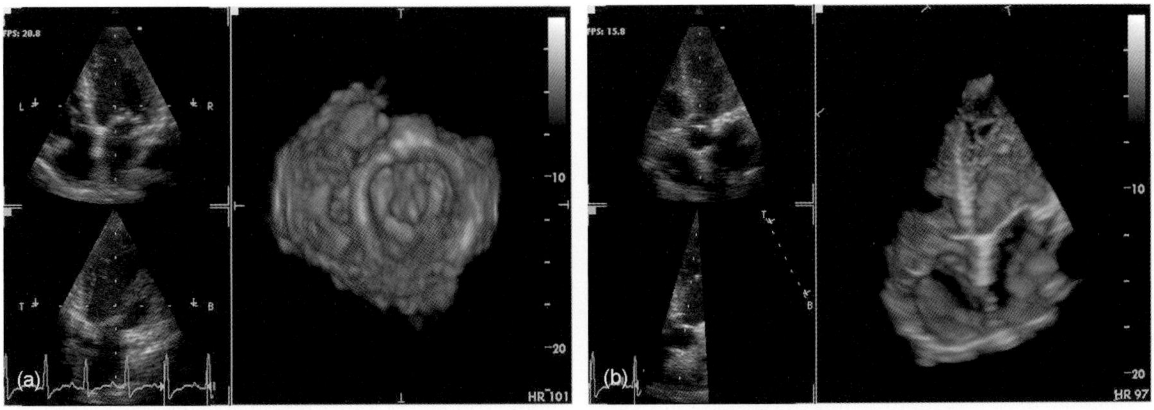

Figure 23.4 (a) Real-time volumetric scan (four cardiac cycles) merged into three-dimensional (3-D) volume data set. This large 3-D volume is not identifiable as a cardiac structure. (b) The full 3-D volume has been 'cropped', revealing the interior right ventricle, tricuspid valve, right atrium, left ventricle, mitral valve and left atrium.

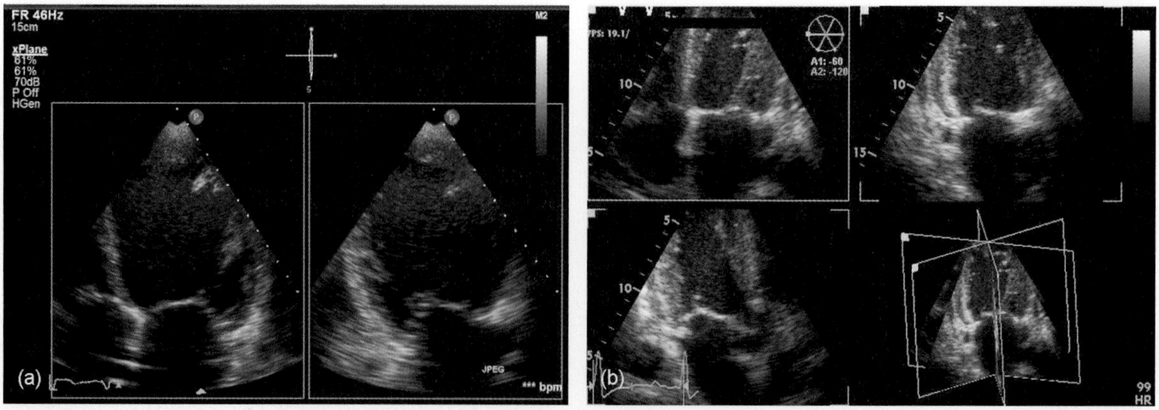

Figure 23.5 (a) True real-time biplane (apical four-chamber and two-chamber views), and (b) triplane (apical four-chamber, two-chamber and apical long-axis views). Note: images obtained without moving the probe.

TRANSTHORACIC (TTE) AND TRANSOESOPHAGEAL ECHOCARDIOGRAPHY

TTE and TOE are complementary ultrasound techniques, each with its own strengths and weakness (Table 23.2). For example, a vegetation imaged on the mitral valve of a septic patient will usually require a TOE to evaluate complications of endocarditis.

TRANSTHORACIC ECHOCARDIOGRAPHY

Recent technological advances such as harmonic imaging have greatly improved transthoracic surface imaging. TTE images may be inadequate in some critically ill patients, especially in intubated mechanically ventilated patients, or patients with chronic lung disease, obesity, chest trauma or surgical wounds. Inability to position such patients appropriately is a further limiting factor.

TRANSOESOPHAGEAL ECHOCARDIOGRAPHY[6,7]

The transducer is mounted at the tip of a flexible gastroscope-like probe which can be manoeuvred to various positions in the oesophagus and stomach close to the heart (Figure 23.6).

The modern multiplane probes allow rotation of the ultrasound scanning plane from 0 to 180°, which provides a mirror-image orientation. Multiple tomographic imaging planes can be obtained without the necessity for further probe manipulation. Compared to TTE, TOE provides additional information in 32–100% of intensive care examinations and unexpected new diagnoses in 38–59%, leading to significant changes in treatment.[8] Approximately 20% of patients with unexplained hypotension require surgery on the basis of new TOE findings.[9,10]

INDICATIONS FOR ECHOCARDIOGRAPHY[11,12]

The indications for echocardiography broadly fall into three categories:

1. morphologic diagnosis of specific cardiac/great-vessel pathology (usually guided by clinical suspicion)
2. haemodynamic assessment and monitoring of cardiac function
3. others, such as evaluation of patients with atrial fibrillation for the presence of left atrial (LA) clot prior to cardioversion

Guidelines for the use of echocardiography are based on expert consensus and observational studies. There are no randomised trials that specifically test the impact of echocardiography on outcome. In intensive care practice, echocardiography is used to evaluate clinical syndromes that suggest a diagnosis or, more often, a number of possible diagnoses. For example, haemodynamic instability in a patient with major blunt chest trauma suggests cardiac contusion or pericardial effusion causing tamponade. Nevertheless, the echocardiographic examination might reveal hypovolaemia with hyperdynamic LV systolic function or valvular damage with severe regurgitation.

Some common syndromes in which echocardiography is especially useful are listed in Table 23.3.

As a general rule, unless there is gross haemodynamic instability or some other overriding reason, the echocardiographic examination should be structured around a basic set of 2-D views. This applies to both TTE and TOE. The focus of the TOE examination should be on the most important specific clinical question. The second priority should be other potential pathology in the differential diagnosis. A printed report should be performed after each echocardiographic examination and should be stored and available for future reference.[13]

Table 23.2 Transthoracic echocardiography (TTE) and transoesophageal echocardiography (TOE): advantages and disadvantages

	TTE	TOE	Comments
Echocardiographic windows	'Unlimited'	'Limited'	
Time lag to diagnosis	(virtually) Instantaneous	Short (min)	
Contraindications	None	Occasional	e.g. oesophageal stricture
Invasive	No	Minimal	
Morbidity	No	Minimal	Low but measurable complication rate with TOE
Mortality	No	Minimal	TOE mortality about 1/10 000
Image quality			
Non-ventilated	Good/excellent	Excellent (usually)	TTE: poor images postop cardiac surgery, chronic airways limitation, obese, etc.
Ventilated	Poor to excellent	Excellent (usually)	
Specific pathology			
Endocarditis			
Native valve	Useful if low index of suspicion	Sensitive and specific	TOE essential for diagnosis of complications, e.g. abscess, etc.
Prosthetic valve	Useful in conjunction with TOE	Essential	
Aortic dissection	?	Essential	TTE occasionally useful for diagnosis. Acute regurgitation can also be assessed
Aortic trauma	±	Essential	
Left atrial appendage clot	No	Essential	
Left ventricle clot	Yes	Yes	TTE more useful than TOE to image LV apical clot
Pericardial effusion	Yes	Yes	TTE essential for guiding needle pericardiocentesis
Localised tamponade (post cardiac surgery)	Occasionally useful	(Usually) essential	TOE especially useful for posterior collections

LV, left ventricular.

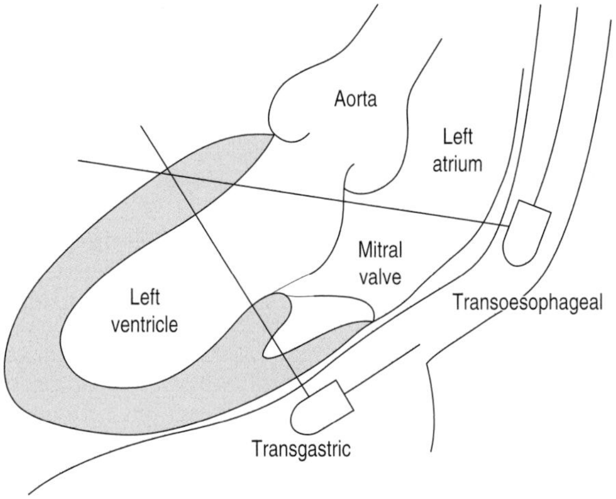

Figure 23.6 Transducer position in transoesophageal echocardiography.

VALVULAR HEART DISEASE[14,15]

Echocardiography is the 'gold standard' for evaluating valvular heart disease. 2-D echocardiography provides excellent imaging of all cardiac valves. Various Doppler techniques allow accurate haemodynamic evaluation of the valves.

VALVULAR STENOSIS

Narrowing or stenosis of any heart valve obstructs blood flow, increasing velocity and causing a pressure gradient across the valve. Evaluation of valvular stenosis requires: (1) imaging of the valve to define the morphology and mobility of the valve cusps; (2) some quantification of the degree of stenosis; and (3) the effect of pressure overload on relevant cardiac chambers. Transvalvular pressure gradients (ΔP) can be estimated by Doppler techniques (see above). Note that in conditions of low cardiac output, pressure gradients will be low, thereby underestimating the severity of stenosis.

Aortic stenosis

The most common aetiology of valvular aortic stenosis is degeneration and calcification of the valve apparatus, although bicuspid aortic valve and rheumatic heart disease may also cause aortic stenosis. Thickening/calcification of relatively immobile valve leaflets causes valvular obstruction and pressure overload, resulting in LV hypertrophy. Severe aortic stenosis may occasionally cause sudden collapse, cardiogenic shock or pulmonary oedema of unknown cause.

Assessment of severity Visual assessment of aortic valve cusp thickness, calcification, mobility and degree of LV hypertrophy will often indicate the physiological significance of the aortic stenosis. Doppler echocardiography

Table 23.3 Indications for echocardiography in the intensive care unit according to clinical syndrome

Clinical syndrome	Findings	Comments
Hypotension		
Acute myocardial infarct		
No murmur	LV RWMA(s)	Usually severe ↓ LV systolic function
	RV RWMA	RV ↓ > LV ↓
	Hypovolaemia	'Empty' LV cavity, systolic function largely preserved
	Acute MR	Often no murmur with normal LA size
New murmur	Papillary muscle rupture (partial or complete)	'Good' LV function with severe MR
	VSD	RWMA. High-velocity left-to-right systolic jet
Rarely	Cardiac rupture/tamponade	Acute pericardial tamponade, usually fatal
	LV pseudoaneurysm	Containment of rupture
Cardiothoracic surgery	Cardiac tamponade	Often localised. There may be no 'echo-free space' due to clot compressing the heart. Cardiac filling pressures may be normal
	(New) RWMA	May be due to graft occlusion, air embolism
	Hypovolaemia	'Empty' LV with RWMA
	Global LV ↓	Stunning or long-standing cardiomyopathy
	Valvular dysfunction	Often long-standing but may be worsened by surgery, e.g. ischaemia to a papillary muscle of mitral valve
Dynamic LVOT obstruction	LVOT pressure gradient, SAM, MR	Inotropes/IABP/hypovolaemia worsen LVOT obstruction
Trauma	Hypovolaemia	'Empty' LV with vigorous contraction
	Cardiac contusion	RWMA (RV > LV)
	Valvular injury	Most common aortic valve (AR) or mitral valve (MR), occasionally tricuspid valve (TR)
	VSD/ASD	Occasionally
	Cardiac tamponade	More common in penetrating chest injuries
	Ruptured thoracic aorta	Widened mediastinum (90%) at isthmus of aorta. TOE required
Sepsis	Often normal LV systolic function with 'empty' LV	Possible global/regional LV depression
	Infective endocarditis – vegetations/abscess/regurgitation	TOE more sensitive than TTE for imaging vegetations/abscess/fistula
'Isolated' hypotension ('hypotension ?cause')	Global LV ↓ or RWMA	Cardiomyopathy or stunning
	Valvular dysfunction	Usually chronic, occasionally acute (e.g. ruptured papillary muscle of mitral valve)
	Dynamic LVOT obstruction	
	Acute cor pulmonale	Pulmonary embolism – usually dilated right heart with depressed systolic function, sometimes with clot in a proximal pulmonary artery
Sepsis (source?)	Vegetations, regurgitation ± abscess	Infective endocarditis until proven otherwise
	Normal TOE examination	Infective endocarditis unlikely. If clinically indicated serial TOE
Systemic emboli (source?)	LA/LAA clot	Usually enlarged LA and atrial fibrillation TOE usually required for diagnosis
	LV clot	Usually associated with RWMA or global LV depression. TTE for apical clot
	Aortic atherosclerotic	TOE essential for diagnosis plaques
	Vegetations – aortic or abscess	Septic?
	Clot – prosthetic aortic or mitral valve	Associated prosthetic valve dysfunction
	Patent foramen ovale with paradoxical embolism	RA pressure > LA pressure (e.g. IPPV with high PEEP). TOE (bubble contrast) usually necessary for diagnosis
	Tumour (e.g. LA myxoma)	Uncommon

Table 23.3 Indications for echocardiography in the intensive care unit according to clinical syndrome—*Continued*

Clinical syndrome	Findings	Comments
Pulmonary oedema (cause?)	↓ LV systolic/diastolic function	Isolated LV diastolic dysfunction not uncommon
	Valvular dysfunction (MR, MS, AR, AS)	If flail leaflet/ruptured papillary muscle suspected then TOE indicated
	Intracardiac shunt	
	Normal	Suggests non-cardiac cause (e.g. ARDS)
Dyspnoea/hypoxia without pulmonary oedema (dyspnoea cause?)	Pulmonary embolism (dilated right heart chambers ± clot in pulmonary artery)	Infers moderate to large clot burden i.e. submassive/massive PE
	Cardiac tamponade	Usually other clinical signs of tamponade present
	Miscellaneous e.g. chronic cor pulmonale, RVH, constrictive pericarditis, diastolic dysfunction, intracardiac shunt, RV volume overload	
Chest pain of uncertain aetiology (chest pain cause?)	RWMA	Infers presence of coronary artery disease
	Dissecting aortic aneurysm (intimal flap, true/false lumen)	TOE more sensitive than TTE
	PE (dilated right heart chambers ± clot in pulmonary artery)	Moderate to large embolus
	Pericarditis	Effusion often too small to diagnose with echocardiography
	Aortic stenosis	Clinical signs of stenosis may be absent

AR, aortic regurgitation; ARDS, acute respiratory distress syndrome; AS, aortic stenosis; ASD, atrial septal defect; IABP, intra-aortic balloon pump; IPPV, intermittent positive-pressure ventilation; LA, left atrium; LAA, left atrial appendage; LV, left ventricle; LVOT, left ventricular outflow tract; MR, mitral regurgitation; MS, mitral stenosis; PE, pulmonary embolism. PEEP, positive end-expiratory pressure; RA, right atrium; RV, right ventricle; RVH, right ventricular haemorrhage; RWMA, regional wall motion abnormality; SAM, systolic anterior motion; TOE, transoesophageal echocardiography; TR, tricuspid regurgitation; VSD, ventricular septal defect.

is essential for assessment of severity: (1) peak aortic velocity; (2) mean transvalvular pressure gradient; (3) aortic valve area; and (4) ratio of LVOT velocity/aortic valve velocity (V_1/V_2).

- *Peak aortic velocity* (normal = 1.7 m/s) (Figure 23.7). In the presence of thickened immobile aortic valve cusps, a peak velocity = 4.5 m/s (i.e. peak pressure gradient 81 mmHg) almost certainly indicates severe stenosis.

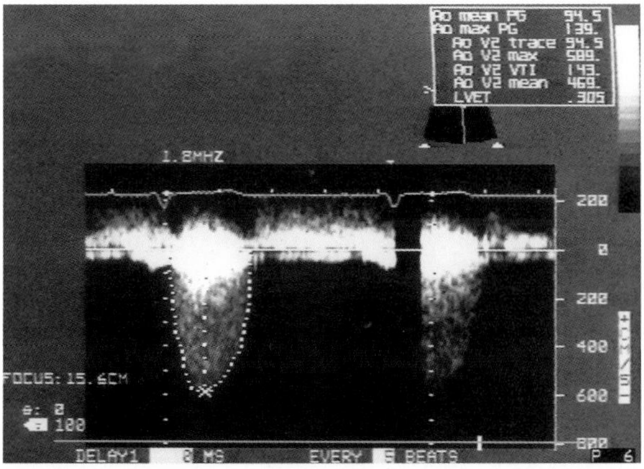

Figure 23.7 Continuous-wave Doppler recording of an aortic stenosis jet in a patient with critical stenosis. The jet velocity is 589 cm/s (5.89 m/s). The calculated maximum pressure gradient is 139 mmHg. Mean pressure gradient is 94 mmHg.

- *Mean transvalvular pressure gradient.* Aortic valve velocity integrated over time is displayed on the monitor and the spectral display traced. A mean pressure gradient of 50 mmHg suggests severe aortic stenosis. From a practical point of view, a patient with normal LV systolic function, a peak aortic velocity gradient of 3.0 m/s and a mean pressure gradient of 30 mmHg is extremely unlikely to have critical aortic stenosis, whereas a patient with thickened aortic leaflets, restricted movement of cusps, aortic velocity > 4.5 m/s and a mean pressure gradient = 50 mmHg will almost certainly have critical aortic stenosis. Difficulties in assessment of aortic stenosis severity arise in patients with depressed LV function and a peak aortic velocity not greatly increased, typically about 3.0–3.5 m/s, and a transvalvular gradient of 25–30 mmHg. Such patients may have mild to moderate aortic stenosis and unrelated LV dysfunction or critical aortic stenosis with severe depression of LV function; dobutamine stress echocardiography is a useful test to distinguish one condition from another.
- *Aortic valve area* (normal 3–4 cm^2). In severe aortic stenosis the aortic valve area is 0.75 cm^2. The aortic valve area is estimated using the continuity equation, which is based on the principle that, if the volume of blood flow upstream from an orifice is known, then measuring the velocity of blood immediately downstream from the orifice allows calculation of its cross-sectional area. According to the formula: $A_1 \times V_1 = A_2 \times V_2$, where A_1 = LVOT cross-sectional area,

V_1 = LVOT VTI, A_2 = aortic valve cross-sectional area, V_2 = aortic VTI. The equation can be rearranged: $A_2 = A_1 \times V_1/V_2$.

- *Ratio of LVOT velocity/aortic valve velocity* (V_1/V_2) provides a 'dimensionless' measurement of aortic stenosis severity which is independent of cardiac output. A velocity ratio (V_1/V_2) of < 0.25 implies an aortic valve area of 0.75 cm^2 (i.e. severe aortic stenosis).

Accurate estimation of maximum aortic jet velocity is best obtained by TTE. However, TOE allows planimetry (tracing) of the aortic valve orifice in the short-axis view which correlates well with catheter-derived aortic valve area.[16] TOE planimetry may be useful in critically ill patients when other data are inconsistent or inconclusive.

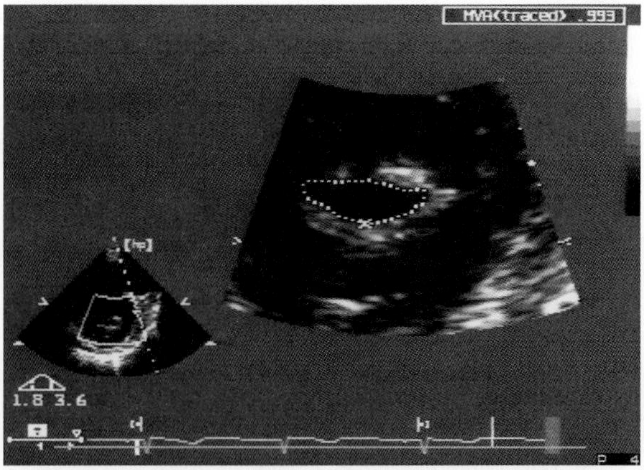

Figure 23.9 Two-dimensional (2-D) echocardiogram of a patient with mitral stenosis. There is diminished separation between the anterior and posterior leaflets, with a typical 'fish-mouth' appearance. The valve area by 2-D planimetry is 0.99 cm^2 (transthoracic echocardiography parasternal short axis).

Mitral stenosis

Significant mitral stenosis can occasionally contribute to haemodynamic instability in critically ill patients. Dyspnoea has usually been present for many years, so that mitral stenosis has been diagnosed prior to admission to intensive care. Mitral stenosis secondary to rheumatic heart disease produces typical M-mode (see Figure 23.1) and 2-D images of thickened and fused mitral valve leaflets with diastolic doming, resulting in a 'hockeystick' appearance of the anterior leaflet, together with an enlarged LA (Figure 23.8). In the short-axis view the mitral valve appears as a 'fish mouth' orifice, the area of which can be estimated (normal 4–6 cm^2) (Figure 23.9) using planimetry.

Assessment of severity In addition to visualisation and planimetry of the valve, accurate assessment of mitral valve stenosis requires Doppler echocardiography: (1) peak velocity (E) across the mitral valve is increased (normal = 1.3 m/s). In severe mitral stenosis, the E velocity is usually > 2 m/s; (2) transvalvular pressure gradient: the mean pressure gradient between the LA and LV is usually > 10 mmHg in severe stenosis; (3) pressure half-time (P_t ½) is the time it takes for the peak pressure gradient to halve. The rate of pressure decline across a stenotic orifice is determined by its cross-sectional area (i.e. the smaller the orifice, the slower the rate of decline). Pressure half-time > 220 ms indicates severe mitral stenosis (mitral valve area = 1 cm^2)[17] (Figure 23.10). Pulmonary artery pressure should also be estimated (see below).

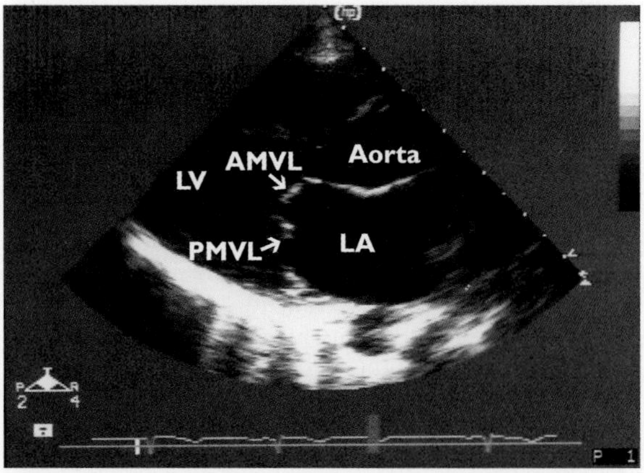

Figure 23.8 Two-dimensional (2-D) echocardiogram of a patient with mitral stenosis. The left atrium (LA) is enlarged. There is doming of both anterior (AMVL) and posterior (PMVL) leaflets with the typical 'hockeystick' appearance of the anterior leaflet (transthoracic echocardiography parasternal long axis). LV, left ventricle.

Tricuspid stenosis and pulmonary stenosis

These disorders can also be diagnosed and quantified using similar echocardiographic techniques.

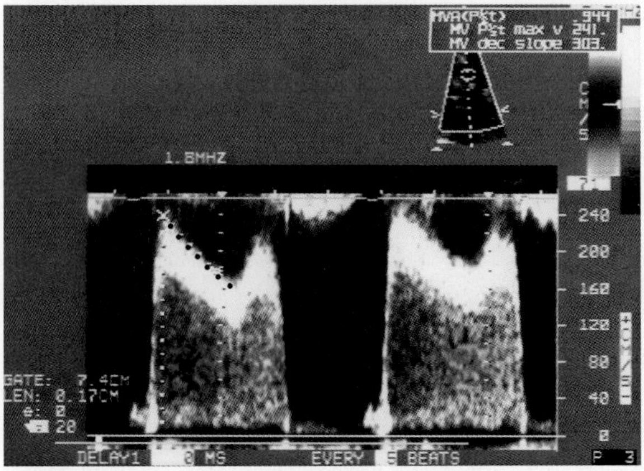

Figure 23.10 Pressure half-time ($Pt_{½}$) measurement in a patient with mitral stenosis. The $Pt_{½}$ corresponds to a valve area of 0.94 cm^2.

VALVULAR REGURGITATION

Evaluation of valvular regurgitation requires: (1) assessment of the valve morphology; (2) estimation of severity of regurgitation; and (3) effects of volume overload on relevant cardiac chambers. Mild valvular regurgitation of the mitral, tricuspid and pulmonary valves is common (70–90%) and such findings have no clinical significance. Trivial aortic regurgitation is found in only about 5% of examinations.

Aortic regurgitation

2-D echocardiography may show the cause of the aortic regurgitation, for example, valve destruction caused by infective endocarditis or a dilated aortic root with aortic dissection or, most commonly, degenerative calcification disease of aortic valve.

Assessment of severity[18] CFD imaging allows some grading of severity of regurgitation by comparing the width of the regurgitant jet to the LVOT area (Figure 23.11). If the jet occupies more than 60% of the LVOT area, then severe aortic regurgitation is probably present.

The velocity of the regurgitant jet is directly related to the pressure gradient between the aortic valve and the left ventricle. In severe aortic regurgitation, especially acute, aortic diastolic pressure falls rapidly and LV end-diastolic pressure increases, resulting in a rapid decay of the pressure gradient: an aortic regurgitant pressure half-time (250 m/s) suggests severe regurgitation. Flow reversal downstream during diastole in the descending aorta indicates severe aortic regurgitation.

Mitral regurgitation As with aortic regurgitation, echocardiography is useful in detecting the aetiology and mechanism of mitral regurgitation, such as annular dilation (poor coaptation of leaflets), endocarditis (leaflet destruction/perforation) and chordal or papillary muscle rupture (inadequate leaflet support). In mitral regurgitation, the left ventricle ejects blood both into the aorta and backwards into the LA. Early in the course of mitral regurgitation the increase in stroke volume is achieved by an increase in LV ejection fraction (EF). Thus, a hyperdynamic normal-sized left ventricle with normal-sized LA implies acute mitral regurgitation. Over time mitral regurgitation causes enlargement of the LA and eventually the left ventricle dilates and LV function becomes less hyperdynamic. This apparent normalisation of LV function suggests impaired contractility and increased LA pressure. Pulmonary artery pressure also increases over time.

Assessment of severity[18] Severity of mitral regurgitation is assessed by CFD imaging of the regurgitant jet. The severity of mitral regurgitation is directly proportional to the size of the regurgitant jet within the LA (Figure 23.12). Mitral valve colour flow jet reaching the posterior wall of the LA suggests severe mitral regurgitation, as does systolic flow reversal in the pulmonary veins. Colour flow mapping of the narrowest cross-sectional area of a regurgitant jet (vena contracta) can estimate the severity of the mitral regurgitation[19] and this can be done in < 1 min.[20] Combining 2-D imaging with spectral Doppler imaging can be used to quantify valvular regurgitation by measuring regurgitant volume (volume of blood that leaks through an incompetent valve) and regurgitant fraction (fraction or percentage of stroke volume that regurgitates).

Another approach for estimating the regurgitant volume is to examine the flow pattern on the LV side of the mitral valve. Proximal isovelocity surface area (PISA): PISA calculations, regurgitant volumes and fractions can be estimated.

Tricuspid regurgitation and pulmonary regurgitation

These disorders can be diagnosed and evaluated using similar principles; for example, severe tricuspid regurgitation causes systolic flow reversal in the hepatic veins.

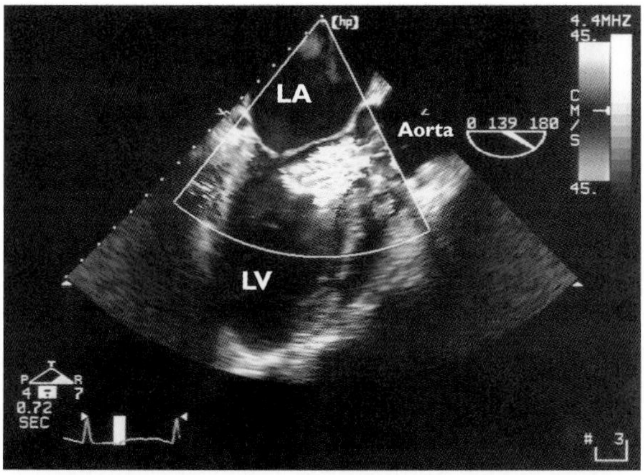

Figure 23.11 Severe aortic regurgitation; aliased jet occupies entire left ventricular (LV) outflow tract (transoesophageal echocardiography long axis). LA, left atrial.

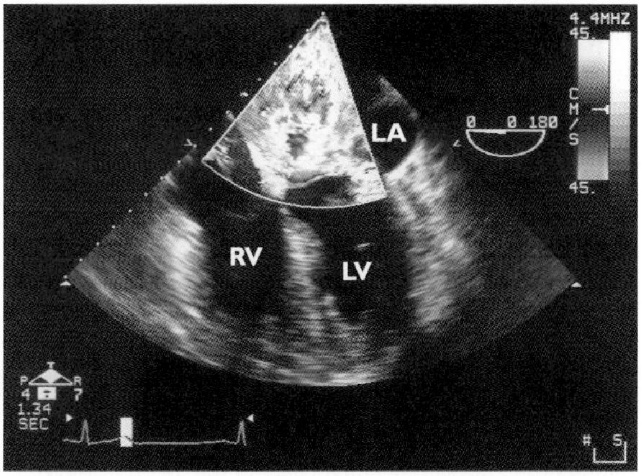

Figure 23.12 Severe mitral regurgitation secondary to flail posterior mitral valve leaflet (transoesophageal echocardiography four-chamber).

INFECTIVE ENDOCARDITIS

Infective endocarditis should be suspected in any critically ill patient with sepsis and no obvious source of infection. The echocardiographic hallmark of endocarditis is the presence of vegetation(s) which appear as an echogenic chaotically moving mass attached to a heart valve (Figure 23.13). The Duke criteria[21–23] integrate clinical, microbiological and echocardiographic information in suspected infective endocarditis. Echocardiographic findings consistent with vegetation or new endocardial infection (abscess, prosthetic valve dehiscence, etc.) are major diagnostic criteria. In some situations, clot, tumour or marantic vegetation may mimic endocarditis. In a patient with endocarditis, echocardiography will: (1) image the vegetation and assess its size; (2) diagnose complications such as paravalvular abscess and fistula; (3) examine underlying valve morphology (e.g. bicuspid aortic valve); (4) diagnose and assess severity of associated valvular regurgitation; (5) assess cardiac function; and (6) image other heart valves. Large vegetations (> 10 mm) increase the risk of embolic events.[24] Despite advances in imaging, TTE is still insensitive compared to TOE[25] for detection of native valve vegetations and fails to demonstrate about 50% of them. TOE accuracy is much better, with a sensitivity and specificity of about 90%. In one study the negative predictive value was 86%.[26] TTE may be adequate to exclude vegetations in patients when clinical suspicion for endocarditis is low[27] provided that image quality is adequate.

About 25% of patients with *Staphylococcus aureus* septicaemia have infective endocarditis, even in the absence of obvious clinical signs.[28] TOE is essential for the diagnosis and detection of associated complications.

PROSTHETIC VALVES

Echocardiographic examination of prosthetic valves requires knowledge of the various types of valves (bioprosthesis, homograft, mechanical). Blood velocity is nearly always increased through normal prosthetic valves and trivial regurgitation is characteristic of most mechanical valves. Such jets are always small, may be multiple and occur within the sewing ring of the valve. Paravalvular leaks are always abnormal and associated with dehiscence; infective endocarditis should always be considered. Suspected prosthetic valve endocarditis mandates TOE and serial examinations are often necessary. A characteristic rocking motion of the valve is diagnostic of dehiscence. TOE is superior to TTE for assessing mitral regurgitation in patients with prosthetic mitral valves, as acoustic shadowing by the mechanical valve of the LA causes poor imaging. In most instances, adequate echocardiographic assessment of prosthetic valves requires combined transthoracic and transoesophageal imaging.

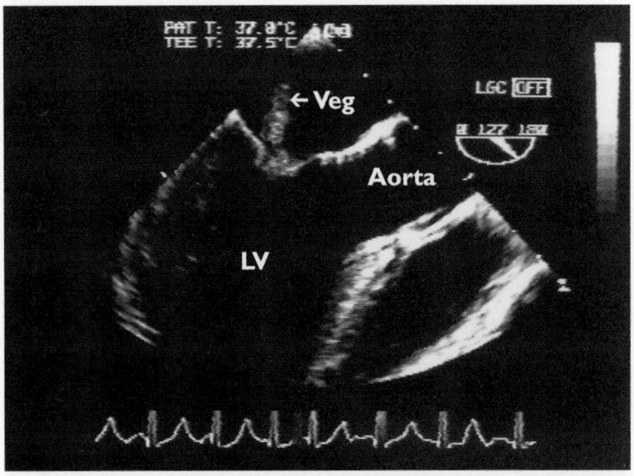

Figure 23.13 Large vegetation (Veg) on the anterior mitral valve leaflet. The patient presented with septic shock and 'meningitis' and no obvious cardiac murmur (transoesophageal echocardiography long axis). LV, left ventricle.

VENTRICULAR FUNCTION AND HAEMODYNAMIC ASSESSMENT

In critically ill patients, echocardiography, especially TOE, has evolved as an independent approach in the assessment and monitoring of cardiovascular haemodynamics. Cardiac systolic function is directly visualised and other parameters can be measured.

LEFT VENTRICLE

2-D and M-mode echocardiography allow accurate measurements of LV dimensions and wall thickness.

Systolic function

Echocardiography provides global and regional estimates of LV performance.

Global LV function

In intensive care patients, the two parameters most frequently used to assess LV global systolic function are EF and cardiac output.

Ejection fraction

The EF is the percentage of the LV diastolic volume that is ejected with each heart beat (normal EF > 50%). It should be appreciated that EF is the result of complex interactions between ventricular loading conditions and contractile state, and may not always reflect true ventricular contractility. Nevertheless, EF is extremely useful and can be estimated using various techniques:

1. Visual inspection of 2-D images. Although widely used, this method is subjective.
2. The American Society of Echocardiography recommends the modified Simpson's rule, where LV volumes are measured in two orthogonal views (apical four-chamber and apical two-chamber) (Figure 23.14a–d). The LV endocardial border is traced at end-diastole and end-systole. The ventricle is considered to be a series of discs which are summated. Calculation of LV end-diastolic and end-systolic volumes, although complicated, is easily computed using modern echocardiographic machines.

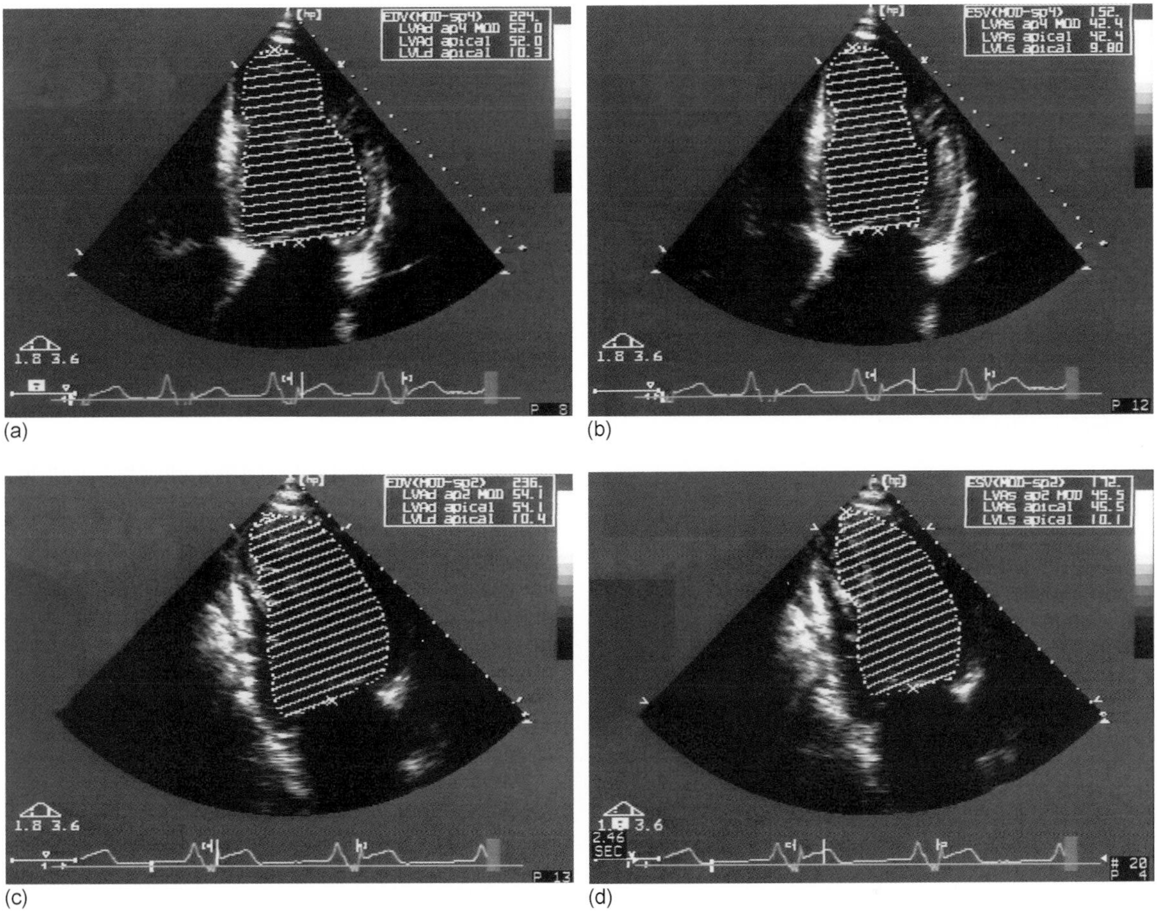

Figure 23.14 Left ventricular (LV) ejection fraction estimation using modified Simpson's rule. The long axis of the LV is divided into a series of discs from base to apex; the LV endocardial border is traced in end-diastole (LVED) and end-systole (LVES) in two orthogonal views: apical (a) LVED, (b) LVES; four-chamber (c) LVED, (d) LVES two-chamber.

$$EF = \frac{EDV - ESV}{EDV} \times 100$$

where EDV = LV end-diastolic volume and ESV = LV end-systolic volume.

Real-time 3-D echocardiography is more accurate than 2-D techniques for the quantification of LV volumes.[29]

Regional left ventricular function[30]

Assessment of LV regional wall motion analysis is based on grading the contractility of individual segments: 1 = normal or hyperkinesis; 2 = hypokinesis; 3 = akinesis; 4 = dyskinesis (paradoxical systolic motion); 5 = aneurysmal. The American Society of Echocardiography divides the LV into 16 segments (six at the base, six at the mid ventricular level and four at the apex) (Figure 23.15).

Real-time 3D echocardiographic imaging is more sensitive than 2-D techniques for the detection of regional LV wall motion abnormalities.[29]

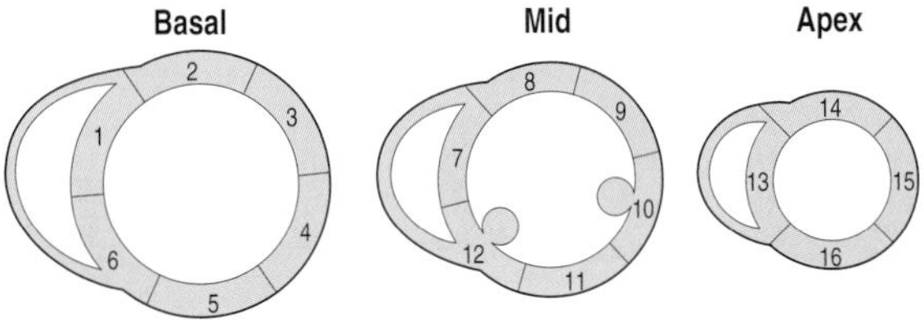

Segment level	AS	Ant	Lat	Post	Inf	Sep
Basal	1	2	3	4	5	6
Mid	7	8	9	10	11	12
Apex	13	14	15	-	16	13

Figure 23.15 Regional wall motion analysis.
AS, Anteroseptum; Ant, anterior; Lat, lateral; post, posterior; Inf, inferior; Sep, septum.

Stroke volume and cardiac output

Doppler-derived blood flow velocities can be used to quantify cardiac output. The technique is based on the principle that the VTI of blood flow multiplied by the cross-sectional area (CSA) of its orifice yields an estimate of stroke volume ($SV = CSA \times VTI$) (Figure 23.16a, b). The LVOT is the most commonly used site for stroke volume and cardiac output estimation. In general, correlations between echocardiographic and thermodilution-derived cardiac output have been reasonable, although neither method is a 'gold standard'.

Real-time 3-D is more accurate than 2-D echocardiography for measurement of LV volumes. Studies comparing 3-D echocardiographic LV volumes with magnetic resonance imaging (MRI) confirm the accuracy of 3-D echocardiography.[29]

Preload (left ventricular end-diastolic volume)

The assessment of LV end-diastolic volume (LVEDV) is often important in critically ill patients. Significant hypovolaemia is inferred by LV end-systolic cavity obliteration. Although a presumptive diagnosis of hypovolaemia can often be made with such echo signs, other causes of end-systolic cavity obliteration, such as decreased systemic vascular resistance, severe mitral or aortic regurgitation, or ventricular septal defect, must be considered. Integrating the clinical picture together with CFD and, if necessary, quantitative assessment of preload, differentiates between the various diagnoses.

Modified Simpson's rule technique is the most accurate echocardiographic method for measuring LVEDV/preload in clinical practice (Figure 23.14a, c).

Afterload

End-systolic wall stress (where wall stress = (pressure $\times$ radius)/2 $\times$ wall thickness), determined by echocardiography, provides an index of LV afterload. This is rarely used in clinical practice.

Diastolic function[31]

The non-invasive assessment of LV diastolic dysfunction has seen major advances in recent years. Diastolic dysfunction is a disorder of LV filling, where the LV is unable to fill to a normal LVEDV without an abnormal increase in end-diastolic pressure. All patients with LV systolic dysfunction have some degree of LV diastolic dysfunction. Some patients with congestive cardiac failure have normal or near-normal LV systolic function with isolated diastolic heart failure. Gandhi *et al.*,[32] using echocardiography, demonstrated that pulmonary oedema in patients with marked systemic hypertension is commonly due to isolated diastolic dysfunction. Mitral and pulmonary inflow patterns are Doppler techniques routinely used to diagnose diastolic dysfunction and assess severity.

E/E^1 ratio. Early diastolic blood flow from LA to LV results in an E-wave. Doppler tissue imaging recordings from the lateral (or medial) mitral annulus during early diastole result in an E^1. E^1 is a good index of LV relaxation. The E/E^1 ratio correlates well with LV filling pressures. An E/E^1 ratio > 15 is associated with LA pressures > 15 mmHg, whereas an $E/E^1 < 8$ is highly specific for normal LA pressure.[31]

RIGHT VENTRICLE (RV)

Evaluation of right-sided heart function is important in critically ill patients.

Chamber size

The normal shape of the RV is a crescent, curving in front of, and concave towards, the LV. A combination of image planes is necessary to assess RV size. Ventricular dilation may be due to right-sided volume overload secondary to conditions such as tricuspid regurgitation, pulmonary regurgitation or atrial septal defect. CFD and occasionally intravenous injection of a contrast agent such as agitated saline will help distinguish the aetiology.

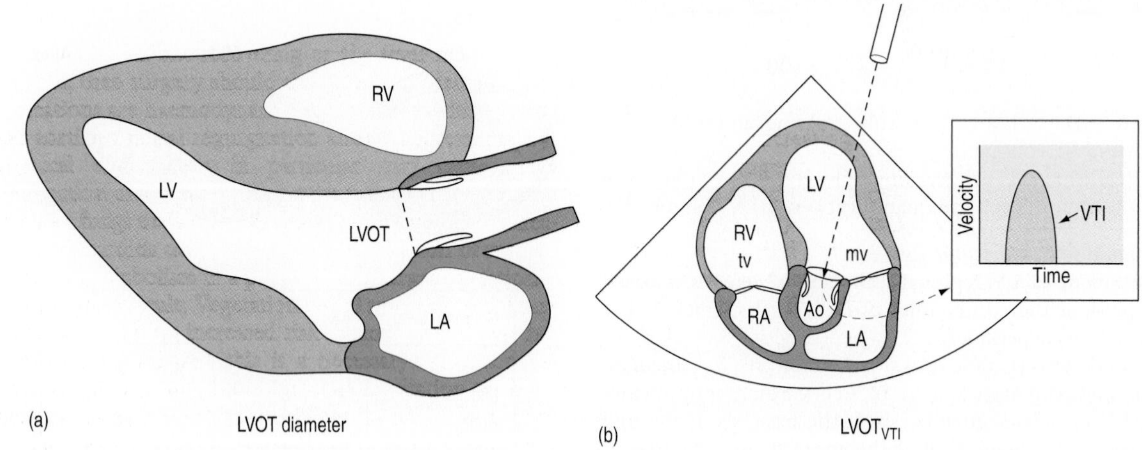

Figure 23.16 Calculation of stroke volume (SV) using the left ventricular outflow tract (LVOT). (a) LVOT diameter ($LVOT_d$) is measured from parasternal long axis view. $LVOT_{CSA} = 0.785 \times (LVOT_d)^2$, where $LVOT_{CSA}$ is the LVOT cross-sectional area. (b) $LVOT_{VTI}$ measured using pulsed-wave Doppler (apical five-chamber or long-axis view), where $LVOT_{VTI}$ is the velocity–time integral. $SV = LVOT_{CSA} \times LVOT_{VTI}$.

Wall thickness

RV hypertrophy (due to pressure overload) leads to increased thickness of the RV free wall.

Systolic function. Right ventricular end-diastolic volume assessment is difficult because the shape of the RV and the presence of prominent trabeculations make the endocardial border difficult to outline. TOE is essential for assessing RV dysfunction following cardiac transplantation.

Detection of regional wall motion abnormalities is a sensitive and specific marker of RV ischaemia or infarction.[33] The diagnosis of cardiac contusion, which occurs commonly after blunt chest trauma, is often unrecognised and can be readily made by TOE.[34]

Pulmonary artery pressure

This is an important and routine part of assessing RV function. Some tricuspid regurgitation is present in > 90% of the adult population. The simplified Bernoulli equation is used: RV systolic pressure is obtained by adding right atrial pressure (RAP) to the transtricuspid gradient derived from the peak tricuspid regurgitation velocity (V_{tr}) measured by Doppler (Figure 23.17). In the absence of pulmonary stenosis, systolic RV pressure = systolic PA pressure.

CARDIOMYOPATHIES

A simple classification of the cardiomyopathies includes: (1) dilated; (2) hypertrophic; and (3) restrictive.

DILATED CARDIOMYOPATHY

All echocardiographic features of dilated cardiomyopathy are non-specific, but LV dilation and reduced global systolic function are characteristic. Both LV end-diastolic and LV end-systolic volumes are increased, with EF and fractional area of change uniformly reduced. Mural thrombus may be present. The RV may also be affected. There may be atrial enlargement. Due to the increased LVEDV, stroke volume and cardiac output may be preserved at rest. Significant mitral regurgitation, secondary to annular dilation and poor coaptation of the mitral leaflets, may be present. Diastolic dysfunction is invariably present and is an important prognostic feature. Pulmonary hypertension estimated from tricuspid regurgitation velocity may predict a poor prognosis.

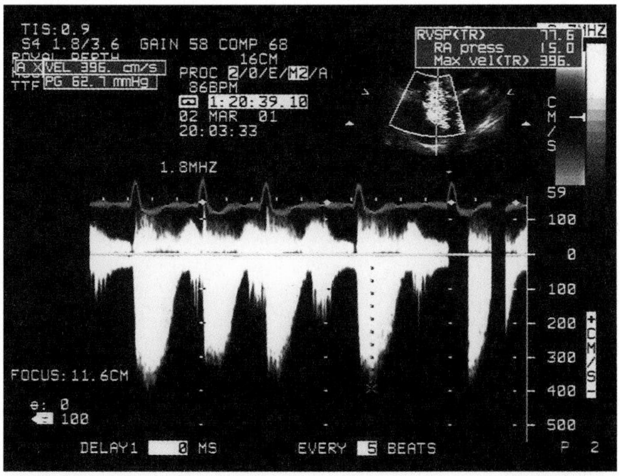

Figure 23.17 Estimation of right ventricular systolic pressure (RVSP) and systolic pulmonary artery pressure (SPAP) in the presence of tricuspid regurgitation (TR). Peak TR velocity (VTR) measured by continuous-wave Doppler is 396 cm/s (3.9 m/s). Right atrial pressure (from central venous pressure) = 15 mmHg. Difference in pressure between RA and RV (using Bernoulli equation) is $4 \times (V_{TR}^2)$ (i.e. $4 \times (3.9)^2 = 62$). Therefore RVSP = 15 + 62 = 77 mmHg. In the absence of pulmonary stenosis, RVSP = SPAP.

HYPERTROPHIC CARDIOMYOPATHY

In critically ill patients, the diagnosis cannot be made without the assistance of echocardiography, where asymmetrical septal hypertrophy, the most common feature, can be readily identified and quantified, as can a variety of other hypertrophic patterns. In the elderly, a normal proximal septal bulge ('sigmoid septum') should not be confused with true hypertrophic cardiomyopathy.

Ventricular outflow tract obstruction

During systole, the anterior leaflet of the mitral valve moves anteriorly toward the interventricular septum and may obstruct the LVOT. The LVOT obstruction is dependent on loading conditions and may be absent at rest. Indeed, the dynamic nature of the LVOT obstruction is one of the hallmarks of this condition. The systolic anterior motion (SAM) of the leaflet distorts the mitral valve, causing mitral regurgitation. CFD (and PW Doppler) not only localise the site of LVOT obstruction, but also quantify the degree of mitral regurgitation. The severity of LVOT obstruction can be estimated by CW Doppler. Although the degree of obstruction may vary, a peak gradient of 50 mmHg indicates significant LVOT obstruction.

Dynamic LVOT obstruction without asymmetrical septal hypertrophy[35]

Dynamic LVOT obstruction with SAM can occur whenever a hyperdynamic state exists, especially in elderly patients with hypovolaemia and a septal bulge ('sigmoid' septum). The haemodynamic effects of this condition are identical to the LVOT obstruction of hypertrophic cardiomyopathy and can cause cardiogenic shock. Dynamic LVOT obstruction may be precipitated or worsened by positive inotropic or vasodilator therapy and intra-aortic balloon pumping. In hypotensive patients, a paradoxical haemodynamic response to conventional inotropic therapy is an indication for TOE. The LVOT gradient can usually be abolished by ensuring adequate volume replacement, avoiding positive inotropic agents and increasing afterload by administration of an agent such as phenylephrine (a pure α-agonist).

RESTRICTIVE CARDIOMYOPATHY

Primary restrictive cardiomyopathy is characterised by impaired LV filling secondary to idiopathic myocardial stiffening. Echocardiographic findings usually include marked biatrial enlargement with normal LV cavity size and wall thickness and normal or slightly reduced systolic function. A characteristic restrictive mitral inflow pattern is present.

Secondary restrictive cardiomyopathy has a similar abnormal diastolic filling pattern secondary to a known myocardial cause (e.g. amyloidosis).

PERICARDIAL DISEASE

PERICARDIAL EFFUSION AND TAMPONADE

Echocardiography is the accepted gold standard for both the diagnosis of pericardial effusion and its haemodynamic significance. Pericardial fluid or blood can be recognised on 2-D as an 'echo-free' space around the heart (Figure 23.18). Whenever a pericardial effusion is imaged, the possibility of tamponade should be considered. When the effusion within the pericardial sac is large enough, intrapericardial pressure exceeds RV diastolic pressure and cardiac tamponade occurs, causing impaired cardiac filling and low cardiac output. 2-D echocardiographic features of cardiac tamponade may include:

1. Moderate to large pericardial effusion (usually). However, it should be appreciated that a small rapidly accumulating effusion (50–100 ml) can increase intrapericardial pressure acutely and tamponade the heart. Conversely, a large, slowly increasing effusion, sometimes over 1 l in volume, may have little effect on intrapericardial pressure and cause no haemodynamic embarrassment.
2. The heart may swing excessively in the pericardial sac. Electrocardiographically this may manifest as electrical alternans.
3. Early diastolic collapse of the RV free wall is more specific (85–100%) but less sensitive (60–90%) for cardiac tamponade than
4. Late diastolic atrial collapse. Sustained (30% of cardiac cycle) RA collapse is more likely to be significant than brief collapse.
5. Respiratory variation in diastolic filling is manifested clinically by pulsus paradoxus. Doppler echocardiography demonstrates a similar phenomenon, namely exaggerated increase in tricuspid and decrease in mitral valve diastolic inflow with inspiration. A tricuspid valve inflow variation > 25% and a mitral valve inflow variation > 15% with respiration is consistent with tamponade. The inferior vena cava is usually dilated and its diameter does not vary with respiration in patients with cardiac tamponade. Doppler examination of the hepatic veins is also very important.

Echocardiography may also be used to guide pericardiocentesis by locating the optimal site for puncture and monitoring the residual effusion after drainage.[36] As 2-D echocardiography is a tomographic imaging technique, the needle tip is often difficult to visualise.

CARDIAC TAMPONADE OCCURRING AFTER CARDIAC SURGERY

The tamponade may be localised with differential compression of the right- or left-sided chambers and the clot is usually 'echo-dense' with little or no 'echo-free' space around the heart (Figure 23.19). Localised tamponade (e.g. of the RA or LA) is not uncommon in such patients. Not surprisingly, standard echocardiographic criteria, such as intermittent chamber collapse, are unreliable in detecting tamponade after cardiac surgery. The presence of 1 cm of pericardial separation (fluid/clot) in a patient with unexplained clinical deterioration (hypotension, decreased cardiac output) appears to be sensitive in

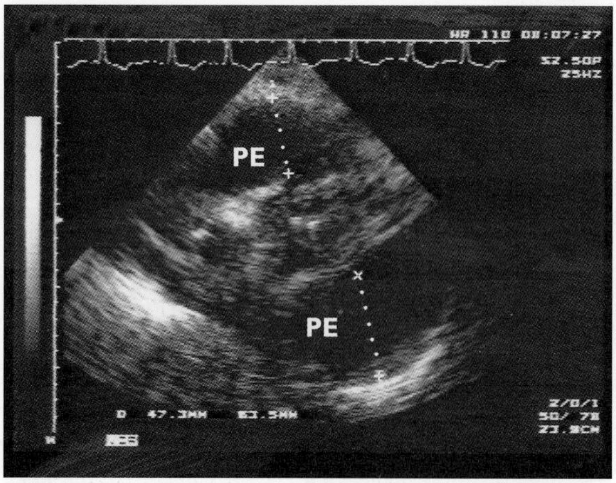

Figure 23.18 Massive (5 cm) pericardial effusion (PE) in a patient with tamponade (transthoracic echocardiography subcostal).

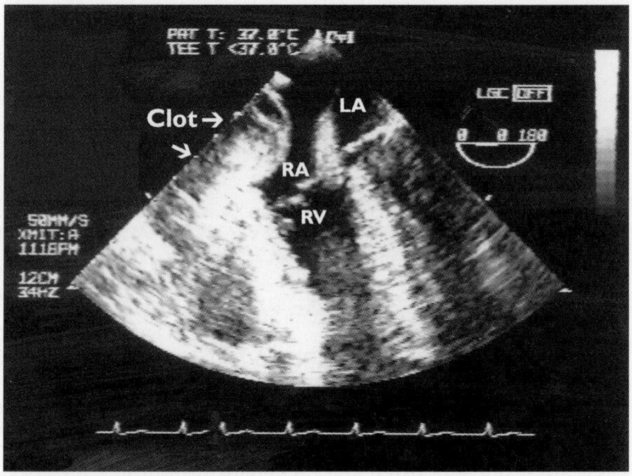

Figure 23.19 Localised clot compressing mainly the right heart in a patient after cardiac surgery (transoesophageal echocardiography four-chamber). LA, left atrium; RA, right atrium; RV, right ventricle.

detecting tamponade.[37] In the absence of tamponade, other causes of hypotension, such as unsuspected hypovolaemia, ventricular dysfunction or LVOT obstruction, may be diagnosed by echocardiography. Indeed, unnecessary reoperation may be prevented in some instances.

CONSTRICTIVE PERICARDITIS

Echocardiography is of value in the diagnosis of constrictive pericarditis. There is often thickening of the pericardium, which may be imaged with 2-D echocardiography. Doppler studies of the tricuspid, mitral and pulmonary veins may show typical findings.

CARDIAC MASSES

Before any diagnosis is made of a cardiac mass, it is essential to rule out pseudomasses (i.e. artefacts or normal cardiac structures). TOE is usually more sensitive than TTE. Intracardiac masses include thrombi, tumours and vegetations.

INTRACARDIAC THROMBUS

Thrombi can occur in any cardiac chamber but are most common in the LV (often at the apex) and the LA (usually in the LA appendage). Low-flow states manifest as spontaneous echocardiographic contrast or echocardiographic 'smoke' and are precursors of clot formation and thromboemboli. LV clot (Figure 23.20), when it occurs after myocardial infarction, is associated with the regional wall motion abnormality. Clot may also occur in patients with dilated cardiomyopathy and severe global depression of LV systolic function. TTE is more sensitive than TOE for detection of LV apical clot. LA clot is much more common than RA clot and usually occurs in the setting of atrial fibrillation or mitral stenosis. TOE provides vastly superior images compared to TTE as LA clot is usually located in or near the LA appendage, which is poorly visualised with TTE. Conventional management for patients with AF = 48 h requires therapeutic anticoagulation for 3 weeks before planned cardioversion. Another approach necessitates LA clot exclusion by TOE. If there is no LA clot, then cardioversion may proceed immediately, otherwise cardioversion is delayed. This TOE-based strategy has been shown to be associated with low embolic rates and a shorter time to cardioversion compared to conventional strategy, but no difference in outcome.[38]

CARDIAC TUMOURS

LA myxoma is by far the most common benign cardiac tumour and can often be imaged by TTE, although superb images can be obtained with TOE. The tumour is usually attached by a pedicle to the interatrial septum. During diastole, the tumour may obstruct the mitral valve orifice. Rarely, other tumours, primary or metastatic, may be visualised.

AORTIC DISEASE

TOE is paramount for diagnosing aortic pathology in critically ill patients because of its accuracy, portability, real-time imaging and low complication rate.

AORTIC DISSECTION[39]

TOE is very useful for diagnosing aortic dissection. The sensitivity and specificity of TOE in diagnosis of aortic dissection are equivalent to that of computed tomography (CT) or MRI.[40] 2-D echocardiography will reveal the intimal flap (Figure 23.21) which is the hallmark of aortic dissection. CFD is useful in differentiating true from false lumen: (1) the false lumen is usually larger with slower flow; (2) the intimal flap pulsates in systole towards the false lumen because of the higher pressure in the true lumen. The entry point of the tear and the presence and extent of aortic regurgitation can also be evaluated.

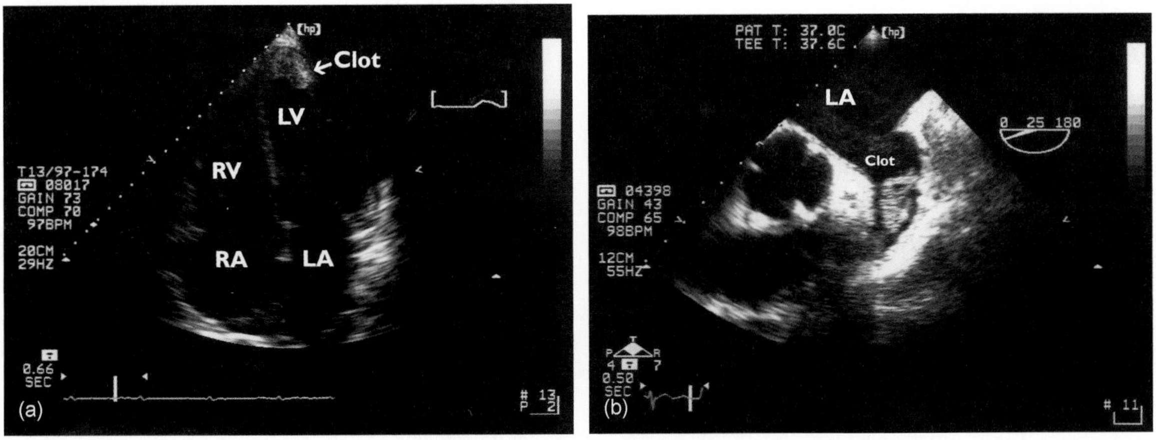

Figure 23.20 (a) Left ventricular (LV) apical clot. There was an associated regional wall motion abnormality (transthoracic echocardiography apical four-chamber). (b) Clot in left atrial appendage. RV, right ventricle; RA, right atrium; LA, left atrium.

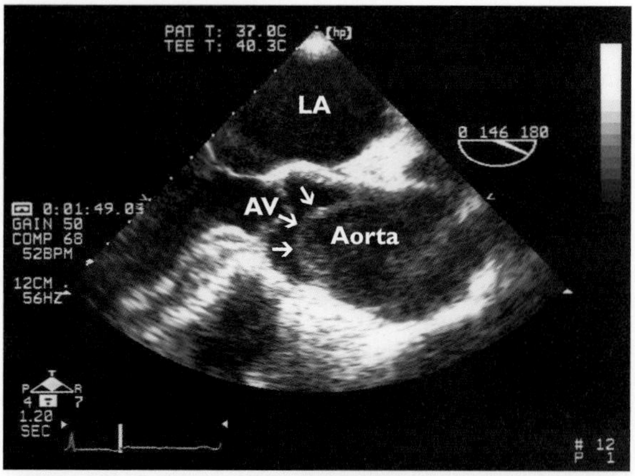

Figure 23.21 Aortic dissection involving the ascending aorta – the intimal flap (arrows) impinges on the aortic valve (AV) cusps during diastole (transoesophageal echocardiography). LA, left atrium.

INTRAMURAL HAEMATOMA (IMH)[41]

IMH represents a variant of aortic dissection with virtually identical clinical presentation. Indeed, it may be an early finding in patients who develop classical aortic dissection or rupture. IMH cannot be diagnosed by angiography as there is no intimal flap. 2-D echocardiography identifies IMH as a (> 0.7 cm) circular or crescentric thickening of the aortic wall or an echolucent zone in the aortic wall. There may be a thrombus-like echo pattern of the aortic wall.

TRAUMATIC AORTIC RUPTURE

TOE is both sensitive and specific for the diagnosis of aortic trauma.[42] The echocardiographic signs of aortic injury may include an intimal flap, aortic wall haematoma, aortic occlusion and fusiform aneurysm. Echocardiographic assessment for aortic injury requires an experienced operator.

AORTIC ATHEROSCLEROSIS

TOE allows imaging of aortic plaques which may be layered and immobile or pedunculated/sessile and liable to embolise systemically. On occasions, the aetiology of stroke, renal failure or peripheral vascular ischaemia in critically ill patients may become apparent after echocardiographic examination of the aorta.

PENETRATING ATHEROSCLEROTIC ULCER

This is an ulceration of an atherosclerotic lesion which penetrates the elastic lamina, resulting in haematoma within the media of the aortic wall. It usually occurs in the descending aorta but may also occasionally occur in the ascending aorta. Aortic pseudoaneurysms or occasionally aortic rupture may be due to progressive penetration of the ulcer. TOE is usually necessary for the diagnosis.

AORTIC ANEURYSM

Aneurysms of the aorta can easily be evaluated with echocardiography. Long-term follow-up of thoracic aneurysms without dissection usually utilises CT or MRI.

PULMONARY EMBOLISM

CT pulmonary angiogram is probably the preferred method for diagnosing pulmonary embolism. Nevertheless, echocardiography is useful to exclude massive or submassive pulmonary embolism in patients with unexplained hypotension. Pulmonary embolism causes acute obstruction of the pulmonary vasculature and haemodynamic compromise. Massive or submassive pulmonary embolism invariably causes acute cor pulmonale. The RV is acutely overloaded, causing distension and 'rounding' of the RV (RV to LV ratio > 0.6 in four-chamber view).[43] The RV hypokinesis is characteristic with sparing of the apex (McConnell's sign).[44] The interventricular septum bulges into the LV cavity, resulting in LV diastolic dysfunction. The LV cavity is usually small and appears 'undervolumed'. Significant RV hypertrophy is absent. Pulmonary hypertension is moderate and its severity can be estimated from the tricuspid regurgitant jet. Clot can also on occasions be directly imaged with TOE in the right heart cavity or proximal pulmonary arteries (Figure 23.22).

It should be appreciated that echocardiography is insensitive for the diagnosis of smaller pulmonary emboli where haemodynamic compromise is usually absent. Echocardiography is useful in assessing the severity of pulmonary embolism, e.g. if there are no signs of RV overload and systolic dysfunction in a patient with pulmonary embolism, then thrombolytics are not indicated.

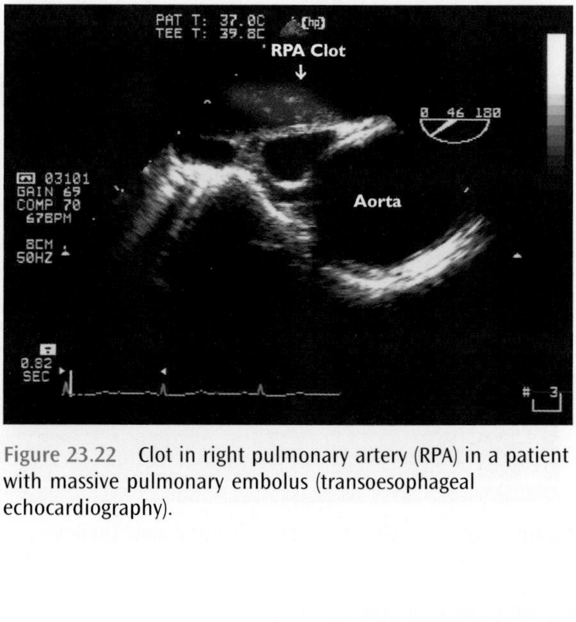

Figure 23.22 Clot in right pulmonary artery (RPA) in a patient with massive pulmonary embolus (transoesophageal echocardiography).

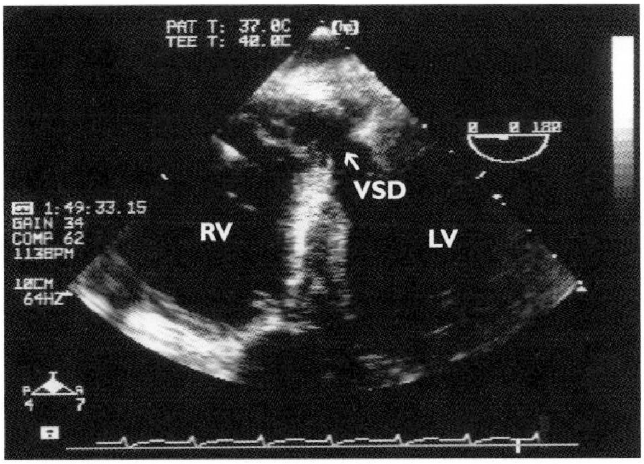

Figure 23.23 Large ventricular septal defect (VSD) in a shocked patient with a recent myocardial infarction (transoesophageal echocardiography deep gastric). RV, right ventricle; LV, left ventricle.

CONGENITAL HEART DISEASE

Echocardiography is essential for the evaluation of patients with known or suspected congenital heart disease. However, it is unusual for adult patients to present to intensive care with undiagnosed haemodynamically significant congenital heart disease. The transoesophageal approach is often necessary in critically ill adult patients with suspected congenital heart disease. Congenital heart abnormalities, such as patent foramen ovale, atrial septal defect, ventricular septal defect, patent ductus arteriosis and coarctation of the aorta, can be diagnosed.

Non-congenital ventricular septal defect (e.g. complicating acute myocardial infarction or trauma) is easily diagnosed using either TTE or TOE (Figure 23.23).

REFERENCES

1. Heidenreich PA. Transesophageal echocardiography (TEE) in the critical care patient. *Cardiol Clin* 2000; **18**: 789–805.
2. Colreavy F, Donovan KD, Lee KY *et al.* Transoesophageal echocardiography in critically ill patients. *Crit Care Med* 2002; **30**: 989–96.
3. Hilton AK. Echocardiography is the best cardiovascular "monitor" in septic shock. *Crit Care Resusc* 2006; **8**: 247–51.
4. Otto CM. Principles of echocardiographic image acquisition and Doppler analysis. In: Otto CM (ed.) *Textbook of Clinical Echocardiography.* Philadelphia: WB Saunders; 2000: 1–29.
5. Quinones MA, Otto CM, Stoddard M *et al.* Recommendations for quantification of Doppler echocardiography. A report from the Doppler Quantification Task Force of the Nomenclature and Standards Committee of the American Society of Echocardiography. *J Am Soc Echocardiogr* 2002; **15**: 167–84.
6. Shanewise JS, Cheung AT, Aronson S *et al.* ASE/SCA guidelines for performing a comprehensive intraoperative multiplane transesophageal echocardiography examination: recommendations of the American Society of Echocardiography Council for Intraoperative Echocardiography and the Society of Cardiovascular Anesthesiologists Task Force for Certification in Perioperative Transesophageal Echocardiography. *J Am Soc Echo-cardiogr* 1999; **12**: 884–900.
7. Flachskampf FA, Decoodt P, Fraser AG *et al.* Guidelines from the working group: recommendations for performing transoesophageal echocardiography. *Eur J Echocardiogr* 2001; **2**: 8–21.
8. Weiss Y, Pollak A, Gilon D. The application of transesophageal echocardiography in critical care medicine. *Curr Opin Crit Care* 1997; **3**: 232–7.
9. Heidenreich PA, Stainback RF, Redberg RF *et al.* Transesophageal echocardiography predicts mortality in critically ill patients with unexplained hypotension. *J Am Coll Cardiol* 1995; **26**: 152–8.
10. Oh JK, Seward JB, Khandheria BK *et al.* Transesophageal echocardiography in critically ill patients. *Am J Cardiol* 1990; **66**: 1492–5.
11. Cheitlin MD, Alpert JS, Armstrong WF *et al.* ACC/AHA guidelines for the clinical application of echocardiography. *Circulation* 1997; **95**: 1686–744.
12. Cheitlin MD, Armstrong WF, Aurigemma GP *et al.* ACC/AHA/ASE 2003 guideline update for the clinical application of echocardiography: summary article. A report of the American College of Cardiology/American Heart Association Task Force on Practice Guidelines (ACC/AHA/ASE Committee to Update the 1997 Guidelines on the Clinical Application of Echocardiography). *J Am Coll Cardiol* 2003; **42**: 954–70.
13. Gardin JM, Adams DB, Douglas PS *et al.* Recommendations for a standardized report for adult transthoracic echocardiography. A report from the American Society of Echocardiography's Nomenclature and Standards Committee and Task Force for a Standardized Echocardiography report. *J Am Soc Echocardiogr* 2002; **15**: 275–90.
14. Bonow RO, Carabello B, de Leon AC *et al.* ACC/AHA practice guidelines: guidelines for the management of patients with valvular heart disease. *Circulation* 1998; **98**: 1949–84.
15. Oh JK, Seward JB, Tajik AJ. Valvular heart disease. In: Oh JK, Seward JB, Tajik AJ (eds) *The Echo Manual.* Philadelphia: Lippincott Williams & Wilkins; 1999: 103–32.
16. Shively BK. Transesophageal echocardiographic (TEE) evaluation of the aortic valve, left ventricular outflow tract, and pulmonic valve. *Cardiol Clin* 2000; **18**: 711–29.
17. Hatle L, Angelsen B, Tromsdal A. Noninvasive assessment of atrioventricular pressure half-time by Doppler ultrasound. *Circulation* 1979; **60**: 1096–104.
18. Zoghbi WA, Enriquez-Sarano M, Foster E *et al.* Recommendations for evaluation of the severity of native valvular regurgitation with two-dimensional

and Doppler echocardiography. A report from the American Society of Echocardiography's Nomenclature and Standards Committee and the Task Force on Valvular Regurgitation, developed in conjunction with The American College of Cardiology Echocardiography Committee, The Cardiac Imaging Committee Council on Clinical Cardiology, The American Heart Association, and The European Society of Cardiology Working Group on Echocardiography. *J Am Soc Echocardiogr* 2003; **16**: 777–802.
19. Hall SA, Brickner E, Willett DL *et al.* Assessment of mitral regurgitation severity by Doppler color flow mapping of the vena contracta. *Circulation* 1997; **95**: 636–42.
20. Thomas JD. How leaky is that mitral valve? Simplified Doppler methods to measure regurgitant orifice area. *Circulation* 1997; **95**: 548–50.
21. Durack DT, Lukes AS, Bright DK. New criteria for diagnosis of infective endocarditis: utilization of specific echocardiographic findings. Duke Endocarditis Service. *Am J Med* 1994; **96**: 200–9.
22. Bayer AS, Ward JI, Ginzton LE *et al.* Evaluation of new clinical criteria for the diagnosis of infective endocarditis. *Am J Med* 1994; **96**: 211–19.
23. Li JS, Sexton DJ, Mick N *et al.* Proposed modifications to the Duke criteria for the diagnosis of infective endocarditis: utilisation of specific echocardiographic findings. Duke Endocarditis Service. *Clin Infect Dis* 2000; **30**: 633–8.
24. Tischler MD, Vaitkus PT. The ability of vegetation size on echocardiography to predict clinical complications: a meta-analysis. *J Am Soc Echocardiogr* 1997; **10**: 562–8.
25. Reynolds HR, Jagen MA, Tunick PA *et al.* Sensitivity of transthoracic versus transesophageal echocardiography for the detection of native valve vegetations in the modern era. *J Am Soc Echocardiogr* 2003; **16**: 67–70.
26. Sochowski RA, Chan KL. Implication of negative results on a monoplane transesophageal echocardiograhpic study in patients with suspected infective endocarditis. *J Am Coll Cardiol* 1993; **21**: 216–21.
27. Lindner JR, Case A, Dent JM *et al.* Diagnostic value of echocardiography in suspected endocarditis. An evaluation based on pretest probability of disease. *Circulation* 1996; **93**: 730–6.
28. Fowler VG, Li J, Corey R *et al.* Role of echocardiography in evaluation of patients with *Staphylococcus aureus* bacteremia: experience in 103 patients. *J Am Coll Cardiol* 1997; **30**: 1072–8.
29. Corsi C, Lang RM, Veronesi F *et al.* Volumetric quantification of global and regional left ventricular function from real-time three-dimensional echocardiographic images. *Circulation* 2005; **112**: 1161–70.
30. Cerqueira MD, Weissman NJ, Dilsizian V *et al.* Standardized myocardial segmentation and nomenclature for tomographic imaging of the heart. A statement for healthcare professionals from the Cardiac Imaging Committee of the Council on Clinical Cardiology of the American Heart Association. American Heart Association Writing Group on Myocardial Segmentation and Registration for Cardiac Imaging. *Circulation* 2002; **105**: 539–42.
31. Khouri SJ, Maly GT, Suh DD *et al.* A practical approach to the echocardiographic evaluation of diastolic function. *J Am Soc Echocardiogr* 2004; **17**: 290–7.
32. Gandhi SK, Powers JC, Nomeir A-M *et al.* The pathogenesis of acute pulmonary edema associated with hypertension. *N Engl J Med* 2001; **344**: 17–22.
33. Goldstein JA. Right heart ischemia: pathophysiology, natural history, and clinical management. *Progr Cardiovasc Dis* 1998; **40**: 324–41.
34. Weiss RL, Brier JA, O'Connor W *et al.* The usefulness of transesophageal echocardiography in diagnosing cardiac contusions. *Chest* 1996; **109**: 73–7.
35. Madu EC, Brown R, Geraci SA. Dynamic left ventricular outflow tract obstruction in critically ill patients: role of transesophageal echocardiography in therapeutic decision making. *Cardiology* 1997; **88**: 292–5.
36. Tsang TS, Barnes ME, Hayes SN *et al.* Clinical and echocardiographic characteristics of significant pericardial effusions following cardiothoracic surgery and outcomes of echo-guided pericardiocentesis for management. Mayo Clinic experience 1979–1998. *Chest* 1999; **116**: 322–31.
37. Bommer WJ, Follette D, Pollock M *et al.* Tamponade in patients undergoing cardiac surgery: a clinical echocardiographic diagnosis. *Am Heart J* 1995; **130**: 1216–23.
38. Klein AL, Grimm RA, Murray RD. Use of transesophageal echocardiography to guide cardioversion in patients with atrial fibrillation. *N Engl J Med* 2001; **344**: 1411–20.
39. Flachskampf FA, Daniel WG. Aortic dissection. *Cardiol Clin* 2000; **18**: 807–17.
40. Armstrong WF, Back DS, Carey LM *et al.* Clinical and echocardiographic findings in patients with suspected acute aortic dissection. *Am Heart J* 1998; **136**: 1051–60.
41. Mohr-Kahaly S, Erbel R, Kearney P *et al.* Aortic intramural hemorrhage visualized by transesophageal echocardiography: findings and prognostic implications. *J Am Coll Cardiol* 1994; **23**: 658–64.
42. Smith MD, Cassidy JM, Souther S *et al.* Transesophageal echocardiography in the diagnosis of traumatic rupture of the aorta. *N Engl J Med* 1995; **332**: 356–62.
43. Jardin F. Dubourg O, Bourdarias J-P. Echocardiographic pattern of acute cor pulmonale. *Chest* 1997; **111**: 209–17.
44. McConnell MV, Solomon SD, Rayan ME *et al.* Regional right ventricular dysfunction detected by echocardiography in acute pulmonary embolism. *Am J Cardiol* 1996; **78**: 469–73.

Part Four

Respiratory Failure

24

Oxygen therapy

Adrian T J Wagstaff

In mammals energy is provided by both anaerobic and aerobic respiration, the former being inadequate to provide adequate energy alone, so oxygen is the key ingredient to survival. Aerobic respiration is the most efficient mechanism for adenosine triphosphate (ATP) production. Absence or lack of ATP results in failure of energy-hungry enzyme systems, loss of cell homeostasis, and initially cellular and later organism death. A substantial part of critical care is targeted at treating and/or preventing hypoxia. An understanding of the common pathways that lead to cellular hypoxia from whatever cause is vital to providing appropriate support and treatment to the acutely unwell patient. This chapter will review the pathophysiology of oxygen delivery from atmosphere to cell; methods of assessment; types of therapy that can be acutely administered; and the potential hazards of oxygen use.

PATHOPHYSIOLOGY OF OXYGEN DELIVERY

The single-cell organism (e.g. amoeba) requires oxygen for its survival and obtains it from the environment from simple diffusion. This relies upon Fick's first law of diffusion:

$$O_2 \text{ diffusion} = K \times A/T \times \Delta P^1$$

where K is the diffusion constant for a particular gas, A is the surface of a membrane, T is the membrane's thickness and ΔP the difference in partial pressure across the membrane. About 600 million years ago single-celled organisms evolved into multicellular organisms. As oxygen is poorly soluble in water, diffusion alone became insufficient to deliver oxygen to the cells, and novel methods of delivery evolved, most notably the cardiovascular system.[2] This provided the means to deliver oxygen around the body.

OXYGEN DELIVERY

Transport of oxygen to the cells can thus be divided into six simple steps reliant only on the laws of physics:

1. convection of oxygen from the environment into the body (ventilation)
2. diffusion of oxygen into the blood (oxygen uptake)
3. reversible chemical bonding with haemoglobin
4. convective transport of oxygen to the tissues (cardiac output: CO)
5. diffusion into the cells and organelles
6. the redox state of the cell

This chain of events is oxygen delivery ($\dot{D}O_2$).

STEP 1: CONVECTION – VENTILATION

The first step occurs in the lung in the form of pulmonary ventilation. At sea level the partial pressure of oxygen in environmental air is approximately 160 mmHg. On inspiration the air is humidified and mixed with exhaled carbon dioxide (CO_2) such that at the alveolus the PaO_2 is 100 mmHg. This will vary in different environments and different conditions (Table 24.1). Much of oxygen therapy is based on increasing oxygen delivery into the lungs, whether it be by masks or other devices.

STEP 2: DIFFUSION – ALVEOLUS TO BLOOD

Oxygen within the alveolus diffuses across the alveolar–capillary membrane. The average thickness of the alveolar capillary membrane is 0.3 μm and the surface area of the respiratory membrane is 50–100 m^2. This leads to a PaO_2 in the pulmonary capillaries of approximately 90 mmHg. Herein lie many of the problems seen in the critically ill where two mechanisms predominate:

1. the thickness and barrier effect of the space between alveolus and capillary
2. the relationship between perfusion and ventilation at alveolar level (V/Q ratio)

Good ventilation and good perfusion is ideal while poor ventilation and poor perfusion is bad. Even in normal lungs the ratios vary across the lung. In disease states the situation is exaggerated. For example, in pneumonia ventilation may be impaired while in pulmonary embolus perfusion is disrupted. Positive-pressure ventilation may further alter the balance of ventilation and perfusion.

STEP 3: HAEMOGLOBIN BINDING

Oxygen is poorly soluble in water, having a solubility of 0.003 082 g/100 g H_2O. Having diffused across the alveolar capillary membrane, the oxygen binds rapidly to the respiratory pigment haemoglobin. The relationship between saturation of haemoglobin with oxygen (SaO_2)

Table 24.1 Clinical significance of some Pao_2 and Sao_2 values

Pao_2 mmHg	kPa	Sao_2 %	Clinical significance
150	20.0	99	Inspired air at sea level
97	12.9	97	Young normal person
80	10.6	95	Young normal person asleep Old normal person awake Inspired air at 19 000 ft (5800 m)
70	9.3	93	Lower limit of normal
60	8.0	90	Respiratory failure (mild) Shoulder of O_2 dissociation curve
50	6.7	85	Respiratory failure (significant) Admit to hospital
40	5.3	75	Venous blood – normal Arterial blood – respiratory failure (severe) Acclimatised person at rest at 9000 ft (2750 m)
30	4.0	60	Unconscious if not acclimatised
26	3.5	50	P50 of haemoglobin
20	2.7	36	Acclimatised mountaineer exercising at 19 000 ft (5800 m) Hypoxic death

and Po_2 is not linear and forms a sigmoidal shape (Figure 24.1). The P50 is the Pao_2 at which 50% of the haemoglobin is saturated. Various factors are known to alter the affinity of haemoglobin for oxygen (Table 24.2). These have teleological advantages as, for example, a low pH or

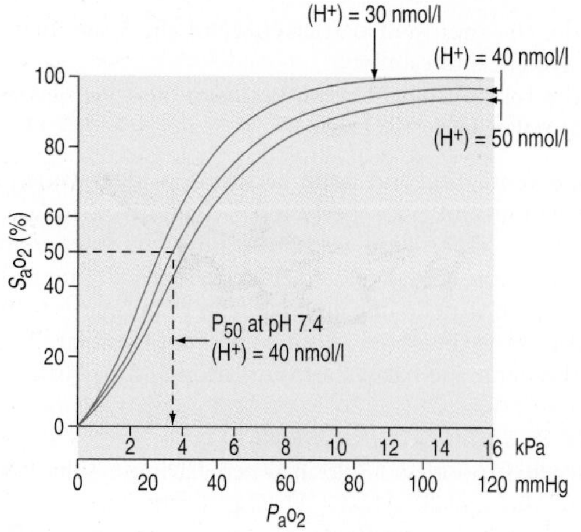

Figure 24.1 Haemoglobin oxygen dissociation curve. Normal curve at 40 nmol/l and shifts to left and right.

Table 24.2 Factors influencing the position of the oxygen dissociation curve

Factors increasing P50 (curve shifts to the right)	Factors decreasing P50 (curve shifts to the left)
Hyperthermia	Hypothermia
Decreased pH (acidaemia)	Increased pH (alkalaemia)
Increased Pco_2 (Bohr effect)	Decreased Pco_2
Increased 2,3-DPG	Decreased 2,3-DPG
	Fetal haemoglobin
	Carbon monoxide
	Methaemoglobin

2,3-DPG, 2,3-diphosphoglycerate.

high CO_2 at tissue level could imply tissue hypoxia, and the reduction in oxygen-binding affinity, may increase oxygen availability. Similarly, hyperthermia (fever), hypercarbia and an increase in the concentration of 2,3-diphosphoglycerate (2,3-DPG) all move the curve to the right and increase oxygen availability. 2,3-DPG is a byproduct of glycolysis and therefore binds haemoglobin in predominantly hypoxic tissues, facilitating a release of oxygen. Conversely hypocarbia, alkalosis and low concentrations of 2,3-DPG result in a leftward shift of the curve and a higher affinity for binding for any given Po_2. Systemic interventions such as alteration in Pco_2 or pH will influence the curve and therefore oxygen dissociation and availability.

STEP 4: CONVECTION – CARDIOVASCULAR

In humans the cardiovascular system is the solitary delivery system of oxygen to the cells. This is achieved by the convection (bulk flow) of oxygen – predominantly bound to haemoglobin (21 ml/100 ml) from the lungs via the heart and out into the systemic circulation by way of the arteries. These branch down to form the capillaries where the oxygen is offloaded to the tissues. Convection of oxygen by the cardiovascular system is influenced mainly centrally by CO and peripherally by local controls of the regional perfusion of the tissues.

The delivery of oxygen also relies on the concentration of oxygen in the blood (Cao_2). This is calculated by the following formula:

$$Cao_2 = ([\text{Hb}](\text{g/dl}) \times 1.34 \times Sao_2) + (0.003 \times Pao_2)$$

1 g of haemoglobin binds 1.34 ml of oxygen. Thus changes in the Sao_2 and haemoglobin concentration are important in determining the oxygen concentration. Delivery of oxygen is therefore summarised by the formula:

$$\text{Delivery of oxygen } (\dot{D}o_2)\ \text{ml/min} = 10 \times \text{CO(1/min)} \times Cao_2$$

The normal resting $\dot{D}o_2$ is approximately 1000 ml/min. Oxygen consumption ($\dot{V}o_2$) at rest is approximately 250 ml/min.

$$\text{Oxygen consumption } (\dot{V}O_2)\ \text{ml/min} = 10 \times CO(1/\text{min}) \times (CaO_2 - C\bar{v}O_2)$$

where $C\bar{v}O_2$ is calculated as $(1.34 \times [Hb] \times S\bar{v}O_2) + (0.003 \times P\bar{v}O_2)$

It can be seen that the amount of oxygen extracted is about 25% of that delivered at rest and that there is a large reserve. This obviously varies between organs. This ratio is referred to as the oxygen extraction ratio (OER).

$$OER = \dot{V}O_2/\dot{D}O_2$$

During exercise this can increase by up to 70–80% at maximum. Oxygen that is not removed by the tissues returns to the heart and lungs. Globally the difference between that delivered and that returning is the consumption. This model can also be used to look at regional consumption. Hence the saturation of mixed venous blood ($S\bar{v}O_2$), which is all the returning blood or central venous blood, can be used as an indicator of global $\dot{V}O_2$ and indirectly the adequacy of $\dot{D}O_2$. If oxygen delivery by the microcirculation and cellular oxygen uptake are adequate, then a $S\bar{v}O_2$ value of 70% usually indicates that global $\dot{D}O_2$ is appropriate. Lower may indicate increased uptake but more often reduced or inadequate delivery. Mixed venous blood is useful for measurement of global $\dot{D}O_2$, but it usually requires the presence of a pulmonary artery catheter. The use of central venous saturations has become an alternative surrogate which is usually adequate and considerably more practical.

The body cannot store large amounts of oxygen and is thus dependent on a continuous supply The excess ability to increase $\dot{D}O_2$ to match changes in $\dot{V}O_2$ is an adaptation that permits sudden changes in demand such as exercise in which $\dot{V}O_2$ can exceed 1500 ml/min in some cases.

STEP 5: DIFFUSION – BLOOD TO MITOCHONDRION

Ninety per cent of cellular aerobic metabolism takes place in the mitochondria. The rate of diffusion of oxygen from bound oxyhaemoglobin to the mitochondria follows similar principles to the diffusion of oxygen into the blood from the alveoli. Namely:

1. Fick's law of diffusion, where the ΔP is dependent on $\dot{D}O_2$ and the rate of cellular uptake and utilisation
2. the position of the oxygen haemoglobin dissociation curve

Once delivered to the cell, oxygen is utilised in the generation of ATP. This is achieved by the production of pyruvate from glucose via glycolysis. This produces only 2 ATP molecules per molecule of glucose. The pyruvate is converted to acetyl coenzyme A and in the mitochondrion enters the citric acid cycle (Krebs cycle), resulting in the production of reducing power to form NADH and $FADH_2$. These molecules are transferred to the electron transport chain and oxidation to water releases the cellular energy currency ATP.[3]

Originally at approximately 160 mmHg, the partial pressure of oxygen at the mouth falls to a PO_2 in some mitochondria which can be as low as 1 mmHg. Below this value, cellular demands for oxygen outweigh its delivery, and ATP production may be reduced.

STEP 6: THE REDOX STATE OF THE CELL

Conventionally oxygen delivery from atmosphere to cell is considered a cascade, implying that a high concentration at one end will cascade down and increase oxygen in the cell. It will increase oxygen available to the cell potentially but the driving force for oxygen to enter the cell and the mitochondrion is the gradient between the partial pressure of oxygen in the cell and outside. Increased oxygen utilisation will reduce that tension and increase the gradient. Conversely, adequate oxygen in the cell will reduce the gradient between the cell and outside and oxygen will not diffuse. The cell determines how much oxygen it uses by creating the gradient that sucks oxygen in – it is not a cascade. Similarly, it is the ATP/adenosine diphosphate (ADP) ratio and probably hydrogen ion concentration that drive ATP production and modify oxygen requirement, i.e. the cell is largely autonomous and uses what it needs.[4] While ensuring adequate oxygen delivery is important, excess oxygen is at least theoretically of no benefit.

PATHOLOGY OF OXYGEN DELIVERY ($\dot{D}O_2$)

Failure of oxygen delivery to the cells leads rapidly to cellular dysfunction, and can lead to cellular death and organ dysfunction, culminating in organism death. Failure of $\dot{D}O_2$ to match $\dot{V}O_2$ ($\dot{V}O_2$ drives the $\dot{D}O_2$ requirement) results in reduction in aerobic metabolism and energy production and necessitates production of ATP by the less efficient glycolytic pathway.

The level of $\dot{D}O_2$ at which $\dot{V}O_2$ begins to decline has been termed the 'critical $\dot{D}O_2$' and is approximately 300 ml/min in an adult (Figure 24.2).[5] 'Shock' is the usual term used in this situation, defined loosely as failure of delivery of oxygen to match the demand of tissue. Commonly this refers to failure of the circulation, but low $\dot{D}O_2$ can result from several pathological mechanisms which can occur as a single problem or in combination. Cellular hypoxia can result from each of the stages of oxygen delivery:

1. reduction in environmental oxygen, e.g. altitude: hypoxic hypoxia
2. failure to ventilate, whether from airway obstruction, loss of respiratory drive from the central nervous system, drugs or muscular failure – neuromuscular disease such as acute inflammatory demyelinating polyneuropathy (Guillain–Barré syndrome): hypoxic hypoxia
3. impaired gas exchange across the alveolar–capillary membrane, e.g. pneumonia, pulmonary embolus, acute asthma, pulmonary oedema: hypoxic hypoxia

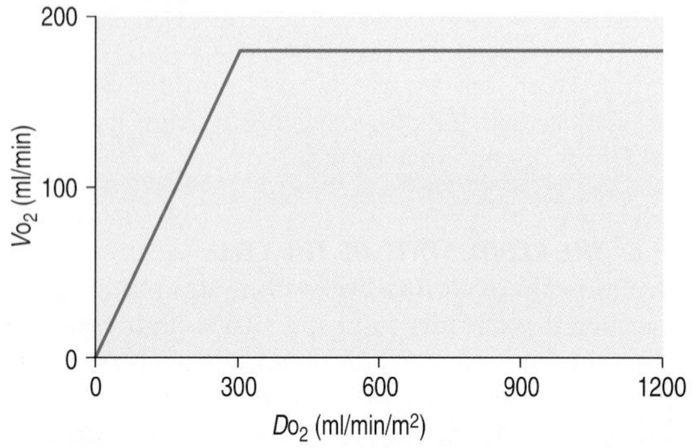

Figure 24.2 The normal relationship between $\dot{V}O_2$ and $\dot{D}O_2$. Above the value of 'critical $\dot{D}O_2$, $\dot{V}O_2$ is independent of oxygen delivery. Below this value, $\dot{V}O_2$ becomes supply-dependent and may be amenable to therapeutic interventions.

4. abnormal or reduced binding to haemoglobin so there is inadequate oxygen carriage, e.g. severe anaemia, carbon monoxide poisoning or methaemoglobinaemia: anaemic hypoxia
5. reduced CO, e.g. left ventricular failure. Failure of oxygen delivery: stagnant or ischaemic hypoxia
6. impaired diffusion at the blood–tissue interface, e.g. tissue oedema due to sepsis: hypoxic hypoxia
7. cytochrome or mitochondrial poisoning. Cyanide, arsenic and some antiretroviral drugs: histotoxic hypoxia

The above is summarised in Table 24.3 as the types of hypoxia.

The impact of a low $\dot{D}O_2$ can be made worse by an increase in oxygen demand. Metabolic rate increases with exercise, inflammation, sepsis, pyrexia, thryotoxicosis, shivering. seizures, agitation, anxiety and pain.[6] Therapeutic interventions such as adrenergic drugs, e.g. adrenaline (epinephrine)[7] and certain feeding strategies can also lead to an increased $\dot{V}O_2$.

In critical illness, where oxygen delivery is considered to be in jeopardy, there has been considerable interest in the relationship between $\dot{D}O_2$ and $\dot{V}O_2$ (see Figure 24.2). The presence of signs or markers of tissue hypoxia such as acidosis implies inadequate tissue oxygenation. This could either be from inadequate delivery failing to meet consumption requirements or due to a reduced ability of the tissues to extract oxygen. The former could be corrected by increasing delivery; the latter is more difficult. Historically this has led to the strategy for delivering 'supranormal' $\dot{D}O_2$ to ensure adequate supply.[8,9] There were some intrinsic problems in this approach. It is irrefutable that, if delivery is inadequate, it should be corrected to meet consumption, but much of the early work was based on the relationship between delivery and consumption trying to reach a point where delivery outstripped consumption. As both values are derived from the same root equation and same data, mathematical linkage was inevitable, so as one increased, so would the other.[10,11] Also the inotropes used to increase delivery also increased consumption.

Clinical studies clearly show that adequate resuscitation to meet oxygen requirements is sensible. In the critically ill going beyond this is not helpful,[12,13] although there may be a place for supraoptimal values in the high-risk surgical patient.[8,9] In the acute situation the combined use of markers of tissue hypoxia, such as acidosis and lactate, in conjunction with surrogates of oxygen delivery, such as $Scv O_2$, and standard haemodynamic measurements of an adequate circulation have proved beneficial.[14,15] So-called early goal-directed therapy is now included in published guidelines for the treatment of severe sepsis (Table 24.4).[16] The benefits of this new approach may well have as much to do with the prompt and aggressive improvements in haemodynamics and resuscitation as the values obtained. Timing is probably the significant difference when compared with other applications of the 'supranormal' technique. Targeted

Table 24.3 Types of hypoxia

Type of hypoxia	Pathophysiology	Examples
Hypoxic hypoxia	Reduced supply of oxygen to the body leading to a low arterial oxygen tension	1. Low environmental oxygen (e.g. altitude) 2. Ventilatory failure (respiratory arrest, drug overdose, neuromuscular disease) 3. Pulmonary shunt: (a) Anatomical – ventricular septal defect with right-to-left flow (b) Physiological – pneumonia, pneumothorax, pulmonary oedema, asthma
Anaemic hypoxia	The arterial oxygen tension is normal, but the circulating haemoglobin is reduced or functionally impaired	Massive haemorrhage, severe anaemia, carbon monoxide poisoning, methaemoglobinaemia
Stagnant hypoxia	Failure of transport of sufficient oxygen due to inadequate circulation	Left ventricular failure, pulmonary embolism, hypovolaemia, hypothermia
Histotoxic hypoxia	Impairment of cellular metabolism of oxygen despite adequate delivery	Cyanide poisoning, arsenic poisoning, alcohol intoxication

Table 24.4 Early goal-directed therapy. A summary of $\dot{D}O_2$ parameters set to achieve in first 6 hours of the diagnosis of severe sepsis with associated hypotension and a plasma lactate concentration of $\geq$ 4 mmol/l

Variable	Parameters
Arterial oxygen saturation (SaO_2)	$\geq$ 93%
Central venous pressure (CVP)	8–12 mmHg
Mean arterial pressure (MAP)	65–90 mmHg
Urine output (UO)	$\geq$ 0.5 ml/kg per hour
Mixed venous oxygen saturations ($S\bar{v}O_2$) or central venous oxygen saturations ($ScvO_2$)	$\geq$ 70%
Haematocrit	$\geq$ 30%

(After Rivers E *et al.* Early goal-directed therapy in the treatment of severe sepsis and septic shock. *N Engl J Med* 2001; **345**: 1368–77.)

Table 24.5 Summary of targeted oxygen delivery

Goal-directed therapy
Supraoptimal values in the critically ill – not recommended
Perioperative optimisation with supranormal values – possibly useful but controversial
Resuscitation against markers of peripheral oxygen use such as $ScvO_2$ and lactate (early goal-directed therapy) – currently advocated

oxygen delivery is a major debate that is still evolving (Table 24.5). Oxygen delivery can be improved in a variety of ways, from the ambient inspired oxygen through the lungs and cardiovascular system to the cell itself, but once at the cell the ability to manipulate delivery ceases.

CELLULAR HYPOXIA

In environments where the $\dot{D}O_2$ is reduced, the human cell can tolerate hypoxia to a certain extent by adapting 'hibernation' strategies to reduce metabolic rate, increased oxygen extraction from surrounding tissues and enzyme adaptations that allow continuing metabolism at low PO_2.[17] Anaerobic metabolism is actively utilised by some tissues. At times of low oxygen concentrations, both myocardial and vascular endothelium upregulate glycolytic enzymes and glucose transport proteins.[18] This is not sustainable.

Local failure of cellular energy production has feedback effects on the local circulation to improve oxygen delivery. This effect is replicated regionally and then systemically with effects on the lungs, heart and circulation to try to meet the oxygen needs. If this fails, the consequences of hypoxia are seen at cellular then regional and finally systemic levels.

REGIONAL HYPOXIA

Much of what has been discussed describes effects of oxygen delivery and uptake for the body as a whole. The reality is far more complex, as not only can each organ system have its $\dot{D}O_2$ manipulated to meet demand, but also within each organ regional demands may vary and can be varied. Few of the clinical methods commonly used for assessing $\dot{D}O_2$ can identify changes in either organ or regional $\dot{D}O_2$. Thus it is possible in critical illness for tissue hypoxia to exist with associated organ dysfunction, despite normal global $\dot{D}O_2$ and $S\bar{v}O_2$ values.[19]

The effects of disordered or diverted regional blood flow can be important. For example, in shock splanchnic blood flow is often reduced with the potential for ischaemia. Clearly detection of gut ischaemia could be used to influence management of oxygen delivery and hopefully reduce the likelihood of multiorgan failure.[20] The control of regional blood flow is itself complex. Methods of increasing global $\dot{D}O_2$ in the hope that it will optimise all tissues often necessitate the use of vasoactive drugs (vasopressors, inotropes and vasodilators). Paradoxically, although such therapy can influence regional flow, it may not necessarily be in the direction sought in individual regions.

DIAGNOSIS AND MONITORING OF $\dot{D}O_2$

The last two decades have shown that the value of correcting markers of tissue hypoperfusion and hypoxia is far greater than that of targeting subjective predictive values for populations. It is important to recognise and treat these problems early so that organ $\dot{D}O_2$ can be preserved.[14] Clinical assessment of $\dot{D}O_2$ and $\dot{V}O_2$, e.g. heart rate, blood pressure or urine output, can be misleading. Particularly in the young patient, the ability of the OER to increase to as high as 70–80% can mean that such variables can change only late in the evolution of diminished $\dot{D}O_2$. However, the assessment of an effective CO (ECO) – normal heart rate, blood pressure and peripheral perfusion with signs of organ function and normal oxygen saturation – must not be excluded in favour of more technical quantitative methods. Rather the technical values must be considered in the clinical context. All assessments of $\dot{D}O_2$, clinical or technical, require continuous re-evaluation to ensure that the treatments being planned or administered are appropriate for the patient's current condition.

SaO_2 and PaO_2

Both these measures are included in the CaO_2 equation (see above), and their importance is clear. However it can be difficult to define what is a 'safe' SaO_2 and/or PaO_2. Measured systemically, they do not alone reflect tissue oxygenation and oxygen extraction mechanisms vary between organs. In general, however, supplementary oxygen is required when Pao_2 falls below 60 mmHg or the Sao_2 is below 90%. The clinical significance of common Pao_2 and Sao_2 values is listed in Table 24.1.

ACID–BASE BALANCE

Many intensive care units use acid–base balance as a simple bedside indicator of global $\dot{D}o_2$. The presence of acidosis and a base deficit of less than –2 may be used to detect evidence of inadequate $\dot{D}o_2$. They can only reflect global perfusion. The use of the plasma lactate concentration is an unreliable indicator of tissue hypoxia. It represents the balance between production and consumption so if used in isolation or as a single value to assess $\dot{D}o_2$ it can easily mislead.[21] The use of lactate as a marker of $\dot{D}o_2$ is best used as a trend using serial measurements.

$S\bar{v}o_2$/$Scvo_2$

In critical illness a falling $\dot{D}o_2$ can be compensated for by an increase in oxygen extraction. This leads to a lower oxygen saturation of haemoglobin returning to the right side of the heart. Analysis of this saturation either in vivo (fibreoptic oximetry) or in vitro (oximetry) allows assessment of the OER. Classically, a low $S\bar{v}o_2$ (<70%), in the face of a normal Sao_2, implies tissue hypoperfusion secondary to a low CO, either hypovolaemia or pump failure. It could however indicate very high $\dot{V}o_2$, which may occur with hyperthermia. Conversely a raised $S\bar{v}o_2$ (> 75%) will imply low demand, e.g. hypothermia, or a cellular utilisation problem, easily explained in cyanide poisoning when the oxidative phosphorylation mechanism is inhibited, but much more difficult to rationalise when it is seen (commonly) in sepsis. In a very-low-output state it could indicate total failure of peripheral perfusion and therefore no oxygen usage. $Scvo_2$ is a reasonable surrogate for $S\bar{v}o_2$ and reduces the need for the more complex pulmonary artery catheter.[15,22] Whichever method of venous oxygen saturation is used, it must be in conjunction with other markers of adequacy of oxygen delivery and clinical context, as outlined in Table 24.4.

MEASUREMENT OF REGIONAL $\dot{D}o_2$

As outlined above, most assessments of $\dot{D}o_2$ are global and do not reflect regional differences between organs or even within differing tissues of the same organ. Current methods of non-invasively assessing individual organ or tissue oxygenation are limited. The measurements are difficult, require specialised techniques and are not widely available. Currently only gastric tonometry and near-infrared spectroscopy (NIRS) have clinical applications in the detection of organ hypoxia.[20] In the future NMR spectroscopy or positron emission tomography may allow direct non-invasive measurement of $\dot{D}o_2$ and tissue oxygenation, but at present the environment for such testing is not easily accessed by the critically ill.

OXYGEN THERAPY APPARATUS AND DEVICES

PRINCIPLES

In the hypoxic self-ventilating patient, delivery of oxygen to the alveoli is usually achieved by increasing the environmental oxygen fraction (Fio_2). Most commonly this involves the application of one of the many varieties of oxygen mask to the face, such that it covers the nose and mouth. There are also other methods, e.g. nasal cannulae, but each method needs to fulfil the same basic requirements.

Most of the simpler oxygen delivery devices, e.g. plastic masks, nasal cannulae, deliver oxygen at relatively low oxygen flow rates relative to peak inspiratory flows (25–100+l/min). The final Fio_2 delivered is heavily influenced by the entrainment of environmental air which dilutes the set Fio_2. From a physics perspective the actual concentration of oxygen delivered is determined by the interaction between the delivery system and the patient's breathing pattern. The actual Fio_2 that reaches the alveolus is therefore unpredictable. Factors that influence this can broadly be divided into patient factors and device factors, which are summarised in Table 24.6.[23]

In the hypoxic patient it is common to find significant increases of inspiratory flow rates as well as an absence of the respiratory pause. This can result in the actual Fio_2 at the alveolus being significantly less than that believed to be being delivered. This is due to a greater proportion of the inhaled gas being entrained air when the patient's inspiratory flow rate increases. The normal peak inspiratory flow rate (PIFR) is between 25 and 35 l/min. In critical illness it can rise to eight times normal (Figure 24.3).[24] The greater the inspiratory flow rate, the lower the alveolar Fio_2. This is particularly true for the variable performance-type masks, but is also seen even in the more 'reliable' Venturi-type masks, particularly when the higher Fio_2 inserts are used. The presence of a valve-controlled reservoir bag on a 'non-rebreather' semirigid plastic mask should compensate for high inspiratory flows, hence the belief that such masks can deliver 100% oxygen. This is not the case, and in models of human ventilation, such masks do not seem to confer significant extra oxygen

Table 24.6 Factors that influence the Fio_2 delivered to a patient by oxygen delivery devices

Patient factors	Device factors
Inspiratory flow rate	Oxygen flow rate
Presence of a respiratory pause	Volume of mask
Tidal volume	Air vent size
	Tightness of fit

(After Leigh J. Variation in performance of oxygen therapy devices. *Anaesthesia* 1970; **25**: 210–22.)

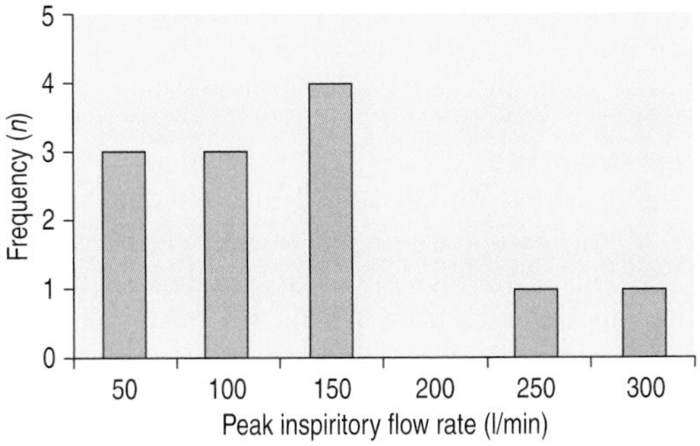

Figure 24.3 Spirometric peak inspiratory flow rates (PIFR) taken from a group of 12 critical care patients with respiratory distress and hypoxia. Most of the patients have a PIFR below 150 l/min. However 2 patients exceed 200 l/min. This will have a negative effect on the concentration of oxygen delivered from a variable-performance system, e.g. Hudson.[24]

delivery ability above that of the semirigid plastic masks without the reservoir bag (Figures 24.4 and 24.5).[25]

The failure of oxygen masks to deliver the desired FiO_2 can be improved by either having a high enough oxygen flow rate and reservoir to compensate for the high inspiratory flow rate, e.g. high-flow nasal cannulae such as the Vapotherm, or sealing the upper airway (nose and mouth)

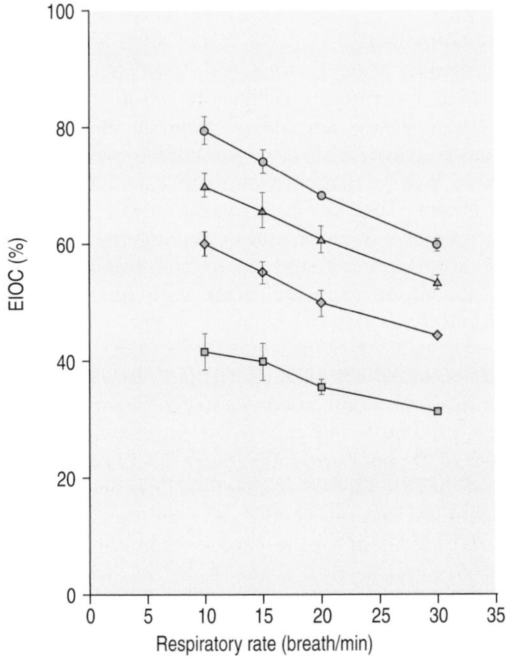

Figure 24.4 The performance of a Hudson mask on a model of human ventilation at a tidal volume of 500 ml and four oxygen flow rates (15 l/min (○), 10 l/min (△), 6 l/min (◇) and 2 l/min (□)). As the respiratory rate increases, so the effective inspired oxygen concentration (EIOC) deteriorates.[25]

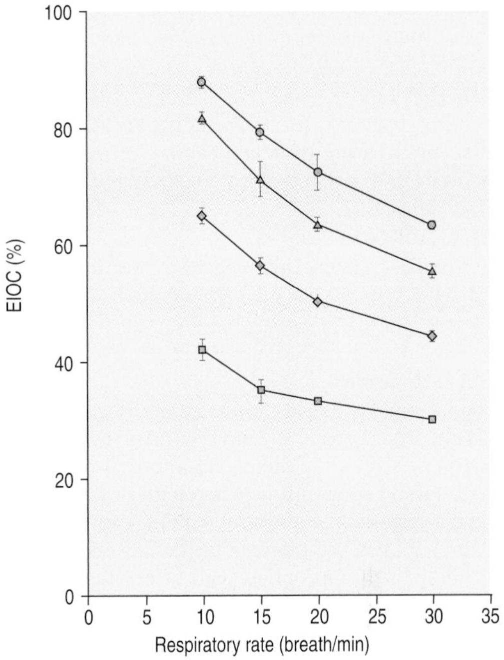

Figure 24.5 The performance of a Hudson non-rebreather mask on a model of human ventilation at a tidal volume of 500 mLs and four oxygen flow rates (15 l/min (○), 10 l/min (△), 6 l/min (◇) and 2 l/min (□)). As the respiratory rate increases, so the effective inspired oxygen concentration (EIOC) deteriorates. Note also how the curves of the graph are similar to the Hudson mask without the reservoir bag, implying no superiority with its addition.[25]

from the environment, e.g. the continuous positive-airways pressure (CPAP) mask. Indeed, there are data to support the hypothesis that some of the improvement in oxygenation seen with CPAP ventilation may be due to the eradication of entrainment of environmental air, rather than the positive airway pressure exerted by the CPAP valve.[24]

In summary, the use of non-sealing oxygen masks and cannulae should be guided by the patient's requirements and response to therapy, rather than a belief that the concentration being delivered is what is reaching the alveolus. This can be particularly important in the treatment of patients whose ventilatory drive is sensitive to PO_2 levels.

OXYGEN DELIVERY DEVICES

Methods of delivering oxygen to conscious patients with no instrumentation to their airway can broadly be divided into four categories:

1. variable-performance systems
2. fixed-performance systems
3. high-flow systems
4. others

With the exception of the intravascular devices, they all consist of similar component parts, as follows.

OXYGEN SUPPLY

Delivery of oxygen can be from pressurised cylinders, hospital supply from cylinder banks, a vacuum-insulated evaporator (VIE) or an oxygen concentrator.

OXYGEN FLOW CONTROL

Oxygen delivery from the supply to the device is controlled by some sort of valve, often with an associated flow meter.

CONNECTING TUBING

The connecting tubing is both from the supply to the flow control and from the flow control to the device. The type and size of the tubing are important. Small-bore tubing can limit oxygen flow when high flow is intended. In some systems the connecting tubing can also act as a reservoir, e.g. Ayre's T-piece. Some devices require specialised tubing with appropriate end attachments, such as the Schräeder valves required for connecting to the wall oxygen supply.

RESERVOIR

All oxygen delivery devices have some sort of reservoir. In the case of the simple oxygen mask it is the mask itself. Some low-flow CPAP circuits have a balloon reservoir. The nasal cannulae utilise the nasopharynx as a reservoir. An oxygen tent uses the volume of the tent as a large reservoir. The effectiveness of the reservoir in storing oxygen ready for the next inspiratory effort is one of the important factors in governing its ability to deliver the desired oxygen concentration. The oxygen tent is a good example of the effectiveness of a large reservoir, as it eliminates air entrainment whatever the patient's PIFR. Thus the oxygen flow rate does not have to be high, just enough to ensure that CO_2 rebreathing is abolished. Indeed it is the retention of CO_2 that can be the major problem if gas is expired into the reservoir.

PATIENT ATTACHMENT

The patient is connected to the oxygen supply and reservoir such that the device delivers oxygen to the airway, by directly covering the upper airway, e.g. plastic mask/head box, or intranasally, or by increasing the oxygen concentration in the wider environment as in an oxygen tent.

EXPIRED-GAS FACILITY

Expired gas from the patient needs to be allowed to dissipate into the environment, and not be retained in the system and be inspired at the next inspiratory effort. Most masks achieve this by having a small reservoir capacity and holes in the plastic to allow the gas to exit. One-way valves, as in the non-rebreather-type reservoir mask, aid in unidirectional flow of gas away from the patient. High-flow T-piece systems like those used in a CPAP system utilise the high flow to remove the gas down an expiratory limb and into the environment.

HUMIDIFICATION

Most systems use the physiological humidification properties of the nasopharynx and trachea. However, high-flow systems may overcome this, leading to drying of the airway and secretions which can be uncomfortable and undesirable. Artificial humidification (and warming) should be employed using devices such as water bath or heat and moisture exchanger (HME).

OXYGEN MONITOR

Some systems have an oxygen monitor incorporated in the apparatus, e.g. a fuel cell. This allows the much more accurate monitoring of F_{IO_2}, but is dependent on where in the system it is placed, and also adds bulk and expense to the oxygen delivery method.

VARIABLE-PERFORMANCE SYSTEMS

Typically these are a non-sealed mask or nasal cannulae system which deliver oxygen at low gas flows (2–15 l/min). The reservoir is usually small, consisting of the volume of the mask in the case of the semirigid type, or the nasopharynx, as in the nasal cannulae. The entrainment of environmental air is important in their delivery capability and has to be considered when being used.

NASAL CANNULAE

The proximity of the reservoir – the nasopharynx – means that these systems are particularly sensitive to changes in inspiratory flow rate and particularly the loss of the respiratory pause. However, for mild hypoxia, they are tolerated well by patients who can eat and drink with them in situ. They can cause drying of the nasal mucosa when used at flow rates, and newer systems are available which can humidify and warm the inspired oxygen. They are cheap and easy to use with no risk of CO_2 retention.

SIMPLE SEMIRIGID PLASTIC MASKS (E.G. HUDSON, MC)

The most commonly used type of oxygen mask, these systems are cheap and easy to administer. The reservoir consists of the mask and rebreathing of CO_2 can therefore occur if they are used at oxygen flow rates below 4 l/min. A maximum F_{IO_2} of 0.6–0.7 can only be achieved, and this will be lower in the presence of respiratory distress.

TRACHEOSTOMY MASKS

These semirigid plastic masks act in the same way as their facial counterparts. However the delivery they achieve is very dependent on the presence of an endotracheal tube and the inflation status of its cuff. If absent or if the cuff is deflated, then air from the nasopharynx will mix with that being delivered to the tracheostomy, and further dilute the F_{IO_2}.

T-PIECE SYSTEM

These simple systems, consisting of an inspiratory limb and expiratory limb forming the bar of the 'T', can be used with endotracheal tubes (oral, nasal or tracheostomy), or with a sealed CPAP-type mask. The oxygen flow rate needs to be high enough to match the patient's PIFR so as to prevent rebreathing of expired gas and thus potential entrainment of air from the expiratory limb. The seal of the mask or tube cuff is also important to prevent entrainment of air.

FIXED-PERFORMANCE SYSTEMS

These systems are so called because their delivery of oxygen is independent of the patient factors outlined above.

VENTURI-TYPE MASKS

Oxygen concentration is determined by the Venturi principle. Oxygen passing through a small orifice entrains air to a predictable dilution. The F_{IO_2} is adjusted by changing the Venturi 'valve' and setting the appropriate oxygen flow rate. Whilst the Venturi effect can deliver 40–60 l/min, this is only possible at the lower F_{IO_2} valves (e.g. at F_{IO_2} of 0.24 the flow rate is approximately 53 l/min at an inflow of 2 l/min), and oxygen flow rate falls as the F_{IO_2} increases. Thus in respiratory distress associated with hypoxia, the reduction in oxygen flow rate can lead to failure despite a higher F_{IO_2} setting. The larger orifice leads to the system behaving more like a simple mask.

ANAESTHETIC BREATHING CIRCUITS

Non-rebreathing systems have one-way valves (e.g. Ambu-bag) and usually closed mask systems so they deliver what is set. Non-rebreathing systems, Mapleson A, B, C, D and E or, in Accident and Emergency, a Waters bag, depend on the gas flows to ensure no rebreathing. No air entrainment is possible but rebreathing occurs readily at low flows (most require flows > 150 ml/kg).

HIGH-FLOW SYSTEMS

As alluded to above, the T-piece system can act as a fixed-performance system if the oxygen flow rate is sufficiently high. Other high-flow systems exist, e.g. Vapotherm, which use flow rates up to 30 l/min nasally. They require humidification and heating of the inspired gas to allow patient tolerance.

POSITIVE-PRESSURE DEVICES

For the purpose of this chapter, non-invasive positive-pressure ventilation (NIPPV) devices are described. NIPPV delivers oxygen with some element of positive pressure exerted during the respiratory cycle. It does not require instrumentation of the airway, and is delivered either by a tight-fitting mask to the face, nose or as a helmet. The simplest CPAP system is a T-piece with a positive-pressure valve attached to the expiratory limb, as with a Mapleson E system. Other methods are also available; some utilise a balloon reservoir rather than a high-flow oxygen generator (Mapleson A). CPAP helps improve functional residual capacity and compliance.[26] There is no air entrainment and is probably why gas exchange initially improves rapidly. Theoretically the positive pressure inhibits alveolar closure which it may do but also to aid recruitment. A potential problem with the T-piece CPAP systems is that the oxygen flow rate has to be adjusted to the patient's PIFR so as to prevent closure of the valve and increasing the inspiratory work of breathing. Other methods of NIPPV such as bilevel positive airway pressure (BPAP) deliver oxygen at flows that should match the patient's demand.

OTHER METHODS OF OXYGEN DELIVERY

Intravascular oxygenation has been used, but not extensively, particularly in the self-ventilating patient population. Extracorporeal membrane oxygenation (ECMO) supporting both heart and lung may be superseded by relatively simple external oxygenators such as the Novolung interventional lung assist (ILA). In these, blood flow may be either 'pumped' or rely on the patient's circulation similar to the haemodiafiltration systems. Currently focused on CO_2 removal there is increasing interest in their oxygenation capabilities.

HAZARDS OF OXYGEN THERAPY

SUPPLY

Medical oxygen supply is a compressed gas. Pipeline supply to the 'wall' is usually at 4 bar of pressure (3040 mmHg). The cylinder supply when full is 137 bar (104 120 mmHg). As such, there are important risks when using oxygen, as explosion is a risk. Direct administration of oxygen at delivery pressures carries a real risk of barotrauma to the airway and alveoli, if not governed by an appropriate pressure-limiting valve, e.g. OHE flow meter.

Oxygen also supports combustion. The possibility of sparks in an oxygen-rich environment must be avoided. Patients must not smoke cigarettes when receiving oxygen therapy, even via nasal cannula. Another example is to ensure that oxygen supplies are removed or turned off when defibrillating, as a spark can occur in such situations.

OXYGEN TOXICITY

CENTRAL NERVOUS SYSTEM TOXICITY (PAUL BERT EFFECT)

Seen in diving, oxygen delivered at high pressure (> 3 atmospheres) can lead to acute central nervous system signs and seizures.

LUNG TOXICITY (LORRIANE SMITH EFFECT)

Exposure to a high FiO_2 results in pulmonary injury. It is known that a progressive reduction in compliance occurs, and is associated with interstitial oedema, leading to fibrosis. The mechanism remains unclear, but is believed to involve direct cellular damage to the lung tissue by highly reactive oxygen free radicals. High concentrations of oxygen produce a higher concentration of free radicals that overwhelm the normal scavenging mechanism lining the respiratory tract. This, possibly associated with loss of surfactant, and increase in sympathetic activity and airway collapse due to the lack of other non respiratory gases, leads to lung damage. Evidence for this mechanism is supported by the worsening of lung damage seen in paraquat poisoning. Paraquat produces large amounts of free oxygen radicals, and the administration of supplemental oxygen worsens its effects. Detecting this problem as the sole aetiology for pulmonary pathology can be difficult, especially as the usual indications for oxygen therapy usually imply some form of pulmonary pathology.

It is reasonable that the risk of oxygen-induced pulmonary toxicity is dependent on concentration and duration of exposure. However, what concentration/duration is likely to cause toxicity is not clear. In some subjects long exposure times and high concentrations do not lead to problems; however, in general, patients should remain below an FiO_2 of 0.5 where possible, and periods above this should be kept to the minimum required. 'Safe' periods of exposure above 0.5 vary from 16 to 30 hours. The clinical signs of oxygen toxicity are listed in Table 24.7. All are relatively non-descript and easily explained by other causes in a critically unwell patient.

BRONCHOPULMONARY DYSPLASIA

First described in 1967, this is a form of chronic lung disease that is associated with neonatal ventilation. Its pathophysiology includes the same factors as the adult form, but with the additional effect of immaturity. The advent of surfactant in the treatment of respiratory distress of the newborn and the addition of maternal steroid therapy to promote pulmonary development have lowered the incidence and reduced the severity of the disease.

Table 24.7 Symptoms and signs of oxygen toxicity

Central nervous system	Pulmonary
Nausea and vomiting	Dry cough
Anxiety	Substernal chest pain
Visual changes	Shortness of breath
Hallucinations	Pulmonary oedema
Tinnitus	Pulmonary fibrosis
Vertigo	
Hiccup	
Seizures	

RETINOPATHY OF PREMATURITY (ROP)

Previously referred to as retrolental fibroplasia, ROP was first described in 1942. It is a vasoproliferative disorder of the eye affecting premature neonates. Similar to the lungs, the completion of development of the retinal vasculature is late in gestation (32–34 weeks).[27] In the 1950s an epidemic of ROP was described and a causal link to uncontrolled oxygen therapy was made.[28] Improved monitoring of oxygen therapy reduced the incidence of ROP, but was associated with an increase in perinatal mortality secondary to respiratory failure.[29] Subsequently, and despite good oxygen control, ROP continues to occur. This is now most likely due to the increased survival of increasingly premature low-birth-weight infants[30] rather than high PaO_2 alone. This suggests both oxygen and non-oxygen-related factors. ROP is a biphasic disease where the relatively hyperoxic environment following delivery initially leads to a slowing or even cessation of retinal vascular development of the premature infant. Additional oxygen may further contribute to this problem, by affecting the expression of vascular growth factors. The second phase of the disease is a hypoxic-induced neovascularisation, similar to that seen in diabetic retinopathy. This leads to fibrous scarring with risk of retinal detachment. How much oxygen is too much remains contentious and further research is required.[31]

HYPERBARIC OXYGEN THERAPY

Oxygen can be delivered to patients at higher than atmospheric pressure (2–3 atmospheres). This serves to increase the amount of oxygen carried in the plasma, rather than bound to haemoglobin. This follows Henry's law that states: 'At a constant temperature, the amount of a given gas dissolved in a given type and volume of liquid is proportional to the partial pressure of that gas in equilibrium with that liquid.' As the partial pressure of oxygen in the environment rises, so the amount of oxygen dissolved in the plasma also rises. Consequently, the contribution of the PaO_2 in the CaO_2 formula (see above) increases. At rest the metabolic demands of an average person can be met by dissolved oxygen alone when breathing 100% at 3 atmospheres.

Hyperbaric oxygen therapy can be delivered either in a monoplace chamber designed for one individual, or in multiplace chambers for 2–10 people. The chambers encompass the whole body, and gas is piped from source, heated and humidified. The common indications for use are listed in Table 24.8.[32,33]

CARBON MONOXIDE POISONING

Carbon monoxide poisoning in particular attracts attention. A common consequence of house fires, it binds to

Table 24.8 Recognised indications for hyperbaric oxygen therapy

Primary therapy	Adjunctive therapy
Carbon monoxide poisoning	Radiation tissue damage
Air or gas embolism	Crush injuries
Decompression sickness (the 'bends')	Acute blood loss
Osteoradionecrosis	Compromised skin flaps or grafts
Clostridial myositis and myonecrosis	Refractory osteomyelitis
	Intracranial abscess
	Enhancement of healing of problem wounds

(After Tibbles PM, Edelsberg JS. Hyperbaric-oxygen therapy. *N Engl J Med* 1996; **334**: 1642–8; and Bennett M. Randomised controlled trials. In: Fledmeier J (ed.) *Hyperbaric Oxygen 2003 – Indications and Results. The UHMS Hyperbaric Oxygen Therapy Committee Report*. Undersea and Hyperbaric Medicine Society: 2003; 1212–37.)

haemoglobin with an affinity 210 times that of oxygen. Its half-life in air is 320 minutes, but this can be reduced to 90 minutes by giving the patient 100% oxygen, or 23 minutes with the addition of 3 atmospheres of hyperbaric therapy. Competitive dissociation of carbon monoxide from the haem-binding site and provision of dissolved oxygen to the tissues is believed to combine to reduce the sequelae of carbon monoxide poisoning, but the mechanisms are likely to be more complex.[34] Some studies have suggested both acute and longer-term benefit,[35,36] but others have been unable to conclude significant benefit.[37,38] Recent investigations have attempted to distinguish those patients more likely to benefit from hyperbaric oxygen therapy. Factors such as increasing age (> 35 years), an exposure time of > 24 hours, an associated loss of consciousness and carboxyhaemoglobin levels greater than 25% appear to result in an increased incidence of neurological sequelae, and probably benefit from hyperbaric oxygen.[39] Geographical distance to an appropriate centre often has a significant influence on hyperbaric usage in the acute setting, but mobile units and some evidence that late therapy may be of benefit should not necessarily preclude its usage.[34,40]

COMPLICATIONS

Hyperbaric therapy is associated with the following complications:

1. barotrauma: middle ear and sinuses, rupture of the oval or round window, gastrointestinal distension, tooth displacement and pain, gas embolism on decompression
2. oxygen toxicity (as above). Especially a problem in the critically ill who may be on high concentrations for longer periods[32]
3. generalised seizures (Paul Bert effect)
4. visual problems: acute myopia, cataract formation

REFERENCES

1. West JB. *Respiratory Physiology, The Essentials*, 6th edn. Philadelphia, PA: Lippincott, Williams & Wilkins: 2000; 171.
2. Hameed S. Oxygen delivery. *Crit Care Med* 2003; **31**: S658.
3. Arthur C, Guyton JH. *Textbook of Medical Physiology*, 10th edn. Philadelphia, PA: Saunders; 2000.
4. Kuper M, Soni N. The oxygen whirlpool. In: Vincent J-L (ed.) *Yearbook of Intensive Care and Emergency Medicine*. New York: Springer; 2004: 656–74.
5. Ronco JJ *et al.* Identification of the critical oxygen delivery for anaerobic metabolism in critically ill septic and nonseptic humans. *JAMA* 1993; **270**: 1724–30.
6. Walsh T. Recent advances in gas exchange measurements in intensive care patients. *Br J Anaesth* 2003; **91**: 120–31.
7. Fellows IW, Bennett T, MacDonald IA. The effects of adrenaline upon cardiovascular and metabolic functions in man. *Clin Sci* 1985; **69**: 215–22.
8. Shoemaker WC *et al.* Prospective trial of supranormal values of survivors as therapeutic goals in high-risk surgical patients. *Chest* 1988; **94**: 1176–86.
9. Boyd O. Optimisation of oxygenation and tissue perfusion in surgical patients. *Intens Crit Care Nurs* 2003; **19**: 171–81.
10. Walsh TS, Lee A. Mathematical coupling in medical research: lessons from studies of oxygen kinetics. *Br J Anaesth* 1998 **81**: 118–20.
11. Vermeij CG, Feenstra BW, Adrichem WJ, Bruining HA. Independent oxygen uptake and oxygen delivery in septic and postoperative patients. *Chest* 1991; **99**: 1438–43.
12. Gattinoni L, Brazzi L, Pelosi P *et al.* A trial of goal-oriented hemodynamic therapy in critically ill patients. $S\bar{v}O_2$ collaborative group. *N Engl J Med* 1995; **333**: 1025–32.
13. Hayes MA, Timmins AC, Yau EH *et al.* Elevation of systemic oxygen delivery in the treatment of critically ill patients. *N Engl J Med* 1994; **330**: 1717–22.
14. Rivers E, Nguyen B, Havstad S *et al.* Early goal-directed therapy in the treatment of severe sepsis and septic shock. *N Engl J Med* 2001; **345**: 1368–77.
15. Rivers EP, Ander DS, Powell D. Central venous oxygen saturation monitoring in the critically ill patient. *Curr Opin Crit Care* 2001; **7**: 204–11.
16. Dellinger RP *et al.* Surviving Sepsis campaign guidelines for management of severe sepsis and septic shock. *Crit Care Med* 2004; **32**: 858–73.
17. Hochachka PW, Buck LT, Doll CJ, Land SC. Unifying theory of hypoxia tolerance: molecular/metabolic defense and rescue mechanisms for surviving oxygen lack. *Proc Natl Acad Sci USA* 1996; **93**: 9493–8.

18. Cartee GD, Douen AG, Ramlal T, Klip A, Holloszy JO. Stimulation of glucose transport in skeletal muscle by hypoxia. *J Appl Physiol* 1991; **70**: 1593–600.
19. Curtis SE, Cain SM. Regional and systemic oxygen delivery/uptake relations and lactate flux in hyperdynamic, endotoxin-treated dogs. *Am Rev Respir Dis* 1992; **145**: 348–54.
20. Gutierrez G, Palizas F, Doglio G *et al.* Gastric intramucosal pH as a therapeutic index of tissue oxygenation in critically ill patients. *Lancet* 1992; **339**: 195–9.
21. Leach RM, Treacher DF. The pulmonary physician in critical care 2: oxygen delivery and consumption in the critically ill. *Thorax* 2002; **57**: 170–7.
22. Wheeler AP, Bernard GR, Thompson BT *et al.* Pulmonary-artery versus central venous catheter to guide treatment of acute lung injury. *N Engl J Med* 2006; **354**: 2213–24.
23. Leigh J. Variation in performance of oxygen therapy devices. *Anaesthesia* 1970; **25**: 210–22.
24. Wagstaff TAJ, Soni N. Arterial oxygenation in respiratory failure: the importance of the CPAP valve. *Br J Anaesth* 2006; **97**: 435P.
25. Wagstaff TAJ, Soni N. Performance of six types of oxygen delivery devices at varying respiratory rates. *Anaesthesia* 2007; **62**: 492–503.
26. Lenique F, Habis M, Lofaso F *et al.* Ventilatory and hemodynamic effects of continuous positive airway pressure in left heart failure. *Am J Respir Crit Care Med* 1997; **155**: 500–5.
27. Roth AM. Retinal vascular development in premature infants. *Am J Ophthalmol* 1977; **84**: 636–40.
28. Campbell K. Intensive oxygen therapy as a possible cause of retrolental fibroplasia; a clinical approach. *Med J Aust* 1951; **2**: 48–50.
29. Avery ME. Recent increase in mortality from hyaline membrane disease. *J Pediatr* 1960; **57**: 553–9.
30. Flynn JT. Acute proliferative retrolental fibroplasia: multivariate risk analysis. *Trans Am Ophthalmol Soc* 1983; **81**: 549–91.
31. Tin W, Gupta S. Optimum oxygen therapy in preterm babies. *Arch Dis Child Fetal Neonatal Ed* 2007; **92**: F143–7.
32. Tibbles PM, Edelsberg JS. Hyperbaric-oxygen therapy. *N Engl J Med* 1996; **334**: 1642–8.
33. Bennett M. Randomised controlled trials. In: Fledmeier J (ed.) Hyperbaric Oxygen 2003 – *Indications and Results. The UHMS Hyperbaric Oxygen Therapy Committee Report*. Flagstaff, AZ: Best; 2003: 1212–37.
34. Stoller KP. Hyperbaric oxygen and carbon monoxide poisoning: a critical review. *Neurol Res* 2007; **29**: 146–55.
35. Weaver LK, Hopkins RO, Chan KJ *et al.* Hyperbaric oxygen for acute carbon monoxide poisoning. *N Engl J Med* 2002; **347**: 1057–67.
36. Hawkins M, Harrison J, Charters P. Severe carbon monoxide poisoning: outcome after hyperbaric oxygen therapy. *Br J Anaesth* 2000; **84**: 584–6.
37. Scheinkestel CD *et al.* Hyperbaric or normobaric oxygen for acute carbon monoxide poisoning: a randomised controlled clinical trial. *Med J Aust* 1999; **170**: 203–10.
38. Juurlink DN, Buckley NA, Stanbrook MB *et al.* Hyperbaric oxygen for carbon monoxide poisoning. *Cochrane Database Syst Rev* 2005; CD002041.
39. Weaver LK, Valentine KJ, Hopkins RO. Carbon monoxide poisoning: risk factors for cognitive sequelae and the role of hyperbaric oxygen. *Am J Respir Crit Care Med* 2007; **176**: 491–7.
40. Lueken RJ, Heffner AC, Parks PD. Treatment of severe carbon monoxide poisoning using a portable hyperbaric oxygen chamber. *Ann Emerg Med* 2006; **48**: 319–22.

25

Airway management and acute upper-airway obstruction

Gavin M Joynt

The primary objective of airway management is to secure unobstructed gas exchange and protect the lungs from soiling. Because of the critical importance of maintaining gas exchange, upper-airway obstruction is a life-threatening emergency. Upper-airway obstruction results from a wide range of pathophysiological processes, and therefore rapid assessment and establishment of a patent airway must take priority, even in the absence of a specific diagnosis. As no single airway management modality is universally applicable, the intensive care unit (ICU) physician must be capable of performing a variety of airway management techniques and instituting them in a logical and systematic way (Figure 25.1).

AIRWAY MANAGEMENT TECHNIQUES

Airway management techniques are generally classified as non-invasive or invasive, depending on whether instrumentation occurs above or below the glottis, surgical or non-surgical, and definitive (Table 25.1). Definitive techniques secure the trachea and provide some protection from macroscopic aspiration and soiling. While bag-and-mask ventilation and direct laryngoscopic tracheal intubation remain the routine methods of airway management in ICU, the use of fibreoptic bronchoscopy is increasingly common, especially in special circumstances. Management of failed intubation and ventilation by various alternative techniques, particularly the use of the intubating laryngeal mask airway (iLMA) and cricothyroidotomy, is well described.[1,2]

The technique of choice will depend on each individual situation and is determined by the interaction of patient and clinical factors, which partially determine the appropriate technique (Table 25.2), and the clinician's experience in applying the chosen technique. Other factors include availability of help, levels of training and supervision and accessibility of equipment. A portable storage unit with a wide choice of equipment appropriate for difficult airway management should be available in every ICU (Table 25.3).

NON-INVASIVE TECHNIQUES

BAG-MASK VENTILATION

Mask ventilation, using a bag-mask resuscitator, is a basic skill that requires time and experience to master. It should be learned using mannekins, simulators and practice in the controlled environment of the operating theatre so that when used in the emergency setting in ICU the skill is already well established. The manually squeezed bag is self-inflating, usually with a simple reservoir bag in series, which, if kept inflated, ensures that a consistent high oxygen concentration can be delivered. The addition of a positive end-expiratory pressure (PEEP) valve may improve arterial oxygenation in patients with lung pathology and help overcome airway obstruction due to laryngospasm. Transparent face masks are recommended as they allow observation of misting during exhalation, assessment of the position of adjunct artifical airways and early observation of gross airway soiling.

Some considerations when performing mask ventilation include the following:

1. *Inadequate ventilation.* Good airway positioning by head tilt and chin lift, or if necessary the jaw thrust manoeuvre, is essential to maintain an open airway. The seal of the mask against the face is important and technically good hand positioning must be learned and practised. A beard may be covered with a large adhesive plastic dressing with a hole cut out for the mouth, or smeared with petroleum jelly or water-based lubricant. Ventilation of edentulous patients may be aided by improving hand position or special masks. Two operators are recommended if a mask face leak is excessive, one to hold the mask and the other to manipulate the bag-mask resuscitator.
2. *Gastric insufflation* is common if high tidal volumes are used and increases the risk of vomiting and aspiration (aim for 300–500 ml). Severe distension may occasionally cause cardiovascular compromise. Carefully applied cricoid may prevent gastric gas insufflation.
3. *Pulmonary aspiration.* In the emergency situation with a full stomach, mask ventilation with cricoid pressure is recommended until the airway can be secured. Passage

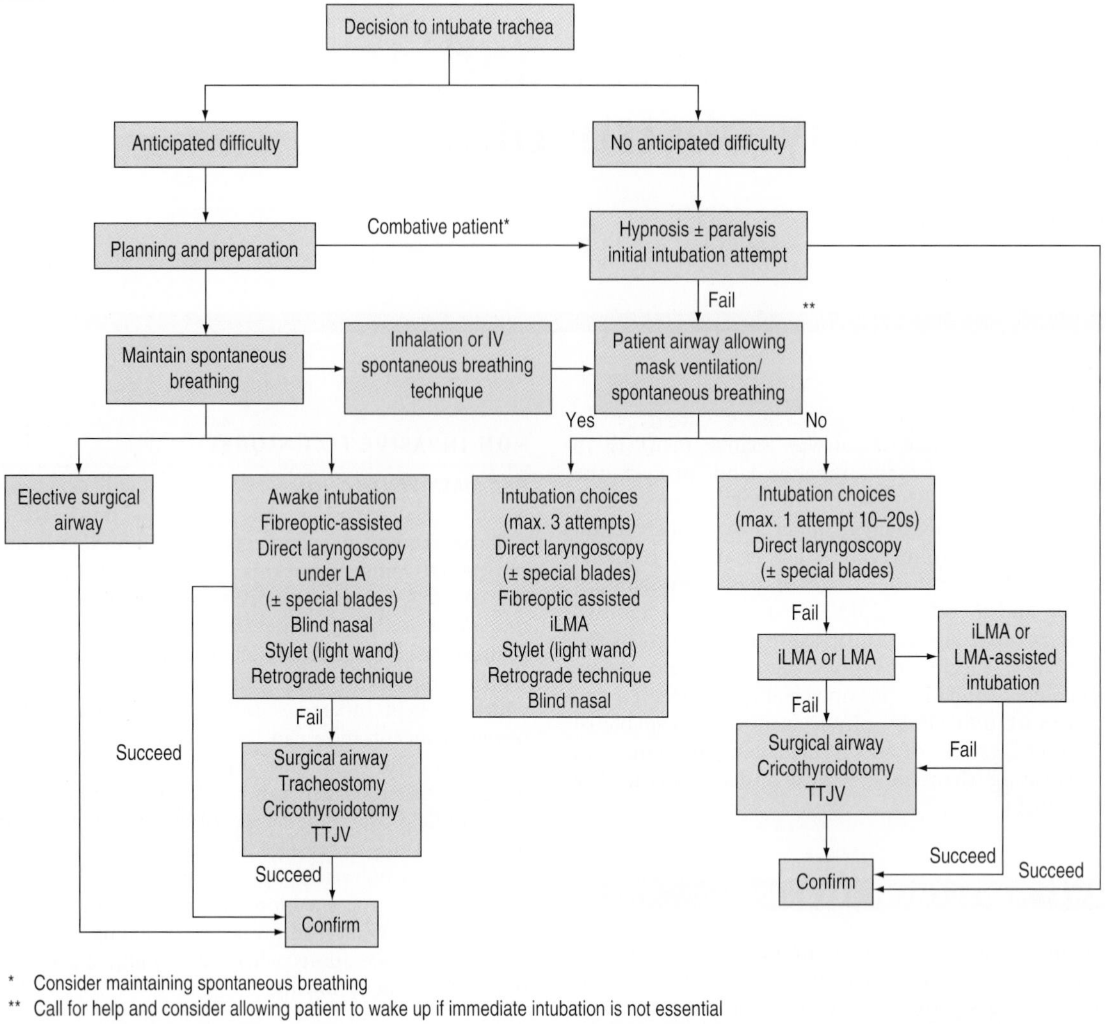

Figure 25.1 Difficult airway algorithm (see text). LMA, laryngeal mask airway; iLMA, intubating laryngeal mask airway; TTJV, transtracheal jet ventilation.

of a nasogastric tube to aspirate gastric contents can be attempted, but with caution as vomiting may be induced.

ORO- AND NASOPHARYNGEAL AIRWAYS

In the unconscious patient, functional obstruction is primarily caused by loss of muscular tone and subsequent inspiratory airway narrowing at the soft palate, epiglottis and tongue base. An oropharyngeal airway can help establish an adequate airway for spontaneous or bag-mask ventilation when proper head positioning is insufficient. It is inserted with the concavity facing the palate and then rotated 180° into the proper position as it is advanced. Complications include mucosal trauma, worsening the obstruction by pressing the epiglottis against the laryngeal outlet if the tongue displaces posteriorly, and occasionally laryngospasm. The following sizes (length from flange to tip) are recommended: large adult: 100 mm (Guedel size 5); medium-sized adult: 90 mm (Guedel size 4); small adult; 80 mm (Guedel size 3).

A nasopharyngeal airway is a soft rubber or plastic tube inserted into the nostril and advanced along the floor of the nose (in the direction of the occiput). Correctly

Table 25.1 Characteristics of airway management techniques

Technique	Experience required	Time required	Definitive
Non-invasive			
Bag-and-mask	+++	Seconds	–
LMA and ILMA	++	< 1min	–
Combitube	–	< 1min	Short-term
Invasive (non-surgical)			
Endotracheal intubation			
Direct laryngoscopy	+++	Variable	+
Bronchoscopic	+++	Minutes	+
Retrograde	+	Minutes	+
Invasive (surgical)			
Jet ventilation	–	<1min	–
Cricothyroidotomy			
Percutaneous	+	Variable	Short-term (if cuffed tube used)
Surgical	+	Minutes	+
Tracheostomy			
Percutaneous	++	Minutes	+
Surgical	+++	Minutes	+

LMA, laryngeal mask airway; ILMA, intubating laryngeal mask airway. It is difficult to gain experience with rarely used techniques such as cricothyroidotomy, jet ventilation and retrograde intubation, but reasonable competence can be achieved using mannekins and simulators.

positioned, the tube traverses the posterior pharynx. It is better tolerated by semiconscious patients than the oropharyngeal airway. Complications include epistaxis, aspiration and, rarely, laryngospasm or oesophageal placement.

LARYNGEAL MASK AIRWAY (LMA) AND INTUBATING LMA

The LMA is a reusable device that consists of a silicone rubber tube connected to a distal elliptical spoon-shaped mask with an inflatable rim, which is positioned blindly into the pharynx to form a low-pressure seal against the laryngeal inlet.[3] LMAs are useful to achieve non-definitive airway patency in many emergency situations (see Figure 25.1), and can be used to provide positive-pressure ventilation.[2] Once positioned the LMA has been used to guide the passage of stylets, bougies, the bronchoscope and an endotracheal tube into the trachea, but with difficulty.[2,4] The iLMA or FasTrach is a modification of the LMA with several features to facilitate intubation once the iLMA is placed.[5] There is a guiding ramp and epiglottic elevating bar at the aperture to direct the endotracheal tube to the glottis. It also has an anatomically curved, rigid shaft and handle to allow easy and firm manipulation during placement and when the endotracheal tube is passed.[6] The iLMA is the laryngeal mask of choice if intubation is required, as is frequently the case in ICU patients.

Although preparation and patient positioning techniques for placement of a LMA and iLMA are similar, the insertion technique is quite different. The mask airway is prepared for insertion by deflating and

Table 25.2 Commonly recommended applications of described airway management techniques. Examples of common alternatives are given in approximate order of choice

	Difficult direct laryngoscopic intubation	With difficult spontaneous/mask ventilation
Awake	Fibreoptic bronchoscopic intubation Direct laryngoscopic intubation* Blind nasal intubation Retrograde intubation	Percutaneous cricothyroidotomy* Surgical tracheostomy*
Anaesthetised or comatose (empty stomach)	Bag-and-mask ventilation Direct laryngoscopic intubation Different blade Fibreoptic bronchoscopic intubation Intubating LMA/LMA Lighted stylet Blind nasal intubation	Laryngeal mask airway (LMA) Transtracheal jet ventilation Rigid ventilating bronchoscope Percutaneous cricothyroidotomy Surgical tracheostomy
(full stomach)	Maintain cricoid pressure with all techniques Intubating LMA/Proseal LMA Combitube	Percutaneous cricothyroidotomy Surgical tracheostomy Combitube

The technique(s) chosen should also depend on the clinician's knowledge and ability. Cricoid pressure should be applied with a force of approximately 30 N, but applied force can be temporarily reduced to assist airway manoeuvres.
*Under local anaesthesia.

Table 25.3 Suggested contents of a portable storage facility for difficult airway management

Masks
Face and nasal masks of differing make and size variety
Airways
Oropharyngeal airways
Nasopharyngeal airways
Airway intubator guide for oral endoscopic intubation
Laryngeal mask airway (LMA) and intubating LMA with appropriate endotracheal tubes
Rigid laryngoscope with a variety of designs and sizes
Short handle or variable angle (Patil-Syracuse) laryngoscope
Curved blades: Macintosh, Bizarri-Guiffrida
Straight blades: Miller
Bent blade: Belscope
Articulating-tip blade: McCoy
Fibreoptic stylet laryngoscope or Bullard laryngoscope
Endotracheal tubes of assorted size
Murphy tubes
Microlaryngoscopy tubes
Endotracheal tube stylets
Gum elastic bougie (Eschmann stylet)
Malleable stylet
Tube changer, hollow tube changer (jet stylet)
Lighted stylet (light wand)
Fibreoptic intubation equipment
Patil endoscopic mask, oral airways or blocks to facilitate oral endoscopic intubation
Fibreoptic endoscopes with light source, adult and paediatric-sized
Combitube
Emergency surgical airway access
Percutaneous cricothyroidotomy set
Transtracheal jet ventilation – cannula and high-pressure O_2 source connectors
Regulated central wall O_2 pressure (Sanders-type injector)
Unregulated central wall O_2 pressure device
Exhaled carbon dioxide monitor
Capnometer/capnograph
Chemical indicators

smoothing out the cuffed rim to be wrinkle-free, and the posterior surface and patient hard palate are lubricated with water soluble jelly. The patient is positioned as for endotracheal intubation, with slight flexion of the neck and extension of the atlanto-occipital joint (sniffing-the-morning-air position). The LMA is inserted with the tip of the cuff continuously applied to the hard palate, and with the right index finger guiding the tube to the back of the tongue until a firm resistance is encountered. The cuff is then inflated with 20–40 ml of air (adult sizes) before attachment of the breathing circuit.

To begin insertion of an iLMA, ensure the curved metal tube is in close proximity to the chin (the metal handle points to the toes) and the mask tip flat against the palate prior to insertion. The mask is inserted and positioned with a circular motion, maintaining contact pressure between the posterior aspect of the mask and the palate and posterior pharynx, until some resistance in the hypopharynx is felt. A laryngoscope can be used to assist placement. Once gas exchange is established, an attempt at intubation can be made. The well-lubricated endotracheal tube is passed down the iLMA tube, rotating gently to distribute the lubricant until the 15-cm marker (or the transverse line on the proprietary LMA Fastrach endotracheal tube). The endotracheal tube tip is now positioned through the epiglottic elevating bar. Gently lift the iLMA about 2–5 cm with the metal handle while the endotracheal tube is advanced into the trachea. Inflate the endotracheal tube cuff and confirm tracheal intubation (see later). Remove the endotracheal tube connector, and position the stabiliser rod on the endotracheal tube opening – this is needed to maintain the tube position in the trachea as the mask is removed. Lastly, gently remove the iLMA over the endotracheal tube/stabiliser assembly. Remove the stabiliser rod, reconfirm tube position and secure.

The successful use of an iLMA requires some familiarity with the equipment and technique, and at least simulated exposure is strongly recommended. Contraindications for using an ILMA or LMA include inability to open the mouth, pharyngeal pathology, airway obstruction at or below the larynx, low pulmonary compliance or high airway resistance. Complications include aspiration, gastric insufflation, partial airway obstruction, coughing, laryngospasm, postextubation stridor and kinking of the shaft of the LMA.

COMBITUBE (OESOPHAGEAL–TRACHEAL DOUBLE-LUMEN AIRWAY)

The oesophageal–tracheal Combitube is a double-lumen tube that is blindly inserted into the oropharynx up to the indicated markings.[7] The oesophageal lumen is blocked at the distal end and has side perforations at the pharyngeal level whereas the tracheal lumen has a hole at the distal end. It has two balloon cuffs, a distal one and a proximal pharyngeal balloon. The patient is ventilated through the oesophageal lumen initially as the Combitube usually enters the oesophagus,[7] with the distal cuff sealing the oesophagus and the proximal balloon sealing the proximal pharynx. Gas exits the perforations and enters the pharynx and larynx. In the event of failure of ventilation, tracheal intubation may have occurred and then the tracheal lumen is ventilated while the distal cuff seals the trachea. Although demonstrated to be a useful airway management adjunct, its role in resuscitation and management of the difficult airway in the ICU environment is yet to be established. Barotrauma, especially oesophageal rupture, has been reported.

INVASIVE TECHNIQUES

ENDOTRACHEAL INTUBATION

Endotracheal intubation remains the 'gold standard' of definitive airway management, allowing for spontaneous and positive-pressure ventilation, with good macroscopic protection from aspiration. Indications include acute airway obstruction, facilitation of tracheal suctioning, protection of the airway in those without protective reflexes, and respiratory failure requiring ventilatory support with high inspired concentrations of oxygen and PEEP.

Preparation

Prior to proceeding with any attempts at intubation, regardless of the technique chosen, preparation and checking of all relevant equipment are essential. Tracheal intubation should be preceded by adequate preoxygenation, particularly in ICU patients who frequently have pulmonary or cardiac pathology. Difficult airway management equipment (see Table 25.3) should also be accessible within a few minutes. Food, vomitus, blood or sputum may obstruct the airway and therefore suction, able to generate at least 300 mmHg (40 kPa) and a flow rate of 30 l/min, should always be available. Excessively vigorous suctioning should be avoided as it can cause laryngospasm, vagal stimulation, mucosal injury and bleeding.

Direct laryngoscopy

Although an essential skill for all intensivists, direct laryngoscopy and intubation is difficult to master.[8] It can be learned by simulation, exposure to patients in a controlled environment such as the operating room and subsequently practised under supervision in the ICU setting. A detailed description of the technique is beyond the scope of this chapter; however certain problems and complications commonly encountered in ICU patients should be anticipated and prevented.

Cricoid pressure is usually required as few ICU patients can be adequately starved prior to intubation. ICU patients are at high risk for severe hypotension following the use of hypnotic or sedative agents used to facilitate intubation. Mechanisms include, but are not limited to, direct drug effects causing myocardial depression and decreases in peripheral vascular resistance, a reduction in venous return and preload following the increase in intrathoracic pressure with positive-pressure ventilation and the removal of sympathetic stimulation once anxiety disappears. It is therefore useful to ensure adequate hydration, availability of inotrope and vasopressor drugs, judicial use of positive ventilatory pressures and close haemodynamic monitoring before and during the intubation period.

Because intubation is often more difficult in ICU patients (see later), excellent technique is needed. All *first* attempts at intubation should incorporate proper head position, the use of techniques such as BURP (backward, upward, rightward pressure) that may be helpful to bring the vocal cords into the field of vision, and, if necessary, the use of a gum elastic bougie or equivalent. A difficult-to-visualise 'anterior larynx' can often be more easily intubated if a gum elastic bougie is advanced in the midline and directed anteriorly into the trachea. The endotracheal tube is then advanced over the guide from an initial 90° anticlockwise-rotated position. Clinical signs of correct tracheal placement of the guide include coughing (in incompletely paralysed patients), a resistance felt before the guide is fully advanced (usually at 45 cm or less from the lips because of resistance at the carina or bronchus) and a sensation of clicks from the tracheal rings. A number of alternative intubating guides are available, including the hollow endotracheal tube changer, which can be attached to a side-stream capnometer, or to an oxygen source. The lighted stylet is less commonly used and has a light at the distal end that results in a characteristic midline transillumination appearance when the light enters the larynx.

If multiple intubation attempts are required, the maximum interruption to ventilation should be about 30 s and adequate ventilation and oxygenation must be provided between attempts. Minimum monitoring should consist of continuous-pulse oximetry, electrocardiogram (ECG) and blood pressure. In ICU patients the largest reasonable endotracheal tube should be chosen to facilitate optimal sputum clearance, access for fibreoptic bronchoscopy and to reduce airway resistance in difficult-to-ventilate patients. Sizes of 8.0–9.0 mm in adult males and 7.0–8.0 mm in adult females are generally used.

The route of intubation may be orotracheal or nasotracheal. The orotracheal route is preferred because it has fewer complications. Nasotracheal intubation is contraindicated in the presence of fracture of the base of skull. Other complications include epistaxis, turbinate cartilage and nasal septal damage, and in the long-term an increased risk of nosocomial pneumonia and sinusitis.[9]

Rigid indirect fibreoptic technique

The Bullard laryngoscope is a rigid, indirect fibreoptic instrument that is shaped to follow the hard palate. The learning curve appears reasonable and it has been shown to be a viable alternative for intubation in the difficult airway and reduces cervical spine movement during laryngoscopy compared with the Macintosh or Miller laryngoscope.[10]

Fibreoptic bronchoscopic technique

This technique offers advantages of direct visualisation, immediate diagnosis of upper-airway lesions and immobility of the neck during the procedure.[11] It also allows reasonably comfortable intubation of a cooperative, awake patient under local anaesthesia, and use of the sitting position. Experience and skill are necessary, especially for dealing with emergent situations, but success rates > 96% are expected.[12] Fibreoptic oral intubation may also be performed in anaesthetised patients, using a modified face mask with diaphragm. Nasal intubation is usually performed through an endotracheal tube placed in the nasopharynx, with the tip just above the glottis. The fibreoptic bronchoscope tip is guided into the trachea and the tube is advanced over the bronchoscope. Correct placement is visually checked before the scope is removed. In ICU the fibreoptic bronchoscope can be used to improve the safety of airway procedures such as endotracheal tube changes and percutaneous tracheostomy.[13,14] A number of specially designed oral airways are available to assist oral fibreoptic intubation. The most common cause of failure is obstructed vision from blood or secretions.

Less commonly used techniques of endotracheal intubation

Blind nasal intubation is less common since the advent of fibreoptic bronchoscopy, but is sometimes considered in spontaneously breathing patients. Possible indications include inability to open the mouth (e.g. mandibular fracture or temporomandibular joint pathology), cervical spine injury and faciomaxillary injury when blood and secretions may obscure a fibreoptic view.

The retrograde intubation technique consists of the percutaneous introduction of a J-tip guidewire through the cricothyroid membrane, which is then advanced into the retropharynx. The tip is retrieved from the oral cavity, and the wire is used to guide an oral endotracheal tube past the obstruction and into the trachea.[15] The procedure is a relatively simple and safe alternative if other techniques fail or are not possible. Commercial kits are available.

Confirmation of tracheal tube placement

Confirming correct intratracheal tube placement is essential. Direct visualisation and measurement of expired CO_2 by capnography are the most reliable methods.[16] Capnography may produce false-positive results with the first few breaths after oesophageal intubation (i.e. detectable end-tidal $P\text{CO}_2$), if gastric insufflation from mask ventilation has occurred. A false-negative (decreased $P\text{CO}_2$, despite correct position) may occur with cardiac arrest and low-cardiac-output states. Position can also be reliably confirmed by fibreoptic confirmation and the use of oesophageal detectors or self-inflating bulbs.[1] Other clinical signs, such as auscultation of breath sounds over both sides of the chest and epigastrium, visualisation of condensed water vapour in the tube and chest wall movement, are less reliable.

Complications of endotracheal intubation

These may be classified into those occurring during intubation (e.g. incorrect tube placement, laryngeal trauma, deleterious cardiovascular response to laryngoscopy and intubation, increase in intracranial pressure, hypoxaemia and aspiration), while the tube is in place (e.g. blockage, dislodgment, tube deformation, damage to larynx and complications of mechanical ventilation), and following extubation (e.g. aspiration and postextubation airway obstruction, laryngeal and tracheal stenosis). Specific techniques should be used to minimise side-effects such as cardiovascular responses and increases in intracranial pressure.

TRANSTRACHEAL JET VENTILATION (TTJV)

Percutaneous TTJV, using a large-bore intravenous (IV) catheter inserted through the cricothyroid membrane, can be used to provide temporary ventilation when other techniques have failed.[17] Ventilation through the cannula with a standard manual resuscitator bag is inadequate, and a jet ventilation system is necessary. A high-pressure (up to 50 psi or 344 kPa) oxygen source is required for adequate ventilation through a 14 FG IV cannula with a manually regulated jet injector. Expiratory gases must be able to escape via the glottis. Appropriate chest movements during expiration must be noted. The consequence of expiratory obstruction is severe and potentially fatal barotrauma.

Complications may be caused by insertion of the IV cannula (e.g. bleeding and oesophageal perforation), use of high-pressure gases (e.g. hyperinflation, barotrauma), catheter kinking or displacement (the latter causing potentially catastrophic subcutaneous emphysema) and failure to protect the airway (i.e. aspiration).

CRICOTHYROIDOTOMY

Cricothyroidotomy, by surgery or percutaneously, is a reliable, relatively safe and easy way of providing an emergency airway.[18] It is the method of choice if severe or complete upper-airway obstruction exists. The simplest, fastest and most proven method uses a horizontal incision through the cricothyroid membrane with the space held wide open by the scalpel handle or forceps. This is followed by insertion of a small tracheostomy or endotracheal tube (Figure 25.2). If available, a small surgical hook is useful to hold down the inferior margin of the incision to facilitate cannulation. Commercial cricothyroidotomy sets, using the Seldinger technique, are available. A tube with internal diameter of 3.0 mm will allow adequate gas flow for self-inflating bag ventilation provided supplemental oxygen is used. Since the diameter of the cricothyroid space is 9×30 mm, tubes of 8.5 mm *outer* diameter or less should avoid laryngeal and vocal cord damage. Commercially available percutaneous tracheostomy sets that meet the above requirements are available. Complications such as subglottic stenosis (1.6%), thyroid fracture, haemorrhage and pneumothorax are acceptably low. Cricothyroidotomy is generally contraindicated in complete laryngotracheal disruption and age < 12 years.

TRACHEOSTOMY

There is little agreement on the indications, best technique or optimal timing of tracheostomy in ICU patients. Suggested indications for tracheostomy include bypass of glottic and supraglottic obstruction, access for tracheal toilet, provision of a more comfortable airway for prolonged ventilatory support and protection of the airways

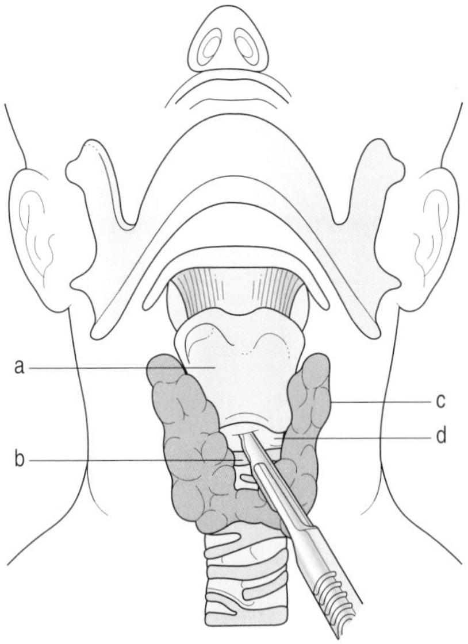

Figure 25.2 Cricothyroidotomy performed with a scalpel. (a) Thyroid cartilage; (b) cricoid cartilage; (c) thyroid gland; (d) cricoid membrane, usually easily palpable subcutaneously.

Table 25.4 Complications of tracheostomy

Immediate
Procedural complications
Haemorrhage
Surgical emphysema, pneumothorax, air embolism
Cricoid cartilage damage
Misplacement in pretracheal tissues or right main bronchus
Compression of tube lumen by cuff herniation
Occlusion of the tip against the carina or tracheal wall
Delayed
Blockage with secretions
Infection of the tracheostomy site, tracheobronchial tree and larynx
Pressure on tracheal wall from the tracheostomy tube or cuff
Mucosal ulceration and perforation
Deep erosion into the innominate artery
Tracheo-oesophageal fistula
Late
Granulomata of the trachea
Tracheal and laryngeal stenosis
Persistent sinus at tracheostomy site
Tracheomalacia and tracheal dilatation

from aspiration.[19] In uncomplicated patients, percutaneous tracheostomy performed by an intensivist at the bedside is at least as safe as surgical tracheostomy performed in the operating room, and is probably associated with a lower incidence of infectious complications.[20,21] The added convenience and cost savings have made percutaneous tracheostomy the procedure of choice in many institutions. However, the percutaneous technique is best avoided in the presence of coagulapathy – an international normalised ratio (INR) > 2 or platelet count $< 40 \times 10^9$/l; significant anatomical abnormality in the anterior neck in the region of the trachea, vessels or thyroid gland; previous tracheostomy scar; or a cervical spinal injury that is considered unstable.

Ciaglia's percutaneous technique was described in 1985.[22] After making an adequate skin incision and using blunt dissection with forceps the trachea is gently exposed. The endotracheal tube is then withdrawn so that its cuff lies just above the vocal cords. The operator confirms tube position to be above the stoma site by palpation of the trachea. A J-wire is placed in the trachea through a needle inserted through the membrane above or below the second tracheal ring. A series of curved dilators is used to enlarge the stoma progressively. A tracheostomy tube is then inserted into the trachea and the endotracheal tube removed. Ciaglia later introduced a modified tapered dilator to avoid the use of multiple dilators. Although quicker, the single dilator may cause more tracheal wall injuries and ring fractures.[22] The Griggs technique utilises a Kelly forceps, modified to allow it to be guided by the J-wire, to dilate the tract before insertion of tracheostomy tube.[23] Although the Griggs technique is marginally faster (by 2–3 minutes) than the Ciaglia technique, most, but not all, prospective studies have suggested that the Griggs technique may cause marginally more bleeding and functional complications, and cannula insertion may be somewhat more difficult.[24,25] Fibreoptic bronchoscopy during percutaneous tracheostomy may help to prevent incorrect guidewire placement and tracheal ring rupture or herniation, but definitive evidence supporting its routine use is lacking. Definitive identification of the best technique still requires further investigation and long-term follow-up.

Minitracheostomy describes the percutaneous insertion of a small 4-mm non-cuffed tracheostomy tube through the cricothyroid membrane or trachea, mainly to facilitate suctioning in patients with poor cough ability.

Complications of tracheostomy are listed in Table 25.4.

LOCAL ANAESTHESIA

Instrumentation of the upper airway in awake patients requires good local anaesthesia to increase comfort, improve cooperation, attenuate cardiovascular responses and reduce the risk of laryngospasm. Rapid transcricoid injection and either sprayed or nebulised lidocaine to the nares, posterior pharynx and tongue are effective (Table 25.5).[26] Nerve block techniques may improve analgesia but are not essential. Cocaine has been a popular choice for its vasoconstrictor properties, but it is toxic and its supply is regulated. Systemic absorption of topically applied lidocaine (maximum dose 4 mg/kg) is variable, and the clinician should be alert for signs and symptoms of toxicity.

Table 25.5 Local anaesthesia of the upper airway in adults

Technique	Drug dosage
Nerve block	
Internal branch of superior laryngeal nerve	Lidocaine 1–2% (2 ml/side)
Glossopharyngeal nerve	Lidocaine 1–2% (3 ml/side)
Topical anaesthesia of the tongue and oropharynx	
Gargle	Lidocaine viscous 4% (5 ml)
Spray	Lidocaine 10% (5–10 sprays = 50–100 mg)
Nebulised	Lidocaine 4%
Topical anaesthesia of the nasal mucosa	
Cocaine spray or paste	Cocaine 4–5% (0.5–2 ml)
Gel	Lidocaine 2% gel (5 ml)
Lidocaine spray	Lidocaine 10% (10 sprays = 100 mg)
Lidocaine + phenylephrine spray	Lidocaine 3% + phenylephrine 0.25% (0.5 ml)
Topical anaesthesia of glottis and trachea	
Spray-as-you-go through bronchoscope	Lidocaine 1–4% (3 mg/kg)
Cricothyroid membrane puncture	Lidocaine 2% (5 ml)
Nebulised	Lidocaine 4% (4 ml) ± phenylephrine 1% (1 ml)

THE DIFFICULT AIRWAY

The difficult airway has been described as one in which a conventionally trained anaesthesiologist experiences difficulty with mask ventilation, tracheal intubation or both. Difficult intubations may be expected in 1–3% of patients presenting for general anaesthesia, and the incidence is likely to be considerably higher in ICU patients.

More than 85% of difficult intubations can be managed successfully by experienced clinicians without resorting to a surgical solution. The experience of the operator is probably the most important factor determining success or failure. Experience implies greater manual skills, better anticipation of problems, use of pre-prepared strategies, and familiarity with multiple techniques. Thus, training of intensivists must specifically include a variety of airway management strategies and skills.

ASSISTANCE AND ENVIRONMENT

Because the patient's condition may rapidly deteriorate as a consequence of a poorly managed airway emergency, the *most senior help available* should be immediately summoned. If the situation allows, the patient should be moved to the best location for emergency airway interventions, usually the operating theatre or ICU, and difficult airway equipment requested (see Table 25.3). A senior assistant can help in gaining IV access, administering drugs, setting up equipment and managing the airway. A skilled intensivist or ear, nose and throat surgeon (gowned and standing by) can help to provide a surgical airway or perform rigid bronchoscopy to remove foreign bodies.

ANTICIPATING AND GRADING A DIFFICULT AIRWAY

Intubation difficulty can be anticipated or predicted by the following (although the sensitivity and specificity of individual features and classifications tend to be low, a combination of features will significantly raise the risk of a difficult airway):

1. Anatomical or pathological features of difficult intubation in subjects who otherwise appear normal:
   (a) short neck, especially if obese or muscular (a thyromental distance < 6 cm)
   (b) limited neck and jaw movements (e.g. as a result of trismus, osteoarthritis, ankylosing spondylitis, rheumatoid arthritis or perioral scarring)
   (c) protruding teeth, small mouth (interincisor distance < 3 cm), long high curved palate or receding lower jaw
   (d) space-occupying lesions of the oropharynx and larynx
   (e) congenital conditions with any of the above features (e.g. Marfan's syndrome)
2. Mallampatti classification[27] of visualising the oropharyngeal structures (a cooperative sitting patient is required for this assessment, and class > 2 predicts possible difficulty):
   (a) class 1: visible soft palate, uvula, fauces and pillars
   (b) class 2: visible soft palate, uvula and fauces
   (c) class 3: visible soft palate and base of uvula
   (d) class 4: soft palate is not visible
3. The degree of difficulty experienced visualising the larynx by direct laryngoscopy should be recorded and is commonly graded by the classification of Cormack and Lehane.[28] Recently grade III has been devided into IIIa (epiglottis is mobile) and IIIb (epiglottis is not mobile) subgrades:
   (a) grade I: complete glottis is visible
   (b) grade II: anterior glottis is not visible
   (c) grade III: epiglottis but not glottis is visible
   (d) grade IV: epiglottis is not visible

FAILED INTUBATION AND VENTILATION ALGORITHMS

A pre-prepared plan in the event of failed intubation and/or ventilation is essential and a number have been described in the form of single or multiple algorithms.[1,2] The algorithm shown here is an example of a single algorithm applicable to some anticipated airway difficulty scenarios in ICU patients (see Figure 25.1). Although not comprehensive, the algorithm is complex and only one or two pathways are applicable to an individual clinical scenario. The relevant pathway should be identified as early as possible in each individual case and then applied. Ultimately effective implementation depends on the skill of the operator and the appropriate use of the airway techniques described above.

If the initial attempt at intubation fails, *call for help immediately*. Repeated attempts at direct laryngoscopy should be avoided unless a more experienced operator intervenes, or a potentially helpful manoeuvre has been carried out (e.g. significant repositioning, externally applied laryngeal pressure or change of laryngoscope blade). Hypoxia will quickly result if the patient is inadequately ventilated between attempts (see above). In addition, oedema and bleeding caused by repeated laryngoscopy attempts may impair both mask ventilation and the use of alternative techniques such as fibreoptic intubation. When indicated to prevent hypoxia a surgical airway should not be delayed (see Figures 25.1 and 25.2).

UPPER-AIRWAY OBSTRUCTION

ANATOMY AND PATHOPHYSIOLOGY

The upper airway begins at the nose and mouth, and ends at the carina. Obstruction is likely to occur at sites of anatomical narrowing, such as the hypopharynx at the base of the tongue, and the false and true vocal cords at the laryngeal opening. Sites of airway obstruction are classified as supraglottic (above the true cords), glottic (involving the true vocal cords) or infraglottic (below the true cords and above the carina).

The upper airway can also be divided into intrathoracic and extrathoracic portions, which behave differently during inspiration and expiration. The intrathoracic airway dilates during inspiration because it is 'pulled outwards' by negative intrapleural pressure. Positive intrapleural pressure during expiration causes compression and narrowing. Conversely the compliant extrathoracic airway, unexposed to intrapleural pressure, collapses during inspiration and expands during expiration. Recalling this phenomenon helps the understanding of typical clinical signs, radiographs and flow–volume loops.

AETIOLOGY

Acute upper-airway obstruction may result from functional or mechanical causes (Table 25.6). Functional causes include central nervous system and neuromuscular dysfunction. Mechanical causes may occur within the lumen, in the wall or extrinsic to the airway.

Table 25.6 Clinical conditions associated with acute upper-airway obstruction

Functional causes
Central nervous system depression
Head injury, cerebrovascular accident, cardiorespiratory arrest, shock, hypoxia, drug overdose, metabolic encephalopathies
Peripheral nervous system and neuromuscular abnormalities
Recurrent laryngeal nerve palsy (postoperative, inflammatory or tumour infiltration), obstructive sleep apnoea, laryngospasm, myasthenia gravis, Guillain–Barré polyneuritis, hypocalcaemic vocal cord spasm
Mechanical causes
Foreign-body aspiration
Infections
Epiglottitis, retropharyngeal cellulitis or abscess, Ludwig's angina, diphtheria and tetanus, bacterial tracheitis, laryngotracheobronchitis
Laryngeal oedema
Allergic laryngeal oedema, angiotensin-converting enzyme inhibitor-associated, hereditary angioedema, acquired C1 esterase deficiency
Haemorrhage and haematoma
Postoperative, anticoagulation therapy, inherited or acquired coagulation factor deficiency
Trauma
Burns
Inhalational thermal injury, ingestion of toxic chemical and caustic agents
Neoplasm
Pharyngeal, laryngeal and tracheobronchial carcinoma, vocal cord polyposis
Congenital
Vascular rings, laryngeal webs, laryngocele
Miscellaneous
Cricoarytenoid arthritis, achalasia of the oesophagus, hysterical stridor, myxoedema

CLINICAL PRESENTATION

The signs of partial airway obstruction are often progressive and begin with hoarseness, other voice changes or coughing, with more severe obstruction being marked by drooling, gagging, choking, inspiratory stridor or noisy respiration. Paradoxical chest wall movements and intercostal and supraclavicular retractions may be marked in severe obstruction. Powerful respiratory efforts may produce dermal ecchymoses and subcutaneous emphysema. Respiratory decompensation may be rapid in onset, and progress to complete obstruction. Lethargy, diminishing respiratory efforts and loss of consciousness are late signs of hypoxaemia and hypercarbia. Bradycardia and hypotension herald impending cardiac arrest.

Signs of sudden complete upper-airway obstruction are characteristic and progress rapidly. The victim cannot breathe, speak or cough, and may hold the throat between the thumb and index finger – the universal choking sign.[29] Agitation, panic and vigorous breathing efforts are rapidly followed by cyanosis. Respiratory efforts diminish as consciousness is lost, and death results within 2–5 min if obstruction is not relieved.

SPECIAL EVALUATION OR INVESTIGATIONS

If the patient remains stable, specific diagnostic evaluation may be undertaken, provided advanced airway management facilities and skilled personnel are immediately available.

LARYNGOSCOPY AND BRONCHOSCOPY

Indirect laryngoscopy in a stable, cooperative patient is useful to diagnose foreign bodies, retropharyngeal or laryngeal masses and other glottic pathology.[30]

Assessment with a flexible fibreoptic bronchoscope or laryngoscope is the evaluation method of choice in ICU patients and enables direct visualisation of upper-airway anatomy and function. The procedure can be performed at most sites without transporting the patient and risking complete obstruction. It can be applied to an awake, spontaneously breathing patient and, with care, should not worsen the obstruction. If indicated, definitive airway control by intubation can usually be achieved, by advancing an endotracheal tube over the bronchoscope into the trachea. Disadvantages are the need for a skilled operator and a cooperative patient, and the poor visual field reduces effectiveness if blood and secretions are copious.

Direct laryngoscopy enables forceps removal of foreign bodies and high-volume suctioning of blood, vomitus and secretions. Endotracheal intubation can rapidly be achieved under direct vision. Disadvantages are the need for general anaesthesia or good local analgesia (often difficult in the emergency setting). Direct laryngoscopy can be traumatic, and may worsen soft-tissue bleeding and oedema.

RADIOGRAPHIC IMAGING

Patients with potentially unstable airways should not be transported from a 'safe' environment like the emergency room, operating theatre or ICU for radiological investigation until the airway is secure. Anteroposterior and lateral plain neck X-rays are useful to detect radiopaque foreign bodies. The lateral view in the upright position in inspiration with the neck fully extended may reveal swelling of the epiglottis and supraglottic tissues. Ballooning of the hypopharynx is a classical signs of epiglottitis, but is not always present. Soft tissues and the extent of space-occupying lesions are best visualised by computed tomography (CT) scan, which can also assess the thyroid, cricoid and arytenoid cartilages and the airway lumen in stable patients, or in those in whom the airway has been secured.[31] Although magnetic resonance imaging (MRI) has been used to image the upper airway, its use in acute airway obstruction is unproven.

GAS FLOW MEASUREMENT

Flow–volume loop measurement reveals characteristic patterns corresponding to different types and position of pathological lesions (Figure 25.3).[32]

MANAGEMENT

PREPARATION

Simplified algorithms to assist the management of partial and complete upper-airway obstruction are shown in Figures 25.4 and 25.5 and an appropriate management path should be chosen. Improvisation may be required for certain difficult problems. Special techniques in patients with suspected cervical spine instability are discussed elsewhere in this volume. Initial management follows:

1. Supplemental oxygen (100%) is immediately administered.
2. A choice of equipment for definitive airway control must be available and ready for use (see Table 25.3).
3. In adults IV access should be secured.

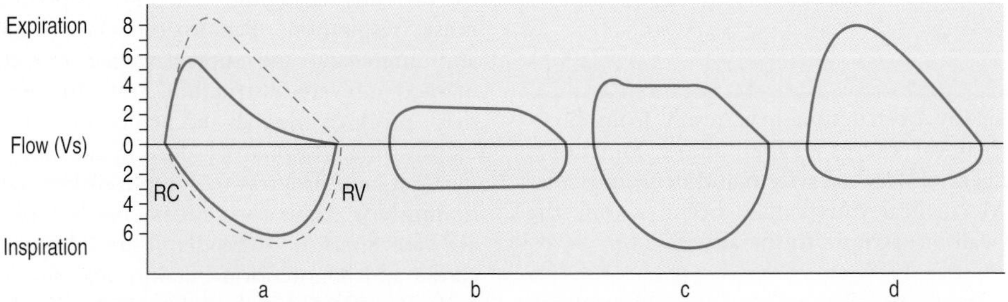

Figure 25.3 Flow–volume loops. Patterns resulting from different pathological lesions: (a) lower-airway obstruction (e.g. chronic obstructive pulmonary disease or asthma); (b) fixed, non-variable upper-airway obstruction (e.g. fibrous ring in trachea); (c) variable upper-airway obstruction, intrathoracic (e.g. tumour in the lower trachea); (d) variable upper-airway obstruction, extrathoracic (e.g. vocal cord tumour or paralysis).

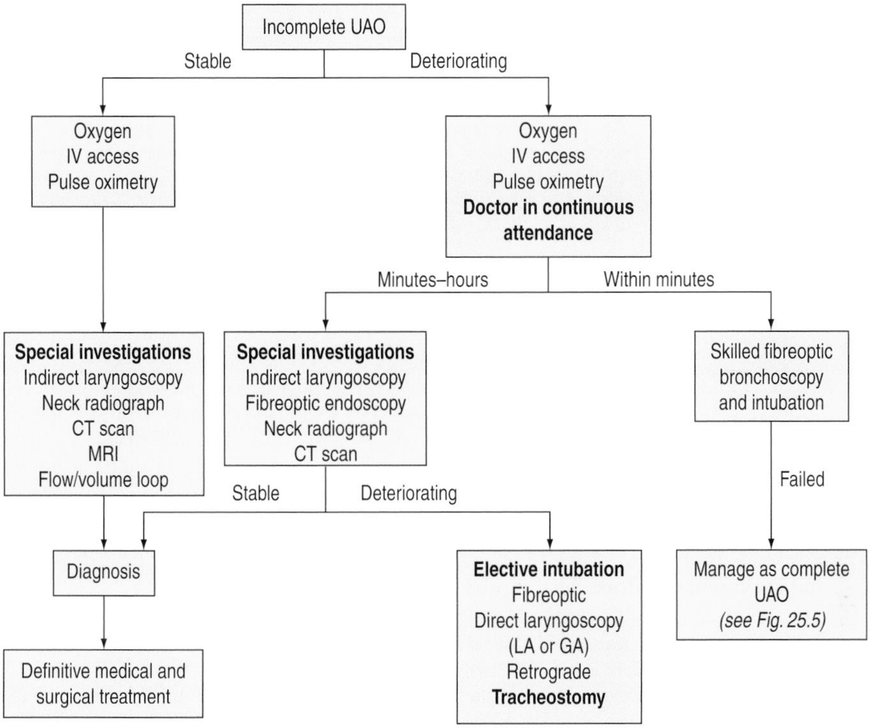

Figure 25.4 Management of partial upper-airway obstruction (UAO). i.v., intravenous; CT, computed tomography; MRI, magnetic resonance imaging; LA, local anaesthesia; GA, general anaesthesia.

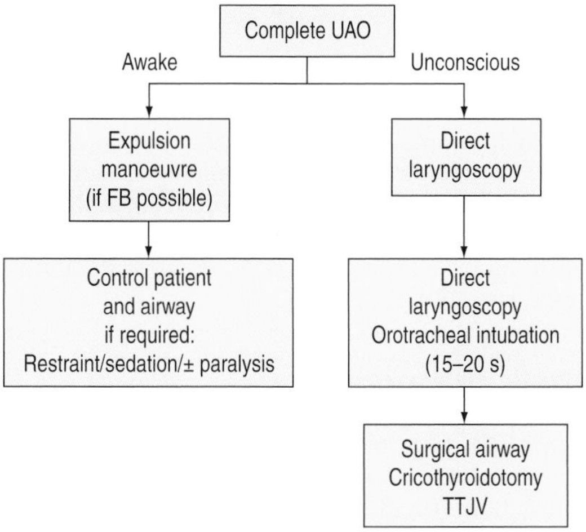

Figure 25.5 Management of complete upper-airway obstruction (UAO). Attempts at orotracheal intubation should not take longer than 10–20 s. FB, foreign body; TTJV, transtracheal jet ventilation.

4. Initiate continuous monitoring of vital signs and pulse oximetry.
5. Patient transport before securing the airway must be carefully considered as it is difficult to provide safe conditions during transport.[30]

AIRWAY MANAGEMENT TECHNIQUES IN AIRWAY OBSTRUCTION

THE UNCONSCIOUS PATIENT

If the upper airway is obstructed by the tongue and retropharyngeal tissues in an unconscious patient, airway patency is initially achieved by using standard airway manoeuvres[33] and oropharyngeal and nasopharyngeal airways. Definitive airway control should follow if consciousness does not immediately return.

ENDOTRACHEAL INTUBATION

1. *Direct laryngoscopic intubation* is the method of choice for the unconscious, apnoeic patient as it allows rapid evaluation of any supraglottic problem and immediate airway security. It can also be attempted in an awake patient after careful application of local anaesthesia. Although there is some risk of loss of the airway after local anaesthesia, complete loss of the airway *under general anaesthesia* is common and may be catastrophic.
2. *Awake fibreoptic intubation* in a spontaneously breathing patient is usually safe, but requires a skilled operator. The procedure will take 2–10 minutes or longer,[34] and urgency of the case must be assessed beforehand with this time frame in mind. Alternatives should be initiated if the obstruction progresses or if intubation fails after a reasonable time. The following

points may assist visualisation in acute upper-airway obstruction:

(a) The procedure is clearly explained to the patient.

(b) Good local anaesthesia and mucosal vasoconstrictors are important. Failure is most commonly due to excessive secretions and bleeding.

(c) If desired, the suction port of the fibrescope can be used to insufflate 100% oxygen or apply local anaesthetic. This also clears the fibrescope tip of secretions. Additional large-bore suction catheters may help.

3. *Blind nasotracheal intubation* provides a patent nasopharyngeal airway during the procedure, but is less useful when fibreoptic laryngoscopy is available.

Once endotracheal intubation is safely accomplished and confirmed, secure fixation of the endotracheal tube is mandatory. The patient's upper limbs may need to be restrained to avoid self-extubation.

SURGICAL AIRWAYS

A surgical airway is indicated when endotracheal intubation is not possible, or when an unstable cervical spine is threatened by available airway techniques. It is the last line of defence against hypoxia. In airway obstruction options include the following:

1. *Cricothyroidotomy* is the method of choice if severe or complete upper-airway obstruction exists.
2. *Percutaneous transtracheal jet ventilation.* The technique must *not* be used in complete upper-airway obstruction because expiratory obstruction can cause severe and potentially fatal barotrauma.
3. *Tracheostomy* in the emergency setting is rarely required, although surgical tracheostomy under local anaesthesia may be reasonable under some controlled conditions (see Figure 25.4).

COMMON CLINICAL CONDITIONS AND THEIR MANAGEMENT

FOREIGN-BODY OBSTRUCTION

Foreign-body obstruction is the most common cause of acute airway obstruction. The elderly, especially those in institutions, are at risk. The use of dentures, alcohol and depressant drugs increases risk. Fatal food asphyxiation or 'café coronary' should be considered in any acute respiratory arrest where the victim cannot be ventilated.[35]

Patients who are still able to cough or speak clearly should be given the opportunity to expel the foreign body spontaneously. If not, expulsion of the foreign body can be attempted with one or a combination of chest thrusts, abdominal thrusts (Heimlich manoeuvre[29]) or back blows applied in rapid sequence in the most convenient order.[33] The abdominal thrust is performed from behind: the rescuer encircles his or her arms around the victim, placing the thumb of one fist between the umbilicus and xiphisternum. The fist is gripped by the other hand, and an inward, upward thrust is applied. Chest thrusts are similar (rescuer's arms should encircle the chest, and a fist placed over midsternum) and are convenient for use in pregnancy and obesity. Unwanted effects, such as vomiting, aspiration, fractured ribs, barotrauma and ruptured organs, have been reported. Extract *visible* solid material with a finger sweep only in unconscious patients.[33] If these manoeuvres fail, management immediately proceeds as shown in Figures 25.4 and 25.5. If cardiac arrest occurs, proceed with cardiopulmonary resuscitation.

EXTRINSIC AIRWAY COMPRESSION

Extrinsic space-occupying lesions can cause upper-airway obstruction. Compression from haematomas may be associated with trauma, neck surgery, central venous catheterisation, anticoagulants and congenital or acquired coagulopathies. Haematomas following surgery should immediately be evacuated by removing skin and subcutaneous sutures. If this fails, an artificial airway must be secured immediately. In patients with coagulation abnormalities, intubation is preferred over a surgical airway. Most haematomas secondary to coagulopathy do not require surgical intervention, and resolve with conservative therapy (i.e. vitamin K and blood component therapy).

Partial airway obstruction caused by retropharyngeal abscess is best managed by drainage under local anaesthesia. Gentle fibreoptic examination and intubation or direct laryngoscopy and intubation in the lateral, head-down position are favored by some.[30] Risks are related to inadvertent rupture of the abscess, with subsequent flooding of the airway.

Ludwig's angina is a mixed infection of the floor of the mouth resulting in an inflammatory mass in the space between the tongue and the muscles and anterior neck fascia. The supraglottic airway is compressed and becomes narrowed.[36] Direct laryngoscopy is difficult, as the tongue cannot be anteriorly displaced. Awake fibreoptic-guided intubation or a surgical airway, along with antibiotic therapy, is required.

INTRINSIC AIRWAY COMPRESSION

Burn inhalation and ingestion injury

Patients with large burn area (more than 40%), or with severe facial burns or inhalation injury (soot in the nostrils, burns of the tongue and pharynx, stridor or hoarseness) are at risk pf developing progressive supraglottic oedema, usually within 24–48 hours. Such patients usually require early prophylactic tracheal intubation. If not prophylactically intubated, subsequent need for tracheal intubation can best be decided by frequent (2–4-hourly), repeated awake fibreoptic laryngoscopy as well as regular charting of known signs and symptoms of obstruction.[37] Careful inspection by direct laryngoscopy is an alternative to fibreoptic laryngoscopy. Ingestion of hot fluids or corrosive agents can also cause delayed oedema and airway swelling and should be managed similarly.[38]

Adult epiglottitis

Epiglottitis is an uncommon but increasingly recognised infectious disease in adults.[39] It involves the epiglottis and supraglottic larynx, causing swelling with consequent airway obstruction. *Haemophilus influenzae, H. parainfluenzae, Streptococcus pneumoniae,* haemolytic streptococci and *Staphylococcus aureus* are common causative organisms. Reported mortality varies in adults (0%–7%), due to difficult diagnosis and non-standardised treatment.[40] Clinical features are sudden onset of sore throat (pain often greater than suggested by clinical findings), muffled voice, dysphagia, stridor, dyspnoea and respiratory distress. Systemic toxaemia is common. Gentle indirect laryngoscopy, fibreoptic laryngoscopy or lateral neck X-ray confirms the diagnosis.

Airway management is controversial.[39–41] Some experts recommend securing a definitive airway on presentation while others suggest close observation in ICU. There are, however, reports of sudden obstruction and death with the latter approach.[40] Onset of dyspnoea is an important sign predicting the need for intubation. Both tracheal intubation and tracheostomy are acceptable, but tracheal intubation may result in better long-term outcome. Prior to securing the airway, patient positioning is important, and changing from a sitting to supine position may induce complete obstruction. In more stable patients, awake fibreoptic intubation is preferable if a skilled operator is available. Endotracheal intubation following gaseous induction is recommended by some authorities, but complete obstruction can occur, even when this procedure is undertaken by a skilled anaesthetist.[41] A skilled assistant, scrubbed and ready to secure a surgical airway, may prevent disaster. Rapid-sequence induction using muscle relaxants is dangerous and should be avoided. Tracheostomy under local anaesthesia is a safe alternative.

Antibiotics are administered as soon as the diagnosis is established. Cefotaxime 2 g IV 6-hourly or ampicillin 1–2 g IV 6-hourly plus chloramphenicol 50 mg/kg per day are empiric regimens; however, patient factors, local bacterial sensitivities and cultures of epiglottal swabs and blood may influence the antibiotic choice. Supportive care includes adequate sedation and tracheobronchial toilet. Abscesses should be surgically drained. There is no good evidence supporting the use of steroids.

Angioedema

Allergic responses involving the upper airway may be localised or part of a systemic anaphylactic reaction. Angioedema is characterised by subepithelial swelling. Angioedema of the lips, supraglottis, glottis and infraglottis may result in airway obstruction. The systemic reaction consists of variable combinations of urticaria (79%), bronchospasm (70%), shock, cardiovascular collapse and abdominal pain.[42] Common causative agents are Hymenoptera stings, shellfish ingestion and drugs. Treatment consists of immediately ensuring an adequate airway (see Figures 25.4 and 25.5), and administration of oxygen, adrenaline (epinephrine) and steroids. As it is likely to recur, the patient should be kept under close supervision and fully investigated.

Hereditary angioedema is a rare, inherited disorder of the complement system, caused by functionless or low levels of C1 esterase inhibitor.[43] Non-pruritic, non-painful angioedema involving skin and subcutaneous tissue occurs in various locations, including the upper airway.[44] Precipitating causes include stress, physical exertion and localised trauma (including dental or maxillofacial surgery and laryngoscopy). Acute attacks do not respond to adrenaline, antihistamines or corticosteroids. Management consists of establishing a secure airway and infusion of C1 esterase inhibitor concentrate (25 U/kg) which has an onset of action of 30–120 minutes.[44,45] If not available, fresh frozen plasma (2–4 units) may be considered. Stanozolol 1–4 mg daily or danazol 50–600 mg/day has been shown to be effective in decreasing frequency and severity of attacks.[46] Antifibrinolytic agents (e.g. tranexamic acid) are less effective. Danazol, C1 esterase inhibitor and fresh frozen plasma (2–4 units) can be used as preoperative prophylaxis.[45]

Angiotensin-converting enzyme inhibitor-related angioedema is increasingly seen and is possibly the result of reduced bradykinin metabolism.[47] Treatment focuses on airway support.

Postextubation laryngeal oedema

Laryngeal oedema following extubation occurs in about 20% of adults, but is not usually severe enough to precipitate reintubation.[48] Risk of severe oedema is increased after excessive airway manipulation, traumatic or prolonged tracheal intubation and if high cuff pressures are used. Treatment in adults is conservative, with close observation and humidified oxygen therapy. Nebulised plain epinephrine (1–2 ml 1:1000 solution diluted with 2 ml saline or undiluted 1:1000 solution 4–5 ml) or racemic epinephrine (0.25–0.5 ml 2.25% solution in 2–4 ml saline) has been used. Nebulisation may need to be repeated every 30–60 minutes. The prophylactic use of steroids to reduce post extubation laryngeal oedema remains controversial. Optimal dose, duration and target groups for prophylaxis have not yet been clearly defined. A recent study demonstrated that methylprednisolone 20 mg IV four-hourly started 12 hours prior to extubation (80 mg total dose) reduced the incidence of early re-intubation in patients intubated for more than 36 hours.[48]

POSTOBSTRUCTION PULMONARY OEDEMA

Postobstruction pulmonary oedema may occur in up to 11% of cases of airway obstruction.[49] Oedema appears to be caused by the markedly decreased intrathoracic and interstitial tissue pressure resulting from forced inspiration against a closed upper airway. The resulting increased hydrostatic gradient causes transudation of fluid from pulmonary capillaries to the interstitium. In addition, increased venous return may increase pulmonary blood flow and pressure, further worsening oedema. Hypoxia and the hyperadrenergic stress state may also affect capillary hydrostatic pressure, although pulmonary capillary occlusion pressure is often normal. The oedema usually occurs within minutes after the relief of the obstruction, but may be delayed up to 2.5 hours.[50] Management includes maintenance of airway patency, oxygen therapy, diuretics, morphine and fluid restriction. Application of continuous positive airways pressure or ventilation with PEEP may be necessary in severe cases. Pulmonary artery catheterisation need only be used for complicated cases.

REFERENCES

1. Practice Guidelines for Management of the Difficult Airway. An updated report by the American Society of Anesthesiologists Task Force on management of the difficult airway. *Anesthesiology* 2003; **98**:1269–77.
2. Henderson JJ, Popat MT, Latto IP *et al.* Difficult Airway Society guidelines for management of the unanticipated difficult intubation. *Anaesthesia* 2004; **59**: 675–94.
3. Brain AIJ. The laryngeal mask: a new concept in airway management. *Br J Anaesth* 1983; **55**: 801–5.
4. McNamee CJ, Meyns B, Pagliero KM. Flexible bronchoscopy via the laryngeal mask: a new technique. *Thorax* 1991; **46**: 141–2.
5. Brain AIJ, Verghese C. *The Intubating Laryngeal Mask (FasTrach) Instruction Manual.* San Deigo, CA: LMA North America; 1998.
6. Ferson DZ, Rosenblatt WH, Johansen MJ *et al.* Use of the intubating LMA-Fastrach in 254 patients with difficult-to-manage airways. *Anesthesiology* 2001; **95**:1175–81.
7. Frass M, Frenzer R, Rauscha F *et al.* Evaluation of esophageal tracheal combitube in cardiopulmonary resuscitation. *Crit Care Med* 1986; **15**: 609–11.
8. Konrad C, Schupfer G, Witlisbach M *et al.* Learning manual skills in anesthesiology: is there a recommended number of cases for anesthetic procedures? *Anesth Analg* 1998; **86**: 635–9.
9. Holzapfel L, Chastang C, Demingeon G *et al.* A randomized study assessing the systematic search for maxillary sinusitis in nasotracheally mechanically ventilated patients. Influence of nosocomial maxillary sinusitis on the occurrence of ventilator-associated pneumonia. *Am J Respir Crit Care Med* 1999; **159**: 695–701.
10. Hastings R, Vigil CA, Hanna R *et al.* Cervical spine movement during laryngoscopy with the Bullard, Macintosh, and Miller laryngoscopes. *Anesthesiology* 1995; **82**: 859–69.
11. Giudice JC, Komansky H, Gordon R *et al.* Acute upper airway obstruction – fibreoptic bronchoscopy in diagnosis and therapy. *Crit Care Med* 1981; **9**: 878–9.
12. Ovassapian A. Fibreoptic assisted airway management. *Acta Anaesthesiol Scand* 1997; **110** (Suppl): 46–7.
13. Bapat P. Use of a fibreoptic bronchoscope to change endotracheal tubes. *Anesthesiology* 1997; **86**: 509.
14. Reilly PM, Schapiro MB, Malcynski JT. Percutaneous dilation tracheostomy under the microscope: justification for intra-procedural bronchoscopy? *Intens Care Med* 1999; **25**: 3–4.
15. McNamara RM. Retrograde intubation of the trachea. *Ann Emerg Med* 1987; **16**: 680–2.
16. Tinker JH, Dull DL, Caplan RA. Role of monitoring devices in prevention of anesthetic mishaps: a closed claim analysis. *Anesthesiology* 1989; **71**: 541.
17. Benumof JL, Scheller MS. The importance of transtracheal jet ventilation in the management of the difficult airway. *Anesthesiology* 1989; **71**: 769–78.
18. Kress TD, Balasubramaniam S. Cricothyroidotomy. *Ann Emerg Med* 1982; **11**: 197–201.
19. Pryor JP, Reilly PM, Schapiro MB. Surgical airway management in the intensive care unit. *Crit Care Clin* 2000; **16**: 473–88.
20. Delaney A, Bagshaw SM, Nalos M. Percutaneous dilatational tracheostomy versus surgical tracheostomy in critically ill patients: a systematic review and meta-analysis. *Crit Care* 2006; **10**: R55.
21. Silvester W, Goldsmith D, Uchino S *et al.* Percutaneous versus surgical tracheostomy: a randomized controlled study with long-term follow-up. *Crit Care Med* 2006; **34**: 2145–52.
22. Ciaglia P, Firsching R, Syniec C. Elective percutaneous dilatational tracheostomy. *Chest* 1985; **87**: 715–19.
23. Griggs WM, Worthley LIG, Gilligan JE *et al.* A simple percutaneous tracheostomy technique. *Surg Gynecol Obstet* 1990; **170**: 543–5.
24. Anon JM, Escuela MP, Gomez V *et al.* Use of percutaneous tracheostomy in intensive care units in Spain. Results of a national survey. *Intens Care Med* 2004; **30**: 1212–5.
25. Nates JL, Cooper DJ, Myles PS *et al.* Percutaneous tracheostomy in critically ill patients: a prospective, randomized comparison of two techniques. *Crit Care Med* 2000; **28**: 3734–9.
26. Gross JB, Hartigan M, Schaffer DW. A suitable substitute for 4% cocaine before blind nasotracheal intubation: 3% lidocaine–0.25% phenylephrine nasal spray. *Anesth Analg* 1984; **63**: 915–18.
27. Mallampatti SR, Gugino LD, Desai SP *et al.* A clinical sign to predict difficult tracheal intubation: a prospective study. *Can J Anaesth* 1985; **32**: 429–34.
28. Cormack RS, Lehane J. Difficult tracheal intubation in obstetrics. *Anaesthesia* 1984; **39**: 1105–11.
29. Heimlich HJ. A life saving maneuver to prevent food-choking. *JAMA* 1975; **234**: 398–401.
30. Bogdonoff DL, Stone DJ. Emergency management of the airway outside the emergency room. *Can J Anaesth* 1992; **39**: 1069–89.
31. Angood PB, Attia EL, Brown RA *et al.* Extrinsic civilian trauma to the larynx and cervical trachea – important predictors of long term morbidity. *J Trauma* 1986; **26**: 869–73.

32. Miller RD, Hyatt RE. Evaluation of obstructing lesions of the trachea and larynx by flow volume loops. *Am Rev Respir Dis* 1973; **108**: 475–81.
33. ECC Committee, Subcommittees and Task Forces of the American Heart Association. 2005 American Heart Association Guidelines for Cardiopulmonary Resuscitation and Emergency Cardiovascular Care. *Circulation* 2005; **112** (Suppl 1): IV1–203.
34. Afilalo M, Guttman A, Stern E *et al.* Fibreoptic intubation in the emergency department: a case series. *J Emerg Med* 1993; **11**: 387–91.
35. Mittleman RE, Wetli CV. The fatal café coronary: foreign body airway obstruction. *JAMA* 1982; **247**: 1285–8.
36. Barakate MS, Jensen MJ, Hemli JM *et al.* Ludwig's angina: report of a case and review of management issues. *Ann Otol Rhinol Laryngol* 2001; **110**: 453–6.
37. Muehlberger T, Kunar D, Munster A *et al.* Efficacy of fibreoptic laryngoscopy in the diagnosis of inhalation injuries. *Arch Otolaryngol Head Neck Surg* 1998; **124**: 1003–7.
38. Joynt GM, Ho KM, Gomersall CD. Delayed upper airway obstruction. A life-threatening complication of Dettol poisoning. *Anaesthesia* 1997; **52**: 261–3.
39. Park KW, Darvish A, Lowenstein E. Airway management for adult patients with acute epiglottitis: a 12-year experience at an academic medical center (1984–1995). *Anesthesiology* 1998; **88**: 254–61.
40. Mayo-Smith M. Fatal respiratory arrest in adult epiglottitis in the intensive care unit. *Chest* 1993; **104**: 964–5.
41. Ames WA, Ward VM, Tranter RM *et al.* Adult epiglottitis: an under-recognized, life-threatening condition. *Br J Anaesth* 2000; **85**: 795–7.
42. Corren J, Schocket AL. Anaphylaxis: a preventable emergency. *Postgrad Med* 1990; **87**: 167–78.
43. Donaldson VH, Evans RR. A biochemical abnormality in hereditary angioneurotic edema: absence of serum inhibitor of C'1-esterase. *Am J Med* 1963; **35**: 37–44.
44. Joynt GM, Abdullah V, Wormald PJ. Hereditary angioedema: report of a case. *Ear Nose Throat J* 2001; **80**: 321–4.
45. Bork K, Barnstedt SE. Treatment of 193 episodes of laryngeal edema with C1 inhibitor concentrate in patients with hereditary angioedema. *Arch Intern Med* 2001; **161**: 714–18.
46. Niels JF, Weiler JM. C1 esterase inhibitor deficiency, airway compromise, and anesthesia. *Anesth Analg* 1998; **87**: 480–8.
47. Agostoni A, Cicardi M, Cugno M *et al.* Angioedema due to angiotensin-converting enzyme inhibitors. *Immunopharmacology* 1999; **44**: 21–5.
48. François B, Bellissant E, Gissot V *et al.* 12-h pretreatment with methylprednisolone versus placebo for prevention of postextubation laryngeal oedema: a randomised double-blind trial. *Lancet* 2007; **369**: 1083–9.
49. Tami TA, Chu F, Wildes TO *et al.* Pulmonary edema and acute upper airway obstruction. *Laryngoscope* 1986; **96**: 506–9.
50. Willms D, Shure D. Pulmonary edema due to upper airway obstruction in adults. *Chest* 1988; **94**: 1090–2.

26

Acute respiratory failure in chronic obstructive pulmonary disease

Matthew T Naughton and David V Tuxen

The terms 'chronic obstructive pulmonary or airways disease' (COPD or COAD) are applied to patients with chronic bronchitis and/or emphysema. COPD affects 5% of the adult population, is the fifth most common cause of death worldwide and is the only major cause of death that is increasing in prevalence.[1] Despite this, when an acute deterioration occurs, most precipitating factors are reversible and the outcome is usually good.[2] This justifies aggressive management in the majority of patients.

AETIOLOGY

The causes of COPD can be divided into environmental and host factors. Environmental factors include tobacco smoke, air pollution, indoor fumes (e.g. indoor cooking with solid biomass fuel) and poor socioeconomic status. The biggest single factor in over 95% of patients with COPD is tobacco smoking (Figure 26.1). However, only approximately 15% of smokers develop COPD. Marijuana smoking may cause premature and quite advanced bullous emphysema compared with tobacco smokers due to extremely hot and toxic inhaled smoke held at peak inspiration for prolonged periods of time.[3] Host factors are the balance between circulating proteases and antiproteases (e.g. alpha-1 antitrypsin deficiency) and the intake of antioxidant vitamins (A, C, E).[4]

PATHOPHYSIOLOGY

Reduced expiratory airflow in COPD is due to both increased airway resistance and reduced lung elastic recoil. Airway resistance is increased by mucosal oedema and hypertrophy, secretions, bronchospasm, airway tortuosity and airflow turbulence and loss of lung parenchymal elastic tissues that normally support the small airways. Loss of lung elastic recoil pressure is due both to loss of lung elastin and loss of alveolar surface tension from alveolar wall destruction.

Reduced lung elastic recoil decreases expiratory airflow by reducing the alveolar pressure driving expiratory airflow and by reducing the intraluminal airway pressure, which normally distends small airways during expiration. Forced expiration increases alveolar driving pressure but also causes dynamic airway compression resulting in no improvement or sometimes reduction in expiratory airflow. These factors are present in varying proportions, depending on the degree of chronic bronchitis and emphysema and the individual patient.

Airflow limitation results in prolonged expiration, pulmonary hyperinflation, inspiratory muscle disadvantage, increased work of breathing and the sensation of dyspnoea. All these factors are worsened during an exacerbation of COPD.

Pulmonary hyperinflation has both static and dynamic components. The static component remains at the end of an expiratory period long enough for all expiratory airflow to cease (30–120 s), enabling the lungs and chest wall to reach their static functional residual capacity (FRC). This component of hyperinflation is due to loss of parenchymal elastic recoil, chest wall adaptation[5] and airway closure that occurs throughout expiration. Dynamic pulmonary hyperinflation is the further increase in hyperinflation due to slow expiratory airflow not allowing completion of expiration before the arrival of the next breath. The extent of dynamic hyperinflation depends on the severity of airflow obstruction, the amount inspired (tidal volume) and the expiratory time.[6] Thus, the degree of hyperinflation may vary in a patient with changes in minute ventilation due to changes in CO_2 production (depending on exercise, diet or the metabolic response to illness) or dead space, as well as with changes in airflow obstruction during an exacerbation.

Chest wall hyperinflation leads to suboptimal muscle length–tension relationships and mechanical disadvantage, thereby predisposing patients to respiratory muscle fatigue, as the work of breathing increases, particularly if associated with myopathic situations (steroids, electrolyte disturbances). Minor reductions in lung function due to infection, mild cardiac failure or atelectasis increase the work of breathing, due to both increases in respiratory impedance and increases in dead space. With acute changes in workload, rapid decompensation with ventilatory failure and acute hypercapnia may occur.

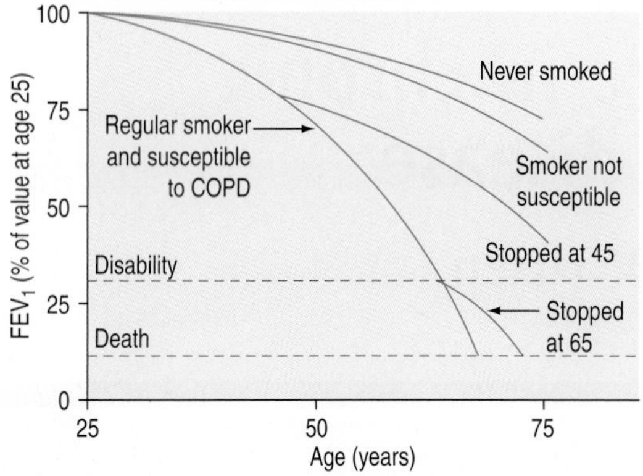

Figure 26.1 Decline in lung function with age in different smoking categories. FEV_1, forced expiratory volume in 1 second; COPD, chronic obstructive pulmonary disease.

Central respiratory drive may also be impaired, or poorly responsive to physiological triggers – hypoxaemia or hypercapnia – and lead to chronic hypercapnia. This may occur in the setting of sleep (i.e. obstructive sleep apnoea), obesity or drugs (sedatives, antiepileptics, alcohol).

Hypoxia and vascular wall changes lead to pulmonary vasoconstriction, pulmonary hypertension, cor pulmonale, V/Q mismatching and the development of shunts.

CHRONIC BRONCHITIS OR EMPHYSEMA?

The value of labelling patients as chronic bronchitis or emphysema is uncertain as the two disease processes usually coexist and the principles of management are similar. Five pathophysiologic processes may be present to varying degrees in each patient with COPD: (1) inflammatory airway narrowing (bronchiolitis); (2) loss of connective tissues tethering airways; (3) loss of alveoli and capillaries; (4) hyperinflation; and (5) increased pulmonary vascular resistance. Early/mild COPD tends to be dominated by bronchiolitis with a minimal component of emphysema (Figure 26.2), whereas when COPD becomes severe, the reverse is true. However, recognition that COPD is dominated by one of these patterns is helpful with regard to clinical pattern and prognosis.

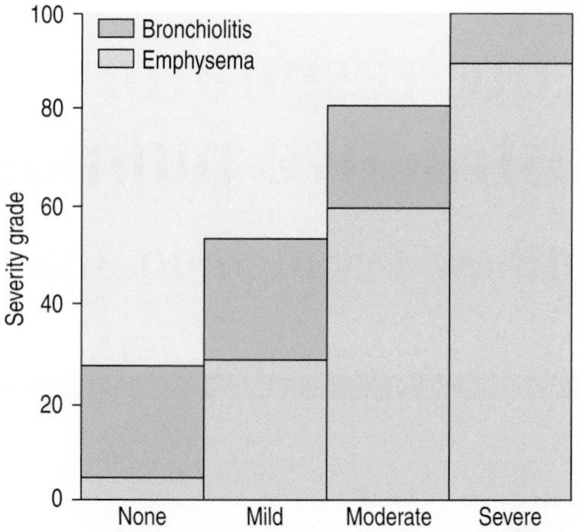

Figure 26.2 Proportional contributions of bronchiolitis and emphysema at different levels of severity of lung disease.

CLINICAL FEATURES OF ACUTE RESPIRATORY FAILURE IN COPD

Acute respiratory failure (ARF) in COPD can present with two distinct clinical patterns[7] (Table 26.1).

Table 26.1 Clinical differences between normocapnic and hypercapnic chronic obstructive pulmonary disease

Normocapnic ($Paco_2$ 35–45 mmHg)	Hypercapnic ($Paco_2$ > 45 mmHg)
Emphysema > chronic bronchitis	Chronic bronchitis > emphysema
Thin	Obese
Pursed-lip breathing	Central nervous system depression: consider the role of oxygen therapy
Accessory muscle use	Alcohol, sedatives, analgesics
Hyperinflated	Sleep-related hypoventilation
Right heart failure late	Right heart failure early

PRECIPITANTS OF ACUTE RESPIRATORY FAILURE

In approximately 50% of patients, there is an infective cause, in 25% heart failure and in the remaining 25% retained secretions, air pollution, coexistent medical problems (e.g. pulmonary embolus, medication compliance or side-effects) or no cause can be identified[8] (Table 26.2).

The most common bacterial isolates are *Streptococcus pneumoniae* and *Haemophilus influenzae* in 80% of exacerbations.[9] *S. viridans*,[10] *Moraxella* (previously *Branhamella*) *catarrhalis*,[11] *Mycoplasma pneumoniae*[12] and *Pseudomonas aeruginosa* may also be found. Viruses can be isolated in 20–30% of exacerbations[13] and include rhinovirus, influenza and parainfluenza viruses, coronaviruses and occasionally adenovirus, and respiratory syncytial virus. Whether these organisms are pathogens or colonisers is often unclear.

PNEUMONIA

Pneumonia has been estimated to account for 20% of presentations requiring mechanical ventilation.[13] It is most commonly caused by *S. pneumoniae* and *H. influenzae* but *Mycoplasma*, *Legionella*, enteric Gram-negatives and viruses are occasional causes.

Table 26.2 Precipitants of acute respiratory failure in chronic obstructive pulmonary disease

Infective (including aspiration)
Left ventricular failure (systolic and diastolic failure)
Sputum retention (postoperative, traumatic)
Pulmonary embolism
Pneumothoraces and bullae
Uncontrolled oxygen
Sedation
Medication – non-compliance or side-effects
Nutritional (K, PO_4, Mg deficiency, CHO excess)
Sleep apnoea

LEFT VENTRICULAR FAILURE

Left ventricular (LV) systolic failure may result from coexisting ischaemic heart disease, fluid overload, tachyarrhythmias or biventricular failure secondary to cor pulmonale. LV diastolic failure occurs commonly and is precipitated by hypoxaemia, tachycardia,[14] pericardial constraint due to intrinsic positive end-expiratory pressure ($PEEP_i$) or right ventricular (RV) dilation. Increased work of breathing related to COPD will also increase by up to 10-fold the amount of blood flow to the respiratory pump muscles,[15] thereby causing an increased demand upon the overall cardiac output. In patients with borderline cardiac status, this may precipitate heart failure. The components of right and LV failure can be accurately distinguished by Doppler echocardiography. Pulmonary congestion can be difficult to diagnose because of the abnormal breath sounds and chest X-ray appearance which are commonly present in COPD. In a recent publication, 51% of patients with acute exacerbation of COPD had echocardiographic evidence of left heart failure (systolic 11%, diastolic 32%, systolic and diastolic 7%).[16]

UNCONTROLLED OXYGEN ADMINISTRATION

This may precipitate acute hypercapnia in patients with more severe COPD, due to: (1) shunting blood to low-$\dot{V}/\dot{Q}$ lung units and increasing dead space; (2) loss of hypoxic drive; (3) dissociation of CO_2 from Hb molecule (Haldane effect); and (4) anxiolysis and reduction in tachypnoea.

DIAGNOSIS AND ASSESSMENT

DIAGNOSIS

The clinical examination findings of COPD depend upon severity.

In mild stable disease (e.g. forced expiratory volume in 1 second (FEV_1) 50–70% predicted normal), an expiratory wheeze on forced expiration and mild exertional dyspnoea may be the only symptoms.

In moderate-severity COPD (e.g. FEV_1 30–50% predicted normal), modest to severe exertional dyspnoea is associated with clinical signs of hyperinflation (ptosed upper border of liver beyond the level of nipple and loss of cardiac percussion) and signs of increased work of breathing (use of accessory muscles and tracheal tug).

In severe stable COPD (e.g. $FEV_1 < 30\%$ predicted normal), marked accessory muscle use is associated with tachypnoea at rest, pursed-lip breathing, hypoxaemia and signs of pulmonary hypertension (RV heave, loud and palpable pulmonary second sound and elevated a-wave in jugular venous pressure (JVP)) and cor pulmonale (elevated JVP, hepatomegaly, ankle swelling).

In severe unstable COPD, there is marked tachypnoea at rest, hypoxaemia and tachycardia, and, in some, signs of hypercapnia (dilated cutaneous veins, blurred vision, headaches, obtunded mentation, confusion).

Clinical examination may also identify associated medical conditions that might have precipitated the exacerbation such as crackles and bronchial breathing due to infection, crackles and cardiomegaly related to heart failure or mediastinal shift related to a pneumothorax.

Basic investigations such as spirometry are very useful in confirming a clinical diagnosis and determining severity of disease. The severity of COPD may be best judged by the reduction in FEV_1 compared with predicted values. Vital capacity (VC) is initially normal and decreases later in the course of the disease, but to a lesser degree than the FEV_1.

An FEV_1/VC ratio $< 70\%$ with an FEV_1 of 50–80% predicted normal without a bronchodilator response usually indicates mild COPD. A significant bronchodilator response, which implies asthma, is regarded as a 12% or greater increase and 200 ml increase in either FEV_1 or VC. An FEV_1 30–50% predicted normal indicates moderately severe COPD and $FEV_1 < 30\%$ predicted normal indicates severe COPD.

Although the diagnosis may be based on spirometry alone, further lung function testing may be useful to characterise the disease. Flow–volume curves demonstrate reduced expiratory flow rates at various lung volumes and show the characteristic concave expiratory flow pattern. Lung volumes measured by either helium dilution or plethysmography show elevated total lung capacity, FRC and residual volume. Characteristically, the residual volume/total lung capacity ratio is $>40\%$ in COPD and represents intrathoracic gas trapping. The total lung carbon monoxide (TLCO) uptake is a measurement of alveolar surface area and its reduction approximates the amount of emphysema present (usually $<80\%$ predicted normal).

A chest X-ray will commonly show hyperinflated lung fields, as suggested by 10 ribs visible posteriorly, six ribs visible anteriorly or large airspace anterior to heart ($> 1/3$ of the length of the sternum), flattened diaphragms (best seen on lateral chest X-ray) and a paucity of lung markings. Pulmonary hypertension is manifest by enlarged proximal and attenuated distal vascular markings and by RV and atrial enlargement. Lung bullae may be evident.

A high-resolution computed tomographic (CT) scan of the chest (1–2-mm slices) can demonstrate characteristic appearance and regional distribution of emphysema. It can also assess for coexistent bronchiectasis, LV failure[17] and pulmonary fibrosis. Such scans are less sensitive than standard chest CT scans (1-cm slice) for detecting pulmonary lesions (e.g. neoplasms). Nuclear ventilation perfusion scans can also provide a characteristic appearance of COPD.

An electrocardiogram (ECG) is commonly normal but may show features of right atrial or RV hypertrophy and RV strain, including P pulmonale, right-axis deviation, dominant R-waves in V1–2, right bundle-branch block, ST depression and T-wave flattening or inversion in V1–3. These changes may be chronic or may develop acutely if there is significant increase in pulmonary vascular resistance during the illness. The ECG may also show coexistent ischaemic heart disease, tachycardia and atrial fibrillation. Occasionally, continuous ECG monitoring is required to identify transient arrhythmias, which may also precipitate acute deterioration. Plasma brain natriuretic peptide (BNP) levels may also assist in the diagnosis of heart failure (elevated BNP) from pulmonary causes (low BNP) in patients under 70 years free of renal impairment.

DIFFERENTIAL DIAGNOSIS

The history of *chronic asthma* is one of long-term dyspnoea, wheeze and cough, usually at night or upon exercise, beginning in childhood with clear-cut precipitating agents (e.g. weather, dust, pets, drugs) and a favourable response to either steroids or inhaled β_2-agonists. Late-onset asthma (>40 years of age) is not uncommon and is often associated with recurrent gastro-oesophageal reflux. In both forms of asthma, TLCO is normal. There is usually a bronchodilator response in the FEV_1 if the patient has unstable asthma. In patients in whom asthma is considered but lung function tests are normal, the FEV_1 response to an inhalational challenge (e.g. methacholine or hypertonic saline) may assist in discriminating asthma from other causes of dyspnoea.

Bronchiolitis obliterans is a condition which presents as a fixed airflow obstruction following a viral illness, inhalation of toxic fumes, following bone marrow or heart/lung transplantation, or related to drugs (e.g. penicillamine). It generally begins as a cough some weeks after insult and insidious onset of dyspnoea. There is a broad spectrum of radiological appearances from normal to reticulonodular to diffuse nodular. Lung tissue via bronchoscopy or by thoracoscopy is required for diagnosis. Histologically, there is a characteristic chronic bronchiolar inflammation appearance, and if granulation tissue extends into the alveoli, it is referred to as bronchiolitis obliterans or organising pneumonia. Removal of the offending agent and instigation of steroids are generally associated with a favourable prognosis.

Bronchiectasis is often associated with fixed mild to moderate airflow obstruction. A chronic productive cough (daily for 2 consecutive years) is characteristic. Clinical features such as clubbing, localised pulmonary crackles and a characteristic appearance on high-resolution CT, with dilated or plugged small airways at least twice the size of accompanying blood vessel, assist in the diagnosis.

Chronic heart failure (CHF) may be a differential diagnosis of COPD, or simply coexist, as both disorders are common in smokers.[14,16] Orthopnoea and paroxysmal nocturnal dyspnoea are features which correlate with heart failure severity. A past history of myocardial ischaemia or atrial fibrillation should alert one to the possibility of heart failure. An echocardiogram and high-resolution CT (looking for shift in interstitial oedema with changes in posture from supine to prone)[17] are sensitive markers of CHF.

DIAGNOSIS OF RESPIRATORY FAILURE

An exacerbation of COPD is usually clinically obvious. However, it is important to diagnose the extent of deterioration. The following may be useful.

BLOOD GASES

Blood gases are mandatory to assess hypoxia, hypercapnia and acid–base status. Chronic hypercapnia may be recognised by a bicarbonate level >30 mmol/l and a base excess >4 mmol/l indicating renal compensation. However, other causes of a high serum bicarbonate need to be excluded (e.g. diuretic therapy, high-dose steroids or high-volume gastric fluid loss) or chronic hypercapnia may be incorrectly assumed and the severity of COPD overestimated. Renal compensation for chronic hypercapnia will increase the serum bicarbonate by approximately 4 mmol/l for each 10 mmHg (1.33 kPa) of chronic $Pa\text{CO}_2$ rise above 40 mmHg (5.3 kPa), in order to return pH to the low-normal range. Irrespective of the COPD patient's usual $Pa\text{CO}_2$ level, an acute increase in $Pa\text{CO}_2$ leads to a decreased arterial pH. This indicates that compensatory mechanisms are exhausted and there is an increased risk of respiratory collapse.

NON-VENTILATORY MANAGEMENT

OXYGEN THERAPY

Oxygen given by low-flow intranasal cannulae or 24–35% Venturi mask should be titrated to achieve a saturation ($Sp\text{O}_2$) of 90 ± 2% as these levels will avoid significant increases in $Pa\text{CO}_2$ in the majority of COPD patients with ARF. Increases in $Pa\text{CO}_2$ are most common in patients with initial $Pa\text{CO}_2$ >50 mmHg and pH <7.35.[18] If the rise in

$Pa\text{CO}_2$ is excessive (>10 mmHg or 1.33 kPa), then $F\text{IO}_2$ should be reduced, titrating $Sp\text{O}_2$ to 2–3% below the previous value, and arterial blood gases should be repeated. If no $Pa\text{CO}_2$ rise occurs with oxygen therapy, then a higher $Sp\text{O}_2$ may be targeted with repeat blood gases.

Inadequate reversal of hypoxia (e.g. $Sp\text{O}_2 < 85\%$) is suggestive of an additional problem such as pneumonia, pulmonary oedema or embolus, or a pneumothorax. Investigation of this should commence and a higher O_2 delivery system should be used (see Chapter 24). Although high levels of O_2 should be avoided, reversal of hypoxia is important and O_2 should not be withheld in the presence of hypercapnia, or withdrawn if it worsens.

BRONCHODILATORS

Bronchodilators are routinely given in all acute exacerbations of COPD because a small reversible component of airflow obstruction is common, and bronchodilators improve mucociliary clearance of secretions.[19] However, a large meta-analysis of 22 large randomised controlled long-term trials of ambulatory COPD patients involving either anticholinergics and/or β_2 agonists (short- and long-acting) over 3–60 months indicates that anticholinergics are more favourable than placebo in terms of acute exacerbations, hospitalisations and respiratory deaths.[20] There were no favourable advantages with β_2-agonists compared with placebo for acute exacerbations or hospitalisations, and placebo was better than β_2-agonists in terms of respiratory death.[20]

ANTICHOLINERGIC AGENTS

Anticholinergic agents, such as ipratropium bromide, have been shown to have a similar or greater bronchodilator action than β-agonists in COPD,[1,21,22] and also to have fewer side-effects and no tachyphylaxis. Anticholinergic agents should be used routinely in COPD with ARF and many now believe them to be the agent of first choice.[1] An ipratropium bromide nebule of 0.5 mg in 2 ml should be nebulised initially 2-hourly, then every 4–6 hours. Long-term use of ipratropium bromide has been shown to reduce the incidence of exacerbations[23] and is therefore recommended for chronic use in ambulatory COPD. Long-acting anticholinergics (e.g. tiotropium) offer potential of once-daily dosing.

NEBULISED β_2-AGONISTS

Nebulised β-agonists are also effective bronchodilators in COPD,[21,22] although they may cause tachycardia, tremor, mild reductions in potassium and $Pa\text{CO}_2$ (due to pulmonary vasodilatation) and tachyphylaxis. Nebulised β-agonists (e.g. salbutamol, terbutaline or fenoterol) given 2–4-hourly should be used routinely in combination with ipratropium. This combination has been shown to be more effective than either agent alone.[1] Parenteral sympathomimetic agents are rarely indicated and not recommended for routine use. In stable patients, long-term use of β-agonists may improve symptoms of dyspnoea, particularly in the subgroup of COPD with an objective bronchodilator response. Long-acting β-agonists may also have a beneficial effect on symptoms, quality of life and exercise capacity in COPD.[24]

AMINOPHYLLINE

Aminophylline is a weak bronchodilator in COPD. It improves diaphragm contractility,[25] stimulates respiratory drive,[26] improves mucociliary transport[27] and right heart function,[28] is anti-inflammatory[29] and is a weak diuretic. Some studies have shown no benefit and significant side-effects,[30] whereas others have shown small benefit[31] instable COPD. Theophylline has a number of additional effects that may also be of benefit in COPD, although the clinical importance of these is not yet established. For an exacerbation, aminophylline (loading dose 5–6 mg/kg IV over 30 min, followed by an infusion of 0.5 mg/kg per h) is commonly also given, despite doubt about its overall benefit. Serum theophylline levels must be monitored regularly to reduce risk of toxicity. The low therapeutic range should be targeted (55–85 mmol/l) for the best ratio of effect to side-effect.[32] The high therapeutic range (85–110 mmol/l) has little additional benefit and a significant increase in side-effects,[32] but is thought necessary for diaphragm contractility and respiratory stimulation effects. There is some evidence in favour of theophylline use in the long-term management[33] of COPD but, due to its narrow therapeutic window, it should be used with caution.

STEROIDS

In acute exacerbations of COPD, short-term steroids have been shown to improve airflow obstruction,[34] including those patients requiring mechanical ventilation for COPD.[35] Doses similar to those for acute asthma should be used. Methylprednisolone 0.5 mg/kg, given 6-hourly for 72 h, was used in the study by Albert *et al.*,[34] demonstrating benefit in patients with an exacerbation of COPD. Current American Thoracic Society guidelines recommend the equivalent to oral prednisolone at 0.5 mg/kg body weight for up to 10 days, then ceasing; however, this will depend upon the response to treatment, and their premorbid use.[1] Steroids should be avoided if the deterioration is clearly due to bacterial pneumonia without bronchospasm.

Longer-term oral steroids in COPD are associated with a substantial increased risk of side-effects (osteoporosis, diabetes, peptic ulcer, myopathy, systemic hypertension, fluid retention, weight gain), which are likely to impair quality of life and precipitate readmission and are therefore not recommended.[1] A small group of patients (15%) may demonstrate a significant bronchodilator response; coexistent asthma is likely in these patients and longer-term high-dose (oral or inhaled) steroids may be necessary. In the majority of patients, long-term inhaled steroids do not improve lung function or survival; however, they do improve quality of life and reduce admissions and are therefore recommended as long-term treatment at low to medium dose.[1]

ANTIBIOTICS

Antibiotics have an accepted role in the treatment of infection-induced exacerbations of COPD. Amoxicillin is a suitable first-line agent against *Haemophilus influenzae* and *Streptococcus pneumoniae* for outpatient exacerbations.[36] Serious exacerbations requiring hospital admission require newer agents such as ciprofloxacin or a third-generation cephalosporin.[37] Antibiotics for pneumonia are discussed elsewhere in this volume.

SECRETION CLEARANCE TECHNIQUES

Clearance of lower respiratory secretions is of crucial importance.

CHEST PHYSIOTHERAPY

Chest physiotherapy should be initiated and regularly repeated as both a curative and preventive measure. Encouragement of coughing and deep breathing are the two most important factors. 'Bubble positive expiratory pressure (PEP)' is an inexpensive method of assisting sputum clearance in patients with retained secretions or those having difficulty expectorating.

NEBULISED MUCOLYTIC AGENTS

Nebulised mucolytic agents, such as acetylcysteine, continue to be proposed, although their benefit has never been established in acute exacerbations of COPD.[38] Oral mucolytics have been shown to reduce cough frequency and severity in stable COPD.[39]

OROPHARYNGEAL/NASOPHARYNGEAL SUCTIONING

Oropharyngeal/nasopharyngeal suctioning can be performed with or without a nasopharyngeal airway. It is desirable but uncommon for the suctioning catheter to enter the trachea; the technique is useful in clearing pharyngeal secretions, stimulating coughing and clearing lower respiratory secretions coughed only as far as the hypopharynx in patients with suppressed conscious states.

FIBREOPTIC BRONCHOSCOPY

Fibreoptic bronchoscopy is occasionally used in COPD with ARF. Although effective in clearing sputum, it is labour-intensive and may be poorly tolerated by a patient with marginal respiratory function. Indications are lobar consolidation, where sputum plug obstruction is suspected, for bronchoalveolar lavage to diagnose pneumonia or to assist difficult secretion clearance.

OTHER MEASURES

Other adjunctive measures are applicable to some patients.

HYDRATION, DIURETICS, DIGOXIN AND VASODILATORS

COPD patients are sensitive to changes in fluid status and intravenous hydration should be undertaken with care and minimised. Diuretics and digoxin are of benefit if LV failure is present. Even if evidence of LV failure is minimal, a trial of diuresis is worthwhile in patients refractory to usual treatment. Digoxin has been shown to improve LV function in patients with cor pulmonale.[40]

Diuretics will reduce fluid overload in cor pulmonale; however, care should be taken with severe pulmonary hypertension where a decrease in RV filling pressure may result in a low-output state. Digoxin is of no established benefit to RV function in cor pulmonale, where the primary problem is increased afterload.[41] Pulmonary hypertension is commonly present in severe COPD and is associated with a poor prognosis. In stable COPD pulmonary vasodilators may have acutely beneficial effects[42] but have not yet been shown to improve outcome.[43] In ARF, pulmonary hypertension invariably increases and may precipitate acute cor pulmonale. Although not clinically proven, pulmonary vasodilators have a rational basis in this setting. Numerous agents have been or are undergoing trials to reduce pulmonary hypertension in COPD. These agents include calcium channel blockers (e.g. nifedipine), endothelin receptor antagonists (e.g. bosentan), phosphodiesterase inhibitors (e.g. sildenafil) and prostacycline analogues (e.g. epoprostenil, iloprost and trepostinil).[42] Side-effects include systemic hypotension, tachycardia, worsening of hypoxia and failure to improve haemodynamics. A trial of vasodilators appears reasonable if cor pulmonale is present with ARF, provided that response to therapy is carefully monitored. The diagnosis and response to treatment of pulmonary hypertension may require a right heart catheter.

ANTICOAGULANTS

Subcutaneous heparin (e.g. 5000 units b.d.) is recommended as a prophylactic measure against venous thromboembolism. There is no evidence for warfarinisation in COPD patients with pulmonary hypertension.

ELECTROLYTE CORRECTION

Electrolyte correction is important. Hypophosphataemia is common and may cause respiratory muscle weakness.[44] Hypomagnesaemia,[45] hypocalcaemia[46] and hypokalaemia may also be present and may impair respiratory muscle function. Hyponatraemia may occur with inappropriate antidiuretic hormone release or with excess use of diuretics and inappropriate intravenous fluids.

HYPOTHYROIDISM

Hypothyroidism is an important condition to be recognised, particularly in the hypercapnic patient group.

INTERCOSTAL DRAINAGE

Intercostal drainage is indicated for pneumothorax and pleural effusions of sufficient volume to compromise respiratory function. Formal intercostal catheter insertion may be required but mandates hospital admission and is associated with infection and discomfort. Simple aspiration of pneumothoraces has been shown to result in few complications, a reduced admission rate and reduced hospital stay.

RESPIRATORY STIMULANTS

Many drugs have been shown to increase respiratory drive and lower $PaCO_2$. These include acetazolamide, medroxyprogesterone, naloxone, doxapram and almitrine. Use of such agents presupposes that the limiting factor is reduced respiratory drive, whereas the majority of ARF is limited by a reduced capacity to deal with an increased load to breathing. Side-effects include increased dyspnoea and fatigue, impaired sleeping, with almitrine, and increased pulmonary hypertension. Respiratory stimulants have not been shown to improve either short-term or long-term outcome. As a result respiratory stimulants are not recommended or used in ARF. Narcotic- or benzodiazepine-induced respiratory depression is best managed with the appropriate antagonist – naloxone or flumazenil.

NUTRITION

Nutrition is important, as patients with severe COPD are often undernourished and suffer a deterioration in nutritional status when hospitalised. This poor nutritional state is associated with decreased respiratory muscle mass and strength, increased risk of fatigue, ARF and death. Enteral feeding is preferred, but parenteral nutrition should be considered if enteral feeding is not tolerated. Excessive carbohydrate calories should be avoided as this increases CO_2 production (by ~15%) and may worsen respiratory failure. Low-carbohydrate/high-fat combinations are preferred in ARF during spontaneous ventilation.

NON-INVASIVE VENTILATION (NIV)

NIV is a technique in which ventilatory support is provided via a nasal or facial mask without endotracheal intubation. There have been several randomised controlled trials of NIV in COPD patients with acute hypercapnic respiratory failure which have demonstrated improved respiratory physiology, reduced mortality (up to 12 months), reduced iatrogenic complications, reduced need for intubation and mechanical ventilation and reduced length of stay in hospital.[47–50] All studies have shown good tolerance of the technique (~80% of patients), with few side-effects, improvements in both oxygenation and $PaCO_2$ compared with medically treated control patients.[51,52]

The goal of this technique is: (1) to unload respiratory muscles and augment ventilation and oxygenation, reduce CO_2 and correct acidosis until the underlying problem can be reversed; (2) when applied intermittently, to offset the adverse effects of sleep or position-induced adverse changes to ventilation, increased upper airway resistance and lung volume.

Indications for NIV are a deterioration of COPD with: (1) acute dyspnoea; (2) respiratory rate > 28 breaths/min; (3) $PaCO_2 > 45$ mmHg with a pH < 7.35, despite optimal medical treatment and not related to excessive supplemental oxygen. Although these indications are for mild exacerbations, most randomised studies have used these as entry guidelines.[47–50] Initial guidelines recommended NIV use to be limited to patients with pH in the range 7.25–7.35; however, recent evidence suggests that NIV is useful even in those patients with lower pH values (to as low as 7.0) and associated more severe hypercapnia (as high as 140 mmHg).[53] Included in the indications are recently extubated patients in whom NIV has been shown to reduce reintubation rates significantly.[54] Recently NIV has been advocated for use in patients with hypoxic respiratory failure,[55] but success is significantly less in the setting of hypoxaemia and either normocapnia or hypocapnia.[56] NIV may also have a role in some patients where mechanical ventilation is considered inappropriate.

Side-effects of NIV have included discomfort, intolerance, skin necrosis, gastric distension and aspiration. Pressure support has been reported as better tolerated than assist/control.[51]

INVASIVE MECHANICAL VENTILATION

OUTCOME OF ARF AND THE DECISION TO VENTILATE INVASIVELY

When respiratory failure progresses or fails to resolve despite aggressive conservative management, including NIV, mechanical ventilatory support may be necessary. The decision to ventilate requires careful consideration in some patients who may have near-end-stage lung disease and whose quality of life may not justify aggressive treatment. This decision requires consideration of the outcome of ARF.

Patients with COPD have a reduced life expectancy compared with an age-matched general population group and this life expectancy decreases in proportion with severity of COPD as assessed by FEV_1 (Figure 26.3).

An episode of ARF further decreases survival (see Figure 26.3). ARF precipitated only by bronchitis has a better outcome,[2] whereas ARF due to more serious causes, such as pneumonia, LV failure and pulmonary embolus, has a worse outcome[57] and studies including all such outcomes have lower survival rates (see Figure 26.3).

If ARF requires invasive mechanical ventilation, survival decreases further still (see Figure 26.3). Although the majority of patients do not require mechanical ventilation, the short-term survival in this more severe subset is still good, with a hospital survival rate in some series as high as 80%,[58] but 2- and 3-year survival is significantly lower (see Figure 26.3).[59,60] The severity of ARF and the severity of underlying COPD based on FEV_1, lifestyle score and dyspnoea score are also predictors of outcome.[13,57] Lifestyle[13] and dyspnoea[61] categories may be the most useful factors in the decision to withhold mechanical ventilation. Lifestyle categories 3 (house-bound and at least partly dependent) and 4 (bed- or chair-bound) indicate both a

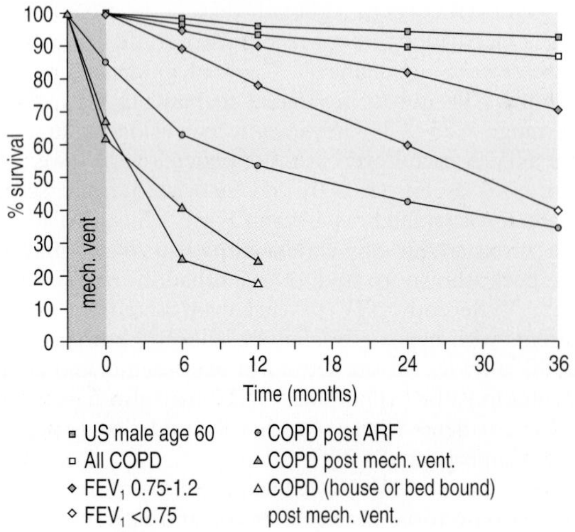

Figure 26.3 Survival curves for various patient groups with chronic obstructive pulmonary disease (COPD). Note: these are approximations only, based on other studies[13,57] with different patient numbers, criteria and study periods. FEV_1, forced expiratory volume in 1 second; ARF, acute respiratory failure.

poor outcome (see Figure 26.3)[13] and quality of life that may not justify aggressive treatment.

Thus invasive mechanical ventilation may be withheld in end-stage lung disease, when low survival, poor quality of life or permanent ventilator dependence are likely. This decision should be based on the following criteria. In general, patients must fulfil all the following criteria for invasive mechanical ventilation to be withheld:

- known severe COPD, which has been assessed and failed to respond to adequate therapy
- severe limitation of lifestyle by dyspnoea with a poor prior quality of life
- no identifiable reversible factors (e.g. pneumonia, sputum retention, LV failure)

If end-stage lung disease is suspected but there is insufficient information, then a trial of aggressive therapy, including invasive mechanical ventilation, should be undertaken and subsequently withdrawn if unsuccessful. Despite this, most patients with COPD who present with ARF do not have end-stage disease and, although their immediate problems may be life-threatening, their short-term outcome is sufficiently good to justify full active treatment.

INDICATIONS FOR INVASIVE MECHANICAL SUPPORT

- The clinical appearance of fatigue and impending respiratory collapse despite non-invasive ventilatory support
- Deteriorating conscious state due to fatigue or hypercapnia or both
- Hypoxia refractory to high levels of inspired O_2
- Deterioration due to failure of secretion clearance
- Respiratory arrest

MECHANICAL VENTILATION TECHNIQUE

The goals of mechanical ventilation in COPD are to support ventilation while reversible components improve, to allow respiratory muscle to rest and recover whilst preventing wasting from total inactivity and to minimise dynamic hyperinflation. This is usually best accomplished with low-level ventilatory support. Patients requiring low-level support may be commenced on 8–15 cmH_2O pressure support, with 3–8 cmH_2O PEEP. Patients who are completely exhausted, postarrest, comatose or not tolerating pressure support alone, should be commenced or transferred to synchronised intermittent mandatory ventilation mode.

Excessive dynamic hyperinflation must be avoided by using a low minute ventilation – 115/ml per kg is a guideline[6] – and allowing adequate time for expiration. This should be achieved by the use of a small tidal volume (8 ml/kg) and a ventilator rate <14 breaths/min.[6,62] Dynamic hyperinflation can be assessed clinically, by visualising the expiratory flow–time curve, and by measuring plateau airway pressure (P_{plat}) or $PEEP_i$. P_{plat} should be measured by applying an end-inspiratory pause of 0.5 s. This should only be applied following a single breath as it shortens expiratory time and, if it is applied to a series of breaths, it increases dynamic hyperinflation, resulting in an increased P_{plat} level and increased risk to the patient. If P_{plat} is >25 cmH_2O, there is likely to be dynamic hyperinflation, and the ventilator rate should be reduced. However, P_{plat} may be high without dynamic hyperinflation if chest wall compliance is low. Intrinsic PEEP measured as a prolonged end-expiratory pause more directly assesses dynamic hyperinflation. Provided $PEEP_i$ is accurately measured, it is a useful tool to follow dynamic hyperinflation. In severe airflow limitation it may be necessary to accept low levels of $PEEP_i$, but as $PEEP_i$ rises above 8–10 cmH_2O, further prolongation of expiratory time must be considered. Although still controversial, the use of a high inspiratory flow rate is recommended,[6,63] as it results in a shorter inspiratory time and hence a longer expiratory time for a given ventilatory rate. It has been shown to reduce dynamic hyperinflation and alveolar pressure[6] further and to improve gas exchange.[63]

If dynamic hyperinflation is excessive and causing circulatory compromise or risk of barotrauma, then minute ventilation should be decreased, hypercapnic acidosis accepted and spontaneous ventilation, which will only increase dynamic hyperinflation, should be discouraged by sedation. Muscle relaxants should be avoided unless essential. When dynamic hyperinflation is critical during controlled mechanical ventilation, $PEEP_i$ increases pulmonary hyperinflation and should not be applied.[64]

If dynamic hyperinflation is not excessive then spontaneous ventilation should be encouraged to promote ongoing respiratory muscle activity and to minimise wasting. Flow-by, pressure support and low-level CPAP may all reduce the work of spontaneous breathing and promote a better ventilatory pattern. CPAP approximately equal to the level of $PEEP_i$ is most commonly recommended.[65] Care must be taken with all of these supports as each can increase dynamic hyperinflation by a different mechanism, leading to circulatory compromise or risk of barotrauma. Flow-by increases resistance through the expiratory valve, pressure support increases tidal volume and may increase inspiratory time and CPAP increases FRC.

WEANING FROM INVASIVE MECHANICAL VENTILATION

Weaning a patient with severe COPD from ventilatory support can be difficult and prolonged. Numerous criteria have been proposed to assess the capacity of the patient to wean;[66] however, the predictive value of any of these individual criteria is limited. The simple criterion of patient respiration rate/tidal volume < 100 breaths/min per litre had the best predictive value for weaning success, but the advantage of this overly simple clinical assessment during weaning is uncertain.[66] Weaning or withdrawal of ventilation is further discussed elsewhere in this volume.

TRACHEOSTOMY

In a small group of patients who have failed extubation despite NIV or who have required long-term ventilatory support, tracheostomy may be beneficial. After 10 days of endotracheal intubation, the risk of trauma and sepsis increases.

A tracheostomy allows long-term ventilatory support, sputum clearance, protection of the upper airway from oral secretions and, off mechanical ventilation, reduced dead space and upper-airway resistance. Compared with naso/orotracheal intubation, tracheostomy is much less intrusive and therefore less sedation is required. Also, it allows direct access to the large airways for the purpose of suctioning and bronchoscopy. However, patients are unable to generate sufficient upper-airway seal to cough, and as such may have ongoing atelectasis until tracheostomy removal and the development of an effective cough. Usually a nasoenteric feeding tube is required. Consider percutaneous endoscopic gastrostomy (PEG) tube feeding if long-term tracheostomy is being considered to avoid nasal trauma and infection and to reduce oesophagitis. Minimal occlusion tracheostomy cuff pressures (usually < 20 cmH_2O) should be checked 8-hourly. Use of double-lumen tracheostomies with adequate humidification is recommended to allow for inner-tube cleaning and the avoidance of occlusion due to dried secretions.

Consider removing the tracheostomy when:

1. there is an absence of upper-airway obstruction (e.g. no granulation tissue or tracheal stenosis)
2. suctioning is becoming less frequent (< 2–4-hourly)
3. the patient is cooperative and has a good capacity to cough, for example, good respiratory muscle strength
4. the patient is able to protect the upper airway from aspiration
5. the patient is less dependent on invasive ventilatory support (e.g. not continuous) and non-invasive ventilatory support is available
6. there is a decreasing oxygenation requirement (e.g. $FiO_2 < 40\%$)

FAILED WEANING

A small group of patients with end-stage lung disease will be unable to wean successfully from ventilator support despite optimisation of all reversible factors. A number of options now exist for such patients:

- long-term institutional or home ventilatory support
- withdrawal of support. Permanent institutional mechanical ventilation for a patient with low general health status represents a poor quality of life and withdrawal of support may be a preferable alternative

POST INTENSIVE UNIT CARE

REHABILITATION

Rehabilitation should be considered for all patients with COPD, particularly those following ARF. There are numerous randomised controlled trials showing improvements in exercise physiology, lung function, quality of life and reduced hospitalisation rates.[67,68] Such programmes include extensive education and aerobic upper and lower-limb and respiratory muscle exercise, usually three times per week over a 6-week period. Patients are recommended to continue with exercises regularly and independently thereafter.

VACCINATION

Vaccination should be considered in all patients with COPD when stable. Annual influenza and 5-yearly pneumococcal vaccination is recommended.[1]

LUNG VOLUME REDUCTION SURGERY

Lung volume reduction surgery is a palliative surgical procedure for patients aged < 75 years, with advanced disabling emphysema. Poorly perfused and poorly ventilated areas of one or both lungs, thought to compress relatively preserved areas of well-functioning lung tissue, are excised by either midline sternotomy or endoscopically, with video assistance.[69] Such areas in the lung, usually apically placed, are determined by *V/Q* scans and high-resolution CT scans. Suitable patients must have undergone a pulmonary rehabilitation programme, be on optimal medical treatment and have disabling dyspnoea and anatomically suitable (apical bullous) emphysema. Patients with profoundly severe emphysema (e.g. FEV_1 or TLCO < 20% predicted) are unlikely to benefit.[69] Group mean data suggest that the mean FEV_1 increases from 0.5 to 0.91 litres, and the mean 6-min walk distance increases from 205 to 290 metres, both associated with significant improvement in quality of life. The peak improvements in physiology occur at 1–2 years and thereafter decline to presurgical levels. Improvements in survival are yet to be determined.[69]

LUNG TRANSPLANTATION

Lung transplantation is another palliative surgical procedure for patients with advanced disabling COPD who are aged < 65 years, are not ventilator-dependent, are on less than 10 mg prednisolone/day and are free of significant coexistent disease. It may be used following lung volume reduction surgery. The current 1-, 2- and 5-year international survival figures are 75, 66 and 50% respectively.[70] Common complications are systemic hypertension, bronchiolitis obliterans, acute rejection, viral infection with cytomegalovirus and neoplasms.[66] Its widespread application in COPD is in doubt because of the very limited supply of donor lungs.[71]

PROGNOSIS

Patients with sufficiently severe COPD to warrant hospital admission incur an inpatient mortality of 7%, and 90-day mortality of 15% in the UK.[72] Predictors of mortality were performance status, age and admission urea, albumin, pH and $Sp\text{O}_2$ plus the presence of respiratory physicians involved in the care.[72] Although in-hospital mortality for hypercapnic COPD patients may reach 62%,[73] in an Australian report, in-hospital mortality for hypercapnic COPD patients treated with NIV was 11% and all deaths were with palliative intent, which followed time to allow for patient and family discussions. In Hong Kong, acute hypercapnic COPD patients have a 12-month readmission rate of 80% and a 49% 1-year mortality.[74] The body mass index, airflow obstruction, dyspnoea and exercise capacity (BODE) index[75] is a 10-point scale made up from the following four variables: (1) body mass index; (2) airflow obstruction; (3) severity of dyspnoea; and (4) exercise capacity, and has been found to be very useful in predicting survival in ambulatory patients with COPD (Table 26.3).

Table 26.3 The body mass index, airflow obstruction, dyspnoea and exercise capacity (BODE) index (maximum is 10)

Score	0	1	2	3
FEV_1 (% predicted)	>65	50–64	36–49	<35
Six-minute walk distance	>350	250–350	150–250	<150
Modified MRC dyspnoea score	0–1	2	3	4
Body mass index	>21	<21		

The 4-year survival rates are 80% for a score of 2, 70% for 3–4, 60% for 5–6 and 20% for scores 7–10. Modified Medical Research Council (MRC) score is from zero (no dyspnoea) to 4 (extreme dyspnoea upon getting dressed or leaving the house).[75]
FEV_1, forced expiratory volume in 1 second.

REFERENCES

1. Pauwels RA, Buist AS, Ma P *et al.* Global strategy for the diagnosis, management, and prevention of chronic obstructive pulmonary disease. NHLBI/WHO global initiative for chronic obstructive lung disease (GOLD) workshop summary. *Am J Respir Crit Care Med* 2001; **163**: 1256–76.
2. Martin T, Lewis S, Albert R. The prognosis of patients with chronic obstructive pulmonary disease after hospitalization for acute respiratory failure. *Chest* 1982; **82**: 310–14.
3. Hii S, Lam J, Thompson BR *et al.* Bullous lung disease due to marijuana. *Respirology* 2008; **13**: 122–7.
4. Britton JR, Pavord ID, Richards KA *et al.* Dietary antioxidant vitamin intake and lung function in the general population. *Am J Respir Crit Care Med* 1995; **151**: 1383–7.
5. Burrows B, Fletcher C, Heard B. The emphysematous and bronchial types of chronic airways obstruction. A clinico-pathological study of patients in London and Chicago. *Lancet* 1966; **7442**: 1830–5.
6. Tuxen D, Lane S. The effects of ventilatory pattern on hyperinflation, airway pressures, and circulation in mechanical ventilation of patients with severe airflow obstruction. *Am Rev Respir Dis* 1987; **136**: 872–9.
7. Fahey P, Hyde R. 'Won't breathe' versus 'can't breathe'. Detection of depressed ventilatory drive in patients with obstructive pulmonary disease. *Chest* 1983; **84**: 19–25.
8. Connors AF Jr, Dawson NV, Thomas C *et al.* Outcomes following acute exacerbations of severe chronic obstructive lung disease. *Am J Respir Crit Care Med* 1996; **154**: 959–67.
9. Schreiner A, Bjerkestrand G, Digrannes A. Bacteriologic findings in the trans-tracheal aspirate from patients with acute exacerbations of chronic bronchitis. *Infection* 1978; **6**: 54–6.
10. Irwin R, Erickson A, Pratter M. Prediction of tracheobronchial colonization in current cigarette smokers with chronic obstructive bronchitis. *J Infect Dis* 1982; **145**: 234–41.
11. Christensen J, Gadeberg O, Bruvn B. *Branhamella catarrhalis*: significance in pulmonary infections and bacteriological features. *Acta Pathol Microbiol Immunol Scand* 1986; **94**: 89–95.
12. Smith CB, Golden CA, Kanner RE *et al.* Association of viral and *Mycoplasma pneumoniae* infections with acute respiratory illness in patients with chronic obstructive

pulmonary disease. *Am Rev Respir Dis* 1980; **121**: 225–32.

13. Menzies R, Gibbons W, Goldberg P. Determinants of weaning and survival among patients with COPD who require mechanical ventilation for acute respiratory failure. *Chest* 1989; **95**: 398–405.
14. Baum GL, Schwartz A, Llamas R *et al.* Left ventricular function in chronic obstructive lung disease. *N Engl J Med* 1971; **285**: 361–5.
15. Robertson C, Foster G, Johnson R. The relationship of respiratory failure to the oxygen consumption of, lactate production by, and distribution of blood flow among respiratory muscles during increasing inspiratory resistance. *J Clin Invest* 1977; **59**: 31–42.
16. Abroug F, Ouanes-Besbes L, Nciri N *et al.* Association of left-heart dysfunction with severe exacerbation of chronic obstructive pulmonary disease: diagnostic performance of cardiac biomarkers. *Am J Respir Crit Care Med* 2006; **174**: 990–6.
17. Kato S, Nakamoto TK, Iizuka M. Early diagnosis and estimation of pulmonary congestion and edema in patients with left-sided heart disease from histogram of pulmonary CT number. *Chest* 1996; **109**: 1439–45.
18. Bone R, Pierce A, Johnson R. Controlled oxygen administration in acute respiratory failure in chronic obstructive pulmonary disease. *Am J Med* 1978; **65**: 896–902.
19. Mossberg B, Strandberg K, Philipson K *et al.* Tracheobronchial clearance and beta-adrenoceptor stimulation in patients with chronic bronchitis. *Scand Respir Dis* 1976; **57**: 281–9.
20. Salpeter SE, Buckley NS, Salpeter EE. Anticholinergics but not beta agonists reduce severe exacerbations and respiratory mortality in COPD. *J Gen Int Med* 2006; **21**: 1011–19.
21. Braun SR, McKenzie WN, Copeland C *et al.* A comparison of effect of ipratropium and albuterol (salbutamol) in chronic obstructive airway disease. *Arch Intern Med* 1989; **149**: 544–7.
22. Karpel JP, Schacter EN, Fanta C *et al.* A comparison of ipratropium and albuterol vs albuterol alone for the treatment of acute asthma. *Chest* 1996; **110**: 611–16.
23. Friedman M, Serby CW, Menjoge SS *et al.* Pharmacoeconomic evaluation of a combination of ipratropium plus albuterol compared with ipratropium alone and albuterol alone in COPD. *Chest* 1999; **115**: 635–41.
24. Boyd G, Morice A, Pounsford J. An evaluation of salmeterol in the treatment of chronic obstructive pulmonary disease. *Eur Respir J* 1997; **10**: 815–21.
25. Aubier M, De Troyer A, Sampson M *et al.* Aminophylline improves diaphragmatic contractility. *N Engl J Med* 1981; **305**: 249–52.
26. Berry RB, Desa MM, Branum JP *et al.* Effect of theophylline on sleep and sleep-disordered breathing in patients with chronic obstructive pulmonary disease. *Am Rev Respir Dis* 1991; **143**: 245–50.
27. Wanner A. Effects of methylxanthines on airway mucociliary function. *Am J Med* 1985; **79**: 16–21.
28. Matthay RA, Berger HJ, Davies R. Improvement in cardiac performance by oral long-acting theophylline in chronic obstructive pulmonary disease. *Am Heart J* 1982; **104**: 1022–6.
29. Pauwels R. New aspects of the therapeutic potential of theophylline in asthma. *J Allergy Clin Immunol* 1989; **83**: 548–53.
30. Rice KL, Leatherman JW, Duane PG *et al.* Aminophylline for acute exacerbations of chronic obstructive pulmonary disease. *Ann Intern Med* 1987; **107**: 305–9.
31. Guyatt GH, Townsend M, Pugsley SO *et al.* Bronchodilators in chronic airflow limitation. Effects on airway function, exercise capacity, and quality of life. *Am Rev Respir Dis* 1987; **135**: 1069–74.
32. Rogers R, Owens G, Pennock B. The pendulum swings again: toward a rational use of theophylline. *Chest* 1985; **87**: 280–2.
33. Chrystyn H, Mulley B, Peake M. Dose response relation to oral theophylline in severe chronic obstructive airways disease. *Br Med J* 1988; **297**: 1506–10.
34. Albert R, Martin T, Lewis S. Controlled clinical trial of methylprednisolone in patients with chronic bronchitis and acute respiratory insufficiency. *Ann Intern Med* 1980; **92**: 753–8.
35. Rubini S, Rampullua C, Nava S. Acute effect of corticosteroids on respiratory mechanics in mechanically ventilated patients with chronic airflow obstruction and acute respiratory failure. *Am J Respir Crit Care Med* 1994; **149**: 306–10.
36. Hosker H, Cooke N, Hawkey P. Antibiotics in chronic obstructive pulmonary disease. *Br Med J* 1994; **308**: 871–2.
37. Basran GS, Joseph J, Abbas AM *et al.* Treatment of acute exacerbations of chronic obstructive airways disease – a comparison of amoxycillin and ciprofloxacin. *J Antimicrob Chemother* 1990; **26** (Suppl. F): 19–24.
38. Siafakas NM, Vermeire P, Pride NB *et al.* Optimal assessment and management of chronic obstructive pulmonary disease (COPD). *Eur Respir J* 1995; **8**: 1398–420.
39. Petty T. The National Mucolytic study. Results of a randomized, double-blind, placebo-controlled study of iodinated glycerol in chronic obstructive bronchitis. *Chest* 1990; **97**: 75–83.
40. Mathur P, Pugsley S, Powles A. Effect of digitalis on left ventricular function in chronic cor pulmonale. *Am Rev Respir Dis* 1980; **121**: 163.
41. Green L, Smith T. The use of digitalis in patients with pulmonary disease. *Ann Intern Med* 1977; **87**: 459–65.
42. Sajkov D, McEvoy R, Cowie R. Felodipine improves pulmonary hemodynamics in chronic obstructive pulmonary disease. *Chest* 1993; **103**: 1354–61.
43. Salvaterra C, Rubin L. Investigation and management of pulmonary hypertension in chronic obstructive pulmonary disease. *Am Rev Respir Dis* 1994; **148**: 1414–7.
44. Aubier M, Murciano D, Lecocguic Y. Effect of hypophosphatemia on diaphragmatic contractility in patients with acute respiratory failure. *N Engl J Med* 1985; **313**: 420–4.

45. Dhingra S, Solven F, Wilson A *et al.* Hypomagnesemia and respiratory muscle power. *Am Rev Respir Dis* 1984; **129**: 497–8.
46. Aubier M, Viires N, Piquet J. Effects of hypocalcemia on diaphragmatic strength generation. *J Appl Physiol* 1985; **58**: 2054–61.
47. Brochard L, Mancebo J, Wysocki M *et al.* Noninvasive ventilation for acute exacerbations of chronic obstructive pulmonary disease. *N Engl J Med* 1995; **333**: 817–22.
48. Bott J, Carroll MP, Conway JH *et al.* Randomised controlled trial of nasal ventilation in acute ventilatory failure due to chronic obstructive airways disease. *Lancet* 1993; **341**: 1555–7.
49. Kramer N, Meyer TJ, Meharg J *et al.* Randomised prospective trial of noninvasive positive pressure ventilation in acute respiratory failure. *Am J Respir Crit Care Med* 1995; **151**: 1799–806.
50. Plant P, Owen J, Elliott M. Early use of noninvasive ventilation for acute exacerbations of chronic obstructive pulmonary disease on general respiratory wards: a multicentre randomised controlled trial. *Lancet* 2000; **355**: 1931–5.
51. Mehta S, Hill NS. Noninvasive ventilation. *Am J Respir Crit Care Med* 2001; **163**: 540–77.
52. Hillberg RE, Johnson DC. Noninvasive ventilation. *N Engl J Med* 1997; **337**: 1746–52.
53. Crummy F, Buchan C, Miller B *et al.* The use of noninvasive ventilation in COPD with severe hypercapnic respiratory acidosis. *Respir Med* 2007; **101**: 53–61.
54. Nava S, Ambrosino N, Clini E *et al.* Noninvasive mechanical ventilation in the weaning of patients with respiratory failure due to chronic obstructive pulmonary disease. A randomized controlled trial. *Ann Intern Med* 1998; **128**: 721–8.
55. Antonelli M, Conti G, Rocco M *et al.* A comparison of noninvasive positive-pressure ventilation and conventional mechanical ventilation in patients with acute respiratory failure. *N Engl J Med* 1998; **339**: 429–35.
56. Wysocki M, Tric L, Wolff MA *et al.* Noninvasive pressure support ventilation in patients with acute respiratory failure. *Chest* 1993; **103**: 907–13.
57. Hudson L. Survival data in patients with acute and chronic lung disease requiring mechanical ventilation. *Am Rev Respir Dis* 1989; **140**: S19–24.
58. Petty T. Acute respiratory failure in chronic obstructive pulmonary disease. In: Sheomaker W, Thompson W, Holbrook P (eds) Textbook of Critical Care. Sydney: WB Saunders; 1984: 264–72.
59. Burk R, George R. Acute respiratory failure in chronic obstructive pulmonary disease (immediate and long term prognosis). *Arch Intern Med* 1972; **132**: 865–8.
60. Admandsson T, Kilburn K. Survival after respiratory failure (145 patients observed 5 to 8.5 years). *Ann Intern Med* 1974; **80**: 54–9.
61. Ferris B. Epidemiology standardization project. *Am Rev Respir Dis* 1978; **118** (Suppl): 1–120.
62. Curtis J, Hudson L. Emergent assessment and management of acute respiratory failure in COPD. *Clin Chest Med (Respir Emerg II)* 1994; **15**: 481–500.
63. Connors A, McCaffree D, Gray B. Effect of inspiratory flow rate on gas exchange during mechanical ventilation. *Am Rev Respir Dis* 1981; **124**: 537–43.
64. Tuxen D. Detrimental effects of positive end-expiratory pressure during controlled mechanical ventilation of patients with severe airflow obstruction. *Am Rev Respir Dis* 1989; **140**: 5–9.
65. Biagorri F, De Monte A, Blanch L. Hemodynamic response to external counterbalancing of auto-positive end expiratory pressure in mechanically ventilated patients with chronic obstructive pulmonary disease. *Crit Care Med* 1994; **22**: 1782–91.
66. Esteban A, Frutos F, Tobin MJ *et al.* A comparison of four methods of weaning patients from mechanical ventilation. *N Engl J Med* 1995; **332**: 345–50.
67. Lacasse Y, Ferreira I, Brooks D *et al.* Critical appraisal of clinical practice guidelines targeting chronic obstructive pulmonary disease. *Arch Intern Med* 2001; **161**: 69–74.
68. Goldstein RS, Gort EH, Stubbing D *et al.* Randomised controlled trial of respiratory rehabilitation. *Lancet* 1994; **344**: 362–8.
69. Stirling GR, Babidge WJ, Peacock MJ *et al.* Lung volume reduction surgery in emphysema: a systematic review. *Ann Thoracic Surg* 2001; **72**: 641–8.
70. Hosenpud JD, Bennett LE, Keck BM *et al.* The registry of the International Society for Heart and Lung Transplantation: seventeenth official report – 2000. *J Heart Lung Transplant* 2000; **19**: 909–31.
71. Snell GI, Griffiths A, Macfarlane L *et al.* Maximising thoracic organ transplant opportunities: the importance of efficient co-ordination. *J Heart Lung Transplant* 2000; **19**: 410–17.
72. Price LC, Lowe D, Hosker HSR *et al.* UK national COPD audit 2003: impact of hospital resources and organisation of care on patient outcome following admission for acute COPD exacerbation. *Thorax* 2006; **61**: 827–42.
73. Squadrone E, Frigerio P, Fogliati C *et al.* Noninvasive vs invasive ventilation in COPD patients with severe acute respiratory failure deemed to require ventilatory assistance. *Intens Care Med* 2004; **30**: 1303–10.
74. Chu CM, Chan VL, Lin AWN *et al.* Readmission rates and life threatening events in COPD survivors treated with non-invasive ventilation for acute hypercapnic respiratory failure. *Thorax* 2004; **59**: 1020–5.
75. Celli BR, Cote CG, Marin JM *et al.* The body-mass index, airflow obstruction, dyspnea and exercise capacity index in chronic obstructive pulmonary disease. *N Engl J Med* 2005; **350**: 1005–12.

27

Mechanical ventilation

Andrew D Bersten

Mechanical ventilation for acute respiratory failure (ARF) is now a routine aspect of patient management in the intensive care unit (ICU). The 1952 Copenhagen polio epidemic introduced the notion of organised areas (ICU) for the provision of positive-pressure ventilation,[1] which was usually applied through a tracheostomy that had been inserted to allow suction of secretions. However, methods of ventilatory assistance without intubation had proliferated prior to the polio epidemic (both negative-pressure chest wall devices and positive-pressure face mask devices), and current trends are to an increased use of non-invasive ventilation (NIV) in patients with respiratory failure.[2]

Almost all of the ventilatory modes that are conventionally applied during *intubated* ventilation (IV) can be applied *non-invasively*; however, IV remains the primary mode of respiratory assistance in critically ill patients. There are also an increasing number of patients receiving chronic ventilatory assistance but, since the majority of these use chronic NIV, this chapter is primarily directed at intubated mechanical ventilation for both ARF and acute-on-chronic respiratory failure.

A PHYSIOLOGICAL APPROACH

During normal spontaneous breathing, contraction of the respiratory muscles overcomes both the elastic recoil and resistance of the respiratory system (lung and chest wall). A fall in regional pleural pressure results in alveolar inflation as gas is forced in under the resultant pressure gradient. Expiration is usually passive but the expiratory muscles may assist the elastic recoil of the respiratory system.

The work (W) performed by the respiratory muscles (W_{mus}) can be measured from the relationship between pressure (P) and volume (V), and partitioned into elastic (W_{el}) and resistive (W_{res}) work:

$$W_{mus} = W_{el} + W_{res} \qquad \textit{Equation 1}$$

Inertial work is negligible, and usually ignored. Further, Equation (1) does not explicitly describe the elastic work required to initiate inspiration when intrinsic positive end-expiratory pressure ($PEEP_i$) is present.

Because volume is constant in Equation (1), it can be simplified to:

$$P_{mus} = P_{el} + P_{res} \qquad \textit{Equation 2}$$

It follows that, during positive-pressure ventilatory assistance, where P_{ao} is the ventilatory pressure applied at the airway:

$$P_{ao} + P_{mus} = P_{el} + P_{res} \qquad \textit{Equation 3}$$

and that when the work is solely applied by the ventilator with no respiratory muscle contraction (controlled mechanical ventilation (CMV)):

$$P_{ao} = P_{el} + P_{res} \qquad \textit{Equation 4}$$

This nomenclature allows physiologic discussion of the different ventilatory modes, from controlled ventilation to spontaneous, unassisted ventilation, and introduces the equation of motion, which is used in the estimation of respiratory mechanics:

$$P_{ao} = E_{rs} \cdot V + R_{rs} \cdot \dot{V} + P_o \qquad \textit{Equation 5}$$

where E_{rs} is the respiratory system (lung and chest wall) elastance (the inverse of compliance), R_{rs} is the respiratory system resistance, $\dot{V}$ is the gas flow rate and P_o is the total PEEP (the sum of extrinsic PEEP [$PEEP_e$] and $PEEP_i$). $PEEP_i$ imposes a threshold load – additional elastic work – as inspiratory muscle contraction must occur without $\dot{V}$ until P_{ao} falls below atmospheric pressure (see section on patient–ventilator interaction, below).

MODES OF VENTILATION

CONTROLLED MECHANICAL VENTILATION

The simplest form of positive-pressure breath occurs in a relaxed subject, and the ventilator provides a constant gas flow during inspiration. The volume delivered will depend upon the inspiratory time (T_i), and P_{ao} during inspiration will reflect E_{rs} and R_{rs} (Figure 27.1). Expiration is a passive, and usually exponential, decline in volume to the relaxation volume of the respiratory system, equal to the functional residual capacity (FRC).

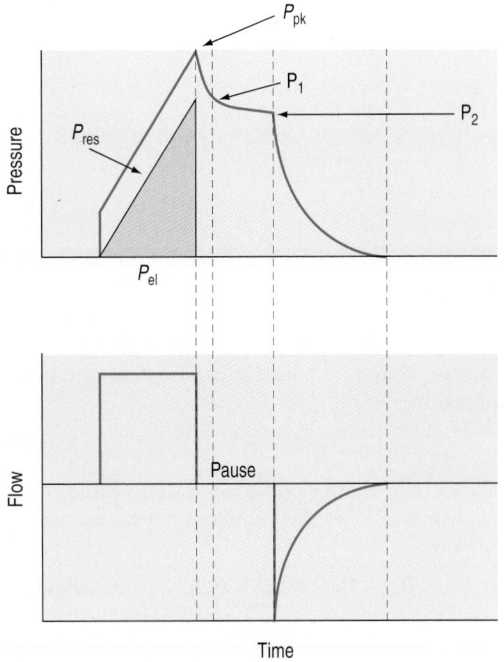

Figure 27.1 Schematic diagram of a volume-controlled breath with constant inspiratory flow. A period of no inspiratory gas flow has been interposed before expiration (pause) to illustrate dissipation of lung resistance as airways resistance (fall from P_{pk} to P_1) and tissue resistance (fall from P_1 to P_2). The inspiratory pressure due to the elastic properties of the respiratory system is illustrated as the filled area (P_{el}), and the lung resistive pressure is labelled as P_{res}. See text for more detail.

CMV is the most basic form of mechanical ventilation; however, it is an extremely useful baseline, and is still commonly used. A preset minute ventilation is made up from a fixed respiratory rate (f) and tidal volume (V_T). Provided that there are not large variations in alveolar dead space, this maintains a preset alveolar ventilation (V_A) and CO_2 clearance. Consequently, CMV is useful in conditions where there is alveolar hypoventilation (e.g. respiratory muscle weakness), when $Pa\text{CO}_2$ needs to be maintained in a fixed range (e.g. raised intracranial pressure) or when the work of breathing must be minimised (e.g. severe cardiorespiratory failure). Because CMV may not match respiratory drive, and spontaneous, supported or assisted breaths are not possible during CMV, sedation, and sometimes muscle paralysis, may be needed. CMV is usually combined with PEEP_e, which can recruit collapsed lung and reduce intrapulmonary shunt. The components are discussed below.

TIDAL VOLUME (V_T)

Although traditional CMV V_T has been 12–15 ml/kg, this may result in excessive lung stretch, particularly in patients with acute lung injury (ALI), leading to ventilator-induced (VILI) – also described as ventilator-associated – lung injury (VALI).[3] The basis for this larger V_T can be traced back to progressive atelectasis and intrapulmonary shunt, when physiologic V_T was used during general anaesthesia. This could be reversed by larger V_T ventilation or intermittent sigh breaths.[4] In patients with ALI, V_T of 6 ml/kg versus 12 ml/kg predicted body weight (i.e. often 4–5 ml/kg versus 9–10 ml/kg true weight) reduced mortality from 40% to 31%.[5] Consequently, lower V_T should be strongly considered during CMV, and other forms of ventilatory assistance in patients with ALI. However, greater levels of PEEP are usually required; similar data are not available for other respiratory diseases. Indeed, although the reduction in V_T is particularly applicable to ALI, excessive lung stretch will be less likely in other patient cohorts that are able to ventilate a greater proportion of the lung (see Chapter 29).

RESPIRATORY RATE (f)

The desired minute ventilation can be selected from the product of V_T and f. Common CMV rates are 10–20 breaths/min in adults. Sufficient expiratory time (T_e) must be allowed to minimise dynamic hyperinflation and PEEP_i. Although high f (up to 35 breaths/min) were allowed in the Acute Respiratory Distress Syndrome (ARDS) Network protocol, and the low-V_T, low-mortality group had a mean f of ~30 breaths/min,[5] laboratory data suggest a possible additive role of high f in VILI.[6]

INSPIRATORY FLOW PATTERN

The simplest form of CMV uses a constant inspiratory flow ($\dot{V}_I$), and in combination with T_i, a preset volume is delivered. This is also called volume-controlled ventilation (VCV), and some ventilators use V_T and T_i to set $\dot{V}_I$. Alternative $\dot{V}_I$ patterns that are commonly available with VCV include a ramped descending flow pattern and a sine pattern. When a time-preset inspiratory pressure is delivered, this is termed pressure-controlled ventilation (PCV).

There are no convincing outcome data differentiating these different modes of CMV and PCV. Although the peak airway pressure (P_{pk}) is lower with PCV than constant-flow CMV, the alveolar distending pressure, which is usually inferred from the plateau pressure (P_{plat}), is no different provided that T_i and V_T are the same.[7] During PCV, P_{res} is dissipated during inspiration so P_{pk} and P_{plat} are equal, and during CMV, P_{res} accounts for the difference between P_{pk} and P_{plat} (Figure 27.2). Similarly, different CMV_I patterns will alter P_{pk} without changing P_{plat} or mean airway pressure (P_{mean}) when T_i and V_T are constant. In ARDS patients, comparing VCV and PCV, there is no difference in haemodynamics, oxygenation, recruited lung volume or distribution of regional ventilation;[7,8] however, PCV may dissipate viscoelastic strain earlier.[8] However, high $\dot{V}_I$ may cause or exacerbate VILI,[9] which may explain why some animal models have found PCV to be injurious compared to VCV, as PCV inherently has a high early $\dot{V}_I$.

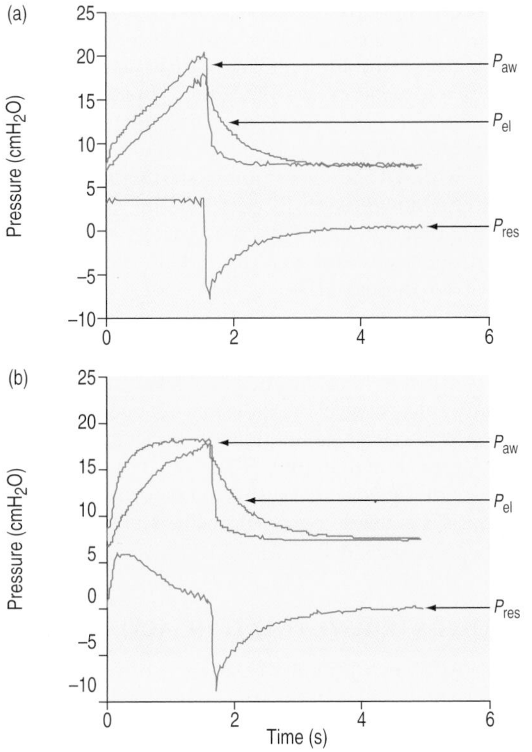

Figure 27.2 Actual pressure–time data from a patient with acute lung injury ventilated with volume-controlled ventilation (panel A), and then with pressure-controlled ventilation (panel B); tidal volume, I:E ratio and respiratory rate are constant. The airway pressure (P_{aw}, bold line) has been broken down to its components, P_{el} and P_{res} (see Figure 27.1). Although there is no inspiratory pause, there is marked similarity between panel A and Figure 27.1, with the inspiratory difference between P_{aw} and P_{el} due to a constant P_{res}. In panel B, the decelerating inspiratory flow pattern seen with pressure-controlled ventilation results in dissipation of P_{res} by end-inspiration. Consequently, during pressure-controlled ventilation $P_{aw} \approx P_{plat}$ obtained during volume-controlled ventilation. In other words, for the same ventilator settings there is no difference in the elastic distending pressure.

Pressure-regulated volume control (PRVC) is a form of CMV where the V_T is preset, and achieved at a minimum pressure using a decelerating flow pattern.

INSPIRATORY PAUSE

An end-inspiratory pause allows examination of the decay in P_{pk}, and measurement of P_{plat}. If T_i and V are maintained constant there is no improvement in oxygenation, and a more rapid $\dot{V}_I$ will be needed. This may alter the distribution of ventilation. Theoretically, an end-inspiratory pause will allow a 32% dissipation of the total energy loss within the respiratory system,[10] which may significantly reduce the forces driving expiration, and this could exacerbate gas trapping in patients with severe airflow limitation.

INSPIRATORY TIME, EXPIRATORY TIME, I:E RATIO

The combination of V_T and inspiratory $\dot{V}$ will determine T_i, which in combination with f sets T_e. A typical T_i is 0.8–1.2 s; with a V_T of 500 ml and inspiratory $\dot{V}$ of 0.5 l/s, the T_i is 1.0 s. During spontaneous ventilation, the distribution of ventilation at low $\dot{V}_I$ is determined by regional E, and at high inspiratory $\dot{V}$ by regional R, leading to greater ventilation of non-dependent lung. In patients with severe airflow limitation high inspiratory flow rates may be used in order to prolong T_e and minimise dynamic hyperinflation.[11]

The I:E ratio is usually set at or below 1:2 to allow an adequate T_e for passive expiration. During inverse-ratio ventilation (IRV), the I:E ratio is greater than 1:1. The putative benefits of a prolonged T_i include recruitment of long time-constant alveoli, and a short T_e results in gas trapping and $PEEP_i$. Early reports of clinical benefit did not control for $PEEP_i$, and when total PEEP, f and V_T are constant,[7,8] pressure control (PC) IRV tends to reduce $Pa\text{CO}_2$ but does not improve oxygenation, may have deleterious haemodynamic effects and may exaggerate regional overinflation.[8]

POSITIVE END-EXPIRATORY PRESSURE

PEEP is an elevation in the end-expiratory pressure upon which all forms of mechanical ventilation may be imposed. When PEEP is maintained throughout the respiratory cycle in a spontaneously breathing subject, the term 'constant positive airway pressure' (CPAP) is used. The primary role of PEEP is to maintain recruitment of collapsed lung, increase FRC and minimise intrapulmonary shunt. PEEP may also improve oxygenation by redistributing lung water from the alveolus to the interstitium, and although there is no direct effect of PEEP to reduce extravascular lung water, this may occur in patients with left ventricular failure due to a reduction in venous return and left ventricular afterload. Further, inadequate PEEP may contribute to VILI by promoting tidal opening and closing of alveoli.[3] PEEP levels of 5–15 cmH_2O are commonly used, and levels up to 25 cmH_2O may be required in patients with severe ARDS. Although a large multicentre study found no benefit of higher PEEP levels when V_T was 6 ml/kg,[12] individual titration may need to be considered.

PEEP titration in ARDS is complex (see Chapter 29), and should aim to improve oxygenation and minimise VILI. Since PEEP reduces venous return, cardiac output and O_2 delivery may fall despite an improvement in $Pa\text{O}_2$; indeed, this concept has been used to optimise PEEP in ARF.[13] However, in addition to recruitment, increasing PEEP may lead to overinflation of non-dependent alveoli which are already aerated at end-expiration.[14,15] This will be less likely if alveolar distending pressure is kept < 30–35 cmH_2O, or the change in driving pressure is < 2 cmH_2O when V_T is constant.[16]

$PEEP_e$ is applied by placing a resistance in the expiratory circuit (Figure 27.3), with most ventilators using a solenoid valve. Independent of the technique, a threshold resistor is preferred since it offers minimal resistance to flow once its opening *P* is reached. This will minimise expiratory work, and avoid barotrauma during coughing or straining.

$PEEP_i$ is an elevation in the static recoil pressure of the respiratory system at end-expiration. $PEEP_i$ arises due to an inadequate T_e, usually in the setting of severe airflow obstruction. However, it may be a desired endpoint during IRV. The sum of $PEEP_e$ and $PEEP_i$ is the total PEEP ($PEEP_{tot}$). The distribution of $PEEP_i$ is likely to be less uniform than an equivalent $PEEP_e$, and this may not have the same physiological effects. When patients with severe airflow obstruction are triggering ventilation, $PEEP_e$ less than $PEEP_i$ may be applied to reduce elastic work (see section on patient–ventilator interaction, below).

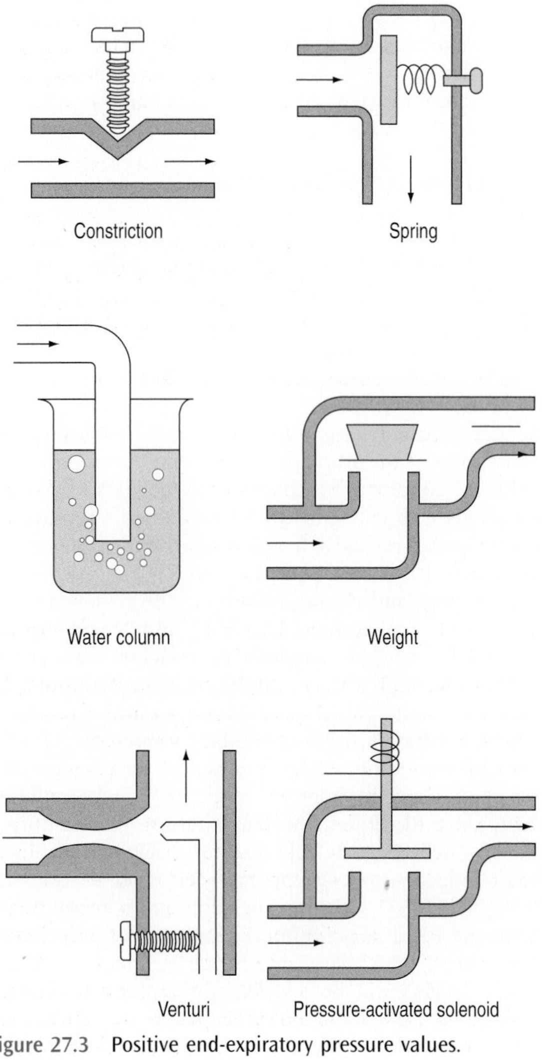

Figure 27.3 Positive end-expiratory pressure values.

FRACTIONAL INSPIRED OXYGEN CONCENTRATION (FiO_2)

Adequate arterial oxygen saturation is achieved through a combination of minute ventilation, PEEP and FiO_2 adjustment. Even patients with normal respiratory systems usually need an $FiO_2 > 0.21$, due to ventilation–perfusion mismatch secondary to positive-pressure ventilation. In patients with ARF it is common to start with an FiO_2 of 1 and titrate down as PEEP and minute ventilation are adjusted. Because high FiO_2s are damaging to the lung, and nitrogen washout may exacerbate atelectasis, it is reasonable to aim at an $FiO_2 \leq 0.6$.

SIGH

Many ventilators have the ability to deliver a breath intermittently at least twice V_T. Sighs may reduce atelectasis, in part through release of pulmonary surfactant,[17] resulting in recruitment and improved oxygenation in ARDS.[18] However, if sighs or recruitment manoeuvres are used, care must be taken to avoid recurrent excessive lung stretch.

ASSIST-CONTROL VENTILATION (ACV)

During ACV, in addition to the set *f*, patient effort can trigger a standard CMV breath (Figure 27.4). This allows greater patient comfort; however, there may be little reduction in respiratory work compared to an unassisted breath at low V_I, because the respiratory muscles continue to contract through much of the breath.[19] The equivalent PCV breath is termed pressure assist-control ventilation (PACV). Differences between triggering modes will be discussed below, in the section on patient–ventilator interaction.

INTERMITTENT MANDATORY VENTILATION (IMV), SYNCHRONISED IMV (SIMV)

IMV was introduced over 20 years ago to aid weaning from CMV by allowing the patient to take unimpeded breaths while still receiving a background of controlled breaths. Proposed advantages include a reduction in sedation, lower mean intrathoracic pressure with less barotrauma and adverse haemodynamic consequences, improved intrapulmonary gas distribution, continued use of respiratory muscles and faster weaning. During SIMV T_i is partitioned into patient-initiated and true spontaneous breaths to avoid breath-stacking. However, during spontaneous breaths the work of breathing imposed by the endotracheal tube, circuit and ventilator must be overcome.[20] In weaning studies comparing SIMV with T-piece trials and pressure support ventilation (PSV), SIMV is the slowest.[21] Many clinicians add PSV during gradual reduction in respiratory rate with SIMV to overcome the added respiratory work imposed by the circuit and endotracheal tube; however, this approach has not been formally compared with other weaning techniques.

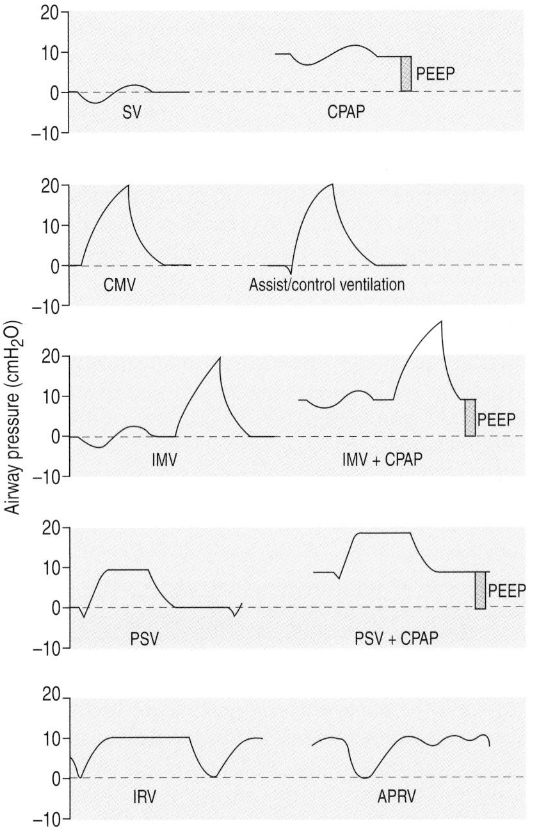

Figure 27.4 Schematic representation of airway pressure versus time for a variety of forms of ventilatory assistance. SV, spontaneous ventilation; CPAP, continuous positive airway pressure; PEEP, positive end-expiratory pressure; CMV, controlled mechanical ventilation; IMV, intermittent mandatory ventilation; PSV, pressure support ventilation; IRV, inverse-ratio ventilation; APRV, airway pressure release ventilation.

PRESSURE SUPPORT VENTILATION

During PSV, each patient-triggered breath is supported by gas flow to achieve a preset pressure, usually designated to be above the $PEEP_e$. This can be explained by referring to the equation of motion where:

$$P_{mus} + P_{ao} = E_{rs} V + R_{rs} \dot{V} + Po \qquad \textit{Equation 6}$$

During PSV, P_{ao} is the targeted variable by the ventilator, which leads to a significant and important reduction in P_{mus} and work of breathing.[22] The detection of neural expiration varies between ventilators, but commonly relies upon a fall in the inspiratory $\dot{V}$ to either 25% of the initial flow rate or to less than 5 l/min: some ventilators allow titration of the percentage reduction in initial flow to allow improved patient–ventilator synchrony. PSV may also be titrated to offset the work imposed by the circuit and endotracheal tube. The absolute level required to offset this will vary with endotracheal tube size and inspiratory $\dot{V}$,[23] but is commonly 5–10 cmH_2O.[24] PSV can be used during weaning, or as a form of variable ventilatory support, with pressures of 15–20 cmH_2O commonly used. Disadvantages include variable V_T, and hence minute ventilation, the potential to deliver an excessive V_T (common in patients recovering from ARDS), and patient-ventilator dyssynchrony (see below).

Volume-assured pressure support (VAPS) is a mode of adaptive PSV where breath-to-breath logic achieves a preset V_T.

PROPORTIONAL ASSIST VENTILATION (PAV)

PAV is a form of partial ventilatory support where inspiratory P is applied in proportion to patient effort. Because this allows the breathing pattern and minute ventilation to be matched to patient effort, it is only suitable if respiratory drive is normal or elevated. In concept this should optimise the patient–ventilator interaction; however, the prescription of PAV requires a greater level of physiological understanding than similar forms of partial ventilatory support such as PSV, since there is no target P, V or $\dot{V}$. PAV is usually prescribed using volume assist (VA) and flow assist (FA), with V and $\dot{V}$ measured continuously. VA generates greater P as V increases, leading to elastic unloading, and FA generates greater P as $\dot{V}$ increases, leading to resistive unloading. Not surprisingly, the units of VA are cmH_2O/L (i.e. an elastance term) and those for FA are cmH_2O/l per second (i.e. a resistance term). This can be illustrated by referring to Equation (6):

$$P_{mus} + P_{ao} = E_{rs} V + R_{rs} = Po$$

where P_{ao} is determined by PAV, where PAV = VA + FA, so:

$$P_{mus} + VA \times V + FA \times \dot{V} = E_{rs} V + R_{rs} \dot{V} + Po \qquad \textit{Equation 7}$$

consequently

$$P_{mus} = (E_{rs} - VA) V + (R_{rs} - FA) \dot{V} + Po \qquad \textit{Equation 8}$$

If E_{rs} and R_{rs} are known, PAV can, at least in principle, be targeted to reduce a specified proportion of either, or both, elastic and resistive respiratory work. For example, when VA and FA are adjusted to counterbalance E_{rs} and R_{rs} so as to achieve normal values, minute ventilation increases, and respiratory drive and work decrease; if $PEEP_i$ is present, work can be further reduced by applying $PEEP_e$.[25] Estimates of respiratory mechanics are relatively hard to measure in spontaneously breathing patients; however, they are now offered on some ventilators. Consequently, PAV is often titrated to patient comfort. Despite a growing body of data demonstrating reduced work of breathing and improved patient–ventilator synchrony with PAV, it is a more difficult technique to use, and definitive studies showing a clinically important outcome difference are awaited.

BILEVEL VENTILATION

Also described as biphasic positive airway pressure (BIPAP), this is a ventilatory mode where two levels of airway pressure are provided. The patient may cycle between these two levels as triggered by their ventilatory effort, in which case inspiratory positive airway pressure (IPAP) and expiratory positive airway pressure (EPAP) are set; however, this is no different to equivalent support with PSV and PEEP. Another use of bilevel ventilation is to allow spontaneous breathing at both levels of airway pressure, with time cycling between both pressure levels (high and low CPAP). An example of this is airway pressure release ventilation (APRV), where minute ventilation and CO_2 excretion are augmented by brief (1–1.5 s) periodic cycling to the lower level of CPAP. As the augmented V_T is dependent upon elastance of the respiratory system, it will be smaller in patients with 'stiff' respiratory systems. APRV without spontaneous breathing has a similar pressure profile to PCIRV.

Adequate ventilatory support can be supplied by both of these forms of bilevel ventilation. Patient-triggered bilevel ventilation is most commonly used during NIV; APRV offers a number of benefits and is usually applied during IV. Spontaneous respiratory efforts may: (1) improve matching of ventilation and perfusion due to increased dependent aeration; (2) increase venous return and hence cardiac output; and (3) promote reduced sedation. However, oxygenation does not immediately improve, and unsupported spontaneous breaths may increase left ventricular afterload and promote ventilator–patient dyssynchrony. APRV is contraindicated in chronic obstructive pulmonary disease, asthma and when deep sedation is required.

HIGH-FREQUENCY VENTILATION (HFV)

HFV encompasses techniques where small V_T (1–3 ml/kg) are delivered at high f (100–300/min). Hazards include inadequate humidification and gas trapping in patients with severe airflow limitation. High-frequency jet ventilation (HFJV) utilises dry gas from a high-pressure source delivered into an intratracheal catheter or specifically manufactured endotracheal tube. High-frequency oscillation (HFO) uses oscillatory flow within the airway to provide active inspiration and expiration at rates of 3–20 Hz. HFO offers benefit over conventional ventilation in neonates and children with respective infant and acute respiratory distress syndrome; data in adults are inconclusive.[26] HFJV has been used with improvement in gas exchange in adults with ARDS.[27]

LIQUID VENTILATION

Perfluorocarbons have a high solubility for both O_2 and CO_2, and reduce surface tension, somewhat analagous to pulmonary surfactant. Partial liquid ventilation is now the most common method of administration, with perfluorocarbon equal to the FRC administered via the endotracheal tube. The non-dependent lung is still ventilated, and may have increased blood flow due to compression of the pulmonary circulation in the dependent lung by the perfluorocarbon. Together with the perfluorocarbon-mediated reduction in surface tension, alveoli are recruited and oxygenation improved. However, when PEEP is applied the perfluorocarbon may be pushed distally and overdistend dependent alveoli.

Small clinical studies have reported improved gas exchange and respiratory mechanics after administration of perfluorocarbons;[28] however, a moderately large clinical study ($n = 311$) found that patients receiving conventional ventilation compared to both low- and high-dose perfluorocarbons had more ventilator-free days and tended to reduce mortality.[29] Consequently, liquid ventilation cannot be recommended.

INDICATIONS AND OBJECTIVES OF MECHANICAL VENTILATION[30]

Institution of mechanical ventilation is a clinical decision; it can only be supported by parameters such as blood gases or measures of respiratory muscle function. Even then, the decision to choose IV over NIV will be influenced by numerous factors, including the likely course of the ARF and its response to treatment. Often there will be an indication for intubation (Table 27.1) and mechanical ventilation; however, if intubation is required to overcome upper-airway obstruction, no ventilatory assistance may be needed despite the increase in respiratory work imposed by the endotracheal or tracheostomy tube.[18]

Table 27.1 Indications and objectives of intubated mechanical ventilation

Endotracheal intubation or tracheostomy

- For airway protection (e.g. coma)
- For suction of secretions
- To assist sedation and neuromuscular paralysis (e.g. to ↓ V_{O_2}, ↓ respiratory distress)
- To overcome upper-airway obstruction.

Mechanical ventilation

- To manipulate alveolar ventilation (V_A) and Pa_{CO_2} (e.g. reverse respiratory acidosis, ↓ cerebral blood flow and intracranial pressure)
- To ↑ Sa_{O_2} and Pa_{O_2} (by ↑ functional residual capacity, ↑end-inspiratory lung volume, ↑ V_A, ↑ Fi_{O_2})
- To ↓ work of breathing (e.g. to overcome respiratory muscle fatigue)
- To ↑ functional residual capacity (e.g. ↑ Pa_{O_2}, ↓ ventilator-induced injury)
- To stabilise the chest wall in severe chest injury

Once the decision has been made to proceed to ventilatory support the choice of mode should be based on a physiological approach, local expertise and simplicity.

Patients who are likely to need ventilatory assistance (e.g. acute severe asthma) should be considered for early ICU admission since this will allow faster responses and avoid cardiorespiratory arrest. Specific issues and methods of ventilatory assistance are dealt with in Chapters 29, 31 and 33. In patients with traumatic brain injury IV is commonly required to protect the airway and control ICP; similarly, patients with severe pancreatitis or serious abdominal infection may need prolonged IV to maintain an adequate FRC, reduce work of breathing, protect their airway and allow suctioning of secretions.

INITIATION OF INTUBATED MECHANICAL VENTILATION

A manual resuscitation circuit, mechanical ventilator and equipment for safe endotracheal intubation (see Chapter 25) should be available. Initial ventilator settings are commonly set to achieve adequate oxygenation and V_A; however, this will depend upon the patient's condition. Common settings are: V_T 6–10 ml/kg, f 10–20 breaths/min, PEEP 5 cmH_2O and Fi_{O_2} of 1.0, and these will need to be adjusted according to a specific patient's pathophysiology and response.

MANUAL RESUSCITATION CIRCUITS

Manual resuscitation circuits are primarily used to provide emergency ventilation when spontaneous effort is absent or inadequate. They may be used with a face or laryngeal mask, or an endotracheal tube. Occasionally they are used to provide a high inspired O_2 concentration during spontaneous breathing; however, this may impose significant additional respiratory work.[31] In the ICU they are commonly used for preoxygenation and manual lung inflation.

Their basic design includes a fresh gas flow of O_2, a reservoir bag and valves to allow spontaneous or positive-pressure breathing. Most manual resuscitation circuits use a self-inflating reservoir bag since this allows the circuit to be used by unskilled personnel and does not require a fresh gas flow. However, circuits using reservoir bags that are not self-inflating are still used in some institutions since they allow a better manual assessment of the respiratory mechanics – the 'educated hand' – and it is clear when there is an inadequate seal with a mask. Oxygen-powered manually triggered devices have been used for many years; however, this has declined markedly since high $\dot{V}$ and P may lead to barotrauma or gastric inflation.

Self-inflating reservoir bags use a series of one-way valves to allow fresh gas flow oxygen and entrained air to fill the bag. Inspired oxygen fractions as high as 0.8 may be achieved with neonatal or paediatric bags when an additional reservoir bag is used to allow fresh gas flow filling during expiration, after the bag has refilled.[32] However, lower Fi_{O_2}s (~0.6) will be obtained with both conventional O_2 flow rates of 8–15 l/min, and usual V_T and f, with an adult bag. Generally the valves are simple flap or duck-bill in nature, and both positive-pressure and spontaneous ventilation are possible. The reservoir bag volume in adults is typically 1600 ml, and V_T can be judged from chest wall movement. It is essential that these devices use standard 15/22-mm connectors to allow rapid connection to standard endotracheal tubes and ventilator circuits.

COMPLICATIONS OF MECHANICAL VENTILATION (TABLE 27.2)[26]

Although mechanical ventilation may be vital, it also introduces numerous potential complications. Monitoring includes a high nurse-to-patient ratio (usually 1:1), ventilator alarms and pulse oximetry. Capnography is recommended to confirm endotracheal tube placement, and may be used to monitor the adequacy of V_A;

Table 27.2 Complications of intubation and mechanical ventilation

Equipment
- Malfunction or disconnection
- Incorrectly set or prescribed
- Contamination

Pulmonary
- Airway intubation (e.g. damage to teeth, vocal cords, trachea; see Chapter 25)
- Ventilator-associated pneumonia (reduced lung defence; see Chapter 32)
- Ventilator-associated lung injury (e.g. diffuse lung injury due to regional overdistension or tidal recruitment of alveoli)
- Overt barotrauma (e.g. pneumothorax)
- O_2 toxicity
- Patient–ventilator asynchrony

Circulation
- ↓ Right ventricular preload → ↓ cardiac output
- ↑ Right ventricular afterload (if the lung is overdistended)
- ↓ Splanchnic blood flow with high levels of positive end-expiratory pressure (PEEP) or mean P_{aw}
- ↑ Intracranial pressure with high levels of PEEP or mean P_{aw}
- Fluid retention due to ↓ cardiac output → ↓ renal blood flow

Other
- Gut distension (air swallowing, hyomotility)
- Mucosal ulceration and bleeding
- Peripheral and respiratory muscle weakness (see Chapter 49)
- Sleep disturbance, agitation and fear (which may be prolonged after recovery)
- Neuropsychiatric complications

however, expired CO_2 is strongly influenced by factors that alter alveolar dead space, such as cardiac output. Intermittent blood gases, $PEEP_i$, airway pressures in volume-preset modes and V_T in pressure-preset modes should be recorded. Individual patients may benefit from more extensive monitoring of their respiratory mechanics or tissue oxygenation.

The patient's airway (i.e. patency, presence of leaks and nature and amount of secretions), breathing (i.e. rate, volume, oxygenation) and circulation (i.e. pulse, blood pressure and urine output) must be monitored. Ventilatory and circuit alarms should be adjusted to monitor an appropriate range of *V*, *P* and temperature. This should alert adjacent staff to changes in *P* and/or *V* that may be caused by an occluded endotracheal tube, tension pneumothorax or circuit disconnection. These alarms may be temporarily disabled while the cause is detected, but never permanently disabled. Sudden difficulties with high *P* during volume-preset ventilation or oxygenation must initiate an immediate search for the cause. This should start with the patency of the airway, followed by a structured approach to both the circuit and ventilator, and to factors altering the *E* and *R* of the lung and chest wall such as bronchospasm, secretions, pneumothorax and asynchronous breathing. In addition to careful clinical examination an urgent chest radiograph and bronchoscopy may be required.

Mechanical ventilation is also associated with a marked increase in the incidence of nosocomial pneumonia due to a reduction in the natural defence of the respiratory tract, and this represents an important advantage offered by NIV. In patients successfully managed with NIV, Girou and colleagues reported a reduction in the incidence of nosocomial pneumonia, associated with improved survival, compared to IV.[33] Erect versus semirecumbent posture[34] also reduces the incidence of ventilator-associated pneumonia.

Although lung overdistension may result in alveolar rupture leading to pulmonary interstitial air, pneumomediastinum or pneumothorax, it may also lead to diffuse alveolar damage similar to that found in ALI and ARDS. Both are termed VILI, and V_T reduction leads to a marked decrease in ALI mortality, due to a reduction in multiple-organ dysfunction.[5] There are also laboratory data suggesting that inadequate PEEP with tidal recruitment and derecruitment of alveoli leads to VILI; however, this has not been proven in a clinical trial. Finally, patient–ventilator asynchrony may result in wasted respiratory work, impaired gas exchange and respiratory distress (see below).

Positive-pressure ventilation elevates intrathoracic pressure, which reduces venous return, right ventricular preload and cardiac output. The impact is reduced by hypervolaemia and partial ventilatory support, where patient effort and a reduction in pleural pressure augment venous return. Secondary effects include a reduction in regional organ blood flow leading to fluid retention by the kidney, and possibly impaired hepatic function. This latter effect is only seen at high levels of PEEP where an increase in resistance to venous return and a reduction in cardiac output may combine to reduce hepatic blood flow.

Sleep disturbance, and agitation and discomfort are common in mechanically ventilated patients. These effects may be reduced with sedation until weaning is planned; however, it is important not to prolong mechanical ventilation due to excessive use of sedatives, which may also depress blood pressure and spontaneous respiratory effort. Finally, complex neuropsychological sequelae have been described in recovering ARDS patients.[35,36] These do not appear to reflect the severity of the acute illness since ARDS patients have a poorer quality of life than patients with a similar severity of illness without ARDS.[37] However, they do correlate with their duration of hypoxaemia. Clearly, this is an important issue that needs further research.

WITHDRAWAL (WEANING) FROM MECHANICAL VENTILATION

Once the underlying process necessitating mechanical ventilation has started to resolve, withdrawal of ventilatory support should be considered; increased duration of ventilation leads to a progressive rise in complications such as ventilator-associated pneumonia. However, other important parameters that must be considered include the neuromuscular state of the patient (ability to initiate a spontaneous breath), adequacy of oxygenation (typically low requirements for PEEP (5–8 cmH_2O) and $FiO_2 < 0.4–0.5$) and cardiovascular stability.[38] Once a patient is considered suitable to wean, a secondary question is whether an artificial airway is still required for airway protection or suction of secretions. Many patients can rapidly make the transition from mechanical ventilation to extubation, but ~20% of patients fail weaning despite meeting clinical criteria.[21] Advanced age, prolonged mechanical ventilation and chronic obstructive pulmonary disease all increase the likelihood that weaning will be difficult.[21]

Weaning failure is usually associated with an increase in respiratory drive and respiratory rate and a fall in V_T which contributes to hypercapnoea;[39] about 10% of patients fail due to central respiratory depression. Various indices such as maximal inspiratory pressure (MIP), minute ventilation (V_E), *f*, V_T *f*/V_T ratio and the compliance, respiratory rate, oxygenation, maximum inspiratory pressure (CROP) index have been investigated as predictors of weaning failure (Table 27.3). They are rarely used alone and careful clinical assessment is often adequate, yielding a reintubation rate as low as 3%,[40] and none of these indices assess airway function following extubation. Although the typical threshold value for the rapid shallow-breathing index (f/V_T ratio) is > 105, a large recent multicentre study reported progressive increase in risk as this increased with a threshold of 57; in addition a

Table 27.3 Sample of measurements that have been used to predict successful outcome from weaning in critically ill patients*

Parameter	Typical threshold value†	Comment
V_E	$\leq$ 15 l/min	Moderate to high sensitivity, low specificity
MIP	≤ -15 cmH_2O	High sensitivity, low specificity
CROP index#	$\geq$ 13	Moderate to high sensitivity, modest specificity
During a spontaneous breathing trial		
f	$\leq$ 38 breaths/min	High sensitivity, low specificity
V_T	$\geq$ 325 ml (4 ml/kg)	High sensitivity, low specificity
f/V_T	$\leq$ 105	High sensitivity, moderate specificity

*See reference 38 for further detail.
†Although threshold values are often used, the data are not dichotonous. For example, as the f/V_T ratio increases, so does the rate of reintubation.[41]
#CROP index = (C_{dyn} × MIP × [Pa_{O_2}/PA_{O_2}]/f).[21]
MIP, maximal inspiratory pressure; CROP, compliance, respiratory rate, oxygenation, maximum inspiratory pressure.

positive fluid balance immediately prior to extubation was a significant risk factor for reintubation.[41] Consequently, weaning indices should not necessarily delay extubation or a weaning trial. However, they may quantitate important issues in the general clinical assessment, and may be directly relevant for a given patient. For example, frequent small V_T, an inadequate vital capacity (less than 8–12 ml/kg), large minute ventilation (= 15 l/min), depressed respiratory drive and reduced respiratory muscle strength (MIP = –15 cmH_2O) or drive should be strongly factored into deciding whether a patient is ready to undergo a trial of weaning safely.

Direct comparisons between T-piece trials, PSV and SIMV as weaning techniques have been performed in patients previously failing a 2-hour trial of spontaneous breathing. In the study by Brochard and colleagues,[42] PSV led to fewer failures and a shorter weaning period. In contrast, Esteban and coworkers[43] found that a once-daily trial of spontaneous breathing resulted in the shortest duration of mechanical ventilation; however, a relatively high proportion of patients required reintubation (22.6%). Viewed together these studies suggest that weaning was slower with SIMV,[19] although SIMV with PSV was not studied, and that either PSV or a T-piece trial is the preferred method for weaning. Since low levels of PSV can help compensate for the additional work of breathing attributable to the endotracheal tube and circuit, some clinicians use low levels of PSV (5–7 cmH_2O) during weaning or during a spontaneous breathing trial. However, the work of breathing following extubation is usually higher than expected, probably due to upper-airway oedema and dysfunction, so that work is similar to that during a T-piece trial.[21]

Reintubation is associated with a 7–11-fold increased risk of hospital death.[19] A number of factors may account for this, including selection of previously unaccounted-for severity of illness as the mortality rate associated with reintubation is much higher in patients whose primary diagnosis was respiratory failure. In addition, complications which may (pneumonia, heart failure) or may not be attributable to extubation contribute to this poor outcome. Hence, an important goal during mechanical ventilation will be to proceed to early and expeditious extubation with a low reintubation rate.

PATIENT–VENTILATOR INTERACTION

This is an extremely important issue in patients with either partial ventilatory support, or those breathing spontaneously through the ventilator. Dyssynchrony can lead to agitation, diaphoresis, tachycardia, hypertension and weaning failure or a failure of NIV. Once this pattern is identified it is crucial that airway complications (partial obstruction, displacement) or a major change in the clinical state (e.g. pneumothorax, acute pulmonary oedema) are excluded before considering problems with patient–ventilator interaction. For simplicity this will be subdivided into: (1) triggering of inspiration; (2) inspiration; and (3) cessation of inspiration; however, difficulties at each of these phases will lead to changes in respiratory drive and effort that may be expressed throughout the respiratory cycle. Importantly, major problems with patient–ventilator dyssynchrony can be identified by carefully observing respiratory effort and ventilator cycling at the bedside and this may be assisted by observing P, V and $\dot{V}$ waveforms displayed by the ventilator.

TRIGGERING OF INSPIRATION

1. $PEEP_i$ is an important hindrance to the triggering of inspiration in patients with severe airflow limitation, since their inspiratory muscles must first reduce P_{ao} below ambient pressure.[44] Consequently P_{mus} must exceed $PEEP_i$ prior to triggering an assisted breath either by reducing airway pressure (pressure trigger) or by reducing circuit flow (flow trigger). This inspiratory threshold load may be up to 40% of the total inspiratory work in ARF with dynamic hyperinflation, and commonly results in ineffective triggering. Triggering can be markedly improved and respiratory work reduced by low levels of CPAP[37,45] – commonly 80–90% of dynamic $PEEP_i$.[46]
2. A fall in P_{ao} has been the most common form of triggering. Pressure is usually sensed at the expiratory block of the ventilator. Sensing at the Y-piece is not superior

since there is a similar delay in sensing as the transducer is usually sited in the ventilator. Flow triggering senses a fall in continuous circuit flow, and was introduced as a method of reducing inspiratory work. However, there has been a marked improvement of both pressure and flow triggering in modern ventilators, with the trigger time delay falling from ~400 to ~100 ms, and a similar improvement in the maximum fall in airway pressure.[47] Attempts to improve the trigger function by oversetting the pressure sensitivity (> –0.5 cmH_2O) may lead to autocycling, which may also occur with overset flow triggering. This is due to the P and $\dot{V}_I$ effects of cardiac oscillations, hiccups, circuit rainout or mask leak with NIV, and has been reported as a cause of apparent respiratory effort in brain-dead patients.[48] Flow triggering reduces the risk of autocycling at a given trigger sensitivity, and reduces respiratory effort a small amount compared to pressure triggering; however, it does not alter the frequency of ineffective efforts,[49] or patient effort following triggering.[40]

INSPIRATION

Once inspiration is triggered or sensed by the ventilator, $\dot{V}$ is determined by P, T_i or V. For example, during PSV ventilation a target P is held until expiration is sensed, and during ACV $\dot{V}$ is held for a set T_i. During ACV there may be continued inspiratory effort, and since inspiratory $\dot{V}$ is fixed, this will be reflected by a scalloping of the P_{ao}–T graph if $\dot{V}$ is inadequate. Again this may be illustrated using the equation of motion:

$$P_{mus} + P_{ao} = E_{rs} V + R_{rs} \dot{V} + Po \qquad \textit{Equation 6}$$

P_{mus} will reflect the difference between P_{ao} due to E,R and P_o and the observed P_{ao}. In contrast, during P-cycled ventilation (PACV), greater patient effort is rewarded, and inspiratory work is lower than during equivalent ACV.[50]

Modern ventilators allow adjustment of inspiratory $\dot{V}$ and $\dot{V}$ pattern, and the rate of rise of P_{ao}. Low inspiratory rates during ACV result in significant inspiratory work, but this may be markedly reduced by increasing inspiratory $\dot{V}$ to 65 l/min.[51] However, these issues are quite complex, and f increases (probably due to a lower respiratory tract reflex) as $\dot{V}_I$ increases,[52] reducing T_e, which may contribute to dynamic hyperinflation in patients with severe airflow obstruction. During PSV and PACV, many ventilators allow adjustment of the rate of rise of P to its target. A steeper P ramp leads to earlier attainment of the P target, greater early rates and reduction of inspiratory drive and work.[53,54]

CESSATION OF INSPIRATION

During PSV, an increase in airways resistance will result in a delayed fall in $\dot{V}_I$. Since this is the trigger for cycling to expiration, the ventilator may continue to provide $\dot{V}_I$ while the patient desires to exhale. This commonly leads to recruitment of expiratory muscles, detected both clinically and as a transient rise in the end-inspiratory P_{ao}.[55] Some modern ventilators allow control of the fall in $\dot{V}_I$ that is sensed as end-inspiration. High levels of PSV ($\geq$ 20 cmH_2O), weak respiratory muscles and mask leak with NIV are other common causes of dyssynchrony at the termination of inspiration. In this last group, PACV, which is time-cycled, allows improved patient–ventilator synchrony at end-inspiration compared to PSV.[56]

REFERENCES

1. Lassen HC. A preliminary report on the 1952 epidemic of poliomyelitis in Copenhagen with special reference to the treatment of acute respiratory insufficiency. *Lancet* 1953; **Jan 3**: 37–41.
2. Mehta S, Hill NS. Noninvasive ventilation. *Am J Respir Crit Care Med* 2001; **163**: 540–7.
3. International Consensus Conference in Intensive Care Medicine. Ventilator-associated lung injury in ARDS. *Am J Respir Crit Care Med* 1999; **160**: 2118–24.
4. Bendixen HH, Hedley-White J, Laver MB. Impaired oxygenation in surgical patients during general anesthesia with controlled ventilation: a concept of atelectasis. *N Engl J Med* 1963; **269**: 991–6.
5. Ventilation with lower tidal volumes as compared with traditional volumes for acute lung injury and the acute respiratory distress syndrome. *N Engl J Med* 2000; **342**: 1301–8.
6. Hotchkiss JR, Blanch L, Murias G *et al.* Effects of decreased respiratory frequency on ventilator-induced lung injury. *Am J Respir Crit Care Med* 2000; **161**: 463–8.
7. Lessard MR, Guerot E, Lorino H *et al.* Effects of pressure-controlled with different I:E ratios versus volume-controlled ventilation on respiratory mechanics, gas exchange, and hemodynamics in patients with adult respiratory distress syndrome. *Anesthesiology* 1994; **80**: 983–91.
8. Edibam C, Rutten AJ, Collins DV *et al.* Effect of inspiratory flow pattern and inspiratory to expiratory ratio on nonlinear elastic behavior in patients with acute lung injury. *Am J Respir Crit Care Med* 2003; **167**: 702–7.
9. Bersten AD, Bryan DL. Ventilator-induced lung injury: do dynamic factors also play a role? *Crit Care Med* 2005; **33**: 907–9.
10. Jonson B, Beydon L, Brauer K *et al.* Mechanics of respiratory system in healthy anesthetized humans with emphasis on viscoelastic properties. *J Appl Physiol* 1993; **75**: 132–40.
11. Tuxen DV, Lane S. The effects of ventilatory pattern on hyperinflation, airway pressures, and circulation in mechanical ventilation of patients with severe airflow obstruction. *Am Rev Respir Dis* 1987; **136**: 872–9.
12. The National Heart, Lung, and Blood Institute ARDS Clinical Trials Network. Higher versus lower positive end-expiratory pressure in patients with the acute respiratory distress syndrome. *N Engl J Med* 2004; **351**: 327–36.
13. Suter PM, Fairley B, Isenberg MD. Optimum end-expiratory airway pressure in patients with acute pulmonary failure. *N Engl J Med* 1975; **292**: 284–9.
14. Gattinoni L, Pelosi P, Crotti S *et al.* Effects of positive end-expiratory pressure on regional distribution of tidal

volume and recruitment in adult respiratory distress syndrome. *Am J Respir Crit Care Med* 1995; **151**: 1807–14.
15. Vieira SRR, Puybasset L, Richecoeur J *et al.* A lung computed tomographic assessment of positive end-expiratory pressure-induced lung overdistension. *Am J Respir Crit Care Med* 1998; **158**: 1571–7.
16. Bersten AD. Measurement of overinflation by multiple linear regression analysis in patients with acute lung injury. *Eur Respir J* 1998; **12**: 526–32.
17. Nicholas TE, Power JHT, Barr HA. The pulmonary consequences of a deep breath. *Respir Physiol* 1982; **49**: 315–24.
18. Pelosi P, Cardringher P, Bottino N *et al.* Sigh in acute respiratory distress syndrome. *Am J Respir Crit Care Med* 1999; **159**: 872–80.
19. Marini JJ, Rodriguez M, Lamb V. The inspiratory workload of patient-initiated mechanical ventilation. *Am Rev Respir Dis* 1986; **134**: 902–9.
20. Bersten AD, Rutten AJ, Vedig AE *et al.* Additional work of breathing imposed by endotracheal tubes, breathing circuits and intensive care ventilators. *Crit Care Med* 1989; **17**: 671–80.
21. Esteban A, Alia I. Clinical management of weaning from mechanical ventilation. *Intens Care Med* 1998; **24**: 999–1008.
22. Brochard L, Harf A, Lorino H *et al.* Inspiratory pressure support prevents diaphragmatic fatigue during weaning from mechanical ventilation. *Am Rev Respir Dis* 1989; **139**: 513–21.
23. Bersten AD, Rutten AJ, Vedig AE. Efficacy of pressure support ventilation in compensating for apparatus work. *Anaesth Intens Care* 1993; **21**: 67–71.
24. Brochard L, Rua F, Lorino H *et al.* Inspiratory pressure support compensates for the additional work of breathing caused by the endotracheal tube. *Anesthesiology* 1991; **75**: 739–45.
25. Appendini L, Purro A, Gudjonsdottir M *et al.* Physiologic response of ventilator-dependent patients with chronic obstructive pulmonary disease to proportional assist ventilation and continuous positive airway pressure. *Am J Respir Crit Care Med* 1999; **159**: 1510–7.
26. Derdak S, Mehta S, Stewart TE *et al.* High-frequency oscillatory ventilation for acute respiratory distress syndrome in adults: a randomized, controlled trial. *Am J Respir Crit Care Med* 2002; **166**: 801–8.
27. Gluck E, Heard S, Patel C *et al.* Use of ultrahigh frequency ventilation in patients with ARDS: a preliminary report. *Chest* 1993; **103**: 1413–20.
28. Hirschl RB, Pranikoff T, Wise C *et al.* Initial experience with partial liquid ventilation in adult patients with the acute respiratory distress syndrome. *JAMA* 1996; **275**: 383–9.
29. Kacmarek RM, Wiedemann HP, Lavin PT *et al.* Partial liquid ventilation in adult patients with acute respiratory distress syndrome. *Am J Respir Crit Care Med* 2006; **173**: 882–9.
30. Slutsky AS. Mechanical ventilation. *Chest* 1993; **104**: 1833–59.
31. Hess D, Hirsch C, Marquis-D'Amico C *et al.* Imposed work and oxygen delivery during spontaneous breathing with adult disposable manual ventilators. *Anesthesiology* 1994; **81**: 1256–63.
32. Agarwal KS, Puliyel JM. A simple strategy to improve first breath oxygen delivery by self inflating bag. *Resuscitation* 2000; **45**: 221–4.
33. Girou E, Schortgen F, Delclaux C *et al.* Association of noninvasive ventilation with nosocomial infections and survival in critically ill patients. *JAMA* 2000; **284**: 2361–7.
34. Drakulovic MB, Torres A, Bauer TT *et al.* Supine body position as a risk factor for nosocomial pneumonia in mechanically ventilated patients: a randomised trial. *Lancet* 1999; **354**: 1851–8.
35. Hopkins RO, Weaver LK, Opep D *et al.* Neuropsychological sequelae and impaired health status in survivors of severe acute respiratory distress syndrome. *Am J Respir Crit Care Med* 1999; **160**: 50–6.
36. Rothenhausler H, Ehrentraut S, Stoll C *et al.* The relationship between cognitive performance and employment and health status in long-term survivors of the acute respiratory distress syndrome: results of an exploratory study. *Gen Hosp Psychiatry* 2001; **23**: 90–6.
37. Davidson TA, Caldwell ES, Curtis JR *et al.* Reduced quality of life in survivors of acute respiratory distress syndrome compared with critically ill control patients. *JAMA* 1999; **281**: 354–60.
38. MacIntyre NR. Evidence-based guidelines for weaning and discontinuing ventilatory support: a collective task force facilitated by the American College of Chest Physicians; the American Association for Respiratory Care; and the American College of Critical Care Medicine. *Chest* 2001; **120**: 375–96S.
39. Tobin MJ, Perez W, Guenther SM *et al.* The pattern of breathing during successful and unsuccessful trials of weaning from mechanical ventilation. *Am Rev Respir Dis* 1986; **134**: 1111–8.
40. Leitch EA, Moran JL, Grealy B. Weaning and extubation in the intensive care unit. Clinical or index-driven approach? *Intens Care Med* 1996; **22**: 752–79.
41. Frutos-Vivar F, Ferguson ND, Esteban A *et al.* Risk factors for extubation failure in patients following a successful spontaneous breathing trial. *Chest* 2006; **130**: 1664–71.
42. Brochard L, Rauss A, Benito S *et al.* Comparison of three methods of gradual withdrawal from ventilatory support during weaning from mechanical ventilation. *Am J Respir Crit Care Med* 1994; **150**: 896–903.
43. Esteban A, Frutos F, Tobin MJ *et al.* A comparison of four methods of weaning patients from mechanical ventilation. *N Engl J Med* 1995; **332**: 345–50.
44. Smith TC, Marini JJ. Impact of PEEP on lung mechanics and work of breathing in severe airflow obstruction. *J Appl Physiol* 1988; **65**: 1488–99.
45. Petrof BJ, Legare M, Goldberg P *et al.* Continuous positive airway pressure reduces work of breathing and dyspnea during weaning form mechanical ventilation in severe chronic obstructive pulmonary disease. *Am Rev Respir Dis* 1990; **141**: 281–9.
46. Ranieri VM, Giuliiani R, Cinnella G *et al.* Physiologic effects of positive end-expiratory pressure in patients

with chronic obstructive pulmonary disease during acute ventilatory failure and controlled mechanical ventilation. *Am Rev Respir Dis* 1993; **147**: 5–13.
47. Alsanian P, El Atrous S, Isabey D *et al.* Effects of flow triggering on breathing effort during partial ventilatory support. *Am J Respir Crit Care Med* 1998; **157**: 135–43.
48. Willatts SM, Drummond G. Brainstem death and ventilator trigger settings. *Anaesthesia* 2000; **55**: 676–7.
49. Sassoon CSH, Foster GT. Patient-ventilator asynchrony. *Curr Opin Crit Care* 2001; **7**: 28–33.
50. Cinnella G, Conti G, Lofaso F *et al.* Effects of assisted ventilation on the work of breathing: volume controlled versus pressure-controlled ventilation. *Am J Respir Crit Care Med* 1996; **153**: 1025–33.
51. Ward ME, Corbeil C, Gibbons W *et al.* Optimization of respiratory muscle relaxation during mechanical ventilation. *Anesthesiology* 1988; **69**: 29–35.
52. Corne S, Gillespie D, Roberts D *et al.* Effect of inspiratory flow rate on respiratory rate in intubated ventilated patients. *Am J Respir Crit Care Med* 1997; **156**: 304–8.
53. Bonmarchand G, Chevron V, Chopin CC *et al.* Increased initial flow rate reduces inspiratory work of breathing during pressure support ventilation in patients with exacerbation of chronic obstructive pulmonary disease. *Intens Care Med* 1996; **22**: 1147–54.
54. Bonmarchand G, Chevron V, Menard JF *et al.* Effects of pressure ramp slope values on the work of breathing during pressure support ventilation in restrictive patients. *Crit Care Med* 1999; **27**: 715–22.
55. Parthasarathy S, Jubran A, Tobin MJ. Cycling of inspiratory and expiratory muscle groups with the ventilator in airflow limitation. *Am J Respir Crit Care Med* 1998; **158**: 1471–8.
56. Calderinin E, Confalonieri M, Puccio PG *et al.* Patient–ventilator asynchrony during noninvasive ventilation: the role of expiratory trigger. *Intens Care Med* 1999; **25**: 662–7.

28

Humidification and inhalation therapy

Andrew D Bersten

The upper airway normally warms, moistens and filters inspired gas. When these functions are impaired by disease, or when the nasopharynx is bypassed by endotracheal intubation, artificial humidification of inspired gases must be provided.

PHYSICAL PRINCIPLES

Humidity, the amount of water vapour in a gas, may be expressed as:

1. *absolute humidity* (AH) – the total mass of water vapour in a given volume of gas at a given temperature (g/m^3)
2. *relative humidity* (RH) – the actual mass of water vapour (per volume of gas) as a percentage of the mass of saturated water vapour, at a given temperature. Saturated water vapour exerts a saturated vapour pressure (SVP). As the SVP has an exponential relation with temperature (Table 28.1), addition of further water vapour to the gas can only occur with a rise in temperature
3. *partial pressure*

PHYSIOLOGY

Clearance of surface liquids and particles from the lung depends on beating cilia, airway mucus and transepithelial water flux. Airway mucus is derived from secretions from goblet cells, submucosal glands and Clara cells, and from capillary transudate. Conducting airways are lined with pseudostratified, ciliated columnar epithelium and numerous fluid-secreting glands. As the airway descends, the epithelium becomes stratified, and then cuboidal and partially ciliated, with very few secretory glands at the terminal airways. The cilia beat in a watery (sol) layer over which is a viscous mucous layer (gel), and move a superficial layer of mucus from deep within the lung toward the glottis (at a rate of 10 mm/min at 37°C and 100% RH). Both cilia function and mucus composition are influenced by temperature and adequate humidification.

The nasal mucosa has a large surface area with an extensive vascular network which humidifies and warms inhaled gas more effectively than during mouth-breathing. Heating and humidification of dry gas are progressive down the airway, with an isothermic saturation boundary (i.e. 100% RH at 37°C or AH of 43 g/m^3) just below the carina.[1] Under resting conditions, approximately 250 ml of water and 1.5 kJ (350 kcal) of energy is lost from the respiratory tract in a day. A proportion (10–25%) is returned to the mucosa during expiration due to condensation.

The minimal moisture level to maintain ciliary function and mucus clearance is uncertain. Although reproducing an isothermic saturation boundary at the carina may be ideal, it does not seem essential in all situations. Mucus flow is markedly reduced when RH at 37°C falls below 75% (AH of 32 g/m^3), and ceases when RH is 50% (AH of 22 g/m^3).[2] This suggests that an AH exceeding 33 g/m^3 is needed to maintain normal function. At this AH level, inspired gas temperature does not appear to be important unless excessive.[3] Mucociliary function is also impaired by upper respiratory tract infection, chronic bronchitis, cystic fibrosis, bronchiectasis, immotile cilia syndrome (including Kartagener's syndrome), dehydration, hyperventilation, general anaesthetics, opioids, atropine and exposure to noxious gases. High fractional inspired oxygen concentrations (FiO_2) may lead to acute tracheobronchitis, with depressed tracheal mucus velocity within 3 h.[4] Inhaled β_2-adrenergic agonists increase mucociliary clearance by augmenting ciliary beat frequency, and mucus and water secretion.[5]

CLINICAL APPLICATIONS OF HUMIDIFICATION

TRACHEAL INTUBATION

The need for humidification during endotracheal intubation and tracheostomy is unquestioned. As the upper airway is bypassed, RH of inspired gas falls below 50% with adverse effects, including:[6]

1. increased mucus viscosity
2. depressed ciliary function
3. cytological damage to the tracheobronchial epithelium, including mucosal ulceration, tracheal inflammation and necrotising tracheobronchitis[7]

Table 28.1 Relationship of temperature and saturated vapour pressure

Temperature (°C)	Saturated vapour pressure (mmHg)	Saturated vapour pressure (kPa)	Absolute humidity (g/m³)
0	4.6	0.6	4.8
10	9.2	1.2	9.3
20	17.5	2.3	17.1
30	31.3	4.2	30.4
34	39.9	5.3	37.5
37	47.1	6.3	43.4
40	55.3	7.4	51.7
46	78.0	10.4	68.7

4. microatelectasis from obstruction of small airways, and reduced surfactant leading to reduced lung compliance
5. airway obstruction due to tenacious or inspissated sputum with increased airway resistance

Metaplasia of the tracheal epithelium occurs over weeks to months in patients with a permanent tracheostomy. These patients do not usually require humidified gas, suggesting that humidification occurs lower down the respiratory tree. Nonetheless, humidification of inspired gas may be needed during an acute respiratory tract infection.

HEAT EXCHANGE

The respiratory tract is an important avenue to adjust body temperature by heat exchange. Humidification of gases reduces the fall in body temperature associated with anaesthesia and surgery.[6] In this setting, active humidifiers are of no benefit over heat and moisture exchangers (HMEs).[8] Excessive heat from humidification may produce mucosal damage, hyperthermia and overhumidification.[9] However, if water content is not excessive, mucociliary clearance is unaffected up to temperatures of 42°C.[3] Overhumidification may increase secretions and impair mucociliary clearance and surfactant activity, resulting in atelectasis.[9]

IDEAL HUMIDIFICATION

The basic requirements of a humidifier should include the following features:[10]

1. The inspired gas is delivered into the trachea at 32–36°C with a water content of 30–43 g/m³.
2. The set temperature remains constant and does not fluctuate.
3. Humidification and temperature remain unaffected by a large range of fresh gas flows, especially high flows.
4. The device is simple to use and to service.
5. Humidification can be provided for air, oxygen or any mixture of inspired gas, including anaesthetic agents.
6. The humidifier can be used with spontaneous or controlled ventilation.
7. There are safety mechanisms, with alarms, against overheating, overhydration and electrocution.
8. The resistance, compliance and dead-space characteristics do not adversely affect spontaneous breathing modes.
9. The sterility of the inspired gas is not compromised.

METHODS AND DEVICES

WATER BATH HUMIDIFIERS

Inspired gas is passed over or through a water reservoir to achieve humidification. Their efficiency is dependent on ambient temperature and the surface area available for gas vaporisation.

COLD-WATER HUMIDIFIERS

These units are simple and inexpensive, but are inefficient, with a water content of around 9 g/m³ (i.e. about 50% RH at ambient temperatures). They are also a potential source of microbiological contamination. Routine use of cold-water humidifiers to deliver oxygen with simple facemasks is unnecessary.

HOT-WATER HUMIDIFIERS (FIGURES 28.1 AND 28.2)

Inspired gas is passed over (i.e. blow-by humidifier, e.g. Fisher–Paykel, Fisher and Paykel Medical, New Zealand) or through (i.e. bubble or cascade humidifier, e.g. Bennett Cascade, Bennett Medical Equipment, USA) a heated-water reservoir. Gas leaving the reservoir theoretically contains high water content. The water bath temperature is thermostatically controlled (e.g. at 45–60°C) to compensate for cooling along the inspiratory tubing targeting an inspired RH of 100% at 37°C. A heated wire may be sited in the inspiratory tubing to maintain preset gas

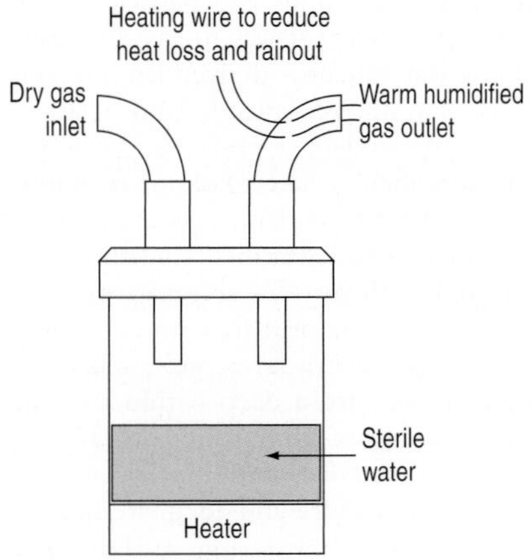

Figure 28.1 Hot-water 'blow-by' humidifier.

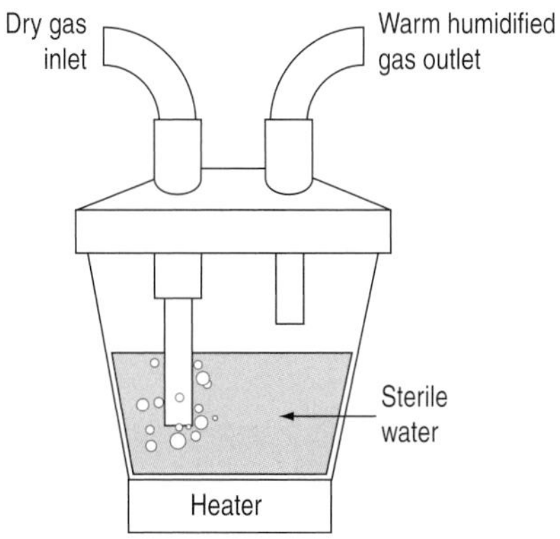

Figure 28.2 Hot-water 'cascade' or 'bubble' humidifier.

temperature and humidity (e.g. Fisher–Paykel humidifier). It is commonly believed that hot-water humidifiers do not produce aerosols, but microdroplets (mostly less than 5 μm diameter) have been reported with bubble humidifiers,[11] and this may be a potential source of infection.

Fisher–Paykel humidifier

This is a commonly used blow-by humidifier. The delivery hose is heated by an insulated heating wire to achieve a manual preset inspired temperature. An additional servo-control unit is available, while more recent models have a dual servo unit which combines this function in the heater base. Audible alarms indicate disconnection and variations over 2°C from the set delivery temperature. The heater base is protected from overheating by a thermostat set at 47°C. If this fails, another safety thermostat operates at 70°C. A disposable humidification chamber is filled manually with water or by a gravity-feed set. To minimise rain-out, the chamber outlet can be set at a temperature below the delivery hose outlet temperature – 2–3°C is usually adequate and does not compromise RH. Temperature alarms are fixed at 41°C and 29.5°C, with a back-up safety set at 66°C for the delivery chamber.

Although these humidifiers are often regarded as providing optimal humidification in ventilated patients, their performance is lower than expected (36 mg/l with MR 850 with the outlet temperature set to 37°C and the delivery hose set at 40°C, and optimal conditions in bench studies, and up to 41.9 mg/l in practice).[12] However, under conditions of high ambient temperature and/or high ventilator output temperature the inlet temperature to the humidification chamber can be high enough that the heater base operates at a low enough temperature that humidification is impaired,with reduction in inspired water content as low as 19 mg/l in bench studies, and 23.4 mg/l in practice.[12] The automatic compensation now available on this humidifier helps compensate for poor performance, which can also be prevented by setting the chamber outlet and hose to 40°C. High minute ventilation is well tolerated, but a small decrease in water content output has also been found with higher respiratory rates.[13]

Counter flow-heated humidifiers

Using the countercurrent principle for gas and heated water, newer designs may further improve performance so that performance is independent of gas flow and respiratory rate, with lower imposed work of breathing.[13]

HEAT AND MOISTURE EXCHANGERS

Modern HMEs are popular intensive care unit (ICU) humidifiers due to their simplicity and increased efficiency. They all work on the basic principle of heat and moisture conservation during expiration, allowing inspired gas to be heated and humidified. HMEs may be hydrophobic or hygroscopic, and may also act as a microbial filter (HMEF). However, since nosocomial pneumonia is primarily due to aspiration of oropharyngeal secretions followed by secondary ventilator tubing colonisation, HMEFs have not been shown to reduce the frequency of nosocomial pneumonia, and the incidence is similar when HMEs and hot-water humidifiers are compared during prolonged ventilation.[14,15]

Modern HMEs are light with a small dead space (30–95 ml), but are varied in their level of humidification. Hygroscopic HMEs adsorb moisture on to a foam or paper-like material that is chemically coated (often calcium chloride or lithium chloride), and this tends to increase their efficiency (i.e. AH around 30 g/m^3) compared to hydrophobic HMEs (i.e. AH 20–25 g/m^3).[16–21] The efficiency of older HMEs decreases with time;[13] however, modern HMEs may retain their ability to humidify for at least 4 days with minimal change in resistance.[22] Consequently, HMEs that achieve relatively high AH may be suitable for long-term mechanical ventilation in selected patients, particularly as the majority of reported HME complications (e.g. thick secretions and endotracheal tube occlusion) occurred with units of lower humidification levels.[23–25] Nevertheless, HMEs increase dead space and imposed work of breathing, and cannot match the humidification offered by hot-water humidifiers, which remain the 'gold standard', particularly if secretions are thick or bloody, minute ventilation is high,[15,19] humidification is necessary for more than 4 days[26] or if used in children and neonates.

COMPLICATIONS OF HUMIDIFICATION

INADEQUATE HUMIDIFICATION

An AH exceeding 30 g/m^3 is recommended in respiratory care.[24] Inadequate humidification is usually only a problem with HMEs. With hot-water humidifiers, however, efficiency is reduced by increasing gas flow rates and rainout. A decrease of about 1°C occurs for each 10 cm of tubing beyond the end of the delivery hose (i.e. the

Y-connector and right-angled connector), and should be catered for. Inadequate humidification in high-frequency ventilation can be overcome by using superheated humidification of the entrained gas with a temperature thermistor built into the endotracheal tube.[23,27]

OVERHUMIDIFICATION

Overheating malfunction of hot-water humidifiers may cause a rise in core temperature, water intoxication, impaired mucociliary clearance and airway burns.[9]

IMPOSED WORK OF BREATHING

The work of breathing imposed by a humidifier, primarily resistive work, is an important additional respiratory load in ICU patients. Consequently their imposed work increases with inspiratory flow rate, and the progressive increase in water content of HMEs is also associated with increased resistance.[28] The Fisher–Paykel humidifier imposes relatively low work compared to the Bennett cascade,[29] and HMEs typically have a resistance of 2.5 cmH_2O/l per second.[19]

INFECTION

Current evidence argues against humidifiers as important factors in nosocomial respiratory tract infection. Although water reservoirs represent a good culture medium for bacteria such as *Pseudomonas* species, it is rare to culture bacteria from humidifiers. Any such positive finding is usually preceded by colonisation of the circuit by the patient's own flora within the first 24 h of use.[30,31] Indeed, the incidence of nosocomial pneumonia is reported to be higher (due to outside contamination) if the circuit is changed too frequently (every 24 h[32] or 48 h[29]).

Many HMEs are also effective bacterial filters, with efficiencies usually greater than 99.9 977%,[15] i.e. less than 23 out of 1 million bacteria will pass through – filters that can exclude all virus particles are not currently available. However, provided that fresh circuits are used for each new patient, filtration does not alter the incidence of ventilator-associated pneumonia or mortality.[33]

ELECTRICAL HAZARDS

See Chapter 75.

INHALATION THERAPY

Therapeutic aerosols are particles suspended in gas that are inhaled and deposited within the respiratory tract. Numerous factors, including particle size, inertia and physical nature, gravity, volume and pattern of ventilation, temperature and humidity, airway geometry, lung disease and the delivery system, alter aerosol deposition. In general, particles of diameter 40 μm deposit in the upper airway, 8–15 μm deposit in bronchi and bronchioles, 3–5 μm deposit in peripheral conducting airways and 0.8–3.0 μm settle in lung parenchyma. Optimal particle size will depend on the clinical indication and agent used (e.g. β_2-adrenergic agonists, anticholinergics, corticosteroids, antibiotics, antivirals, surfactant therapy, sputum induction and water). Obviously, if an HME with filtration characteristics is being used, the aerosol needs to be delivered proximal to the filter.

AEROSOL DELIVERY

Therapeutic aerosols may be delivered by nebuliser (jet or ultrasonic), metered-dose inhaler (MDI) or dry-particle inhaler (DPI). Although each of these methods tends to be less efficient in ventilated patients, provided that care is taken to optimise their performance, each can provide equivalent clinical effect.

NEBULISERS[34]

The most common jet nebulisers are sidestream nebulisers. These use an extrinsic gas flow through a narrow orifice, to create a presure gradient that draws the drug mixture from a liquid reservoir (i.e. Bernoulli's principle; Figure 28.3). The gas is then directed at a baffle to reduce the mean particle size. This extrinsic gas flow (usually 3–10 l/min) adds to the inspiratory flow, and may increase patient tidal volume unless the ventilator automatically compensates, or the preset tidal volume is adjusted. Further, this additional gas flow may impair ventilator triggering since it may prevent the development of a negative pressure or necessary reduction in continuous flow needed. Mainstream nebulisers employ inspiratory gas flow to actuate nebulisation. These are commonly large-volume water nebulisers that entrain air to achieve fresh gas flow rates of 20–30 l/min.

Ultrasonic nebulisers use high-frequency sound waves (typically 1 MHz) to create an aerosol above a liquid reservoir, to produce small uniform droplets (< 5 μm) and a high mist density (i.e. 100–200 g/m^3). Tidal volume is not altered; however, ultrasonic nebulisers may cause overhydration and increased airway resistance.

Nebuliser aerosol deposition is highly variable, with significant rainout in the ventilatory circuit, endotracheal tube and large conducting airways. In a bench study delivery ranged from 6% of nebuliser charge to 37% depending upon humidification and breath activation; parallel in-vivo data were similar but found a 20-fold difference in drug delivery.[35] Numerous factors have been shown to improve aerosol deposition, but only some of these are commonly practised. For example, although heating and humidification reduce aerosol deposition by ~50% due to increase in both droplet size and rainout, regular circuit disconnection and exclusion of humidification prior to nebulisation are not practical. However, placement of the nebuliser in the inspiratory limb of the

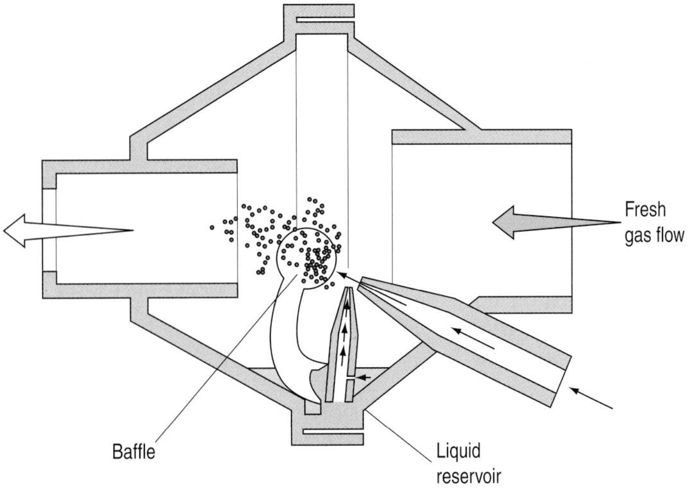

Figure 28.3 Sidestream nebuliser.

circuit less than 30 cm from the endotracheal tube allows this tubing to act as a spacer or aerosol-holding chamber. This reduces aerosol velocity and losses due to impaction. Inspiratory activation of the nebuliser increases deposition by two- and threefold under dry and humidified conditions respectively;[35] use of a large chamber fill, tidal volume of 500 ml or more and minimisation of turbulent inspiratory flow (low flow rate, prolonged inspiratory time) also augment aerosol delivery.[31,36]

METERED-DOSE INHALERS

MDIs suspend micronised crystals of drug in a propellant gas under high pressure, allowing a relatively fixed volume (i.e. dose) to be delivered with each actuation (e.g. 90 μg for salbutamol and 18 μg for ipratropium).[37] Aerosol delivery is approximately 4–6% in ventilated adults,[32] but increases to 11% when a spacer chamber is used, which is similar to optimal no-spacer values reported in the ambulant population.[38] Similar to nebulisers, absence of humidification, inspiratory limb position, inspiratory activation and minimisation of turbulence by lowering inspiratory flow rate and prolonging inspiratory time will increase aerosol delivery. It is important to avoid use of an elbow adapter, because this has been associated with dramatic reductions in aerosol delivery and efficacy. Further hazards of MDIs include a low risk of reaction to chlorofluorocarbons, and the risk of necrotising inflammation of the airway mucosa when large doses of drug are administered with an MDI and catheter system due to oleic acid which is present in some MDI formulations.[39]

DRY-POWDERED INHALERS

DPIs are now in common use in ambulant practice but there is little experience with them in ventilated patients. They could be used in-line with ventilation, but the efficacy of a dry powder in combination with humid gases is unknown.

CLINICAL APPLICATIONS OF INHALATION THERAPY

HUMIDIFICATION

Humidifiers produce gas with a water content dictated by temperature and water vapour pressure, whereas nebulisers produce gas with a water content determined by the aerosol content. The latter can provide water to the respiratory tract, particularly if the water reservoir is heated to increase mist density. However, the risk of infection is increased, as droplets can carry bacteria to the alveoli. Consequently, only sterile water should be used to fill the reservoir, and all units should be regularly changed and sterilised.

MUCOLYTICS

The role of mucolytics to reduce viscosity of secretions in critically ill patients is unknown. Oral mucolytics such as acetylcysteine reduce exacerbations of chronic bronchitis and chronic obstructive pulmonary disease (COPD), although this appears to be isolated to subjects not receiving inhaled steroids.[40] Aerosolised acetylcysteine has also been used as a mucolytic, but may cause bronchospasm. Case reports of recombinant human DNase appear promising when standard regimens fail to clear thick secretions.[36]

BRONCHODILATOR THERAPY

Optimal aerosol delivery and bronchodilator response are extremely important in critically ill patients with severe airflow limitation, and this can be achieved using either a nebuliser or MDI technique provided that care is taken to optimise performance. The response can be judged clinically, and in ventilated patients monitored by changes in peak-to-plateau airway pressure gradient, calculated airways resistance and intrinsic PEEP. Numerous studies show effective bronchodilatation with β_2-agonists and anticholinergic agents such as ipratropium in ventilated patients,[31] and their combination is more effective than a single agent alone.[36] When compared with systemic corticosteroids, inhaled steroids are effective in severe asthma[41] and in exacerbations of COPD.[42]

BRONCHODILATOR DOSING

Standard doses of salbutamol are 2.5 mg administered by a nebuliser or four puffs of an MDI (360 μg), and this can be expected to elicit a bronchodilator response that is slightly shorter-lasting than is usual in ambulatory subjects. Consequently, dosing should be 3–4-hourly. Ipratropium is usually administered as 0.5 mg by a nebuliser or 4 puffs of an MDI. Higher or more frequent drug dosing is often effective when there is severe, reversible airflow obstruction, and continuous nebulisation of a β_2-agonist may be used in acute severe asthma until there has been a clinical response. If the patient is moribund with minimal ventilation or unable to tolerate nebulisation, parenteral administration should be considered; however, under most circumstances there is no particular benefit with this route.[43]

NON-INVASIVE POSITIVE-PRESSURE VENTILATION (NIPPV)

Optimal bronchodilator therapy for patients requiring NIPPV, particularly for acute exacerbations of COPD, is unknown. It is preferable not to interrupt NIPPV for this purpose and both nebulisers and MDIs appear effective during NIPPV.[36] Despite the potential for increased loss of nebulised drug in a high-gas-flow continuous positive-airways pressure circuit, good bronchodilator response with salbutamol has been reported in this setting.[44]

DELIVERY OF ANTIBIOTICS AND ANTIVIRAL AGENTS

Aerosolised antibiotics have been contentious for many years; however, the potential to achieve high concentrations of antibiotics at the site of infection while minimising adverse effects remains appealing. Numerous studies in patients with cystic fibrosis have shown a reduction in sputum volume and density of bacteria, and improved lung function with reduced risk of hospitalisation when inhaled aminoglycosides are used.[45,46] Similar results, including a reduction of markers of airway inflammation, have been reported with bronchiectasis,[47,48] and in mechanically ventilated patients with chronic respiratory failure.[49] Although there has been concern that aerosolised antibiotics will promote the development of resistant organisms,[50] this study examined whole ICU prophylaxis with polymyxin, rather than treatment, and other studies using aminoglycosides have not reported the development of resistance.[39,51] Other antimicrobials that have been safely nebulised include vancomycin, amphotericin B and pentamidine for *Pneumocystis carinii* pneumonia. However, inhaled amphotericin may result in bronchospasm.

In animal models of bronchopneumonia inhaled amikacin[52] and ceftazidime[53] achieved 3–30 times increases in lung tissue concentrations, and better sterilisation of lung when compared to intravenous administration. Using either inhaled gentamicin or vancomycin there appears to be clinical benefit when inhaled antibiotics are added to systemic therapy in ventilator-associated pneumonia.[54] Aerosolised ribavarin is effective for respiratory syncytial virus infection, resulting in a shorter period of ventilation and hospitalisation.[55] However, ribavarin deposition in the circuit may cause valve malfunction, and concerns of teratogenicity in health care personnel have dictated its use with care.[43]

SPUTUM INDUCTION

Nebulised 3% saline is effective in sputum induction for diagnosing *P. carinii* pneumonia in patients with the acquired immunodeficiency syndrome (AIDS), thereby often obviating the need for bronchoscopy.[56] Sputum induction has been used to diagnose a number of other infections, and appears to be safe in patients with severe airflow limitation.[57]

SURFACTANT THERAPY

Surfactant preparations have been delivered by instillation and as an aerosol in neonates with respiratory distress syndrome, and in adults with the acute respiratory distress syndrome. Aerosolised surfactant achieves a more uniform distribution and avoids problems of instilling liquid into injured lungs. However, large amounts are needed for lung deposition, and preferential distribution occurs to less damaged lung areas that receive better ventilation.[58]

PROSTANOIDS[38]

Inhaled prostanoids target selective pulmonary vasodilatation to well-aerated areas, leading to similar improvements in oxygenation as inducible nitrous oxide in patients with the acute respiratory distress syndrome. When delivered systemically these agents lead to impaired oxygenation and to hypotension due to non-selective pulmonary and systemic vasodilatation respectively. Iloprost has a longer half-life (about 20–30 min compared with 3 min for prostacyclin), and is sometimes used for chronic pulmonary hypertension (2.5–5 mg 6–9 times per day), and similar doses can be used in mechanically ventilated patients.

REFERENCES

1. Hedley RM, Allt-Graham J. Heat and moisture exchangers and breathing filters. *Br J Anaesth* 1994; **73**: 227–36.
2. Forbes AR. Humidification and mucus flow in the intubated trachea. *Br J Anaesth* 1973; **45**: 874–8.
3. Forbes AR. Temperature, humidity and mucus flow in the intubated trachea. *Br J Anaesth* 1974; **46**: 29–34.

4. Sackner MA, Landa J, Hirsch J *et al.* Pulmonary effects of oxygen breathing: a six-hour study in normal man. *Ann Intern Med* 1975; **82**: 40–3.
5. LaFortuna CL, Fazio F. Acute effect of inhaled salbutamol on mucociliary clearance in health and chronic bronchitis. *Respiration* 1985; **45**: 111–13.
6. Chalon J, Patel C, Ali M *et al.* Humidity and the anesthetized patient. *Anesthesiology* 1974; **50**: 195–8.
7. Circeo LE, Heard SO, Griffiths E *et al.* Overwhelming necrotizing tracheobronchitis due to inadequate humidification during high-frequency jet ventilation. *Chest* 1991; **100**: 268–9.
8. Linko K, Honkavaara P, Niemenen MT. Heated humidification after major abdominal surgery. *Eur J Anaesthesiol* 1984; **1**: 285–91.
9. Shelley MP, Lloyd GM, Park GR. A review of the mechanisms and methods of humidification of inspired gases. *Intens Care Med* 1988; **14**: 1–9.
10. Chamney AR. Humidification requirements and techniques. *Anaesthesia* 1969; **24**: 602–17.
11. Rhame FS, Streifel A, McComb C *et al.* Bubbling humidifiers produce microaerosols which can carry bacteria. *Infect Control* 1986; **7**: 403–7.
12. Lellouche F, Taillé S, Maggiore SM *et al.* Influence of ambient and ventilator output temperatures on performance of heated-wire humidifiers. *Am J Respir Crit Care Med* 2004; **170**: 1073–9.
13. Schumann S, Stahl CA, Moller K *et al.* Moisturizing and mechanical characteristics of a new counter-flow type heated humidifier. *Br J Anaesth* 2007; **98**: 531–8.
14. Dreyfuss D, Djedaini K, Gros K *et al.* Mechanical ventilation with heated humidifiers or heat and moisture exchangers: effects on patient colonization and incidence of nosocomial pneumonia. *Am J Respir Crit Care Med* 1995; **151**: 986–92.
15. Kollef M, Shapiro S, Boyd V *et al.* A randomized clinical trial comparing an extended-use hygroscopic condenser humidifier with heated-water humidification in mechanically ventilated patients. *Chest* 1998; **113**: 759–67.
16. Jackson C, Webb AR. An evaluation of the heat and moisture exchange performance of four ventilator circuit filters. *Intens Care Med* 1992; **18**: 246–8.
17. Mebius C. Heat and moisture exchangers with bacterial filters: a laboratory evaluation. *Acta Anaesthesiol Scand* 1992; **36**: 572–6.
18. Martin C, Papazian L, Perrin G *et al.* Performance evaluation of three vaporizing humidifiers and two heat and moisture exchangers in patients with minute volumes > 10 l/min. *Chest* 1992; **102**: 1347–50.
19. Shelley M, Bethune DW, Latimer RD. A comparison of five heat and moisture exchangers. *Anaesthesia* 1986; **41**: 527–32.
20. Sottiaux T, Mignolet G, Damas P *et al.* Comparative evaluation of three heat and moisture exchangers during short-term postoperative mechanical ventilation. *Chest* 1993; **104**: 220–4.
21. Unal N, Kanhai JKK, Buijk SLCE *et al.* A novel method of evaluation of three heat-moisture exchangers in six different ventilator settings. *Intens Care Med* 1998; **24**: 138–46.
22. Thomachot L, Boisson C, Arnaud S *et al.* Changing heat and moisture exchangers after 96 hours rather than 24 hours: a clinical and microbiological evaluation. *Crit Care Med* 2000; **28**: 714–20.
23. Misset B, Escudier B, Rivara D *et al.* Heat and moisture exchanger vs heated humidifier during long-term mechanical ventilation: a prospective randomized study. *Chest* 1990; **100**: 160–3.
24. Martin C, Perrin G, Gevaudan MJ *et al.* Heat and moisture exchangers and vaporizing humidifiers in the intensive care unit. *Chest* 1990; **97**: 144–9.
25. Cohen IL, Weinberg PF, Fein IA *et al.* Endotracheal tube occlusion associated with the use of heat and moisture exchangers in the intensive care unit. *Crit Care Med* 1988; **16**: 277–9.
26. AARC clinical practice guideline. Humidification during mechanical ventilation. *Respir Care* 1992; **37**: 887–90.
27. Gluck E, Heard S, Patel C *et al.* Use of high frequency ventilation in patients with ARDS: a preliminary report. *Chest* 1993; **103**: 1413–20.
28. Ploysongsang Y, Branson R, Rashkin MC *et al.* Pressure flow characteristics of commonly used heat-moisture exchangers. *Am Rev Respir Dis* 1988; **138**: 675–8.
29. Oh TE, Lin ES, Bhatt S. Resistance of humidifiers, and inspiratory work imposed by a ventilator-humidifier circuit. *Br J Anaesth* 1991; **66**: 258–63.
30. Craven DE, Goularte TA, Make BJ. Contaminated condensate in mechanical ventilator circuits: a risk factor for nosocomial pneumonia. *Am Rev Respir Dis* 1984; **129**: 625–8.
31. Dreyfuss D, Djedaini K, Weber P *et al.* Prospective study of nosocomial pneumonia and of patient and circuit colonisation during mechanical ventilation with circuit changes every 48 hours versus no change. *Am Rev Respir Dis* 1991; **143**: 738–43.
32. Craven DE, Connolly MG, Lichtenberg DA *et al.* Contamination of mechanical ventilators with tubing changes every 24 or 48 hours. *N Engl J Med* 1982; **306**: 1505–9.
33. Lacherade J-C, Auburtin M, Cerf C *et al.* Impact of humidification systems on ventilator-associated pneumonia: a randomized multicenter trial. *Am J Respir Crit Care Med* 2005; **172**: 1276–82.
34. O'Doherty MJ, Thomas SHL. Nebuliser therapy in the intensive care unit. *Thorax* 1997; **52** (Suppl 2): S5–59.
35. Miller DD, Amin MM, Palmer LB *et al.* Aerosol delivery and modern mechanical ventilation in vitro/in vivo evaluation. *Am J Respir Crit Care Med* 2003; **168**: 1205–9.
36. Dhand R, Tobin MJ. Inhaled bronchodilator therapy in mechanically ventilated patients. *Am J Respir Crit Care Med* 1997; **156**: 3–10.
37. Manthous CA, Hall JB. Administration of therapeutic aerosols to mechanically ventilated patients. *Chest* 1994; **106**: 560–71.
38. Dhand R. Inhalation therapy in invasive and non-invasive mechanical ventilation. *Curr Opin Crit Care* 2007; **13**: 27–38.
39. Spahr-Schopfer IA, Lerman J, Cutz E *et al.* Proximate delivery of a large experimental dose from salbutamol MDI induces epithelial airway lesions in intubated rabbits. *Am J Respir Crit Care Med* 1994; **150**: 790–4.

40. Poole PJ, Black PN. Mucolytic agents for chronic bronchitis or chronic obstructive pulmonary disease. *Cochrane Database Syst Rev* 2006; **3**: CD001287.
41. Rodrigo GJ. Rapid effects of inhaled corticosteroids in acute asthma. an evidence-based evaluation. *Chest* 2006; **130**: 1301–11.
42. Maltais F, Ostinelli J, Bourbeau J *et al.* Comparison of nebulised budesonide and oral prednisolone with placebo in the treatment of acute exacerbations of chronic obstructive pulmonary disease. A randomized controlled trial. *Am J Respir Crit Care Med* 2002; **165**: 698–703.
43. McFadden ER. Acute severe asthma. *Am J Respir Crit Care Med* 2003; **168**: 740–59.
44. Parkes SN, Bersten AD. Aerosol delivery and bronchodilator efficacy during continuous positive airway pressure delivered by face mask. *Thorax* 1997; **52**: 171–5.
45. Ramsey BW, Dorkin HL, Eisenberg JD *et al.* Efficacy of aerosolized tobramycin in patients with cystic fibrosis. *N Engl J Med* 1993; **328**: 1740–6.
46. Ramsey BW, Pepe MS, Quan JM *et al.* Intermittent administration of inhaled tobramycin in cystic fibrosis. Cystic fibrosis inhaled tobramycin study group. *N Engl J Med* 1999; **340**: 23–30.
47. Lin H-C, Cheng H-F, Wang C-H *et al.* Inhaled gentamicin reduces airway neutrophil activity and mucus secretion in bronchiectasis. *Am J Respir Crit Care Med* 1997; **155**: 2024–9.
48. Barker AF, Couch L, Fiel SB *et al.* Tobramycin solution for inhalation reduces sputum *Pseudomonas aeruginosa* density in bronchiectasis. *Am J Respir Crit Care Med* 2000; **162**: 481–5.
49. Palmer LB, Smaldone GC, Simon SR *et al.* Aerosolized antibiotics in mechanically ventilated patients: delivery and response. *Crit Care Med* 1998; **26**: 31–9.
50. Feeley TW, DuMoulin GC, Hedley-White J *et al.* Aerosol polymyxin and pneumonia in seriously ill patients. *N Engl J Med* 1975; **293**: 471–5.
51. Burns JL, Van Dalfsen JM, Shawar RM *et al.* Effect of chronic intermittent administration of inhaled tobramycin on respiratory microbial flora in patients with cystic fibrosis. *J Infect Dis* 1999; **179**: 1190–6.
52. Goldstein I, Wallet F, Nicolas-Robin A *et al.* Lung deposition and efficiency of nebulised amikacin during *Escherichia coli* pneumonia in ventilated piglets. *Am J Respir Crit Care Med* 2002; **166**: 1375–81.
53. Tonnellier M, Ferrari F, Goldstein I *et al.* Intravenous versus nebulised ceftazidime in ventilated piglets with and without experimental bronchopneumonia: comparative effects of helium and nitrogen. *Anesthesiology* 2005; **102**: 995–1000.
54. Palmer LB, Baram D, Duan T *et al.* Ventilator associated pneumonia (VAP) and clinical pulmonary infection score (CPIS): effects of aerosolized antibiotics (AA). *Am J Respir Crit Care Med* 2006; **173**: A525.
55. Committee on Infectious Diseases. Use of ribavarin in the treatment of respiratory syncytial virus infection. *Pediatrics* 1993; **92**: 501–4.
56. Bigby TD, Margolskee D, Curtis JL *et al.* The usefulness of induced sputum in the diagnosis of *Pneumocystis carinii* pneumonia in patients with the acquired immunodeficiency syndrome. *Am Rev Respir Dis* 1986; **133**: 515–18.
57. Vlachos-Mayer H, Leigh R, Sharon RF *et al.* Success and safety of sputum induction in the clinical setting. *Eur Respir J* 2000; **16**: 997–1000.
58. Lewis JF, Jobe AH. Surfactant and the adult respiratory distress syndrome. *Am Rev Respir Dis* 1993; **147**: 218–33.

29

The acute respiratory distress syndrome (ARDS)

Andrew D Bersten

The acute respiratory distress syndrome (ARDS) was first described in 1967 by Ashbaugh and colleagues as the 'acute onset of tachypnea, hypoxemia and loss of compliance after a variety of stimuli'.[1] Continued research examining the underlying mechanisms and management strategies is now translating into improved outcome.

DEFINITIONS

Acute lung injury (ALI) and its more severe subset ARDS describe acute hypoxaemic respiratory failure due to bilateral and diffuse alveolar damage. The most common criteria are the 1994 American–European Consensus Conference definitions[2] (Table 29.1), which are broad and inclusive. However, these fail to specify an acute cause, use a $Pa\text{O}_2/Fi\text{O}_2$ ratio independent of respiratory support and are not specific about the radiographic criteria. The lung injury score (LIS),[3] which uses a four-point score attributed to ranges of $Pa\text{O}_2/Fi\text{O}_2$ ratio, positive end-expiratory pressure (PEEP), respiratory system compliance and the number of quadrants involved on chest radiograph, and the Delphi definition, which demands a $Pa\text{O}_2/Fi\text{O}_2$ ratio ≤ 200 with 10 cmH_2O PEEP, have a greater sensitivity when matched against autopsy evidence of diffuse alveolar damage.[4]

CHEST RADIOGRAPH AND CHEST COMPUTED TOMOGRAPHY IN ACUTE LUNG INJURY

The interpretation of the chest radiograph is central to these definitions of ALI and ARDS. However, there is considerable interobserver variability in both chest radiograph interpretation and in the definition of an infiltrate. In the American–European Consensus Conference definition the infiltrate must be bilateral and consistent with pulmonary oedema,[2] whereas the LIS rates the number of quadrants with alveolar consolidation[3] and the Delphi definition requires bilateral airspace disease. The intention of these descriptions is fairly clear and excludes opacity due to pleural effusion, nodules, masses, collapse and pleural thickening. However, it is desirable to improve interobserver agreement and this will require training and more specific definitions.

Chest computed tomography (CT)[5] has proved extremely helpful in pathophysiological studies of ALI, has demonstrated the heterogeneity of lung inflation and is commonly used to assist clinical management. Autopsy and chest radiographs of ALI show a uniform process affecting both lungs; however, chest CT early in the course of ALI in supine patients demonstrated that there was a dorsal dependent increase in lung density, and that the ventral lung was relatively normal. In addition, CT frequently showed previously undiagnosed pneumothorax, pneumomediastinum and pleural effusion. After the second week of mechanical ventilation CT scans may demonstrate altered lung architecture and emphysematous cysts or pneumatoceles.

CT numbers or Hounsfield units can be assigned to each voxel (~2000 alveoli in a standard 10-mm slice).[5] These data can then be used to assess what proportion of a region of interest is non-aerated, poorly aerated, normally aerated or hyperinflated. Initially a single basal lung slice was studied, but it is clear that far more information can be obtained by studying the whole lung, and by using thinner slices. This allows: (1) reconstruction of the upper and lower lobes (the middle lobe is difficult to separate); (2) the same section of lung to be studied at different levels of inflation or PEEP (the lung also moves in a cephalocaudad direction with respiration); and (3) a broader picture of the lung to be obtained (lung damage is heterogeneous in ALI). However, whole-lung CT demands considerable exposure to ionising radiation, and different information, perhaps more pertinent to mechanical ventilation, is obtained from dynamic CT.

Clinical assessment of chest CT is discussed in Chapter 35, and CT findings in ALI are discussed below, in the section on clinical management.

EPIDEMIOLOGY

Estimates of the incidence and outcome from ALI and ARDS vary widely. In part this has been due to differences

Table 29.1 Definition of acute lung injury (ALI) and acute respiratory distress syndrome (ARDS)[2]

Condition	Timing	Pao_2/Fio_2	Chest radiograph	PAOP
ALI	Acute	≤ 300 mmHg	Bilateral infiltrates	≤ 18 mmHg or no clinical evidence of elevated LAP
ARDS	Acute	≤ 200 mmHg	Bilateral infiltrates	≤ 18 mmHg or no clinical evidence of elevated LAP

PAOP, pulmonary artery occlusion pressure; LAP, left atrial pressure.

in the definitions used, but it also appears likely that case-mix and local factors influence outcome and incidence. Using the 1994 consensus definition the Australian incidence is 34 per 100 000 for ALI and 28 per 100 000 for ARDS;[6] recent US estimates are 79 and 59 per 100 000 respectively[7] – both much greater than many previous estimates. The Australian data equate to 1 in 10 non-cardiothoracic intensive care unit (ICU) patients developing ARDS, which reflects the tendency for clinicians to underestimate the incidence of ALI and ARDS.

Reported mortality rates are also influenced by the definitions used. For many years the mortality for ARDS was reported to be ~60%; the Australian multicentre data reported mortality rates of 32% for ALI and 34% for ARDS,[6] with US mortality rates a little higher at 38.5% and 41%.[7] However, particular diagnostic groups such as multiple trauma have a lower mortality rate than other causes of ARDS, and patients with ALI who have chronic liver disease, non-pulmonary organ dysfunction, sepsis or age greater than 70 years (hazard ratio 2.5)[8] have a higher risk of death. Consequently many factors need to be considered when assessing outcome prediction.

PULMONARY FUNCTION IN SURVIVORS

Respiratory function is most abnormal soon after discontinuation of mechanical ventilation, but usually returns towards normal by 6–12 months. Although a variety of abnormal pulmonary function tests may be found, impaired diffusing capacity is the most common. This is rarely symptomatic, but occasional patients have severe restrictive disease, and this is correlated with their cumulative LIS.[9]

QUALITY OF LIFE IN SURVIVORS

Compared with disease-matched ICU patients who do not develop ARDS, patients with ARDS have a more severe reduction in both pulmonary and general health-related quality of life.[10] Many patients have reduction in exercise tolerance that may be attributable to associated critical-illness neuropathy and myopathy; nerve entrapment syndromes and heterotopic calcification play a role in a minority.[7] Depression, anxiety and posttraumatic stress disorder are also common (20–50% of survivors).[7] However, it is unclear whether neuropsychological disability is a direct consequence of the illness, or related to the associated stress. Finally, most survivors have cognitive impairments such as slowed mental processing, or impaired memory or concentration, and these correlate with the period and severity of desaturation < 90%.[11] Although these data suggest that ARDS confers a specific risk of impaired quality of life, the mechanism is unclear. However, they do caution against permissive hypoxaemia as a strategy to reduce ventilator-induced lung injury (VILI).

PATIENTS AT-RISK FOR ALI AND ARDS

Clinical risk factors for the development of ALI and ARDS can be classified as either direct or indirect (Table 29.2). These identify over 80% of patients who develop ARDS; the most common risk factors are sepsis, pneumonia and aspiration of gastric contents. Multiple risk factors, low pH, chronic alcohol abuse or chronic lung disease substantially increases the incidence of ALI in at-risk patients.

BIOLOGICAL MARKERS AS PREDICTORS OF ALI

In addition to identifying these clinical risk groups, there has been considerable interest in identifying possible biological markers that could be used to predict the development of ALI. Although greater specificity may be gained from sampling the epithelial lining fluid (e.g. using bronchoalveolar lavage fluid), an ideal biological marker would be more simply sampled, such as plasma. Numerous proteins, such as the cytokines interleukin (IL)-1, tumour necrosis factor-α (TNF-α) and IL-10, and von Willebrand's factor antigen are elevated in at-risk

Table 29.2 Clinical risk factors for acute lung injury (ALI) and acute respiratory distress syndrome (ARDS)

Direct	Indirect
Pneumonia (46%)*	Non-pulmonary sepsis (25%)
Aspiration of gastric contents (29%)	Multiple trauma (41%)
Lung contusion (34%)	Massive transfusion (34%)
Fat embolism	Pancreatitis (25%)
Near-drowning	Cardiopulmonary bypass
Inhalational injury	
Reperfusion injury	

*Denotes the approximate percentage of intensive care unit at-risk cases that developed ALI (data from Bersten AD, Hunt T, Nicholas TE et al. Plasma surfactant proteins (SP) as predictors of ARDS: patient demographics from an Australian multicentred study. *Am J Respir Crit Care Med* 2002; **165**: A476) patients and patients with ALI and ARDS; however, they are not predictive. In relatively small studies both ferritin[12] and surfactant protein B[13] have been shown to be predictive of ARDS. Although ferritin likely represents a non-specific oxygen free-radical response, the leakage of surfactant protein B from the alveolus into the blood is lung-specific.

PATHOGENESIS

Although it is well accepted that diffuse alveolar damage with: (1) pulmonary oedema due to damage of the alveolocapillary barrier; (2) a complex inflammatory infiltrate; and (3) surfactant dysfunction are essential components of ALI, the sequence of events is uncertain and probably depends upon the precipitating insult and host response. For example, in endotoxin-induced lung injury, hypoxaemia and reduced lung compliance occur well before recruitment of neutrophils or an increase in lung weight due to an increase in permeability.[14] In addition, surfactant turnover is dramatically increased prior to these changes often thought to be typical of early ALI. Further, epithelial lining fluid sampled immediately following intubation in patients with ALI has markedly increased concentrations of type III procollagen peptide, suggestive of fibrosing alveolitis extremely early in the course of lung damage.

THE ALVEOLOCAPILLARY BARRIER

The normal lung consists of 300 million alveoli with alveolar gas separated from the pulmonary microcirculation by the extremely thin alveolocapillary barrier (0.1–0.2 μm thick). Since the endothelial pore size is 6.5–7.5 nm, and the epithelial pore size is almost one-tenth that, at 0.5–0.9 nm, the epithelium is the major barrier to protein flux.[15] The surface area of the alveoli is estimated to be 50–100 m^2, which is made up predominantly of alveolar type I cells, with the metabolically active type II cells accounting for ~10% of the surface area. In turn, these cells are covered by the epithelial lining fluid, with an estimated volume of 20 ml, ~10% of which is surfactant with the remained filtered plasma water and low-molecular-weight proteins, and a small number of cells, mainly alveolar macrophages and lymphocytes.

In ALI the alveolocapillary barrier is damaged with bidirectional leakage of fluid and protein into the alveolus and leakage of surfactant proteins and alveolar cytokines into the plasma. There is also disruption of the epithelial barrier, surfactant dysfunction and proliferation of alveolar type II cells as the progenitor of type I cells. The outcome of this process must reflect a balance between repair and fibrosing alveolitis. As discussed above, the precise sequence of events causing and maintaining damage of the alveolocapillary barrier is complex and uncertain and likely varies depending on the underlying cause. For example, indirect causes of ALI may initially cause pulmonary endothelial injury followed by recruitment of inflammatory cells and epithelial damage, while direct causes of ALI may initially cause epithelial injury and secondary recruitment of inflammatory cells.

NEUTROPHILS IN ACUTE LUNG INJURY

Neutrophils are the most abundant cell type found in both the epithelial lining fluid (e.g. bronchoalveolar lavage fluid) and alveoli in histological specimens from early in the course of ALI. Although neutrophil migration across the endothelium or epithelium does not cause injury, when activated they release reactive oxygen species, cytokines, eicosanoids and a variety of proteases that may make an important contribution to tissue damage in ALI. Following bone marrow demargination, activated neutrophils adhere to the endothelium on their passage to the alveolus, and this may be accompanied by an early, transient leukopenia. Although neutrophils have an important role in host defence due to their bactericidal activity, there is a marked (50–1000-fold) increase in the release of cytotoxic compounds when they are activated by adherence to the endothelium, epithelium or contact with interstitial extracellular matrix proteins.[16] The factors involved in adhesion of neutrophils are complex and involve the integrin family of proteins, selectins and a number of adhesion molecules.

In models of ALI, antibodies to adhesion molecules (e.g. CD11b/CD18 antibodies) ameliorate lung injury, suggesting a crucial and central role of this cell type. However, ALI occurs in neutropenic patients, and was not more common when granulocyte colony-stimulating factor was administered to patients with pneumonia.[17] Clearly, other cell types play an important role, and neutrophil chemoattractants such as IL-8 must be present in the lung prior to neutrophil accumulation.

OTHER CELL TYPES INVOLVED IN ACUTE LUNG INJURY

Pulmonary endothelial cells, platelets, interstitial and alveolar macrophages and alveolar type II cells also play important roles in alveolar inflammation. Pulmonary endothelial cells express a variety of adhesion molecules and cyclooxygenase-2 (COX-2); secrete endothelin and cytokines, including IL-8;[18] stimulate procoagulant activity; and 'cross-talk' with the alveolar macrophages and type II cells. They will be involved in generalised endothelial activation, and are subject to mechanical stress, secondary to both vascular pressure and to their close association with the alveolus. Von Willebrand's factor antigen is synthesised by vascular endothelial cells, and although this may explain its lack of specificity for ALI, its plasma levels are a good marker of endothelial injury.[19]

Microvascular thrombosis is common in ALI, and contributes to pulmonary hypertension and wasted ventilation. Although platelet aggregation may contribute to ALI through release of thromboxane A_2, serotonin, lysosomal enzymes and platelet-activating factor, they are less important than the other cell types.

Alveolar macrophages are the most common cell type normally found in bronchoalveolar lavage fluid, and, together with interstitial macrophages, play an important role in host defence and modulation of fibrosis. They are capable of releasing IL-6 and a host of mediators, similar to the activated neutrophil, including TNF-α and IL-8 in response to stretch,[20] and may amplify lung injury. However, depletion of alveolar macrophages does not reduce neutrophil recruitment or outcome from tracheal instillation of *Pseudomonas aeruginosa*,[21] questioning the central role of this cell type. Macrophages also release a number of factors such as transforming growth factor-α and platelet-derived growth factor that stimulate fibroblast proliferation, deposition of collagen and glycosaminoglycans, angiogenesis and lung fibrosis.

Alveolar epithelial type II cells are extremely metabolically active; they manufacture and release surfactant, control alveolar water clearance using ion pumps, express cytokines which in turn interact with surfactant production and are the progenitor of type I cells following injury. In response to both stretch and endotoxin, type II cells express IL-8 and TNF-α, with the latter cytokine augmenting Na^+, and hence water, egress from the alveolus.[22]

CHEMOKINES IN ACUTE LUNG INJURY

The expression and secretion of chemokines (chemoattractant cytokines) at sites of inflammation are probably key proximal steps in initiating the inflammatory cascade. IL-8 appears particularly important in initiating ALI because of its ability to induce chemotaxis and activation of neutrophils. IL-8 is elevated in ALI bronchoalveolar lavage fluid within hours of the initiating insult and before recruitment of neutrophils, and in a manner that reflects subsequent morbidity and mortality. In animal models of sepsis and acid aspiration, instillation of antibodies against IL-8 prevents the recruitment of neutrophils and protects the lung. Indeed, the recruitment and retention of neutrophils require the generation and maintenance of a localised chemotactic/haptotactic gradient.[23]

MEDIATORS IN ACUTE LUNG INJURY

From the discussion above it is clear that numerous mediators, derived from a number of different cell types, play important roles in the pathophysiology of ALI. These include cytokines, chemokines, complement, reactive oxygen species, eicosanoids, platelet-activating factor, nitric oxide, proteases, growth factors and lysosomal enzymes. As the alveolocapillary barrier becomes injured, these are no longer compartmentalised in the alveolus, and many of these proteins have been measured in blood as well as in the epithelial lining fluid. Care must be taken when interpreting these data as immunologic levels may not reflect biologic activity; inhibitors or binding proteins may complex with the active protein or epitope and interfere with immunologic detection; and the ultimate biological effect will depend upon a balance of proinflammatory and anti-inflammatory effects.

Although many of the over 40 biologically active cytokines are implicated in ALI, TNF-α, IL-1β, IL-6 and IL-8 are the most important. However, even greater increases are found in their cognate receptors or antagonists, such as the counterregulatory cytokine IL-10, so that their biological impact is markedly reduced.[24] Despite numerous studies, measurement of cytokines in blood or epithelial lining fluid has not proven predictive of the development of ALI or of mortality.

RESOLUTION OF ACUTE LUNG INJURY AND THE DEVELOPMENT OF FIBROSING ALVEOLITIS

Although elevated levels of type III procollagen peptide are found in the epithelial lining fluid soon after diagnosis, histological evidence of fibrosing alveolitis (mesenchymal cells and new vessels in alveoli) is not usually found until at least 5 days following the onset of ALI. In the majority of patients there is clinical resolution of ALI provided that the underlying cause is promptly and effectively treated. Alveolar oedema resolves with active transport of Na^+ by the type II cells followed by passive clearance of water through transcellular aquaporin channels, and repair of the alveolocapillary barrier is associated with improved outcome. Type II cells proliferate and cover the denuded epithelium before differentiating into type I cells. Both proapoptotic and anti-apoptotic (granulocyte colony-stimulating factor (G-CSF) and granulocyte–macrophage colony-stimulating factor (GM-CSF)) factors are found in the alveolus during this phase; however, little is known regarding control over the delicate balance between repair and fibrosis.

CLINICAL MANAGEMENT

The factors leading to ALI must be promptly and appropriately treated. This includes diagnosis and appropriate treatment of infection with drainage of collections and appropriate antimicrobial agents, recognition and rapid resuscitation from shock, splinting of fractures and careful supportive care. Prevention of deep venous thrombosis, stress ulceration and nosocomial infection is important in all critically ill patients. Adequacy of nutrition, often enteral nutrition, must also be considered.

MECHANICAL VENTILATION

Patients present with acute hypoxaemic respiratory failure, and an increase in the work of breathing, usually requiring mechanical ventilation (Table 29.3). The role of non-invasive ventilation in ALI is uncertain as there appears to be a greater complication rate, perhaps due to delayed intubation.[25] However, non-invasive ventilation is worth considering in particular circumstances (see Chapter 33).

Table 29.3 Pathophysiology of acute lung injury (ALI) and adult respiratory distress syndrome (ARDS)

Feature	Cause(s)
Hypoxaemia	True shunt (perfusion of non-ventilated airspaces) Impaired hypoxic pulmonary vasoconstriction *V/Q* mismatch is a minor component
↑ Dependent densities (CT)	Surfactant dysfunction alveolar instability
(Collapse/consolidation)	Exaggeration of normal compression of dependent lung due to ↑ weight (↑ lung water, inflammation)
↑ Elastance (↓ compliance)	Surfactant dysfunction (↑ specific elastance) ↓ Lung volume ('baby lung') ↑ Chest wall elastance Fibrosing alveolitis (late)
↑ Minute volume requirement	↑ Alveolar dead space (V_{Dphys}/V_t often 0.4–0.7) ↑ V_{CO_2}
↑ Work of breathing	↑ Elastance ↑ Minute volume requirement
Pulmonary hypertension	Pulmonary vasoconstriction (thromboxane A_2, endothelin) Pulmonary microvascular thrombosis Fibrosing alveolitis Positive end-expiratory pressure

The method and delivery of ventilatory support must take into account the pathophysiology of ALI and ARDS. For many years laboratory studies have described VILI, and the most important clinical study was the ARDS Network study where 861 ALI patients from 75 ICUs were randomised to receive a tidal volume (V_T) of either 12 or 6 ml/kg predicted body weight.[26] Mortality was reduced by 22% from 40% to 31% in the lower-V_T group. There was a strict PEEP and F_{IO_2} protocol, and patients were ventilated with assist-control ventilation to avoid excessive spontaneous V_T. Meta-regression of five clinical studies trialling different V_T strategies found that a V_T < 7.7 ml/kg predicted body weight (pbw) was protective, and that above 11.2 ml/kg pbw was borderline detrimental.[27] Whether this protective effect of lower V_T is due to lower static distending pressure of the respiratory system is contentious; however, Hager and colleagues[28] found that lower V_T ventilation was protective across all quartiles of plateau pressure (P_{plat}) in the ARDS Network trial, and that no safe upper limit of P_{plat} could be identified.

AVOIDANCE OF OVERSTRETCH AND INADEQUATE RECRUITMENT

The increase in dependent lung density found on chest CT, due to non-aerated and poorly aerated lung, reduces the volume of aerated lung available for tidal inflation. Both PEEP and tidal recruitment will increase aeration of some of these airspaces, but a V_T that is not reduced in proportion to the reduction in aerated lung may lead to overstretch of aerated lung parenchyma, which may lead to further diffuse alveolar damage. Studies where increased chest wall compliance led to increase airway pressure (P_{aw}) have clearly shown that it is lung stretch, not increased P_{aw}, that causes injury;[29] consequently this has been termed volutrauma. In addition, laboratory studies have shown that repeated opening and closing of airspaces by tidal recruitment result in diffuse alveolar damage (atelectrauma). Although data from animal models support both as important mechanisms of VILI, with both resulting in alveolar inflammation and elevated alveolar cytokines (biotrauma),[31] which may 'spill' into the systemic circulation,[30] only VILI due to overstretch is supported by clinical data. CT scans performed during ARDS Network protective ventilation show that tidal inflation occurs primarily in either normally aerated or overinflated compartments, with little tidal recruitment.[31] The pulmonary inflammatory response was associated with tidal overinflation.

OVERSTRETCH

The normal lung is fully inflated at a transpulmonary pressure of ~30 cmH_2O. Consequently, a maximum P_{plat}, the elastic distending pressure, of 30–35 cmH_2O has been recommended to avoid overstretch, and the ARDS Network study targeted $P_{plat} \leq 30$ cmH_2O.[28] The transpulmonary pressure may be lower than expected for a given P_{plat} in patients with a high chest wall elastance (e.g. obesity, abdominal compartment syndrome, postabdominal or thoracic surgery). It is also common for individual patients to show evidence of overinflation at much lower elastic distending pressures (18–26 cmH_2O).[32,33] Finally, inspiratory muscle effort will lower P_{plat} by reducing intrapleural pressure, potentially avoiding detection of an excessive transpulmonary pressure.

This is particularly common when pressure support ventilation is used as a primary mode of ventilatory support: V_T that would produce an unacceptably high P_{plat} during mechanical ventilation will produce the same volutrauma during a spontaneous or supported mode of ventilation, and should be avoided. None of these issues is easily overcome. Although placement of an oesophageal balloon (see Chapter 34) allows measurement of the transpulmonary pressure, it must be correctly placed, have an adequate occlusion pressure ratio, and measurements are preferably performed in a semisitting position in order to lift the mediastinum off the oesophagus. Similarly, static or dynamic volume–pressure curves or quantitative chest CT can be used to determine overinflation, though chest CT cannot determine overstretch.[5] Consequently, unless particular expertise is available, V_T limitation is currently the most practical approach.

ADEQUATE PEEP

PEEP improves PaO_2 by increasing functional residual capacity, and recruiting alveoli. Because PEEP may reduce cardiac output by impairing venous return, Suter and coworkers suggested that maximum oxygen delivery (oxygen content × flow) should be used to optimise PEEP.[33] Other end-points such as either titrating PEEP to a particular PaO_2/FiO_2 ratio or to prevent repeated opening and closing of alveoli have been suggested. The ARDS Network Study protocol[28] titrates PEEP to the PaO_2/FiO_2 ratio, but this results in tidal overinflation in about one-third of patients.[33] Concurrently there is little evidence of tidal recruitment, which may explain why a higher PEEP protocol[34] did not prove beneficial. In patients at risk for ARDS prophylactic PEEP (8 cmH_2O) was not protective.[35]

The lower inflection point of a volume–pressure curve has been used to set PEEP, because early studies suggested that this reflected recruitment of collapsed alveoli. However, in patients with ALI, recruitment occurs well above the lower inflection point, along the entire volume–pressure curve and above the upper inflection point.[36,37] Concurrently, there is frequently evidence of overstretching and hyperinflation on CT scans[33,38] or dynamic volume–pressure analysis.[33] The amount of lung available for recruitment in ARDS is also extremely variable,[39] and does not appear to differ comparing pulmonary with extrapulmonary causes.[40] Although routine CT analysis has been advocated by some, it is cumbersome and has not been shown to influence outcome; non-invasive bedside alternatives are under investigation. Consequently, PEEP titration is often a compromise aiming to minimise both atelectrauma and volutrauma.[41]

Although a protective ventilation strategy using the 'open-lung' approach with PEEP levels above the lower inflection point and frequent recruitment manoeuvres did report a reduction in mortality, the treatment arm also included low V_T and recruitment manoeuvres.[42] Reasonable approaches to PEEP titration include: (1) the use of a scale similar to the ARDS Network protocol; (2) titration of PEEP to PaO_2, aiming for a PEEP of ~15 cmH_2O; or (3) measuring elastic mechanics at the bedside. The delta-PEEP technique is a simple technique that indirectly assesses excessive stress as PEEP is changed at a constant V_T[33] (see Chapter 34).

Recruitment manoeuvres

It is unclear whether additional recruitment manoeuvres are of additional benefit once an adequate level of PEEP is applied. Typically a high level of continuous positive airways pressure (30–40 cmH_2O) is applied for 30–40 seconds in an apnoeic patient, followed by return to a lower level of PEEP and controlled ventilation. This may be followed by a marked improvement in oxygenation. However, this is not a consistent finding, and hypotension may occur due to reduced venous return if there is inadequate fluid loading. Although a recruitment manoeuvre was applied by Amato and colleagues and associated with an improvement in outcome, they also applied a higher level of PEEP and lower V_T in the protective lung strategy group.[42] A number of small trials have shown improvement in oxygenation following recruitment manoeuvres; however, the largest clinical trial[43] failed to show an effect. Grasso and colleagues[44] found that recruitment manoeuvres were only effective early in ARDS and with lower levels of baseline PEEP, probably explaining the variable responses reported.

In addition to physical recruitment of alveoli, lung stretch above resting V_T is the most powerful physiological stimulus for release of pulmonary surfactant from type II cells. This is associated with an increase in lung elastance and improved PaO_2 in the isolated perfused lung,[45] and is a possible explanation for the improvement in oxygenation, recruited lung volume and elastance reported with the addition of three sigh breaths in patients with ARDS.[46] Similarly, in models of lung injury biologically variable or fractal V_T is associated with less lung damage with lower alveolar levels of IL-8,[47] improved oxygenation and lung elastance with greater surfactant release.[48] Again, these data caution against monotonous low V_T ventilation, and suggest that intermittent or variable lung stretch may reduce lung injury.

MODE OF VENTILATION

Non-invasive ventilation should not be routinely used in ALI and ARDS (see Chapter 33) and most patients require intubated mechanical ventilation. Following intubation controlled ventilation allows immediate reduction in the work of breathing and application of PEEP and a high FiO_2. Later in the clinical course assisted or supported modes of ventilation may allow better patient–ventilator interaction (see Chapter 27), and possibly improved oxygenation through better mismatch as a result of diaphragmatic contraction.[49] Withdrawal or weaning from mechanical ventilation is discussed in Chapter 27.

An advantage of assist-control ventilation (as used in the ARDS Network study) is that spontaneous effort cannot generate a greater volume than V_T. Care should be taken with synchronised intermittent mandatory ventilation (SIMV), particularly if pressure support is added to SIMV, as excessive V_T may occur during supported breaths. There is an increasing tendency to use pressure-controlled (PC) ventilation or pressure-regulated volume control (PRVC) as P_{pk} is lower than volume-controlled (VC) ventilation with a constant inspiratory flow pattern. However, the decelerating flow pattern of PC or PRVC means that most of the resistive pressure (P_{res}) during inspiration is dissipated by end-inspiration, which is in contrast to VC with a constant inspiratory flow pattern where Pres is dissipated at end-inspiration (see Chapter 27, Figure 27.2). Consequently, with PC and PRVC $P_{pk} \approx P_{plat}$ which is the same as P_{plat} during VC.[50] In addition oxygenation, haemodynamic stability and mean airway pressure are no different between PC and VC, and a moderately sized randomised study found no difference in outcome.[51] However, there may be differences in lung stress due to greater viscoelastic build up with VC.

Inverse-ratio ventilation, often together with PC, has been used in ARDS. However, when $PEEP_i$ and total PEEP are taken into account, apart from a small decrease in $Pa{CO_2}$, there are no advantages with inverse-ratio ventilation. Mean airway pressure is higher, with a greater risk of both haemodynamic consequences[50] and regional hyperinflation.[52] Consequently, an inspiratory to expiratory ratio less than 1:1 is recommended.

A number of other modes of ventilation (see Chapter 27), including airway pressure release ventilation and high-frequency oscillation, have been proposed for use in ARDS, but without new data there do not appear to be any major advantages over the optimal conventional ventilation.

TARGET BLOOD GASES

As discussed above, there are many variables that need to be considered when choosing target blood gases in ARDS. For example, if a patient also has a traumatic brain injury, it may be inappropriate to accept hypercapnia.

Oxygenation targets and $Fi{O_2}$

There must be a compromise between the major determinants of oxygenation, including the extent of poorly or non-aerated lung, hypoxic pulmonary vasoconstriction and mixed venous oxygen saturation, and the target $Pa{O_2}$. The association between cognitive impairment and arterial saturation ($Sa{O_2}$) < 90%[11] suggests that $Sa{O_2} \geq 90\%$ and usually $Pa{O_2} > 60$ mmHg is a reasonable target. Because positive-pressure ventilation may reduce cardiac output it is also important to consider tissue oxygenation.

In addition to PEEP, increased $Fi{O_2}$ is used to improve $Sa{O_2}$. However, high $Fi{O_2}$ may also cause tissue injury, including diffuse alveolar damage. The balance between increased airway pressure and $Fi{O_2}$ is unknown, but high $Fi{O_2}$ is generally regarded as being less damaging.[53] In part this is because diffuse alveolar damage itself protects the lung against hyperoxia, perhaps through prior induction of scavengers for reactive oxygen species.[54] A reasonable compromise is to start ventilation at a $Fi{O_2}$ of 1 and to titrate down, aiming for an $Fi{O_2} \leq 0.6$. In patients with extreme hypoxaemia, additional measures such as inhaled nitric oxide (iNO) and prone positioning may be tried, along with a lower $Sa{O_2}$ target.

Carbon dioxide target

Low V_T strategies will result in elevations in $Pa{CO_2}$ unless minute ventilation is augmented by an increase in respiratory rate. The ARDS Network protocol aimed at normocapnia, with a maximum respiratory rate of 35 breaths/min, to minimise respiratory acidosis.[28] This exposes the lung to more repeated tidal stretch, and may result in dynamic hyperinflation due to a shortened expiratory time.[55] In addition, allowing the $Pa{CO_2}$ to rise above normal may not be harmful in many patients.

If hypercapnic acidosis occurs slowly, intracellular acidosis is well compensated, and the associated increase in sympathetic tone may augment cardiac output and blood pressure. Although the respiratory acidosis may worsen pulmonary hypertension and induce myocardial arrhythmias, these effects are often small, particularly if there has been time for metabolic compensation. In addition, in an ischaemia–reperfusion model of ALI, therapeutic hypercapnia reduced lung injury and apoptosis.[56] However, clinical studies of permissive hypercapnia must be undertaken before therapeutic hypercapnia is considered. Hypercapnia should be avoided in patients with or at risk from raised intracranial pressure.

ADDITIONAL MEASURES TO IMPROVE OXYGENATION

PRONE POSTURE

In ~ 70% of patients with ARDS, prone positioning will result in a significant increase in $Pa{O_2}$, with a modest increase in $Pa{O_2}$ sustained in the supine position.[57] The mechanisms involved include recruitment of dorsal lung, with concurrent collapse of ventral lung; however, perfusion is more evenly distributed, leading to better matching. Although three large clinical studies[58,59] did not show an improvement in mortality, post-hoc analysis suggests that mortality may be reduced in the most hypoxaemic patients.[57] Although further data are awaited, prone positioning may be used as rescue therapy in life-threatening hypoxaemia.

MANIPULATION OF THE PULMONARY CIRCULATION

iNO and prostacyclin (PGI_2) may be used to reduce pulmonary shunt and right ventricular afterload by reducing pulmonary artery impedance. When hypoxic pulmonary vasoconstriction is active, there is redistribution of pulmonary blood flow away from the poorly ventilated dependent areas to more normally ventilated lung, leading to an increase in $Pa{O_2}$. Both iNO and PGI_2 are potent vasodilators, and since they are delivered as part of the gas mix (iNO) or inhaled (PGI_2), they are delivered to well-ventilated lung. Both act to vasodilate the local pulmonary circulation and increase the redistribution of pulmonary blood flow away from poorly ventilated lung, reducing pulmonary shunt and improving oxygenation. Intravenous almitrine is a selective pulmonary vasoconstrictor that reinforces hypoxic pulmonary vasoconstriction, and although this may improve oxygenation alone, there is a synergistic effect with iNO.

Inhaled NO or PGI_2 may also be used to reduce right ventricular afterload; however a consequent increase in cardiac output is rare in ARDS. Intravenous PGI_2 will improve cardiac output in ARDS; however, there is non-specific pulmonary vasodilation with increased blood flow through poorly ventilated lung zones, resulting in a deterioration in oxygenation.

Inhaled nitric oxide

Nitric oxide is an endothelium-derived smooth-muscle relaxant. It also has other important physiological roles, including neurotransmission, host defence, platelet aggregation, leukocyte adhesion and bronchodilation. Doses as low as 60 parts per billion iNO may improve oxygenation; however, commonly used doses in ARDS are 1–60 parts per million, with the higher doses required for reduction in pulmonary artery pressure. A rise in $Pa\text{O}_2$ exceeding 20% is generally regarded as a positive response, and iNO should be continued at the minimum effective dose.

Inhaled NO may be delivered continuously or using intermittent inspiratory injection. Delivery is usually in the form of medical-grade NO/N_2, and this should be adequately mixed to avoid delivery of variable NO concentrations. It is recommended that inspiratory NO and NO_2 concentrations are measured, either by an electrochemical method or by chemiluminescence. The electrochemical method is accurate to 1 ppm, which is adequate for clinical use, and is less expensive. Local environmental levels of NO and NO_2 are low and predominantly influenced by atmospheric concentrations; however, it is still common practice to scavenge expired gas. Binding to haemoglobin in the pulmonary circulation rapidly inactivates NO, and systemic effects are only reported following high concentrations of iNO. Systemic methaemoglobin levels may be monitored, and are generally less than 5% during clinical use of iNO, but they should be compared to a baseline level. NO may cause lung toxicity through combination with oxygen free radicals, and through metabolism of NO to NO_2, although these do not appear to be major clinical problems.

Only 40–70% of patients with ARDS have improved oxygenation with iNO (responders), and this is likely due to active hypoxic pulmonary vasoconstriction in the remainder. Addition of intravenous almitrine can have an additive effect on oxygenation, and may improve the number of responders. Although clinical trials have shown no improvement in mortality or reversal of ALI, iNO was safe and did significantly improve oxygenation initially (as compared to placebo or no iNO), but this was not sustained beyond 12–24 hours. Consequently iNO cannot be recommended for routine use in ARDS, although in some patients with severe hypoxaemia, perhaps in combination with almitrine, iNO will provide temporary rescue.

Inhaled prostacyclin

PGI_2 (up to 50 ng/kg per min) improves oxygenation as effectively as iNO in ARDS patients. It is continuously jet-nebulised due to its short half-life (2–3 min). Potential advantages include increased surfactant release from stretched type II cells, avoidance of the potential complications of iNO and minimal toxicity. However, PGI_2 is dissolved in an alkaline glycine buffer which alone can result in airway inflammation. Iloprost is a derivative of PGI_2 with similar activity, a longer duration of action, and without an alkaline buffer. However, neither agent has been shown to improve outcome in ARDS patients.

PHARMACOLOGICAL THERAPY

Apart from improved mortality in sepsis following activated protein C,[60] there are no proven pharmacological therapies for ALI or ARDS despite numerous studies. However, the lack of a protective ventilation strategy in many of these studies may have masked a drug effect.

SURFACTANT REPLACEMENT THERAPY

Surfactant dysfunction is an important and early abnormality contributing to lung damage in ALI.[38,61] Pulmonary surfactant reduces surface tension, promoting alveolar stability, reducing work of breathing and lung water. In addition surfactant has important roles in lung host defence. Reactive oxygen species, phospholipases and increased protein permeability lead to inhibition of surfactant function, composition is abnormal and turnover is markedly increased. VILI is difficult to demonstrate without surfactant dysfunction.[56] Consequently, there has been considerable interest in exogenous surfactant replacement therapy.

Recombinant surfactant protein C-based surfactant administered intratracheally improves oxygenation in ARDS without an improvement in mortality.[62] However, as subgroup analysis appeared promising, further clinical trials are under way in direct or pulmonary causes of ARDS.

GLUCOCORTICOIDS

Glucocorticoids may have a role in ARDS through reduction of the intense inflammatory response and their potential to reduce fibroproliferation and collagen deposition, by faster degradation of fibroblast procollagen mRNA. Although a small study, with cross-over, showed a reduction in mortality,[63] a study of 180 patients with persistent ARDS (of at least 7 days' duration) found no improvement in mortality up to 180 days later, but did show an improvement in ventilator-free days and shock-free days.[64] However, this was offset by neuromuscular complications, and patients enrolled at least 14 days after the onset of ARDS had increased 60- and 180-day mortality rates. These data do not support the routine use of steroids in ARDS.

KETOCONAZOLE

Ketoconazole is an antifungal drug that also inhibits thromboxane synthase and 5-lipoxygenase. However, promising results from small studies in at-risk patients have not been confirmed in a larger treatment trial.[65]

OTHER PHARMACOLOGIC THERAPIES

Numerous other therapies, including cytokine antagonism, non-steroidal anti-inflammatory drugs, scavengers of reactive oxygen species and lisofylline[66] have been trialled without success. The complex balance of inflammation and repair in ALI, and the critical additional damage secondary to VILI, may explain these results. However, studies in less heterogeneous groups with minimisation of VILI using standardised ventilation protocols, together with a growing understanding of ALI and ARDS, offer potential pharmacological therapies.

REFERENCES

1. Ashbaugh DG, Bigelow DB, Petty TL *et al.* Acute respiratory distress in adults. *Lancet* 1967; **ii**: 319–23.
2. Bernard GR, Artigas A, Brigham KL *et al.* The American–European Consensus Conference on ARDS: definitions, mechanisms, relevant outcomes, and clinical trial coordination. *Am J Respir Crit Care Med* 1994; **149**: 818–24.
3. Murray JF, Matthay MA, Luce JM *et al.* An expanded definition of the adult respiratory distress syndrome. *Am Rev Respir Dis* 1988; **138**: 720–3. [Erratum, *Am Rev Respir Dis* 1989; **139**: 1065.]
4. Ferguson ND, Frutos-Vivar F, Esteban A *et al.* Acute respiratory distress syndrome: underrecognition by clinicians and diagnostic accuracy of three clinical definitions. *Crit Care Med* 2005; **33**: 2228–34.
5. Gattinoni L, Caironi P, Pelosi P *et al.* What has computed tomography taught us about the acute respiratory distress syndrome? *Am J Respir Crit Care Med* 2001; **164**: 1701–11.
6. Bersten AD, Edibam C, Hunt T *et al.* Incidence and mortality from acute lung injury and the acute respiratory distress syndrome in three Australian states. *Am J Respir Crit Care Med* 2002; **165**: 443–8.
7. Rubenfeld GD, Herridge MS. Epidemiology and outcomes of acute lung injury. *Chest* 2007; **131**: 554–62.
8. Ely EW, Wheeler AP, Thompson BT *et al.* Recovery rate and prognosis in older persons who develop acute lung injury and the acute respiratory distress syndrome. *Ann Intern Med* 2002; **136**: 25–36.
9. McHugh LG, Milberg JA, Whitcomb ME *et al.* Recovery of function in survivors of the acute respiratory distress syndrome. *Am J Respir Crit Care Med* 1994; **250**: 90–4.
10. Davidson TA, Caldwell ES, Curtis SR *et al.* Reduced quality of life in survivors of acute respiratory distress syndrome compared with other critically ill control patients. *JAMA* 1999; **281**: 354–60.
11. Hopkins RO, Weaver LK, Pope D. Neuropsychological sequelae and impaired health status in survivors of severe acute respiratory distress syndrome. *Am J Respir Crit Care* 1999; **160**: 50–6.
12. Connelly KG, Moss M, Parsons PE *et al.* Serum ferritin as a predictor of the acute respiratory distress syndrome. *Am J Respir Crit Care Med* 1997; **155**: 21–5.
13. Bersten AD, Hunt T, Nicholas TE *et al.* Elevated plasma surfactant protein-B predicts development of acute respiratory distress syndrome in patients with acute respiratory failure. *Am J Respir Crit Care Med* 2001; **164**: 648–52.
14. Davidson KG, Bersten AD, Barr HA *et al.* Endotoxin induces respiratory failure and increases surfactant composition and respiration independent of alveolocapillary injury in rats. *Am J Respir Crit Care Med* 2002; **165**: 1516–25.
15. Doyle IR, Nicholas TE, Bersten AD. Partitioning lung and plasma proteins: circulating surfactant proteins as biomarkers of alveolocapillary permeability. *Clin Exp Pharmacol Physiol* 1999; **26**: 185–97.
16. Downey GP, Dong Q, Kruger J *et al.* Regulation of neutrophil activation in acute lung injury. *Chest* 1999; **116**: 46S–54S.
17. Nelson S, Belknap SM, Carlson RW *et al.* A randomized controlled trial of figastrim as an adjunct to antibiotics for treatment of hospitalized patients with community-acquired pneumonia. *J Infect Dis* 1998; **178**: 1075–80.
18. Zimmeraman GA, Albertine KH, Carveth HJ *et al.* Endothelial activation in ARDS. *Chest* 1999; **116**: 18S–24S.
19. Pittet JF, Mackersie RC, Martin TR *et al.* Biological markers of acute lung injury: prognostic and pathogenetic significance. *Am J Respir Crit Care Med* 1997; **155**: 1187–205.
20. Pugin J, Dunn I, Jolliet P *et al.* Activation of human macrophages by mechanical ventilation in vitro. *Am J Physiol* 1998; **275**: L104–50.
21. Cheung DO, Halsey K, Speert DP. Role of pulmonary alveolar macrophages in defense of the lung against *Pseudomonas aeruginosa*. *Infect Immun* 2000; **68**: 4585–92.
22. Rezaiguia S, Garat C, Declauc C *et al.* Acute bacterial pneumonia in rats increases alveolar epithelial fluid clearance by a tumor necrosis-factor-alpha dependent mechanism. *J Clin Invest* 1997; **99**: 325–35.
23. Modelska K, Pittet JF, Folkesson HG *et al.* Acid-induced lung injury. Protective effect of anti-interleukin-8 pretreatment on alveolar epithelial barrier function in rabbits. *Am J Respir Crit Care Med* 1999; **160**: 1450–6.
24. Park WY, Goodman RB, Steinberg KP *et al.* Cytokine balance in the lungs of patients with acute respiratory distress syndrome. *Am J Respir Crit Care Med* 2001; **164**: 1896–903.

25. Delclaux C, L'Her E, Alberti C *et al.* Treatment of acute hypoxemic nonhypercapnic respiratory insufficiency with continuous positive airway pressure delivered by a face mask. A randomized controlled trial. *JAMA* 2000; **284**: 2352–60.
26. Ventilation with lower tidal volumes as compared with traditional tidal volumes for acute lung injury and the acute respiratory distress syndrome. *N Engl J Med* 2000; **342**: 1301–8.
27. Moran JL, Bersten AD, Solomon PJ. Meta-analysis of controlled trials of ventilator therapy in acute lung injury and acute respiratory distress syndrome: an alternative perspective. *Intens Care Med* 2005; **31**: 227–35.
28. Hager DN, Krishnan JA, Hayden DL *et al.* Tidal volume reduction in patients with acute lung injury when plateau pressures are not high. *Am J Respir Crit Care Med* 2005; **172**: 1241–5.
29. Dreyfuss D, Saumon G. Ventilator-induced lung injury: lessons from experimental studies. *Am J Respir Crit Care Med* 1998; **157**: 294–323.
30. Chiumello D, Pristine G, Slutsky AS. Mechanical ventilation affects local and systemic cytokines in an animal model of acute respiratory distress syndrome. *Am J Respir Crit Care Med* 1999; **160**: 109–16.
31. Terragni PP, Rosboch G, Tealdi A *et al.* Tidal hyperinflation during low tidal volume ventilation in acute respiratory distress syndrome. *Am J Respir Crit Care Med* 2007; **175**: 160–6.
32. Bersten AD. Measurement of overinflation by multiple linear regression analysis in patients with acute lung injury. *Eur Respir J* 1998; **12**: 526–32.
33. Suter PM, Fairley B, Isenberg MD. Optimum end-expiratory airway pressure in patients with acute pulmonary failure. *N Engl J Med* 1975; **292**: 284–9.
34. The National Heart, Lung, and Blood Institute ARDS Clinical Trials Network. Higher versus lower positive end-expiratory pressure in patients with the acute respiratory distress syndrome. *N Engl J Med* 2004; **351**: 327–36.
35. Pepe PE, Hudson LD, Carrico CJ. Early application of positive end-expiratory pressure in patients at-risk for adult respiratory distress syndrome. *N Engl J Med* 1984; **311**: 281–6.
36. Jonson B, Richard J-C, Straus R *et al.* Pressure–volume curves and compliance in acute lung injury: evidence for recruitment above the lower inflection point. *Am J Respir Crit Care Med* 1999; **159**: 1172–8.
37. Crotti S, Mascheroni D, Caironi P *et al.* Recruitment and derecruitment during acute respiratory failure: a clinical study. *Am J Respir Crit Care Med* 2001; **164**: 131–40.
38. Malbouisson LM, Muller J-C, Constantin J-M *et al.* Computed tomography assessment of positive end-expiratory pressure-induced alveolar recruitment in patients with acute respiratory distress syndrome. *Am J Respir Crit Care Med* 2001; **163**: 1444–50.
39. Gattinoni L, Caironi P, Cressoni M *et al.* Lung recruitment in patients with the acute respiratory distress syndrome. *N Engl J Med* 2006; **354**: 1775–86.
40. Thille AW, Richard J-C M, Maggiore SM *et al.* Alveolar recruitment in pulmonary and extrapulmonary acute respiratory distress syndrome. Comparison using pressure–volume curve or static compliance. *Anesthesiology* 2007; **106**: 212–17.
41. Rouby JJ, Lu Q, Goldstein I. Selecting the right level of positive end-expiratory pressure in patients with acute respiratory distress syndrome. *Am J Respir Crit Care Med* 2002; **165**: 1182–6.
42. Amato MBP, Barbas CSV, Medeiros DM *et al.* Effect of a protective ventilation strategy on mortality in the acute respiratory distress syndrome. *N Engl J Med* 1998; **338**: 347–54.
43. Brower RG, Morris A, Macintyre N *et al.* Effects of recruitment maneuvers in patients with acute lung injury and acute respiratory distress syndrome ventilated with high positive end-expiratory pressure. *Crit Care Med* 2003; **31**: 2592–7.
44. Grasso S, Mascia L, Del Turco M *et al.* Effects of recruiting maneuvers in patients with acute respiratory distress syndrome ventilated with protective ventilatory strategy. *Anesthesiology* 2002; **96**: 795–802.
45. Nicholas TE, Power JHT, Barr HA. The pulmonary consequences of a deep breath. *Respir Physiol* 1982; **49**: 315–24.
46. Pelosi P, Cadringher P, Bottino N *et al.* Sigh in acute respiratory distress syndrome. *Am J Respir Crit Care Med* 1999; **159**: 872–80.
47. Boker A, Ruth Graham M, Walley KR *et al.* Improved arterial oxygenation with biologically variable or fractal ventilation using low tidal volumes in a porcine model of acute respiratory distress syndrome. *Am J Respir Crit Care Med* 2002; **165**: 456–62.
48. Ingenito EP, Arold S, Lutchen K *et al.* Effects of noisy ventilation (NV) and open lung ventilation (OLV) on lung mechanics, gas exchange, and surfactant content and properties (abstract). *Am J Respir Crit Care Med* 2001; **163**: A483.
49. Wrigge H, Zinserling J, Neumann P *et al.* Spontaneous breathing improves lung aeration in oleic acid-induced lung injury. *Anesthesiology* 2003; **99**: 376–84.
50. Lessard MR, Guerot E, Lorino H *et al.* Effects of pressure-controlled with different I:E ratios versus volume-controlled ventilation on respiratory mechanics, gas exchange, and hemodynamics in patients with adult respiratory distress syndrome. *Anesthesiology* 1994; **80**: 983–91.
51. Esteban A, Alia I, Gordo F *et al.* Prospective randomized trial comparing pressure-controlled ventilation and volume-controlled ventilation in ARDS. For the Spanish Lung Failure Collaborative Group. *Chest* 2000; **117**: 1690–6.
52. Edibam C, Rutten AJ, Collins DV *et al.* Effect of inspiratory flow pattern and inspiratory to expiratory ratio on nonlinear elastic behavior in patients with acute lung injury. *Am J Respir Crit Care Med* 2003; **167**: 702–7.
53. Slutsky AS. Mechanical ventilation. *Chest* 1993; **104**: 1833–59.
54. Frank L, Yam J, Roberts RJ. The role of endotoxin in protection of adult rats from oxygen-induced lung injury. *J Clin Invest* 1978; **61**: 269–75.

55. Richard JC, Brochard L, Breton L *et al.* Influence of respiratory rate on gas trapping during low volume ventilation of patients with acute lung injury. *Intens Care Med* 2002; **28**: 1078–83.
56. Laffey JG, Tanaka M, Engelberts D *et al.* Therapeutic hypercapnia reduces pulmonary and systemic injury following in vivo lung reperfusion. *Am J Respir Crit Care Med* 2000; **162**: 2287–94.
57. Gattinoni L, Tognoni G, Pesenti A *et al.* Effect of prone positioning on the survival of patients with acute respiratory failure. *N Engl J Med* 2001; **345**: 568–73.
58. Guerin C, Gaillard S, Lemasson S *et al.* Effects of systematic prone positioning in hypoxemic acute respiratory failure: a randomized controlled trial. *JAMA* 2004; **292**: 2379–87.
59. Mancebo J, Fernández R, Blanch L *et al.* A multicenter trial of prolonged prone ventilation in severe acute respiratory distress syndrome. *Am J Respir Crit Care Med* 2006; **173**: 1233–9.
60. Bernard GR, Vincent J-L, Laterre P-F *et al.* Efficacy and safety of recombinant human activated protein C for severe sepsis. *N Engl J Med* 2001; **344**: 699–709.
61. Bersten AD, Davidson K, Nicholas TE *et al.* Respiratory mechanics and surfactant in the acute respiratory distress syndrome. *Clin Exp Pharmacol Physiol* 1998; **25**: 955–63.
62. Spragg RG, Lewis JF, Walmrath HD *et al.* Effect of recombinant surfactant protein C-based surfactant on the acute respiratory distress syndrome. *N Engl J Med* 2004; **351**: 884–92.
63. Meduri GU, Headley AS, Golden E *et al.* Effect of prolonged methylprednisolone therapy in unresolving acute respiratory distress syndrome: a randomized controlled trial. *JAMA* 1998; **280**: 159–65.
64. Steinberg KP, Hudson LD, Goodman RB *et al.* Efficacy and safety of corticosteroids for persistent acute respiratory distress syndrome. *N Engl J Med* 2006; **354**: 1671–84.
65. Ketoconazole for early treatment of acute lung injury and acute respiratory distress syndrome. *JAMA* 2000; **283**: 1995–2002.
66. Randomized placebo-controlled trial of lisofylline for early treatment of acute lung injury and acute respiratory distress syndrome. *Crit Care Med* 2002; **30**: 1–6.

30

Pulmonary embolism

Andrew R Davies and David V Pilcher

Pulmonary embolism (PE) is a commonly considered, but relatively uncommonly diagnosed, condition. It is important to have an adequate understanding of the pathophysiology, as well as a rapid and reliable strategy of investigation and management. This is particularly important in critically ill patients where diagnosis can be difficult and PE may be life-threatening.

AETIOLOGY

Deep venous thrombosis (DVT) and PE are components of a single disease termed venous thromboembolism (VTE). Embolisation of DVT to the pulmonary arteries leads to PE, which is the most severe and life-threatening manifestation. VTE occurs in the population at a rate of about 1 in 1000 per year and is more common both with advancing age and in males.

Most PE results from DVT of the lower limbs, pelvic veins or inferior vena cava (IVC), although DVT of the upper limbs, right atrium or ventricle does also occur. Up to 40% of patients with DVT develop PE, although if the DVT is isolated to below the knee, clinically obvious PE is rare.

Predisposing risk factors for VTE involve one or more components of Virchow's triad: (1) venous stasis; (2) vein wall injury; and (3) hypercoagulability of blood. The main factors are immobility (from any cause), surgery, trauma, malignancy, pregnancy and thrombophilia (Table 30.1).

VTE can be recurrent, which should prompt investigation for thrombophilia, which describes a group of conditions which are inherited and associated with a high incidence of VTE. The most important of these is activated protein C resistance, which is mediated by the factor V Leiden mutation. Up to 50% of patients with recurrent VTE episodes (as well as 20% of patients with a single episode) have this condition; however, its association appears to be greater with DVT than with PE.[1] Up to 5% of patients with VTE develop chronic pulmonary hypertension.[2]

PATHOPHYSIOLOGY

The effects of PE range from being incidental and clinically irrelevant to causing severe obstruction to the pulmonary circulation and sudden death. Pulmonary arterial obstruction and the subsequent release of vasoactive agents such as serotonin and thromboxane A_2 from platelets lead to elevated pulmonary vascular resistance and acute pulmonary hypertension.

Acute pulmonary hypertension increases right ventricular (RV) afterload and RV wall tension, which leads to RV dilatation and dysfunction, with coronary ischaemia being a major contributing mechanism.[3] In massive PE, the combination of coronary ischaemia, RV systolic failure, paradoxical interventricular septal shift and pericardial constraint leads to left ventricular (LV) dysfunction and a 'low-cardiac-output' shock state. In patients with underlying cardiorespiratory disease, a small PE can have profound consequences.

Pulmonary arterial obstruction causes a mismatch between lung ventilation and perfusion, which leads to hypoxaemia. The ventilation of lung units which are no longer perfused causes increased dead-space ventilation and a widening of the end-tidal to arterial CO_2 gradient. Alveolar hyperventilation also occurs, leading to hypocapnia. Increased right atrial pressure can open a patent foramen ovale, which often results in right-to-left shunting manifested as either profound hypoxaemia or paradoxical (arterial) embolisation, which commonly presents as a cerebral infarct.

CLINICAL PRESENTATION

PE is relatively uncommon in critically ill patients despite the frequent presence of risk factors for VTE. However, when PE does occur, the diagnosis is frequently overlooked or is difficult to confirm because of the presence of coexistent cardiorespiratory disease. Clinical assessment raises the suspicion of PE but is neither sensitive nor specific. A number of clinical prediction systems have been developed, the most widely reported of which are the Wells' score and the Geneva score.[4] The differential diagnosis is listed in Table 30.2.

SYMPTOMS

Dyspnoea, pleuritic chest pain, and haemoptysis are the classic symptoms of PE. Most patients will have at least

Table 30.1 Risk factors for venous thromboembolism

Primary hypercoagulable states (thrombophilia)
Antithrombin III deficiency
Protein C deficiency
Protein S deficiency
Resistance to activated protein C resistance (inherited factor V Leiden mutation)
Hyperhomocysteinaemia
Lupus anticoagulant (antiphospholipid antibody)
Secondary hypercoagulable states
Immobility
Surgery
Trauma
Malignancy
Pregnancy and the puerperium
Obesity
Smoking
Oestrogen-containing oral contraception or hormone replacement therapy
Indwelling catheters in great veins and the right heart
Burns
Patients with limb paralysis (e.g. spinal injuries)
Heart failure
Increasing age

Table 30.2 Differential diagnosis of pulmonary embolism

Acute myocardial infarction
Acute pulmonary oedema
Pneumonia
Asthma or exacerbation of chronic obstructive pulmonary disease
Pericardial tamponade
Pleural effusion
Fat embolism
Pneumothorax
Aortic dissection
Rib fracture
Musculoskeletal pain
Anxiety

one of these symptoms, with dyspnoea being the most common. The combination of pleuritic chest pain and haemoptysis reflects a late presentation where pulmonary infarction has occurred. If syncope occurs there is a high likelihood that there has been a massive PE. A family history of venous thrombosis raises the possibility of inherited thrombophilia.

PHYSICAL SIGNS

Physical signs can be absent, but the most frequent sign is tachypnoea. Others include tachycardia, fever and signs of RV dysfunction (raised jugular venous pressure, parasternal heave and loud pulmonary component of the second heart sound). If massive PE is present, signs may include hypotension, pale mottled skin and peripheral or even central cyanosis. It is important also to examine for signs of DVT in the legs and arms.

INVESTIGATIONS

The diagnosis of PE requires a high level of clinical suspicion and the appropriate use of investigations. The aim of these investigations is to confirm or exclude the presence of PE and then to stratify treatment accordingly. The optimal investigation strategy depends upon the individual patient and institution as a number of investigations are available. Pulmonary angiography has traditionally been considered the 'gold standard' for the diagnosis of PE. The advent of multidetector row computed tomography (CT) scanning (which compares well with standard pulmonary angiography[5]) has led to the emergence of this as the 'first-line' test in many centres. A suggested investigation algorithm is shown in Figure 30.1.

D-DIMER

The serum D-dimer level is useful for exclusion of VTE, particularly when it is normal and combined with a low-risk clinical assessment.[6] A variety of different assays are available. Negative tests, particularly from enzyme-linked immunosorbent assays (ELISA), are highly predictive of the absence of both DVT and PE.[7] A high D-dimer concentration is also an independent predictive factor associated with mortality.[8]

Unfortunately, positive D-dimer tests are common in intensive care unit (ICU) patients who often suffer from one of the variety of conditions (such as trauma, surgery, diffuse intravascular coagulation, malignancy, acute myocardial infarction, pneumonia and heart failure) which also lead to a raised D-dimer, meaning that other tests are required to confirm or refute the diagnosis of VTE.

TROPONIN, BRAIN NATRIURETIC PEPTIDE (BNP) AND NT-TERMINAL PRO-BNP

Although of little use for diagnosis, measurement of troponin, BNP or NT-terminal Pro-BNP can add to the risk stratification of patients with known PE. The presence of a raised troponin is associated with haemodynamic instability in patients with non-massive PE independently of clinical, echocardiographic and laboratory findings.[9] Raised troponin also predicts a higher mortality.[10] Low levels of BNP and NT-terminal Pro-BNP have been shown to correlate with an uneventful course in patients with known PE.[11] NT-terminal Pro-BNP appears to be a better predictor of outcome than troponin.[12]

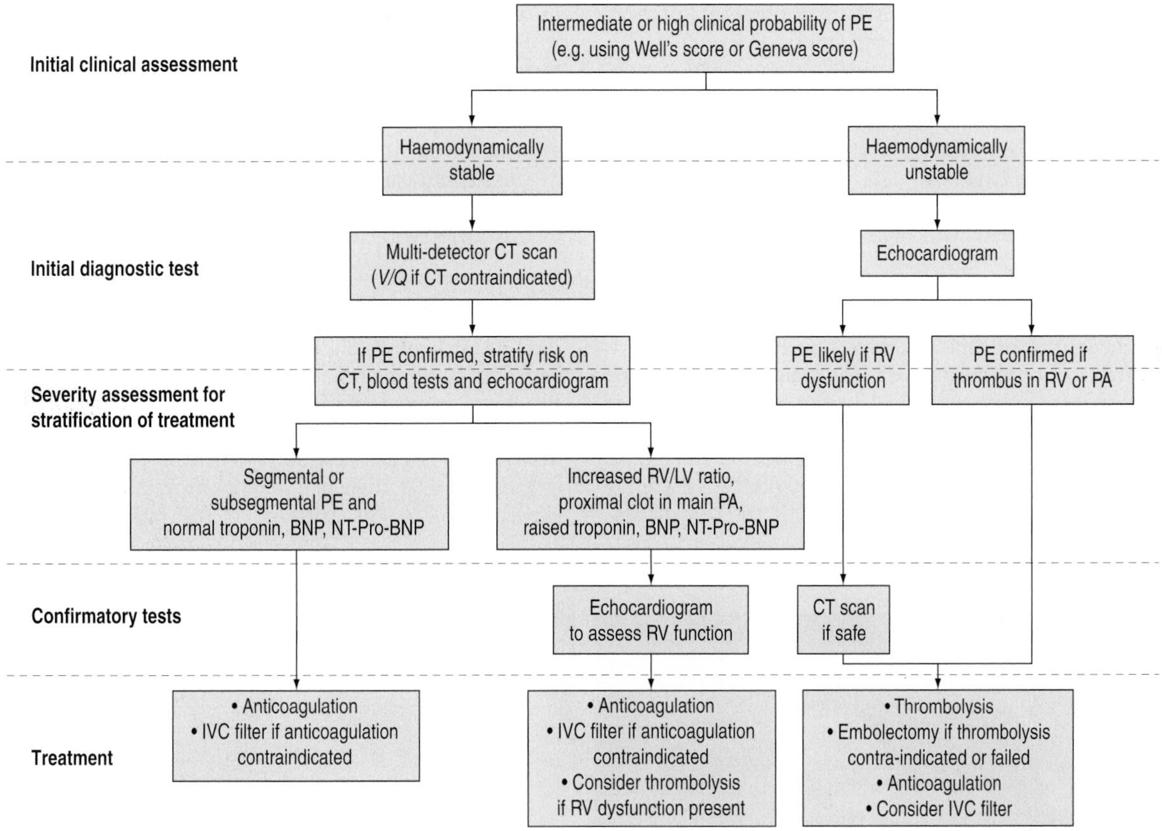

Figure 30.1 Suggested investigation and treatment algorithm for pulmonary embolism (PE). CT, computed tomography; *V/Q*, ventilation/perfusion scan; RV, right ventricular; PA, pulmonary artery; BNP, brain natriuretic peptide; RV/LV, right ventricle/left ventricle; IVC, inferior vena cava.

ARTERIAL BLOOD GASES

A normal arterial blood gas profile does not rule out the diagnosis; however hypoxaemia (with a widened alveolar–arterial oxygen gradient), hypocapnia and an increased end-tidal CO_2 gradient[13] should raise the suspicion of PE, even though there are many other causes of these findings in critically ill patients.[14] Metabolic acidosis may be present if shock from a large PE occurs.

ELECTROCARDIOGRAPH

A normal electrocardiograph (ECG) is found in about one-third of patients. Apart from sinus tachycardia (which is non-specific), the most frequent ECG abnormalities are non-specific S-T depression and T-wave inversion in the anterior leads, reflecting right heart strain. The pattern of a deep S-wave in lead I, and a Q-wave and inverted T-wave in lead III (S1Q3T3) is classical but is infrequently present. Other possible abnormalities include left- or right-axis deviation, P pulmonale, right bundle-branch block and atrial arrhythmias. The ECG is also useful in excluding acute myocardial infarction and pericarditis.

CHEST X-RAY

The chest X-ray is often normal or only slightly abnormal, with non-specific signs such as cardiac enlargement, pleural effusion, elevated hemidiaphragm, atelectasis and localised infiltrates. More specific findings, including focal oligaemia, a peripheral wedge-shaped density above the diaphragm or an enlarged right descending pulmonary artery,[15] are uncommon and difficult for non-radiologists to identify. The chest X-ray is also useful in identifying an alternative diagnosis such as pneumothorax, pneumonia, acute pulmonary oedema, rib fracture and pleural effusion.

COMPUTED TOMOGRAPHY

As CT technology has improved, CT angiography (CTA) has emerged as a cost-effective and clinically reliable alternative to the *V/Q* scan.[16] The single-detector row CT has been superseded by multidetector row CT, which allows imaging of the entire chest with high-resolution images in 'in-plane' and 'through-plane' resolution. High-resolution images to the level of segmental and in some cases subsegmental pulmonary arteries can be obtained in a short time period (often a single breath-hold).

When CTA is compared to conventional angiography it appears reliable, with sensitivity, specificity and accuracy of 100%, 89% and 91% respectively.[5] Adding venography of the leg veins to the CTA (CTA-CTV) further increases the diagnostic certainty.[17] It is therefore recommended that CTA or CTA-CTV should be the principal radiological test for patients with high and moderate probability of PE.[18]

Although the ability of many CT scanners to detect PE at the subsegmental level is limited, it is debatable whether this is of clinical significance. Patients who have negative or indeterminate CT scans and in whom anticoagulation is withheld have low subsequent rates of thromboembolic events.[19]

The advantage of CT is that it can not only diagnose PE but can also be used to assess severity of the condition. Increased RV/LV ratio (> 0.9)[20] and clot in the proximal branches of the pulmonary artery[21] correlate with the clinical severity of PE. Severity stratification is further increased by combining CT with other tests such as troponin[9] and BNP or NT-terminal ProBNP.[11] CT scanning may also identify the causative DVT in the veins of the legs, pelvis and abdomen or detect alternative or additional diagnoses such as a pulmonary mass, pneumonia, emphysema, pneumothorax, pleural effusion or mediastinal adenopathy (Figure 30.2).

ECHOCARDIOGRAPHY

Because of its portability, echocardiography has become increasingly useful in critically ill patients with possible PE. Many patients with PE have an echocardiographic abnormality, the most common being RV dilatation, RV hypokinesis, paradoxical interventricular septal motion toward the LV, tricuspid regurgitation and pulmonary hypertension.[22] The pattern of RV hypokinesis with

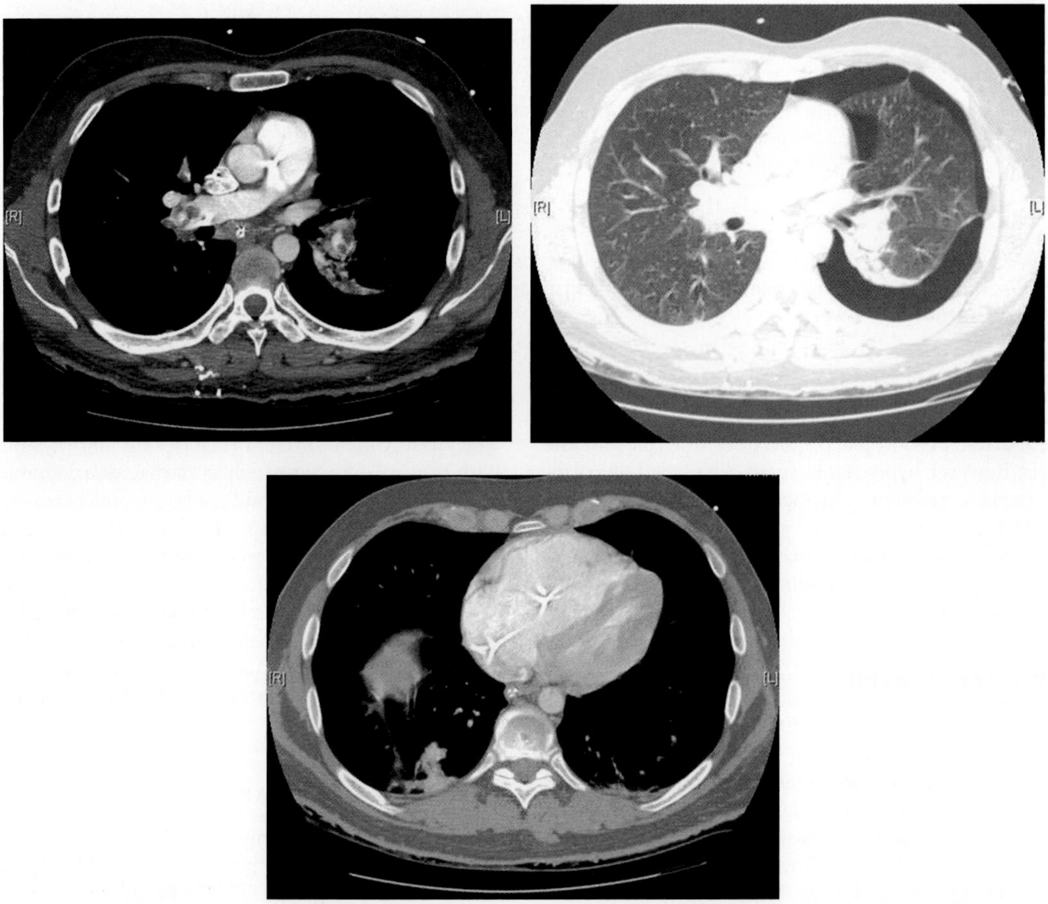

Figure 30.2 Computed tomography (CT) scanning and pulmonary embolism (PE). Three CT images from the same patient demonstrating the ability of CT to detect pulmonary emboli, assess severity and confirm additional diagnoses. Image 1 (mediastinal window): filling defects in the right pulmonary artery and inferior branch of the left pulmonary artery. A pulmonary artery catheter is also in situ. Image 2 (lung window): a left pneumothorax with pleural adhesions, and a small area of left-sided posterior consolidation. Image 3 (mediastinal window): dilatation of the right ventricle relative to the left ventricle.

apical sparing is considered pathognomonic for PE.[23] The presence of RV dysfunction correlates with mortality.[24] Echocardiography is poor at excluding PE, as a negative echocardiogram can miss up to 50% of PEs.[25]

Transthoracic echocardiography will also allow estimation of pulmonary arterial pressure, identification of intracardiac thrombi (which usually requires surgical embolectomy) and aids in differential diagnosis by excluding aortic dissection and pericardial tamponade. Transoesophageal echocardiography has the additional benefit of directly identifying embolus in the proximal pulmonary arteries, which is common in patients with haemodynamically significant PE.[26]

Echocardiography has its best application in haemodynamically unstable patients, where it can be rapidly brought to the patient. If the patient has RV dilatation and hypokinesis in the right clinical setting, PE is extremely likely.

VENTILATION/PERFUSION SCANNING

The lung ventilation/perfusion (*V/Q*) scan is becoming less commonly used with the advent of multidetector row CT. The perfusion scan identifies defects in perfusion which may be classified as single or multiple, and as subsegmental, segmental or lobar. By combining this with ventilation scanning, these perfusion defects can then be labelled as mismatched (normal ventilation in a zone of perfusion defect) or matched defects (ventilation defect corresponds to perfusion defect). The probability of PE is then classified as high, intermediate or low probability for PE, or normal.[27]

A normal lung scan effectively excludes PE and treatment can be safely withheld. A high-probability scan is considered diagnostic for PE. The majority of patients do not have such clear-cut scan results, and even a low-probability scan cannot satisfactorily exclude PE, as a patient with a low-probability scan but with a high level of clinical suspicion has a 40% chance of having a PE.

Despite the increased use of CT, the *V/Q* scan retains a role when CT is either unavailable or contraindicated (e.g. significant renal impairment, anaphylaxis to intravenous contrast or pregnancy).[15] *V/Q* scanning also allows quantification of regional blood flow within the lungs, which may be required in the assessment of chronic pulmonary venous embolism.

MAGNETIC RESONANCE IMAGING

PE may also be diagnosed by gadolinium-enhanced magnetic resonance pulmonary angiography. So far, this has proven more useful in the assessment of chronic VTE.

PULMONARY ANGIOGRAPHY

The pulmonary angiogram is regarded as the only test which can exclude PE with relative certainty. It will detect most PEs even at the subsegmental level. However, it is unavailable in many centres.

SEARCH FOR DEEP VENOUS THROMBOSIS

Doppler ultrasound has been recommended to search for DVT in the leg veins, from where over 90% of emboli originate. If a leg DVT is confirmed, anticoagulation is required unless the DVT is entirely below the knee, where the associated morbidity is low. Ultrasound is highly accurate in symptomatic or proximal DVT, although in asymptomatic patients, ultrasound is much less likely to find DVT, meaning the absence of a DVT does not exclude PE.

Leg venography is a more sensitive test; however, it is invasive and now uncommonly performed.

INVESTIGATION STRATEGY IN HAEMODYNAMICALLY STABLE PATIENTS

- CTA is the preferred initial test and, if positive, the patient should be stratified into high- or low-risk. The presence of clot within pulmonary arteries confirms the diagnosis of PE.
- Echocardiography should then be considered to assess for RV dysfunction for high-risk patients who have:
  - clot within proximal pulmonary arteries
  - raised RV/LV ratio (> 0.9)
  - raised troponin, BNP or NT-terminal Pro-BNP
- If there is a high clinical suspicion of PE and the CT is negative (or the *V/Q* scan is low or intermediate probability), then a pulmonary angiogram is required to exclude PE.

INVESTIGATION STRATEGY IN HAEMODYNAMICALLY UNSTABLE PATIENTS

- Echocardiography (preferably transoesophageal) should be the first test performed.
- If the patient has acute RV dilatation and visible embolus, PE is confirmed.
- If there is RV dilatation but no visible embolus, then a CTA is required depending on how unstable the patient is.
- If there is no RV dilatation, it is unlikely that the haemodynamic instability is caused by PE (although this cannot be excluded completely). Efforts towards finding an alternative diagnosis are the priority.
- If echocardiography is not readily available, a CTA should be performed.

MANAGEMENT

MANAGEMENT PRINCIPLES

Unless there is a serious contraindication, nearly all patients should receive anticoagulation with either unfractionated or low-molecular-weight heparin (LMWH) to prevent VTE recurrence. However removal or destruction of the embolus is a key principle in treatment of the more severe cases of PE based on the importance of RV dysfunction to both the pathophysiology and the outcome of PE.

To assist in planning management, it is worth grading the severity of PE as follows:

MASSIVE PULMONARY EMBOLISM (HAEMODYNAMICALLY UNSTABLE)

Patients with PE and hypotension have a 25–30% mortality rate despite treatment. If cardiopulmonary resuscitation is required, this increases to 65%. These patients have the most to benefit from a strategy that includes attempts at urgent removal of embolus (by administering a thrombolytic agent or performing embolectomy), concurrent haemodynamic support and prevention of further embolisation.

SUBMASSIVE PULMONARY EMBOLISM (HAEMODYNAMICALLY STABLE WITH EVIDENCE OF RIGHT VENTRICULAR DYSFUNCTION)

Patients with PE and evidence of RV dysfunction have higher mortality and recurrence rates than those with normal RV function.[24] They also develop shock and RV thrombi more frequently. These patients require prevention of further embolisation but also warrant strong consideration of removal of embolus using a thrombolytic agent. Thrombolysis appears to improve outcomes,[28] although this appears to be at the expense of a higher bleeding risk.[29] Echocardiogram is not always required to diagnose RV dysfunction as CT-diagnosed RV dilatation has also been shown to predict poor outcomes.[30]

MILD PULMONARY EMBOLISM (HAEMODYNAMICALLY STABLE WITH NO RIGHT VENTRICULAR DYSFUNCTION)

Patients with PE who have normal blood pressure and normal RV function have a low risk of death or recurrence. Methods to remove embolus will therefore be unlikely to confer benefit. Prevention of further embolisation is the major goal.

The major principles of management are therefore:

- prevention of further embolisation (massive, submassive or mild PE)
- removal of emboli (massive or submassive PE)
- concurrent haemodynamic support (massive PE)

A suggested management strategy is outlined in Figure 30.1.

PREVENTION OF FURTHER EMBOLISATION

ANTICOAGULATION

Heparin has been known to prevent recurrence and reduce the mortality from PE for over 35 years. LMWHs are as effective and safe as unfractionated heparin[31] and may even be better.[32] LMWHs offer several advantages over unfractionated heparin, including a longer half-life, increased bioavailability, a more predictable dose–response and less requirement for monitoring and dose adjustments, and can be readily used in the stable patient with PE.

Table 30.3 Weight-based dosing of intravenous heparin (adapted from Raschke *et al.*[33])

Initial dosing			
Loading 80 u/kg			
Maintenance infusion 18 u/kg per h			
Perform APTT in 6 h			
Subsequent dose adjustments			
APTT	Dose change (u/kg per h)	Additional action	Next APTT
< 35	+4	Rebolus of 80 u/kg	6 h
35–45	+2	Rebolus of 40 u/kg	6 h
46–70	0	Nothing	6 h
71–90	−2	Nothing	6 h
> 90	−3	Stop infusion for 1 h	6 h

APTT, activated partial thromboplastin time.

Unfractionated heparin should be used for those patients who have recently had a thrombolytic agent or embolectomy as it can be easily and rapidly reversed. Heparin should be administered by intravenous infusion with a bolus and initial monitoring should be with 6-hourly activated partial thromboplastin time (APTT) testing. Since subtherapeutic levels of anticoagulation increase the risk of recurrence, it is important to achieve therapeutic heparinisation rapidly. Weight-based dosing of heparin should be used as target anticoagulation levels are reached sooner[33] (Table 30.3).

The predominant complications of both unfractionated heparin and LMWHs are haemorrhagic. These include bleeding peptic ulcer, stroke, retroperitoneal haematoma and post surgical wound haemorrhage. Heparin-induced thrombotic thrombocytopenia syndrome (HITTS) can also occur. Bleeding complications and HITTS appear to be less common when LMWHs are being used.

Oral anticoagulants should be started as soon as possible so that heparin can be ceased when the international normalised ratio is > 2.0.

A number of conditions are considered to be relative contraindications to anticoagulant therapy, the major ones are active peptic ulceration, recent surgery, recent trauma and recent cerebral haemorrhage. In each individual patient the risk-to-benefit ratio (taking into account the severity of the PE) should be considered before anticoagulation is withheld from the patient.

INFERIOR VENA CAVA FILTER

IVC filters are another method used to prevent further embolisation. They are indicated for patients in whom anticoagulation is contraindicated, those who experience recurrent PE despite adequate anticoagulation and those undergoing open surgical embolectomy.[34] Insertion is usually performed percutaneously in a radiology department, but it can be done at the bedside.[35] They lower early recurrence rates but increase long-term DVT recurrence rates,[36] although newer retrievable designs may be better.[37] A recent analysis of a multicentre register analysis demonstrated a significant reduction in 90-day mortality associated with IVC filters.[38]

Absolute indications include:

- new or recurrent PE despite anticoagulation
- contraindications to anticoagulation
- complications resulting from anticoagulation

Other recommended indications include:

- patients with extensive DVT
- patients following a surgical embolectomy
- patients with massive PE

REMOVAL OF EMBOLI

THROMBOLYTIC AGENTS

Thrombolytic agents result in dramatic and immediate haemodynamic improvement in some patients by dissolving the embolus and reducing pulmonary arterial obstruction. Experimental studies, clinical observations and randomised trials have consistently demonstrated the favourable effects of thrombolysis on angiographic, haemodynamic and scintigraphic parameters of patients with acute PE. All of the commonly used agents (including streptokinase, urokinase, alteplase and reteplase) can be rapidly effective, although comparisons with patients who received heparin most commonly reveal similar degrees of embolus resolution after a few days to a week.

A large multicentre patient registry found that patients receiving thrombolytic agents (clearly on an ad-hoc basis) had lower rates of mortality and recurrence than patients receiving heparin.[39] Despite this, there has been no randomised study comparing a thrombolytic agent with standard anticoagulation which has found a mortality difference, although the studies have likely been underpowered to detect this.

A meta-analysis found that thrombolytic therapy was associated with a non-significant reduction in recurrent PE or death when compared to heparin in patients with PE. However, when only studies that included massive PE were aggregated, there was indeed a significant reduction in mortality in favour of thrombolysis.[29]

Thrombolytics in patients with submassive PE do not reduce mortality but do significantly reduce clinical deterioration, requiring an escalation of treatment in the ICU.[28]

There is therefore adequate justification for the use of a thrombolytic agent in patients with massive PE unless there is a clear contraindication. There is also strong justification for the use of a thrombolytic in patients with submassive PE (identified by RV dysfunction).

Table 30.4 Recommended doses of thrombolytic agents for pulmonary embolism

Urokinase	4400 u/kg bolus (over 10 min) followed by 4400 u/kg per h for 12 h
Streptokinase	250 000 unit bolus (over 15 min) followed by 100 000 u/h for 24 h
Alteplase	10 mg bolus followed by 90 mg over 2 h
Reteplase	10 unit boluses 30 min apart

Comparative studies between the various thrombolytic agents have been too few to make rational comparison and, although there may be slight differences between thrombolytic agents, the choice of drug is less important than the choice to give a thrombolytic at all. One should be given in the doses recommended in Table 30.4, and this can be administered through either a peripheral or a central venous catheter. In contrast to the use of thrombolytics in acute myocardial infarction, thrombolytics are useful in PE when given up to 14 days after symptoms begin. Once the thrombolytic agent has been ceased, heparin should be commenced.

Haemorrhagic complications are not uncommon and can significantly affect patient morbidity; however it is difficult to predict those patients who are at the highest risk for bleeding. Major clinically significant bleeding can occur in up to 10% of patients, although cerebral haemorrhage is fortunately uncommon (0.5%).[29] Whilst recent surgery is often considered a contraindication, acceptable safety has been demonstrated in these patients. Clearly individual patients should have the risks and the benefits weighed up: in shocked patients with PE the balance appears to be in favour of thrombolytic agents for most patients.

If bleeding occurs, the thrombolytic agent should be ceased, fresh frozen plasma should be given to replace coagulation factors and an antifibrinolytic agent (such as aprotinin) should be commenced.

SURGICAL EMBOLECTOMY

The merit of surgical embolectomy, which has traditionally been seen as a life-saving option for moribund patients with massive PE, has been questioned in the era of increasingly effective thrombolytics. Results of embolectomy surgery vary widely and there has traditionally been an associated perioperative mortality of 25–50%. There is little evidence to compare embolectomy and thrombolytics reliably.

A recent study in an academic centre has documented a perioperative mortality of 6% and a total mortality of 18% when a surgical approach that included rapid diagnosis, prompt surgical intervention and a high frequency of concurrent IVC filter placement was used.[40] Embolectomy was performed in more than half of these patients because either there were contraindications to thrombolytics or the thrombolytic treatment had failed.

Therefore, whilst patients with massive PE who have no contraindications to thrombolysis should receive a thrombolytic agent, surgical embolectomy should be strongly considered in centres with access to cardiothoracic surgeons when a contraindication to thrombolysis exists or the therapy fails.

Indications for embolectomy in patients with PE include:

- massive PE with shock
- patients where thrombolytic agents are contraindicated
- patients who appear to fail thrombolytic agent
- patients with free-floating cardiac thrombus

PERCUTANEOUS EMBOLECTOMY

Percutaneous methods include either embolus extraction techniques (pure percutaneous embolectomy) or embolus disruption techniques (including catheter-directed thrombolysis and percutaneous thrombus fragmentation techniques).[41] Successful embolectomy does not always occur and mortality is still about 20–30%. Rheolytic thrombectomy[42] and methods combining mechanical disruption and thrombolytic therapy[43] have emerged as promising interventions. Whilst awaiting well-designed studies of these interventions, they remain limited to specialised centres.

CONCURRENT HAEMODYNAMIC SUPPORT

Shocked patients with PE need urgent haemodynamic support in addition to the definitive measures mentioned above.

INTRAVENOUS FLUIDS

In patients with moderate or massive PE, volume loading can improve haemodynamic status,[44] although if excessive, fluid therapy worsens RV function which can in turn affect LV function and become detrimental.[45] For this reason cautious amounts of intravenous fluid should be given.

INTRAVENOUS VASOACTIVE AGENTS

Coronary ischaemia is an important component of the pathogenesis of haemodynamic instability in massive PE. A focus on reducing this ischaemia requires elevation of the blood pressure whilst attempts are being made to lower the pulmonary and RV pressures by removal of the embolus (with thrombolytic agent or embolectomy).

An important concept to consider is the RV coronary perfusion pressure (RVCPP), which is estimated by the formula:

$$\text{RVCPP} = \text{MAP} - \text{RVP}_m$$

where

$$\text{RVP}_m = \text{CVP} + 1/3(\text{PAP}_s - \text{CVP})$$

where MAP is the mean arterial pressure, RVP_m is the mean RV pressure, CVP is the central venous pressure and PAP_s is the systolic pulmonary arterial pressure, all in mmHg.

When the RVCPP falls as low as 30 mmHg, RV myocardial blood flow falls substantially, leading to severe RV failure and shock. Efforts to elevate the MAP and reduce the PAP_s will clearly increase the RVCPP and improve coronary blood flow and ischaemia. Vasopressor agents are therefore the most important initial therapy in the shock state due to massive PE as they will predominantly increase MAP, and therefore RVCPP.

Noradrenaline (norepinephrine) is the most appropriate vasopressor, because of its α-adrenoceptor agonist activity. Noradrenaline is preferred to a pure α-agonist, such as phenylephrine, as cardiac output and RV myocardial blood flow effects are greater due to the added β-adrenoceptor agonist action. Dopamine, adrenaline (epinephrine) and vasopressin are appropriate alternatives to noradrenaline.

Although some have suggested using a systemic vasodilator to improve the cardiac output in massive PE, vasodilators can be harmful, as even though cardiac output might improve, the MAP either remains constant or falls and therefore RVCPP is not necessarily improved. Therefore isoprenaline, dobutamine, nitroglycerine, nitroprusside or milrinone should only be considered if MAP is adequate and treatment is focused on cardiac output or pulmonary artery pressure.

Beneficial effects have been shown with intra-aortic balloon counterpulsation in animal studies. In patients apparently dying of PE despite thrombolytics and ongoing resuscitative efforts, this appears a reasonable approach as a method of augmenting RVCPP, as long as it is in association with the use of pressor agents. Extracorporeal membrane oxygenation (ECMO) is an extreme but alternative form of mechanical assistance which may be available in more specialised institutions.[46] Technological advances appear to have reduced the number of procedure-related complications attributed to ECMO.[47]

SELECTIVE PULMONARY VASODILATORS

Inhaled nitric oxide has been used in patients with massive PE based on animal studies and case series,[48] because it selectively decreases pulmonary arterial pressure without influencing systemic haemodynamics. It may have dramatic haemodynamic effects but should be adjunctive to other resuscitative efforts, including elevation of the systemic blood pressure. Inhaled prostacyclin is an alternative, but has limited supporting evidence.[49]

OTHER MANAGEMENT ISSUES

Oxygen should be given to keep an adequate oxygen saturation. High flows may be required because of hyperventilation and the increased dead space. Intubation and mechanical ventilation are often necessary in patients with massive PE.

If chest pain is prominent, morphine should be given. To guide resuscitation, it is useful to have at least a central venous catheter, particularly before a thrombolytic agent is given. Although not essential, if a patient is severely shocked, a pulmonary artery catheter is recommended to assist in the titration of vasoactive agents and measure the pulmonary artery pressure. The pulmonary artery catheter also assists in the estimation of the RVCPP, either through direct measurement of the mean RV pressure using the 20-cm lumen of a pacing pulmonary artery catheter, or by calculation using the formula above. While there is increased risk of bleeding due to the concurrent administration of thrombolytic agents and/or anticoagulants in these patients, this is probably outweighed by the importance of secure venous access and monitoring of the circulation in patients with haemodynamic compromise due to PE.

PREVENTION

Prophylaxis is the most important management aspect of VTE. All ICU patients should have an adequate assessment as to whether prophylaxis is warranted, although

Table 30.5 Prophylaxis of venous thromboembolism

Category of patient	Recommendation
All patients with high bleeding risk	IPC or GCS
General (and other) surgery	
Low-risk	Early mobilisation
Moderate-risk	Heparin bd or LMWH
High-risk	Heparin tds or LMWH
Vascular surgery	
No risk factors	Early mobilisation
Risk factors	Heparin bd or LMWH
Orthopaedic surgery	
Hip replacement	LMWH or fondaparinux or warfarin
Knee arthroplasty	LMWH or fondaparinux or warfarin or IPC
Hip fracture surgery	LMWH or fondaparinux or warfarin or heparin bd
Neurosurgery	
Intracranial surgery	IPC $\pm$ GCS or heparin bd or LMWH
High-risk	GCS/IPC + heparin/LMWH
Trauma patients	
No anticoagulation contraindication	LMWH
Anticoagulation contraindication	IPC $\pm$ GCS
Spinal cord injury	LMWH or IPC + heparin or IPC + LMWH
Burns	Heparin or LMWH
Medical patients	
Risk factors	Heparin or LMWH
Anticoagulation contraindication	GCS or IPC
Risk definitions	
Low-risk surgery	
Minor surgery in patients < 40 years old with no risk factors	
Moderate-risk surgery	
Non-major surgery in patients who are 40–60 years old with no risk factors	
Non-major surgery in patients < 60 years old with risk factors	
Major surgery in patients < 40 years old with no risk factors	
High-risk surgery	
Non-major surgery in patients > 60 years old with or without risk factors	
Major surgery in patients > 40 years old with no risk factors	
Major surgery in patients < 40 years old with risk factors	

IPC, intermittent pneumatic compression device; GCS, graduated compression stockings; heparin bd, 5000 units subcutaneously twice daily; LMWH, low-molecular-weight heparin; heparin tds, 5000 units subcutaneously three times daily.
(Information from Geerts *et al.*[50])

most should receive it.[50] Careful attention to the intervention and dose is required, as omission of prophylaxis[51] and failure of prophylaxis[52] are common. Some groups of surgical patients also appear to benefit from extended out-of-hospital prophylaxis.[53]

Traditional prophylaxis with fixed low-dose subcutaneous unfractionated heparin (i.e. 5000 units twice or three times daily) is now being challenged by both LMWHs and fondaparinux (a factor Xa inhibitor).[50] Both have been shown to be as efficacious as unfractionated heparin in many patient groups and they are associated with less bleeding and less HITTS. Although questions remain about the cost-effectiveness of LMWHs[54] and about comparisons between the various LMWH agents and fondaparinux, LMWHs require less monitoring than unfractionated heparin and are being more commonly recommended.[50]

Aspirin has also been shown to reduce VTE rate and mortality in high-risk patients,[55] although it seems less efficacious than other anticoagulants and is not currently recommended.[50]

Mechanical approaches (including graduated-compression stockings and intermittent pneumatic compression devices[56]) seem best utilised in low-risk patients, patients with contraindications to anticoagulation, or when used in addition to anticoagulation in high-risk patients.

A recommended approach to prophylaxis is included in Table 30.5.[50]

REFERENCES

1. Bounameaux H. Factor V Leiden paradox: risk of deep-vein thrombosis but not of pulmonary embolism. *Lancet* 2000; **356**: 182–3.
2. Kearon C. Natural history of venous thromboembolism. *Circulation* 2003; **107**: I22–30.
3. Kreit JW. The impact of right ventricular dysfunction on the prognosis and therapy of normotensive patients with pulmonary embolism. *Chest* 2004; **125**: 1539–45.
4. Chagnon I, Bounameaux H, Aujesky D *et al.* Comparison of two clinical prediction rules and implicit assessment among patients with suspected pulmonary embolism. *Am J Med* 2002; **113**: 269–75.
5. Winer-Muram HT, Rydberg J, Johnson MS *et al.* Suspected acute pulmonary embolism: evaluation with multi-detector row CT versus digital subtraction pulmonary arteriography. *Radiology* 2004; **233**: 806–15.
6. Fancher TL, White RH, Kravitz RL. Combined use of rapid D-dimer testing and estimation of clinical probability in the diagnosis of deep vein thrombosis: systematic review. *Br Med J* 2004; **329**: 821.
7. Stein PD, Hull RD, Patel KC *et al.* D-dimer for the exclusion of acute venous thrombosis and pulmonary embolism: a systematic review. *Ann Intern Med* 2004; **140**: 589–602.
8. Grau E, Tenias JM, Soto MJ *et al.* D-dimer levels correlate with mortality in patients with acute pulmonary embolism: findings from the RIETE registry. *Crit Care Med* 2007; **35**: 1937–41.
9. Gallotta G, Palmieri V, Piedimonte V *et al.* Increased troponin I predicts in-hospital occurrence of hemodynamic instability in patients with sub-massive or non-massive pulmonary embolism independent to clinical, echocardiographic and laboratory information. *Int J Cardiol* 2008; **124**: 351–7.
10. Becattini C, Vedovati MC, Agnelli G. Prognostic value of troponins in acute pulmonary embolism A meta-analysis. *Circulation* 2007; **116**: 427–33.
11. Kucher N, Goldhaber SZ. Risk stratification of acute pulmonary embolism. *Semin Thromb Hemost* 2006; **32**: 838–47.
12. Maziere F, Birolleau S, Medimagh S *et al.* Comparison of troponin I and N-terminal-pro B-type natriuretic peptide for risk stratification in patients with pulmonary embolism. *Eur J Emerg Med* 2007; **14**: 207–11.
13. Kline JA, Kubin AK, Patel MM *et al.* Alveolar dead space as a predictor of severity of pulmonary embolism. *Acad Emerg Med* 2000; **7**: 611–17.
14. Hedenstierna G, Sandhagen B. Assessing dead space. A meaningful variable? *Minerva Anestesiol* 2006; **72**: 521–8.
15. Piazza G, Goldhaber SZ. Acute pulmonary embolism: part I: epidemiology and diagnosis. *Circulation* 2006; **114**: e28–32.
16. Quiroz R, Schoepf UJ. CT pulmonary angiography for acute pulmonary embolism: cost-effectiveness analysis and review of the literature. *Semin Roentgenol* 2005; **40**: 20–4.
17. Stein PD, Fowler SE, Goodman LR *et al.* Multidetector computed tomography for acute pulmonary embolism. *N Engl J Med* 2006; **354**: 2317–27.
18. Stein PD, Woodard PK, Weg JG *et al.* Diagnostic pathways in acute pulmonary embolism: recommendations of the PIOPED II investigators. *Radiology* 2007; **242**: 15–21.
19. Quiroz R, Kucher N, Zou KH *et al.* Clinical validity of a negative computed tomography scan in patients with suspected pulmonary embolism: a systematic review. *JAMA* 2005; **293**: 2012–17.
20. van der Meer RW, Pattynama PM, van Strijen MJ *et al.* Right ventricular dysfunction and pulmonary obstruction index at helical CT: prediction of clinical outcome during 3-month follow-up in patients with acute pulmonary embolism. *Radiology* 2005; **235**: 798–803.
21. Ghanima W, Abdelnoor M, Holmen LO *et al.* The association between the proximal extension of the clot and the severity of pulmonary embolism (PE): a proposal for a new radiological score for PE. *J Intern Med* 2007; **261**: 74–81.
22. Goldhaber SZ. Echocardiography in the management of pulmonary embolism. *Ann Intern Med* 2002; **136**: 691–700.
23. McConnell MV, Solomon SD, Rayan ME *et al.* Regional right ventricular dysfunction detected by

echocardiography in acute pulmonary embolism. *Am J Cardiol* 1996; **78**: 469–73.
24. Kucher N, Rossi E, De Rosa M *et al.* Prognostic role of echocardiography among patients with acute pulmonary embolism and a systolic arterial pressure of 90 mmHg or higher. *Arch Intern Med* 2005; **165**: 1777–81.
25. Miniati M, Monti S, Pratali L *et al.* Value of transthoracic echocardiography in the diagnosis of pulmonary embolism: results of a prospective study in unselected patients. *Am J Med* 2001; **110**: 528–35.
26. Pruszczyk P, Torbicki A, Kuch-Wocial A *et al.* Diagnostic value of transoesophageal echocardiography in suspected haemodynamically significant pulmonary embolism. *Heart* 2001; **85**: 628–34.
27. The PIOPED investigators. Value of the ventilation/perfusion scan in acute pulmonary embolism Results of the prospective investigation of pulmonary embolism diagnosis (PIOPED). *JAMA* 1990; **263**: 2753–9.
28. Konstantinides S, Geibel A, Heusel G *et al.* Heparin plus alteplase compared with heparin alone in patients with submassive pulmonary embolism. *N Engl J Med* 2002; **347**: 1143–50.
29. Wan S, Quinlan DJ, Agnelli G *et al.* Thrombolysis compared with heparin for the initial treatment of pulmonary embolism: a meta-analysis of the randomized controlled trials. *Circulation* 2004; **110**: 744–9.
30. Schoepf UJ, Kucher N, Kipfmueller F *et al.* Right ventricular enlargement on chest computed tomography: a predictor of early death in acute pulmonary embolism. *Circulation* 2004; **110**: 3276–80.
31. Segal JB, Streiff MB, Hofmann LV *et al.* Management of venous thromboembolism: a systematic review for a practice guideline. *Ann Intern Med* 2007; **146**: 211–22.
32. Hull RD, Raskob GE, Brant RF *et al.* Low-molecular-weight heparin vs heparin in the treatment of patients with pulmonary embolism. American-Canadian Thrombosis Study Group. *Arch Intern Med* 2000; **160**: 229–36.
33. Raschke RA, Reilly BM, Guidry JR *et al.* The weight-based heparin dosing nomogram compared with a "standard care" nomogram. A randomized controlled trial. *Ann Intern Med* 1993; **119**: 874–81.
34. Piazza G, Goldhaber SZ. Acute pulmonary embolism: part II: treatment and prophylaxis. *Circulation* 2006; **114**: e42–47.
35. Sing RF, Jacobs DG, Heniford BT. Bedside insertion of inferior vena cava filters in the intensive care unit. *J Am Coll Surg* 2001; **192**: 570–5.
36. Decousus H, Leizorovicz A, Parent F *et al.* A clinical trial of vena caval filters in the prevention of pulmonary embolism in patients with proximal deep-vein thrombosis. Prevention du Risque d'Embolie Pulmonaire par Interruption Cave Study Group. *N Engl J Med* 1998; **338**: 409–15.
37. Imberti D, Ageno W, Carpenedo M. Retrievable vena cava filters: a review. *Curr Opin Hematol* 2006; **13**: 351–6.
38. Kucher N, Rossi E, De Rosa M *et al.* Massive pulmonary embolism. *Circulation* 2006; **113**: 577–82.
39. Konstantinides S, Geibel A, Olschewski M *et al.* Association between thrombolytic treatment and the prognosis of hemodynamically stable patients with major pulmonary embolism: results of a multicenter registry. *Circulation* 1997; **96**: 882–8.
40. Leacche M, Unic D, Goldhaber SZ *et al.* Modern surgical treatment of massive pulmonary embolism: results in 47 consecutive patients after rapid diagnosis and aggressive surgical approach. *J Thorac Cardiovasc Surg* 2005; **129**: 1018–23.
41. Uflacker R. Interventional therapy for pulmonary embolism. *J Vasc Interv Radiol* 2001; **12**: 147–64.
42. Chauhan MS, Kawamura A. Percutaneous rheolytic thrombectomy for large pulmonary embolism: a promising treatment option. *Catheter Cardiovasc Interv* 2007; **70**: 123–30.
43. Tajima H, Murata S, Kumazaki T *et al.* Hybrid treatment of acute massive pulmonary thromboembolism: mechanical fragmentation with a modified rotating pigtail catheter, local fibrinolytic therapy, and clot aspiration followed by systemic fibrinolytic therapy. *Am J Roentgenol* 2004; **183**: 589–95.
44. Mercat A, Diehl JL, Meyer G *et al.* Hemodynamic effects of fluid loading in acute massive pulmonary embolism. *Crit Care Med* 1999; **27**: 540–4.
45. Wood KE. Major pulmonary embolism: review of a pathophysiologic approach to the golden hour of hemodynamically significant pulmonary embolism. *Chest* 2002; **121**: 877–905.
46. Maggio P, Hemmila M, Haft J *et al.* Extracorporeal life support for massive pulmonary embolism. *J Trauma* 2007; **62**: 570–6.
47. Mielck F, Quintel M. Extracorporeal membrane oxygenation. *Curr Opin Crit Care* 2005; **11**: 87–93.
48. Capellier G, Jacques T, Balvay P *et al.* Inhaled nitric oxide in patients with pulmonary embolism. *Intens Care Med* 1997; **23**: 1089–92.
49. Webb SA, Stott S, van Heerden PV. The use of inhaled aerosolized prostacyclin (IAP) in the treatment of pulmonary hypertension secondary to pulmonary embolism. *Intens Care Med* 1996; **22**: 353–5.
50. Geerts WH, Pineo GF, Heit JA *et al.* Prevention of venous thromboembolism: the Seventh ACCP Conference on Antithrombotic and Thrombolytic Therapy. *Chest* 2004; **126**: 338S–400S.
51. Kahn SR, Panju A, Geerts W *et al.* Multicenter evaluation of the use of venous thromboembolism prophylaxis in acutely ill medical patients in Canada. *Thromb Res* 2007; **119**: 145–55.
52. Goldhaber SZ, Dunn K, MacDougall RC. New onset of venous thromboembolism among hospitalized patients at Brigham and Women's Hospital is caused more often by prophylaxis failure than by withholding treatment. *Chest* 2000; **118**: 1680–4.
53. Eikelboom JW, Quinlan DJ, Douketis JD. Extended-duration prophylaxis against venous thromboembolism after total hip or knee replacement: a

meta-analysis of the randomised trials. *Lancet* 2001; **358**: 9–15.
54. Velmahos GC, Oh Y, McCombs J *et al.* An evidence-based cost-effectiveness model on methods of prevention of posttraumatic venous thromboembolism. *J Trauma* 2000; **49**: 1059–64.
55. Pulmonary Embolism Prevention (PEP) Trial Collaborative Group. Prevention of pulmonary embolism and deep vein thrombosis with low dose aspirin: Pulmonary Embolism Prevention (PEP) trial. *Lancet* 2000; **355**: 1295–302.
56. Urbankova J, Quiroz R, Kucher N *et al.* Intermittent pneumatic compression and deep vein thrombosis prevention. A meta-analysis in postoperative patients. *Thromb Haemost* 2005; **94**: 1181–5.

31

Acute severe asthma

David V Tuxen and Matthew T Naughton

Acute severe asthma is a medical emergency associated with significant morbidity and mortality. The majority of adverse outcomes are attributed to underestimation of severity with delayed and/or inadequate treatment[1–3] and are potentially preventable.

The worldwide prevalence of asthma varies widely (2–37% in children),[4] but it is now clear that the overall prevalence has increased worldwide,[5,6] with life-threatening episodes affecting an estimated 0.5% of asthmatics per year.[7] Australia, New Zealand and the UK have amongst the highest incidences.[7] In Australia, 9% have asthma as a long-term condition[8] and up to 40% of children have asthma symptoms at some time.[5]

Although the prevalence of asthma is increasing, many countries have achieved reductions in hospital presentations and admissions,[9,10] reduced intensive care admissions and reduced overall asthma mortality.[9,10] Improved community management of asthma,[1,2] more widespread use of inhaled corticosteroids[3] and other preventive measures have been given the credit for these improvements.

Despite reducing admissions, significant and potentially preventable mortality continues to occur in those patients who do require intensive care or mechanical ventilation.[11,12]

CLINICAL DEFINITION

Asthma has been defined as a lung disease with the following characteristics:[13]

- airway obstruction that is reversible (completely or partially), either spontaneously or with treatment
- airway inflammation
- increased airway responsiveness to a variety of stimuli

Exacerbations of asthma are characterised by increasing dyspnoea, cough, wheeze, chest tightness and decreased expiratory airflow. Status asthmaticus has had varying definitions. However, for practical purposes, any patient not responding to initial doses of nebulised bronchodilators should be considered to have status asthmaticus.[14]

AETIOLOGY

The pathogenesis of asthma is complex, with both genetic and environmental influences. The increase in asthma prevalence has been attributed to the 'hygiene hypothesis'[15] which suggests that reduced exposure to childhood infections as a result of antibiotics and hygienic lifestyle promotes an imbalance in T-cell phenotype leading to inflammatory cytokine overproduction. Immunoglobulin (Ig) E-dependent mechanisms appear to be particularly important in generating the characteristic state of airway inflammation and bronchial hyperreactivity with the allergens in the local environment dictating the specificity of the antibody response.[16] Triggers of acute asthma can be non-specific (cold air, exercise, atmospheric pollutants), specific allergens (housemite, pollen, animal danders), modifiers of airway control (aspirin, β-blockers) or stress and emotion. No precipitant can be identified in over 30% of patients.

PATHOPHYSIOLOGY

The postmortem airway pathology of patients who die from acute asthma includes bronchial wall thickening from oedema and inflammatory cell infiltrate, hypertrophy and hyperplasia of bronchial smooth muscle and submucosal glands, deposition of collagen beneath the epithelial basement membrane and prominent intraluminal secretions. These secretions may narrow or occlude the small airways and postmortem studies frequently report extensive plugging and atelectasis.[17,18] When interpreting the latter findings it is important to remember that during life in very severe asthma, the lungs are hyperinflated close to total lung capacity (TLC) by maximal inspiratory effort and to beyond TLC during mechanical ventilation. At this time radiological atelectasis is rare, suggesting that most airways are communicating at these high lung volumes, even if airways are very narrowed. Only at death does the prolonged apnoea allow lung deflation, widespread airway closure and alveolar gas absorption to give the postmortem appearance of extensive complete occlusion that was not present to the same degree during life.

In some deaths bronchial mucus is absent; in these cases airway obstruction may be mainly due to intense smooth bronchoconstriction.

This observation may account for two patterns of progression of asthma:

1. Acute severe asthma is the more common group (80–90%), with progression of symptoms over many hours or days, often with a background of poor control and recurrent presentations. The majority of patients in this group are female. Upper respiratory infections are frequent triggers. It responds more slowly to treatment; this may reflect greater contribution from mucous inspissation and chronic bronchial wall inflammation with eosinophilia.[19]
2. Hyperacute, fulminating or asphyxic asthma is where the interval between onset of symptoms and intubation is less than 3 hours.[19–21] This presentation is less common (approximately 10–20% of life-threatening presentations) and tends to occur in younger patients with relatively normal lung function but high bronchial reactivity, and the majority of patients are male. Respiratory allergens, cold air or exercise and psychosocial stress are the most frequent triggers. This pattern typically responds quickly to bronchodilators and is thought to be mainly due to bronchial smooth-muscle contraction.

The characteristic pathology of asthma leads to increased airway resistance and dynamic pulmonary hyperinflation. This has a number of consequences:

- *Increased work of breathing* results from increased airway resistance and reduced pulmonary compliance as a result of high lung volumes. When asthma is severe, dynamic hyperinflation may bring the lung volume close to TLC.[22] This causes a severe mechanical disadvantage of inspiratory muscles with diaphragm flattening and results in a large inspiratory muscle effort affecting a small change in inspiratory pressure. The final outcome can be respiratory muscle failure with insufficient alveolar ventilation and consequent hypercapnia.[23]
- *Ventilation–perfusion mismatch* is the result of airway narrowing and closure. This leads to impaired gas exchange and increases the minute ventilation requirement, further adding to the work of breathing.[23]
- *Adverse cardiopulmonary interactions* are seen when the marked changes in lung volume and pleural pressure impact on the function of both left and right ventricles.[24,25] Spontaneous breathing during acute asthma can generate inspiratory pleural pressures as low as -35 cmH_2O.[24,25] This increases venous return to the right ventricle (RV) and increases RV volume during inspiration. However, increased RV afterload as a result of hypoxic pulmonary vasoconstriction, acidosis, increased lung volume[24,25] and increased pulmonary capacitance decrease return to the left ventricle (LV). These negative intrapleural pressures also cause increased LV afterload[24,25] and increased RV volume with septal shift reduces LV volume,[24,25] further reducing LV output during inspiration. Pulsus paradoxus is the most direct result of these cardiopulmonary interactions in severe asthma. This is a decrease in systolic blood pressure during inspiration of > 10 mmHg (typically 15–25 mmHg, normal = 5 mmHg). The degree of pulsus paradoxus may not correlate with the severity of asthma as it may be reduced by inspiratory muscle weakness or fatigue.

CLINICAL FEATURES AND ASSESSMENT OF SEVERITY

The symptoms of asthma are well known and include wheeze, cough, dyspnoea and chest discomfort or tightness.

Triage and assessment of severity of the acute asthma attack are crucial. Underestimation or non-measurement of asthma severity is associated with increased mortality.[26,27] Assessment has two key features: assessment of initial severity and ongoing assessment of response to treatment.

HISTORY

Any history of prior intubation and mechanical ventilation for asthma is a predictor for life-threatening asthma.[26,27] A history of poor asthma control and multiple recent medical presentations for asthma are recognised risk factors. Other risk factors include a poor response to prior treatments and poor psychosocial circumstances.

PHYSICAL EXAMINATION

The general appearance and level of distress can be an important indicator of severity (Table 31.1). Use of accessory muscles, suprasternal retraction, markedly diminished breath sounds or a silent chest, central cyanosis, inability to speak (sentences, phrases, single words), a disturbance in the level of consciousness, upright posture and diaphoresis all suggest a severe attack.[28] A respiratory rate > 30 breaths/min, pulse rate > 120 beats/min and pulsus paradoxus of > 15 mmHg are associated with severe asthma, though their absence does not preclude life-threatening asthma.

VENTILATORY FUNCTION TESTS

The patient may not be able to perform these due to breathlessness. However, forced expiratory volume in 1 second (FEV_1) and peak expiratory flow rate (PEFR) are useful indicators of severity and response to treatment when done serially. An $FEV_1 < 1.0$ litre or PEFR < 100 l/min indicates very severe asthma at significant risk of requiring mechanical ventilation. In some patients forced expiration may worsen symptoms; these measurements should cease if this occurs.[29]

Table 31.1 Assessment of asthma severity

	Mild	Moderate	Severe
Conscious state	Alert and relaxed	Anxious, difficulty sleeping	Agitated, delirious
Speech	Sentences	Phrases	Words
Accessory muscles	Nil	Mild	Significant sitting upright
Wheeze	Moderate	Loud	Loud or silent
Pulse rate (beats/min)	< 100	100–120	> 120
Peak expiratory flow (% predicted)	$> 80\%$	60–80%	$< 60\%$
$Pa\text{CO}_2$ (mmHg)	< 45	< 45	> 45

Pulsus paradoxus, when present, indicates severe asthma; however it is an unreliable test.

PULSE OXIMETRY

Pulse oximetry ($Sp\text{O}_2$) is usually readily available and provides a rapid assessment of oxygenation. It is also very valuable in regulation oxygen therapy, both for avoiding hypoxia ($Sp\text{O}_2 > 90\%$)[30] and avoiding potential side-effects of hyperoxia ($Sp\text{O}_2 < 95\%$).[31] Of course, pulse oximetry cannot assess arterial $P\text{CO}_2$ or acid–base state or lactate and hence does not replace the need for blood gases

ARTERIAL BLOOD GASES

Arterial hypoxaemia is almost invariably present in a patient with severe asthma breathing room air, though it usually responds well to low-level oxygen supplementation (28–35%).[30] Blood gases should not delay initiation of treatment, and are not required in mild asthma or moderate asthma that is responding well to treatment. They are very important in severe asthma, or moderate asthma with inadequate treatment response. The arterial $Pa\text{CO}_2$ is an important measure of severity and, if hypercapnia is present, an important guide to treatment response.

Ventilation is initially increased in an acute attack, leading to hypocapnia and a respiratory alkalosis.[30] As the asthmatic attack worsens, the work of breathing, *V/Q* mismatch and adverse cardiopulmonary interactions all increase, and the minute ventilation required to maintain the same alveolar ventilation and $Pa\text{CO}_2$ increases. Eventually the patient is incapable of meeting this demand and the $Pa\text{CO}_2$ rises. The presence of hypercapnic acidosis is associated with an FEV_1 of $< 20\%$ predicted and reliably indicates that asthma is severe. A metabolic acidosis may also be present, and this is most commonly due to lactic acidosis[32] associated with intravenous or continuous nebulised β-agonists.[33,34]

CHEST X-RAY

Although not generally helpful in assessing severity,[35] a chest X-ray should be performed when asthma is severe or refractory to treatment, when barotrauma or lower respiratory tract infection is suspected or when the diagnosis is in doubt. It is not required in milder attacks that respond well to treatment.

ASSESSMENT OF TREATMENT RESPONSE

Repeated evaluation of the patient's response to treatment is a valuable tool in assessing severity of acute asthma. The response to the first 2 hours of treatment is an important predictor of outcome.[36] Adverse events are associated with underestimation of severity, inadequate observation after initial assessment and under treatment. Ongoing evaluation of response to therapy is critical. This evaluation should include repeated assessments of:

1. appearance and physical indicators of severity
2. objective measurements: FEV_1 or PEFR, heart rate, respiratory rate, pulsus paradoxus
3. $Sp\text{O}_2$ and oxygen requirements
4. progress of $Pa\text{CO}_2$ or metabolic acidosis if present on blood gases

Admission to intensive care is preferred if the patient fulfils the above criteria for severe asthma. Indications for immediate admission to intensive care include respiratory arrest, altered mental status, arrhythmias or associated myocardial ischaemia.

DIFFERENTIAL DIAGNOSIS

The diagnosis of asthma is usually obvious. However wheeze and dyspnoea may be caused by other illnesses such as left ventricular failure, aspiration, upper-airway obstruction, inhaled foreign body, pulmonary embolism or hyperventilation syndromes. Wheeze and dyspnoea arising in hospitalised patients who were not admitted with asthma are less likely to be due to asthma. Difficult asthma, as opposed to severe asthma, can present acutely and is a diagnostic dilemma. Such patients are well medicated (often self-medicating with high-dose steroids and may appear cushingoid or with high-dose β-agonists with lactic acidosis) and have seen many doctors and attended many hospitals. Lung function may be normal or indicate upper-airway dysfunction, indicative of an underlying vocal cord dysfunction or psychiatric condition, and upon intubation the patient is very easy to ventilate. Clues to another or additional diagnosis include:

1. no past history of asthma
2. sudden onset following vomiting or food intake
3. focal or asymmetrical chest auscultation findings
4. risk factors for thromboembolism
5. onset during hospitalisation when admitted with another condition

MANAGEMENT

ESTABLISHED TREATMENTS

Initial therapy of acute severe asthma should include the following.

OXYGEN

Hypoxaemia contributes to life-threatening events that complicate acute severe asthma.[37] Humidified supplemental oxygen should be titrated to achieve a $Spo_2 > 90\%$. The risk of oxygen-induced increasing hypercapnia with coexisting chronic obstructive pulmonary disease or pre-existing chronic hypercapnia is a well-known reason to maintain a lower Spo_2 (e.g. 90–92%). This phenomenon was not believed to be relevant to the majority of patients with acute asthma; however, there is now emerging evidence that hyperoxia may be harmful to a more widespread group[38] by releasing pulmonary hypoxic vasoconstriction, worsening *V/Q* matching and increasing hypercapnia. A recent randomised controlled trial[31] showed a decrease in $Paco_2$ in a group receiving 28% O_2 and an increase in $Paco_2$ in a group receiving 100% O_2.

β-AGONISTS

Short-acting β-agonists remain the first-line bronchodilator therapy of choice.[6,39–41] Agents include salbutamol (albuterol), terbutaline, isoprenaline and epinephrine. Salbutamol is generally the agent of first choice as it has relative β_2-selectivity, with decreased β_1-mediated cardiac toxicity. Long-acting β-agonists such as salmeterol have no role in status asthmaticus due to slow onset of action and association with fatalities in this setting.[14] Eformoterol is a combined long- and short-acting β-agonist which could theoretically be used for acute asthma; however it is in dry powder form and unlikely to be helpful in intubated and mechanically ventilated patients. β-agonists cause bronchodilatation by stimulation of β_2-receptors on airway smooth muscle and may reduce bronchial mucosal oedema.[42]

β-agonists are best given by metered-dose inhaler (MDI) and a spacer device. There are data to suggest that, in non-intubated patients, MDIs combined with a spacer device are more effective than nebulisers and are cheaper to use.[43,44] In intubated patients both nebulisers and MDIs have been used effectively.[45] The dose per MDI inhalation is 100 μg and this can be given, in severe asthma, in repeated doses at 1–5-minute intervals.

Alternatively, β-agonists can be given by nebuliser in high and repeated doses.[46] The typical adult dose of salbutamol is 5–10 mg (in 2.5–5.0 ml diluent volume) every 2–4 hours but more frequent doses with a higher total dose are often required in severe asthma. It should be noted that less than 10% of the nebulised drug reaches the lung even under ideal conditions.[47] Continuous nebulisation appears to be superior to intermittent doses and is commonly used at the beginning of treatment in severe asthma.[14,48] The nebuliser should be driven by oxygen with the flow at 10–12 l/min and a reservoir volume of 2–4 ml so as to produce particles in the desired 1–3 μm range.[49] The total dose should be modulated by response to treatment and the level of toxic side-effects.

Two-thirds of patients presenting acutely will respond well to inhaled β-agonists,[50] irrespective of the method of administration. The remaining one-third are refractory even to high doses and usually require longer periods of intense treatment, including multiple other agents.

Intravenous β-agonists remain controversial. There is no clear evidence of benefit[51] and significant side-effects. Despite this, intravenous β-agonists have a theoretical benefit of additional access to lung units with severe airflow obstruction and poor nebulised drug delivery, and some studies have demonstrated improved response when intravenous β-agonist is used.[52] Intravenous β-agonists continue to be considered if the patient is not responding to continuous nebulisation.[53] The typical dose is 5–20 μg/min but doses > 10 μg/min should be used with caution because of side-effects, which should be monitored closely. Salbutamol 100–300 μg may also be given intravenously to non-intubated patients in extremis or delivered down an endotracheal tube if there is not time to gain intravenous access.

Side-effects of β-agonists include tachycardia, arrhythmias, hypertension, hypotension, tremor, hypokalaemia, worsening of ventilation–perfusion mismatch and hyperglycaemia,[54] but the most common side-effect of parenteral β-agonist – also occasionally seen with continuous nebulised β-agonists – is lactic acidosis. This occurs in over 70% of patients, has an onset within 2–4 hours of commencing an infusion or following an intravenous statim dose, levels may reach 4–12 mmol/l and may significantly add to respiratory acidosis and respiratory distress.[34,55,56] Parenteral infusions should be initially limited to 10 μg/min and statim doses should not exceed 250 μg. Serum bicarbonate and lactate should be regularly monitored. If lactic acidosis becomes significant, the salbutamol infusion should be reduced or ceased. Lactic acidosis will generally resolve within 4–6 hours of infusion cessation and is seldom a problem with infusions in place for more than 24 hours.

Long-term high-dose β-agonist use has been associated with increased mortality,[57] but whether high-dose β-agonists are a marker of disease severity, an indicator of suboptimal inhaled steroids or a direct cause of death is unclear. These concerns do not apply in the treatment of the acute asthma attack.

ANTICHOLINERGICS

Anticholinergics cause bronchodilatation by decreasing parasympathetic-mediated cholinergic bronchomotor tone.[58] Ipratropium bromide is the most commonly used anticholinergic for asthma and is a quaternary derivative of atropine. A number of studies and meta-analyses now suggest clear additional benefit and few side-effects when ipratropium bromide is added to the β-agonist regimen[59,60] and ipratropium is now considered accepted first-line therapy for acute severe asthma in conjunction with β-agonist therapy. Preservative-induced bronchoconstriction has been reported in a few patients and can be prevented by using preservative-free solutions.[61] The bronchodilatation effect of ipratropium bromide appeared to be maximal with a dose of 250 μg when studied in children between 9 and 17 years of age. The optimal dose is not known in adults; a reasonable regimen would be to add 500 μg ipratropium bromide to the salbutamol nebuliser every 2–6 hours; however, initial dose intervals as low as 10–20 minutes have been recommended.[62]

CORTICOSTEROIDS

The role of corticosteroids in the acute asthma attack has been well established. Systemic steroids should be considered in all but mild exacerbations of asthma.[41] Their benefits include increased β-responsiveness of airway smooth muscle, decreased inflammatory cell response and decreased mucus secretion. Early treatment with corticosteroids has been shown to decrease the likelihood of hospitalisation and decrease the mortality rate from acute asthma. Systematic reviews[41,63] suggest that effects commence within 6–12 hours, that oral administration is as effective as intravenous and that there is little evidence of benefit for initial daily doses exceeding 800 mg/day hydrocortisone (160 mg/day methylprednisolone) given in four divided doses.

Inhaled steroids have established long-term benefit and are believed to be a major factor in asthma mortality reduction.[1–3] There is now emerging evidence that inhaled steroids may also have a role during an acute attack[64,65] and it appears reasonable to use them routinely from day 1 as they may also enable more rapid dose reduction of parenteral steroids, potentially reducing side-effects.

Parenteral corticosteroid dose reductions should commence after 1–3 days according to the severity of the attack, the degree of chronic inflammation and the response to treatment, and should be converted to a reducing dose of oral steroids within 4–7 days (e.g. oral prednisolone starting at 0.5 mg/kg body weight or 40–60 mg/day).

Side-effects of corticosteroids include hyperglycaemia, hypokalaemia, hypertension, acute psychosis and myopathy,[66,67] though they are usually well tolerated acutely. The immunosuppressive effects can increase the risk of infections, including *Legionella*, *Pneumocystis carinii* and varicella,[68,69] especially when the patient is on long-term corticosteroids. Allergic reactions including anaphylaxis have been reported with the use of most corticosteroid preparations.

AMINOPHYLLINE

There have been conflicting reports regarding the efficacy of aminophylline in acute asthma ranging from no benefit[70] to improved lung function and improved outcome.[71] However it is accepted that aminophylline is an inferior bronchodilator, with a narrow therapeutic range and frequent side-effects,[72] including headache, nausea, vomiting and restlessness; cardiac arrhythmias and convulsions can occur at serum levels above 200 μmol/l (40 mg/l).

As a result, aminophylline is not a first-line treatment.[40,41,53] Aminophylline may be given to patients with acute asthma who are not showing a favourable response to full treatment with first-line agents. Careful administration and monitoring are required with an initial loading dose of 3 mg/kg (maximum 6 mg/kg, omitted if the patient is already taking oral theophylline) and an infusion of 0.5 mg/kg per hour. This should be reduced in patients with cirrhosis, cardiac failure or chronic obstructive pulmonary disease and in patients taking cimetidine, erythromycin or antiviral vaccines. Drug levels should be taken after a loading dose (if given), and then 24 hours later, aiming for a level of 30–80 μmol/l (5–12 mg/l). Levels should be repeated daily thereafter until stability has been achieved. The duration should be based on the response to treatment.

NON-ESTABLISHED TREATMENTS

A number of other therapies have reported benefit in acute severe asthma but their role in addition to full standard therapy has not been clearly established and they are not advocated for routine use. However these modes of therapy can be considered in the patient who is in extremis or who remains severe despite conventional treatment.

EPINEPHRINE

Epinephrine has some theoretical advantages over pure β_2-agonists in that its additional α-agonist actions of vasoconstriction and mucosal shrinkage may improve airway calibre. However, in practice, nebulised or subcutaneous epinephrine has not been shown to confer any advantage over nebulised β_2-agonists and is not recommended because of its cardiac side-effects.[62] Epinephrine may be tried in the patient who is failing to respond to conventional treatment. The nebulised dose is 2–4 mg in 2–4 ml (1% solution, 0.05 ml/kg) 1–4-hourly. The subcutaneous dose is 0.2–0.5 mg (0.2–0.5 ml of 1:1000 epinephrine) repeated if necessary 2–3 times at 30-minute intervals. Epinephrine by infusion may avert mechanical ventilation in very severe cases but should be used with caution with electrocardiogram monitoring and preferably with central venous access. An initial intravenous dose of 0.2–1.0 mg (2–10 ml of 1:10 000 epinephrine) is given slowly over 3–5 minutes. This may be followed by a continuous infusion of 1–20 μg/min, which is weaned when the acute attack subsides.[73]

MAGNESIUM SULPHATE

Magnesium sulphate is postulated to block calcium channels, and possibly acetylcholine release at the neuromuscular junction, leading to smooth-muscle relaxation and bronchodilatation. It appeared to be well tolerated in early studies, and a number of randomised, double-blind, prospective trials were performed adding intravenous or nebulised magnesium sulphate to conventional therapy in adults with acute asthma. Some showed benefit whereas others showed no benefit.

Three meta-analyses[74–76] did not support routine use of magnesium and it is not recommended for acute asthma. If given, recommended doses are 5–10 mmol (1.25–2.5 g, 2.5–5.0 ml of 50% solution) given slowly over 20 minutes but doses up to 40–80 mmol (10–20 g) have been given.[77] Side-effects include hypotension, flushing, sedation, weakness, areflexia, respiratory depression and cardiac arrhythmias seen at higher serum levels (> 5 mmol/dl or 12 mg/dl). Serum concentrations should be measured if repeated or high doses are used.

HELIOX

Inhalation of a helium:oxygen mixture reduces gas density and turbulence with reduced airflow resistance. The most effective gas mixture is 70% helium (30% oxygen) and the minimum concentration likely to provide benefit is 60% helium. Work of breathing is decreased and pulmonary access of inhaled bronchodilators may be improved.[78,79] Small case-series and reports have suggested benefit from Heliox, randomised prospective trials have both positive and negative results[80,81] and a recent meta-analysis[82] shows a trend towards improved lung function, but insufficient evidence to recommend use of Heliox in severe asthma. However, it otherwise appears safe and may be tried in critical asthma to avert intubation or during difficult mechanical ventilation providing the patient can tolerate 30–40% O_2.

ANAESTHETIC AGENTS

Ketamine, a dissociative anaesthetic agent, has been used in severe asthma.[83] It may cause bronchodilatation by both sympathomimetic potentiation and a direct effect on airway smooth muscle.[84] Small case-series have suggested some benefit, although a small randomised controlled trial found no benefit with ketamine in the treatment of acute severe asthma.[85] Ketamine may be a useful induction agent for endotracheal intubation (dose 1–2 mg/kg) as it may ameliorate the bronchoconstrictor response to intubation. It has been used as a continuous infusion in the dose range of 0.5–2 mg/kg per hour[85,86] to treat refractory asthma. Side-effects include increased bronchial secretions, a hyperdynamic cardiovascular response and hallucinations; the hallucinations can be reduced with concomitant benzodiazepines.

The volatile inhalational agents, including halothane, isoflurane and enflurane, have been used in mechanically ventilated patients with severe asthma. Clinical data are limited to small case-series and side-effects include direct myocardial depression, arrhythmias and hypotension.[87] The volatile anaesthetic agents should be used with great care and usually only as a prelude to or during invasive ventilation. An anaesthetic machine or custom-fitted ventilator is required for safe administration.

LEUKOTRIENE ANTAGONISTS

Leukotriene antagonists have shown benefit in chronic asthma[88] and there is some evidence of benefit in acute asthma.[89,90] However there is insufficient evidence and these benefits were of insufficient magnitude to recommend these agents for acute severe asthma.

BRONCHOALVEOLAR LAVAGE

Bronchoalveolar lavage has been used in severe refractory asthma to clear mucous plugging during mechanical ventilation.[91] It can transiently worsen bronchospasm and hypoxaemia and should be used when airflow obstruction has stabilised. It may have a role in ventilated patients with resistant mucus impaction, but is rarely used.

THERAPIES NOT RECOMMENDED

Antibiotics are not indicated[92] unless there is evidence of infection. Antihistamines are not effective. Inhaled mucolytics have been shown to have no benefit and may worsen airflow obstruction. Sedation is unsafe in acute asthma. There is a clear association between their use and avoidable deaths.[93] Patients with severe asthma should not be sedated unless being intubated and ventilated or in carefully monitored circumstances.

VENTILATION IN ASTHMA

DYNAMIC HYPERINFLATION

In all degrees of airflow obstruction, slow expiratory airflow results in incomplete exhalation of gas during normal expiratory times. Gas is trapped in the lungs by the arrival of the next breath and the lungs are unable to return their normal passive relaxation volume (functional residual capacity, FRC). Incomplete exhalation of each successive breath causes progressive accumulation of trapped gas, called dynamic hyperinflation (DH; Figure 31.1).[94] This continues until an equilibrium point is reached, where the exhaled volume increases to match the inspired volume (see Figure 31.1).[94] This equilibrium occurs because increasing lung volume increases small-airway calibre and lung elastic recoil pressure, both of which improve expiratory airflow and allow the inspired tidal volume to be exhaled in the expiratory time available. There are three primary determinants of this equilibrium point. Gas trapped at the end of expiration exerts a positive pressure on the alveoli; this pressure is intrinsic positive end-expiratory pressure (PEEPi) or auto-PEEP.[94,95] During expiration, sequential closure of the most severely obstructed

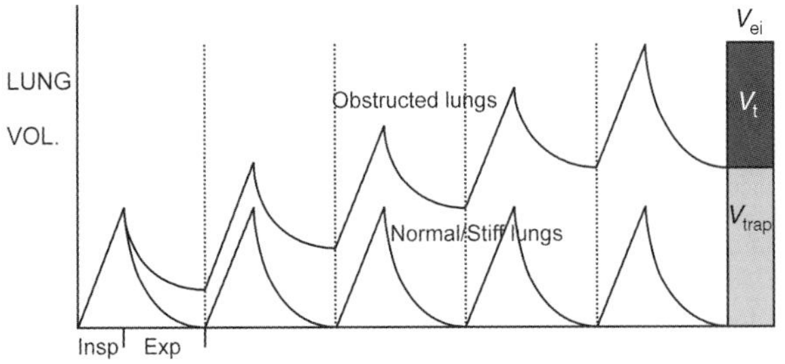

Figure 31.1 Dynamic hyperinflation. The volume history of normal or acutely injured lungs compared with that of obstructed lungs when commenced on controlled mechanical ventilation. This shows initial lung volume to be at the passive relaxation volume of the respiratory system or functional residual capacity (FRC). V_t, tidal volume; V_{trap}, dynamically trapped gas volume above FRC; V_{ei}, end-inspiratory lung volume above FRC.

airways occurs, with only the less obstructed airways remaining in communication with the central airway at the end of tidal expiration.[96] As a consequence, measured $PEEP_i$ underestimates the true magnitude of $PEEP_i$ and is recognised as being insensitive to changes in severity.[96]

In mild airflow obstruction, this process is adaptive as it allows the desired minute ventilation, which could not be achieved at FRC, to be achieved at a higher lung volume (Figure 31.2: 'mild AO'). In mild AO, a normal FRC can still be reached with prolonged passive expiratory period but the mildly narrowed airways undergo airway closure at lower lung volumes, reducing the expiratory reserve capacity (ER Cap) and increasing residual volume (RV; see Figure 31.2). This is in contrast to acute lung injury (ALI), where lung collapse reduces all lung volumes (see Figure 31.2: V_t, ER Cap and RV).

As asthma becomes more severe (see Figure 31.2: 'mod AO'), the static FRC that would be reached with a long expiratory time is elevated above the normal FRC by airway closure (static hyperinflation), there is no ER Cap, DHI further increases lung volume to a level where work of breathing is increased by lower lung compliance and respiratory muscles become less efficient from shortening and mechanical disadvantage. At this level some degree of dyspnoea is expected.

When asthma is severe enough to risk requiring mechanical ventilation, static hyperinflation may increase FRC by 50%[97] and very little DHI is required to reach total lung capacity (see Figure 31.2: 'severe AO'). In this circumstance, the minute ventilation required to maintain normocapnia would cause hyperinflation beyond normal total lung capacity. During spontaneous ventilation, the patient with severe asthma is unable to exceed total lung capacity (see Figure 31.2), has a much lower maximum minute ventilation capacity and as a result must become hypercapnic even at maximum respiratory effort with no fatigue.[14] When mechanical ventilation is commenced, increased tidal volume and rate delivery are easily able to increase minute ventilation and DHI well beyond normal total lung capacity (see Figure 31.2).[94] The consequences of this are commonly hypotension (due to increased intrathoracic pressure and decreased venous return) and barotrauma (Table 31.2).[22,94,97,98]

NON-INVASIVE VENTILATION (NIV)

NIV has been widely used for a variety of respiratory problems.[99] In severe asthma there are a number of potential benefits. Externally applied PEEP may help overcome PEEPi due to gas trapping and thus reduce the inspiratory threshold work of breathing. Augmentation of inspiration with NIV may further decrease the work of

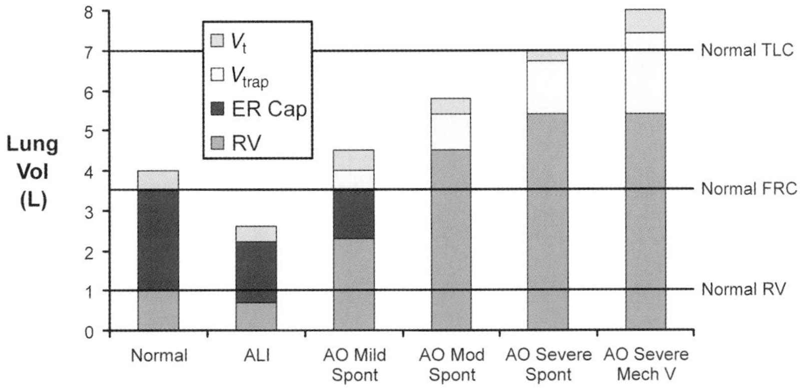

Figure 31.2 Comparison of lung volumes in patients with normal lungs, acute lung injury (ALI), and mild, moderate and severe airflow obstruction (AO). Severe AO is shown during both spontaneous ventilation (Spont) and mechanical ventilation (Mech V). TLC, total lung capacity. Functional residual capacity (FRC) is the static lung volume at the end of expiratory flow (60–90 seconds in severe AO). Expiratory reserve capacity (ER Cap) is the additional gas expired with expiratory effort after FRC has been reached. Residual volume (RV) is the minimum lung volume possible after prolonged expiration and maximum expiratory effort. V_t, tidal volume; V_{trap} is the gas trapped by dynamic hyperinflation during tidal ventilation.

Table 31.2 Comparison of reported mortality associated with the mechanical ventilation of patients with severe asthma over the last five decades

Decade	No. of papers	No. of episodes	No. dead	Mortality		
				Mean	Minimum	Maximum
1960s	8	125	18	14.4%	0%	27%
1970s	7	183	31	16.9%	6%	38%
1980s	10	382	46	12.0%	0%	36%
1990s	12	571	61	10.7%	0%	26%
2000s	3	790	54	6.8%	4%	21%

inspiration and increase tidal volume and minute ventilation. If tidal volume is increased with a shorter inspiratory time, then increased minute ventilation can occur without a proportional increase in dynamic hyperinflation. Both inspiratory augmentation and PEEP may facilitate airspace opening, thus reducing V/Q mismatch.[100,101]

The role of NIV is well established in chronic obstructive pulmonary disease where a number of randomised trials have shown benefit.[102,103] Although there have been no large randomised trials in acute asthma, there is increasing evidence of benefit from NIV for this indication, with all studies reporting positive outcome.[104,105] Non-randomised studies have reported improvements in respiratory acidosis and respiratory rate following the introduction of NIV, and low requirements for invasive ventilation. In a small prospectively randomised study of acute asthma, Soroksky *et al.*[105] showed better lung function and decreased hospitalisation rate with NIV.

A trial of NIV in patients with acute severe asthma and risk of respiratory decompensation is now warranted in patients who are cooperative and can tolerate the face mask. Indications for use are:

1. moderate to severe dyspnoea or respiratory distress
2. hypercapnic acidosis
3. respiratory rate > 25 breaths/min, accessory muscle use or paradoxical breathing[101]

Contraindications to NIV include cardiac or respiratory arrest, a decreased conscious state, severe upper gastrointestinal bleeding, haemodynamic instability, facial trauma or surgery, inability to protect the airway and clear secretions and high risk of aspiration.[100]

Full face masks are used in the acute setting, and with stabilisation nasal masks. All masks must be carefully fitted to achieve comfort and a reliable seal and no leak, without causing redness or breaks to the skin particularly over the nose.

NIV should be commenced with 5 cmH_2O continuous positive airway pressure (CPAP: expiratory positive airway pressure (EPAP) 5 cmH_2O) and 8–10 cmH_2O pressure support (inspiratory positive airway pressure (IPAP) 13–15 cmH_2O). The aim is a respiratory rate < 25 breaths/min and an exhaled tidal volume of 7 ml/kg. CPAP may be increased to 7 or 10 cmH_2O if there is difficulty initiating inspiration or pressure support may be increased if tidal volume is low or respiratory rate remains high. It is not possible to achieve total pressures reliably (IPAP) > 20 cmH_2O. NIV should be undertaken in an area familiar with its use and where close observation is available.

Complications of NIV include nasal bridge ulceration, mask discomfort, nasal congestion, gastric insufflation, aspiration, hypotension and pneumothorax;[101] however hypotension and pneumothorax are uncommon compared with their risk during mechanical ventilation.

INVASIVE VENTILATION

Invasive mechanical ventilation in acute severe asthma may be life-saving, but can be associated with significant morbidity and mortality.[97] Institution of invasive ventilation with endotracheal intubation carries the risk of inadvertent pulmonary hyperinflation[94,95,97] and potential aggravation of bronchospasm, and a significant part of the morbidity and mortality has been attributed to pulmonary hyperinflation.[94,95,97] Despite these risks, the incidence of mechanical ventilation for asthma is decreasing and mortality of patients ventilated for asthma is also decreasing in some series.[9,10]

The decision to intubate depends both on the clinical status of the patient and the natural history of the type of asthma present. Hyperacute asthma may present with marked hypercapnia ($Pa\text{CO}_2$ > 60 mmHg) due to mechanical limitations to ventilation as a result of dynamic hyperinflation. Such patients may not initially be fatigued and may respond rapidly to treatment, thereby avoiding mechanical ventilation. Acute severe asthma that has been progressing for days may have less hypercapnia but will often respond poorly to treatment. The $Pa\text{CO}_2$ may rise despite maximal treatment due to fatigue and the patient may require intubation at a lower $Pa\text{CO}_2$. The general principles are to use NIV early but to avoid mechanical ventilation if safe to do so.

The decision to intubate is based primarily on the degree of respiratory distress as assessed by an experienced clinician and patients themselves. A patient with a high $Pa\text{CO}_2$ (e.g. > 70 mmHg) who is dyspnoeic but not distressed and who may respond to full treatment over a few hours needs close observation but not immediate intubation. Patients are often able to tolerate hypercapnia without requiring invasive ventilation.[106] A patient with a lower $Pa\text{CO}_2$ (e.g. 50–60 mmHg) who has been unwell for days and who has a deteriorating status despite treatment is likely to need intubation. A patient who complains of respiratory exhaustion is likely to need intubation. Absolute indications for intubation include cardiac or respiratory arrest, severe hypoxia or rapid deterioration of conscious state.[14,54]

Once the decision to intubate has been made, a safe option is to perform rapid-sequence intubation using the orotracheal approach. The largest possible endotracheal tube should be used to reduce the work of breathing and to reduce the risk of occlusion by the tenacious secretions that often occur with asthma. Once the endotracheal tube is in place, slow hand ventilation (8–10 breaths/min) should maintain oxygenation until the ventilator can be connected.

INITIAL VENTILATOR SETTINGS

The principles of initial mechanical ventilation are to avoid excessive DHI[107] and hypoventilation (Figure 31.3) by commencing with a minute ventilation < 115 ml/kg per min (< 8 l/min in a 70-kg patient) best achieved with a tidal volume of 5–7 ml/kg, a respiratory rate of 10–12 breaths/min and a short inspiratory time to ensure an expiratory time of ≥ 4 seconds.[22,94,97,98,107] This degree of hypoventilation will usually result in hypercapnic acidosis and continued respiratory distress necessitating heavy sedation, and sometimes requiring 1–2 bolus doses of a neuromuscular-blocking agent (NMBA). During initial controlled hypoventilation, PEEP will further increase lung volume and should not be used.[98]

This use of volume-controlled ventilation is most established for this ventilatory pattern. In volume control, a high inspiratory flow rate (70–100 l/min) is required to achieve a short inspiratory time. This will result in a high peak airway pressure but this will lower DHI and plateau airway pressure (P_{plat}) and reduce barotrauma compared with lower inspiratory flow rates.[94,97] Pressure-controlled or assisted modes have been used[108] without adverse consequences. The theoretical advantage of a safe pressure limit in pressure modes is offset by the fact that equilibrium with the set safe pressure cannot be reached during the short inspiratory times required and thus either a higher pressure must be set or more than necessary hypoventilation may occur. It is not clear if one mode is superior to the other.

If significant hypotension occurs this should be treated by reducing the respiratory rate (thereby reducing dynamic hyperinflation) and intravascular volume loading.

ASSESSMENT OF DYNAMIC HYPERINFLATION

Once mechanical ventilation has started, the degree of DHI should be assessed by measurement of the *plateau airway pressure* (P_{plat}). This is the airway pressure after transient expiratory occlusion at the end of *inspiration*. This may be achieved by an end-inspiratory hold function on most current ventilators, which delays the commencement of the next breath (Figure 31.4a) or by applying a 0.5-second 'plateau' which does not delay the onset of the next breath. The latter should be applied for a single breath only, as application for several breaths in a row will decrease expiratory time and progressively increase DHI. This is the most easily measured estimate of average alveolar pressure at the end of inspiration and is directly proportional to the degree of hyperinflation and should be maintained at < 25 cmH_2O.[94,97]

Intrinsic PEEP is the airway pressure during occlusion of expiratory flow at the end of *expiration* (Figure 31.4b). This also is an automated end-expiratory hold function on most current ventilators. However this measurement is known to underestimate true PEEPi, as a consequence of small-airway closure during expiration, resulting in many higher-pressure alveoli not communicating with the central airway at the end of expiration.[96] Because of this, PEEPi can be used to show the presence of DHI but is not recommended to regulate the mechanical ventilation. Ideally PEEPi should be < 12 cmH_2O, though the exact safe level is unknown.

End-inspiratory lung volume (V_{EI}) (see Figures 31.1 and 31.2) < 20 ml/kg (1.4 litres in a 70-kg patient) has been shown to be a good predictor of complications during mechanical ventilation[97] and to correlate with total lung volume.[22] It is the total exhaled volume during a period of apnoea (30–90 seconds) in a paralysed patient. Although valuable, it is not routinely used as it requires neuromuscular blockade and a volumetric measuring device.

Assessment of the change in blood pressure and central venous pressure during a period of transient ventilator

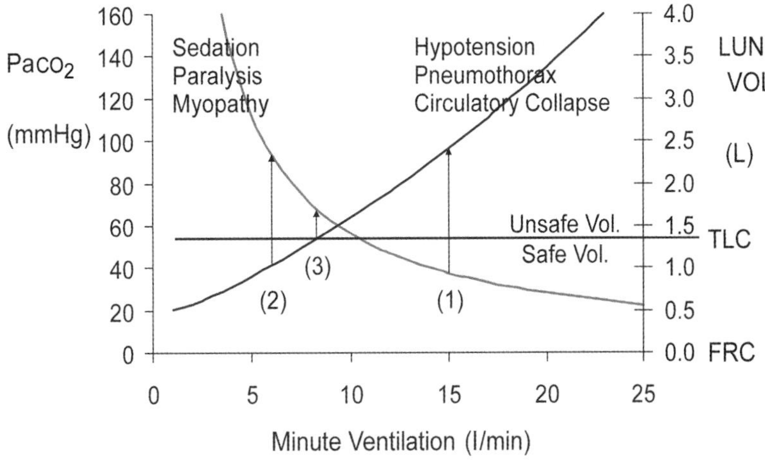

Figure 31.3 The effects of minute ventilation on Pa_{CO_2} and end-inspiratory lung volume above functional residual capacity (FRC) in a typical patient with severe asthma. The minute ventilation required for (1) normocapnia; (2) profound hypoventilation; and (3) optimal hypoventilation.

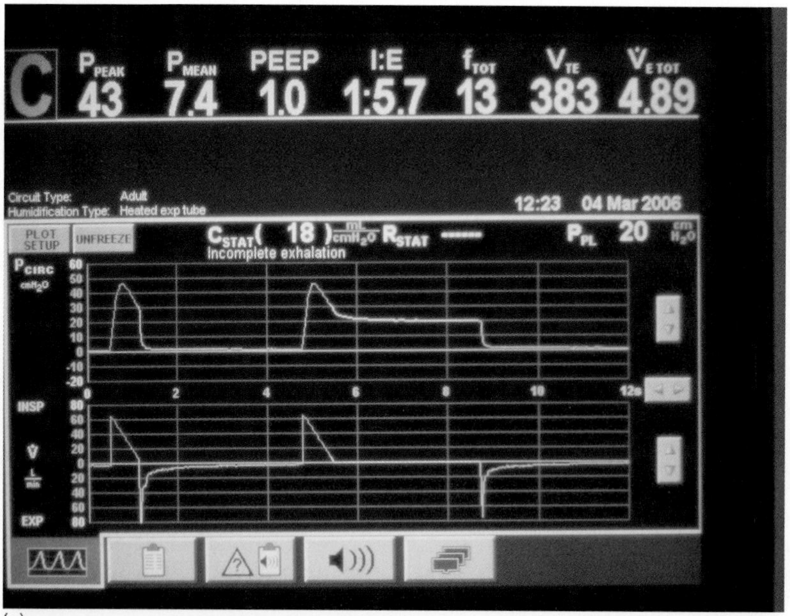

(a)

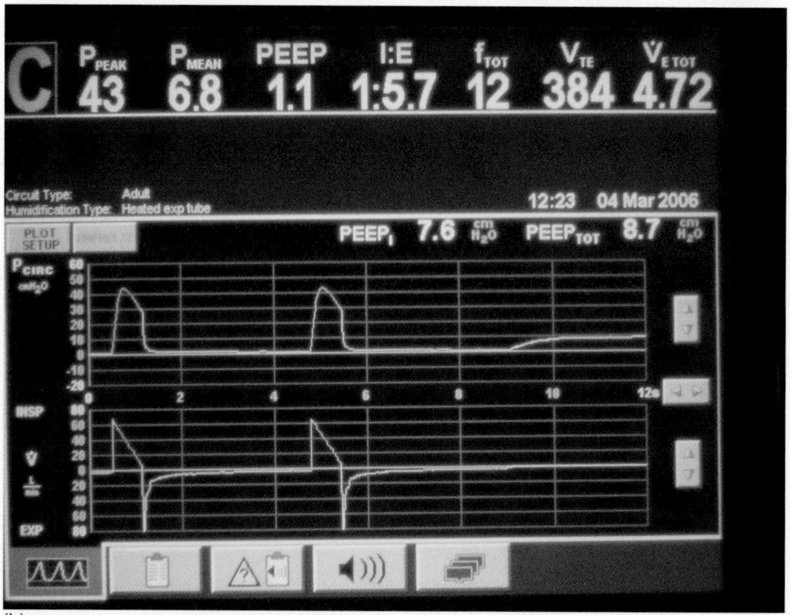

(b)

Figure 31.4 (a) The ventilator circuit pressure and flow traces versus time during controlled ventilation of a patient with severe airflow obstruction. Note the use of a low rate, low tidal volume (V_t), a high inspiratory flow rate (V_i 80 l/min) and hence a short inspiratory time ($t_e < 1$ second). This causes a high peak airway pressure but allows a long expiratory time (> 4 seconds). Expiratory flow is low throughout expiration and appears close to baseline at the onset of the next breath (second on screen), suggesting minimal gas trapping, but when an intrinsic positive end-expiratory pressure ($PEEP_i$) manoeuvre is done (end-expiratory pause) there is a surprising degree of PEEPi present (7.6 cmH_2O). (b) The ventilator circuit pressure and flow traces versus time during controlled ventilation of the same patient as in Figure 31.4b. When a P_{plat} manoeuvre is done (end-inspiratory pause) the P_{plat} is safe (20 cmH_2O) with this ventilator pattern (despite the degree of PEEPi present in Figure 31.4b). Note the low P_{plat} despite the high peak airway pressure.

disconnection (1–2 min) or transient ventilator rate reduction (4–6 breaths/min for 2–4 min): if DHI has been suppressing circulation then a significant increase in blood pressure and reduction in central venous pressure will occur.

ADJUSTMENT OF VENTILATION

Ventilatory patterns with an excessive minute ventilation risk hypotension and barotrauma and are associated with a high mortality. Using profound hypoventilation will guarantee avoidance of these complications but usually necessitates heavy sedation and neuromuscular blockade (see Figure 31.3). This, in association with parenteral steroids, has a high probability of myopathy,[66,109,110] which may cause severe prolonged disability. To minimise the risk of both these complications, DHI should be carefully assessed and the minimum amount of hypoventilation used to achieve a safe level of DHI (see Figure 31.3) in association with less sedation and minimal or no use of NMBAs.

Ventilation should be adjusted based on assessment of DHI, not on $Pa\text{CO}_2$ or pH. If P_{plat} is > 25 cmH$_2$O or circulatory suppression is present, then the ventilator rate should be reduced. If P_{plat} is low, then ventilation can be liberalised by increasing the ventilator rate or reducing sedation and allowing spontaneous ventilation.

Hypercapnia is usually present but is well tolerated[111] and does not appear to depress cardiac function. There is no evidence of benefit from sodium bicarbonate but it may reduce acidaemia-induced respiratory distress and may be given if the pH is less than 7.1.

When airflow obstruction improves (decreasing P_{plat} and PEEPi), sedation may be decreased, ventilator rate reduced and spontaneous ventilation assisted with pressure support ventilation. Pressure support of 10–16 cmH$_2$O may be used. Once spontaneous ventilation has commenced and when DHI is no longer critical, 3–7 cmH$_2$O CPAP may be introduced to assist ventilator triggering and reduce the work of breathing.

COMPLICATIONS OF INVASIVE VENTILATION IN ASTHMA

Hypotension may be caused by sedation, DHI, pneumothoraces or arrhythmias.[94,97] Hypovolaemia may be a contributory factor but is rarely a cause. Hypotension may be mild or life-threatening.[112] Hypotension due to DHI may be diagnosed by recovery of blood pressure during apnoea of 60 seconds (the 'apnoea test')[112] or by a longer period of low ventilator rate (4–6 breaths/min for 2–4 min). If this occurs, ventilation should be continued at a lower rate.

Circulatory arrest with apparent electromechanical dissociation is a recognised complication that may occur within 10 minutes of intubation and can lead to death or severe cerebral ischaemic injury if not managed correctly.[112–114] Standard mechanical ventilation recommendations (minute ventilation 115 ml/kg per min) have been estimated to be safe for 80% of patients requiring mechanical ventilation for acute severe asthma, with the remaining 20% requiring a small to moderate reduction in minute ventilation to return DHI to a safe level.[97] A small percentage of patients with unusually severe asthma can rapidly develop excessive DHI during initial uncontrolled mechanical ventilation, leading to electromechanical dissociation, sometimes despite 'safe' levels of minute ventilation. If the cause of this is not immediately recognised, it can lead to prolonged and unnecessary cardiopulmonary resuscitation, unsafe procedures such as intercostal vascular access needles or pericardial taps and risk cerebral injury and death.[112–114] When this occurs, immediate disconnection from the ventilator for 60–90 seconds (the 'apnoea test'; see above) or profound hypoventilation (2–3 breaths/min)[54] will diagnose and improve this situation. An even smaller percentage of patients may remain hypotensive despite profound hypoventilation with marked hypercapnia, fluid loading and inotropes. These patients may require Heliox delivered by the mechanical ventilator[115] or extracorporeal membrane oxygenation.[114,116,117]

Pneumothoraces were common before the advent of protective ventilatory strategies. DHI during mechanical ventilation was probably the major causative factor involved,[94,97] but pneumothorax may also occur in association with subclavian central venous catheter insertion and as a consequence of intercostal needle insertion for suspected tension pneumothorax during circulatory arrest (see above). The presence of severe airflow obstruction prevents lung collapse and favours gas loss through the ruptured alveoli, with the result that tension is almost always present in the pneumothorax. Once a unilateral tension pneumothorax is present, this will necessarily reduce ventilation to that lung and redistribute ventilation to the contralateral lung, thereby further increasing DHI in the second lung, and bilateral tension pneumothoraces may result with severely adverse consequences.

As soon as a tension pneumothorax is suspected, the ventilator rate should be immediately reduced to decrease the risk to the second lung. Clinical diagnosis of a tension pneumothorax can be difficult as the lungs in severe asthma are already overexpanded and hyperresonant with poor air entry. An urgent chest X-ray is always advisable for confirmation prior to intercostal catheter insertion unless severe hypotension is present. Intercostal catheters should always be inserted by blunt dissection. If intercostal needles are inserted for suspected pneumothorax, an intercostal catheter should always be inserted soon thereafter because if a tension pneumothorax was not present it is highly likely after an intercostal needle.

Acute necrotising myopathy is a serious complication that may occur in patients who are invasively ventilated for asthma and receive NMBAs or very deep sedation.[66,109,110,118,119] It is characterised by weakness with electromyographic evidence of myopathy and increased serum creatine kinase levels. Muscle biopsy reveals two patterns: myonecrosis with muscle cell vacuolisation or predominant type II fibre atrophy.[66,118] Recovery can be slow with prolonged weaning from mechanical ventilation and the need for rehabilitation. Incomplete recovery after 12 months has been reported in a few patients.[119,120] The aetiology of the myopathy appears to be a combination of the effects of corticosteroids and NMBAs with the duration of paralysis a strong predictor of myopathy.[119,120] The type of NMBA used seems to make no difference to the incidence of myopathy.[118] The relative contribution of corticosteroids versus NMBAs in the causation of myopathy is unclear; it seems wise to minimise the dose of parenteral corticosteroids with early introduction of nebulised agents and to minimise or avoid NMBAs if possible.

MORTALITY, LONG-TERM OUTCOME AND FOLLOW-UP

In a summary of 37 papers reporting the outcomes of 1260 patients requiring mechanical ventilation for asthma in the four decades prior to the year 2000[55] there was an overall mortality of 12.4% with a progressive reduction in reported mortality during that period (see Table 31.2). A selection of reports[9,11,12] published since 2000 have shown continued reduction in overall mortality (see Table 31.2) but with mortalities as high as 21% still occurring in one series.[11]

The largest and most comprehensive recent series[9] reported 1899 patients admitted to 22 Australian intensive care units over an 8-year period (1996–2003). This series reported a requirement for mechanical ventilation for 36% of patients admitted with severe asthma and a progressive reduction in annual mortality of the ventilated patients from 10% to 3% over the 8-year period.

The need for invasive ventilation is associated with an increased risk of death[9,11,121] and survivors of these near-fatal episodes of asthma have an increased risk of intensive care readmission and an increased risk of death after hospital discharge.[27]

For these reasons, patients who have an episode of asthma severe enough to require hospitalisation, particularly intensive care admission, need careful follow-up. This should include active identification and avoidance of precipitants, aggressive bronchodilator therapy including inhaled steroids, regular medical review, regular measurement of lung function, management plans for a deteriorating status and ready access to emergency services.[9]

REFERENCES

1. Abramson MJ, Bailey MJ, Couper FJ *et al.* Are asthma medications and management related to deaths from asthma? *Am J Respir Crit Care Med* 2001; **163**: 12–18.
2. McCaul KA, Wakefield MA, Roder DM *et al.* Trends in hospital readmission for asthma: has the Australian National Asthma Campaign had an effect? *Med J Aust* 2000; **172**: 62–6.
3. Suissa S, Ernst P, Benayoun S *et al.* Low-dose inhaled corticosteroids and the prevention of death from asthma. *N Engl J Med* 2000; **343**: 332–6.
4. The International Study of Asthma and Allergies in Childhood (ISAAC) Steering Committee. Worldwide variation in prevalence of symptoms of asthma, allergic rhinoconjunctivitis, and atopic eczema: ISAAC. *Lancet* 1998; **351**: 1225–32.
5. Pearce N, Weiland S, Keil U *et al.* Self-reported prevalence of asthma symptoms in children in Australia, England, Germany and New Zealand: an international comparison using the ISAAC protocol. *Eur Respir J* 1993; **6**: 1455–61.
6. Worldwide variations in the prevalence of asthma symptoms: the international study of asthma and allergies in childhood (ISAAC). *Eur Respir J* 1998; **12**: 315–35.
7. Sly RM. Changing prevalence of allergic rhinitis and asthma. *Ann Allergy Asthma Immunol* 1999; **82**: 233–48; quiz 248–52.
8. Strong K, de Looper M, Magnus P. Asthma mortality in Australia, 1980–1996. *Aust Health Rev* 1998; **21**: 255–63.
9. Stow PJ, Pilcher DV, Wilson J *et al.* Improved outcomes from acute severe asthma in Australian intensive care units (1996–2003). *Thorax* 2007; **62**: 842–7.
10. Wilson DH, Tucker G, Frith P *et al.* Trends in hospital admissions and mortality from asthma and chronic obstructive pulmonary disease in Australia, 1993–2003. *Med J Aust* 2007; **186**: 408–11.
11. Afessa B, Morales I, Cury JD. Clinical course and outcome of patients admitted to an ICU for status asthmaticus. *Chest* 2001; **120**: 1616–21.
12. Gehlbach B, Kress JP, Kahn J *et al.* Correlates of prolonged hospitalization in inner-city ICU patients receiving noninvasive and invasive positive pressure ventilation for status asthmaticus. *Chest* 2002; **122**: 1709–14.
13. US Department of Health and Human Services. *Guidelines for the Diagnosis and Management of Asthma.* Maryland: National Asthma Education Program; 1991.
14. Werner HA. Status asthmaticus in children: a review. *Chest* 2001; **119**: 1913–29.
15. Mattes J, Karmaus W. The use of antibiotics in the first year of life and development of asthma: which comes first? *Clin Exp Allergy* 1999; **29**: 729–32.
16. Busse WW, Lemanske RF, Jr. Asthma. *N Engl J Med* 2001; **344**: 350–62.
17. Bai TR, Cooper J, Koelmeyer T *et al.* The effect of age and duration of disease on airway structure in fatal asthma. *Am J Respir Crit Care Med* 2000; **162**: 663–9.
18. Jeffery PK. Bronchial biopsies and airway inflammation. *Eur Respir J* 1996; **9**: 1583–7.
19. Wasserfallen J, Schaller M, Feihl F *et al.* Sudden asphyxic asthma: a distinct entity? *Am Rev Respir Dis* 1990; **142**: 108–11.
20. Kolbe J, Fergusson W, Garrett J. Rapid onset asthma: a severe but uncommon manifestation. *Thorax* 1998; **53**: 241–7.

21. Woodruff PG, Emond SD, Singh AK *et al.* Sudden-onset severe acute asthma: clinical features and response to therapy. *Acad Emerg Med* 1998; **5**: 695–701.
22. Tuxen D, Williams T, Scheinkestel C *et al.* Use of a measurement of pulmonary hyperinflation to control the level of mechanical ventilation in patients with severe asthma. *Am Rev Respir Dis* 1992; **146**: 1136–42.
23. Evans TW. International Consensus Conferences in Intensive Care Medicine: non-invasive positive pressure ventilation in acute respiratory failure. Organised jointly by the American Thoracic Society, the European Respiratory Society, the European Society of Intensive Care Medicine, and the Société de Réanimation de Langue Française, and approved by the ATS Board of Directors, December 2000. *Intens Care Med* 2001; **27**: 166–78.
24. Pinsky M. Cardiopulmonary interactions associated with airflow obstruction. In: Hall J, Corbridge T, Rodrigo C *et al.* (eds) Acute Asthma: Assessment and Management. New York: McGraw-Hill, 2000: 105–23.
25. Rossi A, Ganassini A, Brusasco V. Airflow obstruction and dynamic hyperinflation. In: Hall J, Corbridge T, Rodrigo C *et al.* (eds) Acute Asthma: Assessment and Management. New York: McGraw-Hill, 2000: 57–82.
26. McFadden ER, Jr. Acute severe asthma. *Am J Respir Crit Care Med* 2003; **168**: 740–59.
27. McFadden ER, Jr., Warren EL. Observations on asthma mortality. *Ann Intern Med* 1997; **127**: 142–7.
28. Brenner B, Abraham E, Simon R. Position and diaphoresis in acute asthma. *Am J Med* 1983; **74**: 1005–9.
29. Lemarchrand P, Labrune S, Herer B *et al.* Cardiorespiratory arrest following peak expiratory flow measurement during attack of asthma. *Chest* 1991; **100**: 1168–9.
30. Carruthers DM, Harrison BD. Arterial blood gas analysis or oxygen saturation in the assessment of acute asthma? *Thorax* 1995; **50**: 186–8.
31. Rodrigo GJ, Rodriquez Verde M, Peregalli V *et al.* Effects of short-term 28% and 100% oxygen on $Pa\text{CO}_2$ and peak expiratory flow rate in acute asthma: a randomized trial. *Chest* 2003; **124**: 1312–7.
32. Mountain R, Heffner J, Brackett N *et al.* Acid–base disturbances in acute asthma. *Chest* 1990; **98**: 651–5.
33. Manthous CA. Lactic acidosis in status asthmaticus: three cases and review of the literature. *Chest* 2001; **119**: 1599–602.
34. Prakash S, Mehta S. Lactic acidosis in asthma: report of two cases and review of the literature. *Can Respir J* 2002; **9**: 203–8.
35. White C, Cole R, Lubetsky H *et al.* Acute asthma: admission chest radiography in hospitalized adult patients. *Chest* 1991; **100**: 14–16.
36. Rodrigo G, Rodrigo C. Assessment of the patient with acute asthma in the emergency department. A factor analytic study. *Chest* 1993; **104**: 1325–8.
37. Beasley R, Pearce N, Crane J *et al.* Asthma mortality and inhaled beta agonist therapy. *Aust NZ J Med* 1991; **21**: 753–63.
38. Chien JW, Ciufo R, Novak R *et al.* Uncontrolled oxygen administration and respiratory failure in acute asthma. *Chest* 2000; **117**: 728–33.
39. National Asthma Campaign. *Asthma Management Handbook 1998.* Melbourne: National Asthma Campaign, 1998.
40. BTS guidelines on asthma management. *Thorax* 2003; **58** (suppl. 1): i1–94.
41. Global Strategy for Asthma Management and Prevention. Global Initiative for Asthma (GINA). *Eur Respir J* 2006; **31**: 143–78.
42. Rossing T, Fanta C, Goldstein D *et al.* Emergency therapy of asthma: comparison of the acute effects of parenteral and inhaled sympathomimetics and infused aminophylline. *Am Rev Respir Dis* 1980; **122**: 365–71.
43. Cates C, Rowe B, Bara A. Holding chamber versus nebulisers for beta-agonist treatment of acute asthma (Cochrane review). Oxford, UK: Cochrane Library: Update Software, 2002.
44. Newman KB, Milne S, Hamilton C *et al.* A comparison of albuterol administered by metered-dose inhaler and spacer with albuterol by nebulizer in adults presenting to an urban emergency department with acute asthma. *Chest* 2002; **121**: 1036–41.
45. Manthous CA, Chatila W, Schmidt GA *et al.* Treatment of bronchospasm by metered-dose inhaler albuterol in mechanically ventilated patients. *Chest* 1995; **107**: 210–13.
46. Rodrigo G. Inhaled therapy for acute adult asthma. *Curr Opin Allergy Immunol* 2003; **3**: 169–75.
47. Bisgaard H. Delivery of inhaled medication to children. *J Asthma* 1997; **34**: 443–67.
48. Papo MC, Frank J, Thompson AE. A prospective, randomized study of continuous versus intermittent nebulized albuterol for severe status asthmaticus in children. *Crit Care Med* 1993; **21**: 1479–86.
49. Dolovich MA. Influence of inspiratory flow rate, particle size, and airway caliber on aerosolized drug delivery to the lung. *Respir Care* 2000; **45**: 597–608.
50. Rodrigo C, Rodrigo G. Therapeutic response patterns to high and cumulative doses of salbutamol in acute severe asthma. *Chest* 1998; **113**: 593–8.
51. Travers AH, Rowe BH, Barker S *et al.* The effectiveness of IV beta-agonists in treating patients with acute asthma in the emergency department: a meta-analysis. *Chest* 2002; **122**: 1200–7.
52. Browne GJ, Penna AS, Phung X *et al.* Randomised trial of intravenous salbutamol in early management of acute severe asthma in children. *Lancet* 1997; **349**: 301–5.
53. Canadian Asthma Consensus Report. Management of patients with asthma in the emergency department and in the hospital. *Can Med Assoc J* 1999; **161** (suppl.): S53–9.
54. Corbridge SJ, Corbridge TC. Severe exacerbations of asthma. *Crit Care Nurs Q* 2004; **27**: 207–28; quiz 229–30.
55. Tuxen D. Mechanical ventilation in asthma. In: Evans T, Hinds C (eds) *Recent Advances in Critical Care Medicine Number 4.* London: Churchill Livingstone, 1996: 165–89.
56. Willmot D. A 24 year old woman admitted to the critical care unit, with 'resistant' asthma and a metabolic acidosis. *Crit Care Resusc* 2000; **2**: 228–9.

57. Spitzer WO, Suissa S, Ernst P *et al.* The use of beta-agonists and the risk of death and near death from asthma. *N Engl J Med* 1992; **326**: 501–6.
58. Beakes DE. The use of anticholinergics in asthma. *J Asthma* 1997; **34**: 357–68.
59. Stoodley RG, Aaron SD, Dales RE. The role of ipratropium bromide in the emergency management of acute asthma exacerbation: a metaanalysis of randomized clinical trials. *Ann Emerg Med* 1999; **34**: 8–18.
60. Rodrigo GJ, Rodrigo C. The role of anticholinergics in acute asthma treatment: an evidence-based evaluation. *Chest* 2002; **121**: 1977–87.
61. Bryant D, Rogers P. Effects of ipratropium bromide nebuliser solution with and without preservatives in the treatment of acute and stable asthma. *Chest* 1992; **102**: 742–7.
62. Rodrigo GJ, Rodrigo C, Hall JB. Acute asthma in adults: a review. *Chest* 2004; **125**: 1081–102.
63. Rowe B, Spooner C, Ducharme F *et al.* Early emergency department treatment of acute asthma with systemic corticosteroids (Cochrane review). Oxford, UK: Update Software, 2002.
64. Rodrigo GJ, Rodrigo C. Triple inhaled drug protocol for the treatment of acute severe asthma. *Chest* 2003; **123**: 1908–15.
65. Edmonds ML, Camargo CA, Jr., Pollack CV, Jr. *et al.* The effectiveness of inhaled corticosteroids in the emergency department treatment of acute asthma: a meta-analysis. *Ann Emerg Med* 2002; **40**: 145–54.
66. Douglass J, Tuxen D, Horne M *et al.* Myopathy in severe asthma. *Am Rev Respir Dis* 1992; **146**: 517–19.
67. Klein-Gitelman MS, Pachman LM. Intravenous corticosteroids: adverse reactions are more variable than expected in children. *J Rheumatol* 1998; **25**: 1995–2002.
68. Abernathy-Carver KJ, Fan LL, Boguniewicz M *et al.* *Legionella* and *Pneumocystis* pneumonias in asthmatic children on high doses of systemic steroids. *Pediatr Pulmonol* 1994; **18**: 135–8.
69. Kasper WJ, Howe PM. Fatal varicella after a single course of corticosteroids. *Pediatr Infect Dis J* 1990; **9**: 729–32.
70. Goodman DC, Littenberg B, O'Connor GT *et al.* Theophylline in acute childhood asthma: a meta-analysis of its efficacy. *Pediatr Pulmonol* 1996; **21**: 211–18.
71. Yung M, South M. Randomised controlled trial of aminophylline for severe acute asthma. *Arch Dis Child* 1998; **79**: 405–10.
72. Parameswaran K, Belda J, Rowe B *et al.* Addition of intravenous aminophylline to beta2-agonists in adults with acute asthma (Cochrane review). Oxford, UK: Update Software, 2002.
73. Tirot P, Bouachour G, Varache N *et al.* Use of intravenous epinephrine in severe acute asthma. *Rev Mal Respir* 1992; **9**: 319–23.
74. Alter HJ, Koepsell TD, Hilty WM. Intravenous magnesium as an adjuvant in acute bronchospasm: a meta-analysis. *Ann Emerg Med* 2000; **36**: 191–7.
75. Rowe BH, Bretzlaff JA, Bourdon C *et al.* Intravenous magnesium sulfate treatment for acute asthma in the emergency department: a systematic review of the literature. *Ann Emerg Med* 2000; **36**: 181–90.
76. Rodrigo G, Rodrigo C, Burschtin O. Efficacy of magnesium sulfate in acute adult asthma: a meta-analysis of randomized trials. *Am J Emerg Med* 2000; **18**: 216–21.
77. Sydow M, Crozier T, Zielman S *et al.* High-dose intravenous magnesium sulfate in the management of life threatening status asthmaticus. *Inten Care Med* 1993; **19**: 467–71.
78. Hess DR, Acosta FL, Ritz RH *et al.* The effect of heliox on nebulizer function using a beta-agonist bronchodilator. *Chest* 1999; **115**: 184–9.
79. Kress JP, Noth I, Gehlbach BK *et al.* The utility of albuterol nebulized with heliox during acute asthma exacerbations. *Am J Respir Crit Care Med* 2002; **165**: 1317–21.
80. Carter E. Quality of writing in manuscripts. *Chest* 1999; **116**: 1494.
81. Kass JE, Terregino CA. The effect of heliox in acute severe asthma: a randomized controlled trial. *Chest* 1999; **116**: 296–300.
82. Rodrigo GJ, Rodrigo C, Pollack CV *et al.* Use of helium-oxygen mixtures in the treatment of acute asthma: a systematic review. *Chest* 2003; **123**: 891–6.
83. Sarma V. Use of ketamine in acute severe asthma. *Acta Anaesthesiol Scand* 1992; **36**: 106–7.
84. Sato N, Matsuki A, Zsigmond E *et al.* Ketamine relaxes and airway smooth muscle contracted by endothelium. *Anesth Analg* 1997; **84**: 900–6.
85. Howton JC, Rose J, Duffy S *et al.* Randomized, double-blind, placebo-controlled trial of intravenous ketamine in acute asthma. *Ann Emerg Med* 1996; **27**: 170–5.
86. Youssef-Ahmed MZ, Silver P, Nimkoff L *et al.* Continuous infusion of ketamine in mechanically ventilated children with refractory bronchospasm. *Intens Care Med* 1996; **22**: 972–6.
87. Tobias JD, Garrett JS. Therapeutic options for severe, refractory status asthmaticus: inhalational anaesthetic agents, extracorporeal membrane oxygenation and helium/oxygen ventilation. *Paediatr Anaesth* 1997; **7**: 47–57.
88. Dockhorn RJ, Baumgartner RA, Leff JA *et al.* Comparison of the effects of intravenous and oral montelukast on airway function: a double blind, placebo controlled, three period, crossover study in asthmatic patients. *Thorax* 2000; **55**: 260–5.
89. Camargo CA, Jr., Smithline HA, Malice MP *et al.* A randomized controlled trial of intravenous montelukast in acute asthma. *Am J Respir Crit Care Med* 2003; **167**: 528–33.
90. Silverman R. Ipratropium bromide in emergency management of acute asthma exacerbation. *Ann Emerg Med* 2000; **35**: 197–8.
91. Smith D, Deshazo R. Bronchoalveolar lavage in asthma. State of the art. *Am Rev Respir Dis* 1993; **148**: 523–32.
92. Graham V, Lasserson T, Rowe B (eds) *Antibiotics for Acute Asthma (Cochrane Review)*. Oxford, UK: Update Software, 2002.

93. Joseph KS, Blais L, Ernst P *et al.* Increased morbidity and mortality related to asthma among asthmatic patients who use major tranquillisers. *Br Med J* 1996; **312**: 79–82.
94. Tuxen D, Lane S. The effects of ventilatory pattern on hyperinflation, airway pressures, and circulation in mechanical ventilation of patients with severe airflow obstruction. *Am Rev Respir Dis* 1987; **136**: 872–9.
95. Pepe P, Marini J. Occult positive end-expiratory pressure in mechanically ventilated patients with airflow obstruction. *Am Rev Respir Dis* 1982; **126**: 166–70.
96. Leatherman J, Ravenscraft S. Low measured auto-positive end-expiratory pressure during mechanical ventilation of patients with severe asthma: hidden auto-positive end-expiratory pressure. *Crit Care Med* 1996; **24**: 541–6.
97. Williams T, Tuxen D, Scheinkestel C *et al.* Risk factors for morbidity in mechanically ventilated patients with acute severe asthma. *Am Rev Respir Dis* 1992; **146**: 607–15.
98. Tuxen D. Detrimental effects of positive end-expiratory pressure during controlled mechanical ventilation of patients with severe airflow obstruction. *Am Rev Respir Dis* 1989; **140**: 5–9.
99. Brochard L. Noninvasive ventilation for acute respiratory failure. *JAMA* 2002; **288**: 932–5.
100. International Consensus Conferences in Intensive Care Medicine: noninvasive positive pressure ventilation in acute respiratory failure. *Am J Respir Crit Care Med* 2001; **163**: 283–91.
101. Mehta S, Hill S. Noninvasive ventilation. *Am J Respir Crit Care Med* 2001; **163**: 540–77.
102. Brochard L, Mancebo J, Wysocki M *et al.* Noninvasive ventilation for acute exacerbations of chronic obstructive pulmonary disease. *N Engl J Med* 1995; **333**: 817–22.
103. Kramer N, Meyer T, Meharg J *et al.* Randomised prospective trial of noninvasive positive pressure ventilation in acute respiratory failure. *Am J Respir Crit Care Med* 1995; **151**: 1799–806.
104. Fernandez MM, Villagra A, Blanch L *et al.* Non-invasive mechanical ventilation in status asthmaticus. *Intens Care Med* 2001; **27**: 486–92.
105. Soroksky A, Stav D, Shpirer I. A pilot prospective, randomized, placebo-controlled trial of bilevel positive airway pressure in acute asthmatic attack. *Chest* 2003; **123**: 1018–25.
106. Mountain R, Sahn S. Clinical features and outcome in patients with acute asthma presenting with hypercapnia. *Am Rev Respir Dis* 1988; **138**: 535–9.
107. Peigang Y, Marini J. Ventilation of patients with asthma and chronic pulmonary disease. *Curr Opin Crit Care* 2002; **8**: 70–8.
108. Mansel J, Stogner S, Petrini M *et al.* Mechanical ventilation in patients with acute severe asthma. *Am J Med* 1990; **89**: 42–8.
109. Hansen-Flaschen J, Cowen J, Raps E. Neuromuscular blockade in the Intensive Care Unit. More than we bargained for. *Am Rev Respir Dis* 1993; **147**: 234–6.
110. Nates J, Cooper D, Tuxen D. Acute weakness syndromes in critically ill patients – a reappraisal. *Anaesth Int Care* 1997; **25**: 502–13.
111. Bellomo R, McLaughlan P, Tai E *et al.* Asthma requiring mechanical ventilation. A low morbidity approach. *Chest* 1994; **105**: 891–6.
112. Rosengarten P, Tuxen D, Dziukas L *et al.* Circulatory arrest induced by intermittent positive pressure ventilation in a patient with severe asthma. *Anaes Int Care* 1990; **19**: 118–21.
113. Kollef M. Lung hyperinflation caused by inappropriate ventilation resulting in electromechanical dissociation: a case report. *Heart Lung* 1992; **21**: 74–7.
114. Mabuchi N, Takasu H, Ito S *et al.* Successful extracorporeal lung assist (ECLA) for a patient with severe asthma and cardiac arrest. *Clin Intens Med* 1991; **2**: 292–4.
115. Gluck E, Onorato D, Castriotta R. Helium–oxygen mixtures in intubated patients with status asthmaticus and respiratory acidosis. *Chest* 1990; **98**: 693–8.
116. King D, Smales C, Arnold A *et al.* Extracorporeal membrane oxygenation as emergency treatment for life threatening acute severe asthma. *Postgrad Med J* 1986; **62**: 555–7.
117. Tajimi K, Kasai T, Nakatani T *et al.* Extracorporeal lung assist (ECLA) for a patient with hypercapnia due to status asthmaticus. *Intens Care Med* 1988; **14**: 588–9.
118. Leatherman J, Fluegel W, David W *et al.* Muscle weakness in mechanically ventilated patients with severe asthma. *Am J Respir Crit Care Med* 1996; **153**: 1686–90.
119. Behbehani NA, Al-Mane F, D'Yachkova Y *et al.* Myopathy following mechanical ventilation for acute severe asthma: the role of muscle relaxants and corticosteroids. *Chest* 1999; **115**: 1627–31.
120. Hirano M, Ott B, Raps E *et al.* Acute quadriplegic myopathy: a complication of treatment with steroids, nondepolarizing blocking agents, or both. *Neurology* 1992; **42**: 2082–7.
121. Marquette C, Saulnier F, Leroy O *et al.* Long-term prognosis of near-fatal asthma. *Am Rev Respir Dis* 1992; **146**: 76–81.

32

Pneumonia

Charles D Gomersall

The management of pneumonia is based on four findings and premises:

1. Pneumonia is associated with a wide range of largely non-specific clinical features.[1]
2. Pneumonia can be caused by over 100 organisms.[2]
3. The relationship between specific clinical features and aetiological organism is insufficiently strong to allow a clinical diagnosis of the causative organism.[3,4]
4. Early administration of appropriate antibiotics is important.[3,5]

The net result is that the differential diagnosis is wide and treatment should be started before the aetiological agent is known. The differential diagnosis and the likely causative organisms can be narrowed by using epidemiological clues, the most important of which are whether the pneumonia is community-acquired or health care-associated and whether the patient is immunocompromised. Note that the flora and antibiotic resistance patterns vary from country to country, hospital to hospital and even intensive care unit (ICU) to ICU within a hospital[6] and this must be taken into account.

COMMUNITY-ACQUIRED PNEUMONIA

Recent evidence-based guidelines have been issued by the Infectious Diseases Society of America (IDSA) and American Thoracic Society (ATS)[7] and the European Respiratory Society.[8] Links to these and other pneumonia-related guidelines can be found at the following link page: http://www.aic.cuhk.edu.hk/web8/Pneumonia guidelines.htm.

DEFINITION

Community-acquired pneumonia is an acute infection of the pulmonary parenchyma that is associated with at least some symptoms of acute infection, accompanied by an acute infiltrate on a chest X-ray (CXR) or auscultatory findings consistent with pneumonia (e.g. altered breath sounds, localised crackles) in a patient not hospitalised or residing in a long-term care facility for $\geq$ 14 days prior to the onset of symptoms.[9]

AETIOLOGY

Table 32.1 gives possible aetiological agents based on epidemiological clues. *Streptococcus pneumoniae* is the most commonly isolated organism. The next most common pathogens in patients admitted to ICU are: *Legionella* species, *Haemophilus influenzae,* Enterobacteriaceae species, *Staphylococcus aureus* and *Pseudomonas* species.[10]

CLINICAL PRESENTATION

Pneumonia produces both systemic and respiratory manifestations. Common clinical findings include fever, sweats, rigors, cough, sputum production, pleuritic chest pain, dyspnoea, tachypnoea, pleural rub and inspiratory crackles. Classic signs of consolidation occur in fewer than 25% of cases. Multiorgan dysfunction or failure may occur depending on the type and severity of pneumonia.

The diagnosis of pneumonia may be more difficult in the elderly. Although the vast majority of elderly patients with pneumonia have respiratory symptoms and signs, over 50% may also have non-respiratory symptoms and over one-third may have no systemic signs of infection.

INVESTIGATIONS[7,8]

Investigations should not delay administration of antibiotics as delays are associated with an increase in mortality.[3] Important investigations include:

1. CXR
2. Arterial blood gases or oximetry
3. Full blood count
4. Serum creatinine, urea and electrolytes
5. Liver function tests
6. Blood cultures ($\times$2) prior to the administration of antimicrobials
7. Sputum (if immediately available) for urgent Gram stain and culture. The usefulness of sputum tests remains debatable because of contamination by upper respiratory tract commensals. However, a single or predominant organism on a Gram stain of a fresh sample or a heavy growth on culture of purulent sputum is likely to be the organism responsible. The finding of many polymorphonuclear cells (PMN) with no bacteria in a patient who has not already received antibiotics can reliably exclude infection by most ordinary bacterial pathogens. Specimens should be obtained by deep cough and be grossly purulent. Ideally the specimen

Table 32.1 Possible aetiological agents based on epidemiological clues[2,3,7,9]

Exposure	Organism
Exposure to animals	
Handling turkeys, chickens, ducks or psittacine birds or their excreta	*Chlamydia psittaci*
Exposure to birds in countries in which avian flu has been identified in birds	Influenza A H5N1
Handling infected parturient cats, cattle, goats or sheep or their hides	*Coxiella burnetii*
Handling infected wool	*Bacillus anthracis*
Handling infected cattle, pigs, goats or sheep or their milk	*Brucella* spp.
Insect bite. Transmission from rodents and wild animals (e.g. rabbits) to laboratory workers, farmers and hunters	*Francisella tularensis*
Insect bites or scratches. Transmission from infected rodents or cats to laboratory workers and hunters	*Yersinia pestis*
Contact with infected horses (very rare)	*Pseudomonas mallei*
Exposure to mice or mice droppings	Hantavirus
Geographical factors	
Immigration from or residence in countries with high prevalence of tuberculosis	*Mycobacterium tuberculosis*
North America. Contact with infected bats or birds or their excreta. Excavation in endemic areas	*Histoplasma capsulatum*
South-west USA	*Coccidiodes* species, Hantavirus
USA. Inhalation of spores from soil	*Blastomyces dermatitidis*
Asia, Pacific, Caribbean, north Australia. Contact with local animals or contaminated skin abrasions	*Burkholderia pseudomallei*
Host factors	
Diabetic ketoacidosis	*Streptococcus pneumoniae, Staphylococcus aureus*
Alcoholism	*Streptococcus pneumoniae, Staphylococcus aureus, Klebsiella pneumoniae,* oral anaerobes, *Mycobacterium tuberculosis, Acinetobacter* spp.
Chronic obstructive pulmonary disease or smoking	*Streptococcus pneumoniae, Haemophilus influenzae, Moraxella catarrhalis, Chlamydia pneumoniae, Legionella* spp., *Pseudomonas aeruginosa*
Sickle-cell disease	*Streptococcus pneumoniae*
Pneumonia complicating whooping cough	*Bordatella pertussis*
Pneumonia complicating influenza	*Streptococcus pneumoniae, Staphylococcus aureus*
Pneumonia severe enough to necessitate artificial ventilation	*Streptococcus pneumoniae, Legionella* spp., *Staphylococcus aureus, Haemophilus influenzae, Mycoplasma pneumoniae,* enteric Gram-negative bacilli, *Chlamydia pneumoniae, Mycobacterium tuberculosis,* viral infection, endemic fungi
Nursing-home residency	Treat as health care-associated pneumonia
Poor dental hygiene	Anaerobes
Suspected large-volume aspiration	Oral anaerobes, Gram-negative enteric bacteria
Structural disease of lung (e.g. bronchiectasis, cystic fibrosis)	*Pseudomonas aeruginosa, Burkholderia cepacia, Staphylococcus aureus*
Lung abscess	Community-acquired methicillin-resistant *Staphylococcus aureus*, oral anaerobes, endemic fungi, *Mycobacterium tuberculosis*, atypical mycobacteria
Endobronchial obstruction	Anaerobes, *Streptococcus pneumoniae, Haemophilus influenzae, Staphylococcus aureus*
Intravenous drug addict	*Staphylococcus aureus*, anaerobes, *Mycobacterium tuberculosis, Streptococcus pneumoniae*
Others	
Epidemic	*Mycoplasma pneumoniae,* influenza virus
Air-conditioning cooling towers, hot tubs or hotel or cruise ship stay in previous 2 weeks	*Legionella pneumophilia*
Presentation of a cluster of cases over a very short period of time	Bioterrorist agents: *Bacillus anthracis, Franciscella tularensis, Yersinia pestis*

should be obtained before treatment with antimicrobials, if this does not delay administration of antibiotics, and be transported to the laboratory immediately for prompt processing to minimise the chance of missing fastidious organisms (e.g. *Streptococcus pneumoniae*). Acceptable specimens (in patients with normal or raised white blood cell (WBC) counts) should contain > 25 PMN per low-power field (LPF) and < 10–25 squamous epithelial cells (SEC)/LPF or > 10 PMN per SEC. These criteria should not be used for *Mycobacterium* and *Legionella* infection. Certain organisms are virtually always pathogens when recovered from respiratory secretions (Table 32.2). Patients with risk factors for tuberculosis (TB) (Table 32.3) and particularly those with cough for more than a month, other common symptoms of TB and suggestive radiographic changes should have sputum examined for acid-fast bacilli (AFB). Sputum cannot be processed for culture for anaerobes due to contamination by the endogenous anaerobic flora of the upper respiratory tract. In addition to the factors listed in Table 32.1, foul-smelling sputum, lung abscess and empyema should raise suspicion of anaerobic infection.

8. Aspiration of pleural fluid for Gram stain, culture, pH and leukocyte count – all patients with a pleural effusion > 1 cm thick on a lateral decubitus CXR.

Table 32.2 Organisms which are virtually always pathogens when recovered from respiratory secretions[9]

Legionella
Chlamydia
Tuberculosis
Influenza, para-influenza virus, respiratory syncytial virus, adenovirus, Hantavirus, severe acute respiratory syndrome (SARS), coronavirus
Stronglyloides stercoralis
Toxoplasma gondi
Pneumocystis carinii
Histoplasma capsulatum
Coccidiodes immitis
Blastomycoses dermatitidis
Cryptococcus neoformans

Table 32.3 Risk factors for pulmonary tuberculosis

Living in or originating from a developing country
Age (< 5 years, middle-aged and elderly men)
Alcoholism and/or drug addiction
Human immunodeficiency virus (HIV) infection
Diabetes mellitus
Lodging-house dwellers
Immunosuppression
Close contact with smear-positive patients
Silicosis
Poverty and/or malnutrition
Previous gastrectomy
Smoking

9. Urinary *Legionella* antigen. This test is specific (> 95%). In patients with severe legionnaire's disease sensitivity is 88–100% for *L. pneumophilia* serogroup 1 (the most commonly reported cause of *Legionella* infection). Thus a positive result is virtually diagnostic of *Legionella* infection but a negative result does not exclude it. In areas where other *Legionella* species are more common, this test is less helpful.
10. Urinary pneumococcal antigen has moderate sensitivity (50–80%) and high specificity (> 90%).
11. Microimmunofluorescence serology for *Chlamydia pneumoniae* immunoglobulin (Ig) M. A titre of 1:16 is significant.
12. Human immunodeficiency virus (HIV) serological status.

Other investigations should be considered in patients with risk factors for infection with unusual organisms. Bronchoalveolar lavage may be useful in immunocompromised patients, those who fail to respond to antibiotics or those in whom sputum samples cannot be obtained.[11]

MANAGEMENT

GENERAL SUPPORTIVE MEASURES

Intravenous fluids may be required to correct dehydration and provide maintenance fluid. A general approach should be made to organ support with an emphasis on correcting hypoxia.

ANTIMICROBIAL REGIMES

Each unit should have its own regimens tailored to the local flora and antibiotic resistance patterns. In the absence of such regimens the regimen outlined in Figure 32.1 may be helpful. This should be modified in the light of risk factors (see Table 32.1). Quinolones may be less appropriate in areas with a high prevalence of TB as their use may mask concurrent TB infection. Appropriate antimicrobial therapy should be administered within 1 hour of diagnosis.[8,14] There is controversy regarding the appropriate change to empiric therapy based on microbiological findings.[7,8] Changing to narrower-spectrum antimicrobial cover may result in inadequate treatment of the 5–38% of patients with polymicrobial infection. Furthermore, dual therapy may be more effective than monotherapy, even when the identified pathogen is sensitive to the agent chosen, particularly in severely ill patients with bacteraemic pneumococcal pneumonia.[15] For the treatment of drug-resistant *Streptococcus pneumoniae*, the regimes in Figure 32.1 are probably suitable for isolates with a penicillin minimum inhibitory concentration (MIC) < 4 mg/l.[7] If the MIC is ≥ 4 mg/l an antipneumococcal fluoroquinolone, vancomycin, teicoplanin or linezolid should be given.[8]

The role of zanamivir and oseltamivir in severe influenza pneumonia is not clear but early treatment of patients with less severe symptoms results in a reduction of the duration of symptoms if treatment is started early (< 48 hours from onset).[16] Oseltamivir is recommended as first-line therapy for patients with suspected avian influenza A/H5N1.[17]

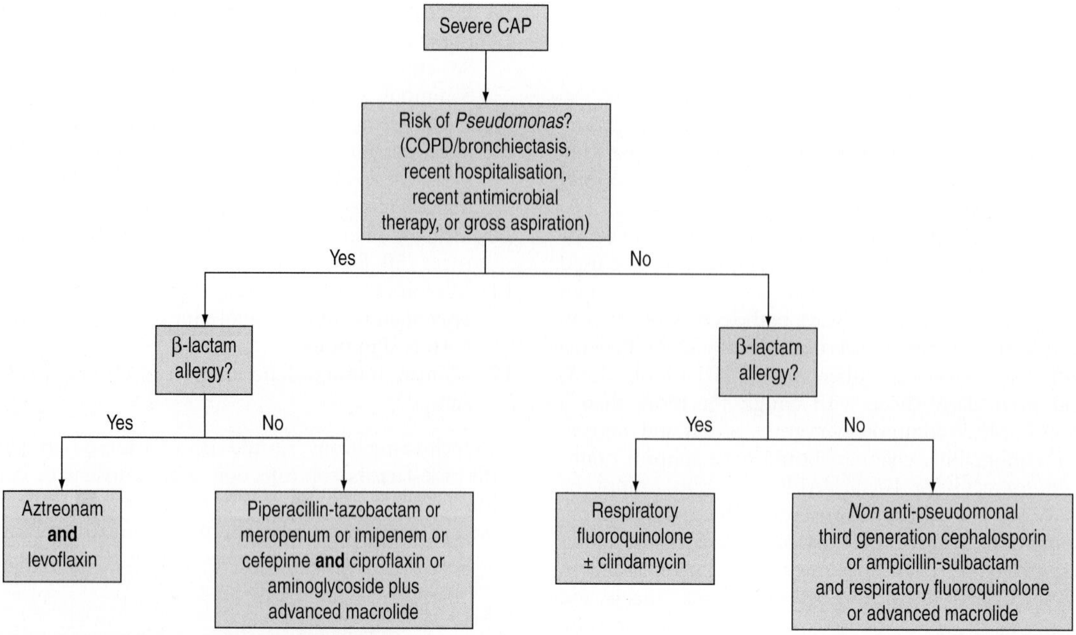

Figure 32.1 Antibiotic regimes for treatment of severe community-acquired pneumonia in critically ill patients.[7,8] Respiratory fluoroquinolones include moxifloxacin and levofloxacin. Advanced macrolides include azithromycin and clarithromycin. Cefotaxime is a suitable non-antipseudomonal third-generation cephalosporin.

Recommended treatment for other pathogens can be found at http://www.journals.uchicago.edu/CID/journal/issues/v44nS2/41620/41620.tb9.html.

DURATION OF THERAPY

There are no clinical trials that have specifically addressed this issue. Courses as short as 5 days may be sufficient[18] but antibiotics should be continued until the patient has been afebrile for 48–72 hours and organ dysfunction has largely resolved.[7] Short courses may be suboptimal for patients with bacteraemic *Staphylococcus aureus* pneumonia, meningitis or endocarditis complicating pneumonia or infection with less common organisms (e.g. *Burkholderia pseudomallei* or fungi) or *Pseudomonas aeruginosa*.

RESPONSE TO THERAPY [7,9,19]

This can be assessed subjectively (a response is usually seen within 1–3 days of starting therapy) or objectively on the basis of respiratory symptoms, fever, oxygenation, WBC count, bacteriology and CXR changes. The average time to defevescence varies with organism, severity and patient age (7 days in elderly patients, 2.5 days in young patients with pneumococcal pneumonia, 6–7 days in bacteraemic patients with pneumococcal pneumonia, 1–2 days in patients with *M. pneumoniae* pneumonia and 5 days in patients with *Legionella* pneumonia). Both blood and sputum cultures are usually negative within 24–48 hours of treatment, although *P. aeruginosa* and *M. pneumoniae* may persist in the sputum despite effective therapy. CXR changes lag behind clinical changes with the speed of change depending on the organism, the age of the patient and the presence and absence of comorbid illnesses. The CXR of most young or middle-aged patients with bacteraemic pneumococcal pneumonia is clear by 4 weeks but resolution is slower in elderly patients and patients with underlying illness, extensive pneumonia on presentation or *L. pneumophilia* pneumonia.

If the patient fails to respond, consider the following questions:

- Does the patient have pneumonia?
- Are there host factors which explain the failure (e.g. obstruction of bronchus by a foreign body or tumour, inadequate host response)?
- Has a complication developed (e.g. empyema, superinfection, bronchiolitis obliterans organising pneumonia)?
- Is the right drug being given in an adequate dose by the right route?
- Is the organism resistant to the drug being given?
- Are there other organisms?
- Is the fever a drug fever?

Useful investigations include computed tomography of the chest, bronchoalveolar lavage (Table 32.4) and transbronchial or open-lung biopsy.

ADMISSION TO ICU

This will largely be determined by the need for organ support and the availability of beds. However the

Table 32.4 Procedure for obtaining microbiological samples using bronchoscopy and protected specimen brushing (PSB) and/or bronchoalveolar lavage (BAL)[12,13]

Infection control	In patients suspected of having a disease which is transmitted by the airborne route (e.g. tuberculosis): • the risk of transmission should be carefully weighed against the benefits of bronchoscopy, which may generate large numbers of airborne particles • perform bronchoscopy in a negative-pressure isolation room • consider the use of a muscle relaxant in ventilated patients, to prevent coughing • staff should wear personal protective equipment which should include a fit-tested negative-pressure respirator (N95, FFP2 or above) as a minimum. Use of a powered air-purifying respirator should be considered
General recommendations	Suction through the endotracheal tube should be performed before bronchoscopy Avoid suction or injection through the working channel of the bronchoscope Perform protected specimen brushing before bronchoalveolar lavage
Ventilated patients	Set F_{IO_2} at 1.0 Set peak pressure alarm at a level that allows adequate ventilation Titrate ventilator settings against exhaled tidal volume Consider neuromuscular blockade in addition to sedation in patients at high risk of complications who are undergoing prolonged bronchoscopy
Protected specimen brushing	Sample the consolidated segment of lung at subsegmental level If purulent secretions are not seen, advance the brush until it can no longer be seen but avoid wedging it in a peripheral position Move brush back and forth and rotate it several times
Bronchoalveolar lavage	Wedge tip of bronchoscope into a subsegment of the consolidated segment of lung Inject, aspirate and collect 20 ml of sterile isotonic saline. Do not use this sample for quantitative microbiology or identification of intracellular organisms. It can be used for other microbiological analysis Inject, aspirate and collect additional aliquots of 20–60 ml The total volume of saline injected should be 60–200 ml
Complications	Hypoxaemia (possibly less with smaller BAL volumes) Arrhythmia Transient worsening in pulmonary infiltrates Bleeding (particularly following PSB) Fever (more common after BAL)
Positive results	>5% of cells in cytocentrifuge preparations of BAL fluid contain intracellular bacteria *or* $\geq 10^3$ colony-forming units/ml in PSB specimen *or* $\geq 10^4$ colony-forming units/ml in BAL fluid

presence of three of the following should prompt referral for admission: systolic blood pressure ≤ 90 mmHg, multilobar disease, P_{aO_2}/F_{IO_2} ratio ≤ 250 (P_{aO_2} in mmHg) or ≤ 33 (P_{aO_2} in kPa), multilobar infiltrates, confusion, urea > 7 mmol/l (20 mg/dl), leukopenia, thrombocytopenia, hypothermia and need for aggressive fluid resuscitation.[7]

HOSPITAL-ACQUIRED PNEUMONIA

Hospital-acquired pneumonia occurs in 0.5–5% of hospital patients, with a higher incidence in certain groups, e.g. postoperative patients and patients in ICU. Diagnosis may be difficult: the clinical features of pneumonia are non-specific and many non-infectious conditions (e.g. atelectasis, pulmonary embolus, aspiration, heart failure and cancer) can cause infiltrates on a CXR. Identification of the organism responsible is even more difficult than in patients with community-acquired pneumonia due to the high incidence of oropharyngeal colonisation by Gram-negative bacteria. Blood cultures are only positive in about 6% of cases of nosocomial pneumonia. Ventilator-associated pneumonia is nosocomial pneumonia arising > 48–72 hours after intubation. It is associated with a higher incidence of multidrug-resistant organisms.[1]

PATHOGENESIS

Nosocomial pneumonia is thought to result from micro-aspiration of bacteria colonising the upper respiratory tract. Other routes of infection include macroaspiration of gastric contents, inhaled aerosols, haematogenous spread, spread from pleural space and direct inoculation from ICU personnel.

CLINICAL DIAGNOSIS

Health care-associated pneumonia is defined on the basis of time of onset (developing more than 48 hours after admission to a health care facility[1]), CXR changes (new or progressive infiltrates) and either clinical features and simple laboratory investigations or the results of quantitative microbiology. Using a clinical approach, pneumonia is diagnosed by the finding of a new infiltrate or a change in an infiltrate on CXR and growth of pathogenic organisms from sputum plus one of the following: WBC count greater than 12×10^5/litre, core temperature ≥ 38.3°C, sputum Gram stain with scores of more than two on a scale of four of polymorphonuclear leukocytes and bacteria.

INVESTIGATIONS

These are broadly similar to those required in community-acquired pneumonia:

- *CXR*: although studies using a histological diagnosis as the gold standard have demonstrated that pneumonia may be present despite a normal CXR, most definitions of nosocomial pneumonia require the presence of new persistent infiltrates on a CXR.
- *Respiratory secretions*: considerable controversy surrounds the issue of whether invasive bronchoscopic sampling (see Table 32.4) of respiratory secretions is necessary. A randomised controlled trial has demonstrated a reduced 14-day mortality amongst patients with ventilator-associated pneumonia who underwent invasive bronchoscopic sampling compared to those who were treated using a non-invasive management strategy.[20] However the important difference between the two groups may have been the use of quantitative microbiological techniques in the former rather than the use of invasive sampling.[21] Previous data have demonstrated a high correlation between the results of quantitative culture of invasive samples and quantitative culture of tracheal aspirates.[22] A more recent trial of non-quantitative culture of bronchoalveolar lavage specimens versus non-quantitative culture of tracheal aspirates revealed no difference in any outcome measures.[23] Although tracheal aspirates may predominantly reflect the organisms colonising the upper airway they may be useful in indicating which organisms are not responsible for the pneumonia, thus allowing the antimicrobial cover to be narrowed.[1] This interpretation is based on the premise that the predominant route of infection is via the upper respiratory tract. From this it can be assumed that if the organism is not present in the upper respiratory tract the probability of it being present in the lung parenchyma is low. Certain organisms are virtually always pathogens when recovered from respiratory secretions (see Table 32.2).
- *Blood cultures* identify the aetiological agent in 8–20% of patients. Bacteraemia is associated with a worse prognosis. In 50% of patients with severe hospital-acquired pneumonia and positive blood cultures there is another source of sepsis.

MANAGEMENT

Management is based on the finding that early treatment with antimicrobials that cover all likely pathogens results in a reduction in morbidity and mortality.[5] If quantitative microbiology is not used the initial selection of antimicrobials is made on the basis of epidemiological clues (Figure 32.2; Table 32.5). Antimicrobials should be administered within 1 hour of diagnosis.[14] The results of microbiological investigations are used to narrow antimicrobial cover later. Treatment should be reassessed after 2–3 days or sooner if the patient deteriorates (Figure 32.3). An outline of management based on an invasive approach is given in Figure 32.4.

DURATION OF THERAPY

Current ATS guidelines recommend 7 days' treatment provided the aetiological agent is not *P. aeruginosa* and the patient has a good clinical response with resolution of clinical features of infection.[1] The outcome of patients who receive appropriate initial empiric therapy for ventilator-associated pneumonia for 8 days is similar to those who receive treatment for 14 days.[24]

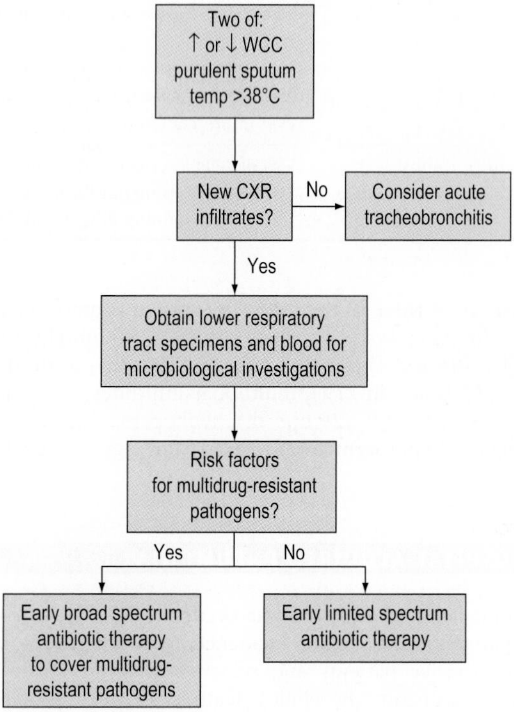

Figure 32.2 An outline of initial management of nosocomial pneumonia based on a non-invasive clinical approach.[1]

Table 32.5 Recommended initial empiric treatment for nosocomial pneumonia[1]*

Situation	Antibiotics
No risk factors for multidrug-resistant pathogens	Cefotaxime *or* Levofloxacin, moxifloxacin or ciprofloxacin *or* Ampicillin/sulbactam *or* Ertapenem
Antimicrobial therapy in previous 90 days *or* Current hospitalisation for ≥ 5 days *or* High frequency of antibiotic resistance in the specific hospital unit *or* Hospitalisation for 2 days or more in previous 90 days *or* Residence in nursing home or extended-care facility *or* Home infusion therapy (including antibiotics) *or* Chronic dialysis within 30 days *or* Home wound care *or* Family member with multidrug-resistant pathogen *or* Immunosuppression *or* Bronchiectasis	One of: Antipseudomonal cephalosporin (cefepime or ceftazidime) *or* Antipseudomonal carbapenem (meropenem or imipenem-cilastin) *or* β-lactam/β-lactamase inhibitor (e.g. piperacillin-tazobactam or cefaperazone-sulbactam) *plus* one of: Aminoglycoside *or* Antipseudomonal quinolone (levofloxacin or ciprofloxacin) *plus* one of the following for patients at high risk of methicillin-resistant *Staphylococcus aureus* (MRSA) infection: Linezolid or vancomycin or teicoplanin

*The use of dual therapy is not well supported by evidence but it does reduce the probability that the pathogen is resistant to the drugs being given. If an extended-spectrum β-lactamase-producing strain or an *Acinetobacter* sp. is suspected, a carbapenem should be given. If *Legionella pneumophilia* is suspected, use a quinolone. Risk factors for MRSA infection in areas with a high incidence of MRSA include diabetes mellitus, head trauma, coma and renal failure.

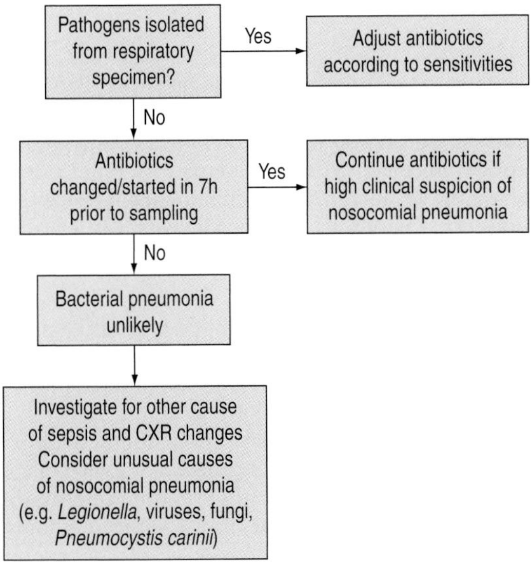

Figure 32.3 Subsequent management of nosocomial pneumonia based on a non-invasive clinical approach.[1]

RESPONSE TO THERAPY

Clinical improvement is usually not apparent for 48–72 hours and therapy should not be changed in this time. The CXR is of limited value for assessing response: initial deterioration is common and improvement often lags behind clinical response. However a rapidly deteriorating CXR pattern with a > 50% increase in size of infiltrate in 48 hours, new cavitation or a significant new pleural effusion should raise concern. If the patient fails to respond consider the diagnosis, host factors (e.g. immunosuppressed, debilitated), bacterial factors (e.g. virulent organism) and therapeutic factors (e.g. wrong drug, inadequate dose). Review the antibiotics and repeat cultures. It may be useful to broaden the antimicrobial cover while waiting for the results of investigations. Consider invasive sampling of respiratory secretions, computed tomography or ultrasound of the chest (to look for an empyema or abscess), another source of infection, open-lung biopsy to establish diagnosis and aetiology, or administration of steroids.

PREVENTION

A number of measures have been shown to reduce the incidence of ventilator-associated pneumonia.[25–31] Measures recommended by the Centers for Disease Control (CDC) include hand-washing, nursing patients in a 30° head-up position, subglottic aspiration of secretions, orotracheal rather than nasotracheal intubation, changing the breathing circuit only when visibly soiled or mechanically malfunctioning and preferential use of non-invasive ventilation. CDC guidelines can be accessed via the link page: http://www.aic.cuhk.edu.hk/web8/Pneumonia guidelines.htm.

TUBERCULOSIS

The main risk factors are listed in Table 32.3. Typical clinical features include fever, sweating, weight loss, lassitude, anorexia, cough productive of mucoid or purulent sputum,

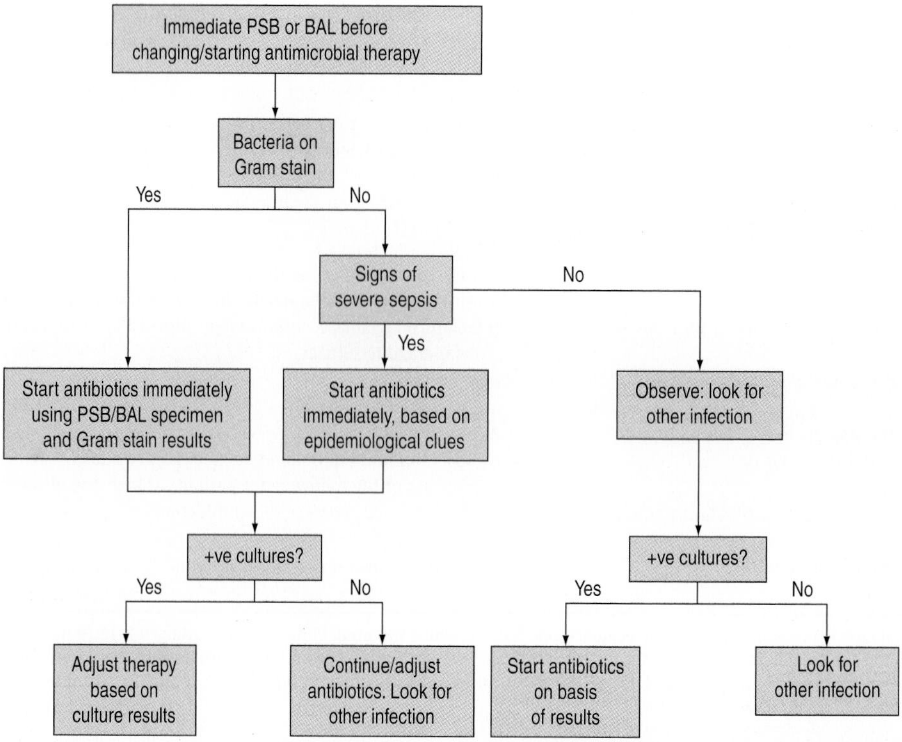

Figure 32.4 Management of suspected nosocomial pneumonia based on invasive sampling of respiratory secretions.

haemoptysis, chest wall pain, dyspnoea, localised wheeze and apical crackles. Patients may also present with unresolved pneumonia, pleural effusions, spontaneous pneumothorax and hoarseness or with enlarged cervical nodes or other manifestations of extrapulmonary disease. Clinical disease is seldom found in asymptomatic individuals, even those with strongly positive tuberculin test (Heaf grade III or IV). Older patients, who may have coexistent chronic bronchitis, can be missed unless a CXR is taken. The outlook for patients with TB who require ICU admission is poor. In one retrospective study the in-hospital mortality for all patients with TB requiring ICU admission was 67% but in those with acute respiratory failure it rose to 81%.[32] The presentation and management of TB in HIV-positive patients is different (see below).

INVESTIGATION OF PULMONARY TUBERCULOSIS

IDENTIFICATION OF MYCOBACTERIA[33]

Multiple (3–6) sputum samples should be collected, preferably on different days, for microscopy for AFB and culture. If sputum is not available bronchial washings taken at bronchoscopy and gastric lavage or aspirate samples should be obtained. Gastric aspirates need to be neutralised immediately on collection. Bronchoscopy and transbronchial biopsy may be useful in patients with suspected TB but negative sputum smear. Pleural biopsy is often helpful and mediastinoscopy is occasionally needed in patients with mediastinal lymphadenopathy. Part of any biopsy specimen should always be sent for culture. Nucleic acid amplification tests on sputum have a sensitivity similar to culture in smear-negative patients with pulmonary TB but have the advantage of a much more rapid result. There is, however, a significant false-negative rate.[34]

CHEST X-RAY

A normal CXR almost excludes TB (except in HIV-infected patients) but endobronchial lesions may not be apparent and early apical lesions can be missed. Common appearances include patchy/nodular shadowing in the upper zones (often bilateral), cavitation, calcification, hilar or mediastinal lymphadenopathy (may cause segmental or lobar collapse), pleural effusion, tuberculomas (dense round or oval shadows) and diffuse fine nodular shadowing throughout the lung fields in miliary TB. Inactivity of disease cannot be inferred from the CXR alone. This requires three negative sputum samples *and* failure of any lesion seen on CXR to progress. CXR appearances in HIV-positive patients with TB differ from non-HIV-infected patients.

TREATMENT OF PULMONARY TUBERCULOSIS[34,35]

The most commonly used regimen consists of a 6-month course of rifampicin 600 mg/day (450 mg for patients < 50 kg) and isoniazid 300 mg/day plus a 2-month course of pyrazinamide 2 g/day (1.5 g for patients < 50 kg) and ethambutol 15 mg/kg daily (streptomycin can be substituted for ethambutol). Ethambutol should only be used in patients who have reasonable visual acuity and who are able to appreciate and report visual disturbances. Visual acuity and colour perception must be assessed (if ethambutol is to be used) and liver and renal function checked before treatment is started. Steroids are recommended for children with endobronchial disease and, possibly, for patients with tuberculous pleural effusions. Pyrazinamide 10 mg/day should be given to prevent isoniazid-induced neuropathy to those at increased risk (e.g. patients with diabetes mellitus, chronic renal failure or malnutrition or alcoholic or HIV-positive patients).

INFECTION CONTROL

Patients admitted to an ICU with infectious TB or suspected of having active pulmonary TB should be managed in an isolation room with special ventilation characteristics, including negative pressure. Patients should be considered infectious if they are coughing or undergoing cough-inducing procedures or if they have positive AFB smears and they are not on or have just started chemotherapy or have a poor clinical or bacteriologic response to chemotherapy.[13,34] Patients with non-drug-resistant TB should be non-infectious after 2 weeks of treatment, which includes rifampicin and isoniazid.[34] As TB is spread through aerosols it is probably appropriate to isolate patients who are intubated even if only their bronchial washings are smear-positive. Staff caring for patients who are smear-positive should wear personal protective equipment including a fit-tested negative-pressure respirator (N95, FFP2 or higher). Use of a powered air-purifying respirator should be considered when bronchoscopy is being performed.[13] Detailed infection control advice can be obtained via the link page http://www.aic.cuhk.edu.hk/web8/Pneumonia guidelines.htm-.

PNEUMONIA IN THE IMMUNOCOMPROMISED

The lungs are amongst the most frequent target organs for infectious complications in the immunocompromised. The incidence of pneumonia is highest amongst patients with haematological malignancies, bone marrow transplant recipients and patients with acquired immunodeficiency syndrome (AIDS).

The speed of progression of pneumonia, the CXR changes (Table 32.6) and the type of immune defect provide clues to the aetiology. Bacterial pneumonias progress rapidly (1–2 days) whereas fungal and protozoal pneumonias are less fulminant (several days to a week or more). Viral pneumonias are not usually fulminant but on occasions may develop quite rapidly. Bronchoscopy is a major component of the investigation of these patients. Empiric management based on CXR appearances is outlined in Table 32.6. There is some evidence that early non-invasive ventilation may improve outcome amongst immunocompromised patients with fever and bilateral infiltrates.[36]

Table 32.6 Causes of chest X-ray changes and empiric treatment of pneumonia in the immunocompromised

Chest X-ray appearance	Causes	Empiric treatment for suspected pneumonia
Diffuse infiltrate	Cytomegalovirus and other herpesviruses *Pneumocystis carinii* Bacteria *Aspergillus* (advanced) *Cryptococcus* (uncommon) Non-infectious causes, e.g. drug reaction, non-specific interstitial pneumonitis, radiation pneumonitis (uncommon), malignancy, leukoagglutinin reaction	Broad-spectrum antibiotics for at least 48 hours (e.g. third-generation cephalosporin and aminoglycoside) Co-trimoxazole Lung biopsy or lavage within 48 hours or full 2-week course of co-trimoxazole (depends on patient tolerance of invasive procedure)
Focal infiltrate	Gram-negative rods *Staphylococcus aureus* *Aspergillus* *Cryptococcus* *Nocardia* *Mucor* *Pneumocystis carinii* (uncommon) Tuberculosis *Legionella* Non-infectious casues (e.g. malignancy, non-specific interstitial pneumonitis, radiation pneumonitis)	Broad-spectrum antibiotics If response seen, continue treatment for 2 weeks If disease progresses, lung biopsy/aspirate within 48–72 hours or empiric trial of antifungal ± macrolide

PNEUMOCYSTIS JIROVECI PNEUMONIA (PCP)[37]

The incidence of this common opportunistic infection has fallen substantially in patients with AIDS who are receiving prophylaxis and effective antiretroviral therapy, with most cases occurring in patients who are not receiving HIV care or among patients with advanced immunosuppression. The onset is usually insidious with dry cough, dyspnoea and fever on a background of fatigue and weight loss. Crackles in the chest are rare. Approximately 15% of patients have a concurrent cause for respiratory failure (e.g. Kaposi sarcoma, TB, bacterial pneumonia). Useful investigations are:

1. *CXR*: classical appearance is diffuse bilateral perihilar interstitial shadowing but in the early stages this is very subtle and easily missed. The initial CXR is normal in 10%. In a further 10% the changes are atypical with focal consolidation or coarse patchy shadowing. None of the changes are specific for PCP and may be seen in other lung diseases asssociated with AIDS. Pleural effusions, hilar or mediastinal lymphadenopathy are unusual in PCP but common in mycobacterial infection or Kaposi's sarcoma or lymphoma.
2. *Induced sputum*: in this technique the patient inhales nebulised hypertonic saline from an ultrasonic nebuliser. This provokes bronchorrhoea and the patient coughs up material containing cysts and trophozoites. The technique is time-consuming, requires meticulous technique and is less sensitive than bronchoscopy but less invasive. The possibility of concurrent TB should be considered and steps taken to minimise the risk of spread of infection.
3. *Bronchoscopy with bronchoalveolar lavage* leads to the diagnosis in over 90% of cases. Specimens should be sent for cytology. Transbronchial biopsy is not necessary in most cases.

Treatment should be started as soon as the diagnosis is suspected. Although there is some suggestion of potential benefit for early retroviral therapy for patients with HIV and PCP, some centres delay initiation of antiretrovirals until completion of PCP treatment in order to reduce the risk of an immune reconstitution syndrome. Treatment of choice is trimethoprim plus sulphamethoxazole (co-trimoxazole) 20 mg/kg per day + 100 mg/kg per day for 3 weeks plus prednisolone 40 mg orally twice daily for 5 days followed by 20 mg twice daily for 5 days and then 20 mg/day until the end of PCP treatment. Side-effects of co-trimoxazole are common in HIV patients (nausea, vomiting, skin rash, myelotoxicity). The dose should be reduced by 25% if the WBC count falls. Patients who are intolerant of co-trimoxazole should be treated with:

- pentamidine 4 mg/kg per day IV *or*
- primaquine with clindamycin *or*
- trimetrexate with leucovorin (± oral dapsone)

Response to treatment is usually excellent, with a response time of 4–7 days. If the patient deteriorates or fails to improve: consider (re-) bronchoscopy (is the diagnosis correct?), treat co-pathogens and consider a short course of high-dose intravenous methylprednisolone and/or diuretics (patients are often fluid-overloaded). Approximately 40% of patients with HIV-related PCP who require mechanical ventilation survive to hospital discharge.[38]

BACTERIAL PNEUMONIA[37]

This is the most common cause of acute respiratory failure in HIV-positive patients. Bacterial pneumonia is more common in HIV-infected patients than in the general population and tends to be more severe. *Streptococcus pneumoniae, Haemophilus influenzae, Pseudomonas aeruginosa* and *Staphylococcus aureus* are the commonest organisms. *Nocardia* and Gram-negatives should also be considered. Atypical pathogens (e.g. *Legionella*) are rare. Response to appropriate antibiotics is usually good but may require protracted courses of antibiotics because of high tendency to relapse. Patients with severe immunodeficiency (CD4$^+$ T-lymphocyte count < 100/μl) and a history of *Pseudomonas* infection or bronchiectasis or neutropenia should receive antibiotics that cover *P. aeruginosa* as well as other Gram-negatives. The possibility of concurrent PCP or TB should be excluded.

TUBERCULOSIS

TB may be the initial presentation of AIDS, particularly in sub-Saharan Africa. The pattern of TB in HIV patients depends on the degree of immunosuppression. In patients with CD4$^+$ T lymphocytes > 350 cells/μl the clinical presentation is similar to TB in non-HIV-infected patients, although extrapulmonary disease is more common. In patients with CD4$^+$ T lymphocytes < 350 cells/μl extrapulmonary disease (pleuritis, pericarditis, meningitis) is common. Severely immunocompromised patients (CD4$^+$ T lymphocytes < 100 cells/μl) may present with severe systemic disease with high fever, rapid progression and systemic sepsis. In these patients lower and middle-lobe disease is more common, miliary disease is common and cavitation is less common. Sputum smears and culture may be positive even with a normal CXR.

Response to treatment is usually rapid. Complex interactions occur between rifamycins (e.g. rifampicin and rifabutin) and protease inhibitors and non-nucleosidase reverse transcriptase inhibitors used to treat patients infected with HIV. The choice of rifampicin or rifabutin depends on a number of factors, including the unique and synergistic adverse effects for each individual combination of rifampicin and anti-HIV drugs and consultation with a physician with experience in treating both TB and HIV is advised.[39] Infectious Diseases Society of America-recommended dosage adjustment for patients receiving antiretrovirals and rifabutin[37] can be obtained via the link page: http://www.aic.cuhk.edu.hk/web8/Pneumonia

guidelines.htm. The optimal time for initiating antiretroviral therapy in patients with TB is controversial. Early therapy may decrease HIV disease progression but may be associated with a high incidence of adverse effects and an immune reconstitution reaction.[37]

CYTOMEGALOVIRUS (CMV) PNEUMONITIS[40,41]

Risk of infection is highest following allogeneic stem cell transplantation, followed by lung transplantation, pancreas transplantation and then liver, heart and renal transplantation and advanced AIDS. If both the recipient and the donor are seronegative then the risk of both infection and disease is negligible. If the recipient is seropositive the risk of infection is approximately 70% but the risk of disease is only 20%, regardless of the serostatus of the donor. However, if the recipient is seronegative and the donor is seropositive, the risk of disease is 70%. If steroid pulses and antilymphocyte globulin are given for treatment of acute rejection the risk of developing disease is markedly increased. Infection may be the result of primary infection or reactivation of latent infection. It is clinically important, but often difficult, to distinguish between CMV infection and CMV disease and a definitive diagnosis can only be made histologically. Detection of CMV-pp65 antigen in peripheral WBCs and detection of CMV DNA or RNA in the blood by quantitative polymerase chain reaction are the most useful tests for demonstrating CMV disease. Using thresholds of 10/300 000–50/200 000 positive circulating peripheral WBC, the positive predictive value for CMV-pp65 ranges from 64% to 82% and the negative predictive value from 70% to 95%.[42–44] Treatment consists of intravenous ganciclovir for at least 14 days. Foscarnet can be used if ganciclovir fails.

FUNGAL PNEUMONIA

Fungi are rare but important causes of pneumonia. They can be divided into two main groups based on the immune response required to combat infection with these organisms. *Histoplasma*, blastomycosis, coccidioidomycosis, paracoccidioidomycosis and *Cryptococcus* require specific cell-mediated immunity for their control and thus, in contrast to infections which are controlled by phagocytic activity, the diseases caused by these organisms can occur in otherwise healthy individuals, although they cause much more severe illnesss in patients with impaired cell-mediated immunity (e.g. patients infected with HIV and organ transplant recipients). With the exception of *Cryptococcus,* these organisms are rarely seen outside North America. *Aspergillus* and *Mucor* spores are killed by non-immune phagocytes and as a result these fungi rarely result in clinical illness in patients with normal neutrophil numbers and function.

CANDIDIASIS

This is effectively a combination of the two types of fungal infection in that impaired cell-mediated immunity predisposes to mucosal overgrowth with *Candida* but impaired phagocytic function or numbers is usually required before deep invasion of tissues occurs. Primary *Candida* pneumonia (i.e. isolated lung infection) is uncommon[40,45,46] and more commonly pulmonary lesions are only one manifestation of disseminated candidiasis. Even more common is benign colonisation of the airway with *Candida*. In most reported cases of primary *Candida* pneumonia amphotericin B has been used. In disseminated candidiasis treatment should be directed to treatment of disseminated disease rather than *Candida* pneumonia per se.[46]

INVASIVE ASPERGILLOSIS[47]

This is a highly lethal condition in the immunocompromised despite treatment and therefore investigation and treatment should be prompt and aggressive. Definitive diagnosis requires both histological evidence of acute-angle branching, septated nonpigmented hyphae measuring 2–4 μm in width and cultures yielding *Aspergillus* species from biopsy specimens of involved organs. Recovery of *Aspergillus* species from respiratory secretions in immunocompromised, but not immunocompetent, patients may indicate invasive disease with a positive predictive value as high as 80–90% in patients with leukaemia or bone marrow transplant recipients. Bronchoalveolar lavage with smear, culture and antigen detection has excellent specificity and reasonably good positive predictive value for invasive aspergillosis in immunocompromised patients. Although radiological features may give a clue to the diagnosis they are not sufficiently specific to be diagnostic. Characteristic CXR features (wedge-shaped pleural-based densities or cavities) occur late. The 'halo sign' (area of low attenuation surrounding a nodular lung lesion) is an early computed tomography finding whereas the 'crescent sign' (an air crescent near the periphery of a lung nodule) is a late feature.

In acutely ill immunocompromised patients intravenous therapy should be initiated if there is suggestive evidence of invasive aspergillosis while further investigations to confirm or refute the diagnosis are carried out. First-line therapy is voriaconazole.[48] Caspofungin and amphotericin are alternatives.

PARAPNEUMONIC EFFUSION

This may be an uncomplicated effusion which resolves with appropriate treatment of the underlying pneumonia or a complicated effusion which develops into an empyema unless drained. Complicated effusions tend to develop 7–14 days after initial fluid formation. They are characterised by increasing pleural fluid volume, continued fever and pleural fluid of low pH (< 7.3) which contains a large number of neutrophils and may reveal organisms on Gram staining or culture. An outline of management is given in Figure 32.5.

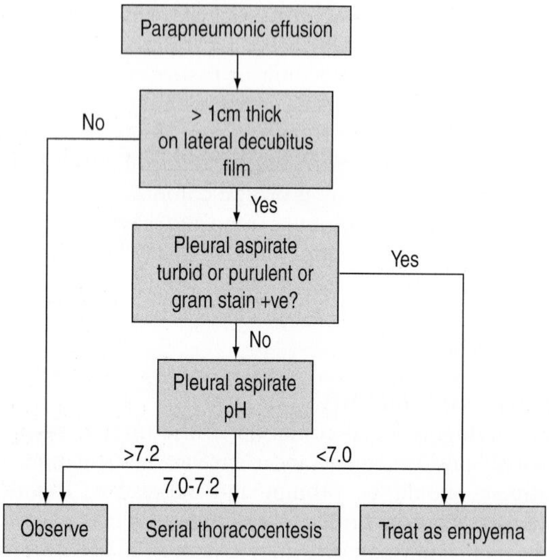

Figure 32.5 An approach to the management of parapneumonic effusions.

EMPYEMA[49]

DEFINITION

An empyema is a collection of pus in the pleural space.

AETIOLOGY

An empyema arises following infection of the structures surrounding the pleural space, including subdiaphragmatic structures, and chest trauma or may be associated with malignancy. Anaerobic bacteria, usually streptococci or Gram-negative rods, are responsible for 76% of cases.

DIAGNOSIS

The diagnosis is simple. The patient is usually septic and may have a productive cough and chest pain. The CXR may show features suggestive of a pleural effusion and underlying consolidation but may also show an abscess cavity with a fluid level, in which case computed tomography scanning will be required to distinguish between an abscess and an empyema. Ultrasound can be useful to confirm the presence of fluid in the pleural space and to determine whether it can be drained by needle aspiration or, if there is debris within the fluid, drainage using an intercostal drain. The diagnosis is confirmed by aspiration of pus.

TREATMENT

The mainstay of treatment is drainage either by intercostal drain or by surgical intervention. Patients who present before the pus is loculated and a fibrinous peel has formed on the lung can usually be treated by simple drainage. The combination with intrapleural fibrinolysis may be beneficial.[50] Optimal surgical management, which consists of decortication (open or thoracoscopic), is indicated if the empyema is more advanced or if simple drainage fails. This is a major procedure and many patients with cardiac or chronic respiratory disease will not tolerate it. Alternatives for these patients are instillation of thrombolytics into the pleural space or thoracostomy. Antibiotics have only an adjunctive role. Broad-spectrum antibiotic regimes with anaerobic cover should be used until the results of microbiological analysis of the aspirated pus are available.

ACKNOWLEDGEMENTS

All tables and figures are reproduced from http://www.aic.cuhk.edu.hk/web8 with permission of the author.

REFERENCES

1. American Thoracic Society and Infectious Diseases Society of America. Guidelines for the management of adults with hospital-acquired, ventilator-associated, and health care associated pneumonia. *Am J Respir Crit Care Med* 2005; **171**: 388–416.
2. Mandell LA, Marrie TJ, Grossman RF *et al.* Canadian guidelines for the initial management of community-acquired pneumonia: an evidence-based update by the Canadian Infectious Diseases Society and the Canadian Thoracic Society. *Clin Infect Dis* 2001; **31**: 383–421.
3. American Thoracic Society. Guidelines for the management of adults with community-acquired pneumonia. *Am J Respir Crit Care Med* 2001; **163**: 1730–54.
4. Fang GD, Fine M, Orloff J *et al.* New and emerging etiologies for community-acquired pneumonia with implications for therapy. A prospective multicenter study of 359 cases. *Medicine (Baltimore)* 1990; **69**: 307–16.
5. Dupont H, Mentec H, Sollet JP *et al.* Impact of appropriateness of initial antibiotic therapy on the outcome of ventilator-associated pneumonia. *Intens Care Med* 2001; **27**: 355–62.
6. Namias N, Samiian L, Nino D *et al.* Incidence and susceptibility of pathogenic bacteria vary between intensive care units within a single hospital: implications for empiric antibiotic strategies. *J Trauma* 2001; **49**: 638–46.
7. Mandell LA, Wunderink RG, Anzueto A *et al.* Infectious Diseases Society of America/American Thoracic Society consensus guidelines on the management of community-acquired pneumonia in adults. *Clin Infect Dis* 2007; **44**: S27–72.
8. Woodhead M, Blasi F, Ewig S *et al.* Guidelines for the management of adult lower respiratory tract infections. *Eur Respir J* 2005; **26**: 1138–80.
9. Bartlett JG, Dowell SF, Mandell LA *et al.* Practice guidelines for the management of community-acquired pneumonia in adults. *Clin Infect Dis* 2000; **31**: 347–82.
10. File TM, Jr. Community-acquired pneumonia. *Lancet* 2003; **362**: 1991–2001.
11. van der Eerden MM, Vlaspolder F, de Graaff CS *et al.* Value of intensive diagnostic microbiological investigation in low- and high-risk patients with

community-acquired pneumonia. *Eur J Clin Micro Infect Dis* 2005; **24**: 241–9.
12. Meduri GU, Chastre J. The standardization of bronchoscopic techniques for ventilator-associated pneumonia. *Chest* 1992; **102**: 557S–64S.
13. Centers for Disease Control and Prevention. Guidelines for preventing the transmission of *Mycobacterium tuberculosis* in health-care settings, 2005. *MMWR Morbid Mortal Week Rep* 2005; **54**: 1–141.
14. Dellinger RP, Carlet JM, Masur H *et al.* Surviving Sepsis Campaign guidelines for management of severe sepsis and septic shock. *Intens Care Med* 2004; **30**: 536–55.
15. Waterer GW, Somes GW, Wunderink RG. Monotherapy may be suboptimal for severe bacteremic pneumococcal pneumonia. *Arch Intern Med* 2001; **161**: 1837–42.
16. Jefferson T, Demicheli V, Deeks J *et al.* Neuraminidase inhibitors for preventing and treating influenza in healthy adults. *Cochrane Database Syst Rev* 2000; CD001265.
17. Gruber PC, Gomersall CD, Joynt GM. Avian influenza (H5N1): implications for intensive care. *Intens Care Med* 2006; **32**: 823–9.
18. Dunbar LM, Wunderink RG, Habib MP *et al.* High-dose, short-course levofloxacin for community-acquired pneumonia: a new treatment paradigm. *Clin Infect Dis* 2003; **37**: 752–60.
19. O'Grady NP, Barie PS, Bartlett JG *et al.* Practice guidelines for evaluating new fever in critically ill adult patients. *Clin Infect Dis* 1998; **26**: 1042–59.
20. Fagon JY, Chastre J, Wolff M *et al.* Invasive and noninvasive strategies for management of suspected ventilator-associated pneumonia. A randomized trial. *Ann Intern Med* 2000; **132**: 621–30.
21. Ruiz M, Torres A, Ewig S *et al.* Noninvasive versus invasive microbial investigation in ventilator-associated pneumonia: evaluation of outcome. *Am J Respir Crit Care Med* 2000; **162**: 119–25.
22. Kirtland SH, Corley DE, Winterbauer RH *et al.* The diagnosis of ventilator-associated pneumonia. A comparison of histologic, microbiologic, and clinical criteria. *Chest* 1997; **112**: 445–57.
23. The Canadian Critical Care Trials Group. A randomized trial of diagnostic techniques for ventilator-associated pneumonia. *N Engl J Med* 2006; **355**: 2619–30.
24. Chastre J, Wolff M, Fagon JY *et al.* Comparison of 8 vs 15 days of antibiotic therapy for ventilator-associated pneumonia in adults: a randomized trial. *JAMA* 2003; **290**: 2588–98.
25. Drakulovic MB, Torres A, Bauer TT *et al.* Supine body position as a risk factor for nosocomial pneumonia in mechanically ventilated patients: a randomised trial. *Lancet* 1999; **354**: 1851–8.
26. Bonten MJ, Kullberg BJ, Van Dalen R *et al.* Selective digestive decontamination in patients in intensive care. *J Antimicrob Chemother* 2000; **46**: 351–62.
27. Liberati A, D'Amico R, Pifferi S *et al.* Antibiotics for preventing respiratory tract infections in adults receiving intensive care (Cochrane Review). The Cochrane Library, Issue 2, 2001 Oxford: Update Software, 2001.
28. Nourdine K, Combes P, Carton MJ *et al.* Does noninvasive ventilation reduce the ICU nosocomial infection risk? A prospective clinical survey. *Intens Care Med* 1999; **25**: 567–73.
29. Guerin C, Girard R, Chemorin C *et al.* Facial mask noninvasive mechanical ventilation reduces the incidence of nosocomial pneumonia. A prospective epidemiological survey from a single ICU. *Intens Care Med* 1997; **23**: 1024–32 [erratum appears in *Intens Care Med* 1998; **24**: 27].
30. Combes P, Fauvage B, Oleyer C: Nosocomial pneumonia in mechanically ventilated patients, a prospective randomised evaluation of the Stericath closed suctioning system. *Intens Care Med* 2000; **26**: 878–82.
31. Valles J, Artigas A, Rello J *et al.* Continuous aspiration of subglottic secretions in preventing ventilator-associated pneumonia. *Ann Intern Med* 1995; **122**: 179–86.
32. Frame RN, Johnson MC, Eichenhorn MS *et al.* Active tuberculosis in the medical intensive care unit: a 15-year retrospective analysis. *Crit Care Med* 1987; **15**: 1012–14.
33. American Thoracic Society, Centers for Disease Control. Diagnostic standards and classification of tuberculosis in adults and children. *Am J Respir Crit Care Med* 2000; **161**: 1376–95.
34. National Collaborating Centre for Chronic Conditions. *Tuberculosis. Clinical Diagnosis and Management of Tuberculosis and Measures for its Prevention.* London: Royal College of Physicians; 2006.
35. Small PM, Fujiwara PI. Management of tuberculosis in the United States. *N Engl J Med* 2001; **345**: 189–200.
36. Hilbert G, Gruson D, Vargas F *et al.* Noninvasive ventilation in immunosuppressed patients with pulmonary infiltrates, fever, and acute respiratory failure. *N Engl J Med* 2001; **344**: 481–7.
37. Benson CA, Kaplan JE, Masur H *et al.* Treating opportunistic infections among HIV-infected adults and adolescents: recommendations from CDC, the National Institutes of Health, and the HIV Medicine Association/Infectious Diseases Society of America. *Clin Infect Dis* 2005; **40**: S131–235.
38. Randall CJ, Yarnold PR, Schwartz DN *et al.* Improvements in outcomes of acute respiratory failure for patients with human immunodeficiency virus-related *Pneumocystis carinii* pneumonia. *Am J Respir Crit Care Med* 2000; **162**: 393–8.
39. Centers for Disease Control. Updated guidelines for the use of rifabutin or rifampicin for the treatment and prevention of tuberculosis among HIV-infected patients taking protease inhibitors or nonnucleoside reverse transcriptase inhibitors. *MMWR Morb Mortal Wkly Rep* 2000; **49**: 185–9.
40. Tamm M. The lung in the immunocompromised patient. Infectious complications part 2. *Respiration* 1999; **66**: 199–207.
41. van der Bij W, Speich R. Management of cytomegalovirus infection and disease after solid-organ transplantation. *Clin Infect Dis* 2001; **33** (Suppl. 1): S32–7.
42. Camargo LF, Uip D, Simpson A *et al.* Comparison between antigenemia and a quantitative-competitive

polymerase chain reaction for the diagnosis of cytomegalovirus infection after heart transplantation. *Transplantation* 2001; **71**: 412–17.
43. Schäfer P, Tenschert W, Cremaschi L *et al.* Area under the viraemia curve versus absolute viral load: utility for predicting symptomatic cytomegalovirus infections in kidney transplant patients. *J Med Virol* 2001; **65**: 85–9.
44. Meyer-Koenig U, Weidmann M, Kirste G *et al.* Cytomegalovirus infection in organ-transplant recipients: diagnostic value of pp65 antigen test, qualitative polymerase chain reaction (PCR) and quantitative Taqman PCR. *Transplantation* 2004; 77: 1692–8.
45. Baughman RP. The lung in the immunocompromised patient. Infectious complications Part 1. *Respiration* 1999; **66**: 95–109.
46. Pappas PG, Rex JH, Sobel JD *et al.* Guidelines for treatment of candidiasis. *Clin Infect Dis* 2004; **38**: 161–89.
47. Stevens DA, Kan VL, Judson MA *et al.* Practice guidelines for diseases caused by *Aspergillus. Clin Infect Dis* 2000; **30**: 696–709.
48. Herbrecht R, Denning DW, Patterson TF *et al.* Voriconazole versus amphotericin B for primary therapy of invasive aspergillosis. *N Engl J Med* 2002; **347**: 408–15.
49. Peek GJ, Morcos S, Cooper G. The pleural cavity. *Br Med J* 2000; **320**: 1318–21.
50. Misthos P, Sepsas E, Konstantinou M *et al.* Early use of intrapleural fibrinolytics in the management of postpneumonic empyema. A prospective study. *Eur J Cardiothoracic Surg* 2005; **28**: 599–603.

33

Non-invasive ventilation

Graeme Duke and Andrew D Bersten

Non-invasive ventilation (NIV) is a valuable therapeutic option in the management of acute and chronic respiratory failure – for some diagnoses it is the preferred option. Successful use of NIV in acute respiratory failure (ARF) was first published in 1936,[1] and the use of NIV predates the introduction of laryngoscopy (early 1900s) and the widespread use of positive-pressure mechanical ventilation (MV) via an endotracheal tube (1950s).[2]

NIV is defined as ventilatory support without an (invasive) endotracheal airway. It has an increasingly important role in the short-term management of readily reversible ARF,[3,4] and in chronic respiratory failure due to obstructive sleep apnoea (OSA) and neuromuscular disease.

NIV may be achieved either through the delivery of positive airway pressure (P_{ao}) or the application of a negative-pressure generator to the chest ('chest box' or cuirass) or body ('iron lung'). A conceptual framework is shown in Figure 33.1. This chapter deals primarily with the use of positive-pressure NIV to treat ARF.

Negative-pressure generators may be used for the management of acute or chronic respiratory disease.[5] Major limitations to the use of negative-pressure generators include the induction of OSA, lack of fractional inspired oxygen ($F\text{IO}_2$) control, equipment bulk and size.[6] However, external negative-pressure generators suit some patients with chronic respiratory failure, particularly as there is no oral or nasal prosthesis.

The clinical efficacy of NIV depends upon: (1) the mode used; and (2) the nature and severity of the underlying respiratory disorder. Correctly applied, NIV can reduce morbidity and mortality, whereas inappropriate application may delay definitive therapy and adversely affect outcome. An understanding of the physiologic rationale for NIV will assist the clinician in understanding the indications and benefits, and predict the side-effects of the various NIV modes.[7,8] Many of the general issues regarding ventilation are discussed in Chapter 27, and this chapter will focus on those issues specific to NIV.

PHYSIOLOGY OF NIV

The physiological benefits of NIV are similar to those of invasive ventilatory support. The application of NIV can reverse many of the physiologic and mechanical derangements associated with respiratory failure through:

- augmentation of alveolar ventilation ($\dot{V}_A$) to reverse respiratory acidosis and hypercarbia
- alveolar recruitment and increased $F\text{IO}_2$ to reverse hypoxia
- reduction in work of breathing (W_{mus}) to reduce or prevent respiratory muscle insufficiency
- stabilisation of the chest wall in the presence of chest trauma or surgery
- reduction in left ventricular (LV) afterload that may lead to an improved cardiac function

The respiratory effort (pressure–volume work) required to achieve a desired minute volume ($\dot{V}_E$) may be viewed as the summation of the individual forces that must be overcome to generate inspiratory flow, namely: elastic work (or 'stretch'; W_{el}), flow-resistive work (airflow obstruction; W_{res}), and threshold work (W_{thres}). Since the volume component is constant the equation of motion can be written as:

$$P_{mus} = P_{el} + P_{res} + P_{thres}$$

See Chapter 27 for a more detailed explanation.

With the addition of a device for ventilatory support, the respiratory muscle effort (P_{mus}) required by the patient is equivalent to the difference between the applied P_{ao} and the total work required to maintain $\dot{V}_E$.

$$P_{mus} = (P_{el} + P_{res} + P_{thres}) - P_{ao}$$

This relationship may be rearranged into its individual components, as follows:

$$P_{mus} + P_{ao} = EV + R\dot{V} + \text{PEEP}$$

where E is the respiratory elastance (inverse of compliance), V is the volume of gas, R is the respiratory and circuit

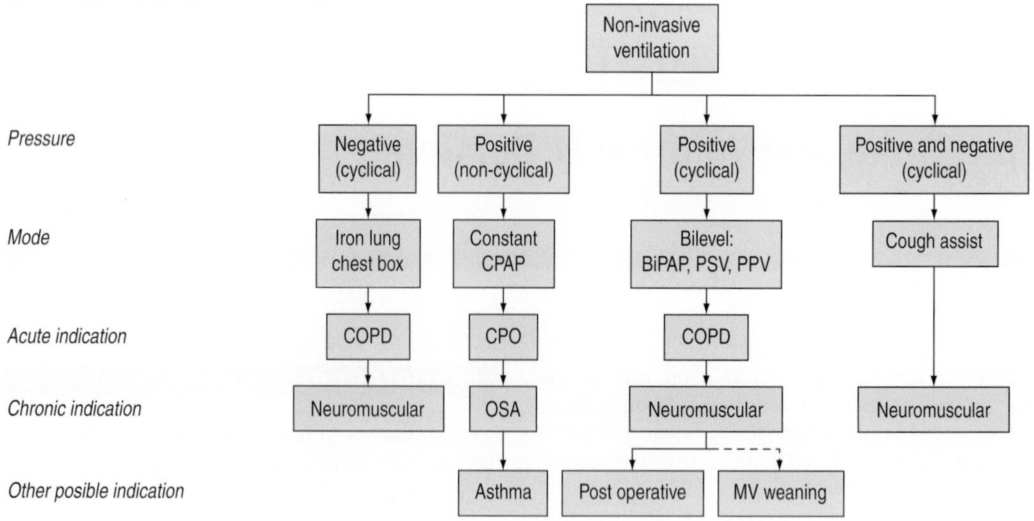

Figure 33.1 Conceptual non-invasive ventilation paradigm. See text for definitions.

flow-resistance, $\dot{V}$ is the inspiratory flow rate and $PEEP_i$ is the sum of the extrinsic and intrinsic PEEP ($\approx P_{thres}$).

It is important to remember that breathing via a circuit will create additional airflow resistance (R) adding to breathing work (P_{mus}), and thus attention to circuit design is important (see below).

$PEEP_i$ is absent in the healthy lung, but common in the presence of tachypnoea, airflow obstruction and dynamic hyperinflation. This threshold load must be counterbalanced by an equivalent amount of inspiratory effort before inspiratory flow can commence. Since threshold load impedes inspiration it will also impede the onset (triggering) of inspiratory support modes (inspiratory positive airway pressure (IPAP) and pressure support ventilation (PSV)).

Respiratory failure occurs when the forces opposing inspiration – namely elastic (P_{el}), resistive (P_{res}) and threshold ($PEEP_i$) work – exceed the respiratory muscle effort (P_{mus}) required to maintain $\dot{V}_E$. Hypermetabolic states (e.g. trauma, sepsis) increase basal $\dot{V}_E$, whereas pulmonary and chest wall diseases increase respiratory workload, and neuromuscular disease impairs respiratory muscle effort. NIV may prevent respiratory failure by counterbalancing the respiratory workload and/or reducing respiratory muscle effort, and thus maintain $\dot{V}_A$.

Although all invasive MV modes may be delivered non-invasively, four are commonly described: continuous positive airway pressure (CPAP); PSV; bilevel or biphasic positive airway pressure (BiPAP); and pressure- or volume-limited intermittent positive-pressure ventilation. Other modes under investigation include high-frequency and proportional assist ventilation.

All NIV modalities utilise closed (or semiclosed) circuits and are thus capable of controlling and delivering high FiO_2. This is an important mechanism by which NIV improves oxygenation, independently of other mechanisms discussed below.

CONTINUOUS POSITIVE AIRWAYS PRESSURE

CPAP is a form of NIV because it provides respiratory support even though the P_{ao} applied is constant throughout the respiratory cycle. This mode can address a number of objectives of ventilatory support, namely:

1. reduction in the work of breathing by:
   - alveolar recruitment leading to reduction in elastic work
   - reducing threshold load created in the presence of $PEEP_i$
2. reversing hypoxia through alveolar recruitment and reduction of intrapulmonary shunt
3. reduction of LV transmural pressure (afterload)[9,10]

INSPIRATORY POSITIVE AIRWAY PRESSURE AND PSV

Positive inspiratory airway pressure, without expiratory pressure (e.g. PSV or IPAP), provides respiratory support by reducing both the elastic and resistive components of respiratory work. This may result in:

- augmentation of tidal volume (V_T) and reduction in $PaCO_2$
- reduction in P_{mus} with reduction or prevention of respiratory muscle insufficiency
- induction of pulmonary surfactant release through alveolar inflation above resting tidal volume[11]

BILEVEL POSITIVE AIRWAY PRESSURE (BPAP)

BPAP allows separate settings for inspiratory (IPAP) and expiratory (EPAP) airway pressure levels, and is conceptually similar to PSV plus CPAP. Respiratory frequency is usually determined by the spontaneous rate but may be time-cycled and independent of patient effort. In some patients BPAP may not be as effective in reducing P_{mus} as the combination of PSV plus CPAP.[2,12]

CONTROLLED VENTILATION

NIV may also be administered as volume- or pressure-limited MV applied via a mask (instead of an endotracheal airway).

PATIENT–VENTILATOR INTERACTION

This is discussed in Chapter 27, and subdivided into: (1) triggering of inspiration; (2) inspiration; and (3) cessation of inspiration. The only aspect that is specific to NIV arises from mask leaks that may interfere with the ability to sense the end of expiration because there is continued 'expiratory' gas flow.

NON-INVASIVE VENTILATION EQUIPMENT

Equipment design varies according to NIV mode and purpose (e.g. critical care or domiciliary setting), and significant variation in performance characteristics have been documented.[12,13] The important characteristics of an efficient NIV circuit include:

- High gas flow that can match the peak inspiratory airflow. Mechanisms to generate high flows include a pressurised gas supply, a gas turbine or a jet Venturi mechanism. A continuous-flow device often imposes less circuit work than a demand flow device.
- An expiratory resistor capable of maintaining the desired PEEP, yet offering a low resistance to expiratory flow to reduce fluctuations in the desired P_{ao}. This may be a threshold resistor or flow resistor. The optimal position for the expiratory valve is as close to the patient's airway as possible.
- Minimal-length, wide-bore tubing to reduce turbulence and flow resistance.
- A flow or pressure sensor for identifying inspiratory effort, and triggering positive inspiratory pressure support (e.g. PSV or IPAP).
- Ability to control and deliver a wide range of F_{IO_2}.
- Other desirable features include the facility to humidify inspired gases and nebulise drugs, and the provision for pressure relief safety valves, battery back-up, apnoea back-up support, acoustic suppression and monitoring of volume and P_{ao}. These features are less important for domiciliary (long-term) NIV equipment.

Many mask designs are also available and the optimal design depends upon the purpose and mode of NIV and patient anatomy and preference. These include intranasal, nasal, oronasal, full-face and helmet (full-head) masks. Desirable features of a mask include light-weight and transparent materials providing a comfortable air-tight seal with minimal dead space and separate inspiratory and expiratory ports to minimise airflow turbulence and rebreathing.[13,14] In lung model studies, expiratory ports over the nasal bridge reduce dead space,[15] which may prove to be clinically advantageous.

Mask discomfort, arising from the mask seal, air leaks, humidification or claustrophobia, is a common cause of poor compliance with NIV. Masks that cover nose and mouth tend to produce more reliable and constant P_{ao} because they are unaffected by mouth breathing, a common problem in the critically ill patient. Nasal masks are less restrictive on the patient's ability to talk, eat/drink and expectorate and have a higher compliance in longer-term and domiciliary applications. To compensate for air leaks effectively, nasal masks should be used with circuits capable of rapidly augmenting and delivering high flows > 100 l/min.

Fibreoptic bronchoscopy can be easily, and often safely, performed during NIV. In addition to the usual precautions regarding fibreoptic bronchoscopy, an orofacial mask with at least two ports is required. One of these can be modified to allow a simple valve for insertion of the bronchoscope, and the other used for NIV. Provided there is adequate NIV flow reserve during suction, this can be performed during all modes of NIV. This technique may allow both diagnostic and therapeutic bronchoscopy without intubation in critically ill patients.

COMPLICATIONS AND ASSESSMENT OF EFFICACY

Contraindications and complications specific to NIV are listed in Table 33.1. Most patients requiring NIV should be managed in a critical care ward with appropriately trained medical and nursing staff. Although the development of sophisticated, portable, non-invasive ventilators makes it

Table 33.1 Contraindications and complications of non-invasive ventilation

Contraindications
• Respiratory arrest
• Unprotected airway (coma, sedation)
• Upper-airway obstruction
• Inability to clear secretions
• Untreated pneumothorax
• Marked hameodynamic instability
Complications
• Mask discomfort, patient intolerance
• Facial or ocular abrasions
• Nasal congestion, sinus pain
• Oronasal dryness
• ↑ Intraocular pressure (particularly in patients with glaucoma)
• ↑ Intracranial pressure (particularly in patients with neurotrauma)
• ↓ Blood pressure (if hypovolaemic)
• Aspiration pneumonia (rare)
• Aerophagy and gastric distension (uncommon; routine gastric decompression is unnecessary)

easy to provide NIV in any environment, its benefits may diminish outside the critical care environment.[16,17]

Following the application of NIV reversal of hypoxia, and transient reduction in respiratory rate and effort are commonly observed irrespective of the underlying disease. Although these are important goals of respiratory support, they are a poor guide to the true efficacy of NIV. More reliable clinical measures of NIV efficacy include reversal of hypercarbia and sustained improvement in respiratory function. Efficacy of NIV should be assessed using outcomes such as rates of compliance, intubation, nosocomial pneumonia and mortality.

NON-INVASIVE VENTILATION AND ACUTE RESPIRATORY FAILURE[2,16,18]

CARDIOGENIC PULMONARY OEDEMA (CPO)[2,8,19]

CPO is a common cause of severe reversible ARF. Since the 1930s, a number of investigators have documented the therapeutic benefits of all modes of NIV – particularly CPAP – in the treatment of CPO. CPO leads to an increase in elastic workload (P_{el}) and, to a less extent, resistive workload (P_{res}) as a consequence of diastolic LV dysfunction, an increase in lung water and impaired surfactant function. CPAP reverses hypoxia, recruits alveoli and reduces intrapulmonary shunt and LV afterload. Redistribution of extravascular lung water from alveoli to the interstitial space is aided by recruitment of alveoli and surfactant production.

Over 20 prospective randomised controlled trials of NIV in CPO have consistently demonstrated physiologic improvements in hypoxic and hypercapnic respiratory failure, and a significant reduction in the need for intubation, hospital length of stay and improved survival (95% confidence interval (CI) relative risk (RR) = 0.38–0.90).[19] Even though the majority of these patients were managed in a critical care setting the average duration of respiratory support was much shorter for NIV (9 ± 11 hours) than those who required MV.[20]

The optimal mode of NIV in CPO appears to be CPAP alone. The optimal P_{ao} level remains to be resolved, although 10 cmH_2O appeared to be safe and effective in the majority of subjects. Whilst the addition of a differential inspiratory pressure (e.g. bilevel[21] and PSV[22,23]) appears to be as effective as CPAP, it does not appear to provide an additional outcome benefit[19] and may increase the rate of myocardial infarction[24,25] (95% CI RR 0.92–2.42).[19] Bilevel NIV and CPAP have equivalent impact on respiratory parameters, but may have different effects on myocardial function.[24,25] CPAP reduces preload and afterload[9,10] and myocardial catecholamine release[26] but the cyclical P_{ao} (of bilevel NIV) may cause preload and afterload to rise and fall during respiration.[2,27]

Current evidence supports the routine use of mask CPAP in moderate or severe CPO as standard therapy and as the first-line option for respiratory support.[16,28]

ACUTE RESPIRATORY FAILURE IN CHRONIC OBSTRUCTIVE PULMONARY DISEASE (COPD)

COPD patients have an elevated resistive work (P_{res}), often coupled with an elevated basal $\dot{V}_E$ and elastic work (P_{el}) as a result of the pre-existing parenchymal damage. Threshold load ($PEEP_i$) is frequently present as a result of airflow obstruction, and is exacerbated during ARF by further increased W_{res} and respiratory rate. Reversible ARF is a common complication of COPD.

Both CPAP and PSV reduce P_{mus} in intubated COPD patients weaning from MV. The importance of NIV in hypercapnic ARF is now supported by at least 14 well-performed prospective randomised controlled studies[18,29–31] in over 600 patients. Most investigators have demonstrated a low incidence of side-effects and a significant decrease in intubation rates and in-hospital mortality.[31] The meta-analysis of NIV trials reveals significant reductions in mortality (95% CI RR = 0.35–0.76) and the need for intubation (95% CI RR = 0.33–0.53) – the number of patients needed to avoid intubation or death were as few as 4 and 10 respectively.[32] Risk reduction appears to be proportional to the severity of respiratory acidosis.[33] The incidence of nosocomial pneumonia is lower with NIV[34–36] and this may explain some of the mortality reduction associated with NIV.[36] Nevertheless, mask intolerance, nursing workload and failure rates are greater than those reported with NIV in CPO.[2]

Current evidence supports the use of NIV in hypercapnic ARF as a component of standard therapy in COPD subjects. This is supported by many respiratory medicine societies throughout the world,[16,28,37] that 'patients hospitalised for exacerbations of COPD with rapid clinical deterioration should be considered for noninvasive positive pressure [ventilatory support] to prevent further deterioration in gas exchange, respiratory workload and the need for endotracheal intubation'.[16]

All modes of NIV have been shown to be effective but there are no comparative trials that address the question of optimal mode or pressure level.[16] Patients with ARF arising predominantly from airflow obstruction (P_{res}) and/or threshold load are likely to respond to CPAP. Most patients also have reduced alveolar ventilation, marked hypercapnia or respiratory muscle insufficiency and are therefore likely to benefit from the addition of inspiratory support, i.e. PSV, IPAP or non-invasive positive-pressure ventilation (NIPPV).

NIV is indicated in the presence of respiratory acidosis ($pH < 7.37$) or persistent breathlessness.[32,38] These patients should be managed in a critical care setting where appropriate equipment and skill are available[2] and reported outcomes appear better.[17,32] The level of inspiratory support (usually 5–15 cmH_2O) should be titrated to improve $\dot{V}_E$, as indicated by improvement in tidal volume and pH, and reductions in respiratory rate and Pa_{CO_2}. Low levels of CPAP (4–8 cmH_2O) should be titrated to minimise the patient effort required to trigger inspiratory assistance and the Fi_{O_2} titrated to reverse hypoxia.

Early predictors of NIV success in COPD patients include the pH and $Pa\text{CO}_2$, but not the $Pa\text{O}_2$, response within the first 2 hours of therapy.[32,39] Predictors of NIV failure include mask intolerance, severe acidosis (pH < 7.25), tachypnoea (> 35/min), impaired conscious state and poor clinical response to initial therapy.[39] Prior to the commencement of NIV the clinician should develop a clear management strategy for those patients who fail a trial of NIV.

Although reported success rates are high (70–90%), NIV failure (i.e. intubation) appears to increase with the severity of respiratory acidosis.[32,38] For the poorly compliant patient, reassurance and explanation together with a trial of different size and/or type of mask, or initiation with lower pressure settings, and brief periods off NIV will sometimes assist. Low-dose anxiolytic drugs may be beneficial where anxiety is a recurrent precipitant of tachypnoea, but should be used with extreme caution because of their respiratory-depressant side-effects.

Late failure (> 48 hours) occurs in 10–20% of patients[18,30,39] despite an initial improvement with NIV. This group of patients has a high mortality risk.[40] Whether their worse outcome is related to the severity of their underlying disease, or from delayed initiation of MV, remains unclear.

ASTHMA

Asthma is an acute inflammatory lung disease that increases resistive (P_{res}) and threshold ($PEEP_i$) respiratory work. Physiological and clinical improvement has been demonstrated in acute asthmatics with the application of CPAP[41–43] and bilevel NIV.[43–45] One randomised controlled trial of bilevel NIV titrated over 30 minutes resulted in significant improvement in forced expiratory volume in 1 second (FEV_1) and a lower hospital admission rate.[46]

The clinical role of NIV in the management of acute asthma and the benefit of differential inspiratory pressure, if any, remains to be clarified. We have found 5 cmH_2O CPAP to be effective in moderate to severe asthma not responding to continuous inhaled bronchodilators. Nebulised drugs can be effectively delivered even in the presence of a high-flow NIV circuit.[47] Controlled clinical studies with robust end-points are awaited.

ACUTE LUNG INJURY (ALI) AND ACUTE RESPIRATORY DISTRESS SYNDROME (ARDS)

Like CPO, ALI leads to increase in elastic workload (P_{el}) and, to a lesser extent, resistive workload (P_{res}) arising from an increase in alveolar–capillary permeability, the release of inflammatory mediators and impaired surfactant function. In contrast to CPO there is little supportive evidence for NIV in ALI and ARDS. Even though the addition of PEEP is important during MV for ALI or ARDS and NIV has a lower prevalence of nosocomial pneumonia,[34–36] current data do not support the routine use of NIV in undifferentiated hypoxaemic ARF.[48,49]

Despite numerous clinical reports of successful use of NIV in the setting of community-acquired pneumonia (without COPD) and other forms of ALI, the failure rate remains high.[31,48,50–53] This may reflect the differences in duration, severity and the pathophysiology of pneumonia, ALI and ARDS compared to CPO. Some studies showing apparent benefit have failed to exclude patients with CPO[54] or COPD[55,56] – specific subgroups known to benefit from NIV.

PNEUMONIA IN THE IMMUNOCOMPROMISED PATIENT

MV is associated with high morbidity and mortality risks in immunocompromised patients.[56–58] These patients may benefit from NIV[2] through a reduction in intubation and MV,[56,57] but it is unclear whether this translates into improved hospital survival[56,58] or not.[36,57] Whether NIV simply avoids a high-morbidity therapy (i.e. MV)[34] or selects those with a more readily reversible form of ARF and those more likely to survive is unclear. Nevertheless it seems reasonable, based on the current data, to offer NIV to these patients.[16] Once again, clear guidelines need to be established for the management of those patients who fail a trial of NIV and those in whom MV is deemed inappropriate or futile.

POSTOPERATIVE AND POSTTRAUMATIC ARF

ARF in postoperative and trauma patients may arise from a number of reversible pathological processes associated with increases in elastic workload (P_{el}) and impaired respiratory muscle function, including dependent atelectasis, impaired chest wall mechanics, poor cough, nosocomial infection, aspiration pneumonitis and non-respiratory trauma or sepsis.

Mask CPAP consistently improves physiological parameters (e.g. oxygenation and respiratory rate) and reduces the risk of intubation in general surgical[59] and cardiothoracic patients[60] with mild postoperative hypoxic respiratory failure, but evidence for an outcome benefit is lacking. It is possible that the addition of inspiratory support (PSV or BiPAP) may improve survival in certain subgroups, such as postoperative lung resection.[61] Many of these patients have underlying COPD, and extrapolation of these results to non-COPD patients awaits further study.

Mask CPAP has been shown to be superior to MV in patients with isolated severe chest trauma,[62,63] but the exact role of NIV is unclear. NIV is contraindicated in the presence of other significant injuries such as neurotrauma and intracranial hypertension and in the presence of an untreated pneumothorax.

NIV-ASSISTED WEANING

As a result of the demonstrable benefits of NIV in COPD and the widespread use of invasive PSV to assist weaning from MV, NIV has also been recommended to expedite weaning from MV by allowing early extubation,[63] and to treat failed or accidental extubation. The putative advantages relate to reduction in the duration and the risks of MV (e.g. nosocomial pneumonia).

For COPD patients, once again, there appears to be a survival benefit,[64] but this is less clear in other groups,[65] where controlled studies do not support an overall benefit.[16] Although NIV is an option for early weaning it is not a substitute for strategies to improve early access to NIV (to reduce the need for MV) and improve weaning success (to reduce the risk of premature extubation).

NIV AND CHRONIC RESPIRATORY DISEASE

NIV is an important modality for short-term assistance and long-term treatment of severe chronic respiratory failure associated with obstructive and central sleep apnoea syndromes,[16,66] and chronic hypoventilation syndromes associated with extrapulmonary disease such as neuromuscular disease,[67] and thoracic deformities.[68] There appears to be less benefit in chronic parenchymal lung disease, such as (stable) COPD and cystic fibrosis.[69]

These patients may require short-term MV or NIV in a critical care environment for respiratory support during an acute illness or as an aid to perioperative care. NIV (plus minitracheostomy for secretion removal) may improve outcome compared to intubation and MV[70] but failure rates appear to be higher than in acute hypercapnic COPD.[71] Alternatively these conditions may be first diagnosed during admission for treatment of severe ARF and, following recovery, will require assessment for long-term NIV.

NIV AND SLEEP APNOEA SYNDROMES[72,73]

Moderate or severe OSA results in nocturnal hypoventilation and episodic hypoxia that can lead to pulmonary and systemic hypertension, cardiac failure, and daytime hypercapnia and somnolence. Many of these complications can be arrested or reversed through the appropriate use of nocturnal CPAP.[16,66,74] Patients with suspected sleep apnoea require accurate assessment by a respiratory physician, including sleep studies, prior to the routine use of domiciliary CPAP. Occasionally bilevel or controlled ventilation will be needed when there is inadequate central respiratory drive. In many patients respiratory drive will improve, and they can then be managed with CPAP after a period of bilevel or controlled ventilation.

Intercurrent illness, surgery or the use of sedatives and opioid analgesics will increase the frequency and duration of hypopnoea, apnoea and hypoxia. CPAP should be available even for those patients who do not require admission to a critical care ward.

NIV AND CHRONIC HYPOVENTILATION SYNDROMES

Domiciliary NIV (predominantly using inspiratory support modes or NIPPV) should be considered in all patients presenting with severe chronic respiratory failure due to neuromuscular disease.[67,69,75] Early referral and consideration of domiciliary NIV are recommended because of improved outcomes[67,76] and quality of life. In cystic fibrosis patients it may have a role simply as a bridge to organ transplantat.[57,68] In direct contrast to the role of NIV in acute exacerbations of COPD, there is little or no benefit of domiciliary NIV in the presence of stable COPD,[16,37,71,77] unless one of the former conditions coexists.

Assessment of these patients for domiciliary NIV includes respiratory function tests, blood gas analysis, sleep studies, together with trials of NIV modes and pressure settings. In general, indications for long-term NIV include the demonstration of symptomatic respiratory failure, daytime hypercapnia and a significantly reduced (< 20% predicted) vital capacity. The use of nocturnal or intermittent NIV has been shown to improve daytime respiratory and cardiac function, to improve exercise endurance, to slow the progression of respiratory dysfunction and to reduce the frequency of hospitalisation.[67,76]

REFERENCES

1. Poulton EP. Left-sided heart failure with pulmonary oedema. Its treatment with the 'pulmonary plus pressure' machine. *Lancet* 1936; **231**: 981–3.
2. Mehta S, Hill NS. Noninvasive ventilation. State of the art. *Am J Respir Crit Care Med* 2001; **163**: 540–77.
3. Carlucci A, Richard JC, Wysocki M *et al.* Noninvasive versus conventional mechanical ventilation. An epidemiologic survey. *Am J Respir Crit Care Med* 2001; **163**: 874–80.
4. Demoule A, Girou E, Richard JC *et al.* Increased use of noninvasive ventilation in French intensive care units. *Intens Care Med* 2006; **32**: 1747–55.
5. Corrado A, Confalonieri M, Marchese S *et al.* Iron lung vs mask ventilation in the treatment of acute on chronic respiratory failure in COPD patients. A multicenter study. *Chest* 2002; **121**: 189–95.
6. Brochard, L. Negative pressure ventilation. *JAMA* 2003; **289**: 983.
7. Duke GJ, Bersten AD. Noninvasive ventilation for acute respiratory failure. Part 1. *Crit Care Resusc* 1999; **1**: 187–98.
8. Duke GJ, Bersten AD. Non-invasive ventilation for adult acute respiratory failure. Part 2. *Crit Care Resusc* 1999; **1**: 199–210.
9. Buda AJ, Pinsky MR, Ingels NB *et al.* The effect of intrathoracic pressure on left ventricular performance. *N Engl J Med* 1979; **301**: 453–9.
10. Naughton MT, Rahman A, Hara K *et al.* Effect of continuous positive airway pressure on intrathoracic and left ventricular transmural pressures in patients with congestive heart failure. *Circulation* 1995; **91**: 1725–31.

11. Nicholas TE, Power JH, Barr HA. The pulmonary consequences of a deep breath. *Respir Physiol* 1982; **49**: 315–24.
12. Calzia E, Lindner KH, Witt S *et al.* Pressure–time product and work of breathing during biphasic continuous positive airway pressure and assisted spontaneous breathing. *Am J Respir Crit Care Med* 1994; **150**: 904–10.
13. Lofaso F, Brochard L, Hang T *et al.* Home versus intensive care pressure support devices. *Am J Respir Crit Care Med* 1996; **153**: 1591–9.
14. Ferguson GF, Gilmartin M. CO_2 rebreathing during BiPAP ventilatory assistance. *Am J Respir Crit Care Med* 1995; **151**: 1125–35.
15. Saatci E, Miller DM, Stell IM *et al.* Dynamic dead space in face masks used with noninvasive ventilators: a lung model study. *Eur Respir J* 2004; **23**: 129–35.
16. American Thoracic Society. International Consensus Conferences in intensive care medicine: noninvasive positive pressure ventilation in acute respiratory failure. *Am J Respir Crit Care* 2001; **163**: 283–91.
17. Plant PK, Owen JL, Parrott S *et al.* Cost effectiveness of ward based non-invasive ventilation for acute exacerbations of chronic obstructive pulmonary disease: economic analysis of randomised controlled trial. *Br Med J* 2003; **326**: 956–61.
18. Meduri GU, Turner RE, Abou-Shala N *et al.* Noninvasive positive pressure ventilation via face mask. First line intervention in patients with acute hypercapnic and hypoxemic respiratory failure. *Chest* 1996; **109**: 179–93.
19. Peter JV, Moran JL, Phillips-Hughes J *et al.* Effect of non-invasive positive pressure ventilation (NIPPV) on mortality in patients with acute cardiogenic pulmonary oedema: a meta-analysis. *Lancet* 2006; **367**: 1155–63.
20. Bersten AD, Holt AW, Vedig AE *et al.* Treatment of severe cardiogenic pulmonary oedema with continuous positive airway pressure delivered by face mask. *N Engl J Med* 1991; **325**: 1825–30.
21. Levitt MA. A prospective, randomized trial of BiPAP in severe acute congestive heart failure. *J Emerg Med* 2001; **21**: 363–9.
22. Nava S, Carbone G, DiBattista N *et al.* Noninvasive ventilation in cardiogenic pulmonary edema. A multicenter randomized trial. *Am J Respir Crit Care Med* 2003; **168**: 1432–7.
23. Bellone A, Vettorello M, Monari A *et al.* Noninvasive pressure support ventilation vs. continuous positive airway pressure in acute hypercapnic pulmonary edema. *Intens Care Med* 2005; **31**: 807–11.
24. Mehta S, Jay GD, Woolard RH *et al.* Randomized, prospective trial of bilevel versus continuous positive airway pressure in acute pulmonary edema. *Crit Care Med* 1997; **25**: 620–8.
25. Sharon A, Shpirer I, Kaluski E *et al.* High-dose intravenous isosorbide-dinitrate is safer and better than BiPAP ventilation combined with conventional treatment for severe pulmonary edema. *J Am Coll Cardiol* 2000; **36**: 832–7.
26. Kaye DM, Mansfield D, Aggarwal A *et al.* Acute effects of continuous positive airway pressure on cardiac sympathetic tone in congestive heart failure. *Circulation* 2001; **103**: 2336–8.
27. Duke GJ. Cardiovascular effects of mechanical ventilation. *Crit Care Resusc* 1999; **1**: 388–99.
28. British Thoracic Society Standards of Care Committee. Non-invasive ventilation in acute respiratory failure. *Thorax* 2002; **57**: 192–211.
29. Bott J, Carroll MP, Keilty SEJ *et al.* Randomised controlled trial of nasal ventilation in acute ventilatory failure due to chronic obstructive airways disease. *Lancet* 1993; **341**: 1555–7.
30. Brochard L, Mancebo J, Wysocki M *et al.* Non-invasive ventilation for acute exacerbations of chronic obstructive pulmonary disease. *N Engl J Med* 1995; **333**: 817–22.
31. Keenan SP, Kernerman PD, Cook DJ *et al.* Effect of noninvasive positive pressure ventilation on mortality in patients admitted with acute respiratory failure: a meta-analysis. *Crit Care Med* 1997; **25**: 1685–92.
32. Ram FSF, Picot J, Lightowler J *et al.* Non-invasive positive pressure ventilation for treatment of respiratory failure due to exacerbations of chronic obstructive pulmonary disease. *Cochrane Database of Systematic Reviews* 2004.
33. Peter JV, Moran JL. Noninvasive ventilation in exacerbations of chronic obstructive pulmonary disease: implications of different meta-analytic strategies. *Ann Intern Med* 2004; **141**: 78–9.
34. Girou E, Brun-Buisson C, Taille S *et al.* Secular trends in nosocomial infection and mortality associated with noninvasive ventilation in patients with exacerbation of COPD and pulmonary edema. *JAMA* 2003; **292**: 2985–91.
35. Nourdine K, Combes P, Carton M-J *et al.* Does non-invasive ventilation reduce the ICU nosocomial infection risk? A prospective clinical survey. *Intens Care Med* 1999; **25**: 567–73.
36. Demoule A, Girou E, Richard JC *et al.* Benefits and risks of success or failure of noninvasive ventilation. *Intens Care Med* 2006; **32**: 1756–65.
37. Abramson MJ, Crockett AJ, Frith PA *et al.* COPDX: an update of guidelines for the management of chronic obstructive pulmonary disease with a review of recent evidence. *Med J Aust* 2006; **184**: 342–5.
38. Lightowler JV, Wedzicha JA, Elliott MW *et al.* Non-invasive positive pressure ventilation to treat respiratory failure resulting from exacerbations of chronic obstructive pulmonary disease: Cochrane systematic review and meta-analysis. *Br Med J* 2003; **326**: 185–90.
39. Confalonieri M, Garuti G, Cattaruzza MS *et al.* A chart of failure risk for noninvasive ventilation in patients with COPD exacerbation. *Eur Respir J* 2005; **25**: 348–55.
40. Moretti M, Cilione C, Tampieri A *et al.* Incidence and causes of non-invasive mechanical ventilation failure after initial success. *Thorax* 2000; **55**: 819–25.

41. Martin JG, Shore S, Engel LA *et al.* Effect of continuous positive airway pressure on respiratory mechanics and pattern of breathing in induced asthma. *Am Rev Respir Dis* 1982; **126**: 812–17.
42. Shivaram U, Miro AM, Cash ME *et al.* Cardiopulmonary responses to continuous positive airway pressure in acute asthma. *J Crit Care* 1993; **8**: 87–92.
43. Fernandez MM, Villagra A, Blanch L *et al.* Noninvasive ventilation in status asthmaticus. *Intens Care Med* 2001; **27**: 486–92.
44. Meduri GU, Cook TR, Turner RE *et al.* Noninvasive positive pressure ventilation in status asthmaticus. *Chest* 1996; **110**: 767–74.
45. Gehlbach B, Kress JP, Kahn J *et al.* Correlates of prolonged hospitalization in inner-city ICU patients receiving noninvasive and invasive positive pressure ventilation for status asthmaticus. *Chest* 2002; **122**: 1709–14.
46. Soroksky A, Stav D, Shpirer I. A pilot prospective, randomized, placebo-controlled trial of bilevel positive airway pressure in acute asthmatic attack. *Chest* 2003; **123**: 1018–25.
47. Parkes SN, Bersten AD. Aerosol kinetics and bronchodilator efficacy during continuous positive airway pressure delivered by face mask. *Thorax* 1997; **52**: 171–5.
48. Delclaux C, L'Her E, Alberti C *et al.* Treatment of acute hypoxemic nonhypercapnic respiratory insufficiency with continuous positive airway pressure delivered by a face mask. A randomized controlled trial. *JAMA* 2000; **284**: 2352–60.
49. Ferrer M, Esquinas A, Leon M *et al.* Noninvasive ventilation in severe hypoxemic respiratory failure: a randomized clinical trial. *Am J Respir Crit Care Med* 2003; **168**: 1438–44.
50. Abou-Shala N, Meduri GU. Noninvasive ventilation in patients with acute respiratory failure. *Crit Care Med* 1996; **24**: 705–15.
51. Jolliet P, Abajo B, Pasquina P *et al.* Non-invasive respiratory support ventilation in severe community-acquired pneumonia. *Intens Care Med* 2001; **27**: 812–21.
52. Phua J, Kong K, Lee KH *et al.* Noninvasive ventilation in hypercapnic acute respiratory failure due to chronic obstructive pulmonary disease vs. other conditions: effectiveness and predictors of failure. *Intens Care Med* 2005; **31**: 533–9.
53. Antonelli M, Conti G, Moro ML *et al.* Predictors of failure of noninvasive positive pressure ventilation in patients with acute hypoxemic respiratory failure: a multi-center study. *Intens Care Med* 2001; **27**: 1718–28.
54. Kramer N, Meyer TJ, Meharg J *et al.* Randomized prospective trial of non-invasive positive pressure ventilation in acute respiratory failure. *Am J Respir Crit Care Med* 1995; **151**: 1799–806.
55. Confalonieri M, Potena A, Carbone G *et al.* Acute respiratory failure in patients with severe community acquired pneumonia. *Am J Respir Crit Care Med* 1999; **160**: 1585–91.
56. Hilbert G, Gruson D, Vargas F *et al.* Noninvasive ventilation in immunosuppressed patients with pulmonary infiltrates, fever and acute respiratory failure. *N Engl J Med* 2001; **344**: 481–7.
57. Antonelli M, Conti G, Bufi M *et al.* Noninvasive ventilation for treatment of acute respiratory failure in patients undergoing solid organ transplantation: a randomized trial. *JAMA* 2000; **283**: 235–41.
58. Confalonieri M, Calderini E, Terraciano S *et al.* Noninvasive ventilation for treating acute respiratory failure in AIDS patients with *Pneumocystis carinii* pneumonia. *Intens Care Med* 2002; **28**: 1233–8.
59. Squadrone V, Coha M, Cerutti E *et al.* Continuous positive air way pressure for treatment of postoperative hypoxemia: a randomized controlled trial. *JAMA* 2005; **293**: 589–95.
60. Richter-Larsen K, Ingwersen U, Thode S *et al.* Mask physiotherapy in patients after heart surgery: a controlled study. *Intens Care Med* 1995; **21**: 469–74.
61. Auriant J, Jallot A, Herve P *et al.* Noninvasive ventilation reduces mortality in acute respiratory failure following lung resection. *Am J Respir Crit Care Med* 2001; **164**: 1231–5.
62. Bolliger CT, Van Eeden SF. Treatment of multiple rib fractures. Randomised controlled trial comparing ventilatory with non-ventilatory management. *Chest* 1990; **97**: 943–8.
63. Gunduz M, Unlugenc H, Ozalevli M *et al.* A comparative study of continuous positive airway pressure (CPAP) and intermittent positive pressure ventilation (IPPV) in patients with flail chest. *Emerg Med J* 2005; **22**: 325–9.
64. Nava S, Ambrosino N, Clini E *et al.* Noninvasive mechanical ventilation in the weaning of patients with respiratory failure due to chronic obstructive pulmonary disease. A randomized, controlled trial. *Ann Intern Med* 1998; **128**: 721–8.
65. Burns KEA, Adhikari NKJ, Meade MO. Noninvasive positive pressure ventilation as a weaning strategy for intubated adults with respiratory failure. *Cochrane Database of Systematic Reviews* 2003, issue 4.
66. American Thoracic Society. Indications and standards for use of nasal continuous positive airway pressure (CPAP) in sleep apnoea syndromes. *Am J Respir Crit Care Med* 1994; **150**: 1738–45.
67. Gomez-Merino E, Bach JR. Duchenne muscular dystrophy: prolongation of life by noninvasive ventilation and mechanically assisted coughing. *Am J Phys Med Rehabil* 2002; **8**: 411–15.
68. National Association for Medical Direction of Respiratory Care. Clinical indications for non-invasive positive pressure ventilation in chronic respiratory failure due to restrictive lung disease, COPD, and nocturnal hypoventilation – a consensus conference report. *Chest* 1999; **116**: 521–34.
69. Madden BP, Kariyawasam H, Siddiqi AJ *et al.* Noninvasive ventilation in cystic fibrosis patients with acute or chronic respiratory failure. *Eur Respir J* 2002; **19**: 310–13.
70. Vianello A, Bevilacqua M , Arcaro G *et al.* Noninvasive ventilatory approach to treatment of acute respiratory failure in neuromuscular disorders. A comparison with endotracheal intubation. *Intens Care Med* 2000; **26**: 384–90.

71. Robino C, Faisy C, Diehl J-L *et al.* Effectiveness of non-invasive positive pressure ventilation differs between decompensated chronic restrictive and obstructive pulmonary disease patients. *Intens Care Med* 2003; **29**: 603–10.
72. Giles Tl, Lasserson TJ, Smith BJ *et al.* Continuous positive airway pressure for obstructive sleep apnoea in adults. *Cochrane Database of Systemic Reviews* 2006, issue 3.
73. Kaneko Y, Floras JS, Usui K *et al.* Cardiovascular effects of continuous positive airway pressure in patients with heart failure and obstructive sleep apnea. *N Engl J Med* 2003; **348**: 1233–41.
74. Granton JT, Naughton MT, Benard DC *et al.* CPAP improves respiratory muscle strength in patients with heart failure and central sleep apnoea. *Am J Respir Crit Care Med* 1996; **153**: 277–87.
75. Annane D, Chevrolet JC, Chevret S *et al.* Nocturnal mechanical ventilation for chronic hypoventilation in patients with neuromuscular and chest wall disorders. *Cochrane Database of Systematic Reviews* 2000, issue 1.
76. Aboussouan LS, Khan SU, Meeker DP *et al.* Effect of noninvasive positive-pressure ventilation on survival in amyotrophic lateral sclerosis. *Ann Intern Med* 1997; **127**: 450–3.
77. Wijkstra PJ, Lacasse Y, Guyatt GH *et al.* Nocturnal non-invasive positive pressure ventilation for stable chronic obstructive pulmonary disease. *Cochrane Database of Systematic Reviews* 2002, issue 2.

34

Respiratory monitoring

Andrew D Bersten

Clinical examination and the trend of vital signs such as respiratory rate (*f*), and quantity and nature of sputum are extremely important in managing patients with respiratory disease. In particular, clinical examination should look for evidence of excessive inspiratory and/or expiratory pleural pressure changes and effort such as accessory muscle use, tracheal tug, supraclavicular and intercostal indrawing, paradoxical abdominal movement (which is suggestive of diaphragmatic fatigue[1]) and pulsus paradoxus. During spontaneous ventilation an excessive fall in blood pressure during inspiration (>10 mmHg) is found in a number of conditions such as cardiac tamponade, cardiogenic shock, pulmonary embolism, hypovolaemic shock and acute respiratory failure. A curvilinear relationship exists between the fall in blood pressure and the change in pleural pressure during inspiration; however, there is marked variation between individuals.[2] Consequently, pulsus paradoxus is most useful in following trends; a reduction in the degree of paradox may be due to improvement and a fall in the negative pleural pressure needed for ventilation, or due to respiratory muscle insufficiency, and an inability to generate the same negative pleural pressure.

Additional information can be gained from blood gases and pulse oximetry (Chapter 14), and capnography, ventilatory pressures and waveform analysis in patients receiving respiratory assistance. This chapter will focus on tests of respiratory function that are directly relevant to critically ill patients.

MONITORING GAS EXCHANGE

OXYGENATION

This is reviewed in Chapter 14, and is only briefly discussed here. Hypoxaemia may be due to a low partial pressure of inspired O_2 (rare), hypoventilation, diffusion impairment (rare), ventilation–perfusion ($\dot{V}/\dot{Q}$) mismatch and shunt. Inert gas analysis has been used to quantitate ($\dot{V}/\dot{Q}$) mismatch, and has demonstrated that hypoxaemia in acute respiratory distress syndrome (ARDS) is predominantly due to alveoli that are perfused but not ventilated (shunt),[3] consistent with computed tomography (CT) scan evidence of increased dependent lung density. However, inert gas analysis remains a research tool, and less direct methods, such as the alveolar gas equation, are used to assess hypoxaemia:

$$PAO_2 = \text{inspired } PO_2 - PaCO_2/\text{respiratory quotient}$$

where PAO_2 is the alveolar PO_2, and this is usually simplified to:

$$PAO_2 = (760 - 47) \times FiO_2 - PaCO_2/0.8$$

where 760 is atmospheric pressure in mmHg, and 47 is the saturated vapour pressure of water at 37 °C since gas at the alveolus is fully humidified. The normal PAO_2 to PaO_2 gradient is less than 7 mmHg, but increases to 14 mmHg in the elderly. This normal A–a gradient is due to some venous admixture through the lungs, and a small right-to-left shunt through both the bronchial veins and the thebesian veins of the coronary circulation. This equation removes hypercarbia as a direct cause of hypoxaemia, and an increase in the A–a gradient will usually be due to ($\dot{V}/\dot{Q}$) mismatch or right-to-left shunt. A commonly used alternative measure of hypoxaemia is the PaO_2/FiO_2 ratio. However, this does not account for the effect of a raised $PaCO_2$, and both measures are influenced by a number of factors (e.g. cardiac output, haemoglobin (Hb), FiO_2) in addition to the extent of venous admixture, which may be estimated from the intrapulmonary shunt equation:

$$\frac{\dot{Q}_s}{\dot{Q}_t} = \frac{Cc'O_2 - CaO_2}{Cc'O_2 - CvO_2}$$

where $\dot{Q}_s$ is the intrapulmonary shunt blood flow, $\dot{Q}_t$ is the total pulmonary blood flow, $Cc'O_2$ is the end-capillary O_2 content calculated from the PAO_2, and CaO_2 and CvO_2 are the O_2 contents of arterial and mixed venous blood respectively.

CARBON DIOXIDE

$PaCO_2$ is determined by alveolar ventilation ($\dot{V}_A$), and CO_2 production ($\dot{V}CO_2$):

$$PaCO_2(\text{mmHg}) = \dot{V}CO_2(\text{ml/min STPD}) \times 0.863/\dot{V}_A(\text{1/min BTPS})$$

where $\dot{V}_A$ is the minute ventilation ($\dot{V}_E$) minus the wasted or dead-space ventilation ($\dot{V}_D$). The modified

Bohr equation (assuming $PACO_2 = PaCO_2$) calculates the proportion of the V_T which is wasted ventilation (i.e. physiological dead space: V_{Dphys}):

$$V_{Dphys}/V_T = PaCO_2 - P\bar{e}CO_2/PaCO_2$$

where $P\bar{e}CO_2$ is the mixed expired $P\bar{e}CO_2$, and V_{Dphys} is composed of anatmical dead space (V_{Danat}) and alveolar dead space (V_{Dalv}) – notionally due to alveoli that are ventilated but not perfused. Normally V_{Dalv} is minimal and V_{Danat} comprises 30% of V_T. Since the volume of an endotracheal tube is less than the mouth or nose, and pharynx, intubation may reduce V_{Danat}; however, when the connection from the endotracheal tube is taken into account there is little change in dead space. Positive-pressure ventilation increases dead space by distension of the airways increasing V_{Danat}, and through a tendency to increase alveoli that are ventilated but not perfused. In patients with ARDS, marked increases in V_{Dalv} lead to marked increases in the V_{Dphys}/V_T ratio (exceeding 0.6), which is an independent prognostic factor.[4]

CAPNOGRAPHY

Capnography measures and displays exhaled CO_2 throughout the respiratory cycle, with sampling usually by a mainstream sensor since sidestream systems tend to become blocked by secretions. However, when capnography is used in non-intubated patients, sidestream sampling is commonly used (e.g. modified nasal cannulae). Infrared spectroscopy measures the fraction of energy absorbed and converts this to a percentage of CO_2 exhaled. During expiration the capnogram initially reads no CO_2, but as anatomical dead space is exhaled there is a rise in the exhaled CO_2 to a plateau which falls to 0% CO_2 with the onset of inspiration. In patients with significant respiratory disease a plateau may never be achieved. The end-tidal CO_2 ($PetCO_2$) is the value at the end of the plateau, and is normally only slightly less than the $PaCO_2$. However, this gradient will increase when alveolar dead space (V_{Dalv}) increases, such as low cardiac output, pulmonary embolism and elevated alveolar pressure. Consequently the $PetCO_2$ may not reflect $PaCO_2$ in critically ill patients. Nevertheless, in a stable patient the gradient will be fairly constant, and can be used to guide $\dot{V}_E$ during transport,[5] and when other factors including the adequacy of minute ventilation are unchanged, sudden changes in the $PetO_2$ may provide an early signal. Indeed, $PetCO_2$ directly correlates with cardiac output, and $PetCO_2$ monitoring has been used to assess adequacy of cardiopulmonary resuscitation, and its prognosis.[6]

The presence of exhaled CO_2 is secondary confirmation of endotracheal tube placement, and is commonly recommended even when the tube is seen to pass through the vocal cords,[7] since clinical assessment is not always reliable. Simple colorimetric devices may be used for this purpose. However, detection of expired CO_2 is not infallible[7] as false positives can rarely occur following ingestion of carbonated liquids, and false negatives may be due to extremely low pulmonary blood flow, or very large alveolar dead space such as pulmonary embolus or severe asthma. Monitoring with capnography has also been recommended for transport[8] and respiratory monitoring[9] in critically ill patients, and should be available for every anaesthetised patient.[10]

GAS TRANSFER (DIFFUSING CAPACITY)

This is a test of the transfer of a gas, typically carbon monoxide (CO), across the alveolocapillary barrier. The transfer factor is calculated as:

$$\text{Volume of CO taken up}/(PA\text{co} - Pc\text{co})$$

and, since CO is so completely taken up by Hb, $Pc\text{co}$ is taken as zero. This test is usually performed as an outpatient, is not usually measured in the intensive care unit (ICU), and diffusion abnormality is rarely a cause of hypoxaemia. The transfer factor is often corrected for lung volume since diseases such as emphysema and pulmonary fibrosis may affect both lung volume and diffusion.

LUNG VOLUME AND CAPACITIES (FIGURE 34.1)

The tidal volume (V_T) is the volume of gas inspired and expired with each breath, with the volume at end-expiration termed the functional residual capacity (FRC). If a forced expiration is performed the expiratory reserve volume (ERV) is expired down to the residual volume (RV). If a maximum inspiratory effort is made from FRC, this is

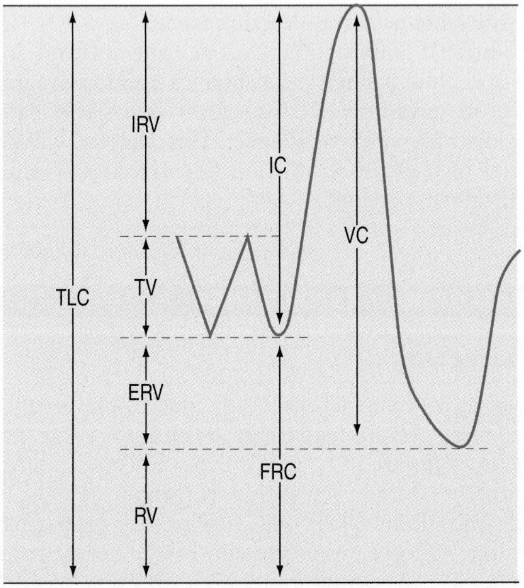

Figure 34.1 Lung volumes and capacities. TLC, total lung capacity; IRV, inspiratory reserve volume; TV, tidal volume; ERV, expiratory reserve volume; RV, residual volume; IC, inspiratory capacity; FRC, functional residual capacity; VC, vital capacity.

termed a vital capacity (VC) manoeuvre when the total lung capacity (TLC) is reached. Clinically, the most important of these are the FRC, V_T and VC, and the latter two are easily measured using a spirometer or integrated from flow.

TIDAL VOLUME

Minute volume is composed of f and V_T – normally ~17 breaths/min and ~400 ml respectively in adults.[11] Rapid shallow breathing is common in patients with respiratory distress, and in those failing weaning. Although a proposed index, an f/V_T ratio > 100 was initially shown to be highly predictive of weaning failure;[12] subsequent studies have reported varying results.

VITAL CAPACITY

At TLC the forces due to the inspiratory muscles are counterbalanced by elastic recoil of the lung and chest wall. Consequently, the TLC is determined by the strength of the inspiratory muscles, the mechanics of the lung and chest wall and the size of the lung, which varies with body size and gender (Table 34.1). Since the VC is the difference between TLC and FRC, factors that reduce FRC, such as increased abdominal chest wall elastance and premature airway closure in chronic obstructive pulmonary disease (COPD), will also reduce it. The normal VC is ~70 ml/kg and reduction to 12–15 ml/kg has previously indicated a probable need for mechanical ventilation. However, many other factors need to be considered, including the patient's general condition, the strength of the patient's expiratory muscles, glottic function and the use of non-invasive ventilation. Indeed, many chronically weak patients are able to manage at home with extremely low VC with the assistance of non-invasive ventilation.

Table 34.1 Factors that decrease vital capacity

Decreased muscle strength
• Myopathy
• Neuropathy
• Spinal cord injury
Increased lung elastance
• Pulmonary oedema
• Atelectasis
• Pulmonary fibrosis
• Loss of lung tissue
Increased chest wall elastance
• Pleural effusion
• Haemothorax
• Pneumothorax
• Kyphoscoliosis
• Obesity
• Ascites
Reduced functional residual capacity
• Atelectasis
• Premature airway closure (e.g. chronic obstructive pulmonary disease)

FUNCTIONAL RESIDUAL CAPACITY

Direct measurement of FRC is rarely measured in ICU; however, techniques such as nitrogen wash-in and wash-out[13] to estimate FRC are becoming available on modern ventilators. When FRC is less than the closing volume, the lung volume at which airway closure collapse is present during expiration, there is a marked increase in $\dot{V}/\dot{Q}$ mismatch. Consequently, positive end-expiratory pressure (PEEP) is commonly used to elevate FRC. Increases in lung volume above resting lung volume can be directly measured from a prolonged expiration to atmospheric pressure using either a spirometer or integration of flow,[14] or by repeated FRC measurements. FRC is decreased in ARDS and pulmonary oedema, in patients with abdominal distension and following abdominal and thoracic surgery. An increase in FRC places the diaphragm at a mechanical disadvantage, and is seen with severe airflow limitation and dynamic overinflation, and when there is loss of elastic recoil (e.g. emphysema).

MEASUREMENT OF LUNG MECHANICS

The forces the respiratory muscles must overcome during breathing are the elastic recoil of the lung and chest wall, and airway and tissue resistance. During controlled mechanical ventilation the ventilatory pressures reflect the work done to overcome these forces; however during partial ventilatory support the pressure at the airway opening reflects both these forces and those generated by the respiratory muscles. Estimates of respiratory mechanics are often readily available, and can assist titration of ventilatory support.

ELASTIC PROPERTIES OF LUNG AND CHEST WALL

The respiratory system (RS) is composed of the lung (L) and chest wall (CW), which is comprised of the ribcage and abdomen. Although it is often convenient to consider respiratory system mechanics as implying information about the lung, abnormal chest wall compliance can markedly influence these measurements.[15–18]

The pressure gradient across the lung (P_L) that generates gas flow is equal to the difference between the pressure at the airway opening (P_{ao}) and the mean pleural pressure (P_{pl}) which is estimated as the oesophageal pressure (P_{es}):

$$P_L = P_{ao} - P_{es}$$

Although the P_{es} is not always an accurate measure of the absolute P_{pl}, the change in P_{es} reflects the change in P_{pl}. However, this requires an appropriately positioned and functioning oesophageal balloon. In spontaneously breathing subjects a thin latex balloon sealed over a catheter is introduced into the lower third of the esophagus and P_{es} and P_{ao} are measured simultaneously during an end-expiratory airway occlusion. A well-positioned oesophageal balloon will have a ratio of $\Delta P_{es}/\Delta P_{ao}$ of ~ 1.[19] This technique is reliable in supine, intubated spontaneously breathing patients,[20] and in paralysed subjects it appears that a similar pressure change, induced by manual rib-cage pressure,[21] can be used to verify oesophageal balloon function.

Chest wall mechanics are derived from P_{es} referenced to atmospheric pressure, and in ventilated relaxed subjects respiratory system mechanics are derived from P_{ao} referenced to atmospheric pressure. It is not surprising then that $P_{RS} = P_L + P_{CW}$. Finally, abdominal mechanics can be estimated as either intravesical or intragastric pressure. However, despite these provisos, useful information can be obtained from respiratory system mechanics.

Measuring the slope of the *V–P* relationship of the lung or respiratory system allows a simple estimate of the elastic properties of the lung. This is termed the *elastance*, which is the inverse of the compliance. The E_{RS} is directly related to its components ($E_{RS} = E_L + E_{CW}$), and $1/C_{RS} = 1/C_L + 1/C_{CW}$. The normal E_{RS} is 10–15 cmH_2O/l and the normal C_{RS} is 60–100 ml/cmH_2O in ventilated patients. Since elastance directly refers to the elastic properties of the lung and respiratory system, mechanics will be described in terms of elastance rather than compliance.

MEASUREMENT OF ELASTANCE

Elastance and resistance are frequency-dependent, and respiratory mechanics depend upon the volume and volume history of the lung.[22] With increasing frequency of breathing, total respiratory system resistance falls and elastance increases, and this is particularly obvious in patients with airflow obstruction.[23,24] Consequently these factors must be taken into account when interpreting respiratory mechanics. In a passively ventilated subject P_{ao} is the sum of: (1) the pressure required to overcome airway, endotracheal tube and circuit resistance (P_{res}); (2) the elastic pressure required to expand the lung and chest wall (P_{el}); (3) the elastic recoil pressure at end-expiration or total PEEP (P_o); and (4) the inertial pressure required to generate gas flow (P_{inert}):

$$P_{ao} = P_{el} + P_{res} + P_o + P_{inert}$$

Since the elastance (E) is equal to $\Delta P/\Delta V$, with the resistance (R) equal to $\Delta P/\Delta \dot{V}$, and ignoring the inertance,[25] this can be rewritten as the single-compartment equation of motion:

$$P_{ao} = E_{RS}V + R_{RS}\Delta\dot{V} + P_o$$

Elastance can then be measured using either static techniques, where cessation of gas flow allows dissipation of P_{res}, or using dynamic techniques where flow is not interrupted.

END-INSPIRATORY OCCLUSION METHOD

The simplest estimate of E_{RS} can be made using a rapid end-inspiratory airway occlusion during a constant-flow breath, provided that the respiratory muscles are relaxed (Figure 34.2). If a plateau is introduced at end-inspiration there is a sudden initial pressure drop due to dissipation of flow resistance ($P_{pk} - P_1$) followed by a slower, secondary pressure drop to a plateau ($P_{dif} = P_1 - P_2$) due to stress relaxation. At least 1–2 seconds are taken for this plateau to be achieved, and P_2 is often called the plateau pressure; however, if P_{plat} is measured too soon it will lie somewhere between P_1 and P_2.

Stress adaptation

Stress relaxation of the respiratory system is due to both tissue viscoelasticity and time-constant inequalities of the respiratory system (pendelluft). In the normal lung pendelluft has a minimal contribution to stress relaxation;[26] however, heterogeneity of regional resistance and elastance can markedly influence stress relaxation.[27] Pulmonary surfactant and its contribution to changes in surface tension, parenchymal factors including elastic fibres in the lung, contractile elements such as the alveolar duct muscle and changes in pulmonary blood volume have all been implicated in the viscoelastic properties of the lung. However, it is not possible to separate either of these factors or the role of pendelluft in stress adaptation.

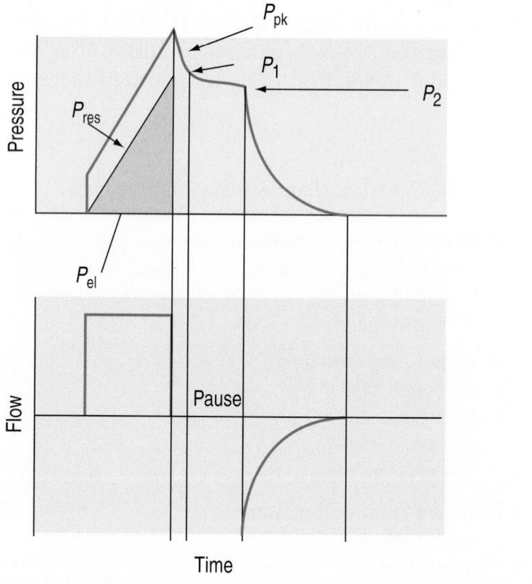

Figure 34.2 Schematic diagram of a volume-controlled breath with constant inspiratory flow. A period of no inspiratory gas flow has been interposed before expiration (pause) to illustrate dissipation of lung resistance as airways resistance (fall from P_{pk} to P_1) and tissue resistance (fall from P_1 to P_2). The inspiratory pressure due to the elastic properties of the respiratory system is illustrated as the filled area, P_{el}), and the lung resistive pressure is labeled as P_{res}. See text for more detail.

Calculation of respiratory mechanics

Returning to Figure 34.2, it is now simple to estimate respiratory system resistance and elastance from P_{ao}. The static elastance ($E_{rs,st}$) and the dynamic elastance ($E_{rs,dyn}$) are calculated as:

$$E_{rs,st} = (P_2 - P_o)/V_T$$

$$E_{rs,dyn} = (P_1 - P_o)/V_T$$

where P_o is the total PEEP (extrinsic plus intrinsic PEEP). The difference between $P_{el,dyn}$ and $P_{el,st}$ is the effective recoil pressure of the respiratory system during mechanical ventilation. Consequently, additional work is performed during inspiration to overcome stress adaptation, and this is stored and dissipated during expiration. This contributes to the hysteresis seen in dynamic volume–pressure curves during mechanical ventilation, and to the generation of expiratory flow. This latter component may be important in patients with airflow obstruction since the imposition of a pause at end-inspiration results in a 32% dissipation of the total energy loss within the respiratory system.[28]

THE STATIC VOLUME–PRESSURE CURVE

The quasistatic volume–pressure (*V–P*) curve has become the de facto 'gold standard' for the measurement of respiratory elastance. However, it is infrequently performed, and the relevance of a measurement performed on a single occasion is questionable when lung mechanics are not constant. Various techniques have been described, but the overall concept is that incremental volume and pressure points are made after a sufficient period of no flow has allowed P_{res} to be dissipated. This allows definition of a sigmoidal-shaped curve with upper and lower inflection points, and a mid-section with relatively linear *V–P* relations, allowing inflation elastance to be measured as this slope at a given lung volume. If similar measures are made during deflation a deflation curve and its hysteresis can also be described.

The *V–P* curve provides an advantage over an end-inspiratory elastance since, with the latter, it is not possible to know which part of the *V–P* curve is being measured. Consequently this 'chord' elastance may span either inflection point, yielding a falsely high figure. The upper inflection point represents a sudden decrease in elastance with increasing volume, and this has been interpreted as lung overinflation. The lower inflection point represents a sudden decrease in elastance with increased volume, and this has been interpreted as recruitment of atelectatic air spaces. Ventilation between these two inflection points should minimise both shearing forces secondary to repetitive collapse and reopening of alveoli, and overstretch of alveoli. However, this interpretation of the *V–P* curve has been questioned. In patients with acute lung injury recruitment occurs well above the lower inflection point, along the entire *V–P* curve and above the upper inflection point.[29,30] An alternative interpretation of these inflection points is that the lower inflection point represents a zone of rapid recruitment, and that the upper inflection point is due to a reduced rate of recruitment.[31]

Conventionally the static *V–P* curve has been measured in ventilated patients with the 'supersyringe' method.[32] In a paralysed patient the respiratory system is progressively inflated from FRC in 100-ml steps up to ~1700 ml or a predefined pressure limit. After each step sufficient time is allowed for a well-defined plateau to become apparent (using a pause of 3–6 seconds). The effects of temperature, humidity, gas compression and ongoing gas exchange during the manoeuvre need to be taken into account,[33,34] and the volume history standardised before it is performed. Since this technique is cumbersome and many patients become hypoxaemic following disconnection from the ventilator and the 60 seconds or so without PEEP, other techniques have been developed. The static *V–P* curve can also be measured by randomly inserting a range of single-volume inflations, followed by a prolonged pause,[35] during normal mechanical ventilation. This is performed in the paralysed state at 0 cmH_2O PEEP. This technique has a number of advantages, including its simplicity, the patient is not disconnected from the ventilator, the volume history is the same for each measurement and gas exchange during the measurement is negligible. However, again, many patients will become hypoxaemic due to prolonged periods without PEEP (this procedure may take ~15 minutes), particularly following a small-volume breath. Finally, an automated low-flow *V–P* curve method allowing subtraction of P_{res} has been described, and is now available on some modern ventilators; this takes around 20 seconds to perform, and seems to correlate well with the static occlusion technique.[36,37]

THE DYNAMIC V–P CURVE

Dynamic P_{ao}, $\dot{V}$ and V are displayed by many ventilators, but the volume signal is not referenced to FRC and the signals are not readily available for quantitative analysis. However, $\dot{V}$ is readily measured with a heated pneumotachograph, and volume can then be derived by simple integration if the signal is collected after analogue-to-digital conversion. If P_{ao} is also collected it is relatively simple to measure dynamic mechanics.

The dynamic *V–P* curve always shows hysteresis, mainly due to the effects of airway and tissue resistance; it is unlikely that hysteresis of the static *V–P* occurs during tidal breathing.[38] In contrast to static *V–P* relations, dynamic mechanics are collected during normal ventilation so they do not interfere with patient care, and they provide a 'functional' description of respiratory mechanics. Indeed the 'effective' alveolar distending pressure is more accurately $P_{el,dyn}$, not $P_{el,st}$. Since dynamic mechanics are potentially continuous they could also be used to servo-control ventilatory strategies.

There a number of ways to analyse dynamic *V–P* data. A line can be drawn between no-flow points at end-inspiration and end-expiration to determine elastance; however, this is relatively inaccurate as it is based on two points that can be hard to identify exactly. Multiple linear regression analysis is now the technique most commonly employed. The patient does not need to be paralysed[39] provided the respiratory muscles are not active during ventilation, and the signal can be split to allow analysis of inspiratory and expiratory mechanics.

Provided the model fit is acceptable, elastance and resistance are accurately and reproducibly calculated using the single-compartment equation of motion:

$$P_{ao} = E_{RS} V + R_{RS} \Delta \dot{V} + P_o$$

Static PEEPi is accurately calculated, as P_o – PEEPe, when compared to either an end-expiratory airway occlusion method,[40] or by direct measurement of end-expiratory alveolar pressure.[41] However, the single-compartment model only approximates the respiratory system, and frequency and volume dependence of the derived mechanics are observed. Provided these factors are recognised and accounted for, it is sound to compare data within and between patients.

A number of techniques have been used to analyse further dynamic V–P data. The most promising of these are the stress index derived from power analysis of the P_{ao}–t curve ($P_{ao} = a^t + c$),[42] and addition of a volume-dependent term to the equation of motion:[13,43]

$$P_{ao} = (E_1 + E_2 V)V + R_{RS} \Delta \dot{V} + P_o$$
$$E_{rs} = E_1 + E_2 V$$

Since power analysis requires a constant inspiratory $\dot{V}$ pattern to discount resistive effects, it is not as versatile as the volume-dependent technique; however, both measures correlate highly with each other, suggesting they measure the same parameter. The volume-dependent technique allows conceptual placement of tidal breathing on a dynamic V–P curve. If the $\%E_2$ is calculated as:

$$\%E_2 = 100 E_2 V / E_{rs}$$

then a $\%E_2 > 30\%$ quantitates high stress, often interpreted as overinflation, and a negative volume dependence (negative $\%E_2$) suggests significant atelectasis during tidal breathing. During constant $\dot{V}$ ventilation, and provided V_T is also constant, the change in either P_{pk} – $PEEP_{tot}$ or P_1 – $PEEP_{tot}$ (the delta pressure: ΔP) 20–30 minutes following a change in PEEP is highly correlated with $\%E_2$.[13] Using the 95% predictive interval for these data, an increase in $\Delta P > 2$ cmH_2O indicates overinflation, a $\%E_2 > 30\%$.

Similarly, a stress index of 0.9–1.1 suggests linear elastic mechanics during inflation; if the stress index is low then this suggests tidal recruitment, and a high stress index suggests overinflation. However, neither the stress index nor volume-dependent elastance has been validated in the clinical setting. High stress may not reflect regional lung hyperaeration; in COPD bullous lung disease is due to a loss of lung tissue and elastic recoil measured on CT as hyperaeration. However the associated wall stress may be high or low, depending upon the degree of inflation.

INTERPRETATION OF ELASTANCE

Elastance may be increased due to a reduction in lung volume or to an increase in specific elastance, the product of E and FRC. Small body size, female gender, lung resection and reduced aerated lung volume are important factors reducing effective lung volume, with this final factor one important reason for the elevated elastance seen in ARDS. Specific elastance is increased pulmonary oedema, pulmonary fibrosis, and reduced or dysfunctional surfactant.

MEASUREMENT OF THE RESISTANCE OF THE LUNG AND CHEST WALL

Lung resistance (R_L) is the sum of airway (R_{aw}) and tissue resistance (R_{ti}). Resistance is flow-, volume- and frequency-dependent, and R_L decreases as f increases. It is also important to compare measurements at similar lung volumes since there is a hyperbolic relation between lung volume and R. This is particularly obvious in ARDS, where the incremental administration of PEEP can result in a decrease in R_{aw} due to concurrent recruitment and an increase in lung volume. Indeed, although the absolute values are increased, when corrected for end-expiratory lung volume R_L, $R_{aw} + R_{ti}$ are unchanged in ARDS.[14] Finally, since gas flow may be a mixture of laminar and turbulent flow, resistance is often flow-dependent.

END-INSPIRATORY OCCLUSION TECHNIQUE

The total inspiratory airways resistance, including the endotracheal tube and associated ventilatory apparatus, can be calculated in a relaxed patient following an inspiratory pause (Figure 34.2) as:

$$R_{aw} = (P_{pk} - P_1)/\dot{V}$$

and R_L calculated by using P_2 instead of P_1. Since the endotracheal tube and apparatus will make a significant contribution to R_{aw} it is best to measure P_{ao} distal to the endotracheal tube with an intratracheal catheter. An alternative approach is to calculate and subtract endotracheal tube resistance using the Rohrer equation ($R = K_1 + K_2$),[44] and this is now automatically included in some ventilators. However, as in vivo endotracheal tube resistance is often greater than in vitro resistance[45] due to the effect of secretions and interaction with the tracheal wall, these corrections may be inaccurate. Despite these provisos, this simple measure of resistance, or the P_{pk} to P_{plat} difference at a constant $\dot{V}$, can be clinically useful in both the diagnosis and monitoring of airflow obstruction.[46]

DYNAMIC TECHNIQUES

Total, inspiratory and expiratory R can also be made, using either multiple linear regression analysis or from linear interpolation of the V–P curve at a constant volume.

However, this latter technique assumes a constant elastance during tidal inflation, and may be inaccurate because it relies on only two measurements. Finally, an average expiratory R can be calculated from the time constant (τ) derived from passive expiration if the E is known, since:

$$\tau = R/E$$

However, the lung does not empty as a single compartment in patients with airflow obstruction, and E is assumed to be constant over the tidal expiration.

OTHER MEASUREMENT TECHNIQUES

The interrupter technique consists of a series of short (100–200 ms) interruptions to relaxed expiration by a pneumatic valve.[47] This results in an expiratory plateau in P_{ao} following equilibration with alveolar pressure. From the V, P and $\dot{V}$ data expiratory elastance and the expiratory P–$\dot{V}$ relationship are measured. This technique does not make assumptions about the behaviour of the respiratory system and can identify dynamic airflow limitation.

Assuming that the respiratory system behaves linearly, it can be analysed following a forced-flow oscillation at the airway opening.[48] The resultant pressure waveform depends upon the impedance of the respiratory system, which can be analysed following Fourier analysis of the P and $\dot{V}$ waveforms into resistance and reactance. This will then allow measurement of R_{aw}, R_{ti}, E_{rs} and inertance, and information can be gained regarding small-airways disease by examining R_{aw} at different oscillatory frequencies.

FORCED EXPIRATORY FLOW

Maximum expiratory flow rates from TLC, the forced vital capacity (FVC), the forced expiratory volume in the first second of expiration (FEV_1) and the peak expiratory flow rate (PEFR) are commonly measured in cooperative subjects with a spirometer or flow meter. The PEFR is cheap but is relatively effort-dependent, and is less specific and reliable than the FEV_1. It is most useful for office or home use. The normal PEFR is 450–700 l/min in males and 300–500 l/min in females. It is reduced with obstructive diseases and gross muscle weakness.

The FEV_1 is usually expressed as a ratio of the FVC since both may be reduced in restrictive disease, with a normal ratio. The FEV_1 is normally 50–60 ml/kg and 70–83% of FVC. In asthma and COPD the FEV_1 is reduced out of proportion to the FVC and the ratio is less than 70%.

MEASUREMENT OF INTRINSIC PEEP

This is an important measurement in critically ill patients. PEEPi: (1) may have unrecognised haemodynamic consequences;[49] (2) adds an elastic load to inspiratory work during partial ventilatory modes, which may be reduced by application of small amounts of PEEPe;[50] and (3) reflects dynamic hyperinflation with the consequent risks of barotrauma[51] and right heart failure. If PEEPi is not taken into account during calculation of chord compliance, an incorrect denominator is used, which may markedly alter the result.[52]

The two most commonly described techniques for measuring PEEPi are end-expiratory airway occlusion in a relaxed subject, and the fall in oesophageal pressure during inspiration prior to initiation of inspiratory $\dot{V}$. However, these are not really comparable measures since static and dynamic PEEPi respectively are measured. Static PEEPi is measured as the plateau P_{ao} that is reached after ~5 seconds following an end-expiratory occlusion. With the cessation of gas flow alveolar pressure equilibrates with P_{ao}. Since the lung is composed of non-homogeneous units, this will represent the average static PEEPi. All respiratory effort must be absent since they may independently influence end-expiratory P_{ao}, and end-expiration must be accurately identified. This is most easily done by the ventilator itself either using an end-expiratory hold manoeuvre or by using the next inspiration, the onset of which is concurrent with expiratory valve closure, to close a valve that directs inspiratory flow to atmosphere and seals the circuit. Static PEEPi is a surrogate measure of dynamic hyperinflation, and this volume may be directly measured using a spirometer[49] or a pneumotachograph[13] during a prolonged expiration.

Dynamic PEEPi is measured as the pressure change required to initiate inflation. In ventilated subjects this will be the change in P_{ao} prior to initiation of inspiratory $\dot{V}$,[50] and in spontaneously breathing subjects the change in oesophageal[48] or transdiaphragmatic[53] pressure from their end-expiratory relaxation values prior to inspiratory $\dot{V}$. Measurement of dynamic PEEPi in spontaneously breathing subjects is not particularly straightforward. The changes in pressure are small and influenced by cardiogenic oscillations which are preferably filtered out.[54] Further dynamic PEEPi is not constant, with breath-to-breath variation probably due to variation in the extent of dynamic hyperinflation, and many patients with airflow obstruction have an active expiration. This 'falsely' increases PEEPi, at least with respect to its elastic load, since cessation of active expiration does not require work, with part of the measured elastic load suddenly dissipated.[55] Consequently, it is preferable to measure intragastric pressure concurrently as a measure of active expiration.

Finally, PEEPi can be measured as P_o from dynamic P, V and $\dot{V}$ data in ventilated subjects. This is thought to be a measure of dynamic PEEPi since static PEEPi systematically yields a slightly greater result,[40] with similar discrepancies reported between other dynamic measures of PEEPi and static PEEPi.[56,57] This systematic difference correlates with, and is thought to be due to, the viscoelastic properties and regional time-constant inequalities of the respiratory system.[56] This has clinical significance since, although matching dynamic PEEPi with PEEPe reduces respiratory work through a decrease in elastic load,[50] it does not counterbalance these forces, which represent an additional elastic load to inspiration.

PATIENT–VENTILATOR DYSSYNCHRONY

Dyssynchrony between the patient and ventilator is common during both intubated and non-invasive ventilatory support. Clinical findings include agitation and anxiety, tachycardia, tachypnoea and increased work of breathing. Failure to trigger the ventilator can be documented by comparing the frequency of ventilator breaths and inspiratory efforts. Bedside analysis of ventilator respiratory waveforms can be used to identify and help match ventilatory assistance to neural drive.[58]

INSPIRATION

TRIGGERING OF INSPIRATION

Ineffective respiratory efforts are best detected from the P_{es} waveform; however, this is rarely monitored. Ineffective triggering due to PEEPi may be detected from the expiratory $\dot{V}$ waveforms as abrupt decrease in $\dot{V}$ at either the onset of inspiratory muscle activity or relaxation of the expiratory muscles. Monitoring of P_{ao} is less sensitive unless the circuit expiratory resistance is increased (e.g. heat and moisture exchanger or poorly functioning expiratory valve) so that small changes in expiratory $\dot{V}$ are reflected in P_{ao}. Inadequate sensitivity may also lead to ineffective triggering with similar but more obvious waveform effects.

Autotriggering, a triggered assisted or supported breath without patient effort, may occur due to excessively low trigger threshold or due to P_{ao} or $\dot{V}$ distortion, as commonly seen with large cardiogenic oscillations, hiccups, condensate in tubing or a circuit leak. Again, waveform analysis may help detect and manage the problem; for example, it may be necessary to reduce trigger sensitivity to prevent cardiogenic oscillations from being detected as inspiratory effort.

INSPIRATION

During an assisted-volume control breath, P_{ao} may fall, often seen as a scalloped shape, if there is excessive inspiratory muscle effort as seen in $\dot{V}$ starvation. Expiratory muscle effort, as may be seen with an excessive V_T or prolonged inspiratory time (T_i), leads to a rise in P_{ao}. During an assisted-pressure control breath or during pressure support, changes in patient effort are detected from the $\dot{V}$ waveform. Finally, excessively rapid development of the set delivered pressure, a rapid rise time, may be detected by an overshoot in P_{ao}; an excessively long rise time will be seen as a rounded inspiratory $\dot{V}$ profile, similar to that seen with continued inspiratory muscle effort.

CESSATION OF INSPIRATION

Mismatch of the mechanical and neural T_i can be detected from waveform changes at the cessation of inspiration.

Mechanical T_i shorter than neural T_i

There will be prolonged inspiratory muscle effort during early expiration; if this leads to a sufficient fall in P_{ao} or $\dot{V}$, an early triggered breath follows. During pressure-cycled ventilation this will lead to a second small V_T breath due to the high baseline lung volume, but in assist-volume control P_{ao} will be excessive. Typically this is seen with a stiff respiratory system, PEEPi or inadequate pressure support.

Mechanical T_i longer than neural T_i

This leads to features of passive inflation such as a linear increase in P_{ao} during assist-volume control ventilation; during pressure-cycled ventilation there may be an increase in P_{ao} due to loss of inspiratory effort, or an unexplained fall in $\dot{V}$.

EXPIRATION

Changes in P_{ao} during expiration are usually small unless expiratory circuit resistance is abnormally high. However, in patients with expiratory flow limitation the expiratory $\dot{V}$ waveform shows a typical 'tick' pattern; there is a rapid spike in expiratory flow due to dynamic compression of large conducting airways at the beginning of expiration, and this is followed by low, slowly declining expiratory $\dot{V}$ due to high $\dot{V}$ expiratory resistance. When PEEPi is present the expiratory $\dot{V}$ fails to cease prior to the inspiratory trigger; however, this may be difficult to detect due to the poor fidelity present on most commercial ventilators.

MONITORING NEUROMUSCULAR FUNCTION

INSPIRATORY OCCLUSION PRESSURE

The pressure 100 ms (P_{100} or $P_{0.1}$) after a random occlusion timed at the beginning of inspiration is a measure of respiratory drive. There is a large range of normal values (1.5–5 cmH_2O), but it is reproducible in an individual patient. In ventilated patients the $P_{0.1}$ correlates with the work of breathing during pressure support ventilation, and changes in the same direction as PEEPe is increased if work is reduced.[59] Consequently, $P_{0.1}$ may prove to be a useful method of titrating PEEPe in patients with dynamic hyperinflation; however, this is not valid when flow triggering is used.

MAXIMUM MOUTH PRESSURES

Maximum inspiratory (MIP) and expiratory (MEP) mouth pressures can be used to estimate the power of the respiratory muscles. MIP is usually measured in ventilated patients using a unidirectional expiratory valve for ~20 seconds.[60] This ensures the procedure is performed from a low lung volume and does not require patient cooperation. However, despite this, the results are quite variable.[61] Normal values vary with age and gender; young females may exceed ~–90 cmH_2O, and young males ~–130 cmH_2O. A MIP <–20 cmH_2O is predictive of weaning failure; however, this is associated with too many false positives and negatives to be useful.[11] MEP may be useful in myopathic patients with expiratory muscle weakness. Transdiaphragmatic pressure is assessed using an oesophageal and gastric balloon to measure the pressure in these two cavities.

WORK OF BREATHING

The work of breathing (W_B) is the sum of elastic work (W_{el}), flow-resistive work (W_{res}) and inertial work (negligible), and can be estimated from *V–P* data during spontaneous or assisted ventilation. An oesophageal balloon is used to examine changes in pleural pressure, $\dot{V}$ is measured with a pneumotachograph and volume is derived as its integral. Although conceptually W_B is the inspiratory area of a *V–P* loop, this needs to be referenced to the chest wall *V–P* curve, and the appropriate area measured from a Campbell diagram.[62]

The normal W_B is ~0.5 J/l of $\dot{V}_E$, and this may be significantly increased in patients with acute respiratory failure, and by additional work imposed by ventilatory apparatus, including the endotracheal tube and connector, humidifier and ventilator circuit.[63] The consequences of a large increase in W_B may include an increase in the O_2 attributable to breathing ($O_{2\ resp}$), respiratory muscle insufficiency, CO_2 retention and acute respiratory failure. However, W_B is rarely measured outside research projects since the Campbell diagram is a relatively tedious approach. Simplifications have been used, but these are not as accurate, and W_B only estimates energy expenditure during muscle shortening, with relatively poor correlation with $O_{2\ resp}$.[64] Consequently, the pressure–time product (PTP), which does correlate with $O_{2\ resp}$,[65] is more commonly measured.[10]

PRESSURE–TIME PRODUCT

PTP is usually calculated from the oesophageal pressure–time integral during inspiration. In mechanically ventilated patients the oesophageal pressure during assisted breathing is compared with that during a controlled breath, or that pressure calculated from the chest wall elastance and lung volume.[10] However, the early correlation of $O_{2\ resp}$ with PTP used the transdiaphragmatic pressure in spontaneously breathing subjects.[62] Using either technique, importantly, the effort expended before $\dot{V}$ occurs due to PEEPi is measured, probably accounting for the better correlation of $O_{2\ resp}$ with PTP than W_B.[62] Although incremental pressure support ventilation may reduce PTP in COPD patients, the effect can be variable, with some patients also showing evidence of expiratory muscle activity due to delayed sensing of neural expiration.[10]

REFERENCES

1. Cohen CA, Zagelbaum G, Gross D *et al.* Clinical manifestations of inspiratory muscle fatigue. *Am J Med* 1982; **73**: 308–16.
2. Martin J, Jardim J, Sampson M *et al.* Factors influencing pulsus paradoxus in asthma. *Chest* 1981; **80**: 543–9.
3. Dantzker DR, Brook CJ, Dehart P *et al.* Ventilation–perfusion distributions in the adult respiratory distress syndrome. *Am Rev Respir Dis* 1979; **120**: 1039–52.
4. Nuckton TJ, Alonso AJ, Kallet RH *et al.* Pulmonary dead-space fraction as a risk factor for death in the acute respiratory distress syndrome. *N Engl J Med* 2002; **346**: 1281–6.
5. Palmon SC, Liu M, Moore LE *et al.* Capnography facilitates tight control of ventilation during transport. *Crit Care Med* 1996; **24**: 608–11.
6. Levine RL. End-tidal CO_2: physiology in pursuit of clinical applications. *Intens Care Med* 2000; **26**: 1595–7.
7. 2005 American Heart Association Guidelines for Cardiopulmonary Resuscitation and Emergency Cardiovascular Care. Advanced cardiovascular life support. *Circulation* 2005; **112**: III-25–54.
8. Joint Faculty of Intensive Care Medicine. *Minimum Standards for Transport of Critically Ill Patients.* Review IC-10. Melbourne: Joint Faculty of Intensive Care Medicine, 2003.
9. Joint Faculty of Intensive Care Medicine. *Minimum Standards for Intensive Care Units.* Review IC-1. Melbourne: Joint Faculty of Intensive Care Medicine, 2003.
10. Australian and New Zealand College of Anaesthetists. *Monitoring During Anaesthesia.* Review PS18. Melbourne: Australian and New Zealand College of Anaesthetists, 2006.
11. Jubran A. Advances in respiratory monitoring during mechanical ventilation. *Chest* 1999; **116**: 1416–25.
12. Yang K, Tobin MJ. A prospective study of indices predicting outcome of trials of weaning from mechanical ventilation. *N Engl J Med* 1991; **324**: 1445–50.
13. Wrigge H, Sydow M, Zinserling J *et al.* Determination of functional residual capacity (FRC) by multibreath nitrogen washout in a lung model and in mechanically ventilated patients. Accuracy depends on continuous dynamic compensation for changes of gas sampling delay time. *Intens Care Med* 1998; **24**: 487–93.
14. Bersten AD. Measurement of overinflation by multiple linear regression analysis in patients with acute lung injury. *Eur Respir J* 1998; **12**: 526–32.
15. Pelosi P, Cereda M, Foti G *et al.* Alterations of lung and chest wall mechanics in patients with acute lung injury: effects of positive end-expiratory pressure. *Am J Respir Crit Care Med* 1995; **152**: 531–7.
16. Mergoni M, Martelli A, Volpi A *et al.* Impact of positive end-expiratory pressure on chest wall and lung pressure–volume curve in acute respiratory failure. *Am J Respir Crit Care Med* 1997; **156**: 846–54.
17. Ranieri VM, Brienza N, Santostasi S *et al.* Impairment of lung and chest wall mechanics in patients with acute respiratory distress syndrome: role of abdominal distension. *Am J Respir Crit Care Med* 1997; **156**: 1082–91.
18. Gattinoni L, Pelosi P, Suter PM *et al.* Acute respiratory distress syndrome caused by pulmonary and extrapulmonary disease. Different syndromes? *Am J Respir Crit Care Med* 1998; **158**: 3–11.
19. Baydur A, Behrakis PK, Zin WA *et al.* A simple method for assessing the validity of the esophageal balloon technique. *Am Rev Respir Dis* 1982; **126**: 788–91.

20. Higgs BD, Behrakis PK, Bevan DR, Milic-Emili J. Measurement of pleural pressure with esophageal balloon in anesthetized humans. *Anesthesiology* 1983; **59**:340–3.
21. Lanteri CJ, Kano S, Sly PD. Validation of esophageal pressure occlusion test after paralysis. *Pediatr Pulmonol* 1994; **17**: 56–62.
22. Fredberg JJ, Stamenovic D. On the imperfect elasticity of lung tissue. *J Appl Physiol* 1989; **67**: 2408–19.
23. Grimby G, Takishima T, Graham W *et al.* Frequency dependence of flow resistance in patients with obstructive lung disease. *J Clin Invest* 1968; **47**: 1455–65.
24. Woolcock AJ, Vincent NJ, Macklem PT. Frequency dependence of compliance as a test for obstruction in the small airways. *J Clin Invest* 1969; **48**: 1097–106.
25. Mead J. Measurement of inertia of the lungs at increased ambient pressure. *J Appl Physiol* 1956; **9**: 208–12.
26. Bates JH, Rossi A, Milic-Emili J. Analysis of the behavior of the respiratory system with constant inspiratory flow. *J Appl Physiol* 1985; **58**: 1840–8.
27. Otis AB, McKerrow CB, Bartlett RA *et al.* Mechanical factors in distribution of pulmonary ventilation. *J Appl Physiol* 1956; **8**: 427–43.
28. Jonson B, Beydon L, Brauer K *et al.* Mechanics of respiratory system in healthy anesthetized humans with emphasis on viscoelastic properties. *J Appl Physiol* 1993; **75**: 132–40.
29. Jonson B, Richard J-C, Straus R *et al.* Pressure–volume curves and compliance in acute lung injury: evidence for recruitment above the lower inflection point. *Am J Respir Crit Care Med* 1999; **159**: 1172–8.
30. Crotti S, Mascheroni D, Caironi P *et al.* Recruitment and derecruitment during acute respiratory failure: a clinical study. *Am J Respir Crit Care Med* 2001; **164**: 131–40.
31. Hickling KG. The pressure–volume curve is greatly modified by recruitment. A mathematical model of ARDS lungs. *Am J Respir Crit Care Med* 1998; **158**: 194–202.
32. Matamis D, Lemaire F, Harf A *et al.* Total respiratory pressure–volume curves in the adult respiratory distress syndrome. *Chest* 1984; **86**: 58–66.
33. Gattinoni L, Mascheroni D, Basilico E *et al.* Volume/pressure curve of total respiratory system in paralysed patients: artefacts and correction factors. *Intens Care Med* 1987; **13**: 19–25.
34. Dall'ava-Santucci J, Armaganidis A, Brunet F *et al.* Causes of error of respiratory pressure–volume curves in paralyzed subjects. *J Appl Physiol* 1988; **64**: 42–9.
35. Levy P, Similowski T, Corbeil C *et al.* A method for studying volume-pressure curves of the respiratory system during mechanical ventilation. *J Crit Care* 1989; **4**: 83–9.
36. Servillo G, Svantesson C, Beydon L *et al.* Pressure–volume curves in acute respiratory failure: automated low flow inflation versus occlusion. *Am J Respir Crit Care Med* 1997; **155**: 1629–36.
37. Lu Q, Vieira SRR, Richecoeur J *et al.* A simple automated method for measuring pressure–volume curves during mechanical ventilation. *Am J Respir Crit Care Med* 1999; **159**: 275–82.
38. Beydon L, Svantesson C, Brauer K *et al.* Respiratory mechanics in patients ventilated for critical lung disease. *Eur Respir J* 1996; **9**: 262–73.
39. Peslin R, da Silva JF, Chabot F *et al.* Respiratory mechanics studied by multiple linear regression in unsedated ventilated patients. *Eur Respir J* 1992; **5**: 871–8.
40. Eberhard L, Guttmann J, Wolff G *et al.* Intrinsic PEEP monitored in the ventilated ARDS patient with a mathematical method. *J Appl Physiol* 1992; **73**: 479–85.
41. Nicolai T, Lanteri C, Freezer N *et al.* Non-invasive determination of alveolar pressure during mechanical ventilation. *Eur Respir J* 1991; **4**: 1275–83.
42. Grasso S, Terragni P, Mascia L *et al.* Airway pressure–time curve profile (stress index) detects tidal recruitment/hyperinflation in experimental acute lung injury. *Crit Care Med* 2004; **32**: 1018–27.
43. Kano S, Lanteri CJ, Duncan AW *et al.* Influence of nonlinearities on estimates of respiratory mechanics using multilinear regression analysis. *J Appl Physiol* 1994; **77**: 1185–97.
44. Sullivan M, Paliotta J, Saklad M. Endotracheal tube as a factor in measurement of respiratory mechanics. *J Appl Physiol* 1976; **41**: 590–2.
45. Wright PE, Marini JJ, Bernard GR. In vitro versus in vivo comparison of endotracheal tube airflow resistance. *Am Rev Respir Dis* 1989; **140**: 10–16.
46. Manthous CA, Hall JB, Schmidt GA *et al.* Metered-dose inhaler versus nebulized albuterol in mechanically ventilated patients. *Am Rev Respir Dis* 1993; **148**: 1567–70.
47. Gottfried SB, Rossi A, Higgs BD *et al.* Noninvasive determination of respiratory system mechanics during mechanical ventilation for acute respiratory failure. *Am Rev Respir Dis* 1985; **131**: 414–20.
48. Peslin R, Fredberg JJ. Oscillation mechanics of the respiratory system. In: Macklem PT, Mead J (eds) *Handbook of Physiology, Respiratory Mechanics.* Bethesda, MD: American Physiological Society; 1986: 145–77.
49. Pepe PE, Marini JJ. Occult positive end-expiratory pressure in mechanically ventilated patients with airflow obstruction: the auto-PEEP effect. *Am Rev Respir Dis* 1982; **126**: 166–70.
50. Petrof BJ, Legare M, Goldberg P *et al.* Continuous positive airway pressure reduces work of breathing and dyspnea during weaning from mechanical ventilation in severe chronic obstructive pulmonary disease. *Am Rev Respir Dis* 1990; **141**: 281–9.
51. Tuxen DV, Lane S. The effects of ventilatory pattern on hyperinflation, airway pressures, and circulation in mechanical ventilation of patients with severe air-flow obstruction. *Am Rev Respir Dis* 1987; **136**: 872–9.
52. Rossi A, Gottfried SB, Zocchi L *et al.* Measurement of static compliance of the total respiratory system in patients with acute respiratory failure during

mechanical ventilation. The effect of intrinsic positive end-expiratory pressure. *Am Rev Respir Dis* 1985; **131**: 672–7.

53. Lessard MR, Lofaso F, Brochard L. Expiratory muscle activity increases intrinsic positive end-expiratory pressure independently of dynamic hyperinflation in mechanically ventilated patients. *Am J Respir Crit Care Med* 1995; **151**: 562–9.
54. Schuessler TF, Gottfried SB, Goldberg P *et al.* An adaptive filter to reduce cardiogenic oscillations on esophageal pressure signals. *Biomed Eng* 1998; **26**: 260–7.
55. Ninane V, Yernault JC, de Troyer A. Intrinsic PEEP in patients with chronic obstructive pulmonary disease. Role of expiratory muscles. *Am Rev Respir Dis* 1993; **148**: 1037–42.
56. Maltais F, Reissmann H, Navalesi P *et al.* Comparison of static and dynamic measurements of intrinsic PEEP in mechanically ventilated patients. *Am J Respir Crit Care Med* 1994; **150**: 1318–24.
57. Yan S, Kayser B, Tobiasz M *et al.* Comparison of static and dynamic intrinsic positive end-expiratory pressure using the Campbell diagram. *Am J Respir Crit Care Med* 1996; **154**: 938–44.
58. Georgopoulos D, Prinianakis G, Kondili E. Bedside waveforms interpretation as a tool to identify patient-ventilator asynchronies. *Intens Care Med* 2006; **32**: 34–47.
59. Mancebo J, Albaladejo P, Touchard D *et al.* Airway occlusion pressure to titrate positive end-expiratory pressure in patients with dynamic hyperinflation. *Anesthesiology* 2000; **93**: 81–90.
60. Caruso P, Friedrich C, Denari SDC *et al.* The unidirectional valve is the best method to determine maximal inspiratory pressure during weaning. *Chest* 1999; **115**: 1096–101.
61. Multz AS, Aldrich TK, Prezant DJ *et al.* Maximal inspiratory pressure is not a reliable test of inspiratory muscle strength in mechanically ventilated patients. *Am Rev Respir Dis* 1990; **142**: 529–32.
62. Banner MJ, Jaeger MJ, Kirby RR. Components of the work of breathing and implications for monitoring ventilator-dependent patients. *Crit Care Med* 1994; **22**: 515–23.
63. Bersten AD, Rutten AJ, Vedig AE *et al.* Additional work of breathing imposed by endotracheal tubes, breathing circuits and intensive care ventilators. *Crit Care Med* 1989; **17**: 671–80.
64. Annat G, Viale J-P. Measuring the breathing workload in mechanically ventilated patients. *Intens Care Med* 1990; **16**: 418–21.
65. Field S, Sanci S, Grassino A. Respiratory muscle oxygen consumption estimated by the diaphragmatic pressure–time index. *J Appl Physiol* 1984; **57**: 44–51.

35

Imaging the chest

Simon P G Padley

RADIOLOGICAL TECHNIQUES

Of the imaging techniques available for investigating patients in the intensive care unit (ICU), the chest radiograph remains the most important, with ultrasound being utilised in a selected group of patients. High-resolution and spiral computed tomography (CT) allow further investigation of these patients in certain situations.

CONVENTIONAL CHEST RADIOGRAPHY

The views of the chest most frequently performed in the ambulant patient are the erect posteroanterior (PA) and lateral projections, taken with the patient breath-holding at total lung capacity. While portable or mobile chest radiography, as undertaken on an ICU, has the obvious advantage that the examination can be done without moving the patient from the ward, there are many disadvantages. These include:

- shorter focus–film distance causing magnification
- limited X-ray output necessitating long exposure times with resultant movement blurring
- difficulties with satisfactory patient positioning

DIGITAL CHEST RADIOLOGY

In the ICU, digital chest radiographs may be obtained utilising conventional X-ray generators, but the image is captured on a reusable photostimulable plate instead of conventional film. The digital information is then manipulated, displayed and stored in whatever format is desired. Traditional systems suffer greatly from the large day-to-day variations in the density of the radiograph due to small differences in exposure. Digital radiographic systems are able to capture and display a standard density image from a much wider range of exposures (Figure 35.1).

COMPUTED TOMOGRAPHY

CT relies on differing absorption of X-rays by tissues with constituents of differing atomic number, so slight differences in X-ray absorption can be interpreted to produce a cross-sectional image. The components of a CT scanner are an X-ray tube, which rotates around the patient, and an array of X-ray detectors opposite the tube. The speed with which a CT scanner acquires an image depends upon the time it takes to rotate the anode around the patient. Modern CT machines have tube rotation times of as little as 0.33 seconds.

Spiral (also known as volume or helical) scanning entails sustained patient exposure by the rotating X-ray tube during continuous movement of the examination couch through the CT gantry aperture. In this way a continuous data set or 'spiral' of information may be acquired in a single breath-hold. The information is reconstructed into axial sections, perpendicular to the long axis of the patient, identical to conventional CT sections. Three-dimensional reconstructions of complex anatomical areas can also be produced.

When short rotation times are coupled with the ability to acquire multiple spirals simultaneously (currently up to 64 slices), the speed of these systems is now so great that breath-holding or suspended ventilation is no longer necessary for high-quality imaging. Furthermore, the detector thickness that determines the minimum slice width of the reconstructed images is now commonly less than 1 mm. Thus a 64-channel scanner can acquire almost 200 submillimetre images per second.

INTRAVENOUS CONTRAST ENHANCEMENT

Because of the high contrast on CT between vessels and surrounding air in the lung, and vessels and surrounding fat within the mediastinum, intravenous contrast enhancement only needs to be given in specific instances, for example to aid the distinction between hilar vessels and a soft-tissue mass. The exact timing of the injection of contrast media depends most on the time the CT scanner takes to scan the thorax. Rapid scanning protocols with automated injectors tend to improve contrast enhancement of vascular structures at the expense of enhancement of solid lesions because of the rapidity of scanning. With spiral CT, it is possible to achieve good opacification of all the thoracic vascular structures with small volumes of contrast media. Optimal contrast enhancement of the pulmonary arteries occurs 10–15 seconds after the start of contrast injection, usually at 3–5 ml/s by a power injector. Timing of image acquisition is vital for accurate diagnosis of pulmonary embolism. However, when examining inflammatory lesions, such as the reaction around an empyema, it may be necessary to delay scanning by 30–40 seconds to allow contrast to diffuse into the extravascular space.

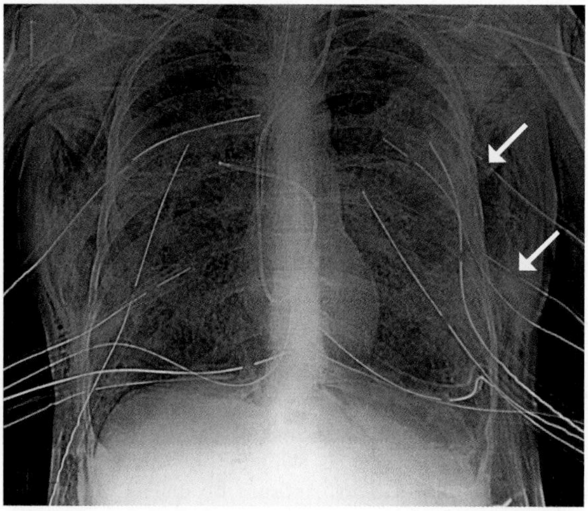

Figure 35.1 Digital radiograph. The image has been edge-enhanced, which makes the multiple chest drains, Swan–Ganz catheter and endotracheal tube position more conspicuous. Note that two of the chest drain side holes lie within the soft tissues of the chest wall (arrows).

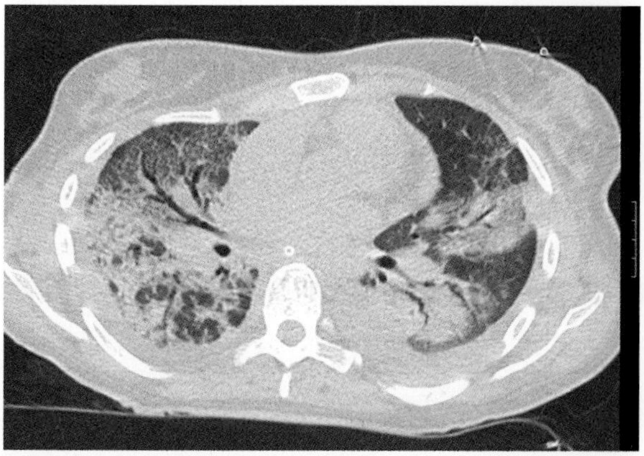

Figure 35.2 Computed tomography of a patient with acute respiratory distress syndrome. Note the marked anterior-to-posterior density gradient. The anterior lung is of almost normal density, becoming of ground-glass attenuation in the mid-part of the lung before fading into consolidation posteriorly. There are also moderate-sized bilateral pleural effusions.

HIGH-RESOLUTION COMPUTED TOMOGRAPHY (HRCT)

Narrow collimation images of the lung correlate closely with the macroscopic appearances of pathological specimens. In diffuse lung disease, HRCT allows a substantial improvement in diagnostic accuracy compared with chest radiography. Narrow section images can be acquired either as part of a volumetric acquisition or as interspaced images, usually 1.5 mm thickness, obtained every 1 cm. The radiation burden to the patient of this interspace or sequential technique is considerably less than with volumetric scanning – typically by a factor of 10 times.

CLINICAL APPLICATIONS OF HRCT IN THE ICU PATIENT

HRCT is increasingly being used to confirm the impression of an abnormality seen on a chest radiograph. HRCT may also be used to achieve a histospecific diagnosis in some patients with obvious but non-specific radiographic abnormalities. Furthermore, HRCT has provided a number of useful insights into chest disease in the severely ill patient in an ICU setting.

HRCT in uncomplicated acute respiratory distress syndrome (ARDS):[1]

- reveals that the apparently homogeneous opacification apparent on the chest radiograph has an anterior-to-posterior graded increase in density – an appearance referred to as a gravitational gradient (Figure 35.2)
- demonstrates early dilatation of the smaller airways within areas of ground-glass density, an appearance that suggests development of fibrosis, and may prompt anti-inflammatory treatment
- demonstrates that a shift from the supine to the prone position results in redistribution of the previously dependent dense parenchymal opacification to the now dependent anterior lung, a phenomenon that may be accompanied by improvements in patient oxygenation

HRCT of complications of ARDS[2,3]

- Infection is common in ARDS. Diagnosis may be difficult. Radiographically there may be a lack of specific findings, often due to superimposition of changes attributable to ARDS. This is a particular problem in the critically ill patient when the usual indicators of pneumonia are also unreliable. Although the diagnosis may still be in question following HRCT, associated pneumonic changes such as abscess formation, empyema and mediastinal disease, as well as development of non-dependent areas of consolidation, are all useful pointers to superadded infection (see Figure 35.2).
- Barotrauma – mediastinal and interstitial emphysema, as well as pneumothorax, are all increasingly common at higher levels of peak end-expiratory pressure (PEEP). The incidence of barotrauma has been reported to be as high as 50%.
- HRCT delineates early change and allows exact location of loculated air collections to be defined.

NORMAL RADIOGRAPHIC ANATOMY

THE MEDIASTINUM, CENTRAL AIRWAYS AND HILAR STRUCTURES

Appreciation of abnormality requires a sound grasp of normal radiological anatomy. The mediastinum is delimited by the lungs on either side, the thoracic inlet above, the diaphragm below and the vertebral column posteriorly. Because the various structures that make up the mediastinum are superimposed on each other on the chest radiograph, they cannot be separately identified. Nevertheless, because a chest radiograph is usually the first imaging investigation, it is necessary to have an appreciation of the normal appearances of the mediastinum, together with variations due to the patient's body habitus and age. Key points include:

- Only the outline of the mediastinum and the air-containing trachea and bronchi (and sometimes oesophagus) are clearly seen on a normal chest radiograph.
- The right superior mediastinal border is formed by the right brachiocephalic vein and superior vena cava, and becomes less distinct as it reaches the thoracic inlet. The right side of the superior mediastinum can appear to be considerably widened in patients with an abundance of mediastinal fat.
- The left mediastinal border above the aortic arch is the result of summation of the left carotid and left subclavian arteries together with the left brachiocephalic and jugular veins.
- The left cardiac border comprises the left atrial appendage which merges inferiorly with the left ventricle. The silhouette of the heart should always be sharply outlined. Any blurring of the border is due to loss of immediately adjacent aerated lung, usually by collapse or consolidation.
- The density of the heart shadow to the left and right of the vertebral column should be identical and any difference indicates pathology (for example, an area of consolidation or a mass in a lower lobe).
- The trachea and main bronchi should be visible through the upper and middle mediastinum.
- In older individuals, the trachea may be displaced by a dilated aortic arch. In approximately 60% of normal subjects, the right wall of the trachea (the right paratracheal stripe) can be identified as a line of uniform thickness (less than 4 mm in width); when it is visible it excludes the presence of an adjacent space-occupying lesion, most usually lymphadenopathy.
- The carinal angle is usually less than 80 °. Splaying of the carina is an insensitive sign of subcarinal disease, either in the form of massive subcarinal lymphadenopathy, or a markedly enlarged left atrium.
- The origins of the lobar bronchi, where they are projected over the mediastinal shadow, can usually be identified but the segmental bronchi within the lungs are not generally seen on plain radiography.
- Normal hilar shadows on a chest radiograph represent the summation of the pulmonary arteries and veins.
- The hila are approximately the same size and the left hilum normally lies between 0.5 cm and 1.5 cm above the level of the right hilum. The size and shape of the hila show remarkable variation in normal individuals, making subtle abnormalities difficult to identify.

THE PULMONARY FISSURES, VESSELS AND BRONCHI

The two lungs are separated by the four layers of pleura behind and in front of the mediastinum. The resulting posterior and anterior junction lines are often visible on chest radiographs as nearly vertical stripes, the posterior junction line lying higher than the anterior. The junction lines are not invariably seen and their presence or absence is not usually of significance (Figure 35.3).

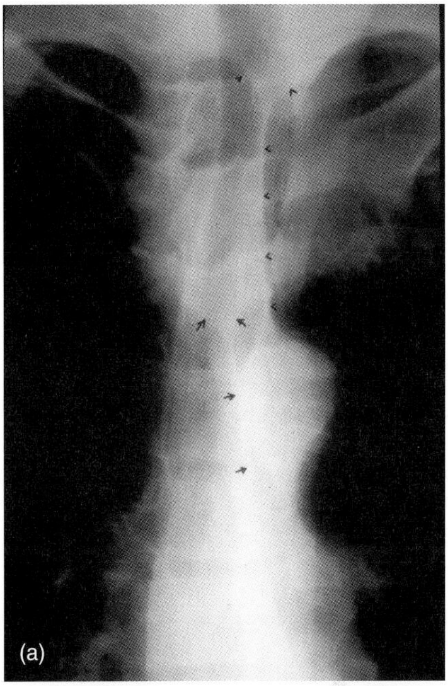

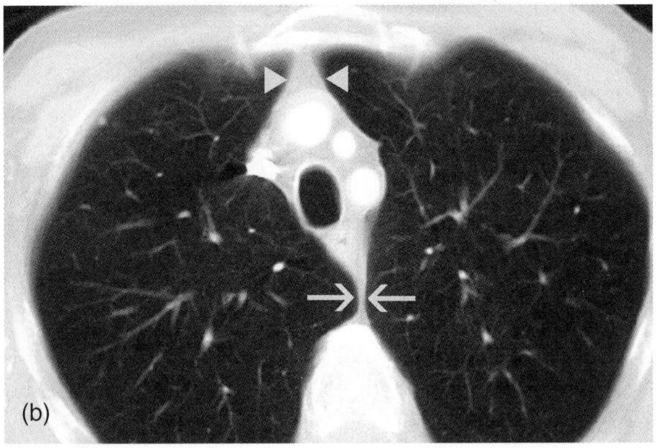

Figure 35.3 (a) Close-up of the mediastinum of a patient in whom both the anterior and posterior junction lines are evident. The anterior junction line is more inferior and slants from right to left (short arrows), whereas the posterior junction line is more vertical, superior and is delineated by the arrowheads. (b) Computed tomography scan through the upper mediastinum demonstrating the anterior (arrowheads) and posterior (arrows) junction lines in a different patient.

The upper and lower lobes of the left lung are separated by the major (or oblique) fissure. The upper, middle and lower lobes of the right lung are separated by the major fissure and the minor (horizontal or transverse) fissure. The minor fissure is visible in over half of normal PA chest radiographs. The major fissures are not visible on a frontal radiograph and are inconstantly identifiable on lateral radiographs. In a few individuals, fissures are incompletely developed; a point familiar to thoracic surgeons performing a lobectomy, because of incomplete cleavage between lobes. Accessory fissures are occasionally seen.

All of the branching structures seen within normal lungs on a chest radiograph represent pulmonary arteries or veins. It is often impossible to distinguish arteries from veins in the lung periphery. On a chest radiograph taken in the erect position, there is a gradual increase in the diameter of the vessels, at equidistant points from the hilum, travelling from lung apex to base; this gravity-dependent effect disappears if the patient is supine or in cardiac failure.

THE DIAPHRAGM AND THORACIC CAGE

The interface between aerated lung and the hemidiaphragms is sharp and the highest point of each dome is normally medial to the mid-clavicular line. The right dome of the diaphragm is higher than the left by up to 2 cm in the erect position unless the left dome is elevated by air in the stomach (Figure 35.4).

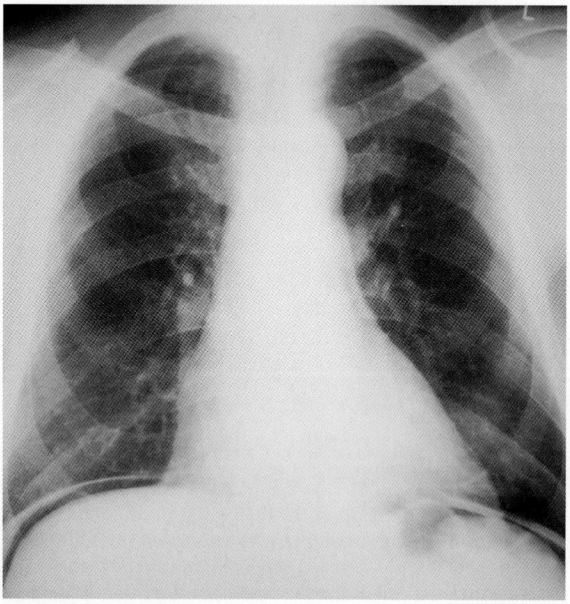

Figure 35.4 Erect chest radiograph of a patient with a pneumoperitoneum demonstrating the normal thickness in position of the hemidiaphragms. The right lies slightly higher than the left.

Filling-in or blunting of these costophrenic angles usually represents pleural disease, either pleural thickening or an effusion.

POSITIONING OF TUBES AND LINES[4]

CENTRAL VENOUS CATHETERS (CVC)

The end of a CVC needs to be intrathoracic, and is ideally in the superior vena cava. CVCs may be introduced via an antecubital, subclavian or jugular vein. Subclavian venous puncture carries a risk of pneumothorax and mediastinal hematoma. Rarely, perforation of the subclavian vein leads to fluid collecting in the mediastinum or pleura. All catheters have a potential risk of coiling, misplacement, knotting and fracture (Figure 35.5). The tip should not abut the vessel wall at an obtuse angle.

PULMONARY ARTERY FLOTATION CATHETERS

Ideally the end of the catheter should be maintained 5–8 cm (2–3 inches) beyond the bifurcation of the main pulmonary artery in either the right or left pulmonary artery (see Figure 35.5). When the pulmonary artery occlusion pressure is measured the balloon is inflated, and the flow of blood carries the catheter tip peripherally, to an occluded position. After the measurement has been

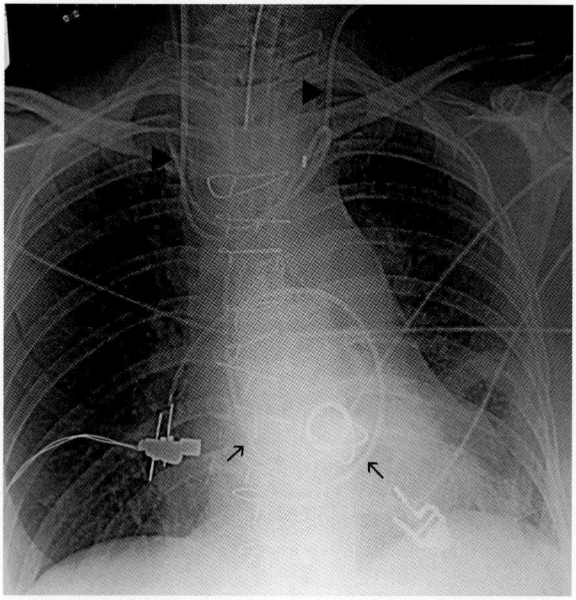

Figure 35.5 Intensive care unit patient with multiple tubes and lines in place. The endotracheal tube tip position is satisfactory, and there are sternotomy wires, an intra-aortic balloon pump (radiopaque tip) and a prosthetic heart valve. The central line inserted into the left internal jugular vein passes into the right internal jugular vein. The Swan–Ganz catheter, which has been inserted via the right internal jugular vein, loops into the left brachiocephalic vein, before taking a satisfactory course through the cardiac chambers (black arrows).

made the balloon is deflated and the catheter returns to a central position; otherwise there is a risk of pulmonary infarction. The inflation balloon is radiolucent. The balloon should normally be kept deflated.

NASOGASTRIC TUBES

These should reach the stomach but may coil in the oesophagus or occasionally are inserted into the tracheobronchial tree (Figure 35.6).

ENDOTRACHEAL TUBES

Extension and flexion of the neck may make the tip of an endotracheal tube move by as much as 5 cm. With the neck in neutral position the tip of the tube should ideally be about 5–6 cm above the carina. A tube that is inserted too far usually passes into the right bronchus, with the risk of non-ventilation or collapse of the left lung (Figure 35.7).

TRACHEOSTOMY TUBES

The tube tip should be situated centrally in the airway at the level of T3. Acute complications of tracheostomy include pneumothorax, pneumomediastinum and subcutaneous emphysema. Long-term complications include tracheal ulceration, stenosis and perforation.

PLEURAL TUBES

These are used to treat pleural effusions and pneumothoraces. A radiopaque line usually runs along pleural tubes, and is interrupted where there are side holes. It is important to check that all the side holes are within the thorax. Tracks may remain on the chest X-ray following removal of chest tubes, causing tubular or ring shadows. When doubt remains about tube position, then CT scanning should be considered (Figure 35.1 and 35.8).

MEDIASTINAL DRAINS

These are usually present following sternotomy. Apart from their position, they look like pleural tubes.

INTRA-AORTIC BALLOON PUMP

These are used in patients with cardiogenic shock, often following cardiac surgery. The ideal position of the catheter tip is just distal to the origin of the left subclavian artery (Figure 35.9). If the catheter tip is advanced too far it may occlude the left subclavian artery, and if it is

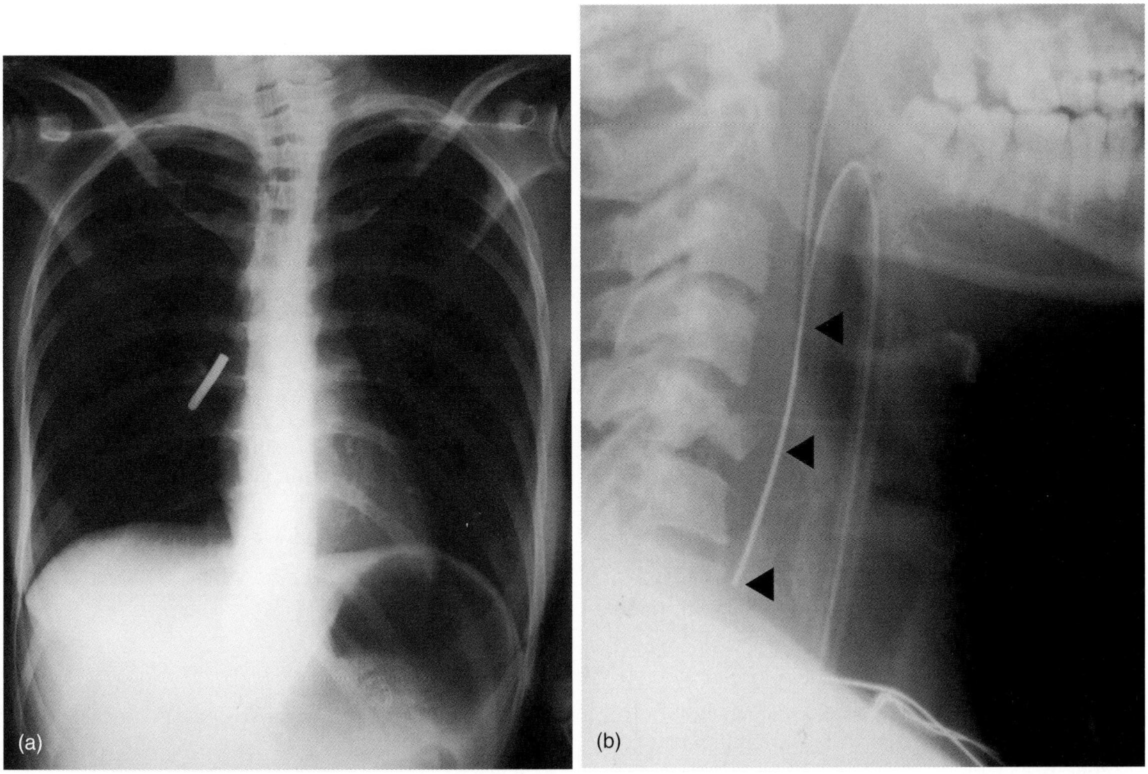

Figure 35.6 Misplaced nasogastric tube. (a) The tip of the tube is in the bronchus intermedius. (b) The tube is looped in the oesophagus (black arrowheads) before passing into the trachea, as demonstrated on this lateral spine view. Note the anterior wedge fracture of C5.

Continued

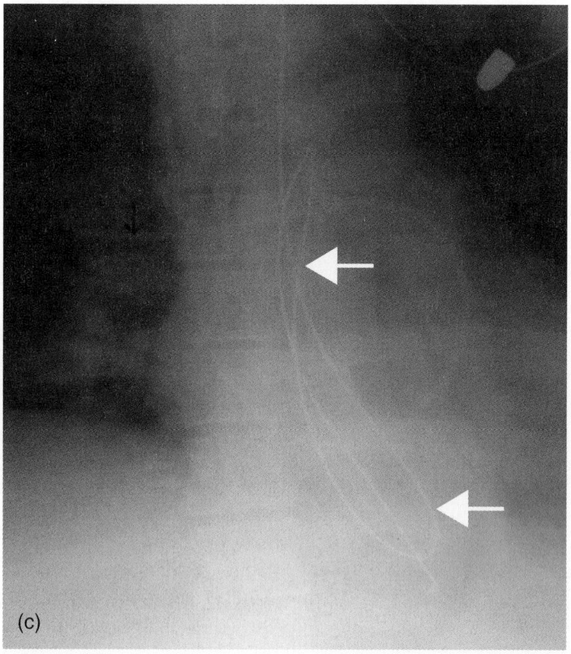

Figure 35.6 *Continued* (c) The tube is coiled in the oesophagus without passing into the stomach. Note the bullet projected over the left upper zone and the adequately positioned Swan–Ganz catheter (white arrow).

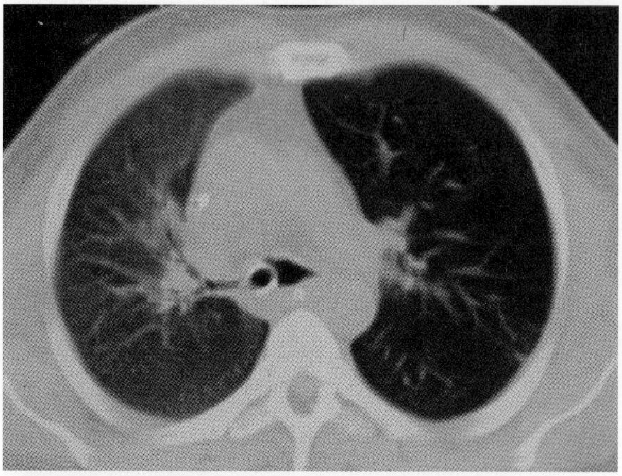

Figure 35.7 Endotracheal tube inserted into the right main bronchus as demonstrated on computed tomography. This image, obtained in expiration, demonstrates air trapping in the left lung.

too distal the balloon may occlude branches of the abdominal aorta. The intra-aortic balloon pump may only be visible by its radiopaque tip (see Figure 35.5).

PACEMAKERS

These may be permanent or temporary (Figure 35.10). Temporary epicardial wires are sometimes inserted

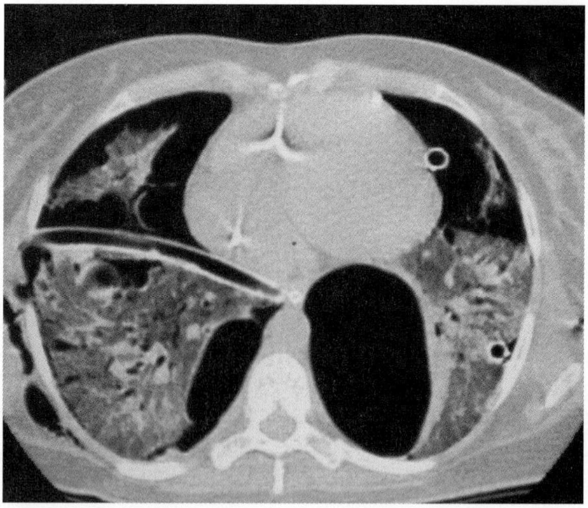

Figure 35.8 Computed tomography scan demonstrating loculated pneumothoraces in a patient with acute lung injury. The posteromedial pneumothorax on the left is not being drained by the multiple chest tubes.

during cardiac surgery, and may be seen as thin, almost hair-like metallic opacities overlying the heart. Temporary pacing electrodes are usually inserted transvenously via a subclavian or jugular vein. If a patient is not pacing properly, a chest X-ray may reveal that the position of the electrode tip is unstable, or a fracture in the wire may be seen.

RADIOGRAPHIC SIGNS OF PATHOLOGY

CONSOLIDATION

Consolidation, or synonymously air space shadowing, is due to opacification of the air-containing spaces of the lung, usually without a change in volume of the affected area. It is not possible to tell what the air space filling is due to in the absence of a clinical history, except perhaps for shadowing due to cardiogenic alveolar oedema, when there will be associated signs of cardiac failure. Typical features of all forms of consolidation (Figure 35.11) include:

- ill-defined margins, except where it directly abuts a pleural surface
- sharply demarcated by fissures
- loss of vascular markings
- air bronchograms – the bronchi, usually invisible, may become apparent in negative contrast to the air space opacification
- acinar opacities, due to individual acini or secondary pulmonary lobules being opacified but still surrounded by normally aerated lung, usually seen at the periphery of a more confluent area of consolidation, and 0.5–1 cm in diameter

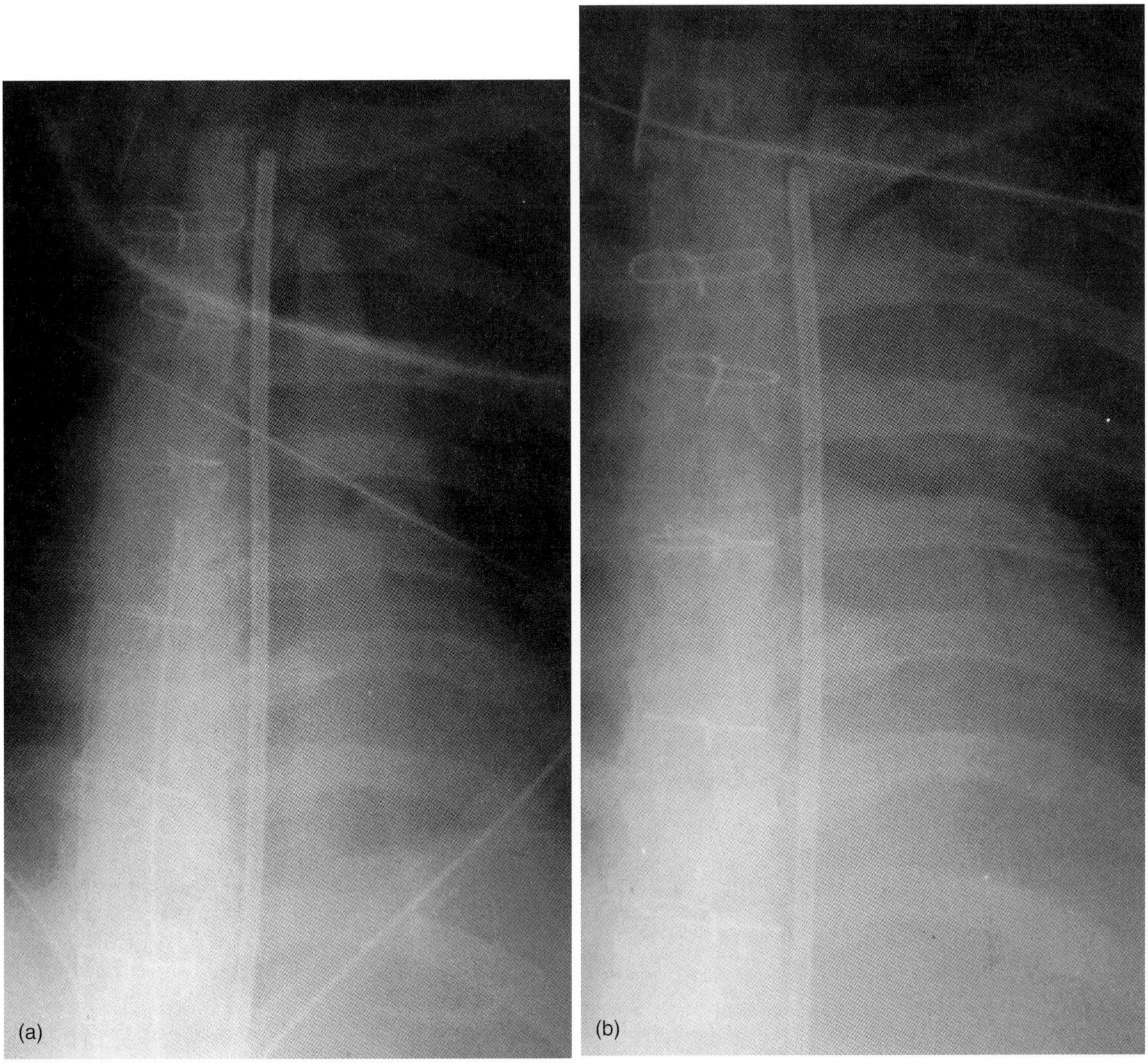

Figure 35.9 Intra-aortic balloon pump. Two chest radiographs in the same patient demonstrating the balloon pump during the inflated (a) and deflated (b) phases. The tip of this balloon pump will be impinging upon the origin of the left subclavian artery and is slightly too high.

- ground-glass opacification, when consolidation has caused only partial filling of the air spaces
- silhouette sign – consolidation abutting a soft-tissue structure causes the silhouette of that structure to be lost

When an area of consolidation undergoes necrosis, either due to infection or infarction, then liquefaction may result, and if there is either a gas-forming organism or communication with the bronchial tree, then an air–fluid level may develop in addition to cavity formation.

COLLAPSE

When there is partial or complete volume loss in a lung or lobe this is referred to as collapse or atelectasis, implying a diminished volume of air in the lung with associated reduction of lung volume. There are several different mechanisms for lung or lobar collapse, for example relaxation or passive collapse, when fluid or air accumulates in the pleural space, cicatrisation collapse when volume loss is associated with pulmonary fibrosis, adhesive collapse as in ARDS, or resorption collapse, as in bronchial obstruction.

The radiographic appearance in pulmonary collapse depends upon a number of factors. These include the mechanism of collapse, the extent of collapse, the presence or absence of consolidation in the affected lung and the pre-existing state of the pleura. This latter factor includes the presence of underlying pleural tethering or thickening and the presence of pleural fluid.

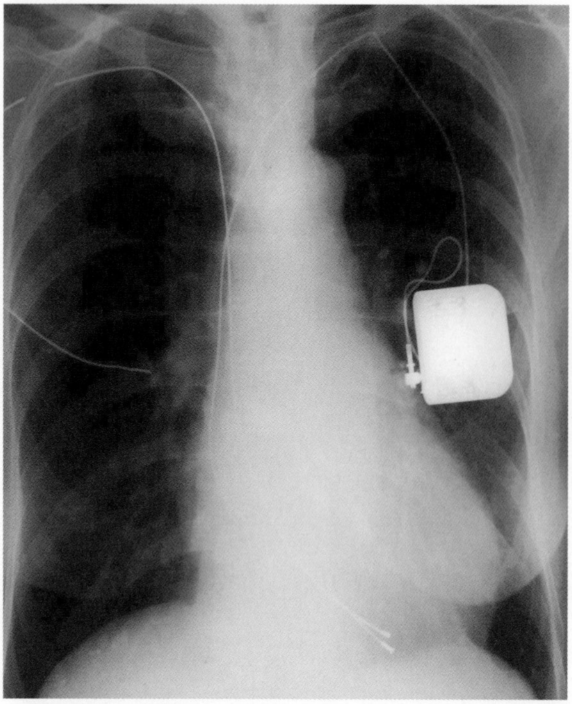

Figure 35.10 There is a fracture in the now redundant pacing wire on the right side. The functioning pacing wire is sharply kinked as it passes over the first rib and is at increased risk of subsequent fracture.

The direct signs of collapse include:

- displacement of interlobar fissures
- loss of aeration resulting in increased density or the presence of the silhouette sign
- crowding of vessels and bronchi

The indirect signs of collapse include:

- elevation of the hemidiaphragm, especially with lower lobe collapse
- mediastinal displacement, especially in upper lobe collapse
- hilar displacement, where the hilum is elevated in upper lobe collapse and depressed in lower lobe collapse
- compensatory hyperinflation of remaining normal lung, resulting in increased transradiancy or herniation across the midline from the normal side
- crowding of the ribs reflecting diminished overall volume of the affected hemithorax

COMPLETE LUNG COLLAPSE

Complete collapse (Figure 35.12) will cause complete opacification of the hemithorax, with displacement of the mediastinum to the affected side and elevation of the hemidiaphragm. Compensatory hyperinflation of the contralateral lung with herniation across the midline may be apparent. Herniation may occur in the retrosternal space, anterior to the ascending aorta, or may be posterior to the heart.

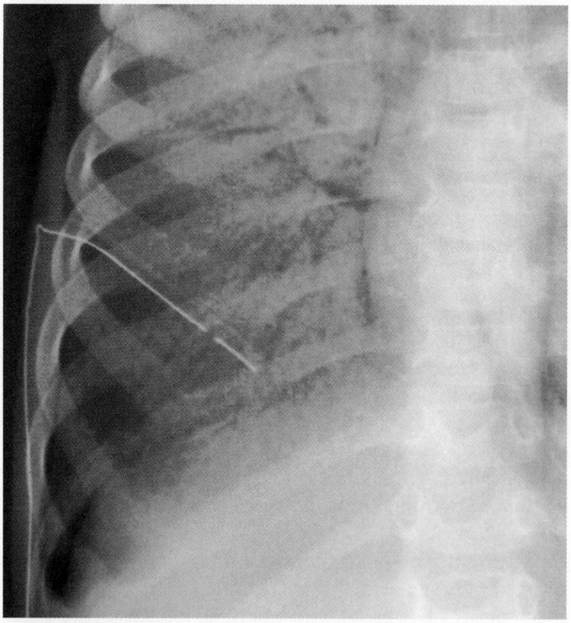

Figure 35.11 Close-up view of an area of consolidation adjacent to the right heart border, which is obscured. Air bronchograms can be identified passing through this area. A chest tube is in situ.

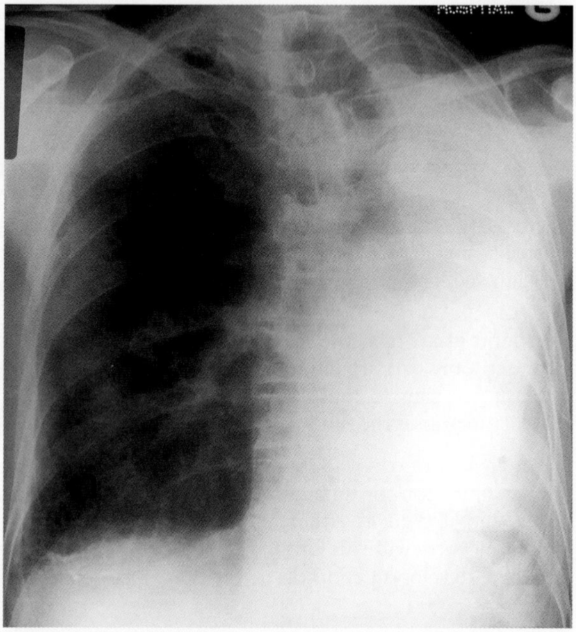

Figure 35.12 Complete lung collapse. The left hemithorax is opaque and the mediastinum has shifted to that side, together with deviation of the trachea. There was an obstructing tumour in the left main stem bronchus.

INDIVIDUAL OR COMBINED LOBAR COLLAPSE

In any situation, some or all of the signs may be present.

Right upper lobe collapse (***Figure 35.13***)

- horizontal fissure moves upwards and medially towards the superior mediastinum
- trachea deviates to the right
- compensatory hyperinfiation of the right middle and lower lobes

Middle lobe collapse (***Figure 35.14***)

- horizontal fissure and lower half of the oblique fissure move towards each other – best seen on the lateral projection
- frontal radiograph changes may be subtle, with obscuration of the right heart border
- indirect signs of volume loss are rarely obvious

Right lower lobe collapse

- partial depression of the horizontal fissure
- triangular opacity of the collapsed lower lobe on the frontal projection, usually obscuring the diaphragm but preserving the right heart border
- eventually a completely collapsed lower lobe may be so small that it flattens and merges with the mediastinum, producing a thin, wedge-shaped shadow

Left lower lobe collapse (***Figure 35.15***)

- collapsed lobe may be obscured by the heart and a penetrated view may be required

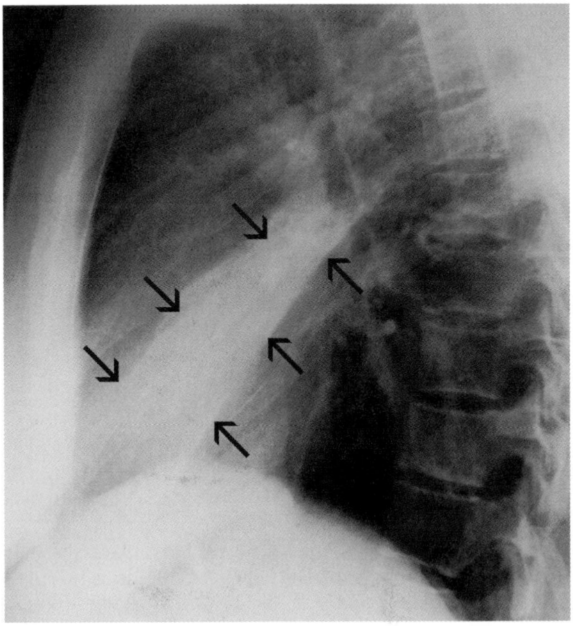

Figure 35.14 Middle lobe collapse. The horizontal fissure is depressed and demarcates the collapsed middle lobe as a wedge-shaped density best demonstrated on the lateral (arrows).

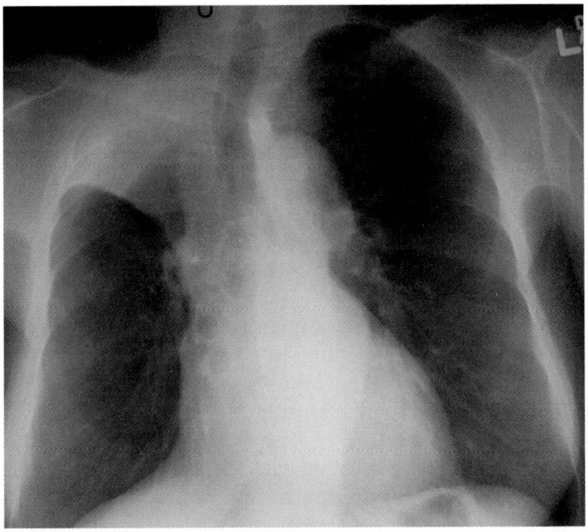

Figure 35.13 Right upper lobe collapse. The horizontal fissure has become elevated and the right upper lobe has become a wedge-shaped density extending from the hilum to the right lung apex. There is evidence of volume loss with shift of the trachea to the right side.

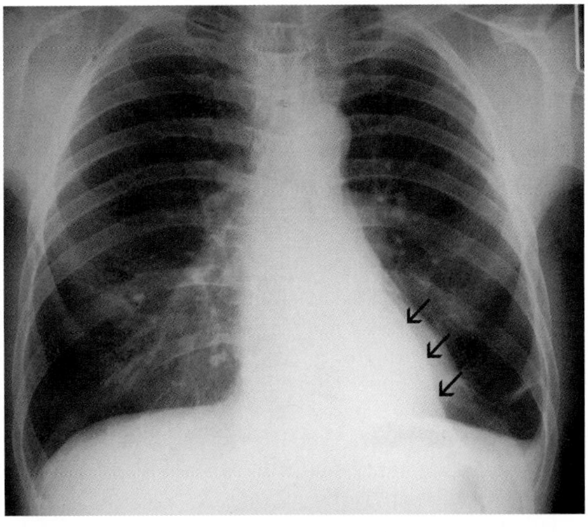

Figure 35.15 Left lower lobe collapse. The left lower lobe has become a wedge-shaped density behind the heart forming a double left heart border (arrows). The left hilar vessel to the lower lobe has disappeared as a result of collapse.

- mediastinal structures and the diaphragm adjacent to the non-aerated lobe are obscured
- extreme volume loss may cause the lobe to be so small as to be invisible as a separate opacity
- loss of lower lobe artery silhouette at the hilum

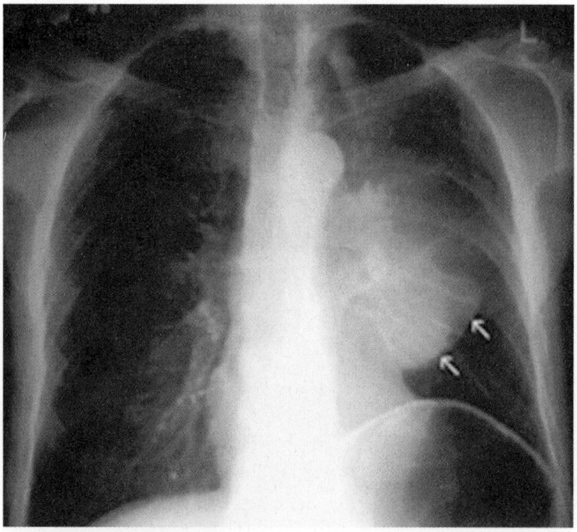

Figure 35.16 Left upper lobe collapse. A hazy opacity extends from the hilum towards the left lung apex. It is sharply demarcated inferiorly and laterally (white arrows) due to the presence of a large tumour at the left hilum which is obstructing the left upper lobe bronchus. Note the signs of volume loss, particularly the elevation of the left hemidiaphragm.

Lingula collapse

- often involved in collapse of the left upper lobe
- may collapse individually
- radiographic features are similar to those of middle lobe collapse

Left upper lobe collapse **(*Figure 35.16*)**

- Lateral view demonstrates anterior displacement of the entire oblique fissure, oriented almost parallel to the anterior chest wall, demarcating the posterior surface of the upper lobe as an elongated opacity extending from the apex almost reaching the diaphragm and lying anterior to the hilum.
- Eventually the upper lobe retracts posteriorly and loses contact with the anterior chest wall.
- Frontal radiograph demonstrates an ill-defined hazy opacity in the upper, mid and sometimes lower zones, with loss of hilar clarity.
- Hilum is often elevated, and the trachea deviated to the left.

COMBINED COLLAPSE

Right lower and middle lobe collapse is the most common pairing since a lesion may occur in the bronchus intermedius. The appearances are similar to right lower lobe collapse except that the horizontal fissure is not apparent, and the opacification reaches the lateral chest wall on the frontal radiograph, and similarly extends to the anterior chest wall on the lateral view.

Right upper and middle lobe collapse is much less common because of the distance between the origins of their bronchi, and can generally be taken to imply the presence of more than one lesion. This combination will produce appearances almost identical to those of left upper lobe collapse (see Figure 35.16). On occasion isolated right upper lobe collapse will also produce appearances that are identical to left upper lobe collapse.

UNILATERAL INCREASED TRANSRADIANCY

The commonest causes are technical and include:

- patient rotation
- poor beam centring
- offset grid

Pathological causes include:

- chest wall changes
- mastectomy
- congenital unilateral absence of pectoral muscles, known as Poland's syndrome
- reduced vascularity when interruption or significant reduction in the blood supply to one lung may cause that lung to be of increased transradiancy
- lung hyperexpansion due to air trapping or asymmetric emphysema

When there is relative increased transradiancy of one hemithorax for which there is no obvious cause then the possibility of generalised increase in radiopacity of the opposite side should be considered – for example, the posterior layering of a pleural effusion in a supine patient. Usually hypertransradiancy due to technical factors can be identified by comparison of the soft tissues around the shoulder girdle, and particularly over the axillae.

ABNORMALITIES OF THE MEDIASTINUM

Pneumomediastinum or mediastinal emphysema is the presence of air between the tissue planes of the mediastinum (see section on injuries to the mediastinum, below). Chest radiography may show vertical translucent streaks in the mediastinum, representing air separating the soft-tissue planes. The air may extend up into the neck and over the chest wall, causing subcutaneous emphysema, and also over the diaphragm. The mediastinal pleura may be displaced laterally and then be visible as a thin stripe alongside the mediastinum.

Acute mediastinitis is usually due to perforation of the oesophagus, pharynx or trachea and chest radiograph usually shows widening of the mediastinum and pneumomediastinum.

Mediastinal haemorrhage may occur from venous or arterial bleeding (Figure 35.17). The mediastinum appears widened, and blood may be seen tracking over the lung apices. It is imperative to identify a life-threatening cause such as aortic rupture.

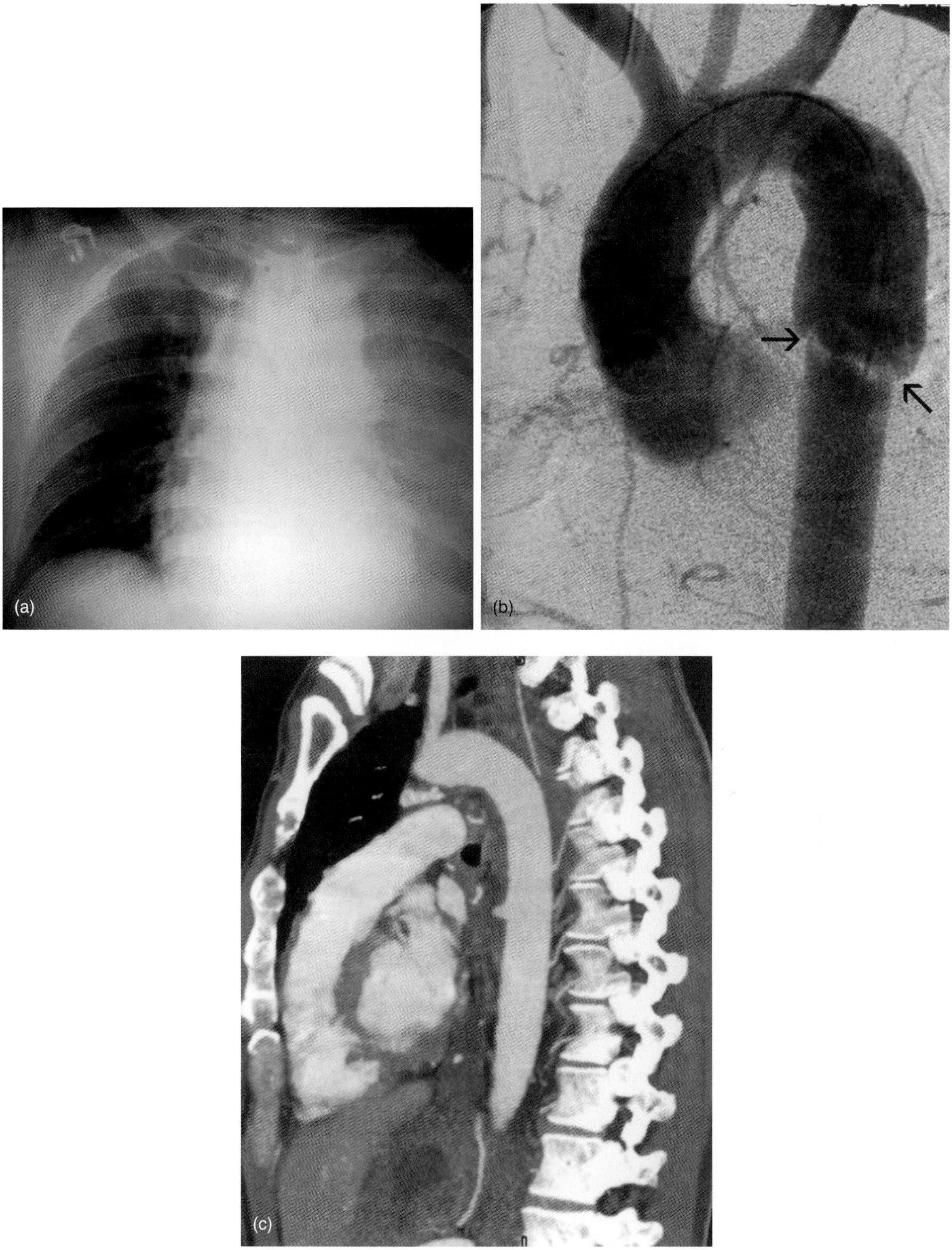

Figure 35.17 Aortic rupture. (a) There is opacification of the left hemithorax due to a large haemothorax which is layering posteriorly in this supine patient. There is widening of the mediastinum due to mediastinal haemorrhage. (b) Arch aortogram demonstrating widening of the descending thoracic aorta due to the aortic wall rupture. The point of return to normal calibre is demarcated by the arrows. (c) Computed tomography angiography of a different patient demonstrating a penetrating ulcer resulting in an aorto-oesophageal fistula that caused massive haematemesis. Note the local irregularity in the otherwise smooth anterior aortic wall on this oblique sagittal reformat.

PLEURAL FLUID

The most dependent recess of the pleural space is the posterior costophrenic angle and this is where a small effusion will tend to collect. As little as a few millilitres of fluid may be detected using decubitus views with a horizontal beam, ultrasound or CT. Larger volumes of fluid eventually fill in the costophrenic angle on the frontal view, and with increasing fluid a homogeneous opacity spreads upwards, obscuring the lung base (Figure 35.18). The fluid usually demonstrates a concave upper edge, higher laterally than medially, and obscures the diaphragm. Fluid may track into the fissures. A massive effusion may cause complete opacification of a hemithorax with passive atelectasis. The space-occupying effect of the effusion may push the mediastinum towards the opposite side, especially when the lung does not collapse significantly. Effusions in a supine patient redistribute into the paravertebral sulcus and produce an even increased density throughout that hemithorax.

Lamellar effusions are shallow collections between the lung surface and the visceral pleura, sometimes sparing the costophrenic angle, and occur early in heart failure.

Subpulmonary effusions accumulate between the diaphragm and undersurface of a lung, mimicking elevation of the hemidiaphragm, altering the diaphragmatic contour so the apex moves more laterally than usual. When left-sided, there is increased distance between the gastric air bubble and lung base.

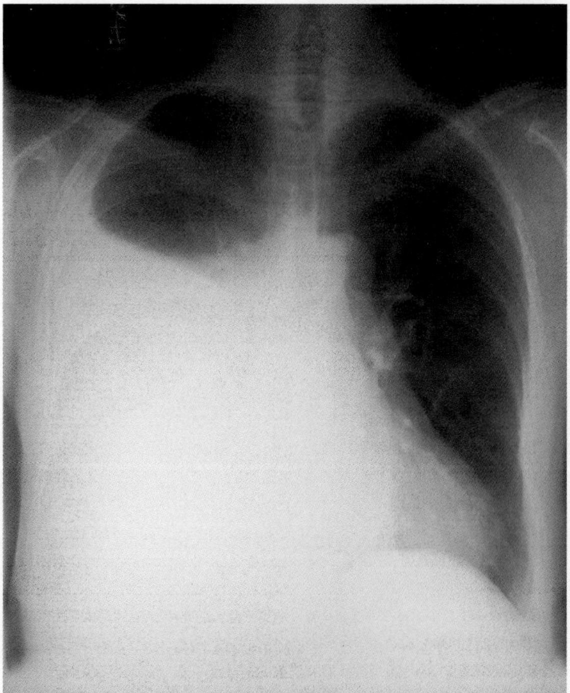

Figure 35.18 A large right pleural effusion is present in this patient. There is a typical configuration of its upper border, a meniscus extending up the lateral chest wall.

Fluid may become loculated in the interlobar fissures and is most frequently seen in heart failure. Loculated interlobar effusions may disappear rapidly and are sometimes known as pulmonary pseudotumours.

Differentiation between a simple effusion and a complicated parapneumonic effusion or an empyema usually requires thoracentesis. Loculation is best demonstrated with ultrasound.

PNEUMOTHORAX

In an erect patient, air will usually collect at the apex (Figure 35.19). The lung retracts towards the hilum and on a frontal chest film the sharp white line of the visceral pleura will be visible, separated from the chest wall by the radiolucent pleural space, which is devoid of lung markings. This should not be confused with a skin fold, which mostly occurs in supine or recumbent patients. The lung usually remains aerated, although perfusion is reduced in proportion to ventilation and therefore the radiodensity of the partially collapsed lung remains relatively normal. A large pneumothorax may lead to complete retraction of the lung, with some mediastinal shift towards the normal side. Because it is a medical emergency, tension pneumothorax is often treated before a chest radiograph is obtained. However, if a radiograph is taken in this situation it will show marked displacement of the mediastinum. Radiographically the lung may be squashed against the mediastinum, or herniate across the midline, and the ipsilateral hemidiaphragm may be depressed. A supine pneumothorax may produce increased transradiancy towards the diaphragm, and a deep sulcus sign.

COMPLICATIONS OF PNEUMOTHORAX

Pleural adhesions may limit the distribution of a pneumothorax and result in a loculated or encysted pneumothorax (see Figure 35.8). The usual appearance is an ovoid air collection adjacent to the chest wall, and it may be radiographically indistinguishable from a thin-walled subpleural pulmonary cyst or bulla. Pleural adhesions are occasionally seen as line shadows stretching between the two pleural layers, preventing relaxation of the underlying lung. Rupture of an adhesion may produce a haemopneumothorax. Collapse or consolidation of a lobe or lung in association with a pneumothorax is important because they may delay re-expansion of the lung.

Since the normal pleural space contains a small volume of fluid, blunting of the costophrenic angle by a short fluid level is commonly seen in a pneumothorax. In a small pneumothorax this fluid level may be the most obvious radiological sign. A larger fluid level usually signifies a complication and represents exudate, pus or blood, depending on the aetiology of the pneumothorax. A hydropneumothorax is a pneumothorax containing

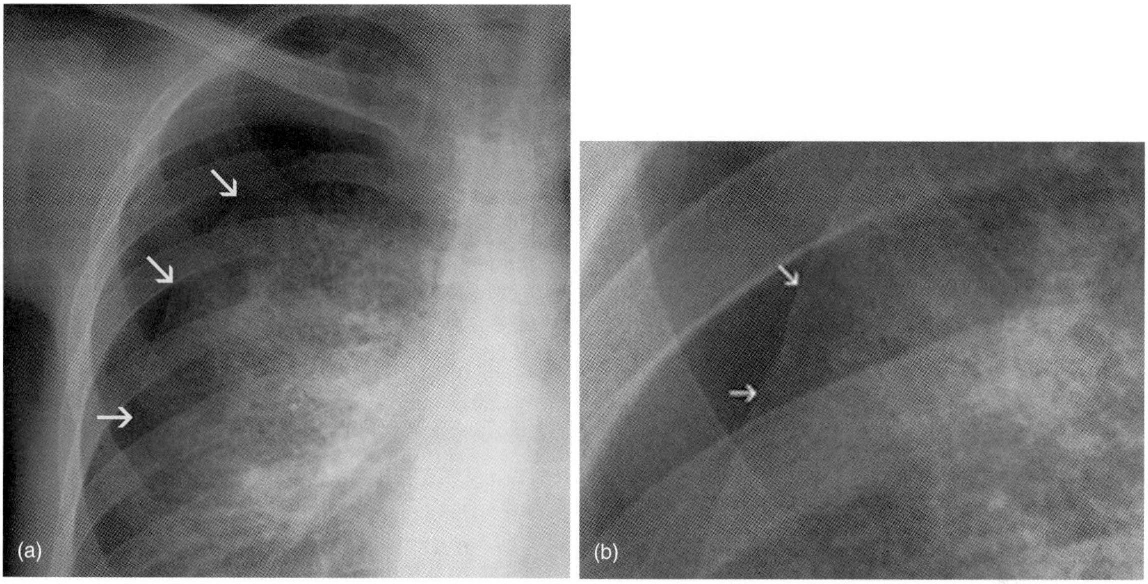

Figure 35.19 Pneumothorax. (a) This patient, with underlying lung abnormality, has developed a pneumothorax. The fine white line that represents the visceral pleura delineates the edge of the lung. (b) Close-up of the pleural line. Note how there are no vascular markings beyond this point.

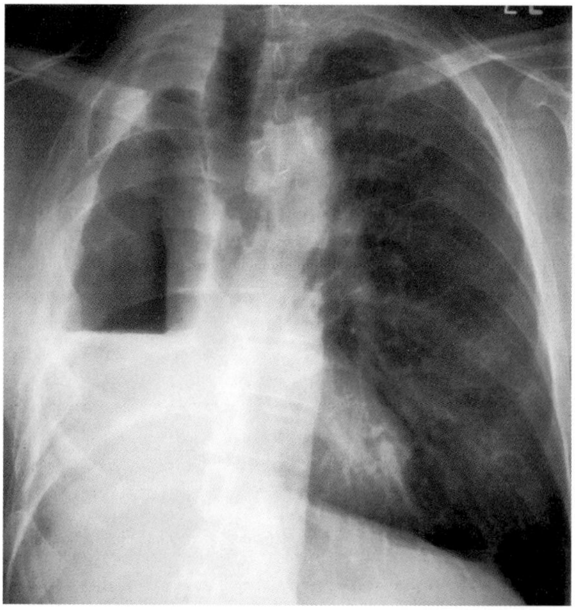

Figure 35.20 Hydropneumothorax developing in a patient who has had a previous pneumonectomy on the right for carcinoma. Spontaneous development of a bronchopleural fistula has occurred.

a significant amount of fluid (Figure 35.20). On a radiograph obtained with a horizontal beam, a fluid level is evident. A hydro- or pyopneumothorax may arise as a result of a bronchopleural fistula, and may be a complication of surgery, tumour or infection.

PULMONARY EMBOLISM

CT diagnosis of pulmonary embolism is becoming routinely available, and depends upon the ability to acquire, within a single breath-hold, a volume of data large enough to include the entire thorax. This rapid acquisition allows excellent contrast opacification of the pulmonary arterial tree for the duration of the scan, revealing any thrombus within the central pulmonary vessels (Figure 35.21). There are numerous studies evaluating helical and electron beam CT in the diagnosis of acute pulmonary embolus, with excellent reported sensitivity and specificity for the detection of clot down to the segmental level.[5–8] Most of these studies also allow other diagnoses to be made that explain the symptoms of chest pain or dyspnoea, even when no pulmonary embolism is present.

TRAUMA AND THE ICU PATIENT

SKELETAL INJURY[9]

Following trauma rib fractures are common and may be single, multiple, unilateral or bilateral. In cases of chest trauma, the chest X-ray is more important in detecting a complication of rib fracture than the fracture itself. Fracture of one of the first three ribs is often associated with major intrathoracic injury, and fracture of the lower three ribs may be associated with important hepatic, splenic or renal injury. Complications of rib fracture include a flail segment, pneumothorax, haemothorax and subcutaneous emphysema. A flail segment is usually apparent clinically

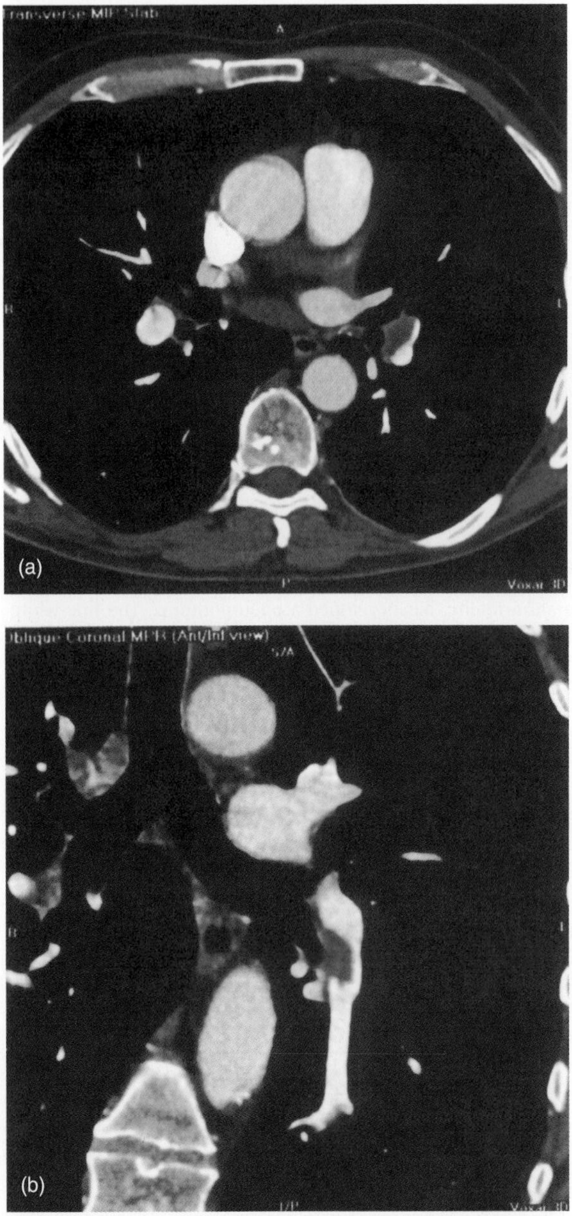

Figure 35.21 (a) Large pulmonary embolus in the right lower lobe pulmonary artery demonstrated by spiral computed tomography scanning. Both pulmonary arteries are outlined by contrast except for the embolus itself. (b) Coronal reformat in the same case, domonstrating thrombus in the lower lobe artery.

and radiologically. The fractured ends of ribs may penetrate underlying pleura and lung and cause a pneumothorax, haemothorax, haemopneumothorax or intrapulmonary haemorrhage. Air may also escape into the chest wall and cause subcutaneous emphysema. Fractures of the sternum usually require a lateral film or CT for visualisation. Fractures of the thoracic spine may be associated with a paraspinal shadow, which represents haematoma. Fractures of the clavicle may be associated with injury to the subclavian vessels or brachial plexus, and posterior dislocation of the clavicle at the sternoclavicular joint may cause injury to the trachea, oesophagus, great vessels or nerves of the superior mediastinum.

DIAPHRAGMATIC INJURY[10]

Laceration of the diaphragm may result from penetrating or non-penetrating trauma to the chest or abdomen. Rupture of the left hemidiaphragm is encountered more frequently in clinical practice than rupture on the right (Figure 35.22). The typical plain film appearance is of obscuration of the affected hemidiaphragm and increased shadowing in the ipsilateral hemithorax due to herniation of stomach, omentum, bowel or solid viscera, although such herniation may be delayed. Ultrasound may demonstrate diaphragmatic laceration and free fluid in both the pleura and peritoneum. Barium studies may be useful to confirm herniation of stomach or bowel into the chest.

PLEURAL INJURY[9,11]

Pneumothorax may be a complication of rib fracture, and is then usually associated with a haemothorax. If no ribs are fractured, pneumothorax is secondary to a pneumomediastinum, pulmonary laceration or penetrating chest injury. Pneumothorax due to a penetrating injury is liable

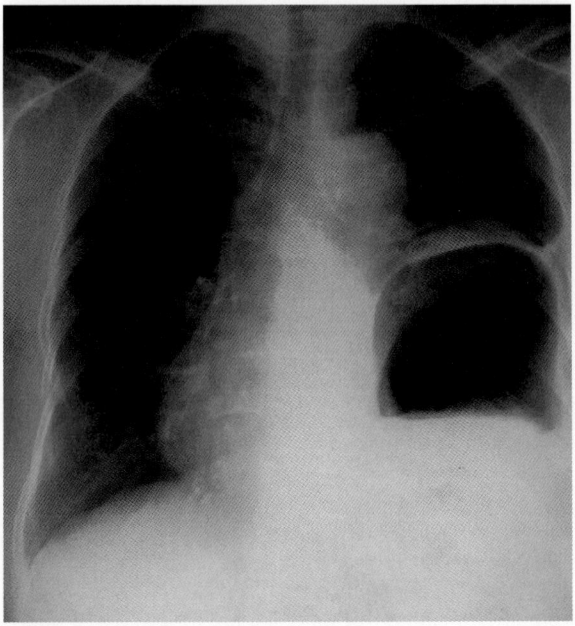

Figure 35.22 Ruptured left hemidiaphragm. Previous trauma resulted in rupture of the hemidiaphragm. A chest radiograph obtained some months later demonstrates herniation of the stomach into the left hemithorax.

to develop increased pressure, resulting in a tension pneumothorax, which may require emergency decompression. Haemothorax may also occur with or without rib fractures, and is due to laceration of intercostal or pleural vessels. If a pneumothorax is also present a fluid level will be seen on a horizontal-beam film. Pleural effusion may also result from trauma. Open injuries to the pleura are prone to infection and development of an empyema.

INJURIES TO THE LUNG[12–14]

Pulmonary contusion is due to haemorrhagic exudation into the alveoli and interstitial spaces and appears as patchy, non-segmental consolidation within the first few hours of penetrating or non-penetrating trauma. There is usually improvement within 2 days and clearance within 3–4 days. Pulmonary lacerations may be obscured by pulmonary contusion, but, as this resolves, the laceration will become evident. If filled with blood it appears as a homogeneous round opacity, and if partly filled with blood it may show a fluid level. Such pulmonary haematomas or blood cysts gradually decrease in size, but may take a few months to resolve completely. Fat embolism is a rare complication of multiple fractures, with poorly defined nodular opacities throughout both lungs, which resolve within a few days.

INJURIES TO THE TRACHEA AND BRONCHI[13,15]

Laceration or rupture of a major airway is an uncommon result of severe chest trauma. Fracture of the first three ribs and mediastinal emphysema and pneumothorax may also be evident. The injury is usually in the trachea just above the carina, or in a main bronchus just distal to the carina. If the bronchial sheath is preserved there may be no immediate signs or symptoms, but tracheostenosis or bronchiectasis may occur later. CT may be helpful in diagnosis, but bronchoscopy is the best diagnostic method in the acute stage.

INJURIES TO THE MEDIASTINUM[16]

Pneumomediastinum and mediastinal emphysema, discussed above, are the presence of air between the tissue planes of the mediastinum. Air may reach here as a result of pulmonary interstitial emphysema, perforation of the oesophagus, trachea or bronchus, or from a penetrating chest injury. Pulmonary interstitial emphysema is a result of alveolar wall rupture due to high intra-alveolar pressure, and may occur during violent coughing, severe asthma or crush injuries, or be due to positive-pressure ventilation. Air dissects centrally along the perivascular sheath to reach the mediastinum. Rarely, air may dissect into the mediastinum from a pneumoperitoneum. A pneumomediastinum may extend beyond the thoracic inlet into the neck, and over the chest wall. Pneumothorax is a common complication of pneumomediastinum, but the converse rarely occurs. Pneumomediastinum usually produces vertical translucent streaks in the mediastinum. This represents gas separating and outlining the soft-tissue planes and structures of the mediastinum. Gas shadows may extend up into the neck, or dissect extrapleurally over the diaphragm, or extend into the soft-tissue planes of the chest wall, causing subcutaneous emphysema. The mediastinal pleura may be displaced laterally, and become visible as a linear soft-tissue shadow parallel to the mediastinum. If mediastinal air collects beneath the pericardium the central part of the diaphragm may be visible, producing the 'continuous diaphragm' sign. Mediastinal haemorrhage may result from penetrating or non-penetrating trauma, and be due to venous or arterial bleeding. Many cases are probably unrecognised, as clinical and radiographic signs are absent. Important causes include automobile accidents, aortic rupture and dissection, and introduction of CVCs. There is usually bilateral mediastinal widening, but a localised haematoma may occur.

ACUTE AORTIC INJURY

Aortic rupture (see Figure 35.17)[17] is usually the result of an automobile accident. Most non-fatal aortic tears occur at the aortic isthmus, the site of the ligamentum arteriosum. Only 10–20% of patients survive the acute episode, but a small number may develop a chronic aneurysm at the site of the tear. The commonest acute radiographic signs are widening of the superior mediastinum, and obscuration of the aortic knuckle. Other radiographic signs include deviation of the left main bronchus anteriorly, inferiorly and to the right, and rightward displacement of the trachea, a nasogastric tube or the right parasternal line. A left apical extrapleural cap or a left haemothorax may be visible. Although aortography is the definitive investigation, CT, transoesophageal echocardiography or magnetic resonance imaging may be diagnostic. In everyday practice, many departments will have emergency access to a CT scanner, but will not be centres of cardiothoracic surgery. A properly conducted CT scan demonstrating a normal mediastinum has a very high negative predictive value for aortic rupture. However, if CT is equivocal or shows a mediastinal haematoma then generally angiography will be required prior to surgery.

CARDIAC INJURY[18]

This is rare but may result from penetrating or blunt trauma. Penetrating injuries are usually rapidly fatal but may cause tamponade, ventricular aneurysm or septal defects. Blunt trauma may cause myocardial contusion and infarction and may be associated with transient or more permanent rhythm disturbance.

OESOPHAGEAL RUPTURE[19]

This is usually the result of instrumentation or surgery, but occasionally occurs in penetrating trauma, and is rarely spontaneous and due to sudden increase of intraoesophageal pressure (Boerhaave syndrome). Clinically there is acute mediastinitis; radiographically there are signs of pneumomediastinum, with or without a pneumothorax or hydropneumothorax, which is usually left-sided. The diagnosis should be confirmed by a swallow. This should initially be with water-soluble contrast medium in order to avoid the small risk of granuloma formation in the mediastinum that has been described following barium leakage. Chylothorax due to damage to the thoracic duct may become apparent hours or days after trauma. Thoracic surgery is the commonest cause.

THE POSTOPERATIVE CHEST

THORACIC COMPLICATIONS OF GENERAL SURGERY

ATELECTASIS

Atelectasis is the commonest pulmonary complication of thoracic or abdominal surgery. The chest X-ray usually shows elevation of the diaphragm, due to a poor inspiration. Linear opacities are present in the lower zones, and represent a combination of subsegmental volume loss and consolidation. The shadows usually appear about 24 hours postoperatively and resolve within 2–3 days.

PLEURAL EFFUSIONS

Pleural effusions are common immediately following abdominal surgery and usually resolve within 2 weeks. They may be associated with pulmonary infarction. Effusions due to subphrenic infection usually occur later.

PNEUMOTHORAX

Pneumothorax, when it complicates extrathoracic surgery, is usually a complication of positive-pressure ventilation or central venous line insertion. It may complicate nephrectomy.

ASPIRATION PNEUMONITIS

Aspiration pneumonitis is common during anaesthesia, but fortunately is usually insignificant. When significant, patchy consolidation appears within a few hours, usually basally or around the hila. Clearing occurs within a few days, unless there is superinfection.

PULMONARY OEDEMA

In the postoperative period oedema may be cardiogenic or non-cardiogenic.

PNEUMONIA

Postoperative atelectasis and aspiration pneumonitis may be complicated by pneumonia. Postoperative pneumonias, therefore, tend to be associated with bilateral basal shadowing.

SUBPHRENIC ABSCESS

Subphrenic abscess usually produces elevation of the hemidiaphragm, pleural effusion and basal atelectasis. Loculated gas may be seen below the diaphragm, and fluoroscopy may show splinting of the diaphragm. Subphrenic abscess can be demonstrated by CT or ultrasound.

PULMONARY EMBOLISM

Pulmonary embolism may produce pulmonary shadowing, pleural effusion or elevation of the diaphragm, but is not excluded by a normal radiograph. In the ICU setting the radiological investigation of choice is spiral CT scanning.

THORACIC COMPLICATIONS OF CARDIAC SURGERY

Most cardiac operations are performed through a sternotomy incision, and wire sternal sutures are often seen on the postoperative films. Mitral valvotomy is now rarely performed via a thoracotomy incision, but this route is still used for surgery of coarctation of the aorta, patent ductus arteriosus, Blalock–Taussig shunts and pulmonary artery banding.

Widening of the cardiovascular silhouette is usual, and represents bleeding and oedema. Marked or progressive widening of the mediastinum suggests significant haemorrhage (Figure 35.23). Some air commonly remains in the pericardium following cardiac surgery, so that the signs of pneumopericardium may be present.

Left basal shadowing is almost invariable, representing atelectasis. This shadowing usually resolves over a week or two. Small pleural effusions are also common in the immediate postoperative period.

Pneumoperitoneum is sometimes seen, due to involvement of the peritoneum by the sternotomy incision. It is of no pathological significance (see Figure 35.4).

Violation of left or right pleural space may lead to a pneumothorax. Damage to a major lymphatic vessel may lead to a chylothorax or a more localised chyloma. Phrenic nerve damage may cause paresis or paralysis of a hemidiaphragm.

Surgical clips or other metallic markers have sometimes been used to mark the ends of coronary artery bypass grafts. Prosthetic heart valves are usually visible radiographically, but they may be difficult to see on an underpenetrated film.

Sternal dehiscence may be apparent radiographically by a linear lucency appearing in the sternum and alteration in position of the sternal sutures on consecutive films. The diagnosis is usually made clinically and may be associated with osteomyelitis. A first or second rib may be fractured when the sternum is spread apart. The importance of this observation is that it may explain chest pain in the postoperative period.

Acute mediastinitis may complicate mediastinal surgery, although it is more commonly associated with oesophageal perforation or surgery. Radiographically there may be mediastinal widening or pneumomediastinum, and these features are best assessed by CT scan.

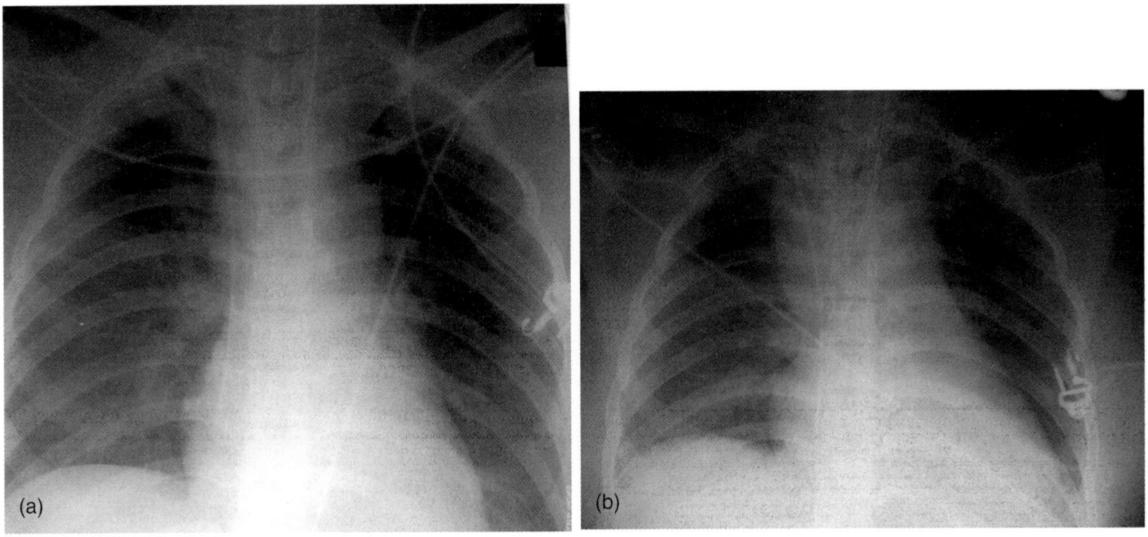

Figure 35.23 Following cardiac surgery (a) the postoperative chest radiograph appears satisfactory. A few hours later (b) the mediastinum has widened considerably, due to mediastinal haemorrhage.

REFERENCES

1. Desai SR. Acute respiratory distress syndrome: imaging of the injured lung. *Clin Radiol* 2002; **57**: 8–17.
2. Chastre J, Trouillet J-L, Vuagnat A *et al.* Nosocomial pneumonia in patients with acute respiratory distress syndrome. *Am J Respir Crit Care Med* 1998; **157**: 1165–72.
3. Gillette MA, Hess DR. Ventilator-induced lung injury and the evolution of lung-protective strategies in acute respiratory distress syndrome. *Respir Care* 2001; **46**: 130–48.
4. Knutstad K, Hager B, Hauser M. Radiologic diagnosis and management of complications related to central venous access. *Acta Radiol* 2003; **44**: 508–16.
5. Task force report. Guidelines on the diagnosis and management of acute pulmonary embolism. *Eur Heart J* 2000; **21**: 1301–36.
6. Monreal M, Suarez C, Fajardo JA *et al.* Management of patients with acute venous thromboembolism: findings from the RIETE registry. *Pathophysiol Haemost Thromb* 2004; **33**: 330–4.
7. Baile EM, King GG, Muller NL *et al.* Spiral computed tomography is comparable to angiography for the diagnosis of pulmonary embolism. *Am J Respir Crit Care Med* 2000; **161**: 1010–15.
8. Wildberger JE, Mahnken AH, Das M *et al.* CT imaging in acute pulmonary embolism: diagnostic strategies. *Eur Radiol* 2005; **15**: 919–29.
9. Wicky S, Wintermark M, Schnyder P *et al.* Imaging of blunt chest trauma. *Eur Radiol* 2000; **10**: 1524–38.
10. Eren S, Kantarci M, Okur A. Imaging of diaphragmatic rupture after trauma. *Clin Radiol* 2006; **61**: 467–77.
11. Miller LA. Chest wall, lung, and pleural space trauma. *Radiol Clin North Am* 2006; **44**: 213–24.
12. Nelson LD. Ventilatory support of the trauma patient with pulmonary contusion. *Respir Care Clin North Am* 1996; **2**: 425–47.
13. Wanek S, Mayberry JC. Blunt thoracic trauma: flail chest, pulmonary contusion, and blast injury. *Crit Care Clin* 2004; **20**: 71–81.
14. Keough V, Pudelek B. Blunt chest trauma: review of selected pulmonary injuries focusing on pulmonary contusion. *AACN Clin Issues* 2001; **12**: 270–81.
15. Kiser C, O'Brien SM, Detterbeck FC. Tracheobronchial injuries: treatment and outcomes. *Ann Thorac Surg* 2001; **71**: 2059–65.
16. Ketai L, Brandt MM, Schermer C. Nonaortic mediastinal injuries from blunt chest trauma. *J Thorac Imaging* 2000; **15**: 120–7.
17. Mirvis SE. Diagnostic imaging of acute thoracic injury. *Semin Ultrasound CT MR* 2004; **25**: 156–79.
18. Bansal MK, Maraj S, Chewaproug D *et al.* Myocardial contusion injury: redefining the diagnostic algorithm. *Emerg Med J* 2005; **22**: 465–9.
19. Younes Z, Johnson DA. The spectrum of spontaneous and iatrogenic esophageal injury: perforations, Mallory–Weiss tears, and hematomas. *J Clin Gastroenterol* 1999; **29**: 306–17.

Part Five

Gastrointestinal Emergencies

36

Acute gastrointestinal bleeding

Joseph J Y Sung

Acute gastrointestinal (GI) bleeding is a common admission to the intensive care unit (ICU) and a major cause of morbidity and mortality. Peptic ulcer disease accounts for 75% of upper GI bleeding.[1,2] Bleeding from varices, oesophagitis, duodenitis and Mallory–Weiss syndrome each account for between 5% and 15% of cases. About 20% of GI bleeding arises from the lower GI tract. Common aetiological causes for GI bleeding are listed in Table 36.1. Mortality from upper GI bleeding has remained at approximately 10% for decades, but recent reports suggest that mortality from bleeding ulcers has fallen substantially to about 5%.[3] On the other hand, variceal bleeding has a much higher mortality of about 30%. Risk factors for mortality include old age, associated medical problems, coagulopathy and magnitude of bleeding.

UPPER GASTROINTESTINAL BLEEDING

CLINICAL PRESENTATION

The patient may or may not present with a history of upper GI problems. There may be pain but bleeding ulcers can be painless, especially in elderly patients and users of non-steroidal anti-inflammatory drugs. Frequently, the symptoms of hypovolaemia such as tachycardia, pallor, sweating, cyanosis, mental confusion and oliguria may be present, especially in massive GI bleeding. A history of vomiting and retching preceding haematemesis suggests Mallory–Weiss syndrome.

Haematemesis and melaena are the most common presentations of acute upper GI bleeding. Haematochezia is the passage of bright red or maroon blood from the rectum, in the form of pure blood or admixed with stool. It usually represents a lower intestinal source of bleeding, but can also be a feature of massive upper GI bleeding.

INVESTIGATION

ENDOSCOPY OR BARIUM STUDY

As history and physical examination are seldom useful in identifying the source of bleeding, investigations are necessary in most cases of GI bleeding. Endoscopy has replaced barium studies as the investigation of choice. It should be performed as soon as the patient is haemodynamically stabilised, and adequate supportive personnel are available. Endoscopy is preferred to barium X-rays for the following reasons:

- Endoscopy allows more precise identification of the site and nature of bleeding.
- Endoscopic appearance often predicts the risk of recurrent bleeding from ulcer and varices (see below).
- Lesions such as gastritis, portal hypertensive gastropathy and duodenitis are difficult to diagnose by barium X-ray.
- Treatments such as injecting ulcers may be instigated during endoscopy (see below).
- Barium X-ray is notoriously unreliable in patients with previous gastric surgery.

However, endoscopy can induce serious hypoxia in patients with cardiorespiratory diseases. Continuous monitoring of blood pressure, pulse and oxygen saturation with a pulse oximeter is mandatory. Oxygen should be administered by nasal cannula when necessary.

ANGIOGRAPHY

Angiography is seldom used for the diagnosis of upper GI bleeding. Theoretically, when the bleeding is very brisk and obscures the endoscopic view, angiography may help to identify the sources of bleeding and may sometimes be used to embolise the bleeding point. In practice, however, most patients with this degree of haemorrhage should be considered for emergency laparotomy.

MANAGEMENT OF NON-VARICEAL UPPER GI BLEEDING

The goals of managing a patient with acute GI bleeding are first, to resuscitate; second, to control active bleeding; and third, to prevent recurrence of haemorrhage.

RESUSCITATION

Blood and plasma expanders should be given through large-bore intravenous cannulae. Vital signs should be closely monitored. In patients with hypovolaemic shock, central venous pressure and hourly urine output should also be observed (see Chapter 11). Following adequate resuscitation, management is directed to identify the

Table 36.1 Common causes of acute gastrointestinal bleeding

Upper gastrointestinal bleeding
Peptic ulcers (DU:GU 3:1)
Varices (oesophageal varices:gastric varices 9:1)
Portal hypertensive gastropathy
Mallory–Weiss syndrome
Gastritis, duodenitis and oesophagitis
Lower gastrointestinal bleeding
Diverticular bleeding
Angiodysplasia and arteriovenous malformation
Colonic polyps or tumours
Meckel's diverticulum
Inflammatory bowel diseases

DU, duodenal ulcer; GU, gastrointestinal ulcer.

lesion and distinguish the high-risk patient, who is likely to require early endoscopic or surgical treatment.

THE HIGH-RISK PATIENT

Significant GI bleeding is indicated by syncope, haematemesis, systolic blood pressure below 100 mmHg (13.3 kPa), postural hypotension and, if more than 4 units of blood have to be transfused in 12 hours, to maintain blood pressure. Patients over 60 years old and with multiple underlying diseases are at even higher risk.[3] Those admitted for other medical problems (e.g. heart or respiratory failure, or cerebrovascular bleed) and who have GI bleeding during hospitalisation also have a higher mortality.

THE HIGH-RISK ULCER

Peptic ulcers that are actively bleeding or have bled recently may show stigmata of haemorrhage on endoscopy. These include localised active bleeding (i.e. pulsatile, arterial spurting or simple oozing), an adherent blood clot, a protuberant vessel or a flat pigmented spot on the ulcer base. Stigmata of haemorrhage are important predictors of recurrent bleeding (Table 36.2). The proximal postero inferior wall of the duodenal bulb and the high lesser curve of the stomach are common sites for severe recurrent bleeding, due probably to their respective large arteries (gastroduodenal and left gastric arteries).

TREATMENT

Pharmacological control

Acid-suppressing drugs such as H_2-receptor antagonists and proton pump inhibitors are very effective drugs to

Table 36.2 Stigmata of haemorrhage and risk of recurrent bleeding in peptic ulcers

Stigmata of haemorrhage	% recurrent bleeding
Spurter or oozer	85–90
Protuberant vessel	35–55
Adherent clot	30–40
Flat spot	5–10
None	5

promote ulcer healing. An acidic environment impairs platelet function and haemostasis. Therefore, reducing the secretion of gastric acid should reduce bleeding and encourage ulcer healing. A recent study has shown that potent acid suppression using intravenous proton pump inhibitors reduces recurrent bleeding after endoscopic therapy.[4] Proton pump inhibitors should be recommended in high-risk peptic ulcer bleeding patients as an adjuvant to endoscopic therapy. In contrast, antifibrinolytic agents such as tranexamic acid have not been effective in reducing the operative rate and mortality of acute GI haemorrhage. Recent studies show that in patients at high risk of recurrent bleeding, pharmacologic control without endoscopic hemostasis is inadequate.[5] Thus a combination of endoscopic and pharmacologic therapy offers the best therapy for ulcer bleeding patients.[6,7]

Endoscopic therapy

Most patients with acute upper GI haemorrhage stop bleeding spontaneously and have an uneventful recovery. No specific intervention is required in these patients. Endoscopic haemostasis should be used in patients with a high risk of persistent or recurrent bleeding. In the last two decades, endoscopic haemostasis, with its high efficacy and low morbidity, has resulted in a dramatic decrease in emergency surgery, and has reduced the mortality of ulcer bleeding. The three most popular methods of haemostasis are as follows.

Adrenaline (epinephrine) injection Endoscopic injection of adrenaline (1:10 000 dilution) at 0.5–1.0-ml aliquots (up to 10–15 ml) into and around the ulcer bleeding point has achieved successful haemostasis in over 90% of cases.[6] Debate exists as to whether the haemostatic effect is a result of local tamponade by the volume injected, or vasoconstriction by adrenaline. Absorption of adrenaline into the systemic circulation has been documented, but without any significant effect on the haemodynamic status of the patient.[8] Adrenaline injection is an effective, cheap, portable and easy-to-learn method of haemostasis, and has acquired worldwide popularity.

Coaptive coagulation This method uses direct pressure and heat energy (heater probe) or electrocoagulation (bipolar coagulation probe (BICAP)) to control ulcer bleeding. The depth of tissue injury induced by these devices is minimised, as the bleeding vessel is tamponaded prior to coagulation. The overall efficacy of the adrenaline injection, heater probe and BICAP probe methods is comparable.[9] Occasionally, it is not possible to obtain a view en face of the bleeding ulcers, particularly those on the lesser curve or on the posterior wall of the duodenal bulb. In these situations, direct pressure cannot be applied, and the failure rate of coaptive coagulation in these situations is expected to be higher.

Haemoclips Endoscopic clipping of a bleeding vessel is an appealing alternative treatment which has gained popularity in recent years. The advantage of haemoclips over thermocoagulation is that there is no tissue injury induced and hence the risk of perforation is reduced. Studies comparing haemoclips against injection and thermocoagulation have shown favourable results.[10,11] However, the application of haemoclips in certain sites, for example lesser curve, gastric fundus and posterior wall of the duodenum, is technically difficult. Loading of clips on to the application device is cumbersome and time-consuming and transfer of torque from the handle to the tip of the device is limited.

SURGERY

Surgery remains the most definitive method of stopping haemorrhage. However, there is little agreement on the exact indications and best timing for surgical intervention. These issues are even less clear now that endoscopic treatment is so effective. Accordingly, good cooperation among intensivists, gastroenterologists and surgeons is essential. Indications for surgery can be:

- arterial bleeding that cannot be controlled by endoscopic haemostasis
- massive transfusion (i.e. total of 6–8 units of blood) required to maintain blood pressure
- recurrent clinical bleeding after initial success in endoscopic hemostasis
- evidence suggestive of GI perforation

Surgical procedures include underrunning of the ulcer, underrunning plus vagotomy and drainage, and various types of gastrectomy. The overall mortality of emergency surgery for GI bleeding is about 15–20%. In a study investigating the best salvage treatment for patients with recurrent bleeding after endoscopic therapy, surgery was found to be comparable to repeating endoscopic treatment in securing hemostasis.[12] However, morbidity is significantly higher in surgical patients than in endoscopic patients. Early surgery should be considered in patients with hypovolaemic shock and/or large peptic ulcer with protuberant vessels. A protocol to manage bleeding peptic ulcer is shown in Figure 36.1.[13]

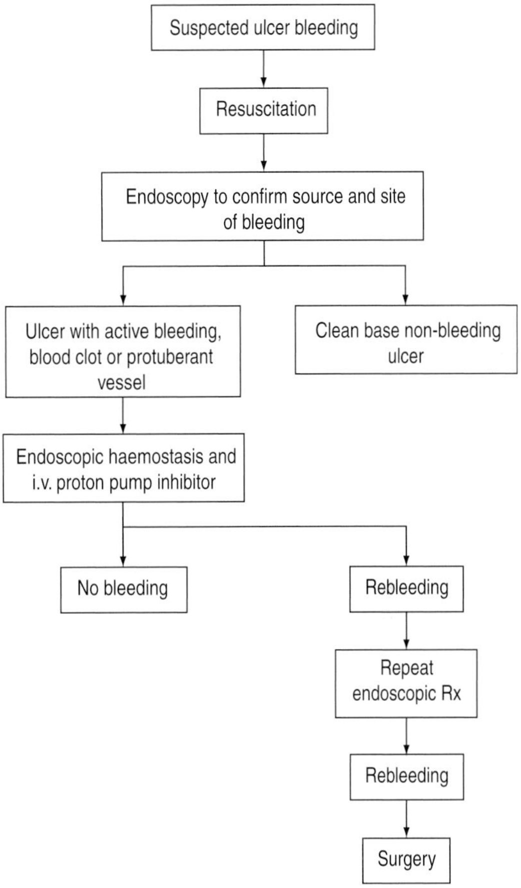

Figure 36.1 Management of peptic ulcer bleeding.

ACUTE STRESS ULCERATION

Acute stress ulceration is associated with shock, sepsis, burns, multiple trauma, head injuries, spinal injuries and respiratory, renal and hepatic failure. Lesions are most commonly seen in the gastric fundus, and range from mild erosions to acute ulcerations. The exact mechanism leading to acute mucosal erosion/ulceration in critically ill patients is still unclear. Hypoxia and hypoperfusion of the gastroduodenal mucosa are probably the most important factors. Besides haemodynamic instability, respiratory failure and coagulopathy are also strong independent factors in critically ill patients. The incidence of stress-related mucosal bleeding in ICU patients has reported to range from 8 to 45%.[14] It has been declining in the last decade as a result of highly effective management of hypotension and hypoxaemia. Bleeding may be occult or overt, from 'coffee-grounds' aspirates to frank haemorrhage.

PROPHYLAXIS AND TREATMENT

Significant ulcerations are managed as above. Minor bleeding and prophylactic treatment are considered together. Prophylactic treatment aims for gastric alkalinisation (gastric pH > 3.5), with the rationale that gastric acidity is the main cause of stress ulceration.[14] The incidence of stress ulcerations appears to be lower with prophylactic gastric alkalinisation than with placebos, although an improvement in survival has not been shown.[15,16] Gastric bacterial overgrowth and the associated nosocomial pneumonia have been concerns, but have not been substantiated by existing data. On balance, prophylactic treatment should probably be reserved only for at-risk patients. Scoring systems to estimate the risk of stress-ulcer bleeding have been proposed, for example Zinner and Tryba scores.[17,18] The mainstay of prophylaxis and treatment for minor bleeding remains supportive – optimise oxygenation and tissue perfusion and control of infection. There is little consensus among critical care experts in the choice of prophylactic treatment used.[19] Drugs given include the following:

Antacids

Antacids given hourly via a nasogastric tube can maintain gastric alkalinisation. Gastric pH monitoring is necessary. Antacids contain magnesium, aluminium, calcium or sodium, and complications may arise from excessive intake of these minerals. Bowel stasis and diarrhoea can also be problems. They are used less commonly now.

Sucralfate

This is a basic aluminium salt of sucrose octasulphate. It is effective in healing ulcers by increasing mucus secretion, mucosal blood flow and local prostaglandin production. These effects promote mucosal resistance against acid and pepsin (i.e. they are cytoprotective). As it does not alter gastric pH, Gram-negative bacterial colonisation of gastric juice is less likely. The incidence of nosocomial pneumonia may be less with sucralfate than with antacids or H_2-receptor antagonists, but this is debatable and there is a potential risk of aspiration.[15] Sucralfate is given via a nasogastric tube as 1.0 g every 4–6 hours. Constipation is a side-effect, and aluminium toxicity may arise from renal dysfunction.

H_2-receptor antagonists

These drugs suppress acid secretion by competing for the histamine receptor on the parietal cell. Cimetidine is less potent and has interactions with anticonvulsants, theophyllines and warfarin. Famotidine and nizatidine are newer agents but have no particular advantage over ranitidine. The problem of H_2-receptor antagonists is the development of tachyphylaxis after the first day of administration, leading to reduction of effectiveness in acid suppression. At least one meta-analysis showed that ranitidine did not confer any protection against stress ulcer in intensive care patients.[21]

Proton pump inhibitors

These are potent acid-suppressing agents as they block the final common pathway of acid secretion by the parietal cell, namely the proton pump. All proton pump inhibitors (omeprazole, lansoprazole, pantoprazole and rabeprazole) can be given as oral medication. Omeprazole and pantoprazole are also available in intravenous form for those who cannot be fed orally. In two non-randomized studies, intravenous omeprazole has been shown to protect critically ill patients who required ventilation from the development of stress-related mucosal bleeding from the upper GI tract.[20] Yet, there are no prospective data indicating which are the high-risk patients who might benefit from this treatment.

VARICEAL BLEEDING

Acute variceal bleeding is a serious complication of portal hypertension, with a high mortality. About 50% of patients with bleeding varices have had an earlier bleed during hospitalisation. The degree of liver failure, using Child–Pugh's classification (see Chapter 38), is the most important prognostic factor for early rebleeding and survival.

RESUSCITATION

Immediate resuscitation with whole blood and fluid is mandatory. Overtransfusion may cause a rebound increase in portal pressure (with a consequent increased risk of rebleeding) and must be avoided. Fresh frozen plasma and platelet concentrates transfusion may be indicated. A nasogastric cannula is often inserted for the removal of blood (and also drug administration). Forceful aspiration through the nasogastric tube should be discouraged as bleeding may be induced. Lactulose (15–30 ml every 4–6 hours) should be given to prevent or correct hepatic encephalopathy. A colonic wash-out can be used, but a magnesium-containing enema should be avoided in the presence of renal failure. Close attention must be given to haemodynamic monitoring.

When the patient is haemodynamically stable, upper endoscopy should be performed to identify the source of bleeding. Patients with portal hypertension could bleed from oesophageal or gastric varices, peptic ulcers and portal hypertensive gastropathy.

PHARMACOLOGICAL CONTROL

Vasopressin (0.2–0.4 U/min) used to be the most widely used agent to reduce portal blood pressure and control variceal bleeding. Adverse effects of vasopressin such as cardiac ischaemia (in about 10% of patients) and worsening coagulopathy (by release of plasminogen activator) have discouraged the use of this drug in recent years. Terlipressin, a triglycyl synthetic analogue of vasopressin, has a longer half-life and fewer cardiac side-effects and appears more effective and safe when used in combination with glyceryl trinitrate.[22] Infusion of somatostatin and its analogue (octreotide, vapreotide) reduces portal blood pressure and azygous blood flow. They are safe and effective vasoactive agents to be used in acute variceal bleeding.[23] The benefit is more prominent if these vasoactive agents are given early, even before endoscopy.[22,24] Octreotide has also been shown to be effective when used as an adjuvant therapy in combination with endoscopic therapy.[25] Recurrent bleeding episodes and hence requirement of transfusion are significantly reduced.

ENDOSCOPIC SCLEROTHERAPY

Endoscopic injection sclerotherapy is the mainstay of treatment. At endoscopy, sclerosants can be injected directly into the variceal columns (intravariceal injection) or into the mucosa adjacent to the varices (paravariceal injection) to cause venous thrombosis and inflammation, and tissue fibrosis. Commonly used sclerosants are ethanolamine oleate, sodium tetradecyl sulphate (1–3%), polidocanol and ethyl alcohol. None has appreciable advantage over the others and the choice is very much a personal preference of the endoscopist, and depends also on availability. Endoscopic sclerotherapy controls 80–90% of acute variceal bleeding. Complications such as ulcer formation, fever, chest pain and mediastinitis are common. Bleeding from gastric varices is more difficult to control by injection sclerotherapy because of difficult access. Butylcyanoacrylate (Histoacryl) has recently been used for gastric variceal injections, with a claimed superior haemostatic effect. It is mixed with lipiodol to delay the rate of polymerisation and allow radiological monitoring of the injection.

ENDOSCOPIC VARICEAL LIGATION

Endoscopic variceal ligation was introduced in the late 1980s as a mechanical method to control bleeding from varices. Rubber bands mounted on the banding device at the tip of the endoscope are released to strangulate the bleeding varices. Numerous studies comparing endoscopic variceal ligation with endoscopic sclerotherapy showed that the technique is as effective as injection sclerotherapy in acute bleeding.[9] Procedure-related complications are significantly fewer, as there is no tissue chemical irritation. An overtube to facilitate banding avoids aspiration during the procedure, but may result in serious oesophageal injury if used improperly. The tunnel vision produced by the banding device as originally designed restricts visibility, and thus makes the procedure technically difficult when bleeding is heavy. With the introduction of multiple banding devices which are loaded with 5–10 rubber bands, and the use of transparent caps, the problems of overtube injury and tunnel vision have been overcome. In many centres, endoscopic variceal ligation has replaced injection sclerotherapy as the first choice for variceal haemorrhage. Many have combined the two endoscopic treatments together in an attempt to improve the outcome. Existing data so far do not support this combined therapy to be better. Combined endoscopic therapy cannot be recommended.

BALLOON TAMPONADE

Variceal bleeding can be controlled by exerting pressure directly on the bleeding point using a balloon. The Sengstaken–Blackmore tube has been replaced by the four-lumen Minnesota tube which allows aspiration of gastric and oesophageal contents. Inflation of the gastric balloon (by 250–350 ml of water) is often sufficient to stop the bleeding by occluding the feeding veins to the oesophageal varices. If bleeding continues, the oesophageal balloon can be inflated by air and kept at a pressure of 50–60 mmHg (6.7–8.0 kPa). Duration of using balloon tamponade should be limited to 24 hours to avoid tissue pressure necrosis. Because of available effective pharmacological and endoscopic therapies, balloon tamponade should only be used in the exceptional cases when these therapies fail to effect control of bleeding.

TRANSJUGULAR INTRAHEPATIC PORTOSYSTEMIC SHUNT (TIPS)

Using a transjugular approach, a catheter is inserted into the hepatic vein, and advanced under fluoroscopic guidance into a branch of the portal vein.[26] By means of a guidewire and dilators, a self-expandable metal stent is introduced to create an intrahepatic portosystemic shunt. In good hands, success can be achieved in over 90% of cases. This procedure significantly reduces portal blood pressure and thus bleeding from varices. Major complications include intra-abdominal haemorrhage and stent occlusion. Hepatic encephalopathy has been reported in 25–60% of patients. Nevertheless, this is an effective salvage treatment for uncontrolled variceal bleeding. Meta-analysis comparing TIPS with endoscopic therapy showed that the former has secure haemostasis but at the cost of increasing risk of hepatic encephalopathy.[27]

A number of markers of outcome after TIPS have been under investigation, including the Acute Physiology, Age and Chronic Health Evaluation (APACHE) score, presence of hyponatraemia and Child C liver disease, hepatic encephalopathy before TIPS, presence of ascites and serum albumin. Before a reliable marker of outcome can be identified, TIPS should be reserved for the subset of patients who continue to bleed or develop recurrent bleeding after endoscopic therapy. Unlike shunt surgery, TIPS will not reduce the chance of future liver transplantation.

SURGERY

Surgical treatments for variceal bleeding include direct devascularisation of the lower oesophagus plus the proximal stomach and a variety of surgical shunts. The role of surgery has diminished since the advent of endoscopic treatment and TIPS.[28] Surgery is now used as a second-line treatment, when bleeding continues or recurs after two sessions of injection sclerotherapy or banding ligation. Both staple transection of the oesophagus and portocaval shunt surgery are highly effective emergency measures. Despite successful control of bleeding, long-term survival is not significantly improved. Hepatic encephalopathy is one of the major complications of shunting operations. Expectations that the Warren distal splenorenal shunt will preserve antegrade portal flow and avoid accelerated deterioration of liver function have not been realised. The Warren shunt is technically more difficult, especially if performed as an emergency. Choice of surgery should be carefully made in those who are potential transplant candidates, as it may complicate subsequent surgery. A protocol to manage variceal bleeding is shown in Figure 36.2.

LOWER GASTROINTESTINAL BLEEDING

Lower GI bleeding arises from a source distal to the ligament of Treitz. It accounts for 10–20% of acute GI bleeding. Common causes of colonic bleeding include diverticular haemorrhage and angiodysplasia (both occur on the right-sided colon), colonic polyps and carcinoma, and inflammatory bowel diseases.

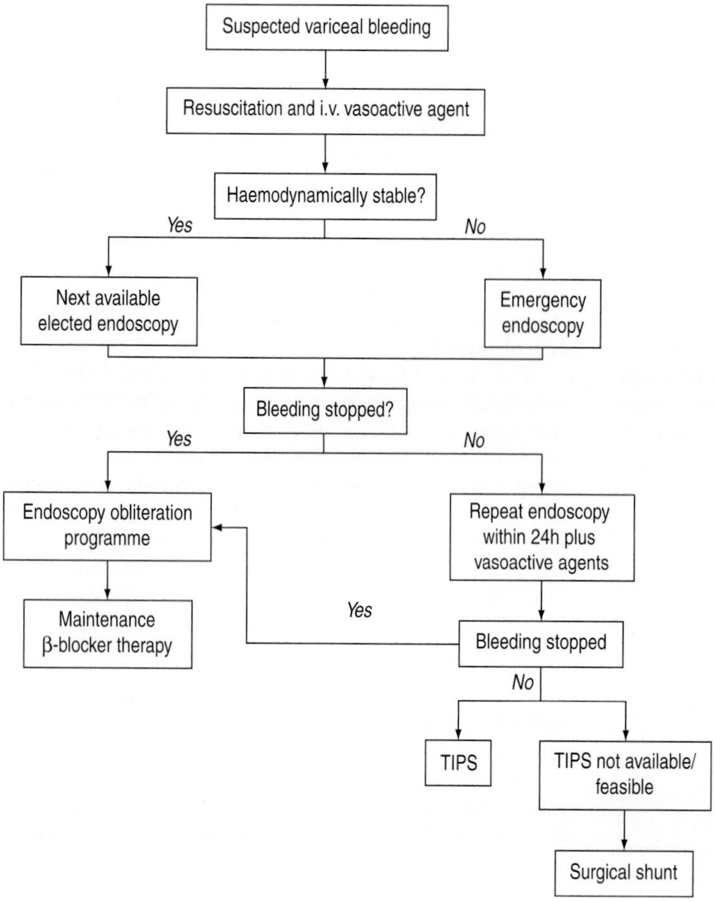

Figure 36.2 Management of variceal haemorrhage. TIPS, transjugular intrahepatic portosystemic shunt.

CLINICAL PRESENTATION

Haematochezia (bright-red blood) is the most common presentation of lower GI bleeding. However, bleeding from small intestine and right colon may also present as melaena. Abdominal pain preceding a massive bleeding episode suggests either ischaemia or inflammatory bowel disease. Painless massive bleeding is common in diverticulosis, angiodysplasia or from a Meckel's diverticulum. In a patient with portal hypertension, haemorrhoids may present with massive haematochezia.

INVESTIGATIONS

Haemorrhoids and rectal tumour can easily be identified by proctosigmoidoscopy, which should always be performed. Since upper GI bleeding is about five times as common as lower GI bleeding, the former should be excluded. When both proctosigmoidoscopy and gastroscopy are negative, the lower GI tract should be examined by colonoscopy, angiography or radionucleotide scan. Barium enema plays no role in the management of acute rectal bleeding.

COLONOSCOPY

Patients with mild-to-moderate haematochezia can be examined safely by colonoscopy. Colonoscopy is difficult in an actively bleeding patient, and may carry an increased risk of perforation. Visualisation is often unsatisfactory due to the dark discoloration of blood. Colonoscopy yields much better results with adequate bowel preparation once bleeding has stopped.

ANGIOGRAPHY OR RADIONUCLIDE SCAN

The diagnostic efficacy of radionuclide scan and angiography varies in different studies. ^{99m}Tc sulphur colloid is quickly removed from the blood stream after injection. Its diagnostic yield is low because of its short circulatory half-life. ^{99m}Tc labelling of red cells prolongs the duration of radioactivity in the body. Red cell scan has been reported to detect the source of active bleeding in over 80% of cases.

Diagnostic angiography is helpful in two situations: (1) when the view of endoscopy is completely obscured by active haemorrhage; (2) in defining abnormal vasculatures, where angiography is more sensitive even if extravasation of contrast material is not seen. These lesions include angiodysplasia, arteriovenous malformation and various inherited vascular anomalies (e.g. Rendu–Osler–Weber syndrome, pseudoxanthoma elasticum and Ehlers–Danlos syndrome). Angiography may localise the site of bleeding in 80–85% of patients when the bleeding rate is more than 0.5 ml/min. Both superior and inferior mesenteric angiograms are often needed.

MANAGEMENT

ENDOSCOPY

Bleeding from vascular anomalies can be treated by electrocoagulation, heater probe and laser photocoagulation, unless the anomalies are too large or too diffuse. Bleeding colonic polyps can be removed by polypectomy or coagulated by hot biopsy forceps. Bleeding from colonic diverticula can also be controlled with thermocoagulation through colonoscopy.[29]

ANGIOGRAPHY

Angiographic intra-arterial infusion of vasopressin or occlusion of the bleeding artery with embolic agents such as an absorbable gelatin sponge (Gelfoam) may be used in lower GI bleeding pathologies. Both diverticular bleeding and bleeding from angiodysplasia can be stopped by vasopressin infusion during angiography, but recurrence of bleeding frequently occurs with diverticular disease.

SURGERY

Diverticular bleeding usually arises from a relatively large vessel, and may be difficult to control with endoscopic or angiographic therapy. Partial resection of the colon is warranted after localisation of the bleeding site. Surgery is also indicated in vascular anomalies when endoscopic treatment fails. When an obvious and refractory massive lower GI bleeding is not identified by endoscopic or angiographic examinations, immediate laparotomy with possible subtotal colectomy should be offered. A protocol to manage lower GI bleeding is shown in Figure 36.3.

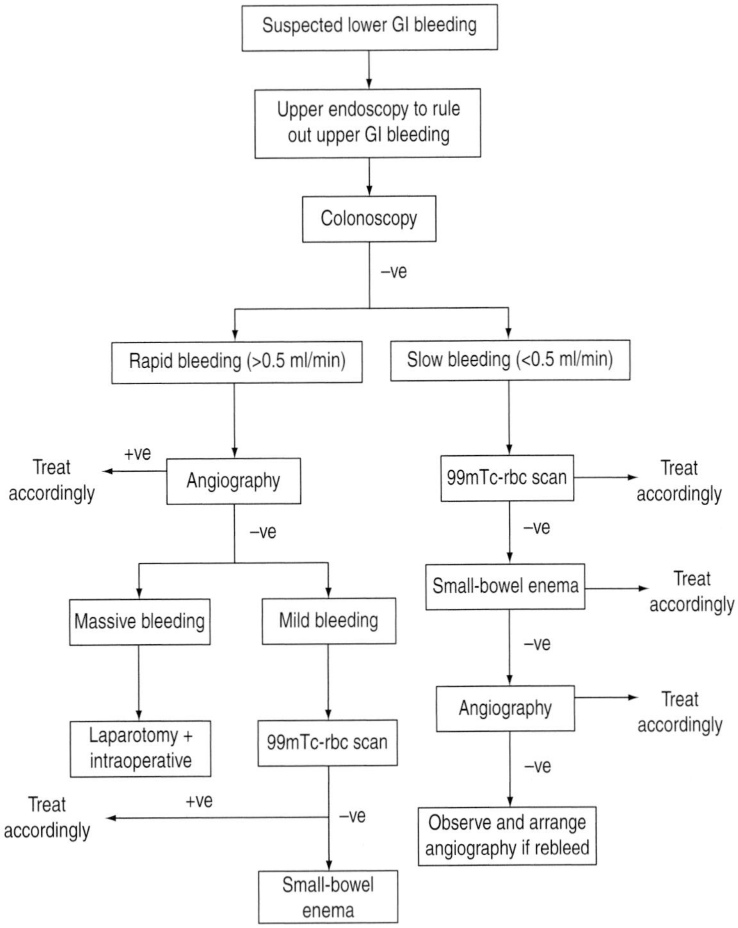

Figure 36.3 Management of lower gastrointestinal (GI) bleeding.

REFERENCES

1. Silverstein FE, Gilbert DA, Tedesco FJ *et al.* The national ASGE survey on upper gastrointestinal bleeding. I. Study design and baseline data. *Gastrointest Endosc* 1981; **27**: 73–9.
2. Silverstein FE, Gilbert DA, Tedesco FJ *et al.* The national ASGE survey on upper gastrointestinal bleeding. II. Clinical prognostic factors. *Gastrointest Endosc* 1981; **27**: 80–93.
3. Holman RA, Davis M, Gough KR *et al.* Value of a centralised approach in the management of haematemesis and melaena: experience in a district general hospital. *Gut* 1990; **31**: 504–8.
4. Lau JYW, Sung JJY, Lee KKC *et al.* A comparison of high-dose omeprazole infusion to placebo after endoscopic hemostasis to bleeding peptic ulcer. *N Engl J Med* 2000; **343**: 310–16.
5. Lau JY, Sung JJ, Lee KK *et al.* Effect of intravenous omeprazole on recurrent bleeding after endoscopic treatment of bleeding peptic ulcers [see comment]. *N Engl J Med* 2000; **343**: 310–16.
6. Chung SS, Lau JY, Sung JJ *et al.* Randomised comparison between adrenaline injection alone and adrenaline injection plus heat probe treatment for actively bleeding ulcers [see comment]. *Br Med J* 1997; **314**: 1307–11.
7. Sung JJY, Chan FKL, Lau JYW *et al.* The effect of endoscopic therapy in patients receiving omeprazole for bleeding ulcers with nonbleeding visible vessels or adherent clots: a randomized comparison. *Ann Intern Med* 2003; **139**: 237–43.
8. Sung JY, Chung SC, Low JM *et al.* Systemic absorption of epinephrine after endoscopic submucosal injection in patients with bleeding peptic ulcers. *Gastrointest Endosc* 1993; **39**: 20–2.
9. Laine L, Cook D. Endoscopic ligation compared with sclerotherapy for treatment of esophageal variceal bleeding. A meta-analysis [see comment]. *Ann Intern Med* 1995; **123**: 280–7.
10. Chung IK, Ham JS, Kim HS *et al.* Comparison of the hemostatic efficacy of the endoscopic hemoclip method with hypertonic saline-epinephrine injection and a combination of the two for the management of bleeding peptic ulcers. *Gastrointestin Endosc* 1999; **49**: 13–18.
11. Cipolletta L, Bianco MA, Marmo R *et al.* Endoclips versus heater probe in preventing early recurrent bleeding from peptic ulcer: a prospective and randomized trial. *Gastrointest Endosc* 2001; **53**: 147–51.
12. Lau JY, Sung JJ, Lam YH *et al.* Endoscopic retreatment compared with surgery in patients with recurrent bleeding after initial endoscopic control of bleeding ulcers. *N Engl J Med* 1999; **340**: 751–6.
13. Sung JJY. Current management of peptic ulcer bleeding. *Nature Clin Pract Gastro Hepatol* 2006; **3**: 24–32.
14. Cook DJ, Fuller HD, Guyatt GH *et al.* Risk factors for gastrointestinal bleeding in critically ill patients. Canadian Critical Care Trials Group. *N Engl J Med* 1994; **330**: 377–81.
15. Tryba M. Sucralfate versus antacids or H_2-antagonists for stress ulcer prophylaxis: a meta-analysis on efficacy and pneumonia rate. *Crit Care Med* 1991; **19**: 942–9.
16. Cook DJ, Witt LG, Cook RJ *et al.* Stress ulcer prophylaxis in the critically ill: a meta-analysis. *Am J Med* 1991; **91**: 519–27.
17. Zinner MJ, Zuidema GD, Smith P *et al.* The prevention of upper gastrointestinal tract bleeding in patients in an intensive care unit. *Surg Gynecol Obstet* 1981; **153**: 214–20.
18. Tryba M. Risk of acute stress bleeding and nosocomial pneumonia in ventilated intensive care unit patients: sucralfate versus antacids. *Am J Med* 1987; **83**: 117–24.
19. Lam NP, Le PD, Crawford SY *et al.* National survey of stress ulcer prophylaxis [see comment]. *Crit Care Med* 1999; **27**: 98–103.
20. Lasky MR, Metzler MH, Phillips JO. A prospective study of omeprazole suspension to prevent clinically significant gastrointestinal bleeding from stress ulcers in mechanically ventilated trauma patients. *J Trauma-Inj Infect Crit Care* 1998; **44**: 527–33.
21. Messori A, Trippoli S, Vaiani M *et al.* Bleeding and pneumonia in intensive care patients given ranitidine and sucralfate for prevention of stress ulcer: meta-analysis of randomised controlled trials. *Br Med J* 2000; **321**: 1103–6.
22. Levacher S, Letoumelin P, Pateron D *et al.* Early administration of terlipressin plus glyceryl trinitrate to control active upper gastrointestinal bleeding in cirrhotic patients. *Lancet* 1995; **346**: 865–8.
23. D'Amico G, Politi F, Morabito A *et al.* Octreotide compared with placebo in a treatment strategy for early rebleeding in cirrhosis. A double blind, randomized pragmatic trial. *Hepatology* 1998; **28**: 1206–14.
24. Avgerinos A, Nevens F, Raptis S *et al.* Early administration of somatostatin and efficacy of sclerotherapy in acute oesophageal variceal bleeds: the European Acute Bleeding Oesophageal Variceal Episodes (ABOVE) randomised trial [see comment]. *Lancet* 1997; **350**: 1495–9.
25. Sung JJ, Chung SC, Lai CW *et al.* Octreotide infusion or emergency sclerotherapy for variceal haemorrhage. *Lancet* 1993; **342**: 637–41.
26. Rossle M, Haag K, Ochs A *et al.* The transjugular intrahepatic portosystemic stent-shunt procedure for variceal bleeding [see comment]. *N Engl J Med* 1994; **330**: 165–71.
27. Papatheodoridis GV, Goulis J, Leandro G *et al.* Transjugular intrahepatic portosystemic shunt compared with endoscopic treatment for prevention of variceal rebleeding: a meta-analysis. *Hepatology* 1999; **30**: 612–22.
28. Bornman PC, Krige JE, Terblanche J. Management of oesophageal varices. *Lancet* 1994; **343**: 1079–84.
29. Jensen DM, Machicado GA, Jutabha R *et al.* Urgent colonoscopy for the diagnosis and treatment of severe diverticular hemorrhage. *N Engl J Med* 2000; **342**: 78–82.

37

Severe acute pancreatitis

Duncan L A Wyncoll

Acute inflammation of the pancreas produces a spectrum of symptoms, which may be mild and self-limiting, or reflect severe disease that leads rapidly to multiple-organ failure and death. In a majority of patients a treatable underlying cause is identified. Although mild, interstitial, oedematous pancreatitis is more common, it is the more severe form, acute necrotising pancreatitis (ANP), that accounts for the associated mortality. Two decades ago the mortality was frequently quoted to be 25–35%, even in the best centres.[1] However, more recently published series have suggested a lower mortality (15%).[2] Management of patients with severe ANP is time-consuming, and labour- and resource-intensive. Long-term follow-up suggests that, although some survivors suffer permanent exocrine and endocrine insufficiency, most maintain a good quality of life.[3]

In the last 20 years there has been a gradual move towards aggressive supportive therapy for ANP. Numerous putative therapeutic interventions have been tried, but few have provided any objective evidence of clinical benefit.

AETIOLOGY

Biliary disease and alcohol remain the two commonest causes of acute pancreatitis worldwide, accounting for 70% of cases. Although no discernible cause is found in many of the remaining cases, there are well-established associations with a number of infections, certain drugs, hyperlipidaemias and trauma. See Table 37.1 for a more exhaustive list.

RANSON'S CRITERIA

Although the overall mortality rate for acute pancreatitis is approximately 10%, the vast majority of deaths occur in those with the severe form of the disease. Since 1974 the standard means of documenting the severity of disease and risk of mortality has been by Ranson's criteria (Table 37.2).[4] These factors were determined following the analysis of 100 patients with predominantly alcohol-induced pancreatitis using clinical and laboratory data obtained on admission and after 48 hours, and the number of positive criteria should predict outcome. A decade later these criteria were re-evaluated and the first eight were found to be most predictive – this is now known as the Glasgow criteria, or Imrie score.[5]

SCORING

The Acute Physiology and Chronic Health Evaluation (APACHE) II scoring system has also been used in predicting the severity of pancreatitis, and can be used daily throughout the patient's hospital admission rather than solely within the first 48 hours, thus potentially documenting progress or deterioration. However, such scoring systems are complex to perform and have only been evaluated prospectively 24–48 hours after the onset of pancreatitis, which means that the criteria may not be valid for patients subsequently admitted to the intensive care unit (ICU). Those factors with most predictive value for mortality include advanced age, presence of renal or respiratory insufficiency and presence of shock.

The scoring of patients with acute pancreatitis is important for a number of reasons. Firstly, the clinician can be alerted to the presence of potentially severe disease. Secondly, comparisons of severity can be made both within and between patient series; and thirdly, rational selection of patients can be made for inclusion in trials of potential new treatments or interventions. Unfortunately the scoring systems used at present are often inadequate in patients with severe ANP, which is characterised by rapidly progressive multiple-system organ dysfunction. In this setting the Ranson criteria and APACHE score do not take account of the effects of treatment upon measured parameters. The way forward may be to use a combination of the Ranson score, the radiological scoring systems (see below) and a descriptive organ failure score such as the Sepsis-related Organ Failure Assessment.[6]

THE MANAGEMENT OF SEVERE PANCREATITIS

IMAGING

Dynamic contrast-enhanced computed tomography (CT) provides the best means of accurately visualising the pancreas and diagnosing pancreatitis and its local

Table 37.1 Aetiology of acute pancreatitis

Excess alcohol ingestion
Biliary tract disease
Idiopathic
Metabolic
Hyperlipidaemia
Hyperparathyroidism
Diabetic ketoacidosis
End-stage renal failure
Pregnancy
Post renal transplant
Mechanical disorders
Posttraumatic, postoperative, post endoscopic retrograde cholangiopancreatography
Penetrating duodenal ulcer
Duodenal obstruction
Infections
Human immunodeficiency virus, mumps, Epstein–Barr virus, *Mycoplasma, Legionella, Campylobacter*, ascariasis
Vascular
Necrotising vasculitis – systemic lupus erythematosus, thrombotic thrombocytopenia
Atheroma
Shock
Drugs
Azathioprine, thiazides, furosemide, tetracyclines, oestrogens, valproic acid, metronidazole, pentamidine, nitrofurantoin, erythromycin, methyldopa, ranitidine
Toxins
Scorpion venom, organophosphates, methyl alcohol

Table 37.2 Adverse prognostic factors in acute pancreatitis: Ranson's score[4]

On admission	Age > 55 years
	White cell count > 16 000/mm^3
	Glucose > 11 mmol/l
	Lactate dehydrogenase > 400 IU/l
	Aspartate transaminase > 250 IU/l
Within 48 hours of hospitalisation	Decrease in haematocrit > 10%
	Increase in blood urea > 1.8 mmol/l
	Calcium < 2 mmol/l
	Pa_{O_2} < 8 kPa
	Base deficit > 4 mmol/l
	Fluid deficit > 6 litres
Risk factors	**Mortality rate**
0–2	< 1%
3–4	≅ 15%
5–6	≅ 40%
> 6	≅ 100%

Blamey *et al.*[5] found only eight variables (not lactate dehydrogenase, base deficit and fluid deficit) were predictive and are often referred to as the Glasgow criteria or Imrie score.

complications. It may also be used for guiding percutaneous catheter drainage. Guidelines have been suggested for the efficacious use of CT scanning and these are shown in Table 37.3.[7]

In severe acute pancreatitis, there is lack of normal enhancement to contrast of the gland or a portion thereof. This is consistent with pancreatic necrosis, defined as diffuse or focal areas of non-viable parenchyma. Microscopically, there is evidence of damage to the parenchymal network, acinar cells and pancreatic ductal system and necrosis of perilobular fat. Areas of necrosis are often multifocal and rarely involve the whole gland, and may be confined to the periphery with preservation of the core. Necrosis develops early in the course of the disease and is usually established 96 hours after the onset of symptoms.[8] The extent of pancreatic necrosis and the degree of peripancreatic inflammation have been used to determine outcome. A grading system combining the two CT prognostic indicators (the extent of necrosis and the grade of peripancreatic inflammation) has been developed to give the 'CT severity index'. Most complications of acute pancreatitis occur in patients in whom the initial diagnosis is based upon peripancreatic fluid collections, and a strong correlation has been established between the CT depiction of necrosis and the development of complications and death.[9] For patients with necrosis in the pancreatic head, the outcome is as severe as when the entire pancreas is affected. By contrast, for patients with necrosis in only the distal portion of the gland, the outcome is favourable, with few complications.[10] The mechanism may be that necrosis in the pancreatic head causes obstruction of the pancreatic duct, and produces a rise in pressure in the acinar cells leading to damage and leakage of activated destructive proteases.

Following the initial CT scan, additional scanning is only indicated if the patient's clinical condition deteriorates, usually through the development of pancreatic necrosis, abscess or pancreatic pseudocyst, haemorrhage, or colonic ischaemia or perforation.

Ultrasonography in acute pancreatitis is less useful since visualisation of the gland may be obscured by 'gas-filled' bowel. Moreover, the degree of necrosis, which determines prognosis, cannot be assessed. However, there may be a role for this mode of imaging in

Table 37.3 Guidelines for efficacious use of computed tomography scanning in suspected acute pancreatitis[6]

Patients in whom the clinical diagnosis is in doubt
Patients with hyperamylasaemia and severe clinical pancreatitis, abdominal distension, tenderness, high fever (> 39°C) and leukocytosis
Patients with Ranson score > 3 or APACHE II > 8
Patients showing lack of improvement after 72 hours of initial conservative therapy
Acute deterioration following initial clinical improvement

APACHE, Acute Physiology, Age and Chronic Health Evaluation.

demonstrating gallstones, or in the subsequent management when ultrasound-guided fine-needle aspiration (FNA) of the pancreas or surrounding tissue may help to establish the presence of infection.

SURGERY IN SEVERE PANCREATITIS

The role of surgery remains a controversial area in the management of severe ANP.[11] During the 1980s, most patients with acute pancreatitis of even moderate severity underwent operative intervention. The results were poor, with mortality rates in excess of 50%, although this was without ICU facilities. In 1991, Bradley and Allen introduced the concept of a conservative, non-surgical approach to severe ANP.[12] During the past decade, targeting surgical intervention according to infection status, based on Gram stain and culture of CT-guided FNA, has refined this conservative approach with beneficial results.[13]

A laparotomy for an acute abdomen is essential when the diagnosis of pancreatitis is in doubt. Surgery may increase the incidence of subsequent infection, but this risk is outweighed by the dangers of delaying the diagnosis and treatment of other serious intra-abdominal conditions. Accepted and controversial indications for surgery in severe ANP are summarised in Table 37.4. If severe acute pancreatitis is an unsuspected 'chance' finding at laparotomy, a T-tube should be inserted into the common bile duct, particularly if it has been explored and the opportunity taken for placement of a feeding jejunostomy tube. Some surgeons oppose this approach, as opening a hollow viscus risks peritonitis.

INFECTED PANCREATIC NECROSIS

The presence of infected pancreatic necrosis seems to be an undisputed indication for urgent surgery. A contrast-enhanced CT scan documents necrosis, and infection is proven by FNA of localised fluid collections or of the necrotic tissue. All such patients require some form of surgical treatment, although whether this should consist of debridement and gravity drainage, continuous closed lavage of the lesser sac, staged repeated laparotomy or open packing remains to be established. Current surgical practice is not based on well-designed clinical trials and numerous surgical techniques have been described. Minimally invasive surgical techniques are gaining in popularity, but no firm recommendations can be made at this stage.

Table 37.4 Indications for surgery in severe acute pancreatitis

Accepted	Controversial
Differential diagnosis	Stable but persistent necrosis
Persistent biliary pancreatitis	Deterioration in clinical course
Infected pancreatic necrosis	Organ system failure
Pancreatic abscess	Abdominal compartment syndrome

STERILE PANCREATIC NECROSIS

The observation that some patients with severe ANP survive without becoming infected and avoid surgery is well documented. Moreover, operating upon such patients may hypothetically increase the risk of subsequent infection and its associated mortality. This is the basis of the critical decision as to whether patients with sterile ANP should undergo operative intervention. Currently a conservative approach is recommended, but with regular surveillance looking for evidence of pancreatic infection.[14]

PANCREATIC ABSCESSES

Pancreatic abscesses are circumscribed collections of pus containing little or no pancreatic necrosis, which arise as a later consequence of acute pancreatitis or pancreatic trauma. They commonly occur about 3–4 weeks after the onset of severe pancreatitis, and CT scan most accurately makes the diagnosis. If the appropriate expertise is available, percutaneous catheter drainage may be successful. Some series report effective drainage of intra-abdominal collections with a single treatment in 70% of patients, increasing to 82% with a second attempt, although proceeding to open surgical drainage is more frequently required in pancreatic abscess, especially if complicated by yeast infection.[15]

ENDOSCOPIC RETROGRADE CHOLANGIOPANCREATOGRAPHY (ERCP)

ERCP represents an alternative approach, particularly for patients with severe biliary pancreatitis. A number of prospective randomised studies have been carried out to compare early ERCP with conservative treatment in acute biliary pancreatitis. Although the studies are not entirely consistent, ERCP and papillotomy seem to be beneficial in confirmed or suspected severe biliary pancreatitis if undertaken by a skilled operator, whereas in mild pancreatitis the risks of intervention probably outweigh the benefits. This observation is confirmed by both a systematic review of the four ERCP trials,[16] and by the recommendations of the 2004 International Consensus Conference on the management of severe acute pancreatitis in the critically ill.[17]

TREATMENT WITH PHARMACOLOGICAL AGENTS

Theories regarding the pathogenesis of acute pancreatitis have promoted the concept that autodigestion of the gland and peripancreatic tissue by activated pancreatic enzymes is a central component. This has led to the suggestion that the reduction of pancreatic exocrine secretion, thereby 'resting the pancreas', might improve outcome. The problem is that the secretory status of the pancreas in severe ANP is not known. Consequently, it is not clear whether inhibition of secretion actually occurs or whether this is beneficial. Therapies designed to inhibit pancreatic secretion, such as H_2-blockers, atropine, calcitonin, glucagon and fluorouracil, do not alter the course of the disease. However, other pharmacological therapies, such as aprotonin and gabexate mesilate, both protease inhibitors, and somatostatin and octreotide, are in widespread use in the hope of improving the outcome.

SOMATOSTATIN AND OCTREOTIDE

Somatostatin and its long-acting analogue octreotide are potent inhibitors of pancreatic secretion. They also stimulate activity of the reticuloendothelial system and play a regulatory role, mostly inhibitory, in the modulation of the immune response via autocrine and neuroendocrine pathways. Both are cytoprotective with respect to the pancreas.[18] Other effects include:

- Somatostatin also blocks the release of tumour necrosis factor and interferon-γ by peripheral mononuclear cells.
- Octreotide increases the phagocytotic activity of monocytes.

These actions may be important in the modulation of the pathogenesis of acute respiratory distress syndrome (ARDS) and septic shock, both of which can complicate severe ANP. Both agents are effective in experimental pancreatitis, and in the prevention of complications in patients undergoing surgery for chronic pancreatitis.[19] Potential difficulties include:

- Pre-emptive administration is not possible in the acute situation.
- Both agents are powerful splanchnic vasoconstrictors.
- The development of pancreatic necrosis has been linked to hypoperfusion of the gland and vasoconstrictors worsen the histological severity of experimental pancreatitis.[20]

Consequently, these agents have both beneficial and detrimental effects.

Systematic evaluation suggests that there is insufficient evidence at present to support the use of octreotide or somatostatin in the treatment of patients with moderate to severe acute pancreatitis.[21] Additionally, the therapeutic effect of octreotide, if present at all, is probably very small and therefore unlikely to have any significant impact on the management of ANP.

PROTEASE INHIBITORS

A further pathogenic mechanism involved in acute pancreatitis is autodigestion of the pancreas by the activation of proteases. More accurately, there is an imbalance between proteases and antiproteases. Aprotinin and gabexate mesilate are proteolytic enzyme inhibitors that act on serine proteases such as trypsin, phospholipase A_2, kallikrein, plasmin, thrombin and C1r and C1s esterases.

The only two prospective, randomised studies of the protease inhibitor gabexate mesilate in patients with moderate or severe pancreatitis, when combined, showed no significant reduction in mortality or the need for surgery.[22]

The reason why these agents, in clinical practice, do not have the expected beneficial effect on outcome may be the lag time between the onset of pancreatitis and administration. Additionally, derangement to the microvascular control of the pancreas combined with increased vascular permeability may contribute. Continuous regional arterial infusion or intraperitoneal administration may be more advantageous, but so far trials using these modes of administration have only involved small numbers of patients. At present, there is insufficient evidence to recommend protease inhibitors in ANP.[23]

ANTI-INFLAMMATORY THERAPY

Patients with ANP exhibit a generalised uncontrolled inflammatory response. Potentially there is a therapeutic window between the onset of symptoms and the development of organ failure during which anti-inflammatory therapy might be successful. Potential targets include tumour necrosis factor-α, interleukin (IL)-1β, IL-6, IL-8, IL-10, platelet-activating factor and intracellular adhesion molecules.[24] Although many have been studied in animals, there are limited human data. Recombinant human activated protein C (rh-APC) has proven effectiveness in reducing mortality in severe sepsis.[25] Sixty-two patients with pancreatitis were enrolled in the PROWESS trial; mortality was 24% in the placebo arm and 15% in those receiving rh-APC.[17] All patients had a known or suspected source infection, which is not the case in many patients with ANP. There are currently no studies of rh-APC in patients without a documented source of infection, yet it seems that these patients demonstrate the same low levels of activity of protein C, antithrombin III, and higher concentrations of D-dimer and plasminogen activator inhibitor that are associated with poor outcome in patients with severe sepsis.[26]

It is also fascinating to observe that there is a constellation of changes in hypopituitary–adrenal axis hormone levels that strongly suggest that the existence of relative adrenocortical insufficiency in patients with ANP is very comparable to that of severe sepsis and multiple-organ failure.[27] There are currently no published trials of corticosteroid therapy in patients with ANP.

PROPHYLACTIC ANTIBIOTICS

Bacterial infection of necrotic pancreatic tissue occurs in approximately 40–70% of patients with ANP, and infection is the major cause of morbidity and mortality.[28] Early studies investigating the role of antibiotics in acute pancreatitis showed no benefit, but most included patients with mild disease and employed agents (e.g. ampicillin) with inefficient penetration of pancreatic tissue. Subsequent studies are more encouraging.

Carbapenems have exceptional penetration into pancreatic tissues and broad activity against most of the common pathogens encountered in this disease. One study compared imipenem with placebo in patients with early necrotising pancreatitis.[29] The incidence of septic complications was significantly reduced in the treated group (12.2 versus 30.3%), although there was only a trend towards decreased mortality (7 versus 12%). In another study of ethanol-induced ANP, cefuroxime was compared to placebo.[30] There were more infectious complications in the non-antibiotic group (mean per patient 1.8 versus 1.0; $P < 0.01$) and mortality was also higher (7 versus 1 death; $P = 0.03$). The most recent meta-analysis of the only three adequately controlled studies of prophylactic antibiotics in patients with contrast-enhanced CT proven ANP strongly suggests benefit, with a reduction in sepsis of 21%, and a reduced mortality of 12.3%.[31]

Patients with mild pancreatitis do not benefit from antibiotics.

PROPHYLACTIC ANTIFUNGAL THERAPY

The incidence of fungal infection correlates with the extent of pancreatic necrosis, as well as the severity of disease on admission. Antibiotic administration has been claimed to promote fungal infection; however, up to 25% of patients with ANP who do not receive antibiotics also develop fungal infection with an associated mortality rate of up to 84%.[32] One small, randomised study suggested fluconazole reduced the rate of fungal infection, but had no effect on mortality. Advocates of prophylactic antifungal therapy argue that it may delay the need for surgery, which is associated with a better outcome.[33]

SELECTIVE DECONTAMINATION OF THE GUT

The original selective digestive decontamination (SDD) strategy contained three components: oropharyngeal and gastric decontamination with polymyxin E, tobramicin, and amphotericin B and intravenous cefotaxime for 4 days.[34] There is ongoing debate as to the effectiveness of this strategy and results are conflicting regarding any reduction in mortality, particularly when applied to a general critically ill population. However, more promising results have been seen in specific patient populations.

Severe acute pancreatitis may be one clinical situation which supports the hypothesis that gut hypoperfusion promotes bacterial translocation, leading to infection of the inflamed pancreas and peripancreatic tissue.[35] The only controlled trial of SDD in pancreatitis was performed in 102 patients,[36] who were randomised to receive SDD: oral colistin, amphotericin and norfloxacin with addition of a daily dose of the three drugs given as a rectal enema and systemic cefotaxime until Gram-negative bacteria were successfully eliminated from the oral cavity and rectum. Surveillance samples were taken regularly to assess whether any subsequent infection was of exogenous or endogenous origin. There were 18 deaths (35%) in the control group, compared with 11 (22%) in the SDD group ($P < 0.05$). This difference was caused by a fall in late mortality due to significant reduction in the incidence of Gram-negative pancreatic infection. There was also a reduction in the mean number of laparotomies in the SDD patients. Since the SDD regimen used in this study incorporated intravenous cefotaxime it could be argued that the improvement in outcome was not due to the colistin, amphotericin or norfloxacin components, but merely due to a systemic antibiotic effect.

Meta-analyses of SDD suggest that there are clear trends towards a reduction in mortality in critically ill patients.[37] However, the perhaps unfounded fear of the emergence of resistant Gram-positive cocci prevents widespread adoption of this strategy.

NUTRITIONAL SUPPORT IN ACUTE NECROTISING PANCREATITIS

The provision of nutritional support for the patient with ANP is an essential component of supportive therapy, especially since many patients with pancreatitis are nutritionally depleted prior to their illness and face increased metabolic demands throughout the course of their disorder. Failure to reverse or prevent malnutrition, and a prolonged negative nitrogen balance, increases mortality rates. The route by which nutrition is administered is, none the less, still debated. In the last two decades there has been a trend away from the use of total parenteral nutrition (TPN) in favour of enteral nutrition (EN) in supporting the critically ill. Studies suggest that early EN started within 24 hours of admission to ICU, compared with TPN, is associated with reduced infective complications and hospital length of stay.[38]

TOTAL PARENTERAL NUTRITION

Severe pancreatitis is often quoted as an absolute contraindication to EN, and TPN is considered 'standard' therapy in some recently reported trials. This is largely because it is regarded as a way of 'resting the pancreas', based on the assumption that the necrotic pancreas is still a secretor of activated enzymes. In fact, the secretory state of the pancreas has never been prospectively studied in severe necrosis. Several retrospective and prospective evaluations of TPN in acute pancreatitis have failed to demonstrate conclusively an effect on survival, or on the incidence and severity of organ failure.

ENTERAL NUTRITION

An increasing number of reports on the use of EN in severe ANP continue to challenge the persisting dogma regarding the use of TPN in this condition. When EN is given it has been suggested that it should be delivered distal to the ligament of Treitz, below the area of the cholecystokinin (CCK) cells distal to the third part of the duodenum, as CCK stimulation may worsen the course of the disease. Intragastric delivery of nutrients results in an increased volume of pancreatic protein and bicarbonate secretion. By contrast, jejunal nutrient delivery is not associated with any increase in pancreatic exocrine secretion.

Consequently, jejunal tube feeding as far distally as possible in the upper gastrointestinal tract conforms to the concept of 'pancreatic rest'. A number of comparisons of EN with TPN have been made in mild and severe acute pancreatitis, all suggesting that EN is well tolerated without adverse effects on the course of the disease.[39] Patients who received EN experienced fewer total complications and were at lower risk of developing septic complications than those receiving TPN.[40] EN seems to modulate the inflammatory and sepsis response beneficially, and if tolerated, may be superior to TPN.[41] In spite of the enthusiasm for EN of some clinicians, in ANP where there is often an ileus and slow bowel transit time, some patients will not tolerate it.[42] It is not uncommon to be faced with the option of no nutrition or TPN; in this situation TPN enriched with glutamine should be used.[43]

A number of recommendations can be made:

1. Most patients with mild uncomplicated pancreatitis do not benefit from nutritional support.
2. In moderate to severe pancreatitis, let hyperacute inflammation settle, then start a trial of EN via a jejunal tube.
3. In patients who require surgery for diagnosis or treatment, a jejunal tube should be placed, either pulled down from the stomach, or a separate jejunostomy.
4. TPN (enriched with glutamine) is only indicated if a 5–7-day trial of EN is not tolerated.
5. In all patients, whether fed enterally or parenterally, a protocol ensuring strict glycaemic control is recommended.

CONCLUSION

The main determinant of outcome in severe acute pancreatitis is the extent of pancreatic necrosis and the subsequent risk for the development of infected necrosis. A thorough assessment using appropriate scoring systems and the early use of dynamic contrast-enhanced CT will highlight those patients likely to benefit from early critical care. Despite numerous suggested specific therapies there is still no incontrovertible evidence that any one confers a significant mortality benefit. However, general supportive measures should include vigorous replacement of fluid losses to correct circulating volume, correction of electrolyte and glucose abnormalities, and respiratory, cardiovascular and renal support as necessary. Those patients with infected pancreatic necrosis should probably undergo surgery. Patients with sterile necrosis should receive a broad-spectrum prophylactic antibiotic that adequately penetrates pancreatic tissue. Due attention should also be paid to nutritional support, for which a jejunal feeding tube with EN is recommended prior to initiation of TPN.

REFERENCES

1. Banerjee AK, Kaul A, Bache E *et al.* An audit of fatal acute pancreatitis. *Postgrad Med J* 1995; **71**: 472–5.
2. Malangoni MA, Martin EL. Outcome of severe pancreatitis. *Am J Surg* 2005; **189**: 273–7.
3. Cinquepalmi L, Boni L, Dionigi G *et al.* Long-term results and quality of life of patients undergoing sequential surgical treatment for severe acute pancreatitis complicated by infected pancreatic necrosis. *Surg Infect* 2006; 7: S113–16.
4. Ranson JHC, Rifkind KM, Roses DF *et al.* Prognostic signs and the role of operative management in acute pancreatitis. *Surg Gynaecol Obstet* 1974; **139**: 69–81.
5. Blamey SL, Imrie CW, O'Neill J *et al.* Prognostic factors in acute pancreatitis. *Gut* 1984; **25**: 1340–6.
6. Halonen KI, Pettila V, Leppaniemi AK *et al.* Multiple organ dysfunction associated with severe acute pancreatitis. *Crit Care Med* 2002; **30**: 1274–9.
7. Balthazar E, Freeny P, van Sonnenberg E. Imaging and intervention in acute pancreatitis. *Radiology* 1994; **193**: 297–306.
8. Isenmann R, Buchler M, Uhl W *et al.* Pancreatic necrosis: an early finding in severe acute pancreatitis. *Pancreas* 1993; **8**: 358–61.
9. Casas JD, Diaz R, Valderas G *et al.* Prognostic value of CT in the early assessment of patients with acute pancreatitis. *Am J Roentgenol* 2004; **182**: 569–74.
10. Kemppainen E, Sainio V, Haapianen L *et al.* Early localization of necrosis by contrast-enhanced computed tomography can predict outcome in severe acute pancreatitis. *Br J Surg* 1996; **83**: 924–9.
11. Uhl W, Warshaw A, Imrie C *et al.* IAP guidelines for the surgical management of acute pancreatitis. *Pancreatology* 2002; **2**: 565–73.
12. Bradley EL, Allen K. A prospective longitudinal study of observation versus surgical intervention in the management of necrotizing pancreatitis. *Am J Surg* 1991; **161**: 19–25.
13. Buchler MW, Gloor B, Muller CA *et al.* Acute necrotizing pancreatitis: treatment strategy according to the status of infection. *Ann Surg* 2000; **232**: 619–26.
14. Hartwig W, Maksan SM, Foitzik T *et al.* Reduction in mortality with delayed surgical therapy of severe pancreatitis. *J Gastrointest Surg* 2002; **6**: 481–7.
15. Cinat ME, Wilson SE, Din AM. Determinants for successful percutaneous image-guided drainage of intra-abdominal abscess. *Arch Surg* 2002; **137**: 845–9.
16. Sharma VK, Howden CW. Metaanalysis of randomised controlled trials of endoscopic retrograde cholangiography and endoscopic sphincterotomy for the treatment of acute biliary pancreatitis. *Am J Gastroenterol* 1999; **94**: 3211–4.
17. Nathens AB, Curtis JR, Beale RJ *et al.* Management of the critically ill patient with severe acute pancreatitis. *Crit Care Med* 2004; **32**: 2524–36.
18. Van Hagen PM, Krenning EP, Kwekkeboom DJ *et al.* Somatostatin and the immune and haematopoietic system: a review. *Eur J Clin Invest* 1994; **24**: 91–9.
19. Friess H, Beger HG, Sulkowski U *et al.* Randomised controlled multicentre study of the prevention of complications by octreotide in patients undergoing surgery for chronic pancreatitis. *Br J Surg* 1995; **82**: 1270–3.

20. Klar E, Rattner DW, Compton C *et al.* Adverse effect of therapeutic vasoconstrictors in experimental acute pancreatitis. *Ann Surg* 1991; **214**: 168–74.
21. Cavallini G, Frulloni L. Somatostatin and octreotide in acute pancreatitis: the never-ending story. *Dig Liver Dis* 2001; **33**: 192–201.
22. Heinrich S, Schafer M, Rousson V *et al.* Evidenced-based treatment of acute pancreatitis. A look at established paradigms. *Ann Surg* 2006; **243**: 154–68.
23. Seta T, Noguchi Y, Shimada T *et al.* Treatment of acute pancreatitis with protease inhibitors: a meta-analysis. *Eur J Gastroenterol Hepatol* 2004; **16**: 1287–93.
24. Bhatia M. Novel therapeutic targets for acute pancreatitis and associated multiple organ dysfunction syndrome. *Curr Drug Targets Inflamm Allergy* 2002; **1**: 343–51.
25. Bernard GR, Vincent JL, Laterre PF *et al.* Efficacy and safety of recombinant human activated protein C for severe sepsis. *N Engl J Med* 2001; **344**: 699–709.
26. Radenkovic D, Bajec D, Karamarkovic A *et al.* Disorders of hemostasis during the surgical management of severe necrotizing pancreatitis. *Pancreas* 2004; **29**: 152–6.
27. Muller CA, Vogeser M, Belyaev O *et al.* Role of endogenous glucocorticoid metabolism in human acute pancreatitis. *Crit Care Med* 2006; **34**: 1060–6.
28. Beger HG, Rau B, Mayer J *et al.* Natural course of acute pancreatitis. *World J Surg* 1997; **21**: 130–5.
29. Pederzoli P, Bassi C, Vesentini S *et al.* A randomised multicenter trial of antibiotic prophylaxis of septic complications in acute necrotizing pancreatitis with imipenem. *Surg Gynaecol Obstet* 1993; **176**: 480–3.
30. Sainio V, Kemppainen E, Puolakkainen P *et al.* Early antibiotic treatment in acute necrotizing pancreatitis. *Lancet* 1995; **346**: 663–7.
31. Sharma VK, Howden CW. Prophylactic antibiotic administration reduces sepsis and mortality in acute necrotizing pancreatitis: a meta-analysis. *Pancreas* 2001; **22**: 28–31.
32. Gotzinger P, Wamser P, Barlan M *et al. Candida* infection of local necrosis in severe acute pancreatitis is associated with increased mortality. *Shock* 2000; **14**: 320–3.
33. Eggiman P, Jamdar S, Siriwardena AK. Pro/con debate: antifungal prophylaxis is important to prevent fungal infection in patients with acute necrotizing pancreatitis receiving broad-spectrum antibiotics. *Crit Care* 2006; **10**: 229.
34. Stoutenbeek C, van Saene H, Miranda D *et al.* The effects of selective decontamination of the digestive tract on colonisation and infection rate in multiple trauma patients. *Intens Care Med* 1984; **10**: 185–92.
35. Lee TK, Medich DS, Melhem MF *et al.* Pathogenesis of pancreatic sepsis. *Am J Surg* 1993; **165**: 46–50.
36. Luiten EJT, Hop WCJ, Lange JF *et al.* Controlled clinical trial of selective decontamination for the treatment of severe acute pancreatitis. *Ann Surg* 1995; **222**: 57–65.
37. D'Amoco R, Pifferi S, Leonetti C *et al.* Effectiveness of antibiotic prophylaxis in critically ill adult patients: systematic review of randomised controlled trials. *Br Med J* 1998; **316**: 1275–85.
38. Peter JV, Moran JL, Phillips-Hughes J. A metaanalysis of treatment outcomes of early enteral versus early parenteral nutrition in hospitalised patients. *Crit Care Med* 2005; **33**: 213–20.
39. McClave SA, Chang W-K, Dhaliwal R *et al.* Nutritional support in acute pancreatitis: a systematic review of the literature. *JPEN* 2006; **30**: 143–56.
40. Abou-assi S, Craig K, O'Keefe SJ. Hypocaloric jejunal feeding is better than total parenteral nutrition in acute pancreatitis: results of a randomised comparative study. *Am J Gastroenterol* 2002; **97**: 2255–62.
41. Windsor AC, Kanwar S, Li AG *et al.* Compared with parenteral nutrition, enteral feeding attenuates the acute phase response and improves disease severity in acute pancreatitis. *Gut* 1998; **42**: 431–5.
42. Wan X, Gong Z, Wu K *et al.* Gastrointestinal dysmotility in patients with acute pancreatitis. *J Gastroenterol Hepatol* 2003; **18**: 57–62.
43. Dechelotte P, Hasselmann M, Cynober L *et al.* L-alanyl-L-glutamine dipeptide-supplemented total parenteral nutrition reduces infectious complications and glucose intolerance in critically ill patients: the french controlled, randomized, double-blind, multicenter study. *Crit Care Med* 2006; **34**: 598–604.

38

Acute liver failure

Elizabeth Sizer and Julia Wendon

DEFINITION AND AETIOLOGY

Acute liver failure (ALF) is a complex multisystemic illness that evolves after significant liver insult. The liver damage is manifest by the development of coagulopathy and encephalopathy within days or weeks of the liver injury. ALF is a heterogeneous condition incorporating a range of clinical syndromes. The dominant factors that give rise to this heterogeneity are the variable aetiology, the age of the patient and concomitant comorbidity and the duration of time over which the disease evolves. There are multiple definitions used in this disease but the one used by O'Grady *et al.* is most commonly used, utilising the description of acute, hyperacute and subacute.[1] This system uses a trigger of jaundice and encephalopathy whilst others have used symptoms of encephalopathy. All the definitions used recognise that the syndrome may have a rapid presentation or a somewhat slower presentation, and the clinical features and outcomes are significantly different in the two presentations.

The O'Grady *et al.* definitions are given below.

- *hyperacute*: the onset of encephalopathy is within 7 days of the development of jaundice
- *acute*: encephalopathy develops 8–28 days after the onset of jaundice
- *subacute*: encephalopathy develops 4–26 weeks after the onset of jaundice

HYPERACUTE DISEASE

Prevalent aetiologies in hyperacute disease include:

- paracetamol (acetaminophen)
- ischaemic
- viral
- toxins

This group will frequently demonstrate the greatest degree of coagulopathy, encephalopathy, organ dysfunction and cerebral oedema but also carries the greatest chance of spontaneous survival.

SUBACUTE DISEASE

The aetiology is more frequently seronegative or idiopathic and drug-related, e.g. non-steroidal. Jaundice is inevitable but the transaminitis is often less pronounced than in the former group. Patients frequently present with established ascites and so may be clinically difficult to distinguish from chronic liver disease (CLD). Encephalopathy is often late and carries a lower risk of cerebral oedema and intracranial hypertension. Once they develop poor prognostic criteria the chances of effective liver regeneration and thus of spontaneous recovery are low: the prognosis is very poor without liver transplantation.

The aetiology of ALF must always be sought, not just for prognosis but for treatment options (Table 38.1).

The relative incidence of aetiologies varies across the world. Paracetamol is common in the UK, USA and Denmark, whereas hepatitis B is more common in France. A recent paper from the USA Acute Liver Failure group highlights the increasing incidence of paracetamol toxicity and also the potential role it plays as a covert agent in patients with no history of excess ingestion and non-specific symptoms that would otherwise be attributed to the seronegative group.[2] The rate of hepatitis B virus-induced ALF is decreasing with immunisation but is still highly prevalent and should always be considered.

A good history and review of the results of blood tests over the preceding weeks can be essential to the diagnosis. Any new drug ingestion (prescribed, recreational or over-the-counter) should be considered a potential culprit and discontinued if possible. In addition any treatments that may be detrimental to liver recovery should be avoided.

Acute viral hepatitis accounts for 40–70% of patients with ALF worldwide. Clinical characteristics are shown in Table 38.2. Acute hepatitis A (HAV) infection rarely leads to ALF (0.35% of infections), but continues to account for up to 10% of cases; morbidity increases with the age of infection. It is hoped that the rate will decrease with improving hygiene standards generally and the uptake of vaccination. It is diagnosed by the presence of the immunoglobulin (Ig) M antibody to HAV. HAV-related ALF has a relatively good prognosis, although age and comorbidity are relevant.

Acute hepatitis B (HBV) has been the cause of 25–75% of instances of ALF from viral hepatitis. The liver injury is immunologically mediated with active destruction of infected hepatocytes. Diagnosis is by the

Table 38.1 Causes of liver failure

Cause	Agent responsible
Viral hepatitis	Hepatitis A, B, D, E, cytomegalovirus, herpes simplex virus, seronegative hepatitis (14–25% of cases in the UK)
Drug-related	Dose-related, e.g. paracetamol, and idiosyncratic reactions, e.g. antituberculous drugs, statins, recreational drugs, anticonvulsants, non-steroidal anti-inflammatory drugs, cyproterone and many others
Toxins	Carbon tetrachloride, *Amanita phalloides*
Vascular events	Ischaemic hepatitis, veno-occlusive disease, Budd–Chiari Heatstroke
Other	Pregnancy-related liver diseases, Wilson's disease, lymphoma, carcinoma, trauma

presence of the IgM antibody (HBcAb) to hepatitis B core antigen. Hepatitis B surface antigen (HbsAg) is frequently negative by the time of presentation. Hepatitis B DNA should also be assayed. ALF may also be seen with hepatitis D, as either a coinfection or suprainfection. Reactivation of hepatitis B is an increasing cause of ALF and should always be considered in a patient who has received steroids or chemotherapy. High-risk patients should be screened for sAg and HBV DNA and treated with antiviral agents if they are positive. This is a recognised problem in oncology and haematology but it is also a potential risk to patients in intensive care where steroids may be administered.

Hepatitis C (HCV) infection is commonly associated with CLD. It is detected by the presence of antibodies to HCV in serum. It rarely if ever results in ALF.

Hepatitis E (HEV), like hepatitis A, is transmitted via the faecal–oral route. It is particularly prevalent in the Indian subcontinent and Asia generally and is responsible for sporadic instances of ALF in the western world. It can be diagnosed by the detection of antibodies to HEV in serum.

Other viruses, such as herpes simplex 1 and 2, varicella-zoster virus, cytomegalovirus, Epstein–Barr virus and measles virus, may all rarely cause ALF, but may be seen especially in the immunocompromised patient. Diagnosis is by serological and polymerase chain reaction (PCR) testing. Rift Valley fever, dengue, yellow fever, lassa fever and the haemorrhagic fevers should be considered in those who are at risk.

Seronegative hepatitis (so called) is seen in patients in whom there are no identifiable viral causes nor obvious candidate drugs. Such patients may present with a prodromal illness and with acute or subacute maniifestations of the disease. Prognosis is less good than those with an identifiable virus and once they have poor prognostic criteria the chances of survival without liver transplant are exceptionally small. A subgroup may represent an acute autoimmune form of ALF, although many will not have any positive immmune markers such as elevated IgG or positive smooth-muscle or liver kidney antibodies. The pattern of markers shows an increased incidence of autoantibody positivity in seronegative cases and viral cases with elevated IgM in viral causes.[2,3]

Table 38.2 Aetiology of acute liver failure and initial investigations

Hepatitis A (HAV)	Immunoglobulin M (IgM) anti-HAV
Hepatitis B + D (HBV, HDV)	HBsAg, IgM anti-core, HBeAg, HBeAb, HBV DNA, delta antibody
Hepatitis E (HEV)	IgM antibody
Seronegative hepatitis	All tests negative: diagnosis of exclusion
Paracetamol	Drug levels in blood and clinical pattern of disease – may be negative on third or subsequent days after overdose; markedly elevated aspartate and alanine serum transaminase (often > 10 000)
Idiosyncratic drug reactions	Eosinophil count may be elevated, although most diagnoses are based on temporal relationship
Ecstasy	Blood, urine, hair analysis and history
Autoimmune	Autoantibodies, immunoglobulin profile
Pregnancy-related syndromes	
Fatty liver	Uric acid elevated, neutrophilia, often first pregnancy, history, CT scan for rupture and assessment of vessels
HELLP syndrome	Platelet count, disseminated intravascular coagulation a prominent feature; CT scan as above
Liver rupture	May be seen in association with pre-eclampsia, fatty liver and HELLP
Wilson's disease	Urinary copper, ceruloplasmin (although low in many causes of acute liver failure), present up to second decade of life, Kayser–Fleischer rings, low alkaline phosphate levels
Amanita phalloides	History of ingestion of mushrooms, diarrhoea
Budd–Chiari syndrome	Ultrasound of vessels (HV signal lost, reverse flow in portal vein), CT angiography, ascites, prominent caudate lobe on imaging, haematological assessment
Malignancy	Imaging and histology; increased alkaline phosphate and LDH; often imaging may be interpretated as normal
Ischemic hepatitis	Clinical context, marked elevation of transaminases (often > 5000); may demonstrate diated hepatic veins on ultrasound, echocardiogram
Heatstroke	Myoglobinuria and rhabdomyolysis are often prominent features

CT, computed tomography; HELLP, *h*aemolysis (microangiopathic haemolytic anaemia), *e*levated *l*iver enzymes and *l*ow *p*latelets; HIV, human immunodeficiency virus; LDH, lactate dehydrogenase.

Drug-induced hepatitis is responsible for approximately 15–25% of cases of ALF. In some patients there appears to be a true hypersensitivity reaction, and symptoms develop after a sensitisation period of 1–5 weeks, recur promptly with readministration of the drug and may be accompanied by fever, rash and eosinophilia. In others the clinical pattern is less acute. Some herbal remedies are implicated as putative hepatotoxins but their role is made more difficult to assess by the variable nature of the constituent parts. Halothane hepatitis is now almost unheard of.

Paracetamol, taken intentionally or inadvertently, remains one of the commonest forms of acute hepatotoxicity. The early signs of nausea and vomiting after overdose are followed by signs of liver failure 48–72 hours after paracetamol ingestion. Treatment is with *N*-acetylcysteine, which increases hepatic stores of glutathione and metabolism of the toxic metabolite.

The recommended dosage schedule is 150 mg/kg in 5% dextrose over 15 minutes, followed by 50 mg/kg in 5% dextrose over 4 hours, followed by 100 mg/kg in 5% dextrose over 16 hours.

Even late administration of *N*-acetylcysteine (up to 36 hours after ingestion) may improve outcome. Predisposition to paracetamol-induced hepatotoxicity may occur in the following instances:

- heavy chronic alcohol ingestion
- enzyme-inducing agents
- glutathione-depleted, e.g. anorexics

Mushroom poisoning can be seen even when only very small amounts have been ingested, e.g *Amanita phalloides*. The initial presentation is often with diarrhoea. Patients subsequently develop signs of hepatic necrosis at 2–3 days after ingestion. The liver injury is caused by amatoxins. Forced diuresis may be helpful as large amounts of toxin are excreted in urine, but inadvertent dehydration may result in renal failure. Thioctic acid, silibinin and penicillin have been advocated as therapy, but have not been subjected to controlled trials.

RECREATIONAL DRUGS AND ACUTE LIVER FAILURE

Ecstasy (methylenedioxymethamphetamine) may cause ALF although, given the amount of exposure to the drug, the incidence is presumably low. Proposed mechanisms of injury include immune mechanisms and/or heatstroke. Cocaine may result in an ischaemic hepatitis. Yellow phosphorus, carbon tetrachloride, chloroform, trichloroethylene and xylene (in glue sniffers) are very rare causes of ALF.

Miscellaneous causes account for a small proportion of cases of ALF but are very important to recognise.

FULMINANT WILSON'S DISEASE

The characteristic features are those of cirrhosis, seen on imaging, with concomitant problems such as thrombocytopenia which may be long-standing, Kayser–Fleischer rings on examination and frequently non-immune-mediated haemolysis.

Pregnancy-related liver failure includes HELLP (*h*aemolysis (microangiopathic haemolytic anaemia), *e*levated *l*iver enzymes and *l*ow *p*latelets), acute fatty liver of pregnancy and liver rupture, often in association with pre-eclampsia. The prognosis of pregnancy-related ALF is usually good, although some develop severe liver injury with small-vessel disease, liver ruptures may require packing and occasionally transplantation is required (Figure 38.1).

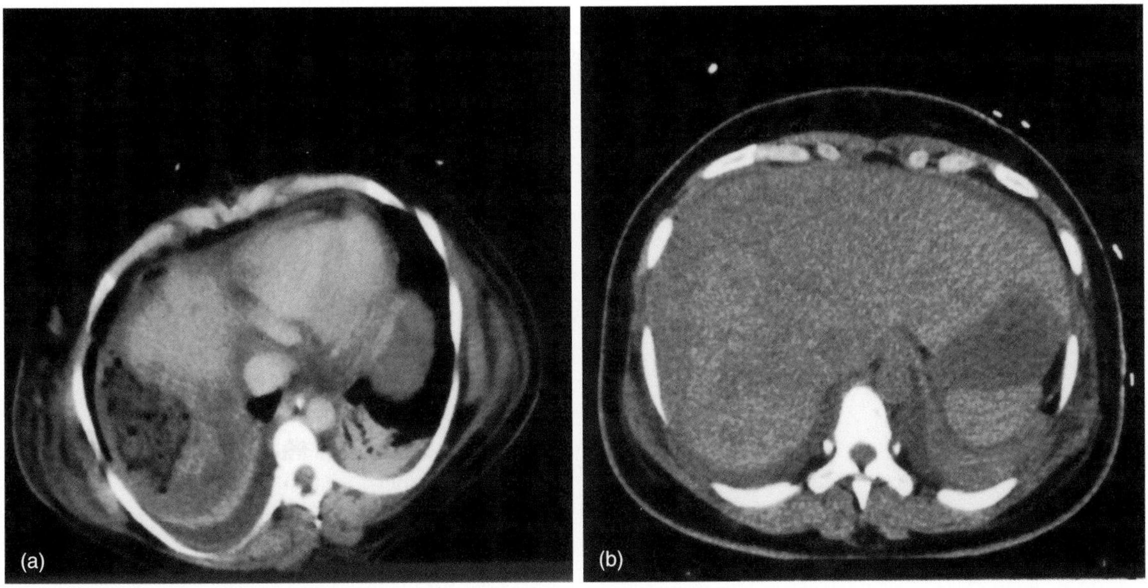

Figure 38.1 Liver CT in pregnancy related liver disease demonstrating abnormal perfusion (a and b) with rupture, packing (a) and associated areas of infarction. Major bleeding into the liver.

Heat shock injury is now relatively rarely seen but the ischaemic hepatitides remain relatively common. They are normally associated with a congested liver that is subjected to a secondary insult – hypoxia or decreased-flow arterial inflow. This is seen with hypoxaemic respiratory failure, cardiac arrhythmias and hypotension.

Hepatic venous obstruction (Budd–Chiari syndrome) may cause ALF. There are symptoms and signs of liver of necrosis, often with capsular pain from congestion and ascites. In Asia this may be associated with anatomical anomalies of the inferior vena cava, whereas in Europe and the USA the experience is normally of thrombosis of the hepatic veins, often with an underlying procoagulant condition (Figures 38.2 and 38.3).

Malignancy may also present with ALF, albeit rarely. The clinical pattern normally is that of elevated biliary enzymes in addition to the transaminases. This pattern of disease may be seen in those with hepatic lymphoma, often with an elevated lactate dehydrogenase or indeed with diffuse infiltration with other malignancies.

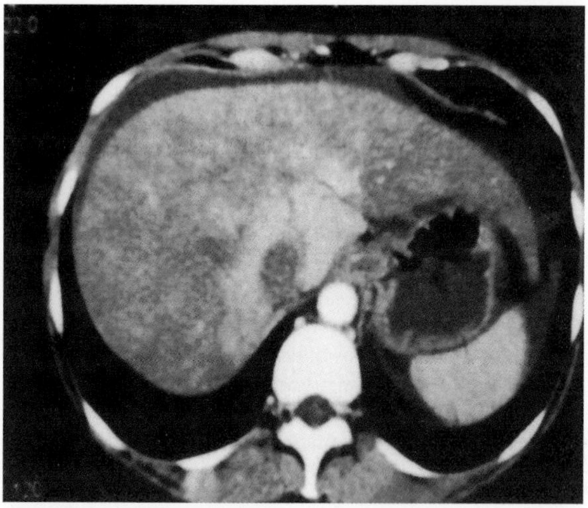

Figure 38.2 CT of Budd Chiari demonstrating arterio portal shunting and clot in Hepatic veins and IVC.

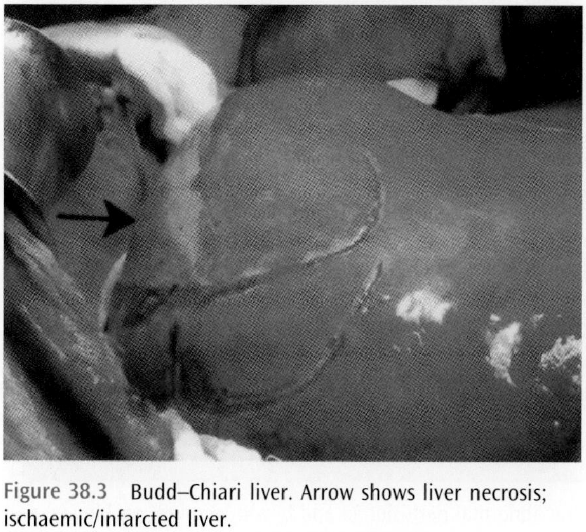

Figure 38.3 Budd–Chiari liver. Arrow shows liver necrosis; ischaemic/infarcted liver.

DIAGNOSIS

The aetiology of ALF must be accurately identified; some specific investigations are outlined in Table 38.2. History and clinical examination are paramount in this disease and the clinical course of biochemical and haematological parameters is important in assessing course and management. All patients should have routine chemistry, haematology and coagulation assessment; viral and autoimmune profiles should similarly be undertaken in all.

Ultrasound should be used to assess both the nature of the liver and its vascular pattern and will show the presence of ascites and splenomegaly if present.

Nodularity of the liver should not be assumed to represent cirrhosis and CLD. The imaging pattern of subacute liver failure, with focal areas of collapse and regeneration, may be inappropriately considered cirrhosis. The contribution of histology to the assessment of ALF is controversial. Histologic features may suggest specific diagnoses, including malignant infiltration, Wilson's disease (cirrhosis) and autoimmune features. Confluent necrosis is the commonest histological finding, which is not diagnostic. Its severity has been used to assess prognosis: $> 50\%$ necrosis is associated with poor prognosis. However, nodules of regeneration may occur randomly, particularly in subacute liver failure, and sampling error may thus make this a less than ideal tool for predicting outcome. Diagnostic clues may sometimes be found, however, and it is especially relevant if there is any concern with regard to lymphoma or other malignant process.

The biopsy is normally undertaken by the transjugular route.

SPECIFIC TREATMENTS

The management of ALF is largely supportive, providing an optimal environment for either regeneration or stability until a suitable liver becomes available.

SPECIFIC CONSIDERATIONS

N-acetylcysteine is administered for paracetamol-induced ALF, as mentioned above. Its role in non-paracetamol-induced ALF remains undefined and a US trial is at present assessing this.

Chelating agents are not of benefit in patients with established ALF secondary to Wilson's disease but play an important role in chronic presentations. Withdrawal of such treatments, or indeed non-compliance, especially in teenagers, may precipitate ALF.

Antiviral therapy has a predominant role in preventing reactivation of hepatitis B in patients exposed to chemotherapy and steroids.

Thrombolytic therapies may be of benefit in patients with early acute Budd–Chiari syndrome, although increasingly the treatment option would be to undertake a transhepatic portosystemic shunt (TIPS) shunt, decompressing the liver with a stent passed either through the hepatic vein (if the clot is soft enough) or via the inferior vena cava and through to the portal vein. Such procedures should be undertaken in units with the facilities to transplant as there is a risk of precipitating ALF. Chemotherapy may be offered to those with lymphoma involving the liver and in these instances tissue is paramount, either of liver or from another diagnostic site.

Steroid therapy is beneficial in acute autoimmune hepatitis but its role in autoimmune ALF has been less clear. A recent publication from the Paris group suggests that steroids for those with established ALF are potentially detrimental.[4]

CLINICAL COURSE, COMPLICATIONS AND MANAGEMENT

ENCEPHALOPATHY

This is part of the syndrome of ALF. The spectrum extends from mild confusion progressing to deep coma, cerebral oedema and raised intracranial hypertension. ALF is also associated with renal, cardiovascular and respiratory failure along with significant metabolic disarray and coagulopathy.

COAGULOPATHY

Coagulopathy is the hallmark of ALF, with prolongation predominantly of the prothrombin time and to lesser degrees the activated partial thromboplastin ratio (APTR). In a small percentage of patients the coagulopathy will respond, at least partially, to vitamin K. Intravenous vitamin K 10 mg is normally administered. Thrombocytopenia is frequent and normally consumptive in nature. Bleeding is rare, although may be seen in those with severe prolongation of APTR, low fibrinogen and severe thrombocytopenia. Coagulation or repletion of coagulation factors is necessary for clinical bleeding and prophylactically before major invasive procedures. Coagulation support is normally not given routinely so that the international normalised ratio (INR) can be monitored with regard to prognosis.

ENCEPHALOPATHY

Hepatic encephalopathy encompasses a wide spectrum of neuropsychiatric disturbances associated with both acute and chronic liver dysfunction. Importantly, encephalopathy in ALF may be complicated by cerebral oedema and progress from minor levels to deep levels of coma with great rapidity. This has to be considered when transferring patients with ALF between hospitals. Intubation and sedation prior to undertaking any transfer should be considered in any patient with progressive encephalopathy.

Encephalopathy is a clinical diagnosis, graded from 1 to 4 depending on clinical severity (Table 38.3). The development of encephalopathy is essential for the diagnosis of ALF. Patients with acute and hyperacute liver failure are at greatest risk of developing grade IV coma and cerebral oedema.

Clear aetiological factors in the development of encephalopathy remain under discussion but it is believed that there is a build-up of putative toxins, of which ammonia is thought to be most pertinent, resulting in glutamine intracerebral accumulation and the development of cerebral oedema.[5–7] In ALF there is a clear relationship between the development of higher grades of coma and arterial ammonia levels (cut-off between 150 and 200 μmol/l) renal dysfunction and aetiology.[8–10] The relationship in CLD exists but is less clear.

The development of cerebral oedema and intracranial hypertension in patients with ALF is thought to relate, amongst other things, to the speed of onset. In patients with CLD, adaptation occurs and there is improved control of intracellular osmolarity (myoinositol) so that cellular oedema is rare and of low grade.[11]

Table 38.3 Modified Parsons–Smith scale of hepatic encephalopathy

Grade	Clinical features	Neurological signs	Glasgow Coma Score
0/subclinical	Normal	Only seen on neuropsychometric testing	15
1	Trivial lack of awareness, shortened attention span	Tremor, apraxia, incoordination	15
2	Lethargy, disorientation, personality change	Asterixis, ataxia, dysarthria	11–15
3	Confusion, somnolence to semistupor, responsive to stimuli	Asterixis, ataxia	8–11
4	Coma	± Decerebration	< 8

The association between the development of encephalopathy and markers of inflammation is well demonstrated, both in regard to systemic inflammatory response syndrome (SIRS) markers and inflammatory mediators such as tumour necrosis factor.[12,13] Curiously, a similar relationship between inflammation and encephalopathy is seen in patients with CLD.[14] What is not yet clear is whether treatments that modulate the inflammatory response will be of benefit. This and other avenues proposed from basic animal research may well result in several novel approaches to the treatment of cerebral oedema and possibly encephalopathy over the forthcoming years.

Cerebral blood flow shows marked variability in patients with ALF. Hyperaemia has increased prevalence in those who develop intracranial hypertension. The role of hyperventilation has not been shown to be beneficial in routine management but plays a role in the treatment of increased intracranial pressure (ICP) with associated hyperaemia.[15]

The clinical management of the cerebral complications of ALF has been developed pragmatically and by the extrapolation of data from the neurosurgical literature rather than from the results of large randomised controlled clinical trials. Patients whose conscious level deteriorates to grade 3/4 coma should undergo elective intubation, sedation and ventilation. Sedation may be undertaken with a variety of compounds but the standard would be to utilise an opiate and a sedative such as propofol.

Cerebral perfusion pressure of greater than 60 mmHg has been suggested as optimal. It is of note that patients with ALF often do not autoregulate to pressure and consequently increases in blood pressure may be associated with increased cerebral blood flow and potentially increased ICP, particularly if they are at a critical point on their pressure–volume curve. This promotes the use of ICP monitoring in patients requiring pressor agents.[8] Cardiovascular failure necessitates invasive monitoring to optimise treatment and to determine the optimal therapeutic agents. The issue of noradrenaline (norepinephrine) versus vasopressin or terlipressin is difficult. In one study terlipressin resulted in a significant increase in ICP but in another there were no such detrimental effects.[14,16] It may be that the effects of terlipressin are highly individual and potentially time course-dependent, again supporting the role of ICP monitoring in these situations.

CARBON DIOXIDE

In most patients normocapnia is ideal as the relationship between cerebral blood flow and arterial CO_2 is maintained.

The complexity of these patients defines the importance of multimodule monitoring being considered in all patients with ALF who develop grade III/V coma, and especially those who are deemed high-risk. These include those with respiratory dysfunction, of young age, hyperacute and acute presentations, renal failure, fever and other SIRS markers or any patients on vasopressors.

Arterial ammonia – both the level (levels greater than 150–200 μmol/l) and the failure of this level to fall with treatment – may help in prognostication.[8,10] The monitoring may comprise reverse jugular monitoring, middle cerebral artery Doppler measurements and ICP monitoring. ICP monitoring is more controversial as it has not been shown specifically to improve outcome (few monitoring devices in isolation have altered outcome). A recent retrospective study from the US Acute Liver Failure group showed that ICP monitoring carried a complication rate of 10%: half of the complications were serious and two-thirds possibly contributed to mortality. Monitoring did result in more treatment interventions being undertaken.[17]

Coagulation problems and the risk of bleeding associated with monitoring may be minimised by a combination of coagulation support at the time of placement and technical expertise. Some centres support coagulation at the time of insertion with plasma products and platelets whilst others utilise recombinant factor VII.

A standard baseline approach to the management of patients with ALF and grade III/IV coma would be as follows.

Appropriate sedation and ventilation – hypercarbia should be avoided, although in the setting of acute lung injury, lung-protective strategies should be undertaken, probably in conjunction with cerebral monitoring so as to ensure optimal manipulation of the physiological variables.

Hyponatraemia and hyperammonaemia have been shown to be detrimental, whereas a randomised controlled trial showed benefit to the patients whose serum Na was maintained between 140 and 150 mmol/l. (Bolus hypertonic saline, 30%, was used for episodes of ICP greater than 25 mmHg.)[18]

Cerebral perfusion pressure should be optimised using ICP monitoring to ensure that changes in mean arterial pressure do not compromise cerebral perfusion pressure.

Sustained ICP rises beyond 25 mmHg require treatment. First-line treatment remains mannitol 0.5 g/kg given as a bolus with an appropriate subsequent diuresis. It is essential that serum osmolarity is maintained at less than 320 mosmol to avoid damage to the blood–brain barrier and worsening of vasogenic oedema. Increasingly hypertonic saline may also be utilised in this setting.

Some patients remain resistant to treatment and in these cases other therapies may be considered. Hypothermia has been shown to decrease cerebral blood flow, decrease ICP and decrease cerebral ammonia uptake in one clinical study.[19,20] The role of hypothermia as an early preventive intervention in grade III/IV coma is contentious and, given the problems of hypothermia in the neurosurgical arena, the results of controlled studies are awaited. Fever should be avoided in these patients and hypothermia reserved for intracranial hypertension that is resistant to standard treatment.

Other treatment options that have been shown to be potentially beneficial are thiopental and intravenous indometacin (0.5 mg/kg).[21] Potential monitoring and treatment algorithms, as used by this unit, are seen in Figure 38.4.

SEPSIS

Sepsis is common in ALF and both culture-positive and negative SIRS are seen in ALF patients. They are functionally immunosuppressed in terms of impaired cell-mediated immunity, complement levels and phagocytosis.[22] Functional immmunoparesis can only be observed and depression of human leukocyte antigen (HLA) DR expression correlates with prognosis and severity of liver injury.[23,24] As such, scrupulous attention with regard to hand-washing and line care needs to be applied to decrease the risk of nosocomial infection. Regular culture screens are required and antimicrobials are indicated in patients with any clinical suggestion of sepsis. Prophylactic intravenous antifungals should be considered, especially in those listed for transplantation. The choice of antimicrobial agent should be driven by local resistance patterns. Antimicrobial therapy should be reviewed in the light of culture results on a daily basis.

CARDIOVASCULAR

Patients with ALF develop a hyperdynamic circulation with peripheral vasodilation and central volume depletion. Hypotension is common and may initially respond to volume repletion. Assessment of volume reponsiveness in the clinical setting may be difficult and pressure measurements are a poor indicator of volume status. Hypotension that does not respond to volume will normally require some form of invasive haemodynamic monitoring and frequently institution of vasopressor agents. Increasingly it is recognised that volume responsiveness, as in general intensive care unit patients is best determined by dynamic rather than static variables.

The requirement for pressor agents should raise the possibility of adrenal dysfunction. Patients with ALF have been demonstrated to have impaired response to adrenocorticotrophic hormone (ACTH).[25 26] The response at 30 and 60 minutes in terms of cortisol should be examined following 250 μg ACTH in all patients with ALF who are requiring pressor agents. A subnormal response should result in consideration of hydrocortisone replacement therapy, normally given for a period of 10 days. Interestingly, adrenal dysfunction has similarly been reported in acute-on-chronic liver failure and steroid replacement may result in improved outcome.[26,27]

Elevated troponin levels can be observed in patients with liver failure, especially those with cardiovascular failure.[28]

RESPIRATORY

Ventilatory support is frequently required in patients with ALF, usually because of decreased conscious level rather than hypoxia, at least in the initial stages of disease.

Common respiratory complications are pleural effusions, atelectasis and intrapulmonary shunts. Acute respiratory distress syndrome (ARDS) and acute lung injury may be seen and can be precipitated by extrapulmonary sepsis or inflammation.

Ventilatory strategies are influenced by both the respiratory and the multiorgan involvement that is characteristic of ALF. Thus patients with deep levels of coma and at risk of cerebral oedema will require close attention to CO_2 levels and tailored sedation regimens. Hypercapnia may have to be tolerated in patients progressing to ARDS. This requires balancing against the cerebral needs of these patients as hypercarbia and increased cerebral blood flow will tend to increase ICP. Pleural effusions may require drainage if they are impeding ventilation. Weaning may be facilitated by undertaking tracheostomy during the recovery period of ALF.

RENAL

Renal failure is common, with an incidence as high as 50%. This is particularly the case with paracetamol-induced liver failure, where the drug may also exert a directly toxic effect on the renal tubule. The aetiology of acute renal dysfunction is frequently multifactorial, with hepatorenal failure being a rare occurrence. Acute tubular necrosis and prerenal renal failure are more common precipitants. As such, volume therapy and maintenance of intrathoracic blood volume are essential in the management of such patients, as is the avoidance of nephrotoxins. Intra-abdominal hypertension is frequent and may reduce renal perfusion pressure and contribute to renal dysfunction; the measurement of intra-abdominal pressure may be a valuable component of monitoring.

Established renal failure requires the institution of renal replacement therapy (RRT). In patients with ALF early consideration should be given to RRT to control fluid balance and acid–base disturbances and to avoid rapid changes in osmolarity. It may limit or control elevations of arterial ammonia and retard the development of cerebral complications. The haemodynamic instability and associated cerebral complications of this patient group have resulted in the application of continuous modes of RRT rather than intermittent haemodialysis. Inability of the liver to metabolise and utilise lactate or acetate buffer solutions results in the use of bicarbonate buffers. Extrapolation from data in critically ill patients with acute renal failure suggests that the optimal filtration rate is 35 ml/kg per hour.

ANTICOAGULATION AND COAGULOPATHY

A balance needs to be achieved between risk of bleeding and platelet protection across an extracorporeal filter. A prostaglandin such as epoprostenol may be advantageous

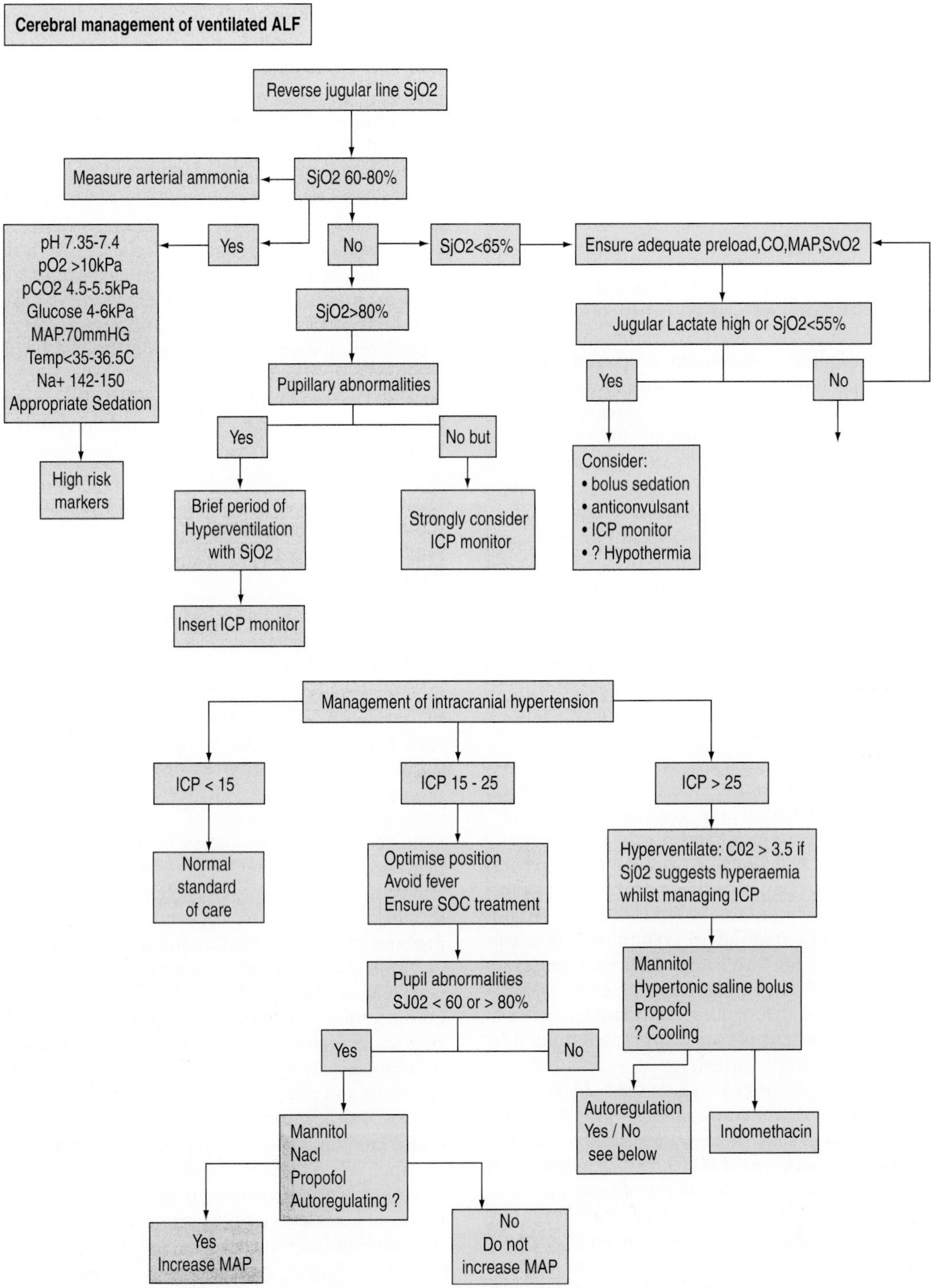

Figure 38.4 Treatment of raised intracranial pressure.

in terms of decreasing bleeding and prolonging filter life. Alternatively, circuits may be run without anticoagulation, with regional heparin or citrate or low-dose systemic heparin. In patients with thrombocytopenia consideration should be given to the diagnosis of heparin-induced thrombocytopenia and, if confirmed, heparin should be withdrawn and circuits primed with an alternative agent, e.g. lepirudin.

METABOLIC AND FEEDING

Enteral nutrition should commence as soon as feasible after admission if there are no contraindications. In patients with large aspirates (> 200 ml/4 hours) a prokinetic agent should be commenced: erythromycin (250 mg intravenously 6-hourly) appears to be more effective than metoclopromide. Endoscopic placement of a postpyloric feeding tube should be considered in refractory cases, although this may need to delayed in patients with or at risk of cerebral oedema. In patients with profound coagulopathy, placement of a nasogastric tube may be associated with nasal/pharyngeal bleeding and oral tube placement may be preferred in ventilated patients. The optimal nature of enteral feed used has not been investigated but metabolic data on these patients demonstrate increased calorific requirements.[27,29] Patients with ALF demonstrate both peripheral and hepatological insulin resistance.[30] Tight glycaemic control would seem reasonable in this population.

Metabolic acidosis is a relatively frequent occurrence that may relate to lactic acidosis, hyperchloraemic acidosis or renal failure.

Hyperlactataemia may be secondary to volume depletion and hence will resolve with appropriate fluid loading or may reflect the inability of the liver to metabolise the lactate produced. A failure of blood lactate to normalise following volume loading is associated with a poor prognosis.[30,31] Metabolic acidosis may be a secondary effect of other drugs ingested as part of an episode of self-harm. Falls in serum phosphate levels are seen in ALF associated with liver regeneration and are associated with a good prognosis in paracetamol-induced ALF.[32] Pancreatitis is a common complication of ALF and should be actively sought.

SPECIFIC TREATMENTS

Very few specific treatments are of proven benefit. *N*-acetylcysteine is useful for paracetamol-related liver failure. There are specific antiviral therapies to prevent reactivation of hepatitis B in at-risk individuals.

Therapies should aim to provide an environment for liver regeneration or stability until a suitable liver is available for orthotopic transplantation. The role of extracorporeal liver support systems remains a hope for the future but at present no system has been shown to have a definitive survival benefit in a controlled trial.

PROGNOSIS

Prognostication is important in the management of ALF. It is essential to identify those patients who will not survive without liver transplant but also to identify those who will succumb even if offered such a procedure.[33] Several risk stratification systems are presented in Table 38.4. The most commonly used are those of O'Grady and Clichy. The model for end-stage liver disease (MELD) has also been examined with regard to prognosis in ALF and may be particularly useful in non-paracetamol cases.[34] It is essential that such systems are rigorously applied and in the context of paracetamol are only utilised at least 24 hours postingestion and following appropriate volume resuscitation.

CIRRHOSIS AND ACUTE-ON-CHRONIC LIVER DISEASE

This is the commonest form of liver disease presenting to the intensive care environment. The commonest precipitants are:

- encephalopathy
- sepsis
- renal failure
- variceal bleeding
- cardiorespiratory failure

Table 38.4 Prognostic criteria for acute liver failure

O'Grady criteria
Paracetamol-related
Acidosis (pH < 7.3) *or*
Prothrombin time of > 100 seconds (INR > 6.5), creatinine > 300 mol/l and grade III/IV encephalaopthy – all occurring within a 24-hour time frame
Non-paracetamol-related
Any three of the following in association with encephalopathy:
Age less than 10 or greater than 40 years
Bilirubin > 300 mol/l
Time from jaundice to encephalopathy > 7 days
Aetiology: either non-A, non-B (seronegative hepatitis) or drug-induced
Prothrombin time > 50 seconds
or
Prothrombin time > 100 seconds/INR > 6.5
French criteria (Clichy criteria)
The criteria are the presence of encephalopathy (coma or confusion) *and*
Age < 20 years with factor V level < 20%
or
Factor V levels < 30% if greater than 30 years of age[59]

INR, international normalised ratio.

The cause of decompensation should be sought in all cases when it is not clinically apparent. Common causes include sepsis, dehydration, drug therapies, e.g. opiates and sedatives, hepatocellular carcinoma (HCC) and portal vein thrombosis.

Ultrasound should be undertaken in all patients, examining the hepatic veins and portal veins for patency. Signs of an HCC should be sought on ultrasound, alpha-fetoprotein and frequently axial imaging techniques. The therapies available for HCC have improved dramatically in recent years and prognosis can be good, especially with the option of cure with liver transplantation.

Sepsis should be actively sought and treated. In patients with ascites a diagnostic tap should always be undertaken for microbiological culture and cell count (a polymorphonuclear count > $250/mm^3$ is indicative of bacterial peritonitis).

Alcoholic hepatitis is a frequent cause of decompensation and requires aggressive treatment. The severity can be assessed using the Glasgow score or Madrey score and in high-risk patients steroid therapy may be considered.[36,37] Response to steroids over the first 7 days is associated with improved outcome.[38] The role of antioxidants has been examined but no benefit was seen.[39,40] Another approach has been to look at the value of enteral feeding, which was comparable with steroid treatment over a 4-week period, albeit in a small study.[41] The use of pentoxifylline has been reported in a single-centre study to decrease the risk of developing hepatorenal failure and hence impacting on outcome.[42]

ENCEPHALOPATHY

This is frequently seen in patients with cirrhosis and a systemic inflammatory response – sepsis should be sought and treated. Unlike ALF, this group does not normally develop intracranial hypertension and as such the main thrust for managing encephalopathy is determined by control of the airway and prevention of aspiration.

Therapies to alleviate encephalopathy aim to decrease ammonia levels and thus focus on bowel cleansing with agents such as lactulose. There is little evidence-based research to support any particular avenue of treatment. A recent trial examining the role of albumin dialysis in the management of encephalopathy has been recently completed. [43]

As noted previously, the role of inflammation seems of importance in the development of encephalopathy.[44,45] The role of feeding and encephalopathy has always caused controversy. Recent guidance suggests that protein restriction is not appropriate and a study examining early versus slow introduction of protein into enteral nutrition showed no increase in encephalopathy and indeed appeared beneficial in respect of nitrogen balance.[46,47]

VARICEAL HAEMORRHAGE

The management of variceal haemorrhage remains that of basic resuscitation and care of the airway. Coagulation factors require appropriate supplementation along with other blood products. The role of sepsis in variceal haemorrhage has become clearer, with sepsis being a frequent precipitant of bleeding. Cultures should be taken and all patients with variceal haemorrhage should be given antibiotics and this has been shown to decrease the risk of rebleeding.[48,49] Splanchnic vasoconstrictors, such as glypressin, are beneficial in controlling oesophageal haemorrhage but their role in gastric variceal haemorrhage per se has not been examined.[50,51] Banding ligation therapy remains the treatment of choice for oesophageal haemorrhage, with tissue adhesives being utilised in gastric varices. Failure to control variceal bleeding after two endoscopic sessions should result in consideration of TIPS insertion.[52,53] In patients in whom TIPS might be considered to be of benefit in controlling variceal bleeding, consideration needs to be given to the severity of the underlying liver disease that may in its own right make TIPS ill advised.[54]

RENAL FAILURE

Hepatorenal failure is seen in cirrhosis – the rapidly progressive form is more commonly seen in the critical care environment. It should be noted that this is a diagnosis of exclusion of other causes. The evidence base for colloid therapy (to ensure adequate central volume repletion) along with splanchnic vasoconstrictor therapy (glypressin) is reasonable but more recently data suggest that constrictors such as noradrenaline may be equally applied.[51,55–57] Prevention of renal failure should also be considered with appropriate volume resuscitation in patients with sepsis and bacterial peritonitis. Ascitic drainage should be undertaken with appropriate albumin loading if large-volume drainage is undertaken or in patients at risk of central volume depletion.[58]

Paracetamol-related hepatotoxicity should also be considered for transplantation if arterial lactate remains elevated following volume resuscitation (> 3.5 mmol/l) and serum phosphate is elevated.

It should be noted that these criteria were not developed in patients with acute Budd–Chiari syndrome, Wilson's disease or pregnancy-related liver failure. Nor have they been or should they be applied in the setting of trauma-related liver failure. Although these criteria demonstrate that being a child (age < 10 years) is a poor prognostic feature, the decision to transplant children is not normally derived from these criteria.

In children the finding of an isolated INR > 4.5 suggests the need for transplantation, assuming that the child has not ingested paracetamol (in this setting the paracetamol criteria would be applied).

The Pittsburgh data suggest that a poor outcome is associated with a liver volume of less than 1000 ml and greater than 50% hepatocyte necrosis of biopsy. The latter may be difficult to interpret due to sampling error.

In acute Budd–Chiari syndrome the combination of encephalopathy and renal failure should lead to consideration for transplantation. Increasingly, TIPS shunts have a place in the earlier management of acute Budd–Chiari syndrome. Such an undertaking should be performed at a centre providing transplantation since a proportion of patients will decompensate with encephalopathy and severe ALF, requiring urgent transplantation.

REFERENCES

1. O'Grady JG, Schalm SW, Williams R. Acute liver failure: redefining the syndromes. *Lancet* 1993; **342**: 273–5.
2. Lee WM. Acute liver failure in the United States. *Semin Liver Dis* 2003; **23**: 217–26.
3. Bernal W, Ma Y, Smith HM *et al.* The significance of autoantibodies and immunoglobulins in acute liver failure: a cohort study. *J Hepatol* 2007; **47**: 664–70.
4. Ichai P, Duclos-Vallee JC, Guettier C *et al.* Usefulness of corticosteroids for the treatment of severe and fulminant forms of autoimmune hepatitis. *Liver Transpl* 2007; **13**: 996–1003.
5. Jalan R, Olde Damink SW, Hayes PC *et al.* Pathogenesis of intracranial hypertension in acute liver failure: inflammation, ammonia and cerebral blood flow. *J Hepatol* 2004; **41**: 613–20.
6. Rose C, Ytrebo LM, Davies NA *et al.* Association of reduced extracellular brain ammonia, lactate, and intracranial pressure in pigs with acute liver failure. *Hepatology* 2007; **46**: 1883–92.
7. Tofteng F, Hauerberg J, Hansen BA *et al.* Persistent arterial hyperammonemia increases the concentration of glutamine and alanine in the brain and correlates with intracranial pressure in patients with fulminant hepatic failure. *J Cereb Blood Flow Metab* 2006; **26**: 21–7.
8. Bernal W, Hall C, Karvellas CJ *et al.* Arterial ammonia and clinical risk factors for encephalopathy and intracranial hypertension in acute liver failure. *Hepatology* 2007; **46**: 1844–52.
9. Bhatia V, Singh R, Acharya SK. Predictive value of arterial ammonia for complications and outcome in acute liver failure. *Gut* 2006; **55**: 98–104.
10. Clemmesen JO, Larsen FS, Kondrup J *et al.* Cerebral herniation in patients with acute liver failure is correlated with arterial ammonia concentration. *Hepatology* 1999; **29**: 648–53.
11. Shawcross DL, Balata S, Olde Damink SW *et al.* Low myo-inositol and high glutamine levels in brain are associated with neuropsychological deterioration after induced hyperammonemia. *Am J Physiol Gastrointest Liver Physiol* 2004; **287**: G503–9.
12. Rolando N, Wade J, Davalos M *et al.* The systemic inflammatory response syndrome in acute liver failure. *Hepatology* 2000; **32**: 734–9.
13. Vaquero J, Polson J, Chung C *et al.* Infection and the progression of hepatic encephalopathy in acute liver failure. *Gastroenterology* 2003; **125**: 755–64.
14. Shawcross DL, Davies NA, Mookerjee RP *et al.* Worsening of cerebral hyperemia by the administration of terlipressin in acute liver failure with severe encephalopathy. *Hepatology* 2004; **39**: 471–5.
15. Strauss GI, Moller K, Holm S *et al.* Transcranial Doppler sonography and internal jugular bulb saturation during hyperventilation in patients with fulminant hepatic failure. *Liver Transpl* 2001; **7**: 352–8.
16. Eefsen M, Dethloff T, Frederiksen HJ *et al.* Comparison of terlipressin and noradrenalin on cerebral perfusion, intracranial pressure and cerebral extracellular concentrations of lactate and pyruvate in patients with acute liver failure in need of inotropic support. *J Hepatol* 2007; **47**: 381–6.
17. Vaquero J, Fontana RJ, Larson AM *et al.* Complications and use of intracranial pressure monitoring in patients with acute liver failure and severe encephalopathy. *Liver Transpl* 2005; **11**: 1581–9.
18. Murphy N, Auzinger G, Bernel W *et al.* The effect of hypertonic sodium chloride on intracranial pressure in patients with acute liver failure. *Hepatology* 2004; **39**: 464–70.
19. Jalan R, Damink SW, Deutz NE *et al.* Moderate hypothermia for uncontrolled intracranial hypertension in acute liver failure. *Lancet* 1999; **354**: 1164–8.
20. Jalan R, Olde Damink SW, Deutz NE *et al.* Restoration of cerebral blood flow autoregulation and reactivity to carbon dioxide in acute liver failure by moderate hypothermia. *Hepatology* 2001; **34**: 50–4.
21. Tofteng F, Larsen FS. The effect of indomethacin on intracranial pressure, cerebral perfusion and extracellular lactate and glutamate concentrations in patients with fulminant hepatic failure. *J Cereb Blood Flow Metab* 2004; **24**: 798–804.
22. Wade J, Rolando N, Philpott-Howard J *et al.* Timing and aetiology of bacterial infections in a liver intensive care unit. *J Hosp Infect* 2003; **53**: 144–6.
23. Antoniades CG, Berry PA, Davies ET *et al.* Reduced monocyte HLA-DR expression: a novel biomarker of disease severity and outcome in acetaminophen-induced acute liver failure. *Hepatology* 2006; **44**: 34–43.
24. Clapperton M, Rolando N, Sandoval L *et al.* Neutrophil superoxide and hydrogen peroxide production in patients with acute liver failure. *Eur J Clin Invest* 1997; **27**: 164–8.
25. Harry R, Auzinger G, Wendon J. The clinical importance of adrenal insufficiency in acute hepatic dysfunction. *Hepatology* 2002; **36**: 395–402.
26. Marik PE. Adrenal-exhaustion syndrome in patients with liver disease. *Intens Care Med* 2006; **32**: 275–80.
27. Fernandez J, Escorsell A, Zabalza M *et al.* Adrenal insufficiency in patients with cirrhosis and septic shock: effect of treatment with hydrocortisone on survival. *Hepatology* 2006; **44**: 1288–95.
28. Parekh NK, Hynan LS, De Lemos J *et al.* Elevated troponin I levels in acute liver failure: is myocardial injury an integral part of acute liver failure? *Hepatology* 2007; **45**: 1489–95.
29. Walsh TS, Wigmore SJ, Hopton P *et al.* Energy expenditure in acetaminophen-induced fulminant hepatic failure. *Crit Care Med* 2000; **28**: 649–54.
30. Clark SJ, Shojaee-Moradie F, Croos P *et al.* Temporal changes in insulin sensitivity following the

development of acute liver failure secondary to acetaminophen. *Hepatology* 2001; **34**: 109–15.
31. Bernal W, Donaldson N, Wyncoll D *et al.* Blood lactate as an early predictor of outcome in paracetamol-induced acute liver failure: a cohort study. *Lancet* 2002; **359**: 558–63.
32. Schmidt LE, Dalhoff K. Serum phosphate is an early predictor of outcome in severe acetaminophen-induced hepatotoxicity. *Hepatology* 2002; **36**: 659–65.
33. Blei AT. Selection for acute liver failure: have we got it right? *Liver Transpl* 2005; **11** (Suppl. 2): S30–4.
34. Yantorno SE, Kremers WK, Ruf AE *et al.* MELD is superior to King's College and Clichy's criteria to assess prognosis in fulminant hepatic failure. *Liver Transpl* 2007; **13**: 822–8.
35. Schiodt FV, Rossaro L, Stravitz RT *et al.* Gc-globulin and prognosis in acute liver failure. *Liver Transpl* 2005; **11**: 1223–7.
36. Forrest EH, Evans CD, Stewart S *et al.* Analysis of factors predictive of mortality in alcoholic hepatitis and derivation and validation of the Glasgow alcoholic hepatitis score. *Gut* 2005; **54**: 1174–9.
37. Forrest EH, Morris J, Stewart S *et al.* The Glasgow alcoholic hepatitis score identifies patients who may benefit from corticosteroids. *Gut* 2007; **56**: 1743–6.
38. Mathurin P, Abdelnour M, Ramond MJ *et al.* Early change in bilirubin levels is an important prognostic factor in severe alcoholic hepatitis treated with prednisolone. *Hepatology* 2003; **38**: 1363–9.
39. Phillips M, Curtis H, Portmann B *et al.* Antioxidants versus corticosteroids in the treatment of severe alcoholic hepatitis – a randomised clinical trial. *J Hepatol* 2006; **44**: 784–90.
40. Stewart S, Prince M, Bassendine M *et al.* A randomized trial of antioxidant therapy alone or with corticosteroids in acute alcoholic hepatitis. *J Hepatol* 2007; **47**: 277–83.
41. Cabre E, Rodriguez-Iglesias P, Caballeria J *et al.* Short- and long-term outcome of severe alcohol-induced hepatitis treated with steroids or enteral nutrition: a multicenter randomized trial. *Hepatology* 2000; **32**: 36–42.
42. Akriviadis E, Botla R, Briggs W *et al.* Pentoxifylline improves short-term survival in severe acute alcoholic hepatitis: a double-blind, placebo-controlled trial. *Gastroenterology* 2000; **119**: 1637–48.
43. Hassanein TI, Tofteng F, Brown RS *et al.* Randomized controlled study of extracorporeal albumin dialysis for hepatic encephalopathy in advanced cirrhosis. *Hepatology* 2007; **46**: 1853–62.
44. Shawcross DL, Davies NA, Williams R *et al.* Systemic inflammatory response exacerbates the neuropsychological effects of induced hyperammonemia in cirrhosis. *J Hepatol* 2004; **40**: 247–54.
45. Shawcross DL, Wright G, Olde Damink SW *et al.* Role of ammonia and inflammation in minimal hepatic encephalopathy. *Metab Brain Dis* 2007; **22**: 125–38.
46. Marchesini G, Bianchi G, Rossi B *et al.* Nutritional treatment with branched-chain amino acids in advanced liver cirrhosis. *J Gastroenterol* 2000; **35** (Suppl. 12): 7–12.
47. Alvarez MA, Cabre E, Lorenzo-Zuniga V *et al.* Combining steroids with enteral nutrition: a better therapeutic strategy for severe alcoholic hepatitis? Results of a pilot study. *Eur J Gastroenterol Hepatol* 2004; **16**: 1375–80.
48. Hou MC, Lin HC, Liu TT *et al.* Antibiotic prophylaxis after endoscopic therapy prevents rebleeding in acute variceal hemorrhage: a randomized trial. *Hepatology* 2004; **39**: 746–53.
49. Fernandez J, Ruiz del Arbol L, Gomez C *et al.* Norfloxacin vs ceftriaxone in the prophylaxis of infections in patients with advanced cirrhosis and hemorrhage. *Gastroenterology* 2006; **131**: 1049–56; quiz 285.
50. Escorsell A, Ruiz del Arbol L, Planas R *et al.* Multicenter randomized controlled trial of terlipressin versus sclerotherapy in the treatment of acute variceal bleeding: the TEST study. *Hepatology* 2000; **32**: 471–6.
51. Gluud LL, Kjaer MS, Christensen E. Terlipressin for hepatorenal syndrome. *Cochrane Database Syst Rev* 2006; **4**:CD005162.
52. Khan S, Tudur Smith C, Williamson P *et al.* Portosystemic shunts versus endoscopic therapy for variceal rebleeding in patients with cirrhosis. *Cochrane Database Syst Rev* 2006; **4**: CD000553.
53. Thabut D, Bernard-Chabert B. Management of acute bleeding from portal hypertension. *Best Pract Res Clin Gastroenterol* 2007; **21**: 19–29.
54. Schepke M, Roth F, Fimmers R *et al.* Comparison of MELD, Child–Pugh, and Emory model for the prediction of survival in patients undergoing transjugular intrahepatic portosystemic shunting. *Am J Gastroenterol* 2003; **98**: 1167–74.
55. Alessandria C, Ottobrelli A, Debernardi-Venon W *et al.* Noradrenalin vs terlipressin in patients with hepatorenal syndrome: a prospective, randomized, unblinded, pilot study. *J Hepatol* 2007; **47**: 499–505.
56. Moreau R, Durand F, Poynard T *et al.* Terlipressin in patients with cirrhosis and type 1 hepatorenal syndrome: a retrospective multicenter study. *Gastroenterology* 2002; **122**: 923–30.
57. Moreau R, Lebrec D. The use of vasoconstrictors in patients with cirrhosis: type 1 HRS and beyond. *Hepatology* 2006; **43**: 385–94.
58. Moreau R, Asselah T, Condat B *et al.* Comparison of the effect of terlipressin and albumin on arterial blood volume in patients with cirrhosis and tense ascites treated by paracentesis: a randomised pilot study. *Gut* 2002; **50**: 90–4.
59. Bernuau J, Goudeau A, Poynard T *et al.* Multivariate analysis of prognostic factors in fulminant hepatitis B. *Hepatology* 1986; **6**: 648–51.

39

Abdominal surgical catastrophes

Stephen J Streat

Intra-abdominal surgical catastrophes are common conditions in intensive care units (ICUs)[1] and typically occur in elderly patients with comorbidity and reduced physiological reserve. They are often associated with sepsis, either primarily or secondarily, and with subsequent multiple-organ failure. Overall mortality is high[2,3] and those who do survive usually require a long period in intensive care. The long-term health outcomes of patients with these conditions may be poor, particularly if severe comorbidity and functional impairment were present before the catastrophe. These factors inevitably lead treating clinicians to consider carefully the costs and benefits[4,5] of various treatment strategies during an illness which often has many of the characteristics of a tragic saga.[6] The clinical issues alone are complex and decision-making is often hampered by the lack of controlled trials of various strategic approaches. These many difficulties create the potential for conflict to arise between intensivists and other involved clinicians, particularly surgeons, who inhabit different moral economies[6] and often have differing opinions of what are realistic goals and reasonable strategies,[7] particularly for patients who are near the end of life.[8,9] It is in the care of these patients that the particular day-to-day work skills of the intensivist[10,11] ('seeing the big picture', providing meticulous bedside care, and negotiating and maintaining consensus, good communication and teamwork between various clinicians and the family) are tested to the limits. In this chapter, vascular catastrophes, intra-abdominal sepsis and a few serious abdominal complications are discussed. Gastrointestinal bleeding and pancreatitis are covered elsewhere (Chapters 36 and 37).

VASCULAR CATASTROPHES

ABDOMINAL AORTIC ANEURYSM (AAA)

AAA is a disease of the elderly, which is up to six times more common in men than women.[12] Rupture of an AAA is the most common vascular catastrophe seen in ICUs and accounts for 2% of all deaths in men over 60 years of age.[13] The prevalence of AAA (defined as infrarenal aortic diameter of 30 mm or more), as detected by screening in men, rises from less than 1% at age 50 to around 4% at aged 60, between 5 and 10% at age 70 and around 10% at age 80. Ultrasound screening of elderly men for AAA reduces mortality and is probably cost-effective.[14] Aortic diameter is the strongest predictor of the risk of rupture, which is below 1% per year with aortic diameter < 5 cm and about 17% per year with aortic diameter of 6 cm or more.[13] The risk of rupture is higher in women (who have faster aneurysm growth rates than men[15]) and is increased by current smoking and hypertension. Aortic aneurysm expansion is around 0.3 cm/year for aneurysms smaller than 5 cm and around 0.5 cm/year for those larger than 5 cm and this rate may be able to be reduced by a short course of macrolide or by stopping smoking. Perioperative mortality for open elective aneurysm repair is ~5% – somewhat higher when there is significant preoperative respiratory or renal dysfunction.[16] Increasingly endovascular repair is performed because of lower perioperative mortality (~1.5%), although 2-year survival is the same (~90%) after either open or endovascular repair.[17] A higher proportion of patients treated endovascularly will experience long-term complications (predominantly endoleaks, rupture and graft thrombosis), with associated increase in cost.[18] Endovascular repair does not improve survival in patients judged medically unfit for open repair.[19]

Operative mortality is increased to around 15% in urgently repaired (non-ruptured) aneurysms[20] and around 50% in ruptured aneurysms repaired as an emergency.[20] Ruptured aneurysm may lead to death before hospital admission in around 30% of cases,[21] is almost always lethal without repair[22] and not all patients are offered repair. Vascular surgeons are less selective (~10% non-operative) than general surgeons (~60% non-operative), without an increase in mortality in operated patients.[22]

These results have led to recommendations for population screening by ultrasound at age 65, continued surveillance for small aneurysms[23] and elective open (or endovascular) repair in patients without severe comorbidity when aneurysm diameter exceeds 5 or 6 cm.[24]

RUPTURE OF AN ABDOMINAL AORTIC (OR ILIAC ARTERY) ANEURYSM

The clinical features of rupture include the sudden onset of shock and back pain or abdominal pain or tenderness in a patient typically over the age of 70. Most ruptures are, initially at least, retroperitoneal with intraperitoneal rupture resulting in greater physiological disturbance and much higher subsequent operative mortality.[25] The correct clinical diagnosis is often not made by the first attending doctor[26] as a pulsatile abdominal mass is commonly not detectable[25] and many patients do not have shock when first seen. Although immediate bedside ultrasound may sometimes be able to confirm the clinical diagnosis without increasing delay, others have found that this investigation commonly delayed vascular surgical referral and subsequent operation without diagnostic benefit.[27] The diagnosis of ruptured aneurysm is confirmed (by computed tomography (CT) angiography) in only half of the patients in whom it is suspected[28] but CT carries a significant risk of sudden deterioration outside the operating room. It may sometimes be inappropriate to proceed to operation (very severe comorbidity, poor quality of life) and this decision should be very carefully considered.[29] Lack of physiological reserve (often associated with advanced age) predicts high operative mortality and long periods of intensive care and hospitalisation in survivors. Open repair remains the current treatment of choice but successful endovascular repair (sometimes with subsequent laparotomy for evacuation of haematoma[30]) is also possible in some of these aneurysms[31] and is the subject of an ongoing randomised controlled trial.[28] A very small number of patients with aortic aneurysm have infection of the aneurysm, usually with *Staphylococcus* or *Salmonella*, which is often diagnosed at rupture.[32] A period of postoperative intensive care is appropriate for most patients. During this time common physiological abnormalities (e.g. hypothermia, dilutional coagulopathy, minor bleeding, circulatory shock, renal tubular dysfunction) can be corrected and serious complications can be sought and if possible treated (Table 39.1).

Rapid ventilator weaning and extubation are recommended, perhaps with thoracic epidural anaesthesia[33] if coagulation allows. Abdominal decompression in these particular patients may not be helpful.[34] Finally, an assessment of overall progress should be made after 24–48 hours. Severe or progressive multiple-organ failure[35] or major visceral or limb infarction should lead to a reappraisal of the appropriateness of continued intensive therapies. Persistent renal failure occurs more commonly after acute renal failure in this context than in other intensive care patients. Massive upper gastrointestinal haemorrhage (usually aortoduodenal) is a rare complication, usually resulting from infection of a previous aortic repair and less commonly from primary infection in an aortic aneurysm. Some of these patients can be rescued surgically.

Table 39.1 Some complications of a ruptured aortic aneurysm

Major bleeding
Renal failure
Myocardial infarction
Acute lung injury
Peripheral ischaemia
Stroke
Pulmonary embolism
Persistent ileus
Mesenteric ischaemia
Pancreatitis
Acalculous cholcystitis
Increased abdominal pressure – compartment syndrome

ACUTE AORTIC OCCLUSION

This is an uncommon syndrome, usually due to thrombotic occlusion (of a stenotic or aneursymal aorta) or to saddle embolism. Presentation is with painful lower-limb paraparesis or paraplegia and absent distal circulation. Minimising delay to emergency revascularisation is of the essence but mortality and multisystem morbidity remain high.[36]

MESENTERIC INFARCTION

This uncommon syndrome presents with an acute abdomen, may develop in critically ill patients and is commonly due to non-occlusive arterial ischaemia, arterial embolism or atherosclerotic arterial thrombosis and less often to venous occlusion, low-flow or hypercoagulable states.[37] Despite surgery (usually including gut resection), mortality is high. Successful endovascular revascularisation has been reported.[38]

AORTIC DISSECTION

Aortic dissection[39] has an incidence of 5–30 per million per year. The typical patient is elderly, has a history of hypertension[40] and presents with pain in a distribution corresponding to the site of dissection. Cases have been reported in young people and after circumstances suggesting acute situational hypertension. Pericardial tamponade, haemothorax, myocardial infarction, stroke, paraplegia due to spinal cord ischaemia, anuria or an acute abdomen may be present. Most aortic dissections originate in the ascending thoracic aorta. Some dissections extend to involve the abdominal aorta but spontaneous dissection of the abdominal aorta alone is rare. Mortality remains high but is falling in association with earlier diagnosis and treatment.[39]

SPONTANEOUS RETROPERITONEAL HAEMORRHAGE

Excluding rupture of an aortic aneurysm, spontaneous retroperitoneal haemorrhage is uncommon. It is usually associated with vascular or malignant disease of the kidney or adrenal gland and, less commonly, with spontaneous rupture of the retroperitoneal veins or with anticoagulant therapy, including warfarin, unfractionated heparin and low-molecular-weight heparin. The presentation is most often with acute abdominal pain, shock and a palpable abdominal or groin mass and CT will confirm the diagnosis.[41] Correction of coagulopathy and interventional radiologic embolisation may control some situations but surgery may be required in others, either to stop bleeding or to relieve associated intra-abdominal hypertension.

INTRA-ABDOMINAL SEPSIS

OVERVIEW

Intra-abdominal sepsis is very common in the ICU. In our own experience the abdomen (including continuous ambulatory peritoneal dialysis (CAPD) peritonitis) was the most common septic site in patients admitted to ICU with severe sepsis and accounted for 583 (35.9%) of the 1624 such admissions over the 17 years from 1984 to 2000.[42] The incidence of sepsis in ICUs is reported to be increasing[43] and our experience reflects this. The mortality of intensive care patients with severe intra-abdominal infections is variously reported between 25 and 80% but varies greatly depending on the extent of comorbidity[43] and the severity of the acute illness.

The general principles of the treatment of severe sepsis are to support oxygen transport as required, if possible to remove the septic source[44] and to give appropriate antimicrobial therapy. Sepsis should be thought of as a time-critical condition[45] wherein delay in the execution of these principles is likely to worsen outcome. The place of other therapies remains controversial.[46,47] The issue of severe sepsis in general is covered in Chapter 61.

In the critically ill patient with intra-abdominal sepsis, effective source control usually involves surgery, although occasionally interventional procedures may suffice. Laparotomy without delay or further investigation is recommended for most patients presenting acutely with shock and clinical evidence of peritonitis. Diagnostic peritoneal aspiration or lavage, abdominal CT scanning or laparoscopy may have limited applicability in unusual circumstances that do not mandate immediate laparotomy.

Common syndromes include:

- faecal peritonitis
- primarily – diverticular disease or colonic malignancy
- secondarily – after prior anterior resection
- perforated upper abdominal viscus (usually of a gastric or duodenal ulcer)
- biliary obstruction (sometimes with perforation)
- intestinal infarction without perforation (usually adhesive, less commonly ischaemic)
- appendicitis (which is more often perforated in older patients)

Less common syndromes include localised intra-abdominal abscess, acalculous cholecystitis, toxic megacolon, perforation of a fallopian tube abscess, spontaneous bacterial peritonitis (SBP, in nephrotic syndrome or end-stage liver disease) and CAPD-associated peritonitis (not all of which is non-surgical).

SURGICAL SOURCE CONTROL

Surgical source control should involve definitive control of the septic site at the first ('damage control') operation but definitive surgical therapy for the underlying disease may not always be feasible or desirable at this time. Initial surgery[44] involves:

- removal of all peritoneal contamination (both macroscopically and by generous lavage)
- drainage of abscesses
- resection of devitalised tissue
- defunctioning the gut to prevent ongoing contamination

The abdomen may be left open (with a temporary fascial closure) if required for intra-abdominal hypertension or to facilitate repeat laparotomy. Successful primary colonic anastomosis (even left-sided) after resection in the presence of sepsis is supported by several case series.[44]

Failure of the sepsis syndrome to settle ('failure to thrive') after apparently definitive surgical source control should suggest ongoing contamination or ischaemia or the development of abscess. Repeat laparotomy on clinical grounds is recommended when early postoperative progress is unsatisfactory,[3] whereas CT scanning followed by either directed laparotomy[48] or interventional radiologic drainage are more successful strategies for late abscess formation.

INTESTINAL-SOURCE PERITONITIS

Peritonitis secondary to contamination by intestinal contents usually results in mixed aerobic and anaerobic infection and recommended antibiotic regimens,[42,49] therefore usually involve either combination therapy with an aminoglycoside (or aztreonam) and metronidazole (or clindamycin) or alternatively monotherapy with a carbapenem. Similar antibiotic regimens are appropriate in sepsis following intestinal infarction without perforation. An agent active against *Staphylococcus aureus*[50] should probably be included in patients with peritonitis following gastric or duodenal perforation.

BILIARY SEPSIS

Biliary ultrasound followed by endoscopic sphincteromy and stone removal is recommended for critically ill patients with cholangitis. Antibiotic regimens should cover enterococci and aerobic Gram-negative bacilli.

ACALCULOUS CHOLECYSTITIS

Acalculous cholecystitis is a rare but serious condition in ICUs. A small number of patients with the syndrome of acute cholecystitis will have acalculous cholecystitis but these patients have low mortality and do not present to ICUs. Of greater concern are the perhaps half of all cases of acalculous cholecystitis that develop insidiously in intensive care patients who are already critically ill for another reason (e.g. recent trauma or surgery) and can therefore go unrecognised until gangrene, perforation or abscess develops. The gallbladder histology in such patients usually includes prominent ischaemia and arteriosclerosis and low cardiac output may predispose to the condition. A high index of suspicion should be had in an intensive care patient who develops new abdominal pain or clinical signs of sepsis. Although a variety of investigations, including scintigraphy, CT scanning, ultrasound and laparoscopy, have been used to help establish the diagnosis, none performs reliably[51] and many surgeons advocate a low threshold to exploratory laparotomy on clinical grounds where suspicion exists. Percutaneous cholecystostomy[44] has been used successfully whereas early cholecystectomy is advocated by others[52] as infarction or perforation of the gallbladder is commonly found at laparotomy.

TOXIC MEGACOLON

Toxic megacolon[53] is now a rare indication for intensive care admission. It is characterised by systemic toxicity accompanying a dilated, inflamed colon and is usually due to inflammatory bowel disease. Infection by *Clostridium difficile*, cytomegalovirus (in patients with human immunodeficiency virus (HIV) disease or immunosuppression) or rarely other organisms may also precipitate toxic megacolon. The diagnosis should be considered in patients with diarrhoea and abdominal distension. Limited colonoscopy (despite the risk of perforation) and biopsy may both yield important microbiological information and help in the decision to operate. Supportive therapy in an ICU is usually recommended and includes both antibiotics as for colonic perforation and steroids (equivalent of ~300 mg/day of hydrocortisone). Other immunosuppression (tacrolimus or anti-tumour necrosis factor (anti-TNF) monoclonal antibody) has also been used. Frequent surgical reassessment and abdominal X-rays are used to monitor progress. Intravenous nutrition may help to reduce the activity of Crohn's disease but does not reduce hospital stay or the need for surgery in ulcerative colitis. A period of several days of careful observation may be reasonable to assess the response to medical treatment but urgent surgery (subtotal colectomy with end-ileostomy) is indicated for increasing colonic dilatation, perforation, bleeding or progressive systemic toxicity.[54] Parenteral metronidazole may be effective in severe pseudomembranous colitis without megacolon (but early surgery is often recommended if megacolon develops).

RUPTURE OF A TUBO-OVARIAN ABSCESS

Rupture of a tubo-ovarian abscess is a rare cause of peritonitis presenting to ICUs and is best treated with surgical extirpation. Antibiotic therapy should include activity against anaerobic organisms.

SPONTANEOUS BACTERIAL PERITONITIS

SBP is usually a monomicrobial infection (usually with *Escherichia coli*, *Klebsiella pneumoniae*, pneumococci or enterococci and rarely with anaerobes).[42] The development of SBP in patients with end-stage liver disease is a grave prognostic sign – hepatic decompensation and multiple-organ failure commonly develop and the median survival in such patients (without liver transplantation) is short. Early albumin supplementation has been shown to reduce both renal failure and mortality in SBP associated with end-stage liver disease.[55] Treatment with a broad-spectrum beta-lactam antibiotic should be followed by secondary oral antibiotic prophylaxis.

CAPD-ASSOCIATED PERITONITIS

Peritonitis is not uncommon in CAPD patients but is rarely a cause of intensive care admission. The development of (extrarenal) organ failure is an ominous sign and usually reflects delay in effective treatment, abscess formation, the presence of unusual organisms (including a variety of fungi), or an unrecognised gastrointestinal septic source.[56]

TERTIARY PERITONITIS

Tertiary peritonitis – 'peritonitis in the critically ill patient that persists or recurs at least 48 hours after the apparently adequate management of primary or secondary peritonitis'[57] – occurs occasionally in severely ill patients with prior laparotomy. It is commonly due to *Staphylococcus epidermidis*, enterococci, *Enterobacter*, *Pseudomonas* or *Candida albicans*[42,57] and initial empiric treatment should include amoxicillin, gentamicin and metronidazole until culture results are available. When infection is due to *Candida* spp. other antimicrobial agents should be discontinued, any foreign bodies removed if possible, and treatment with amphotericin B given for at least 4 weeks.[58]

COMPLICATIONS

INTRA-ABDOMINAL HYPERTENSION AND THE ABDOMINAL COMPARTMENT SYNDROME

These phenomena occur uncommonly in critically ill patients, particularly after surgery for trauma or sepsis and in association with excessive crystalloid fluid administration. A recent consensus conference has defined intra-abdominal hypertension as intra-abdominal pressure (IAP) >12 mmHg and abdominal compartment syndrome as IAP >20 mmHg with associated organ dysfunction.[59] IAP can be conveniently and easily measured via intravesical pressure,[34,59] is normally 5–7 mmHg in critically ill adults and is increased in patients with increased body mass index. Physiological impairment (including cardiorespiratory, renal, splanchnic and neurological) can occur with acute increases in IAP to levels above 12 mmHg. However, in the absence of evidence from randomised controlled trials, expert opinion[60] suggests that the development of the abdominal compartment syndrome (IAP > 20 mmHg with associated organ dysfunction) should prompt a search for decompressive measures. Traditionally this has involved urgent decompressive laparotomy and temporary fascial closure; however other measures include:

- avoidance of the prone position
- gastric and colonic decompression
- neostigmine or other prokinetic agents
- neuromuscular blockade

Diuresis or ultrafiltration or percutaneous drainage of intraperitoneal fluid or gas may be effective in some patients and should also be considered.[60] Despite abdominal decompression, mortality for such patients remains high (~50%).[34]

THE OPEN ABDOMEN AND STAGED ABDOMINAL REPAIR

The use of synthetic materials to provide temporary fascial closure has facilitated the care of the patient with an open abdomen and allowed repeat laparotomy and staged abdominal repair to proceed in a timely and unhurried manner. Our own practice[34] has been to use polypropylene mesh alone for this purpose if the period of open abdomen is likely to be short (less than a week) and the mesh can be removed before significant adhesion occurs. Two or more drains on moderate suction are laid over the mesh and then covered with a clear plastic adhesive dressing to provide a sterile waterproof seal and allow continual removal of ascites. If a longer period is required with an open abdomen, then a non-adherent plastic material should be used either under or instead of the mesh to prevent adherence and minimise the risk of gut perforation and fistula during removal of the material and fascial closure. The management of fistulation in the open abdomen remains problematic as proximal defunctioning is often impossible and control of wound contamination is not ideal with soft-catheter intubation of the small bowel via the fistulous tract.

ENTEROCUTANEOUS FISTULAS – INTESTINAL, BILIARY AND PANCREATIC

These are rare complications in intensive care patients but they usually present formidable problems because of their common associations with serious gastrointestinal comorbidity, e.g. inflammatory bowel disease, intestinal malignancy and pancreatitis as well as concurrent severe sepsis. In addition complex fistulation with multiple collections, fistulation through an open abdomen, inability to proximally defunction or distal obstruction are commonly present. A standard approach to fistula management should apply.[61]

This may include:

- attention to drainage of sepsis
- control of the fistula by drainage
- if necessary, by proximal defunctioning
- protection of the skin from the deleterious effects of the fistula fluid
- nutritional support
- replacement of fluid and electrolyte losses

Although somatostatin analogues have been shown to reduce high-output small-bowel fistula losses and they and H_2-blockers are commonly recommended in fistulas of intestinal or pancreatic origin, their efficacy in achieving closure is less clear.[62] Parenteral nutrition is usually recommended for proximal small-bowel fistulas but more distal intestinal, biliary or pancreatic fistulas can probably be safely treated with a trial of enteral nutrition. Treatment with an anti-TNF antibody has been shown to be effective in chronic enterocutaneous fistulas in (non-ICU) patients with Crohn's disease.[63] Persistent high-output fistula should lead to investigation of possible causes, including complete disruption of the gut lumen, distal obstruction or persistent intra-abdominal sepsis. Definitive operative treatment for fistulas that do not close should await clinical recovery and, if possible, nutritional repletion.

COLONIC PSEUDO-OBSTRUCTION

Colonic pseudo-obstruction (Ogilvie's syndrome, a severe form of colonic ileus) is not uncommon in critically ill patients. The syndrome may contribute to ventilatory difficulty, intra-abdominal hypertension and failure of enteral feeding. It carries a small risk of spontaneous perforation with high resultant mortality. Conventional conservative treatment includes nasogastric drainage, intravenous fluid replacement and avoidance of opioids and anticholinergic agents. Treatment with neostigmine has been found to be highly effective[64] but may cause symptomatic bradycardia. Colonoscopy or surgery may be required if these measures fail.[65]

REFERENCES

1. Streat SJ, Plank LD, Hill GL. Overview of modern management of patients with critical injury and severe sepsis. *World J Surg* 2000; **24**: 655–63.
2. McLauchlan GJ, Anderson ID, Grant IS *et al.* Outcome of patients with abdominal sepsis treated in an intensive care unit. *Br J Surg* 1995; **82**: 524–9.
3. Hutchins RR, Gunning MP, Lucas DN *et al.* Relaparotomy for suspected intraperitoneal sepsis after abdominal surgery. *World J Surg* 2004; **28**: 137–41.
4. Sznajder M, Aegerter P, Launois R *et al.* A cost-effectiveness analysis of stays in intensive care units. *Intens Care Med* 2001; **27**: 146–53.
5. Heyland DK, Konopad E, Noseworthy TW *et al.* Is it 'worthwhile' to continue treating patients with a prolonged stay (>14 days) in the ICU? An economic evaluation. *Chest* 1998; **114**: 192–8.
6. Cassell J. *Life and Death in Intensive Care.* Philadelphia: Temple University Press, 2005.
7. Cassell J, Buchman TG, Streat S *et al.* Surgeons, intensivists, and the covenant of care: administrative models and values affecting care at the end of life – updated. *Crit Care Med* 2003; **31**: 1551–7.

8. Rabow MW, Hardie GE, Fair JM *et al.* End-of-life care content in 50 textbooks from multiple specialties. *JAMA* 2000; **283**: 771–8.
9. Streat S. When do we stop? *Crit Care Resuscitation* 2005; 7: 227–32.
10. Fisher MM. Critical care. A specialty without frontiers. *Crit Care Clin* 1997; **13**: 235–43.
11. Curtis JR, Patrick DL, Shannon SE *et al.* The family conference as a focus to improve communication about end-of-life care in the intensive care unit: opportunities for improvement. *Crit Care Med* 2001; **29** (Suppl.): N26–33.
12. Vardulaki KA, Walker NM, Day NE *et al.* Quantifying the risks of hypertension, age, sex and smoking in patients with abdominal aortic aneurysm. *Br J Surg* 2000; **87**: 195–200.
13. Law M. Screening for abdominal aortic aneurysms. *Br Med Bull* 1998; **54**: 903–13.
14. Cosford P, Leng G. Screening for abdominal aortic aneurysm. *Cochrane Database Syst Rev* 2007; **2**: CD002945.
15. Mofidi R, Goldie VJ, Kelman J *et al.* Influence of sex on expansion rate of abdominal aortic aneurysms. *Br J Surg* 2007; **94**: 310–14.
16. Brady AR, Fowkes FG, Greenhalgh RM *et al.* Risk factors for postoperative death following elective surgical repair of abdominal aortic aneurysm: results from the UK Small Aneurysm Trial. On behalf of the UK Small Aneurysm Trial participants. *Br J Surg* 2000; **87**: 742–9.
17. Blankensteijn JD, de Jong SE, Prinssen M *et al.* Two-year outcomes after conventional or endovascular repair of abdominal aortic aneurysms. *N Engl J Med* 2005; **352**: 2398–405.
18. EVAR trial participants. Endovascular aneurysm repair versus open repair in patients with abdominal aortic aneurysm (EVAR trial 1): randomised controlled trial. *Lancet* 2005; **365**: 2179–86.
19. EVAR trial participants. Endovascular aneurysm repair and outcome in patients unfit for open repair of abdominal aortic aneurysm (EVAR trial 2): randomised controlled trial. *Lancet* 2005; **365**: 2187–92.
20. Sayers RD, Thompson MM, Nasim A *et al.* Surgical management of 671 abdominal aortic aneurysms: a 13 year review from a single centre. *Eur J Vasc Endovasc Surg* 1997; **13**: 322–7.
21. Johansson G, Swedenborg J. Ruptured abdominal aortic aneurysms: a study of incidence and mortality. *Br J Surg* 1986; **73**: 101–3.
22. Basnyat PS, Biffin AH, Moseley LG *et al.* Mortality from ruptured abdominal aortic aneurysm in Wales. *Br J Surg* 1999; **86**: 765–70.
23. The UK Small Aneurysm Trial Participants. Mortality results for randomised controlled trial of early elective surgery or ultrasonographic surveillance for small abdominal aortic aneurysms. *Lancet* 1998; **352**: 1649–55.
24. Scott RA, Ashton HA, Lamparelli MJ *et al.* A 14-year experience with 6 cm as a criterion for surgical treatment of abdominal aortic aneurysm. *Br J Surg* 1999; **86**: 1317–21.
25. Aburahma AF, Woodruff BA, Stuart SP *et al.* Early diagnosis and survival of ruptured abdominal aortic aneurysms. *Am J Emerg Med* 1991; **9**: 118–21.
26. Rose J, Civil I, Koelmeyer T *et al.* Ruptured abdominal aortic aneurysms: clinical presentation in Auckland 1993–1997. *ANZ J Surg* 2001; **71**: 341–4.
27. Acheson AG, Graham AN, Weir C *et al.* Prospective study on factors delaying surgery in ruptured abdominal aortic aneurysms. *J R Coll Surg Edinb* 1998; **43**: 182–4.
28. Hoornweg LL, Wisselink W, Vahl A *et al.* The Amsterdam Acute Aneurysm Trial: suitability and application rate for endovascular repair of ruptured abdominal aortic aneurysms. *Eur J Vasc Endovasc Surg* 2007; **33**: 679–83.
29. Prance SE, Wilson YG, Cosgrove CM *et al.* Ruptured abdominal aortic aneurysms: selecting patients for surgery. *Eur J Vasc Endovasc Surg* 1999; **17**: 129–32.
30. Greenberg RK, Srivastava SD, Ouriel K *et al.* An endoluminal method of hemorrhage control and repair of ruptured abdominal aortic aneurysms. *J Endovasc Ther* 2000; 7: 1–7.
31. Peppelenbosch N, Yilmaz N, van Marrewijk C *et al.* Emergency treatment of acute symptomatic or ruptured abdominal aortic aneurysm. Outcome of a prospective intent-to-treat by EVAR protocol. *Eur J Vasc Endovasc Surg* 2003; **26**: 303–10.
32. Muller BT, Wegener OR, Grabitz K *et al.* Mycotic aneurysms of the thoracic and abdominal aorta and iliac arteries: experience with anatomic and extra-anatomic repair in 33 cases. *J Vasc Surg* 2001; **33**: 106–13.
33. Rodgers A, Walker N, Schug S *et al.* Reduction of postoperative mortality and morbidity with epidural or spinal anaesthesia: results from overview of randomised trials. *Br Med J* 2000; **321**: 1493–7.
34. Torrie J, Hill AA, Streat S. Staged abdominal repair in critical illness. *Anaesth Intens Care* 1996; **24**: 368–74.
35. Meesters RC, van der Graaf Y, Vos A *et al.* Ruptured aortic aneurysm: early postoperative prediction of mortality using an organ system failure score. *Br J Surg* 1994; **81**: 512–16.
36. Surowiec SM, Isiklar H, Sreeram S *et al.* Acute occlusion of the abdominal aorta. *Am J Surg* 1998; **176**: 193–7.
37. Newman TS, Magnuson TH, Ahrendt SA *et al.* The changing face of mesenteric infarction. *Am Surg* 1998; **64**: 611–16.
38. Gartenschlaeger S, Bender S, Maeurer J *et al.* Successful percutaneous transluminal angioplasty and stenting in acute mesenteric ischemia. *Cardiovasc Intervent Radiol* 2008; **31**: 398–400.
39. Erbel R, Alfonso F, Boileau C *et al.* Diagnosis and management of aortic dissection. *Eur Heart J* 2001; **22**: 1642–81.
40. Meszaros I, Morocz J, Szlavi J *et al.* Epidemiology and clinicopathology of aortic dissection. *Chest* 2000; **117**: 1271–8.
41. Nazarian LN, Lev-Toaff AS, Spettell CM *et al.* CT assessment of abdominal hemorrhage in coagulopathic patients: impact on clinical management. *Abdom Imaging* 1999; **24**: 246–9.

42. Thomas MG, Streat SJ. Infections in intensive care patients. In: Finch, Greenwood *et al.* (eds) *Antibiotic and Chemotherapy.* London: Harcourt, 2001.
43. Angus DC, Linde-Zwirble WT, Lidicker J *et al.* Epidemiology of severe sepsis in the United States: analysis of incidence, outcome, and associated costs of care. *Crit Care Med* 2001; **29**: 1303–10.
44. Marshall JC, Maier RV, Jimenez M *et al.* Source control in the management of severe sepsis and septic shock: an evidence-based review. *Crit Care Med* 2004; **32** (Suppl.): S513–26.
45. Rivers E, Nguyen B, Havstad S *et al.* Early goal-directed therapy in the treatment of severe sepsis and septic shock. *N Engl J Med* 2001; **345**: 1368–77.
46. Eichacker PQ, Natanson C, Danner RL. Surviving sepsis – practice guidelines, marketing campaigns, and Eli Lilly. *N Engl J Med* 2006; **355**: 1640–2.
47. Poulton B. Advances in the management of sepsis: the randomised controlled trials behind the Surviving Sepsis Campaign recommendations. *Int J Antimicrob Agents* 2006; **27**: 97–101.
48. Bunt TJ. Non-directed relaparotomy for intra-abdominal sepsis. A futile procedure. *Am Surg* 1986; **52**: 294–8.
49. Wong PF, Gilliam AD, Kumar S *et al.* Antibiotic regimens for secondary peritonitis of gastrointestinal origin in adults. *Cochrane Database Syst Rev* 2005; **2**: CD004539.
50. Brook I, Frazier EH. Microbiology of subphrenic abscesses: a 14-year experience. *Am Surg* 1999; **65**: 1049–53.
51. Kalliafas S, Ziegler DW, Flancbaum L *et al.* Acute acalculous cholecystitis: incidence, risk factors, diagnosis, and outcome. *Am Surg* 1998; **64**: 471–5.
52. Shapiro MJ, Luchtefeld WB, Kurzweil S *et al.* Acute acalculous cholecystitis in the critically ill. *Am Surg* 1994; **60**: 335–9.
53. Sheth SG, LaMont JT. Toxic megacolon. *Lancet* 1998; **351**: 509–13.
54. Ausch C, Madoff RD, Gnant M *et al.* Aetiology and surgical management of toxic megacolon. *Colorectal Dis* 2006; **8**: 195–201.
55. Sort P, Navasa M, Arroyo V *et al.* Effect of intravenous albumin on renal impairment and mortality in patients with cirrhosis and spontaneous bacterial peritonitis. *N Engl J Med* 1999; **341**: 403–9.
56. Carmeci C, Muldowney W, Mazbar SA *et al.* Emergency laparotomy in patients on continuous ambulatory peritoneal dialysis. *Am Surg* 2001; **67**: 615–18.
57. Marshall JC, Innes M. Intensive care unit management of intra-abdominal infection. *Crit Care Med* 2003; **31**: 2228–37.
58. British Society for Antimicrobial Chemotherapy Working Party. Management of deep *Candida* infection in surgical and intensive care unit patients. *Intens Care Med* 1994; **20**: 522–8.
59. Malbrain ML, Cheatham ML, Kirkpatrick A *et al.* Results from the International Conference of Experts on Intra-abdominal Hypertension and Abdominal Compartment Syndrome. I. Definitions. *Intens Care Med* 2006; **32**: 1722–32.
60. Cheatham ML, Malbrain ML, Kirkpatrick A *et al.* Results from the International Conference of Experts on Intra-abdominal Hypertension and Abdominal Compartment Syndrome. II. Recommendations. *Intens Care Med* 2007; **33**: 951–62.
61. Hill GL. *Disorders of Nutrition and Metabolism in Clinical Surgery – Understanding and Management.* Edinburgh: Churchill Livingstone, 1992.
62. Li-Ling J, Irving M. Somatostatin and octreotide in the prevention of postoperative pancreatic complications and the treatment of enterocutaneous pancreatic fistulas: a systematic review of randomized controlled trials. *Br J Surg* 2001; **88**: 190–9.
63. Present DH, Rutgeerts P, Targan S *et al.* Infliximab for the treatment of fistulas in patients with Crohn's disease. *N Engl J Med* 1999; **340**: 1398–405.
64. Ponec RJ, Saunders MD, Kimmey MB. Neostigmine for the treatment of acute colonic pseudo-obstruction. *N Engl J Med* 1999; **341**: 137–41.
65. Saunders MD, Kimmey MB. Systematic review: acute colonic pseudo-obstruction. *Aliment Pharmacol Ther* 2005; **22**: 917–25.

Part Six

Acute Renal Failure

40

Acute renal failure

Rinaldo Bellomo

Acute renal failure (ARF) remains a major diagnostic and therapeutic challenge for the critical care physician. The term 'ARF' describes a syndrome characterised by a rapid (hours to days) decrease in the kidney's ability to eliminate waste products. Such loss of function is clinically manifested by the accumulation of end-products of nitrogen metabolism such as urea and creatinine. Other typical clinical manifestations include decreased urine output (not always present), accumulation of non-volatile acids and an increased potassium and phosphate concentration.

Depending on the criteria used to define its presence, ARF has been reported to occur in 15–20% of intensive care unit (ICU) patients.[1] Recently a consensus definition and classification for ARF have been developed and validated in hospital and ICU patients.[2–4] This definition, which goes by the acronym of RIFLE, divides renal dysfunction into the categories of risk, injury and failure (Figure 40.1) and is likely to be the dominant approach to defining ARF in ICUs for the next 5–10 years. Using this classification, the incidence of some degree of renal dysfunction has reported to be up to 67% in a recent study of > 5000 ICU patients.[3] In hospital patients, the development of failure (in the RIFLE classification) increases the odds ratio of death 10 times.[4]

ASSESSMENT OF RENAL FUNCTION

Renal function is complex (control of calcium and phosphate, acid–base balance, water balance, tonicity, erythropoiesis, disposal of some cytokines, lactate removal). In the clinical context, however, monitoring of renal function is reduced to the indirect assessment of glomerular filtration rate (GFR) by the measurement of urea and creatinine in blood. These waste products are insensitive markers of GFR and are heavily modified by nutrition, the use of steroids, the presence of gastrointestinal blood, muscle mass, age, gender or muscle injury. Furthermore, they start becoming abnormal only when more than 50% of GFR is lost, they do not reflect dynamic changes in GFR and are grossly modified by aggressive fluid resuscitation. The use of creatinine clearance (2- or 4-hour collections) or of calculated clearance by means of formulae might increase the accuracy of GFR estimation, but rarely changes clinical management. The use of more sophisticated radionuclide-based tests is cumbersome in the ICU and only useful for research purposes.

DIAGNOSIS AND CLINICAL CLASSIFICATION

The most practically useful approach to the aetiological diagnosis of ARF is to divide its causes according to the probable source of renal injury: prerenal, renal (parenchymal) and postrenal.

PRERENAL RENAL FAILURE

This form of ARF is by far the most common in ICU. The term indicates that the kidney malfunctions predominantly because of systemic factors, which decrease GFR. For example, GFR may be decreased if renal blood flow is diminished by decreased cardiac output, hypotension or raised intra-abdominal pressure. Raised intra-abdominal pressure can be suspected on clinical grounds and confirmed by measuring bladder pressure with a urinary catheter. A pressure of > 25–30 mmHg above the pubis should prompt consideration of decompression. If the systemic cause of renal failure is rapidly removed or corrected, renal function improves and relatively rapidly returns to near-normal levels. However, if intervention is delayed or unsuccessful, renal injury becomes established and several days or weeks are then necessary for recovery. Several tests (measurement of urinary sodium, fractional excretion of sodium and other derived indices) have been promoted to help clinicians identify the development of such 'established' ARF. Unfortunately, their accuracy is doubtful.[5] The clinical utility of these tests in ICU patients who receive vasopressors, massive fluid resuscitation and loop diuretic infusions is low. Furthermore, it is important to observe that prerenal ARF and established ARF are part of a continuum, and their separation has limited clinical implications. The treatment is the same – treatment of the cause while promptly resuscitating the patient using invasive haemodynamic monitoring to guide therapy.

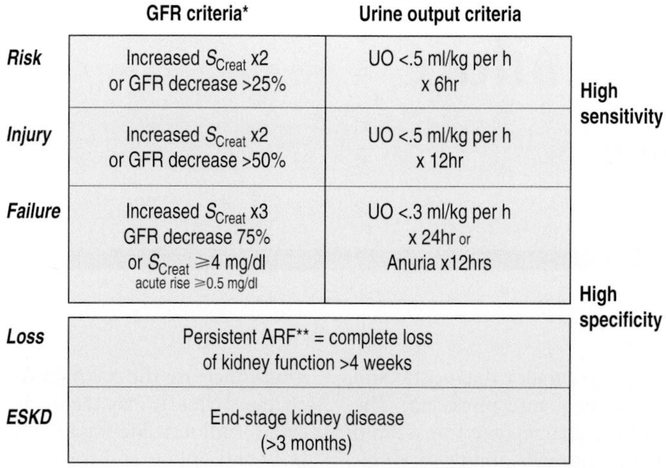

Figure 40.1 RIFLE (risk injury failure loss end-stage) classification scheme for acute renal failure. The classification system includes separate criteria for creatinine and urine output. The criteria, which lead to the worst possible classification, should be used. Note that RIFLE-F (F = failure) is present even if the increase in serum creatinine concentration (S_{Creat}) is less than threefold as long as the new S_{Creat} > 4.0 mg/dl (350 μmol/l) in the setting of an acute increase of at least 0.5 mg/dl (44 μmol/l). The designation RIFLE-F_C should be used in this case to denote 'acute-on-chronic' disease. Similarly, when RIFLE-F classification is reached by urine output criteria only, a designation of RIFLE-F_O should be used to denote oliguria. The shape of the figure denotes the fact that more patients (high sensitivity) will be included in the mild category, including some who do not actually have 'renal failure' (less specificity). In contrast, at the bottom, the criteria are strict and therefore specific, but some patients with renal dysfunction might be missed. GFR, glomerular filtration rate; ARF, acute renal failure; UO, urine output.

PARENCHYMAL RENAL FAILURE

This term is used to define a syndrome where the principal source of damage is within the kidney and where typical structural changes can be seen on microscopy. Disorders which affect the glomerulus or the tubule can be responsible (Table 40.1).

Among these, nephrotoxins are particularly important, especially in hospital patients. The most common nephrotoxic drugs affecting ICU patients are listed in Table 40.2. Many cases of drug-induced ARF rapidly improve upon removal of the offending agent. Accordingly, a careful history of drug administration is *mandatory* in all patients with ARF. In some cases of parenchymal ARF, a correct working diagnosis can be obtained from history, physical examination and radiological and laboratory investigations. In such patients one can proceed to a therapeutic trial without the need to resort to renal biopsy. However, if immunosuppressive therapy is considered, renal biopsy is recommended. Renal biopsy in ventilated patients under ultrasound guidance does not carry additional risks compared to standard conditions.

More than a third of patients who develop ARF in ICU have chronic renal dysfunction due to factors such as age-related changes, long-standing hypertension, diabetes or atheromatous disease of the renal vessels. Such chronic renal dysfunction may be manifest by a raised serum creatinine. However, this is not always the case. Often, what may seem to the clinician to be a relatively trivial insult, which does not fully explain the onset of ARF in a normal patient, is sufficient to unmask lack of renal functional reserve in another.

Table 40.1 Causes of parenchymal acute renal failure

Glomerulonephritis
Vasculitis
Interstitial nephritis
Malignant hypertension
Pyelonephritis
Bilateral cortical necrosis
Amyloidosis
Malignancy
Nephrotoxins

Table 40.2 Drugs which may cause acute renal failure in the intensive care unit

Radiocontrast agents
Aminoglycosides
Amphotericin
Non-steroidal anti-inflammatory drugs
β-lactam antibiotics (interstitial nephropathy)
Sulphonamides
Acyclovir
Methotrexate
Cisplatin
Cyclosporin A
FK-506 (tacrolimus)

HEPATORENAL SYNDROME

This condition is a form of ARF, which occurs in the setting of severe liver dysfunction in the absence of other known causes of ARF. Typically, it presents as progressive oliguria with a very low urinary sodium concentration (< 10 mmol/l). Its pathogenesis is not well understood. It is important to note, however, that, in patients with severe liver disease, other causes of ARF are much more common. They include sepsis, paracentesis-induced hypovolaemia, raised intra-abdominal pressure due to tense ascites, diuretic-induced hypovolaemia, lactulose-induced hypovolaemia, alcoholic cardiomyopathy, and any combination of these. The avoidance of hypovolaemia by albumin administration in patients with spontaneous bacterial peritonitis has been shown to decrease the incidence of renal failure in a recent randomised controlled trial (RCT).[6] These causes must be looked for and promptly treated. Recent small studies suggest that a vasopressin derivative called terlipressin may improve GFR in this condition.[7]

RHABDOMYOLYSIS-ASSOCIATED ARF

This condition accounts for close to 5–10%[8] of cases of ARF in ICU depending on the setting. Its pathogenesis involves prerenal, renal and postrenal factors. It is now typically seen following major trauma, drug overdose with narcotics, vascular embolism, and in response to a variety of agents which can induce major muscle injury. The principles of treatment are based on retrospective data, small series and multivariate logistic regression analysis, because no RCTs have been conducted. They include prompt and aggressive fluid resuscitation, elimination of causative agents, correction of compartment syndromes, the alkalinisation of urine (pH > 6.5) and the maintenance of polyuria (> 300 ml/h). The role of mannitol is controversial.

POSTRENAL RENAL FAILURE

Obstruction to urine outflow is the most common cause of functional renal impairment in the community,[9] but is uncommon in the ICU. Typical causes of obstructive ARF include bladder neck obstruction from an enlarged prostate, ureteric obstruction from pelvic tumours or retroperitoneal fibrosis, papillary necrosis or large calculi. The clinical presentation of obstruction may be acute or acute-on-chronic in patients with long-standing renal calculi. It may not always be associated with oliguria. If obstruction is suspected, ultrasonography can be easily performed at the bedside. However, not all cases of acute obstruction have an abnormal ultrasound and, in many cases, obstruction occurs in conjunction with other renal insults (e.g. staghorn calculi and severe sepsis of renal origin). Assessment of the role of each factor and overall management should be conducted in conjunction with a urologist. Finally the sudden and unexpected development of anuria in an ICU patient should always suggest obstruction of the urinary catheter as the cause. Appropriate flushing or changing of the catheter should be implemented in this setting.

PATHOGENESIS OF ACUTE RENAL FAILURE

The pathogenesis of obstructive ARF involves several humoral responses as well as mechanical factors. The pathogenesis of parenchymal renal failure is typically immunological. It varies from vasculitis to interstitial nephropathy and involves an extraordinary complexity of immunological mechanisms. The pathogenesis of prerenal ARF is of greater direct relevance to the intensivist. Several mechanisms have been reported to play a major role in the development of renal injury:

1. ischaemia of outer medulla with activation of the tubuloglomerular feedback[10]
2. tubular obstruction from casts of exfoliated cells[11]
3. interstitial oedema secondary to back-diffusion of fluid[11]
4. humorally mediated afferent arteriolar renal vasconstriction[11]
5. inflammatory response to cell injury and local release of mediators[11]
6. disruption of normal cellular adhesion to the basement membrane[11]
7. radical oxygen species-induced apoptosis[11]
8. phospholipase A_2-induced cell membrane injury[12]
9. mitogen-activated protein kinase-induced renal injury[13]

In septic patients with hyperdynamic circulations, ARF may occur in the setting of increased renal blood flow, with the loss of GFR being secondary to decreased intraglomerular pressure induced by efferent arteriolar vasodilatation.[14]

No studies exist to tell us which of the above mechanism/s are pathogenetically most important in ICU patients with or without sepsis and when they might be active in the course of a patient's illness.

THE CLINICAL PICTURE

The most common clinical picture seen in ICU is that of a patient who has sustained or is experiencing a major systemic insult (trauma, sepsis, myocardial infarction, severe haemorrhage, cardiogenic shock, major surgery and the like). When the patient arrives in the ICU, resuscitation is typically well under way or surgery may have just been completed. Despite such efforts, the patient is already anuric or profoundly oliguric, the serum creatinine is rising and a metabolic acidosis is developing. Potassium and phosphate levels may be rapidly rising as well. Accompanying multiple-organ dysfunction (mechanical ventilation and need for vasoactive drugs) is common. Fluid resuscitation is typically undertaken in the ICU under the guidance of invasive hemodynamic monitoring.

Vasoactive drugs are often used to restore mean arterial pressure (MAP) to 'acceptable' levels (typically > 65–70 mmHg). The patient may improve over time and urine output may return with or without the assistance of diuretic agents. If urine output does not return, however, renal replacement therapy needs to be considered.

If the cause of ARF has been removed, and the patient has become physiologically stable, slow recovery occurs (from 4–5 days to 3–4 weeks). In some cases, urine output can be above normal for several days. If the cause of ARF has not been adequately remedied, the patient remains gravely ill, the kidneys do not recover and death from multiorgan failure may occur.

PREVENTING ACUTE RENAL FAILURE

The fundamental principle of ARF prevention is to treat its cause. If prerenal factors contribute, these must be identified and haemodynamic resuscitation quickly instituted.

RESUSCITATION

Intravascular volume must be maintained or rapidly restored, and this is often best done using invasive hemodynamic monitoring (central venous catheter, arterial cannula and pulmonary artery catheter or pulse contour cardiac output catheters in some cases). Oxygenation must be maintained. An adequate haemoglobin concentration (at least > 70 g/l) must be maintained or immediately restored. Once intravascular volume has been restored, some patients remain hypotensive (MAP < 70 mmHg). In these patients, autoregulation of renal blood flow may be lost. Restoration of MAP to near-normal levels may increase GFR.[15,16] Such elevations in MAP, however, require the addition of vasopressor drugs.[15,16] In patients with hypertension or renovascular disease, a MAP of 75–80 mmHg may still be inadequate. The nephroprotective role of additional fluid therapy in a patient with a normal or increased cardiac output and blood pressure is questionable. Despite these resuscitation measures renal failure may still develop if cardiac output is inadequate. This may require a variety of interventions from the use of inotropic drugs to the application of ventricular assist devices.

NEPHROPROTECTIVE DRUGS

Following haemodynamic resuscitation and removal of nephrotoxins, it is unclear whether the use of additional pharmacological measures is of further benefit to the kidneys.

'RENAL DOSE' OR 'LOW-DOSE' DOPAMINE

Evidence of the efficacy or safety of its administration in critically ill patients is lacking. However, this agent is a tubular diuretic and occasionally increases urine output. This may be incorrectly interpreted as an increase in GFR. Furthermore, a recent large phase III trial in critically ill patients showed low-dose dopamine to be as effective as placebo in the prevention of renal dysfunction.[17]

MANNITOL

A biological rationale exists for the use of mannitol, as is the case for dopamine. However, no controlled human data exist to support its clinical use. The effect of mannitol as a renal-protective agent remains questionable.

LOOP DIURETICS

These agents may protect the loop of Henle from ischaemia by decreasing its transport-related workload. Animal data are encouraging, as are ex-vivo experiments. There are no double-blind RCTs of suitable size to prove that these agents reduce the incidence of renal failure. However, there are some studies which support the view that loop diuretics may decrease the need for dialysis in patients with developing ARF.[18] They appear to achieve this by inducing polyuria, which results in the prevention or easier control of volume overload, acidosis and hyperkalaemia, the three major triggers for renal replacement therapy in the ICU. Because avoiding dialysis simplifies treatment and reduces cost of care, loop diuretics are occasionally used in patients with renal dysfunction, especially in the form of continuous infusion.

OTHER AGENTS

Other agents, such as *theophylline*, *urodilatin* and *anaritide* (a synthetic atrial natriuretic factor), have also been proposed. Studies so far, however, have been experimental, too small or have shown no beneficial effect. In a randomised double-blind, placebo-controlled trial, *fenoldopam* has been shown to attenuate the deterioration in serum creatinine typically seen in septic patients.[19] Studies of this agent in other situations, however, have failed to show a benefit.[20] Its role in ARF remains uncertain. Similarly, in a single-centre study, rhANF has been shown to attenuate renal injury in higher-risk patients having cardiac surgery[21] but a large multicentre study of ARF failed to show a benefit.[22] Many more investigations are needed in this field.

RADIOCONTRAST NEPHROPATHY

In patients receiving radiocontrast an RCT suggested that saline infusion to maintain intravascular fluid expansion is superior to the addition of mannitol or furosemide. Several RCTs of similar patients demonstrated a beneficial effect of *N-acetylcysteine* treatment before and after radiocontrast administration, as confirmed in a recent meta-analysis.[23] Since these preventive interventions have minimal toxicity, they should be considered whenever a patient is scheduled for the administration of intravenous radiocontrast. Their effectiveness in ICU patients who have already been fluid-resuscitated remains unknown.

DIAGNOSTIC INVESTIGATIONS

An aetiological diagnosis of ARF must always be established. Such diagnosis may be obvious on clinical grounds. However, in many patients, it is best to consider all possibilities and exclude common treatable causes by simple investigations. Such investigations include the examination of urinary sediment and exclusion of a urinary tract infection (in most, if not all, patients), the exclusion of obstruction when appropriate (some patients) and the careful exclusion of nephrotoxins (all patients).

In specific situations, other investigations are necessary to establish the diagnosis, such as creatine kinase and free myoglobin for possible rhabdomyolysis. A chest radiograph, a blood film, the measurement of non-specific inflammatory markers and the measurement of specific antibodies (antiglomerular basement membrane, antineutrophil cytoplasm, anti-DNA, antismooth-muscle) are useful screening tests to help support the diagnosis of vasculitis or of certain types of collagen disease or glomerulonephritis. If thrombotic thrombocytopenic purpura is suspected, the additional measurement of lactic dehydrogenase, haptoglobin, unconjugated bilirubin and free haemoglobin is needed. In some patients, specific findings (cryoglobulins, Bence Jones proteins) are almost diagnostic. In a few rare patients, the clinical picture, laboratory investigations and radiological investigations are not sufficient to make a causative diagnosis with sufficient certainty. In such patients a renal biopsy might become necessary.

MANAGEMENT OF ESTABLISHED ACUTE RENAL FAILURE

The principles of management of established ARF are the treatment or removal of its cause and the maintenance of physiological homeostasis while recovery takes place. Complications such as encephalopathy, pericarditis, myopathy, neuropathy, electrolyte disturbances or other major electrolyte, fluid or metabolic derangement should never occur in a modern ICU. Their prevention may include several measures, which vary in complexity from fluid restriction to the initiation of extracorporeal renal replacement therapy.

Nutritional support must be started early and must contain adequate calories (30–35 kcal/kg per day) as a mixture of carbohydrates and lipids. Adequate protein (at least 1–2 g/kg per day) must be administered. There is no evidence that specific renal nutritional solutions are useful. Vitamins and trace elements should be administered at least according to their recommended daily allowance. The role of newer immunonutritional solution remains controversial. The enteral route is preferred to the use of parenteral nutrition.

Hyperkalaemia (> 6 mmol/l) must be promptly treated with insulin and dextrose administration, the infusion of bicarbonate if acidosis is present, the administration of nebulised salbutamol, or all of the above together. If the 'true' serum potassium is > 7 mmol/l or electrocardiographic signs of hyperkalaemia appear, calcium chloride (10 ml of 10% solution intravenously) should also be administered. The above measures are temporising actions while renal replacement therapy is being set up. The presence of hyperkalaemia is a major indication for the immediate institution of renal replacement therapy.

Metabolic acidosis is almost always present but rarely requires treatment per se. Anaemia requires correction to maintain a haemoglobin of at least > 70 g/l. More aggressive transfusion needs individual patient assessment.[24] Drug therapy must be adjusted to take into account the effect of the decreased clearances associated with loss of renal function. Stress ulcer prophylaxis is advisable and should be based on H_2-receptor antagonists or proton pump inhibitors in selected cases. Assiduous attention should be paid to the prevention of infection.

Fluid overload can be prevented by the use of loop diuretics in polyuric patients. However, if the patient is oliguric, the only way to avoid fluid overload is to institute renal replacement therapy at an early stage (see Chapter 41). Marked azotaemia ([urea] > 40 mmol/l or [creatinine] > 400 μmol/l) is undesirable and should probably be treated with renal replacement therapy unless recovery is imminent or already under way and a return toward normal values is expected within 24–48 hours. It is recognized, however, that no RCTs exist to define the ideal time for intervention with artificial renal support.

PROGNOSIS

The mortality of critically ill patients with ARF remains high (40–80% depending on case-mix). It is frequently stated that patients die *with* renal failure rather than *of* renal failure. However, growing evidence suggests that better uraemic control and more intensive artificial renal support may improve survival by perhaps 30%.[25,26] Such evidence supports a careful and proactive approach to the treatment of patients with ARF, which is based on the prevention of uncontrolled uraemia and the maintenance of low urea levels throughout the patient's illness.

REFERENCES

1. Chew SL, Lins RL, Daelemans R *et al.* Outcome in acute renal failure. *Nephrol Dial Transplant* 1993; **8**: 101–7.
2. Bellomo R, Ronco C, Kellum JA *et al.* Acute renal failure – definition, outcome measures, animal models, fluid therapy and information technology needs: the Second International Consensus Conference of the Acute Dialysis Quality Initiative (ADQI) Group. *Crit Care* 2004; **8**: R204–10.

3. Hoste EAJ, Clermont G, Kersten A *et al.* RIFLE criteria for acute kidney injury are associated with hospital mortality in critically ill patients: a cohort analysis. *Crit Care* 2006; **10**: R73–83.
4. Uchino S, Bellomo R, Goldsmith D *et al.* An assessment of the RIFLE criteria for acute renal failure in hospitalized patients. *Crit Care Med* 2006; **34**: 1913–17.
5. Langenberg C, Wan L, Bagshaw SM *et al.* Urinary biochemistry in experimental septic acute renal failure. *Nephrol Dial Transplant* 2006; **21**: 3389–97.
6. Sort P, Navasa M, Arroyo V *et al.* Effect of intravenous albumin on renal impariment and mortality in patients with cirrhosis and spontaneous bacterial peritonitis. *N Engl J Med* 1999; **341**: 403–9.
7. Fabrizi F, Dixit V, Martin P. Meta-analysis: terlipressin therapy for the hepatorenal syndrome. *Aliment Pharmacol Ther* 2006; **24**: 935–44.
8. Uchino S, Kellum J, Bellomo R *et al.* Acute renal failure in critically ill patients – a multinational, multicenter study. *JAMA* 2005; **294**: 813–18.
9. Feest TG, Round A, Hamad S. Incidence of severe acute renal failure in adults: results of a community-based study. *Br Med J* 1993; **306**: 481–3.
10. Brezis M, Rosen SN, Silva P *et al.* Selective vulnerability of the medullary thick ascending limb to anoxia in the isolated perfused rat kidney. *J Clin Invest* 1984; **73**: 182–90.
11. Bonventre JV. Mechanisms of ischemic acute renal failure. *Kidney Int* 1993; **43**: 1160–78.
12. Portilla D, Mandel LJ, Bar-Sagi D *et al.* Anoxia induces phospholipase A_2 activation in rabbit renal proximal tubules. *Am J Physiol* 1992; **262**: F354–60.
13. Di Mari JF, Davis R, Safirstein RL. MAPK activation determines renal epithelial cell survival during oxidative injury. *Am J Physiol* 1999; **277**: F195–203.
14. Langenberg C, Wan L, Egi M *et al.* Renal blood flow in experimental septic acute renal failure. *Kidney Int* 2006; **69**: 1996–2002.
15. Bellomo R, Kellum JA, Wisniewski SR *et al.* Effects of norepinephrine on the renal vasculature in normal and endotoxemic dogs. *Am J Respir Crit Care Med* 1999; **159**: 1186–92.
16. Bersten AD, Holt AW. Vasoactive drugs and the importance of renal perfusion pressure. *N Horizons* 1995; **3**: 650–61.
17. ANZICS Clinical Trials Group. Low-dose dopamine in patients with early renal dysfunction: a placebo-controlled randomised trial. *Lancet* 2000; **356**: 2139–43.
18. Majumdar S, Kjellstrand CM. Why do we use diuretics in acute renal failure? *Semin Dialysis* 1996; **9**: 454–9.
19. Morelli A, Ricci Z, Bellomo R *et al.* Prophylactic fenoldopam for renal protection in sepsis: a randomized double-blind, placebo-controlled trial. *Crit Care Med* 2005; **33**: 2451–6.
20. Bove T, Landoni G, Calabro MG *et al.* Renoprotective action of fenoldopam in high-risk patients undergoing cardiac surgery: a prospective double-blind randomized clinical trial. *Circulation* 2005; **111**: 3230–5.
21. Sward K, Valsson F, Odencrants P *et al.* Recombinant human atrial natriuretic peptide in ischemic acute renal failure: a randomized placebo-controlled trial. *Crit Care Med* 2004; **32**: 1310–15.
22. Chertow GM, Lazarus JM, Paganini EP *et al.* Predictors of mortality and the provision of dialysis in patients with acute tubular necrosis: the Auriculin Anaritide Acute Renal Failure Study Group. *J Am Soc Nephrol* 1998; **9**: 692–8.
23. Birck R, Krzossok S, Markowetz F *et al.* Acetylcysteine for prevention of contrast nephropathy. *Lancet* 2003; **362**: 598–603.
24. Hebert P, Wells G, Blajchman MA *et al.* A multicenter randmized controlled clinical trial of transfusion requirements in critical care. *N Engl J Med* 1999; **340**: 409–17.
25. Saudan P, Niederberger M, De Seigneux S *et al.* Adding dialysis dose to continuous hemofiltration increases survival in patients with acute renal failure. *Kidney Int* 2006; **70**: 1312–17.
26. Ronco C, Bellomo R, Homel P *et al.* Effects of different doses in continuous veno-venous haemofiltration on outcomes of acute renal failure: a prospective randomized trial. *Lancet* 2000; **355**: 26–30.

41

Renal replacement therapy

Rinaldo Bellomo

When acute renal failure (ARF) is severe, resolution can take several days or weeks. During this time, the kidneys cannot maintain homeostasis of fluid, potassium, metabolic acid and waste products. Life-threatening complications frequently develop. In these patients, extracorporeal techniques of blood purification must be applied to prevent such complications. Such techniques, broadly named renal replacement therapy (RRT), include continuous haemofiltration (HF), intermittent haemodialysis (IHD) and peritoneal dialysis (PD), each with its technical variations. All of these techniques rely on the principle of removing unwanted solutes and water through a semipermeable membrane. Such membrane is either biological (peritoneum) or artificial (haemodialysis or HF membranes), and each offers several advantages, disadvantages and limitations.

PRINCIPLES

The principles of RRT have been extensively studied and described.[1–3] This is a summary of some aspects which are relevant to the critical care physician.

WATER REMOVAL

The removal of unwanted solvent (water) is therapeutically as important as the removal of unwanted solute (acid, uraemic toxins, potassium and the like). During RRT, water is removed through a process called ultrafiltration. This process is essentially the same as that performed by the glomerulus; it requires a driving pressure to move fluid across a semipermeable membrane. This pressure is achieved by:

1. generating a transmembrane pressure (as in HF or during IHD) which is greater than oncotic pressure
2. increasing osmolarity of the dialysate (as in PD)

SOLUTE REMOVAL

The removal of unwanted solute can be achieved by:

1. creating an electrochemical gradient across the membrane using a flow-past system with toxin-free dialysate (diffusion), as in IHD and PD
2. creating a transmembrane pressure-driven 'solvent drag', where solute moves together with solvent (convection) across a porous membrane, is discarded and then replaced with toxin-free replacement fluid, as in HF

The rate of diffusion of a given solute depends on its molecular weight, the porosity of the membrane, the blood flow rate, the dialysate flow rate, the degree of protein binding and its concentration gradient across the membrane. If standard, low-flux, cellulose-based membranes are used, middle molecules of >500 daltons (D) molecular weight (MW) cannot be removed. If synthetic high-flux membranes are used (cut-off at 10–20 kiloDaltons (kD) in MW), larger molecules can be removed. With these membranes convection is superior to diffusion in achieving the clearance of middle molecules.

INDICATIONS FOR RENAL REPLACEMENT THERAPY

In the critically ill patient, RRT should be initiated early, prior to the development of complications. Fear of early dialysis stems from the adverse effects of conventional IHD with cuprophane membranes, especially haemodynamic instability, and from the risks and limitations of continuous or intermittent PD.[4–5] However, continuous RRT (CRRT)[6,7] or slow low-efficiency daily dialysis (SLEDD)[8] minimises these effects. The criteria for the initiation of RRT in patients with chronic renal failure may be inappropriate in the critically ill.[9,10] A set of modern criteria for the initiation of RRT in the intensive care unit (ICU) is presented in Table 41.1.

With IHD, CRRT or SLEDD there are limited data on what is 'adequate' intensity of dialysis. However, this concept should include maintenance of homeostasis at all levels,[10] and better uraemic control may translate into better survival.[11,12] An appropriate target urea might be 15–25 mmol/l, with a protein intake around 1.5 g/kg per day. This can be easily achieved using CRRT at urea clearances of 35–45 l/day depending on patient size and catabolic rate. If intermittent therapy is used, daily and extended treatment as described with SLEDD becomes desirable.[13]

Table 41.1 Modern criteria for the initiation of renal replacement therapy (RRT) in the intensive care unit*

Oliguria (urine output < 200 ml/12 h)
Anuria (urine output: 0–50 ml/12 h)
[Urea] > 35 mmol/l
[Creatinine] > 400 μmol/l
[K^+] > 6.5 mmol/l or rapidly rising†
Pulmonary oedema unresponsive to diuretics
Uncompensated metabolic acidosis (pH < 7.1)
[Na^+] < 110 and > 160 mmol/l
Temperature > 40°C
Uraemic complications (encephalopathy/myopathy/neuropathy/pericarditis)
Overdose with a dialysable toxin (e.g. lithium)

*If one criterion is present, RRT should be considered. If two criteria are simultaneously present, RRT is strongly recommended.
†Please be aware of differences between plasma versus serum measurement in your laboratory.

MODE OF RENAL REPLACEMENT THERAPY

There is a great deal of controversy as to which mode of RRT is 'best' in the ICU, due to the lack of randomised controlled trials comparing different techniques. In their absence, techniques of RRT may be judged on the basis of the following criteria:

1. haemodynamic side-effects
2. ability to control fluid status
3. biocompatibility
4. risk of infection
5. uraemic control
6. avoidance of cerebral oedema
7. ability to allow full nutritional support
8. ability to control acidosis
9. absence of specific side-effects
10. cost

CRRT and SLEDD offer many advantages over PD and conventional IHD (3–4 h/day, 3–4 times/week),[13] and whereas CRRT is almost exclusively used in some centres,[14] only a minority of American ICU patients receive CRRT. Some salient aspects of CRRT, IHD and PD require discussion.

CONTINUOUS RENAL REPLACEMENT THERAPY

First described in 1977, CRRT has undergone several technical modifications. Initially, it was performed as an arteriovenous therapy (continuous arteriovenous HF: CAVH). The need to cannulate an artery, however, is associated with 15–20% morbidity. Accordingly, double-lumen catheters and peristaltic blood pumps have come into use (continuous venovenous HF: CVVH) with or without control of ultrafiltration rate. Ultrafiltration rates of 2 l/h yield urea clearances >30 ml/min. Diagrams illustrating typical HF circuits are presented in Figures 41.1–41.3.

In a venovenous system, dialysate can also be delivered countercurrent to blood flow (continuous veno-venous haemodialysis/haemodiafiltration) to achieve either almost pure diffusive clearance or a mixture of diffusive and convective clearance.

No matter what technique is used, the following outcomes are predictable:

1. continuous control of fluid status
2. haemodynamic stability
3. control of acid–base status
4. ability to provide protein-rich nutrition while achieving uraemic control
5. control of electrolyte balance, including phosphate and calcium balance
6. prevention of swings in intracerebral water
7. minimal risk of infection
8. high level of biocompatibility

However, CRRT mandates the presence of specifically trained nursing and medical staff 24 hours a day. Small ICUs often cannot provide such level of support. If CRRT is only used 5–10 times a year, the cost of training may be unjustified and expertise may be hard to maintain. Furthermore, depending on the organisation of patient care, CRRT may be more expensive than IHD. Finally, the issues of continuous-circuit anticoagulation and the potential risk of bleeding have been a major concern.

DOSE OF CRRT AND CIRCUIT ANTICOAGULATION

The optimal dose (expressed as effective effluent per kilogram per hour) of CRRT remains unknown. Several studies suggest that higher dose may translate into better outcome.[12,15] However such studies have been single-centre in nature and require confirmation in multicentre randomised controlled trials. Such trials are now under way (see below).[16] It seems wise to wait for the results of larger studies before making any changes to the typical dose of approximately 25 ml/kg per hour currently delivered in Australia and New Zealand.

The flow of blood through an extracorporeal circuit causes activation of the coagulation cascade and promotes clotting of the filter and circuit itself. In order to delay such clotting and achieve acceptable operational lives (approximately 24 hours) for the circuit, anticoagulants are frequently used.[17] However, circuit anticoagulation increases risk of bleeding. Therefore, the risks and benefits of more or less intense anticoagulation and alternative strategies (Table 41.2) must be considered.

In the vast majority of patients, low-dose heparin (< 500 IU/h) is sufficient to achieve adequate filter life, is easy and cheap to administer and has almost no effect on the patient's coagulation tests. In some patients, a higher dose is necessary. In others (pulmonary embolism, myocardial ischaemia), full heparinisation may actually be concomitantly indicated. Regional citrate anticoagulation is very effective but requires a special dialysate or replacement fluid.[18] Regional heparin/protamine anticoagulation is also somewhat complex but may be useful if frequent filter clotting occurs and further anticoagulation

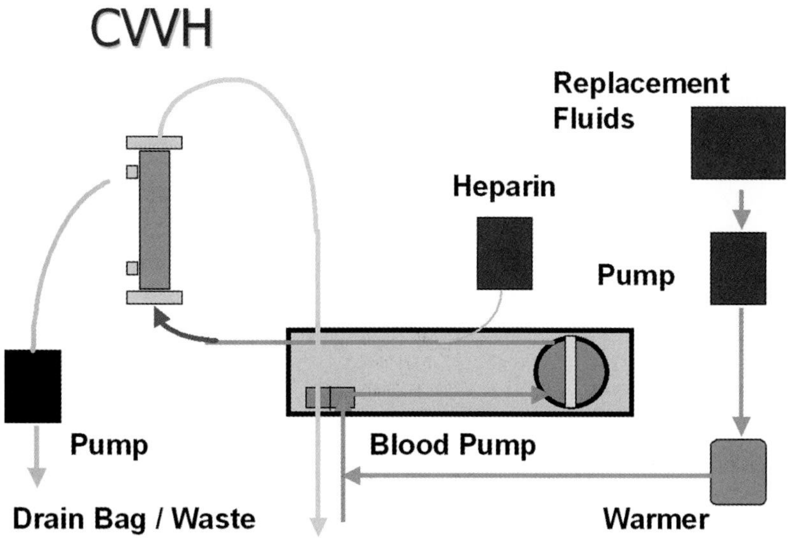

Figure 41.1 Diagrams illustrating a continuous venovenous haemofiltration circuit (CVVH).

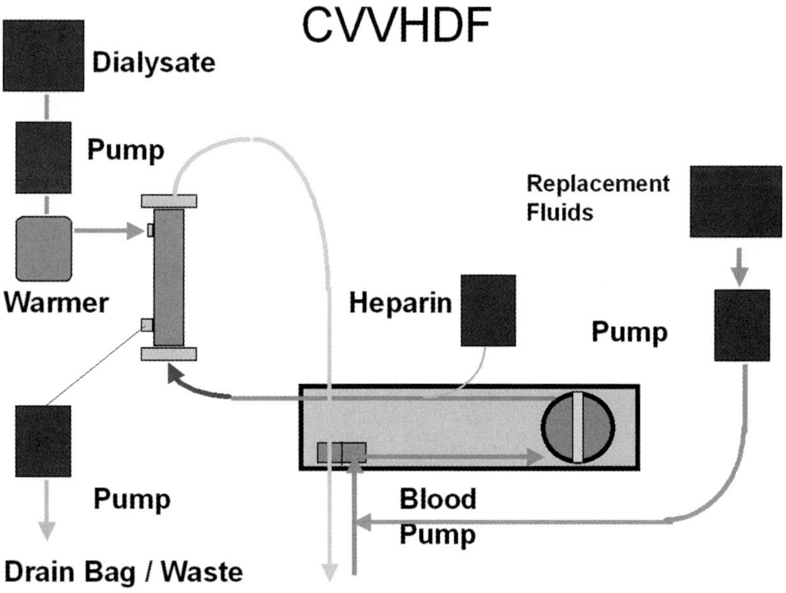

Figure 41.2 Diagrams illustrating a continuous venovenous haemodiafiltration circuit (CVVHDF).

of the patient is considered dangerous. Low-molecular-weight heparin is also easy to give but more expensive. Its dose must be adjusted for the loss of renal function. Heparinoids and prostacyclin may be useful if the patient has developed heparin-induced thrombocytopoenia and thrombosis. Finally, in perhaps 10–20% of patients anticoagulation is best avoided because of endogenous coagulopathy or recent surgery. In such patients adequate filter life can be achieved provided that blood flow is kept at about 200 ml/min and vascular access is reliable.[19]

Many circuits clot for mechanical reasons (inadequate access, unreliable blood low from double-lumen catheter depending on patient position, kinking of catheter). Responding to frequent filter clotting by simply increasing anticoagulation without making the correct aetiological diagnosis (checking catheter flow and position, taking a history surrounding the episode of clotting, identifying the site of clotting) is often futile and exposes the patient to unnecessary risk. Particular attention needs to be paid to the adequacy or ease of flow through the double-lumen catheter. Smaller (11.5 Fr) catheters in the subclavian position are a particular problem. Larger catheters (13.5 Fr) in the femoral position appear to function more reliably.

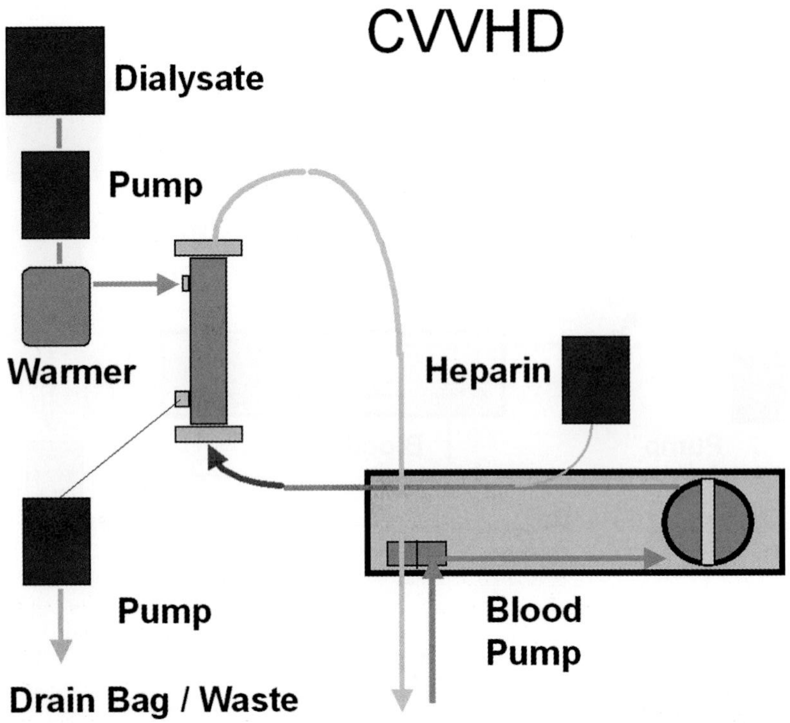

Figure 41.3 Diagram illustrating a continuous venovenous haemodialysis circuit (CVVHD).

Table 41.2 Strategies for circuit anticoagulation during continuous renal replacement therapy

No anticoagulation
Low-dose prefilter heparin (< 500 IU/h)
Medium-dose prefilter heparin (500–1000 IU/h)
Full heparinisation
Regional anticoagulation (prefilter heparin and postfilter protamine, usually at a 100 IU:1 mg ratio)
Regional citrate anticoagulation (prefilter citrate and postfilter calcium – special calcium-free dialysate needed)
Low-molecular-weight heparin
Prostacyclin
Heparinoids
Serine proteinase inhibitors (nafamostat mesylate)

CRRT TECHNOLOGY

The increasing use of venovenous CRRT has led to the development of a field of CRRT technology which offers different kinds of machines to facilitate its performance.[20] Some understanding of these devices is important to the successful implementation of CRRT in any ICU. One can a have simple blood pump with safety features (air bubble trap and pressure alarms) and use widely available volumetric pumps to control replacement or dialysate flow and effluent flow. Such adaptive technology is inexpensive, but is not user-friendly. Also, volumetric pumps have an inherent inaccuracy of about 5%, which, in a system exchanging up to 50 l/day, can cause problems. Various manufacturers have now produced custom-made machines for HF. These machines are safer and have much more sophisticated pump control systems, alarms and graphic displays. They are much more user-friendly, especially with the set-up procedure.

The choice of membrane is also a matter of controversy. There are no controlled studies to show that one confers a clinical advantage over the others. The AN 69 is the most commonly used CRRT membrane in Australia. The issue of membrane size is also controversial as no controlled studies have compared different membrane surface sizes. If high-volume haemofiltration is planned, however, the membrane surface needs to be in the 1.6–2 m^2 range.

INTERMITTENT HAEMODIALYSIS

Vascular access is typically by double-lumen catheter, as in continuous HF. The circuit is also the same. Countercurrent dialysate flow is used as in CVVHD. The major differences are that standard IHD uses high dialysate flows (300–400 ml/min), generates dialysate by mixing purified water and concentrate and treatment is applied for short periods of time (3–4 hours), usually every second day. These differences have important implications. Firstly, volume has to be removed over a short period of time and this may cause hypotension. Repeated hypotensive episodes may delay renal recovery.[4] Secondly, solute removal is episodic. This translates into inferior uraemic control[21] and acid–base control. Limited fluid and uraemic control imposes unnecessary limitations on nutritional support. Furthermore, rapid solute shifts increase brain water content and raise intracranial pressure.[22] Finally, much controversy has surrounded the issue of membrane bioincompatibility. Standard low-flux dialysing membranes made of cuprophane are known to trigger the activation of several inflammatory pathways, when compared to high-flux synthetic membranes (also used for continuous HF). It is possible that such proinflammatory effect contributes to further renal damage and delays recovery or even affects mortality. Given the minimal difference in cost between biocompatible and bioincompatible low-flux membranes, biocompatible membranes (polysulfone) are now preferred.

The limitations of applying 'standard' IHD to the treatment of ARF[9] has led to the development of new approaches (so-called 'hybrid techniques') such as SLEDD.[13] These techniques seek to adapt IHD to the clinical circumstances and thereby increase its tolerance and its clearances.

PERITONEAL DIALYSIS

This technique is now uncommonly used in the treatment of adult ARF in developed countries.[14] However, it may be an adequate technique in developing countries or in children where the peritoneal membrane has a greater relative surface or alternatives are considered too expensive, too invasive, or are not available. Typically access is by the insertion of an intraperitoneal catheter. Glucose-rich dialysate is then inserted into the peritoneal cavity and acts as the 'dialysate'. After a given 'dwell time' it is removed and discarded with the extra fluid and toxins that have moved from the blood vessels of the peritoneum to the dialysate fluid. Machines are also available which deliver and remove dialysate at higher flows, providing intermittent treatment or higher solute clearances. Several major shortcomings make PD relatively unsuited to the treatment of adult ARF:

1. limited and sometimes inadequate solute clearance
2. high risk of peritonitis
3. unpredictable hyperglycaemia
4. fluid leaks
5. protein loss
6. interference with diaphragm function

There have not been any reports of the sole use of PD for the treatment of adult patients with ARF in the last 15 years. A randomised trial comparing PD to CVVH found that PD was associated with increased mortality.[23]

OTHER BLOOD PURIFICATION TECHNIQUES

HAEMOPERFUSION

During haemoperfusion, blood is circulated through a circuit similar to one used for CVVH. However, a charcoal cartridge is perfused with blood instead of a dialysis membrane. In some cases an ion exchange resin (Amberlite) has been used. Charcoal microcapsules effectively remove molecules of 300–500 D MW, including some lipid-soluble and protein-bound substances. Heparinisation is necessary to prevent clotting. Attention must also be paid to changes in intravascular volume at the start of therapy because of the large priming volume of the cartridge (260 ml). Glucose absorption is significant and monitoring of blood glucose is necessary to avoid hypoglycaemia. Also thrombocytopenia is common, and can be marked. The role of haemoperfusion is controversial, as no controlled trials have ever shown it to confer clinically significant advantages. It may be useful, however, in patients with life-threatening theophylline overdose because it removes the agent effectively.

PLASMAPHERESIS OR PLASMA EXCHANGE

With this technique, plasma is removed from the patient and exchanged with fresh frozen plasma (FFP) and a mixture of colloid and crystalloid solutions. This technique can also be performed in an ICU familiar with CRRT techniques. A plasmafilter (a filter that allows the passage of molecules up to 500 kD) instead of a haemofilter is inserted in the CVVH circuit, and the filtrate (plasma) is discarded. Plasmapheresis can also be performed with special machines using the principles of centrifugation. The differences, if any, between centrifugation and filtration technology are unclear. Replacement (postfilter) will occur as in CVVH using, for example, a 50/50 combination of FFP and albumin. Plasmapheresis has been shown to be effective treatment for thrombotic thrombocytopenic purpura and for several diseases mediated by abnormal antibodies (Guillain–Barré syndrome, cryoglobulinaemia, myasthenia gravis, Goodpasture's syndrome) in which antibody removal appears desirable. Its role in the treatment of sepsis remains uncertain.[24]

BLOOD PURIFICATION TECHNOLOGY OUTSIDE ARF

There is growing interest in the possibility that blood purification may provide a clinically significant benefit in patients with severe sepsis/septic shock by removing circulating 'mediators'. A variety of techniques, including plasmapheresis, high-volume HF, very-high-volume HF, coupled plasma filtration adsorption[24–27] and large-pore HF,[27] are being studied in animals and in phase I/II studies in humans. Initial experiments support the need to continue exploring this therapeutic option. However, no suitably powered randomised controlled trials have yet been reported. Also, blood purification technology in combination with bioreactors containing either human or porcine liver cells is under active investigations as a form of artificial liver support for patients with fulminant liver failure or for patients with acute-on-chronic liver failure. Albumin-based dialysis has been developed to deal with protein-bound toxins in patients with liver failure.

Table 41.3 Drug dosage during dialytic therapy*

Drug	CRRT	IHD
Aminoglycosides	Normal dose q 36 h	50% normal dose q 48 h – 2/3 redose after IHD
Cefotaxime or ceftazidime	1 g q 8–12 h	1 g q 12–24 h after IHD
Imipenem	500 mg q 8 h	250 mg q 8 h and after IHD
Meropenem	500 mg q 8 h	250 mg q 8 h and after IHD
Metronidazole	500 mg q 8 h	250 mg q 8 h and after IHD
Co-trimoxazole	Normal dose q 18 h	Normal dose q 24 h after IHD
Amoxicillin	500 mg q 8 h	500 mg daily and after IHD
Vancomycin	1 g q 24 h	1 g q 96–120 h
Piperacillin	3–4 g q 6 h	3–4 g q 8 h and after IHD
Ticarcillin	1–2 g q 8 h	1–2 g q 12 h and after IHD
Ciprofloxacin	200 mg q 12 h	200 mg q 24 h and after IHD
Fluconazole	200 mg q 24 h	200 mg q 48 h and after IHD
Acyclovir	3.5 mg/kg q 24 h	2.5 mg/kg per day and after IHD
Gancyclovir	5 mg/kg per day	5 mg/kg per 48 h and after IHD
Amphotericin B	Normal dose	Normal dose
Liposomal amphotericin	Normal dose	Normal dose
Ceftriaxone	Normal dose	Normal dose
Erythomycin	Normal dose	Normal dose
Milrinone	Titrate to effect	Titrate to effect
Amrinone	Titrate to effect	Titrate to effect
Catecholamines	Titrate to effect	Titrate to effect
Ampicillin	500 mg q 8-hourly	500 mg daily and after IHD

CRRT, continuous renal replacement therapy; IHD, intermittent haemodialysis.
*The above values represent approximations and should be used as a general guide only. Critically ill patients have markedly abnormal volumes of distribution for these agents which will affect dosage. CRRT is conducted at variable levels of intensity in different units, also requiring adjustment. The values reported here relate to continuous venovenous haemofiltration at 2 l/h of ultrafiltration. Vancomycin is poorly removed by continuous venovenous haemofiltration. IHD may also differ from unit to unit. The values reported here relate to standard IHD with low-flux membranes for 3–4 hours every second day.

This system, known as MARS (molecular adsorption recirculating system), has shown benefits in patients with elevated intracranial pressure and/or acute-on-chronic liver failure, but not in patients with fulminant liver failure.[28]

DRUG PRESCRIPTION DURING DIALYTIC THERAPY

ARF and RRT profoundly affect drug clearance. A comprehensive description of changes in drug dosage according to the technique of RRT, residual creatinine clearance and other determinants of pharmacodynamics is beyond the scope of this chapter and can be found in specialist texts.[29] Table 41.3 provides general guidelines for the prescription of drugs commonly used in the ICU.

SUMMARY

The field of RRT has undergone remarkable changes over the last 10 years and is continuing to evolve rapidly. Technology is being improved to facilitate clinical application and new areas of research are developing. CRRT is now firmly established throughout the world as perhaps the most commonly used form of RRT. Conventional dialysis, however, which was slowly losing ground, is reappearing in the form of extended, slow-efficiency treatment, especially in the USA. Two large phase IV trials (> 1000 patients) are under way in the USA and in Australia/New Zealand to compare different dialytic strategies (IHD or SLEDD or CRRT) or to define the optimal dose of CRRT and the results should be available in 2008. In the meantime the use of novel membranes, of sorbents and of different intensities of treatment is being explored in the area of sepsis management and liver support. Intensivists need to keep abreast of this rapid evolution if they are to offer their patients the best of care.

REFERENCES

1. Sargent J, Gotch F. Principles and biophysics of dialysis. In: Maher J (ed.) *Replacement of Renal Function by Dialysis*. Dordrecht: Kluwer Academic; 1989: 87–102.
2. Henderson L. Biophysics of ultrafiltration and hemofiltration. In: Maher J (ed.) *Replacement of Renal Function by Dialysis*. Dordrecht: Kluwer Academic; 1989: 300–32.
3. Nolph KD. Peritoneal dialysis. In: Brenner BM, Rector FC (eds) *The Kidney*. Philadelphia: WB Saunders; 1986: 1791–845.
4. Conger JD. Does hemodialysis delay recovery from acute renal failure? *Semin Dial* 1990; **3**: 145–6.
5. Howdieshell TR, Blalock WE, Bowen PA *et al.* Management of post-traumatic acute renal failure with peritoneal dialysis. *Am Surg* 1992; **58**: 378–82.
6. Bellomo R, Boyce N. Continuous venovenous hemodiafiltration compared with conventional dialysis in critically ill patients with acute renal failure. *ASAIO J* 1993; **39**: M794–7.
7. Gettings LG, Reynolds HN, Scalea T. Outcome in post-traumatic acute renal failure when continuous renal replacement therapy is applied early vs. late. *Intens Care Med* 1999; **25**: 805–81.
8. Chatoth DK, Shaver MJ, Marshall MR *et al.* Daily 12-hour sustained low-efficiency hemodialysis (SLED) for the treatment of critically ill patients with acute renal failure: initial experience. *Blood Purif* 1999; **17**: abstract 16.
9. Paganini EP. Dialysis is not dialysis is not dialysis! Acute dialysis is different and needs help! *Am J Kidney Dis* 1998; **32**: 832–3.
10. Bellomo R, Ronco C. Adequacy of dialysis in the acute renal failure of the critically ill: the case for continuous therapies. *Int J Artif Organs* 1996; **19**: 129–42.
11. Kanagasundaram NS, Paganini EP. Critical care dialysis – a Gordian knot (but is untying the right approach?). *Nephrol Dial Transplant* 1999; **14**: 2590–4.
12. Ronco C, Bellomo R, Homel P *et al.* Effects of different doses in continuous veno-venous haemofiltration on outcomes of acute renal failure: a prospective randomized trial. *Lancet* 2000; **356**: 26–30.
13. Marshall MR, Golper TA, Shaver MJ *et al.* Hybrid renal replacement modalities for the critically ill. *Contrib Nephrol* 2001; **132**: 252–7.
14. Cole L, Bellomo R, Silvester W *et al.* A prospective, multicenter study of the epidemiology, management and outcome of severe acute renal failure in a 'closed' ICU system. *Am J Respir Crit Care Med* 2000; **162**: 191–6.
15. Saudan P, Niederberger M, De Seigneux S *et al.* Adding a dialysis dose to continuous hemofiltration increases survival in patients with acute renal failure. *Kidney Int* 2006; **70**: 1312–17.
16. Bellomo R. Do we know the optimal dose for renal replacement therapy in the intensive care unit? *Kidney Int* 2006; **70**: 1202–4.
17. Mehta R, Dobos GJ, Ward DM. Anticoagulation procedures in continuous renal replacement. *Semin Dial* 1992; **5**: 61–8.
18. Naka T, Egi M, Bellomo R *et al.* Low-dose citrate continuous veno-venous hemofiltration and acid–base balance. *Int J Artif Organs* 2005; **28**: 222–8.
19. Tan HK, Baldwin I, Bellomo R. Hemofiltration without anticoagulation in high-risk patients. *Intens Care Med* 2000; **26**: 1652–7.
20. Ronco C, Brendolan A, Bellomo R. Current technology for continuous renal replacement therapies. In: Ronco C, Bellomo R (eds) *Critical Care Nephrology*. Dordrecht: Kluwer Academic; 1998: 1327–34.
21. Macias WL, Clark WR. Azotemia control by extracorporeal therapy in patients with acute renal failure. *N Horizons* 1995; **3**: 688–93.
22. Davenport A. The management of renal failure in patients at risk of cerebral edema/hypoxia. *N Horizons* 1995; **3**: 717–24.
23. Phu NH, Hien TT, Mai NT *et al.* Hemofiltration and peritoneal dialysis in infection-associated acute renal failure in Vietnam. *N Engl J Med* 2002; **347**: 895–902.
24. Reeves JH, Butt WW, Shann F *et al.* Continuous plasmafiltration in sepsis syndrome. *Crit Care Med* 1999; **27**: 2096–104.
25. Bellomo R, Baldwin I, Ronco C. High-volume hemofiltration. *Contrib Nephrol* 2001; **132**: 375–82.
26. Brendolan A, Bellomo R, Tetta C *et al.* Coupled plasma filtration adsorption in the treatment of septic shock. *Contrib Nephrol* 2001; **132**: 383–91.
27. Uchino S, Bellomo R, Morimatsu H *et al.* Cytokine dialysis: an ex-vivo study. *ASAIO J* 2002; **48**: 650–3.
28. Mitzner SR, Stange J, Klammt S *et al.* Extracorporeal detoxification using the molecular adsorbent recirculating system for critically ill patients with liver failure. *J Am Soc Nephrol* 2001; **12**: S755–82.
29. Buckmaster J, Davies AR. Guidelines for drug dosing during continuous renal replacement therapies. In: Ronco C, Bellomo R (eds) *Critical Care Nephrology*. Dordrecht: Kluwer Academic; 1998: 1327–34.

Part Seven

Neurological Disorders

42

Disorders of consciousness

Balasubramanian Venkatesh

NEUROANATOMY AND PHYSIOLOGY OF WAKEFULNESS

A normal level of consciousness depends on the interaction between the cerebral hemispheres and the rostral reticular activating system (RAS) located in the upper brainstem. Although the RAS is a diffuse projection, the areas of RAS of particular importance to the maintenance of consciousness are those located between the rostral pons and the diencephalon. In contrast, consciousness is not focally represented in any of the cerebral hemispheres and is in many ways related to the mass of functioning cortex. Thus anatomical bilateral hemispheric lesions or brainstem lesions may result in an altered conscious state.[1] Large unilateral hemispheric lesions may produce impairment of consciousness by compression of the upper brainstem. In addition metabolic processes may result in coma from interruption of energy substrate delivery or alteration of neuronal excitability. Disorders of consciousness are characterised by an alteration in either the level or content of consciousness (Table 42.1). The last few conditions described in Table 42.1 are a frequent source of confusion and require further discussion (Table 42.2). These neurological states are seen more frequently in modern-day clinical practice partly because of the advances in therapy of severe brain injury and intensive care which have led to the survival of many patients who would otherwise have died.

DIFFERENTIAL DIAGNOSIS OF COMA

Although the aetiology of coma is invariably multifactorial, the differential diagnosis of coma can be broadly grouped into three classes:

1. diseases that produce focal or lateralising signs
2. coma without focal or lateralising signs, but with signs of meningeal irritation
3. coma without focal or lateralising signs or signs of meningeal irritation

These are considered in greater detail in Table 42.3.

CLINICAL EXAMINATION OF THE COMATOSE PATIENT

The neurological examination of the comatose patient is of crucial importance to assess the depth of coma and to locate the site of lesion. Although the detailed neurological examination which can be carried out in a conscious patient is not possible in a comatose individual, useful information can be obtained by performing a thorough general examination and a neurological examination, particularly evaluating the level of consciousness, brainstem signs and motor responses in coma.

GENERAL EXAMINATION

General examination of the patient may point to the aetiology of coma. Skin changes may be seen in carbon monoxide poisoning (cherry-red discoloration of skin), alcoholic liver disease (telangiectasia, clubbing), hypothyroidism (puffy facies) and hypopituitarism (sallow complexion). The presence of cutaneous petechiae or ecchymoses may point to meningococcaemia, rickettsial infection or endocarditis as possible causes of coma. Needle puncture marks may suggest substance abuse. Bullous skin lesions are a feature of barbiturate overdose. An excessively dry skin may indicate diabetic ketoacidosis or anticholinergic overdose.

Periorbital haematomas (raccoon eyes) indicate an anterior basal skull fracture, particularly if there is associated cerebrospinal fluid rhinorrhoea. The other signs of a basal skull fracture include Battle's sign and cerebrospinal fluid otorrhoea. Nuchal rigidity may be seen in meningoencephalitis and subarachnoid haemorrhage, although this sign may not be present in the elderly and in patients in deep coma.

The presence of hepatomegaly or stigmata of chronic liver disease may suggest hepatic encephalopathy. Bilateral enlarged kidneys may indicate polycystic kidney disease and should prompt one to consider subarachnoid haemorrhage as a possible aetiology of coma. The breath may smell of alcohol or other poisons (organophosphates). The smell of ketones on the breath is an unreliable sign and hepatic and uraemic foetor are rare.

Table 42.1 Disorders of consciousness

Consciousness	An awake individual demonstrates full awareness of self and environment
Confusion	Inability to think with customary speed and clarity, associated with inattentiveness, reduced awareness and disorientation
Delirium	Confusion with agitation and hallucination
Stupor	Unresponsiveness with arousal only by deep and repeated stimuli
Coma	Unarousable unresponsiveness
Locked-in syndrome	Total paralysis below third cranial nerve nuclei; normal or impaired mental function
Persistent vegetative state	Prolonged coma > 1 month, some preservation of brainstem and motor reflexes
Akinetic mutism	Prolonged coma with apparent alertness and flaccid motor tone
Minimally conscious state	Preserved wakefulness, awareness and brainstem reflexes, but poorly responsive

LEVEL OF CONSCIOUSNESS

This is assessed by the Glasgow Coma Scale (GCS),[2] which takes into account a patient's response to command and physical stimuli. The GCS (Table 42.4) which was originally developed to grade the severity of head injury and prognosticate outcome, has now been extended for all causes of impaired consciousness and coma. Although it is a simple clinical score, easily performed by both medical and nursing staff by the bedside, there are a number of caveats:

1. The GCS should always be determined prior to administration of sedative drugs or endotracheal intubation.
2. It should also be defined with regard to a patient's vital signs, namely blood pressure, heart rate and temperature.
3. The GCS must be interpreted in the light of previous or concomitant drug therapy.
4. The presence of alcohol in the breath or in the serum should always be documented.
5. Because of the considerable interobserver variation in scoring, it is important to define the responses in descriptive terms rather than emphasising the numerical score associated with each response.
6. Measurement of awareness by the GCS is limited. Subtle changes in brainstem reflexes are not adequately assessed by the GCS.

PUPILLARY RESPONSES IN COMA[3]

The presence of normal pupils (2–5 mm and equal in size and demonstrating both direct and consensual light reflexes) confirms the integrity of the pupillary pathway (retina, optic nerve, optic chiasma and tracts, midbrain and third cranial nerve nuclei and nerves). The size of the pupil is a balance between the opposing influences of both sympathetic (causing dilatation) and parasympathetic (causing constriction) systems. Pupillary abnormalities have localising and diagnostic value in clinical neurology (Table 42.5). When the pupils are miosed, the light reaction is difficult to appreciate and may require a magnifying glass.

OPHTHALMOSCOPY IN COMA

The pupils *should never be dilated pharmacologically* without prior documentation of the pupillary size and the light reflex. The presence of papilloedema suggests the presence of intracranial hypertension, but is frequently absent when the lesion is acute. Subhyaloid and vitreous haemorrhages are seen in patients with subarachnoid haemorrhage.[4]

EYE MOVEMENTS IN COMA[5]

Horizontal eye movements to the contralateral side are initiated in the ipsilateral frontal lobe and closely coordinated with the corresponding centre in the contralateral pons. To facilitate conjugate eye movements, yoking of the third-, fourth- and sixth-nerve nuclei is achieved by the medial longitudinal fasciculus.

To look to the left, the movement originates in the right frontal lobe and is coordinated by the left pontine region and vice versa. In contrast to horizontal gaze, vertical eye movements are under bilateral control of the cortex and upper midbrain.

The position and movements of the eyes are observed at rest. The presence of spontaneous roving eye movements excludes brainstem pathology as a cause of coma. In a paralytic frontal-lobe pathology, the eyes will deviate towards the side of the lesion, whilst in pontine pathologies, the eyes will deviate away from the side of the lesion. Ocular bobbing, an intermittent downward jerking eye movement, is seen in pontine lesions due to loss of horizontal gaze and unopposed midbrain controlled vertical gaze activity.[6] Skew deviation (vertical separation of the ocular axes) occurs with pontine and cerebellar disorders.[7]

The presence of full and conjugate eye movements in response to oculocephalic and oculovestibular stimuli demonstrates the functional integrity of a large segment of the brainstem. Corneal reflexes are preserved until late in coma. Upward rolling of the eyes after corneal stimulation (Bell's phenomenon) implies intact midbrain and pontine function.

Table 42.2 Coma-like syndromes and related states

Syndrome	Features	Site of lesion	EEG	Metabolism (% of normal)[35]	Comments
Locked-in syndrome[31] (de-efferented state)	Alert and aware, vertical eye movements present, and able to blink. Quadriplegic, lower cranial nerve palsies, no speech, facial or pharyngeal movements	Bilateral anterior pontine lesion which transects all descending motor pathways, but spares ascending sensory and reticular activating systems	Normal	90–100%	Similar state seen with severe polyneuropathies, myasthenia gravis and neuromuscular blocking agents
Persistent vegetative state (PVS)[32,33] (apallic syndrome, neocortical death)	Previously comatose, who now appear to be awake. Spontaneous limb movements, eye movements and yawning seen. However patient inattentive, no speech, no awareness of environment and total inability to respond to commands	Extensive damage to both cerebral hemispheres with relative preservation of the brainstem	Polymorphic delta or theta waves, sometimes alpha	40–60%	When vegetative state lasts longer than 4 weeks, it is termed persistent. PVS lasting for longer than 2 weeks implies a poor prognosis
Akinetic mutism[34] (coma vigile)	Partially or fully awake patient, immobile and silent	Lesion in bilateral frontal lobes or hydrocephalus or third ventricular masses	Diffuse slowing	40–80%	'Abulia' is the term applied to milder forms of akinetic mutism
Catatonia	Awake patients, sometimes a fixed posture, muteness with decreased motor activity	Usually of psychiatric origin	Non-specific EEG patterns associated with associated medical conditions	Variable metabolic changes in prefrontal cortex	May be mimicked by frontal lobe disease and drugs
Minimally conscious state[35]	Globally impaired responsiveness, limited but discernible evidence of self and environment	Global neuronal damage	Theta and alpha waves	40–60%	Differs from PVS in that patients diagnosed with minimally conscious state have some level of awareness

EEG, electroencephalogram.

LIMB MOVEMENTS AND POSTURAL CHANGES IN COMA

Restlessness, crossing of legs and spontaneous coughing, yawning, swallowing and localising movements suggest only a mild depression of the conscious state. Choreoathetotic or ballistic movements suggest a basal ganglion lesion. Myoclonic movements indicate a metabolic disorder, usually of postanoxic origin. Asterixis is seen with metabolic encephalopathies. Hiccup is a non-specific sign and does not have any localising value.

Decerebrate rigidity is characterised by stiff extension of the limbs, internal rotation of the arms and plantar flexion of the ankles. With severe rigidity, opisthotonos and jaw clenching may be observed. These movements may be unilateral or bilateral, and spontaneous or in response to a noxious stimulus. Whereas animal studies suggest that the lesion is usually in the midbrain or caudal diencephalon (leading to exaggeration of antigravity reflexes), in humans such posturing may be seen in a variety of disease states: midbrain lesion, certain metabolic disorders such as hypoglycaemia, anoxia, hepatic coma and in drug intoxication.

Table 42.3 Differential diagnosis of coma

Category	Specific disorder	Features in history and examination	Investigations	Comments
Coma with focal signs	*Trauma* – extradural, subdural and parenchymal haemorrhage, concussions	History of trauma, findings of fracture at base of skull, scalp haematoma, other associated body injuries	Usually an abnormal CT	Exclude coexisting drug or alcohol ingestion
	Vascular –intracerebral haemorrhage	Sudden onset, history of headaches or hypertension, neck stiffness may be present	Abnormal CT scan	Consider causes of secondary hypertension in young hypertensives
	Vascular – thromboembolic	Sudden onset, atrial fibrillation, vascular bruits, endocarditis	An abnormal CT after a few days	Consider echocardiography to diagnose cardiac sources of emboli
	Brain abscess	Subacute onset, look for ENT and dental sources of infection	Abnormal CT and CSF	Consider infective endocarditis and suppurative lung disease as sources of sepsis
Coma without focal signs, but with meningeal irritation	Infection, meningitis, encephalitis	Onset of illness over a few hours to days, neck stiffness, rash of meningococcaemia	Abnormal CSF	Consider underlying immunosuppressive states
	Subarachnoid haemorrhage	Onset usually sudden, subhyaloid haemorrhages on fundoscopy	Abnormal CT and CSF	Consider polycystic kidney disease in subarachnoid haemorrhage
Coma without focal signs and no meningeal irritation	Metabolic causes Hyponatraemia Hypoglycaemia Hyperglycaemia Hypoxia Hypercapnia Hypo- and hyperthermia Hyper- and hypo-osmolar states	History might point to the cause of metabolic disturbance, asterixis a feature of hypercapnia-induced coma	Abnormal blood results	Rapid correction of hyponatraemia and osmolality should be avoided
	Endocrine causes Myxoedema Adrenal insufficiency Hypopituitarism	Puffy facies, may be hypothermic	Abnormal electrolyte profile, hypoglycaemia	Multiple disorders may be present in the same patient
	Seizure disorders	History typical	Abnormal EEG, check anticonvulsant levels	CT scan to exclude an underlying space-occupying lesion
	Organ failure Hepatic Renal	History of jaundice, chronic alcohol ingestion, stigmata of liver disease, asterixis	Abnormal hepatic and renal functions	Presence of A-V fistula may be a pointer to chronic renal failure
	Toxic/drug Sedatives Narcotics Alcohol Psychotropic	History, may be hypothermic at presentation except in psychotropic drug overdose	Metabolic screen is usually normal	Rapid improvement in conscious states with antidotes

Continued

Table 42.3 Differential diagnosis of coma—*Continued*

Category	Specific disorder	Features in history and examination	Investigations	Comments
	Carbon monoxide Poisons			
	Behavioural Sleep deprivation Pseudocoma	No typical features	No specific diagnostic tests	Diagnosis of exclusion

CT, computed tomography; CSF, cerebrospinal fluid; ENT, ear, nose and throat; EEG, electroencephalogram; A-V, arteriovenous.

Table 42.4 Glasgow Coma Scale

Eye opening	Points
Spontaneous	4
To speech	3
To pain	2
Nil	1
Best verbal response	
Oriented	5
Confused	4
Inappropriate	3
Incomprehensible	2
Nil	1
Intubated	T
Best motor response	
Obeys commands	6
Localises to pain	5
Withdraws to pain	4
Abnormal flexion	3
Extensor response	2
Nil	1

Decorticate posturing is characterised by flexion of elbows and wrists and extension of the lower limbs. The lesion is usually above the midbrain in the cerebral white matter.

RESPIRATORY SYSTEM[8]

Abnormal respiratory rate and patterns have been described in coma, but their precise localising value is uncertain. As a general rule, at lighter levels of impaired consciousness tachypnoea predominates, whereas respiratory depression increases with the depth of coma. Some of the commonly observed respiratory abnormalities are summarised in Table 42.6. Respiratory failure in comatose patients may result from hypoventilation, aspiration pneumonia and neurogenic pulmonary oedema, a sympathetic nervous system-mediated syndrome seen in acute brain injury.

BODY TEMPERATURE IN COMA

The presence of altered core body temperature is a useful aid in the diagnosis of coma. Hypothermia (< 35°C) is frequently observed with alcohol or barbiturate intoxication, sepsis with shock, drowning, hypoglycaemia, myxoedema, coma and exposure to cold. Severe hyperthermia may be seen in pontine haemorrhage, intracranial infections, heat stroke and anticholinergic drug toxicity.

RECOGNITION OF BRAIN HERNIATION[9,10]

When patients with impaired level of consciousness deteriorate, it is important to consider brain herniation as a possible cause of worsening. Brain herniation results from the downward displacement of the upper brainstem (central herniation) with or without involvement of the uncus (lateral herniation). The clinical signs of a central herniation are progressive obtundation, Cheyne–Stokes respiration, small pupils followed by extensor posturing and medium-sized fixed dilated pupils. Uncal herniation differs from central herniation in that pupillary dilatation occurs early in the process because of third-nerve compression. The traditional Cushing's response of hypertension and bradycardia is not always a feature of herniation and any heart rhythm may be present.

DIFFERENTIATING TRUE COMA FROM PSEUDOCOMA

Patients feigning coma resist passive eye opening and may even hold their eyes tightly closed. They may blink in response to a threat and do not demonstrate spontaneous roving eye movements. In contrast, they move the eyes concomitantly with head rotation and, with cold caloric testing, they may wake up or demonstrate preservation of the fast component of nystagmus. They also demonstrate avoidance of 'self-injury'. In addition, the pattern of clinical 'abnormalities' does not fit any specific neurological syndromes.

MANAGEMENT OF THE COMATOSE PATIENT

EMERGENT THERAPEUTIC MEASURES

Irrespective of the aetiology of coma, certain emergent therapeutic measures apply to the care of all patients. These take precedence over any diagnostic investigation.

Table 42.5 Pupillary abnormalities in coma

Abnormality	Cause	Neuroanatomical basis
Miosis (< 2 mm in size)		
Unilateral	Horner's syndrome	Sympathetic paralysis
	Local pathology	Trauma to sympathetics
Bilateral	Pontine lesions	
	Thalamic haemorrhage	Sympathetic paralysis
	Metabolic encephalopathy	
	Drug ingestion	
	Organophosphate	Cholinesterase inhibition
	Barbiturate	
	Narcotics	Central effect
Mydriasis (> 5 mm in size)		
Unilateral fixed pupil	Midbrain lesion	Third-nerve damage
	Uncal herniation	Stretch of third nerve against the petroclinoid ligament
Bilateral fixed pupils	Massive midbrain haemorrhage	Bilateral third-nerve damage
	Hypoxic cerebral injury	Mesencephalic damage
	Drugs	
	Atropine	Paralysis of parasympathetics
	Tricyclics	Prevent local reuptake of catecholamines by nerve endings
	Sympathomimetics	Stimulation of sympathetics

Table 42.6 Disorders of respiratory rate and pattern in coma

Abnormality	Significance
Bradypnoea	Drug-induced coma, hypothyroid coma
Tachypnoea	Central neurogenic hyperventilation (midbrain lesion), metabolic encephalopathy
Cheyne–Stokes respiration	Deep cerebral lesions, metabolic encephalopathy (hyperpnoea alternating regularly with apnoea)
Apneustic breathing (an inspiratory pause)	Pontine lesions
Ataxic breathing	Medullary lesions
(Ataxic breathing normally progresses to agonal gasps and terminal apnoea)	

1. Ensure adequate airway and oxygenation.
2. Secure intravenous access and maintain circulation.
3. Administer 50% dextrose after drawing a sample of blood for serum glucose levels. Although there are theoretical concerns about augmentation of brain lactic acid production[11,12] in anoxic coma, the relatively good prognosis for hypoglycaemic coma when treated expeditiously far outweighs any potential risks of glucose administration.
4. Thiamine must always be administered in conjunction with dextrose to prevent precipitation of Wernicke's encephalopathy.
5. Consideration should be given to administering naloxone when there is a suspicion of narcotic overdose with impending respiratory arrest.
6. If hypertension, bradycardia and fixed dilated pupils are present at the time of the initial presentation, suggestive of marked intracranial hypertension and tentorial herniation, 20% mannitol at a dose 0.5–1 g/kg body weight should be administered. Consideration should be given to the emergency placement of an external ventricular drain.
7. Treat suspected meningitis with antibiotics even if cerebrospinal fluid results are not available. A combination of penicillin and ceftriaxone is usually recommended for community-acquired bacterial meningitis.
8. Control of seizures must be achieved as outlined in Chapter 43.
9. Treat extreme body temperatures.

INVESTIGATIONS

The order of investigation depends on the clinical circumstances. In the majority of cases, history and examination will provide enough information to be able to perform specific cause-related investigation. In general, the investigations can be grouped as follows.

ROUTINE INVESTIGATIONS

Measurements of serum glucose, electrolytes, arterial blood gases, liver and renal function tests, osmolality, blood count and blood film are part of the routine investigations. When drug overdose is suspected, a toxicology screen for alcohol, paracetamol, salicylates, benzodiazepines and tricyclic antidepressants should be performed. A sample of serum should be stored for later analysis for uncommon drug ingestions.

NEUROIMAGING

COMPUTED TOMOGRAPHY (CT) SCAN

The most commonly used radiological investigation for evaluation of the comatose patient is CT scan of the brain. This is useful for diagnosing central nervous system trauma, subarachnoid and intracerebral haemorrhage, haemorrhagic and non-haemorrhagic strokes, cerebral oedema, hydrocephalus and the presence of a space-occupying lesion (SOL) (Figures 42.1–42.10). Frequently a CT is performed prior to a lumbar puncture (LP) to exclude rather than confirm the presence of severe cerebral oedema or an SOL. Its other advantages include lower cost, easy availability, short examination time and safety in the presence of pacemakers, surgical clips and other ferromagnetic substances. The advent of helical CT whereby multiple images are possible has reduced scanning times and is suitable for the uncooperative patient. Limitations of a CT scan include:

1. the need to transfer the patient to a site where resuscitation and monitoring facilities are limited
2. the need to sedate and possibly endotracheally intubate patients who are agitated
3. its low sensitivity to demonstrate an abnormality in the acute phase of a stroke
4. its low sensitivity for detecting brainstem lesions
5. the need to administer intravenous contrast agents . The two major side-effects of intravenous contrast include anaphylaxis (with an approximate death rate of 1 in 40 000) and renal failure. The use of *N*-acetylcysteine, sodium bicarbonate and haemodialysis has been reported to reduce the incidence of contrast-induced nephropathy, although data in critically ill patients are minimal.[13]

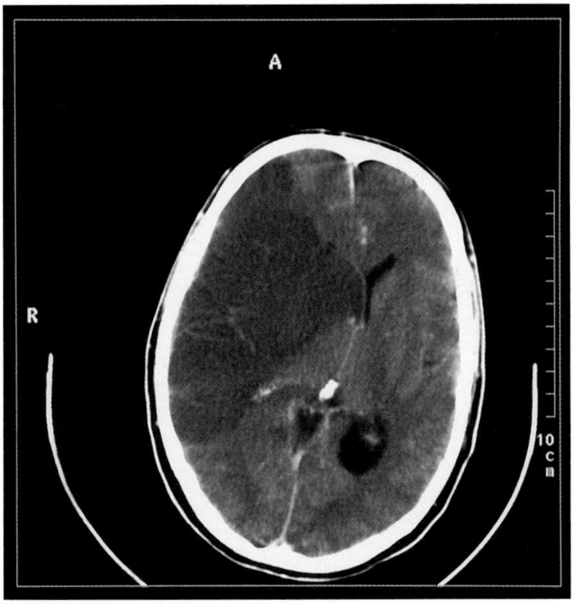

Figure 42.1 Right middle cerebral artery infarct. There is anterior and posterior sparing. Loss of right lateral ventricle. Moderate mass effect with midline shift.

MAGNETIC RESONANCE IMAGING (MRI)

MRI scans provide superior contrast and resolution of the grey and white matter as compared to CT scans, thus facilitating easy identification of the deep nuclear structures within the brain. MRI is more sensitive than CT for the detection of acute ischaemia, diffuse axonal injury and cerebral oedema, tumour and abscess. Brainstem and posterior fossa structures are better visualised (Figures 42.11–42.13). It can also show vasculature (see Figure 42.13b and c). The other advantage of MRI is the use of non-ionising energy. The use of gadolinium, a paramagnetic agent, as a contrast agent permits sharp definition of lesions. MR coupled with angiography (MRA) may enable diagnosis of vascular lesions. MRI is however limited by:

1. the need for special equipment
2. long imaging times
3. the need to transfer the patient to a site where resuscitation and monitoring facilities are limited
4. the need to sedate and possibly endotracheally intubate patients who are agitated
5. the risk of dislodgement of metal clips on blood vessels and resetting of pacemakers

PET AND SPECT SCANS

Newer nuclear medicine scans such as single-photon emission with computed tomography (SPECT) and positron emission tomography (PET) are useful for the assessment of cerebral blood flow and oxygenation and in the prognostication of neurotrauma, but have little role to play in the management of acute disorders of consciousness. In PET scans, positron-emitting isotopes such as ^{11}C, ^{18}F and ^{15}O are incorporated into biologically active compounds such as deoxyglucxose or fluorodeoxyglucose which are metabolised in the body. By determining the concentration of the various tracers in the brain and constructing tomographic images, cerebral blood flow and metabolism can be measured by PET scanning.

SPECT scans use iodine-containing isotopes incorporated into biologically active compounds and, like PET scans, their cranial distribution is determined after a dose

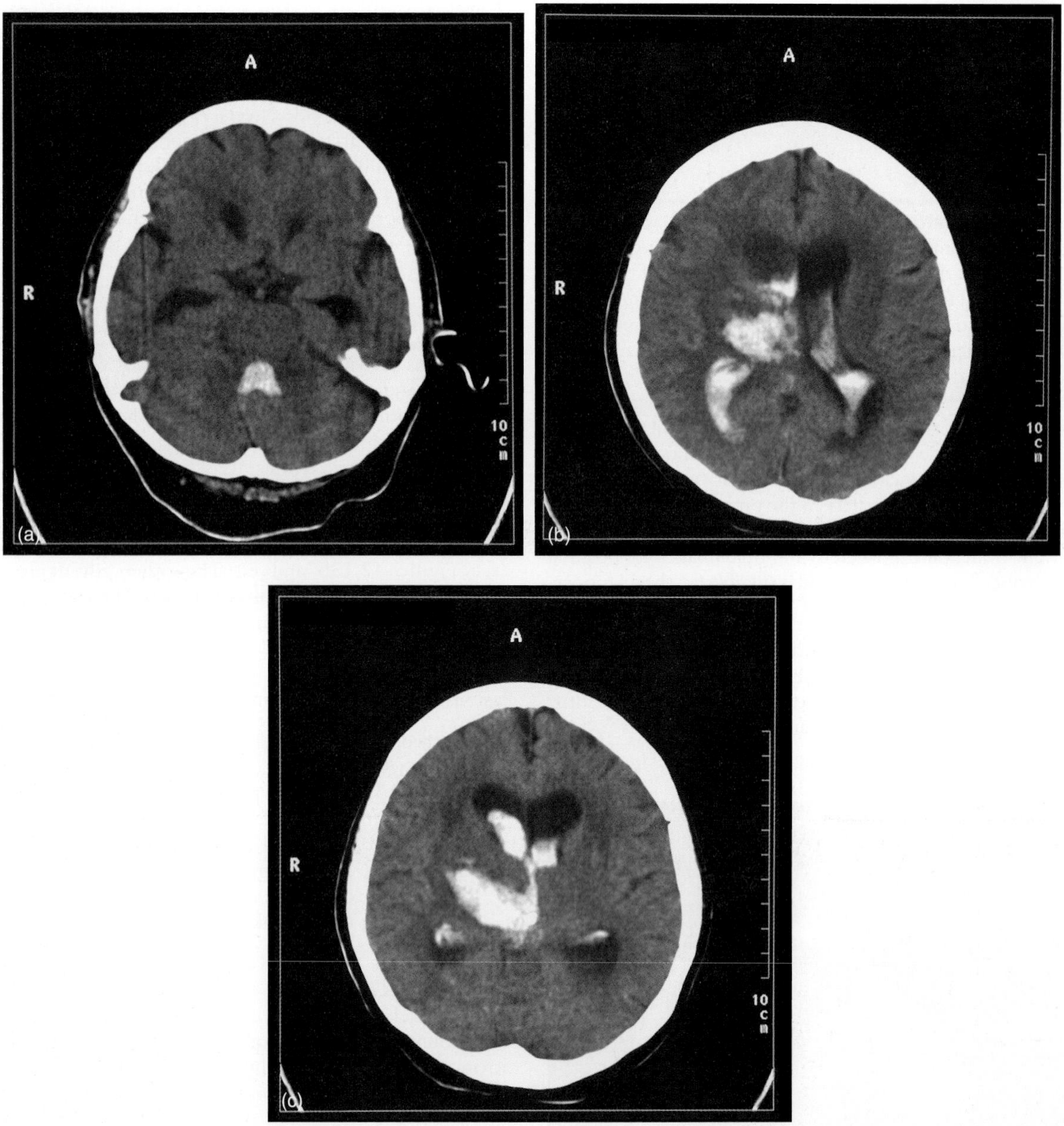

Figure 42.2 Blood. Right thalamic intraparenchymal bleed with subarachnoid blood. (a) Fourth ventricle; (b) both lateral ventricles; (c) ventricles and intraparenchymal blood.

of tracer. Information on cerebral blood flow and metabolism can be obtained from SPECT scans. The advantage of a PET scan is that it does not require a cyclotron for the generation of isotopes. Despite their many advantages, both these technologies continue to be research tools and are not routinely available in many medical centres.

LUMBAR PUNCTURE[14]

Cerebrospinal fluid is most commonly obtained by means of an LP. This should be performed after ensuring that raised intracranial pressure has been excluded clinically or radiologically. The major use of an LP is to diagnose an intracranial infection and to detect abnormal cytology

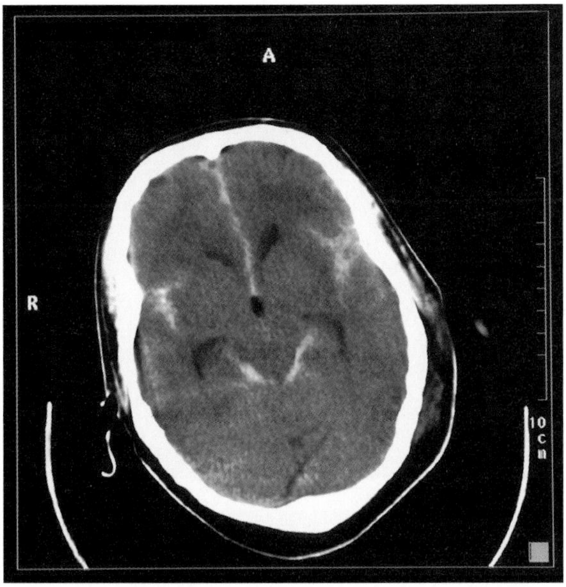

Figure 42.3 Subarachnoid haemorrhage. Blood in the Sylvian fissure and in basal cisterns.

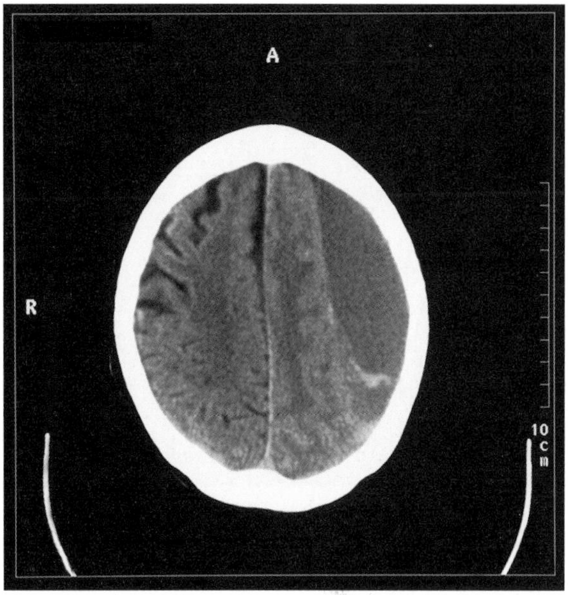

Figure 42.5 Chronic left subdural haematoma. Isodense fluid filling space. The small white area may suggest a recent acute bleed.

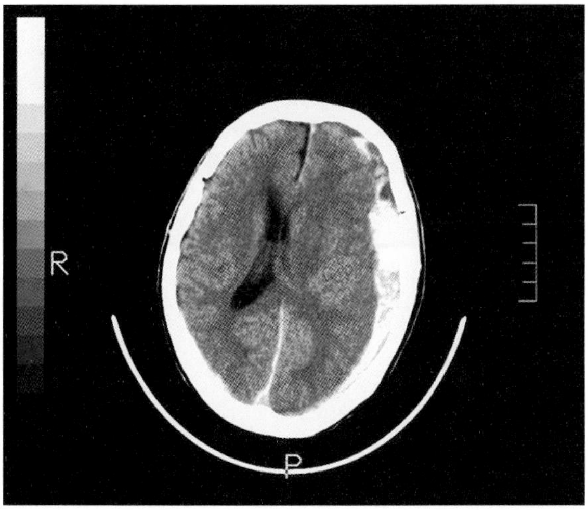

Figure 42.4 Acute left subdural haematoma. Crescenteric pattern within the skull with high attenuation. Loss of ventricle.

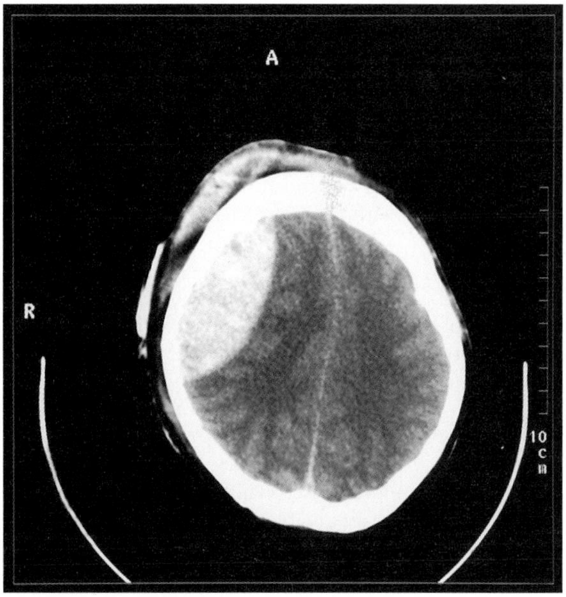

Figure 42.6 Right extradural haematoma. Note soft-tissue swelling.

in cases of suspected malignant meningeal infiltration. The advent of CT scans has diminished the role of LP in the diagnosis of subarachnoid haemorrhage. Some of the commonly reported complications post-LP include postpuncture headache (12–39%) and traumatic tap (15–20%). Brain herniation is a rare potential complication seen with conditions associated with raised intracranial pressure due to an SOL.

ELECTROENCEPHALOGRAM (EEG) IN COMA[15,16]

The usefulness of EEG in coma is summarised in Table 42.7. Continuous EEG monitoring in the intensive care unit (ICU) has been reported to be useful in the

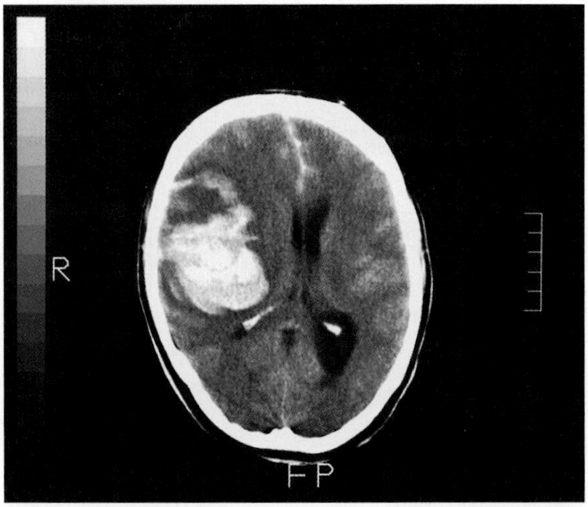

Figure 42.7 Right frontoparietal bleed. Note oedema, loss of lateral ventricle and minor midline shift.

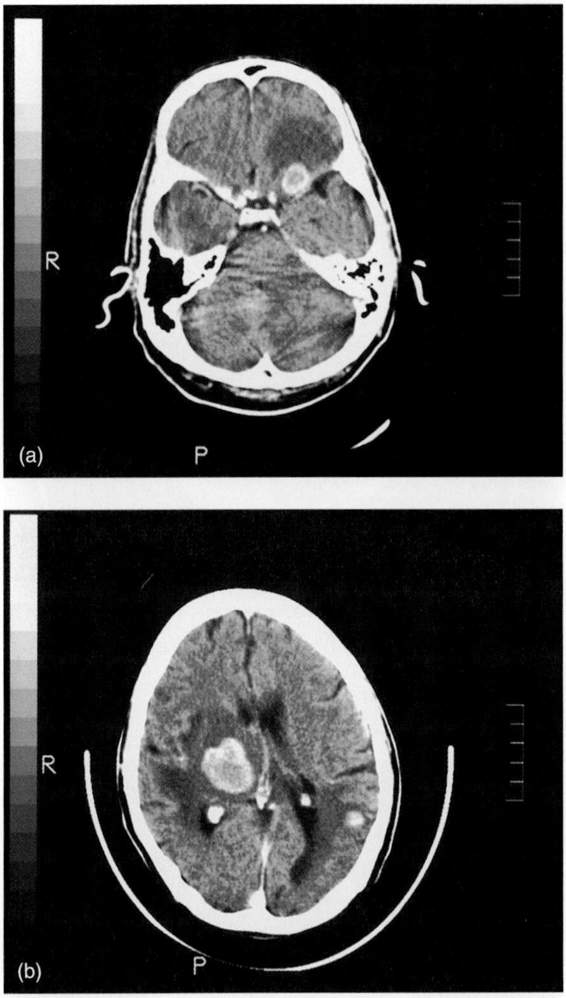

Figure 42.8 Multiple enhanced lesions – metastases. (a) Left frontal lesion; (b) right thalamic lesion.

identification of acute cerebral ischaemia and non-convulsive seizures.

EVOKED POTENTIALS

Visual, brainstem and somatosensory evoked potentials test the integrity of neuroanatomical pathways within the brain and the spinal cord. They may be used in the diagnosis of blindness in comatose patients and in the assessment of locked-in states. There are data to suggest that they have better prognostic value than clinical judgement in patients with anoxic coma.[17]

BIOCHEMICAL ABNORMALITIES[18]

A number of biomarkers of brain injury have been evaluated as predictors of severity of brain injury and to assess progression of injury severity from traumatic and non-traumatic aetiologies. These include neurone-specific enolase (cytoplasm of neurons), S-100 B protein (astroglial cells), CK-BB fraction (astrocytes), glial fibrillary acidic protein (glial origin), calpain and caspase. Whilst early studies showed S-100B to be a reliable marker of traumatic brain injury, concerns remain about their sensitivity and specificity for assessment of severity and prediction of outcome.

CARE OF THE COMATOSE PATIENT

AIRWAY

As mentioned before, assessment of airway adequacy should take precedence over any diagnostic investigation in comatose patients. This is best done by assessing the patient's response to command and physical stimulation, and whether a gag reflex is present. Securing the airway will depend on the level of consciousness. This may entail simple manoeuvres such as jaw thrust, chin lift, use of oropharyngeal airways or in the comatose patient mandate endotracheal intubation. All of these patients are at risk of pulmonary aspiration and there must be a low threshold for establishing a definitive airway.

As a general rule, patients presenting with medical causes of coma may be nursed on their side (in the coma position) if the airway is adequate. However, all traumatised patients should be assumed to have a potential cervical spine injury and must be nursed with the cervical spine in the neutral position and/or with a rigid collar until an injury is excluded by definitive radiological views. All

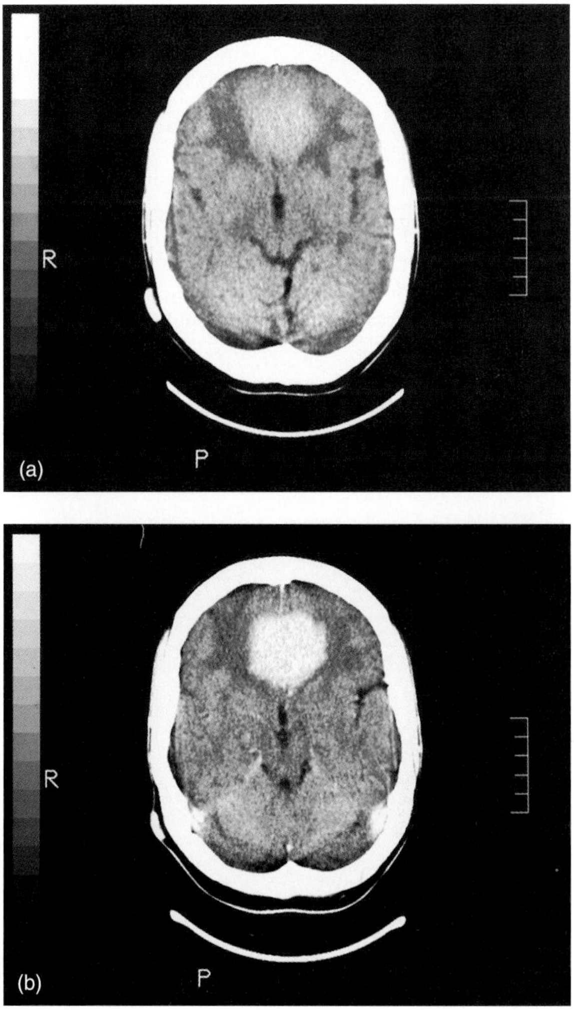

Figure 42.9 Frontal meningioma. (a) Precontrast; (b) postcontrast.

patients with disordered consciousness must receive supplemental oxygen.

VENTILATION

It is important to ensure optimal gas exchange and avoid hypoxia and hypercapnia. Generally a $Pa\text{O}_2$ of > 80 torr and $P\text{CO}_2$ of 35–40 torr is desirable. If spontaneous ventilatory efforts are not adequate to achieve these levels of arterial blood gases, mechanical ventilatory support may be necessary.

CIRCULATION

Adequacy of circulation should be assessed by conventional clinical endpoints. The goals of circulatory therapy in coma include prompt restoration of appropriate mean arterial blood pressure, correction of dehydration and hypovolaemia and urgent attention to life-threatening causes of shock.

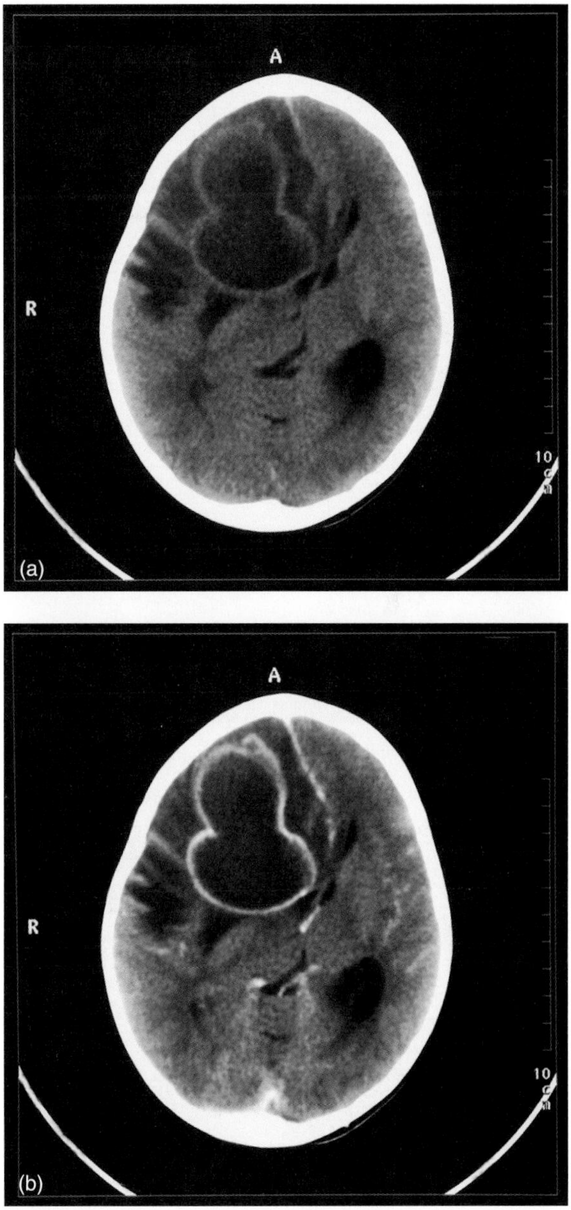

Figure 42.10 Abscess. (a) Precontrast; (b) postcontrast.

SPECIFIC TREATMENT

This will depend on the underlying aetiology of the coma and is discussed in the relevant chapters. Avoidance of

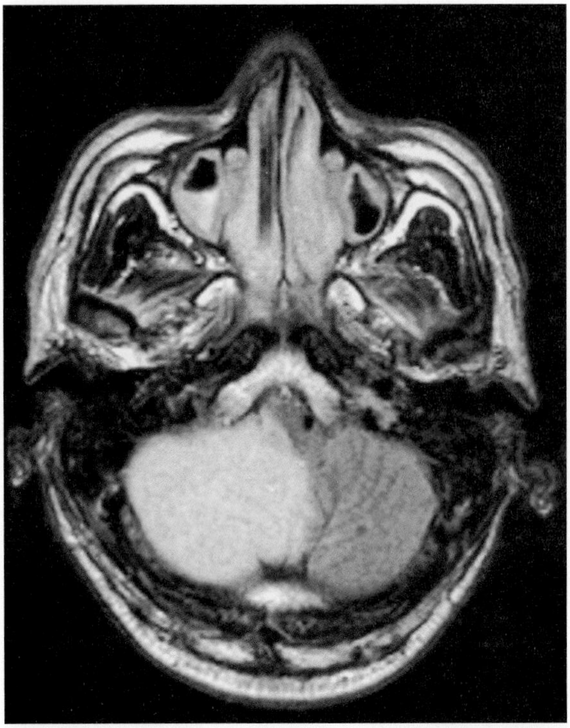

Figure 42.11 Cerebellar infarct.

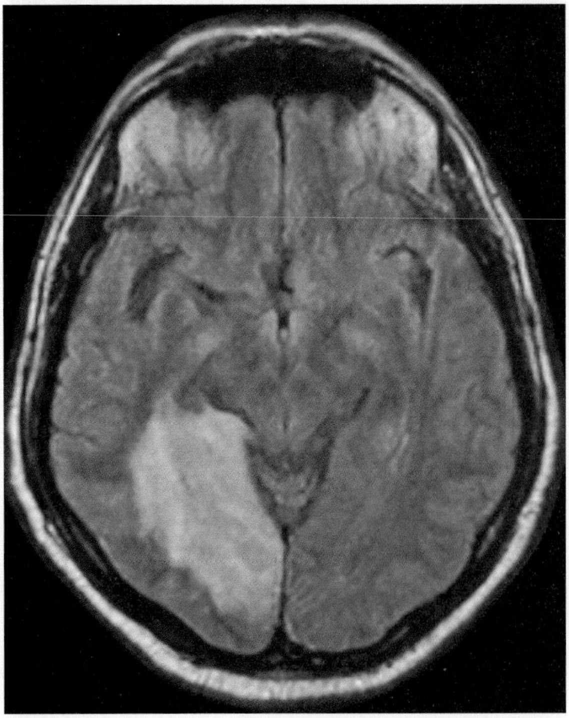

Figure 42.12 Posterior cerebral bleed.

secondary insults is of paramount importance in the management of these patients.[19]

NURSING CARE

Meticulous eye and mouth care, regular changes in limb position, limb physiotherapy, bronchial toilet and psychological support are mandatory. Nosocomial infections and iatrogenic complications are associated with an increased mortality and morbidity in these patients and must be promptly diagnosed and treated. The rational use of daily investigations, invasive procedures and antibiotic prescription is essential.

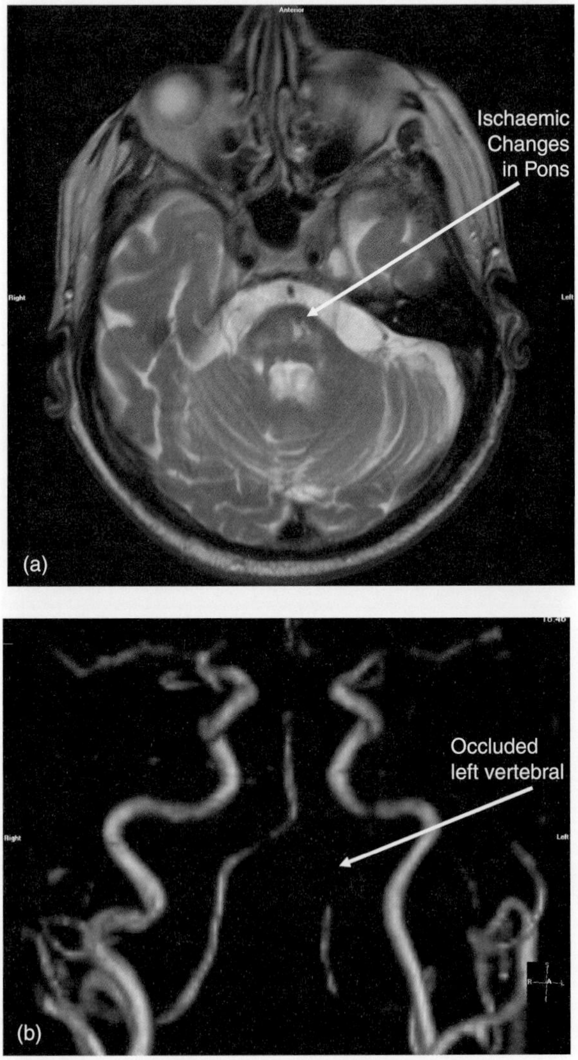

Figure 42.13 (a) Pontine ischaemia seen on magnetic resonance imaging (MRI). MRI can also be used to show vasculature. (b) Ocluded left vertebral artery;

Continued

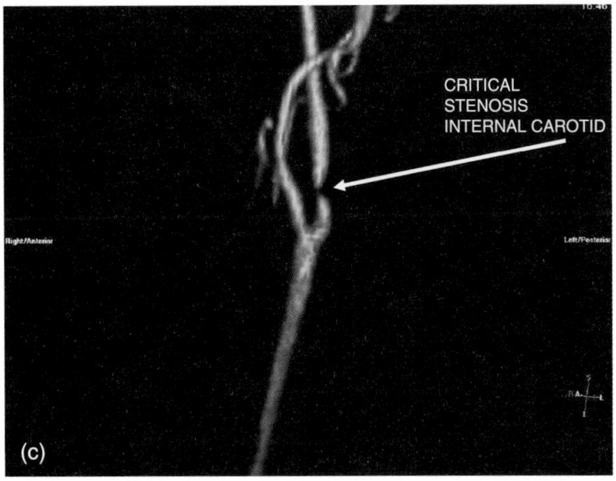

Figure 42.13 *Continued* (c) critical stenosis of left internal carotid artery.

Table 42.7 Usefulness of electroencephalogram in coma

Identification of non-convulsive status epilepticus
Diagnosis of hepatic encephalopathy
Presence of paroxysmal triphasic waves
Assessing severity of hypoxic encephalopathy
Presence of theta activity
Diffuse slowing
Burst suppression (seen with more severe forms)
Alpha coma (seen with more severe forms)
Herpes encephalitis
Periodic sharp spikes

OTHER THERAPY

Stress ulcer and deep-vein thrombosis prophylaxis should be instituted. Early establishment of enteral feeding via a nasoenteric tube is preferable. It is important to exclude a basal skull fracture before insertion of a nasoenteric tube.

ANOXIC COMA/ENCEPHALOPATHY

Cardiac arrest is the third leading cause of coma resulting in ICU admission after trauma and drug overdose. The symptomatology and clinical outcome of patients with anoxic brain damage depend on the severity and duration of oxygen deprivation to the brain. A number of criteria have been developed to prognosticate outcome in anoxic coma. Although a number of laboratory and imaging criteria contribute to the prognostic assessment, clinical signs still have major prognostic impact. The important clinical predictors of outcome are listed in Table 42.8. However there are data to suggest that electrophysiological studies using evoked potential have far greater prognostic accuracy compared to clinical assessment.[20]

Table 42.8 Clinical and laboratory predictors of unfavourable prognosis in anoxic coma[17,36–38]

Clinical predictor	Unfavourable prognosis
Duration of anoxia (time interval between collapse and initiation of CPR)	8–10 min
Duration of CPR (time interval between initiation of CPR and ROSC)	> 30 min
Duration of postanoxic coma	> 72 hours
Pupillary reaction	Absent on day 3
Motor response to pain (absent = a motor response worse than withdrawal)	Absent on day 3
Roving spontaneous eye movements	Absent on day 1
Elevated neuron specific enolase	> 33 μg/l
SSEP recording	Absent N20

CPR, cardiopulmonary resuscitation; ROSC, restoration of spontaneous circulation; SSEP, somatosensory evoked potential.

THE CONFUSED/ENCEPHALOPATHIC PATIENT IN THE ICU

'Encephalopathy' is a term used to describe the alteration in the level or content of consciousness due to a process extrinsic to the brain. Metabolic encephalopathy, particularly of septic aetiology, is the most common cause of altered mental status in the ICU setting.[21] A number of processes can lead to metabolic encephalopathy (Table 42.9). A number of features in the history and examination help to differentiate metabolic from structural causes of altered conscious states (Table 42.10).

Owing to their increased frequency in and exclusiveness to the critical care setting, two types of encephalopathy will be considered in detail: septic encephalopathy and ICU syndrome.

Table 42.9 Aetiology of metabolic/toxic encephalopathy[39–41]

Hepatic failure
Renal failure
Respiratory failure
Sepsis
Electrolyte abnormalities: hyponatraemia, hypernatraemia, hypercalcaemia
Hypoglycaemia and hyperglycaemia
Acute pancreatitis
Endocrine – addisonian crisis, myxoedema coma, thyroid storm
Drug withdrawal – benzodiazepine, opiates
Hyperthermia
Toxins: alcohols, glycols, tricyclic antidepressants
Intensive care unit syndrome
D-lactic acidosis

Table 42.10 Distinguishing features of structural and metabolic encephalopathy[41]

Feature	Structural	Metabolic
State of consciousness	Usually fixed level of depressed conscious state, may deteriorate progressively	Milder alteration of conscious state, waxing and waning of altered sensorium
Fundoscospy	May be abnormal	Usually normal
Pupils	May be abnormal, either in size or response to light	Usually preserved light response (although pupil shape and reactivity affected in certain overdoses: see above)
Eye movements	May be affected	Usually preserved
Motor findings	Asymmetrical involvement	Abnormalities usually symmetrical
Involuntary movements	Not common	Asterixis, tremor, myoclonus frequently seen

Sepsis-associated encephalopathy (SAE) has been reported to occur in 8–80% of patients with sepsis.[22] The criteria to diagnose SAE include presence of impaired mental function, evidence of an extracranial infection and absence of other obvious aetiologies for the altered conscious state. Although the precise mechanism of damage to the brain has not been delineated, the pathogenesis of the encephalopathy is thought to be multifactorial: alteration in cerebral blood flow induced by mediators of inflammation, generation of free radicals by activated leukocytes resulting in erythrocyte sludging in the microcirculation, breakdown of the blood–brain barrier resulting in cerebral oedema, reduced brain oxygen consumption induced by endotoxin and cytokines, neuronal degeneration and increased neuronal apoptosis, increases in aromatic amino acids resulting in altered neurotransmitter function and increased gamma-aminobutyric acid (GABA)-mediated neurotransmission leading to general inhibition of the central nervous system. Hypotension may contribute to the encephalopathy. The asterixis, tremor and myoclonus – features of other metabolic encephalopathies – are uncommon in sepsis. The presence of lateralising signs are extremely rare in SAE and warrant exclusion of other causes, such as stroke. The mortality of patients with SAE is higher than in those with sepsis without encephalopathy.[23] Therapy is largely directed at the underlying septic process.

ICU ENCEPHALOPATHY OR ICU SYNDROME[24,25]

This is a term used to describe behavioural disorders which develop in patients 5–7 days after admission to intensive care. Clinically this may present as agitation, restlessness and frank delirium. The causes are multifactorial: prolonged ventilation, sleep deprivation,[26,27] distortion of perception with loss of day–night cycles, immobilisation, noisy environment and monotony. Coupled with administration of multiple sedatives and neurological consequences of the underlying disease, these factors can precipitate psychotic behaviour in the ICU. It is important to bear in mind that *this is a diagnosis of exclusion and that all other reversible causes are looked for (see Table 42.7)* before this diagnostic label is applied.

Abnormal behaviour can increase patient morbidity (self-extubation, ripping of catheters, soft-tissue damage). It is important to identify the underlying cause of the abnormal behaviour to institute appropriate therapy. Management of this condition may require the use of restraints, sedation and major tranquillisers. Improvement of sleep quality (minimising interruption of nocturnal sleep, adjusting lighting in the ICU), reducing patient boredom by the use of television and music and better communication with the patient may reduce the incidence and severity of this syndrome.

PROGNOSIS IN COMA

Drug-induced comas usually have a good prognosis unless hypoxia and hypotension have resulted in severe secondary insults. Coma following head injury has a statistically better outcome compared to non-traumatic coma (coma occurring during the course of a medical illness). In non-traumatic coma lasting for 6 hours or greater, only 15% of the patients make a meaningful recovery to be able to return to their premorbid state of health.[28] The prognosis following anoxic coma has been described in a separate section. Within the non-traumatic coma category, coma resulting from infection, metabolic causes and multiple-organ dysfunction syndrome has a better outcome compared to anoxic coma.[29] A number of outcome scales have been developed to assess neurological recovery following brain injury.[30] These include the Barthel index, Rankin scale and the Glasgow Outcome Scale (GOS). The GOS is widely used to assess recovery after traumatic brain injury. It has five broad categories: 1 = good recovery; 2 = moderate disability; 3 = severe disability; 4 = persistent vegetative state; and 5 = death. It is simple, easy to administer and has been reported to have good interrater agreement.

REFERENCES

1. Ropper A, Martin J. Coma and other disorders of consciousness. In: Isselbacher K (ed.) *Harrison's Principles of Internal Medicine.* Maidenhead and New York: McGraw Hill; 1994: 146–52.
2. Teasdale G, Jennett B. Assessment of coma and impaired consciousness. A practical scale. *Lancet* 1974; **2**: 81–4.
3. Adams R, Victor M, Ropper A. Coma and related disorders of consciousness. In: *Principles of Neurology.* New York: McGraw Hill; 1997: 344–66.
4. Keane JR. Retinal hemorrhages. Its significance in 100 patients with acute encephalopathy of unknown cause. *Arch Neurol* 1979; **36**: 691–4.
5. Keane J. Eye movements in coma. In: Jakbiec AA (ed.) *Principles and Practice of Ophthalmology.* Philadelphia, PA: WB Saunders; 2000: 4075–83.
6. Fisher C. Ocular bobbing. *Arch Neurol* 1964; **11**: 543.
7. Keane JR. Ocular skew deviation. Analysis of 100 cases. *Arch Neurol* 1975; **32**: 185–90.
8. North JB, Jennett S. Abnormal breathing patterns associated with acute brain damage. *Arch Neurol* 1974; **31**: 338–44.
9. Kernohan J, Woltman H. Incisura of the crus due to contralateral brain tumour. *Arch Neurol Psych* 1929; **21**: 274.
10. McNealy D, Plum F. Brainstem dysfunction with supratentorial mass lesions. *Arch Neurol* 1962; **7**: 10.
11. De Salles AA, Muizelaar JP, Young HF. Hyperglycemia, cerebrospinal fluid lactic acidosis, and cerebral blood flow in severely head-injured patients. *Neurosurgery* 1987; **21**: 45–50.
12. Penney DG. Hyperglycemia exacerbates brain damage in acute severe carbon monoxide poisoning. *Med Hypotheses* 1988; **27**: 241–4.
13. Van Den Berk G, Tonino S, De Fjtjer C *et al.* Bench to bedside review: preventive measures for contrast induced nephropathy in critically ill patients. *Crit Care* 2005; **9**: 361–70.
14. Venkatesh B, Scott P, Ziegenfuss M. Cerebrospinal fluid in critical illness. *Crit Care Resuscit* 2000; **2**: 43–55.
15. Bauer G. Coma and brain death. In: Niedermeyer E, Da Silva F (eds) *Electroencephalogrpahy: Basic Principles, Clinical Applications and Related Fields.* Baltimore, Williams & Wilkins; 1999, 459–75.
16. Nuwer MR. Continuous EEG monitoring in the intensive care unit. *Electroencephalogr Clin Neurophysiol* 1999; **50** (Suppl.): 150–5.
17. Zandbergen EG, de Haan RJ, Stoutenbeek CP *et al.* Systematic review of early prediction of poor outcome in anoxic-ischaemic coma. *Lancet* 1998; **352**: 1808–12.
18. Berger RP. The use of serum biomarkers to predict outcome after traumatic brain injury in adults and children. *J Head Trauma Rehabil* 2006; **21**: 315–33.
19. Chesnut RM, Marshall LF, Klauber MR *et al.* The role of secondary brain injury in determining outcome from severe head injury. *J Trauma* 1993; **34**: 216–22.
20. Kaplan PW. Electrophysiological prognostication and brain injury from cardiac arrest. *Semin Neurol* 2006; **26**: 403–12.
21. Stevens RD, Pronovost PJ. The spectrum of encephalopathy in critical illness. *Semin Neurol* 2006; **26**: 440–51.
22. Wilson JX, Young GB. Progress in clinical neurosciences: sepsis associated encephalopathy: evolving concepts. *Can J Neurol Sci* 2003; **30**: 98–105.
23. Eidelman LA, Putterman D, Putterman C *et al.* The spectrum of septic encephalopthy. Definiitons, etiologies and mortalities. *JAMA* 1996; **275**: 470–3.
24. McGuire BE, Basten CJ, Ryan CJ *et al.* Intensive care unit syndrome: a dangerous misnomer. *Arch Intern Med* 2000; **160**: 906–9.
25. Pun BT, Ely EW. The importance of diagnosing and managing ICU delirium. *Chest* 2007; **132**: 624–36.
26. Granberg Axell AI, Malmross CW, Bergbom IL *et al.* Intensive care unit syndrome/delirium is associated with anemia, drug therapy and duration of ventilation. *Acta Anaesthesiol Scand* 2002; **46**: 726–31.
27. Shilo L, Dagan Y, Smorjik Y *et al.* Patients in the intensive care unit suffer from severe lack of sleep associated with loss of normal melatonin secretion pattern. *Am J Med Sci* 1999; **317**: 278–81.
28. Plum F, Levy DE. Outcome from severe neurological illness; should it influence medical decisions? *Ciba Found Symp* 1979; **69**: 267–77.
29. Levy DE, Bates D, Caronna JJ *et al.* Prognosis in nontraumatic coma. *Ann Intern Med* 1981; **94**: 293–301.
30. Kasner SE. Clinical interpetation and use of stroke scales. *Lancet Neurol* 2006; **5**: 603–12.
31. Nordgren RE, Markesbery WR, Fukuda K *et al.* Seven cases of cerebromedullospinal disconnection: the 'locked-in' syndrome. *Neurology* 1971; **21**: 1140–8.
32. Multi Society Task Force on PVS. Medical aspects of the persistent vegetative state (1). *N Engl J Med* 1994; **330**: 1499–508.
33. Jennett B, Plum F. Persistent vegetative state after brain damage. A syndrome in search of a name. *Lancet* 1972; **1**: 734–7.
34. Cairns H, Oldfield R, Pennybacker K. Akinetic mutism with an epidermoid cyst of the third ventricle. *Brain* 1941; **64**: 273.
35. Stevens RD, Bhardwaj A. Approach to the comatose patient. *Crit Care Med* 2006; **34**: 31–41.
36. Berek K, Jeschow M, Aichner F. The prognostication of cerebral hypoxia after out-of-hospital cardiac arrest in adults. *Eur Neurol* 1997; **37**: 135–45.
37. Levy DE, Caronna JJ, Singer BH *et al.* Predicting outcome from hypoxic–ischemic coma. *JAMA* 1985; **253**: 1420–6.
38. Wijducks EF, Hijdra A, Young GB *et al.* Practice parameter; prediction of outcome in comatose survivors after cardiopulmonary resuscitation (an evidence based review): report of the quality standards subcommittee of the American Academy of Neurology. *Neurology* 2006; **67**: 203–10.

39. Surtees R, Leonard JV. Acute metabolic encephalopathy: a review of causes, mechanisms and treatment. *J Inherit Metab Dis* 1989; **12** (Suppl. 1): 42–54.
40. Uribarri J, Oh MS, Carroll HJ. D-lactic acidosis. A review of clinical presentation, biochemical features, and pathophysiologic mechanisms. *Medicine (Baltimore)* 1998; 77: 73–82.
41. Plum F. Sustained impairment of consciousness. In: Bennett CPF (ed.) *Cecil Textbook of Medicine*. Philadelphia: PA: WB Saunders; 1996: 1970–8.

43

Status epilepticus

Helen Ingrid Opdam

Status epilepticus (SE) is a medical emergency requiring prompt intervention to prevent the development of irreversible brain damage.

The duration of seizure activity required to define SE has not been universally agreed upon. Most authors have defined SE as more than 30 minutes' duration of either a single seizure, or intermittent seizures with no regaining of consciousness between seizures.[1–4] This definition is most useful for epidemiological research and is based on experimental studies that show that irreversible neuronal damage occurs after 30 minutes of seizure activity.[5,6]

More recently an operational definition of SE as 5 minutes of continuous seizure activity, or two or more discrete seizures with no intervening recovery of consciousness, has been used.[7] This definition promotes earlier diagnosis and treatment of SE. It has arisen from the generally accepted need to initiate treatment for SE rapidly and the observation that seizures persisting beyond this duration are unlikely to remit spontaneously.[8]

Refractory SE is defined as failure of initial therapy, such as benzodiazepines and phenytoin, with seizures persisting beyond 1–2 hours and usually requiring agents that induce general anaesthesia to control them.[9,10] Refractory SE is associated with a worse prognosis.[9,11]

SE is commonly separated into two categories:

1. Generalised convulsive SE (GCSE). Seizures are primary or secondarily generalised and the patient has generalised tonic and/or clonic convulsive movements with loss of consciousness.
2. Non-convulsive SE (NCSE). There is altered consciousness without convulsive movements but electroencephalography (EEG) evidence of seizures. NCSE may evolve from GCSE when electrical seizure activity continues with loss of motor manifestations. NCSE includes absence SE and complex partial SE.

The incidence of SE is U-shaped, being greatest under 1 year and over 60 years of age.[2]

PATHOPHYSIOLOGY

Ongoing or recurrent seizures result from failure of normal seizure-terminating mechanisms or excessive excitation causing seizure activity to persist. The major inhibitory mechanism in the brain is γ-aminobutyric acid A ($GABA_A$) receptor-mediated inhibition. Glutamatergic excitatory synaptic transmission is important in sustaining SE.[12]

The pathophysiological effects of seizures on the brain are thought to result from both direct excitotoxic neuronal injury and secondary injury due to systemic complications such as hypotension, hypoxia and hyperthermia. Ongoing excitation results in excessive intracellular calcium flux through the opening of NMDA (*N*-methyl-D-aspartate) receptor-mediated calcium channels, inducing a cascade of intracellular neurochemical events that damage or kill the cell.

AETIOLOGY

SE may occur de novo (approximately 60% of presentations) or, less commonly, in a previously diagnosed epileptic.[2] The aetiologies of SE, in decreasing order of frequency as they occur in adults, are given in Table 43.1.[2]

For SE that has its onset in the intensive care unit (ICU), the following should be considered as possible causes:

- drug withdrawal (narcotics, benzodiazepines, omission of anticonvulsant medications)
- metabolic disturbance (hyponatraemia, hypocalcaemia, hyperglycaemia, hypoglycaemia, uraemia, hepatic encephalopathy)
- drug toxicity (pethidine, theophylline, ciclosporin, tacrolimus, antibiotics, e.g. penicillins, cephalosporins, ciprofloxacin, imipenem in renal failure)
- stroke – vascular occlusion or haemorrhage

GENERALISED CONVULSIVE STATUS EPILEPTICUS

GCSE is the most common and dangerous type of SE and accounts for approximately 75% of cases.[2] It encompasses a broad spectrum of clinical presentations, from overt generalised tonic-clonic seizures to subtle convulsive movements in a profoundly comatose patient.[13]

Table 43.1 Causes of status epilepticus in adults

Low antiepileptic drug levels (poor compliance, recent dose reduction or discontinuation)
Temporally remote causes (previous central nervous system injury e.g. stroke, trauma, tumour, meningitis)
Stroke – vascular occlusion or haemorrhage
Cerebral hypoxia/anoxia
Metabolic disturbances (electrolyte abnormalities, uraemia, hyperglycaemia, hypoglycaemia)
Alcohol – withdrawal or intoxication
Central nervous system tumours – primary or secondary
Systemic infection
Idiopathic
Central nervous system infection – meningitis, encephalitis
Head trauma
Drug toxicity (tricyclic antidepressants, phenothiazines, theophylline, isoniazid, cocaine, amphetamine)

Table 43.2 Physiological changes in generalised convulsive status epilepticus[18,56]

Hypoxia
Respiratory acidosis
Lactic acidosis
Hyperpyrexia
Hypertension (early)/hypotension (late)
Hyperglycaemia (early)/hypoglycaemia (late)
Tachycardia
Cardiac arrhythmias
Blood leukocytosis
Cerebrospinal fluid pleocytosis, increased cerebrospinal fluid protein
Intracranial hypertension
Neurogenic pulmonary oedema
Aspiration pneumonitis
Rhabdomyolysis

CLINICAL

Typically, early in the evolution of seizures, patients are unresponsive with obvious tonic (sustained contractions) and/or clonic (rhythmic jerking) movements (overt GCSE). Motor manifestations may be symmetrical or asymmetrical.

With time, the clinical manifestations may become subtle, and patients have only small-amplitude twitching movements of the face, hands or feet or nystagmoid jerking of the eyes (late or subtle GCSE).[13]

Later still some patients will have no observable repetitive motor activity and the detection of ongoing seizures requires EEG (electrical GCSE). Most authors classify this as a form of NCSE.[14–16] Such patients are still at risk of central nervous system (CNS) injury and require prompt treatment.

EEG CHANGES

Just as there is a progression from overt to increasingly subtle motor manifestations, there is also a predictable sequence of EEG changes during untreated GCSE. Initially, discrete electrographic seizures merge to a waxing and waning pattern of seizure activity, followed by continuous monomorphic discharges, which become interspersed with increasing periods of electrographic silence and, eventually, periodic epileptiform discharges on a relatively flat background.[13,17] The presence of any of these EEG patterns should suggest the diagnosis of GSCE.

ENDOCRINE AND METABOLIC EFFECTS

Early in GCSE there is a marked increase in plasma catecholamines, producing systemic physiologic changes that resolve if SE is stopped early (Table 43.2). However, if seizures continue, many of these early physiologic changes reverse and the resultant hypotension and hypoglycaemia may exacerbate neurological injury.[18]

Hyperthermia is due to both muscle activity and central sympathetic drive, and thus may still occur when paralysing agents prevent motor activity. In early SE, both cerebral metabolic activity and cerebral blood flow (CBF) are increased. In late SE, although cerebral metabolic activity remains high, CBF may fall due to hypotension and loss of cerebral autoregulation, leading to cerebral ischaemia.

PSEUDOSEIZURES

An important differential diagnosis of generalised convulsive epilepsy is pseudoseizures. These can occur in patients with or without a history of epilepsy.[19] Clinical features suggestive of pseudoseizures are listed in Table 43.3. Distinction between the two may be extremely difficult, and can only be made with complete certainty using EEG monitoring.[19] Pseudo-status, misdiagnosed as true SE, is often refractory to initial therapy and can lead to patients receiving general anaesthesia and mechanical ventilation.

Table 43.3 Features suggestive of pseudoseizures

Lack of stereotyped seizures, with behavioural manifestations varying from event to event
Lack of sustained convulsive activity – 'on–off' appearance
Increase in movement if restraint is applied
Abolition of motor movements with reassurance or suggestion
Resistance to eye opening and gaze aversion
Poor response to treatment, refractory status epilepticus
Absence of pupillary dilatation
Normal tendon reflexes and plantar responses immediately after convulsion
Lack of metabolic consequences despite some hours of apparent fitting

NON-CONVULSIVE STATUS EPILEPTICUS

This may account for approximately 25% of SE, though its incidence is probably underestimated because of failure to recognise and diagnose the condition.

The diagnosis of NCSE should be considered in any patient with an unexplained altered conscious state, particularly those with CNS injury, metabolic disturbance, hepatic encephalopathy and sepsis. Series where EEG has been performed in critically ill patients with an unexplained depressed conscious state have found a high incidence of NCSE (8–18%).[20–22] EEG monitoring is required in patients with GCSE who do not recover consciousness after resolution of overt convulsive activity; in one study more than 14% of such patients had NCSE.[14]

Considerable debate exists regarding the precise criteria for diagnosing NCSE and published reports often describe diverse cohorts of patients. The diagnosis of NCSE generally requires a change in behaviour and/or mentation from baseline for at least 30 minutes, no overt seizure activity and an EEG with epileptiform discharges. A response to intravenous antiepileptic drugs (e.g. benzodiazepines), with clinical improvement and resolution or improvement in EEG epileptic activity, is helpful in confirming the diagnosis.[23]

Various classifications for NCSE have been suggested.[4,23–25] Traditionally NCSE is divided into absence SE (ASE) and complex partial SE (CPSE), though it may not always be possible to differentiate between the two types.[23,24]

ASE is characterised by bilateral diffuse synchronous seizures.[23] Typical ASE has generalised 3-Hz spike-wave discharge EEG activity occurring with altered behaviour or loss of responsiveness and is seen in children with idiopathic generalised epilepsy who are otherwise normal. This form of SE is relatively benign. Atypical ASE is a heterogeneous syndrome occurring in patients with mental retardation and epilepsy with multiple seizure types, or with other forms of diffuse cerebral dysfunction. The prognosis is usually poor and is related to the underlying condition.

CPSE, also referred to as 'epileptic twilight state' and 'temporal-lobe SE', is accompanied by lateralised seizure activity on EEG.[23] A wide variety of clinical features and degree of impairment of consciousness is possible and includes confusion, agitation, bizarre or aggressive behaviour and coma. Behavioural accompaniments such as lip smacking, automatisms and gaze deviation may occur, depending on the seizure origin within the brain. Debate exists over whether the seizure activity causes brain injury and much of the morbidity appears attributable to the underlying illness.

NCSE is often mistaken for other conditions, resulting in a delay in diagnosis and treatment. A high index of suspicion must therefore be present to trigger investigation with an EEG.

The differential diagnosis of NCSE is:

- metabolic encephalopathy
- drug intoxication
- cerebrovascular disease
- psychiatric syndromes (dissociative reactions, acute psychosis)
- postictal confusion

EPILEPTIFORM ENCEPHALOPATHIES

Some variants of SE deserve mention, such as comatose patients with epileptiform patterns on EEG who do not fit into the traditional classification of NCSE. Some of these cases may be late GCSE but many occur without prior clinical convulsions. In such situations it is unclear whether the abnormal discharges seen on the EEG are responsible for, or contribute to, the altered consciousness and abnormal movements, or are merely a reflection of a severe cerebral insult.[24]

Myoclonic SE that follows a hypoxic insult falls into this category. Patients have incessant, at times asynchronous, rhythmic jerks that may involve the entire body. This clinical appearance after an anoxic insult is associated with an extremely poor outcome.[26]

INVESTIGATIONS

Not all of the investigations listed in Table 43.4 need to be performed in every patient. The selection of tests depends on both the patient's history and presentation.

NEUROIMAGING

Most patients with SE should have a computed tomography (CT) scan of the brain performed at some point. Many patients with established epilepsy who have already been thoroughly evaluated do not require another brain-imaging procedure after an episode of SE.[1] However, if there is reason to suspect a new problem, and when the need for imaging is not urgent, magnetic resonance

Table 43.4 Investigations in status epilepticus

Initial studies
Blood glucose, electrolytes (sodium, potassium, calcium, magnesium), urea
Oximetry Spo_2 or arterial blood gases
Anticonvulsant drug levels
Full blood count
Urinalysis
Further investigations after stabilisation
Liver function tests, lactate, creatine kinase
Toxicology screen
Lumbar puncture
Electroencephalogram
Brain imaging with computed tomography or magnetic resonance imaging

imaging (MRI) may be preferable because it occasionally reveals abnormalities not visualised on CT scans. In children, emergent imaging is required if there is a persisting neurological deficit or abnormal mental state, and electively for focal seizures. Imaging should only be performed after control of SE and patient stabilisation.[27]

LUMBAR PUNCTURE

In any patient, especially in young children with fever and SE, CNS infection and lumbar puncture along with blood cultures should be considered. Meningitis is an uncommon cause of SE in adults and, unless the suspicion of CNS infection is high, brain imaging should be performed before a lumbar puncture. Contraindications to lumbar puncture include intracranial hypertension, mass lesion and hydrocephalus. If meningitis is suspected but a lumbar puncture cannot be performed expediently, antibiotics should be administered immediately rather than delayed. Approximately 20% of patients have a modest CSF white cell count pleocytosis after SE and such patients should be treated for suspected meningitis until the diagnosis is excluded by culture or other means.[1]

MANAGEMENT

GENERALISED CONVULSIVE STATUS EPILEPTICUS

An accurate history should be obtained, with particular emphasis on eye-witness accounts of the onset and nature of the seizures, and a full physical examination performed. However, neither should delay initial emergency management. There is evidence that the longer SE goes untreated, the harder it is to control with drugs.[28,29]

Management of SE involves termination and prevention of recurrence of seizures, treating precipitating causes and underlying conditions, and avoidance of complications.

Few controlled data are available to support the use of any particular agents. The most useful evidence comes from a randomised, double-blind clinical trial for treatment of GCSE which found that lorazepam, phenobarbital or diazepam followed by phenytoin are all acceptable as initial treatment, but that phenytoin alone was not as effective as lorazepam.[29] Another randomised controlled trial in the pre-hospital setting found intravenous lorazepam and diazepam to be equally effective and superior to placebo in terminating GCSE.[7]

The EEG goal of treatment for refractory SE remains controversial, with some advocating EEG background suppression (isoelectric) and others suppression of seizures regardless of the EEG background activity.[10,16,30]

Various protocols for SE management have been suggested.[1,16,30] One approach is outlined in Box 43.1.

NON-CONVULSIVE STATUS EPILEPTICUS

Patients with NCSE are a heterogeneous group who are likely to vary in their response to treatment depending on the underlying aetiology.[23]

There is considerable debate as to whether NCSE presents the same degree of risk of neurological injury as GCSE.[25] Prompt treatment is generally recommended and the use of additional non-anaesthetising anticonvulsants, such as phenobarbital and valproate, prior to embarking on general anaesthesia has been suggested.[16,23] Others recommend that, for comatose patients with NCSE, a similar treatment approach to GCSE be taken.[30]

The potential side-effects of aggressive treatment (hypotension, immunosuppression) need to be balanced against the potential neurologic morbidity of NCSE.[24,31] Particularly in elderly patients, aggressive treatment and anaesthesia may be associated with more risk than benefit and result in a worse outcome.[31,32]

Prognosis is most closely related to the underlying aetiology.[33]

DRUGS FOR STATUS EPILEPTICUS

BENZODIAZEPINES

Benzodiazepines are fast-acting antiseizure drugs and are therefore preferred as initial therapy. They act mainly by enhancing the neuroinhibitory effects of $GABA_A$. The efficacy of benzodiazepines may diminish with prolonged use in SE due to reduced receptor affinity for benzodiazepines.[12]

Diazepam is a highly lipid-soluble drug with rapid CNS penetration, but with a short duration of action. It can be administered intravenously or by the rectal route. Rectal administration can be achieved using a specially formulated rectal gel or the intravenous preparation can be diluted with an equal amount of saline and flushed into the rectum. Rectal administration should be considered when vascular access is delayed and may be particularly useful in the pre-hospital setting.

Lorazepam is less lipid-soluble than diazepam and after intravenous injection, brain and CSF levels rise at a slower rate than those of diazepam. However, a double-blind, randomised comparison of intravenous diazepam and lorazepam in SE in the pre-hospital setting found both drugs to be equally safe and effective.[7] Despite their equivalence as initial therapies, lorazepam has a longer duration of antiseizure effect than diazepam, and has a lower incidence of seizure recurrence when used alone.[1]

Midazolam has a short duration of action that may allow earlier assessment of the patient's postictal neurologic condition than longer-acting benzodiazepines. Midazolam has the advantage of being able to be administered via buccal, intranasal and intramuscular routes.

Box 43.1 **Protocol for management of status epilepticus**

1. Assess A, B, C, GCS
2. Give O_2 and consider need for intubation/ventilation
3. Monitor blood pressure, ECG, pulse oximetry
4. Obtain IV access and draw blood for investigations
5. If patient is hypoglycaemic, or if blood glucose estimation is not available, give glucose:
   Adults: give thiamine 100 mg IV and 50 ml of 50% glucose IV
   Children: give 2 ml/kg of 25% glucose IV
6. Seizure control:

   A. Give benzodiazepine,* for example:
      Diazepam 0.2 mg/kg IV at 5 mg/min up to total dose of 20 mg
      Lorazepam 0.1 mg/kg IV at 2 mg/min up to total dose of 10 mg
      Clonazepam 0.01–0.02 mg/kg IV at 0.5 mg/min up to total dose of 4 mg
      If diazepam stops the seizures, phenytoin should be given next to prevent recurrence
      Repeat dose every 2–5 min if required. Note: risk of respiratory depression with cumulative doses
   B. If seizures persist, give phenytoin:
      Phenytoin 15–20 mg/kg (adults ≤ 50 mg/min; children ≤ 1 mg/kg per min) or fosphenytoin 15–20 phenytoin equivalents (PE) mg/kg IV (adults ≤ 150 mg/min; children ≤ 3 mg/kg per min)
      Additional doses of 5 mg/kg IV, to a maximum dose of 30 mg/kg, can be given for persistent seizures
      Monitor blood pressure and ECG during infusion. If hypotension or arrhythmias develop, stop or slow the rate of the infusion
   C. If seizures persist (refractory status epilepticus), intubate and ventilate patient. Give either:
      Thiopental: slow bolus 3–5 mg/kg IV, followed by infusion 1–5 mg/kg per h *or*
      Propofol: slow bolus 1–2 mg/kg IV, followed by infusion 2–5 mg/kg per h† *or*
      Midazolam: slow bolus 0.1–0.2 mg/kg, followed by infusion 0.1–1.0 mg/kg per h
      Titrate doses based on clinical and electrographic evidence of seizures, targeting electrographic suppression of seizures or EEG background suppression (isoelectric)
      Monitor BP and maintain normotension by reducing infusion rate and/or giving fluids/pressor agents
   D. Insert nasogastric tube and administer usual anticonvulsant medications if patient is receiving treatment for pre-existing epilepsy
   E. Beware of ongoing unrecognised seizures
      Use EEG monitoring until seizures are controlled and then for 1–2 h after seizures stop. Continue to monitor the EEG continuously, or for periods of more than 30 min every 2 h, during the maintenance phase
      Avoid muscle relaxants (use continuous EEG if giving repeated doses of muscle relaxants)
   F. Discontinue midazolam or thiopental, or start reducing propofol, approximately 12 h after resolution of seizures. Use continuous EEG monitoring and observe for further clinical and/or EEG seizure activity. If seizures recur, reinstate the infusion and repeat this step at 12–24-h intervals or longer if the patient's seizures remain refractory

In addition:
Look for and treat cause and precipitant‡
Look for and treat complications: hypotension, hyperthermia, rhabdomyolysis

*If IV access is not obtainable, consider rectal diazepam, buccal/sublingual or intranasal or intramuscular midazolam, intramuscular fosphenytoin.
†High infusion rates for prolonged periods require caution.
‡In refractory status epilepticus, consider giving pyridoxine for children < 18 months or if isoniazid toxicity is suspected in adults.
GCS, Glasgow Coma Score; ECG, electrocardiogram; IV, intravenous; EEG, electroencephalogram; BP, blood pressure.

Intranasal midazolam is as effective as intravenous diazepam in children[34] and buccal midazolam is as effective as rectal diazepam in prolonged seizures.[35] Whereas intramuscular administration of diazepam and lorazepam is not recommended owing to their slow absorption, intramuscular midazolam is rapidly absorbed and in one study it was equally efficacious as intravenous diazepam in treating motor seizures in children.[36] These alternative routes of administration may be more convenient and acceptable than intravenous and rectal administration, particularly in the pre-hospital setting and when intravenous access is difficult.

Midazolam administered by bolus and infusion may terminate seizures when other agents have failed. It may also have fewer side-effects than alternative agents available for the treatment of refractory SE.[37] A limiting factor in its use is tachyphylaxis, which may necessitate a several-fold increase in the dose to maintain seizure control.[30] There is a wide variation in recommended infusion rates, from 0.1–0.4 mg/kg per hour[16] to 0.2–2.9 mg/kg per hour.[10]

Clonazepam has a longer duration of action than diazepam and is given by intravenous bolus. Early reports suggested that it has better efficacy and fewer side-effects than diazepam, though there are no published comparisons.

PHENYTOIN

Phenytoin is useful for maintaining a prolonged antiseizure effect after rapid termination of seizures with a benzodiazepine, or when benzodiazepines fail. When used alone as initial therapy phenytoin is not as efficacious as benzodiazepines for terminating seizures.[29]

The recommended intravenous loading dose is 20 mg/kg. The common practice of giving a standard loading dose of 1000 mg of phenytoin may provide inadequate therapy for some adults.

When phenytoin is infused at the maximal adult recommended rate of 50 mg/min, hypotension occurs in up to 50% of patients and cardiac rhythm disturbance occurs in 2%. These adverse effects are more common in older patients and those with cardiac disease and are due to the phenytoin itself as well as the propylene glycol diluent. Blood pressure and the ECG should be monitored during infusion of phenytoin and the infusion slowed or stopped if cardiovascular complications occur.

Intramuscular administration of phenytoin is not recommended as absorption is erratic and it can cause local tissue reactions.

Fosphenytoin, a new water-soluble prodrug of phenytoin, is converted to phenytoin by endogenous phosphatases.[38] Doses of fosphenytoin are expressed as phenytoin equivalents (PE). Fosphenytoin can be administered at rates of up to 150 PE mg/min, since it is not formulated with propylene glycol, allowing therapeutic serum concentrations of fosphenytoin to be attained within 10 minutes. However, this may not necessarily result in more rapid CNS penetration and onset of action.[39]

Systemic side-effects are similar for phenytoin and fosphenytoin, although reactions at the infusion site are less common with fosphenytoin.[38]

Fosphenytoin can also be administered intramuscularly, though absorption is slower than intravenous administration, and this route should only be used when intravenous access is not possible.

SODIUM VALPROATE

There are reports of intravenous valproate being used to treat both GCSE and NCSE in adults and children. It is non-sedating and it appears to be well tolerated with few reports of hypotension or respiratory depression.[40] An initial dose of 25–45 mg/kg administered at a maximum rate of up to 6 mg/kg per min has been recommended.[16] The exact role of valproate in the management of SE remains to be established and there are insufficient data to recommend its use before phenytoin.

BARBITURATES

Phenobarbital is a potent anticonvulsant with a long duration of action. The usual dose is 15–20 mg/kg intravenously. It has equal efficacy to benzodiazepines and phenytoin when used first-line, but may cause greater depression of respiration, blood pressure and consciousness and therefore is often only used if these agents fail. However, many would advocate alternative and more aggressive measures for treatment of refractory SE at this point as the likelihood of phenobarbital controlling seizures when these other agents have failed is small.[10,15]

Thiopental is an intravenous anaesthetic agent used for refractory SE. A dose of 3–5 mg/kg is usually given for intubation, followed by repeated doses of 0.5–1 mg/kg until seizures are controlled. Following bolus intravenous administration, the drug is rapidly redistributed into peripheral fat stores and an infusion of 1–5 mg/kg per hour is required for ongoing suppression of seizures. Once lipid stores are saturated the duration of action is prolonged and recovery may take hours to days. Prolonged therapy requires the use of EEG monitoring to ensure that the seizures remain suppressed and to allow titration to the lowest dose that achieves the EEG target of seizure and/or EEG background suppression. Side-effects include hypotension, myocardial depression and immunosuppression with increased risk of infection.

Pentobarbital (the first metabolite of thiopental) is available in the USA as the alternative to thiopental.

Compared with other agents used in refractory SE (midazolam and propofol), barbiturates may result in a lower frequency of short-term treatment failure and breakthrough seizures but more hypotension and slower recovery from anaesthesia.[41]

PROPOFOL

Propofol (2,6-diisopropylphenol) is an anaesthetic agent that has become increasingly popular for the treatment of refractory SE. It is administered as an intravenous bolus followed by infusion and intubation and ventilation are required.

Compared with high-dose barbiturates (pentobarbital) in adult patients with refractory SE, propofol has been found to control seizures more quickly and, because of its shorter duration of action, allows earlier re-emergence from anaesthesia.[42] However, seizures tend to recur with sudden discontinuation of propofol, necessitating recommencement of the infusion and a more gradual tapering of the dose, such that both drugs may ultimately result in similar duration of ventilation and ICU stay.[42]

There is concern that prolonged high-dose propofol use (e.g. > 5 mg/kg per hour) may result in myocardial failure, hypoxia, metabolic acidosis, lipaemia, rhabdomyolysis and death (propofol infusion syndrome).[43] Initial reports were in children but later also adults and, as such, its use requires caution. There are series, however, of prolonged high-dose propofol use in adults with SE without major adverse effects.[44]

NEUROMUSCULAR-BLOCKING AGENTS

Paralysis is indicated if uncontrolled fitting causes difficulty with providing adequate ventilation or severe lactic acidosis. Neuromuscular blockade should only be used if continuous EEG monitoring is available, as the clinical expression of seizure activity is abolished.

OTHER AGENTS OF POTENTIAL USE IN REFRACTORY STATUS EPILEPTICUS

Ketamine may be a useful adjuvant in the treatment of refractory SE.[45] The newer antiepileptic drugs such as topiramate may also have a role in refractory SE treatment.[46] Inhalational anaesthetic agents such as isoflurane may also be useful.[47]

SURGERY

Surgery has occasionally been used in refractory SE with procedures based on standard epilepsy surgery techniques. Some success has been reported with focal resections, subpial transection, corpus callosotomy, hemispherectomy and vagus nerve stimulation.[48–50]

INTENSIVE CARE MONITORING

Monitoring using ECG, intra-arterial and central venous catheters, capnography and pulse oximetry should be considered in patients with, or at risk of, cardiorespiratory compromise. Indications for EEG monitoring are listed in Table 43.5. Cerebral function monitors are useful in titrating doses of anaesthetic agents to EEG background suppression, but may not have sufficient sensitivity to detect seizure activity at other times. Intracranial pressure monitoring should be considered if elevated intracranial pressure is suspected.

Table 43.5 Indications for electroencephalogram (EEG) monitoring[14]

Refractory status epilepticus, to aid the titration of anticonvulsant anaesthetic drugs (minimising dose and toxicity) and ensure suppression of seizure activity*
Patients receiving neuromuscular blockade*
Patients who continue to have a poor conscious state after apparent cessation of seizures
Suspected non-convulsive status epilepticus in a patient with an altered conscious state
Suspected pseudoseizures

*Continuous or regular intermittent EEG monitoring is recommended.

OUTCOME

The prognosis of patients with SE is most strongly related to age and aetiology.[3,33] Overall 30-day mortality is 15–20%.[3,4] Children have a much lower mortality of 3%[51] whereas those aged over 65 years have a mortality rate of 30%.[3,4] SE that is precipitated by low antiepileptic drug levels or systemic infection has a very low mortality.[3] Patients who develop SE secondary to an acute CNS or systemic metabolic insult have a higher mortality than those who develop SE without a clear precipitant.[3] SE precipitated by hypoxia is usually fatal.[26] NCSE detected in comatose critically ill patients, despite recognition and treatment, has a poor outcome.[22,32] Refractory SE carries a worse prognosis that is mainly determined by the underlying cause.[9,11]

The duration of SE and time to provision of adequate treatment are also important factors that may influence the ease with which seizures can be controlled, the risk of residual neurological deficits and mortality.[9,28,29] The degree of impairment of consciousness at presentation may also be an important factor influencing outcome.[4]

The EEG may provide useful prognostic information, with periodic epileptiform discharges present at any time during or after SE being associated with a worse outcome.[52]

Neurone-specific enolase (NSE) is a well-studied marker of brain injury and high serum levels have been found in GCSE and NCSE, particularly CPSE.[53] Elevated levels may reflect either the severity of brain injury resulting from SE, the underlying brain pathology, or both. Increases in serum NSE have been correlated with the duration and prognosis of GCSE.[53]

STATUS EPILEPTICUS IN CHILDREN

The majority of paediatric cases of SE occur in young children, with 80% occurring in those below 4 years of age.[51] The vast majority of cases are convulsive and generalised.[27]

The distribution of causes is highly age dependent, with febrile SE and that due to acute neurological disease (e.g. CNS infection) being more common in children under 4 years. Remote symptomatic causes and SE in a child with previously diagnosed epilepsy are more common in older children.[51] The most frequent aetiologies of SE in children are listed in Table 43.6.[27,51]

The likelihood of bacterial meningitis is much higher (12%) in febrile children presenting with a first-ever episode of SE as opposed to a brief seizure (1%) and a high index of suspicion is required to investigate and treat for meningitis.[51]

Table 43.6 Causes of status epilepticus in children[27,51]

Febrile (previously neurologically normal, temperature > 38°C, central nervous system infection excluded)
Acute symptomatic – meningitis, encephalitis, trauma, metabolic derangement, hypoxia, drug-related, cerebrovascular disease
Remote symptomatic causes – previous traumatic brain injury or cerebral insult, central nervous system malformation, cerebral palsy
Progressive neurologic conditions
Cryptogenic

Treatment of SE in children is essentially the same as in adults.[54]

The underlying cause is the main determinant of mortality, which is negligible for prolonged febrile seizures and 12–16% for acute symptomatic causes.[55] Similarly, the risk of subsequent epilepsy is low in neurologically normal children but higher than 50% in those with acute or remote symptomatic causes.[55]

REFERENCES

1. Treatment of convulsive status epilepticus. Recommendations of the Epilepsy Foundation of America's Working Group on Status Epilepticus. *JAMA* 1993; **270**: 854–9.
2. DeLorenzo RJ, Hauser WA, Towne AR *et al.* A prospective, population-based epidemiologic study of status epilepticus in Richmond, Virginia. *Neurology* 1996; **46**: 1029–35.
3. Logroscino G, Hesdorffer DC, Cascino G *et al.* Short-term mortality after a first episode of status epilepticus. *Epilepsia* 1997; **38**: 1344–9.
4. Rossetti AO, Hurwitz S, Logroscino G *et al.* Prognosis of status epilepticus: role of aetiology, age, and consciousness impairment at presentation. *J Neurol Neurosurg Psychiatry* 2006; **77**: 611–15.
5. Meldrum BS, Brierley JB. Prolonged epileptic seizures in primates. Ischemic cell change and its relation to ictal physiological events. *Arch Neurol* 1973; **28**: 10–17.
6. ILAE Commission Report. The epidemiology of the epilepsies: future directions. International League Against Epilepsy. *Epilepsia* 1997; **38**: 614–18.
7. Alldredge BK, Gelb AM, Isaacs SM *et al.* A comparison of lorazepam, diazepam, and placebo for the treatment of out-of-hospital status epilepticus [see comment] [erratum appears in *N Engl J Med* 2001; **345**: 1860]. *N Engl J Med* 2001; **345**: 631–7.
8. Shinnar S, Berg AT, Moshe SL *et al.* How long do new-onset seizures in children last? *Ann Neurol* 2001; **49**: 659–64.
9. Mayer SA, Claassen J, Lokin J *et al.* Refractory status epilepticus: frequency, risk factors, and impact on outcome. *Arch Neurol* 2002; **59**: 205–10.
10. Bleck TP. Refractory status epilepticus. *Curr Opin Crit Care* 2005; **11**: 117–20.
11. Rossetti AO, Logroscino G, Bromfield EB. Refractory status epilepticus: effect of treatment aggressiveness on prognosis. *Arch Neurol* 2005; **62**: 1698–702.
12. Macdonald RL, Kapur J. Acute cellular alterations in the hippocampus after status epilepticus. *Epilepsia* 1999; **40**: S9–20; discussion S21–2.
13. Treiman DM. Electroclinical features of status epilepticus. *J Clin Neurophysiol* 1995; **12**: 343–62.
14. DeLorenzo RJ, Waterhouse EJ, Towne AR *et al.* Persistent nonconvulsive status epilepticus after the control of convulsive status epilepticus. *Epilepsia* 1998; **39**: 833–40.
15. Dhar R, Mirsattari SM. Current approach to the diagnosis and treatment of refractory status epilepticus. *Adv Neurol* 2006; **97**: 245–54.
16. Meierkord H, Boon P, Engelsen B *et al.* EFNS guideline on the management of status epilepticus. *Eur J Neurol* 2006; **13**: 445–50.
17. Kaplan PW. The EEG of status epilepticus. *J Clin Neurophysiol* 2006; **23**: 221–9.
18. Walton NY. Systemic effects of generalized convulsive status epilepticus. *Epilepsia* 1993; **34**: S54–8.
19. Betts T. Pseudoseizures: seizures that are not epilepsy. *Lancet* 1990; **336**: 163–4.
20. Towne AR, Waterhouse EJ, Boggs JG *et al.* Prevalence of nonconvulsive status epilepticus in comatose patients. *Neurology* 2000; **54**: 340–5.
21. Claassen J, Mayer SA, Kowalski RG *et al.* Detection of electrographic seizures with continuous EEG monitoring in critically ill patients. *Neurology* 2004; **62**: 1743–8.
22. Pandian JD, Cascino GD, So EL *et al.* Digital video-electroencephalographic monitoring in the neurological–neurosurgical intensive care unit: clinical features and outcome. *Arch Neurol* 2004; **61**: 1090–4.
23. Kaplan PW. The clinical features, diagnosis, and prognosis of nonconvulsive status epilepticus. *Neurologist* 2005; **11**: 348–61.
24. Krumholz A. Epidemiology and evidence for morbidity of nonconvulsive status epilepticus. *J Clin Neurophysiol* 1999; **16**: 314–22; discussion 353.
25. Kaplan PW. No, some types of nonconvulsive status epilepticus cause little permanent neurologic sequelae (or: "the cure may be worse than the disease"). *Neurophysiol Clin* 2000; **30**: 377–82.
26. Wijdicks EF, Hijdra A, Young GB *et al.* Practice parameter: prediction of outcome in comatose survivors after cardiopulmonary resuscitation (an evidence-based review): report of the Quality Standards Subcommittee of the American Academy of Neurology. *Neurology* 2006; **67**: 203–10.
27. Riviello JJ Jr, Ashwal S, Hirtz D *et al.* Practice parameter: diagnostic assessment of the child with status epilepticus (an evidence-based review): report of the Quality Standards Subcommittee of the American Academy of Neurology and the Practice Committee of the Child Neurology Society. *Neurology* 2006; **67**: 1542–50.

28. Lowenstein DH, Alldredge BK. Status epilepticus at an urban public hospital in the 1980s. *Neurology* 1993; **43**: 483–8.
29. Treiman DM, Meyers PD, Walton NY *et al.* A comparison of four treatments for generalized convulsive status epilepticus Veterans. Affairs Status Epilepticus Cooperative Study Group. *N Engl J Med* 1998; **339**: 792–8.
30. Marik PE, Varon J. The management of status epilepticus. *Chest* 2004; **126**: 582–91.
31. Walker MC. Status epilepticus on the intensive care unit. *J Neurol* 2003; **250**: 401–6.
32. Litt B, Wityk RJ, Hertz SH *et al.* Nonconvulsive status epilepticus in the critically ill elderly. *Epilepsia* 1998; **39**: 1194–202.
33. Shneker BF, Fountain NB. Assessment of acute morbidity and mortality in nonconvulsive status epilepticus. *Neurology* 2003; **61**: 1066–73.
34. Mahmoudian T, Zadeh MM. Comparison of intranasal midazolam with intravenous diazepam for treating acute seizures in children. *Epilepsy Behav* 2004; **5**: 253–5.
35. Scott RC, Besag FM, Neville BG. Buccal midazolam and rectal diazepam for treatment of prolonged seizures in childhood and adolescence: a randomised trial. *Lancet* 1999; **353**: 623–6.
36. Chamberlain JM, Altieri MA, Futterman C *et al.* A prospective, randomized study comparing intramuscular midazolam with intravenous diazepam for the treatment of seizures in children. *Pediatr Emerg Care* 1997; **13**: 92–4.
37. Prasad A, Worrall BB, Bertram EH *et al.* Propofol and midazolam in the treatment of refractory status epilepticus. *Epilepsia* 2001; **42**: 380–6.
38. Browne TR. Fosphenytoin (Cerebyx). *Clin Neuropharmacol* 1997; **20**: 1–12.
39. Walton NY, Uthman BM, El Yafi K *et al.* Phenytoin penetration into brain after administration of phenytoin or fosphenytoin. *Epilepsia* 1999; **40**: 153–6.
40. Limdi NA, Shimpi AV, Faught E *et al.* Efficacy of rapid IV administration of valproic acid for status epilepticus. *Neurology* 2005; **64**: 353–5.
41. Claassen J, Hirsch LJ, Emerson RG *et al.* Treatment of refractory status epilepticus with pentobarbital, propofol, or midazolam: a systematic review. *Epilepsia* 2002; **43**: 146–53.
42. Stecker MM, Kramer TH, Raps EC *et al.* Treatment of refractory status epilepticus with propofol: clinical and pharmacokinetic findings. *Epilepsia* 1998; **39**: 18–26.
43. Vasile B, Rasulo F, Candiani A *et al.* The pathophysiology of propofol infusion syndrome: a simple name for a complex syndrome. *Intens Care Med* 2003; **29**: 1417–25.
44. Rossetti AO, Reichhart MD, Schaller MD *et al.* Propofol treatment of refractory status epilepticus: a study of 31 episodes. *Epilepsia* 2004; **45**: 757–63.
45. Nathan BN, Smith TL, Bleck TP. The use of ketamine in refractory status epilepticus. *Neurology* 2002; **58**: A197.
46. Towne AR, Garnett LK, Waterhouse EJ *et al.* The use of topiramate in refractory status epilepticus. *Neurology* 2003; **60**: 332–4.
47. Mirsattari SM, Sharpe MD, Young GB. Treatment of refractory status epilepticus with inhalational anesthetic agents isoflurane and desflurane. *Arch Neurol* 2004; **61**: 1254–9.
48. Ma X, Liporace J, O'Connor MJ *et al.* Neurosurgical treatment of medically intractable status epilepticus. *Epilepsy Res* 2001; **46**: 33–8.
49. Duane DC, Ng YT, Rekate HL *et al.* Treatment of refractory status epilepticus with hemispherectomy. *Epilepsia* 2004; **45**: 1001–4.
50. Winston KR, Levisohn P, Miller BR *et al.* Vagal nerve stimulation for status epilepticus. *Pediatr Neurosurg* 2001; **34**: 190–2.
51. Chin RF, Neville BG, Peckham C *et al.* Incidence, cause, and short-term outcome of convulsive status epilepticus in childhood: prospective population-based study. *Lancet* 2006; **368**: 222–9.
52. Nei M, Lee JM, Shanker VL *et al.* The EEG and prognosis in status epilepticus. *Epilepsia* 1999; **40**: 157–63.
53. DeGiorgio CM, Heck CN, Rabinowicz AL *et al.* Serum neuron-specific enolase in the major subtypes of status epilepticus. *Neurology* 1999; **52**: 746–9.
54. Prasad AN, Seshia SS. Status epilepticus in pediatric practice: neonate to adolescent. *Adv Neurol* 2006; **97**: 229–43.
55. Raspall-Chaure M, Chin RF, Neville BG *et al.* Outcome of paediatric convulsive status epilepticus: a systematic review. *Lancet Neurol* 2006; **5**: 769–79.
56. Simon RP. Physiologic consequences of status epilepticus. *Epilepsia* 1985; **26**: S58–66.

44

Acute cerebrovascular complications

Bernard Riley

Cerebrovascular disease is common and its acute manifestations, known as stroke, produce considerable morbidity and mortality. Stroke is defined as an acute focal neurological deficit caused by cerebrovascular disease, which lasts for more than 24 hours or causes death before 24 hours. Transient ischaemic attack (TIA) also causes focal neurology, but this resolves within 24 hours. In the UK, stroke is responsible for 12% of all deaths and is the most common cause of physical disability in adults. The incidence in most developed countries is about 1–2/1000 population per year.[1] The main causes of stroke are cerebral infarction as a consequence of thromboembolism and spontaneous intracranial haemorrhage (either intracerebral or subarachnoid haemorrhage (SAH)), causing about 85% and 15% of strokes, respectively. The main risk factors are increasing age, hypertension, ischaemic heart disease, atrial fibrillation, smoking, obesity, some oral contraceptives and raised cholesterol or haematocrit. The manifestations of stroke are:

- cerebral infarction
  - thrombosis
  - embolism
- spontaneous intracranial haemorrhage
  - intracerebral haemorrhage
  - SAH

PROGNOSIS IN ACUTE CEREBROVASCULAR DISEASE

Mortality after stroke averages 30% within a month, with more patients dying after SAH or intracerebral haemorrhage than after cerebral infarction, although survival to 1 year is slightly better in the haemorrhagic group. In all types of stroke about 30% of survivors remain disabled to the point of being dependent on others. Risk of stroke increases with age, so that it rises from 3/100 000 in the third and fourth decades to 300/100 000 in the eighth and ninth decades.[2] Thus stroke is often accompanied by significant age-related medical comorbidity. In the past this may have been partially responsible for a relatively non-aggressive approach to the treatment of stroke patients, so that the gloomy prognosis of stroke becomes a self-fulfilling prophecy. The challenge for intensivists is to identify those patients who are most likely to survive and not to offer aggressive therapy to those who are not. It has been suggested that, by regarding stroke as a medical emergency, a 'brain attack' analogous to 'heart attack', and ensuring early intensive care support, outcome may be improved.[3,4]

CEREBRAL INFARCTION

Infarction of cerebral tissue occurs as a result of inadequate perfusion from occlusion of cerebral blood vessels in association with inadequate collateral circulation. It may occur due to cerebral thrombosis or embolism.

AETIOLOGY AND PATHOLOGY

CEREBRAL THROMBOSIS

Atherosclerosis is the major cause of major arterial occlusion and most often produces symptoms if it occurs at the bifurcation of the carotid artery or the carotid syphon. Progressive plaque formation causes narrowing and forms a nidus for platelet aggregation and thrombus formation. Ulceration and rupture of the plaque expose its thrombogenic lipid core, activating the clotting cascade. Hypertension and diabetes mellitus are common causes of smaller arterial thrombosis. Rarer causes of thrombosis include any disease resulting in vasculitis, vertebral or carotid artery dissection (either spontaneous or posttraumatic) or carotid occlusion by strangulation or systemic hypotension after cardiac arrest. Cerebral venous thrombosis, responsible for less than 1% of strokes, may occur in hypercoagulable states such as dehydration, polycythaemia, thrombocythaemia, some oral contraceptive pills, protein C or S deficiency or antithrombin III deficiency, or vessel occlusion by tumour or abscess. Cerebral infarction may also result from sustained systemic hypotension from any cause, particularly if associated with hypoxaemia.

CEREBRAL EMBOLISM

Embolism commonly occurs from thrombus or platelet aggregations overlying arterial atherosclerotic plaques, but 30% of cerebral emboli will arise from thrombus in the left atrium or ventricle of the heart. This is very likely in the presence of atrial fibrillation, left-sided valvular disease, recent myocardial infarction, chronic atrial enlargement or ventricular aneurysm. The presence of a patent foramen ovale or septal defects allows paradoxical embolism to occur. Iatrogenic air embolism may occur during cardiopulmonary bypass, cardiac catheterisation or cerebral angiography. Embolisation may also occur as a complication of attempted coil embolisation of cerebral aneurysms or arteriovenous malformations (AVMs) after SAH.

CLINICAL PRESENTATION

In cerebral thrombosis, there is initially no loss of consciousness or headache and the initial neurological deficit develops over several hours. Cerebral embolism may be characterised by sudden onset and rapid development of complete neurological deficit. No single clinical sign or symptom can reliably distinguish a thrombotic from an embolic event. Where infarction occurs in a limited arterial territory the clinical signs are often characteristic. The commonest site involves the middle cerebral artery, which classically produces acute contralateral brachiofacial hemiparesis with sensory or motor deficits, depending on the precise area of infarction.

- Infarction of the middle cerebral territory leads to a dense contralateral hemiplegia, contralateral facial paralysis, contralateral hemianopia and ipsilateral eye deviation.
- Dominant left-hemisphere lesions result in language difficulties from aphasia, dysphasia, dysgraphia and dyscalculia.
- Non-dominant right hemispheric lesions cause the patient to neglect the left side, and may not communicate with anyone approaching from that side.
- In strokes involving the posterior fossa the precise pattern of symptoms depends on the arterial territories involved and the presence or absence of collaterals. The onset of symptoms such as gait disturbance, headache, nausea, vomiting and loss of consciousness may be very rapid.
- Venous thrombosis may occur particularly in the cerebral veins, sagittal or transverse dural sinuses, causing headache, seizures, focal neurology and loss of consciousness.

Other cognitive effects of stroke include memory impairment, anxiety, depression, emotional lability, aprosody and spatial impairment. Bilateral brainstem infarction after basilar artery thrombosis may produce deep coma and tetraparesis. Pontine stroke may produce the 'locked-in' syndrome. The precise clinical presentation depends on the size of the infarcted area and its position in the brain.

INVESTIGATIONS

A full history and examination of the patient are required, and the results of this will produce a differential diagnosis that will require specific investigations. The aim is to make the diagnosis, establish the nature, size and position of the pathology, so that correct treatment can be administered to compensate for the effects of the primary injury, and prevent extension of the lesion or complications occurring.

BLOOD TESTS

Haemoglobin, white cell count and platelets are determined to look for polycythaemia, infection or thrombocythaemia. A raised erythrocyte sedimentation rate or C-reactive protein level may indicate vasculitis, infection or carcinoma, warranting further appropriate investigations.

Coagulation screen should be taken together with serum cholesterol, triglyceride and syphilis serology. Specific investigation for thrombophilia due to protein C, protein S, Leiden factor V and antithrombin III abnormalities should be undertaken in patients with venous thrombosis or patients with otherwise unexplained cerebral infarction or TIA.

ELECTROCARDIOGRAPHY

This may demonstrate atrial fibrillation or other arrhythmia, or recent myocardial infarct.

ECHOCARDIOGRAPHY

Either transthoracic or transoesophageal echocardiography (TOE) may demonstrate mural or atrial appendage thrombus as a source of embolism. TOE is more effective in detecting patent foramen ovale, aortic arteriosclerosis or dissection.

COMPUTED TOMOGRAPHY (CT) OR MAGNETIC RESONANCE IMAGING (MRI) SCANNING

These techniques are used to distinguish infarction from haemorrhage. Tumour, abscess or subdural haematoma may also produce the symptoms and signs of stroke. Ideally, the scans should be undertaken as soon as possible to exclude conditions that are treatable by neurosurgery. Early scanning is vital if interventional treatment such as thrombolysis, anticoagulation, antiplatelet therapy or surgery is planned.

The CT scan may be normal or show only minor loss of grey/white matter differentiation in the first 24 hours after ischaemic stroke but haemorrhage is seen as areas of increased attenuation within minutes. After a couple of weeks the CT appearances of an infarct or haemorrhage become very similar and it may be impossible to distinguish them if CT is delayed beyond this time. CT angiography will often demonstrate vascular abnormalities and vasospasm but multimodal MRI, a combination of diffusion and perfusion-weighted MRI and MR angiography (MRA), is much more sensitive in demonstrating small areas of ischaemia and targeting those patients most suitable for thrombolysis.[5] Where cerebral infarction has occurred as a result of venous thrombosis, the best imaging technique is MRA. Other imaging techniques are appropriate to identify the source of stroke in specific areas. Any patient with a stroke or TIA in the internal carotid artery territory should have duplex Doppler ultrasonography which may demonstrate stenosis, occlusion or dissection of the internal carotid. Where trauma is an aetiological factor reconstruction CT bone window views.

MANAGEMENT

Ideally, treatment for stroke patients should be coordinated within a stroke unit, as there is a 28% reduction in mortality and disability at 3 months compared to patients treated on general medical wards.[6] In general only those patients with a compromised airway due to depressed level of consciousness or life-threatening cardiorespiratory disturbances require admission to medical or neurosurgical ICUs. In either case, attention to basic resuscitation, involving stabilisation of airway, breathing and circulation, is self-evident.

AIRWAY AND BREATHING

Patients with Glasgow Coma Scores (GCS) of 8 or less or those with absent gag will require intubation to preserve their airway and prevent aspiration. Where this requirement is likely to be prolonged, early tracheostomy should be considered. Adequate oxygenation and ventilation should be confirmed by arterial blood gas analysis, and supplemental oxygen prescribed if there is any evidence of hypoxia. If hypercarbia occurs then ventilatory support to achieve normocarbia is necessary to prevent exacerbation of cerebral oedema. Ventilatory support in such cases has been shown to result in improved prognosis.[7]

CIRCULATORY SUPPORT

A large number of stroke patients will have raised blood pressure on admission, presumably as an attempt by the vasomotor centre to improve cerebral perfusion. Hypertensive patients may have impaired autoregulation and regional cerebral perfusion may be very dependent on blood pressure.[8] The patient's clinical condition and neurological status should determine treatment rather than an arbitrary level of blood pressure. Control of even very high blood pressure (220/120 mmHg; 29.3/16.0 kPa) is not without risk and may result in progression of ischaemic stroke, so reduction should be monitored closely.[9] It would seem reasonable on physiological grounds to avoid drugs that cause cerebral vasodilatation in that they may aggravate cerebral oedema, although there is no hard evidence for this. Animal experiments have suggested that haemodilution could improve blood flow by reducing whole blood viscosity but a recent multicentre study has failed to identify any clinical benefit.[10] Cardiac output should be maintained and any underlying cardiac pathology such as failure, infarction and atrial fibrillation treated appropriately.

METABOLIC SUPPORT

Both hypo- and hyperglycaemia have been shown to worsen prognosis after acute stroke, therefore blood sugar levels should be maintained in the normal range.[11] In the long term, nutritional support must not be neglected and early enteral feeding instituted by nasogastric intubation. In the longer term, particularly where bulbar function is reduced, percutaneous endoscopic gastrostomy is necessary.

ANTICOAGULATION

In theory, the use of anticoagulation reduces the propagation of thrombus and should prevent further embolism. In practice, the reduction in risk of further thromboembolic stroke is offset by a similar number of patients dying from cerebral or systemic haemorrhage as a result of anticoagulation.[12,13] Anticoagulation can only be recommended in individuals where there is a high risk of recurrence, such as in those patients with prosthetic heart valves, atrial fibrillation with thrombus or those with thrombophilic disorders. A CT scan must be obtained prior to commencing therapy to exclude haemorrhage, and careful monitoring used. In patients with large infarcts there is always the risk of haemorrhage (haemorrhagic conversion) into the infarct and early heparinisation is best avoided.

THROMBOLYSIS

Systemic thrombolysis with streptokinase carries a very high risk of cerebral haemorrhage and should not be used.[14] There is some evidence that intravenous recombinant tissue plasminogen activator (alteplase) has a better safety/efficacy profile. The National Institute of Neurological Disorders and Stroke (NINDS) trial showed a significant improvement in those patients given alteplase rather than placebo within 3 hours of acute stroke.[15] This benefit was not found to be statistically significant in two European trials[16,17] and the ATLANTIS trial showed no significant benefit at 90 days in the alteplase group together with an increased risk of intracranial haemorrhage.[18] The 2006 Cochrane Library database states that thrombolysis appears to result in a significant net reduction in the proportion of patients dead or dependent in activities of daily living. However, there appears to be an increase in deaths within the first 7–10 days, symptomatic intracranial haemorrhage and deaths at follow-up at 3–6 months. The data from trials using intravenous recombinant tissue plasminogen activator, from which there is the most evidence on thrombolytic therapy so far, suggest that it may be associated with less hazard and more benefit. There is heterogeneity between the published trials for some outcomes so that the optimum criteria to identify patients most likely to benefit and least likely to be harmed, the latest time window, the agent, dose and route of administration are all unclear. Nevertheless, the data are promising and may justify the use of thrombolytic therapy with intravenous recombinant tissue plasminogen activator in experienced centres in highly selected patients where a licence exists. However, the data do not support the widespread use of thrombolytic therapy in routine clinical practice at this time, but suggest that further trials are needed to identify which patients are most likely to benefit from treatment and the environment in which it may best be given.[19]

CEREBRAL PROTECTION

Various agents such as free-radical scavengers, calcium antagonists, magnesium, amino-3-hydroxy-5-methyl-4-isoxazolepropionate (AMPA) antagonists, glutamate antagonists and γ-aminobutyric acid antagonists have been used in attempts to limit the deleterious effects of the biochemical changes that occur intracellularly following ischaemia. No agent has been shown to be effective in placebo-controlled phase III trials.

DECOMPRESSIVE CRANIOTOMY

This is an option in young patients with large middle cerebral artery territory infarcts in the non-dominant hemisphere. Untreated, these normally have a mortality of 80% and it is suggested that this procedure can reduce mortality to around 30%, but with residual neurological deficit. This procedure is limited to specialist centres. Other forms of surgical intervention proven to be effective in making more intracranial space and reducing intracranial pressure are drainage of secondary hydrocephalus by extraventricular drain (EVD) insertion or evacuation of haemorrhage into infarcted areas, resulting in new compressive symptoms. This is especially useful in the posterior fossa where the room for expansion of mass lesions is limited by its anatomy.

COMPLICATIONS

Local complications include cerebral oedema, haemorrhage into infarcted areas or secondary hydrocephalus. General complications include bronchopneumonia, aspiration pneumonia, deep-vein thrombosis, urinary tract infections, pressure sores, contractures and depression. A team approach of specialist nursing, physiotherapists, occupational and speech and language therapists is best able to avoid these complications.

SPONTANEOUS INTRACRANIAL HAEMORRHAGE

Spontaneous intracranial haemorrhage producing stroke may occur from either intracerebral haemorrhage (10%) or SAH (5%).

INTRACEREBRAL HAEMORRHAGE

The incidence of intracerebral haemorrhage is about 9/100 000 of the population, mostly in the age range of 40–70 years, with an equal incidence in males and females.

AETIOLOGY AND PATHOLOGY

The commonest cause is the effect of chronic systemic hypertension. This results in degeneration of the walls of vessels or microaneurysms, by the process of lipohyalinosis, and these microaneurysms then suddenly rupture. This may also occur in:

- malignant tumour neovasculature
- vasculitis
- mycotic aneurysms
- amyloidosis
- sarcoidosis
- malignant hypertension
- primary haemorrhagic disorders
- overanticoagulation

Occasionally, cerebral aneurysms or AVMs may cause intracerebral haemorrhage without SAH. Where intracerebral haemorrhage occurs in young patients the most likely cause is an underlying vascular abnormality. In some areas this is also associated with the abuse of drugs with sympathomimetic activity such as cocaine. The rupture of microaneurysms tends to occur at the bifurcation of small perforating arteries. Common sites of haemorrhage are the putamen (55%), cerebral cortex (15%), thalamus (10%), pons (10%) and cerebellum (10%). Haemorrhage is usually due to rupture of a single vessel, and the size of the haemorrhage is influenced by the anatomical resistance of the site into which it occurs. The effect of the haemorrhage is determined by the area of brain tissue that it destroys. Cortical haemorrhages tend to be larger than pontine bleeds but the latter are much more destructive owing to the anatomical density of neural tracts and nuclei.

CLINICAL PRESENTATION

Usually, there are no prodromal symptoms and a sudden onset of focal neurology or depressed level of consciousness occurs. Headache and neck stiffness will occur in conscious patients if there is subarachnoid extension by haemorrhage into the ventricles. Where intraventricular extension occurs there may be a progressive fall in GCS as secondary hydrocephalus occurs, and this may be accompanied by ocular palsies, resulting in 'sunset eyes'. As with ischaemic stroke, focal neurology is determined by which area of the brain is involved. The only way to differentiate absolutely between ischaemic, intracerebral or SAH is by appropriate imaging. The symptoms relate to tissue destruction, compression and raised intracranial pressure which, if progressive, will result in brainstem ischaemia and death.

INVESTIGATIONS

The general investigations are essentially those listed previously for ischaemic stroke, since it is difficult to distinguish between the two in the early stages. In addition, CT and/or MRI should be performed at the earliest opportunity. Lumbar puncture may be performed to exclude infection if mycotic aneurysm is suspected, but only after CT has excluded raised intracranial pressure or non-communicating hydrocephalus. Digital subtraction angiography will enable localisation of the source of the haemorrhage and will facilitate any surgical intervention for aneurysm or AVM (see Figures 42.7, 44.1 and 44.2).

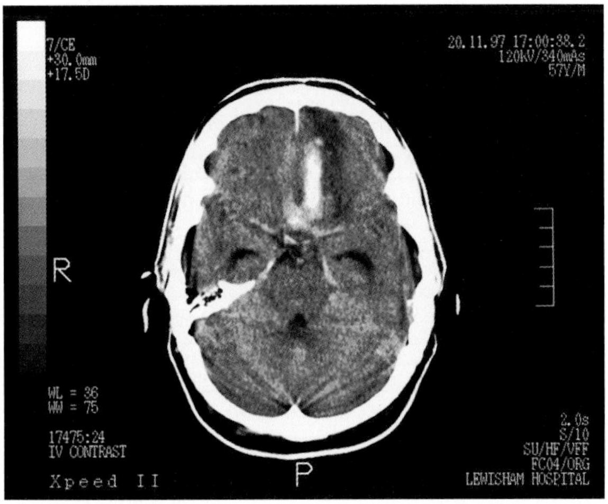

Figure 44.1 Left frontal intraparenchmal bleed with local oedema.

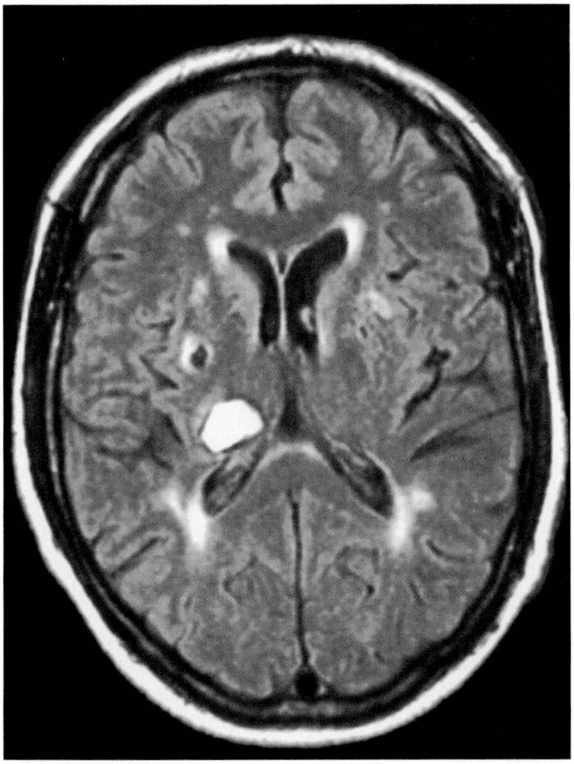

Figure 44.2 Magnetic resonance imaging: thalamic bleed.

MANAGEMENT

The general management principles are identical to those for ischaemic stroke. There is, of course, no place for anticoagulation or thrombolysis, and reversal of any coagulation defect either primary or secondary to therapeutic anticoagulation must be undertaken as a matter of urgency. A full coagulation screen must be performed and the administration of vitamin K, fresh frozen plasma, cryoprecipitate, etc. directed by the results. Where intraventricular extension has occurred the insertion of an EVD may increase conscious level, particularly in the presence of secondary hydrocephalus. The EVD level should be set such that the cerebrospinal fluid (CSF) drains at around 10 mmHg. The normal production of CSF should produce an hourly output and a sudden fall in output to zero should alert staff to the possibility that the drain has blocked. This is particularly likely if the CSF is heavily blood-stained. The meniscus of the CSF within the drain tubing should be examined for transmitted vascular pulsation or the level of the drain temporally lowered by a few centimetres to see if drainage occurs. If the drain is blocked, secondary hydrocephalus will recur. Because of the risk of introducing infection and causing a ventriculitis, the drain must be unblocked in a sterile manner by the neurosurgeons. Operative decompression of the haematoma should only be undertaken in neurosurgical centres and safe transfer must be assured if this is considered. This is a controversial treatment as the most recently published trial shows that patients with spontaneous supratentorial intracerebral haemorrhage in neurosurgical units show no overall benefit from early surgery when compared with initial conservative treatment.[20] Subgroup analysis showed that those patients with intracerebral haemorrhage less than 1 cm from the cortical surface benefited from early surgery. Patients presenting with a GCS of less than 8/15 had an almost universally poor outcome. Not all intracerebral haematomata are amenable to surgery, and the CT scans should be reviewed by the Neurosurgical Unit, preferably prior to transfer by digital image link. Ideally clot evacuation within 6 hours maximum should be the goal.

The management of hypertension following spontaneous intracerebral haemorrhage may be difficult as too high a blood pressure may provoke further bleeding whereas too low a blood pressure may result in ischaemia. The Stroke Council of the American Heart Association has recommended that in patients with chronic hypotension the mean arterial pressure should not exceed 130 mmHg and that, if systolic blood pressure falls to 90 mmHg, then vasopressors should be used.[21] The administration of mannitol prior to transfer should be discussed with the Neurosurgical Unit. There is no place for steroids, and hyperventilation to Pa_{CO_2} of 30 mmHg (4 kPa) or less to control raised intracranial pressure will have detrimental effects on cerebral blood flow in other areas of the brain.

SUBARACHNOID HAEMORRHAGE

SAH refers to bleeding which occurs principally into the subarachnoid space and not into the brain parenchyma. The incidence of SAH is around 6/100 000: the apparent decrease, compared with earlier studies, is due to more frequent use of CT scanning which allows exclusion of other types of haemorrhage. Risk factors are the same as for stroke, but SAH patients are usually younger, peaking in the sixth decade, with a female-to-male ratio of 1.6:1. Black people have twice the risk for SAH as whites. Between 5 and 20% of patients with SAH have a positive family history, with first-degree relatives having a three- to sevenfold risk, whereas second-degree relatives have the same degree of risk as the general population. Specific inheritable disorders are rare and account for only a minority of all patients with SAH.[22] The only modifiable risk factors for SAH are smoking, heavy drinking and hypertension, which increase the risk odds ratio by 2 or 3.[23] Overall mortality is 50%, of which 15% die before reaching hospital, with up to 30% of survivors having residual deficit producing dependency.

AETIOLOGY AND PATHOLOGY

The majority of cases of SAH are caused by ruptured saccular (berry) aneurysms (85%), the remainder being caused by non-aneurysmal perimesencephalic haemorrhage (10%) and rarer causes such as arterial dissection, cerebral or dural AVMs, mycotic aneurysm, pituitary apoplexy, vascular lesions at the top of the spinal cord and cocaine abuse. Saccular aneurysms are not congenital, almost never occur in neonates and young children and develop during later life. It is not known why some adults develop aneurysms at arterial bifurcations in the circle of Willis and some do not. It was thought that there was a congenital weakness in the tunica media, but gaps in the arterial muscle wall are equally as common in patients with or without aneurysms and once the aneurysm is formed, the weakness is found in the wall of the sac and not at its neck.[24] The association with smoking, hypertension and heavy drinking would suggest that degenerative processes are involved. Sudden hypertension plays a role in causing rupture, as shown by SAH in patients taking crack cocaine or, rarely, with sulfenidil.

CLINICAL PRESENTATION

Classically, there is a 'thunderclap' headache developing in seconds, with half of patients describing its onset as instantaneous. This is followed by a period of depressed consciousness for less than an hour in 50% of patients, with focal neurology in about 30% of patients.[25] About a fifth of patients recall similar headaches and these may have been due to 'warning leaks'. The degree of depression of consciousness depends upon the site and extent of the haemorrhage. Meningism – neck stiffness, photophobia, vomiting and a positive Kernig's sign – is common in those patients with higher GCS. The clinical severity of SAH is often described by a grade, the most widely used being that described by the World Federation of Neurological Surgeons (WFNS),[26] which is summarised in Table 44.1.

Table 44.1 Clinical neurological classification of subarachnoid haemorrhage

Grade	Signs
I	Conscious patient with or without meningism
II	Drowsy patient with no significant neurological deficit
III	Drowsy patient with neurological deficit – probably intracerebral clot
IV	Deteriorating patient with major neurological deficit (because of large intracerebral clot)
V	Moribund patient with extensor rigidity and failing vital centres

WFNS grade	GCS	Motor deficit
I	15	Absent
II	14–13	Absent
III	14–13	Present
IV	12–7	Present or absent
V	3–6	Present or absent

WFNS, World Federation of Neurological Surgeons; GCS, Glasgow Coma Score.

This grading, together with the extent of the haemorrhage and the age of the patient, gives some indication of the prognosis, in that the worse the grade the bigger the bleed, and the older the patient, the less likely a good prognosis.

COMPLICATIONS

The clinical status of the patient may be complicated by factors other than the physical effect of initial bleed, and factors such as acute hydrocephalus, early rebleeding, cerebral vasospasm, parenchymal haematoma, seizures and medical complications must be considered.

ACUTE HYDROCEPHALUS

This may occur within the first 24 hours postictus and is often characterised by a one-point drop in the GCS, sluggish pupillary responses and bilateral downward deviation of the eyes ('sunset eyes'). If these signs occur, CT scan should be repeated and, if hydrocephalus is confirmed, or there is a large amount of intraventricular blood, then a ventricular drain may be inserted. This is not without risk as it may provoke more bleeding and introduce infection. Only observational studies exist and these are

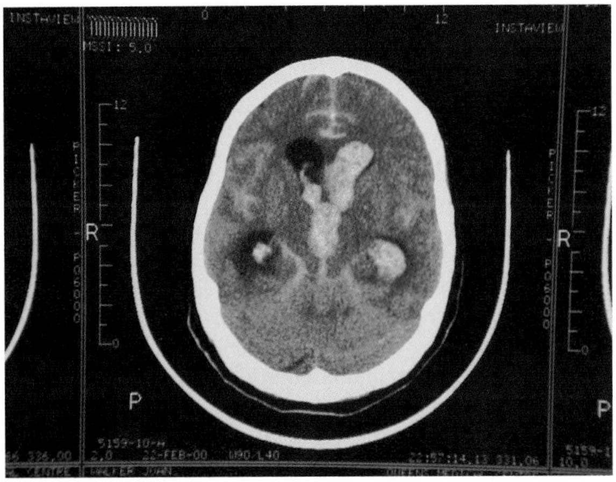

Figure 44.3 Spontaneous subarachnoid haemorrhage and secondary hydrocephalus.

contradictory so no firm recommendation can be made (Figure 44.3).

REBLEEDING

This may occur within the first few hours after admission and 15% of patients may deteriorate from their admission status.[26] They may require urgent intubation and resuscitation but not all rebleeds are unsurvivable and such deterioration should be treated. The chance of rebleeding is dependent on the site of the aneurysm, presence of clot, degree of vasospasm, age and sex of the patient. A preliminary report of the Co-operative Aneurysm Study gave the rebleeding rate in the first 2 weeks after the initial SAH was reported as 19% cumulative and then approximately 1.5% per day for the next 13 days in 1983.[27,28]

CEREBRAL VASOSPASM

This is the term used to describe narrowing of the cerebral blood vessels in response to SAH seen on angiography. It occurs in up to 70% of patients, but not all of these patients will have symptoms.[29] Use of transcranial Doppler (TCD) to estimate middle cerebral artery blood velocity has shown that a velocity of more than 120 cm/s correlates with angiographic evidence of vasospasm. This technology allows diagnosis in the ICU and provides a means of monitoring the success of treatment to reduce vasospasm, which is undertaken to reduce the severity of delayed neurological deficit secondary to vasospasm. The problem is that not all patients who have angiographic vasospasm or high Doppler velocities have symptoms. If there is evidence of a depressed level of consciousness in the absence of rebleeding, hydrocephalus or metabolic disturbances, but there is evidence of vasospasm on TCD or angiogram, then it would seem appropriate to initiate treatment to reduce the vasospasm. If vasopasm occurs at the time of angiography or coiling, then intravascular vasodilators such as papaverine have been used.

Table 44.2 Types of medical complication seen in patients with subarachnoid haemorrhage

Medical complication	Incidence
Arrhythmias	35%
Liver dysfunction	24%
Neurogenic pulmonary oedema	23%
Pneumonia	22%
ARDS and atelectasis	20%
Renal dysfunction	5%

ARDS, acute respiratory distress syndrome.

PARENCHYMAL HAEMATOMA

This may occur in up to 30% of SAH following aneurysm rupture and has a much worse prognosis than SAH alone.[29] If there is mass effect with compressive symptoms then evacuation of haematoma and simultaneous clipping of the aneurysm may improve outcome.

MEDICAL COMPLICATIONS

During the placebo-controlled study of nicardipine in WFNS grade I and II SAH patients, there was a 40% incidence of at least one life-threatening medical complication in the placebo group.[30] The mortality due to medical complications was almost the same as that due to the combined effects of the initial bleed, rebleeds and vasospasm. The types of medical complication seen are shown in Table 44.2.

INVESTIGATIONS

The general investigations for stroke should be performed and early CT imaging is mandatory. Blood appears characteristically hyperdense on CT and the pattern of haemorrhage may enable localisation of the arterial territory involved. Very rarely, a false-positive diagnosis may be made if there is severe generalised oedema resulting in venous congestion in the subarachnoid space. Small amounts of blood may not be detected and the incidence of false-negative reports is around 2%.[31] It may be difficult to distinguish between post-traumatic SAH and primary aneurysmal SAH, which precipitates a fall in the level of consciousness that provokes an accident or fall.[32] MR scanning is particularly effective for localising the bleed after 48 hours when extravasated blood is denatured, and provides a good signal on MRI.[33]

Lumbar puncture is still necessary in those patients where the suspicion of SAH is high despite a negative CT, or there is a need to exclude infection. There must be no raised intracranial pressure and at least 6 hours should have passed to give time for the blood in the CSF to lyse, enabling xanthochromia to develop.

Angiography via arterial catheterisation is still the most commonly used investigation for localising the aneurysm or other vascular abnormality prior to surgery. It is generally performed on patients who remain, or become, conscious after SAH. It is not without risk and aneurysms may rupture during the procedure and a meta-analysis has shown a complication rate of 1.8%.[34] Other methods under investigation include CT angiography and MR angiography, and it is likely that these techniques may replace catheter angiography for diagnosis, although intra-arterial catheterisation would still be needed for endovascular therapy.[35,36]

Intracranial pressure monitoring is of limited use in SAH patients except in those where hydrocephalus or parenchymal haematoma is present and early detection of pressure increases may be the trigger for drainage or decompressive surgery.

Transcranial Doppler studies may be useful in detecting vasospasm or those patients in whom autoregulation is impaired.[37] The technique is dependent on there being a 'window' of thin temporal bone allowing isonation of the Doppler signal along the middle cerebral artery. It is very user-dependent and 15% of patients do not have an adequate bone window.

MANAGEMENT

GENERAL CARE

The initial management of SAH is influenced by the grading, medical comorbidity or complications, and the timing or need for surgery. Patients with decreased GCS may need early intubation and ventilation, simply for airway protection, whereas those with less severe symptoms require regular neurological observation, analgesia for headache and bedrest prior to investigation and surgery. Other management options are:

- stress ulcer prophylaxis
- deep-vein thrombosis prophylaxis using compression stockings or boots
- seizures control with phenytoin or barbiturates

If the patent is sedated and ventilated, the use of an analysing cerebral function monitor should be considered to detect subclinical seizure activity.

Hyponatraemia is a common finding and adequate fluid therapy with normal saline is required with electrolyte levels maintained in the normal range. Occasionally, as in other types of brain injury, excessive natriuresis occurs and may result in hyponatraemic dehydration – cerebral salt-wasting syndrome (CSWS). Its aetiology is not known but some suggest increased levels of atrial natriuretic peptide. It usually occurs within the first week after insult and resolves spontaneously in 2–4 weeks. Failure to distinguish CSWS from the syndrome of inappropriate secretion of antidiuretic hormone (SIADH) could lead to inappropriate treatment by fluid restriction, which would have adverse effects on cerebral perfusion. Urine sodium concentrations are usually elevated in both SIADH and CSWS (> 40mmol/l) but urinary sodium excretion, urine sodium concentration [Na mmol/l] × urine volume [l/24 hours] is high in CSWS and normal in SIADH. If CSWS does not respond to fluid replacement with saline or is not self-limiting then fludricortisone therapy may be useful.

BLOOD PRESSURE CONTROL

Elevation of blood pressure is commonly seen after SAH and there are no precise data on what constitutes an unacceptably high pressure that is likely to cause rebleeding. Equally, there are no precise data on a minimum level of pressure below which infarction is likely to occur, since this will depend on the patient's normal pressure, degree of cerebral oedema and the presence or absence of intact autoregulation. One observational study has demonstrated reduced rebleeding but higher rates of infarction in newly treated compared with untreated post-SAH hypertensive patients.[38] If blood pressure exceeds 200 mmHg (26.6 kPa) systolic or 100 mmHg (13.3 kPa) diastolic, then empirically it would seem wise to reduce this pressure in SAH patients who have unclipped aneurysms. β-adrenergic blockers or calcium antagonists are the most widely used agents, since drugs producing cerebral vasodilation may increase intracranial pressure.

VASOSPASM

Angiographic demonstration of vasospasm may be seen in about 70% of SAH patients but only about 30% develop cerebral symptoms related to vasospasm. Transcranial Doppler-derived flow velocities in the middle cerebral arteries of more than 120 cm/s are accurate in predicting ischaemia.[37] Symptoms tend to occur between 4 and 14 days postbleed, which is the period when cerebral blood flow is decreased after SAH.

One method of pre-empting vasospasm is the prescription of oral nimodipine at 60 mg given 4-hourly for 21 days, which has been shown to achieve a reduction in the risk of ischaemic stroke of 34%.[39] Intravenous nimodipine should be used in the patients who are not absorbing, but it must be titrated against blood pressure to avoid hypotension. Other calcium antagonists, notably nicardipine and the experimental drug AT877, reduce vasospasm but do not improve outcome.

Low cerebral blood flow is known to worsen outcome and this resulted in the development of prophylactic hypertensive hypervolaemic haemodilution – so-called triple-H therapy.[40] As originally described, the therapy involved the use of fluid loading to achieve haemodilution and vasopressor therapy to increase cerebral blood flow, and was combined with surgery within 24 hours if possible. The therapy was continued for 21 days and all patients remained neurologically stable or improved as a result, apparently, of the absence of vasospasm. Very few centres use the strict protocol as originally described, but fluid loading rather than fluid restriction is the norm and inotropes or vasopressors are used subsequently if neurological function decreases. Despite its widespread use, there remains no prospective randomised trial that demonstrates its utility.

The use of intravascular catheters to deliver papaverine into vasospastic vessels remains experimental. Where symptoms develop it is important to exclude other causes such as rebleeding, hydrocephalus or metabolic disorder.

SURGERY

Clipping of the aneurysm is the surgical treatment of choice, with wrapping, proximal ligation or bypass grafting being used if the aneurysm is inaccessible to Yasargil clipping. The timing of surgery remains debatable. Early surgery, within 3 days of the bleed, has the advantage of fewer deaths occurring from rebleeding but is technically difficult due to the friability of associated tissues. Delayed surgery, around 10–12 days postbleed, gives better operating conditions but allows some patients to suffer a rebleed. There is no type 1 evidence but an observational study suggested that there is no difference in outcome after early or late operation.[41]

ENDOVASCULAR COILING

The development of detachable microcoils made of platinum by Gugliemi in 1990 has resulted in endovascular embolisation of aneurysms or AVMs by interventional radiology.[42] A microcatheter is passed from the femoral artery to the cerebral aneurysm and the coils positioned sequentially in the lumen of saccular aneurysms to occlude it. Rupture of the aneurysm or adjacent vessel occlusion, causing ischaemia, is the most frequent complication.[43] The International Subarachnoid Aneurysm Trial (ISAT) of neurosurgical clipping versus endovascular coiling in 2143 patients with ruptured intracranial aneurysms – a randomised comparison of effects on survival, dependency, seizures, rebleeding, subgroups and aneurysm occlusion – has come down in favour of coiling over the open surgical technique at 1-year follow-up. In patients with ruptured intracranial aneurysms suitable for both treatments, endovascular coiling is more likely to result in independent survival at 1 year than neurosurgical clipping; the survival benefit continues for at least 7 years. The risk of late rebleeding is low, but is more common after endovascular coiling than after neurosurgical clipping.[44] Additional complications of coiling include rupture during catheter placement in the aneurysm, coil embolisation and vasopasm. Not all aneurysms, particularly those with wide necks, multiple filling vessels or giant aneurysms, are suitable for coiling.

NEUROPROTECTIVE THERAPY

There has been a great deal of research on the cellular and biochemical responses to brain injury and several drugs have been investigated to try and reduce mortality in SAH. The 21-amino steroid tirilizad, nicaraven and ebselen, all free-radical scavengers, have been the most widely investigated. None has been shown to improve outcome consistently in all types of patient with SAH.

THERAPY OF MEDICAL COMPLICATIONS

This is obviously specific to the type of complication. Pneumonia may require continuous positive airways pressure or ventilatory support together with directed antimicrobial therapy; acute respiratory distress syndrome requires lung-protective/recruitment ventilatory strategies; and renal failure necessitates an appropriate means of renal replacement therapy. Arrhythmias require correction of trigger factors such as hypovolaemia and electrolyte or acid–base disturbances prior to the appropriate antiarrhythmic drug or DC cardioversion. Neurogenic pulmonary oedema may be associated with severe cardiogenic shock, which may require inotropic support or even temporary intra-aortic balloon counterpulsation. The cardiogenic shock is reversible and patients can make a good recovery despite the need for aggressive support.[45]

REFERENCES

1. Wolfe CDA. The impact of stroke. *Br Med Bull* 2000; **56**: 275–6.
2. Bonita R. Epidemiology of stroke. *Lancet* 1992; **339**: 342–4.
3. Treib J, Grauer MT, Woessner R *et al.* Treatment of stroke on an intensive stroke unit: a novel concept. *Intens Care Med* 2000; **26**: 1598–11.
4. Wolfe C, Rudd A, Dennis M *et al.* Taking acute stroke care seriously. *Br Med J* 2001; **323**: 5–6.
5. Jansen O, Schellinger P, Fiebach J *et al.* Early recanalisation in acute ischaemic stroke scar tissue at risk defined by MRI. *Lancet* 1999; **353**: 2036–7.
6. Stroke Trialists Collaboration. Collective systematic review of the randomised trials of organised inpatient (stroke unit) care after stroke. *Br Med J* 1997; **314**: 1151–9.
7. Steiner T, Mendoza G, De Gorgia M *et al.* Prognosis of stroke patients requiring mechanical ventilation in a neurological critical care unit. *Stroke* 1997; **28**: 711–15.
8. Fujii K, Satoshima S, Okada Y *et al.* Cerebral blood flow and metabolism in normotensive and hypotensive patients with transient neurological deficits. *Stroke* 1990; **21**: 283–90.
9. Treib J, Haa BA, Stoll M *et al.* Monitoring and management of antihypertensive therapy induced deterioration in acute ischaemia stroke. *Am J Hypertens* 1996; **9**: 513–14.
10. Aichner FT, Fazehar F, Bainin M *et al.* Hypervolaemic hemodilution in acute ischaemic stroke. The Multicenter Austrian Hemodilution Stroke Trial (MAHST). *Stroke* 1998; **29**: 743–9.
11. Jorgensen HS, Nakayam H, Raaschon HO *et al.* Effect of blood pressure and diabetes on stroke in progression. *Lancet* 1994; **344**: 156–9.
12. International Stroke Trial Collaborative Group. The International Stroke Trial (IST): a randomised trial of aspirin, subcutaneous heparin, both or neither among

19435 patients with acute ischaemic stroke. *Lancet* 1997; **349**: 1564–5.
13. The Publications Committee for the Trial ORG 10172 in Acute Stroke Treatment (TOAST). Low molecular weight heparinoid ORG 10172 (Danaparoid) and outcome after acute ischaemic stroke. *JAMA* 1998; **279**: 1265–72.
14. Multicentre Acute Stroke Trial – Europe Study Group. Thrombolytic therapy with streptokinase in acute ischaemic stroke. *N Engl J Med* 1996; **335**: 145–50.
15. National Institute of Neurological Disorders and Stroke rt-PA Stroke Study Group. Tissue plasminogen activator for acute ischaemic stroke. *N Engl J Med* 1996; **333**: 1–7.
16. Hacke W, Kaste M, Fieschi C *et al.* Intravenous thrombolysis with recombinant tissue plasminogen activator for acute hemispheric stroke. The European Co-operative Acute Stroke Study (ECASS) *JAMA* 1995; **274**: 1017–25.
17. Hacke W, Kaste M, Fieschi C *et al.* Randomised double blind placebo-controlled trial of thrombolytic therapy with intravenous alteplase in acute ischaemic stroke (ECASS II). *Lancet* 1998; **352**: 1245–51.
18. Clark WM, Wissman S, Albers GW *et al.* Recombinant tissue type plasminogen activator (alteplase) for ischaemic stroke 3 to 5 hours after symptom onset. The ATLANTIS study: a randomised controlled trial. Alteplase thrombolysis for acute non-interventional therapy in ischaemic stroke. *JAMA* 1999; **282**: 2019–26.
19. Wardlow JM, del Zoppo G, Yamaguchi T *et al.* Thrombolysis for acute ischaemic stroke. *Cochrane Database of Systematic Reviews* 2003; **3**: CD000213.
20. Siddique MS, Mendelow AD. Early surgery versus initial treatment in patients with spontaneous supratentorial haematomas in the International Surgical Trial in Cerebral Haemorrhage (STITCH): a randomised trial. *Lancet* 2005; **365**: 361–2.
21. Broderick JP, Adams HP Jr, Barsan W *et al.* Guidelines for the management of spontaneous intracerebral hemorrhage: a statement for healthcare professionals from a special writing group of the Stroke Council, American Heart Association. *Stroke* 1999; **30**: 905–15.
22. Van Gijn J, Rinkel GJE. Subarachnoid haemorrhage: diagnosis, causes and management. *Brain* 2001; **124**: 248–9.
23. Teunissen LL, Rinkel GJE, Algra A *et al.* Risk factors for subarachnoid haemorrhage – a systematic review. *Stroke* 1996; **27**: 544–9.
24. Stehbens WE. Etiology of intracranial berry aneurysms. *J Neurosurg* 1989; **70**: 823–31.
25. Linn FH, Rinkel GJ, Algra A *et al.* Headache characteristics in subarachnoid haemorrhage and benign thunderclap headache. *J Neurol Neurosurg Psychiatry* 1998; **65**: 791–3.
26. Drake CG, Hunt WE, Kassell NF *et al.* Report of the World Federation of Neurological Surgeons Committee on a universal subarachnoid haemorrhage grading scale. *J Neurosurg* 1996; **84**: 985–6.
27. Fujii Y, Takeuchi S, Sasaki O *et al.* Ultra-early rebleeding in spontaneous subarachnoid haemorrhage. *J Neurosurg* 1996; **84**: 35–42.
28. Kassell NF, Torner JC. Aneurysmal rebleeding: a preliminary report from the Cooperative Aneurysm Study. *Neurosurgery* 1983; **13**: 479–81.
29. Weir B, MacDonald L. Cerebral vasospasm. *Clin Neurosurg* 1992; **40**: 40–5.
30. Hauerberg J, Eskesen V, Rosenova J. The prognostic significance of intracerebral haematoma as shown on CT scanning after subarachnoid haemorrhage. *Br J Neurosurg* 1994; **8**: 333–9.
31. Solenski NJ, Haley EC, Kassell NF *et al.* Medical complications of aneurysmal subarachnoid haemorrhage: a report of the multicenter cooperative aneurysm study. *Crit Care Med* 1995; **25**: 1007–17.
32. Van der Wee N, Rinkel GJ, Hasan D *et al.* Detection of subarachnoid haemorrhage on early CT: is lumbar puncture still needed after a negative scan? *J Neurol Neurosurg Psychiatry* 1995; **58**: 357–9.
33. Vos PE, Zwienenberg M, O'Hannion KL *et al.* Subarachnoid haemorrhage following rupture of an ophthalamic artery aneurysm presenting as traumatic brain injury. *Clin Neurol Neurosurg* 2000; **102**: 29–32.
34. Noguchi K, Ogawa T, Seto H *et al.* Sub-acute and chronic subarachnoid haemorrhage: diagnosis with fluid attenuated inversion – recovery MR imaging. *Radiology* 1997; **203**: 257–62.
35. Cloft HJ, Joseph GJ, Dion JE. Risk of cerebral angiography in patients with subarachnoid haemorrhage, cerebral aneurysm and arteriovenous malformation: a meta-analysis. *Stroke* 1999; **30**: 317–20.
36. Wardlaw JM, White PM. The detection and management of unruptured intracranial aneurysms. *Brain* 2000; **123**: 205–21.
37. Hashimoto H, Iida J, Hironaka Y *et al.* Use of spiral CT angiography in patients with subarachnoid haemorrhage in whom subtraction angiography did not reveal cerebral aneurysms. *J Neurosurg* 2000; **92**: 278–83.
38. Vora YY, Suarez-Almazor M, Steinke DE, *et al.* Role of transcranial Doppler in the diagnosis of cerebral vasospasm after subarachnoid haemorrhage. *Neurosurgery* 1999; **44**: 1237–47.
39. Wijdicks EF, Vermeulen M, Murray GD *et al.* The effects of treating hypertension following aneurysmal subarachnoid haemorrhage. *Clin Neurol Neurosurg* 1990; **92**: 111–17.
40. Pickard JD, Murray GD, Illingworth R *et al.* Effect of oral nimodipine on cerebral infarction and outcome after subarachnoid haemorrhage: British Aneurysm Nimodipine Trial (BRANT). *Br Med J* 1989; **298**: 636–42.
41. Origatano TC, Wascher TM, Reichman OU *et al.* Sustained increased cerebral blood flow with prophylactic hypertensive hemodilution ('triple-H' therapy) after subarachnoid haemorrhage. *Neurosurgery* 1990; **27**: 729–40.

42. Kassell NF, Torner JC, Jane JA *et al.* The International Cooperative Study on the Timing of Aneurysm Surgery. Part 2: surgical results. *J Neurosurg* 1990; **73**: 18–36.
43. Guglielmi G, Vinuela F, Duckwriter G *et al.* Endovascular treatment of posterior circulation aneurysms by electrothrombosis using electric-ally detachable coils. *J Neurosurg* 1992; 77: 515–24.
44. Molyneux AJ, Kerr RSC, Yu LM *et al.* The International Sub Arachnoid Aneurysm Trial (ISAT) of neurosurgical clipping versus endovascular coiling in 2143 patients with ruptured intracranial aneurysms: a randomised comparison of effects on survival, dependency, seizures, rebleeding, subgroups and aneurysm occlusion. *Lancet* 2005; **366**: 809–17.
45. Parr MJ, Finfer SR, Morgan MK. Reversible cardiogenic shock complicating subarachnoid haemorrhage. *Br Med J* 1996; **313**: 681–3.

45

Cerebral protection

Victoria Heaviside and Michelle Hayes

The cerebral circulation is arguably the most important and most vulnerable in the body. Arrest of the circulation for only a few minutes can cause neuronal death. The concept of cerebral protection has been engaged across a broad spectrum of clinical scenarios. It has been incorporated into the prophylaxis, treatment and subsequent management of ischaemia and infarction and even into attempts to ameliorate postischaemic or anoxic damage following cardiorespiratory resuscitation. A complete review is beyond the scope of this chapter, but an understanding of the current approaches to cerebral protection is certainly helpful in the management of cerebral insults.

NORMAL BRAIN PHYSIOLOGY

The brain has a high energy requirement, utilisng approximately 3–5 ml O_2/min per 100 g tissue (45–75 ml O_2/min per 1500 g brain) and 5 mg glucose/min per 100 g tissue (75 mg glucose/min per 1500 g brain). It has little ability to store precursors of metabolism and thus depends on a constant supply of nutrients from the blood.

At a cerebral blood flow (CBF) of 50 ml/min per 100 g tissue (750 ml/min per 1500 g brain) and a normal oxygen content of 20 ml O_2/100 ml blood, the brain receives approximately 150 ml O_2/min per 1500 g brain, or 2–3 times the amount needed for normal brain activity.

At the same CBF of 50 ml/min per 100 g tissue and a blood glucose concentration of 5.5 mmol/l (100 mg/100 ml blood), there is 50 mg/min per 100 g tissue (750 mg/min per 1500 g brain) delivery of glucose. Glucose extraction by the brain, at 5 mg/min per 100 g brain tissue, is a tenth of that delivered – minimal compared with oxygen.

Cerebral injury has many aetiologies, but the mechanisms of injury are thought to be few. The most common is lack of the essential nutrients, oxygen and glucose, either separately with preserved blood flow (i.e. hypoxia or hypoglycaemia), or together, because of reduced or absent perfusion (i.e. ischaemia or infarction). A reduction in these energy precursors is a major contributor in the mechanism of brain injury, regardless of the aetiology.

NATURAL PROTECTIVE MECHANISMS

The importance of the brain to the whole being is highlighted by the mechanisms in place to protect the cerebral elements from ischaemia.

COLLATERAL BLOOD SUPPLY

An elaborate vascular architecture is designed to ensure adequate CBF. The anterior cerebral circulation is provided by bilateral internal carotid arteries as they each divide into anterior and middle cerebral arteries. They provide approximately 70% of the cerebral circulation and supply the anterior cerebrum (frontal, parietal and temporal lobes) and anterior diencephalon (basal ganglia and hypothalamus). The remaining 30% of the cerebral circulation is provided posteriorly by the vertebrobasilar system which runs the length of the posterior fossa, supplying the brainstem, cerebellum and posterior portion of the cerebrum (occipital lobes) and diencephalon (thalamus). These two circulations are joined by communicating arteries, ultimately forming the circle of Willis (Figure 45.1). This joining of the anterior and posterior circulations at the base of the brain is the major component of cerebral vasculature in humans. Between these arterial distributions are watershed zones fed by leptomeningeal connections. In addition, persistent fetal arteries can infrequently provide collateral routes between the anterior and posterior arterial systems in the brain.

CEREBRAL BLOOD FLOW

CEREBRAL PERFUSION PRESSURE

The amount of blood delivered to the brain is highly regulated and is determined by several factors. CBF is determined in part by the perfusion pressure across the brain, called cerebral perfusion pressure (CPP). CPP, is the difference between the arterial pressure in the feeding arteries as they enter the subarachnoid space and the pressure in the draining veins before they enter the major dural sinuses. Because these pressures are difficult to measure, CPP is derived from the difference between the systemic mean arterial pressure (MAP) and the intracranial pressure (ICP), which is an estimate of tissue pressure.

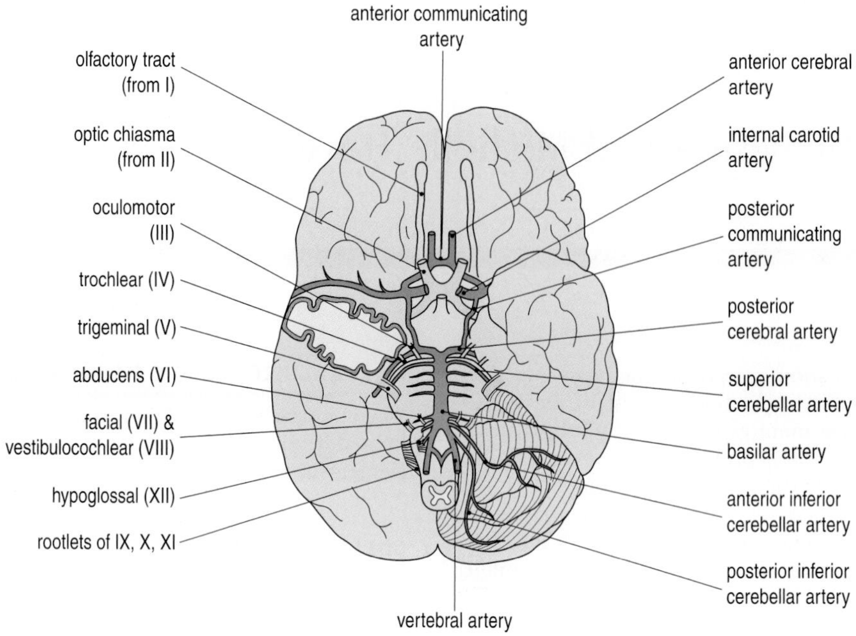

Figure 45.1 Circle of Willis.

The cerebral vessels change diameter inversely with changing perfusion pressure: as CPP rises, the vessels constrict and as CPP falls the vessels dilate, such that blood flow is kept constant over a wide range of CPP (Figure 45.2a). This pressure autoregulation is thought to be controlled by local myogenic responses of the vessel wall to changes in intra-arterial pressure. At pressures above and below this range of 6.7–20 kPa (50–150 mmHg), cerebral perfusion becomes pressure-passive and increases or decreases in direct proportion to changes in CPP. The autoregulatory range varies with age, being shifted to the left in newborns and to the right in those with chronic hypertension. The latter is important to remember to avoid overtreating systolic blood pressure in such patients and thus incur the risk of cerebral ischaemia at the lower limits of autoregulation. Alternatively, cerebral perfusion above normal can be caused by acute hypertension overcoming the upper limits of autoregulation. This may lead to cerebral oedema secondary to increased hydrostatic pressures (hypertensive encephalopathy) and potentially lead to seizures or cerebral haemorrhage.

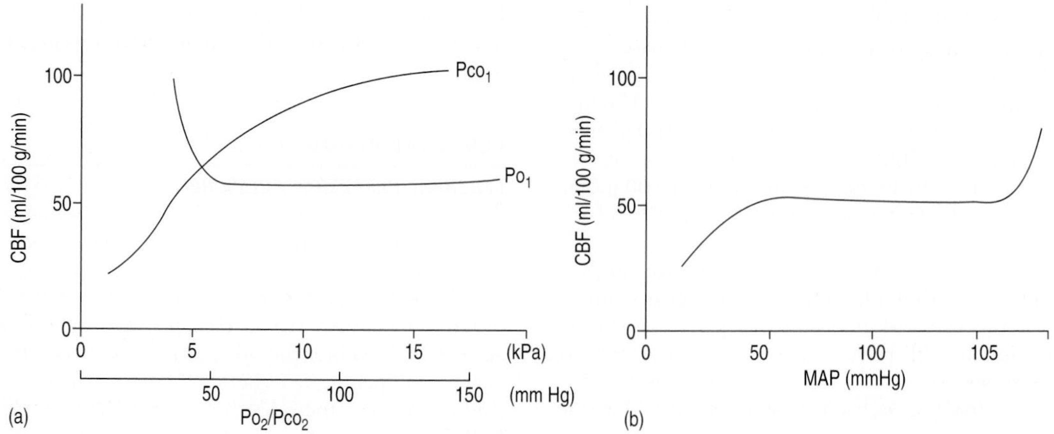

Figure 45.2 (a) The relationship between the partial pressure of oxygen ($P\text{o}_2$) and carbon dioxide ($P\text{co}_2$) and cerebral blood flow (CBF). (b) The relationship between mean arterial pressure (MAP) and cerebral blood flow under normal circumstances, illustrating the range of autoregulation.

Pao_2 AND $Paco_2$ EFFECTS

A second group of factors control CBF through an influence on the local metabolic milieu. Prominent in this mechanism are oxygen and carbon dioxide. Arterial content or partial pressure of oxygen in the normal or hyperoxic ranges causes very little change in CBF. Perhaps this represents a demand for another nutrient (i.e. glucose) or a need to remove waste products (i.e. carbon dioxide or metabolic acid). With the onset of hypoxaemia (Pao_2 60 mmHg or 8 kPa), there is a prompt increase in CBF proportional to the decrease in blood oxygen content, in order to maintain oxygen delivery constant (Figure 45.2b).

There is also a direct relationship between CBF and $Paco_2$, such that cerebral perfusion increases with increasing $Paco_2$ (Figure 45.2b). This probably represents the need of the brain to maintain homeostatic pH by removing metabolic breakdown products more efficiently by increased blood flow. Unlike the response to oxygen, the CBF response to changes in $Paco_2$ is dramatic in the physiological range, such that for every 0.13 kPa (1.0 mmHg) change in $Paco_2$ there is a 1–2 ml/min per 100 g tissue change in CBF. Therefore, an increase in $Paco_2$ to 10.6 kPa (80 mmHg) will increase CBF to approximately 100 ml/min per 100 g and a decrease in $Paco_2$ to 2.7 kPa (20 mmHg) will decrease CBF to 25 ml/min per 100 g. Thus:

- doubling $Paco_2$ doubles CBF
- halving $Paco_2$ halves CBF within this range

Understanding this basic physiology will make treatment logical (see below), as increases in CBF often lead to increases in cerebral blood volume, which in turn can increase ICP – a common cause of cerebral ischaemia.

CEREBRAL INJURY

Vascular insufficiency or disruption, trauma, tumour, infection, inflammation and metabolic and nutritional derangement can all cause damage. Whatever the cause, the mechanism of injury is usually hypoxic and/or ischaemic injury.

- Hypoxia is lack of oxygen.
- Ischaemia is lack of flow.

Therefore, it is possible to have high flow but no oxygen or, alternatively, no flow but plenty of oxygen. At the cellular level the consequence is the same.

The protective mechanisms afforded by the ability to increase CBF manifold in response to hypoxaemia and the generous oversupply of nutrients under normal conditions allow for sufficient blood flow, with maintenance of oxygen delivery and supply of other nutrients in many cases. Limitation in the ability to alter CBF, whether through cerebrovascular disease restricting perfusion or intracranial masses, oedema and increased ICP exerting excess local pressure, and altering blood flow, will cause hypoxic/ischaemic injury. Systemic problems such as severe or prolonged hypoxaemia will eventually disturb systemic circulatory homeostasis, leading to hypotension and eventual ischaemia. Thus hypoxic and ischaemic injury may be considered synonymous, although there may be aetiological differences between them. A more important distinction is to be made between global and focal hypoxic or ischaemic insults.

GLOBAL HYPOXIC/ISCHAEMIC INSULTS

These types of insult are caused by hypoxaemia and cardiovascular insufficiency or arrest, respectively. These are usually sudden, short and severe. If there is to be recovery, prompt return of oxygen delivery and spontaneous circulation are necessary. The recovery may be variable, depending on the severity and duration of the insult and the selective vulnerability of the cell types involved. Different mechanisms are responsible for reversible loss of cellular function and for irreversible cell death and there are also differences between the mechanisms that cause death of neurones, glia and endothelial cells. After 4–6 minutes of complete global ischaemia, there are signs of permanent histological damage in selective neuronal populations and the beginnings of neurological deficits in survivors. Outcome worsens significantly after 15 minutes of global ischaemia.[1]

FOCAL HYPOXIC/ISCHAEMIC INSULTS

These insults often occur suddenly but are usually of more prolonged duration. Only a subtotal of the brain is affected and the injury may be less severe if the surrounding brain is preserved by collateral blood supply.

The area of the focal ischaemia supplied by end-arteries will result in cell death unless reperfusion is established rapidly. The periphery of an infarcted area is the ischaemic penumbra. Here, CBF is greater than at the infarcted core, but less than in the normal tissue around it. Animal studies suggest that the time course for infarction and irreversible damage to brain from a focal hypoxic/ischaemic event is around 30–60 minutes. The focus of therapeutic intervention is the penumbral area, on the basis that if blood flow can be normalised in this region, or pharmacological agents can be delivered despite the reduced blood flow, there is a potential for recovery. Conversely, failure to maintain this area will result in a coalescing of the penumbra into the infarcted area, as the ischaemic stimulus continues.

It is likely that the ongoing ischaemic penumbral area of a focal insult and transient whole-brain ischaemia (e.g. during early cardiac arrest, low-flow cardiopulmonary resuscitation (CPR) or elevated ICP states) are subject to similar pathophysiological processes. As pretreatment is usually impossible, prevention and treatment of the secondary insults are the focus in neuroprotection and tissue salvage strategies.

BRAIN ISCHAEMIC AND INFARCTION PROCESSES

Changes in normal physiology begin to occur when blood flow is reduced.

- At CBF below 50 ml/min per 100 g neurological function is impaired and there is slowing of the electroencephalogram (EEG).
- A CBF of 15–25 ml/min per 100 g results in loss of electrical activity.
- A CBF between 10 and 15 ml/min per 100 g can maintain adenosine triphosphate (ATP) levels sufficiently to support ionic pump function for a time, despite the lack of electrical activity and normal neurological function.
- At a CBF of 10 ml/min per 100 g membrane failure occurs, due to a critical loss of ATP, which causes ionic imbalance between the cell and the extracellular milieu. If prolonged or worsened, CBF at this level will lead to permanent neurological impairment as a result of cell death.

EFFECTS OF ISCHAEMIA

Ischaemia results in reduced available oxygen and glucose to support aerobic production of ATP. Levels of ATP are depleted within 2–3 minutes of complete ischaemia (animal studies). There is little brain storage of either glucose or oxygen, and ATP production during ischaemia relies on anaerobic glycolysis for as long as stores last. This results in continued ATP use, but suboptimal production of ATP to fuel aerobic metabolism, so a lactic acidosis develops. Loss of ATP causes failure of membrane ionic pump function, leading to an efflux of potassium and an influx of sodium, calcium and chloride ions, the beginnings of cytotoxic oedema.

This begins a cascade of events resulting in eventual cell death:

- Potassium leakage causes cell depolarisation, ion channel opening and the release of excitatory amino acid (EAA) neurotransmitters (glutamate and aspartate and others).
- EAA cause further depolarisation of neighbouring cells and distal, otherwise unaffected, parts of the brain which result in:
- sodium and chloride influx via kainate (K) and quisqualate (Q) receptors (with water worsening intracellular oedema)
- calcium influx via *N*-methyl-D-aspartate (NMDA) receptors
- release of excitatory transmitters
- conversion of phosphorylases, uncoupling of oxidative phosphorylation, activation of proteases, degradation of cystosolic protein and stimulation of lipases. Lipases liberate arachidonic acid and other free fatty acids that cause tissue damage via production of oxygen radicals and prostaglandins

Other effects within the cell influence DNA and RNA production, hence inhibiting protein production. This may explain why cellular and clinical recovery is partial, even with restoration of ionic equilibrium and near-normal ATP levels after successful reperfusion. Necrosis is thought to occur in the core of the cerebral infarct following acute vascular occlusion, with further neurodegeneration occurring more slowly in the penumbra, by apoptosis or release of various immunological mediators.[2]

EXTRACELLULAR EFFECTS

Leukocytes are thought to be major contributors to reperfusion injury in that:

- they may plug up small capillaries under conditions of low blood flow and prevent reflow in certain areas, thus hindering restoration of perfusion
- they may enhance production of oxygen radicals and begin a cascade of inflammatory mediators, which may potentiate cell destruction in injured tissue

This results in tissue oedema, which may affect the core lesion by narrowing blood vessels and worsening chances of reperfusion. Local mechanical compression of tissue or its blood supply can cause deterioration in neighbouring tissue. The alteration in volume is of extreme importance in the adult brain because the cranial vault is non-distensible, preventing accommodation to an expanding lesion. This will impede CBF both locally and globally.

Hypoxic/ischaemic insults are rarely predictable, so that the process is usually well established when clinicians intervene. It is therefore highly likely that the injury will be only partially remediable.

MANAGEMENT

In neurological injury, the initial aims are to provide basic support. Assessment of the airway and respiration are the first priority, closely followed by optimisation of the circulation.

In cases of head trauma, it is very important to prevent secondary brain injury. Reviews of intensive care practice have resulted in recommendations for treatment in this group of patients.[3] These involve:

- institution of monitoring
- early treatment of hypotension, hypoxia, hyperthermia and intracranial hypertension
- maintenance of CPP

Following stroke, it is also important to optimise homeostasis and address any hypertension, hyperglycaemia, hyperthermia and intracranial hypertension, as these are independent factors of a poor prognosis.

HYPERTENSION

Most patients have elevated blood pressure in the early phase after an acute ischaemic stroke. The mechanism and effects of this blood pressure elevation are not well understood and the benefits of intervention remain debated. Most experts would not advocate antihypertensive treatment in the acute phase after stroke, unless the blood pressure is particularly high. Currently hypertension (systolic blood pressure > 180 mmHg) should be treated if thrombolytics are to be administered, based on the trials involving these agents in which the blood pressure was lowered prior to treatment.[4] Ongoing studies such as Blood Pressure in Acute Stroke Collaboration (BASC) should help define optimal management.

HYPERGLYCAEMIA

Hyperglycaemia has also been associated with an increased mortality and reduced functional outcome after stroke irrespective of whether the patient has a diabetic history or not.[5] Proposed explanations for this are:

- Hyperglycaemia may be directly toxic to the ischaemic brain.
- Decreased levels and reduced peripheral uptake of insulin in these patients result in increased cerebral glucose availability which may impair endothethelial-dependent vasodilatation.
- Hyperglycaemia may indicate dysglycaemia, which is associated with vascular disease and endothelial dysfunction, both of which may exacerbate ischaemic damage at the time of stroke.

Hyperglycaemia may result in a hypercoaguable state, with decreased plasma fibrinolytic activity, which may delay reperfusion and increase haemorrhagic infarct conversion in tissue plasminogen activator-treated patients.[6]

Insulin, as well as having a glucose-lowering effect, has also been shown to be directly neuroprotective and this is the subject of a number of ongoing trials[7] (Treatment of Hyperglycaemia in Ischaemic Stroke (THIS) trial, the Glucose Regulation in Acute Stroke Patients (GRASP) trial and the Glucose Insulin Stroke Trial UK (GIST-UK).

HYPERTHERMIA

An increased temperature increases cerebral metabolism, oxygen requirements, CBF and ICP. Hyperpyrexia following acute stroke adversely influences stroke severity, infarct size, functional outcome and mortality.[8] A raised temperature should, therefore, be treated aggressively and any evidence of infection identified early and treated with appropriate antibiotics.

REVASCULARISATION

For global ischaemia following cardiac arrest, the theoretical principles are to re-establish systemic blood pressure and to consider the no-reflow phenomenon in certain areas of the brain. Current research is addressing attempts to increase blood pressure during CPR and to open up capillaries that may have collapsed during the arrest period.

For focal cerebral ischaemia:

- Start treatment as early as possible.
- Increase local CBF (fibrinolysis).
- Try to ameliorate ischaemic cascade (neuroprotection).

Ischaemic neuronal degeneration follows the onset of perfusion failure so that interventional therapy must begin immediately. Diagnostic imaging is required before using thrombolytic agents. For acute ischaemic stroke the National Institute of Neurological Disorders and Stroke (NINDS study) suggested efficacy if intravenous thrombolytic therapy is initiated within the first 3 hours of stroke symptoms (using recombinant tissue plasminogen activator).[9]

Current issues in implementing this treatment include:

- diagnosis, including imaging within this time frame
- the potential risks of thrombolysis
- accurately selecting patients eligible for thrombolysis

HAEMODILUTION

Current practice includes the use of hypervolaemic haemodilution and deliberate hypertension with augmentation of cardiac output using vasopressors and inotropic agents, particularly in the treatment of delayed ischaemic deficits after subarachnoid haemorrhage related to vasospasm. This therapy can be administered safely with intensive monitoring, but benefits are anecdotal, as it has not been tested with concurrent controls.[10]

Decreasing haematocrit and viscosity by haemodilution may improve flow and hence blood and oxygen delivery to areas with impaired arterial supply. Benefit in animal models of ischaemia has not been found in clinical trials of stroke. Trials of normovolaemic[11] and hypervolaemic haemodilution[12] have had complications from volume therapy in patients with associated heart disease.

Theoretical neuroprotective benefits of human haemoglobin-derived blood substitutes have not translated into clinical benefit, largely due to adverse events, and therefore clinical development of substitutes were discontinued.[13]

INTRACRANIAL PRESSURE

Raised ICP can cause global ischaemia. Treating ICP requires knowledge of the three compartments contributing to ICP within a fixed cranium:

1. blood
2. relatively non-compliant brain tissue
3. cerebrospinal fluid (CSF)

The relationship between ICP and intracranial volume is described by a non-linear pressure–volume curve. At lower intracranial volumes the ICP remains low and reasonably constant. Any increases in intracranial volume are compensated for by decreases in intracerebral blood or CSF volume. If greater intracranial volumes persist, this compensation is lost and ICP rises considerably, despite relatively small increases in intracerebral blood volume. Eventually at high levels of ICP cerebrovascular responses are lost, ICP equals MAP and CPP is very low.[14]

To maintain adequate cerebral perfusion, treatment should be targeted at ensuring an adequate perfusion pressure and a reduction in ICP. MAP should be raised to a level at or above the usual pressure for that patient, within the zone of pressure autoregulation – hence knowledge of premorbid blood pressure is important. If the majority of the vasculature is autoregulating, raising the blood pressure may decrease vascular diameter and reduce blood volume within the cranium. If the cause of the raised ICP cannot be corrected (e.g. blood clot or brain tumour), then the focus should be to prevent secondary injury around the lesion. An increased ICP can cause further ischaemia, and a reduction in ICP may facilitate adequate perfusion to areas at risk. Whenever possible, the offending compartment should be treated primarily (e.g. tumour removal, blood evacuation, drainage of hydrocephalus and, on occasion, craniectomy). If this is not advisable, reducing the relative volumes of other compartments may improve compliance overall and reduce the ICP.

MONITORING OF ICP (FIGURE 45.3)

ICP-monitoring devices have been ranked by the Brain Trauma Foundation[14] on their accuracy, stability and ability to drain CSF. Intraventricular and intraparenchymal catheters are seen as most favourable, followed by subdural, subarachnoid and epidural devices.

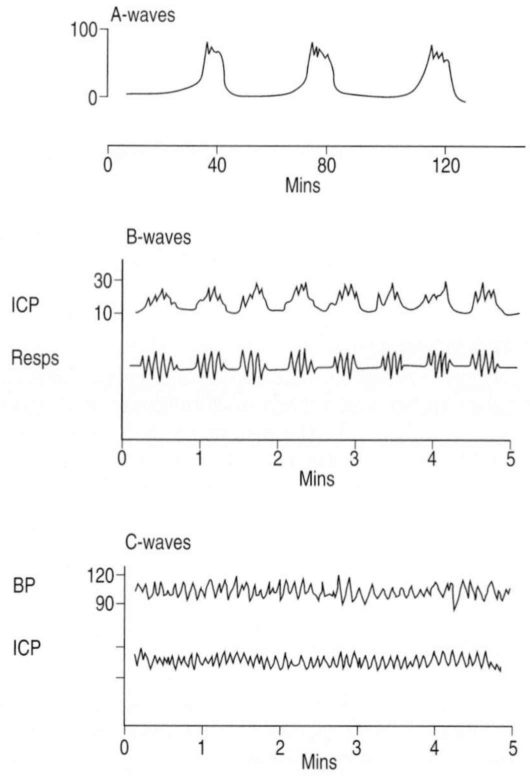

Figure 45.3 Intracranial pressure (ICP) waveforms. A-waves are plateau waves of 50-100 mmHg, sustained for 5–15 minutes, associated with raised ICP and compromised cerebral blood flow. B-waves are small changes in pressure every 0.5–2 minutes, often associated with breathing patterns and possibly due to local variations in the partial pressure of oxygen and carbon dioxide. C-waves are low-amplitude oscillations with a frequency of about 5 per minute, associated with variation in vasomotor tone. Resps, respirations; BP, blood pressure.

INTRAVENTRICULAR DEVICES

ICP is measured from an external pressure transducer attached to an intraventricular catheter inserted in one of the lateral ventricles using the external auditory meatus as the reference point. This device allows CSF sampling for culture or therapeutic drainage, the administration of antibotics and the ability to rezero following insertion. The main disadvantage is the high infection rate associated with their use.[14,15] Infection rates increase significantly after 5 days of catheter insertion and with repeated use of the device's flushing system. The use of antibiotic-impregnated catheters may lower the infection rate. Air, blood, tissue debris and ventricular collapse can all adversely affect measurement.

INTRAPARENCHYMAL DEVICES

ICP can be measured by either a miniature strain gauge pressure transducer mounted at the end of a thin catheter or by a fibreoptic cable which directs light to a miniature mirror at the end of the cable placed in brain tissue. These monitors are advantageous when lateral ventricles have collapsed secondary to raised ICP. This system is not dependent on fluid coupling for pressure transduction so waveform damping and artefacts are avoided. The infection rates are very low. Its main disadvantages include lack of recalibration in vivo, a tendency for baseline drift requiring transducer replacement, the inability to drain CSF and the ability to measure only localised pressure which may not be representative of the global ICP.[15]

Alternative invasive ICP monitoring includes epidural, subarachnoid and subdural devices, although these are not as accurate. All invasive ICP monitoring devices are associated with a risk of parenchymal damage with the potential for parenchymal and subdural bleeding. When it is not possible to insert an ICP-monitoring device, e.g. because of severe coagulopathy, ICP can be estimated from non-invasive alternatives, e.g. transcranial Doppler examination. However all ICP-monitoring devices have their limitations. Clarification should be sought by computed tomographic (CT) scanning if there is doubt about whether to intervene with treatment of an elevated ICP.

REGULATION OF INTRACRANIAL PRESSURE

BRAIN COMPARTMENT

Reduction in the parenchymal compartment depends on removal of either free water or the lesion causing the raised ICP.

Free water must be moved across an intact blood–brain barrier. Mannitol increases plasma osmolarity and reduces brain oedema. In addition, it may have a beneficial effect on microcirculatory flow. It is also thought to have antioxidant effects, although these may not be clinically important. Hypertonic saline has reduced ICP in patients with haemorrhagic shock and traumatic brain injury when used for volume resuscitation (7.5%), and also for treatment of raised ICP refractory to mannitol (23.4%).[16]

Removal of tumour or blood clot, drainage of abscesses and extirpation of infarcted brain are all therapies aimed at improving compliance. Mounting evidence now suggests that there is a penumbra of functionally impaired but potentially reversible neuronal injury surrounding a haematoma. Indications for clot removal, despite numerous studies performed over the last four decades, has been controversial. The Surgical Trial in Intracerebral Haemorrhage (STICH) compared early surgical evacuation of haematoma with initial conservative treatment, but found no significant difference in outcomes between the two treatments.[17]

The rationale for removing part of the skull overlying the stroke in patients with or at risk of developing cerebral oedema and intracranial hypertension is simply to decompress the brain swelling and prevent herniation. Decompressive craniectomy has been assessed in experimental cerebral infarction and was effective in reducing death and neurological impairment whether performed 1 hour or 24 hours after induction of permanent middle cerebral artery occlusion.[18] An uncontrolled trial comparing patients with hemicraniectomy with historical controls found that mortality rates were reduced from 80% to 35% in the surgical group.[19] These non-randomised studies are clearly at risk of bias and properly controlled trials of craniectomy for malignant middle cerebral artery infarction are required.

BLOOD COMPARTMENT

Although a small component of intracranial volume, the blood compartment is the most compliant. Reduction in blood volume is useful in the treatment of raised ICP, especially in the acute setting. As explained above, hypoxia and hypercarbia can lead to hyperaemia and an increase in cerebral blood volume, potentially worsening ICP. Alternatively, induced hypocarbia leads to very rapid changes in blood flow and blood volume. Hyperventilation for raised ICP is controversial. Up until 10 years ago, patients were often aggressively hyperventilated to a $Pa\text{CO}_2$ of 25 mmHg in order to reduce ICP rapidly as a result of arteriolar vasoconstriction. Unfortunately, the resultant reduction in cerebral blood volume may be accompanied by a fall in global CBF, which may result in ischaemia and a worsened outcome. The Brain Trauma Foundation guidelines in the 1990s recommended that chronic hyperventilation ($Pa\text{CO}_2$ = 25 mmHg) should not be instituted in severe traumatic brain injury in patients with a normal ICP and that prophylactic hyperventilation to a $Pa\text{CO}_2$ of 35 mmHg should also be avoided in the first 24 hours after a severe traumatic brain injury, as it can reduce cerebral perfusion during a time of reduced CBF. Current studies suggest that ICP reduction, as a result of moderate hyperventilation within the first 24 hours and the resultant decrease in CBF, do not compromise cerebral metabolism.[20] It is recommended that a secondary treatment be instituted as soon as possible to allow slow withdrawal of hyperventilation.[21] If adaptation to hypocapnia has not occurred, hyperventilation can be reinstituted with the same effect. Prevention of seizures and hyperthermia lower the cerebral metabolic demand and reduce CBF and volume.

CEREBROSPINAL FLUID COMPARTMENT

CSF drainage can be used to reduce ICP but is only possible if there is a ventricular catheter in place. Care is taken regarding the route and rate of CSF drainage to avoid herniation of a mass lesion, either towards the other side of the brain or through the tentorium. In recent years there has been a move towards the use of less invasive methods to measure ICP. However, the Brain Trauma Foundation guidelines for the management of severe head injury provide some evidence supporting the increased use of CSF drainage for ICP control.[22]

HYPOTHERMIA

Injury to the central nervous system is temperature-dependent. Fever can make an existing neurological dysfunction more apparent and may worsen an ongoing dysfunction. Potential mechanisms by which hyperthermia worsens cerebral ischaemia may include:

- neurotransmitter and oxygen free radical production
- blood–brain barrier failure
- damaging depolarisations in the ischaemic penumbra
- impaired recovery of energy metabolism
- cytoskeletal proteolysis[23]

Hyperthermia is harmful so treatment of fever should be aggressive, using cooling blankets, cool water, cool intravenous fluids, fans and antipyretic medications.

Hypothermia has been known to offer protection for years. In particular, drowning victims who were hypothermic have survived long periods of ischaemia. The mechanism of ICP reduction is unknown but may be due to a reduction in intracranial blood volume secondary to cerebral vasoconstriction or to alterations in metabolism. The protective effect of cooling appears to be much greater than that explained by changes in metabolism alone.

In contrast to preventing hyperthermia, the use of induced hypothermia is more complex. It has been used for protection extensively in coronary artery bypass surgery where hypothermia (28–30°C) is commonplace and deep hypothermia (< 20°C) has allowed prolonged circulatory arrest for surgery such as high thoracic and giant cerebral aneurysms. Animal work suggests that moderate, systemic hypothermia reduces the cerebral oedema and death after injury to the cerebral cortex. In several centres cooling has been used as therapy for severe head injuries. Unfortunately, a study which evaluated the efficacy of hypothermia in head injuries was halted after the enrolment of 392 patients because the treatment was ineffective.[24] Cooling patients to 33°C within 8 hours after injury and maintaining hypothermia for 48 hours were not effective in improving the clinical outcome at 6 months and patients older than 45 years of age had a poorer outcome. This contrasted with two earlier studies,[25,26] both of which demonstrated an improvement in outcome with cooling to 32°C.

In conclusion, at present:

- There is no evidence that hypothermic therapy after traumatic brain injury reduces risk of death or neurological outcome.
- Hypothermia may put the patient at more harm, with the risk of pneumonia, arrhythmias and coagulopathies.
- It may be more problematic in patients over 45 years of age.

In stroke patients there are no randomised controlled trials of hypothermia. Animal models suggest that hypothermia reduces ischaemic stroke lesion size.[27] A small uncontrolled study of moderate hypothermia found reduced mortality from an expected value of 78% to 44% in patients with severe middle cerebral artery infarction.[28] There are ongoing studies such as the Nordic Cooling Stroke Study (NOCSS).

In cardiac arrest the situation is changing. Although 50 years ago therapeutic hypothermia was used post cardiac arrest, it was abandoned because of the uncertain benefit. In the 1980s, animal studies indicated benefit with mild (32–35°C) rather than moderate or deep hypothermia. Two randomised clinical trials of hypothermia, after witnessed out-of-hospital cardiac arrest, demonstrated improved survival and neurological outcome after 12 or 24 hours of hypothermia at 33°C.[29,30] The evidence from these two relatively small trials has led to recommendations as set out by the International Liaison Committee on Resuscitation:

> *Unconcious adult patients with spontaneous circulation after out-of-hospital cardiac arrest should be cooled to 32°C to 34°C for 12 to 24 hours when the initial rhythm is ventricular fibrillation (VF).*

It has also been suggested, currently without evidence, that hypothermia may be beneficial for other rhythms or for in-hospital cardiac arrest. It is not recommended in patients with severe cardiogenic shock, life-threatening arrhythmias, pregnant patients or those with a coagulopathy.[31]

The uptake of these recommendations is variable. Recently, in the UK, a survey suggested that only 26% of units currently undertook therapeutic hypothermia after cardiac arrest. The main reasons for not using therapeutic hypothermia appeared to be due to logistical or resource issues and a perceived lack of evidence or lack of consensus within individual intensive care unit teams.[32]

There is currently insufficient evidence to recommend therapeutic hypothermia in children resuscitated from cardiac arrest. Neonatal animal studies, however, have shown promising results with regard to neuroprotection offered by posthypoxic hypothermia, although it has been shown that the protective effects of hypothermia are lost without adequate sedation.[33]

ANAESTHETIC AGENTS

Barbiturates have shown convincing benefit, especially for focal ischaemia in many animal species. In one small clinical study of induced barbiturate coma during coronary bypass surgery, there was a reduction in focal deficits.[34] Barbiturate-mediated neuroprotection was initially attributed to suppression of cerebral metabolic rate but more recently to redistribution of CBF to injured areas, the blockade of glutamate receptors and sodium channels, inhibition of free radical formation and potentiation of GABAergic activity.[35] At present barbiturates are not commonly used either in coronary bypass surgery or in situations of global ischaemia. Barbiturates are now less commonly used in head-injured patients but can play a role in those patients who have intractable intracranial hypertension.

Propofol has been shown to be neuroprotective in vivo, in focal and global models of cerebral ischaemia. It decreases cerebral metabolic rate and hence CBF. It has been shown to have antioxidant properties, potentiate GABA-A-mediated inhibition of synaptic transmission and inhibit glutamate release. It delays neuronal death by being a free radical scavenger, preventing lipid peroxidation and modulating apoptosis-regulating proteins.[35,36] Its side-effects include hypotension with a reducing CPP and hyperlipidaemia when an infusion of 200 μg/kg per min is used to produce burst suppression.[37] This latter problem has been lessened by the introduction of a more concentrated formulation.

Inhalational agents have significant neuroprotective effects but the precise mechanism by which they reduce cerebral injury is unclear.[36] It is possible that isoflurane may attenuate excitotoxicity by inhibiting glutamate release and its postsynaptic responses at both anaesthetic and EEG burst supression concentrations. The neuroprotection provided by volatile agents may also be attributable to their effect at GABA-A receptors and an ability to reduce the sympathetic vascular response to ischaemia. Certainly their effect on reducing cerebral metabolic rate is not sufficient to explain their neuroprotective properties.[35,36] These potential benefits in adults are offset by recent studies which have suggested that in neonatal animal studies there may be disturbing increases in cerebral apoptosis, although this has yet to be confirmed. There is an increasing interest in xenon, which presently looks promising.

Nitrous oxide exhibits the neuroprotective and neurotoxic features of an NMDA antagonist. Studies, however, have shown that, when combined with an opioid, e.g. fentanyl, its neuroprotective effect during incomplete cerebral ischaemia is still inferior when compared to volatile agents.[36]

Midazolam reduces the cerebral metabolic rate for oxygen, CBF and volume. It does not produce burst suppression or an isoelectric EEG, even in large doses.

Neuromuscular blockade is often used in head-injured patients to prevent any coughing on the tracheal tube and subsequent rise in ICP. Their use is not associated with better outcome despite the improvements in ICP control.

CALCIUM ANTAGONISTS

The influx of calcium from the extracellular space and from intracellular organelles has been implicated as the common mediator of cell death from a variety of causes. Calcium antagonists were among the first neuroprotective agents studied to prevent cerebral ischaemia. Despite the effects seen in animal models, human studies in both global and focal ischaemia have been disappointing. Two large trials of intravenous nimodipine in patients with acute ischaemic stroke were terminated early as neurological and functional outcome were significantly poorer in the nimodipine group.[38,39] A close relationship was found between a reduction in diastolic and mean blood pressure in the group treated with nimodipine and an unfavourable neurological outcome. A review of 29 randomised acute stroke trials involving calcium antagonists concluded that the use of calcium antagonists could not be justified in patients with ischaemic stroke and that, although the published trials showed no overall effect on death and dependency, unpublished trials were associated with a statistically significant worse outcome.[40] Nimodipine, however, has become the standard prophylactic treatment for cerebral vasospasm after subarachnoid haemorrhage, with a consequent decrease in cerebral infarction and better patient outcome.[41] Benefits appear to be due to an effect on smaller penetrating vessels not seen by angiography, or a neuroprotective effect at the cellular level, rather than cerebral vasodilatation identifiable by angiography.

Nimodipine was shown to be neuroprotective in head-injured patients with traumatic subarachnoid haemorrhage.[42] Regrettably, further studies to test the neuroprotective effect of nimodipine in severely head-injured patients with traumatic subarachnoid haemorrhage (including the multicentre study, HIT IV) failed to confirm the beneficial effects of nimodipine. A small group of patients with a Glasgow Coma Score < 9 did appear to be a have a better outcome in the nimodipine-treated group;[43] however, a recent systematic review concluded that there was no beneficial effect on outcome.[44] Its use therefore remains contentious.

STEROIDS

Glucocorticoids were used for over 30 years in the treatment of head injury despite the fact that randomised trials had failed to demonstrate their effectiveness reliably. They were thought to decrease cerebral oedema associated with breakdown of the blood–brain barrier (i.e. vasogenic oedema) and show improvement in central nervous system function with brain tumours and abscesses.[45,46]

The Corticosteroid Randomisation After Significant Head injury (CRASH) trial investigated the effects of a 48-hour infusion of methylprednisolone on death within 14 days or disability at 6 months in 10 008 adults with clinically significant head injury. The trial was stopped early, as at interim analysis, the steroid-treated subjects had significantly higher all-cause 2-week mortality (21.1% versus 17.9%, $P = 0.0001$). The 6-month mortality was also higher in steroid-treated subjects (25.7% versus 22.3%, $P = 0.0001$), with a trend toward increases in the combined endpoint of death or severe disability (38.1% versus 36.3%, $P = 0.08$). In neither report did the results differ by injury severity or time since injury.[47] The cause for the increased mortality is unclear.

In subarachnoid and primary intracerebral haemorrhage, corticosteroids have also been commonly used. In 2005, a Cochrane Review concluded that there was no evidence to support the use of mineralocorticoids or glucocorticoids in subarachnoid haemorrhage or to support the use of glucocorticoids in primary intracerebral haemorrhage. Corticosteroid use may also be associated with adverse events.[48]

In acute spinal cord injury, high-dose methylprednisolone for 24 hours has been shown to offer a small but significant benefit, provided treatment begins within 8 hours of injury (National Spinal Cord Injury Study (NASCIS) II trial).[49,50] This is still controversial. Adverse side-effects such as sepsis and poor wound healing were associated with the use of methylprednisolone, although some of these side-effects did not reach statistical significance. Currently steroid therapy in spinal cord injury is an unproven standard of care.[51]

EXPERIMENTAL THERAPY – THE FUTURE

There are a range of laboratory studies which have identified numerous potential therapeutic interventions for the treatment of head injury and stroke, some of which have progressed to clinical trials:

- Glutamate receptor antagonists. Dizocilpine (MK-801) is a non-competitive glutamate antagonist acting at the NMDA receptor. No clinical trials have been performed because of fears regarding hippocampal neurotoxicity.

- Free radical scavengers. In high concentrations free radicals react with almost all cellular structures and ultimately cause cell damage and cell death. Free radical scavengers attempt to attenuate this effect by a direct antioxidant effect or by providing a free radical degradation enzyme. Polyethylene glycol-conjugated superoxide dismutase (PEG-SOD) converts these harmful molecules into harmless metabolites. Neither mechanism has yet had clinically useful results.[43]
- Ciclosporin A may protect against traumatically induced mitochondrial damage by blocking mitochondrial permeability pores and preventing influx and efflux of harmful ions and free radicals. It is neuroprotective in animal models and phase II studies are currently ongoing.

In stroke, several classes of cerebral protective agents have been investigated in phase II and III trials.

- Gavestinel, an antagonist of the glycine site of the NMDA receptor, was administered in acute ischaemic or haemorrhagic stroke (Glycine Antagonist In Neuroprotection: GAIN) with no improvement in functional outcome.[52]
- Magnesium acts as an endogenous vasodilator of brain circulation and is a non-competitive antagonist of NMDA receptors and of the voltage-dependent calcium channels. The phase III trial (Intravenous Magnesium Efficacy in Acute Stroke: IMAGES) found no benefit in administration of magnesium within 12 hours of stroke.[53] An ongoing trial is evaluating whether giving magnesium within 2 hours of stroke is beneficial (Field Administration of Stroke Therapy–Magnesium: FAST-MAG).[54]
- Topiramate is a gamma-aminobutyric acid (GABA) agonist and an anticonvulsant that stabilises the cell membrane through increased chloride conductivity and might be useful in traumatic brain injury. As a GABA agonist, it acts as a stabiliser by hyperpolarising the cell membrane.[43] Clomethiazole is another GABA agonist.[55]
- A sodium channel and nitric oxide blocker (lubeluzole) is also being trialled.[56] Lubeluzole inhibits glutamate release in the penumbra area and decreases postischaemic excitotoxicity.
- Albumin, 25%, at 1.25–2.5 g/kg reduces infarct volume and brain swelling in rats. It has been suggested that the protective effect is not just due to haemodilution but rather to the multiple actions of the albumin molecule in binding to free fatty acids, inhibiting oxygen free radical production and supporting endothelial function.[57]

Intracerebral haemorrhage is the least treatable form of stroke and is associated with a high morbidity and mortality. Recombinant activated factor VIIa (rFV11a) administered within 4 hours of onset and within 1 hour of a diagnostic CT scan has been shown in one trial to limit haematoma growth, reduce mortality and improve 90-day functional outcome. There was, however, a small increase in the frequency of thromboembolic events.[58]

Thrombolysis within the first few hours has been effective following ischaemic stroke. The search continues for safe neuroprotective strategies to use in ischaemic stroke which can be used alone or in combination with thrombolysis.

To date the completed trials have yielded disappointing efficacy results and some have shown safety problems. Despite this, it is believed that, with the increased understanding of the mechanism of cell death and new targets for drug treatment, it is only a matter of time before an effective cerebral protective agent will become available.

REFERENCES

1. Bedell S, Delbanco T, Cook E *et al.* Survival after cardiopulmonary resuscitation in the hospital. *N Engl J Med* 1983; **309**: 569–76.
2. Dirnagi U, Iadecola C, Moskowitz MA. Pathobiology of ischaemic stroke: an integrated view. *Trends Neurosci* 1999; **22**: 391–7.
3. Maas AIR, Dearden M, Teassdale GM *et al.* EBIC guidelines for management of severe head injury in adults. *Acta Neurochir* 1997; **139**: 286–94.
4. Brott T, Lu M, Kothari R *et al.* Hypertension and its treatment in the NINDS rt-PA stroke trial. *Stroke* 1998; **29**: 1504–9.
5. Capes SE, Hunt D, Malmberg K *et al.* stress hyperglycaemia and prognosis of stroke in nondiabetic and diabetic patients; a systematic overview. *Stroke* 2001; **32**: 2426–32.
6. Ribo M, Molina C, Montaner J *et al.* Acute hyperglycaemia state is associated with lower t-PA-induced recanalisation rates in stroke patients. *Stroke* 2005; **36**: 1705–9.
7. Strong AJ, Fairfield JE, Monteiro E *et al.* Insulin protects cognitive function in experimental stroke. *J Neurol Neurosurg Psychiatry* 1990; **53**: 847–53.
8. Reith J, Jorgensen HS, Pedersen PM *et al.* Body temperature in acute stroke: relation to stroke severity, infarct size, mortality and outcome. *Lancet* 1996; **347**: 422–5.
9. The National Institute of Neurological Disorders and Stroke rt-PA Stroke Study Group. Tissue plasminogen activator for acute ischaemic stroke. *N Engl J Med* 1995; **333**: 1581–7.
10. Solomon R, Fink M, Lennihan L. Early aneurysm surgery and prophylactic hypervolemic, hypertensive therapy for the treatment of aneurysmal subarachnoid hemorrhage. *Neurosurgery* 1988; **23**: 699–704.
11. Italian Acute Stroke Study Group. Haemodilution in acute stroke: results of the Italian haemodilution trial. *Lancet* 1988; **1**: 318–21.
12. The Hemodilution in Stroke Study Group. Hypervolemic hemodilution treatment of acute stroke. Results of a randomised multicenter trial using pentastarch. *Stroke* 1989; **20**: 317–23.

13. Saxena R, Wijnhoud AD, Carton H *et al.* Controlled safety study of a haemoglobin-based oxygen carrier, DCL Hb, in acute ischaemic stroke. *Stroke* 1999; **30**: 993–6.
14. Brain Trauma Foundation. Available online at: www2.braintrauma.org/.
15. Steiner LA, Andrews PDJ. Monitoring the injured brain: ICP and CBF. *Br J Anaesth* 2006; **97**: 26–38.
16. Qureshi AI, Suarez JI. Use of hypertonic saline solutions in treatment of cerebral oedema and intracranial hypertension. *Crit Care Med* 2000; **28**: 3301–13.
17. Mendelow AD, Gregson BA, Fernandes HM *et al.* Early surgery versus initial conservative treatment in patients with spontaneous supratentorial intracerebral haematomas in the International Surgical Trial in Intracerebral Haemorrhage (STICH): a randomised trial. *Lancet* 2005; **365**: 387–97.
18. Forsting M, Reith W, Shabitz W-R *et al.* Decompressive craniectomy for cerebral infarction. An experimental study in rats. *Stroke* 1995; **26**: 259–64.
19. Rieke K, Schwab S, Horn M *et al.* Decompressive surgery in space occupying hemispheric infarction: results of an open, prospective trial. *Crit Care Med* 1995; **23**: 1576–87.
20. Oertel M, Kelly DF, Lee JH *et al.* Efficacy of hyperventilation, blood pressure elevation, and metabolic suppression therapy in controlling intracranial pressure after head injury. *J Neursurg* 2002; **97**: 1045–53.
21. Muizelaar JP, Marmarou A, Ward JD *et al.* Adverse effects of prolonged hyperventilation in patients with severe head injury: a randomized clinical trial. *J Neurosurg* 1991; **75**: 731–9.
22. Bullock MR, Povilshock JT. Indications for intracranial pressure monitoring. *J Neurotrauma* 1996; **13**: 667–9.
23. Ginsberg MD, Busto R. Combating hyperthermia in acute stroke: a significant clinical concern. *Stroke* 1998; **29**: 529–34.
24. Clifton GL, Miller ER, Choi SC *et al.* Lack of effect of induction of hypothermia after acute brain injury. *N Engl J Med* 2001; **344**: 556–63.
25. Clifton GL, Allen S, Barrodale P *et al.* A phase II study of moderate hypothermia in severe brain injury. *J Neurotrauma* 1993; **10**: 263–71.
26. Marion DW, Obrist WD, Carlier PM *et al.* The use of moderate therapeutic hypothermia for patients with severe head injuries: a preliminary report. *J Neurosurg* 1993; **79**: 354–62.
27. Baker J, Onesti T, Solomon R. Reduction by delayed hypothermia of cerebral infarction following middle cerebral artery occlusion in the rat: a time-course study. *J Neurosurg* 1992; **77**: 438–44.
28. Schwab S, Schwartz S, Spranger M *et al.* Moderate hypothermia in the treatment of patients with severe middle cerebral artery infarction. *Stroke* 1998; **29**: 2461–6.
29. The Hypothermia after Cardiac Arrest Study Group. Mild therapeutic hypothermia to improve the neurological outcome after cardiac arrest. *N Engl J Med* 2002; **346**: 549–56.
30. Bernard SA, Gray TW, Buist MD *et al.* Treatment of comatose survivors of out-of-hospital cardiac arrest with induced hypothermia. *N Engl J Med* 2002; **346**: 557–63.
31. Nolan JP, Morley PT, Vanden Hoek TV *et al.* Therapeutic hypothermia after cardiac arrest: an advisory statement by the Advanced Life Support Task Force of the International Liaison Committee on Resuscitation. *Circulation* 2003; **108**: 118–21.
32. Laver SR, Padkin A, Atalla A *et al.* Therapeutic hypothermia after cardiac arrest: a survey of practice in intensive care units in the United Kingdom. *Anaesthesia* 2006; **61**: 873–7.
33. Tooley JR, Satas S, Porter H *et al.* Head cooling with mild systemic hypothermia in anaesthetised piglets is neuroprotective. *Ann Neurol* 2003; **53**: 65–72.
34. Nussmeier NA, Arlund C, Slogoff S. Neuropsychiatric complications after cardiopulmonary bypass: cerebral protection by a barbiturate. *Anesthesiology* 1986; **64**: 165–70.
35. Kawagughi M, Furuya H, Patel PM. Neuroprotective effects of anaesthetic agents. *J Anesth* 2005; **19**: 150–6.
36. Sanders RD, Ma D, Maze M. Anaesthesia induced neuroprotection. *Best Pract Res Clin Anaesthesiol* 2005; **19**: 461–74.
37. Menon DK. Cerebral protection in severe brain injury: physiological determinants of outcome and their optimisation. *Br Med Bull* 1999; **55**: 226–58.
38. Wahlgren NG, MacMahon DG, De Keyser J *et al.* Intravenous Nimodipine West European Stroke Trial (INWEST) of nimodipine in the treatment of acute ischaemic stroke. *Cerebrovasc Dis* 1994; **4**: 20–10.
39. Bridgers S, Koch G, Munera C *et al.* Intravenous nimodipine in acute stroke: interim analysis of randomised trial. *Stroke* 1991; **22**: 29.
40. Horn J, Limburg M. Calcium antagonists for ischaemic stroke: a systematic review. *Stroke* 2001; **32**: 570–6.
41. Pickard JD, Murray GD, Illingworth R *et al.* Effect of oral nimodipine on cerebral infarction and outcome after subarachnoid haemorrhage: British aneurysm nimodipine trial. *Br Med J* 1989; **298**: 636–42.
42. Harders A, Kakarieka A, Braakman R *et al.* Traumatic subarachnoid haemorrhage and its treatment with nimodipine. *J Neurosurg* 1996; **85**: 82–5.
43. Clausen T, Bullock R. Medical treatment and neuroprotection in traumatic brain injury. *Curr Pharm Design* 2001; **7**: 1517–32.
44. Vergouwen MD, Vermeulen M, Roos YB. Effect of nimodipine on outcome in patients with traumatic subarachnoid haemorrhage: a systematic review. *Lancet Neurol* 2006; **5**: 1029–32.
45. Reulen H. Vasogenic brain oedema. New aspects in its formation, resolution and therapy. *Br J Anaesth* 1976; **48**: 741–52.
46. French LA, Galicich JH. The use of steroids for control of cerebral oedema. *Clin Neurosurg* 1964; **10**: 212–23.
47. CRASH trial collaborators. Final results of the MRC CRASH trial, a randomised placebo-controlled trial of

intravenous corticosteroid in adults with head injury-outcomes at 6 months. *Lancet* 2005; **365**: 1957–9.
48. Feigin V.L, Anderson N, Rinkel GJE *et al.* Corticosteroids for aneurysmal subarachnoid haemorrhage and primary intracerebral haemorrhage. *Cochrane Database of Systematic Reviews* 2005; **3**: CD004583.
49. Bracken M, Shepard M, Collins W *et al.* Methylprednisolone or naloxone treatment after acute spinal cord injury: one-year follow-up data. *J Neurosurg* 1992; **76**: 23–31.
50. Bracken MB, Shepard MJ, Collins W *et al.* A randomized, controlled trial of methylprednisolone or naloxone in the treatment of acute spinal-cord injury. Results of the second national acute spinal cord injury study. *N Engl J Med* 1990; **322**: 1405–11.
51. Hurlbert R. Strategies of a medical intervention in the management of acute spinal cord injury. *Spine* 2006; **31** (suppl.): S16–21.
52. Sacco RL, DeRosa JT, Clarke Haley Jr E *et al.* Glycine antagonist in neuroprotection for patients with acute stroke. GAIN Americas: a randomised controlled trial. *JAMA* 2001; **285**: 1728–9.
53. Meloni BP, Zhu H, Knuckey NW. Is magnesium neuroprotective following global and focal ischaemia? A review of published studies. *Magnesium Res* 2006; **19**: 123–37.
54. Saver JL, Kidwell C, Eckstein M *et al.* Prehospital neuroprotective therapy for acute stroke: results of the Field Administration of Stroke Therapy–Magnesium (FAST-MAG) pilot trial. *Stroke* 2004; **35**: 106–8.
55. Wahlgren NG, for the CLASS study group. The Clomethiazole Acute Stroke Study (CLASS): results of a randomised controlled trial of clomethiazole versus placebo in 1360 acute stroke patients. *J Stroke* 1999; **230**: 21–8.
56. Diener HC, for the European and Australian Lubelozole Ischaemic Stroke Study Group. Multinational randomised controlled trial of lubelozole in acute ischaemic stroke. *Cerebrovasc Dis* 1998; **8**: 172–81.
57. Ginsberg MD. Adventures in the pathophysiology of brain ischaemia: penumbra, gene expression, neuroprotection. The 2002 Thomas Willis lecture. *Stroke* 2003; **34**: 214–23.
58. Mayer SA, Brun NC, Begtrup K *et al.* Recombinant activated factor VII for acute intracerebral hemorrhage. *N Engl J Med* 2005; **352**: 777–85.

46

Brain death

Marcus Peck and Martin Smith

Most people die a 'conventional' death when their heart stops beating. In others the advent of intensive organ support has complicated the diagnosis of death. Patients who have sustained irreversible structural brain damage as a result of head injury, subarachnoid haemorrhage, stroke or cerebral anoxia lie in a deep coma without the capacity to breathe. Prompt medical attention may have taken over ventilation, but recovery is impossible. It therefore became necessary to reappraise death based on the integrity of the central nervous system.[1–3] Brain death describes a state of irreversible loss of brain function, including loss of brainstem function. The ability to certify death under such circumstances allows intensivists to withdraw treatment on ethical, humanitarian and utilitarian grounds. Relatives are relieved of unnecessary prolonged anxiety and false hopes, and the burden on expensive medical resources is reduced. A further benefit for society is the availability of organs for transplantation from heart-beating donors.

DEFINITION OF DEATH

Three distinct mechanisms of death are recognised – cardiac arrest, respiratory arrest and brain death. This distinction is artificial. Cardiorespiratory arrest only results in inevitable death if the period of arrest has been long enough to result in irreversible damage to the brainstem due to lack of perfusion with oxygenated blood. Shorter periods of cardiac or respiratory arrest may result in survival with differing degrees of brain damage. As the neurones of the brainstem are the most resistant to anoxia, patients may retain the ability to breathe but survive with severe, irreversible cortical damage (the persistent vegetative state: PVS). The key feature of both cardiorespiratory death and brainstem death is irreparable brain damage. Death of the brainstem, whether caused by intracranial events or extracranial phenomena such as hypoxia, represents death of a person as a whole.

Dying is a process but death is an event that can be defined in a number of ways. In the UK there is no statutory definition of death, but English law has adopted widely accepted criteria and considers death to be the 'the irreversible loss of the capacity for consciousness, combined with the irreversible loss of the capacity to breathe'. In Australia, for the purpose of organ harvest, the statutory definition is 'irreversible cessation of all brain function'.

Brain death results from massive swelling of the traumatised brain, a sustained rise in intracranial pressure equal to or above systemic arterial pressure causing cessation of cerebral circulation, and brainstem herniation. The principal causes in adults are traumatic brain injury (50%), subarachnoid haemorrhage (30%) and severe hypoxic–ischaemic injury (20%). Complete and irreversible loss of brainstem function may also be seen in isolated brainstem injury without the typical features of herniation (e.g. brainstem infarction), which may or may not be accompanied by complete loss of hemispheric function.

PERSISTENT VEGETATIVE STATE

Severe brain damage is distinct from brain death. Comatose patients with severe brain damage may recover, albeit with varying degrees of disability, or remain in persistent coma. PVS is an irreversible condition in patients who have lost cortical activity. Coma has progressed to a state of wakefulness without detectable awareness and the patient is able to breathe spontaneously. PVS is therefore compatible with life if supportive care is provided. This is in contrast to brain death, where there is irreversible loss of the capacity to breathe and independent survival is impossible. PVS is not recognised as death in any jurisdiction and, in most, withdrawal of support to patients with PVS requires legal authority.

ROLE OF THE BRAINSTEM

There is sometimes a lack of clarity between brain death and brainstem death and this reflects differing diagnostic practices.[4] In the USA the Uniform Determination of Death Act describes brain death as death of the *whole* brain and states: 'an individual who has sustained irreversible cessation of all functions of the entire brain, including the brainstem, is dead'.[5] This formulation is one of the most commonly applied worldwide and forms the basis of the legal status in many countries. A notable exception exists in the UK, where a brainstem-based definition of death is in place.[2]

The brainstem contains the cranial nerve nuclei and respiratory and cardiovascular control centres. It is also the conduit for all ascending and descending pathways that connect the cortex with the rest of the body and is an essential part of the reticulo-activating system (RAS). Awareness depends on the integrity of the RAS. The mechanism of loss of consciousness in brainstem death is related to disruption of the RAS. After onset of brainstem death, brainstem reflexes are lost sequentially in a craniocaudal direction. This process may take several hours to become complete but finally results in apnoea due to failure of the medulla oblongata. Because of the fundamental controlling role of the brainstem, myocardial and other systemic physiological functions deteriorate after the onset of brainstem death.[6] Without cardiovascular support most patients confirmed as brain-dead progress to asystolic cardiac arrest within 24–48 hours.

ESTABLISHMENT OF BRAIN DEATH CRITERIA

Brain death was first described in 1959 by Mollaret and Goulon,[7] two French physicians, who coined the phrase 'coma dépassé' (meaning literally a state beyond coma) to describe 23 unconscious apnoeic patients who had lost brainstem reflexes.

In 1968 an ad hoc committee of the Harvard Medical School defined irreversible coma, or brain death, as unresponsiveness and lack of receptivity, the absence of movement and breathing, the absence of brainstem reflexes and coma whose cause has been identified (the Harvard criteria).[1] In the following year the committee indicated that brain death could be diagnosed on clinical grounds alone. This was affirmed in 1971 by two neurosurgeons (Mohandas and Chou) who described irreversible loss of brainstem function as the 'point of no return' (the Minnesota criteria).[8] At this time it was reiterated that brain death could be diagnosed on clinical judgement alone, without the need for a confirmatory electroencephalogram (EEG), so long as certain aetiological preconditions were present.

In 1976 a memorandum from the Conference of Medical Colleges and their Faculties in the UK stated that 'permanent functional death of the brainstem constitutes brain death' and that this could be diagnosed clinically in the context of irremediable structural brain damage after certain specified conditions had been excluded.[2] The memorandum established a set of guidelines and clinical tests for the diagnosis of brainstem death that became the foundation of practice worldwide. A subsequent memorandum in 1979 concluded that the identification of brain death means that the patient is dead, whether or not the function of some organs, such as the heart beat, is still maintained by artificial means. A further memorandum in 1983 made additional recommendations about the timing of the clinical tests and who should perform them. It also confirmed that there may be circumstances in which it is impossible or inappropriate to carry out every one of the tests and it is for the doctor at the bedside to decide when the patient is dead.

Simultaneously to the guidance being issued in the UK, other countries were formalising practice. In the USA, the 1981 Report to the President's Commission confirmed the requirement for the irreversible cessation of brain and brainstem functions to diagnose death.[5] Because death of the whole brain is diagnosed in the USA, this report recommended that confirmatory tests be used to support the clinical diagnosis and reduce the required time of observation.

CRITERIA FOR THE DIAGNOSIS OF BRAIN DEATH

Common to the determination of brain death in the UK and USA is the confirmation of the absence of clinical function of the brainstem, i.e. loss of consciousness, unresponsiveness, coma and loss of brainstem reflexes, including the capacity to breathe. The UK criteria form the basis of the clinical diagnosis of brain death in other countries and will be used as an exemplar of clinical testing. The diagnostic algorithm has three sequential but interdependent steps. Certain preconditions and exclusions must be fulfilled before clinical tests of brainstem function are performed.[9]

PRECONDITIONS

- The patient should be in apnoeic coma, i.e. unresponsive and dependent on mechanical ventilation.
- The patient's condition must be due to structural brain damage that is consistent with the diagnosis of brainstem death.
- The underlying disorder that has led to this state must be established.

In all cases a cranial computed tomography (CT) scan and full neurological examination are essential. Establishing the causative diagnosis is relatively straightforward in the case of head injury or intracranial haemorrhage but may take longer in coma arising from hypoxia or other causes.

EXCLUSIONS

Reversible causes of coma must be excluded. These include:

- *Alcohol intoxication or drug overdose.* Drug history must be reviewed and, in case of any doubt, a toxicology screen obtained.
- *The effects of therapeutic depressant drugs.* Narcotics, hypnotics and tranquillisers are likely to have been administered in the period leading up to brain death. These can have lengthy and unpredictable elimination

times, particularly in critically ill patients. The drug's type, dose, pharmacokinetics, half-life and the presence of organ dysfunction are all factors that contribute to duration of effect. Adequate time must be allowed for the residual sedative effects of these drugs to be excluded and, in the absence of organ dysfunction, a period of 3–4 times the half-life of the drug is recommended. Most commonly used drugs are cleared within 10–12 hours. Measurement of plasma concentration of active drug or metabolite will indicate whether drug levels are below the usual therapeutic range. However, plasma concentration does not always correlate with therapeutic effect in critically ill brain-injured patients. The use of specific pharmacological antagonists may be used in certain circumstances.

- *Residual action of neuromuscular-blocking agents.* This must be excluded by confirmation of the absence of deep tendon reflexes or lack of response to peripheral nerve stimulation.
- *Hypothermia.* Extreme hypothermia (< 28°C) invariably results in depressed brainstem reflexes but higher temperatures (32–34°C) can also have effects on conscious level. Core temperature should be > 35°C prior to testing brainstem reflexes.
- *Metabolic and endocrine disturbances.* There must be no profound abnormality of serum urea and electrolytes, acid–base status or blood glucose.
  - Serum sodium values < 115 mmol/l and > 160 mmol/l should be corrected prior to testing brainstem reflexes. Diabetes insipidus (DI) is a regular sequela of brain death and significant hypernatraemia is common. The 1998 UK Code of Practice allows differentiation between abnormalities which arise as a consequence of brainstem failure (e.g. hypernatraemia due to DI) from causative abnormalities of endocrine or biochemical function.[9]
  - Blood glucose should be between 2 and 20 mmol/l.
  - Potassium must be greater than 2 mmol/l to avoid effects on neuromuscular function.
  - Coexistent endocrine disorders must be excluded or treated before testing brainstem reflexes.
- *Neurological conditions that can mimic brainstem death.* These should be excluded by careful clinical examination (see below).

CLINICAL TESTS

These demonstrate the absence of brainstem reflexes and confirm the presence of persistent apnoea. They should be performed only when the preconditions and exclusions have been met. Confirmation of absence of the occulocephalic reflex ('doll's-eye' movements) is not part of the UK criteria. However, the presence of this reflex confirms that brainstem function persists and that further tests are inappropriate. Examination for 'doll's-eye' movement is a part of protocols in other countries. Facial trauma or obstruction to external ear canals may make assessment of brainstem reflexes difficult, but injury preventing bilateral examination does not invalidate the diagnosis.

CRANIAL NERVE EXAMINATION

The following signs of brainstem areflexia must be present to confirm the diagnosis of brainstem death:[3,9]

- Both pupils should be fixed in diameter and unresponsive to bright light. Pupil size is irrelevant but usually dilated – tests optic (II) and occulomotor (III) nerves.
- Corneal reflexes are absent during firm pressure over the cornea with a gauze swab – tests trigeminal sensory (V) and facial (VII) nerves.
- A standardised painful stimulus in the three areas of trigeminal nerve distribution (e.g. supraorbital pressure or jaw thrust) should not elicit a motor response in cranial or somatic distributions. Peripheral stimulation such as nailbed pressure should also not result in facial grimacing, although somatic spinal reflexes may persist – tests trigeminal (V) and facial (VII) nerves.
- There should be no gag or cough reflex in response to pharyngeal, laryngeal or tracheal stimulation – tests glossopharyngeal (IX) and vagus (X) nerves.
- The occulovestibular reflexes (caloric response) must be absent. Ice-cold water (50 ml) is injected slowly into each auditory meatus over 1 minute with the head flexed at 30°. There is absence of tonic deviation of the eyes towards the side being tested. Clear access to each tympanic membrane must first be confirmed by visual access – tests oculomotor (III), abducens (VI) and vestibulocochlear (VIII) nerves.

APNOEA TEST

The apnoea test confirms the absence of spontaneous respiratory effort despite $Paco_2$ at a level above the threshold for stimulation of respiration (usually 6.5 kPa). Severe hypoxaemia, excessive hypercarbia and changes in arterial blood pressure can occur if the apnoea test is not carried out correctly. To minimise the risk of further damage to potentially recoverable brain tissue, the apnoea test should not be performed if any of the preceding tests confirm the presence of brainstem reflexes. The following method describes a safe method for conduct of the apnoea test. The patient should be preoxygenated with 100% for 10 minutes. Arterial blood gases (ABGs) are checked to ensure correlation with end-tidal CO_2 ($EtCO_2$) and oxygen saturation (Sao_2). When Sao_2 is above 95%, minute ventilation is reduced until $EtCO_2$ rises to 6.5 kPa. ABGs are then checked to ensure that $Paco_2$ is also > 6.5 kPa and pH < 7.35. In patients with CO_2 retention the $Paco_2$ may need to be higher to achieve the target pH. If blood pressure is stable, this state should be maintained for 10 minutes, after which the patient is disconnected from the ventilator. Oxygenation is maintained by endotracheal insufflation of oxygen at 5 l/min via a suction catheter. Prior recruitment manoeuvres and continuous positive airway pressure may be necessary if maintenance of oxygenation is difficult. The patient should be observed for spontaneous ventilatory effort during the following 5 minutes. If there is no respiratory effort, absence of respiratory centre activity is confirmed and documented after repeat ABG analysis demonstrates that $PaCO_2$ remains > 6.5 kPa. After testing, normal minute ventilation should be restored to return ABGs to pretesting values.

Table 46.1 Indications for confirmatory tests to diagnose brain death

- No clear cause for coma exists
- Possible drug or metabolic effect on coma that cannot be excluded
- Cranial nerves cannot be adequately tested bilaterally
- Cervical cord injury is present or suspected
- Cardiorespiratory instability that precludes testing for apnoea

OTHER ISSUES DURING CLINICAL TESTING

In some jurisdictions, including the UK, Australia and some states in the USA, two medical practitioners are required to confirm the diagnosis of brain death.[10] The base speciality is not important but each doctor must be competent in carrying out such an assessment. It is often recommended that the apnoea test be supervised by an anaesthetist or intensivist. The doctors should be senior and not involved in organ transplantation programmes. Although the two doctors may carry out the tests together or independently, two sets of tests are recommended to demonstrate irreversibilty. The interval between the two sets of tests is not proscribed for adults in the UK but other jurisdictions set minimum time limits between the tests.[10] Although death is confirmed by the second set of brainstem tests in the UK, the legal time for certification of death is that of the initial testing. In other countries, such as Australia, the time of death for certification purposes is the time after the second confirmatory examination.

The confidence in application of clinical criteria for the diagnosis of brainstem death comes from over 30 years of experience. There is no report in the world literature of response during the second tests in a patient who has satisfied the clinical criteria for brain death during the first tests. Furthermore, there has been no subsequent recovery in those in whom ventilation was not discontinued.

Despite robust guidelines for the diagnosis of brainstem death, interpretation of this guidance varies widely.[11] In a study examining compliance with guidelines in the UK, marked differences in the timing of testing, the exclusion of residual sedative agents, the management of deranged biochemistry and the conduct of the caloric and apnoea test were noted.[12]

SUPPLEMENTARY DIAGNOSTIC TECHNIQUES

Clinical tests are the gold standard for assessment of brainstem function and supplementary tests are not required in the UK, Australia or New Zealand. They are required by law in some European countries where the diagnosis of whole brain death is made.[13] They are optional in the USA, but recommended if special circumstances limit clinical assessment or render it unreliable.

Supplementary investigations do not test brainstem function but are surrogate markers of cortical function. Many have been validated against clinical diagnosis and are not 100% specific or sensitive. They are therefore usually recommended as confirmatory rather than absolute tests.[14,15] Ancillary tests are of assistance if brainstem function cannot be adequately assessed clinically (Table 46.1). They are also required in very young children.

ASSESSMENT OF BLOOD FLOW IN THE LARGER CEREBRAL ARTERIES

Investigations of cerebral blood flow are independent of confounding variables such as sedation, metabolic disturbance or hypothermia. However, the presence of residual cerebral blood flow does not preclude a diagnosis of brain death. These techniques may therefore produce false-negative results and this is particularly likely in the presence of decompressive craniectomy, skull fracture or cerebrospinal fluid drains.

- *Four-vessel cerebral angiography:* injection of contrast into both vertebral and carotid arteries confirms no filling of the intracerebral vessels. Absence of flow beyond the foramen magnum will be observed in the posterior circulation and no flow beyond the petrosal portion of the carotid artery in the anterior circulation. Isolated or minimal filling necessitates repeat examination. Cerebral angiography is invasive, time-consuming and readily available only in the radiology suites of neuroscience units. However, it is reliable and easy to interpret and the gold-standard confirmatory test for brain death in some jurisdictions.
- *Magnetic resonance or CT angiography:* this is non-invasive but has similar logistical problems to formal angiography.
- *Transcranial Doppler ultrasonography (TCD):* TCD is a non-invasive, bedside investigation that is being increasingly used as a confirmatory test during diagnosis of brain death. Blood flow through both middle cerebral and vertebral arteries is compared with that through extracranial vessels. Absence of signal may be artefactual and should not be taken as diagnostic. Typical findings after brain death include diastolic reverberating flow and little or no forward systolic flow. TCD has 91–99% sensitivity with 100% specificity in skilled hands. However the technique has significant operator dependence and previous surgery or the presence of a ventricular drain may make waveform interpretation difficult.

ASSESSMENT OF BRAIN TISSUE PERFUSION

- *Contrast-enhanced CT cerebral perfusion:* These techniques are becoming more widely available and their use to confirm brain death is likely to increase.
- *Single-photon emission computed tomography:* This technique is sensitive and specific, although interpretation can be difficult.
- *Positron emission tomography (PET)*: PET is accurate and unambiguous but access to this technique is limited to a few centres.
- *Nuclear imaging*: brain images obtained sequentially up to 2 hours after injection of radionuclide confirm the absence of intracerebral uptake.

ASSESSMENT OF NEUROPHYSIOLOGICAL FUNCTION

- *EEG*: EEG is a widely used confirmatory test. However, specialist expertise is required for interpretation. Absence of cortical electrical activity is demonstrated by recordings from 16 or 18 channels for over 30 minutes using high sensitivity. Artefacts from the intensive care unit (ICU) environment are common because of the high levels of sensitivity required. A silent EEG in the absence of metabolic or drug effects suggests cortical death but cannot confirm or exclude brainstem activity. Equally, electrical activity in some cortical cells does not mean that the brain as a whole is alive. Confirmatory EEG is mandatory in many European countries. In the USA the choice of supportive test is at the discretion of the attending physician, but confirmatory EEG is strongly recommended because loss of whole-brain function must be demonstrated.
- *Somatosensory evoked potentials (SSEPs) and brainstem auditory evoked potemtials (BAEPs)*: SSEPs and BAEPs demonstrate successive loss of function of various afferent pathways of the brainstem. Multimodality evoked potentials are non-invasive, relatively unaffected by sedative agents and increasingly used as a confirmatory test.

DIAGNOSING BRAIN DEATH IN SPECIAL CIRCUMSTANCES

HIGH CERVICAL CORD INJURY

Confirmation of apnoea is fundamental to the clinical diagnosis of brain death. The possibility that apnoea may be related to high cervical cord injury may bring some difficulty to the diagnosis.[16] It is important to quantify the degree of any spinal cord injury clinically, structurally and functionally by meticulous clinical examination, magnetic resonance imaging and electrophysiological tests, including SSEPs and motor evoked potentials. Confirmatory tests may also assist the clinician in being confident that the patient is brain-dead.

NEUROLOGICAL CONDITIONS

Some rare neurological conditions may mimic brain death.[3] In the 'locked-in syndrome' the patient is tetraplegic but conscious, with preservation of conjugate vertical gaze and the ability to blink. Cranial nerve involvement and respiratory paralysis are associated with Guillain–Barré syndrome and may lead to diagnostic confusion[17] but pupil dilatation in this condition is rare. Brainstem reflexes may also be absent in brainstem encephalitis but the patient is usually drowsy rather than comatose. The preconditions for diagnosis of brain death are not met in these neurological conditions. Meticulous application of the clinical criteria and careful clinical examination will ensure that these neurological conditions cannot be mistaken for brain death.

BARBITURATES

There has been resurgence in the use of barbiturates to treat intractable intracranial hypertension and some patients will progress to brain death. The usual exclusion criteria apply but previous barbiturate infusion brings particular problems to the diagnosis of brain death because of its long and unpredictable action. Plasma barbiturate levels may not reflect clinical effect, particularly in the context of brain injury, and there is no consensus regarding an acceptable minimal plasma concentration.[18] Access to the assay may also be restricted and there is often a delay in obtaining the results. Another option is to wait an arbitrary period of time to allow the barbiturate effects to wear off: a period of between 2 and 5 days has been recommended. However, this 'best-guess' approach represents an inefficient use of ICU resource and represents additional pressures for relatives because of delays. The effects of high-dose barbiturates can mimic brain death, particularly in the presence of hypothermia. However, except in children, this is exceptionally rare and some aspect of brainstem function, such as the pupil response to light, often remains intact. In the presence of other stigmata of brain death, such as dilated unreactive pupils, characteristic cardiovascular changes and DI, the diagnosis is rarely in doubt. Confirmatory tests, particular cerebral angiography or BAEPs, may also be of assistance.

CHILDREN

Special care is recommended in diagnosing brain death in children less than 5 years of age.[19] The general criteria are the same as for adults but the period of observation should be longer and confirmatory investigations, such as EEG or cerebral angiography, are often conducted. A higher $Pa\text{CO}_2$ target is also recommended during the apnoea test.[20]

- *Less than 37 weeks' gestation:* apnoea and coma are common in this age group and the development of brainstem reflexes is uncertain. In the UK it has been suggested that the concept of brain death is inappropriate in this age group and decisions to withdraw intensive support should be made on the basis of futility.[21]
- *37 weeks to 2 months.* coma in this age group may occur for a wide variety of reasons, but hypoxic–ischaemic encephalopathy, sustained in utero or at the time of birth, is common. Making a diagnosis of brain death at this age can be difficult. Because associated severe multisystem failure is common at such a young age, it

may not be appropriate or necessary to confirm brain death if care can be withdrawn on the grounds of futility. In the USA two sets of clinical tests are conducted 48 hours apart in the presence of an isoelectric EEG.

- *Children older than 2 months:* in the UK and USA the clinical criteria for assessing brainstem death in adults are applicable to this age group. However, the clinical tests should always be carried out by two senior doctors, one of whom should be a paediatrician and one not primarily involved with the child's care.

INTERNATIONAL DIFFERENCES IN BRAIN DEATH CRITERIA

Whilst the fundamentals of the guidance for the diagnosis of brain death are common worldwide, specific criteria and requirements are often inconsistent.[4] The guidelines for the diagnosis of brain death in 80 countries encompassing a broad diversity of culture and religious belief were reviewed in 2002.[10] Only 88% had national guidelines and those that did showed considerable variation. Criteria for the clinical testing of brainstem areflexia were identical in all national guidelines but there were marked differences in other areas of practice (Table 46.2).

Table 46.2 International differences in the diagnosis of brain death in 80 countries

	National practice	No. of countries
National guidelines in place		70
Confirmation of brainstem areflexia by clinical testing		70
Apnoea testing	With $Pa\text{CO}_2$ target	41
	Without $Pa\text{CO}_2$ target	20
	Not required	19
Confirmatory tests	Not required or optional	52
	Mandatory	28
Number of physicians required to make clinical diagnosis	1	31
	2	24
	>2	11
	Unspecified	14
Minimum observation time prior to testing (hours)	2	4
	3	2
	6	20
	12	8
	24	8
	Unspecified	38

(Modified from Wijdicks E. Brain death worldwide – accepted fact but no global consensus in diagnostic criteria. *Neurology* 2002; **58**: 20–5.)

SUMMARY

The care of the injured brain has advanced since the clinical criteria for the diagnosis of brain death were first established. Lack of worldwide agreement on how to diagnose brain death and brainstem death remains a problem. There is an urgent need for international consensus for the diagnosis of brain death. This should retain clinical tests as fundamental but include confirmatory investigations when appropriate. Flexibility should be maintained and, as in other areas of medicine, the clinical findings should be interpreted with common sense by an experienced and humane physician.[22]

REFERENCES

1. Ad Hoc Committee of the Harvard Medical School. A definition of irreversible coma. Report of the ad hoc committee of the Harvard Medical School to examine the definition of brain death. *JAMA* 1968; **205**: 337–40.
2. Working group of the conference of Medical Royal Colleges and their Faculties in the United Kingdom. Diagnosis of death. *Br Med J* 1976; **ii**: 1187–8.
3. Wijdicks EFM. The diagnosis of brain death. *N Engl J Med* 2001; **344**: 1215–21.
4. Baron L, Shemie SD, Teitelbaum J *et al.* Brief review: history, concept and controversies in the neurological determination of death. *Can J Anesth* 2006; **53**: 602–8.
5. Guidelines for the determination of death. Report of the medical consultants on the diagnosis of death to the President's Commission for the Study of Ethical Problems in Medicine and Biomedical and Behavioural Research. *JAMA* 1981; **246**: 2184–6.
6. Smith M. Physiological changes during brainstem death – lessons for management of the organ donor. *J Heart Lung Transplant* 2004; **23** (Suppl.): S217–22.
7. Mollaret P, Goulon M. Le coma dépassé. *Rev Neurol* 1959; **101**: 3–15.
8. Mohandas A, Chou SN. Brain death – a clinical and pathological study. *J Neurosurg* 1971; **35**: 211–18.
9. Department of Health. *A Code of Practice for the Diagnosis of Brainstem Death.* London: Department of Health, 1998.
10. Wijdicks E. Brain death worldwide – accepted fact but no global consensus in diagnostic criteria. *Neurology* 2002; **58**: 20–5.
11. Powner DJ, Hernandez M, Rives TE. Variability among hospital policies for determining brain death in adults. *Crit Care Med* 2004; **32**: 1284–8.
12. Bell MD, Moss E, Murphy PG. Brainstem death testing in the UK – time for reappraisal? *Br J Anaesth* 2004; **92**: 533–40.
13. Haupt WF, Rudolf J. European brain death codes: a comparison of national guidelines. *J Neurol* 2000; **246**: 432–7.
14. Young GB, Shemie SD, Doig CJ *et al.* Brief review: the role of ancillary tests in the neurological determination of death. *Can J Anaesth* 2006; **53**: 620–7.

15. Young GB, Lee D. A critique of ancillary tests for brain death. *Neurocrit Care* 2004; **4**: 499–508.
16. Waters CE, French G, Burt M. Difficulty in brainstem death testing in the presence of high spinal cord injury. *Br J Anaesth* 2004; **92**: 760–4.
17. Vargas F, Hilbert G, Gruson D *et al.* Fulminant Guillain–Barré syndrome mimicking cerebral death: case report. *Intens Care Med* 2000; **6**: 623–7.
18. Pratt OW, Bowles B, Protheroe RT. Brainstem death testing after thiopental use: a survey of UK neurocritical care practice. *Anaesthesia* 2006; **61**: 1075–8.
19. Banasiak KJ, Lister G. Brain death in children. *Curr Opin Pediatr* 2003; **15**: 288–93.
20. Shemie SD, Pollack MM, Morioka M *et al.* Diagnosis of brain death in children. *Lancet Neurol* 2007; **6**: 87–92.
21. Working Party of the British Paediatric Association. *Diagnosis of brain stem death in infants and children.* London: British Paediatric Association, 1991.
22. Shaner DM, Orr RD, Drought T *et al.* Really, most sincerely dead: policy and procedure in the diagnosis of death by neurologic criteria. *Neurology* 2004; **62**: 1683–6.

47

Meningitis and encephalomyelitis

Angus M Kennedy

Infections of the cranial contents can be divided into those which affect the meninges (meningitis) and those which affect the brain parenchyma (encephalitis). Chronic, insidious or rare infections are beyond the scope of this chapter, which will focus on acute bacterial and viral causes of meningitis and encephalomyelitis.

- *Meningitis*: defined as infection or inflammation of the meninges and subarachnoid space. The infection can be caused by viruses, bacteria, fungi or protozoa. Meningeal inflammation may be caused by subarachnoid haemorrhage or vaccination or be a manifestation of other multiorgan diseases, such as systemic lupus erythematosus, sarcoidosis, lymphoma or meningeal micrometastases from a disseminated carcinoma.
- *Aseptic meningitis*: aseptic meningitis is a generic term for cases of meningitis in which bacteria cannot be isolated from the cerebrospinal fluid (CSF). The differential diagnosis in this situation includes: (1) viral meningitis; (2) partially treated bacterial meningitis; (3) tuberculous meningitis; (4) fungal meningitis; (5) lymphoma; (6) sarcoidosis; and (7) other collagen vascular diseases. The most common causes of aseptic meningitis are due to viral infection most often due to an enterovirus or coxsackie infection.
- *Encephalitis*: encephalitis is an infection of the brain parenchyma. The patient may have a history of preceding seizures together with cognitive or behavioural symptoms.
- *Tuberculous mengingitis*: this causes a subacute lymphocytic meningitis. Patients may have a non-specific prodromal phase, including symptoms such as headache, vomiting and fever.
- *Subdural empyema*: subdural empyema is a suppurative process in the space between the pia and dura mata.
- *Brain abscess*: brain abscess is a collection of pus within the brain tissue.

BACTERIAL MENINGITIS

GENERAL POINTS

Bacterial meningitis is an inflammatory response due to infection of the leptomeninges and subarachnoid space. This is characterised by the clinical syndrome of fever, headache, neck stiffness and CSF pleocytosis. Despite the existence of antibiotic therapy, patients continue to suffer significant morbidity and mortality.

The bacterial organisms are usually not confined to the brain and meninges and frequently cause systemic illness, for example, severe sepsis, shock, acute respiratory distress syndrome, and bleeding disorders such as disseminated intravascular coagulation.[1,2]

A variety of other pathogens cause meningeal inflammation, resulting in very similar clinical presentations. Bacterial infections must be treated urgently and appropriately to limit ongoing central nervous system (CNS) damage. It is also important to treat the complications of meningitis such as seizures and raised intracranial pressure (ICP).

Where possible, spinal fluid examination following a lumbar puncture is required in order to confirm the diagnosis and establish the pathogenic organism responsible. A CSF examination may be contraindicated if there are signs of raised ICP, including:

- papilloedema
- focal neurological signs
- seizures

These features raise the possibility of an undiagnosed cerebral mass lesion which, in turn, could cause cerebral herniation if lumbar puncture is performed. A computed tomography (CT) brain scan is required prior to CSF examination in order to explore this possibility and lessen but not obviate the risk of cerebral herniation. Even if the CT brain scan is normal, ICP may still be raised. The importance of performing a safe CSF examination must be balanced against the need to commence immediate treatment in each individual patient.[3,4]

AETIOLOGY

The main causes of meningitis are spread by droplet infection or exchange of saliva. Meningitis may occur when pathogenic organisms colonise the nasopharynx and reach the blood–brain barrier. Meningitis can occur as a result of infection in the middle ear, sinus or teeth, leading to secondary meningeal infection. Most bacteria obtain entry into the CNS via the haematogenous route. As the organisms multiply, they release cell wall products and lipopolysaccharide, and generate a local inflammatory reaction which in itself also releases inflammatory mediators. The net result of the release of cytokines, tumour necrosis factor and other factors is associated with a significant inflammatory response. Vasculitis of CNS vessels, thrombosis, cell damage and exudative material all contribute to vasogenic and cytotoxic oedema, altered blood flow and cerebral perfusion pressure. Later on infarction and raised ICP occur.[5]

The inflammatory events seen with infection are summarised in Figure 47.1.

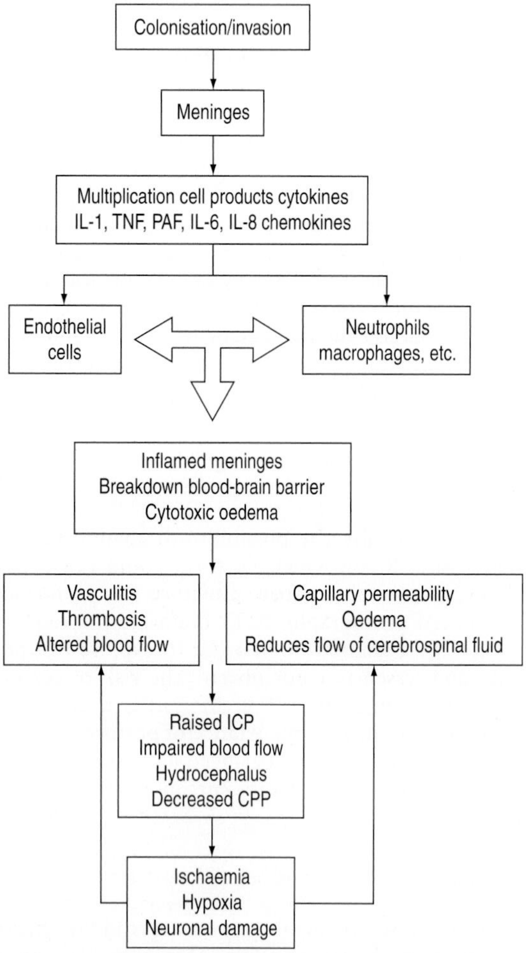

Figure 47.1 Cascade of events in meningitis. IL-1, interleukin-1; TNF, tumour necrosis factor; PAF, platelet-activating factor; ICP, intracranial pressure; CPP, cerebral perfusion pressure.

ORGANISMS

Acute bacterial meningitis can be caused by many species of bacteria, although three organisms are commonly reported:

1. *Haemophilus influenzae*
2. *Streptococcus pneumoniae*
3. *Neisseria meningitidis* (which accounts for 70% of cases in the neonatal period)

Until the advent of the meningitis vaccination programme, *H. influenzae* type B was the most common cause of bacterial meningitis. Recently *S. pneumoniae* and *N. meningitidis* have been considered the main causes, although one study suggested that *Listeria monocytogenes* is the second most common isolate in adult population. The occurrence of pneumococcal strains which are resistant to penicillin has also influenced the epidemiology of meningitis.[6]

NOSOCOMIAL INFECTIONS

Common systemic nosocomial pathogens such as *Escherichia coli, Pseudomonas* spp., *Klebsiella* and *Acinetobacter* spp. account for a high percentage of nosocomial infections of the meninges.

IMMUNOCOMPROMISED HOSTS

In the immunocompromised patient with meningitis (e.g. human immunodeficiency virus: HIV), fungal viral and cryptocococal meningitis should be considered.[7]

NEUROSURGERY AND TRAUMA

Infections following skull trauma are frequently caused by *Staphylococcus aureus* and *S. epidermidis,* which should be considered in those with shunts or other intracranial devices.

CLINICAL PRESENTATION

The history may reveal evidence of trauma or infection. Meningitis usually presents with an acute onset of:

- fever
- headache
- neck stiffness
- photophobia
- altered conscious level
- irritabilty
- seizures (paediatric)

However, in the immunocompromised, elderly or infant patient, non-specific features such as a low-grade fever or mild behavioural change may be all that is apparent. Many of the classic symptoms are late manifestations of meningitis: preceding trivial early symptoms such as leg pain or cold hands may not immediately suggest the more serious underlying diagnosis.

It is important to identify from the history reported about preceding trauma, upper respiratory tract infection or ear infection. Symptoms may develop over hours or days. Specific infections relate partly to an individual's age.

Neurological signs can be present with meningitis but signs such as nuchal rigidity, or a positive Kernig's sign (pain and hamstring spasm resulting from attempts to straighten, the leg with the hip fiexed) are not universally found. A number of recent studies have shown that the classic signs were present in less than 50% of cases. Systemic signs may occur most often in meningococcal disease, where a haemorrhagic, petechial or purpuric rash may be observed. Digital gangrene or skin necrosis may occur. Some patients are severely septic, with acute respiratory distress syndrome and disseminated intravascular coagulation.

Approximately 25% of patients have a seizure during the course of the illness. Differential diagnosis may include subarachnoid haemorrhage, migraine, encephalitis and tumour.

INVESTIGATIONS

The patient with suspected bacterial meningitis requires immediate blood cultures and should be given empirical intravenous (IV) antibiotics if there is likely to be any delay in further assessment (Table 47.1).

CEREBROSPINAL FLUID FINDINGS

A CSF examination is a vitally important investigation which may definitively confirm the diagnosis of bacterial meningitis. In this regard its value should should not be dismissed. Concern about the risks of coning following lumbar puncture should be considered in the context of patients' symptoms where the presence of seizures, focal neurological signs and papilloedema may suggest raised ICP. Neuroimaging may provide some level of reassurance that it is safe to proceed with a lumbar puncture; however, the clinican should be aware that all factors need to be taken into consideration.

Bacterial meningitis is suggested when there is:

- polymorph leukocytosis
- low CSF glucose relative to the plasma value
- raised CSF protein concentration

An urgent Gram stain and microbiological culture are mandatory. The Gram stain is usually positive in approximately 50–60% of cases. A CSF examination shortly after empirical antibiotics does not necessarily decrease the diagnostic sensitivity of CSF culture. Polymerase chain reaction (PCR) techniques can be used to detect different organisms. A throat swab should be routinely taken. The clinical decision-making process that determines whether somebody does or does not have bacterial meningitis cannot be modelled easily and depends on multiple factors including clinical, laboratory findings and observation of the patient over time.

Blood cultures comprise an important investigation in patients with meningitis, as spread is haematogenous, and a number of sets of cultures should be sent. It is advisable to check routinely a full blood count clotting profile (to exclude disseminated intravascular coagulation) and biochemistry, including blood glucose level. A chest X-ray and blood gases should be performed to identify systemic involvement. Obviously, relevant areas such as infected sinuses or ears should be examined if there is an indication that they are implicated.

MANAGEMENT

Antibiotics should be started as early as possible and broad-spectrum coverage is recommended until bacterial identifcation is made (Table 47.2). The selection of antibiotics is influenced by the clinical situation in conjunction with known allergies or local patterns of antibiotic resistance and the CSF findings. Delays in administering antibiotics are a significant risk factor for a poor prognosis. In the absence of a known organism, empirical choice for antibiotics has been complicated by the development of resistant strains. Penicillin G, ampicillin and third-generation cephalosporins are typical first-line agents. Until recently, ampicillin was appropriate for pneumococcal, meningococcal and *Listeria* infections. The emergence of resistant strains influences local antibiotic practice. If there is a history of recent head injury, a broad-spectrum cephalosporin may be indicated with vancomycin. Discussions with local

Table 47.1 Cerebrospinal fluid changes in meningitis

	Normal	Bacterial	Viral
Appearance	Clear	Turbid/purulent	Clear/turbid
White cell count	< 5 per mm^3 mononuclear	200–10 000 per mm^3 predominantly polymorphonuclear	< 500 per mm^3 mainly lymphocytes
Protein	0.2–0.4 g/l	0.5–2.0 g/l	0.4–0.8 g/l
Glucose	Blood glucose	$\leq$ Blood glucose	Blood glucose pressure is usually raised

Table 47.2 Empiric antibiotics for meningitis

Indication	Antibiotic	Dose
<50 years	Ceftriaxone or cefotaxime	2–4 g q 24 h 2 g q 4 h
>50 years or impaired cell immunity	Ceftriaxone or cefotaxime Cefotaxime + ampicillin or penicillin G	2–4 g q 24 h 2 g q 4 h 2 g q 4 h or 3–4 MU q 4 h
Drug-resistant *Streptococcus pneumoniae*	Ceftriaxone + rifampicin or vancomycin	2–4 g q 8 h 2 g q 4 h 0.5 g q 6 h
Neurosurgery shunts trauma	Ceftazidime + nafcillin *or* Vancomycin + aminoglycoside (gentamicin 5–7 mg/kg stat)	2 g q 8 h 2 g q 4 h 0.5 g q 6 h 2 mg / kg q 8 h

microbiology services are recommended. If the CSF examination identifies the organism, then specific regimens can be prescribed (Table 47.3).

It is more difficult to select an appropriate empirical antibiotic in the immunocompromised patient. When the organism has been identified and sensitivity results are available, it may be necessary either to change the antibiotic or to rationalise those being given.[8]

In all cases, it is important to monitor the clinical response to therapy and, if necessary, antibiotics should be reviewed and appropriately altered once antibiotic sensitivities are known or a patient is not considered to be improving. A repeat CSF examination should be performed if there is concern about antibiotic sensitivity or selection. In those with penicillin-resistant pneumococcal meningitis, a CSF examination 48 hours after presentation is recommended to ensure bacteriological improvement. Antibiotics should be given for 10–14 days, although a shorter course may be adequate in some circumstances. Intrathecal antibiotics are not recommended.

STEROID ADMINISTRATION

The benefit of steroid administration in adult meningitis has been debated. Clear guidance is now available to support its routine use from the Cochrane Database, including 1800 adults and children, which demonstrated a reduction in mortality, hearing loss and neurological complications. Some concerns remain, including the possibility that dexamethasone may adversely affect CSF penetration or cause longer-term cognitive problems.[9] A longer and more established literature exists for the use of steroids in bacterial meningitis in children. These studies confirm a benefit for those with *Haemophilus infiuenzae* type B infection and reduce the frequency of postmeningitis deafness.

RECOMMENDATIONS IN ADULTS

Dexamethasone is an adjuvant treatment and should be given with the first dose of antibiotics and continued 6-hourly for 4 days (0.6 mg/kg daily).

Table 47.3 General recommendation for known organisms*

Organism	Antibiotic	Second line or allergy
Streptococcus pneumoniae (Penicillin-resistant)	Ceftriaxone + vancomycin or rifampicin	Vancomycin + rifampicin
Streptococcus pneumoniae (Penicillin-sensitive)	Penicillin G	Ceftriaxone or chloramphenicol
β-haemolytic streptococcus	Penicillin or ampicillin	Cefotaxime or chloramphenicol or vancomycin
Haemophilus influenzae	Ceftriaxone or cefotaxime	Chloramphenicol
Neisseria meningitidis	Penicillin G	Ceftriaxone or chloramphenicol
Listeria monocytogenes	Ampicillin + gentamicin	Trimethoprim + sulfamethoxazole
Enterobacteriaceae	Ceftriaxone + gentamicin	Quinolones
Pseudomonas aeruginosa	Ceftazidime + tobramycin	Quinolones

*Always check local sensitiviity as resistance patterns are variable.

ANTICONVULSANTS

Focal or generalised seizures should be treated immediately with IV benzodiazepines to stop the seizures and the individual should then subsequently be loaded with IV phenytoin. The possibility of the following should be considered:

- raised ICP
- cerebritis
- cerebral abscess
- venous thombosis

The development of seizures may be indicative of a poor prognosis.

INTRACRANIAL PRESSURE

Intracranial hypertension is a common complication of meningitis. ICP monitoring may be required and standard measures such as hyperventilation, mannitol infusion or CSF drainage may be considered. Depending upon the particular circumstance, serial lumbar punctures or external ventricular drainage should be implemented.

GENERAL MANAGEMENT CONSIDERATIONS[10]

INTRAVENOUS FLUID THERAPY

Normal haemodynamics should be maintained. Currently, there is emphasis on maintaining the cerebral perfusion pressure at around 70 mmHg. Inappropriate antidiuretic hormone secretion may occur in meningitis.

RESPIRATORY SUPPORT

It is important to secure the airway and respiratory support may be required for those with severe shock or profound coma. Attention should be paid to management of the unconscious patient with appropriate mouth and eye care. Physiotherapy will be required in order to prevent the onset of pressure sores. Surgical evaluation may be needed for skin necrosis.[11,12]

PUBLIC HEALTH

Meningitis prophylaxis is commended for close (kissing contacts) associates and for those medical personnel with close contact. A 2-day course of oral rifampicin 600 mg 12-hourly is recommended. There should be procedures for alerting infectious disease team.

PROGNOSIS

Untreated, bacterial meningitis is usually fatal. Appropriate therapy significantly reduces the mortality rate; however, recent studies still show that the overall mortality is approximately 18%. Mortality is slightly higher in those who have seizures and when there have been delays introducing treatment, or if the patient is elderly or very young[12,13] (see Table 47.3).

VIRAL MENINGITIS

The majority of cases of viral meningitis are benign, usually self-limiting conditions which are often caused by enterovirus or coxsackie infection. Some are caused by arboviruses. The same viruses that produce meningitis can also cause encephalitis. Herpes simplex virus type 1 (HSV 1) usually produces encephalitis but rarely causes meningitis. Other viruses causing CNS infections include echoviruses, mumps, polio and HIV. Patients with migrainous headaches often receive a lumbar puncture to rule out viral meningitis, which may prolong their hospital stay with a post lumbar puncture headache and migraine.

CLINICAL PRESENTATION

Patients usually present with symptoms of meningeal irritation, fever, headache, neck stiffness, retrobulbar pain, photophobia, vertigo, nausea and vomiting which are less severe than those with bacterial meningitis. The presence of intellectual impairment, focal neurological symptoms or seizures suggests that the brain parenchyma is involved and, consequently, these are due to meningoencephalitis. True viral meningitis develops over hours to days but rarely lasts longer than 7–10 days. A variety of associated symptoms, such as nausea, vomiting and generalised malaise, may accompany this condition.[14]

INVESTIGATIONS

A CSF examination is important and usually shows:

- a mild to moderate lymphocytic pleocytosis
- a mildly elevated CSF protein concentration
- normal glucose concentration

Staining for microorganisms, including bacteria, *Mycobacterium tuberculosis* and cryptococcal meningitis, is necessary. Sites for culture include the mucous membranes, throat, skin and rectum.

MANAGEMENT

Acute viral meningitis is usually a self-limiting condition and only supportive therapy is required, with analgesia and bedrest. Viral meningitis caused by HSV 1 or 2 may require IV aciclovir. Acute HIV infection causing meningitis may respond to retroviral therapy.

ENCEPHALITIS

Encephalitis is a viral infection of the brain. HSV 1 is the most common and serious cause of focal encephalitis, which usually affects the temporal and frontal lobes. There are a large number of arboviruses that cause epidemics of encephalitis. These are usually borne by arthropod vectors, such as mosquitoes and ticks, and therefore are considered as airborne viruses.[15] West Nile virus is now the most common cause of epidemic viral encephalitis in some countries. Neuroimaging changes in basal ganglia may suggest the diagnosis but the CSF pleocytosis may have a predominance. Specific CSF antibodies can be sent for West Nile virus.

CLINICAL PRESENTATION

The key clinical pointer of encephalitis is the presence of focal neurological symptoms, indicating involvement of the brain parenchyma. In particular, the presence of speech disturbance, seizures, altered cognition and disturbance of conscious level suggests this.

Diagnosis can be difficult.

- Abnormalities on cranial imaging, such as T2-weighted magnetic resonance imaging (MRI), may support this diagnosis (Figure 47.2)
- Electroencephalogram (EEG) studies may show slow-wave activity or epileptiform discharges in temporal lobe.
- PCR examination of the CSF examination may confirm the virus at a later date.

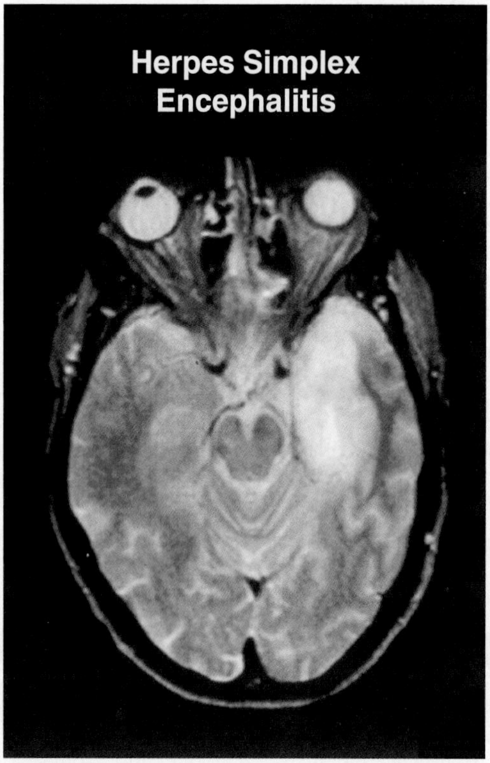

Figure 47.2 Enhanced temporal lobe with herpes encephalitis.

TREATMENT

Specific treatment for HSV encephalitis requires IV aciclovir at a dose of 30 mg/kg per day for 14 days. Left untreated, the mortality of HSV encephalitis is approximately 70% but there is still a 25% mortality in patients treated with optimal therapy. Patients can be left with significant disability in terms of cognitive dysfunction or seizures. Most patients with significant cerebral oedema receive empirical steroids, although there are no clinical trials to support this therapy. Aciclovir can cause renal impairment and the patient should be hydrated intravenously and renal function monitored.[16] Aggressive treatment of seizures is important.

Cytomegalovirus (CMV) infection requires antiviral therapy with ganciclovir or valganciclovir. CMV may cause a ganglionitis and polyradiculitis, which may suggest this diagnosis clinically in an immunocompromised patient.

Most CNS viruses cause neuronal damage but chronic JC virus infection in oligodendrocytes causes the syndrome of progressive multifocal leukoencephalopathy (PML). This condition presents with a subacute onset of confusion, weakness and visual symptoms, usually in an immunosuppressed individual. The MRI scan is usually suggestive but CSF examination with PCR amplification of the JC virus particles may be required. Currently, no specific therapy for PML exists. The survival of HIV patients with associated PML is poor, averaging 6 months in 90% of individuals.

Viral infection with HIV 1, measles and rubella can also cause chronic CNS infection, leading to chronic encephalitides.

A number of systemic neurological conditions (e.g. lymphoma, Lyme disease, sarcoidosis and vasculides such as Behçet's disease) may present with aseptic meningitis. It is therefore important to consider these systemic conditions in those presenting with viral meningitis or encephalitis.

TUBERCULOUS MENINGITIS

Tuberculous meningitis has a variable natural history with a range of different clinical presentations. This and the lack of specific and sensitive tests hinders the diagnosis of this condition. Approximately 10% of individuals with tuberculosis develop meningeal involvement. A variety of risk factors, such as HIV, diabetes mellitus and recent steroid use, may increase the risk of tuberculous meningitis.[17]

CLINICAL FEATURES

Tuberculous meningitis has a very varied clinical presentation. Often, it is heralded by a non-specific prodromal phase, frequently but not necessarily including headache, vomiting and fever. Of one case series which included those admitted to an intensive care unit, only 65% had fever, 52% had focal neurology and 88% had signs of meningism. A variety of cranial nerve palsies can occur but other presentations include those seen with stroke, hydrocephalus and tuberculoma.

DIAGNOSIS

An investigation of the differential diagnosis of tuberculous meningitis is important. PCR amplification of mycobacterial DNA has not been fully evaluated in this technique which, in the case of tuberculous meningitis, usually requires a lumbar puncture examination. Those who are immunosuppressed may have atypical CSF appearance, including normal CSF examinations in occasional HIV individuals. Tuberculosis culture from CSF is required but may take up to 6 weeks before a positive culture result is available. Imaging studies may show a basal meningitis and hydrocephalus but these features are non-specific.[18]

Current advice suggests that the first 2 months of treatment should comprise quadruple therapy:

- Isoniazid oral/IV 10 mg/kg per day up to 300 mg. It is bactericidal and has good CNS penetration.
- Pyrazinamide oral/IV 25 mg/kg per day up to 2.5 g/day.
- Rifampicin high dosage as poor penetration, 10 mg/kg per day up to 600 mg.
- Ethambutol IV high dosage, as it is highly protein-bound and therefore has poor penetration.

Streptomycin is used rarely. The toxicity of the agents must be monitored in terms of renal and liver function and the effect on other organs such as the eye.

There is increasing multidrug-resistant tuberculous meningitis, especially in the HIV-positive population, and so sensitivity is important. Some clinical trials suggest that steroids have a beneficial effect in some groups of patients.[19] Patients may require neurosurgical intervention for the treatment of hydrocephalus.

SUBDURAL EMPYEMA

This is a collection of pus between the dural and arachnoid space and is usually a consequence of middle-ear or sinus disease. It may follow cranial osteomyelitis related to previous neurosurgery. Head trauma can also be responsible.

Individuals present acutely with headache, fever, neck stiffness, seizures and focal neurological symptoms. Meningeal signs and evidence of hemispheric dysfunction with sinusitis should suggest the diagnosis.

DIAGNOSIS

CT and MRI are both effective in demonstrating a fluid collection.

Surgical intervention, drainage and appropriate antibiotic regimes are required. Both Gram-positive *Staphylococcus* and *Streptococcus* and Gram-negative organisms may be implicated. Initial broad-spectrum cover should be narrowed to targeted treatment when the organism or organisms are known.

PROGNOSIS

If left untreated, this condition is invariably fatal. With treatment, mortality is in the order of 20% and neurological sequelae are common.

EPIDURAL INFECTION

Cranial and spinal epidural abscess is an infection between skull and dura, often as a consequence of osteomyelitis, from an orbital infection or malignancy. There is a very low but occasional incidence following an epidural. It is similar to subdural empyema. The organism involved where a catheter or drain is implicated is often the same as that found at the skin; hence, *Staphylococcus aureus* is frequently responsible.

PRESENTATION

Epidural infection commonly presents on the back, and may be generalised to the area of the back involved. There may be local tenderness over the site associated with redness of the catheter insertion site. Fever is common. Initially mild neurological deficit may rapidly progress, leading to para/quadriparesis.

Blood cultures may be positive and may indicate the organism.

DIAGNOSIS

CT and MRI are both effective in diagnosis.

Spinal decompression and drainage are urgently required. This is usually a nosocomial infection and therefore resistant organisms are commonly found. Antibiotics should be specific for the organisms involved and may need to be continued for prolonged periods, often weeks, to eradicate the infection.

Where there have been neurological symptoms and signs prior to surgery, residual deficit is common. In one series, the recovery rate for patients with paresis/plegia after lumbar epidural abscess was 50%, while no patients with paresis/plegia following a thoracic abscess recovered. The majority of long-term survivors had severe neurological deficits.

CEREBRAL VENOUS AND SAGITTAL SINUS THROMBOSIS

Venous and sinus thrombosis may occur in the context of infection; in particular meningitis, and epidural or subdural abscess. It may also be secondary to facial or dental

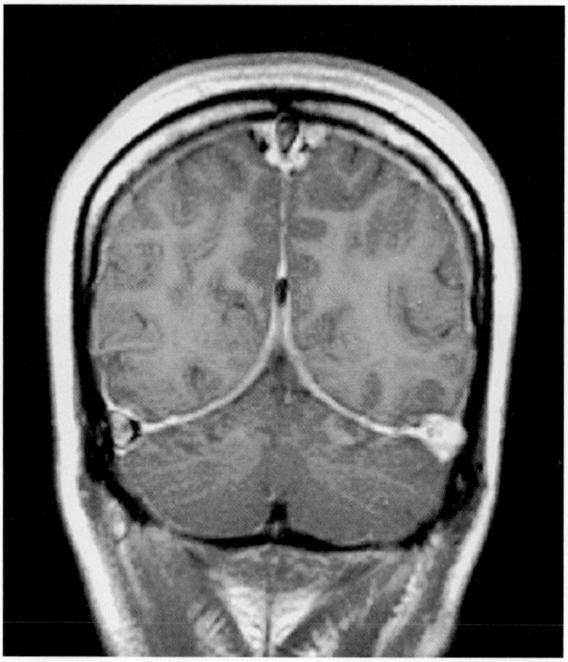

Figure 47.3 Magnetic resonance imaging (MRI) of superior sagittal sinus thrombosis. Coronal T1-weighted postcontrast MRI. Patient developed a sinus thrombosis following protracted labour and delivery.

infection. It may have no septic aetiology but can occur either as an isolated event or in association with prothrombotic problems such as diabetic ketoacidosis, methylenedioxymethamphetamine (MDMA) abuse (ectsasy), oral contraceptives and hereditary prothrombotic conditions in pregnancy.[20]

Clinical signs at presentation include:

- headache
- focal neurological deficits – in particular, cranial nerves
- seizures
- papilloedema

The diagnostic sensitivities of CT, MRI and digital subtract angiography are 59%, 86% and 100%, respectively, but MRI with magnetic resonance angiography reaches 96% (Figure 47.3).

TREATMENT

- Treat the primary infection if present.
- Anticoagulants are the mainstay of treatment. Paradoxically, there are often areas of intracerbral haemorrhage in a patient with sinus thrombois. The presence of such haemorrhages is not a contraindication to anticoagulation.

BRAIN ABSCESS

AETIOLOGY

A brain abscess may spread directly from bone or dura or spread may be haematogenous. Predisposition includes cranial trauma, neurosurgery, chronic ear or sinus disease, suppurative lung disease, congenital heart disease and recurrent sepsis. Immunological compromise may predispose to more exotic organisms: more common organisms include *Staphylococcus* spp. associated with trauma, and *Streptococcus*, *Bacteroides* and Gram-negative bacteria, which are common with lung disease or recurrent sepsis.

PRESENTATION

The presentation is severe headache, vomiting, obtundation, seizures and focal neurological signs. Neck stiffness is often absent. Clinical sepsis may not be obvious.

DIAGNOSIS (FIGURE 47.4)

- An obvious primary source of infection
- Evidence of raised ICP
- Focal cerebral or cerebellar signs

INVESTIGATIONS

- Lumbar puncture is potentially dangerous and is contraindicated.
- CT scan: contrast will usually show ring-enhancing lesions.
- MRI.
- Assessment of a patient's immune status.
- Specific blood tests, such as HIV and *Toxoplasma* serology.

TREATMENT

Indications for surgery include large single lesions, relief of raised ICP and the need for tissue diagnosis.

Antibiotics are the mainstay of therapy. If the organism is known, then the treatment should be specific. In the absence of a definitive organism, penicillin plus chloramphenicol (as for meningitis) and metronidazole 500 mg IV 8-hourly or 500 mg rectally 12-hourly should be empirical therapy. Cefotaxime 1–2 g can be given IV 6–8-hourly and metronidazole 500 mg IV 8-hourly. If there is a recent history of trauma or neurosurgery, then a regimen that will cover *Staphylococcus* should be used. Antibiotics should be continued for 3–6 weeks.

Supportive therapy limits morbidity, which is nevertheless high. Mortality from cerebral abscesses is still 10–20%.[21]

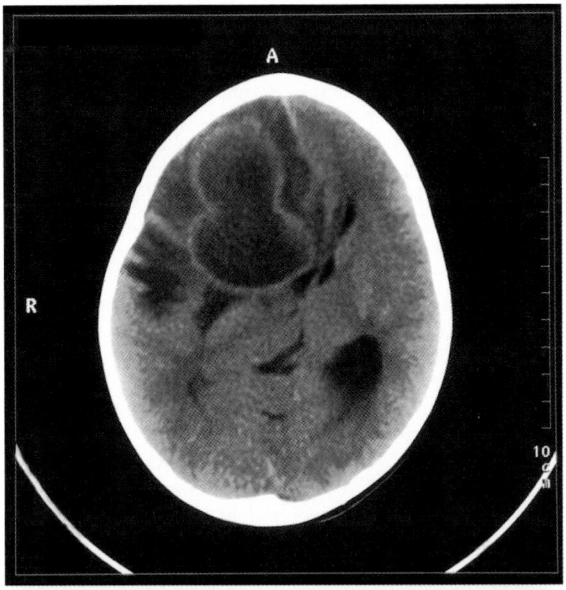

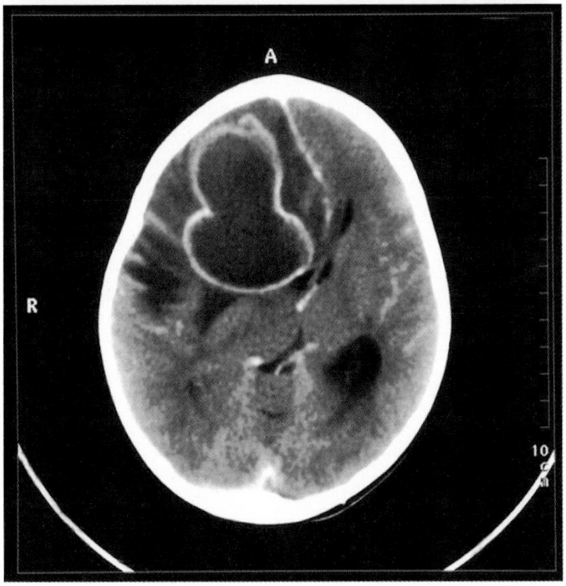

Figure 47.4 Abscess: (a) precontrast and (b) postcontrast.

LYME DISEASE

This is a tickborne multisystem disease with dermatological, cardiological, rheumatological and neurological effects caused by the spirochaete *Borrelia burgdorferi*.

Lyme disease usually presents as an acute febrile illness with gastrointestinal upset, but it may present in a variable fashion neurologically, including as a cranial neuropathy (commonly a facial palsy) or as a meningoencephalitis or radiculopathy. It may also cause a lymphocytic meningitis and may have been diagnosed as a 'viral' meningitis in the past. A variety of longer-term neurological sequelae have been described.[22]

INVESTIGATIONS

CEREBOSPINAL FLUID

White cell count is equivocal but may be raised. Protein is normal or marginally raised and sugar is normal or marginally low. Serology and enzyme-linked immunosorbent assay may be difficult. PCR may be helpful. It may have characteristic MRI appearances. Vaccination is the only empirically demonstrated method of preventing Lyme disease.

TREATMENT

β-lactam antibacterials, such as penicillin V, amoxicillin and cefuroxime, are effective first-line treatment. The optimal duration of treatment is not known, but 10–21 days is recommended.[23,24] Practice parameters for the treatment of nervous system Lyme disease state that nervous system infection responds favourably to penicillin, ceftriaxone, cefotaxime and doxycycline. Prolonged treatment with antibiotic appears to have no benefit in preventing post-Lyme syndrome.

OTHER DISEASES

There are several other diseases that may have an encephalopathic component. Cerebral malaria is dealt with elsewhere. *Legionella* may lead to subclinical or clinical neurological manifestations, ranging from headache to coma or encephalopathy, usually seen in conjunction with pneumonia, in addition to possible renal impairment. Similarly, *Mycoplasma* has been associated with an encephalitic picture characterised by impaired consciousness and seizures, and by normal or non-specific neuroradiological findings. Occasionally, symmetrical lesions in the putamen and its external surrounding areas have been seen.

Septic encephalopathy has been described as a common complication in the critically ill, presenting in a panoply of ways, from the agitated confused state seen in acute sepsis through to profound loss of consciousness. The aetiology is almost certainly multifactorial, involving changes in cerebral blood flow, alteration in oxygen extraction, cerebral oedema, disruption of the blood–brain barrier, the presence and effects of diverse inflammatory mediators and abnormal neurotransmitter activity. Deranged liver and renal function contribute. It is a syndrome of exclusion based on observation and circumstantial evidence. The EEG is usually abnormal with decreased fast activity and an increase of slow-wave activity, but the findings are not pathognomonic. There are no specific treatments. In general terms, outcome appears to correlate with the management of the underlying sepsis.[25]

REFERENCES

1. Isenberg H. Bacterial meningitis: signs and symptoms. *Antibiot Chemother* 1992; **45**: 79–95.
2. Spach DH, Jackson LA. Bacterial meningitis. *Neurol Clin* 1999; **17**: 711–35.
3. Roos KL. Acute bacterial meningitis. *Semin Neurol* 2000; **20**: 293–306.
4. Anderson M. Management of cerebral infection. *J Neurol Neurosurg Psychiatry* 1993; **56**: 1243–58.
5. Pfister HW, Fontana A, Tauber MG *et al.* Mechanisms of brain injury in bacterial meningitis: workshop summary. *Clin Infect Dis* 1994; **19**: 463–79.
6. van Deuren M, Brandtzaeg P, van der Meer JW. Update on meningococcal disease with emphasis on pathogenesis and clinical management. *Clin Microbiol Rev* 2000; **13**: 144–66.
7. Gottfredsson M, Perfect JR. Fungal meningitis. *Semin Neurol* 2000; **20**: 307–22.
8. Vandecasteele SJ, Knockaert D, Verhaegen J *et al.* The antibiotic and anti-inflammatory treatment of bacterial meningitis in adults: do we have to change our strategies in an era of increasing antibiotic resistance? *Acta Clin Belg* 2001; **56**: 225–33.
9. Van de Beek D, de Gans J, McIntyre P *et al.* Corticosteroids for acute bacterial meninigitis (review). *Cochrane Collaboration* 2007.
10. Raser K, Deziel PJ. The danger of bacterial meningitis in the adult. *JAAPA* 2001; **14**: 16–18, 21–4.
11. Hussein AS, Shafran SD. Acute bacterial meningitis in adults. A 12-year review. *Medicine (Baltimore)* 2000; **79**: 360–8.
12. Durand ML, Calderwood SB, Weber DJ *et al.* Acute bacterial meningitis in adults. A review of 493 episodes. *N Engl J Med* 1993; **328**: 21–8.
13. Pfister HW, Feiden W, Einhaupl KM. Spectrum of complications during bacterial meningitis in adults. Results of a prospective clinical study. *Arch Neurol* 1993; **50**: 575–81.
14. Robert HA. Viral meningitis. *Semin Neurol* 2000; **20**: 277–92.
15. Schmutzhard E. Viral infections of the CNS with special emphasis on herpes simplex infections. *J Neurol* 2001; **248**: 469–77.
16. Gutierrez KM, Prober CG. Encephalitis. Identifying the specific cause is key to effective management. *Postgrad Med* 1998; **103**: 123–5, 129–30, 140–3.
17. Thwaites G, Chau TT, Mai NT *et al.* Tuberculous meningitis. *J Neurol Neurosurg Psychiatry* 2000; **68**: 289–99.
18. Roos KL. *Mycobacterium tuberculosis* meningitis and other etiologies of the aseptic meningitis syndrome. *Semin Neurol* 2000; **20**: 329–35.
19. Prasad K, Volmink J, Menon GR. Steroids for treating tuberculous meningitis. *Cochrane Database Syst Rev* 2000; **3**: Cd002244.
20. de Bruijn SF, Stam J, Koopman MM *et al.* Case-control study of risk of cerebral sinus thrombosis in oral contraceptive users and in carriers of hereditary prothrombotic conditions. The Cerebral Venous Sinus Thrombosis Study Group. *Br Med J* 1998; **316**: 589–92.
21. Yildizhan A, Pasaoglu A, Ozkul MH *et al.* Clinical analysis and results of operative treatment of 41 brain abscesses. *Neurosurg Rev* 1991; **14**: 279–82.
22. Halperin JJ, Shapiro D, Logigia N *et al.* Practice parameter: treatment of nervous system Lyme disease: report of the Quality Standards Subcommittee of the American Academy of Neurology. *Neurology* 2007: **69**: 91–102.
23. van Dam AP. Recent advances in the diagnosis of Lyme disease. *Exp Rev Mol Diagn* 2001; **1**: 413–27.
24. Glaser C, Lewis P, Wong S. Pet-, animal-, and vector-borne infections. *Pediatr Rev* 2000; **21**: 219–32.
25. Papadopoulos MC, Davies DC, Moss RF *et al.* Pathophysiology of septic encephalopathy: a review. *Crit Care Med* 2000; **28**: 3019–24.

48

Tetanus

Jeffrey Lipman

Tetanus is a preventable, often Third-World disease, frequently requiring expensive First-World technology to treat. It is an acute, often fatal disease caused by exotoxins produced by *Clostridium tetani,* and is characterised by generalised muscle rigidity, autonomic instability and sometimes convulsions.

EPIDEMIOLOGY

Recently, tetanus has become a disease of the elderly and debilitated in developed countries, as younger people are likely to have been immunised.[1] In the USA, its incidence decreased from 0.23 per 100 000 in 1955 to 0.04 per 100 000 in 1975, and remained stable thereafter.[1] The annual world mortality from tetanus is estimated to be 400 000–2 000 000. Tetanus claimed the lives of over 433 000 infants in 1991, and accounts for 5 deaths for every 1000 live births in Africa. It is geographically prevalent in rural areas with poor hygiene and medical services. Thus, tetanus remains a significant public health problem in the developing world, primarily because of poor access to immunisation programmes. In addition, modern management requires intensive care unit (ICU) facilities, which are rarely available in the most severely afflicted populations.[2] Therefore, tetanus will continue to afflict developing populations in the foreseeable future.

PATHOGENESIS

C. tetani is an obligate anaerobic, spore-bearing, Gram-positive bacillus. Spores exist ubiquitously in soil and in animal and human faeces. After gaining access to devitalised tissue, spores proliferate in the vegetative form, producing toxins, tetanospasmin and tetanolysin. Tetanospasmin is extremely potent; an estimated 240 g could kill the entire world population,[3] with 0.01 mg being lethal for an average man. Tetanolysin is of little clinical importance.

C. tetani is non-invasive. Hence, tetanus occurs only when the spores gain access to tissues to produce vegetative forms. The usual mode of entry is through a puncture wound or laceration, although tetanus may follow surgery, burns, gangrene, chronic ulcers, dog bites, injections such as with drug users, dental infection, abortion and childbirth. Tetanus neonatorum usually follows infection of the umbilical stump. The injury itself may be trivial, and in 20% of cases there is no history or evidence of a wound.[1] Germination of spores occurs in oxygen-poor media (e.g. in necrotic tissue), with foreign bodies, and with infections. *C. tetani* infection remains localised, but the exotoxin tetanospasmin is widely distributed via the blood stream, taken up into motor nerve endings and transported into the nervous system. Here it affects motor neurone end-plates in skeletal muscle (to decrease release of acetylcholine), the spinal cord (with dysfunction of polysynaptic reflexes) and the brain (with seizures, inhibition of cortical activity and autonomic dysfunction). Tetanus is not communicable from person to person.

The symptoms of tetanus appear only after tetanospasmin has diffused from the cell body through the extracellular space, and gained access to the presynaptic terminals of adjacent neurons.[1] Tetanospasmin spreads to all local neurons, but is preferentially bound by inhibitory interneurons, i.e. glycinergic terminals in the spinal cord, and γ-aminobutyric acid (GABA) terminals in the brain.[2] Its principal effect is to block these inhibitory pathways. Hence stimuli to and from the central nervous system (CNS) are not 'damped down'.

ACTIVE IMMUNOPROPHYLAXIS[1,3]

Natural immunity to tetanus does not occur. Tetanus may both relapse and recur. Victims of tetanus must be *actively immunised.* Tetanus toxoid is a cheap and effective vaccine which is thermally stable.[3] It is a non-toxic derivative of the toxin which, nevertheless, elicits and reacts with antitoxic antibody. By consensus, an antibody titre of 0.01 u/ml serum is protective.[4] None the less, tetanus has been reported in a few victims with much higher serum antibody titres.[1]

In adults, a full immunisation course consists of three toxoid doses, given at an optimal interval of 6–12 weeks between the first and second doses, and 6–12 months between the second and third doses. A single dose will offer no immediate protection in the unimmunised, but a full course should never be repeated. Neonates have immunity from maternal antibodies. Children over 3 months should be actively immunised, and need four doses in total. Two or more doses to child-bearing females over 14 years will protect any child produced within the next 5 years. Pregnant females who are not immunised should thus be given two spaced-out doses 2 weeks to 2 months before delivery. Booster doses should be given routinely every 10 years.

Side-effects of tetanus toxoid are uncommon and not life-threatening. They are associated with excessive levels of antibody due to indiscriminate use.[5] Common reactions include urticaria, angioedema and diffuse, indurated swelling at the site of injection.

CLINICAL PRESENTATION[1,4,6]

The incubation period (i.e. time from injury to onset of symptoms) varies from 2 to 60 days. The period of onset (i.e. from first symptom to first spasm) similarly varies. Nearly all cases (90%), however, present within 15 days of infection.[6] The incubation period and the period of onset are of prognostic importance, with shorter times signifying more severe disease.

Presenting symptoms are pain and stiffness. Stiffness gives way to rigidity, and there is difficulty in mouth-opening – trismus or lockjaw. Most cases (75%) of non-neonatal generalised tetanus present with trismus.[6] Rigidity becomes generalised, and facial muscles produce a characteristic clenched-teeth expression called risus sardonicus. The disease progresses in a descending fashion. Typical spasms, with flexion and adduction of the arms, extension of the legs and opisthotonos, are very painful, and may be so intense that fractures and tendon separations occur.[1] Spasms are caused by external stimuli, e.g. noise and pressure. As the disease worsens, even minimal stimuli produce more intense and longer-lasting spasms. Spasms are life-threatening when they involve the larynx and/or diaphragm.

Neonatal tetanus presents most often on day 7 of life,[4] with a short (1-day) history of failure of the infant to feed. The neonate displays typical spasms that can easily be misdiagnosed as convulsions of another aetiology. In addition, because these infants vomit (as a result of the increased intra-abdominal pressure) and are dehydrated (because of their inability to swallow), meningitis and sepsis are often considered first.

Autonomic dysfunction occurs in severe cases,[6–8] and begins a few days after the muscle spasms. (The toxin has further to diffuse to reach the lateral horns of the spinal cord.) There is increased basal sympathetic tone, manifesting as tachycardia and bladder and bowel dysfunction. Also, episodes of marked sympathetic overactivity involving both α- and β-receptors occur. Vascular resistance, central venous pressure and, usually, cardiac output are increased, manifesting clinically as labile hypertension, pyrexia, sweating, and pallor and cyanosis of the digits.[7] These episodes are usually of short duration and may occur without any provocation. They are caused by reduced inhibition of postsynaptic sympathetic fibres in the intermediolateral cell column, as evidenced by very high circulating noradrenaline (norepinephrine) concentrations.[1,8] Other postulated causes of this variable sympathetic overactivity include loss of inhibition of the adrenal medulla with increased adrenaline (epinephrine) secretion, direct inhibition by tetanospasmin of the release of endogenous opiates and increased release of thyroid hormone.[1,2]

The role of the parasympathetic nervous system is debatable. Episodes of bradycardia, low peripheral vascular resistance, low central venous pressure and profound hypotension are seen, and are frequently preterminal.[7] Sudden and repeated cardiac arrests occur, particularly in intravenous drug abusers.[8] These events have been attributed to total withdrawal of sympathetic tone, since it is unresponsive to atropine.[9] However they may be caused by catecholamine-induced myocardial damage[8,10] or direct brainstem damage.[8] Whatever the mechanism, patients afflicted with the autonomic dysfunction of tetanus are at risk of sudden death.

Local tetanus is an uncommon mild form of tetanus with a mortality of 1%. The signs and symptoms are confined to a limb or muscle, and may be the result of immunisation. *Cephalic tetanus* is also rare. It results from head and neck injuries, eye infections and otitis media. The cranial nerves, especially the seventh, are frequently involved, and the prognosis is poor. This form may progress to a more generalised form. Tetanus in heroin addicts seems to be severe, with a high mortality, but numbers are small.[8,11]

DIAGNOSIS

The diagnosis is clinical and often straightforward. There are no laboratory tests specific to tetanus. *C. tetani* is cultured from the wound only in a third of cases. The most common differential diagnosis is dystonic reaction to tricyclics. Other differential diagnoses include strychnine poisoning, local temporomandibular disease, local oral disease, convulsions, tetany, intracranial infections or haemorrhage and psychiatric disorders.

MANAGEMENT

Initial objectives of treatment are to neutralise circulating toxin (i.e. passive immunisation) and prevent it from entering peripheral nerves (i.e. wound care), as well as eradicating the source of the toxin (i.e. extensive surgery, hygiene, wound care and antibiotics). Treatment then aims to minimise the effect of toxin already bound in the nervous system, and to provide general supportive care.

PASSIVE IMMUNISATION[1,12]

Human antitetanus toxin has now largely replaced antitetanus serum (ATS) of horse origin, as it is less antigenic. Antitetanus toxin will at best neutralise only circulating toxin, but does not affect toxins already fixed in the CNS, i.e. it does not ameliorate symptoms already present. Although never prospectively tested, present recommendations for human antitetanus toxin in tetanus are 3000–6000 units intravenously (IV). It has been suggested that unimmunised patients or those whose immunisation status is unknown should be given human rich antiserum on presentation with contaminated wounds. No controlled study has shown this to be more effective than wound toilet and penicillin administration.

Intrathecal administration of antitetanus toxin is still controversial. A large meta-analysis reported it to be ineffective.[13] A recent trial comparing intrathecal antitetanus immunoglobulin showed better clinical progression than those treated by the intramuscular route with no difference in mortality.[14] Moreover, suitable intrathecal preparations are not widely available. Side-effects of human antitetanus toxin include fever, shivering and chest or back pains. Cardiovascular parameters need to be monitored, and the infusion may need to be stopped temporarily if significant tachycardia and hypotension present.[1,5,12] If human antiserum is not available, equine ATS can be used after testing and desensitisation.[1]

ERADICATION OF THE ORGANISM

WOUND CARE

Once human antitetanus toxin has been given, the infected site should be thoroughly cleaned and all necrotic tissue extensively debrided.

ANTIBIOTICS

Tetanus spores are destroyed by antibiotics. The vegetative form (bacillus) is sensitive to antibiotics in vitro. However, in vivo efficacy depends on the antibiotic concentration at the wound site, and large doses may be required, Recommended antibiotic regimens include:

1. Metronidazole 500 mg IV 8-hourly for 10 days: The drug has a spectrum of activity against anaerobes, is able to penetrate necrotic tissue and has been shown to be more effective than penicillin in this situation.[15]
2. Penicillin G 1–3 Mu IV at 6-hourly intervals for 10 days: penicillin is a GABA antagonist in the CNS,[16] and may aggravate the spasms. Nevertheless, it is still often used in this situation.
3. Erythromycin has been used, but should not be routinely used.

SUPPRESSION OF EFFECTS OF TETANOSPASMIN

CONTROLLING MUSCLE SPASMS

In the early stages of tetanus, the patient is most at risk from laryngeal and other respiratory muscle spasm. Therefore, if muscle spasms are present, airway should be urgently secured by endotracheal intubation or tracheostomy. If respiratory muscles are affected, mechanical ventilation should be instituted. In severe tetanus, spasms usually preclude effective ventilation, and muscle relaxants may be required. Any muscle relaxant can be used.[17] Heavy sedation alone may prevent muscle spasms and improve autonomic dysfunction (see below).

MANAGEMENT OF AUTONOMIC DYSFUNCTION

Autonomic dysfunction manifests in increased basal sympathetic activity[18] and episodic massive outpourings of catecholamines.[18–20] During these episodes, noradrenaline and adrenaline may be up to 10 times basal levels.[18,19] The clinical picture is variable.[20] Hypertension, tachycardia and sweating do not always occur concurrently.

Traditionally, a combination of α- and β-adrenergic blockers has been used to treat sympathetic overactivity. Phenoxybenzamine, phentolamine, bethanidine and chlorpromazine have been used as α-receptor blockers. Ganglion blockers and nitroprusside have occasionally been used. Propranolol and labetalol have had limited success.[21–23] However, unopposed β-adrenergic blockade cannot be advised. Deaths from acute congestive cardiac failure have resulted.[21,22] Removal of β-mediated vasodilatation in limb muscle causes a rise in systemic vascular resistance, and β-blocked myocardium may not be able to maintain adequate cardiac output. Also, with β-blockade, hypotension follows when sympathetic overactivity abates. Esmolol, a very-short-acting β-adrenergic blocker given IV, has been reported to be useful.[24] However, although sympathetic crises can be controlled by esmolol, catecholamine levels remain raised.[20] This raises concern, because excessive catecholamine secretion is associated with myocardial damage.[10]

From above, it appears more logical to decrease catecholamine output. This can be done with sedatives. Benzodiazepines and morphine are successfully used.[19] Morphine and diazepam act centrally to minimise the effects of tetanospasmin. Morphine probably acts by replacing deficient endogenous opioids.[1] Benzodiazepines increase the affinity and efficacy of GABA.[1] Very large doses of these agents, e.g. diazepam 3400 mg/day[19] and morphine 235 mg/day,[25] may be required, and are well tolerated.

Magnesium has been used as an adjunct to sedation,[19,26] now confirmed by a large trial.[27] Magnesium sulphate infusions to keep serum concentrations between 2.5 and 4.0 mmol/l have decreased systemic vascular resistance and pulse rate, with a small decrease in cardiac output.[19,26] In animal studies, magnesium inhibits release of adrenaline and noradrenaline, and reduces the sensitivity of receptors to these neurotransmitters. Magnesium also has a marked neuromuscular-blocking effect, and may reduce the intensity of muscle spasms. Nevertheless, it could not be shown to decrease the need for mechanical ventilation.[27] However, magnesium sulphate must be used with sedatives,[19] and calcium supplements may be needed when it is infused. Anecdotally, clonidine, a central α_2-stimulant, has successfully produced sedation with control of autonomic dysfunction.[28] It seems sensible to attempt to make use of the central nervous system effects of an α_2-adrenergic agonist, namely sedation and vasodilatation.[29] Intrathecal baclofen has produced similar beneficial results in a series of cases, but significant respiratory depression occurred in a third.[30] When given intrathecally, baclofen can diminish spasms and spasticity, allowing for a reduction in sedative and paralysis requirements.[31]

SUPPORTIVE TREATMENT

Steps should be taken to prevent contractures, nosocomial pneumonias and deep-vein thrombosis. The patient (including the mother if a neonate is afflicted) must be actively immunised. Where possible, supportive psychotherapy should be offered to both patient and family.

COMPLICATIONS[1,4,6,10,32]

Muscle spasms disappear after 1–3 weeks, but residual stiffness may persist. Although most survivors recover completely by 6 weeks, cardiovascular complications, including cardiac failure, arrhythmias, pulmonary oedema and hypertensive crises, can be fatal. No obvious cause of death can be found at autopsy in up to 20% of deaths. Other complications include those associated with factors shown in Table 48.1.

OUTCOME

Recovery from tetanus is thought to be complete. However, in 25 non-neonatal patients followed for up to 11 years,[33] 15 were reported to have one or more abnormal neurological features, such as intellectual or emotional changes, fits and myoclonic jerks, sleep disturbance, and decreased libido. Of the 10 apparently normal survivors, 6 had electroencephalogram changes. Some of these symptoms resolved within 2 years.

Mortality figures depend on the availability of intensive care. In neonates, the mortality from African countries with no ICU facilities can be up to 80% of cases, but falls to about 10% when artificial ventilation is used. In the USA, mortality in non-neonates relates directly to age, with rates from 0% in patients under 30 years rising to 50% in those 60 years or older. An average of 10% mortality would seem to be reasonable for most ICUs. However, as this disease is easily and completely preventable, loss of life is unacceptable.

Table 48.1 Factors contributing to death in tetanus

Hypoxia
Complications of mechanical ventilation
Myoglobinuria and its attendant problems
Sepsis, particularly pneumonia
Fluid and electrolyte problems (including inappropriate antidiuretic hormone secretion)
Deep-vein thrombosis and embolic phenomena
Bed sores
Bony fractures

REFERENCES

1. Bleck TP. Tetanus: pathophysiology, management and prophylaxis. *Dis Mon* 1991; **37**: 556–603.
2. Ackerman AD. Immunology and infections in the pediatric intensive care unit. Part B: Infectious diseases of particular importance to the pediatric intensivist. In: Rogers MC (ed.) *Textbook of Pediatric Intensive Care.* Baltimore: Williams and Wilkins; 1987: 866–75.
3. Editorial. Prevention of neonatal tetanus. *Lancet* 1983; **1**: 1253–4.
4. Stoll BJ. Tetanus. *Pediatr Clin North Am* 1979; **26**: 415–31.
5. Editorial. Reactions to tetanus toxoid. *Br Med J* 1974; **1**: 48.
6. Alfery DD, Rauscher LA. Tetanus: a review. *Crit Care Med* 1979; 7: 176–81.
7. Kerr JH, Corbett JL, Prys-Roberts C *et al.* Involvement of the sympathetic nervous system in tetanus. *Lancet* 1968; **2**: 236–41.
8. Tsueda K, Oliver PB, Richter RW. Cardiovascular manifestations of tetanus. *Anesthesiology* 1974; **40**: 588–92.
9. Kerr J. Current topics in tetanus. *Intens Care Med* 1979; **5**: 105–10.
10. Rose AG. Catecholamine-induced myocardial damage associated with phaeochromocytomas and tetanus. *S Afr Med J* 1974; **48**: 1285–9.
11. Sun KO, Chan YW, Cheung RT *et al.* Management of tetanus: a review of 18 cases. *J R Soc Med* 1994; **87**: 135–7.
12. Annotation. Antitoxin in treatment of tetanus. *Lancet* 1976; **1**: 944.
13. Abrutyn E, Berlin JA. Intrathecal therapy in tetanus: a meta-analysis. *JAMA* 1991; **266**: 2262–7.
14. Miranda-Filho Dde B, Ximenes RA, Barone AA *et al.* Randomised controlled trial of tetanus treatment with antitetanus immunoglobulin by the intrathecal or intramuscular route. *Br Med J* 2004; **328**: 615–17.
15. Ahmadsyah I, Salim A. Treatment of tetanus: an open study to compare the efficacy of procaine penicillin and metronidazole. *Br Med J* 1985; **291**: 648–50.
16. Clarke G, Hill RG. Effects of a focal penicillin lesion on responses of rabbit cortical neurones to putative neurotransmitters. *Br J Pharmacol* 1972; **44**: 435–41.

17. Spelman D, Newton-John H. Continuous pancuronium infusion in severe tetanus. *Med J Aust* 1980; **1**: 676.
18. Domenighetti GM, Savary G, Stricker H. Hyperadrenergic syndrome in severe tetanus: extreme rise in catecholamines responsive to labetalol. *Br Med J* 1984; **288**: 1483–4.
19. Lipman J, James MFM, Erskine J *et al.* Autonomic dysfunction in severe tetanus: magnesium sulphate as an adjunct to deep sedation. *Crit Care Med* 1987; **15**: 987–8.
20. Beards SC, Lipman J, Bothma P *et al.* Esmolol in a case of severe tetanus: adequate haemodynamic control despite markedly elevated catecholamine levels. *S Afr J Surg* 1994; **32**: 33–5.
21. Buchanan N, Smit L, Cane RD *et al.* Sympathetic overactivity in tetanus: fatality associated with propranolol. *Br Med J* 1978; **2**: 254–5.
22. Wesley AG, Hariparsad D, Pather M *et al.* Labetalol in tetanus. *Anaesthesia* 1983; **38**: 243–9.
23. Edmondson RS, Flowers MW. Intensive care in tetanus: management, complications and mortality in 100 cases. *Br Med J* 1979; **1**: 1401–4.
24. King WW, Cave DR. Use of esmolol to control autonomic instability of tetanus. *Am J Med* 1991; **91**: 425–8.
25. Rocke DA, Wesley AG, Pather M *et al.* Morphine in tetanus – the management of sympathetic nervous system overactivity. *S Afr Med J* 1986; **70**: 666–8.
26. James MFM, Manson EDM. The use of magnesium sulphate infusions in the management of very severe tetanus. *Intens Care Med* 1985; **11**: 5–12.
27. Thwaites CL, Yen LM, Loan HT *et al.* Magnesium sulphate for treatment of severe tetanus: a randomised controlled trial. *Lancet* 2006; **368**: 1436–43.
28. Sutton DN, Tremlett MR, Woodcock TE *et al.* Management of autonomic dysfunction in severe tetanus: the use of magnesium sulphate and clonidine. *Intens Care Med* 1990; **16**: 75–80.
29. Kamibayashi T, Maze M. Clinical uses of alpha$_2$-adrenergic agonists. *Anesthesiology* 2000; **93**: 1345–9.
30. Saissy JM, Demaziere J, Vitris M *et al.* Treatment of severe tetanus by intrathecal injections of baclofen without artificial ventilation. *Intens Care Med* 1992; **18**: 241–4.
31. Boots RJ, Lipman J, O'Callaghan J *et al.* The treatment of tetanus with intrathecal baclofen. *Anaesth Intens Care* 2000; **28**: 438–42.
32. Potgieter PD. Inappropriate ADH secretion in tetanus. *Crit Care Med* 1983; **11**: 417–18.
33. Illis LS, Taylor FM. Neurological and electroencephalographic sequelae of tetanus. *Lancet* 1971; **1**: 826–30.

49

Neuromuscular disorders in intensive care

George A Skowronski

A number of disorders producing generalised neuromuscular weakness can require admission to the intensive care unit (ICU), or complicate the course of ICU patients. These may involve:

- spinal anterior horn cells – motor neurone disease, poliomyelitis
- peripheral nerve conduction – Guillain–Barré syndrome (GBS) and related disorders
- the neuromuscular junction – myasthenia gravis (MG), botulism
- muscle contraction – critical-illness myopathy, periodic paralysis

Table 49.1 lists a differential diagnosis of muscle weakness in critically ill patients.

GUILLAIN–BARRÉ SYNDROME AND RELATED DISORDERS

In 1834 James Wardrop reported a case of ascending sensory loss and weakness in a 35-year-old man, leading to almost complete quadriparesis over 10 days, and complete recovery over several months.[1] In 1859, Landry described an acute ascending paralysis occurring in 10 patients, 2 of whom died. Guillain, Barré and Strohl in 1916[2] reported 2 cases of motor weakness, paraesthesiae and muscle tenderness in association with increased protein in the cerebrospinal fluid (CSF: lumbar puncture for CSF examination was first described only in the 1890s).

Many variants of this syndrome have since been reported, and this has resulted in confusion in nomenclature. The lack of specific diagnostic criteria has also been a problem. Clinical, electrical and laboratory criteria for the predominant variant – acute inflammatory demyelinating polyradiculopathy (AIDP) – are now well described,[3] though 10–15% of cases do not fit these criteria, and GBS is best regarded as a heterogeneous group of immunologically mediated disorders of peripheral nerve function.

INCIDENCE

Since the incidence of poliomyelitis has declined markedly due to mass immunisation programmes, GBS has become the major cause of rapid-onset flaccid paralysis in previously healthy people, with an incidence of approximately 1.7 per 100 000. Epidemics have occurred in large populations exposed to viral illness or immunisation.[4] Immunosuppression and concurrent autoimmune disease may also be predisposing factors.[5] The disorder is slightly commoner in males, and up to four times commoner in the elderly. No consistent seasonal or racial predilection has been demonstrated.

AETIOLOGY

Most recent evidence supports the proposition that GBS is caused by immunologically mediated nerve injury.[6] Cell-mediated immunity, in particular, probably plays a significant role, and inflammatory cell infiltrates are often seen in association with demyelination, which is generally regarded as the primary pathologic process. Antibodies to a number of nervous system components have been demonstrated in GBS patients, with most interest in recent years focusing on antiganglioside antibodies.

Although the precise mechanism of sensitisation is not known, clinical associations suggest that antecedent viral infections or immunisations are commonly involved. Infective agents implicated include influenza A, parainfluenza, varicella-zoster, Epstein–Barr, chickenpox, mumps, human immunodeficiency virus (HIV),[7] measles virus and *Mycoplasma*. *Campylobacter jejuni* gastroenteritis now appears to be the most common predisposing infection and may be associated with a more severe clinical course; 26–41% of GBS patients show evidence of recent *C. jejuni* infection.[8] Cytomegalovirus infection accounts for a further 10–22% of cases.[9] Immunisations against viral infections, tuberculosis, tetanus and typhoid have all preceded the development of GBS. Most of these associations are anecdotal and of doubtful aetiological significance, but 65% of patients present within a few weeks of minor respiratory (43%) or gastrointestinal (21%) illness.

PATHOGENESIS[6]

The peripheral nerves of patients who have died of GBS show infiltration of the endoneurium by mononuclear cells in a predominantly perivenular distribution. The inflammatory process may be distributed throughout

Table 49.1 Differential diagnosis of muscle weakness in critically ill patients

Cerebral cortex
Vascular event
Metabolic or ischaemic encephalopathy
Brainstem
Lower pontine hemorrhage or infarction (locked-in state)
Spinal cord
Transverse myelitis
Compression by tumour, abscess or hemorrhage
Carcinomatous or lymphomatous meningitis
Peripheral nerve
Critical-illness polyneuropathy
Phrenic nerve injury during thoracic surgery
Guillain–Barré syndrome
Ingested toxins, including arsenic, thallium, cyanide
Neuromuscular junction
Delayed reversal of neuromuscular blockade
Myasthenia gravis
Lambert–Eaton syndrome
Botulism
Pesticide poisoning
Skeletal muscle
Acute necrotising myopathy
Steroid myopathy
Severe hypokalaemia, hypophosphataemia and/or hypomagnesaemia
Acute alcoholic myopathy
Polymyositis or dermatomyositis
Toxic myopathy (colchicine, lovastatin, cocaine, bumetanide, amiodarone and others)

Adapted from Hansen-Flaschen J. Neuromuscular disorders of critical illness. *UpToDate* 2006; version 14.3.

the length of the nerves, but with more marked focal changes in the nerve roots, spinal nerves and major plexuses. Electron micrographs show macrophages actively stripping myelin from the bodies of Schwann cells and axons. In some cases, wallerian degeneration of axons is also seen, and failure of regeneration in these cases may correspond with a poor clinical outcome.

The underlying immune response is complex and poorly understood, but serum from GBS patients produces myelin damage in vitro when complement is present.[10] Although antibodies to various glycolipids have been demonstrated in GBS, these are generally in low titre and can occasionally be seen in controls. Patients with recent *C. jejuni* infection have a high incidence of antibodies to the ganglioside GM1.[8] Antibodies to GD1a and GQ1b gangliosides are associated with the rarer acute motor axonal neuropathy (AMAN) and acute motor sensory axonal neuropathy (AMSAN) variants (see below).[11] The basis of the effectiveness of plasma exchange and immunoglobulin therapy is likely to be blocking of demyelinating antibodies by several mechanisms.[12]

CLINICAL PRESENTATION

The majority of patients describe a minor illness in the 8 weeks prior to presentation, with a peak incidence 2 weeks beforehand. Approximately half the patients initially experience paraesthesiae, typically beginning in the hands and feet. One-quarter complain of motor weakness, and the remainder have both.[13] Motor weakness proceeds to flaccid paralysis, which becomes the predominant complaint. Objective loss of power and reduction or loss of tendon reflexes usually commence distally and ascend, but a more haphazard spread may occur. Cranial nerves are involved in 45% of cases, most commonly the facial nerve, followed by the glossopharyngeal and vagus nerves. One-third of patients require ventilatory support.

In the Miller–Fisher syndrome, a variant of GBS,[14] cranial nerve abnormalities predominate, with ataxia, areflexia and ophthalmoplegia as the main features. This is strongly associated with recent *C. jejuni* infection and with the presence of GQ1b antibodies.

Another subgroup of patients presents with a primarily axonal neuropathy – AMSAN. In these cases motor and sensory axons appear to be the primary targets of immune attack, rather than myelin. These patients have a more fulminant and severe course, and there is again a strong association with *C. jejuni* infection.

Sensory loss is generally mild, with paraesthesiae or loss of vibration and proprioception, but occasionally sensory loss, pain or hyperaesthesia can be prominent features. Autonomic dysfunction is common, and a major contributor to morbidity and mortality in ventilator-dependent cases.[15] Orthostatic or persistent hypotension, paroxysmal hypertension and bradycardia are all described, as are fatal ventricular tachyarrhythmias. Sinus tachycardia is seen in 30% of cases. Paralytic ileus, urinary retention and abnormalities of sweating are also commonly seen.

DIFFERENTIAL DIAGNOSIS

Most of the important alternative diagnoses are listed as exclusion criteria in Table 49.2. In patients with prolonged illness, the possibility of chronic inflammatory demyelinating polyradiculopathy (CIDP) should be considered.[16] In this condition, which is usually distinguished from GBS, preceding viral infection is uncommon, the onset is more insidious and the course is one of slow worsening or stepwise relapses. Corticosteroids and plasma exchange are possibly effective in this disorder, but adequate studies of immunosuppressive drugs have not been carried out.

An intermediate *subacute* polyradiculopathy (SIDP) as well as a recurrent form of GBS are also described, and all of these variants may be part of the spectrum of a single condition. However, a purely motor axonal neuropathy (AMAN), which causes seasonal childhood epidemics mimicking classical GBS in China and elsewhere,[17] appears to be a distinct entity. Once again, this is strongly associated with *C. jejuni* infection.

Table 49.2 Diagnostic criteria for typical Guillain–Barré syndrome[3]

Features required for diagnosis
Progressive weakness in both arms and both legs
Areflexia
Features strongly supportive of the diagnosis
Progression over days to 4 weeks
Relative symmetry of symptoms
Mild sensory symptoms or signs
Cranial nerve involvement, especially bilateral weakness of facial muscles
Recovery beginning 2–4 weeks after progression ceases
Autonomic dysfunction
Absence of fever at onset
High concentration of protein in cerebrospinal fluid protein, with fewer than 10×10^6 cells/l
Typical electrodiagnostic features
Features excluding diagnosis
Diagnosis of botulism, myasthenia, poliomyelitis or toxic neuropathy
Abnormal porphyrin metabolism
Recent diphtheria
History or evidence of lead intoxication
Purely sensory syndrome, without weakness

INVESTIGATIONS

In over 90% of patients, CSF protein is increased (greater than 0.4 g/l), within a week of onset of symptoms. The level does not correlate with the clinical findings. A pleocytosis with lymphocytes and monocytes in the CSF may be seen in a small proportion of patients, especially later in the disease. Nerve conduction studies typically demonstrate reduced conduction velocity and prolonged distal latencies,[18] but there is no consensus on precise electrophysiological criteria for the various subtypes.[11] Severely reduced distal motor amplitude and a predominantly axonal pattern are associated with more severe disease and a guarded prognosis.

MANAGEMENT

The management of the patient with severe and protracted GBS provides a major challenge, as the prognosis is generally excellent if complications can be treated early or avoided. These complications may be life-threatening, affect any of the major organ systems or result in permanent disability, and can be prevented only by meticulous attention to detail.

SPECIFIC THERAPY

Plasma exchange (plasmapheresis) is of value in GBS. Two large controlled trials showed a reduction in patients requiring mechanical ventilation, reduced duration of mechanical ventilation for those who required it, reduced time to motor recovery and time to walking without assistance.[19] Mortality, however, was not altered. Plasma exchange was most effective when carried out within 7 days of onset of symptoms. The plasma exchange schedules consisted of three to five exchanges of 1–2 plasma volumes each, over 1–2 weeks. Adverse events are common, and some relate to the disease itself. Fresh frozen plasma is reported to have more side-effects than albumin as the replacement fluid.

Immunoglobulin therapy was as effective as plasmapheresis[20] and previous concerns of higher recurrence rates are probably unfounded. Because of its ease of use, many authorities now advocate immunoglobulin as the treatment of choice. A dose of 0.4 g/kg body weight intravenously, daily for 5 days, was used in the most recent trials.

About 10% of patients relapse after initial treatment with either plasmapheresis or immunoglobulin; most respond well to a further course.

A recent Cochrane review confirms that low- or high-dose corticosteroids are of no value,[21] and may even slow recovery. The combination of high-dose steroids with immunoglobulin may hasten recovery, but does not affect the long-term outcome.

SUPPORTIVE CARE

RESPIRATORY

In the spontaneously breathing patient, chest physiotherapy and careful monitoring of respiratory function are of paramount importance. Regular measurement of vital capacity is probably the best way to predict respiratory failure, and is more reliable than arterial blood gases.[22] The latter nevertheless remain a useful guide. Any patient with a vital capacity less than 15 ml/kg or 30% of the predicted level, or a rising arterial $P\text{CO}_2$ is likely to require mechanical ventilation.

Bulbar involvement should be carefully sought, as there is a significant risk of aspiration of upper-airway secretions, gastric contents or ingested food. The cough reflex may be inadequate, and airway protection by tracheal intubation or tracheostomy is then required. Oral feeding should be stopped in any patient in whom bulbar involvement is suspected.

Mechanical ventilation is mandatory if coughing is inadequate, pulmonary collapse or consolidation develop, arterial blood gases are significantly abnormal, vital capacity is less than predicted tidal volume (approximately 10 ml/kg) or the patient is dyspnoeic, tachypnoeic or appears exhausted. Mechanical ventilation, if necessary, will probably be required for several weeks (although there is wide variation), and early tracheostomy should be considered.

CARDIOVASCULAR

Cardiac rhythm and blood pressure should be monitored. Sinus tachycardia is the commonest autonomic manifestation of GBS and usually requires no active treatment.

Table 49.3 Drugs associated with cardiovascular instability in Guillain–Barré syndrome

Exaggerated hypotensive response
Phentolamine
Nitroglycerine
Edrophonium
Thiopental
Morphine
Furosemide
Exaggerated hypertensive response
Phenylephrine
Ephedrine
Dopamine
Isoprenaline
Arrhythmias
Suxamethonium
Cardiac arrest
General anaesthesia

(Modified from Dalos NO, Borel C, Hanley DF. Cardiovascular autonomic dysfunction in Guillain–Barré syndrome. Therapeutic implications of Swan Ganz monitoring. *Arch Neurol* 1988; **45:** 115–17, with permission.)

Induction of anaesthesia appears particularly likely to induce serious arrhythmias. Use of suxamethonium may contribute significantly to this,[23] and, as with many other neuromuscular disorders, should be avoided. Endotracheal suctioning has also been associated with serious arrhythmias. Cardiovascular instability may also be exacerbated by a number of other drugs (Table 49.3). These, likewise, should be avoided or used with great care.

Mild hypotension and bradycardia may require no treatment, particularly if renal and cerebral function are maintained. However, blood volume expansion or inotropic drugs may be required in some cases. Hypertension is often transient, but occasionally requires appropriate drug therapy. Hypoxia, hypercarbia, pain and visceral distension should be excluded as causes.

FLUIDS, ELECTROLYTES AND NUTRITION

Paralytic ileus is not uncommon, especially immediately following the institution of mechanical ventilation, and a period of parenteral nutrition may be required. However, wherever possible, nasoenteric feeding should be instituted because of its significantly greater safety. Energy and fluid requirements are considerably reduced in these patients.

SEDATION AND ANALGESIA

In non-ventilated patients, sedation should be avoided because of the potential for worsening respiratory and upper-airway function. In ventilated patients, sedation becomes less necessary as the patient becomes accustomed to the ventilator, but night sedation may help to preserve diurnal rhythms. Limb pain, particularly with passive movement, is very common and often quite severe. Quinine, minor and non-steroidal analgesics and antidepressant drugs may all be tried, but the pain can be difficult to control and opioids are often required. Methadone, transdermal fentanyl, gabapentin and tramadol have all been advocated.

GENERAL AND NURSING CARE

A comprehensive programme of physiotherapy should be implemented by nurses and physiotherapists, with careful attention to pressure area care, the maintenance of joint mobility and pulmonary function. Opportunistic infection should be actively sought with culture of urine and respiratory secretions at least twice weekly. Sites of vascular access should be inspected frequently, and changed whenever necessary. It may be possible to manage stable long-term patients without venous access. Care should be taken to prevent corneal ulceration and faecal impaction.

Prophylaxis against venous thromboembolism should be given, and enterally administered low-dose warfarin may be preferable to twice-daily heparin injections in long-stay patients. Psychological problems, especially depression, are common, and some patients are helped by antidepressant drugs. Good communication and rapport between the patient and staff, involvement of allied health practitioners, the provision of television, radio and reading aids, and, where possible, occasional trips out of the ICU are all of great value.

PROGNOSIS

The nadir of the disease is reached within 2–4 weeks, and gradual resolution follows over weeks to months. Of those who survive the acute illness, 70% are fully recovered within 1 year, and a further 20% are left with only minor limitation. Poor prognostic features include age over 60 years, rapid progression to quadriparesis in less than 7 days, the need for mechanical ventilation (except for children), and a preceding diarrhoeal illness. Even in patients ventilated for more than 2 months, gradual improvement may continue for 18 months to 2 years.[24] These severely affected patients require a protracted period of rehabilitation.

Death in up to 25% of GBS patients has been reported in those requiring intensive care.[25] Many of these deaths were due to potentially avoidable problems such as respiratory arrest, ventilator malfunction and intercurrent sepsis, and considerably better results have been achieved. A more representative estimate of the overall mortality is 5–8%.[26]

WEAKNESS SYNDROMES COMPLICATING CRITICAL ILLNESS[27]

A number of neuromuscular disorders specifically associated with critical illness have been described over the last 30 years, and remain poorly understood. They are probably much more common than previously appreciated, demonstrable to some degree in up to 50% of patients.[28] These include neuropathies, myopathies and combinations of both. Variations in nomenclature, the lack of a satisfactory classification or diagnostic test, and confusion with other disorders, such as GBS and corticosteroid-induced myopathy, have further complicated this area. There is also considerable overlap among the various subtypes. Sepsis, neuromuscular-blocking agents (NMBA), disuse atrophy, asthma, corticosteroids and the multiple-organ dysfunction syndrome (MODS) have all been implicated. Although the two major subgroups are outlined below, a number of rarer variants have also been described. No specific therapies are available, but most patients improve after a period of supportive care.

CRITICAL-ILLNESS POLYNEUROPATHY

This acute, diffuse, mainly motor neuropathy is probably the commonest of these disorders. It usually presents in the recovery phase of a severe systemic illness with persistent quadriparetic weakness, hyporeflexia and difficulty in weaning from respiratory support. There appears to be a specific association with severe sepsis and MODS. Histological and electrophysiological features are consistent with axonal degeneration. The mortality in this group is high, presumably reflecting that of the underlying condition. However, among those who survive the acute illness, the outlook for recovery of function appears quite good, with 70% recovering completely over an average of 4–5 months.[29]

CRITICAL-ILLNESS MYOPATHY

This disorder is linked with asthma and with the use of corticosteroids, NMBA and, less convincingly, aminoglycosides and β-adrenergic agonists. Reflexes are preserved except in severe cases, as is sensation. Elevated blood creatine phosphokinase (CPK) concentrations are often seen. A few patients have a more severe, fulminant form with very high CPK levels, frank rhabdomyolysis and, rarely, renal failure. Electrophysiological findings are somewhat variable, though muscle necrosis is usually apparent on histology. Although steroidal muscle relaxants (pancuronium or vecuronium)[30] have been particularly implicated, the disorder has also been seen with other types of NMBA. On the basis of two small case series, the outlook for functional recovery appears good.[30]

DIFFERENTIAL DIAGNOSIS

The influence of drugs, metabolic abnormalities and hyperthermia should always be excluded when unexplained neuromuscular weakness appears in an intensive care patient. The possibility of a coincident illness such as the Eaton–Lambert syndrome, MG, vasculitis or GBS must also be carefully considered. Severe catabolism and disuse atrophy are common in many of these patients and can themselves result in significant weakness.

MYASTHENIA GRAVIS

MG is an autoimmune disorder caused by antibodies directed against acetylcholine (ACh) receptors in skeletal muscle. Despite its relative rarity, it is the most studied and best-understood clinical disorder of neuroreceptor function, and arguably the best-understood organ-specific autoimmune disease. It is characterised clinically by weakness or exaggerated fatigability on sustained effort. Intensive care is most commonly required because of severe involvement of the bulbar or respiratory muscles, which may be the result of a spontaneous exacerbation of the disease, a complication of drug therapy, intercurrent illness or surgery or following surgical thymectomy – a definitive treatment for many patients.

INCIDENCE

The incidence of MG is approximately 1 in 20 000 in the USA. There is no racial or geographic predilection. Although MG can occur at any age, it is very rare in the first 2 years of life, and the peak incidence is in young adult females. Overall, females are affected about twice as often as males. This sexual predilection decreases with increasing age, and there is a smaller, second incidence peak in elderly males.[31]

AETIOLOGY AND PATHOPHYSIOLOGY

In 75% of cases, there is histological evidence of thymic abnormality. Thymic hyperplasia is present in the majority of patients, but approximately 10% have a thymoma. The latter appears more common in the older age group. The precise role of the thymus is uncertain, but ACh receptors are present in the myoid cells of the normal thymus, and there is evidence that anti-ACh receptor antibody production is mediated by both B and T lymphocytes of thymic origin. Other organ-specific autoimmune disorders, most commonly thyroid disease,[32] but also rheumatoid arthritis, lupus erythematosus and pernicious anaemia, are significantly associated with MG, and autoantibodies to other organs may be seen in MG patients without evidence of disease.

Children born to mothers with MG demonstrate transient weakness ('neonatal MG') in about 15% of cases. A number of congenital myasthenic syndromes exist, in which symptoms develop in infancy, without evidence of autoantibody production.[33] A familial tendency is more common in this group, and structural changes at the neuromuscular junction have been demonstrated.

The stimulus to autoantibody production is not known, but these can be detected in about 90% of patients with generalised myasthenia. They may interfere with neuromuscular transmission by competitively blocking receptor sites, by initiating immune-mediated destruction of receptors, or by binding to portions of the receptor molecule which are not part of the ACh receptor site, but which, nevertheless, are important in allowing ACh to bind.

CLINICAL PRESENTATION

Ptosis and diplopia are the most common initial symptoms, and in 20% of cases, the disorder remains confined to the eye muscles (ocular MG).[34] Bulbar muscle weakness is common and may result in nasal regurgitation, dysarthria and dysphagia. Limb and trunk weakness can occur with varying distribution, and is usually asymmetrical. Some patients complain of fatigue rather than weakness, and may be misdiagnosed as having psychiatric problems. However, weakness can be elicited by sustained effort of an involved muscle group, e.g. sustained upward gaze is often worse at the end of the day and improves with rest.

INVESTIGATIONS

Impairment of neuromuscular transmission may be confirmed by a positive edrophonium (Tensilon) test. However, this traditional test is waning in popularity as it has high sensitivity but rather poor specificity.[35] Atropine 0.6 mg is given intravenously to prevent muscarinic side-effects, and this is followed by 1 mg edrophonium. If there is no obvious improvement within 1–2 minutes, a further 5 mg may be given. Some authors recommend the use of a saline placebo injection, and the presence of a second doctor as a 'blinded' observer. Resuscitation facilities should be available, as profound weakness may ensue, especially in patients already receiving anticholinesterase drugs. Intramuscular neostigmine, 1–2 mg, may produce a positive response in 5–10% of patients who do not respond to edrophonium.

The presence of autoantibodies against ACh receptors is quite specific, but false positives may occur in patients with penicillamine-treated rheumatoid disease, other autoimmune diseases and in some first-degree relatives of myasthenic patients.[36] About 20% of patients are seronegative.

Electromyography shows characteristic changes in 90% of patients with generalised MG, and also in many patients with ocular symptoms only.

A syndrome of myasthenic weakness occurs in association with malignancy and other autoimmune diseases (Eaton–Lambert syndrome). Although fatigability is present, the pelvic and thigh muscles are predominantly affected, whereas ocular and bulbar involvement is rare. Tendon reflexes are reduced or absent, and there are specific eletromyographic changes.

MANAGEMENT

1. *Symptomatic treatment* is provided by anticholinesterase drugs which potentiate the action of ACh at receptor sites. Pyridostigmine (Mestinon) is the most commonly used, and is usually commenced at a dose of 60 mg orally four times daily. Considerable adjustment of dosage may be required.
2. *Corticosteroids* are effective in approximately 70% of patients, and give best results when high doses (e.g. prednisolone 50–100 mg/day) are used initially, and then gradually reduced. However, transient exacerbation upon commencement of steroids is very common,[37] and severely affected patients are often hospitalised for the initiation of therapy with gradually increasing doses. Older patients are more likely to respond, but an average of 4 months' treatment is required to achieve clinical stability, and the majority will require continuing treatment indefinitely.[38]
3. *Azathioprine and cyclophosphamide* are both effective adjuncts to corticosteroid therapy. Overall, 80% of patients are helped, but improvement may be seen only after some months. A few patients may achieve complete remission.[39] Ciclosporin is also effective, and patients may show benefit more quickly than with azathioprine.[40]
4. *Thymectomy* offers the best chance of long-term, drug-free remission and, despite the lack of unequivocal clinical trial evidence, early thymectomy is now advocated in most patients, particularly those under 60, with more than mild disease, regardless of the presence of a thymoma.[41] Compared with medical therapy, thymectomy results in an earlier onset of remission, lower mortality and greater delay in the appearance of extrathymic recurrences.

   Preoperative optimisation of neuromuscular function is essential, using anticholinesterase drugs and steroids, supplemented by plasma exchange if necessary. Though anticholinesterase requirements are usually reduced in the immediate postoperative period to about three-quarters of the preoperative dose, sustained improvement following thymectomy may not be seen for months or even years. A transcervical approach has been advocated, but doubts remain about the completeness of excision by this route. A thoracoscopic approach may achieve equivalent results with less short-term morbidity, but the traditional sternotomy approach continues to be much more widely used.[42]
5. *Plasma exchange* is effective in producing short-term clinical improvement. It is mainly used in myasthenic crisis or to improve severely affected patients before thymectomy. Its use should be considered, particularly in patients with severe respiratory failure refractory to conventional therapy (see below).[43] Typically, five exchanges of 3–4 litres each are performed over a 2-week period, and this results in improvement within days. However, the benefits are short-lived, lasting only weeks.[44]
6. *Intravenous γ-globulin* has similar effects to those of plasma exchange. A dose of 400 mg/kg per day is usually given for 5 successive days, and occasional patients derive long-term benefit. Interestingly, γ-globulin has

no consistent effect on ACh receptor antibody concentrations, and its mechanism of action is unknown. Clinical trial evidence suggests that γ-globulin is as effective as plasmapheresis,[45] but some clinical experts continue to favour the latter, claiming the clinical response is more rapid.

MYASTHENIC AND CHOLINERGIC CRISIS

Patients with known MG may undergo life-threatening episodes of acute deterioration affecting bulbar and respiratory function. These may occur spontaneously, or may follow intercurrent infection, pregnancy, surgery, the administration of various drugs (Table 49.4)[46] or attempts to reduce the level of immunosuppression. Such episodes, known as myasthenic crises, usually resolve over several weeks, but occasionally last months. The incidence of myasthenic crisis increases markedly with age.

Rarely, a patient may deteriorate due to excessive dosage of anticholinesterase drugs ('cholinergic crisis'). Abdominal cramps, diarrhoea, excessive pulmonary secretions, sweating, salivation and bradycardia may be present, but these can also occur in patients with myasthenic crisis on high doses of pyridostigmine. Though the two situations may be difficult to distinguish, myasthenic crisis is far more likely unless extremely large doses of pyridostigmine, at least 120 mg every 3 hours, have been administered.

A Tensilon test is now considered an unreliable method of distinguishing between these two possibilities, may be hazardous, and is generally not recommended.

Patients with myasthenic crisis should be admitted directly to the ICU, as there is a significant risk of pulmonary aspiration due to bulbar involvement, bacterial pneumonia due to stasis, acute respiratory failure or cardiorespiratory arrest. After initial stabilisation and resuscitation, every effort should be made to identify and correct reversible causes, especially respiratory infections and electrolyte disturbances.

Frequent estimations of vital capacity and maximum inspiratory force should be made and recorded. Tracheal intubation and mechanical ventilation should be considered in patients with significant bulbar involvement or clinical evidence of worsening respiratory failure. As with other neuromuscular disorders, deterioration of blood gases may occur late, and is an unreliable sign of progressive respiratory failure. Aggressive chest physiotherapy, urinary drainage and nasogastric feeding may be required. Hypokalaemia, hypocalcaemia and hypermagnesaemia should be avoided, as all may exacerbate muscle weakness.

If the patient's clinical status cannot be rapidly improved by the adjustment of anticholinesterase dosage and aggressive treatment of intercurrent illness, high-dose corticosteroids and plasma exchange should be commenced simultaneously, and may produce some benefit within as little as 24 hours.[47]

Table 49.4 Drugs which may exacerbate myasthenia gravis

Antibiotics
Streptomycin
Kanamycin
Tobramycin
Gentamicin
Polymyxin group
Tetracycline
Antiarrhythmics
Quinidine
Quinine
Procainamide
Local anaesthetics
Procaine
Lidocaine
General anaesthetics
Ether
Muscle relaxants
Curare
Suxamethonium
Analgesics
Morphine
Pethidine

PERIOPERATIVE MANAGEMENT

MG patients often require intensive care in relation to surgery for intercurrent illness or, more often, thymectomy. Unstable patients should be admitted to hospital some days in advance for stabilisation. In severely affected patients, preoperative high-dose corticosteroids and/or plasma exchange may be used to improve the patient's fitness for surgery. It may be prudent to omit premedication, and an anaesthetic technique which avoids the use of non-depolarising muscle relaxants is usually advocated, though vecuronium and atracurium are probably acceptable in reduced dosage.[48,49] Suxamethonium can be used safely in normal dosage.[50]

Up to one-third of patients require continuing mechanical ventilation postoperatively following thymectomy. Predictive factors include a long preoperative duration of myasthenia, coexistent chronic respiratory disease, high anticholinesterase requirements (e.g. pyridostigmine >750 mg/day), and a preoperative vital capacity of less than 2.9 litres.[51] In those cases requiring mechanical ventilation, some authors advocate temporary cessation of anticholinesterase drugs to reduce respiratory secretions but in all other cases they should be continued, though dosage requirements must be reassessed carefully and repeatedly.

MOTOR NEURONE DISEASE (AMYOTROPHIC LATERAL SCLEROSIS, LOU GEHRIG'S DISEASE)[52]

Motor neurone disease refers to a large group of related disorders (Table 49.5), a few of which are clearly genetically determined, while most arise sporadically, are of completely unknown aetiology and are generally untreatable. The most common variant is the sporadic form known as amyotrophic lateral sclerosis (ALS), a relentlessly progressive degenerative disease which most commonly affects males over 50 years of age. In North America the term 'ALS' is often used more generically, essentially equivalent to the broader term 'motor neurone disease'.

PATHOGENESIS

The disease affects both upper and lower motor neurones. The involvement of either can predominate early on, giving rise to several clinically recognisable subgroups (see Table 49.5). The cerebral cortex as well as the anterior horns of the spinal cord are involved, with shrinkage, degenerative pigmentation and, eventually, disappearance of the affected cells accompanied by gliosis of the lateral columns ('lateral sclerosis'). As muscles are denervated, there is progressive atrophy of muscle fibres ('amyotrophy'), but, remarkably, sensory neurones as well as those concerned with autonomic function, coordination and higher cerebral function are all spared. The precise cause remains unknown. Postulated pathogenetic causes include oxygen free radicals, viral or prion infection, excess excitatory neurotransmitters and growth factors, and immunological abnormalities.[53] Heavy-metal exposure has also been implicated. The only established clinical risk factors are age and family history.

CLINICAL PRESENTATION

The earliest symptoms are those of insidiously developing limb weakness, often asymmetrical, accompanied by obvious muscle wasting. This classically affects the small muscles of the hand and may be accompanied by fasciculation. As time passes, the disease becomes more generalised and more symmetrical, with a mixture of upper and lower motor neurone signs (i.e. spasticity and hyperreflexia in addition to gross wasting), eventually involving bulbar and respiratory muscles. Awareness and intellect were previously thought to be preserved, but it is now recognised that up to half the patients have evidence of cognitive dysfunction.[54] Death occurs in 50% of cases within 3–5 years, usually due to respiratory infection, aspiration or ventilatory failure from profound weakness. However, there is wide variability, and a few patients may survive for many years.

Table 49.5 Degenerative motor neurone diseases

Amyotrophic lateral sclerosis
Spinal muscular atrophy
Bulbar palsy
Primary lateral sclerosis
Pseudobulbar palsy
Heritable motor neurone diseases
Autosomal-recessive spinal muscular atrophy
Familial amyotrophic lateral sclerosis
Other
Associated with other degenerative disorders

(Modified from Beal MF, Richardson EP, Martin JB. Degenerative diseases of the nervous system. In: Wilson JD, Braunwald E, Isselbacher KJ *et al.* (eds) *Harrison's Principles of Internal Medicine.* New York: McGraw-Hill; 1991: 2060–75, with permission.)

DIAGNOSIS

There are no specific investigations, and the diagnosis must be made on clinical grounds together with electromyogram (EMG) evidence of denervation in at least three limbs. Experienced neurologists correctly diagnose the condition with 95% accuracy.[55] The most important differential diagnosis is multifocal motor neuropathy. The distinction is of clinical importance, as the latter is amenable to treatment. Poliomyelitis can also result in a syndrome of progressive weakness, wasting and fasciculation, beginning many years after the initial illness (the post-polio syndrome), and leading occasionally to respiratory failure and death.[56]

MANAGEMENT

Treatment is essentially symptomatic and supportive. No benefit has been shown with antioxidants, growth factors and immunosuppressants.[53] However, the centrally acting glutamate antagonist riluzole has been shown to slow slightly the progression of ALS.[57] Admission to ICU is sometimes requested when these patients present with an acute deterioration or intercurrent illness. The intensivist may be asked to assist with ambulatory or home respiratory support for gradually worsening chronic respiratory failure. Such cases present major ethical as well as clinical problems, but the provision of assisted ventilation can result in an improved quality of life, and possibly prolonged survival for carefully selected individuals.[58] Respiratory support may be given by facemask, nasal mask or, rarely, by tracheostomy using simple, compact ventilators. Some patients require only intermittent support, particularly at night or during periods of acute deterioration due to intercurrent illness. Long-term respiratory support outside the ICU is a major undertaking, requiring specific equipment and extensive liaison with the patient, the family and numerous specialised support services.

RARE CAUSES OF ACUTE WEAKNESS IN THE ICU

PERIODIC PARALYSIS[59]

This term describes a group of rare primary disorders, mostly inherited as autosomal-dominant traits, producing episodic weakness. They must be distinguished from other causes of intermittent weakness, including electrolyte abnormalities, MG and transient ischaemic attacks. In the inherited disorders, the underlying abnormality is a defect of skeletal muscle ion channels. Symptoms begin early in life (before age 25), and follow rest or sleep rather than exertion. Alertness during attacks is completely preserved, and muscle strength between attacks is normal. Treatment is usually successful in preventing both the attacks and the chronic weakness, which can develop after many years in untreated patients.

The *hypokalaemic* form of periodic paralysis is predominantly inherited, but can also arise sporadically in association with thyrotoxicosis. Involvement of bulbar or respiratory muscles occurs rarely, as can cardiac arrhythmias. The degree of hypokalaemia during attacks is mild, but patients rapidly respond to potassium administration. Effective prophylaxis is conferred by acetazolamide, but not by oral potassium.

The *hyperkalaemic* form is milder, almost always inherited and virtually never requires intensive care. During attacks the serum potassium may be modestly elevated or normal. Patients respond to carbohydrate administration, and thiazide diuretics or acetazolamide provide effective prophylaxis.

BOTULISM[60]

Botulism is a widespread but very uncommon potentially lethal disease caused by exotoxins produced by *Clostridium botulinum* – an anaerobic, spore-forming Gram-positive bacillus. The vast majority of botulism is *food-borne* and outbreaks are largely due to home-preserved vegetables (type A toxin), meat (type B) or fish (type E), but high-risk foods also include low-acid fruit and condiments. Signs and symptoms are caused by toxin produced in vitro and then ingested.

Wound botulism arises rarely, when wounds (typically open fractures) are contaminated by soil containing type A or B organisms. Intravenous drug abusers are an increasing source of this condition through infected injection sites.

Infantile botulism arises in infants under 6 months of age, and is due to the active production of toxin by organisms in the gut rather than the direct ingestion of toxin.

Hidden botulism describes the adult equivalent of infantile botulism, and is a rare complication of various gastrointestinal abnormalities.

Inadvertent botulism is the most recently described form, and occurs as a complication of the medical or cosmetic use of botulinum toxin.

Inhalational botulism is the form that would occur as a result of aerosolised toxin released in the context of bioterrorism.

In most cases, exogenously produced exotoxin is absorbed (primarily in the upper small intestine), and carried by the blood stream to cholinergic nerves at the neuromuscular junction, postganglionic parasympathetic nerve endings and autonomic ganglia, to which it irreversibly binds. The toxin enters the nerve endings to interfere with ACh release.

Most patients become ill about 3 days after ingestion of toxin, with gastrointestinal symptoms (nausea, vomiting, abdominal pain, diarrhoea or constipation), dryness of the eyes and mouth, dysphagia and generalised weakness, which progresses in a symmetrical, descending fashion, with ventilatory failure in severe cases. Cranial nerve dysfunction is manifested by ptosis and diplopia, facial weakness and impaired upper-airway reflexes.

The differential diagnosis includes food poisoning from other causes, MG and GBS. Botulism can be confirmed by the presence of toxin (either in the patient's serum or stool, or in contaminated food) in about two-thirds of cases.

Treatment is mainly supportive, with airway protection and mechanical ventilation when required. Clearance of toxin from the bowel with enemas and cathartics has been advocated. Guanidine hydrochloride, which enhances the release of ACh from nerve terminals, has been reported to improve muscle strength, especially in ocular muscles, and may be useful in milder cases. Antibiotics have not been clearly shown to be useful. Equine antitoxins are available, but side-effects are common and their efficacy is limited. A human-derived antitoxin has been shown to be effective in *infantile botulism*,[61] and the US Defense Department has a pentavalent antitioxin, which is not available for public use. In *wound botulism*, antibiotics (penicillin or metronidazole) and aggressive debridement are recommended.

Most patients begin to improve after a week or so, but hospitalisation is usually required for 1–3 months. The mortality is low (5–8%) with good supportive care, including mechanical ventilation. Mild weakness and constipation may persist for many months.

REFERENCES

1. Wardrop J. Clinical observations on various diseases. *Lancet* 1834; **1**: 380.
2. Guillain G, Barré JA, Strohl A. Sur un syndrome de radiculo-névrites avec hyperalbuminose du liquide cephalorachidren sans réaction cellulaire. Remarques sur les caractères cliniques et graphiques des reflexes tendineaux. *Bull Soc Med Hop Paris* 1916; **40**: 1462.
3. Asbury AK, Aranson BG, Karp HR *et al.* Criteria for diagnosis of Guillain–Barré syndrome. *Ann Neurol* 1998; **3**: 565–6.
4. Sliman NA. Outbreak of Guillain–Barré syndrome associated with water pollution. *Br Med J* 1978; **1**: 751–2.
5. Korn-Lubetzki I, Abramsky O. Acute chronic demyelinating inflammatory polyradiculoneuropathy: association with auto-immune diseases and lymphocyte response to human neuritogenic protein. *Arch Neurol* 1986; **43**: 604–8.
6. Giovannoni G, Hartnung H-P. The immunopathogenesis of multiple sclerosis and Guillain–Barré syndrome. *Curr Opin Neurol* 1996; **9**: 165–77.

7. Simpson DM, Olney RK. Peripheral neuropathies associated with human immunodeficiency virus infection. *Neurol Clin* 1992; **10**: 685–711.
8. Jacobs BS, van Doorn PA, Schmitz PIM *et al.* *Campylobacter jejuni* infection and anti-GM1 antibodies in Guillain–Barré syndrome. *Ann Neurol* 1996; **40**: 181–7.
9. Visser LH, van der Meché FGA, Meulste J *et al.* Cytomegalovirus infection and Guillain–Barré syndrome: the clinical, electrophysiological and prognostic features. *Neurology* 1996; **47**: 668–73.
10. Sawant S, Clark MB, Koski CL. In vitro demyelination by serum antibody from patients with immune complexes. *Ann Neurol* 1991; **29**: 397–404.
11. Hughes RAC, Cornblath DR. Guillain–Barré syndrome. *Lancet* 2005; **366**: 1653–66.
12. Slater RA, Rostomi A. Treatment of Guillain–Barré syndrome with intravenous immunoglobulin. *Neurology* 1998; **51** (Suppl. 5): S9–15.
13. Loffel NB, Rossi LN, Mumethaler M *et al.* Landry–Guillain–Barré syndrome: complications, prognosis and natural history in 123 cases. *J Neurol Sci* 1977; **33**: 71–9.
14. Fisher CM. Unusual variant of acute idiopathic polyneuritis (syndrome of ophthalmoplegia, ataxia and areflexia). *N Engl J Med* 1956; **255**: 57–65.
15. Truax BT. Autonomic disturbances in the Guillain–Barré syndrome. *Semin Neurol* 1984; **4**: 462–8.
16. Hughes RA. The spectrum of acquired demyelinating polyradiculopathy. *Acta Neurol Belg* 1994; **94**: 128–32.
17. McKhann GM, Cornblath DR, Griffin JW *et al.* Acute motor axonal neuropathy: a frequent cause of acute flaccid paralysis in China. *Ann Neurol* 1993; **33**: 333–42.
18. Olney RK, Aminoff MJ. Electrodiagnostic features of the Guillain–Barré syndrome: the relative sensitivities of different techniques. *Neurology* 1990; **40**: 471–5.
19. The Guillain–Barré study group. Plasmapheresis and acute Guillain–Barré syndrome. *Neurology* 1985; **35**: 1096–104.
20. Plasma Exchange/Sandoglobulin Guillain–Barré Syndrome Trial Group. Randomised trial of plasma exchange, intravenous immunoglobulin and combined treatments in Guillain–Barré syndrome. *Lancet* 1997; **349**: 225–30.
21. Hughes RA, Swan AV, van Koningsveld R *et al.* Corticosteroids for Guillain–Barré syndrome. *Cochrane Database Syst Rev* 2006; **2**: CD001446.
22. Hund EF, Borel CO, Cornblath DR *et al.* Intensive management and treatment of severe Guillain–Barré syndrome. *Crit Care Med* 1993; **21**: 433–66.
23. Fergusson RJ, Wright DJ, Willey RJ *et al.* Suxamethonium is dangerous in polyneuropathy. *Br Med J* 1981; **282**: 298–9.
24. Ropper AH. Severe acute Guillain–Barré syndrome. *Neurology* 1986; **36**: 429–32.
25. Scott IA, Seeley G, Wright M *et al.* Guillain–Barré syndrome: a retrospective review. *Aust NZ J Med* 1988; **18**: 149–55.
26. Ng KKP, Howard RS, Fish DR *et al.* Management and outcome of severe Guillain–Barré syndrome. *Q J Med* 1995; **88**: 243–50.
27. Sliwa JA. Acute weakness syndromes in the critically ill patient. *Arch Phys Med Rehabil* 2000; **81**: S45–52.
28. Deem S, Lee CM, Curtis JR. Acquired neuromuscular disorders in the intensive care unit. *Am J Respir Crit Care Med* 2003; **168**: 735–9.
29. Op de Cool AAW, Verheul GAM. Leijten ACM *et al.* Critical illness polyneuropathy after artificial respiration. *Clin Neurol Neurosurg* 1991; **93**: 27–33.
30. Margolis B, Kachikian D, Friedman Y *et al.* Prolonged reversible quadriparesis in mechanically ventilated patients who received long-term infusions of vecuronium. *Chest* 1991; **100**: 877–8.
31. Kurtze JF, Kurland LT. The epidemiology of neurologic disease. In: Joynt RJ (ed.) *Clinical Neurology*, vol. 4. Philadelphia: JB Lippincott; 1992: 80–8.
32. Osserman KE, Tsairis P, Weiner LB. Myasthenia gravis and thyroid disease. Clinical and immunological correlation. *Mt Sinai J Med* 1967; **34**: 469–83.
33. Engel AG, Ohno K, Sine SM. Congenital myasthenic syndromes. *Arch Neurol* 1999; **56**: 163–7.
34. Sharp HR, Degrip A, Mitchell D *et al.* Bulbar presentations of myasthenia gravis in the elderly patient. *J Laryngol Otol* 2001; **115**: 1–13.
35. Meriggioli MN, Sanders DB. Myasthenia gravis: diagnosis. *Semin Neurol* 2004; **24**: 31–9.
36. Vincent A, Newsom-Davis J. Acetylcholine receptor antibody as a diagnostic test for myasthenia gravis: results in 153 validated cases and 2967 diagnostic assays. *J Neurol Neurosurg Psychiatry* 1986; **48**: 1246–52.
37. Johns TR. Long-term corticosteroid treatment of myasthenia gravis. *Ann NY Acad Sci* 1987; **505**: 568–83.
38. Sghirlanzoni A, Peluchetti D, Mantegazza R *et al.* Myasthenia gravis: prolonged treatment with steroids. *Neurology* 1984; **34**: 170–4.
39. Niakan E, Harati Y, Rolak LA. Immunosuppressive drug therapy in myasthenia gravis. *Arch Neurol* 1986; **43**: 155–6.
40. Schalke BCG, Kappos L, Rohrbach E *et al.* Cyclosporine A vs azathioprine in the treatment of myasthenia gravis: final results of a randomised, controlled double-blind clinical trial. *Neurology* 1988; **38** (suppl. 1): 135.
41. Busch C, Machens A, Pichlmeier U *et al.* Long-term outcome and quality of life after thymectomy for myasthenia gravis. *Ann Surg* 1996; **224**: 225–32.
42. Younger DS, Jaretzky A III, Penn AS *et al.* Maximum thymectomy for myasthenia gravis. *Ann NY Acad Sci* 1987; **505**: 832–5.
43. Gracey DR, Howard FM, Divertie MB. Plasmapheresis in the treatment of ventilator-dependent myasthenia gravis patients. Report of four cases. *Chest* 1984; **85**: 739–43.
44. Drachman DB. Myasthenia gravis. *N Engl J Med* 1994; **330**: 1797–810.
45. Gajdos P, Chevret S, Clair B *et al*, Myasthenia Gravis Clinical Study Group. Clinical trial of plasma exchange

and high-dose intravenous immunoglobulin in myasthenia gravis. *Ann Neurol* 1997; **41**: 789–96.
46. Wittbrodt ET. Drugs and myasthenia gravis. *Arch Intern Med* 1997; **157**: 399–408.
47. Berroschot J, Baumann I, Kalischewski P *et al.* Therapy of myasthenic crisis. *Crit Care Med* 1997; **25**: 1228–35.
48. Bell CF, Florence AM, Hunter JM *et al.* Atracurium in the myasthenic patient. *Anaesthesia* 1984; **39**: 691–8.
49. Eisenkraft JB, Sawkney RK, Papatestas AE. Vecuronium in the myasthenic patient. *Anaesthesia* 1986; **41**: 666–7.
50. Wainwright AP, Broderick PM. Suxamethonium in myasthenia gravis. *Anaesthesia* 1987; **42**: 950–7.
51. Eisenkraft JB, Papatestas AE, Kahn CH *et al.* Predicting the need for postoperative mechanical ventilation in myasthenia gravis. *Anaesthesiology* 1986; **65**: 79–82.
52. Rowland LP, Shneider NA. Amyotrophic lateral sclerosis. *N Engl J Med* 2001; **344**: 1688–700.
53. Jerusalem F, Pohl Ch, Karitzky J *et al.* ALS. *Neurology* 1996; **47** (Suppl. 4): S218–220.
54. Ringholz GM, Appel SH, Bradshaw M *et al.* Prevalence and patterns of cognitive impairment in sporadic ALS. *Neurology* 2005; **65**: 586–90.
55. Rowland LP. Diagnosis of amyotrophic lateral sclerosis. *J Neurol Sci* 1998; **160** (Suppl. 1): S6–24.
56. Fisher DA. Poliomyelitis: late respiratory complications and management. *Orthopedics* 1985; **8**: 891–4.
57. Bensimon G, Lacomblez L, Meininger V *et al.* A controlled trial of riluzole in amyotrophic lateral sclerosis. *N Engl J Med* 1994; **330**: 585–91.
58. Edwards PR, Howard P. Methods and prognosis of non-invasive ventilation in neuromuscular disease. *Monaldi Arch Chest Dis* 1993; **48**: 176–82.
59. Gutman L. Periodic paralyses. *Neurol Clin* 2000; **18**: 195–202.
60. Cherington M. Clinical spectrum of botulism. *Muscle Nerve* 1998; **21**: 701–10.
61. Arnon SS, Schechter R, Maslanka SE *et al.* Human botulism immune globulin for the treatment of infant botulism. *N Engl J Med* 2006; **354**: 462–71.

Part Eight

Endocrine Disorders

50

Diabetic emergencies

Richard T Keays

Diabetes mellitus is due to an absolute or relative deficiency of insulin. The sustained effect of poor glycaemic control results in a wide array of end-organ damage as a consequence of small- and large-vessel pathology. Mortality and morbidity are related to the progress of this damage but often there are acute metabolic deteriorations that can be life-threatening. Diabetic ketoacidosis (DKA) and hyperosmolar hyperglycaemic state (HHS) are two of the most common acute complications of diabetes, both accompanied by hyperglycaemia. The pathophysiologic changes that occur in both disease states represent an extreme example of the superfasted state. Coma may also result from severe hypoglycaemia due to overtreatment, usually with insulin.

DIABETES MELLITUS

TYPE 1

Insulin-dependent diabetes mellitus (IDDM) has a peak incidence in the young, rising from 9 months to 14 years and declining thereafter. In 25% of patients the presentation is with ketoacidosis, especially in those under 5 years of age.[1] Usually the fasting plasma glucose is > 7.8 mmol/l and glucose and ketones may be present in the urine. In the asymptomatic patient with equivocal fasting plasma glucose an impaired glucose tolerance test may be demonstrated.

TYPE 2

Non-insulin-dependent diabetes mellitus (NIDDM) is prevalent in the elderly but can occur at any age. Truncal obesity is a risk factor and there is ethnic variation in susceptibility. Diagnosis is often delayed and may be incidental from blood or urine sugar screening.[2] It may present with classical symptoms, as a diabetic emergency, with complications of organ damage or vascular disease.

EPIDEMIOLOGY

Diabetes mellitus affects about 6% of the world's population and is set to rise to 300 million sufferers by 2025.[3] Most of these (97%) will have type 2 diabetes but the resources required to treat the complications of type 1 diabetes are such that health-care costs are equivalent between the two groups. The annual incidence of DKA is 4.6–8 episodes per thousand patients with type 1 diabetes and in the USA it has been estimated that about $1 billion is spent each year in treating DKA. HHS represents approximately 1% of primary admissions to hospital with diabetes as compared with DKA. An interplay of both genetic and environmental factors contributes to disease development. In type 1 diabetes there is some evidence for genetic susceptibility, but environmental factors play a greater part. It varies across race and regions, being highest in northern Europe and the USA and lowest in Asia and Australasia.[4] Genetic factors in type 2 diabetes are evidently crucial, with a concordance between monozygotic twins approaching 100%.

PATHOGENESIS

Normal carbohydrate metabolism depends upon the presence of insulin (Figure 50.1). However, different tissues handle glucose in different ways; for example, red blood cells lack mitochondria and therefore lack pyruvate dehydrogenase and the enzymes involved in β-oxidation, whereas liver parenchymal cells are able to perform the full range of glucose disposal (Figure 50.2). Both DKA and HHS result from a reduction in the effect of insulin with a concomitant rise in counterregulatory hormones such as glucagon, catecholamines, cortisol and growth hormone. Hyperglycaemia occurs as a consequence of three processes: (1) increased gluconeogenesis; (2) increased glycogenolysis; and (3) reduced peripheral glucose utilisation. The increase in glucose production occurs in both the liver and the kidneys as there is a high availability of gluconeogenic precursors such as amino acids (protein turnover shifts from balanced synthesis and degradation to reduced synthesis and increased degradation). Lactate and glycerol also become available due to an increase in skeletal muscle glycogenolysis and an increase in adipose tissue lipolysis respectively. Lastly, there is an increase in gluconeogenic enzyme activity, enhanced further by stress hormones. Whilst hepatic gluconeogenesis is the main mechanism for producing hyperglycaemia, a significant proportion can be produced by the kidneys.[5] What is unclear is the temporal relationship of these changes,

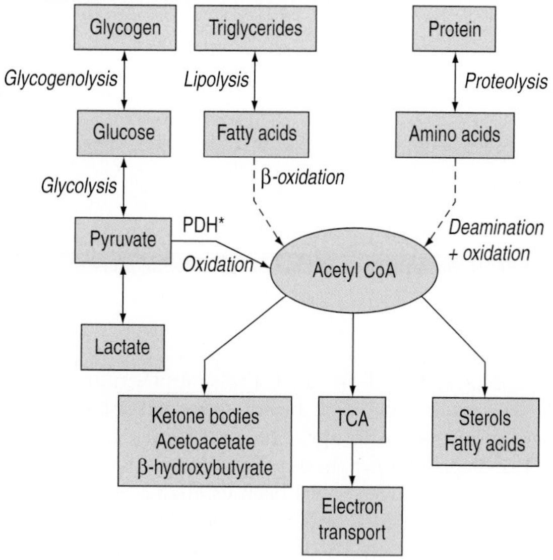

Figure 50.1 Sources and fate of acetyl coenzyme A (CoA). *Pyruvate conversion by pyruvate dehydrogenase (PDH) is essentially irreversible, therefore no net conversion of fatty acids to carbohydrates can occur. TCA, tricarboxylic acid.

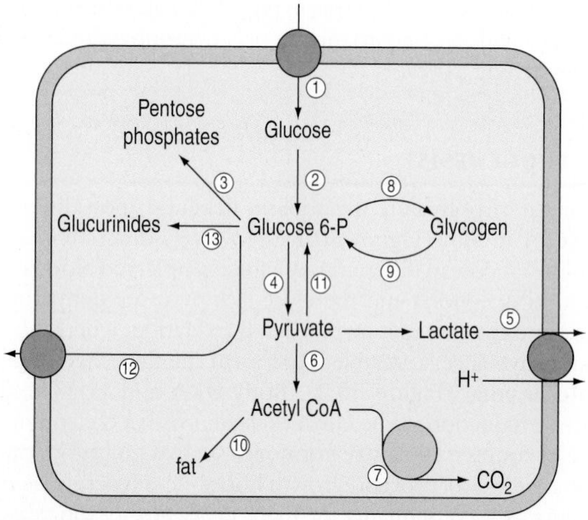

Figure 50.2 Glucose metabolism within hepatocyte. (1) Glucose transport: GLUT-1. (2) Hexokinase phosphorylation. (3) Pentose phosphate pathway (hexose monophosphate shunt). (4) Glycolysis. (5) Lactate transport out of cell. (6) Pyruvate decarboxylation. (7) Tricarboxylic acid (TCA) cycle. (8) Glycogenesis. (9) Glycogenolysis. (10) Lipogenesis. (11) Gluconeogenesis. (12) Glucose-6-phosphate (G-6-P) hydrolysis and release of glucose. (13) Glucuronidation.

although an increase in both catecholamines and the glucagon/insulin ratio are early features.[6]

Decreased insulin and increased adrenaline (epinephrine) levels activate adipose tissue lipase, causing a breakdown of trigylcerides into glycerol and free fatty acids (FFAs). Once again glucagon is implicated, as hepatic oxidation of FFAs to ketone bodies is predominantly stimulated by its inhibitory effect on acetyl-coenzyme A (CoA) carboxylase. The resultant reduced synthesis of malonyl-CoA causes a disinhibition of acyl-carnitine synthesis and subsequent promotion of fatty acid transport into mitochondria, where ketone body formation occurs. Both cortisol and growth hormone are capable of increasing FFA and ketone levels and once again the exact contribution of insulin deficiency or stress hormone increase to ketogenesis is undetermined. As ketone bodies are comparatively strong acids, a large hydrogen ion load is produced due to their dissociation at physiologic pH. The need to buffer hydrogen ions depletes the body's alkali reserves and ketone anions accumulate, accounting for the elevated plasma anion gap.

By contrast HHS does not share the ketogenic features of DKA and it is of interest in what ways these two conditions differ. Reduced levels of FFAs, glucagon, cortisol and growth hormone have been demonstrated in HHS relative to DKA, although this is by no means a consistent observation. However, the presence of higher levels of C-peptide in HHS (with lower levels of growth hormone) relative to DKA suggests there is just enough insulin present in HHS to prevent lipolysis but not enough to promote peripheral glucose utilisation.[7]

Hyperosmolarity, which is a prominent feature of HHS, is caused by the prolonged effect of an osmotic diuresis with impaired ability to take adequate fluids. It has been shown that, even when well, patients who have suffered from HHS have impaired thirst reflexes. However the hyperosmolarity seen in about one-third of patients with DKA results from a shorter osmotic diuresis and to variable fluid intake due to nausea and vomiting – often ascribed to the brainstem effects of ketones.

Interestingly, hyperglycaemia, with or without ketoacidosis, leads to a significant increase in proinflammatory cytokine production, which resolves when insulin therapy is commenced.[8] This has led others to postulate a wider beneficial anti-inflammatory effect attributable to insulin therapy.

CLINICAL PRESENTATION

DKA and HHS represent the two extremes of presentation due to the absolute or relative deficiency of insulin. However, up to one-third of cases can present with mixed features.[9] DKA develops over a shorter time period whereas HHS appears more insidiously (Table 50.1). Polyuria, polydipsia and weight loss are experienced for a variable period prior to admission and, in patients with DKA, nausea and vomiting are also common symptoms. Abdominal pain is commonly seen in children and occasionally in adults and may mimic an acute abdomen. Dehydration presents with loss of skin turgor, dry mucous membranes, tachycardia and hypotension. Mental obtundation occurs more frequently in HHS than DKA as more patients, by definition, are hyperosmolar

Table 50.1 Comparison of DKA and HHS

Presentation	DKA	HHS
Prodromal Illness	Days	Weeks
Coma	++	+++
Blood glucose	++	+++
Ketones	+++	0 or +
Acidemia	+++	0 or +
Anion Gap	++	0 or +
Osmolality	++	+++
Typical deficits		
Total water (litres)	6	9
Water (ml/kg)	100	100–200
Na^+ (mEq/kg)	7–10	5–13
Cl^- (mEq/kg)	3–5	5–15
K^+ (mEq/kg)	3–5	4–6
PO_4 (mEq/kg)	5–7	3–7
Mg^{2+} (mEq/kg)	1–2	1–2
Ca^{2+} (mEq/kg)	1–2	1–2

and the presence of stupor or coma in patients who are not hyperosmolar requires consideration of other potential causes for altered mental status.[10] However, loss of consciousness is not a common presentation with DKA or HHS (< 20%). Most hospitalisations are caused by infection (29%) or non-compliance with medication (17%) in previously diagnosed diabetics; however, in some patients it is the first presentation with undiagnosed diabetes (17%).[11] Given that there is a high likelihood of concurrent infection, most patients have a normal or low temperature and most patients also have a leukocytosis, whether there is infection present or not.

DIABETIC KETOACIDOSIS

DKA tends to occur more often in patients with type 1 diabetes. Rapid, deep breathing due to acidosis (Kussmaul breathing) may be present, as may the breath odour that is characteristic of ketones, which is somewhat like nail polish remover. A history of insulin therapy omission is common, and patients using continuous insulin delivery devices are particularly at risk due to the use of short-acting insulin which provides no insulin reserve if the pump fails. Diagnostic criteria include pH < 7.3, HCO_3^- <15 mmol/l and blood glucose >14 mmol/l. Increasing acidaemia, ketonaemia and deteriorating conscious level indicate increasing severity. Blood glucose per se is not a good determinant of severity and euglycaemic ketoacidosis is possible, depending on the hepatic glycogen stores *prior* to the onset of DKA – a patient who has not been eating well in the recent past may well have a minimally elevated blood glucose. A high amylase is frequently seen and may be extrapancreatic in origin. It should be interpreted cautiously as evidence of pancreatitis.

HYPEROSMOLAR HYPERGLYCAEMIC SYNDROME

HHS is more often seen in patients with type 2 diabetes and the dominant feature is hyperosmolarity (> 320 mosmol/kg). HHS is typically observed in elderly patients with NIDDM, although it may rarely be a complication in younger patients with IDDM, or those without diabetes following severe burns,[12] parenteral hyperalimentation, peritoneal dialysis or haemodialysis. Patients receiving certain drugs, including diuretics, corticosteroids, β-blockers, phenytoin and diazoxide, are at increased risk of developing this syndrome. HHS may be caused by lithium-induced diabetes insipidus.[13] Not only may mental obtundation occur but occasionally focal neurological features or seizures are present.

MANAGEMENT

Intensive care unit admission is indicated in the management of DKA, HHS and mixed cases in the presence of cardiovascular instability, inability to protect the airway, altered sensoria, the presence of acute abdominal signs or symptoms suggestive of acute gastric dilatation.

INITIAL ASSESSMENT

These conditions are medical emergencies and a prompt and thorough history and physical examination should be obtained, with special attention paid to airway patency, conscious level, cardiovascular and renal status, possible sources of infection and state of hydration. Some assessment of the severity of DKA is also aided by the degree of acidosis. The majority of patients have a leukocytosis irrespective of whether they have a source of sepsis or not.

FLUID REQUIREMENTS

Dehydration and sodium depletion develop as a result of the osmotic diuresis that accompanies hyperglycaemia in both DKA and HHS. In DKA there is an additional ketoanion excretion which is approximately half that of glucose. This obligates cation (sodium, potassium and ammonium) excretion and contributes to the electrolyte losses. Despite the dual osmotic load of glucose and ketones in DKA, dehydration is often worse in HHS due to the more prolonged onset. Insulin itself also promotes salt, water and phosphate reabsorption in the kidney and its lack can contribute further to these losses. The total osmolar load on the kidney in DKA can be as much as 2000 mosmol/day.[14] Fluid resuscitation is initially directed to repleting the intravascular volume, and colloids achieve this more rapidly than crystalloids. There is individual variation as to how much fluid will be required and simple vital signs, such as heart rate, blood pressure and peripheral perfusion, should guide the resuscitation. Fluid challenges with assessment of response may be less likely to avoid the problems of fluid overload. The usual urinary sodium concentration is 60–70 mmol/l, which is roughly similar to half-normal saline, and this is the logical fluid to use for rehydration.[15] This avoids too great a sodium load and is less likely to produce a hyperchloraemic acidosis which, if rhabdomyolysis occurs, will further acidify the urine and promote precipitation of myoglobin in the renal tubule. As insulin therapy is commenced extracellular water is driven into the intracellular compartment, exacerbating hypovolaemia.

Inappropriate fluid replacement can lead to problems. Studies of DKA and cerebral oedema are limited but there is some evidence that overly aggressive replacement of water losses can precipitate cerebral and other forms of oedema. Water losses do not need to be corrected rapidly and hyperosmolality should not be corrected more rapidly than 3 mosmol/kg H_2O per hour. Inappropriate resuscitation fluid can also lead to further overshoot in plasma sodium levels and a further increase in plasma osmolarity which has been associated with pontine myelinolysis.[16]

General guidelines are given in Figure 50.3, but it must be remembered that each case needs individual tailoring of treatment. It is mostly agreed that the first litre should be isotonic saline, even in patients with marked hypertonicity. This should be given over the first hour. If there is any evidence of cardiovascular compromise due to hypovolaemia, plasma expansion with colloids should also be given as a matter of urgency. For the next 2 hours 0.45% saline can be given if the serum sodium is normal or high. If the corrected sodium is low, then 0.9% saline should be continued. When the blood glucose falls to 15 mmol/l or below, then a combination of 5% dextrose solution (100–250 ml/h) with some further saline-containing solution should be commenced. Assuming cardiovascular stability, the aim should be to correct the remaining fluid deficit gradually over the next 24–48 hours whilst also taking account of ongoing urinary losses.

INSULIN THERAPY

It is now clear that an initial bolus dose of 0.15 U/kg followed by low-dose (0.1 U/kg per hour) insulin infusions and gradual correction of hyperglycaemia in DKA results in a reduced mortality.[17] This is because there are fewer therapy-induced episodes of hypoglycaemia and hypokalaemia. Intravenous rather than subcutaneous or intramuscular delivery is preferable as glucose decrement is the same whatever route is chosen, but intravenous insulin reduces ketone body production faster. It is mandatory to use the intravenous route where hypovolaemic shock is present. Appropriate rehydration also acts to reduce blood glucose levels by increased glomerular filtration and a reduction in counterregulatory hormone levels. Inadequate glucose decrement may indicate inadequate fluid resuscitation. Severe insulin resistance occurs in 10% of cases and will necessitate the use of higher doses.

ELECTROLYTE THERAPY

Potassium

Hyperosmolarity causes a shift of potassium from within cells to the extracellular space and this potassium is lost as a result of the osmotic diuresis. Renal losses are augmented by secondary hyperaldosteronism and ketoanion

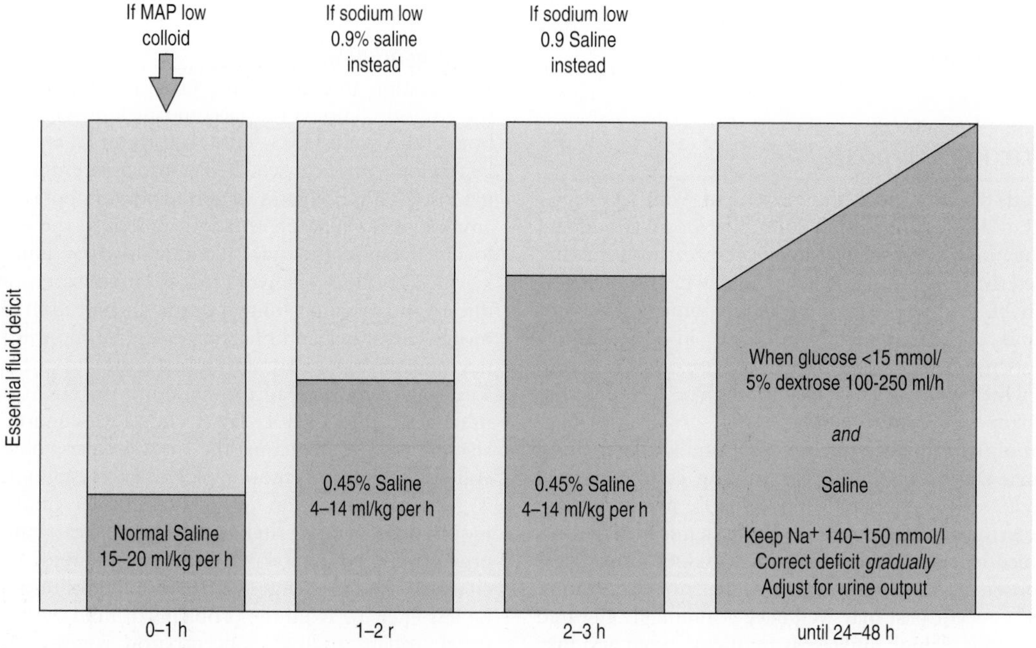

Figure 50.3 Fluid regimen in hyperglycaemic emergencies. There are no major differences between diabetic ketoacidosis (DKA) and hyperosmolar hyperglycaemic state (HHS), except glucose supplement needs to be given at an earlier stage of correction in HHS when the blood glucose is 17 mmol/l or less. MAP, mean arterial pressure.

excretion as potassium salts. Typical total body deficits are shown in Table 50.1. Serum potassium levels may initially be high and potassium replacement should not commence until this has fallen to < 5.5 mmol/l. Potassium can be replaced as a combination of the chloride and phosphate salt, as this can avoid hyperchloraemia and hypophosphataemia. Occasionally the presenting potassium level will be low (< 3.3 mmol/l), which represents profound potassium depletion (600–800 mmol), and replacement should commence immediately and before insulin therapy is initiated. If the patient is in between these two levels then 20–40 mmol of potassium may be given in the first hour – this should not generally be exceeded. Further decisions regarding potassium replacement need to be adjusted with respect to serum levels and the urine output, but usually 20–30 mmol/h is required. Electrocardiogram monitoring has been recommended where potassium replacement is required for hypokalaemia or cardiac rhythms other than sinus tachycardia.[7]

Phosphate

A total body phosphate deficit of greater than 1 mmol/kg is typical. Once again the shift is from the intracellular compartment with subsequent urinary loss; however, serum levels are typically normal or increased. Insulin causes an intracellular shift of phosphate and, although hypophosphataemia rarely results in adverse complications, muscle weakness, haemolytic anaemia and impaired cardiac systolic performance can occur. Routine phosphate replacement has not been shown to be beneficial in DKA[18] but correction of severely low levels (< 0.4 mmol/l) may be necessary. Excessive phosphate replacement leads to hypocalcaemia and serum calcium should be monitored.

Magnesium

A chronic magnesium deficiency may be present in type 1 or 2 diabetes and may be exacerbated by renal impairment. The benefits of magnesium replacement have not been demonstrated in diabetic emergencies, but the principles of magnesium supplementation are similar to other critical care situations.

CORRECTION OF ACIDOSIS

This occurs more slowly than the correction of blood glucose but the use of bicarbonate in DKA remains controversial. In most studies the use of sodium bicarbonate fails to provide any haemodynamic benefit that could not be attributed purely to osmotic load of sodium administered.[19] There is no doubt that blood pH can be improved, but at the expense of worsening the intracellular acidosis.[20] In addition to cerebrospinal fluid acidosis, sodium bicarbonate is associated with other side-effects that may overshadow any potential benefits, such as increased CO_2 production, hypokalaemia, rebound alkalosis, volume overload and altered tissue oxygenation. In the context of DKA sodium bicarbonate also delays the clearance of ketones and may further enhance hepatic production, even when insulin and glucose are being delivered.[21] At pH > 7.0 insulin will block lipolysis and ketoacid production; however, when the pH is between 6.9 and 7.1 it remains uncertain whether bicarbonate is beneficial or otherwise. Below pH 6.9 most authorities would recommend the use of bicarbonate to correct the pH partially. The threshold for correction is debatable (between pH 6.9 and 7.15) but life-threatening hyperkalaemia is an undisputed indication for bicarbonate therapy.

Sometimes there is a persistent acidosis without ketosis. Regeneration of bicarbonate in DKA once insulin activity has been restored occurs via two mechanisms: renal and hepatic. The latter requires a metabolisable substrate, typically ketones, which are lost to the body, especially if the diuresis is substantial. The former is slow and hyperchloraemia may persist, particularly when a high chloride-containing fluid such as normal saline is used.[22]

UNDERLYING CAUSE

Attention must also focus on any underlying precipitant. The two major factors involved are inadequate insulin treatment and infection causing a change in insulin responsiveness. The latter must be actively looked for in the management of these patients.

MONITORING

The following monitoring parameters are also undertaken as investigations on presentation:

1. Blood glucose concentration: initially every hour, then less frequently.
2. Blood urea and creatinine concentrations: on admission and then at least daily. Creatinine assays that rely on a colorimetric method may be interfered with by the presence of acetoacetate, giving a falsely elevated value.
3. Serum electrolytes:
   - (a) *Serum sodium*: on admission and at least daily. It represents the relative water and electrolyte losses and cannot be used to infer a state of hydration. It may be normal (50% of cases), raised or lowered. Each 1.0 mmol/l rise in blood glucose will decrease serum sodium by 0.3 mmol/l, so hypernatraemia represents a profound loss of water.
   - (b) *Serum potassium*: initially every hour, then less frequently (every 2–4 hours). DKA patients have a K^+ deficit of 3–5 mmol/kg. However, serum concentrations are usually normal or raised because of a shift from the intracellular to the extracellular compartment due to acidaemia, insulin deficiency and hypertonicity. Hypokalaemia on admission represents severe potassium depletion (> 600–800 mmol) and requires potassium administration before starting insulin therapy.
   - (c) *Serum chloride*: as indicated.
   - (d) *Serum phosphate*: on admission and every 1–2 days. Routine replacement is not of any benefit. Despite evidence that hypophosphataemia leads to a decrease in 2,3-diphosphoglycerate levels, subsequent correction has no impact on the oxyhaemoglobin dissociation curve, and dangerous hypocalcaemia may result.[18]

(e) *Serum magnesium*: on admission and every 1–2 days. Chronic hypomagnesaemia may be present and may contribute to insulin resistance, carbohydrate intolerance and hypertension. Severe uncontrolled diabetes also results in magnesium depletion. Although the benefits of replacement therapy have not been demonstrated, correction may be necessary if arrhythmias are present.

4. Serum ketones (if available): on admission. This test relies on the nitroprusside reaction and, because it does not measure β-hydroxybutyrate (which is the main ketoacid in DKA), it consequently underestimates the degree of ketoacidosis.
5. Urinary glucose and ketones: 4-hourly. Ketonuria may persist up to 2 days after the correction of acidosis due to the presence of acetone, which is not an acid anion and is highly lipid-soluble.
6. Arterial blood gases: frequently as indicated.
7. Serum osmolality and anion gap: initially and as indicated. Serum osmolality can be measured with an osmometer or estimated from the equation:

$$\text{Osmolality (normal 285} - \text{300 mosmol/l)} = 2(\text{Na}^+ + \text{K}^+) + \text{glucose} + \text{urea (all values in mmol/l)}$$

The anion gap is calculated by the equation:

$$\text{Anion gap (normal 10} - \text{17 mmol)} = (\text{Na}^+ + \text{K}^+) - (\text{Cl}^- + \text{HCO}_3^-)\text{(all values in mmol/l)}$$

8. Serum lactate: if acidosis is severe and anion gap is large.
9. Full blood count and coagulation studies: daily and as indicated. Leukocytosis with left shift may occur in the absence of sepsis.
10. Chest X-ray.
11. Blood cultures, urine and sputum microscopy and culture and culture of relevant specimens as indicated.
12. Pulse oximetry continuously.
13. Electrocardiogram – 12-lead recording and continuous monitoring.
14. Invasive haemodynamic monitoring as indicated.
15. Neurological status and observations: including Glasgow Coma Score and computed tomography scans as indicated for persistent coma or worsening neurological state.
16. Other investigations as indicated (e.g. liver function tests, serum amylase, cardiac enzymes and creatinine clearance).

COMPLICATIONS

EARLY

The commonest early complications are hypoglycaemia due to overtreatment with insulin, hypokalaemia due to inadequate replacement and hyperglycaemia due to interruption of insulin. A hyperchloraemic acidosis can develop in about 10% of patients with DKA. It can be exaggerated by excessive saline use and is not usually clinically significant except in cases of acute renal failure or extreme oliguria.

Clinically apparent cerebral oedema is a rare (0.5–1%) but extremely serious complication of DKA, occurring predominantly in children. Recent studies have suggested a subclinical incidence approaching 50%.[23] Risk factors for developing cerebral oedema include: degree of hypocapnia and dehydration, the failure of serum sodium to rise with treatment and the use of sodium bicarbonate.[24] It does also occur in young adults and may be associated with rapid deterioration in conscious level with or without seizures. If progressive signs of brainstem herniation are present the mortality is high, with only 7–14% likely to make a complete recovery. The risks of brain herniation are related to the degree of acidosis and the volume of initial fluid resuscitation. Oedema formation most likely occurs due to a vasogenic mechanism,[25] and cerebral hyperaemia with loss of autoregulation is evident, which can take up to 36 hours to resolve.[26,27] It has been recommended that plasma osmolality is slowly reduced and that glucose must be added to the hydrating fluids when the plasma glucose has fallen to 15 mmol/l in DKA, and possibly before this in HHS. Fatal cases of cerebral oedema have been reported in HHS as well, and treatment is aimed at maintaining plasma osmolality with intravenous mannitol.

Some degree of brain dysfunction is apparent even in those patients who are not comatose but who have severe DKA, as measured by sensory evoked potentials. This reverts to normal with correction of the ketoacidosis.[28]

Hypoxia and non-cardiogenic pulmonary oedema can also occur, and the increase in lung water and resultant reduced lung compliance are again attributed to the reduction in colloid oncotic pressure. Myocardial infarction can also occur, particularly in the elderly.

INTERMEDIATE

A reversible critical-illness motor weakness syndrome has been described in HHS, and led to slowness to wake up and reversible tetraplegia.[29] Deep-venous thrombosis and pulmonary embolism occur more frequently in DKA and are a significant cause of mortality in HHS.[30,31] Prophylaxis with subcutaneous heparin is advisable.

LATE

Various movement disorders can rarely persist after recovery from HHS.[32] The effects of neuroglycopenia can result in an array of late complications ranging from amnesia to optic atrophy.

PROGNOSIS

In a series of 610 patients with DKA or HHS the overall mortality was 6.2%. HHS is a more serious disease and has an associated mortality 2–3 times higher than DKA; nevertheless DKA is approximately six times commoner. A retrospective analysis of causes of death in this group of patients revealed that pneumonia was the commonest cause of death (37%), followed by myocardial infarction (21%), with mesenteric or iliac thrombosis accounting for 16% of deaths.[33] Rhabdomyolysis has been reported in both DKA and HHS and, when present, increases the mortality.[34] The likelihood of a poorer outcome in HHS was associated with older age, low blood pressure, low sodium, pH and bicarbonate plasma levels, and high urea plasma levels, of which urea has the strongest association.[35] Mortality is also age-related in DKA. Pregnant women with type 1 diabetes are more likely to have worse outcome from DKA than non-pregnant diabetic women who develop DKA. The presence of hypothermia is also a poor prognostic sign.

Survival depends upon establishing a high index of suspicion and making a rapid diagnosis.[36]

HYPOGLYCAEMIC COMA

This results from overtreatment with insulin, and is the commonest cause of diabetic coma. Clinically, there is confusion and agitation, progressing to coma and fitting. Tremor, tachycardia and sweating may be blunted by diabetic autonomic neuropathy. It may be precipitated in known type 1 diabetic patients (up to 10% of patients per year) by missed meals, exercise and overdose of insulin or oral hypoglycaemic agents. Changing therapy or insulin periods are susceptible periods and there is an increased risk associated with long-acting sulphonylurea agents. Alcoholic ketoacidosis is a syndrome of hypoglycaemia, ketoacidosis and dehydration associated with starvation, vomiting, upper abdominal pain and neurological changes, including seizures and coma. Hypoglycaemia may complicate other disease states (e.g. liver and renal failure, or adrenocortical insufficiency).

Severe hypoglycaemia (blood glucose < 1 mmol/l) is a medical emergency. Brain metabolism uses half the glucose produced by the liver and neuronal stores of glycogen are depleted in 2 minutes, after which the brain is susceptible to damage. Urgent glucose infusion (50 ml of 50% glucose) is required and leads to rapid resolution of coma. Intramuscular glucagon is an alternative that is especially suited to out-of-hospital circumstances, but achieves a slower result when compared to intravenous glucose.[37] Hypoglycaemia due to long-acting insulins or oral hypoglycaemic agents will require ongoing glucose infusion.

REFERENCES

1. Pinkey JH, Bingley PJ, Sawtell PA *et al.* Presentation and progress of childhood diabetes mellitus: a prospective population-based study. The Bart's-Oxford Study Group. *Diabetologia* 1994; **37**: 70–4.
2. Harris MI. Undiagnosed NIDDM: clinical and public health issues. *Diabetes Care* 1993; **16**: 642–52.
3. Adeghate E, Schattner P, Dunn E. An update on the etiology and epidemiology of diabetes mellitus. *Ann N Y Acad Sci* 2006; **1084**: 1–29.
4. Karvonen M, Tuomilehto J, Libman I *et al.* A review of the recent epidemiological data on the worldwide incidence of type 1 (insulin-dependent) diabetes mellitus. World Health Organization DIAMOND Project Group. *Diabetologia* 1993; **36**: 883–92.
5. Meyer C, Stumvoll M, Nadkarni V *et al.* Abnormal renal and hepatic glucose metabolism in type 2 diabetes mellitus. *J Clin Invest* 1998; **102**: 619–24.
6. Schade DS, Eaton RP. The temporal relationship between endogenously secreted stress hormones and metabolic decompensation in diabetic man. *J Clin Endocrinol Metab* 1980; **50**: 131–6.
7. Kitabchi AE, Umpierrez GE, Murphy MB *et al.* Management of hyperglycemic crises in patients with diabetes. *Diabetes Care* 2001; **24**: 131–53.
8. Stentz FB, Umpierrez GE, Cuervo R *et al.* Proinflammatory cytokines, markers of cardiovascular risks, oxidative stress, and lipid peroxidation in patients with hyperglycemic crises. *Diabetes* 2004; **53**: 2079–86.
9. Magee MF, Bhatt BA. Management of decompensated diabetes. Diabetic ketoacidosis and hyperglycemic hyperosmolar syndrome. *Crit Care Clin* 2001; **17**: 75–106.
10. Umpierrez GE, Khajavi M, Kitabchi AE. Review: diabetic ketoacidosis and hyperglycemic hyperosmolar nonketotic syndrome. *Am J Med Sci* 1996; **311**: 225–33.
11. Wachtel TJ, Tetu-Mouradjian LM, Goldman DL *et al.* Hyperosmolarity and acidosis in diabetes mellitus: a three-year experience in Rhode Island. *J Gen Intern Med* 1991; **6**: 495–502.
12. Inglis A, Hinnie J, Kinsella J. A metabolic complication of severe burns. *Burns* 1995; **21**: 212–14.
13. Hyperosmolar coma due to lithium-induced diabetes insipidus. *Lancet* 1995; **346**: 413–17.
14. DeFronzo RA, Goldberg M, Agus ZS. The effects of glucose and insulin on renal electrolyte transport. *J Clin Invest* 1976; **58**: 83–90.
15. Hillman K. Fluid resuscitation in diabetic emergencies – a reappraisal. *Intens Care Med* 1987; **13**: 4–18.
16. McComb RD, Pfeiffer RF, Casey JH *et al.* Lateral pontine and extrapontine myelinolysis associated with hypernatremia and hyperglycemia. *Clin Neuropathol* 1989; **8**: 284–8.
17. Wagner A, Risse A, Brill HL. Therapy of severe diabetic ketoacidosis. Zero-mortality under very-low-dose insulin application. *Diabetes Care* 1999; **22**: 674–7.
18. Fisher JN, Kitabchi AE. A randomized study of phosphate therapy in the treatment of diabetic ketoacidosis. *J Clin Endocrinol Metab* 1983; **57**: 177–80.
19. Cooper DJ. Hemodynamic effects of sodium bicarbonate. *Intens Care Med* 1994; **20**: 306–7.
20. Forsythe SM, Schmidt GA. Sodium bicarbonate for the treatment of lactic acidosis. *Chest* 2000; **117**: 260–7.
21. Okuda Y, Adrogue HJ, Field JB *et al.* Counterproductive effects of sodium bicarbonate in diabetic ketoacidosis. *J Clin Endocrinol Metab* 1996; **81**: 314–20.

22. Matz R. Severe diabetic ketoacidosis. *Diabetes Med* 2000; **17**: 329.
23. Glaser NS, Wootton-Gorges SL, Buonocore MH *et al.* Frequency of sub-clinical cerebral edema in children with diabetic ketoacidosis. *Pediatr Diabetes* 2006; **7**: 75–80.
24. Glaser N, Barnett P, McCaslin I *et al.* Risk factors for cerebral edema in children with diabetic ketoacidosis. *N Engl J Med* 2001; **344**: 264–9.
25. Figueroa RE, Hoffmann WH, Momin Z *et al.* Study of subclinical cerebral edema in diabetic ketoacidosis by magnetic resonance imaging T2 relaxometry and apparent diffusion coefficient maps. *Endocrinol Res* 2005; **31**: 345–55.
26. Roberts JS, Vavilala MS, Schenkman KA *et al.* Cerebral hyperemia and impaired cerebral autoregulation associated with diabetic ketoacidosis in critically ill children. *Crit Care Med* 2006; **34**: 2217–23.
27. Hyperglycemic crises in patients with diabetes mellitus. *Diabetes Care* 2001; **24**: 154–61.
28. Eisenhuber E, Madl C, Kramer L *et al.* Detection of subclinical brain dysfunction by sensory evoked potentials in patients with severe diabetic ketoacidosis. *Intens Care Med* 1997; **23**: 587–9.
29. Kennedy DD, Fletcher SN, Ghosh IR *et al.* Reversible tetraplegia due to polyneuropathy in a diabetic patient with hyperosmolar non-ketotic coma. *Intens Care Med* 1999; **25**: 1437–9.
30. Ceriello A. Coagulation activation in diabetes mellitus: the role of hyperglycaemia and therapeutic prospects. *Diabetologia* 1993; **36**: 1119–25.
31. Whelton MJ, Walde D, Havard CW. Hyperosmolar non-ketotic diabetic coma: with particular reference to vascular complications. *Br Med J* 1971; **1**: 85–6.
32. Lin JJ, Chang MK. Hemiballism-hemichorea and non-ketotic hyperglycaemia. *J Neurol Neurosurg Psychiatry* 1994; **57**: 748–50.
33. Hamblin PS, Topliss DJ, Chosich N *et al.* Deaths associated with diabetic ketoacidosis and hyperosmolar coma. 1973–1988. *Med J Aust* 1989; **151**: 439–44.
34. Wang LM, Tsai ST, Ho LT *et al.* Rhabdomyolysis in diabetic emergencies. *Diabetes Res Clin Pract* 1994; **26**: 209–14.
35. Pinies JA, Cairo G, Gaztambide S *et al.* Course and prognosis of 132 patients with diabetic non ketotic hyperosmolar state. *Diabetes Metab* 1994; **20**: 43–8.
36. Small M, Alzaid A, MacCuish AC. Diabetic hyperosmolar non-ketotic decompensation. *Q J Med* 1988; **66**: 251–7.
37. Patrick AW, Collier A, Hepburn DA *et al.* Comparison of intramuscular glucagon and intravenous dextrose in the treatment of hypoglycaemic coma in an accident and emergency department. *Arch Emerg Med* 1990; **7**: 73–7.

51

Diabetes insipidus and other polyuric syndromes

Craig Carr

Diabetes insipidus (DI: literal translation, 'tasteless siphon') refers to a syndrome characterised by pathological polyuria, excessive thirst and polydipsia. Polyuria is arbitrarily defined as a urine loss of > 3 l/day in an adult of normal mass. The urine produced in DI is inappropriately dilute, having both low specific gravity and low osmolality in the face of a high or normal plasma osmolality.

Three subtypes of DI are recognised:

1. *nephrogenic DI (NDI)* – caused by insensitivity of the kidney to antidiuretic hormone (ADH)
2. *central/hypothalamic/neurogenic DI* – caused by reduced or absent production of ADH
3. *gestational DI (GDI)* – caused by an increase in the placental production of vasopressinase or as a variant of central or NDI developing during pregnancy

A separate disorder is occasionally classified as a fourth form of DI – *primary polydipsia* (also called psychogenic or neurogenic polydipsia or polydipsic DI). This is caused by excessive water ingestion, usually due to psychological disturbance but occasionally associated with a lesion of the hypothalamus. In the context of hospital inpatients, a similar iatrogenic condition is created by overenthusiastic administration of intravenous solutions of dextrose 5% or hypotonic saline. Whilst water overload will reduce plasma osmolality and reduce the ability of the kidney to concentrate urine maximally, the diuresis of hypo-osmolar urine seen with water overload is not pathological but physiological and appropriate. In this instance, plasma osmolality is low or in the low-normal range and the body is attempting to restore plasma osmolality to normality by reducing water reabsorption in the kidneys and inducing a water diuresis.

In critically ill patients, polyuria may be the sole part of the DI syndrome apparent to the clinician. Patients are seldom in control of their own fluid intake and are frequently unable to report thirst. The recognition of DI is important as failure to recognise and treat the syndrome appropriately will result in severe dehydration and hyperosmolality with a significant risk of morbidity and mortality. As there are many causes of polyuria in the critically ill (Table 51.1), it is important to adopt a systematic approach to the clinical assessment, investigations, diagnosis and management of such patients.

The classification as a solute or water diuresis is not always absolute; the table provides a convenient structure but a diuresis should be considered in terms of the individual patient and both physical and biochemical examinations. A diuresis may frequently represent the clearance of both an excess of water and solute, such as is usually the case following the resolution of septic shock with multiorgan failure.

BACKGROUND PHYSIOLOGY AND ANATOMY

OSMOLALITY

Osmolality is the measure of osmoles of solute per kilogram of solvent and includes both permeant (e.g. urea) and impermeant solutes (e.g. sodium) and thus osmolality may change due to both water movement and the movement of permeant solute. *Osmolarity* is the measure of osmoles per litre of solute and thus is temperature-dependent. *Osmolality* is temperature-independent. Normal plasma osmolality is in the range of 275–295 mosmol/kg. Plasma osmolality can be estimated from several equations.[1] The formula of Worthley *et al.*[2] below is both simple and correlates well with measured values.[3]

$$\text{Plasma osmolality (mOsm/kg)} = 2\,[\text{Na}^+] + [\text{Urea}] + [\text{Glucose}]$$

All units of solute are mmol/l.

Where a patient is markedly uraemic, a value of 8 mmol/l is substituted for the actual urea. Actual osmolality may differ markedly from estimated osmolality in the presence of unmeasured, osmotically active solutes such as mannitol, ethanol, bicarbonate, lactate and amino acids. Whenever concern exists that a patient may be hyper- or hypo-osmolal, osmolality should be measured by assessing the freezing-point depression of the plasma or urine. Increasing the osmolality results in depression of the freezing point.

The osmolal gap is the difference between the calculated and measured osmolality in plasma or urine.

Table 51.1 Causes of polyuria

Water diuresis
Pathological
Diabetes insipidus: cranial, nephrogenic, gestational
Physiological
Psychogenic polydipsia (excess drinking is pathological but the diuresis is not)
Iatrogenic – excessive administration of hypotonic solutions, e.g. 5% dextrose solution, 0.45% saline, 0.18% saline 4% dextrose solutions
Solute diuresis
Pathological
Fanconi's syndrome
Renal tubular acidosis
Glomerulonephritis
Hyperaldosteronism
Anorexia nervosa
Migraines
Paroxysmal tachycardia (via increased atrial natriuretic peptide release)
Poisons/drugs:
Ethanol
Methanol
Ethylene glycol
Mannitol
Loop diuretics
Thiazide diuretics
Hyperglycaemia
Physiological
Resolving sepsis (redistribution of fluid into the vascular compartment from the third space)
Iatrogenic – excessive administration of isotonic or hypertonic solutions, e.g.
0.9% saline
Hypertonic saline
Hartmann's solution
Gelofusin

The normal osmolal gap is < 10 mosmol/l. An increased osmolal gap indicates the presence of an unmeasured osmotically active solute.

TONICITY

Tonicity describes the ability of a solution of impermeant solute (such as sodium) to cause the movement of water between itself and another fluid compartment. It may be considered an index of the water concentration rather than the solute concentration as the solute is impermeant. The tonicity of plasma is largely determined by its sodium content, the main solute in extracellular fluid, which is not freely permeable to cross into the intracellular space. This characteristic facilitates the control of extracellular fluid volume through the regulation of sodium balance.

It is possible for a solution to be both hypotonic and iso-osmolar. Dextrose solution 5% is an example of this; the solution contains no impermeant solute (assuming no absence of insulin, glucose freely enters the cell), but is iso-osmolar with the intracellular milieu.

SOLUTE AND WATER INTAKE AND LOSSES

In order to understand disorders of osmolality, tonicity, fluid balance and urine output, it is necessary to be aware of the essential physiological mechanisms which maintain the fluid and osmolal states of the body in health. Assuming a normal diet, in a 75-kg man, every day there is an obligatory loss of around 800 mmol of solute – approximately 300 mmol of urea and 500 mmol of cations and anions. The maximum concentrating ability of the healthy kidney is around 1200 mosmol/kg; consequently, a minimum of 666 ml of urine a day is required to excrete osmotically active solutes. Additionally, insensible losses of water (respiratory water, faecal water and sweat) approximate to 10 ml/kg per day and this rises markedly with fever and hot dry climates. Thus obligatory water losses of around 1.5 l/day arise due to insensible losses and obligatory solute excretion.

NORMAL URINARY OSMOLALITY

In health, urinary osmolality is usually maintained between 500 and 700 mosmol/kg. As the obligatory solute load to be excreted is relatively constant in value, urine osmolality will fall in response to an increased intake in free water and rise in response to dehydration or water restriction (Figure 51.1). The minimum osmolality of urine achievable in

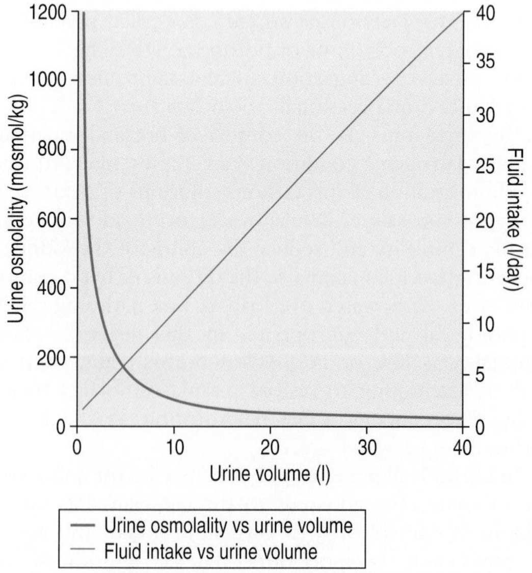

Figure 51.1 Urine output rises and urine osmolality falls in health as a function of increasing water intake. Assuming normal solute ingestion, normal solute excretion (around 800 mmol/day) is preserved between water intakes of 1.5 and 32 litres/day.

humans is around 25 mosmol/kg. Diuresis refers to the passage of a high volume of urine (> 1.5 ml/kg per hour) and may be transient or persistent, physiological or pathological. The production of > 3 l/day is arbitrarily defined as polyuria. Water diuresis occurs when the total solute in the urine excreted per day is within the normal range but the osmolality of the urine passed is low. An osmotic or solute diuresis occurs when the total solute passed per day is higher than normal, and the urine passed is usually iso-osmolar to plasma if the extracellular fluid volume is expanded or hyperosmolar if the patient is hypo- or euvolaemic.

PLASMA OSMOLALITY AND PLASMA VOLUME REGULATION

Changes in plasma osmolality and changes in plasma volume can occur in tandem or independently of one another. Although normal plasma osmolality lies in a population range of 275–295 mosmol/kg (265–285 mosmol/kg in pregnancy), individuals tend to vary less than ± 1% around their set value. In pregnancy this set value falls but the limited variability around it does not. The body regulates osmolality and volume by separate mechanisms. Water balance and osmolality are maintained via osmoreceptors which mediate their control via control of thirst and ADH production. Control of the plasma volume is maintained via volume receptors and sodium receptors, which mediate their actions through the sympathetic nervous system, the renin–angiotensin–aldosterone system and atrial natriuretic peptide (ANP). Additionally, the volume receptors have inputs to the hypothalamus via which they too can mediate ADH release and the sensation of thirst.

THIRST

In health fluid intake is determined by the sensation of thirst and the subsequent ingestion of fluid; a plasma osmolality of > 290 mosmol, elevated angiotensin II concentration, sympathetic nervous system activation and circulating volume depletion of 5–10% are all associated with the onset of thirst. Fluid and solute excretion are largely regulated through the kidney, although some solutes such as ethanol and glucose are largely cleared through metabolism rather than excretion.

In the intensive care unit (ICU), the patient loses control over intake of fluids and solute and frequently has impaired excretory mechanisms. Thus both volume and solute homeostasis may become heavily dependent upon the skills of attending clinicians.

OSMORECEPTORS AND OTHER INPUTS TO THE SUPRAOPTIC AND PARAVENTRICULAR NUCLEI

Detection of osmolality occurs largely at osmo- (Na^+) receptors sited around the anterior aspect of the third ventricle of the brain. These are sensitive to plasma osmolality and cerebrospinal fluid sodium concentration. Hypertonic saline is a more potent stimulus than equi-isotonic equiososmolar solutions of other solutes.[4] These osmoreceptors link to the cells of the paraventricular nuclei (PVN) and supraoptic nuclei (SON), the sites of ADH synthesis. The axons of the cells in the PVN and SON form part of the pituitary stalk linking the hypothalamus to the pituitary gland in which they terminate. A smaller proportion of the axons terminate in the median eminence where they release ADH and oxytocin, which is transported to the anterior lobe of the pituitary by portal vessels. The ADH and oxytocin so released cause release of adrenocorticotrophic hormone (ACTH) and prolactin respectively; the ADH acts synergistically with corticotrophin-releasing factor (CRF) but is also believed to have ACTH secretagogue properties in its own right.[5,6]

Direct inputs from the sympathetic nervous system to the PVN and SON can stimulate ADH release via α-adrenoreceptors. Other central osmoreceptors lie outside the blood–brain barrier in the subfornical organ and come into contact with plasma. It is believed that ANP and angiotensin II[7] act via these receptors to inhibit or elicit ADH synthesis and ADH release and to modify the sensation of thirst. Additional osmoreceptors in the mouth, stomach and liver are believed to play a role in the anticipation of an osmolal load following ingestion of food and can pre-emptively stimulate ADH synthesis in the hypothalamus.

As the baroreceptor and osmoreceptor inputs to the PVN and SON are distinct, it is possible to lose the normal ADH response to hyperosmolality but maintain a normal ADH response to hypovolaemia.[8] Additionally, in animal experiments, when hypotension increases the basal plasma ADH concentration, there is a simultaneous resetting of the osmomolality–plasma ADH response curve in an attempt to preserve osmoregulatory function from the new higher baseline.[9] If this did not occur, the ADH response to hypotension would always result in the development of a hypo-osmolal state in addition to causing vasoconstriction.

The normal response of osmoreceptors to changing plasma osmolality in terms of ADH is illustrated in Figure 51.2. At plasma osmolalities of < 275 mosmol/kg, the osmoreceptors remain hyperpolarised and virtually no ADH release occurs via them. At osmolalities > 295 mosmol/kg, the osmoreceptors are maximally depolarised and plasma concentrations of ADH of > 5 pg/ml are attained. Other inputs and influences upon ADH release are summarised in Figure 51.3 and Table 51.2.

ANTIDIURETIC HORMONE/ARGININE VASOPRESSIN (AVP)

ADH (8-arginine vasopressin) is a nine-amino-acid peptide which differs from oxytocin at only two residues but shares the disulphide bond between the first and sixth ones. This similar structure and conformation results in some cross-reactivity at receptors and in function.[10] It is synthesised in the SON and PVN, bound to neuorophysin, transferred through axons to the posterior pituitary gland and stored in granules prior to release. Synthesis

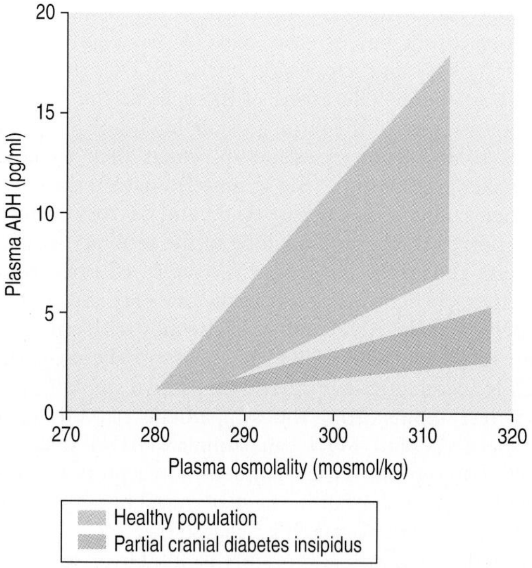

Figure 51.2 Plasma antidiuretic hormone (ADH) and plasma osmolality in health and partial cranial diabetes insipidus.

Table 51.2 Factors influencing antidiuretic hormone (ADH) release

Increased ADH release with:
Hyperosmolality
Hypovolaemia
Hypotension
Hypoxia
Hypothyroidism
Hyperthermia
Positive-pressure ventilation
Pain
Emotional stress
Exercise
Nausea
Nicotine
Trauma/surgery
Decreased ADH release with:
Hypo-osmolality
Hypervolaemia
Hypertension
Ethanol
Cranial diabetes insipidus

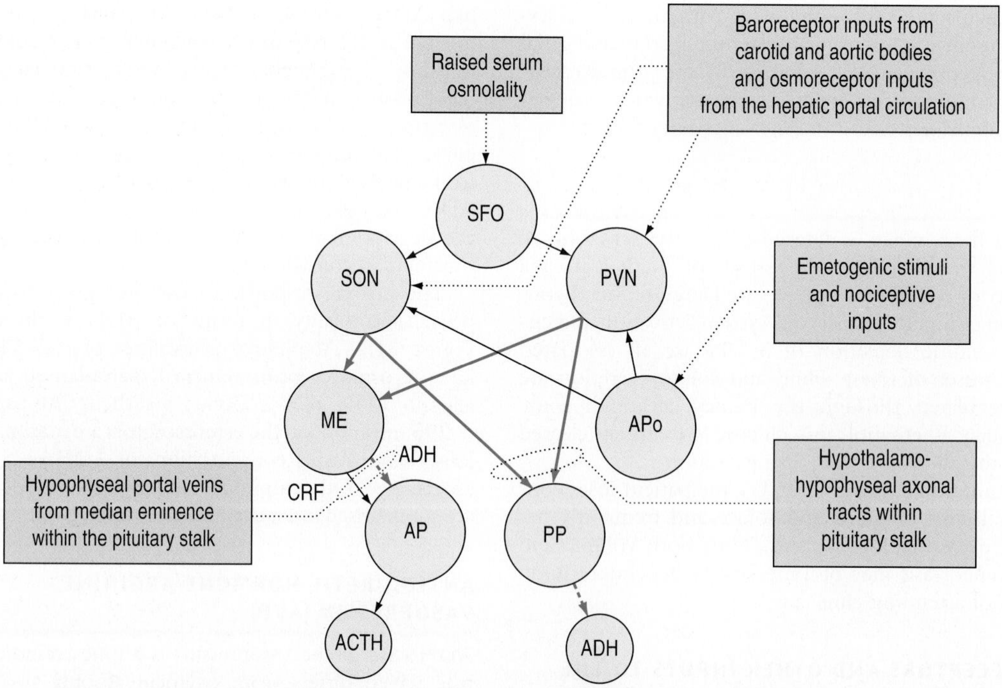

Figure 51.3 A schematic representation of anatomical and physiological connections of the supraoptic and paraventricular nuclei (SON and PVN), the principal sites of antidiuretic hormone (ADH) synthesis within the hypothalamus. Blue arrows represent the transport of ADH or its precursor between anatomically distinct sites. Baroreceptor inputs into these nuclei travel via the vagus nerve to reach the central nervous system. Whilst the majority of ADH produced in the SON and PVN is transported to the posterior pituitary (PP) for storage, some is transported to the median eminence (ME) then onwards to the anterior pituitary (AP), where it acts synergistically as a secretagogue for adrenocorticotropic hormone (ACTH). APo, area postrema; SFO, subfornical organ; CRF, corticotrophin-releasing factor.

to replace any released stores is a rapid process (1–2 hours from synthesis to storage) and patients with damage to the pituitary can achieve near-normal plasma concentrations of ADH, in terms of osmoregulatory function, via release of newly synthesised ADH via the axons terminating in the median eminence. However, the higher plasma concentrations associated with hypovolaemia cannot be achieved. Normal osmoregulatory plasma ADH concentrations are in the range of 1–8 pg/ml but rise as high as 40 pg/ml in hypovolaemic patients under the influence of the sympathetic nervous system, baroreceptor responses and angiotensin II.

Once released from the pituitary, ADH has a plasma half-life of around 10–35 minutes.[11] It is metabolised by hepatic and renal vasopressinases and around 10% of the active hormone is excreted unchanged in the urine.

ACTIONS OF ADH

ADH has antidiuretic, vasopressor, haemostatic and ACTH secretagogue actions. Additionally, it has roles in memory, water permeability of the blood–brain barrier, nociception, splenic contraction and thermoregulation. These actions are mediated through V_1, V_2 and V_3 receptors. It also has actions on the uterus and mammary tissue mediated through oxytocin receptors. Cardiac inotropic effects are reported to be mediated through purinergic P_2 receptors but this remains controversial.[12]

Antidiuresis

ADH binds to V_2 receptors on the basal membranes of the principal cells of the collecting duct and distal tubule. The activated receptor induces production of cyclic adenosine monophosphate (cAMP) by adenylate cylase and this in turn activates protein kinases which effect the integration into the luminal membrane of vesicles containing aquaporin-2 highly selective water channels. The production of prostaglandin E_2 (PGE_2) inhibits cAMP production. PGE_2 synthesis is stimulated by the action of ADH on V_1 receptors on the luminal membrane of the collecting duct.[13] Thus, a form of autoregulatory limitation of the antidiuretic effect of ADH may exist. Hypokalaemia, lithium and hypercalcaemia also anatagonise the renal actions of ADH.

ADH also increases the urinary concentrating ability of the kidney by increasing the expression of urea transport proteins in the collecting duct and reducing renal medullary blood flow (V_1-mediated), facilitating an increase in medullary interstitial hypertonicity. This hypertonicity additionally depends upon intact functioning of the ascending loop of Henle where sodium and chloride are reabsorbed without absorption of water at the same time. Interference with this process reduces the osmolal gradient between the collecting duct and the interstitium and reduces water absorption even in the presence of ADH and functioning aquaporin-2.

In low dose, administration of exogenous ADH may paradoxically cause a diuresis in patients with septic shock.[14] Whether this is due to increased renal perfusion pressure and raised glomerular filtration rate (GFR) is unclear.

Vasoconstriction

At higher concentrations (> 40 pg/ml), ADH activates not only V_2 receptors but also V_1 receptors, through which it causes preferential vasoconstriction in muscle, skin and fat with relative sparing of coronary, cerebral and mesenteric circulations. However, these relative sparing effects are controversial, with some authors reporting relative sparing and others reporting significant vasoconstriction.[15–18] Activation of V_1 receptors activates phospholipase C and increases inositol triphosphate intracellularly. Ultimately this increases intracellular free calcium and leads to smooth-muscle constriction in the blood vessel wall.

In brain-dead organ donors, a failure to produce ADH may result in the development of both hypotension and cranial DI (CDI) with disturbances of osmolality and organ function. Treatment with α-adrenoreceptor agonists may restore organ perfusion pressure but cause ischaemic damage too. The use of low-dose ADH infusions at 0.5–3 U/h titrated against urine output reduces the need for catecholamine support and also reduces perturbations in plasma osmolality and fluid balance. 1-deamino-8-O-arginine vasopressin (DDAVP) has similar benefits but causes less vasoconstriction. It is preferred for the treatment of CDI associated with brainstem death where hypotension is not a concomitant feature.

Coagulation

ADH increases circulating levels of tissue plasminogen activator, factor VIII and von Willebrand factor.[19] These effects may be mediated by V_2 receptors but this remains controversial. At high but physiological concentrations it can act as a platelet-aggregating agent.[20,21] Platelet aggregation is mediated through activation of platelet V_1 receptors.[22] ADH and its analogue DDAVP are used as first-line treatments in patients with von Willebrand's disease, and may be used in bleeding associated with renal failure and platelet dysfunction.

ACTH secretion

ADH transported via the portal venous system between the median eminence and the anterior pituitary acts upon V_3 receptors in the anterior pituitary to stimulate release of ACTH which in turn increases plasma cortisol. The ADH both increases the efficacy of CRF in releasing ACTH and also has independent efficacy in stimulating ACTH release itself. In septic shock, it is possible that ADH insufficiency partially accounts for the relative adrenal insufficiency noted in certain patients. The relative importance and potency of ADH compared with CRF in stimulating ACTH release in humans are unclear.

VOLUME RECEPTORS

Volume homeostasis takes precedence over sodium homeostasis and so rises and falls in sodium will occur in order to preserve the circulating volume. In euvolaemic patients sodium homeostasis is maintained. Sodium concentration is detected by both the osmoreceptors of the subfornical organ outside the blood–brain barrier and also by the juxtaglomerular apparatus which secretes renin in response to reduced GFR and a lower sodium load in the tubule.[23]

The predominant determinants of sodium balance, however, are the high-pressure baroreceptors in the pulmonary veins, left atrium, carotid sinus and aortic arch.[24] Reduced stretch of these receptors increases sympathetic nervous system activity and activation of the renin–angiotensin–aldosterone system, resulting in reduced sodium excretion (via reduced GFR) and increased reabsorption of sodium in the proximal and distal convoluted tubules. Additionally, release of ADH can be stimulated, resulting in concomitant water retention. Conversely, stretch of the baroreceptors will result in a fall in sodium retention through reduced activity of the sympathetic nervous and renin–angiotensin–aldosterone systems. Stretch additionally results in the release of ANP and a natriuresis through reduced sodium reabsorption in the distal convoluted tubule and collecting duct. ADH release is reduced by the fall in sympathetic nervous tone from the baroreceptors. ADH secretion may also be inhibited by the action of ANP on cerebral osmoreceptors lying outside the blood–brain barrier.[25]

The role of low-pressure baroreceptors in the systemic venous circulation and right atrium is less clearly defined. When venodilatation occurs, as is seen in sepsis, or when there is a reduction in cardiac output, reduced baroreceptor signalling in the high-pressure system will result in both sodium and water retention, as outlined previously. This will expand the extracellular fluid compartment and potentially cause tissue oedema. As sepsis resolves, venous tone is restored, capillary leak reduces, an increase in the loading of the high-pressure baroreceptors results and a natriuresis takes place. Patients may become transiently polyuric as they clear the excess salt and water accumulated whilst shocked. During this physiological diuresis, plasma osmolality remains tightly within the normal range, provided that renal concentrating mechanisms have not been injured during the septic episode or by drug administration.

CRANIAL DIABETES INSIPIDUS

CONGENTIAL CDI

Congenital CDI is rare and usually inherited as an autosomal-dominant characteristic which results from mutations of the gene encoding an ADH precursor – prepro-vasopressin neurophysin II. The onset of the disease may occur anywhere between 1 year of age and middle adult life and is associated with the final destruction of the ADH-producing cells due to an accumulation of the abnormal ADH precursor. Until the destruction of the SON and PVN cells occurs, ADH secretion (facilitated by expression of the normal gene) and regulation of plasma osmolality are often unaffected.

ACQUIRED CDI

Acquired CDI may be transient or permanent and can arise due to an absolute (complete) or relative (incomplete) lack of ADH. Complete central DI is usually associated with lesions above the level of the median eminence in the SON or PVN or of the neurohypophyseal stalk whereby the production of ADH in the hypothalamus is terminated.[26] Permanent central DI tends to be associated with transecting, obliterating or chronic inflammatory lesions, whereas transient DI is more likely to be associated with acute inflammatory or oedematous lesions with some recovery of ADH secretion occurring as the inflammation or oedema resolves. An exception to this is the transient DI seen following excision or destruction of the posterior pituitary; ADH produced in the hypothalamus can still be released into the systemic circulation from capillaries in the median eminence.

In the past the majority of acquired non-traumatic CDI was categorised as idiopathic but it has become apparent that the majority of these cases are associated with abnormality of the inferior hypophyseal arterial system[27] or autoimmune reactivity against ADH-producing cells.[28] These findings may indicate causality or association.

When the normal release of ADH into the circulation in response to rising plasma osomolality is reduced or absent, inappropriately high urine volumes are passed and the urine osmolality becomes inappropriately low for the state of water depletion being suffered by the patient. Where ADH is entirely absent from the circulation, over 20 litres of very dilute urine (25–200 mosomol/kg) per day may be produced. If patients are unable to drink freely (most ICU patients) or their thirst mechanisms are impaired, profound dehydration will result very rapidly unless appropriate interventions are made by the physician.

Where ADH deficiency is relative rather than absolute, it is possible for the patient to concentrate the urine partially and values of 500–800 mosmol/kg would not be atypical. However, these osmolalities are inappropriately low relative to the plasma osmolality. In partial ADH deficiency volumes of urine as low as 3 l/day may be evidenced. These are still inappropriately high when assessed in terms of the solute excretion of the patient but are more difficult to recognise as being due to DI as there are many other causes of diureses of this magnitude. Additionally, extrinsic stimulants of ADH release (see Table 51.2) may have an antidiuretic effect, further complicating the diagnosis.

The plasma osmolality measured in central DI is usually in the higher regions of the normal range or very slightly supranormal. It is remarkably constant in those with free access to water and intact thirst mechanisms as they will drink huge quantities of water to regulate and maintain their water balance. Hyperosmolality or hypernatraemia suggest impaired sensation of thirst or inability to access water (see water deprivation test later) and can also be seen if patients are administered large quantities of isotonic saline or Hartmann's solution to replace their hypotonic urine losses. If unrecognised and untreated, hyperosmolality and hypernatraemia may result in death.

CDI is usually associated with reduced production of ADH or damage to the normal release mechanisms of ADH. However, there can be dysfunction of the osmolality-sensing mechanism at receptor or intracellular signalling levels whilst actual ADH production and storage are normal. It is possible to have a normal release of ADH in response to baroreceptor detection of hypotension but subnormal release in response to hyperosmolality. This has been described in association with chronic hypernatraemia.[29]

The main recognised causes of central DI are listed in Table 51.3. A particularly common cause of DI seen in the ICU is traumatic or postsurgical brain injury.

Table 51.3 Causes of cranial diabetes insipidus

Acquired
Idiopathic
Autoimmune
Tumours (especially suprasellar, lung, breast, lymphoma and leukaemia)
Surgery (especially transsphenoidal surgery)
Traumatic head injury (strongly associated with base-of-skull fracture*)
Hypoxic brain injury
Brainstem death
Electrolyte disturbance – profound hyponatraemia
Radiotherapy
Drugs – amiodarone, lithium (lithium more likely to cause nephrogenic diabetes insipidus)
Inflammatory/infectious diseases
Sickle-cell disease
Tuberculosis
Abscesses
Encephalitis
Meningitis
Sarcoidosis (may also cause nephrogenic diabetes insipidus)
Wegener's granulomatosis
Histiocytosis X
Vascular disease
Ischaemic or haemorrhagic strokes
Aneurysmal bleeds (especially anterior communicating artery subarachnoid haemorrhage)
Sheehan's syndrome
Pituitary apoplexy
Congenital
Autosomal-dominant mutations of antidiuretic hormone expression (despite the dominant expression of the gene, the onset of clinical diabetes insipidus may take up to 30 years to develop)†
Wolfram syndrome – autosomal-recessive condition characterised by diabetes insipidus, diabetes mellitus, optic atrophy and deafness

*Doczi T, Tarjanyi J, Kiss J. Syndrome of inappropriate antidiuretic syndrome after head injury. *Neurosurgery* 1982; **10:** 685–8.
†Repaske DR, Medlej R, Gulteken EK *et al.* Heterogeneity in clinical manifestation of autosomal dominant neurohypophyseal diabetes insipidus caused by a mutation encoding Ala^1-Val in the signal peptide of the arginine vasopressin/neurophysin II/copeptin precursor. *J Clin Endocrinol Metab* 1997; **82:** 51–6.

Transsphenoidal surgery for treatment of suprasellar tumours can result in DI in 10–70% of patients; the frequency parallels the magnitude of the tumour being removed. Additionally, transcranial surgery may cause the development of DI in the absence of a fall in plasma ADH. This is postulated to be due to the release of a hypothalamic ADH precursor which acts as a competitive antagonist of both ADH and synthetic analogues. The presence of a competitive antagonist effectively creates an endocrinologice picture similar to NDI with normal or high plasma ADH levels but an inappropriate diuresis of dilute urine.

Following surgery or traumatic brain injury, several different patterns of polyuria can be seen: immediate permanent or transient polyuria, initial normal or low urine production followed by transient or permanent polyuria, or initial low followed by normal urine output. Additionally, a classical triphasic pattern of urine output may be observed with:

1. transient polyuria due to transient impairment of the release of ADH (0–5 days in duration), then
2. a phase of normal or reduced urine output; the ADH previously stored in the pituitary gland is gradually released into the circulation as the cells storing it involute (3–6 days in duration)
3. persistent polyuria as the pituitary stores exhaust and no replacement hormone from the hypothalamus is produced

During the second phase of this pattern, administration of fluids may result in volume overload and hyponatraemia as the ADH release is not under feedback control from osmoreceptors but occurring in an uncontrolled manner as a result of pituitary degeneration. Effectively, there is a transient syndrome of inappropriate ADH (SIADH) secretion. The triphasic pattern is usually associated with sudden severe damage to the hypothalamus or pituitary from trauma, surgery or intracranial bleed, and careful, regular clinical and biochemical assessment is essential to ensure normal water balance and osmolality during this transition from DI to SIADH and back to DI again.

The exact nature of the urinary pattern seen in DI is relatively unimportant and gradual resolution may occur over several months in those with transient DI. What is essential is that meticulous assessments of patients and their plasma and urinary biochemistry as well as fluid inputs and outputs are made to prevent the development of unnecessary fluid and solute imbalances which could lead to worsening morbidity or mortality.

It is important to maintain a high level of suspicion for the development of DI in anyone who is suffering from pituitary disease or who has suffered a pituitary injury as the symptoms may have gradual onset. Anterior pituitary failure can lessen the impact of central DI because of the deficiency of ACTH and cortisol, which reduces GFR and free water loss. Additionally, the loss of feedback inhibition may stimulate increased release of ADH from the median eminence. Thus in Sheehan's syndrome and pituitary apoplexy, the presenting symptoms tend not to be those of DI with polyuria. However, once corticosteroid therapy is commenced, polyuria indicating DI may become apparent or exacerbated. Conversely, patients with persistent DI of idiopathic origin should have long-term endocrine follow-up as a number will go on to develop tumours of the pituitary several years following the diagnosis of DI.[30,31]

TREATMENT OF CDI

Four separate problems have to be addressed when treating CDI:

1. Associated anterior pituitary dysfunction needs to be considered.
2. Hypernatraemia must be recognised and treated with painstaking care.
3. Any deficit of total body water must be recognised and addressed (this may be urgent if the patient is shocked).
4. The underlying deficiency of ADH causing the polyuria must be addressed.

In all ICU patients with DI, hourly urine measurements, hourly fluid losses and fluid inputs and at least twice-daily urine and plasma osmolalities are recommended. In shocked patients and those with hypernatraemia, hourly monitoring of plasma sodium is recommended to prevent worsening of hyperosmolality or over-rapid correction of hypernatraemia.

ANTERIOR PITUITARY DYSFUNCTION

If this is present, it requires recognition and treatment. In the emergent situation with a shocked patient, hydrocortisone 100 mg can be administered as an intravenous bolus, and steroid replacement continued if needed. Steroid administration may worsen the diuresis but will improve cardiovascular stability in patients with pituitary ablation.

HYPERNATRAEMIA

If the patient with CDI and ongoing water diuresis has had restricted access to fluids and has developed hyperosmolality/hypertonicity or alternatively has developed hypertonicity through replacement of dilute urine with equal volumes of isotonic (to plasma) intravenous fluids, then sudden reduction in plasma tonicity may result in pontine myelonecrosis and permanent neurological damage. When a euvolaemic state is present, AVP or DDAVP may be administered to reduce urine output (see below). At the same time, fluid restriction should be imposed and replacement of the previous hour's urine output undertaken with an appropriate fluid to avoid a fall in concentration of sodium by more than 0.5 mmol/h.[32] Absolute safety data are not available to determine the ideal rate of reduction of plasma sodium. However, a fall of more than 5 mmol/l in any 24-hour period should be avoided.

DEHYDRATION AND HYPOVOLAEMIA

If associated with shock, hypovolaemia requires rapid resuscitation. If hypovolaemia is also associated with hypernatraemia, extreme caution is required in the resuscitation, which should take place with isotonic saline solution and frequent reassessments of plasma sodium and cardiovascular and neurological status. Where the hypernatraemia is very marked (>155 mmol/l), consideration of a combination of isotonic (0.9%) and hypertonic saline should be given to reduce the rate of sodium reduction. In the face of hypertonicity of the plasma, cells reduce their chloride and potassium conductance and synthesise intracellular osmolytes such as amino acids, taurine and sorbitol. If 0.9% saline (effective osmolality 290 mosmol/kg when diluted by plasma proteins) is infused rapidly into hypertonic plasma with a sodium of 160 mmol/l, an effective osmolality of 330 mosmol/kg, a rapid drop in plasma osmolality may cause cerebral and other organ oedema; seizures and death. By reducing the tonicity of the plasma gradually, the cells have time to downregulate their synthesis of intracellular osmolytes and increase potassium and chloride conductance to reduce swelling as plasma tonicity falls.

CORRECTION OF POLYURIA AND ADH DEFICIENCY

At mild levels of polyuria (2–3 ml/kg per hour) where there is an expectation that the condition may resolve, it may be appropriate merely to replace the previous hour's urine output with an appropriate fluid (usually 5% dextrose or 0.18% saline/4% dextrose) whilst undertaking regular measurements of plasma and urine osmolality and electrolytes. Care must be taken not to give so much dextrose as to result in hyperglycaemia, hyperosmolality and osmotic diuresis.

Where polyuria is expected to be persistent or is excessive, either ADH or its synthetic analogue DDAVP may be administered. DDAVP is a selective V_2 receptor agonist and thus is less likely to cause hypertension. It is also longer-acting, resisting breakdown by vasopressinases, and is usually administered once or twice daily. The usual daily dose rate, when administered intravenously, intramuscularly or subcutaneously, is 1–4 μg daily. ADH may be administered subcutaneously or by intravenous infusion and DDAVP may be presented intranasally, subcutaneously, intravenously or orally. In the acute situation, an ADH infusion (0.1–3 U/h) can be conveniently titrated against urine output. The use of the infusion ensures 100% bioavailability and facilitates re-establishment of the hypertonic renal medullary interstitium before changing the patient to the longer-acting DDAVP. The dose of ADH or DDAVP is often higher during the acute-onset phase of CDI – this may be due to the loss of hypertonicity in the medullary interstitium or due to biologically inactive ADH precussors released from the damaged hypothalamic–pituitary tract which act as competitive antagonists at the V_2 renal receptors.

The dose of ADH or DDAVP used is the minimum dose required to control urine output to an acceptable rate. Excessive administration can result in water retention and the development of hypo-osmolal syndromes.

Other drugs may also be used to reduce the polyuria of CDI. Provided there is some residual ADH synthesis, chlorpropamide, clofibrate and carbamazepine are all reported to enhance ADH release and also increase the renal responsiveness to ADH. Thiazide diuretics can also be used effectively. Whilst these agents all reduce urine output, there is little place for them in the modern management of CDI in the ICU where DDAVP and ADH have excellent safety profiles and are more easily titrated to effect. These alternative drugs are discussed later in the treatment of NDI.

NEPHROGENIC DIABETES INSIPIDUS

NDI may be congenital or acquired (Table 51.4). As the majority of congenital cases present in the first week of life, the majority of cases seen in the adult ICU are acquired. The commonest of these are lithium toxicity due to long-term drug treatment, hypercalcaemia and postobstructive uropathy following relief of ureteric or urtethral obstruction.

CONGENITAL NDI

Some 80–90% of patients with congenital NDI have an X-linked recessive abnormality of the *AVPR*$_2$ gene coding for the V_2 receptor. Different mutations of the gene are described but the majority result in trapping of the V_2 receptor intracellularly, unable to integrate into the membrane of the collecting duct cell. Drugs have been developed which can facilitate receptor integration into the membrane, restoring some of the urine-concentrating abilities of ADH.[33] The sex linkage results in the vast majority of affected patients being male. However, female children can also present less severe polyuria and polydipsia due to expression of the abnormal gene.

Non-sex-linked genetic abnormalities can also cause NDI. Approximately 10% of cases of congenital NDI have mutations of the *AQP*$_2$ (acquaporin 2) gene which codes for the AQP_2 channel. Over 40 mutations, both autosomal-dominant and recessive, have been described to date.

The remainder of cases of congenital NDI have a variety of pathologies which result in failure to generate a hypertonic renal medulla, with inability to reabsorb water even if the V_2 receptor and acquaporin$_2$ channels are normal.

A lack of the Kidd antigen (a blood group antigen) results in an inability to concentrate urine to more than 800 mosmol/kg even with water deprivation and exogenous ADH administration. This is because the antigen is also expressed in the collecting duct epithelium where it functions as a urea transporter (urea transport B protein) and facilitates movement of urea from urine into the medullary interstitium maintaining some of the gradients required to facilitate water reabsorption. Similarly, patients with mutations in chloride channel genes, potassium channel genes or the sodium–potassium–chloride co-transporter gene resulting in the Bartter syndrome are unable to generate a hypertonic medullary interstium. However, in these patients the defect is more marked and urine can rarely be concentrated above 350 mosmol/kg.

With congenital NDI, early diagnosis and management are essential as avoidance of hypernatraemia and dehydration facilitates the achievement of normal developmental milestones and avoids the cerebral damage once commonly accepted as an inevitable association of NDI.

Table 51.4 Causes of Nephrogenic DI

Acquired
(i) lithium toxicity
(ii) post-obstructive diuresis
(iii) hypercalacemia
(iv) hypoklaemia
(v) hypoproteinameia
(vi) Sjogren's syndrome
(vii) Amyloid
(viii) sickle cell disease
(ix) poly-cystic kidney disease
(x) other drugs: amiodarone, amphotericin B, clozapine, demeclocycline, foscarnet, gentamicin, loop diuretics, rifampicin
Congenital
(i) x-linked recessive – $AVPR_2$ gene mutations
(ii) autosomal recessive or dominant – AQP_2 gene mutations
(iii) Bartter's syndrome
(iv) Gitelman's syndrome
(v) Urea Transport Protein B (Kidd Ag) deficiency/absence

ACQUIRED NDI

Lithium-associated nephrotoxicity remains the commonest form of acquired NDI with more than 20% of patients on chronic lithium therapy developing polyuria. Lithium is taken up into the principal cells of the collecting duct via sodium channels and inhibits intracellular adenylate cylcase antagonising the effects of ADH. Additionally, it reduces the medullary interstitial hypertonicity, possibly through reducing expression of urea transport protein B. If patients with early lithium-related NDI are prescribed amiloride, some reversal of both the polyuria and lithium-mediated toxicity is possible. Amiloride's natriuretic action is achieved through closure of the luminal sodium channels in the collecting duct; the sodium channels through which lithium enters the cells.[34] Indomethacin increases intracellular cAMP and counteracts the diminution of this and AQP_2 caused by lithium, resulting in a marked and immediate drop in urine output. However, care is required as non-steroidal anti-inflammatory drugs (NSAIDs) may worsen renal failure, reducing GFR and lithium excretion, thereby worsening toxicity.

Hypercalcaemia, hypokalaemia, release of ureteric or urethral obstruction and hypoproteinaemia are also recognised as causing NDI and are associated with reduced expression of AQP_2 channels, urea transport proteins and a loss of interstitial hypertonicity. These defects normally cause milder polyuria than that associated with lithium toxicity.

TREATMENT OF NDI

The treatment of NDI aims to minimise the occurrence of hypernatraemia and hypovolaemia and wherever possible to remove the underlying cause.

1. Correct reversible causes:
   (a) Stop any drugs suspected in the aetiology.
   (b) Correct hypokalaemia, hypercalcaemia and hypoproteinaemia.
2. Reduce solute load. As urine output is determined by the solute load to be excreted, reducing the solute intake will reduce the urine volume accordingly; if maximum urine concentration is 250 mosmol/kg, a solute intake of 750 mosmol/day requires production of at least 3 litres of urine to clear the solute whereas if intake is reduced to 500 mmol. 2 litres of urine will suffice. In ICU, the reduction of solute can be difficult as many drugs and diluents have a high solute load. Additionally, patients may be catabolic and have a high protein requirement. It may be more appropriate not to aim to restrict solute intake for certain patients but to closely monitor fluid balance and ensure adequate appropriate replacement.
   (a) Regulate salt intake (aiming at < 100 mmol/day).
   (b) Reduce protein intake, aiming to provide the minimum daily requirement including essential amino acids – this should be done with specialist dietetic advice and requires careful follow-up to avoid protein malnutrition. It is not appropriate to protein-restrict children as this may adversely affect normal growth and development.
3. Diuretics – thiazides and amiloride:
   (a) Thiazides – whereas DI loses water in excess to solute, rendering the plasma hyperosmolal and resulting in intracellular dehydration to maintain the intravascular volume, thiazide diuretics cause solute loss in excess of water and lead to a drop in intravascular volume. This causes activation of the sympathetic nervous system, the renin–angiotensin–aldosterone system and a fall in glomerular filtration and ANP. Additionally, thiazides are associated with an increased expression of AQP_2 channels in the collecting duct.[35] There is an increase in proximal tubular reabsorption of sodium and water and an increase in ADH release. Thus, less ultrafiltrate reaches the collecting duct and urine volume can fall by as much as 30%. Combined with a solute-reduced diet, the fall in urine production can be as high as 50%.
   (b) Amiloride – this is a useful adjunct to thiazide diuretics in NDI where it causes a further slight reduction in urine output and combats the hypokalaemia associated with the thiazides. It may have benefit in its own right in lithium-associated nephrotoxicity, where it blocks the sodium channels through which lithium enters the principal cells. If administered before lithium damage becomes irreversible, it can both reduce the damage to the cells themselves and reverse the antagonism of lithium on the effects of ADH.

   Loop diuretics are not effective in reducing the diuresis of NDI, as although they reduce intravascular volume and stimulate the sympathetic nervous system in a similar manner to thiazides, they also reduce interstitial medullary sodium concentrations and hypertonicity, thus reducing water reabsorption by the collecting duct rather than enhancing it.
4. ADH. Where NDI is not absolute (most cases of acquired NDI), supplementing endogenous ADH to create supraphysiological concentrations in the plasma can result in a fall of urine production by up to 25%. This effect may occur by antagonising the effects of any V_2 receptor antagonists or by causing greater receptor occupation. Care is required with long-term use as hypertension and its associated complications may result.
5. NSAIDs. NSAIDs reduce the formation of renal PGE_2 which increases GFR and urine flow and decreases intracellular cAMP and thus aquaporin expression. Reduction of PGE_2 using NSAIDs alone may reduce urine output by up to 50%.[36] Combination with low-solute diet and a thiazide diuretic may provide additional antidiuretic benefit.[37] However, the use of NSAIDs has to be weighed against their long-term complications. This is particularly true in the ICU population who are at increased risk of both renal impairment and gastric erosions. Indomethacin is cited to have greater treatment benefit than other NSAIDs in NDI.[38] It is also more likely to produce unwanted adverse effects.
6. Chlorpropamide. This oral hypoglycaemic agent enhances both ADH release and the sensitivity of the kidney to it. It is suggested to act via increasing the hypertonicity of the renal medulla. Doses of 250 mg od or bd are prescribed but are likely to cause hypoglycaemia.[39] Its use is therefore reserved for severe refractory cases of partial NDI.
7. Clofibrate. This oral lipid-lowering agent is reported to enhance ADH release and increase renal sensitivity to ADH.[40] Its use in CDI has largely stopped because of the efficacy and safety of DDAVP. Its use in treatment of DI has been associated with myopathy.[41] If considered for treatment of partial NDI, biochemical markers of myopathy should be measured regularly.
8. Carbamazepine. Carbamazepine can also be tried as a treatment in partial NDI, although it is more effective in treating partial CDI. It increases the renal responsiveness to ADH but requires a dose rate three times higher than that effective as an antiepileptic. This high dose rate limits its usefulness in therapy.

9. Molecular chaperones. Novel drugs described as 'molecular chaperones' are being developed to treat NDI where the V_2 receptor is functional and intact but confined to the intracellular space, unable to integrate into the basolateral membrane of the principal cell. The drugs are membrane-permeable V_2 receptor antagonists and are believed to cause refolding of the receptor in a form that allows normal processing of the receptor into the membrane.[42] These are showing some success in animal models of congenital NDI and with human V_2R mutations associated with NDI in in vitro testing. Early studies in humans report some success.[43]

GESTATIONAL DIABETES INSPIDUS (TABLE 51.5)

In pregnancy the normal range of plasma osmolalities falls to 265–285 mosmol/kg and the plasma sodium is < 140 mmol/l. The reduction in osmolality is attributed to a resetting of the central osmostat.[44,45] The retention of water and sodium is mediated by reduced baroreceptor stimulation.[46] During pregnancy, the placenta produces vasopressinases, which increase ADH metabolism up to fourfold, and relaxin, which contributes to the 50% increase in GFR and venodilatation.[47] Aldosterone concentrations rise up to fivefold. Solute elimination also rises so a small reduction in urine-concentrating ability may have a more marked effect. The volume of urine passed per day increases as a result of passage of an increased solute load (including urinary proteins, glucose and amino acids), increased drinking and a raised GFR. A diagnosis of DI therefore requires careful differentiation from a physiological polyuria or potentially pathological polyuria of separate aetiology (e.g. gestational diabetes) in pregnancy.

GDI can result from:

1. Increased destruction of ADH by excessive production of placental vasopressinases.[48] This may be unresponsive to exogenous ADH administration as it too is rapidly metabolised. DDAVP can be used instead as it is resistant to degradation by placental vasopressinase.
2. Permanently deficient reserve of ADH secretion, which in the non-pregnant state is asymptomatic but which in the pregnant state is unmasked by the higher vasopressinase activity which cannot be compensated for by increased secretion.[49] This condition responds to treatment with ADH.
3. Central DI associated with acute fatty liver of pregnancy,[50] Sheehan's syndrome and pituitary apoplexy. Sheehan's syndrome is commonest, and is usually preceded by major bleeding or hypotension at the time of delivery. Pituitary apoplexy has been described antenatally too.[51]
4. Gestational NDI of unknown aetiology, which is resistant to both ADH and DDAVP, with resolution in the postnatal period, has also been described.[52]

Table 51.5 Causes of Gestational DI

(i)	Sheehan's Syndrome
(ii)	Pituitary Apoplexy
(iii)	Acute fatty liver of pregnancy
(iv)	Vasopressinase release by placenta
(v)	Idiopathic gestational NDI (resolves post-partum)

The treatment of GDI varies depending on the underlying cause. In all cases, it is important not to allow the patient to become hypernatraemic and hyperosmolal as this is likely to have adverse effects on both mother and child. Where hypernatraemia and hyperosmolality do occur, careful correction is required in a closely monitored, very gradual, stepwise fashion. A lowering of sodium by as little as 10 mmol/day has been associated with pontine myelinolysis.[53]

POLYDIPSIA (PSYCHOGENIC/NEUROGENIC)

Polydipsia may result from:

1. a psychiatric disorder or disturbance[54]
2. drugs which give the sensation of dry mouth[55] or airways, e.g. oxygen therapy, phenothiazines, anticholinergics
3. hypothalamic lesions which directly disturb the thirst centre,[56] e.g. sarcoidosis

In all three of the above causes of polydipsia, excessive drinking is associated with the production of large quantities of urine of appropriate osmolality. If the fluid ingested is largely hypotonic, the urine will be hypo-osmolal and result from a fall in ADH secretion. If the fluid ingested is hypertonic, the urine will have high osmolality but remain of high volume because of the interplay of ADH production (determined by osmoreceptors and volume receptors) and ANP production (determined by volume receptors) resulting in a solute diuresis.

Polydipsia may also result from the appropriate detection by osmoreceptors of a raised plasma osmolality due to raised glucose or sodium. The glycosuria itself will cause an osmotic diuresis and plasma osmolality may be normal or raised depending on the severity of the hyperglycaemia and any accompanying ketoacidosis and dehydration.

SOLUTE DIURESIS

Just as failure to reabsorb water can result in polyuria, failure to reabsorb solute can result in an osmotic load in the tubule which opposes water absorption in the convoluted tubules and collecting duct. The commonest cause of this in the general patient population is glycosuria. In the ICU setting a solute diuresis may also be associated with the administration of diuretic drugs, high-protein feeds (increased urea load), supranormal quantities of sodium and other solutes through fluids, feeds and drugs, recovery from acute renal failure with tubular inability to reabsorb solute, and drug-induced tubular damage.

To differentiate a solute diuresis from a water diuresis it is advisable to measure the 24-hour excretion of solute in the urine. Normally, between 600 and 900 mosmol/day of solute is excreted in the urine. Values higher than this indicate a solute diuresis. A spot urine osmolality may be measured; osmolality higher than 300 mosmol/kg, is suggestive of a solute diuresis. It would not be uncommon in the critically ill patient to encounter simultaneous impairment of both water reabsorption and impaired solute handling in the nephron. In this instance, 24-hour solute excretion may be increased but the urine may remain hypo-osmolal.

THE DIAGNOSIS OF POLYURIC SYNDROMES

MEASURE AND CALCULATE PLASMA OSMOLALITY AND URINE OSMOLALITY

A high urine osmolality in the presence of a high plasma osmolality is appropriate and, if the plasma osmolality is higher than 295 mosmol/l, urine osmolality should reach 1000–1200 mosmol/kg. Urine osmolalities of less than this imply that there is a urine-concentrating defect and lead to consideration of the causes of DI and also the use of medications that might reduce renal interstitial hypertonicity, such as loop diuretics. Urine osmolalities of < 150 mosmol/kg in this circumstance are sufficient to make the diagnosis of DI provided there is not obvious gross fluid and solute overload of the patient.

Where the patient is polyuric with a high plasma osmolality and maximum urine osmolalities are being achieved, an osmotic diuresis is implied. The diuresis may be inappropriate in as much as it is leading to dehydration but appropriate in that the kidneys are retaining as much water as they can for the large solute load being excreted. If there is a normal *osmolal gap* (the difference between measured and calculated plasma osmolality, normal < 10 mosmol/kg), then hyperglycaemia, hypernatraemia or hyperkalaemia is implied. If the osmolal gap is greater than 10 mosmol/kg, investigation should be undertaken to look for an unmeasured solute such as ethanol, mannitol, ethylene glycol, sorbitol or methanol.

If plasma osmolality is less than 280 mosmol/kg, urine osmolality would also be expected to be lower than this as the body attempts to clear free water. This picture implies water overload which may be iatrogenic or patient-mediated. Low plasma osmolality with high urine osmolality implies SIADH and would not normally be associated with polyuria.

WATER DEPRIVATION AND ADH TESTS

In health, being deprived of water rapidly results in an increase in plasma osmolality which causes ADH release and an increase in urine osmolality to between 1000 and 1200 mosmol/kg in order to preserve water and reduce plasma osmolality back towards its normal value. When the cause of polyuria is unclear and the patient is not already clinically dehydrated, a water deprivation test may be useful to determine the cause of the diuresis. In patients with severe polyuria, the test is potentially dangerous as dehydration and hyperosmolality can develop very rapidly, resulting in permanent cerebral damage and cardiovascular collapse. It is therefore wise to undertake the test under very close supervision during daylight hours.

The limitations of the test should also be appreciated:

1. In acute CDI, release of ADH precursors from injured brain tissue may render interpretation of ADH tests unreliable and cross-react with ADH measurement assays.
2. At high concentrations of ADH, the urine concentrations achieved in partial NDI and primary polydipsia may be similar.
3. Patients with partial CDI may occasionally become hypersensitive to relatively small rises in ADH which may be induced by the rise in osmolality associated with water deprivation and thus maximally concentrate urine once osmolality is raised, leading to an erroneous diagnosis of primary polydipsia.[57]
4. In patients with chronic hypernatraemia and CDI secondary to osmoreceptor dysfunction, hypovolaemia with water deprivation may cause sufficient baroreceptor stimulus to release ADH and suggest normal urine-concentrating abilities:[58]

Step 1: Plasma and urine osmolalities and plasma ADH are measured at time zero and access to intravenous/oral fluids is denied.

Step 2: Plasma and urine osmolalities are measured hourly until either three consecutive urine osmolalities are within 50 mosmol/kg of one another or plasma osmolality is > 295 mosmol/kg. At this time, plasma ADH is measured again.

Step 3: If plasma osmolality is > 295 mosmol/kg and urine osmolality is < 1000 mosmol/kg, ADH (5 units AVP subcutaneously or 4 μg DDAVP subcutanesously) is administered to the patient and urine osmolality is measured hourly for 3 hours (this time is necessary to allow time for at least partial recovery of the medullary interstitial hypertonic gradient in patients with primary polydipsia).

[DDAVP is preferred to AVP as it avoids misinterpretation of results in the presence of vasopressinases which would rapidly metabolise AVP and suggest a diagnosis of NDI rather than CDI. Although neither is the correct diagnosis if vasopressinases are present, the treatment is as for CDI, i.e. the administration of DDAVP.]

Step 4: Urine osmolality is then plotted against plasma osmolality (Figure 51.4).

Step 5: Plasma and urine osmolalities are plotted against plasma ADH concentrations (Figure 51.5).

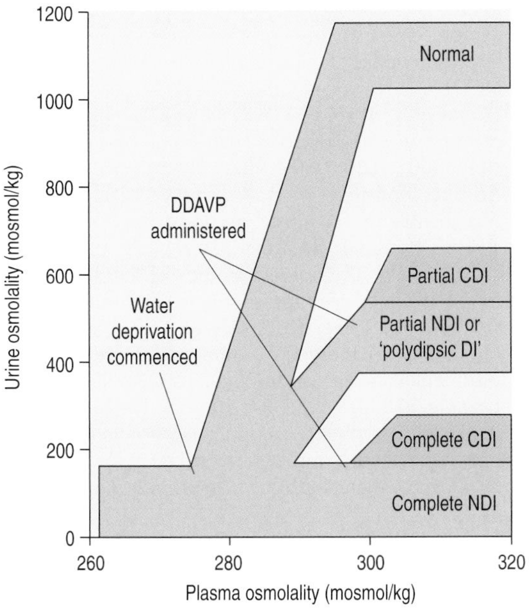

Figure 51.4 Urine versus plasma osmolality during water deprivation testing. DDAVP, 1-deamino-8-0-arginine vasopressin; CDI, cranial diabetes insipidus; NDI, nephrogenic diabetes insipidus. Adapted from Sands JM, Bichet DG. Ann Intern Med 2006; 144: 186–94.

INTERPRETATION OF THE TESTS (SEE FIGURES 51.4 AND 51.5)

In complete DI, plasma osmolality will rise but urine osmolality will not rise above 300 mosmol/kg. Upon administration of ADH, patients with complete CDI will raise their urine osmolality to 500 mosmol/kg or higher whereas there will be no rise in urine osmolality in complete NDI.

In complete CDI, the original plasma ADH measurement will be zero, whereas in complete NDI, the initial ADH measurement will be normal or high depending on the corresponding plasma osmolality at the time of measurement.

In partial DI, plasma osmolality will rise and urine osmolality will also increase but usually plateaus between 400 and 800 mosmol/kg. In partial CDI the ADH will initially be normal or low and will rise with increasing plasma osmolality but is unlikely to rise above 4–5 pg/ml. In partial NDI, the ADH will initially be normal or high and will increase with plasma osmolality to > 8 pg/ml but without achieving a correspondingly appropriate rise in urine concentration.

Following administration of ADH or DDAVP, urine osmolality is expected to double at least in complete CDI and rise by 10–50% in partial CDI or NDI. In complete NDI, there will be no rise in urine osmolality. Partial CDI may be inferentially differentiated from partial NDI on the basis of urine osmolality alone; in the former, urine osmolality rises above plasma osmolality whereas in partial NDI it tends to remain hypo-osmolal or iso-osmolal to

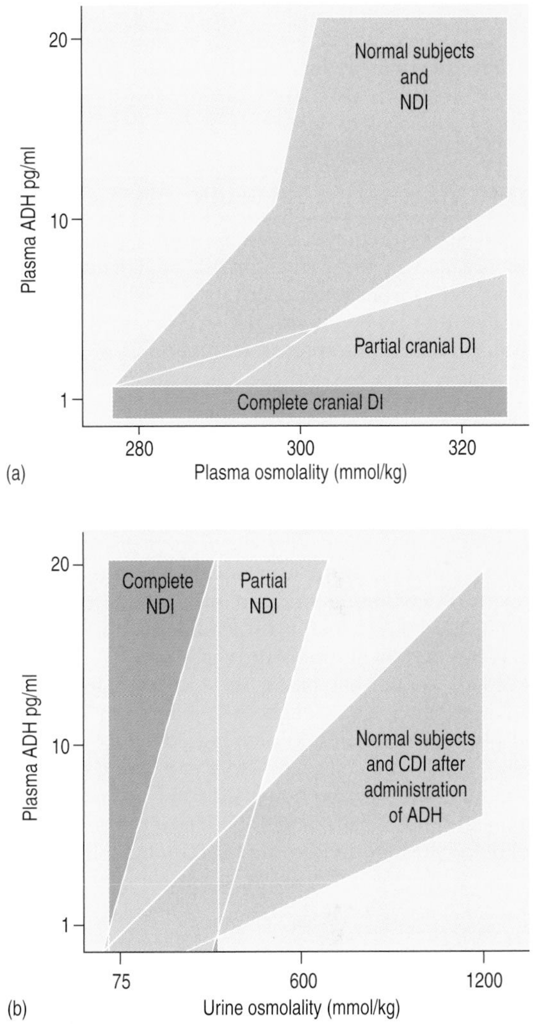

Figure 51.5 (a) As plasma osmolality increases as a result of water deprivation or hypertonic saline infusion, the measured concentration of antidiuretic hormone (ADH) should rise. Failure to do so suggests cranial diabetes insipidus. (b) At a given value of plasma ADH, whether endogenous or exogenous in origin, urine osmolality is expected to lie within a corresponding range of osmolality. However, the range of expected osmolalities is high as osmoreceptors adjust regulation around the basal level of ADH, which is also partly determined by volume receptors. In nephrogenic diabetes insipidus (NDI), the urine osmolality remains low even when high plasma ADH concentrations are measured.

plasma following ADH/DDAVP administration. However, this generalisation is indicative only and for greater certainty, it is preferred to have measured sequential ADH concentrations to assess hypothalamic–pituitary function independently of the renal concentrating ability.

Water deprivation tests should not be conducted in infants or patients with pre-existing hypovolaemia or hyperosmolality. In the latter two categories, treatment of the fluid deficit and/or solute excess should precede further investigations. In infants and in adults with equivocal water deprivation test results, an infusion of hypertonic saline should be considered.

HYPERTONIC SALINE INFUSION

In patients with equivocal results from a water deprivation test and in those at high risk of dehydration and hypovolaemia from water deprivation, a hypertonic saline infusion test may be undertaken to establish the cause of a water diuresis. Interpretation of the test is as for the water deprivation test but there is a clearer demarcation between partial CDI and primary polydipsia and the risk of missing a diagnosis of CDI secondary to osmoreceptor dysfunction is reduced.[59]

Hypertonic saline is available in multiple different concentrations. Care is required in calculating the appropriate infusion rate to use for the test as this varies with the concentration of the hypertonic preparation stocked. Hypertonic sodium chloride solution (0.0425 mmol/kg per min) is infused for up to 3 hours or until a plasma osmolality of 300 mosmol/kg is achieved.

Blood samples are taken 30 minutes before and at 30-minute intervals throughout the duration of the test and plasma sodium, osmolality and ADH are measured. Urine samples are collected before and where possible at 60-minute intervals throughout the test period and measurements of osmolality and sodium are performed. Thirst and blood pressure are recorded at 30-minute intervals.

REFERENCES

1. Dorwart WV, Chalmers L. Comparison of methods for calculating serum osmolality from chemical concentrations and the prognostic value of such calculations. *Clin Chem* 1975; **21**: 190–4.
2. Worthley LI, Guerin M, Pain RW. For calculating osmolality, the simplest formula is the best. *Anaesth Intens Care* 1987; **15**: 199–202.
3. Rasouli M, Kalantair KR. Comparison of methods for calculating serum osmolality: multivariate linear regression analysis. *Clin Chem Lab Med* 2005; **43**: 635–40.
4. McKinely MJ, Denton DA, Weisinger RS. Sensors for antidiuresis and thirst – osmoreceptors or CSF sodium detectors? *Brain Res* 1978; **141**: 89–103.
5. Keller-Wood M. ACTH responses to CRF and AVP in pregnant and non-pregnant ewes. *Am J Physiol Regulat Integr Comp Physiol* 1998; **274**: 1762–8.
6. Kalogeras KT, Nieman LK, Friedman TC *et al.* Inferior petrosal sinus sampling in healthy human subjects reveals a unilateral corticotropin-releasing hormone-induced arginine vasopressin release associated with ipsilateral adrenocorticotropin secretion. *J Clin Invest* 1996; **97**: 2045–50.
7. Stricker EM, Sved AF. Thirst. *Nutrition* 2000; **16**: 821–6.
8. Halter JB, Goldberg AP, Robertson GL *et al.* Selective osmoreceptor dysfunction in the syndrome of chronic hypernatraemia. *J Clin Endocrinol Metab* 1977; **44**: 609–16.
9. Holmes CL, Patel BM, Russell JA *et al.* Physiology of vasopressin relevant to management of septic shock. *Chest* 2001; **120**: 989–1002.
10. Antunes-Rodrigues J, de Castro M, Elias LLK *et al.* Neuroednocrine control of body fluid metabolism. *Physiol Rev* 2004; **84**: 169–208.
11. Czaczkes JW. Physiologic studies of antidiuretic hormone by its direct measurement in human plasma. *J Clin Invest* 1964; **43**: 1625–40.
12. Holmes CL, Landry DW, Granton JT. Science review: vasopressin and the cardiovascular system parts 1 and 2. *Crit Care* 2003; **7**: 427–34; 2004; **8**: 15–23.
13. Bankir L. Antidiuretic action of vasopressin: quantitative aspects and interaction between V1a and V2 receptor mediated effects. *Cardiovasc Res* 2001; **51**: 372–90.
14. Landry DW, Levin HR, Gallant EM *et al.* Vasopressin pressor hypersensitivity in vasodilatory septic shock. *Crit Care Med* 1997; **95**: 1122–5.
15. Maturi MF, Martin SE, Markle D *et al.* Coronary vasoconstriction induced by vasopressin. Production of myocardial ischaemia in dogs by constriction of non-diseased small vessels. *Circulation* 1991; **83**: 2111–21.
16. Vanhoutte PM, Katusic ZS, Shepherd JT. Vasopressin induces endothelium-dependent relaxations of cerebral and coronary but not of systemic arteries. *J Hypertens* 1984; **2** (Suppl.): S421–2.
17. Okamurat T, Ayajiki K, Fujiokah H *et al.* Mechanisms underlying arginine vasopressin induced relaxation in isolated monkey coronary arteries. *J Hypertens* 1999; **17**: 673–8.
18. Sellke FW, Quillen JE. Altered effects of vasopressin on the coronary circulation after ischaemia. *J Thorac Cardiovasc Surg* 1992; **104**: 357–63.
19. Nussey SS, Bevaqn DH, Ang VT *et al.* Effects of arginine vasopressin (AVP) infusions on circulating concentrations of platelet AVP, factor VIII:C and von Willebrand factor. *Thromb Haemost* 1986; **55**: 34–6.
20. Haslam RJ, Rosson GM. Aggregation of human blood platelets by vasopressin. *Am J Physiol* 1972; **223**: 958–67.
21. Wun T, Paglieroni T, Lanchant NA. Physiological concentrations of arginine vasopressin activate human platelets in vitro. *Br J Haematol* 1996; **92**: 968–72.
22. Filep J, Rosenkranz B. Mechanisms of vasopressin induced platelet aggregation. *Thromb Res* 1987; **45**: 7–15.
23. Vander AJ. *Renal Physiology*, 5th edn. McGraw Hill, USA; 1995: 116–44.
24. Schrier RW. Water and sodium retention in edematous disorders: role of vasopressin and aldosterone. *Am J Med* 2006; **119**: S47–53.
25. Richard D, Bourque CW. Atrial natriuretic peptide modulates synaptic transmission from osmoreceptor afferents to the supraoptic nucleus. *J Neurosci* 1996; **16**: 7526–32.

26. Shucart WA, Jackson I. Management of diabetes insipidus in neurosurgical patients. *J Neurosurg* 1976; **44**: 65–71.
27. Maghnie M, Altobelli M, di Iorgi N *et al.* Idiopathic central diabetes insipidus is associated with abnormal blood supply to the posterior pituitary gland caused by vascular impairment of the inferior hypophyseal artery system. *J Endocrinol Metab* 2004; **89**: 1891–6.
28. Pivonello R, De Bellis A, Faggiano A *et al.* Central diabetes insipidus and autoimmunity: relationship between the occurrence of antibodies to arginine vasopressin-secreting cells and clinical, immunological and radiological features in a large cohort of patients with central diabetes insipidus of unknown etiology. *J Clin Endocrinol Metab* 2003; **88**: 1629–36.
29. Halter JB, Goldberg AP, Robertson GL *et al.* Selective osmoreceptor dysfunction in the syndrome of chronic hypernatraemia. *J Clin Endocrinol Metab* 1977; **44**: 609–16.
30. Charmandari E, Brook CG. 20 years of experience in idiopathic central diabetes insipidus. *Lancet* 1999; **353**: 2212–13.
31. Sudha LM, Anthony JB, Grumbach MM *et al.* Idiopathic hypothalamic diabets insipidus, pituitary stalk thickening and the occult intracranial germinoma in children and adolescents. *J Clin Endocrinol Metab* 1997; **82**: 1362–7.
32. Blum D, Brasser D, Kahn A *et al.* Safe oral rehydration of hypertonic dehydration. *J Pediatr Gastroenterol Nutr* 1986; **5**: 232–5.
33. Robben JH, Sze M, Knoers NV *et al.* Functional rescue of vasopressin V2 receptor mutants in MDCK cells by pharmacochaperones: relevance to therapy of nephrogenic diabetes insipidus. *Am J Physiol Renal Physiol* 2007; **292**: F253–60.
34. Battle DC, von Riotte AB, Gaviria M *et al.* Amelioration of polyuria by amiloride in patients receiving long-term lithium therapy. *N Engl J Med* 1985; **312**: 408–14.
35. Kim GH, Lee JW, Oh YK *et al.* Nephrogenic diabetes insipidus is associated with up-regulation of aquaporin-2, Na-Cl cotransporter and epithelieal sodium channel. *J Am Soc Nephrol* 2004; **15**: 2836–43.
36. Lam SS, Kjellstrand C. Emergency treatment of lithium-induced diabetes insipidus with non-steroidal anti-inflammatory drugs. *Renal Fail* 1997; **19**: 183–8.
37. Hochberg Z, Even L, Danon A. Amelioration of polyuria in nephrogenic diabetes insipidus due to aquaporin-2 deficiency. *Clin Endocrinol* 1998; **49**: 39–44.
38. Libber S; Harrison H; Spector D. Treatment of nephrogenic diabetes insipidus with prostaglandin synthesis inhibitors. *J Pediatr* 1986; **108**: 305–11.
39. Thompson P Jr, Erll JM, Schaaf M. Comparison of clofibrate and chlorpropamide in vasopressin responsive diabetes insipidus. *Metabolism* 1977; **26**: 749–62.
40. Moses AM, Howanitz J, vanGemert M *et al.* Clofibrate-induced antidiuresis. *J Clin Invest* 1973; **52**: 535–42.
41. Matsukura S, Matsumoto J, Chihara K *et al.* Clofibrate-induced myopathy in patients with diabetes insipidus. *Endocrinol Jpn* 1980; **27**: 401–3.
42. Wuller S, Wiesner B, Loffler A *et al.* Pharmacochaperones post-translationally enhance cell surface expression by increasing conformational stability of wild type and mutant vasopressin V2 receptors. *J Biol Chem* 2004; **279**: 47254–63.
43. Bernier V, Morello JP, Zarruk A *et al.* Pharmacologic chaperones as a potential treatment for X-linked nephrogenic diabetes insipidus. *J Am Soc Nephrol* 2006; **17**: 232–43.
44. Durr JA, Stamoutsos B, Lindheimer MD. Osmoregulation during pregnancy in the rat. Evidence for resetting of the threshold for vasopressin secretion during gestation. *J Clin Invest* 1998; **68**: 337–46.
45. Lindheimer MD, Davison JM. Osmoregulation, the secretion of arginine vasopressin and its metabolism during pregnancy. *Eur J Endocrinol* 1995; **132**: 133–43.
46. Schrier RW, Durr J. Pregnancy: an overfill or underfill state. *Am J Kidney Dis* 1987; **9**: 284–9.
47. Dschietzig T, Stangl K. Relaxin: a pregnancy hormone as central player of body fluid and circulation homeostasis. *Cell Mol Life Sci* 2003; **60**: 688–700.
48. Durr JA, Haggard JG, Hunt JM *et al.* Diabetes insipidus in pregnancy associated with abnormally high circulating vasopressin activity. *N Engl J Med* 1987; **316**: 1070–4.
49. Iwasaki Y, Osio Y, Kondo K *et al.* Aggravation of subclinical diabetes insipidus during pregnancy. *N Engl J Med* 1991; **324**: 522–6.
50. Cammu H, Velkeniers B, Charels K *et al.* Idiopathic acute fatty liver of pregnancy associated with transient diabetes insipidus. *Br J Obstet Gynaecol* 1987; **94**: 173–8.
51. de Heide LJM, van Tol KM, Doorenbos B. Pituitary apoplexy presenting during pregnancy. *Netherl J Med* 2004; **62**: 393–6.
52. Jin-no Y, Kamiya Y, Okado M *et al.* Pregnant woman with transient diabetes insipidus resistant to 1-desamino-8-D-arginine vasopressin. *Endocrinol J* 1998; **45**: 693–6.
53. Hoashi S, Margey R, Haroum A *et al.* Gestational diabetes insipidus, severe hypernatraemia and hyperemesis gravidarum in a primigravid pregnancy. *Endocrinol Abstr* 2004; 7: 297.
54. de Leon J. Polydipsia: a study in a long-term psychiatric unit. *Eur Arch Psychiatry Clin Neurosci* 2003; **253**: 37–9.
55. Rao KJ, Miller M, Moses A. Water intoxication and thioridazine. *Ann Intern Med* 1975; **82**: 61–5.
56. Martin JB, Riskind PN. Neurologic manifestations of hypothalamic disease. *Prog Brain Res* 1992; **93**: 31–40.
57. Zerbe RL, Robertson GL. A comparison of plasma vasopressin measurements with a standard indirect test in the differential diagnosis of polyuria. *N Engl J Med* 1981; **305**: 1539–46.
58. Bayliss PH, Robertson GL. Osmoregulation of vasopressin secretion in health and disease. *Clin Endocrinol* 1988; **29**: 549–76.
59. Mohn N, Acerini CL, Cheetham TD *et al.* Hypertonic saline test for the investigation of posterior pituitary function. *Arch Dis Child* 1998; **79**: 431–4

52

Thyroid emergencies

Jonathan Handy

Thyroid emergencies are a rare cause for admission to critical care. However, mortality is high unless specific treatment is provided in an expeditious manner. Abnormal thyroid function tests are commonly encountered during critical illness; numerous factors must be considered before interpreting these findings as indicating thyroid disease.

BASIC PHYSIOLOGY

Thyroid hormones affect the function of virtually every organ system and must be constantly available for these functions to continue. The two biologically active hormones are tetraiodothyronine (thyroxine or T_4) and triiodothyronine (T_3). These are synthesised by incorporating iodine into tyrosine residues, a process which occurs in thyroglobulin contained within the lumena of the thyroid gland. Stimulation of hormone release by thyroid-stimulating hormone (TSH) results in endocytosis of thyroglobulin from the lumen into the follicular cells, followed by hydrolysis to form T_4 and T_3, which are released into the circulation.[1]

Both T_4 and T_3 contain two iodine atoms on their inner (tyrosine) ring. They differ in that T_4 contains two further iodine atoms on its outer (phenol) ring, whereas T_3 contains only one. T_4 is produced solely by the thyroid gland whereas the majority of T_3 is synthesised peripherally by the removal of one iodine atom (deiodination) from the outer ring of T_4. If deiodination of an inner-ring iodine atoms occurs, the metabolically inert reverse-T_3 (rT_3) is formed. This is produced in preference to T_3 during starvation and many non-thyroidal illnesses, and the ratio of inactive (rT_3) to active T_3 synthesis appears to play an important role in the control of metabolism.[2] Numerous factors can affect the peripheral deiodination process (Table 52.1). Both T_4 and T_3 are highly protein-bound in the serum, predominantly to thyroid-binding globulin (TBG), but to a lesser extent to albumin and prealbumin. Changes in concentration of these serum-binding proteins have a large effect on total T_4 and T_3 serum concentrations. Such protein changes do not, however, affect the concentration of free hormone or their rates of metabolism. The serum-binding proteins act as both a store and a buffer to allow an immediate supply of the metabolically active free T_4 (fT_4) and free T_3 (fT_3). In addition, protein binding reduces the glomerular filtration and renal excretion of the hormones.

On reaching the target organs, fT_4 and fT_3 enter the cells predominantly by diffusion. Here, microsomal enzymes deiodinate the fT_4 to form fT_3. This varies in differing tissues, the majority occurring in the liver, kidneys and muscles. The fT_3 subsequently diffuses into the nucleus where it binds nuclear receptors and exerts its effect through stimulation of messenger RNA (mRNA) with subsequent synthesis of polypeptides, including hormones and enzymes. The role of thyroid hormones in development and homeostasis is widespread and profound: the most obvious effects are to stimulate basal metabolic rate and sensitivity of the cardiovascular and nervous systems to catecholamines.

The regulation of thyroid function is predominantly determined by three main mechanisms, the latter two providing physiological control. Firstly, availability of iodine is crucial for the synthesis of the thyroid hormones. Dietary iodide is absorbed and rapidly distributed in the extracellular fluid, which also contains iodide released from the thyroid gland and from peripheral deiodination processes. This becomes trapped within thyroid follicular cells, from which it is actively transported into the lumen to be oxidised into iodine and subsequently combined with tyrosine.[3] Other ions, such as perchlorate and pertechnetate, share this follicular cell active transport mechanism, acting as competitive inhibitors for the process.

Secondly, thyroid hormone release is controlled by a closed feedback loop with the anterior pituitary. Diminished levels of circulating hormones trigger secretion of TSH which acts on the follicular cells of the thyroid gland, causing them to release thyroglobulin-rich colloid from the lumen, which is hydrolysed to form T_4 and T_3 for systemic release. Increased levels of T_4 and T_3 cause diminished TSH secretion, resulting in the follicular cells becoming flat and allowing increased capacity for colloid storage. As a result, less thyroglobulin is mobilised and hydrolysed with less T_4 and T_3 release. The degree to which TSH is secreted in response to changes in circulating thyroid hormones is dependent on the hypothalamic

Table 52.1 States associated with decreased deiodination of thyroxine to triiodothyronine

- Systemic illness
- Fasting
- Malnutrition
- Postoperative state
- Trauma
- Drugs: propylthiouracil; glucocorticoids; propranolol; amiodarone
- Radiographic contrast agents (ipodate, ipanoate)

hormone thyrotrophin-releasing hormone (TRH), which is itself modulated by feedback from the thyroid hormones. TRH secretion is inhibited by dopamine, glucocorticoids and somatostatin.

Lastly, further regulation occurs during the enzyme-dependent peripheral conversion of fT_4 to fT_3. It is this latter stage that provides the rapid and fine control of local fT_3 availability. All of these mechanisms may be altered by drugs, and in pathological states.

THYROID CRISIS (THYROID STORM)

Thyrotoxic storm is arguably the most serious complication of hyperthyroidism, with reported mortality ranging from 10 to 75% in hospitalised patients.[4,5] Crisis most commonly occurs as a result of unrecognised or poorly controlled Graves disease; however, other underlying diseases may be the cause.[6,7] Females outnumber males. Laboratory findings are inconsistent due to acute disruption of the normal steady state of the circulating hormones, and there is no definitive value that separates thyrotoxicosis from thyroid storm. The latter is a clinical diagnosis and a scoring system has been proposed to guide the likelihood of the diagnosis (Figure 52.1).[8] Precipitating factors are not always present, though many have been identified (Table 52.2).

CLINICAL PRESENTATION (TABLE 52.3)

The classic signs of thyroid crisis include fever, tachycardia, tremor, diarrhoea, nausea and vomiting.[9] However presentation is extremely variable and may range from apathetic hyperthyroidism (apathy, depression, hyporeflexia and myopathy)[10] to multiple-organ dysfunction.[11,12] Differential diagnosis includes sepsis and other causes of hyperpyrexia such as adrenergic and anticholinergic syndromes.

FEVER

This is the most characteristic feature. Temperature may rise above 41°C. There have been suggestions that pyrexia is present in all cases of thyroid storm,[13] though normothermia has been reported.[11] Pyrexia is rare in uncomplicated thyrotoxicosis and should always raise suspicion of thyroid storm. It is not clear whether this febrile response is due to alteration of central thermoregulation or elevation of basal metabolic thermogenesis beyond the body's ability to lose heat.

CARDIOVASCULAR FEATURES

Fluid requirements may be substantial in some patients, whereas diuresis may be required in those with severe cardiac congestion. Cardiac decompensation can occur in young patients with no known antecedent cardiac disease. Systolic hypertension with widened pulse pressure is common initially; however hypotension supervenes later. Cardiogenic shock with vascular collapse is a preterminal sign.[14] Arrhythmias are common and include atrial and polymorphic ventricular tachycardias. The latter may result from prolonged QTc interval, the presence of which may complicate and contraindicate the use of amiodarone therapy.

NEUROMUSCULAR FEATURES

Tremor is a common early sign, but as 'storm' progresses, central nervous dysfunction evolves with progression to encephalopathy or even coma.[15] Thyroid storm has been reported in association with status epilepticus and cerebrovascular accident.[16] Weakness may be a feature, particularly with apathetic thyrotoxicosis.[10] Thyrotoxic myopathy and rhabdomyolysis may be present,[11,17] the latter being differentiated from the former by its association with markedly elevated creatine phosphokinase levels. A number of other syndromes of neuromuscular weakness have been described, including hypokalaemic periodic paralysis[18] and myasthenia gravis.[19]

GASTROINTESTINAL FEATURES

Diarrhoea, nausea and vomiting are common, though the patient may present with symptoms of an acute abdomen.[20] Severe abdominal tenderness should raise the possibility of an abdominal emergency. Liver function tests may be abnormal due to congestion or necrosis and tenderness over the hepatic area may be present. Hepatosplenomegaly may be present. The presence of jaundice is a poor prognostic sign.[14]

RESPIRATORY CONSIDERATIONS

Dyspnoea at rest or on exertion may be present for a number of reasons. Oxygen consumption and carbon dioxide production are increased with subsequent increase in the respiratory burden. This may be exacerbated by pulmonary oedema, respiratory muscle weakness and tracheal obstruction from enlarged goitre (rare).

LABORATORY FINDINGS

Numerous abnormalities may be found:

- fT_4 and fT_3 are usually increased, though this does not correlate with clinical severity: TSH is undetectable

Temperature (°C)	Pulse	Cardiac failure	CNS effects	GI symptoms	Score
Normal	<99	Absent	Normal	Normal	0
37.2–37.7	99–109	Pedal oedema	-	-	5
37.8–38.2	110–119	Bibasal crepitations Atrial fibrillation	Agitation	Diarrhoea Nausea Vomiting Abdominal pain	10
38.3–38.8	120–129	Pulmonary oedema	-	-	15
38.9–39.3	130–139	-	Delirium	Unexplained jauntice	20
39.4–39.9	>140	-	-	-	25
>40	-	-	Seizure Coma	-	30

Calculations:

- Add the scores for each of the five clinically observed parameters
- Add a furthr *10 points* if *atrial fibrillation* is present
- Add a furthr *10 points* if an identifiable *precipitating factor* is present

- Total score of *45* or greater is highly suggestive of thyroid storm
- Total score of *25–44* supports impending crisis
- Total score of less than *25* makes thyroid storm unlikely

Figure 52.1 Severity assessment in thyroid crisis. CNS, central nervous system; GI, gastrointestinal. (Adapted from Tewari K, Balderston KD, Carpenter SE *et al.* Papillary thyroid carcinoma manifesting as thyroid storm of pregnancy: case report. *Am J Obstet Gynecol* 1998; **179**: 818–19.)

- hyperglycaemia in non-diabetics
- leukocytosis with a left shift, even in the absence of infection (leukopenia may be present in patients with Graves disease)
- abnormal liver function tests and hyperbilirubinaemia
- hypercalcaemia due to haemoconcentration and the effect of thyroid hormones on bone resorption
- hypokalaemia and hypomagnesaemia (particularly in apathetic thyrotoxicosis)
- serum cortisol should be elevated. If low values are found, adrenal insufficiency should be considered and treated. Adrenal reserve in thyrotoxic patients is often exceeded in the absence of absolute adrenal insufficiency

MANAGEMENT

Treatment is aimed at:

- control and relief of adrenergic symptoms
- correction of thyroid hormone abnormalities
- the precipitating cause
- investigation and treatment of the underlying thyroid disease
- supportive measures

β-ADRENERGIC BLOCKADE

This is the mainstay of controlling adrenergic symptoms.[21] Intravenous propranolol titrated in 0.5–1-mg increments,

Table 52.2 Factors associated with precipitating thyroid storm

- Infection; sepsis
- Withdrawal of antithyroid treatment
- Surgery; trauma
- Parturition
- Diabetic ketoacidosis
- Radioactive iodine therapy
- Iodinated contrast dyes
- Hypoglycaemia
- Excessive palpation of the thyroid gland
- Emotional stress
- Burn injury
- Pulmonary thromboembolism
- Cerebrovascular accident; seizure disorder (including eclampsia)
- Thyroid hormone overdose

Table 52.3 Clinical features of hyperthyroidism/thyroid crisis

- **Fever**
- **Cardiovascular**
  - Tachycardia, atrial fibrillation, ventricular arryhthmias
  - Heart failure
  - Hypertension (early), hypotension (late)
- **Neuromuscular**
  - Tremor
  - Encephalopathy, coma
  - Weakness
- **Gastrointestinal**
  - Diarrhoea, nausea and vomiting
- **Respiratory**
  - Dyspnoea
  - Increased oxygen consumption and carbon dioxide production
- **Goitre (possible airway compromise)**
- **Laboratory abnormalities**

while monitoring cardiovascular response, diminishes the systemic hypersensitivity to catecholamines. In addition it inhibits peripheral conversion of T_4 to T_3.[22] Concurrent administration of enteral propranolol is the norm, with doses as high as 60–120 mg 4–6-hourly often being necessary due to enhanced elimination during thyroid crisis.[23] An alternative regimen uses intravenous esmolol with a loading dose of 250–500 μg/kg followed by infusion at 50–100 μg/kg per min. This allows rapid titration of β-blockade while minimising adverse reactions.[24] β_1-selective antagonists such as metoprolol may be of use, particularly in the presence of reactive airways and heart failure. These agents do not inhibit conversion of T_4 to T_3 to the extent of non-selective β-antagonists and should be combined with other therapy. Patients who exhibit resistance to β-adrenergic blockade may be successfully treated with reserpine or guanethidine, though their onset of action is slow and side-effects may be significant.

DIGOXIN

Control of heart rate and rhythm may result in significant improvement in cardiac performance. Electrolyte imbalance, particularly hypokalaemia and hyomagnesaemia, should be corrected prior to drug therapy. Relative resistance to digoxin may occur due to increased renal clearance[25] and increased Na/K-ATPase units in cardiac muscle.[26] Arterial thromboembolic phenomena are common (10–40%) in thyrotoxicosis-related atrial fibrillation. This may be due to a procoagulant state or an increased incidence of mitral valve prolapse. Anticoagulation is controversial given the increased sensitivity to warfarin and potential for bleeding; however it should be considered in the management of these patients.

AMIODARONE

Amiodarone has theoretical benefits in thyrotoxicosis as it inhibits peripheral conversion of T_4 to T_3 and reduces the concentration of T_3-induced adrenoceptors.[27] It does however cause profound (and sometimes physiologically irrelevant) changes to thyroid function tests and should not therefore be used as the first-line agent. The presence of prolonged QTc interval should be excluded before commencing therapy.

THIONAMIDES

These drugs block de novo synthesis of thyroid hormones within 1–2 hours of administration, but have no effect on the release of preformed glandular stores of thyroid hormones. Transient leukopenia is common (20%) and agranulocytosis can rarely occur with carbimazole use.

Propylthiouracil

This is usually considered the drug of choice in thyroid storm due to its ability to block partially peripheral conversion of T_4 to T_3. Its main mechanism of action is to block the iodination of tyrosine. Only enteral preparations are available and absorption may be unpredictable during thyroid crisis. Rectal administration has been reported. Loading dose is 100 g followed by 100 mg every 2 hours.

Methimazole

Methimazole lacks peripheral effects, but has a long duration of action, making administration easier and more reliable. It may be used in combination with drugs that block peripheral T_4-to-T_3 conversion (such as iopanoate or ipodate). Only enteral preparations are available, though rectal administration has been reported. Loading dose is 100 g followed by 20 g every 8 hours.

Carbimazole

This is metabolised to methimazole and is rarely associated with agranulocytosis. Only enteral preparations are available.

IODINE

The release of preformed glandular thyroid hormones is inhibited by administering either inorganic iodine or lithium. Enterally administered iodides include Lugol's solution and sodium or potassium iodide. Intravenous infusion of sterile sodium iodide may be used at a dose of 1 g 12-hourly; however, this is not always available commercially. If not, it may be prepared by the hospital pharmacy. Iodine therapy should not commence without prior thionamide administration. Used alone, it will enrich hormone stores within the thyroid gland and exacerbate thyrotoxicosis.

Iodine-containing contrast media (e.g. ipodate and iopanoate) may be used instead of the simple iodides; the former blocking T_4-to-T_3 conversion and inhibiting the cardiac effects of T_4. Ipodate is administered orally as a loading dose of 3 g followed by 1 g daily. As with the iodides, treatment should always be preceded by thionamide administration.

LITHIUM

Lithium carbonate has a similar, though weaker, action to iodine and can be used in patients with iodine allergy. An initial dose regime of 300 mg 6-hourly has been used with subsequent dosage adjusted to maintain serum drug levels at about 1 mmol/l.[28] Renal and neurological toxicity tends to limit its use.

STEROIDS

Glucocorticoids reduce T_4-to-T_3 conversion and may modulate any autoimmune process underlying the thyroid crisis (e.g. Graves disease). In addition, relative glucocorticoid deficiency may be a feature of the crisis. An adrenocorticotrophic hormone (ACTH) stimulation test is desirable prior to administration of hydrocortisone (100 mg 6–8-hourly); alternatively dexamethasone (4 mg 6-hourly) can be administered until the test has been performed. Combination therapy with iodides can produce rapid results. Glucocorticoids are the most effective treatment for type 2 amiodarone-induced thyrotoxicosis.[29]

OTHER THERAPIES

Plasmapharesis, charcoal haemoperfusion and dantrolene have all been used as novel therapies in thyroid storm; however their use is not established or proven.

SUPPORTIVE THERAPY

Fluid management

Fluid management may be extremely difficult in patients suffering from thyroid storm, particularly the elderly. Fluid losses may be profound due to diarrhoea, vomiting, pyrexia and reduced intake. However, cardiac failure may also develop as a result of the high cardiac demand. Echocardiography and cardiac output monitoring may be invaluable in guiding therapy for such patients.

Nutrition

Thyrotoxic patients have high energy expenditure and may present with a significant energy, vitamin and nitrogen deficit. Nutritional requirements should take account of any deficit and the ongoing hypercatabolic state. Thiamine is usually supplemented.

Drug therapy

Consideration should be given to the enhanced metabolism and elimination of drugs that occur in thyrotoxic patients. Salicylates and furosemide should be avoided as they both displace thyroid hormones from their binding proteins and can rapidly exacerbate systemic symptoms.

Precipitating factors

Both the precipitating factors and the disease process underlying the thyroid crisis should be sought and treated aggressively. Infection is the leading precipitant of crisis; thus early microbiological cultures and antibiotic therapy should be considered.

MYXOEDEMA COMA

Myxoedema coma is the extreme manifestation of hypothyroidism which, although rare, carries a mortality ranging from 30% to 60%. The term is a misnomer in that the majority of patients present with neither the non-pitting oedema, known as myxeodema, nor coma.[30] The condition should be considered in any patient presenting with reduced level of consciousness and hypothermia. The crisis occurs most commonly in elderly women with long-standing undiagnosed or undertreated hypothyroidism in whom an additional significant stress is experienced. Numerous precipitating factors have been identified (Table 52.4).

Table 52.4 Factors precipitating myxoedema coma

- Infection
- Cold environmental temperatures/hypothermia
- Burns
- Stroke
- Surgery
- Trauma
- Chronic heart failure
- Carbon dioxide retention
- Gastrointestinal haemorrhage
- Hypoglycaemia
- Carbon dioxide retention
- Gastrointestinal haemorrhage
- Hypoglycaemia
- Medications
    - Amiodarone
    - Anaesthetic agents
    - Analgesics/narcotics
    - Beta-blockers
    - Diuretics
    - Lithium
    - Phenytoin
    - Rifampicin
    - Sedatives/tranquillisers

CLINICAL PRESENTATION (TABLE 52.5)

Myxoedema coma can be defined when decreased mental status, hypothermia and clinical features of hypothyroidism are present (see Table 52.5). When these features are present, diagnosis is straightforward; however, asymptomatic or atypical presentation (e.g. decreased mobility) may occur.[31]

NEUROMUSCULAR

Alteration of conscious or mental state is present in all patients. This can range from personality changes to coma, with about 25% of patients experiencing seizures prior to the onset of coma. Electroencephalogram usually reveals non-specific changes. Weakness is common and skeletal muscle dysfunction may develop secondary to increased membrane permeability. The latter can lead to a rise in creatine phosphokinase. Hyponatraemia is present in up to 50% of patients and may contribute to alterations in conscious level (see below). Lumbar puncture often reveals elevated protein levels and a high opening pressure.

Table 52.5 Clinical features of myxoedema coma

- **Neuromuscular**
  - Abnormal conscious level
  - Psychiatric alterations
  - Weakness
  - Slow relaxing reflexes
  - Fatigue
- **Hypothermia**
- **Cardiovascular**
  - Diastolic hypertension
  - Bradycardia
  - Low cardiac output
  - Pericardial effusions
  - Electrocardiogram alterations
- **Respiratory**
  - Diminshed central response to hypoxia and hypercapnia
  - Respiratory alkalosis
  - Respiratory muscle weakness
  - Increased sensistivity to sedative drugs
  - Pleural effusions
  - Sleep apnoea
- **Airway**
  - Deep voice, goitre, vocal cord oedema, macroglossia
- **Gastrointestinal**
  - Gastric atony, distension, paralytic ileus, faecal impaction and megacolon (late)
  - Weight gain
  - Malabsoprtion
  - Ascites (rare)
- **Bladder dystension, urinary retention**
- **Cold intolerance**
- **Coarse hair**
- **Dry, pale, cool skin**
- **Laboratory abnormalities**

HYPOTHERMIA

Hypothermia represents the decrease in thermogenesis that accompanies reduced metabolism and is exacerbated by low ambient temperatures. Mortality is proportional to the degree of hypothermia. A low-reading thermometer should be used during assessment.

CARDIOVASCULAR FEATURES

Diastolic hypertension is due to increased systemic vascular resistance and blood volume reduction;[32] however myxoedema is associated with bradycardia and impaired myocardial contractility, with reduced cardiac output and hypotension a common feature. While pericardial effusions may occur, tamponade is uncommon. Creatine phosphokinase may be elevated, though this more commonly originates from skeletal rather than cardiac muscle. Acute coronary syndrome must nevertheless be excluded as a precipitant of the crisis. Electrocardiographic changes include bradycardia, decreased voltage, non-specific ST and T changes, varying types of block and prolonged QT interval. All of the cardiovascular abnormalities are reversible with thyroid hormone treatment.[33]

RESPIRATORY FEATURES

Hypothyroidism causes numerous respiratory alterations (see Table 52.5). There is a propensity to respiratory alkalosis, particularly during artificial ventilation. This is due to low metabolic rate, which may be compounded by iatrogenic hyperventilation.[34] Diaphragmatic weakness may occur due to abnormalities of the phrenic nerve; as a result, exercise tolerance may be significantly reduced. These abnormalities improve with thyroid hormone replacement, though full recovery can take several months.

LABORATORY FINDINGS

Thyroid function tests will reveal low T_4 and T_3; TSH is raised in primary and low in secondary and tertiary hypothyroidism. Hyponatraemia is common and usually develops due to free water retention resulting from excess vasopressin secretion or impaired renal function.[35] It may be severe and can contribute to diminished mental function. Although total body water is increased, intravascular volume is usually decreased. Hypoglycaemia may result from hypothyroidism alone, or as a result of concurrent adrenal insufficiency (Schmidt's syndrome). The mechanism is probably reduced gluconeogenesis, but infection and starvation may contribute. Azotaemia and hypophosphataemia are common; renal function may be severely abnormal due to low cardiac output and vasoconstriction. Mild leukopenia and normocytic anaemia are frequently present, though macrocytic and pernicious anaemia due to autoimmune dysfunction may occur. Arterial blood gases often reveal respiratory acidosis, hypoxia and hypercapnia.

MANAGEMENT

The mainstay of therapy consists of thyroid hormone replacement, steroid replacement and supportive measures. Once clinical diagnosis has been made or is suspected, blood should be collected for thyroid function and plasma cortisol tests. This should be followed by thyroid hormone treatment, which should not be delayed to await laboratory results. Consideration should be given to identifying and treating precipitating factors and complications of the crisis.

THYROID HORMONE THERAPY

All patients with suspected myxoedema coma should receive presumptive treatment with thyroid hormone. The optimum speed, type, route and dose of thyroid hormone replacement in myxedema coma are unknown due to the rarity of the condition and paucity of trials. The severity of clinical presentation does not correlate with the doses of replacement hormone required. Rapid replacement can result in life-threatening myocardial ischaemia or arrhythmias; delayed therapy exposes patients to prolonged risk of complications from the crisis. Both scenarios are associated with increased mortality.

Some experts favour administration of T_3 as it is biologically more active; has more rapid onset of action; and bypasses the impaired deiodination of T_4 to T_3 which occurs in hypothyroidism and non-thyroidal illness. High serum T_3 concentration has, however, been associated with increased mortality[36] and T_3 is expensive and may be difficult to obtain. T_3 may be administered orally or intravenously and has been combined with T_4 therapy.[37]

Most authorities recommend use of T_4 alone[38,39] as the delayed conversion to T_3 allows more gradual replacement of the deficient hormone. Bioavailability of orally administered T_4 is unpredictable given the high incidence of gastrointestinal dysfunction; therefore intravenous administration is more frequently used. A loading dose of intravenous levothyroxine 100–500 mcg is recommended[38] as this saturates the binding proteins. This should be followed by 50–100 mcg daily until conversion to the bioequivalent oral formulation is possible. The doses must be adjusted to allow for patient age, weight and cardiovascular risk factors; the lower doses should be administered to patients who are elderly, frail or have comorbidities (particularly cardiovascular disease).

CORTICOSTEROIDS

Corticosteroids are an important part of treatment as relative or absolute hypoadrenalism may occur concurrently with hypothyroid disease. A random serum cortisol level should be collected prior to commencing hydrocortisone therapy at 100 mg 8-hourly. If ACTH stimulation test is warranted, dexamethasone 4 mg 6-hourly should be commenced with conversion to hydrocortisone or cessation of treatment once the results are known. If random serum cortisol levels return at normal levels, steroid treatment can be discontinued.

SUPPORTIVE THERAPY

Hypothermia should be treated by passive rewarming where possible but active measures may be required. Appropriate cardiovascular, temperature gradient, electrolyte and acid–base monitoring should be provided during the rewarming phase in order to prevent haemodynamic and metabolic compromise.

Numerous alterations in respiratory physiology occur, including hypoventilation and altered response to arterial oxygen and carbon dioxide tensions. In addition, anatomical changes to the airway, delayed gastric empyting and increased sensitivity to sedative drugs may be present. These changes should be considered when mechanical ventilation is required, particularly during intubation and the weaning process.[34]

Patients usually present with intravascular fluid depletion despite peripheral oedema. Cardiac output monitoring may help guide fluid resuscitation and therapy. Echocardiography is useful in identifying cardiac dysfunction and pericardial effusions and assisting in assessment of intravascular volume status. Cardiac monitoring should be used to alert to the presence of arrhythmias. Inotropes and vasopressors should be avoided where possible due to their potential to precipitate cardiac arrhythmias. Where inotropes are required, increased dosage may be necessary as reduction in β-adrenoceptors is common. α-adrenoceptor function is usually preserved.

Hyponatraemia is reversible with thyroid hormone treatment, but severe abnormalities contributing to neurological dysfunction may require more expeditious correction. Free water intake should be restricted and hypertonic saline solutions may be required. Hypotonic fluid therapy should be avoided. If glucose therapy is required, hypertonic solutions (20–50%) should be infused via a central venous catheter.

Precipitating factors must be considered. As with all critically ill patients, microbial cultures should be collected and antibiotic therapy commenced unless cultures are negative. Prophylaxis against venous thromboembolism and peptic ulceration should be considered. Enteral feeding should be attempted but may be unsuccessful if gastrointestinal dysfunction and stasis are present.

NON-THYROIDAL ILLNESS

Non-thyroidal illness describes the phenomenon of starved or systemically unwell patients with abnormal serum thyroid function tests but with no apparent thyroidal illness. Low T_3, T_4 and TSH are commonly found; the degree of abnormality correlates with the severity of illness. Variants of these hormone levels are well described. Low serum T_3 is a frequent finding and occurs due to downregulation of the monodeiodinase enzyme that converts T_4 to T_3, while rT_3 may increase due to increased activity of the T_4-to-rT_3 monodeiodinase.[40]

Serum T_4 is also commonly low in the critically ill. This is due to a decrease in the concentration of thyroid

Table 52.6 Changes in thyroid hormone concentrations

	fT4	T_3	TSH
Euthyroid	N	N	N
Hyperthyroid	↑	↑	↓
Hypothyroid	↓	↓ N	↑
Non-thyroidal illness	↑ N ↓	↓	N ↓

fT4, free tetraiodothyronine; T_3, triiodothyronine; TSH, thyroid-stimulating hormone; N, normal; ↑ increased; ↓ decreased.

hormone-binding proteins and the presence of inhibitors that reduce T_4 binding to these proteins. There is also the suggestion that T_4 entry into cells may be impaired.[41] Free T_4 levels should be normal in less severe illness; however, in severe illness, the level may be low due to inadequate correction during the fT_4 assay.[42]

Low serum TSH levels were previously thought to be associated with the euthyroid state; however more recent work suggests that acquired transient central hypothyroidism is present in these patients.[43] Cytokines such as tumour necrosis factor-α are known to inhibit TSH secretion. Such phenomena are probably evolutionary adaptations to conserve protein and energy during severe illness. Elevated TSH may also occur in non-thyroidal illness, but few of these patients prove to have hypothyroidism following recovery from their acute illness.

Changes in thyroid function test are well described during starvation, sepsis, bone marrow transplantation, surgery, myocardial infarction, coronary artery bypass surgery and probably any critical illness. However, replacement of thyroid hormone in these patients is of no benefit and may be harmful;[44] hence thyroid function should not be assessed in critically ill patients unless there is a strong clinical indication to do so. A number of specific non-thyroidal illnesses are associated with abnormal thyroid function tests. These include: some psychiatric illnesses; hepatic disease; nephritic syndrome; acromegaly; acute intermittent porphyria; and Cushing's syndrome.[45] Where assays are performed, TSH should not be interpreted in isolation as low values will not discriminate between true thyroid and non-thyroidal disease. If low T_4 is also present, non-thyroidal illness is likely. If T_4 is elevated then hyperthyroidism is the likely diagnosis, though elevated T_4 has been documented in non-thyroidal illness.

Given the alterations in these hormones and difficulties with their assay during critical illness, thyroid hormone replacement should not be undertaken on the strength of thyroid function test results alone: additional laboratory and clinical indications must also be present (Table 52.6).

REFERENCES

1. Kopp P. Thyroid hormone synthesis. In: Braverman LE, Utiger RD (eds) *The Thyroid: Fundamental and Clinical Text*, 9th edn. Philadelphia: Lippincott Williams and Wilkins; 2005: 52.
2. Marshall W, Bangert S. The thyroid gland. In: Marshall W, Bangert S (eds) *Clinical Chemistry*, 5th edn. Mosby, Elsevier; 2004: 161–75.
3. Spitzweg C, Heufelder AE, Morris JC. Thyroid iodine transport. *Thyroid* 2000; **10**: 321.
4. Dillman WH. Thyroid storm. *Curr Ther Endocrinol Metab* 1997; **6**: 81–5.
5. Tietgens ST, Leinung MC. Thyroid storm. *Med Clin North Am* 1995; **79**: 169–84.
6. Tewari K, Balderston KD, Carpenter SE *et al.* Papillary thyroid carcinoma manifesting as thyroid storm of pregnancy: case report. *Am J Obstet Gynecol* 1998; **179**: 818–19.
7. Naito Y, Sone T, Kataoka K *et al.* Thyroid storm due to functioning metastatic thyroid carcinoma in a burn patient. *Anaesthesiology* 1997; **87**: 433–5.
8. Burch HB, Wartofsky L. Life-threatening thyrotoxicosis. Thyroid storm. *Endocrinol Metab Clin North Am* 1993, **22**: 263.
9. Waldstein SS, Slodki SJ, Kaganiec GI. A clinical study of thyroid storm. *Ann Intern Med* 1960; **52**: 626–42.
10. Yi-Sun Y, Chong-Jen Y, Fen-Yu T. Apathetic hyperthyroidism associated with thyroid storm. *Geriatr Geron-tol Int* 2004; **4**: 255–8.
11. Jiang Y-Z, Hutchinson A, Bartelloni P *et al.* Thyroid storm presenting as multiple organ dysfunction syndrome. *Chest* 2000; **118**: 877–9.
12. Rufener S, Arunachalam V, Ajluni R *et al.* Thyroid storm precipitated by infection. *Endocrinologist* 2005; **15**: 111–14.
13. Mazzaferri MEL, Skillman TG. Thyroid storm: a review of 22 episodes with special emphasis on the use of guanethadine. *Arch Intern Med* 1969; **124**: 684–90.
14. Wartofsky L. Thyroid storm. In: Wass JAH, Shalet SM, Gale E (eds) *Oxford Textbook of Endocrinology and Diabetes.* Oxford: Oxford University Press; 2002: 481–5.
15. Aiello DP, DuPlessis AJ, Pattishall EG III *et al.* Thyroid storm presenting with coma and seizures. *Clin Pediatr* 1989; **28**: 571–4.
16. Lee TG, Ha CK, Lim BH. Thyroid storm presenting as status epilepticus and stroke. *Postgrad Med J* 1997; **73**: 61.
17. Lichstein DM, Arteaga RB. Rhabdomyolysis associated with hyperthyroidism. *Am J Med Science* 2006; **332**: 103–5.
18. Dias Da Silva MR, Cerutti JM *et al.* A mutation in the KCNE3 potassium channel gene is associated with susceptibility to thyrotoxic hypokalaemic periodic paralysis. *J Clin Endocrinol Metab* 2002; **87**: 4881–4.
19. Marino M, Ricciardi R, Pinchera A *et al.* Mild clinical expression of myasthenia gravis associated with autoimmune thyroid diseases. *J Clin Endocrinol Metab* 1997; **82**: 438–43.
20. Bhattacharyya A, Wiles PG. Thyrotoxic crisis presenting as acute abdomen. *J R Soc Med* 1997; **90**: 681–2.
21. Das G, Kreiger M. Treatment of thyrotoxic storm with intravenous administration of propranolol. *Ann Intern Med* 1969; **70**: 985.

22. Perrild H, Hansen JM, Skovsted L *et al.* Different effects of propranolol, alprenolol, sotalol, atenolol, and metoprolol on serum T3 and rT3 in hyperthyroidism. *Clin Endocrinol* 1983; **18**: 139.
23. Feely J, Forrest A, Gunn A *et al.* Propranolol dosage in thyrotoxicosis. *J Clin Endocrinol Metab* 1980; **51**: 658–61.
24. Brunette DD, Rothong C. Emergency department management of thyrotoxic crisis with esmolol. *Am J Emerg Med* 1991; **9**: 232.
25. Shenfield GM, Thompson J, Horn DB. Plasma and urinary digoxin in thyroid dysfunction. *Eur J Clin Pharmacol* 1977; **12**: 437–43.
26. Chaudhury S, Ismail-Beigi F, Gick GG *et al.* Effect of thyroid hormone on the abundance of Na,K adenosine triphosphate-subunit messenger ribonucleic acid. *Mol Endocrinol* 1987; **1**: 83–9.
27. Perret G, Yin YL, Nicolas P *et al.* Amiodarone decreases cardiac beta-adrenoceptors through an antagonistic effect on 3,5,3′triodothyronine. *J Cardiovasc Pharmacol* 1992; **19**: 541–5.
28. Boehm TM, Burman KD, Barnes S *et al.* Lithium and iodine combination therapy for thyrotoxicosis. *Acta Endocrinol (Copenh)* 1980; **94**: 174–83.
29. Bartalena L, Brogioni S, Grasso L *et al.* Treatment of amiodarone-induced thyrotoxicosis, a difficult challenge: results of a prospective study. *J Clin Endocrinol Metab* 1996; **81**: 2930–3.
30. Nicoloff JT, LoPresti JS. Myxedema coma. A form of decompensated hypothyroidism. *Endocrinol Metab Clin North Am* 1993; **22**: 279–90.
31. Mintzer MJ. Hypothyroidism and hyperthyroidism in the elderly. *J Fla Med Assoc* 1992; **79**: 231–5.
32. Streeten DHP, Anderson GH Jr, Howard T *et al.* Effects of thyroid function on blood pressure. *Hypertension* 1988; **11**: 78.
33. Shenoy MM, Goldman JM. Hypothyroid cardiomyopathy. Echocardiographic documentation of reversibility. *Am J Med Sci* 1987; **294**: 1.
34. Behnia M, Clay A, Farber M. Management of myedematous respiratory failure: review of ventilation and weaning principles. *Am J Med Sci* 2000; **320**: 368–73.
35. Iwasaki Y, Oisa Y, Yamauchi K *et al.* Osmoregulation of plasma vasopressin in myxedema. *J Clin Endocrinol Metab* 1990; **70**: 751.
36. Hylander B, Rosenqvist U. Treatment of myxoedema coma – factors associated with fatal outcome. *Acta Endocrinol (Copenh)* 1985; **108**: 65.
37. Wartofsky L. Myxedema coma. In: Braverman LE, Utiger RD (eds) *The Thyroid.* Philadelphia: Lippincott-Raven; 1996: 871.
38. Rodriguez I, Fluiters E, Perez-Mendez LF *et al.* Factors associated with mortality of patients with myxoedema coma: prospective study of 11 cases treated in a single institution. *J Endocrinol* 2004; **180**: 347.
39. Smallridge RC. Metabolic and anatomic thyroid emergencies: a review. *Crit Care Med* 1992; **20**: 276–91.
40. Peeters RP, Wouters PJ, Kaptein E *et al.* Reduced activation and increased inactivation of thyroid hormone in tissues of critically ill patients. *J Clin Endocrinol Metab* 2003; **88**: 3202.
41. De Groot LJ. Dangerous dogmas in medicine: the nonthyroidal illness syndrome. *J Clin Endocrin Metab* 1999; **84**: 151–64.
42. Chopra IJ, Solomon DH, Hepner GW *et al.* Misleading low free T4 index (FT4I) and usefulness of reverse T3 (rT3) measurement in nonthyroidal illness. *Ann Intern Med* 1979; **90**: 905.
43. Chopra IJ. Euthyroid sick syndrome: Is it a misnomer? *J Clin Endocrinol Metab* 1997; **82**: 329.
44. Utiger RD. Altered thyroid function in nonthyroidal illness and surgery. To treat or not to treat? *N Engl J Med* 1995; **333**: 1562.
45. Ross DS. Thyroid function in nonthyroidal illness. *Up To Date* 2006; version 14.2.

53

Adrenocortical insufficiency in critical illness

Balasubramanian Venkatesh and Jeremy Cohen

The adrenal glands form an essential part of the organism's response to stress. Hence, in intensive care, an adequate adrenal response is considered to be of prime importance. Whilst primary adrenal insufficiency (AI) is a well-recognised but rare condition in intensive care, secondary, or RAI, is thought to be more prevalent. Adrenocortical insufficiency may present as an insidious, occult disorder, unmasked by conditions of stress, or as a catastrophic syndrome that may result in death.

PHYSIOLOGY

The adrenal glands are functionally divided into medulla and cortex; the cortex is responsible for the secretion of three major classes of hormones: glucocorticoids, mineralocorticoids and sex hormones. The major pathogenic effects of disease result from cortisol and aldosterone deficiency.

Cortisol, the major glucocorticoid synthesised by the adrenal cortex, plays a pivotal role in normal metabolism. It is necessary for the synthesis of adrenergic receptors, normal immune function, wound healing and vascular tone. These actions are mediated by the glucocorticoid receptor, a member of the nuclear hormone receptor superfamily. The activated receptor migrates to the nucleus and binds to specific recognition sequences within target genes, but also interacts with numerous transcription factors and cytosolic proteins. Numerous isoforms of the glucocorticoids receptor have now been described; the alpha subtype, a 777-amino-acid polypeptide chain, was initially felt to be the primary mediator of glucocorticoid action. In contrast the beta isoform, a 742-amino-acid chain was felt to have no physiological activity. More recently it appears that the beta subtype has a negative effect on alpha-mediated gene transactivation, the physiological relevance of which remains controversial. Furthermore, additional isoforms have now been described, suggesting that glucocorticoid receptor diversity may be an important factor in understanding the complex effects of corticosteroid action.[1]

Under normal circumstances, cortisol is secreted in pulses, and in a diurnal pattern.[2] The normal basal output of cortisol is estimated to be 15–30 mg/day, producing a peak plasma cortisol concentration of 110–520 nmol/l (4–19 μg/dl) at 8–9 a.m., and a minimal cortisol level of $<$ 140 nmol/l ($<$ 5 μg/dl) after midnight. The daily output of aldosterone is estimated to be 100–150 μg/day.

Secretion is under the control of the hypothalamic–pituitary axis. There are a variety of stimuli to secretion, including stress, tissue damage, cytokine release, hypoxia, hypotension and hypoglycaemia. These factors act upon the hypothalamus to favour the release of corticotrophin-releasing hormone (CRH) and vasopressin. CRH is synthesised in the hypothalamus and carried to the anterior pituitary in portal blood, where it stimulates the secretion of adrenocorticotrophic hormone (ACTH), which in turn stimulates the release of cortisol, mineralocorticoids (principally aldosterone) and androgens from the adrenal cortex. CRH is the major (but not the only) regulator of ACTH release and is secreted in response to a normal hypothalamic circadian regulation and various forms of 'stress'. Vasopressin, oxytocin, angiotensin II and β-adrenergic agents also stimulate ACTH release while somatostatin, β-endorphin and enkephalin reduce it. Cortisol has a negative feedback on the hypothalamus and pituitary, inhibiting hypothalamic CRH release induced by stress, and pituitary ACTH release induced by CRH. During periods of stress, trauma or infection, there is an increase in CRH and ACTH secretion and a reduction in the negative-feedback effect, resulting in increased cortisol levels, in amounts roughly proportional to the severity of the illness.[3–5]

The majority of circulating cortisol is bound to an α-globulin called transcortin (corticosteroid-binding globulin, CBG). At normal levels of total plasma cortisol (e.g. 375 nmol/l or 13.5 μg/dl) less than 5% exists as free cortisol in the plasma; however it is this free fraction that is biologically active. Circulating CBG concentrations are approximately 700 nmol/l. In normal subjects CBG can bind approximately 700 nmol/l (i.e. 25 g/dl).[6] At levels greater than this, the increase in plasma cortisol is largely in the unbound fraction. The affinity of CBG for synthetic corticosteroids, with the exception of prednisolone, is negligible. CBG is a substrate for elastase, a polymorphonuclear enzyme that cleaves CBG, markedly decreasing its affinity for cortisol.[7] This enzymatic cleavage results in the liberation of free cortisol at sites of inflammation. CBG levels have been documented to fall during critical illness,[8–10] and these changes are postulated to increase the amount of circulating free cortisol.

Cortisol has a half-life of 70–120 minutes. It is primarily eliminated by hepatic metabolism and glomerular filtration. The excretion of free cortisol through the kidney represents 1% of the total secretion rate. Currently, available routine assays measure only total cortisol levels – bound and free.

The metabolic effects of cortisol are complex and varied. In the liver, cortisol stimulates glycogen deposition by increasing glycogen synthase and inhibiting the glycogen-mobilising enzyme glycogen phosphorylase.[11] Hepatic gluconeogenesis is stimulated, leading to increased blood glucose levels. Concurrently, glucose uptake by peripheral tissues is inhibited.[12] Free fatty acid release into the circulation is increased, and triglyceride levels rise.

In the circulatory system, cortisol increases blood pressure both by direct actions upon smooth muscle, and via renal mechanisms. The actions of pressor agents such as catecholamines are potentiated, whilst nitric oxide-mediated vasodilation is reduced.[13,14] Renal effects include an increase in glomerular filtration rate, and sodium transport in the proximal tubule, and sodium retention and potassium loss in the distal tubule.[15]

The primary effects of cortisol upon the immune system are anti-inflammatory and immunosuppressive. Lymphocyte cell counts decrease, whilst neutrophil counts rise.[15] Accumulation of immunologically active cells at inflammatory sites is decreased. The production of cytokines is inhibited, an effect that is mediated via nuclear factor (NF)-κB. This occurs both by induction of NF-κB inhibitor and by direct binding of cortisol to NF-κB, thus preventing its translocation to the nucleus. Whilst the well-defined effects of cortisol upon the immune system are primarily inhibitory, it is also suggested that normal host defence function requires some cortisol secretion. Cortisol has been described as having a positive effect upon immunoglobulin synthesis, potentiation of the acute-phase response, wound healing and opsonisation.[16]

CLASSIFICATION

AI may be considered to be primary, secondary or relative. Primary AI, otherwise known as Addison's disease, results from hypofunction of the adrenal cortex. Secondary AI occurs when there is suppression or absence of ACTH secretion from the anterior pituitary. RAI describes a situation of inadequate cortisol response to stress in the setting of critical illness.

PRIMARY ADRENAL INSUFFICIENCY

Primary AI or Addison's disease is a rare disorder. In the western world its estimated prevalence is 120 per million.[17] In adulthood, the commonest cause is autoimmune, but in the intensive care setting, consideration should be given to other causes of adrenal gland destruction (Table 53.1). These include infection, haemorrhage and infiltration. Tuberculosis is the commonest infective cause worldwide, but rarer infections such as histoplasmosis, coccidiomycosis and cytomegalovirus (especially in patients with human immunodeficiency virus (HIV)) have also been implicated. Haemorrhage into the glands is associated with septicaemias, particularly meningococcal (Waterhouse–Friedrichsen syndrome). Asplenia and the antiphospholipid syndrome may also be associated with adrenal haemorrhage. Adrenal gland destruction may also be secondary to infiltration with tumour, or amyloid.

Drugs may impair adrenal function either by inhibiting cortisol synthesis (etomidate, ketoconazole) or by inducing hepatic cortisol metabolism (rifampicin, phenytoin). High levels of circulating cytokines are also reported to have a suppressive effect upon ACTH release.[18]

Table 53.1 Causes of primary adrenal insufficiency

Infections
Tuberculosis
Histoplasmosis
Coccidiomycosis
Cytomegalovirus
Autoimmune-mediated
Haemorrhagic
Sepsis (especially meningococcal)
Antiphospholipid syndrome
Trauma
Surgery
Coagulation disorders
Infiltrative
Tumour
Amyloid
Sarcoidosis
Haemochromatosis
Drug-related
Etomidate
Fluconazole
Ketoconazole
Metyrapone
Suramin
Rifampicin
Phenytoin
Congenital
Adrenal dysgenesis
Adrenoleukodystrophy
Impaired steroidogenesis
Cytokine-mediated

PRESENTATION (Table 53.2)

The disease is often unrecognised in its early stages as the presenting features are ill-defined. Symptoms include tiredness and fatigue, vomiting, weight loss, anorexia and postural hypotension. Hyperpigmentation is seen in non-exposed areas (such as palmar skin creases) and is due to the hypersecretion of melatonin, a breakdown product from the ACTH precursor pro-opiomelanocortin (POMC).

Presentation to an intensive care physician is likely to be in the form of adrenal crisis. This may be precipitated by concurrent illness or surgery, or by failure to take replacement medication. Classically adrenal crisis will present as refractory shock with a poor response to inotropic or pressor agents. Abdominal or flank pain is often present and may lead to an erroneous diagnosis of an acute surgical abdomen.

Treatment should consist of immediate supportive measures, fluid resuscitation and high-dose intravenous glucocorticoid therapy. A standard dose would be 100 mg hydrocortisone 6-hourly, or as an infusion. At these doses separate mineralocorticoid replacement is not required.[19]

Adrenal crisis should be suspected in cases of undifferentiated shock not responding to standard management. Suggestive features would include a history of symptomatology consistent with the diagnosis, hyperpigmentation on examination, and demonstration of hyponatraemia, hyperkalaemia and peripheral blood eosinophilia. A random plasma total cortisol taken during a crisis will be low (below 80 nmol/l) and in the acute phase ACTH stimulation testing is not required.

Table 53.2 Clinical features of Addison's disease

Symptoms
Muscular weakness
Fatigue
Abdominal pain
Vomiting
Diarrhoea
Salt craving
Weight loss
Arthralgia and myalgia
Mood change
Headache
Sweating
Syncope
Signs
Hyperpigmentation – skin creases, buccal mucosa
Postural hypotension
Associated vitiligo
Decreased axillary and pubic hair
Auricular calcification
Vasodilated shock (in crisis)

SECONDARY ADRENAL INSUFFICIENCY

The commonest cause of ACTH deficiency is sudden cessation of exogenous glucocorticoid treatment. Patients who have been taking more than 30 mg/day hydrocortisone or equivalent for more than 3 weeks are at risk of adrenal suppression.[20] Other causes include pituitary surgery, pituitary infarction (Sheehan's syndrome) or pituitary tumour.

Presentation is similar to that of primary AI. The major distinguishing characteristics are a lack of hyperpigmentation, and the absence of mineralocorticoid deficiency; hence hyperkalaemia is not a feature of secondary AI, although hyponatraemia may still be present due to increased vasopressin levels.

INVESTIGATION OF ADRENAL INSUFFICIENCY

In a stable patient suspected AI is routinely investigated by an ACTH stimulation test. The test is performed by administering 250 μg of a synthetic ACTH molecule comprising the first 24 amino acids – tetracosactrin (Synacthen). Plasma total cortisol is measured at 0 and 30 minutes after administration, and a normal response is defined as a cortisol measurement over 525 nmol/l.[21] However, it should be noted that current immunoassays exhibit a significant degree of variability, and thus local laboratory reference ranges should be used.[22] The test cannot be performed if the patient is currently being prescribed hydrocortisone as this will cross-react with the assays; an alternative replacement therapy such as dexamethasone should be used in these cases.

Secondary AI may be differentiated from primary by a prolonged ACTH test. This is performed by the use of a depot preparation or an intravenous infusion of tetracosactrin for 24–48 hours. Patients with secondary hypoadrenalism show a greater plasma cortisol response at 24 hours than at 4 hours; alternatively measurement of a baseline ACTH level may be used. In patients with primary AI this will be elevated.

Other biochemical tests that may be used in investigation of AI include the insulin hypoglycaemia test, the overnight metyrapone test and the CRH stimulation test. These investigations are not normally necessary in uncomplicated cases. In addition the use of the low-dose ACTH stimulation test has been advocated, in which only 1 mcg of tetracosactrin is used. This approach has not yet gained widespread acceptance.

RELATIVE ADRENAL INSUFFICIENCY

The term *relative AI* (RAI) was coined to describe a syndrome where the adrenal gland partially responds to stress but the magnitude of response is not commensurate.

Annane *et al.* prospectively studied 189 patients with septic shock and detailed a three-level classification system based upon the basal cortisol level and response to ACTH.[23] Mortality was found to be highest in those patients with a basal cortisol level above 34 μg/dl (938 nmol/l) and

Table 53.3 Controversies in the diagnosis of adrenal insufficiency in the critically ill

Limitations of a random cortisol
In the critically ill there is a marked fluctuation in plasma cortisol concentration limiting the utility of a random cortisol[30]
The 'normal' range of cortisol in critical illness is not defined
There is no consensus 'cut-off' value below which adrenal insufficiency is present
Limitations of total cortisol
Free cortisol is the bioactive fraction of cortisol
There is a large variation in total cortisol assay results when the same specimen is tested in different laboratories and using different assays[22]
Peripheral tissue-specific glucocorticoid resistance is not tested
Limitations of the conventional Synacthen test
The HDSST results in plasma Synacthen concentrations that are supraphysiological
Published data may have overestimated the incidence of adrenal insufficiency, as many studies have not excluded patients who received etomidate
The low-dose SST may be more a better predictor of outcome

HDSST, high-dose short Synacthen test; SST, short Synacthen test.

response to ACTH of less than 9 μg/dl (248 nmol/l). Patients with a basal cortisol above 34 μg/dl but a cortisol response greater than 9 μg/dl did better, whilst the best prognosis was seen in the group with a lower basal cortisol level and high response to ACTH. This pattern – a high basal cortisol and blunted response to ACTH,[24–27] which is associated with increasing mortality – has now come to be referred to as RAI. The significance of this observation, however, is not clear. It has been suggested either to represent a partially suppressed adrenal axis, implying a role for cortisol replacement therapy, or alternatively as indicating an 'overstressed' axis, in which case steroid treatment would be inappropriate. Treatment of septic patients fulfilling RAI criteria with hydrocortisone has been shown to improve outcome in one study,[28] but these results have not been widely accepted (see below). Alternative diagnostic criteria, relying on baseline plasma cortisol levels without ACTH stimulation, have been proposed,[29] but the lack of a consistently observed relationship between cortisol levels and mortality means that the optimal diagnostic criteria for RAI remain controversial (Table 53.3). Possible explanations for the difficulties in assessing adrenal function in this patient group include spontaneous fluctuations in the measured cortisol values,[30] increased variability of assays,[22] and changes in CBG levels affecting free cortisol values.[10,31]

STEROID THERAPY IN CRITICAL ILLNESS

Steroids have an established role in the management of a number of critical illnesses, as outlined in Table 53.4.

Table 53.4 Proven role for steroids in critical illness

Addisonian crisis
Anaphylaxis
Asthma
Bacterial meningitis
Chronic obstructive pulmonary disease with acute respiratory failure
Croup
Fulminant vasculitis
Hypercalcaemia
Idiopathic thrombocytopenic purpura
Myasthenic crisis
Myxoedema coma
Organ transplantation
Pneumocystis carinii pneumonia
Thyroid storm

However their use in other conditions has not been without controversy.

SPINAL INJURY

High-dose methylprednisolone has been advocated in the management of patients with spinal cord injury following the publication of the National Acute Spinal Cord Injury Study (NASCIS) II and III trials. The major criticism of these studies is the lack of a demonstrable improvement in the primary outcome measures. For a more detailed review of the use of steroids in spinal cord injury, the reader is referred to Chapter 70.

HEAD INJURY

The role of steroids in the management of cerebral oedema secondary to tumours is well documented and accepted. However, their role in the management of head injury has been the subject of intense debate. Several prospective studies have not been able to prove any benefit with steroids in head trauma. However, these studies were not adequately powered to detect a difference. The recent Corticosteroid Randomization After Significant Head Injury (CRASH) trial, with nearly 10 000 patients, clearly demonstrated the lack of any benefit with steroids in head injury.[32]

ACUTE RESPIRATORY DISTRESS SYNDROME (ARDS)

The first clinical trial to report a beneficial effect of steroids in ARDS was the one by Meduri *et al.* in 1998.[33] In a randomised, placebo-controlled, cross-over single-centre trial enrolling 24 patients, steroids were shown to improve lung injury score and reduce mortality. The ARDS clinical trial network published the results of its multicentre study where corticosteroids were administered to patients with ARDS persisting beyond 7 days. Although steroid use was associated with earlier ventilatory wean, improved arterial oxygenation and increased respiratory compliance, there was a higher rate of return to assisted ventilation and neuromuscular weakness.[34] No overall mortality difference was demonstrable between steroid and placebo groups. Commencement of steroids more than 2 weeks after onset of ARDS led to almost a fourfold increase in mortality as compared to the placebo group. Consequently, steroids cannot be routinely recommended for persistent ARDS and may be harmful in late-stage ARDS.

SEPTIC SHOCK

Since the first reported use of steroids in sepsis in 1951, therapy with this drug has undergone several transformations from 'steroid success' in sepsis and malaria in the 1970s and early 1980s to 'steroid excess' (30 mg/kg methylprednisolone) in severe sepsis in the mid to late 1980s, to total abandonment in the early 1990s and finally a resurgence of its use in the new millennium. The results of the only prospective randomised trial of steroids in septic shock by Annane *et al.*,[28] which found a beneficial effect, have not been widely accepted owing to problems of randomisation, change of protocol and the use of etomidate (an adrenal suppressant drug) in the study. A recently published European multicenter randomised trial of steroids in septic shock Corticosteroid Therapy of Septic Shock (CORTICUS), did not demonstrate a mortality difference between steroids and placebo. However, this study has in turn been criticised for potential selection bias.

SIDE-EFFECTS OF STEROID THERAPY

Steroid therapy is associated with numerous side-effects. Those that would be of particular relevance to intensive care are discussed below. A full list is given in Table 53.5.

1. Suppression of the adrenal axis (discussed above). Patients who have been receiving steroid treatment for less than a week are unlikely to be affected.
2. Hyperglycaemia – this may be associated with adverse outcomes in critically ill patients.[35]
3. Myopathy: steroid therapy has been known to be associated with muscle weakness since 1932, but has only more recently been shown to be an independent risk factor for developing muscle paresis acquired in the intensive care unit.[36] This has significant clinical implications for weaning patients from mechanical ventilation.
4. Hypokalaemia.
5. Leukocytosis: corticosteroids increase the neutrophil count by a shift from the marginating to the circulating pool. This effect may lead to concerns that the patient has developed an occult infection.
6. Poor wound healing.
7. Immunosupression.
8. Pancreatitis.

Table 53.5 Side-effects of corticosteroid therapy

Adrenal suppression
Hypokalaemia
Glucose intolerance
Truncal obesity
Myopathy
Mood alterations, including psychosis
Hypertension
Osteoporosis
Peptic ulcer disease
Glaucoma
Hyperlipidaemia
Aseptic necrosis of femoral/humeral head

ROLE OF FLUDROCORTISONE IN SEPSIS

The role of fludrocortisone in septic shock also remains controversial. The study by Annane *et al.*, quoted above, included a dose of 50 μg fludrocortisone administered orally.[28] It has been argued, however, that doses of cortisol above 50 mg/day provide sufficient mineralocorticoid cover, and thus separate supplementation is unnecessary.[19]

Furthermore, the oral route of administration is unreliable in critically ill patients. A study comparing fludrocortisone plus hydrocortisone versus hydrocortisone alone in septic patients is currently recruiting.

REFERENCES

1. Yudt MR, Cidlowski JA. The glucocorticoid receptor: coding a diversity of proteins and responses through a single gene. *Mol Endocrinol* 2002; **16**: 1719–26.
2. Weitzman ED, Fukushima D, Nogeire C *et al.* Twenty-four hour pattern of the episodic secretion of cortisol in normal subjects. *J Clin Endocrinol Metab* 1971; **33**: 14–22.
3. Esteban NV, Loughlin T, Yergey AL *et al.* Daily cortisol production rate in man determined by stable isotope dilution/mass spectrometry. *J Clin Endocrinol Metab* 1991; **72**: 39–45.
4. Barton RN, Stoner HB, Watson SM. Relationships among plasma cortisol, adrenocorticotrophin, and severity of injury in recently injured patients. *J Trauma* 1987; **27**: 384–92.
5. Chernow B, Alexander HR, Smallridge RC *et al.* Hormonal responses to graded surgical stress. *Arch Intern Med* 1987; **147**: 1273–8.
6. Williams G, Dluhy R. Disorders of the adrenal cortex. In: Braunwald E, Fauci A, Kasper D *et al.* (eds) *Harrison's Principles of Internal Medicine.* New York: McGraw-Hill; 2001: 2001–84.
7. Pemberton PA, Stein PE, Pepys MB *et al.* Hormone binding globulins undergo serpin conformational change in inflammation. *Nature* 1988; **336**: 257–8.
8. Beishuizen A, Thijs LG, Vermes I. Patterns of corticosteroid-binding globulin and the free cortisol index

during septic shock and multitrauma. *Intens Care Med* 2001; **27**: 1584–91.
9. le Roux CW, Chapman GA, Kong WM *et al.* Free cortisol index is better than serum total cortisol in determining hypothalamic–pituitary–adrenal status in patients undergoing surgery. *J Clin Endocrinol Metab* 2003; **88**: 2045–8.
10. Hamrahian AH, Oseni TS, Arafah BM. Measurements of serum free cortisol in critically ill patients [see comment]. *N Engl J Med* 2004; **350**: 1629–38.
11. Stalmans W, Laloux M. Glucocorticoids and hepatic glycogen metabolism. In: JD Baxter, GG Rousseau, eds. *Glucocorticoid Hormone Action.* New York: Springer-Verlag; 1979: 518–33.
12. Olefsky JM. Effect of dexamethasone on insulin binding, glucose transport, and glucose oxidation of isolated rat adipocytes. *J Clin Invest* 1975; **56**: 1499–508.
13. Grunfeld JP, Eloy L. Glucocorticoids modulate vascular reactivity in the rat. *Hypertension* 1987; **10**: 608–18.
14. Saruta T, Suzuki H, Handa M *et al.* Multiple factors contribute to the pathogenesis of hypertension in Cushing's syndrome. *J Clin Endocrinol Metab* 1986; **62**: 275–9.
15. Larsen P, Kronenburg H, Melmed S *et al. Williams Textbook of Endocrinology*, 10th edn. Philadelphia, PA: WB Saunders; 2003: 219–25.
16. Burchard K. A review of the adrenal cortex and severe inflammation: quest of the 'eucorticoid' state. *J Trauma* 2001; **51**: 800–14.
17. Willis AC, Vince FP. The prevalence of Addison's disease in Coventry, UK. *Postgrad Med J* 1997; **73**: 286–8.
18. Bateman A, Singh A, Kral T *et al.* The immune–hypothalamic–pituitary–adrenal axis. *Endocrinol Rev* 1989; **10**: 92–112.
19. Shenker Y, Skatrud JB. Adrenal insufficiency in critically ill patients. *Am J Respir Crit Care Med* 2001; **163**: 1520–3.
20. Larsen P, Kronenberg H, Melmed S *et al. Williams Textbook of Endocrinology*, 10th edn. Philadelphia, PA: WB Saunders; 2003: 1009–16.
21. Clark PM, Neylon I, Raggatt PR *et al.* Defining the normal cortisol response to the short Synacthen test: implications for the investigation of hypothalamic–pituitary disorders [see comment]. *Clin Endocrinol* 1998; **49**: 287–92.
22. Cohen J, Ward G, Prins J *et al.* Variability of cortisol assays can confound the diagnosis of adrenal insufficiency in the critically ill population. *Intens Care Med* 2006; **32**: 1901–5.
23. Annane D, Sebille V, Troche G *et al.* A 3-level prognostic classification in septic shock based on cortisol levels and cortisol response to corticotropin. *JAMA* 2000; **283**: 1038–45.
24. Bollaert PE, Fieux F, Charpentier C *et al.* Baseline cortisol levels, cortisol response to corticotropin, and prognosis in late septic shock. *Shock* 2003; **19**: 13–15.
25. Aygen B, Inan M, Doganay M *et al.* Adrenal functions in patients with sepsis. *Exp Clin Endocrinol Diabetes* 1997; **105**: 182–6.
26. Soni A, Pepper GM, Wyrwinski PM *et al.* Adrenal insufficiency occurring during septic shock: incidence, outcome, and relationship to peripheral cytokine levels. *Am J Med* 1995; **98**: 266–71.
27. Moran JL, Chapman MJ, O'Fathartaigh MS *et al.* Hypocortisolaemia and adrenocortical responsiveness at onset of septic shock. *Intens Care Med* 1994; **20**: 489–95.
28. Annane D, Sebille V, Charpentier C *et al.* Effect of treatment with low doses of hydrocortisone and fludrocortisone on mortality in patients with septic shock [see comment]. *JAMA* 2002; **288**: 862–71.
29. Cooper MS, Stewart PM. Corticosteroid insufficiency in acutely ill patients. *N Engl J Med* 2003; **348**: 727–34.
30. Venkatesh B, Mortimer RH, Couchman B *et al.* Evaluation of random plasma cortisol and the low dose corticotropin test as indicators of adrenal secretory capacity in critically ill patients: a prospective study. *Anaesth Intens Care* 2005; **33**: 201–9.
31. Ho JT, Al-Musalhi H, Chapman MJ *et al.* Septic shock and sepsis: a comparison of total and free plasma cortisol levels. *J Clin Endocrinol Metab* 2006; **91**: 105–14.
32. Roberts I, Yates D, Sandercock P *et al.* Effect of intravenous corticosteroids on death within 14 days in 10008 adults with clinically significant head injury (MRC CRASH trial): randomised placebo-controlled trial. *Lancet* 2004; **364**: 1321–8.
33. Meduri GU, Headley AS, Golden E *et al.* Effect of prolonged methylprednisolone therapy in unresolving acute respiratory distress syndrome: a randomized controlled trial. *JAMA* 1998; **280**: 159–65.
34. Steinberg KP, Hudson LD, Goodman RB *et al.* Efficacy and safety of corticosteroids for persistent acute respiratory distress syndrome. *N Engl J Med* 2006; **354**: 1671–84.
35. van den Berghe G, Wouters P, Weekers F *et al.* Intensive insulin therapy in the critically ill patients. *N Engl J Med* 2001; **345**: 1359–67.
36. De Jonghe B, Sharshar T, Lefaucheur JP *et al.* Paresis acquired in the intensive care unit: a prospective multicenter study. *JAMA* 2002; **288**: 2859–67.

54

Acute calcium disorders

Balasubramanian Venkatesh

Calcium is an important cation and the principal electrolyte of the body. A total of 1–2 kg is present in the average adult, of which 99% is found in bone. Of the remaining 1%, nine-tenths is present in the cells and only a tenth in the extracellular fluid. In plasma, 50% of the calcium is ionised, 40% bound to plasma proteins, mainly to albumin, and the remaining 10% is chelated to anions such as citrate, bicarbonate, lactate, sulphate phosphate and ketones.[1] The chelated fraction is usually of little clinical importance, but is increased in conditions where some of these anionic concentrations might be elevated, as in renal failure. Whilst most calcium inside the cell is in the form of insoluble complexes, the concentration of intracellular ionised calcium is about 0.1 μmol/l, creating a gradient of 10 000:1 between plasma and intracellular fluid levels of ionised calcium.[2] A schematic illustration of calcium distribution within the various body compartments is shown in Figure 54.1.

Because ionised calcium is the biologically active component of extracellular fluid calcium with respect to physiological functions (Table 54.1) and is also the reference variable for endocrine regulation of calcium homeostasis, its measurement is recognised as being one of prime importance in the management of disorders of calcium homeostasis.

HORMONAL REGULATION OF CALCIUM HOMEOSTASIS[1,3]

The concentration of ionised calcium in the plasma is subject to tight hormonal control, particularly parathyroid hormone (PTH). A G-protein-coupled calcium receptor plays a significant role in the maintenance of calcium homeostasis. This receptor, responsible for sensing extracellular calcium concentration, is present on the cell membrane of the chief cells of the parathyroid and in bone, gut and the kidney. In response to ionised hypocalcaemia, PTH secretion is stimulated, which in turns serves to restore serum calcium levels back to normal by increasing osteoclastic activity in the bone and renal reabsorption of calcium and stimulating renal synthesis of 1,25 $OH\text{-}D_3$ (calcitriol – the active metabolite of vitamin D), which increases gut absorption of calcium.

Calcitriol production is stimulated by hypocalcaemia, and vice versa. Calcitriol increases serum calcium by largely promoting gut reabsorption, and to a lesser extent renal reabsorption of calcium.

Calcitonin, a hypocalcaemic peptide hormone produced by the thyroid, acts as a physiological antagonist to PTH. Although calcitonin has been shown to reduce serum calcium levels in animals by increasing renal clearance of calcium and inhibiting bone resorption, its role in humans is less clear. Despite extreme variations in calcitonin levels, for example total lack in patients who have undergone total thyroidectomy, or excess plasma levels as seen in patients with medullary carcinoma of the thyroid gland, no significant changes in calcium and phosphate metabolism are seen. Calcitonin is useful as a pharmacological agent in the management of hypercalcaemia.

METABOLIC FACTORS INFLUENCING CALCIUM HOMEOSTASIS

Alterations in serum protein, pH, serum phosphate and magnesium closely impact on serum calcium concentrations. Total plasma calcium levels vary with alterations in plasma protein concentration. A correction is made for hypoalbuminaemia by adding 0.2 mmol/l to the measured serum calcium concentration for every 10 g/l decrease in serum albumin concentration below normal (40 g/l). The corresponding correction factor for globulins is – 0.04 mmol/l of serum calcium for every 10 g/l rise in serum globulin.

Changes in pH alter calcium protein binding. An increase in pH by 0.1 pH units results in a decrease in ionised calcium by approximately 0.1 mmol/l.[4]

Calcium and phosphate are closely linked by the following reaction in the extracellular fluid: $HPO_4^{2-} + Ca^{2+} = CaHPO_4$. Increases in serum phosphate shift the reaction to the right. When the calcium phosphate solubility product exceeds the critical value of 5 mmol/l, calcium deposition occurs in the tissues, resulting in a fall in serum calcium concentration and a secondary increase in PTH secretion. Reductions in phosphate concentration lead to corresponding changes in the opposite direction.

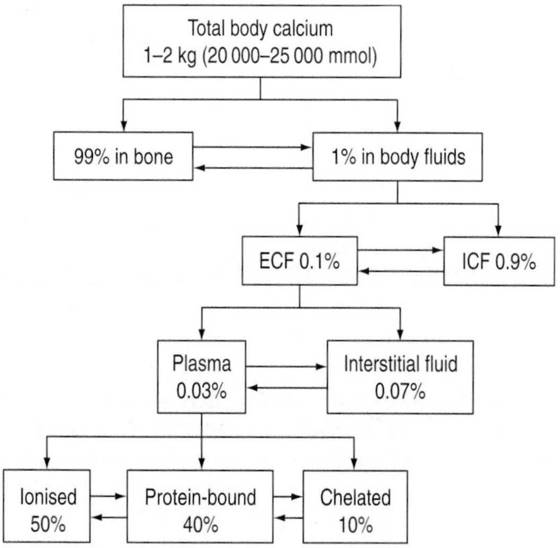

Figure 54.1 Distribution of body calcium. ECF, extracellular fluid; ICF, intracellular fluid.

Table 54.1 Functions of calcium[1,15]

Excitation – contraction coupling in cardiac, skeletal and smooth muscle
Cardiac action potentials and pacemaker activity
Release of neurotransmitters
Coagulation of blood
Bone formation and metabolism
Hormone release
Ciliary motility
Catecholamine responsiveness at the receptor site[7]
Role as a strong cation
Regulation of cell growth and apoptosis

As magnesium is required for PTH secretion and end-organ responsiveness, alterations in serum magnesium have an impact on serum calcium concentration.

Turnover of calcium in the bone is predominantly under the control of PTH and calcitriol, although prostaglandins and some of the cytokines also play a role in it. Bone resorption is mediated by osteoclasts, whereas osteoblasts are involved in bone formation. The daily calcium balance is summarised in Table 54.2.

MEASUREMENT OF SERUM CALCIUM

Most hospital laboratories measure total serum calcium. The normal plasma concentration is 2.2–2.6 mmol/l. However, the ionised form (1.1–1.3 mmol/l) is the active fraction and its measurement is not routine in many laboratories, although most state-of-the-art blood gas analysers can measure serum ionised calcium concentrations. Estimation of ionised calcium from total serum calcium

Table 54.2 Daily calcium balance

Gastrointestinal tract	
Diet	600–1200 mg/day
Absorbed	200–400 mg/day
Secreted	150–800 mg/day
Renal	
Filtered	11 000 mg/day
Reabsorbed (97% in the proximal convoluted tubule)	10 800 mg/day
Urinary calcium	200 mg/day
Bone	
Turnover	600–800 mg/day

concentration using mathematical algorithms is unreliable in critically ill patients.[5–7] Heparin forms complexes with calcium and decreases ionised calcium.[8] A heparin concentration of < 15 units/ml of whole blood is therefore recommended for the measurement of ionised calcium.[9] Anaerobic collection of the specimen is recommended, as CO_2 loss from the specimen may result in alkalosis and reduction in ionised calcium concentration. Calcium levels are also reduced by a concomitant lactic acidosis owing to chelation by lactate ion.[10] Free fatty acids (FFAs) increase calcium binding to albumin and may form a portion of the calcium-binding site.[11] Increases in FFAs may be seen in relation to stress, use of steroids, catecholamines and heparin. The impact of pH on calcium measurements has been described above. The normal reference levels of serum calcium are reduced in pregnancy and in the early neonatal period.[12]

HYPERCALCAEMIA IN CRITICALLY ILL PATIENTS

The frequency of hypercalcaemia in critically ill patients is not well established, although it is not as common as hypocalcaemia. Depending on the patient population, the reported incidence ranges from 3–5% to as high as 32%.[13,14] Admission to the intensive care unit (ICU) with a primary diagnosis of a hypercalcaemic crisis is uncommon. Although a number of aetiologies has been described (Table 54.3), in the critical care setting it is usually due to malignancy-related hypercalcaemia, renal failure or posthypocalcaemic hypercalcaemia.[15] Before undertaking a work-up for hypercalcaemia, it is important to exclude false-positive measurements. This is usually the result of inadvertent haemoconcentration during venepuncture and elevation in serum protein, although ionised calcium levels are not reported to be affected by haemoconcentration.[16] *Pseudohypercalcaemia* has also been described in the setting of essential thrombocythaemia. The erroneous result is thought to be due to in vitro release of calcium from platelets, analogous to the pseudohyperkalaemia seen in the same condition.[17]

Table 54.3 Causes of hypercalcaemia

Common causes of hypercalcaemia in the critically ill patient
Complication of malignancy
Bony metastases
Humoral hypercalcaemia of malignancy
Posthypocalcaemic hypercalcaemia
Recovery from pancreatitis[15]
Recovery from acute renal failure following rhabdomyolysis[37–41]
Primary hyperparathyroidism
Adrenal insufficiency[23,24]
Prolonged immobilisation[18–21]
Disorders of magnesium metabolism
Use of total parenteral nutrition[42]
Hypovolaemia
Iatrogenic calcium administration
Less common causes of hypercalcaemia in the critically ill patient
Granulomatous diseases – sarcoidosis, tuberculosis, berylliosis
Vitamin A and D intoxication
Multiple myeloma
Endocrine
Thyrotoxicosis
Acromegaly
Phaeochromocytoma
Lithium – chronic therapy
Rare association between drugs and hypercalcaemia
Theophylline, omeprazole and growth hormone therapy

From a pathophysiological standpoint, hypercalcaemia may be due to an elevation in PTH, in which case the homeostatic regulatory and feedback mechanisms are preserved, and this is termed *equilibrium hypercalcaemia*. Alternatively, it could be a non-parathyroid-mediated hypercalcaemia with associated breakdown of homeostatic mechanisms, and this situation is termed *dysequilibrium hypercalcaemia*.

MECHANISMS OF HYPERCALCAEMIA

Malignancy-related hypercalcaemia might arise from bony metastases or humoral hypercalcaemia of malignancy. In the latter (seen with bronchogenic carcinoma and hypernephroma), tumour osteolysis of bone resulting from the release of PTH-like substances (these cross-react with PTH in the radioimmunoassay, but are not identical to PTH), calcitriol, osteoclast-activating factor and prostaglandins is thought to be the major underlying mechanism. Aggravating factors include dehydration, immobilisation and renal failure.

Posthypocalcaemic hypercalcaemia is a transient phenomenon seen in patients following a period of hypocalcaemia.[15] This has been attributed to a parathyroid hyperplasia which develops during the period of hypocalcaemia, resulting in a rebound hypercalcaemia following resolution of the underlying hypocalcaemic disorder.

Immobilisation hypercalcaemia results from an alteration in balance between bone formation and resorption.[18–21] This leads to loss of bone minerals, hypercalcaemia, hypercalciuria and increased risk of renal failure. In patients with normal bone turnover, immobilisation rarely causes significant hypercalcaemia. However, in patients with rapid turnover of bone (children, postfracture patients, hyperparathyroidism, Paget's disease, spinal injuries and Guillain–Barré syndrome), this may result in severe hypercalcaemia.

Intravascular volume depletion reduces renal calcium excretion by a combination of reduced glomerular filtration and increased tubular reabsorption of calcium. Hypercalcaemia further compounds this problem by causing a concentrating defect in the renal tubules, thus creating a polyuria and further aggravating the hypovolaemia.

Extrarenal production of calcitriol by lymphocytes in granulomata is thought to be the predominant mechanism of hypercalcaemia in granulomatous diseases.[22]

Only 10–20% of patients with adrenal insufficiency develop hypercalcaemia.[23,24] The aetiology of this is thought to be multifactorial: intravascular volume depletion, haemoconcentration of plasma proteins and the loss of antivitamin D effects of glucocorticoids.

For rarer causes of hypercalcaemia, the reader is referred to a recent review.[25]

MANIFESTATIONS OF HYPERCALCAEMIA

The clinical manifestations of hypercalcaemia (commonly encountered when total serum calcium exceeds 3 mmol/l) are outlined in Table 54.4. *Hypercalcaemic crisis* is defined as severe hypercalcaemia (total serum Ca > 3.5 mmol/l) associated with acute symptoms and signs.

INVESTIGATIONS

A detailed diagnostic algorithm is outside of the scope of this chapter. The basic work-up should include serum calcium, phosphorus and alkaline phosphatase estimation, PTH assay, renal function assessment and a skeletal survey.

THERAPY OF HYPERCALCAEMIA AND HYPERCALCAEMIC CRISIS

Mild asymptomatic hypercalcaemia does not require emergent treatment. Therapy is usually directed at the underlying cause.

The management of hypercalcaemic crisis consists of two principal components:

1. increasing urinary excretion of calcium
2. reducing bone resorption

INCREASING URINARY EXCRETION OF CALCIUM

As almost all patients with hypercalcaemia are volume-depleted, the initial therapy consists of rehydration with normal saline followed by diuresis with furosemide. Rehydration with normal saline improves intravascular volume,

Table 54.4 Clinical manifestations of hypercalcaemia*

Cardiovascular	
Hypertension	
Arrhythmias	
Digitalis sensitivity	
Catecholamine resistance	
Urinary system	
Nephrocalcinosis	
Nephrolithiasis	
Tubular dysfunction	
Renal failure	
Gastrointestinal	
Anorexia/nausea/vomiting	
Constipation	
Peptic ulcer	
Pancreatitis	
Neuromuscular	
Weakness	
Neuropsychiatric	
Depression	
Disorientation	
Psychosis	
Coma	
Seizures	

*Ectopic calcification is usually seen with chronic hypercalcaemia.

reduces serum calcium by extracellular dilution and saliuresis promotes calcium loss in the urine. Volume expansion should be titrated to clinical endpoints and central venous pressure monitoring. A urine output of 4–5 litres should be aimed for in these patients to promote calciuresis. In many patients, these measures would achieve a reduction in serum calcium by about 0.4–0.5 mmol/l. Hypokalaemia, hypomagnesaemia and calcium stone formation in the urine are potential side-effects of this mode of treatment.

In patients with established renal failure in whom forced diuresis cannot be instituted, dialysis against a dialysate with zero or low calcium concentrations should be the treatment of choice.

REDUCING BONE RESORPTION

Measures to increase urinary excretion of calcium should be followed up with administration of agents minimising bone resorption. A number of agents are available and these are listed in Table 54.5.

Disodium ethylenediaminetetraacetic acid (EDTA) at a dose of 15–50 mg/kg intravenously rapidly lowers serum calcium. However, its propensity to reduce serum calcium rapidly coupled with its nephrotoxic effects limits its usefulness in life-threatening hypercalcaemia. Other therapeutic modalities include the use of non-steroidal anti-inflammatory drugs and parathyroidectomy. Calcimimetics are agents which increase the activation of the calcium receptor, thus reducing serum PTH concentrations. Cinacalcet is a first-generation calcimimetic which has shown promise in early randomised trials for the management of hypercalcaemia. However, their role in the management of acute hypercalcaemia needs to be established.[26]

At the present time, several newer and more potent biphosphonates are under development. Their efficacy, combined with a relative lack of side-effects, makes them the agents of choice for the treatment of malignancy-related hypercalcaemia.

Other drugs that have been used in the management of hypercalcaemia include prostaglandin inhibitors for cancer-related hypercalcaemia, ketoconazole and chloroquine (for sarcoid-induced hypercalcaemia).[27]

ADJUNCT MEASURES IN THE MANAGEMENT OF HYPERCALCAEMIA

Monitoring of cardiorespiratory function and biochemical status is mandatory during therapy of hypercalcaemia. Thiazide diuretics, vitamin D and absorbable antacids should be avoided. Hypercalcaemia potentiates digitalis effect and dosage should be adjusted accordingly. Endocrinologists should be consulted for further management.

HYPOCALCAEMIA

Hypocalcaemia is more common than hypercalcaemia in critically ill patients, with an estimated incidence of around 70–90%.[5] As the ionised calcium is the biologically active moiety, it is important to look at ionised hypocalcaemia. The frequency of this is far more varied, ranging from 15 to 70%.[5,28,29] Spurious hypocalcaemia may be seen in the following circumstances: a) prolonged storage of specimens prior to analysis (resulting in CO_2 loss from specimens) or b) if the blood sample is drawn with a syringe containing large doses of heparin as an anticoagulant or c) inadvertent collection of the blood sample into EDTA containing tubes (due to calcium chelation). Gadolinium agents (used as contrast for MRI) may also cause a pseudohypocalcaemia if a colorimetric assay is used for the measurement of calcium.

AETIOLOGIES

The aetiology of ionised hypocalcaemia based on the predominant pathophysiological mechanism is listed in Table 54.6. The other contributory mechanisms of hypocalcaemia in each of the conditions are shown in brackets.

Although a long list of causes exists for hypocalcaemia, calcium chelation and hypoparathyroidism constitute the common mechanisms of ionised hypocalcaemia in intensive care. Frequently, hypocalcaemia is accompanied by a number of other biochemical abnormalities; thus a pattern recognition approach towards the cause of hypocalcaemia will point to its aetiology and save a considerable amount of investigations for the patient. Common diagnostic patterns are listed in Table 54.7.

Whilst alkalosis is frequently associated with ionised hypocalcaemia, the presence of a metabolic acidosis in the face of a low serum ionised calcium narrows the differential diagnosis even further (Table 54.8).

Table 54.5: Therapeutic agents for reducing bone restorption

Therapy	Indications	Dose	Onset time/ duration	Limitations	Mechanism of action	Comments
Bi-Phosponates* Etidronate (first-generation)	Malignancy-related hypercalcaemia	5 mg/kg per day	1–2 days, lasts 5–7 days	Hyperphosphataemia, short duration of action	Inhibit osteoclast activity, may have some effect on osteoblasts	High-potency group. Pamidronate lowers Ca levels more rapidly than etidronate
Pamidronate (second-generation)		90 mg as an infusion every 4 weeks	1–2 days, lasts 10–14 days	Hypophosphataemia, fever and hypomagnesaemia		
Calcitonin	Hypercalcaemia, Paget's disease	Initial IV dose 3–4 U/kg followed by 4 U/kg SC 12-hourly	Hours, lasts 2–3 days	Nausea, abdominal pain, flushing, tachyphylaxis, limited efficacy	Inhibit osteoclast activity, reduces renal tubular reabsorption of calcium	Tachyphylaxis minimised by concomitant steroid therapy
Glucocorticoids	Vitamin D toxicity, myeloma, lymphoma, granulomata	IV hydrocortisone 200–400 mg/day	Days, lasts days to weeks	Glucocorticoid side-effects	Inhibit inflammatory cell production of calcitriol, reduce gut absorption of calcium	Improve the efficacy of calcitonin
Gallium nitrate	Malignancy-related hypercalcaemia	100–200 mg/m^2 per day for 5–7 days	5–6 days, lasts 7–10 days	Nephrotoxic	Inhibits bone resorption and alters bone crystal structure	Recent phase II data suggest equivalent efficacy with pamidronate[43]
Plicamycin	Malignancy-related hypercalcaemia	25 μg/kg IV	Rapid onset, lasts for a few days	Hepatotoxic, nephrotoxic and thrombocytopoenia	Inhibits cellular RNA synthesis	Side-effect profile limits the use of this drug
Intravenous phosphates	Limited clinical role	10–15 mmol as an infusion repeated at regular intervals	Hours, lasts 24–48 hours after cessation	Ectopic calcification, severe hypocalcaemia	Ectopic calcification, reduce gut absorption, inhibition of bone resorption	Use superseded by the other modalities described

*Other biphosphonates include ibandronate, risedronate and zoledronate. As compared to pamidronate, zoledronate has the advantage of simplicity of administration and better control of hypercalcemia.
IV, intravenous; SC, subcutaneous.

Table 54.6 Aetiology of ionised hypocalcaemia

Calcium chelation
Alkalosis (increased binding of calcium by albumin)
Citrate toxicity (calcium chelation)
Hyperphosphataemia (calcium chelation, ectopic calcification, reduced vitamin D_3 activity)
Pancreatitis (calcium soap formation, reduced parathyroid secretion)
Tumour lysis syndrome (hyperphosphataemia)
Rhabdomyolysis (hyperphosphataemia and reduced levels of calcitriol)
Hypoparathyroidism
Hypo- and hypermagnesaemia
Sepsis (decreased parathyroid hormone secretion, calcitriol resistance, intracellular shift of calcium)
Burns (decrease in parathyroid hormone secretion)
Neck surgery (removal of parathyroid gland, calcitonin release during thyroid surgery and 'hungry-bone' syndrome postparathyroidectomy)
Hypovitaminosis D
Inadequate intake
Malabsorption
Liver disease (impaired 25-hydroxylation of cholecalciferol)
Renal failure (impaired 1-hydroxylation of cholecalciferol, hyperphosphataemia)
Reduced bone turnover
Osteoporosis
Elderly
Cachexia
Drug-induced
Phenytoin (accelerated metabolism of vitamin D_3)
Diphosphonates (see under hypercalcaemia)
Propofol
Ethylenediaminetetraacetic acid (EDTA: calcium chelation)
Ethylene glycol (formation of calcium oxalate crystals in the urine)
Cis-platinum (renal tubular damage leading to hypermagnesuria)
Protamine
Gentamicin (hypermagnesuria leading to hypomagnesaemia and therefore hypocalcaemia)

CLINICAL MANIFESTATIONS OF HYPOCALCAEMIA

Mild degrees of hypocalcaemia are usually asymptomatic. Ionised calcium levels less than 0.8 mmol/l may cause neuromuscular irritability and result in clinical symptoms. The clinical manifestations of hypocalcaemia are summarised in Table 54.9. The manifestations listed in Table 54.9 are by no means a comprehensive list of all the clinical features, but include the ones most commonly seen in the critical care setting.

When eliciting tetany, Trousseau's sign (carpopedal spasm) is more specific for hypocalcaemia than Chvostek's

Table 54.8 Hypocalcaemia with metabolic acidosis

Acute renal failure
Tumour lysis
Rhabdomyolysis
Pancreatitis
Ethylene glycol poisoning
Hydrofluoric acid intoxication

Table 54.9 Clinical manifestations of hypocalcaemia

Central nervous system
Circumoral and peripheral paraesthesia
Muscle cramps
Tetany
Seizures
Extrapyramidal manifestations: tremor, ataxia, dystonia
Proximal myopathy
Depression, anxiety, psychosis
Cardiovascular
Arrhythmias
Hypotension, inotrope unresponsiveness
Prolonged QT intervals, T-wave inversion
Loss of digitalis effect
Respiratory
Apnoea
Laryngospasm
Bronchospasm

Table 54.7 Pattern recognition in the diagnosis of common causes of hypocalcaemia

Aetiology of hypocalcaemia	Clinical/biochemical patterns
Low serum albumin	Reduced total calcium, normal ionised calcium
Alkalosis	Normal total calcium, reduced ionised calcium
Hypomagnesaemia	Reduced ionised calcium and hypokalaemia
Pancreatitis	Hypocalcaemia, elevated serum lipase and glucose
Renal failure	Elevated blood urea nitrogen, elevated phosphate
Rhabdomyolysis	Hypocalcaemia, elevated phosphate, creatine kinase and urinary myoglobin
Tumour lysis syndrome	Hypocalcaemia, elevated phosphate, potassium and urate

sign (facial twitch in response to facial nerve stimulus – present in 10–30% of the normal population). Electrocardiogram changes do not correlate well with the degree of hypocalcaemia. The symptoms of hypocalcaemia are exacerbated by a coexisting hypokalaemia and hypomagnesaemia.

The laboratory work-up should include serum calcium, phosphorus, magnesium and alkaline phosphatase, PTH and vitamin D assays and renal function assessment.

APPROACH TO THE TREATMENT OF ASYMPTOMATIC AND SYMPTOMATIC HYPOCALCAEMIA

ARGUMENTS FOR AND AGAINST CORRECTION OF ASYMPTOMATIC HYPOCALCAEMIA

As stated before, it is not clear if asymptomatic hypocalcaemia needs correction. Based on published data which suggest that critical care hypocalcaemia is associated with a higher mortality and increased length of stay in intensive care,[30–32] it is advocated that ionised hypocalcaemia be corrected routinely, irrespective of the level. However, arguments exist against the routine correction of asymptomatic ionised hypocalcaemia. Increases in cytosolic calcium lead to disruption of intracellular processes and activation of proteases and can lead to ischaemia and reperfusion injury.[33] Also, there are data suggesting that ionised calcium is an important participant in the pathogenesis of coronary and cerebral vasospasm.[34] In rodent models of endotoxic shock, there are also data demonstrating an increased mortality when these rats were administered intravenous calcium.[35] Most clinicians agree that an ionised calcium level of < 0.8 mmol/l needs correction, even if asymptomatic.

MANAGEMENT OF ACUTE SYMPTOMATIC HYPOCALCAEMIA

Acute symptomatic hypocalcaemia is a medical emergency that requires immediate therapy. In addition to treatment of underlying cause and support of airway, breathing and circulation, the definitive treatment includes administration of intravenous calcium. Intravenous calcium is available as a calcium salt of chloride or gluconate or acetate. The main difference between these formulations is the amount of elemental calcium available at equivalent volumes of drug (Table 54.10). The dose of calcium required should be based on the elemental calcium.[36] Intravenous calcium can be administered as a bolus or as an infusion. Rapid administration of calcium may cause nausea, flushing, headache and arrhythmias. Digitalis toxicity may be precipitated. Extravasation of calcium may lead to tissue irritation, particularly with the chloride salt.

Calcium chloride may be better than calcium gluconate for the management of hypocalcaemia, if there is concomitant alkalosis. Following an initial bolus, an infusion may be commenced at a rate of 1–2 mg/kg per hour of elemental calcium to maintain target levels of ionised calcium. With correction of the underlying disorder and restoration of calcium to normal levels, the infusion can be tapered and stopped. Adequacy of calcium therapy can be monitored clinically and by performing serial determinations of ionised calcium. Failure of ionised calcium to increase after commencement of intravenous calcium may indicate an underlying magnesium deficiency. This can be corrected by administration of 10 mmol of intravenous magnesium over 20 minutes. Administration of calcium in the setting of hyperphosphataemia may result in calcium precipitation in the tissues. Calcium salts should not be administered with bicarbonate since the two precipitate. The other indications for calcium administration are listed in Table 54.11. Other therapy for hypocalcaemia consists of oral calcium supplements and calcitriol administration, although these are usually used in the management of chronic hypocalcaemia.

Table 54.10 Commonly used intravenous calcium preparations

Preparation	Dosage	Elemental calcium/gram
Calcium gluconate	10 ml	93 mg (2.3 mmol)
Calcium chloride	10 ml	272 mg (6.8 mmol)

Table 54.11 Indications for calcium administration

Absolute
Symptomatic hypocalcaemia
Ionised Ca < 0.8 mmol/l
Hyperkalaemia
Calcium channel blocker overdose
Relative
β-blocker overdose
Hypermagnesaemia
Hypocalcaemia in the face of high inotrope requirement
Massive blood transfusion post cardiopulmonary bypass to augment cardiac contractility

REFERENCES

1. Bourdeau J, Attie M. Calcium metabolism. In: Narins R (ed.) *Clinical Disorders of Fluid and Electrolyte Metabolism*, 5th edn. New York: McGraw-Hill; 1994: 243–50.
2. Zaloga GP. Hypocalcemia in critically ill patients. *Crit Care Med* 1992; **20**: 251–62.
3. Holick M, Krane S, Potts J. Calcium, phosphorus and bone metabolism: calcium-regulating hormones. In: Fauci AS (ed.) *Principles of Internal Medicine*. New York: McGraw Hill; 1998.
4. Watchko J, Bifano EM, Bergstrom WH. Effect of hyperventilation on total calcium, ionized calcium,

and serum phosphorus in neonates. *Crit Care Med* 1984; **12**: 1055–6.
5. Zaloga GP, Chernow B, Cook D *et al.* Assessment of calcium homeostasis in the critically ill surgical patient. The diagnostic pitfalls of the McLean–Hastings nomogram. *Ann Surg* 1985; **202**: 587–94.
6. Vincent JL, Jankowski S. Why should ionized calcium be determined in acutely ill patients? *Acta Anaesthesiol Scand* 1995; **107** (suppl.): 281–6.
7. Toffaletti J. Physiology and regulation. Ionized calcium, magnesium and lactate measurements in critical care settings. *Am J Clin Pathol* 1995; **104** (Suppl. 1): 88–94.
8. Landt M, Hortin GL, Smith CH *et al.* Interference in ionized calcium measurements by heparin salts. *Clin Chem* 1994; **40**: 565–70.
9. Sachs C, Rabouine P, Chaneac M *et al.* In vitro evaluation of a heparinized blood sampler for ionized calcium measurement. *Ann Clin Biochem* 1991; **28**: 240–4.
10. Toffaletti J, Abrams B. Effects of in vivo and in vitro production of lactic acid on ionized, protein-bound, and complex-bound calcium in blood. *Clin Chem* 1989; **35**: 935–8.
11. Zaloga GP, Willey S, Tomasic P *et al.* Free fatty acids alter calcium binding: a cause for misinterpretation of serum calcium values and hypocalcemia in critical illness. *J Clin Endocrinol Metab* 1987; **64**: 1010–14.
12. Aggarwal R, Upadhyaya M, Deorari AK *et al.* Hypocalcemia in the new born. *Ind J Pediatr* 2001; **68**: 973–5.
13. Forster J, Querusio L, Burchard KW *et al.* Hypercalcemia in critically ill surgical patients. *Ann Surg* 1985; **202**: 512–18.
14. Lind L, Ljunghall S. Critical care hypercalcemia – a hyperparathyroid state. *Exp Clin Endocrinol* 1992; **100**: 148–51.
15. Zaloga GP. Calcium homeostasis in the critically ill patient. *Magnesium* 1989; **8**: 190–200.
16. McMullan AD, Burns J, Paterson CR. Venepuncture for calcium assays: should we still avoid the tourniquet? *Postgrad Med J* 1990; **66**: 547–8.
17. Howard MR, Ashwell S, Bond LR *et al.* Artefactual serum hyperkalemia and hypercalcemia in essential thrombocythaemia. *J Clin Pathol* 2000; **53**: 105–9.
18. Massagli TL, Cardenas DD. Immobilization hypercalcemia treatment with pamidronate disodium after spinal cord injury. *Arch Phys Med Rehabil* 1999; **80**: 998–1000.
19. Sato Y, Fujimatsu Y, Kikuyama M *et al.* Influence of immobilization on bone mass and bone metabolism in hemiplegic elderly patients with a long-standing stroke. *J Neurol Sci* 1998; **156**: 205–10.
20. Kedlaya D, Brandstater ME, Lee JK. Immobilization hypercalcemia in incomplete paraplegia: successful treatment with pamidronate. *Arch Phys Med Rehabil* 1998; **79**: 222–5.
21. Evans RA, Lawrence PJ, Thanakrishnan G *et al.* Immobilization hypercalcaemia due to low bone formation and responding to intravenous sodium sulphate. *Postgrad Med J* 1986; **62**: 395–8.
22. Sharma OP. Hypercalcemia in granulomatous disorders: a clinical review. *Curr Opin Pulm Med* 2000; **6**: 442–7.
23. Miell J, Wassif W, McGregor A *et al.* Life-threatening hypercalcaemia in association with Addisonian crisis. *Postgrad Med J* 1991; **67**: 770–2.
24. Vasikaran SD, Tallis GA, Braund WJ. Secondary hypoadrenalism presenting with hypercalcaemia. *Clin Endocrinol (Oxf)* 1994; **41**: 261–4.
25. Jacobs TP, Bilezikian JP. Clinical review. Rare causes of hypercalcemia. *J Clin Endocrinol Metab* 2005; **90**: 6316–22.
26. Steddon SJ, Cunningham J. Calcimimetics and calcilytics – fooling the calcium receptor. *Lancet* 2005; **365**: 2237–9.
27. Sharma OP. Hypercalcemia in granulomatous disorders: a clinical review. *Curr Opin Pulm Med* 2000; **6**: 442–7.
28. Zaloga GP, Chernow B. The multifactorial basis for hypocalcemia during sepsis. Studies of the parathyroid hormone–vitamin D axis. *Ann Intern Med* 1987; **107**: 36–41.
29. Desai TK, Carlson RW, Geheb MA. Prevalence and clinical implications of hypocalcemia in acutely ill patients in a medical intensive care setting. *Am J Med* 1988; **84**: 209–14.
30. Chernow B, Zaloga G, McFadden E *et al.* Hypocalcemia in critically ill patients. *Crit Care Med* 1982; **10**: 848–51.
31. Desai TK, Carlson RW, Thill-Baharozian M *et al.* A direct relationship between ionized calcium and arterial pressure among patients in an intensive care unit. *Crit Care Med* 1988; **16**: 578–82.
32. Broner CW, Stidham GL, Westenkirchner DF *et al.* Hypermagnesemia and hypocalcemia as predictors of high mortality in critically ill pediatric patients. *Crit Care Med* 1990; **18**: 921–8.
33. Cheung JY, Bonventre JV, Malis CD *et al.* Calcium and ischemic injury. *N Engl J Med* 1986; **314**: 1670–6.
34. Lemmer JH Jr, Kirsh MM. Coronary artery spasm following coronary artery surgery. *Ann Thorac Surg* 1988; **46**: 108–15.
35. Zaloga GP, Sager A, Black KW *et al.* Low dose calcium administration increases mortality during septic peritonitis in rats. *Circ Shock* 1992; **37**: 226–9.
36. Stratta P, Soragna G, Morellini V *et al.* The patient whose hypocalcaemia worsened after prompt intravenous calcium replacement therapy. *Lancet* 2006; **367**: 273.
37. Meneghini LF, Oster JR, Camacho JR *et al.* Hypercalcemia in association with acute renal failure and rhabdomyolysis. Case report and literature review. *Miner Electrolyte Metab* 1993; **19**: 1–16.
38. Akmal M, Bishop JE, Telfer N *et al.* Hypocalcemia and hypercalcemia in patients with rhabdomyolysis with and without acute renal failure. *J Clin Endocrinol Metab* 1986; **63**: 137–42.
39. Leonard CD, Eichner ER. Acute renal failure and transient hypercalcemia in idiopathic rhabdomyolysis. *JAMA* 1970; **211**: 1539–40.
40. Prince RL, Hutchison BG, Bhagat CI. Hypercalcemia during resolution of acute renal failure associated with

rhabdomyolysis: evidence for suppression of parathyroid hormone and calcitriol. *Aust NZ J Med* 1986; **16**: 506–8.

41. Sperling LS, Tumlin JA. Case report: delayed hypercalcemia after rhabdomyolysis-induced acute renal failure. *Am J Med Sci* 1996; **311**: 186–8.
42. Izsak EM, Shike M, Roulet M *et al.* Pancreatitis in association with hypercalcemia in patients receiving total parenteral nutrition. *Gastroenterology* 1980; **79**: 555–8.
43. Cvitkovic F, Armand JP, Tubiana-Hulin M *et al.* Randomized, double-blind, phase II trial of gallium nitrate compared with pamidronate for acute control of cancer-related hypercalcemia. *Cancer J* 2006; **12**: 47–53.

Part Nine

Obstetric Emergencies

55

Pre-eclampsia and eclampsia

Warwick D Ngan Kee and Tony Gin

Pre-eclampsia is a syndrome specific to pregnancy. It has no definitive biomarkers and is diagnosed clinically by new onset of hypertension and proteinuria after 20 weeks' gestation (Table 55.1). Oedema and hyperreflexia typically also occur. Diagnostic criteria have varied among countries and over time, although in recent years international working groups have worked towards consensus.[1,2] There is overlap among pre-eclampsia, pre-existing hypertension, pre-eclampsia superimposed on pre-existing hypertension and non-proteinuric gestational hypertension. Eclampsia describes the occurrence in a pre-eclamptic woman of seizures not attributable to other causes.

Pre-eclampsia complicates 2–7% of pregnancies in developed countries and is a leading cause of maternal deaths.[2,3] Associated maternal mortality is 1.5 per 100 000 live births in the USA.[4] The incidence of eclampsia is 0.04–0.1% in the USA and UK,[5] with maternal mortality in the UK of 1.8% and fetal/neonatal mortality of around 7%.[6] Incidence and mortality for both pre-eclampsia and eclampsia are much higher in developing countries.[5]

Factors associated with increased maternal risk include:

- onset at $\leq$ 32 weeks' gestation
- greater maternal age and parity
- pre-existing hypertension or medical complications
- Afro-Caribbean descent
- nausea and vomiting and epigastric pain
- abnormal laboratory tests, including raised liver enzymes, increased serum creatinine and increased serum uric acid[7,8]

Patients may be referred to the intensive care unit (ICU) for poorly controlled hypertension or convulsions, postoperative care or following complications such as pulmonary oedema, renal failure, haemorrhage, coagulopathy and stroke.

AETIOLOGY

The cause of pre-eclampsia is unknown. As yet, there is no satisfactory single unifying aetiological hypothesis. Although there is a genetic predispostion, the exact mode of inheritance is unclear and there may be multiple phenotypes.[9] Immunologic factors such as an abnormal maternal response to fetopaternal antigens have been implicated. Pre-eclampsia is more common in primigravidae, multiple gestation, obesity, black race, molar pregnancy, when there is pre-existing hypertension, underlying disease (e.g. autoimmune disease, renal disease, diabetes and thrombophilias) and when there is a previous or family history of pre-eclampsia.[10] A change in partner has been considered a risk factor but this may be partially related to increased risk associated with extended intervals between pregnancies.[11]

PATHOGENESIS

Pre-eclampsia is a systemic disease that affects most organ systems. Many theories of pathogenesis have been proposed,[12–14] but a common concept is that of a two-stage disease with an initial stage of abnormal placentation followed by a second stage of clinical disease. Initially, there is inadequate endovascular invasion of fetal trophoblast into the spiral arteries with reduced dilatation of uterine spiral arteries and placental hypoxia. This acts as a precipitating factor that leads to a generalised inflammatory response, of which diffuse endothelial dysfunction is a prominent component. The result is an increase in sensitivity to vasoactive substances, a decrease in endothelial synthesis of vasodilator substances such as prostaglandin and nitric oxide, activation of platelet and coagulation and an increase in capillary permeability. This causes widespread vasoconstriction, fluid extravasation, proteinuria, decreased intravascular volume, haemoconcentration and decreased organ perfusion. The link between placental triggering and the systemic response is unknown, but has been theorised to involve oxidative stress and circulating cytotoxic factors. Candidates for the latter include circulating angiogenic factors such as vascular endothelial growth factors, placental growth factor and fms-like tyrosine kinase-1 (sFlt1).[13,14]

CLINICAL PRESENTATION

Pre-eclampsia is a syndrome with a spectrum of presentations. Although hypertension is the cardinal sign, some women present with convulsions, abdominal pain or general

Table 55.1 Basic diagnostic criteria for pre-eclampsia

Hypertension	Systolic arterial pressure > 140 mmHg *or* Diastolic arterial pressure* > 90 mmHg
and	
Proteinuria	≥ 300 mg protein in a 24-hour collection

*Korotkoff phase V.
A rise in blood pressure above baseline and oedema are now not usually included.
A positive dipstick test for proteinuria should be confirmed by 24-hour urine collection.

Table 55.2 Clinical features suggestive of severe pre-eclampsia

Blood pressure	Systolic arterial pressure > 160 mmHg Diastolic arterial pressure > 110 mmHg
Renal	Proteinuria ≥ 2 g/24 h Oliguria < 500 ml/24 h Serum creatinine > 0.09 mmol/l
Hepatic	Epigastric or right-upper-quadrant pain Elevated bilirubin and/or transaminases
Neurological	Persistent headaches Visual disturbances
	Convulsions (eclampsia)
Haematological	Thrombocytopenia Deranged coagulation tests Haemolysis
Cardiac/respiratory	Pulmonary oedema Cyanosis

malaise[15] and some complications may be life-threatening without a marked increase in blood pressure. Features typical of severe disease are listed in Table 55.2. Rarely, cocaine intoxication and phaeochromocytoma may be confused with pre-eclampsia.

Haemodynamic changes of pre-eclampsia consist of hypertension, increased systemic vascular resistance and decreased intravascular volume. Cardiac output is usually decreased, usually secondary to changes in preload and afterload rather than contractility.[16] Sympathetic activation occurs, and this may account for observations of increased cardiac output in the early stage.[17] Pulmonary oedema may occur because of iatrogenic fluid overload, decreased left ventricular function, increased capillary permeability and narrowing of the colloid osmotic–pulmonary capillary wedge pressure gradient; this is more likely to occur after delivery. Sudden ventricular tachycardia may occur during hypertensive crises.

Neurological complications include eclamptic convulsions, cerebral oedema, raised intracranial pressure and stroke. Intracranial haemorrhage is an important cause of death.[3]

Renal changes include reduced glomerular filtration rate and renal plasma flow, which are associated with the characteristic lesion of glomeruloendotheliosis. Hyperuricaemia is associated with increased prenatal risk, particularly if serum uric acid concentration rises rapidly.

Haemostatic abnormalities include thrombocytopenia, which may be associated with decreased platelet function. Associated coagulation abnormalities may occur but are unlikely unless the platelet count is $< 100\,000 \times 10^9/l$.[18,19]

Hepatic complications include liver oedema, hepatocellular necrosis, periportal and subcapsular haemorrhage, hepatic infarcts and rupture. Patients with HELLP syndrome (see below) are particularly at risk.

The leading causes of maternal death in pre-eclampsia/eclampsia are intracranial haemorrhage, pulmonary oedema and hepatic complications.[3,4] Fetal morbidity results from placental insufficiency, prematurity and abruptio placentae.

MANAGEMENT

The treatment of pre-eclampsia is delivery of the placenta and fetus. Before delivery, and during the immediate postpartum period, management is supportive and focused on control of blood pressure, prevention of seizures, maintenance of placental perfusion and prevention of complications. If complications are avoided, the disease normally resolves completely after delivery. Transfer of the mother to a tertiary centre before delivery should be considered if a level III neonatal unit is not available (see Chapter 1). Pregnant and postnatal women may have special requirements which not all staff are experienced with.[20] Admission into an ICU before delivery may be appropriate in severe cases, or when the labour ward lacks the expertise or equipment for intensive monitoring. Because prematurity is a major cause of neonatal morbidity, expectant management to prolong pregnancy has been described in patients < 34 weeks' gestation.[21] This requires careful balancing of the maternal and perinatal risks. After delivery, severe cases should preferably be managed in an ICU for 24–72 hours.

GENERAL MEASURES

Before delivery, patients should be kept in the lateral or semilateral position and the fetal heart rate should be monitored. Regular oral or intravenous histamine H_2 antagonists will decrease gastric acidity and volume. Prophylactic dexamethasone or betamethasone should be considered for fetal lung maturity if gestation is less than 34 weeks and early delivery is anticipated. Routine monitoring should include frequent clinical assessment, blood pressure, electrocardiogram (ECG) and fluid balance. Pulse oximetry aids the detection of incipient pulmonary oedema.[22] Central venous pressure (CVP) monitoring, preferably via an antecubital vein, and/or pulmonary artery catheterisation may assist in fluid balance (see below). Full blood count, coagulation screen, electrolytes, uric acid, renal function, liver function and urinalysis should be performed serially to monitor disease progression.

ANTIHYPERTENSIVE THERAPY

The aim of antihypertensive therapy is to prevent maternal complications (intracerebral haemorrhage, cardiac failure and abruptio placentae) while maintaining placental blood flow. It is important to appreciate that hypertension is a marker and not a causal factor in pre-eclampsia. Therefore, although controlling hypertension reduces the risk of complications, it does not ameliorate the underlying pathological process. Acute treatment is indicated when blood pressure is greater than 160 mmHg systolic or 105–110 mmHg diastolic. Reduction of systolic pressure is particularly important for the prevention of stroke.[23] Initially, systolic blood pressure should only be reduced by about 20–30 mmHg and diastolic pressure by 10–15 mmHg while monitoring the fetus.[1] Concomitant plasma expansion reduces the risk of sudden hypotension when vasodilators are used.[1] Recommended antihypertensive drugs for acute treatment are summarised in Table 55.3 and described below.[1,2] The most commonly used drugs are hydralazine, labetalol and nifedipine; insufficient data are currently available to prove which of these is superior.[24]

HYDRALAZINE

Hydralazine is a direct arteriolar vasodilator with a long history of use in pre-eclampsia. It has a relatively slow onset of action of 10–20 minutes and a duration of action of 6–8 hours. Comcomitant volume expansion may reduce the incidence of associated hypotension and fetal distress. Adverse effects include headache, tachycardia, tremor, nausea and rare cases of neonatal thrombocytopenia.

Table 55.3 Main drugs used for acute management of hypertension in pre-eclampsia

Drug	Dosage guide
Hydralazine	*Bolus* 5 mg IV followed by 5–10 mg every 20 min to maximum of 40 mg
Labetalol	*Bolus* 20–40 mg IV every 10–15 min to a maximum of 220 mg *Infusion* 1–2 mg/min, reducing to 0.5 mg/min or less after blood pressure is controlled
Nifedipine	*Orally* 10 mg, repeated after 30 min as required

IV, intravenously.

LABETALOL

Labetalol is a non-selective β-adrenergic receptor blocker with some α_1-blocking effect. When given intravenously, it rapidly reduces blood pressure without decreasing uteroplacental blood flow,[25] and does not cause reflex tachycardia, headache or nausea. Although labetalol crosses the placenta, neonatal bradycardia and hypoglycaemia are rarely seen. Duration of action is variable. It should not be given to patients with asthma or myocardial dysfunction.

NIFEDIPINE

Nifedipine is a calcium-channel blocker that directly relaxes arterial smooth muscle. In pre-eclamptic patients with severe hypertension it causes a steady decrease in blood pressure and systemic vascular resistance within 30 minutes with a concomitant increase in maternal cardiac index and heart rate.[26] Nifedipine is recommended to be given orally. It is also effective sublingually or chewed but this may be associated with sudden hypotension and fetal compromise. Hypotension and potentiation of neuromuscular block have been reported in patients receiving magnesium sulphate. Nifedipine causes relaxation of uterine muscle which may increase the risk of postpartum haemorrhage. Mild side-effects include headache, flushing, and nausea.

OTHER AGENTS

Sodium nitroprusside (initial dose 0.25 μg/kg per min, maximum dose 5 μg/kg per min) can be used to reduce blood pressure rapidly in a hypertensive emergency[3] but care should be taken in patients with depleted intravascular volume and duration should be limited to < 4 hours to avoid fetal cyanide poisoning.[3] *Nitroglycerine* infusion (initial dose 5 μg/min, maximum dose 100 μg/min) may be useful in cases complicated by pulmonary oedema. *Methyldopa* is often used for mild cases but its slow onset time makes it unsuitable for acute treatment. *Diazoxide, ketanserin, nimodipine* and *magnesium* are not recommended as first-line agents.[24] *Beta-blockers* other than labetalol may cause decreased uteroplacental perfusion, fetal bradycardia and decreased fetal tolerance to hypoxia. *Angiotensin-converting enzyme inhibitors* and *angiotensin antagonists* should not be used before delivery because of adverse fetal effects.[1,3] *Diuretics* should be avoided since pre-eclamptic patients have reduced plasma volume.

ANTICONVULSANT THERAPY

Anticonvulsants are used to prevent recurrent convulsions in eclampsia or to prevent initial convulsions in pre-eclampsia. Magnesium sulphate is the drug of choice, although it may not be effective in all cases.[27–29]

MAGNESIUM SULPHATE

There is universal agreement that patients with eclampsia should receive magnesium sulphate. However, because only a small proportion of patients with pre-eclampsia progress to eclampsia, the effectiveness and risk–benefit and cost–benefit ratios of prophylactic administration in pre-eclampsia are controversial.[30–32] The authors' practice is to start magnesium when there are clinical signs of severe pre-eclampsia, although the concept that eclampsia follows on from severe pre-eclampsia has been questioned.[33] The mechanism of action of magnesium for preventing eclamptic seizures is unknown. Although abnormal electroencephalograms are frequent in pre-eclampsia and eclampsia, they are not altered by magnesium sulphate. Part of magnesium's action has been considered to be reduction of cerebral vasospasm via antagonism of calcium at membrane channels or intracellular sites. However, the cerebral vasodilator nimodipine was shown to be ineffective for preventing seizures.[34] Magnesium amplifies release of prostacyclin by vascular endothelium, and this may inhibit platelet aggregation and vasoconstriction. Doppler ultrasonography suggests that magnesium vasodilates smaller-diameter intracranial blood vessels, and some of its effects may be from relieving cerebral ischaemia. Part of the anticonvulsant activity of magnesium may be mediated by blockade or suppression of *N*-methyl-D-aspartate (NMDA) receptors. Magnesium has tocolytic effects and mild general vasodilator and antihypertensive actions and increases renal and uterine blood flow.

Guidelines for administration of magnesium sulphate are summarised in Table 55.4. An intravenous loading dose followed by an infusion is preferred, although intramuscular administration is an alternative. Magnesium is rapidly excreted by the kidney. The half-life in patients with normal renal function is 4 hours and 90% of the dose is excreted by 24 hours after the infusion.[35] When there is renal impairment or oliguria the dose should be reduced and serum concentration should be monitored. Suggested target serum concentration for severe pre-eclampsia is 2–3.5 mmol/l (4–7 mEq/l or 4.8–8.4 mg/dl). Magnesium toxicity is associated with muscle weakness and may lead to respiratory paralysis (> 7.5 mmol/l). Increased conduction time with increased PR and QT intervals and QRS duration can lead to sinoatrial and atrioventricular block (> 7.5 mmol/l) and cardiac arrest in diastole (> 12.5 mmol/l). Toxicity is unlikely when deep tendon reflexes are present (the upper limb should be used during epidural analgesia). Magnesium toxicity can be treated with small intravenous doses of calcium. Other reported adverse effects of magnesium include death from overdose, increased bleeding, slowed cervical dilatation and increased risk of pulmonary oedema. Magnesium crosses the placenta and can cause neonatal flaccidity and respiratory depression.

Table 55.4 Dosage regimens for magnesium sulphate

Intravenous regimen	Loading dose: 4–6 g over 20 min Maintenance: 1–2 g/h
Intramuscular regimen	4 g every 4 h

Renal function and tendon reflexes should be monitored. Reduce dose and monitor serum concentrations in oliguria or renal impairment. (1 g magnesium sulphate = 98 mg = 4.06 mmol = 8.12 mEq elemental magnesium).

OTHER ANTICONVULSANTS

If repeated seizures occur despite therapeutic levels of magnesium, conventional anticonvulsants can be considered, but it is important to exclude other causes of convulsions. Although *phenytoin* is inferior to magnesium for preventing eclamptic seizures,[36] it may be considered when there is renal failure. An initial intravenous loading dose of 10 mg/kg is followed 2 hours later by 5 mg/kg. Doses are diluted in normal saline and given no faster than 50 mg/min. Electrocardiogram and arterial pressure should be monitored. Maintenance doses of 200 mg orally or intravenously are started 12 hours after the second bolus and given 8-hourly. Similarly, intravenous infusion of *diazepam* has been used (40 mg diazepam in 500 ml normal saline titrated to keep patients sedated but rousable).[37]

ECLAMPSIA

Eclampsia may occur without marked preceding hypertension or without proteinuria,[33] and up to one-third of cases occur postpartum, often more than 48 hours after delivery.[38] Priorities in the management of eclamptic seizures are airway protection, oxygenation, and termination and prevention of seizures. Delivery of the fetus should be considered after maternal stabilisation. Patients should be placed in the left lateral position and given oxygen. Magnesium should be given if not already started. Approximately 10% of eclamptic patients will have a recurrent seizure despite receiving magnesium.[39] Prolonged seizures can be terminated by diazepam 5–10 mg intravenously. If seizures are refractory, thiopental and suxamethonium should be given and the airway secured. Recurrent convulsions or prolonged unconsciousness may indicate additional cerebral pathology (e.g. cerebral oedema, intracerebral haemorrhage, venous thrombosis) and a computed tomographic (CT) scan should be done. Intensive neurological management, aimed at controlling intracranial pressure and optimising cerebral perfusion, has significantly reduced mortality in unconscious eclamptic patients.[40]

FLUID BALANCE

Fluid management in pre-eclampsia is controversial. Pre-eclamptic patients usually have reduced circulating intravascular volume and oliguria is common in patients with pre-eclampsia. Therefore, fluid loading with crystalloid or colloid solution has been advocated. However, the effectiveness of this is uncertain and, because of the risk of pulmonary oedema, this practice can be questioned.[41] A suggested fluid regimen is to start maintenance crystalloid at 75–125 ml/h intravenously, aiming for urine output > 0.5 ml/kg per hour, averaged over 3–4 hours. When there is oliguria or other signs of poor perfusion, repeated fluid challenge with 250–500 ml crystalloid or 100–200 ml colloid may be given, while monitoring with a pulse oximeter and examining for fluid overload. Urinary sodium < 20 mmol/l, osmolality > 500 mosmol/kg or fractional excretion of sodium of < 1 supports a prerenal cause for oliguria. Renal failure in pre-eclampsia is uncommon. Some patients with persistent oliguria and a rising serum creatinine concentration may require a period of continuous renal replacement therapy but the majority of cases recover. However, the risk of irreversible renal damage is greater when there is associated abruptio placentae, disseminated intravascular coagulation (DIC), hypotensive shock, or sepsis.[15] Low-dose dopamine (3 μg/kg per min) and furosemide (5 mg/h) infusions have been used after correction of hypovolaemia to improve urine output and renal function in oliguric pre-eclamptic patients,[42] but whether this reduces the need for dialysis is undetermined.

There is controversy over the effectiveness of CVP and pulmonary capillary wedge pressure (PCWP) for assisting fluid management in pre-eclamptic patients. CVP and PCWP have poor correlation, especially when CVP is greater than 6 mmHg (0.8 kPa).[43] Optimal CVP and PCWP values are unknown but the measured response to fluid challenge may be informative and useful. Pulmonary artery catheterisation has risks in patients who are oedematous and coagulopathic and should only be considered when there are clear indications (e.g. refractory hypertension, pulmonary oedema and refractory oliguria).[43] Pulmonary oedema is unlikely with a CVP less than 6 mmHg, but when it occurs, should be managed with oxygen therapy, positive end-expiratory pressure with or without ventilation, inotropes, vasodilators, morphine or diuretics as indicated.

POSTPARTUM CARE

Patients are frequently referred to an ICU for postpartum care, particularly after caesarean delivery. The risk of pulmonary oedema is greatest after delivery and most maternal deaths occur then.[44] After delivery, there is often an initial improvement with a relapse in the first 24 hours. Magnesium should be continued for 24–48 hours. Antihypertensive drugs may be reduced according to the blood pressure. Some patients may require a change to oral medication which may need to be continued for several weeks. Psychological support is important, especially if there has been an adverse neonatal outcome. Full recovery from the organ dysfunction of pre-eclampsia is normally expected within 6 weeks.

HELLP SYNDROME AND HEPATIC COMPLICATIONS

HELLP syndrome is a particularly high risk form of pre-eclampsia characterised by more pronounced hepatic rather than cerebral or renal involvement. Diagnosis is based on laboratory findings showing *h*aemolysis (microangiopathic haemolytic anaemia), *e*levated *l*iver enzymes and *l*ow *p*latelets, although exact criteria vary.[45,46] Clinical presentation is variable. Many patients have nonspecific signs such as right-upper-quadrant or epigastric pain, nausea, malaise or headache. Although most patients will have hypertension and proteinuria, these can be mild or absent. Important differential diagnoses include idiopathic thrombocytopenic purpura, systemic lupus erythematosus, thrombotic thrombocytopenic purpura, haemolytic–uraemic syndrome and acute fatty liver of pregnancy.[45,46] Typically, HELLP syndrome presents at early gestational ages and is more common in white and multiparous women.[47] In about 30% of cases, it first presents in the postpartum period, sometimes with no evidence of pre-eclampsia before delivery.[46] After delivery, patients usually show a continuing deterioration in platelet count and liver enzymes, with a peak in severity 24–48 hours after delivery followed by gradual resolution and complete recovery if complications are avoided. Complications of HELLP syndrome include DIC, abruptio placentae, acute renal failure, pulmonary oedema, severe ascites, pleural effusion, liver haemorrhage or failure, acute respiratory distress syndrome (ARDS), sepsis and stroke.[46]

Patients with HELLP should be managed aggressively, similarly to pre-eclampsia, with an emphasis on stabilisation and delivery. Expectant management of patients with gestation less than 34 weeks has been described but the relative benefits and risks of this are controversial.[45,46] Use of high-dose intravenous corticosteroids (e.g. dexamethasone 10 mg 6-hourly for 2 doses, then 6 mg 6-hourly for 2 doses) has been reported to accelerate recovery, but this is also controversial.[45,46,48] Plasma exchange with fresh frozen plasma has been described for postpartum patients with delayed resolution of HELLP with variable response.[49]

Life-threatening hepatic complications may occur in pre-eclampsia, particularly in patients with HELLP syndrome.[45,46] These include segmental hepatic infarction, parenchymal haemorrhage and subcapsular haemotoma with or without rupture. If suspected, patients should have an urgent CT scan.[46] Hepatic rupture is a surgical emergency. Hepatic haemorrhage without rupture has been managed conservatively.[45]

ANAESTHESIA AND ANALGESIA

Platelet count and coagulation tests should be checked before regional anaesthesia. Epidural analgesia in labour reduces fluctuations in arterial pressure and improves placental blood flow.[50] For caesarean section, the use of epidural or spinal anaesthesia avoids the risks of aspiration, difficult intubation from airway oedema, exaggerated hypertensive response to intubation and magnesium-induced sensitivity to muscle relaxants associated with general anaesthesia. If general anaesthesia is required, smaller-size endotracheal tubes may be required. The hypertensive response to intubation should be attenutated with drugs such as fentanyl (2.5 μg/kg), alfentanil (10 μg/kg), magnesium sulphate (40 mg/kg), a combination of alfentanil (7.5 μg/kg) with magnesium sulphate (30 mg/kg), or remifentanil (1 μg/kg). Occasionally, awake intubation under topical anaesthesia may be necessary when there is airway obstruction.

REFERENCES

1. Brown MA, Hague WM, Higgins J *et al.* The detection, investigation and management of hypertension in pregnancy: executive summary. *Aust NZ J Obstet Gynaecol* 2000; **40**: 133–8.
2. Report of the National High Blood Pressure Education Program Working Group on High Blood Pressure in Pregnancy. *Am J Obstet Gynecol* 2000; **183**: S1–22.
3. Confidential Enquiry into Maternal and Child Health. *Why Mothers Die 2000–2002: The Sixth Report of the Confidential Enquiries into Maternal Death in the United Kingdom.* London: RCOG Press, 2004.
4. MacKay AP, Berg CJ, Atrash HK. Pregnancy-related mortality from preeclampsia and eclampsia. *Obstet Gynecol* 2001; **97**: 533–8.
5. Aagaard-Tillery KM, Belfort MA. Eclampsia: morbidity, mortality, and management. *Clin Obstet Gynecol* 2005; **48**: 12–23.
6. Douglas KA, Redman CW. Eclampsia in the United Kingdom. *Br Med J* 1994; **309**: 1395–400.
7. Mattar F, Sibai BM. Eclampsia. VIII. Risk factors for maternal morbidity. *Am J Obstet Gynecol* 2000; **182**: 307–12.
8. Martin JN Jr, May WL, Magann EF *et al.* Early risk assessment of severe preeclampsia: admission battery of symptoms and laboratory tests to predict likelihood of subsequent significant maternal morbidity. *Am J Obstet Gynecol* 1999; **180**: 1407–14.
9. Lachmeijer AM, Dekker GA, Pals G *et al.* Searching for preeclampsia genes: the current position. *Eur J Obstet Gynecol Reprod Biol* 2002; **105**: 94–113.
10. Duckitt K, Harrington D. Risk factors for pre-eclampsia at antenatal booking: systematic review of controlled studies. *Br Med J* 2005; **330**: 565.
11. Skjaerven R, Wilcox AJ, Lie RT. The interval between pregnancies and the risk of preeclampsia. *N Engl J Med* 2002; **346**: 33–8.
12. Pridjian G, Puschett JB. Preeclampsia. Part 1: clinical and pathophysiologic considerations. *Obstet Gynecol Surv* 2002; **57**: 598–618.
13. Redman CW, Sargent IL. Latest advances in understanding preeclampsia. *Science* 2005; **308**: 1592–4.
14. Noris M, Perico N, Remuzzi G. Mechanisms of disease: pre-eclampsia. *Nat Clin Pract Nephrol* 2005; **1**: 98–114.
15. Walker JJ. Pre-eclampsia. *Lancet* 2000; **356**: 1260–5.
16. Lang RM, Pridjian G, Feldman T *et al.* Left ventricular mechanics in preeclampsia. *Am Heart J* 1991; **121**: 1768–75.
17. Easterling TR. The maternal hemodynamics of pre-eclampsia. *Clin Obstet Gynecol* 1992; **35**: 375–86.
18. Leduc L, Wheeler JM, Kirshon B *et al.* Coagulation profile in severe preeclampsia. *Obstet Gynecol* 1992; **79**: 14–18.
19. Sharma SK, Philip J, Whitten CW *et al.* Assessment of changes in coagulation in parturients with preeclampsia using thromboelastography. *Anesthesiology* 1999; **90**: 385–90.
20. Pollock WE. Caring for pregnant and postnatal women in intensive care: what do we know? *Aust Crit Care* 2006; **19**: 54–65.
21. Haddad B, Sibai BM. Expectant management of severe preeclampsia: proper candidates and pregnancy outcome. *Clin Obstet Gynecol* 2005; **48**: 430–40.
22. Walker JJ. Care of the patient with severe pregnancy induced hypertension. *Eur J Obstet Gynecol Reprod Biol* 1996; **65**: 127–35.
23. Martin JN Jr, Thigpen BD, Moore RC *et al.* Stroke and severe preeclampsia and eclampsia: a paradigm shift focusing on systolic blood pressure. *Obstet Gynecol* 2005; **105**: 246–54.
24. Duley L, Henderson-Smart DJ, Meher S. Drugs for treatment of very high blood pressure during pregnancy. *Cochrane Database Syst Rev* 2006; **3**: CD001449.
25. Jouppila P, Kirkinen P, Koivula A *et al.* Labetalol does not alter the placental and fetal blood flow or maternal prostanoids in pre-eclampsia. *Br J Obstet Gynaecol* 1986; **93**: 543–7.
26. Visser W, Wallenburg HC. A comparison between the haemodynamic effects of oral nifedipine and intravenous dihydralazine in patients with severe pre-eclampsia. *J Hypertens* 1995; **13**: 791–5.
27. Lucas MJ, Leveno KJ, Cunningham FG. A comparison of magnesium sulfate with phenytoin for the prevention of eclampsia. *N Engl J Med* 1995; **333**: 201–5.
28. Collaborative Eclampsia Trial. Which anticonvulsant for women with eclampsia? Evidence from the Collaborative Eclampsia Trial. *Lancet* 1995; **345**: 1455–63.
29. Sibai BM. Magnesium sulfate prophylaxis in pre-eclampsia: evidence from randomized trials. *Clin Obstet Gynecol* 2005; **48**: 478–88.
30. The Magpie Trial Collaborative Group. Do women with pre-eclampsia, and their babies, benefit from magnesium sulphate? The Magpie Trial: a randomised placebo-controlled trial. *Lancet* 2002; **359**: 1877–90.
31. Simon J, Gray A, Duley L. Cost-effectiveness of prophylactic magnesium sulphate for 9996 women with pre-eclampsia from 33 countries: economic evaluation of the Magpie Trial. *Br J Obstet Gynaecol* 2006; **113**: 144–51.

32. Sibai BM. Magnesium sulfate prophylaxis in preeclampsia: lessons learned from recent trials. *Am J Obstet Gynecol* 2004; **190**: 1520–6.
33. Katz VL, Farmer R, Kuller JA. Preeclampsia into eclampsia: toward a new paradigm. *Am J Obstet Gynecol* 2000; **182**: 1389–96.
34. Belfort MA, Anthony J, Saade GR *et al.* A comparison of magnesium sulfate and nimodipine for the prevention of eclampsia. *N Engl J Med* 2003; **348**: 304–11.
35. Lu JF, Nightingale CH. Magnesium sulfate in eclampsia and pre-eclampsia: pharmacokinetic principles. *Clin Pharmacokinet* 2000; **38**: 305–14.
36. Duley L, Henderson-Smart D. Magnesium sulphate versus phenytoin for eclampsia. *Cochrane Database Syst Rev* 2003; **4**: CD000128.
37. Crowther C. Magnesium sulphate versus diazepam in the management of eclampsia: a randomized controlled trial. *Br J Obstet Gynaecol* 1990; **97**: 110–17.
38. Chames MC, Livingston JC, Ivester TS *et al.* Late postpartum eclampsia: a preventable disease? *Am J Obstet Gynecol* 2002; **186**: 1174–7.
39. Sibai BM. Diagnosis, prevention, and management of eclampsia. *Obstet Gynecol* 2005; **105**: 402–10.
40. Richards AM, Moodley J, Graham DI *et al.* Active management of the unconscious eclamptic patient. *Br J Obstet Gynaecol* 1986; **93**: 554–62.
41. Duley L, Williams J, Henderson-Smart DJ. Plasma volume expansion for treatment of pre-eclampsia. *Cochrane Database Syst Rev* 1999; **4**: CD001805.
42. Keiseb J, Moodley J, Connolly CA. Comparison of the efficacy of continuous furosemide and low-dose dopamine infusion in preeclampsia/eclampsia-related oliguria in the immediate postpartum period. *Hypertens Pregnancy* 2002; **21**: 225–34.
43. Clark SL, Cotton DB. Clinical indications for pulmonary artery catheterization in the patient with severe preeclampsia. *Am J Obstet Gynecol* 1988; **158**: 453–8.
44. Sibai BM, Mabie BC, Harvey CJ *et al.* Pulmonary edema in severe preeclampsia-eclampsia: analysis of thirty-seven consecutive cases. *Am J Obstet Gynecol* 1987; **156**: 1174–9.
45. O'Brien JM, Barton JR. Controversies with the diagnosis and management of HELLP syndrome. *Clin Obstet Gynecol* 2005; **48**: 460–77.
46. Sibai BM. Diagnosis, controversies, and management of the syndrome of hemolysis, elevated liver enzymes, and low platelet count. *Obstet Gynecol* 2004; **103**: 981–91.
47. Saphier CJ, Repke JT. Hemolysis, elevated liver enzymes, and low platelets (HELLP) syndrome: a review of diagnosis and management. *Semin Perinatol* 1998; **22**: 118–33.
48. Visser W, Wallenburg HC. Temporising management of severe pre-eclampsia with and without the HELLP syndrome. *Br J Obstet Gynaecol* 1995; **102**: 111–17.
49. Martin JN Jr, Files JC, Blake PG *et al.* Postpartum plasma exchange for atypical preeclampsia-eclampsia as HELLP (hemolysis, elevated liver enzymes, and low platelets) syndrome. *Am J Obstet Gynecol* 1995; **172**: 1107–25.
50. Jouppila P, Jouppila R, Hollmén A *et al.* Lumbar epidural analgesia to improve intervillous blood flow during labor in severe preeclampsia. *Obstet Gynecol* 1982; **59**: 158–61.

56

General obstetric emergencies in the ICU

Tony Gin and Warwick D Ngan Kee

The intensive care unit (ICU) will receive obstetric patients with the usual range of medical and surgical emergencies, and also provide supportive care for patients who suffer specific obstetric complications. The pattern of admission varies widely among countries with different standards of obstetric care, but complications of hypertensive disorders and haemorrhage usually make up a large proportion of cases,[1] while respiratory failure and sepsis are also common.[2] The proportion of obstetric patients in most ICUs is still low, and this may lead to relative inexperience in management and teamwork between the intensivist and obstetrician. The latest report of the UK Confidential Enquiries into Maternal Deaths noted that one-third of mothers who died had some intensive care involvement.[3] Unfortunately, major problems identified on the ward were:

- failure to recognise the severity of disease
- late referral to the ICU
- inadequate management of the ill patient while awaiting ICU admission

Maternal outcome is usually favourable because patients are often young and healthy. Scoring systems appear to be valid when the primary problem is medical, but overestimate mortality when the problem is obstetric.[1] This is partly because normal pregnant physiological variables are scored as abnormal.

PATHOPHYSIOLOGY

Two important points to recognise in treating obstetric patients are:

1. During pregnancy, the normal ranges for physiological variables change[4] (Table 56.1). This may modify the presentation of the problem, the normal physiological variables used to guide treatment and also the response to treatment. The majority of physiological changes revert to normal several days after delivery.
2. Both mother and fetus are affected by the pathology and subsequent treatment.

AIRWAY AND VENTILATION

Several factors may complicate tracheal intubation in pregnancy:

- altered anatomy in pregnancy predisposes to a potentially difficult airway
- oedematous tissues
- delayed gastric emptying
- increased oxygen consumption

Intensivists must be familiar with the difficult airway algorithm and the use of the laryngeal mask airway.[36,37] Avoidance of intubation and the use of non-invasive ventilation may be a good option in selected cases.

Some causes of respiratory failure are modified by pregnancy (e.g. aspiration of gastric contents, viral pneumonia) and some are unique to pregnancy (e.g. amniotic fluid embolism (AFE), pre-eclampsia).[5] Pregnant patients are more susceptible to pulmonary oedema because of the increased blood volume and lower oncotic pressure. Mechanical ventilation can be more problematic in the pregnant patient.[6] Respiratory alkalosis is normal during pregnancy and fetal gas exchange must be considered when titrating respiratory support. Although the changes in anatomy and lung compliance present no difficulty to the mechanics of ventilation, strategies for managing adult respiratory distress syndrome (ARDS) such as permissive hypercapnia may be more difficult to implement[5,7] (see below).

CIRCULATION

ALTERED SIGNS

Tachycardia, low blood pressure, increased cardiac output and warm peripheries are normal in late pregnancy, but these can mask early signs of sepsis and hypovolaemia. After 20 weeks' gestation, aortocaval compression by the gravid uterus can decrease uterine perfusion and venous return to the heart. This is best prevented by using the full left lateral position, but a left lateral tilt or manual displacement of the uterus may be more practicable.

Haemodynamic support should generally start with good hydration, and assessment should take into account the altered cardiovascular variables in pregnancy. Non-invasive cardiac output monitoring is inaccurate and

Table 56.1 Changes in physiological variables during late pregnancy

Systolic arterial pressure	−5 mmHg
Mean arterial pressure	−5 mmHg
Diastolic arterial pressure	−10 mmHg
Central venous pressure	No change
Pulmonary capillary wedge pressure	No change
Heart rate	+15%
Stroke volume	+30%
Cardiac output	+45%
Systemic vascular resistance	−15%
Pulmonary vascular resistance	−30%
Tidal volume	+40%
Respiratory rate	+10%
Minute volume	+50%
Oxygen consumption	+20%
pH	No change
$Pa{O_2}$	+10 mmHg
$Pa{CO_2}$	−10 mmHg
$HCO3^-$	−4 mmol/l
Total blood volume	+40%
Haematocrit	−0.06
Plasma albumin	−5 g/l
Oncotic pressure	−3 mmHg

invasive monitoring with pulmonary artery catheters may be helpful in severe pre-eclampsia, pulmonary oedema and cardiac disease.[8] The uterine vascular bed is considered maximally dilated but still responsive to stimuli that cause vasoconstriction, such as circulating catecholamines. Ephedrine has traditionally been the vasoconstrictor used in obstetrics because it was thought to preserve uterine blood flow better than pure alpha-agonists. However, alpha-agonists such as phenylephrine are more effective and not associated with fetal acidosis when used to manage hypotension during caesarean delivery.[9] There is no evidence favouring any particular inotrope.

COAGULATION

Pregnancy is associated with a fivefold increase in thromboembolism, and patients should be given prophylaxis for thromboembolism, typically with unfractionated heparin or low-molecular-weight heparin (LMWH) and elastic compression stockings.

MOTHER AND FETUS

The mother's welfare usually takes precedence over fetal concerns, especially as fetal survival is dependent on optimal maternal management. However, the possibility of fetal viability also creates ethical dilemmas. In the critically ill it is important to monitor the fetus because of the problems associated with:

- premature labour
- the placental transfer of drugs
- maintenance of placental perfusion and oxygenation

An obstetric opinion should be sought as soon as possible regarding cardiotocography, ultrasound examination and timing of delivery. Nutrition is also very important for the fetus and adequate maternal feeding should be started as soon as possible. Perineal and breast nursing care should not be neglected.

CARDIOPULMONARY RESUSCITATION[10]

Cardiac arrest is rare in pregnancy and estimated to occur once in every 30 000 deliveries.

At more advanced gestation, one must consider potential fetal viability and recognise that the aetiology of cardiac arrest may include particular obstetric complications, such as AFE or drug toxicity from magnesium sulphate and local anaesthetics. As soon as the cardiac arrest call is activated, an obstetrician should be notified and preparations made for perimortem caesarean delivery if appropriate (see below).

Normally, external cardiac massage produces only 30% of cardiac output and this is reduced further if there is vena caval compression. After about 20 weeks' gestation it becomes increasingly necessary to relieve aortocaval compression during basic life support (BLS). Left lateral tilt decreases the efficiency of closed-chest compression, but a wedge providing an angle of 27° gives significant relief of vena caval obstruction while allowing 80% of the maximal force for chest compression.[11] During BLS, aortocaval compression may be minimised by manually displacing the uterus using a wedge, or positioning the pregnant patient's back on the rescuer's thighs. Chest compression should be performed with a slightly higher hand position (slightly above centre of sternum). Early tracheal intubation after cricoid pressure will facilitate ventilation and decrease the risk of acid aspiration. During advanced life support (ALS), drugs are given and defibrillation performed according to the normal protocols. Apical placement of the paddle may be difficult because of position and breast enlargement, and adhesive defibrillation pads are preferred.

Fetal or uterine monitors should be removed before defibrillation.

Case reports at advanced gestation indicate that both maternal and fetal survival from cardiac arrest may depend on prompt caesarean delivery to relieve the effects of aortocaval compression. The European Resuscitation Council Guidelines[12] and International Liaison Committee on Resuscitation (ILCOR) advisory statement[13] suggest that, if there is no immediate response to ALS, perimortem caesarean delivery should be considered. The decision must be made quickly because the surgery should start within 4 minutes of the arrest, with the aim of delivering the infant within 5 minutes of the arrest. There is no need to perform the delivery if the fetus is less than 20 weeks because aortal caval compression is not problematic then.

There is now some experience with somatic support after brain death to allow the fetus to mature.[10]

TRAUMA

Trauma occurs in approximately 6–7% of all pregnancies but only requires hospital admission in 0.3–0.4% of pregnancies. Trauma is the leading non-obstetric cause of maternal mortality and survivors have a high rate of fetal loss.[14] Head injuries and haemorrhagic shock account for most maternal deaths, while placental abruption and maternal death are the most frequent causes of fetal death.[15] Most injuries occur as the result of motor vehicle accidents, but other common causes are suicide (usually postpartum), falls and assaults.

Initial resuscitation should follow the normal plan of attention to airway, breathing and circulation.[16] Oxygen 100% should be given and cricoid pressure applied during tracheal intubation. Blood volume is increased during pregnancy and hypotension may not be evident until 35% or more of total blood volume is lost. Uterine blood flow is not autoregulated and may be decreased despite normal maternal haemodynamics, so that slight overhydration may be preferred to underhydration. Excessive resuscitation with crystalloids or non-blood colloids may increase the mortality from severe haemorrhage.

Treatment of hypotension always includes positioning or manual uterine displacement to avoid aortocaval compression. Drug treatment of modest hypotension can be started with ephedrine, but more potent vasopressors should be used if necessary. AFE has been reported after blunt abdominal trauma.

Assessment of trauma should note the increased significance of pelvic fractures for uterine injury and retroperitoneal haemorrhage.

- Ultrasound is the investigation of choice.
- Diagnostic peritoneal lavage, if performed, should be through an open surgical incision above the fundus.
- Chest drains are placed slightly higher than normal, in the third or fourth intercostal space.
- It is important to exclude herniation of abdominal contents through a ruptured diaphragm.

Necessary radiological investigations should be performed as indicated because radiation hazard to the fetus is very unlikely, except in the early first trimester, where exposure to more than 50–100 mGy is a cause for concern. A chest X-ray delivers less than 5 mGy to the lungs and very little to the shielded abdomen. The fetal radiation dose from abdominal examinations can range from 1 mGy for a plain film, up to 20–50 mGy for an abdominal pelvic computed tomography (CT) with fluoroscopy.[17]

Cardiotocographic monitoring is considered essential, but there is wide variation in practice and in the recommended duration of monitoring. Premature labour and placental abruption may not be diagnosed unless regular monitoring is continued for at least 6 hours and even 24 hours if indicated.[18] Rh immune globulin 300 g should be considered for all Rh D-negative within 72 hours of injury. The Kleihauer–Betke test can be used to detect fetal blood in the maternal circulation and give an estimate of the volume of transplacental haemorrhage.

BURNS

Serious burns during pregnancy are seen more commonly in the developing world. Although the women are usually young and healthy, pregnancy is already a hypermetabolic state and the fetus is at great risk from many complications.[19]

- Severe burns and sepsis are associated with high levels of prostaglandins that may cause preterm labour.
- Replacement of fluid loss from burns must keep in mind the normally increased circulating volume of pregnancy.
- Inhalational injuries with hypoxia and carbon monoxide are especially detrimental to the fetus.
- Infection is responsible for many of the maternal and fetal deaths but prophylactic antibiotic policies are controversial.

Patients of advanced gestation should not be kept supine and nutritional support for the fetus is necessary early. Topical povodine-iodine solution should be avoided because the iodine may be absorbed and affect fetal thyroid function. Premature delivery may have to be considered, especially with extensive burns.

SEVERE OBSTETRIC HAEMORRHAGE

Severe bleeding is the most important cause of maternal death worldwide. Peripartum haemorrhage contributes to 15% of maternal deaths, but if one includes ectopic pregnancy, 25% of maternal deaths are a result of haemorrhage. It seems obvious that the treatment of massive haemorrhage requires sufficient intravenous access and the logistic capability to replace circulating volume quickly with warmed fluids, blood and clotting factors. Adequate preparation may even require the use of cell saver technology and operating in the angiography suite after the placement of catheters in preparation for embolisation. Unfortunately, many deaths have occurred because blood loss was often underestimated and volume replacement delayed. Conversely, excessive resuscitation with crystalloids or non-blood colloids when blood is required may increase the mortality from severe haemorrhage.

Antepartum haemorrhage is mostly from placenta praevia or placental abruption and both are ultimately managed by delivery. In placenta praevia, the placenta implants in advance of the presenting part and classically presents as painless bleeding during the second or third trimester. Placenta praevia is relatively common (1 in 200 pregnancies) but severe haemorrhage is relatively rare. In placental abruption, a normally implanted placenta separates from the uterine wall. The incidence of placental abruption is low (0.5–2%) but perinatal mortality may be as high as 50%. Several litres of blood may be concealed in the uterus as a retroplacental clot. Bleeding may continue after delivery for a variety of reasons, including:

- uterine atony
- lacerations to cervix or vagina
- disseminated intravascular coagulation
- placenta accreta

Postpartum haemorrhage is usually from uterine atony or placenta accreta. In an emergency, the aorta can be compressed against the vertebral column by a fist pressed on the abdomen above the umbilicus. The control of haemorrhage allows time for resuscitation and more definitive surgical treatment.

Uterine atony is managed initially with bimanual compression, uterine massage and intravenous oxytocin given intravenously by bolus (5 units) or infusion (20 units). Oral misoprostol (0.6–1.0 mg) can also be used, while methylergonovine (0.2 mg) or 15-methyl-prostaglandin $F_{2\alpha}$ (0.25 mg) is given intramuscularly or intramyometrially for persistent atony. Recombinant factor VIIa has also been used but the place of this therapy is still unclear.[38,39] If bleeding persists, tamponade techniques using gauze packs or balloons may be useful. Otherwise specific invasive management such as angiographic arterial embolisation, surgical ligation of the uterine, ovarian or internal iliac arteries or hysterectomy may be required.[20]

With massive bleeding and transfusion, there should be no need to wait for a coagulation profile before giving coagulation factors. Disseminated intravascular coagulation still develops in 10–30% of cases, partly because tissue thromboplastin is released during abruption. Blood should be sent for measurement of fibrinogen and fibrin degradation products and blood component therapy, and cryoprecipitate given as appropriate.

SEPSIS AND SEPTIC SHOCK[21,22]

Although sepsis is a major problem in intensive care, maternal sepsis and septic shock are relatively uncommon and the prognosis is usually better than in the general population. The most common sources of infection are chorioamnionitis, postpartum endometritis, urinary tract infections, pyelonephritis and septic abortion. The physiological changes of pregnancy may influence the course and presentation of septic shock. Animal studies suggest that pregnancy increases the susceptibility to endotoxin, and that metabolic acidosis and cardiovascular collapse occur earlier.

Management of septic shock follows normal guidelines with eradication of the infectious source, although the normal range for haemodynamic variables may be different. Gram-negative organisms are the frequent causative organisms but streptococci and *Bacteroides* may also be present. Antimicrobial therapy is dependent on hospital prevalence and susceptibility patterns, but empirical broad-spectrum therapy should be started early. Typical combinations are ampicillin, gentamicin and clindamycin, or imipenem, cilastatin and vancomycin. Tetracyclines and quinolones should not be used in pregnancy.

Newer approaches such as insulin therapy, corticosteroids and activated protein C have not been properly evaluated in pregnancy.[2]

VENOUS THROMBOEMBOLISM[23]

Pulmonary thromboembolism is a common cause of maternal death, accounting for 15–25% of maternal mortality. Pregnancy is associated with a fivefold increase in thromboembolism because of:

- venous stasis
- hypercoagulable state
- vascular injury associated with delivery.

Patients with acquired and hereditary thrombophilias have an even greater risk.

Accurate diagnosis of venous thromboembolism is crucial because of the long-term implications for therapy. Symptoms of dyspnoea or pain in the leg or chest require accurate diagnosis, especially in the immediate postpartum period. Although contrast venography is the gold-standard test for diagnosing deep-vein thrombosis, the radiation exposure and invasive nature of the test mean that duplex Doppler ultrasonography is the usual first choice. D-dimer testing may also be useful but a positive test must be interpreted in the clinical context because D-dimer values normally increase throughout pregnancy. Venography, perfusion lung scanning, pulmonary angiography and helical CT scan should not be avoided if indicated.[2]

There are various reviews summarising the guidelines for anticoagulant therapy during pregnancy.[24,25] Although LMWH has gradually replaced unfractionated heparin for the prophylaxis and treatment of deep-venous thrombosis and pulmonary embolism in pregnancy, there is not adequate evidence for a definitive recommendation in pregnancy. Patients with suspected or proven deep-vein thrombosis or pulmonary embolus should be given full anticoagulant therapy that is continued throughout pregnancy. Warfarin should not be used before delivery so heparin is continued until labour begins and restarted in the postpartum patient for at least 6–12 weeks.

With life-threatening massive pulmonary embolus, surgical treatment or thrombolysis must be considered. Thrombolysis was thought to be relatively contraindicated during pregnancy because of the risk of maternal and fetal haemorrhagic complications. No controlled trials are feasible and outcome data must be extracted from case reports. A recent review found that thrombolytic therapy was associated with a low maternal mortality rate of 1%, with a 6% rate of fetal loss and 6% rate of premature delivery.[26] The fetal risks appear to be lower than that obtained with surgical intervention in pregnant patients, and maternal risks lower than reported risks for surgery, thrombolysis or transvenous filters in non-pregnant patients. Although heparin remains the treatment of choice, thrombolysis appears to be a viable option except during the immediate postpartum period.

AMNIOTIC FLUID EMBOLISM

AFE remains largely an unpredictable and unpreventable disease of uncertain pathophysiology.[27,28] Most of the information about AFE has been derived from case reports, maternal mortality reviews and reports from national registries of AFE, such as those in the USA[29] and UK.[30] The incidence of AFE varies between 1 in 8000 and 1 in 80 000 deliveries, although there must be undetected and unsuspected cases where minimal amounts of amniotic fluid produce few symptoms. AFE is the cause of 5–10% of maternal deaths, and 25–50% of patients with suspected or proven AFE die within the first hour. The overall maternal mortality has been as high as 86% in symptomatic patients, with a perinatal and neonatal mortality up to 40% and significant neurological problems in surviving neonates. However, recent figures of 26–37% mortality are more encouraging and this may be the result of early suspicion of AFE and early intensive care support.

AFE was thought to be associated with vigorous labour and the use of oxytocics, but it may occur in any parturient. The exact pathogenic factors for the syndrome of AFE remain unclear.[31] Amniotic fluid is thought to enter the maternal circulation through endocervical or uterine lacerations, uterine veins at the site of placental separation or placental abruption. Amniotic fluid normally contains prostaglandins, leukotrienes, endothelin and fetal debris that can cause complement activation, pulmonary vasoconstriction and physical blockage of pulmonary capillaries, with resultant damage and release of further mediators. By these mechanisms, AFE has more in common with anaphylaxis and septic shock than other embolic diseases.

The initial diagnosis of AFE is made on clinical grounds and is often one of exclusion. Classically, patients may present with severe dyspnoea, cyanosis, sudden cardiovascular collapse, coma or convulsions during labour but AFE may occur earlier during pregnancy, during delivery or in the early puerperium. Some patients may present with bleeding and most patients eventually develop a coagulopathy.

Animal studies indicate that AFE causes a biphasic haemodynamic response. The early phase probably lasts less than half an hour and is characterised by severe hypoxia and right heart failure as a result of pulmonary hypertension from vasoconstriction or vessel damage. Patients who survive this first phase develop left ventricular failure with return of normal right ventricular function. Left ventricular failure may be a result of the initial hypoxia or the depressant effects of mediators. Disseminated intravascular coagulation is present in most patients but the mechanism is unknown. It could be caused by a specific activator of factor X, tissue factor or other substances, such as trophoblasts, in the amniotic fluid. Traditionally, AFE is confirmed by detection of squamous cells and fetal debris in the pulmonary circulation either at autopsy or in blood samples from a pulmonary artery catheter, but squamous cells are a contaminant that can be found in other parturients and even in non-pregnant patients.

No specific therapy is available. Immediate cardiopulmonary resuscitation and 100% oxygen are necessary. Assessment of central venous pressure may be misleading, and early pulmonary artery catheterisation has been advocated in a series reporting 100% survival in 5 patients by treating left ventricular failure aggressively.[32] The differential diagnoses must be evaluated quickly because urgent delivery of the fetus by caesarean section may improve resuscitation and prevent further AFE. Patients who survive the first few hours will continue to require supportive treatment for their acute lung injury. Blood component therapy is given as necessary to manage the coagulopathy. Cryoprecipitate has sometimes provided significant improvement in patient oxygenation, and recombinant factor VIIa has also been used. Survivors of AFE regain normal cardiorespiratory function but may have neurological sequelae.

ACUTE RESPIRATORY FAILURE

Asthma is the commonest respiratory condition complicating pregnancy but specific concerns are mainly related to the possibility of fetal toxicity from pharmacologic therapy. However there is no evidence that systemic corticosteroids or short-term use of beta-agonists are associated with adverse fetal outcomes.[6]

Pulmonary oedema is more likely in the pregnant patient (1:1000 pregnancies) because of the increased cardiac output and blood volume, and the decreased plasma oncotic pressure. The principles of treatment are relatively straightforward in terms of determining the cause of the oedema and improving oxygenation, although it can be difficult to distinguish between hydrostatic and permeability oedema.[2,7]

The prevalence of acute respiratory distress syndrome during pregnancy has been estimated at 16–70 cases per 100 000 pregnancies, with mortality rates from 23 to 50%.[5,7] Some of the recommended strategies for managing this condition may be problematic. Low tidal volumes make it difficult to maintain the increased ventilatory requirements of pregnancy, and higher tidal volumes and alveolar plateau pressures up to 35 cmH_2O (0.34 kPa) may be necessary. Transfer of CO_2 across the placenta requires a gradient of 10 mmHg (1.33 kPa). Permissive hypercapnia may cause fetal respiratory acidosis that will reduce the ability of fetal haemoglobin to bind oxygen, and Pa_{CO_2} should probably be kept below 45 mmHg (6.0 kPa) and Pa_{O_2}

above 70 mmHg (9.3 kPa).[5] If conventional ventilation fails, the effectiveness of alternative strategies is unknown. There are no data on the prone position and only a few reports of inhaled nitric oxide.

Unlike in other obstetric-related conditions, delivery of the fetus does not appear to result in marked improvement of maternal respiratory failure.

ACID ASPIRATION (MENDELSON'S SYNDROME)

Obstetric patients are at increased risk of acid aspiration because of decreased gastric emptying, increased gastric acidity and volume and increased intra-abdominal pressure. Aspiration of acidic material will cause acute lung injury, the severity being related to the amount, content and acidity of the aspirate.

The initial presentation is hypoxaemia and bronchospasm. Chemical pneumonitis and increased permeability pulmonary oedema develop over several hours.

Treatment includes standard respiratory support. Rigid bronchoscopy may be required to remove large food particles. Bronchoalveolar lavage and steroids are not useful and antibiotics should only be given for proven infection.

TOCOLYTIC THERAPY AND PULMONARY OEDEMA[33]

Pulmonary oedema is an uncommon (1 in 400 pregnancies) but serious complication of tocolytic therapy with beta-adrenergic agonists. The underlying mechanism for pulmonary oedema is unclear, but it is probably related to fluid overload and the cardiovascular effects of beta-adrenergic agonists leading to increased pulmonary capillary hydrostatic pressure. The initial management of pulmonary oedema is discontinuation of the beta-adrenergic agonist and oxygen therapy, with further monitoring, diuretics and respiratory support as necessary. This problem should disappear as alternative tocolytics such as nifedipine and atosiban are used.

COCAINE TOXICITY[34]

Cocaine abuse during pregnancy has become a significant problem in the USA, affecting more than 30 million people, with 90% of the women of child-bearing age. Cocaine has local anaesthetic and sympathomimetic actions and can cause:

- hypertension, dysrhythmias, myocardial ischaemia and infarction
- tachycardia and increased cardiac output, but decreased uterine blood flow
- increased uterine contractility

Patients commonly present with chest pain. cardiovascular complications or placental abruption and fetal distress. Acute toxicity may also mimic pre-eclampsia by presenting with cerebral haemorrhage or convulsions.

For the treatment of hypertension, the drug of choice is controversial. Although hydralazine is often used in obstetrics to treat maternal hypertension, labetalol is also widely used. However, concerns about beta-blockers allowing unopposed alpha-adrenergic stimulation may also apply to a lesser extent with labetalol, and calcium-channel antagonists and nitroglycerine have also been advocated. Nitroglycerine and benzodiazepines have been recommended for the treatment of cocaine-related myocardial ischaemia and infarction.

OVARIAN HYPERSTIMULATION SYNDROME[35]

Ovarian hyperstimulation syndrome (OHSS) remains a significant but unpredictable and incompletely understood complication of ovarian stimulation. The syndrome is typically associated with:

- exogenous human chorionic gonadotrophin (hCG) regimens, used to induce ovulation in assisted reproduction techniques
- increased capillary permeability, leading progressively to hypovolaemia with haemoconcentration, oedema and accumulation of fluid in the abdomen and pleural spaces

The pathophysiology of OHSS has not been fully determined. A likely mediator is vascular endothelial growth factor, but many interacting cytokines and endocrine factors may be involved.

OHSS is most severe at several days to a week after a stimulated cycle, but early signs and symptoms can often be seen during the stimulatory phase. Fertility clinics will have their own protocols to try and minimise the incidence of OHSS and to detect its early stages. In general, symptoms resolve spontaneously over 2 weeks, in parallel with the decline in hCG from the last doses given. However, a successful pregnancy implantation will increase endogenous hCG and may temporarily worsen OHSS. Although subclinical OHSS may be found in most patients, only a small percentage require ward admission for careful fluid management to restore circulating volume with saline or albumin, prevention of thrombosis with heparin, and treatment of ascites by ultrasound-guided paracentesis as necessary. Severe OHSS may cause renal failure, respiratory failure or thromboembolism, which requires supportive intensive care therapy. Invasive monitoring is essential for fluid management.

REFERENCES

1. Zeeman GG. Obstetric critical care; a blueprint for improved outcomes. *Crit Care Med* 2006; **34** (Suppl.): S208–214.
2. Martin SR, Foley MR. Intensive care in obstetrics: an evidence-based review. *Am J Obstet Gynecol* 2006; **195**: 673–89.

3. Clutton-Brock T. Maternal deaths from anaesthesia. An extract from Why Mothers Die 2000-2002, the Confidential Enquiries into Maternal Deaths in the United Kingdom. Chapter 17: Trends in intensive care. *Br J Anaesth* 2005; **94**: 424–9. [Full report available at http://www.cemach.org.uk/.].
4. Chamberlain G, Broughton-Pipkin F. *Clinical Physiology in Obstetrics*, 3rd edn. Oxford: Blackwell Science; 1998.
5. Cole DE, Taylor TL, McCullough DM *et al.* Acute respiratory distress syndrome in pregnancy *Crit Care Med* 2005; **33** (Suppl.): S269–78.
6. Campbell LA, Klocke RA. Implications for the pregnant patient. *Am J Respir Crit Care Med* 2001; **163**: 1051–4.
7. Bandi VD, Munnur U, Matthay MA. Acute lung injury and acute respiratory distress syndrome in pregnancy. *Crit Care Clin* 2004; **20**: 577–607.
8. Fujitani S, Baldisseri MR. Hemodynamic assessment in a pregnant and peripartum patient. *Crit Care Med* 2005; **33** (Suppl.): S354–61.
9. Macarthur A, Riley ET. Obstetric anesthesia controversies: vasopressor choice for postspinal hypotension during cesarean delivery. *Int Anesthesiol Clin* 2007; **45**: 115–32.
10. Mallampalli A, Guy E. Cardiac arrest in pregnancy and somatic support after brain death. *Crit Care Med* 2005; **33** (Suppl.): S325–31.
11. Rees GAD, Willis BA. Resuscitation in late pregnancy. *Anaesthesia* 1988; **43**: 347–9.
12. Soar J, Deakin CD, Nolan JP *et al.* European Resuscitation Council Guidelines for Resuscitation 2005. Section 7. Cardiac arrest in special circumstances. *Resuscitation* 2005; **67** (Suppl. 1): S135–70.
13. Kloeck W, Cummins RO, Chamberlain D *et al.* Special resuscitation situations. An advisory statement from the International Liaison Committee on Resuscitation. *Circulation* 1997; **95**: 2196–210.
14. Mattox KL, Goetzl L. Trauma in pregnancy. *Crit Care Med* 2005; **33** (Suppl.): S385–9.
15. Rogers FB, Rozycki GS, Osler TM *et al.* A multi-institutional study of factors associated with fetal death in injured pregnant patients. *Arch Surg* 1999; **134**: 1274–7.
16. Tsuei BJ. Assessment of the pregnant trauma patient. *Injury* 2006; **37**: 367–73.
17. Goldman SM, Wagner LK. Radiological management of abdominal trauma in pregnancy. *Am J Radiol* 1996; **166**: 763–7.
18. Curet MJ, Schermer CR, Demarest GB *et al.* Predictors of outcome in trauma during pregnancy: identification of patients who can be monitored for less than 6 hours. *J Trauma* 2000; **49**: 18–25.
19. Polko LE, McMahon MJ. Burns in pregnancy. *Obstet Gynecol Surv* 1998; **53**: 50–6.
20. American College of Obstetricians and Gynecologists. ACOG Practice Bulletin: Clinical management guidelines for obstetrician-gynecologists number 76, October 2006. Postpartum hemorrhage. *Obstet Gynecol* 2006; **108**: 1039–47.
21. Sheffield JS. Sepsis and septic shock in pregnancy. *Crit Care Clin* 2004; **20**: 651–60.
22. Fernández-Pérez ER, Salman S, Pendem S *et al.* Sepsis during pregnancy. *Crit Care Med* 2005; **33** (Suppl.): S286–93.
23. Stone SE, Morris TA. Pulmonary embolism during and after pregnancy: maternal and fetal issues. *Crit Care Med* 2005; **33** (Suppl.): S294–300.
24. Krivak TC, Zorn KK. Venous thromboembolism in obstetrics and gynecology. *Obstet Gynecol* 2007; **109**: 761–77.
25. Andres RL, Miles A. Venous thromboembolism and pregnancy. *Obstet Gynecol Clin North Am* 2001; **28**: 613–30.
26. Ahearn GS, Hadjiliadas D, Govert JA *et al.* Massive pulmonary embolism during pregnancy successfully treated with recombinant tissue plasminogen activator: a case report and review of treatment options. *Arch Intern Med* 2002; **162**: 1221–7.
27. O'Shea A, Eappen S. Amniotic fluid embolism. *Int Anaesthesiol Clin* 2007; **45**: 17–28.
28. Davies S. Amniotic fluid embolus: a review of the literature. *Can J Anaesth* 2001; **48**: 88–98.
29. Clark SL, Hankins GDV, Dudley DA *et al.* Amniotic fluid embolism: analysis of the national registry. *Am J Obstet Gynecol* 1995; **172**: 1158–69.
30. Tuffnell DJ. United Kingdom amniotic fluid embolism register. *Br J Obstet Gynaecol* 2005; **112**: 1625–9.
31. Moore J, Baldisseri MR. Amniotic fluid embolism. *Crit Care Med* 2005; **33** (Suppl.): S279–85.
32. Clark SL, Cotton DB, Gonik B *et al.* Central hemodynamic alterations in amniotic fluid embolism. *Am J Obstet Gynecol* 1988; **158**: 1124–6.
33. Lamont RF. The pathophysiology of pulmonary oedema with the use of beta-agonists. *Br J Obstet Gynaecol* 2000; **107**: 439–44.
34. Kuczkowski KM. Peripartum care of the cocaine-abusing parturient: are we ready? *Acta Obstet Gynecol Scand* 2005: **84**: 108–16.
35. Avecillas JF, Falcone T, Arroliga AC. Ovarian hyperstimulation syndrome. *Crit Care Clin* 2004; **20**: 679–95.
36. Vasdev GM, Harrison BA, Keegan MT, Burkle CM. Management of the difficult and failed airway in obstetric anesthesia. *J Anesth* 2008; **22**: 38–48.
37. Kuczkowski KM, Reisner LS, Benumof JL. Airway problems and new solutions for the obstetric patient. *J Clin Anesth* 2003; **15**: 552–63.
38. Welsh A, McLintock C, Gatt S *et al.* Guidelines for the use of recombinant activated factor VII in massive obstetric haemorrhage. *Aust NZ J Obstet Gynaecol* 2008; **48**: 12–6.
39. Platt F, Van de Velde M. Recombinant factor VIIa should be used in massive obstertric haemorrhage. *Int J Obstet Anesth* 2007; **16**: 354–9. (Report on debate: Platt F, Proposer, pp 354–7 and Van de Velde M, Opposer, pp 357–9).

57

Severe pre-existing disease in pregnancy

Steve M Yentis

The two main sources of information about the spectrum of pre-existing conditions that result in severe morbidity in pregnancy are national or local registries/databases and published case series of admissions to intensive care, high-dependency units or obstetric units. Information about mortality comes from registries of maternal death such as the Confidential Enquiries into Maternal and Child Health (CEMACH; formerly Reports on Confidential Enquiries into Maternal Deaths) in the UK, or from individual case series. Taken together, the most important pre-existing conditions likely to lead to intensive care unit (ICU) admission and/or death overall are cardiac disease, respiratory disease, neurological disease, psychaiatric disease (including drug addiction) and haematological, connective tissue and metabolic disease.

With increasingly successful medical care during childhood and early adulthood, the number of women with severe disease who survive to child-bearing age has increased. Part of such women's wishes to live a normal life includes the desire to have children, and this places increasing demands on obstetric, anaesthetic and ICU services, as well as on women's physiological reserves.

It is important that women with severe disease are appropriately counselled before pregnancy since the risks to both them and their fetuses may be considerable. This early counselling should ideally include anaesthetic input.

CARDIAC DISEASE

There are more maternal deaths in the UK from cardiac disease than from pre-eclampsia and haemorrhage combined.[1] Over the last 20–40 years, there has been a shift away from acquired cardiac disease (mainly rheumatic heart disease) towards congenital heart disease as modern techniques of cardiac surgery in early life enable female babies with previously fatal conditions to reach maturity. More recently, there has been an increase in prevalence of ischaemic heart disease resulting from increased obesity, maternal age and smoking. Mortality varies from less than 1% in uncomplicated conditions to over 40% in Eisenmenger's syndrome, even with modern methods of medical management.[2]

PHYSIOLOGY AND PATHOPHYSIOLOGY

The physiological changes of pregnancy are discussed in Chapter 56. The changes most relevant to cardiac disease are:

- susceptibility to aortocaval compression
- reduction in systemic vascular resistance
- increases in blood volume and cardiac output by up to 40–50% by the 20th week of gestation, with a potential further increase in cardiac output (up to 50%) during labour

In patients whose cardiac function is already impaired, such as those with cardiomyopathy or valvular stenoses, inability to meet these challenges may result in cardiac failure. If there is a right-to-left shunt, the fall in systemic vascular resistance encourages blood to bypass the lungs; this, together with the increasing demands of the fetus and the reduced maternal pulmonary reserve, may lead to severe exacerbation of hypoxaemia.

GENERAL ANTEPARTUM AND PERIPARTUM MANAGEMENT

Antepartum management consists mainly of regular assessments and measures to reduce cardiac workload, for example, by reducing activity and treating arrhythmias/cardiac failure.

Electrocardiography, chest X-ray and echocardiography are the most useful investigations. Flow gradients across stenosed valves can be expected to increase in pregnancy because of the increase in cardiac output that occurs, and echocardiographic measurement of valve areas provides a more consistent and useful measure of severity in such cases. Pulse oximetry is a simple, non-invasive tool for monitoring the degree of right-to-left shunt and can easily be repeated during pregnancy.

An obstetric and anaesthetic plan should be prepared and the intensivists informed of the anticipated delivery date. Antithromboembolic prophylaxis should be considered since cardiac patients are more at risk, even without prolonged bedrest. Low-molecular-weight heparins are now standard for prophylaxis, although both heparin and warfarin have been used for patients with prosthetic heart valves, the main decision being between the better safety profile of heparin for the fetus but with greater risk of thrombosis in the mother, and the more effective anticoagulation achieved with warfarin but with greater risk of fetal complications.[3] The requirements for heparin increase in pregnancy, so greater doses than normal are usually required.

The principles of peripartum management have moved over the last few years towards vaginal delivery unless caesarean section is indicated for obstetric indications. Elective caesarean section has been advocated in the past as a matter of course, traditionally under general anaesthesia, but the stresses and complications of surgery are now generally felt to exceed those of a well-controlled vaginal delivery. Low-dose epidural regimens using weak solutions of local anaesthetic (e.g. 0.1% bupivacaine or less) with opioids such as fentanyl have been found to be effective and cardiostable.[4] Combined spinal epidural analgesia using similar low concentrations are also suitable, and continuous spinal analgesia has also been described. In patients with marked exercise intolerance, outlet forceps or ventouse delivery is usually recommended to limit pushing and the duration of the second stage. If caesarean section is required, both regional and general anaesthesia have their advocates,[5,6] but either is acceptable so long as due care is taken.

Peripartum complications such as bleeding, pulmonary oedema, arrhythmias and sudden increases in pulmonary vascular resistance or drops in systemic vascular resistance may be tolerated badly by patients with limited reserves.

Oxytocin analogue (Syntocinon) has marked cardiovascular effects[7,8] that, although tolerable in normal patients, may cause a calamitous drop in systemic vascular resistance with hypotension, tachycardia and worsening of shunt in susceptible patients. If Syntocinon is required it should be diluted and given very slowly (e.g. 5 units infused over 10–20 minutes). Withholding of oxytocics altogether may be a problem as such patients may be especially sensitive to acute blood loss. In patients with fixed cardiac outputs and no pulmonary hypertension, ergometrine may be preferable. At caesarean section, mechanical compression of the uterus with a 'brace' suture may be used to reduce or avoid the need for oxytocics.[9] Exacerbation of right-to-left shunt is manifested by worsening hypoxaemia, which may be improved by vasoconstrictors such as phenylephrine – the chronotropic and inotropic effects of ephedrine are often undesirable in patients with cardiac disease.

Monitoring ranges from simple non-invasive methods to peripheral arterial, central venous and pulmonary arterial cannulation, depending on the severity of the underlying disease.[10] Arterial cannulation is usually straightforward but central venous cannulation is often difficult because of the increased maternal body weight and fluid retention, and the inability to lie flat, let alone head-down. The antecubital fossa should be considered as a route for cannulation first. Scrupulous attention must be paid to avoiding intravascular air in patients with right-to-left shunts, because of the risk of systemic embolism.

Table 57.1 Common peripartum problems in patients with pre-existing cardiac disease

- Arrhythmias
- Cardiac failure/pulmonary oedema
- Pulmonary embolism
- Bacterial endocarditis
- Increased susceptibility to the effects of haemorrhage
- Increased risk of cardiovascular collapse in response to iatrogenic reductions in systemic vascular resistance, e.g. regional anaesthesia, intravenous bolus of oxytocin
- Myocardial ischaemia (certain lesions)
- Increased risk from air embolism (certain lesions)

The principles of haemodynamic support are generally the same as in non-pregnant patients, remembering that pregnant women have a propensity to acute lung injury if overloaded with fluid. The physiological changes of pregnancy, especially tachycardia and increased cardiac output, should be remembered. The risk from aortocaval compression is often forgotten and this must be reinforced at all times, with the woman placed in the lateral or supine wedged position. If a pregnant woman requires intensive care before the baby is born, there may be a conflict between the maternal need for vasopressors and/or inotropes and the adverse effects of these drugs on uteroplacental blood flow. Similarly, attempts to prolong pregnancy with steroids and β_2-adrenergic agonists such as terbutaline or salbutamol may cause adverse cardiovascular effects (primarily pulmonary oedema) in the mother.

Common peripartum complications are summarised in Table 57.1.

POSTPARTUM COMPLICATIONS

Women may continue to be at risk from bleeding, arrhythmias and cardiac failure postpartum. Specific problems need to be considered:

- If oxytocin has been withheld, postpartum haemorrhage may become a problem.
- Pulmonary embolism is a particular risk in the postpartum period, and the risks and benefits of anticoagulant therapy must be weighed up in each individual case.
- Patients with Eisenmenger's syndrome typically die on or around the 10th postpartum day of pulmonary haemorrhage, embolism or both.[11]
- Endocarditis should be prevented with appropriate antibacterial drugs (typically amoxicillin and gentamicin, or vancomycin if allergic to penicillin). The threat of endocarditis should always be considered.
- There is susceptibility to chest infection and its effects (and those of wound or other infection) may be devastating; thus a high index of suspicion and aggressive early management are required.

RESPIRATORY DISEASE

The most common respiratory causes of morbidity and mortality in pregnancy are pneumonia, asthma and cystic fibrosis; thus the latter two conditions are the most common pre-existing respiratory diseases that cause mothers to present to ICUs.[1,12–14]

Asthma is very common but rarely causes serious morbidity in its own right, although there is a higher risk of maternal and neonatal morbidity.[12]

Cystic fibrosis is relatively rare but is more likely to be associated with poor outcomes.[13,14] Studies suggest that pregnancy itself does not increase mortality in women with mild cystic fibrosis and that the risk factors are the same as in non-pregnant patients (pre-pregnancy forced expiratory volume in 1 second (FEV_1) < 50–60% of predicted; colonisation with *Burkholderia cepacia*; and pancreatic insufficiency). Overall mortality has been reported as 5% within 2 years of pregnancy, 10–20% within 5 years of pregnancy and 20–21% within 10 years. Psychological support is an important consideration. The decision to have a child, with the risk of passing on the cystic fibrosis gene and the adverse effect that pregnancy might have on the mother, is one that imposes a great deal of stress on the mother, her partner and their relatives.

PHYSIOLOGY AND PATHOPHYSIOLOGY

If respiratory function is already impaired, the physiological effects of pregnancy add an extra burden on the respiratory system that may precipitate respiratory failure:

- reduced functional residual capacity
- splinting of the diaphragm
- increased oxygen demand

In cystic fibrosis, an additional stress is the increased nutritional demand in a patient who may already be malnourished because of malabsorption. In addition, chronic hypoxaemia may lead to chronic pulmonary vasoconstriction, cor pulmonale and pulmonary hypertension.

GENERAL MANAGEMENT AND COMPLICATIONS

Antepartum management comprises regular assessment and adjustment of medical treatment when required. Patients may be taking a variety of drugs, including steroids. This is particularly relevant in asthma, in which there is a trend nowadays towards aggressive treatment of acute exacerbations of asthma, with early use of steroids. Although prednisolone is about 90% metabolised by the placenta, large doses have been associated with neonatal adrenal suppression.

Regional analgesia is indicated in patients with moderate or severe functional limitation, in order to reduce the demands of labour. If caesarean section is required, regional anaesthesia is thought to reduce the risk of postoperative pulmonary complications, although objective evidence is lacking. Care is required, for if regional anaesthesia extends too high, ventilation and the ability to cough may be impaired.

In cystic fibrosis, the principles of intensive care are generally the same as in non-pregnant patients. Assessment of patients with respiratory disease requires knowledge of the physiological changes induced by pregnancy and parameters such as blood gases need to be considered in that context. An arterial partial pressure of carbon dioxide of 45 mmHg (6 kPa) represents a much greater deviation from the normal value in pregnancy than in non-pregnant patients. The mainstay of supportive treatment is regular physiotherapy and antibiotic therapy. It is important to know whether the patient has been previously colonized with unusual and/or resistant organisms, for example, *Burkholderia cepacia*. The biggest single hazard for the mother is an acute infective exacerbation in the middle/third trimester provoking incipient respiratory failure. Infection has to be treated both early and aggressively. Exhaustion and respiratory failure have been managed with non-invasive ventilatory techniques with some success.

Problems with intermittent positive-pressure ventilation during an acute exacerbation in severe disease appear to relate to widely disparate compliance in different lung areas. This produces $\dot{V}/\dot{Q}$ mismatch with a large effective physiological dead space. The key to management is control and clearance of the underlying infection but this can be very difficult.

The beneficial effect of delivery on maternal oxygenation is usually immediate, although pain following caesarean section may limit deep inspiration and encourage basal atelectasis. Fatigue can also be a problem. Just because the baby has been delivered, scrupulous respiratory support cannot be forgone.

NEUROLOGICAL DISEASE

Epilepsy has been highlighted as an important cause of maternal death, often related to poor medical control secondary to altered pharmacodynamics and pharmacokinetics of anticonvulsant drugs in pregnancy. A convulsion while in the bath is a particular risk. In terms of pre-existing neurological disease leading to admission to the ICU during or shortly after pregnancy, no single condition stands out, although those potentially affecting respiratory function (e.g. myasthenia gravis, multiple sclerosis and high spinal cord lesions) might be expected to cause particular problems.

GENERAL MANAGEMENT

Until recently, regional analgesia and anaesthesia was traditionally avoided in most neurological disease, for fear of exacerbating the condition, or being blamed for an exacerbation should it occur. Nowadays, most authorities actively encourage regional analgesia for labour since it

Table 57.2 Guide to converting oral to systemic medication in mothers with myasthenia gravis. Approximate conversion doses are given

Drug	Oral dose	Intramuscular dose	Intravenous dose
Neostigmine	15 mg	0.7–1.0 mg	0.5 mg
Pyridostigmine	60 mg	3–4 mg	2 mg

reduces the physiological demand and thus the risk of respiratory insufficiency or excess fatigue. Similarly, regional anaesthesia for caesarean section avoids the problems of excessive postoperative sedation and how or whether to use neuromuscular-blocking drugs, including suxamethonium. Initial fears about an increased relapse rate of multiple sclerosis following regional anaesthesia have fortunately not been borne out by large prospective series.[15]

If there is raised intracranial pressure, the use of regional techniques is more controversial. On the one hand, labour and vaginal delivery without effective analgesia can result in marked increases in intracranial pressure; on the other, accidental dural puncture can be disastrous. Even if successfully placed, rapid epidural injection may be associated with increases in intracranial pressure.[16] This risk still exists with epidural analgesic techniques continued into the postoperative period.

Management of conditions in which there are spinal abnormalities is also controversial. Spina bifida and other lesions have been successfully managed using regional techniques, although in each case a careful balance between risk and benefit must be achieved. These patients are unlikely to present to intensivists unless they are associated with respiratory impairment.

Myasthenia gravis poses a particular problem because of the need for regular medication throughout labour and after delivery. Gastric emptying may be decreased during labour, especially if systemic opioids are given, although this effect can also occur (albeit to a lesser extent) with boluses of epidural opioids. It is therefore important to consider alternative routes of administering the mother's drug therapy if opioids are given in this way. A useful guide is offered in Table 57.2. Epidural analgesia can be very helpful in limiting maternal fatigue during and after labour. The mother needs watching carefully for signs of increasing weakness up to 7–10 days postpartum.

PSYCHIATRIC DISEASE (INCLUDING DRUG ADDICTION)

Psychiatric disease features consistently in surveys of maternal morbidity and mortality, for example through parasuicide or suicide, violence or the complications of drug addiction. In recent CEMACH reports, suicide and psychiatric disease are relatively common causes of death overall.[1] Psychiatric patients may be more vulnerable to becoming pregnant, and pregnant women more vulnerable to suffering from psychiatric disease either during or after pregnancy.

Abuse of drugs poses similar problems to those in the non-pregnant population, with the additional effect of fetal addiction and retarded growth. In particular, cocaine is commonly abused in parts of the developed world and has been implicated in causing placental abruption and maternal convulsions, hypertension and tachycardia, with increased morbidity and mortality for both mother and fetus.[17] Unplanned operative intervention for delivery is more likely, which may contribute to an increased requirement for intensive care. The combination of substance abuse and human immunodeficiency virus (HIV) infection poses a particular challenge in the obstetric patient.

Management in terms of intensive care is usually similar to that in non-pregnant patients, with special attention to the effects of maternal drugs on the fetus (if antepartum), for example those taken in overdose or those used for sedation and as antidotes.

HAEMATOLOGICAL, CONNECTIVE TISSUE AND METABOLIC DISEASE

Several haematological conditions may predispose to critical illness in pregnancy, sickle-cell disease being one of the most common. Patients with coagulopathy are clearly at increased risk of haemorrhage but, in general, ICU management of patients with haematological disease is as for non-pregnant patients. It is important that all staff appreciate that significant amounts of blood may be lost into the uterus or vagina without its being visible externally.

Connective tissue disease rarely presents to the intensivist unless there is widespread and severe systemic involvement. Cardiac and pulmonary manifestations are the usual culprits, and these may be exacerbated by pregnancy because of the increased demands. Such patients are also at risk of obstetric complications such as bleeding (including postpartum).

Diabetes mellitus is the most important pre-existing metabolic disease in pregnancy. It is well known to increase both maternal and fetal morbidity but usually features in the ICU as a contributory factor to other conditions, for example, sepsis. Anecdotal reports suggest that diabetic coma presenting in pregnancy may be particularly difficult to treat and stability of blood glucose may only be achieved after delivery of the fetus.

REFERENCES

1. Lewis G (ed). The Confidential Enquiry into Maternal and Child Health (CEMACH). Saving mothers' lives: reviewing maternal deaths to make motherhood safer 2003–2005. The seventh report on confidential

enquiries into maternal deaths in the united kingdom. London, CEMACH: 2007.

2. Uebing A, Steer PJ, Yentis SM *et al.* Pregnancy and congenital heart disease. *Br Med J* 2006; **332**; 401–6.
3. Bates SM, Greer IA, Hirsh J *et al.* Use of antithrombotic agents during pregnancy: the Seventh ACCP Conference on Antithrombotic and Thrombolytic Therapy. *Chest* 2004; **126** (Suppl. 3): 627S–44S.
4. Suntharalingam G, Dob D, Yentis SM. Obstetric epidural analgesia in aortic stenosis: a low-dose technique for labour and instrumental delivery. *Int J Obstet Anesth* 2001; **10**: 129–34.
5. Brighouse D. Anaesthesia for caesarean section in patients with aortic stenosis: the case for regional anaesthesia. *Anaesthesia* 1998; **53**: 107–9.
6. Whitfield A, Holdcroft A. Anaesthesia for caesarean section in patients with aortic stenosis: the case for general anaesthesia. *Anaesthesia* 1998; **53**: 109–12.
7. Weis FR, Markello R, Mo B *et al.* Cardiovascular effects of oxytocin. *Obstet Gynecol* 1975; **46**: 211–14.
8. Pinder AJ, Dresner M Calow C *et al.* Haemodynamic changes caused by oxytocin during caesarean section under spinal anaesthesia. *Int J Obstet Anesth* 2002; **11**: 156–9.
9. Hayman RG, Arulkumaran S, Steer PJ. Uterine compression sutures: surgical management of postpartum hemorrhage. *Obstet Gynecol* 2002; **99**: 502–6.
10. Fujitani S, Baldisseri M. Hemodynamic assessment in a pregnant and peripartum patient. *Crit Care Med* 2005; **33**: 10 (suppl.) S354–61.
11. Yentis SM, Steer P, Plaat F. Eisenmenger's syndrome in pregnancy: maternal and fetal mortality in the 1990s. *Br J Obstet Gynaecol* 1998; **105**: 921–2.
12. Kwon HL, Belanger K, Bracken MB. Effect of pregnancy and stage of pregnancy on asthma severity: a systematic review. *Am J Obstet Gynecol* 2004; **190**: 1201–10.
13. McMullen AH, Pasta DJ, Frederick PD *et al.* Impact of pregnancy on women with cystic fibrosis. *Chest* 2006; **129**: 706–11.
14. Gillet D, de Braekeleer M, Bellis G *et al.* Cystic fibrosis and pregnancy. Report from French data (1980–1999). *Br J Obstet Gynaecol* 2002; **109**: 912–18.
15. Confavreux C, Hutchinson M, Hours MM *et al.* Rate of pregnancy-related relapse in multiple sclerosis. *N Engl J Med* 1998; **339**: 285–91.
16. Hilt H, Gramm HJ, Link J. Changes in intracranial pressure associated with extradural anaesthesia. *Br J Anaesth* 1986; **58**: 676–80.
17. Ludlow JP, Evans SF, Hulse G. Obstetric and perinatal outcomes in pregnancies associated with illicit substance abuse. *Aust NZ J Obstet Gynaecol* 2004; **44**: 302–6.

Part Ten

Infections and Immune Disorders

58

Anaphylaxis

Malcolm McD Fisher

Anaphylaxis is a symptom complex accompanying the acute reaction to a chemical recognised as hostile. In the classical reaction the patient has been previously sensitised (immediate hypersensitivity or type 1 hypersensitivity), although the sensitising agent may be unknown. The term 'anaphylactoid reaction' is used to describe reactions clinically indistinguishable from anaphylaxis, in which the mechanism is non-immunological, or has not been determined. Recent consensus meetings have suggested the use of the term 'anaphylactoid' be discontinued and 'anaphylaxis' used to describe the symptom complex which may be either 'non-immune' or 'immune'.[1] Non-immune anaphylaxis may be produced by direct drug effects, physical factors or exercise, and a causative agent cannot always be determined. The mediators involved are the same as those in other acute inflammatory responses such as sepsis, but the rate of release is more rapid and of shorter duration.

AETIOLOGY

Clinical anaphylaxis in hospital commonly follows injection of drugs, blood products, plasma substitutes, contrast media, or exposure to latex products or chlorhexidine. Outside hospital, ingestion of foods or food additives (especially peanut products) or insect stings may be more common causes than drugs.

Neugut *et al.*[2] estimated 1400–1500 deaths per year in the USA and between 3.3 and 40.9 million patients at risk. They estimated radiocontrast media and penicillin to be the greatest cause of death, with food and stings the next groups. In contrast a postmortem study of 56 deaths in the UK[3] attributed 19 deaths to venoms, 16 to foods and 19 to drugs and radiocontrast media.

In anaphylaxis, sensitisation occurs following exposure to an allergenic substance, which either alone, or by combination with a protein or hapten, stimulates the synthesis of immunoglobulin E (IgE). Some IgE binds to the surface of mast cells and basophils. Later, re-exposure to antigen produces an antigen–cell surface IgE antibody interaction where two IgE molecules are bridged. This results in mast cell degranulation, and the release of histamine and other mediators, including interleukin, prostaglandins and platelet-activating factor. Histamine is responsible for the early signs and symptoms, but is rapidly cleared from plasma. The overall effects of the mediators are to produce vasodilatation, smooth-muscle contraction, increased glandular secretion and increased capillary permeability. The mediators act both locally and upon distant target organs.

Anaphylactoid reactions may be due to a direct histamine-releasing effect of drugs or other triggers on basophils and mast cells. The symptom complex may also be produced by other mechanisms. Some intravenous drugs and X-ray contrast media may activate the complement system. Plasma protein and human serum albumin reactions may be induced by either albumin aggregates or stabilising agent-modified albumin molecules. Other reactions, including those to dextrans and gelatin preparations, may be activated by non-IgE antibody already present in the plasma or osmotic factors (dextrose, mannitol).

The direct histamine-releasing effects of some drugs may produce reactions due to the effect of histamine alone, and such reactions are related to volume, rate and amount of infusion. Recent work suggests that the site of release of histamine may be important in its clinical effects. Drugs such as morphine and Haemaccel release histamine from skin alone,[4] and are unlikely to produce symptoms such as bronchospasm, whereas drugs which produce release from lung mast cells (e.g. atracurium, vecuronium and propofol) may be more likely to produce bronchospasm.[5] Direct histamine release is usually a transient phenomenon, but in some patients severe manifestations may occur, particularly with Haemaccel and vancomycin.

Anaphylactic reactions are usually seen in fit and well patients. It is likely that the adrenal response to stress 'pretreats' sick patients, and blocks the release and effects of anaphylactic mediators. The exception to this appears to be patients with asthma, in whom reactions to the additives in steroid and aminophylline preparations may occur, and this may be related to the reduced catecholamine response in asthma.[6] Patients on β-blockers and with epidural blockade may be more likely to develop adverse responses due to histamine release, and this may also be related to reduced catecholamine responsiveness. Reactions occurring in these groups are more difficult to treat.

CLINICAL PRESENTATION

The latent period between exposure and development of symptoms is variable, but usually occurs within 5 minutes if the provoking agent is given parenterally. Reactions may be transient or protracted (lasting days), and may vary in severity from mild to fatal. Recurrent anaphylaxis is described. Cutaneous, cardiovascular, respiratory or gastrointestinal manifestations may occur singly or in combination.

Cutaneous features include piloerection, erythematous flush, generalised or localised urticaria, angioneurotic oedema, conjunctival injection, pallor and cyanosis. Awake patients may experience an aura, warning of an impending reaction. Cardiovascular system involvement occurs most commonly and may occur as a sole clinical manifestation.[7] It is characterised by initial bradycardia then sinus tachycardia, hypotension and the development of shock.

In patients reacting due to venom desensitization, bradycardia may be severe and require treatment.[8] Respiratory manifestations include rhinitis, bronchospasm and laryngeal obstruction. Gastrointestinal symptoms of nausea, vomiting, abdominal cramps and diarrhoea may be present. Other features include apprehension, metallic taste, choking sensation, coughing, paraesthesiae, arthralgia, convulsions, clotting abnormalities and loss of consciousness. Pulmonary oedema is a rare sign. Rarely, some women develop a profuse, watery, vaginal discharge 3–5 days after anaphylaxis. It is self-limiting.

Anaphylaxis is rare in the intensive care unit (ICU), probably because of the protective effects of the adrenal response to stress. However, use of the mast cell tryptase assay (see below) may detect anaphylaxis as an unsuspected cause of shock in intensive care.

PATHOPHYSIOLOGY OF CARDIOVASCULAR CHANGES

The traditional concept of the cardiovascular changes in clinical anaphylaxis is that of an initial vasodilatation, followed by capillary leak of plasma which produces endogenous hypovolaemia, reduced venous return and lowered cardiac output.

Whether or not cardiac function is impaired has been controversial. Although most anaphylactic mediators adversely affect myocardial function in vitro, most case reports of anaphylaxis in which invasive cardiovascular monitoring has been used suggest minimal impairment of cardiac function. Patients with normal cardiac function before the reaction rarely show evidence of cardiac failure or arrhythmias other than supraventricular tachycardia, but the incidence of serious arrhythmias and cardiac failure increases in those with prior cardiac disease.[7] Echocardiography in anaphylaxis usually shows an 'empty', normally contracting heart. Troponins are elevated after anaphylaxis, but these elevations do not normally predict coronary artery disease requiring intervention. A recent study of patients with anaphylaxis during venom desensitisation showed that bradycardia requiring treatment was a common finding.[8] Two reactions in patients with no previous cardiac disease, where the major manifestation was prolonged global myocardial dysfunction, and the use of a balloon counterpulsator was life-saving, have been reported.[9]

TREATMENT

There are no randomised controlled trials of treatment in anaphylaxis, and the unexpected onset, rapid course and usual rapid response to treatment preclude performing such trials. Treatment recommendations are based on historical practice, case reports, series of cases and animal models.

OXYGEN

Oxygen is given by facemask. Endotracheal intubation may be required to facilitate ventilation, especially if angioedema or laryngeal oedema is present. Oedema of the upper airway is more common when anaphylaxis is due to foods than to drugs.[3] Mechanical ventilation is indicated for severe bronchospasm, apnoea or cardiac arrest.

ADRENALINE (EPINEPHRINE)

Epinephrine is universally recommended as the drug of choice for severe reactions. In the community epinephrine may be given intramuscularly in a dose of 0.3–1.0 mg early in anaphylaxis. Intramuscular epinephrine produces higher levels earlier in stable allergic patients than subcutaneous epinephrine.[10] In severe shock or in patients in whom muscle blood flow is thought to be compromised by shock, intravenous injection of 3–5 ml of 1:10 000 epinephrine is given. A second dose is necessary in 35%[11] and an infusion in 10%.

Epinephrine, by increasing intracellular levels of cyclic adenosine monophosphate (cAMP) in leukocytes and mast cells, inhibits further release of histamine. It has beneficial effects on myocardial contractility, peripheral vascular tone and bronchial smooth muscle, and stabilises mast cells. A common management error is not to institute external cardiac massage (ECM) as the arrhythmia is 'benign'. If the patient is pulseless, ECM should be instituted irrespective of rhythm, although there are no data to support its efficacy.

There has been controversy regarding the best route of administration of epinephrine outside hospital. Both case reports and patients self-injecting show efficacy for intramuscular epinephrine when given early. Intravenous epinephrine may rarely cause arrhythmias and myocardial infarction, particularly in unmonitored patients. In our series it seems to be more hazardous when the diagnosis of anaphylaxis is incorrect. Recent recommendations endorse the use of intramuscular epinephrine.[12]

OTHER SYMPATHOMIMETIC AMINES

Other sympathomimetic drugs may reverse the symptoms, but appear (albeit in the absence of any randomised trials) to be less effective than epinephrine. Norepinephrine by infusion may be life-saving in the absence of a response to fluid loading and epinephrine. Vasopressin has been described as effective in one patient with hypotension refractory to norepinephrine.

COLLOIDS

Plasma expanders are given rapidly to correct the hypovolaemia consequent to acute vasodilatation and leakage of fluid from the intravascular space.[13] The author favours plasma protein solution or gelatin preparations rather than crystalloids, as they remain in the vascular compartment earlier and for longer. There are, however, no data showing improved outcomes from colloid over crystalloid, and there are many patients who have been successfully resuscitated with crystalloid alone. Greater volumes of crystalloid are necessary and on occasions very large volumes of fluid may be required; central venous pressure monitoring and measurement of haematocrit are helpful.

BRONCHOSPASM

Epinephrine should be given. Nebulised salbutamol should be given for severe asthma. Aminophylline 5–6 mg/kg intravenously may be given over 30 minutes, if bronchospasm is unresponsive to epinephrine alone. Aminophylline increases intracellular cAMP by phosphodiesterase inhibition, and its effect on inhibiting histamine and interleukin release is theoretically additive to that of epinephrine. Adverse responses have not been observed in our series but a recent comprehensive review[14] suggested safer agents with proven efficacy should be preferred. Volatile anaesthesia, ketamine and magnesium sulphate may produce improvement in some patients with severe asthma.

CORTICOSTEROIDS

Steroids have no proven benefit, particularly early, and should be reserved for refractory bronchospasm. Conversely, steroids are often given and there is no evidence of harm.

ANTIHISTAMINES

Antihistamines are the treatment of choice in localised non-severe reactions. In severe reactions they are only indicated in protracted cases or in those with angioneurotic oedema which may recur. The data on antihistamines are not conclusive, but in protracted anaphylaxis, improvement is often reported with H_2-blockers.

DIAGNOSIS

The most important advance in the diagnosis of anaphylaxis has been the introduction of an assay for mast cell tryptase. The mast cell enzyme is elevated 1 hour after a reaction begins, and the elevation may persist for up to 4 hours. It can also be used to diagnose anaphylaxis from postmortem specimens.[15,16] The assay is highly specific and sensitive for anaphylaxis, although elevated levels are found with direct histamine release, and at postmortem in some patients with myocardial infarction. A negative mast cell tryptase assay does not exclude anaphylaxis as the diagnosis. Mast cell tryptase has been used to diagnose anaphylaxis postmortem.

FOLLOW-UP

Following successful acute management, the drug or agent responsible should be determined by in vitro or in vivo testing if possible. Hyposensitisation should be considered for food, pollen and bee venom allergy. A medic alert bracelet should be worn and the patient should be given a letter stating the nature of the reaction to the particular causative agent.

If re-exposure to the allergen is likely at home, patients or their relatives should be instructed in the use of epinephrine, salbutamol inhalation and antihistamines. Clinical anaphylaxis may be modified by pretreatment with disodium cromoglicate, corticosteroids, antihistamines, salbutamol and isoprenaline.

In patients with recurrent anaphylaxis in whom no cause can be found corticosteroids on alternate days reduce the incidence and severity of attacks.

REFERENCES

1. Sampson HA, Munoz-Furlong A, Campbell RL *et al.* Second symposium on the definition and management of anaphylaxis: summary report. Second National Institute of Allergy and Infectious Disease/Food Allergy and Anaphylaxis Network symposium. *J Allerg Clin Immunol* 2006; **117**: 391–17.
2. Neugut AL, Ghatak AT, Miller RL. Anaphylaxis in the United States: an investigation into its epidemiology. *Arch Intern Med* 2001; **161**: 15–21.
3. Pumphrey RS, Roberts IS. Postmortem findings after fatal anaphylactic reactions. *J Clin Pathol* 2000; **53**: 273–6.
4. Tharp MD, Kagey-Sobotka A, Fox CC *et al.* Functional heterogeneity of human mast cells from different anatomic sites: in vitro responses to morphine sulphate. *J Allergy Clin Immunol* 1987; **79**: 646–53.
5. Stellato C, de Paulis A, Cirillo R *et al.* Heterogeneity of human mast cells and basophils in response to muscle relaxants. *Anesthesiology* 1991; **74**: 1078–86.
6. Ind PW, Causon RC, Brown MJ *et al.* Circulating catecholamines in acute asthma. *Br Med J* 1985; **290**: 267–9.

7. Fisher MM. Clinical observations on the pathophysiology and treatment of anaphylactic cardiovascular collapse. *Anaesth Intens Care* 1986; **14**: 17–21.
8. Brown SG, Blackman KE, Stenlake V *et al.* Insect sting anaphylaxis; prospective evaluation of treatment with intravenous adrenaline and volume resuscitation. *Emerg Med J* 2004; **21**: 149–54.
9. Raper RF, Fisher MM. Profound reversible myocardial depression following human anaphylaxis. *Lancet* 1988; **8582**: 386–8.
10. Simons FE, Roberts JR, Gu X *et al.* Epinephrine absorption in children with a history of anaphylaxis. *J Allergy Clin Immunol* 1988; **101**: 33–7.
11. Korenblat P, Lundie MJ, Dankner RE *et al.* A retrospective study of epinephrine administration for anaphylaxis: how many doses are needed. *Allergy Asthma Proc* 1988; **20**: 83–6.
12. Project team of the Resuscitation Council UK. Emergency medical treatment of anaphylactic reactions. *Resuscitation* 1999; **41**: 93–9.
13. Fisher MM. Blood volume replacement in acute anaphylactic cardiovascular collapse related to anaesthesia. *Br J Anaesth* 1977; **49**: 1023–6.
14. Ernst ME, Graber MA. Methylxanthine use in anaphylaxis: what does the evidence tell us? *Ann Pharmacother* 1999; **33**: 1001–4.
15. Yunginger JW, Nelson DR, Squilace DL. Laboratory investigation of deaths due to anaphylaxis. *J Forensic Sci* 1991; **36**: 857–65.
16. Fisher MM, Baldo BA. The diagnosis of fatal anaphylactic reactions during anaesthesia: employment of immunoassays for mast cell tryptase and drug-reaction IgE antibodies. *Anaesth Intens Care* 1993; **21**: 353–7.

59

Host defence mechanisms and immunodeficiency disorders

Steve Wesselingh and Martyn A H French

There is a coordinated immunological response to infection involving both cellular and humoral components. The outcome of an infection will be determined by the balance between the body's ability to eliminate invading microorganisms and the microorganism's virulence. Humans have diverse host defence mechanisms to protect the different anatomical compartments of the body from a great variety of microorganisms (Table 59.1). There are many ways in which the immune system can be defective, leading to an increased propensity to infections. The immune response also needs to be controlled to avoid inappropriate and excessive activation, which may damage the host. A certain degree of host damage is inevitable during the response to infection, particularly if there is systemic activation resulting in disseminated intravascular coagulation (DIC) and an excessive inflammatory response.

INNATE IMMUNE RESPONSES

The immune system is capable of reacting to microorganisms without having been previously exposed to antigens from those microorganisms. This innate immune system consists of plasma proteins, including alternative-pathway components of the complement system and mannose-binding lectin (MBL), a subset of lymphocytes with cytotoxic activity (natural killer or NK cells), and some macrophage functions. Innate immune responses provide a first line of defence against many pathogenic microorganisms.

ACUTE-PHASE REACTION

The acute-phase reaction is a response of the haematopoietic and hepatic systems, involving at least 20 plasma proteins and the cellular components of the blood. The reaction occurs within hours of acute physical stress or infection. The functions of many of these acute-phase proteins remains unclear, but teleologically, they should be assumed to be beneficial to the patient. The falls in haemoglobin, serum iron and albumin are all normal in the acute-phase reaction. Most of the proteins are inflammatory mediators or inhibitors of transport proteins. Fibrinogen, the bulk protein of the coagulation system, is one of the plasma proteins to show the greatest rise in the acute-phase reaction, and is responsible for the elevation in the erythrocyte sedimentation rate. The fall in albumin is due to redistribution and decreased synthesis and generally does not require supplementation.

THE ADAPTIVE IMMUNE SYSTEM

Adaptive immune responses are characterised by specificity, memory, amplification and diversity. The specificity of an immune response against a particular antigenic component of a microorganism, and the memory which results in a prompt response on subsequent exposures, is determined by lymphocytes and antigen receptors on their surface. Amplification and diversity of immune responses are regulated by cytokines, which are secreted by lymphocytes and other cells, and through the effects of various lymphocyte surface molecules, including adhesion molecules and co-stimulatory molecules. Cytokines have various activities, the most important of which are cell activation (e.g. interferon-gamma (IFN-γ)), regulation of immune responses (e.g. interleukin (IL)-10) and proinflammatory effects (e.g. tumour necrosis factor (TNF)) and lymphotoxins).

ANTIGEN PRESENTATION

The most important events in the initiation of an immune response are the processing and presentation of fragments of the microorganism in a form which makes the fragments antigenic to lymphocytes. Major histocompatibility complex (MHC) class I (human leukocyte antigen (HLA)-A, B, C) and class II (HLA-DR, DP, DQ) molecules are the major cell-surface antigen presentation molecules. These molecules also determine the nature of the subsequent response against the antigen. Class I MHC molecules are present on most nucleated cells, and present processed endogenous peptides (such as fragments of viruses) to the antigen receptor (T-cell receptor;

Table 59.1 Host defence mechanisms

Physical barriers
Skin and mucosal surfaces
Cilia
Fever
Lysozyme
Lactoferrin
Acute-phase proteins, e.g. C-reactive protein
Fibronectin
Immune system, including secondary mediators
Other mediators of inflammation
Kinins
Vasoactive amines
Coagulation system

TcR) of T cells expressing CD8 molecules. Class II MHC molecules present antigenic fragments of microorganisms which are exogenous to cells and have been taken into the cell by phagocytosis, in the case of macrophages and monocytes, or by binding to antigen-specific surface immunoglobulins (the B-cell antigen receptor), in the case of B cells. Antigens presented on class II MHC molecules bind to TcRs on CD4+ T cells.

T CELLS AND B CELLS

CD8+ T cells have a cytotoxic effect on cells expressing class I MHC-associated viral antigens, resulting in the death of the cell and inhibition of viral replication. Antigen-induced stimulation of CD4+ T cells results in activation of the T cell and the expression of cell-surface molecules and secretion of cytokines with immunoregulatory effects. These immunoregulatory molecules augment the functions of many other cells, including B cells, T cells and macrophages (T-cell help). A response to an antigen directed by CD4+ T cells may also elicit macrophage activation and killing of the microorganism expressing that antigen. Activation of macrophages by CD4+ T cells is critically dependent on the production of IFN-γ.

The activation and proliferation of T cells occur under the influence of cytokines and other regulatory molecules, including co-stimulatory molecules such as the ligand of the B-cell membrane molecule CD40 (CD40L). Proliferating B cells differentiate into plasma cells, which secrete immunoglobulins with antibody activity against the initiating antigen. Nine isotypes of immunoglobulin can be produced, each of which has a different function.

IMMUNOGLOBULINS AND ANTIBODIES

Immunoglobulin M (IgM) is a large pentameric molecule, which is particularly effective as a bacterial agglutinator and activator of the complement system, and has its major effect within the circulation. IgA_1 and IgA_2 are produced at secretory surfaces, such as the mucosa of the gut and respiratory tract, and also in the breast, where IgA is a major constituent of the colostrum and provides secretory antibody to the gut of the neonate. IgE antibodies are also produced at mucosal surfaces where they form an important part of the immune response against parasitic infections. Antibodies of the IgG_1 and IgG_3 subclass are particularly effective at activating the complement system and binding to Fc receptors on phagocytic cells. IgG_2 antibodies are mainly active against polysaccharide antigens, such as those present in bacterial cell walls. The functions of IgG_4 antibodies are unclear.

SECONDARY ANTIBODY FUNCTION

The elimination of a microorganism by antibodies usually requires the activation of a secondary effector mechanism, of which there are several. Antibodies complexed with antigens activate the complement system through the classical pathway. The complement system may also be activated directly by components of microorganisms through the alternative pathway or MBL pathway. Activation of the complement system results in the generation of biologically active molecules, such as C3b, which is an important opsonin, and the activation of the membrane attack complex (MAC), which lyses bacterial cell walls. Like C3b, antibodies of the IgM, IgG_1 and IgG_3 isotype are also important opsonins. These molecules, when bound to the surface of a microorganism, facilitate their opsonisation and phagocytosis. These effects of complement and antibody are mediated through complement receptors (CRs) and receptors for the Fc portion of the immunoglobulin molecules (Fc receptors) on the surface of phagocytic cells such as neutrophils and macrophages.

DIVERSITY OF IMMUNE RESPONSES

The type of immune response produced against a microorganism varies according to the nature of the infecting organism. Thus, virus-infected cells elicit a cytotoxic CD8+ T-cell response; intracellular pathogens such as mycobacteria and protozoa elicit a CD4+ T-cell response, which results in macrophage activation; encapsulated bacteria elicit an opsonising antibody response; and some bacteria such as *Neisseria* spp. elicit a complement-activating antibody response, which lyses the cell wall of the bacterium. The nature of the immune response is regulated by cytokines, which provide T-cell help (Th) in the course of an immune response. Thus, IL-2, IL-12 and IFN-γ production induces a predominantly cellular immune response (Th1), whereas the production of IL-4 and IL-13 induces a predominantly antibody-mediated immune response (Th2).

IMMUNE DEFECTS UNDERLYING IMMUNODEFICIENCY DISORDERS

Defects of the immune system may give rise to immunodeficiency disorders, which are generally of five types: antibody deficiency, complement deficiency, cellular immunodeficiency, combined immunodeficiency (T cells, B cells and NK cells) and phagocyte dysfunction.

ANTIBODY DEFICIENCY

A deficient systemic antibody response most commonly results in a lack of opsonising antibody, and a propensity to infections with encapsulated bacteria such as pneumococci or *Haemophilus influenzae*. Recurrent respiratory tract infections including sinusitis are therefore the most common complication of this type of immune defect. Chronic echovirus infections of the nervous system and infection with some mycoplasmas may also occur in patients with severe primary immunoglobulin deficiency (agammaglobulinaemia).

Deficient secretory antibody responses are common in patients with IgA deficiency, but most affected individuals are able to produce compensatory secretory IgM or IgG antibody responses and do not suffer from infections.

CELLULAR IMMUNODEFICIENCY

Impairment of cell-mediated immune responses leads to an increased propensity to infection with microorganisms which are normally controlled by cellular immune responses (Table 59.2). These microorganisms are often pathogens that replicate intracellularly (intracellular pathogens) and cause persistent (latent) infections that reactivate when the cellular immune response against them becomes ineffective.

COMPLEMENT COMPONENT DEFICIENCY

Complement-mediated lysis of bacterial cell walls is a critical mechanism in the immune response against certain bacteria, especially *Neisseria* spp. and related bacteria such as *Moraxella* spp. and *Acinetobacter* spp. Deficiency of complement components, particularly MAC components (C5–C9), may therefore result in infection with these bacteria. C3b is an important opsonin and C3 deficiency will often impair phagocytosis of bacteria. Deficiency of classical pathway components may also result in impaired antibody responses.

Table 59.2 Microorganisms that most commonly cause disease in patients with cellular immunodeficiency

Mycobacteria	*Mycobacterium tuberculosis*
	Non-tuberculous mycobacteria
Bacteria	*Salmonella* spp.
	Shigella spp.
	Listeria monocytogenes
Fungi and yeasts	*Candida* spp. (mucosal infections)
	Pneumocystis jiroveci
	Cryptococci
	Aspergillus spp.
Protozoa	*Toxoplasma gondii*
	Cryptosporidia
Viruses	Herpes simplex viruses
	Cytomegalovirus
	Varicella-zoster virus
	Epstein–Barr virus
	Molluscum contagiosum virus
	JC virus (cause of progressive multifocal leukoencephalopathy)

PHAGOCYTE DEFECTS

Depletion or functional impairment of phagocytes results in an increased propensity to bacterial and fungal infections, particularly infection with *Staphylococcus aureus*, Gram-negative enteric bacteria, *Candida* spp. and *Aspergillus* spp. Fungal and yeast infections are often systemic in patients with severe neutropenia, indicating the importance of phagocytes in the systemic immune response against these microorganisms.

Phagocytosis of a bacterium or fungus by a neutrophil leukocyte or macrophage is dependent on chemotactic attraction of phagocytes to the site of infection, their adhesion to endothelial cells via adhesion molecules such as integrins, binding to opsonins on the microorganism, ingestion and intracellular killing. Intracellular killing involves both oxidative and non-oxidative mechanisms. Primary or acquired defects of phagocytes may result in localised pyogenic infections or pneumonia. However, in the neutropenic patient, localised infections may show little inflammatory reaction and overwhelming systemic infections are common.

IMMUNODEFICIENCY DISORDERS

Immunodeficiency disorders are classified as primary or acquired. Primary immunodeficiency disorders are the result of a developmental anomaly or a genetically determined defect of the immune system. Genetically determined defects are usually of two types:

1. the consequence of an absent or non-functional gene product, which is critical for the normal development or function of a component of the immune system
2. aberrant regulation of lymphocyte differentiation, which is probably determined by the products of several genes and possibly by environmental factors

Immunodeficiency disorders caused by the latter type of defect usually present later in life than congenital immunodeficiency caused by a non-functioning gene product.

Acquired immunodeficiency disorders are more common than primary immunodeficiency disorders and may present at any time after early childhood. Most result from an immune defect that is a consequence of a disease process, infection or complication of a therapeutic procedure such as splenectomy, immunosuppressant therapy or haemopoietic stem cell transplantation (HSCT).

Table 59.3 Tests of immunocompetence

Antibody-mediated immunity	
	Serum immunoglobulins, including IgG subclasses
	Systemic antibody responses (after vaccination if necessary)
	Polysaccharide antigens, e.g. pneumococcal
	Protein antigen, e.g. tetanus toxoid
	Blood B-cell (CD19+) counts
Cell-mediated immunity	
	Delayed-type hypersensitivity (DTH) skin test responses to antigens
	Blood T-cell (CD3+) and T-cell subset (CD4+ or CD8+) counts
Phagocyte function	
	Blood neutrophil numbers
	Tests of oxidative killing mechanisms, e.g. NBT test
	Leukocyte expression of CR3 (a CD18 integrin)
	Neutrophil migration assays
	Bacteria or *Candida* killing assays
Complement system	
	Immunochemical quantitation of individual components
	Functional assays of the classical pathway (CH50) or alternative pathway (AH50)

IgG, immunoglobulin G; NBT, nitroblue tetrazolium.

Diagnosis of an immunodeficiency disorder in a patient with an abnormal propensity to infections is dependent on the demonstration of an immune defect, as indicated in Table 59.3.

ANTIBODY DEFICIENCY

PRIMARY ANTIBODY DEFICIENCY DISORDERS

Failure of B-cell production or the presence of immature B cells due to a defect of differentiation is the cause of most primary antibody deficiency disorders.[1] B cells are absent from blood and secondary lymphoid tissues in patients with X-linked agammaglobulinaemia (XLA) because mutations of the *Btk* gene on the X-chromosome result in the absence of a B-cell tyrosine kinase necessary for the maturation of pre-B cells to B cells in the bone marrow. In the hyper-IgM immunodeficiency syndrome, B cells are able to differentiate into plasma cells secreting IgM, but not IgG or IgA. The X-linked form of this condition results from mutations in the gene encoding CD40L, which is critical in delivering a T-cell signal to differentiating B cells.

Common variable immunodeficiency (CVID) and IgA deficiency appear to be the consequence of immunoregulatory defects which result in impaired B-cell differentiation. Severe immunoglobulin deficiency (hypogammaglobulinaemia) and systemic antibody deficiency are characteristic of CVID, whereas most individuals with IgA deficiency are asymptomatic. Those IgA-deficient patients who suffer from recurrent infections often have a defect of systemic antibody responses, which commonly manifests as deficiency of an IgG subclass and/or impairment of antibody responses to polysaccharide antigens.[2]

The immunoregulatory defect underlying CVID and IgA deficiency sometimes results in an increased propensity to autoimmunity, which can include the production of anti-IgA antibodies. These antibodies may be a cause of anaphylactoid reactions to blood products containing IgA.

ACQUIRED ANTIBODY DEFICIENCY DISORDERS

B-cell chronic lymphocytic leukaemia or lymphoma and myeloma are commonly associated with reduced synthesis of normal immunoglobulins, which may result in immunoglobulin and antibody deficiency resulting in bacterial infections.[3] A thymoma is a rare cause of immunoglobulin and antibody deficiency, and should be considered in a patient presenting with primary immunoglobulin deficiency after the age of 40.[4] Impaired production of antibodies against polysaccharide antigens contributes to the susceptibility of asplenic patients to infection with encapsulated bacteria, such as pneumococci and meningococci, particularly in patients who had haematological malignancy.[5]

Drugs occasionally affect B-cell differentiation and cause immunoglobulin deficiency, particularly IgA deficiency. The most common offender is phenytoin. Most patients do not have antibody deficiency severe enough to cause infections. Intensive plasmapheresis may also cause severe immunoglobulin deficiency if immunoglobulin replacement is not used.

TREATMENT OF ANTIBODY DEFICIENCY DISORDERS

Infections can be prevented by regular infusions of intravenous immunoglobulin (IVIg) in patients with primary or acquired antibody deficiency. The usual dose is 300–500 mg/kg given monthly. Acute infections should be treated with appropriate antibiotics. The use of IVIg as an adjunct in the management of sepsis, particularly pneumococcal infections, has been suggested. In the absence of documented antibody deficiency there is no evidence to support this practice.

CELLULAR IMMUNODEFICIENCY

PRIMARY CELLULAR IMMUNODEFICIENCY

Complete or partial absence of the thymus gland resulting in depletion of T cells from blood and lymphoid tissue is the characteristic immunological abnormality in children with the Di George syndrome.[6] Infections of the type listed in Table 59.2 occur from birth onwards. A less severe defect of cellular immunity is present in patients with chronic mucocutaneous candidiasis. This usually occurs in patients with the autoimmune polyendocrinopathy–candidiasis–ectodermal dystrophy syndrome (APECED) syndrome, which results from a disorder of T-cell-processing in the thymus.[7]

ACQUIRED CELLULAR IMMUNODEFICIENCY

Acquired defects of cellular immunity are by far the most common cause of cellular immunodeficiency. Infection of cells of the immune system by human immunodeficiency viruses (HIVs) 1 and 2 is the most common (see Chapter 60). Less commonly, Hodgkin's disease, T-cell lymphomas and sarcoidosis may also be complicated by opportunistic infections occurring as a consequence of cellular immunodeficiency. A thymoma is a rare cause of chronic mucocutaneous candidiasis which, like thymoma and immunoglobulin deficiency, occurs later in life.[4]

Suppression of cellular immune responses is an intended effect of many immunosuppressant drugs used to treat allograft rejection, graft-versus-host disease (GvHD), autoimmune diseases and vasculitis. However, opportunistic infections may be a complication of this type of immunodeficiency, and may cause severe morbidity and death.

TREATMENT OF CELLULAR IMMUNODEFICIENCY DISORDERS

Since most infections complicating cellular immunodeficiency are reactivated latent infections, an important aspect of management is prevention of infection by the use of prophylactic antimicrobial drugs, as exemplified by HIV-induced immunodeficiency.[8] In circumstances of acquired cellular immunodeficiency it is essential to take into account the severity and duration of immunodeficiency. It is possible to predict the likelihood of infection and the likely pathogens by determining the degree of cellular immunodeficiency. This allows for appropriate decisions to be made regarding investigations, treatment and prophylaxis.

Acquired cellular immunodeficiency may be corrected, at least temporarily, by removing its cause (e.g. by suppressing HIV infection or ceasing immunosuppressive therapy). Thymus transplantation may be effective in children with thymus aplasia.

COMPLEMENT COMPONENT DEFICIENCY

Deficiency of complement components is an uncommon but often overlooked cause of recurrent bacterial infections.

PRIMARY COMPLEMENT DEFICIENCY

Congenital deficiency of C3 is extremely rare and usually causes a propensity to severe pyogenic infections. Deficiency of MAC components (C5–9) is more common, and should be considered in patients with meningococcal infections, particularly when the infections are recurrent.[9] Deficiency of classical pathway components (C1, C2, C4) may also result in an increased propensity to infection with meningococci and some other bacteria, but most affected individuals do not experience recurrent infections.

ACQUIRED COMPLEMENT DEFICIENCY

Disease processes that cause persistent activation of the complement system may cause depletion of complement components, particularly classical pathway components. This can result in infections with *Neisseria* spp. or related bacteria, and sometimes overwhelming septicaemia when the complement deficiency is severe. Systemic lupus erythematosus, myeloma and chronic atrioventricular shunt infections are rare causes of complement component deficiency.

MANAGEMENT OF PATIENTS WITH COMPLEMENT DEFICIENCY

An awareness of the possibility of complement deficiency is the most important aspect of management. Replacement therapy is not available. If a complement component deficiency is identified, screening of family members should be considered.

PHAGOCYTE DISORDERS

PRIMARY DISORDERS OF PHAGOCYTOSIS

Congenital neutropenias are rare. Defects of phagocyte function usually affect chemotaxis, adhesion or intracellular killing, either alone or in combination. The best-characterised defect of phagocyte adherence results from a congenital absence of the β-subunit of CD18 integrins in patients with leukocyte adhesion deficiency syndrome type 1.[10] Defects of intracellular killing are usually caused by a deficiency of microbicidal enzymes. In chronic granulomatous disease (CGD), deficiency of a phagosome enzyme (NADPH oxidase) results in ineffective oxidative killing mechanisms.[11] CGD usually presents in childhood but may present in adults, even as late as the seventh decade.[12] It should be considered in patients with recurrent abscesses or suppurative lymphadenitis, and in patients with pneumonia caused by *Staphylococcus aureus* or *Aspergillus* spp. infection.

ACQUIRED DISORDERS OF PHAGOCYTOSIS

Severe neutropenia may be complicated by bacterial or fungal infections. There are many causes of neutropenia, including autoimmune neutropenia, drug therapy and haematological diseases such as cyclic neutropenia, myelodysplastic syndromes and aplastic anaemia. Cytotoxic chemotherapy, used to treat various malignancies, commonly causes neutropenia, which is often complicated by severe bacterial and fungal infections.

MANAGEMENT OF PHAGOCYTE DISORDERS

Acquired neutropenia may be corrected by removing the underlying cause and/or use of granulocyte colony-stimulating factor (G-CSF). Febrile neutropenia requires investigation for the source of sepsis and empirical antibiotics. If fever persists antifungals should be added. IFN-γ therapy may be effective in patients with CGD.

COMBINED IMMUNODEFICIENCY DISORDERS

Several immunodeficiency disorders result from a combination of immune defects. Some combinations of congenital immune defects are so severe that death is a common occurrence, unless the defect can be corrected. Such conditions are classified as severe combined immune deficiency (SCID) syndromes.

PRIMARY COMBINED IMMUNODEFICIENCY

There are many primary combined immunodeficiency syndromes, which present in early childhood.[13] Some are still classified descriptively, but the molecular defects have now been demonstrated for many of them. For example, defective expression of MHC class II molecules, adenosine deaminase (ADA) deficiency, and deficiency of the common γ-chain of the receptor for several interleukins (IL-2, 4, 7, 9, 15, 21) all result in a deficiency and/or functional impairment of B cells, T cells and sometimes NK cells. Deficiency of the interleukin receptor common γ-chain results from mutations of its gene on the X-chromosome and is the underlying defect of X-linked SCID.

TREATMENT OF PRIMARY COMBINED IMMUNODEFICIENCY

HSCT is the treatment of choice for many types of primary SCID, though enzyme replacement therapy can be effective in ADA deficiency and gene replacement therapy has been used to treat X-linked SCID. Antibody replacement with IVIg therapy and prophylaxis for opportunistic infections are also important in primary SCID.

ACQUIRED COMBINED IMMUNODEFICIENCY

Combined immune defects are a characteristic of several acquired immunodeficiency disorders.

Haemopoietic stem cell transplantation

Combined immune defects may result in severe infections in patients who have received an HSCT.[14] Following transplantation, the recipient's immune system is reconstituted with donor cells. A degree of immunocompetence is passively transferred from the donor to recipient by antigen-specific lymphocytes, but as this and any residual immunocompetence of the recipient declines, an immunodeficient state exists until the donor immune system is established. Consequently, both antibody-mediated and cell-mediated immunity are deficient in the first 3–4 months after transplantation and may remain deficient for a longer period of time in patients with GVHD. This combined immune defect is often compounded by neutropenia and/or the effects of corticosteroid or immunosuppressant therapy for GVHD. Defective antibody responses may persist for several years after transplantation, particularly antibody responses against polysaccharide antigens.

Critical illness

Many patients who are critically ill as a result of surgery, trauma, thermal injury or overwhelming sepsis also have acquired immune defects.[15] These defects include abnormalities of cellular immunity, immunoglobulin deficiency and impaired neutrophil function. They appear to be associated with an increased propensity to infections and arise from abnormalities that are complex and multifactorial. Impairment of cell-mediated immune responses usually manifests as decreased T-cell proliferation and impaired delayed-type hypersensitivity responses, and probably results from a combination of factors, including the effects of anaesthetic drugs, blood transfusion, negative nitrogen balance and serum suppressor factors, including cytokines such as TNF. Phagocyte defects are mostly due to impairment of neutrophil chemotaxis by serum factors, and impaired intracellular killing. Deficiency of serum immunoglobulins also occurs, especially IgG deficiency, and may be associated with antibody deficiency. Serum leakage is a factor in patients with thermal injuries, and reduced synthesis and increased catabolism of immunoglobulins occur in many critically ill patients.

The correction of immune defects in critically ill patients has been intensely investigated, but no effective treatment regimen has been defined. General measures such as adequate nutrition, achieving a positive nitrogen balance and excision of thermally injured tissue are effective. Biological response modifiers, cytokine and mediator inhibitors, and IVIg therapy have all been evaluated. The number of acute infections, particularly pneumonia, can be reduced by the use of IVIg therapy, but patient survival is not increased. G-CSF levels are increased during critical illnesses and correlate with the severity of illness. Administration of G-CSF has been shown to be safe in intensive care patients with no apparent increases in acute respiratory distress syndrome or multiple-organ dysfunction. However there is no current evidence that the administration of G-CSF improves outcome and until further evidence is presented, G-CSF is not indicated in the treatment of critically ill intensive care unit patients.

Asplenia and hyposplenism

The spleen is an important part of the immune system's response to infections, particularly blood stream infections. The most important splenic functions in this context are removal of opsonised microorganisms from the blood by splenic macrophages and production of an early antibody response to the polysaccharide antigens of encapsulated bacteria by IgM memory B cells (also known as mantle-zone B cells). In those people in whom the spleen is removed or does not function, best-practice guidelines recommend lifelong education, vaccination and appropriate use of antibiotics. The risk of severe life-threatening infection related to splenectomy alone is in the order of 1 in 500 per annum with 50% mortality. The most common organisms identified with overwhelming postsplenectomy infection (OPSI) include encapsulated bacteria, such as pneumococcus, *Haemophilus infiuenzae* and meningococcus, for which vaccines are available. Other bacteria, which are sometimes important, include group A *Streptocccus*, *Capnocytophagia canimorsus* following dog bites, *Salmonella*, *Enterococcus* and *Bacteroides*.

Pneumococcus, *Haemophilus infiuenzae* and meningococcus vaccines including regular boosters and annual infiuenza vaccine are recommended. This is consistent with US guidelines and broadly with UK guidelines, which make the last bacterial vaccine optional. Second, chemoprophylaxis with penicillin for at least 2 years after splenectomy, if the patient is not allergic, should be considered.

SUMMARY: APPROACH TO THE IMMUNODEFICIENT PATIENT

1. Determine: (a) type of immunodeficiency; (b) degree of immunodeficiency; and (c) duration of immunodeficiency.
2. Predict: (a) the likelihood of infection; and (b) the type of infection.
3. Commence: (a) empirical; and (b) prophylactic therapy.
4. Targeted diagnostic tests.

REFERENCES

1. Buckley RH. Primary immunodeficiency diseases due to defects in lymphocytes. *N Engl J Med* 2000; **343**: 1313–24.
2. French MA, Denis K, Dawkins RL *et al.* Infection susceptibility in IgA deficiency: correlation with low polysaccharide antibodies and deficiency of IgG_2 and/or IgG_4. *Clin Exp Immunol* 1995; **100**: 47–53.
3. Tsiodras S, Samonis G, Keating MJ *et al.* Infection and immunity in chronic lymphocytic leukemia. *Mayo Clin Proc* 2000; **75**: 1039–54.
4. Tarr PE, Sneller MC, Mechanic LJ *et al.* Infections in patients with immunodeficiency with thymoma (Good syndrome). Report of 5 cases and review of the literature. *Medicine (Baltimore)* 2001; **80**: 123–33.
5. Cherif H, Landgren O, Konradsen HB *et al.* Poor antibody response to pneumococcal polysaccharide vaccination suggests increased susceptibility to pneumococcal infection in splenectomized patients with hematological diseases. *Vaccine* 2006; **24**: 75–81.
6. Hong R. The DiGeorge anomaly. *Clin Rev Allergy Immunol* 2001; **20**: 43–60.
7. Collins SM, Dominguez M, Ilmarinen T *et al.* Dermatological manifestations of autoimmune polyendocrinopathy–candidiasis–ectodermal dystrophy syndrome. *Br J Dermatol* 2006; **154**: 1088–93.
8. Kovacs JA, Masur H. Prophylaxis against opportunistic infections in patients with human immunodeficiency virus infection. *N Engl J Med* 2000; **342**: 1416–29.
9. Fijen CA, Kuijper EJ, te Bulte MT *et al.* Assessment of complement deficiency in patients with meningococcal disease in The Netherlands. *Clin Infect Dis* 1999; **28**: 98–105.
10. Bunting M, Harris ES, McIntyre TM *et al.* Leukocyte adhesion deficiency syndromes: adhesion and tethering defects involving beta 2 integrins and selectin ligands. *Curr Opin Hematol* 2002; **9**: 30–5.
11. Winkelstein JA, Marino MC, Johnston RB Jr *et al.* Chronic granulomatous disease. Report on a national registry of 368 patients. *Medicine (Baltimore)* 2000; **79**: 155–69.
12. Schapiro BL, Newburger PE, Klempner MS *et al.* Chronic granulomatous disease presenting in a 69 year old man. *N Engl J Med* 1991; **325**: 1786–90.
13. Buckley RH. Advances in the understanding and treatment of human severe combined immunodeficiency. *Immunol Res* 2001; **22**: 237–51.
14. Ninin E, Milpied N, Moreau P *et al.* Longitudinal study of bacterial, viral, and fungal infections in adult recipients of bone marrow transplants. *Clin Infect Dis* 2001; **33**: 41–7.
15. Napolitano LM, Faist E, Wichmann MW *et al.* Immune dysfunction in trauma. *Surg Clin North Am* 1999; **79**: 1385–416.

60

HIV and the acquired immunodeficiency syndrome

Steve Wesselingh and Martyn A H French

HIV REPLICATION

Human immunodeficiency viruses (HIVs) 1 and 2 are retroviruses of the Lentivirus group. Like other lentiviruses, they exhibit tropism for cells of the immune system and cause immunological disorders, particularly immunodeficiency. Infection of immune cells in the nervous system may also cause neurological disease. Entry of HIV into cells of the immune system is via cell surface receptors. The major receptor is the CD4 molecule but the chemokine receptors CCR5 and CXCR4 play an important role as co-receptors. Inside the cell, the viral RNA is reverse-transcribed into DNA by a viral reverse transcriptase enzyme, and the DNA is integrated into the DNA of the host cell as proviral DNA by a viral integrase enzyme. The proviral DNA remains there until the cell is activated, when it is transcribed into RNA, which provides the template for assembly of new HIVs under the control of viral enzymes such as proteases. Budding of new virus from the cell is followed by infection of new cells and a repeat of the replication cycle.

PRIMARY HIV INFECTION

Initial infection by HIV-1 is associated with a primary HIV infection syndrome (also known as a seroconversion illness) in 50–70% of patients. This syndrome is similar to infectious mononucleosis, being characterised by fever, lymphadenopathy, headache, photophobia, fatigue and myalgia. However, mucocutaneous lesions, neurological disease and even transient immunodeficiency may also occur and, when present, this differentiates it from infectious mononucleosis. It may take a number of weeks for HIV antibody (detected by enzyme-linked immunosorbent assay (ELISA)) to become positive during seroconversion; however the level of plasma HIV RNA is very high. The diagnostic test of choice during this period is the measurement of HIV viral load utilising HIV RNA RT/PCR (reverse transcription of HIV RNA and amplification by polymerase chain reaction). HIV RNA peaks at a median of 10 days.[1]

CHRONIC HIV INFECTION

The viraemia associated with primary HIV infection is controlled by a cellular and antibody-mediated immune response, which results in resolution of symptoms. However, even though the great majority of people become asymptomatic, HIV replication continues to take place. This results in activation of the immune system, depletion of CD4+ T cells and immunodeficiency, especially cellular immunodeficiency. These abnormalities develop at different rates in different individuals. In untreated patients the median time to develop the acquired immunodeficiency syndrome (AIDS) after acquiring HIV infection is 9 years. However, about 5% of HIV-infected individuals have no abnormalities after 15 years and are referred to as long-term non-progressors.

Early in the course of chronic HIV infection, virus is present in lymphoid tissues where it is bound to follicular dendritic cells. There is a persistent immune response against the HIV but, as this fails, viral replication increases and the viral load increases and other cells become infected, including macrophages, microglial cells of the nervous system and CD4+ T cells.

Chronic HIV infection may cause weight loss, fevers and diarrhoea, though such symptoms are more likely to be caused by an opportunistic infection in immunodeficient patients. Effects of worsening HIV infection are an immunodeficiency syndrome, which results in the development of opportunistic infections, tumours and neurological disease. Neurological disease is a consequence of HIV infection of macrophages and microglial cells in the central and peripheral nervous system.

DIAGNOSIS

A diagnosis of HIV infection can usually be made by demonstrating anti-HIV antibodies in the patient's serum. However, the serological diagnosis of HIV infection can sometimes be problematic. A small minority of individuals who are not infected by HIV have serum antibodies which are reactive with some HIV proteins, and give false-positive results with some ELISAs. Many laboratories use two different types of ELISA to identify such sera. To ensure that HIV infection is not incorrectly diagnosed, an antibody test should only be considered positive if antibody is also detected according to defined criteria, using a confirmatory antibody test such as a Western blot immunoassay.[2] Anti-HIV antibodies may be absent from the serum of patients with primary HIV infection. They are usually detectable by 2–6 weeks after infection, and almost always detectable by 12 weeks. After this time, absence of HIV antibodies excludes HIV infection in all but the most advanced cases of AIDS, or in a patient with an antibody deficiency disorder.

VIROLOGICAL MONITORING

It could be argued that HIV has been one of the major driving forces in the development of modern virology. For the first time HIV viral load monitoring has enabled the clinician to predict outcome, and monitor therapy during a viral infection.

HIV VIRAL LOAD MEASUREMENT

The major advance in viral diagnostics has been the development of polymerase chain reaction (PCR) and the application of this to the detection and quantification of viral nucleic acid in body fluids. Measurement of the blood 'HIV load' can be done by quantitating HIV RNA in plasma. Knowledge of the HIV load is useful in prognostication and essential when making decisions to commence and optimise therapy[3] (Figure 60.1).

GENOTYPING HIV TO DETECT DRUG RESISTANCE MUTATIONS

Drug susceptibility testing of HIV from a clinical specimen is performed in order to detect mutations in the genome of HIV that predict failure of individual antiviral therapeutic agents. The predominant genotype from an individual's plasma or cerebrospinal fluid sample is determined by sequencing the reverse transcriptase and protease genes of complementary DNA (cDNA) obtained following RT/PCR. This information is used to assist the clinician and patient in the choice of an antiretroviral drug combination with the best chance of successful suppression of HIV replication, especially where resistance is suspected, i.e. in a failing regimen.[4]

IMMUNOLOGICAL MONITORING

Immunodeficiency and neurological disease caused by HIV infection usually develop gradually over months to years. It is important to monitor their severity to determine when to commence therapy, and when the patient is susceptible to various disease manifestations.

The blood CD4+ T-cell count or percentage is the best indicator of the severity of HIV-induced immunodeficiency and, therefore, of the patient's susceptibility to opportunistic infections. Measurement of the blood CD4+ T-cell count or percentage is therefore critical in determining if the symptoms of an HIV-infected patient are likely to be caused by an opportunistic infection, and if so, what type of infection (Figure 60.2; and see text below).[5]

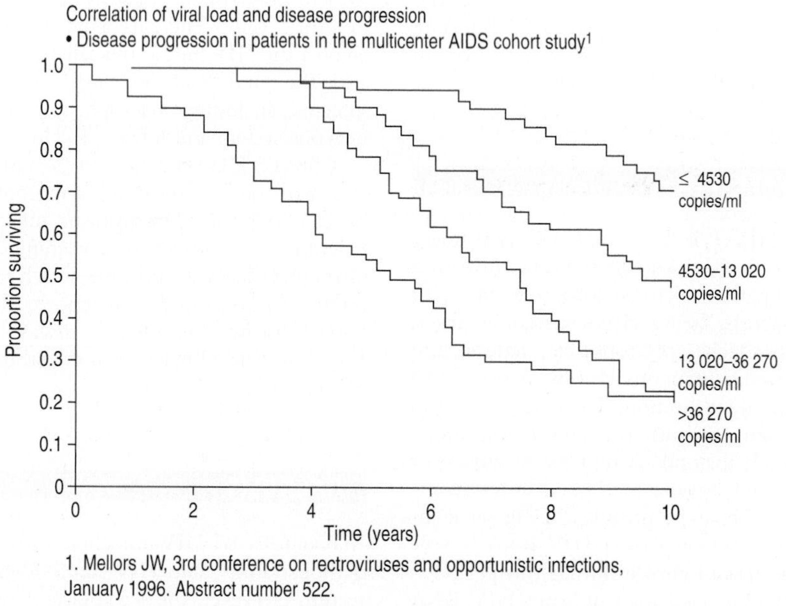

Figure 60.1 Correlation of viral load with disease progression. AIDS, acquired immunodeficiency syndrome. (From Mellors JW, Rinaldo CR, Gupta P *et al.* Prognosis in HIV-1 infection predicted by the quantity of virus in plasma. *Science* 1996; **272**: 1167–70. Copyright: American Association for the Advancement of Science; reproduced with permission.)

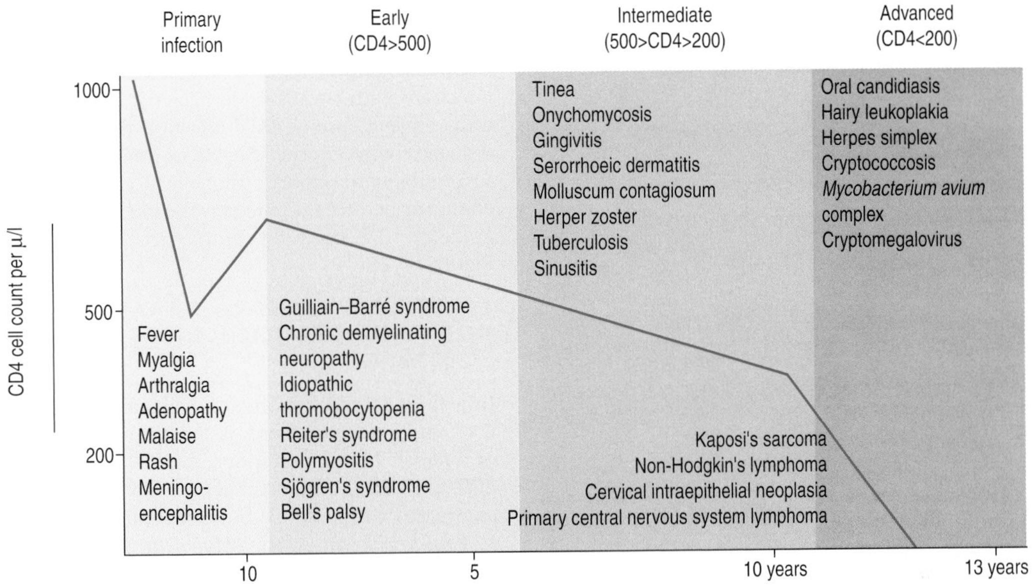

Figure 60.2 Chronological framework for understanding human immunodeficiency virus (HIV) disease and its management. (From Stewart G. Managing HIV. *Med J Aust* 1997; 5, reproduced with permission.)

MANAGEMENT OF THE HIV-INFECTED PATIENT

The impact of combination antiretroviral therapy on the morbidity and mortality associated with HIV infection has been dramatic. The HIV Outpatient Study demonstrated a stepwise reduction in opportunistic infections and mortality with increasing intensity of antiretroviral therapy.[6] In Australia, a comparison of cohorts before and after the introduction of combination antiretroviral therapy documented the effectiveness of these agents in reducing the risk of progression to AIDS and death.[7] This reflects similar epidemiological studies conducted in Switzerland,[8] France[9] and the USA.[10] A 70–80% reduction in mortality over 5 years has been the norm. AIDS-defining illnesses in Australia now occur predominantly in those without a past diagnosis of HIV infection.

Six classes of antiretroviral drugs are currently in use (Table 60.1). Fusion inhibitors block fusion of the virus with the cell membrane and CCR5 inhibitors block binding of CCR5-tropic strains of virus with CCR5, a co-receptor for HIV. Reverse transcriptase inhibitors are of three types. Firstly, nucleoside analogues and nucleotide analogues act by substituting for natural nucleosides or nucleotides during HIV replication, thereby inhibiting DNA chain elongation and the effects of the reverse transcriptase enzyme. Secondly, non-nucleoside reverse transcriptase inhibitors inhibit the reverse transcriptase enzyme by a different mechanism. Thirdly, integrase inhibitors block integration of viral DNA into host DNA and protease inhibitors inhibit the viral protease. All antiretroviral drugs have a limited duration of efficacy if used alone because HIV eventually develops resistance to them. The use of drug combinations is much more effective than single drugs, partly because drug resistance develops more slowly. Adherence to antiretroviral therapy is critical for the success of treatment.

DRUG TOXICITY

With decreased rates of HIV morbidity and mortality, attention has now become focused on the toxicities of treatments. Adverse effects of antiretroviral drugs are common, and are a cause of significant morbidity and even mortality.

Recently, nucleoside analogue reverse transcriptase inhibitors (NRTIs) have been implicated in the development of syndromes that include fatigue, fat wasting, lactic acidosis and peripheral neuropathy. It has been suggested that these symptoms may be due to an inhibition of mitochondrial DNA (mtDNA) synthesis.[11,12] Pancreatitis has occurred uncommonly with ddI (5–7%) and d4T (1–2%).

The most common adverse effect of NNRTIs is a skin rash. This occurs in up to 25% of subjects started on nevirapine and can range from a mild rash to Stevens–Johnson syndrome. Combination antiretroviral therapy is associated with a syndrome characterised by redistribution of fat (lipodystrophy) and fat atrophy (lipoatrophy). The biological mechanism responsible for the development of this syndrome is still unclear,[13] although protease inhibitors in association with d4T have been implicated.

The use of antiretroviral therapy is also associated with hepatotoxicity in about 10% of patients.[14] Co-infection with hepatitis C virus is one risk factor for hepatotoxicity and at least some cases are probably a type of immune

Table 60.1 Antiretroviral drugs used to treat human immunodeficiency virus (HIV) infection

Fusion inhibitors
Enfuvirtide (T20)
CCR5 inhibitors
Maraviroc
Nucleoside/nucleotide analogue reverse transcriptase inhibitors
Nucleoside analogues
Abacavir (ABV)
Didanosine (ddI)
Emtricitabine (FTC)
Lamivudine (3TC)
Stavudine (d4T)
Zidovudine (AZT)
Nucleotide analogues
Tenofovir (TNF)
Nucleoside/nucleotide fixed-dose combination tablets
Combivir (AZT + 3TC)
Trizivir (AZT + 3TC + ABV)
Kivexa (ABV + 3TC)
Truvada (TNF + FTC)
Non-nucleoside reverse transcriptase inhibitors
Delavirdine
Efavirenz
Nevirapine
Integrase inhibitors
Raltegravir
Protease inhibitors
Atazanavir*
Darunavir*
Fosamprenavir*
Indinavir*
Lopinivir*
Nelfinavir
Saquinavir*
Tipranavir*

*Administered with low-dose ritonavir to increase serum levels (lopinavir + low-dose ritonavir are co-formulated as Kaletra).

restoration disease.[15] Restoration of immune responses against pathogens also appears to be a cause of other types of inflammatory disease after the use of combination antiretroviral therapy.[16,17]

HIV-INDUCED IMMUNODEFICIENCY

Patients who are not treated with antiretroviral therapy or whose antiretroviral therapy is ineffective, for whatever reason, often become immunodeficient. Both CD4+ T-cell depletion and the effects of other immune defects lead to the development of an immunodeficiency syndrome. This syndrome is characterised by impaired cellular immunity and an increased propensity to opportunistic infections. In addition, some patients have impaired antibody responses and phagocyte dysfunction, which results in infections with encapsulated bacteria. As mentioned previously, during chronic HIV infection there is a strong relationship between the degree of immunodeficiency and susceptibility to opportunistic infections. The CD4+ T-cell count (or percentage) predicts the likely pathogens and is a guide to the need for prophylactic antimicrobials (see Figure 60.2).

MILD IMMUNODEFICIENCY (CD4 T-CELL COUNT > 200/ml, 20%)

Infectious complications of cellular immunodeficiency may occur when there is relatively mild impairment of cellular immune responses (CD4+ T-cell counts of 200–500/ml). Mucocutaneous infections occur most commonly (Table 60.2) but infections with bacteria such as *Campylobacter jejuni*, *Salmonella* spp. or *Shigella* spp. are a cause of diarrhoea, and occasionally bacteraemia. Bacteraemic pneumococcal disease is also more common in this group. Most of these infections are not restricted to patients with HIV infection, and are therefore not considered to be AIDS-defining opportunistic infections. However, when they present atypically, are severe or are recurrent, they may be the first indication of underlying HIV-induced immunodeficiency. In contrast to the other infections, oral hairy leukoplakia (due to Epstein–Barr virus infection of epithelial cells) is almost always indicative of HIV infection.

MODERATE IMMUNODEFICIENCY (CD4 T-CELL COUNT 50–200/UL, 10–20%)

Cellular immunodeficiency which is severe enough to result in an increased propensity to systemic opportunistic infections is usually associated with a CD4 T-cell count of < 200/ml. Such infections are considered to be indicative of the presence of AIDS. Infection with many different microorganisms may occur, including infection with unusual microorganisms. Only the most common are described here.

Table 60.2 Mucocutaneous opportunistic infections in patients with human immunodeficiency virus (HIV)-induced immunodeficiency

Herpes zoster (varicella-zoster virus infection)
Mucosal candidiasis
Oral hairy leukoplakia (Epstein–Barr virus infection)
Seborrhoeic dermatitis (*Pityrosporon* spp. yeast infection)
Molluscum contagiosum (poxvirus infection)
Genital and cutaneous warts (human papillomavirus infection)
Fungal infections of the skin and nails
Recurrent mucocutaneous herpes simplex virus infections
Folliculitis (*Staphylococcus aureus, Pityrosporon* spp.)

PNEUMOCYSTIS JIROVECI PNEUMONITIS

Infection of the lungs by *Pneumocystis jiroveci* causes an interstitial pneumonitis. Patients with this condition usually have a history of subacute progressive dyspnoea, cough, fever and weight loss. Examination often reveals basal pulmonary crackles. The chest X-ray usually shows interstitial infiltrates but is occasionally normal. Other findings which would support a diagnosis of *P. jiroveci* pneumonitis (PJP) are hypoxaemia, an increased serum lactate dehydrogenase (LDH) concentration, diffuse uptake of radiolabelled gallium into the lungs on a gallium scan, ground-glass pulmonary opacities on a high-resolution computed tomographic (CT) scan of the lungs, and detection of *Pneumocystis* by smear or DNA by PCR in induced sputum specimens. A definitive diagnosis can be made by demonstrating *Pneumocystis* cysts in an induced sputum specimen, bronchoalveolar lavage fluid or a transbronchial biopsy.[18]

PJP is treated with co-trimoxazole (trimethoprim-sulfamethoxazole), given orally or intravenously depending on disease severity. However, many patients develop a hypersensitivity reaction to co-trimoxazole which is usually mild and transient but, if systemic and severe, alternative medications, including oral dapsone and trimethoprim or intravenous pentamidine, can be used with equal efficacy. Steroid therapy should also be used if the Pao_2 is < 70 mmHg (9.3 kPa)[19] with an Fio_2 of 0.21.

Pneumocystis infection can be prevented by prophylactic medications, which should be offered to all patients with a CD4 T-cell count of < 200/ml. The most effective drug is co-trimoxazole. Alternatives for patients who are sensitive to co-trimoxazole include dapsone (with or without pyrimethamine) or inhaled pentamidine.[20]

OESOPHAGEAL CANDIDIASIS

Candida infection of the oesophageal mucosa presents with odynophagia and dysphagia. The occurrence of such symptoms in association with oral candidiasis is usually sufficient to make a presumptive diagnosis of oesophageal candidiasis and to start treatment. Endoscopy is required for a definitive diagnosis. Treatment is usually with an azole, such as fluconazole. However, in patients with severe immunodeficiency, resistance to azoles is not uncommon and treatment with intravenous amphotericin may be required.

CRYPTOCOCCAL MENINGITIS

Meningitis is the most common manifestation of infection with *Cryptococcus neoformans* in patients with AIDS. It usually presents with headache and fever, but sometimes confusion or behavioural abnormalities are the predominant abnormalities. Neck stiffness is often minimal or absent. Cerebrospinal fluid examination may reveal little evidence of inflammation, particularly in the most severe cases, but cryptococcal antigen is virtually always present in both serum and cerebrospinal fluid and cultures for cryptococci are positive.[21] Most patients also have cryptococcal antigen in their serum. Intravenous amphotericin is the treatment of choice, and must be followed by suppressive therapy or oral fluconazole, until immune reconstitution is achieved with antiretroviral therapy, to prevent relapses.[22]

TOXOPLASMA *ENCEPHALITIS*

Reactivation of *Toxoplasma gondii* infection most commonly presents as a focal encephalitis. This may cause headaches, fever, focal neurological deficits, convulsions and even coma. One or more brain lesions may be present. They usually produce ring-enhancing lesions with surrounding oedema on a contrast brain CT scan, and can occur in many sites, with a predilection for the basal ganglia. Serological evidence of previous *Toxoplasma* infection is present in virtually all patients, and absence of serum *Toxoplasma* antibody is strongly against the diagnosis. Treatment is with intravenous sulfadiazine or clindamycin and oral pyrimethamine. Hypersensitivity reactions to sulfadiazine and clindamycin are common, and an alternative drug regimen may be necessary. A brain CT scan should be repeated after 2–3 weeks of therapy, and an alternative diagnosis considered if there has been no resolution of the lesions. Cerebral lymphoma can produce very similar lesions to *Toxoplasma* encephalitis. A brain biopsy is often necessary to make the diagnosis.[23]

SEVERE IMMUNODEFICIENCY (CD4 T CELLS < 50/UL, 10%)

CYTOMEGALOVIRUS (CMV) DISEASE

CMV disease most often occurs in patients with very severe immunodeficiency (CD4 T-cell count < 50/ml). The most common site for reactivation of CMV infection is the retina. CMV retinitis usually presents with unilateral blurred vision, visual field loss or 'floaters'. Diagnosis is by fundoscopy and should be confirmed by an ophthalmologist. Treatment is with intravenous ganciclovir or foscarnet or oral valganciclovir, followed by suppressive therapy to prevent relapses until there is immune reconstitution following the use of combination antiretroviral therapy.

CMV infection less commonly presents with disease of other organs, particularly the oesophagus, bile ducts or colon. Biopsy of affected tissue is necessary to make a definitive diagnosis. High or increasing CMV viral load in blood provides support for a diagnosis of CMV infection. In addition, CMV load can be utilised to monitor the response to therapy and early identification of resistance.

CRYPTOSPORIDIOSIS

Infection of the gastrointestinal tract by *Cryptosporidium parvum* causes a severe and intractable secretory diarrhoea, which is often associated with a malabsorption syndrome. It can also cause cholangitis. Diagnosis is by demonstrating *Cryptosporidium* oocysts in faeces and/or a rectal or duodenal biopsy. There is no satisfactory treatment, but nitozoxanide is of use in some patients. Resolution is common following successful antiretroviral therapy.

MYCOBACTERIUM AVIUM COMPLEX (MAC) INFECTION

Infection with MAC is usually disseminated and affects blood leukocytes, liver, spleen and lymph nodes, and the gastrointestinal tract. This infection often results in weight loss, fatigue, fevers, anaemia and diarrhoea. The diagnosis is usually made by culturing MAC from blood, but sometimes stool microscopy and culture or biopsy of affected tissues are necessary. Treatment with multiple-drug therapy is often successful. Commonly used drugs are clarithromycin, rifabutin and ethambutol. Suppressive therapy should be continued until there is immune reconstitution following the use of combination antiretroviral therapy.[24] An unusual painful necrotising lymphadenopathy following initiation of antiretroviral therapy has been identified as MAC immune restoration disease.[16,17]

AIDS-RELATED NEOPLASMS

Certain neoplasms are a characteristic complication of cellular immunodeficiency, including HIV-induced immunodeficiency. 'Opportunistic' virus infections resulting from the immunodeficiency are involved in the pathogenesis of these neoplasms.

Kaposi's sarcoma (KS) is an angioproliferative tumour which originates from vascular endothelium, and is a complication of human herpesvirus-8 (HHV-8) infection. It usually presents as skin lesions, which have a reddish-brown colour. They vary in extent from one or two small papules to numerous bulbous lesions. The mucosal surface of the gastrointestinal tract, lymph nodes and, rarely, internal organs may also be involved. A clinical diagnosis of KS can be confirmed by biopsy of a lesion. KS may present at any degree of immunodeficiency but occurs most often, and is more severe, in patients with moderate to severe immunodeficiency. New antimitotic agents plus antiretroviral therapy have resulted in KS essentially disappearing as a clinical problem in treated individuals.

Lymphomas are also a complication of HIV-induced immunodeficiency. The great majority are B-cell lymphomas (non-Hodgkin's), and reactivation of Epstein–Barr virus infection is implicated in the pathogenesis of many cases. Primary cerebral lymphoma or extracerebral lymphoma, which often has extranodal involvement, is common in patients with severe immunodeficiency. These lymphomas are usually high-grade with poor prognosis (stage 3/4, CD4 < 100, median survival 44 weeks).[25]

Cervical intraepithelial neoplasia is more common in women with HIV infection. This is presumably because human papillomavirus infection is more likely to be present in women with HIV infection, and the cellular immunodeficiency permits human papillomavirus replication. As a consequence, the incidence of cervical carcinoma appears to be increased in HIV-infected women. Anal neoplasia is also increased in males.

HIV-RELATED NEUROLOGICAL DISEASE

In addition to the opportunistic infections of the nervous system discussed above, HIV infection of macrophages and microglial cells in the nervous system often results in neurological disease by incompletely understood mechanisms. Encephalopathy, myelopathy and peripheral neuropathy are all possible. In a small number of patients, the neurological disease is more problematic than the immunodeficiency. The encephalopathy usually develops insidiously in individuals with advanced immunodeficiency and eventually results in cognitive, motor and behavioural abnormalities. Myelopathy, which is now rare, results in an ataxic spastic paraparesis.[26]

Investigation of HIV patients with space-occupying cerebral lesions requires analysis of serology, cerebrospinal fluid and neuro-imaging investigations. Analysis of cerebrospinal fluid includes PCR for Epstein–Barr virus (indicative of lymphoma), herpes simplex virus, CMV, varicella-zoster virus (viral encephalitis), JC virus (indicative of progressive multifocal leukoencephalopathy), toxoplasmosis and *Mycobacterium tuberculosis*.[27]

HIV/AIDS AND ADMISSION TO THE INTENSIVE CARE UNIT (ICU)

HIV infection remains an incurable condition but is controllable by antiretroviral therapy for long periods of time. The prognosis has improved significantly over the past 10 years, with mathematical models indicating a median survival of 30 years. The admission of a patient with AIDS to an ICU is therefore often indicated.[28,29]

The most common indications are:

- respiratory failure complicating *Pneumocystis carinii* pneumonia or other infective pulmonary conditions
- coma or convulsions complicating opportunistic infections or tumours of the brain
- non-HIV-related conditions, such as self-poisoning and postoperative management

Respiratory failure complicating PJP has been the most common reason for admitting an HIV-infected patient to an ICU. Survival following ventilation for PJP was poor in the early 1980s, but improved with treatment advances. In recent years, survival has worsened again in some cohorts, particularly for patients with a CD4 T-cell count of < 50/ml and for those who develop pneumothorax as a result of barotrauma. The poor outcome in recent years may reflect the fact that patients are living longer because of improved therapy, and are hence often more immunodeficient when PJP develops. A first episode of PJP, a CD4 T-cell count of > 50/ml and no previous antiretroviral therapy are all favourable factors for survival. Furthermore, ventilation may be avoided by the use of continuous positive airways pressure (CPAP) or bilevel positive airways pressure (BPAP), thereby reducing the risks of a pneumothorax, airway obstruction and nosocomial infection. Prolonged illness antedating

ICU admission, low serum albumin and few options for antiretroviral therapy should be considered when assessing predictors of survival.

Drug–drug interactions are of particular importance, especially when ART includes protease inhibitors or efaverenz (metabolised via P450 hepatic enzyme system). Web-based guidelines are very useful (www.HIV-druginteractions.org) when prescribing antimicrobials, antiemetics and lipid-lowering drugs.

NEEDLESTICK INJURIES AND POSTEXPOSURE PROPHYLAXIS

Patients with unrecognised HIV infection or AIDS may also be admitted to an ICU with the first manifestation of HIV disease. It is therefore important for all ICU staff to practise stringent infection control procedures at all times.

HIV transmission from needlesticks occurs at a rate of approximately 0.3%, and from mucosal exposure at a rate of approximately 0.009%. There have been no reported seroconversions after skin exposure. The major risk factors for infection after a needlestick injury are: (1) deep injury; (2) visible blood on device; (3) needle placement in a vein or artery; and (4) a source patient with late-stage HIV/AIDS (high viral load).

There is evidence that antiretroviral prophylaxis is associated with a reduction in transmission rates. On the basis of this, antiretroviral prophylaxis guidelines have been published.[30] A protocol for dealing with blood and body fluid exposure should therefore be developed for every health-care institution.

REFERENCES

1. Tindall B, Cooper DA. Primary HIV infection: host responses and intervention strategies. *AIDS* 1991; **5**: 1–14.
2. Robertson P, Dwyer D. Western blot assay. In: Lee N (ed.) *Clinical Microbiology Update* no. 35. Sydney: University of New South Wales; 1993: 9–16.
3. Mellors JW, Rinaldo CR, Gupta P *et al.* Prognosis in HIV-1 infection predicted by the quantity of virus in plasma. *Science* 1996; **272**: 1167–70.
4. Durant J, Clevenbergh P, Halfon P *et al.* Drug resistance genotyping in HIV-1 therapy: the VIRADAPT randomised controlled trial. *Lancet* 1999; **353**: 2195–9.
5. Mellors JW, Munoz A, Giogi JV *et al.* Plasma viral load and CD4+ lymphocytes as prognostic markers of HIV-1 infection. *Ann Intern Med* 1997; **126**: 946–54.
6. Palella FJ, Delaney KM, Moorman AC *et al.* Declining morbidity and mortality among patients with advanced human immunodeficiency virus infection. *N Engl J Med* 1998; **338**: 853–60.
7. Correll PK, Law MG, McDonald AM *et al.* HIV disease progression in Australia at the time of combination antiretroviral therapies. *Med J Aust* 1998; **169**: 469–72.
8. Egger M, Hirschel B, Francioli P *et al.* Impact of new antiretroviral combination therapies in HIV infected patients in Switzerland: prospective multicentre study: HIV cohort study. *Br Med J* 1997; **315**: 1194–9.
9. Mouton Y, Alfandari S, Valette M *et al.* Impact of protease inhibitors on AIDS defining events and hospitalizations in 10 French AIDS reference centres. *AIDS* 1997; **11**: F101–5.
10. Dore GJ, Cooper DA. HAART's first decade: success brings further challenges. *Lancet* 2006; **368**: 427–8.
11. Brinkman K, Smeitink JA, Romijn JA *et al.* Mitochondrial toxicity induced by nucleoside-analogue reverse-transcriptase inhibitors is a key factor in the pathogenesis of antiretroviral-therapy-related lipodystrophy. *Lancet* 1999; **354**: 1112–15.
12. Carr A, Miller J, Law M *et al.* A syndrome of lipoatrophy, lactic acidaemia and liver dysfunction associated with HIV nucleoside analogue therapy: contribution to protease inhibitor-related lipodystrophy syndrome. *AIDS* 2000; **14**: F25–32.
13. Carr A, Cooper DA. Adverse effects of antiretroviral therapy. *Lancet* 2000; **356**: 1423–30.
14. Monforte Ade A, Bugarini R, Pezzotti P *et al.* The ICONA (Italian Cohort of Naive for Antiretrovirals) Study Group. Low frequency of severe hepatotoxicity and association with HCV coinfection in HIV-positive patients treated with HAART. *J Acquir Immune Defic Syndr* 2001; **28**: 114–23.
15. John M, Flexman J, French MA. Hepatitis C virus-associated hepatitis following treatment of HIV-infected patients with HIV protease inhibitors: an immune restoration disease? *AIDS* 1998; **12**: 2289–93.
16. French MA, Lenzo N, John M *et al.* Immune restoration disease after the treatment of immunodeficient HIV-infected patients with highly active antiretroviral therapy. *HIV Med* 2000; **1**: 107–15.
17. French MA. Disorders of immune reconstitution in patients with HIV infection responding to antiretroviral therapy. *Curr HIV/AIDS Rep* 2007; **4**: 16–21.
18. Frame P, Wilkin A. *Pneumocystis carinii* pneumonia. In: Crowe S, Hoy J, Mills J (eds) Management of the HIV-Infected Patient. London: Martin Dunitz; 2002: 421–42.
19. Consensus statement on the use of corticosteroids as adjunctive therapy for *Pneumocystis* pneumonia in the acquired immunodeficiency syndrome. The National Institutes of Health University of California expert panel for corticosteroids as adjunctive therapy for *Pneumocystis* pneumonia. *N Engl J Med* 1990; **323**: 500–4.
20. Kovacs JA, Masur H. Prophylaxis against opportunistic infections in patients with human immunodeficiency virus infection. *N Engl J Med* 2000; **342**: 1416–29.
21. Dismukes WE. Cryptococcal meningitis in patients with AIDS. *J Infect Dis* 1998; **157**: 624–8.
22. Powderly WG, Sagg MS, Cloud GA *et al.* A controlled trial of fiuconazole or amphotericin B to prevent relapse of cryptococcal meningitis in patients with the acquired immunodeficiency syndrome. *N Engl J Med* 1992; **326**: 793–8.

23. Porter SB, Sande M. Toxoplasmosis of the central nervous system in the acquired immunodeficiency syndrome. *N Engl J Med* 1992; **327**: 1643–8.
24. Aberg A J, Yajko DM, Jacobson MA. Eradication of AIDS-related disseminated *Mycobacterium avium* complex infection after twelve months of antimycobacterial therapy combined with highly active antiretroviral therapy. *J Infect Dis* 1998; **178**: 1446–9.
25. Straus DJ, Huang J, Testa MA *et al.* Prognostic factors in the treatment of human immunodeficiency virus-associated non-Hodgkin's lymphoma: analysis of AIDS Clinical Trials Group Protocol 142-low-dose versus standard-dose m-BACOD plus granulocyte-macrophage colony-stimulating factor. *J Clin Oncol* 1998; **16**: 3601–6.
26. McArthur JC, Brew B, Nath A. Neurological complications of HIV infection. *Lancet Neurol* 2005; **4**: 543–55.
27. Antinori A, Ammassari A, De Luca A *et al.* Diagnosis of AIDS-related focal brain lesions: a decision-making analysis based on clinical and neuroradiologic characteristics combined with polymerase chain reaction assays in CSF. *Neurology* 1997; **48**: 687–94.
28. Nickas G, Wachter RM. Outcomes of intensive care for patients with human immunodeficiency virus infection. *Arch Intern Med* 2000; **169**: 541–7.
29. Gill JK, Greene L, Miller R *et al.* ICU admission in patients infected with the human immunodeficiency virus – a multicentre survey. *Anaesthesia* 1999; **4**: 727–32.
30. Young TN, Arens FJ, Kennedy GE *et al.* Antiretroviral post-exposure prophylaxis (PEP) for occupational HIV exposure. *Cochrane Database Syst Rev* 2007; **1**: CD002835.

61

Severe sepsis

A Raffaele De Gaudio

The incidence of sepsis has increased steadily over the last three decades, at least in part because of ageing western populations.[1] Nearly 15% of patients in intensive care have severe sepsis and two-thirds of them have septic shock.[2,3] Despite our increased understanding, improved support and more powerful antibiotic therapy, severe sepsis is consistently reported as a leading cause of death in non-cardiac intensive care units (ICUs). Mortality remains high[3,4] and severe sepsis claims far more lives than the common diseases of western countries such as acute myocardial infarction, stroke and trauma.[1,4]

DEFINITION

In 1991 the American College of Chest Physicians and Society of Critical Care Medicine convened a consensus conference with the goal of providing a uniform definition for sepsis and its sequelae, using common clinical findings such as alteration in body temperature, tachycardia, tachypnoea and abnormalities in the white blood cell count that were identifiable at the bedside or early in the clinical process.[5] They proposed to differentiate systemic inflammation from the inflammatory response itself, and advocated a model in which *sepsis* is defined as infection in association with a state of systemically activated inflammation (Table 61.1). To differentiate illness severity further, *severe sepsis* was defined as sepsis with organ dysfunction and *septic shock* as sepsis with haemodynamic collapse.[5]

These consensus definitions delineate gradations of mortality risk, but they do not adequately stratify patients into homogeneous groups with respect to the underlying pathophysiology or potential to respond to therapy. They define concepts, but do not identify patients with a single disease.[6,7] For these reasons, a new consensus conference held in 2001 presented a new framework of consensus definitions and a staging system. This system, called *PIRO* (Table 61.2), includes domains for *predisposition* (premorbid illness), *insult/infection* (site, bacteriology of infection, severity of other insults such as trauma), *response* (hypotension, severity of illness measures such as such as Acute Physiology, Age and Chronic Health Evaluation – APACHE), and *organ dysfunction* (aggregate organ dysfunction scores such as multiple-organ dysfunction syndrome and Sequential Organ Failure Assessment – SOFA).[6,7]

PATHOGENESIS

Severe sepsis and septic shock evolve from a systemic inflammatory and coagulation response to a documented infection. Gram-negative bacilli (mainly *Escherichia coli*, *Klebsiella* spp. and *Pseudomonas aeruginosa*) and Gram-positive cocci (mainly staphylococci and streptococci) are the pathogens most commonly associated with the development of sepsis, although fungi, viruses and parasites cause the syndrome. Fungi, mostly *Candida*, account for only 5% of all cases of severe sepsis.[7,8]

The pathophysiology of bacterial sepsis is initiated by the outer-membrane components of both Gram-negative organisms (lipopolysaccharide, lipid A, flagellin and peptidoglycan) and Gram-positive organisms (teichoic acid, lipoteichoic acid, peptidoglycan). These outer-membrane components and other cell wall components are able to bind to the CD14 receptor, a protein anchored in the outer leaflet of the surface of monocytes. Recently, some coreceptors called Toll-like receptors were identified and it was demonstrated that bacterial components also interact with them. Ten members of the Toll-like receptor family have been identified, each of which shows a degree of specificity for pathogenic microorganisms and cellular products (e.g. TLR2 for peptidoglycan, lipoteichoic acid or TLR4 for lipopolysaccharide).[7,8]

Binding of Toll-like receptors activates intracellular signalling pathways that trigger transcription factors, such as nuclear factor-κB, which in turn control the expression of immune response genes, resulting in the release of cytokines (Figure 61.1). They secrete either cytokines with inflammatory properties (including tumour necrosis factor-α (TNF-α), interleukin-1 (IL-1), IL-2, IL-6) or cytokines with anti-inflammatory properties (IL-4 and IL-10).[7,8]

A network of inflammatory mediators activates leukocytes, promotes leukocyte–vascular endothelium adhesion and induces endothelial damage.[6] This endothelial damage, in turn, leads to tissue factor expression and activation of the tissue factor-dependent clotting cascade with subsequent formation of thrombin, so that microaggregates of fibrin,

Table 61.1 Sepsis definitions from the 1991 American College of Chest Physician and Society of Critical Care Medicine Consensus Conference[5]

Systemic inflammatory response syndrome (SIRS)	At least two among the following: Temperature < 36°C or > 38°C Heart rate > 90 beats/min Respiratory rate > 20 breaths/min *or* Pa_{CO_2} < 32 mmHg or mechanically ventilated Leukocyte count < 4000/µl *or* > 12 000/µl *or* > 10% immature band forms
Sepsis	SIRS + confirmed or presumed infection
Severe sepsis	Sepsis + organ hypoperfusion or dysfunction
Septic shock	Sepsis with refractory hypotension (systolic arterial blood pressure < 90 mmHg, mean arterial pressure < 70 mmHg) or vasopressor dependency after adequate volume resuscitation

Table 61.2 The PIRO sepsis staging system[6]

Predisposition	Previous illness with reduced probability of short-term survival Age Genetic polymorphisms in components of inflammatory response
Insult/infection	Culture and sensitivity of infecting pathogens Disease amenable to source control Gene transcript profiles
Response	Systemic inflammatory response syndrome (SIRS) Sepsis Severe sepsis Septic shock Markers of activated inflammation (C-reactive protein, procalcitonin, interleukin-6) Markers of impaired host responsiveness (human leukocyte antigen (HLA)-DR) Detection of therapy target (protein C, tumour necrosis factor, platelet-activating factor)
Organ dysfunction	Number of failing organs Composite scores

platelets, neutrophils and red blood cells impair capillary blood flow, thereby decreasing oxygen and nutrient delivery.[6–8]

In particular, early inflammatory cytokines increase the expression of the enzyme-inducible nitric oxide synthase (iNOS) in endothelial cells; increased synthesis of the potent vasodilator nitric oxide leads to a decrease in systemic vascular resistance characteristic of shock. Inflammatory cytokines such as TNF also contribute to disruption of the tight junctions between endothelial cells, resulting in increased permeability to plasma proteins and fluid with generalised tissue oedema.[7,9] IL-6 alters hepatocyte protein synthesis, inducing the synthesis of acute-phase reactants and promoting anaemia. The acute-phase response also results in downregulation of the production of albumin and anticoagulant proteins such as protein C.[7,9] Microcirculatory dysfunction plays a key role in the development of organ dysfunction in septic patients.[10] As a result of the vicious cycle of inflammation and coagulation, cardiovascular insufficiency (due to the myocardial-depressant effect of TNF, vasodilation and capillary leak) and multiple-organ failure occur, often leading to death (see Figure 61.1).

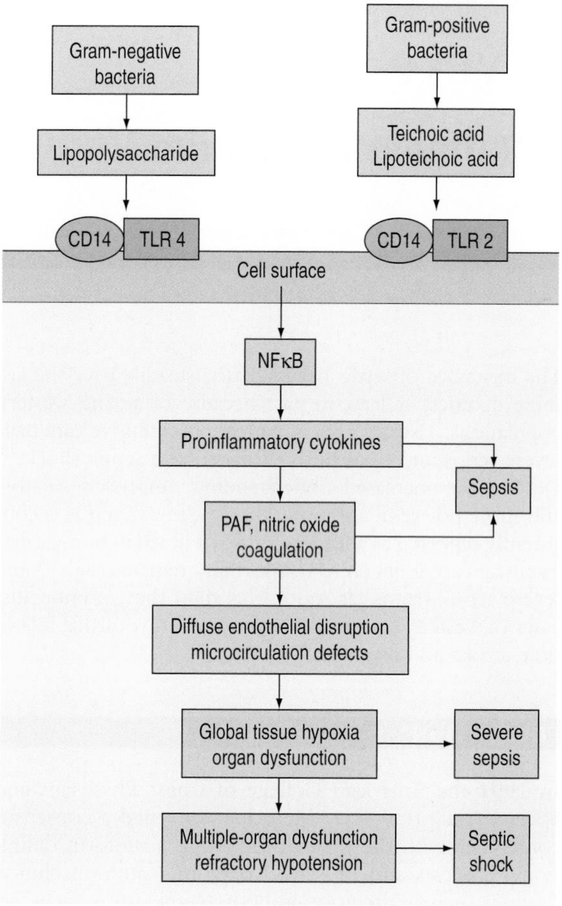

Figure 61.1 Pathogenesis of bacterial sepsis.

DIAGNOSIS

The initial presentation of severe sepsis and septic shock is often non-specific and its severity is cryptic. Diagnosis

Table 61.3 Diagnosis of sepsis-associated organ dysfunctions

Cardiovascular	Systolic arterial blood pressure < 90 mmHg Decrease in systolic blood pressure > 40 mmHg Mean arterial blood pressure < 70 mmHg Decreased capillary refill or mottling
Respiratory	$Pao_2/Fio_2 < 300$
Renal	Creatinine increase > 60 μmol/l from baseline Creatinine increase > 60 μmol/l within last 24 hours Urine output < 0.5 ml/kg per hour for 2 hours despite fluid resuscitation
Coagulation	Activated partial thromboplastin time > 60 seconds International normalised ratio > 1.5 Platelets < 100 000/μl
Liver	Bilirubin > 70 mmol/l
Acid–base	Lactate > 2.1 mmol/l

requires the presence of a presumed or known site of infection, evidence of a systemic inflammatory response syndrome and acute sepsis-associated organ dysfunction (Table 61.3).

Clinical signs include fever or hypothermia, tachycardia, tachypnoea, mental status changes and signs of peripheral vasodilation, that are manifestations of the systemic inflammatory response syndrome.

Laboratory and invasive haemodynamic measurements include:

1. increased cardiac output with normal or low systemic vascular resistance
2. increased oxygen consumption (low $Scvo_2$)
3. leukocytosis or leukopenia
4. lactic acidosis
5. impaired renal or liver function

PULMONARY DYSFUNCTION

Detection of sepsis is facilitated by the nearly universal presence of tachypnoea and hypoxaemia. Pulmonary dysfunction requires a high-volume ventilation, precisely when compliance of the lungs is diminished, airway resistance is increased and muscle efficiency is impaired. Respiratory failure often progresses rapidly; sustained high respiratory rate is usually a sign of impending ventilatory collapse, even if arterial oxygen levels are normal.

CARDIOVASCULAR FAILURE

Cardiovascular failure is caused by an inadequate supply or inappropriate use of metabolic substrate. There is increasing evidence that sepsis is accompanied by a hypermetabolic state, with enhanced glycolysis and hyperlactataemia that do not necessarily indicate tissue hypoxia.[11] Hypotension is frequently the result of low systemic vascular resistance. Shock is typically defined as a systolic pressure lower than 90 mmHg that is unresponsive to fluids or that requires vasoactive drugs.

RENAL DYSFUNCTION

Oliguria is related to hypotension. Anuria is rare. Volume deficit correction reverses oliguria but does not always prevent moderate increases in the serum creatinine level. Renal failure requiring dialysis occurs in about 5% of patients.

LIVER DYSFUNCTION

The liver is a mechanical and immunologic filter for portal blood and may be a major source of cytokines. An increase in aminotransferase and bilirubin levels is common,[12] but hepatic failure is rare.

COAGULATION ABNORMALITIES

Subclinical coagulopathy, with a mild elevation of the prothrombin or partial thromboplastin time, or a moderate reduction in platelet count or an increase in plasma fibrinogen degradation and D-dimer levels may occur. Coagulopathy is caused by deficiencies of the coagulation system proteins (antithrombin III, protein C, tissue factor pathway inhibitor and the kinin system) (Figure 61.2). Simultaneous activation of coagulation by inflammatory cytokines and reduced production of anticoagulant proteins contribute to disseminated intravascular coagulation.[12]

SEPSIS-ASSOCIATED ENCEPHALOPATHY

A diffuse cerebral dysfunction is often present in sepsis and may ensue even before signs of other organ failure. It is better defined as 'sepsis-associated encephalopathy' (SAE), in order to stress the absence of direct infection of the central nervous system. The main sign of SAE is an altered mental status. Electroencephalography is the most sensitive diagnostic test, and allows the grading of the severity of cerebral dysfunction that is related to outcome. SAE is potentially reversible, but always worsens the prognosis. The pathophysiology of SAE is still not completely understood, and it is probably multifactorial. Indeed, brain dysfunction in sepsis may be related to microorganism toxin activity, to the effects of inflammatory mediators, to metabolic alterations and to abnormalities in cerebral circulation.[13,14]

BIOLOGICAL MARKERS

More than 80 biological markers of sepsis have been proposed for diagnosis and prognosis (including C-reactive protein, IL-6, procalcitonin). At the moment lack of availability, non-standardised assays and cut-off values limit their practical use.[12]

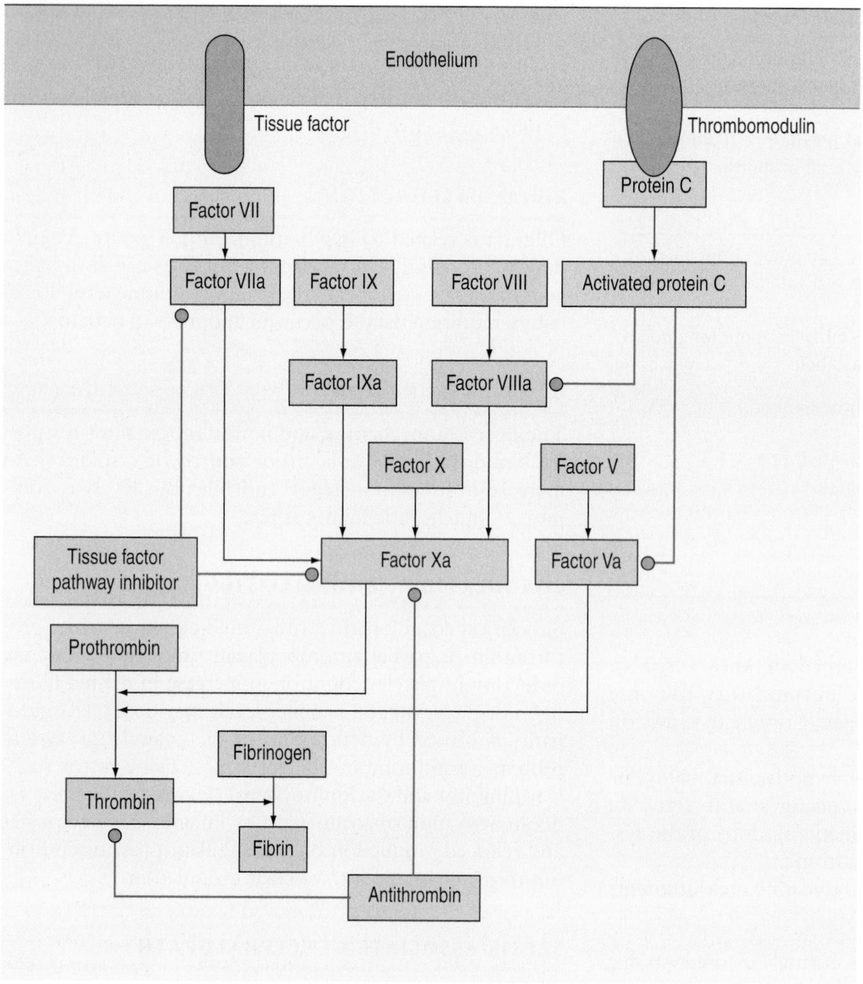

Figure 61.2 Coagulation cascade and its inhibition by activated protein C, antithrombin and tissue factor pathway inhibitor.

TREATMENT

Timely and proper care of the patient with severe sepsis is essential and includes: (1) treatment of the infection with source control and antimicrobial agents; (2) supportive measures such as fluid therapy and vasoactive agents; and (3) adjuvant therapies (Table 61.4).

During the past few years, several randomised controlled trials in patients with severe sepsis and septic shock have demonstrated significant reductions in mortality rates with new applied therapies. Concurrently, antimicrobial resistance to several agents has emerged and changed considerations about empirical therapy. Advances in imaging and non-invasive interventional techniques have also led to new diagnostic and therapeutic strategies for early source control. Some of the new approaches to management of severe sepsis appear to be time-dependent, suggesting a 'golden hour' and a 'silver day' perspective on the management of this syndrome.[15]

SURVIVING SEPSIS CAMPAIGN

In order to improve the standard of care offered to patients with sepsis, the Society of Critical Care Medicine, the European Intensive Care Society and the International Sepsis Forum launched the Surviving Sepsis Campaign (SSC) with a founding statement that became known as the 'Barcelona declaration'.[16] All aspects of management of the patient with severe sepsis were covered and recommendations or bundles, depending on the available level of evidence, were developed for each category[16] (Table 61.5).

However, at the moment, there is no evidence that their beneficial effects are synergistic.[17,18]

SOURCE CONTROL OF INFECTION

Adequate source control of infection is as important as appropriate antimicrobial therapy. All patients presenting with the clinical syndrome of sepsis should be evaluated for

Table 61.4 Management of severe sepsis/septic shock

Monitoring of heart rate, blood pressure, pulse oximetry and urine output
Investigation of the infection source
Laboratory tests for organ dysfunction and global tissue hypoxia (lactate)
Empiric broad-spectrum antibiotics
Central venous access and early goal-directed therapy in patients with lactate > 4 mmol/l or systolic arterial pressure < 90 mmHg even after 20–40 ml/kg fluid challenge
Source control (abscess drainage, tissue debridement, prothesis removal)
Fluid therapy, vasoactive and inotrope drugs
Consider adjuvant therapies
Additional general treatment components

Table 61.5 Issues considered by the Surviving Sepsis Campaign Guidelines[16]

Diagnosis
Intial resuscitation
Antibiotic therapy
Fluid therapy
Vasopressors
Inotropic therapy
Steroids
Activated protein C
Blood product administration
Mechanical ventilation
Sedation/analgesia
Glucose control
Renal replacement
Bicarbonate therapy
Deep-vein thrombosis prophylaxis
Stress ulcer prophylaxis
Consideration regarding limitation of life support

the possible presence of a focus of infection amenable to treatment by source control measures. A source of infection should be rapidly sought by integration of the clinical history, physical examination and results of focused diagnostic tests and imaging examinations.[7] Advances in diagnostic or interventional radiology and surgical procedure have revolutionised the management of many intra-abdominal infections: Specifically, the diagnostic impact of abdominal computed tomography (CT) scan has been significant in patients with multiple potential causes of their acute abdominal pain or sepsis of unknown origin.[15]

Source control includes removal of infected foreign bodies (such as intravascular catheters, vascular draft); incision and drainage (open or percutaneous) of abscesses or fluid collections; the debridement of infected necrotic tissue and the definitive management of anatomical derangements that permit ongoing microbial contamination. For patients with necrotising fasciitis mortality and extent of tissue loss are directly related to the rapidity of surgical intervention.[7]

ANTIMICROBIAL THERAPY

The site of infection and causative organisms are often unknown. Appropriate antimicrobial therapy must be administered empirically in these cases, guided by knowledge of the most common site of infection and most common infecting organisms. Specimens for culture and sensitivity testing should be obtained before empiric wide-spectrum antibiotic therapy is started.

If cultures do not support a diagnosis of infection as the cause of a systemic inflammatory response within 3 days, systemic antibiotics should be discontinued to reduce the risk of superinfection with resistant species, and the patient re-evaluated.

Observational studies suggest a significant reduction in mortality when antibiotics are administered within 4 and 8 hours of hospital admission.[19] Current SSC recommendations are to administer antibiotics within 1 hour of sepsis diagnosis.[16] Specific antibiotic strategies may be found in Chapter 64.

EARLY HAEMODYNAMIC RESUSCITATION (FIRST 6 HOURS)

Haemodynamic resuscitation to normal physiological parameters has been trialled as early goal-directed therapy (EGDT), which revealed a statistically significant mortality reduction of 16.5%.[20] EGDT aims to restore the balance between oxygen supply and demand within the first 6 hours. The strategy involves obtaining adequate oxygen delivery by optimisation of intravascular volume (preload) with the use of: (1) central venous pressure (CVP) monitoring; (2) blood pressure (afterload) with mean arterial pressure monitoring; (3) contractility monitoring to avoid tachycardia; and (d) restoration of the balance between systemic oxygen delivery and oxygen demand to resolve global tissue hypoxia (guided by $Scvo_2$).[15,21,22] A low $Scvo_2$ (< 70%), coupled with an elevated lactate level, suggests a mismatch between systemic oxygen delivery and oxygen consumption of the tissues. When a low $Scvo_2$ is identified, therapies to augment the components of oxygen delivery are recommended to restore the balance between systemic oxygen delivery and consumption (oxygen-carrying capacity, arterial oxygen saturation and cardiac output). $Scvo_2$ can be measured intermittently from venous gas samples taken from the distal port of a standard central venous catheter.[23] At the moment, EGDT appears to decrease ICU pulmonary artery catheter utilisation.[23,24] In any case, the pulmonary artery catheter remains effective as a measurement site, although outcome benefit from its use remains to be demonstrated.[23,24]

Resuscitation goals proposed in SSC[16] include: central venous pressure of 8–12 mmHg, mean arterial pressure $\geq$ 65 mmHg, urine output $\geq$ 0.5 ml/kg per hour, central venous (superior vena cava) oxygen saturation $\geq$ 70% or mixed venous $\geq$ 65%.

FLUID THERAPY

Initial resuscitation efforts should incorporate intravenous fluid therapy. The first goal of volume therapy of sepsis is repletion of the patient's intravascular volume. The selection of crystalloid versus colloid solutions has been vigorously debated. At the moment no randomised controlled trial or systemic review has definitively shown a benefit in the critically ill septic patient for the use of colloid or crystalloid fluid.[25,26] A larger volume of crystalloids (2–3 times) is usually required. A smaller volume of colloid will produce a similar improvement in volume status, but these fluids are more expensive and may alter blood coagulation. Intravenous fluid therapy should begin with 1000 ml crystalloid fluid challenge or 500 ml colloids over 30 min.[16] Rapid and repeated 500-ml boluses of either crystalloid or colloid fluid may be necessary up to an initial resuscitation volume of 20–40 ml/kg body weight.[15,21]

VASOACTIVE AGENTS AND INOTROPES

Organ perfusion cannot be maintained with fluids alone. Vasoactive agents (Table 61.6) should be administered when hypotension is persistent or mean arterial blood pressure is less than 65 mmHg, after a crystalloid challenge of 20–40 ml/kg.[15,21] However, existing evidence does not clearly support the superiority of one vasopressor over another.[27] Both noradrenaline (norepinephrine) and dopamine have been advocated as first-line vasopressor agents in cases of sepsis,[15,21] although some prefer norepinephrine.[28] Norepinephrine and phenylephrine, agents with more alpha-agonist effects, may be preferable for patients with tachycardia or ischaemic cardiac diseases. The combination of noradrenaline plus low-dose dobutamine has been shown to prevent gastric mucosal perfusion in comparison with adrenaline (epinephrine) or dopamine.[28,29]

Inotropic support with dobutamine may treat the myocardial depression, improving contractility.[15] When hypotension persists, a vasopressin deficiency may be considered. Exogenously administered vasopressin in physiologic replacement doses may act synergistically with other vasopressor agents.[18,23] The SSC[16] recommends vasopressin infusion for refractory shock and in limited doses.

ADMINISTRATION OF ERYTHROCYTES

The patient's oxygen-carrying capacity may be augmented by the administration of packed erythrocytes to achieve a haematocrit above 30%, with a more restrictive transfusion strategy in the convalescent phase of the disease.[16,30]

DECREASING OXYGEN CONSUMPTION

Strategies to minimise oxygen demand should consider: intubation, analgo-sedation, control of fever with antipyretic, mechanical ventilation to reduce the work of breathing and oxygen consumption by respiratory muscles.[21]

ADJUVANT THERAPIES

Several additional therapies initiated early after identification of severe sepsis can improve the patient's outcome, and reduce the mortality rate. At the moment there is no consensus in these issues.

ACTIVATED PROTEIN C (APC)

During sepsis the APC pathway serves as a major system for controlling thrombosis, inhibiting thrombin formation, limiting inflammatory responses and potentially decreasing endothelial cell apoptosis. Recombinant APC (rhAPC) could also improve microcirculatory blood flow in septic patients, as recently measured in vivo.[10] There are concerns about the effects of rhAPC, although it has been shown to yield a 6.1% absolute reduction in 28-day all-cause mortality when administered to a heterogeneous group of patients with severe sepsis (Protein C Worldwide Evaluation in Severe Sepsis (PROWESS) trial).[31] This was supported by the open-label extended evaluation of recombinant human protein C (ENHANCE study).[32] However, a second large randomised controlled trial that compared rhAPC with placebo in patients with less severe sepsis was terminated early, when there appeared to be no mortality benefit for this patient population (Administration of Drotrecogin alfa (activated) in Early Stage Severe Sepsis (ADDRESS) trial).[33]

Table 61.6 Vasopressors and inotropes used for severe sepsis/septic shock

Agent	Receptor pharmacology				Cardiovascular effect		Dose
	α_1	β_1	β_2	Dopaminergic	CO	SVR	
Dopamine	0	+	0	++	+	+	0.5–2 μg/kg per min
	+	++	0	++	+	+	5–10 μg/kg per min
	++	++	0	++	+	++	10–20 μg/kg per min
Dobutamine	0/+	+++ +	++	0	++	-	2.5–20 μg/kg per min
Adrenaline (epinephrine)	+++	+++	++	0	++	0/+	1–10 μg/min
Noradrenaline (norepinephrine)	+++	++	0	0	0/+	++	0.5–1.5 μg/kg per min
Phenylephrine	+++	0	0	0	0/+	++	1–10 μg/kg/min

CO, cardiac output; SVR, systemic vascular resistance.

The SSC recommends rhAPC in patients at high risk of death (APACHE II $\geq$ 25), sepsis-induced multiple-organ failure, septic shock or sepsis-induced acute respiratory distress syndrome (ARDS) and with no absolute contraindication related to bleeding risk or relative contraindication that outweighs the potential benefit of rhAPC.[16] This may not seem the most reliable method for choosing patients because the use of this drug has not been validated in this context, and there are numerous variables in the calculation of the APACHE II score, including age.[18] Further studies are necessary to optimise the use of this drug; many uncertainties remain and it must also be taken into account that the drug is expensive, carries an elevated risk of bleeding and that its introduction was accompanied by more than the usual amount of scientific debate.[7,34,35]

STEROIDS

Steroid administration in severe sepsis and septic shock remains controversial. The SSC recommends the use of intravenous corticosteroids in patients with septic shock who, despite adequate fluid replacement, require vasopressor therapy to maintain blood pressure.[16]

The use of large doses of methylprednisolone has not been shown to be beneficial.[36] Recently, the concept of inadequate adrenal reserve, or relative adrenal insufficiency (RAI), has led to the consideration of administering moderate doses of steroids. The administration of low doses of hydrocortisone (200–300 mg/day for 7 days) plus fludrocortisone (50 μg orally per day for 7 days) to patients with septic shock decreased their requirements for vasopressors and lowered their mortality rate.[37–39] In other studies RAI was diagnosed using the 250-μg adrenocorticotrophin test to identify patients who would benefit more from steroid administration.[37–39]

Recently, in a multicentre, randomised, double-blind, placebo-controlled trial on about 500 patients, hydrocortisone did not improve survival or reversal of septic shock, either overall or in patients who did not have a response to corticotrophin.[40]

TIGHT BLOOD GLUCOSE CONTROL

When conservative glycaemic control was compared with tight control in a multicentre randomised clinical trial, tight control led to a significant reduction in mortality and improved morbidity at 1 year.[41] Other advantages included shorter intensive care stay, a reduced risk of renal failure and a much lower incidence of critical-illness polyneuropathy. The study involved cardiac surgery patients. A recent trial by the same group in medical critically ill patients showed no significant difference.[42] As it is not clear if slightly less stringent control has the same advantages, it is necessary to carry out meticulous monitoring of blood glucose in order to prevent the risk of hypoglycaemia, particularly in unstable septic patients.

Insulin has anti-inflammatory effects that may contribute to its beneficial action in sepsis. Other characteristics of insulin (i.e. prevention of apoptosis) that may be responsible for its most important therapeutic effect in these patients should also be considered.

PROTECTIVE LUNG STRATEGIES

High tidal volumes coupled with high plateau pressures should be avoided in those patients who develop acute lung injury (ALI) or ARDS as a consequence of severe sepsis.[43] Mechanical ventilation with large tidal volume can stretch lung tissue to excess (volume trauma), exacerbating the inflammatory response and leading to ALI. In one study patients with ALI or ARDS were randomised to receive ventilation with tidal volumes of 12 ml/kg predicted body weight (control) or 6 ml/kg predicted body weight (treatment), with plateau pressure maintained at < 30 cm H_2O. An absolute reduction of 9.9% in 28-day mortality was demonstrated in the low tidal volume group,[44] with fewer days on ventilatory support and lower levels of circulating IL-6.

EXTRACORPOREAL BLOOD PURIFICATION TECHNIQUES

These techniques may hold promise for the treatment of sepsis.[45] At the moment definitive studies have yet to be performed. Dialysis does improve survival among patients with sepsis who have established renal insufficiency. It is not certain that dialysis, plasmapheresis or plasma exchange will improve outcomes in patients with sepsis who do not have renal failure. Studies in animals and humans examining this issue have been inconclusive. There is also a potential for harm, since this therapy could remove beneficial compounds or molecules as well.[46]

ADDITIONAL GENERAL TREATMENT COMPONENTS

Additional components in the care of severe sepsis include:

1. adequate early nutrition that is best accomplished via the enteral route, to avoid catheter-related blood stream infections and to maintain gut mucosa integrity
2. deep-venous thrombosis prevention that can be accomplished with the use of subcutaneous heparin or continuous use of pneumatic compression stockings
3. gastric ulcer prophylaxis that may be accomplished with sucralfate, an H_2-receptor antagonist or a proton pump inhibitor
4. prevention of nosocomial infection (adopting selective antimicrobial decontamination of digestive tract,[47] removing catheters)

OUTCOME

The overall hospital mortality rate for patients with severe sepsis is high. Since this disease is reversible, prompt recognition and resuscitation are key to optimising outcome. Studies focused on novel targets, mechanism of action and combination therapy may also improve outcome.[48]

REFERENCES

1. Finfer S, Bellomo R, Lipman J *et al.* Adult population incidence of severe sepsis in Australian and New Zealand intensive care units. *Intens Care Med* 2004; **30**: 527–9.
2. Martin GS, Mannino DM, Eaton S *et al.* The epidemiology of sepsis in the United States from 1979 through 2000. *N Engl J Med* 2003; **348**: 1546–54.
3. Brun Buisson C. Epidemiology of severe sepsis. *Presse Med* 2006; **35**: 513–20.
4. Angus DC, Linde-Zwirble WT, Lidicker J *et al.* Epidemiology of severe sepsis in the United States: analysis of incidence, outcome and associated costs of care. *Crit Care Med* 2001; **29**: 1303–10.
5. Bone RC, Balk RA, Cerra F *et al.* Definition for sepsis and organ failure and guidelines for use of innovative therapies in sepsis: American College of Chest Physicians/Society of Critical Care Medicine. *Chest* 1992; **101**: 1644–55.
6. Levy MM, Fink M, Marshall JC *et al.* SCCM/ESICM/ACCP/ATS/SIS international sepsis definitions conference. *Crit Care Med* 2003; **34**: 1250–6.
7. Marshall JC. Sepsis: current status, future prospects. *Curr Opin Crit Care* 2004; **10**: 250–64.
8. Bochud PY, Calandra T. Pathogenesis of sepsis: new concepts and implications for future treatment. *Br Med J* 2003; **326**: 262–6.
9. Opal SM, Esmon CT. Bench-to-bedside review: functional relationships between coagulation and the innate immune response and their respective roles in the pathogenesis of sepsis. *Crit Care* 2003; **7**: 23–38.
10. Hoffmann JN, Fertmann JM, Jauch KW. Microcirculatory disorders in sepsis and transplantation: therapy with natural coagulatory inhibitors antithrombin and activated protein C. *Curr Opin Crit Care* 2006; **12**: 426–30.
11. Levy B. Lactate and shock state: the metabolic view. *Curr Opin Crit Care* 2006; **1**: 315–21.
12. Marshall JC. Inflammation, coagulopathy, and the pathogenesis of the multiple organ dysfunction syndrome. *Crit Care Med* 2001; **29**: S106.
13. Gren R, Scott LK, Minagar A *et al.* Sepsis associated encephalopathy (SAE): a review. *Front Biosci* 2004; **9**: 1637–41.
14. Consales G, De Gaudio AR. Sepsis associated encephalopathy. *Minerva Anestesiol* 2005; **71**: 39–52.
15. Nguyen BN, Rivers EP, Abraham FM *et al.* Severe sepsis and septic shock: review of the literature and emergency department management guidelines. *Ann Emerg Med* 2006; **48**: 1–54.
16. Dellinger RP, Levy M, Carlet J. Surviving Sepsis Campaign: international guidelines for management of severe sepsis and septic shock: 2008. *Intens Care Med* 2008; **34**: 17–60.
17. Poulton B. Advances in the management of sepsis: the randomised controlled trials behind the Surving Sepsis campaign recommendations. *Int J Antimicrob Agents* 2006; **27**: 97–101.
18. Vincent JL. Is the current management of severe sepsis and septic shock really evidence based? *Plos Med* 2006; **3**: 346–50.
19. Houck PM, Bratzler DW. Administration of first hospital antibiotics for community-acquired pneumonia: does timeliness affect outcomes? *Curr Opin Infect Dis* 2005; **18**: 151–6.
20. Rivers E, Nguyen B, Havstad S *et al.* Early goal-directed therapy in the treatment of severe sepsis and septic shock. *N Engl J Med* 2001; **345**: 1368–77.
21. Rivers EP, McIntyre L, Morro DC *et al.* Early and innovative interventions for severe sepsis and septic shock: taking advantage of a window of opportunity. *CMAJ* 2005; **173**: 1054–65.
22. Hollenberg SM, Ahrens TS, Annane D *et al.* Practice parameters for hemodynamic support of sepsis in adult patient: 2004 update. *Crit Care Med* 2004; **32**:1928–48.
23. Trzeciak S, Dellinger RP, Abate NL *et al.* Translating research to clinical practice: a 1-year experience with implementing early goal-directed therapy for septic shock in the emergency department. *Chest* 2006; **129**: 225–32.
24. Harvey S, Harrison DA, Singer M *et al.* Assessment of the clinical effectiveness of pulmonary artery catheters in management of patients in intensive care. *Lancet* 2005; **366**: 472–7.
25. Finfer S, Bellomo R, Boyce N *et al.* A comparison of albumin and saline for fluid resuscitation in the intensive care unit. *N Engl J Med* 2004; **350**: 2247–56.
26. Boldt J. Do plasma substitutes have additional properties beyond correcting volume deficits? *Shock* 2006; **25**: 103–16.
27. Sessler CN, Perry JC, Varney KL. Management of severe sepsis and septic shock. *Curr Opin Crit Care* 2004; **10**: 354–63.
28. Leone M, Vallet B, Teboul J *et al.* Survey of the use of catecholamines by French physicians. *Intens Care Med* 2004, **30**: 984–8.
29. Zhou SX, Qiu HB, Huang YZ *et al.* Effects of norepinephrine, epinephrine, and epinephrine – dobutamine on systemic and gastric mucosal oxygenation in septic shock. *Acta Pharmacol Sin* 2002; **23**: 654–8.
30. Vincent J L., Baron JF, Reinhart K *et al.* Anemia and blood transfusion in critically ill patients. *JAMA* 2002; **288**: 1499–507.
31. Bernard GR, Vincent JL, Laterre PF *et al.* Efficacy and safety of recombinant human activated protein C for severe sepsis. *N Engl J Med* 2001; **344**: 699–709.
32. Vincent JL, Bernard GR, Beale R *et al.* Drotrecogin alfa (activated) treatment in severe sepsis from the global open-label trial ENHANCE. *Crit Care Med* 2005; **33**: 2266–77.
33. Abraham E, Laterre PF, Garg R *et al.* Administration of Drotrecogin alfa (activated) in Early Stage Severe Sepsis (ADDRESS) study group: drotrecogin alfa (activated) for adults with severe sepsis and a low risk of death. *N Engl J Med* 2005; **353**: 1332–41.

34. Warren HS, Suffredini AF, Eicchacker PQ *et al.* Risks and benefits of activated protein C treatment for severe sepsis. *N Engl J Med* 2002; **347**: 1027–30.
35. Eichacker PQ, Natanson C. Increasing evidence that the risks of rhAPC may outweigh its benefits. *Intens Care Med* 2007; **33**: 396–9.
36. Hotchkiss RS, Karl IE. The pathophysiology and treatment of sepsis. *N Engl J Med* 2003; **348**: 138–50.
37. Briegel J, Forst H, Haller M *et al.* Stress doses of hydrocortisone reverse hyperdynamic septic shock: a prospective, randomized, double-blind, single-center study. *Crit Care Med* 1999; **27**: 723–32.
38. Annane D, Sebille V, Charpentier C *et al.* Effect of treatment with low doses of hydrocortisone and fludrocortisone on mortality in patients with septic shock. *JAMA* 2002; **288**: 862–71.
39. Annane D, Bellissant E, Bollaert P *et al.* Corticosteroids for treating severe sepsis and septic shock. *Cochrane Database Syst Rev* 2004; **1**: CD002243.
40. Sprung CL, Annane D, Keh D *et al.* Hydrocortisone therapy for patients with septic shock. *N Engl J Med* 2008; **358**: 111–24.
41. Van den Berghe G, Wouters P, Weekers F *et al.* Intensive insulin therapy in the critically ill patient. *N Engl J Med* 2001; **345**: 1359–67.
42. Van den Berghe G, Wilmer A, Hermans G *et al.* Intensive insulin therapy in the medical ICU. *N Engl J Med* 2006; **354**: 449–61.
43. Frank JA, Matthay MA. Science review: mechanisms of ventilator-induced injury. *Crit Care* 2003; **7**: 233–41.
44. The Acute Respiratory Distress Syndrome Network. Ventilation with lower tidal volumes as compared with traditional tidal volumes for acute lung injury and the acute respiratory distress syndrome. *N Engl J Med* 2000; **342**: 1301–8.
45. Ronco C, Brendolan A, Lonnemann G *et al.* A pilot study of coupled plasma filtration with adsorption in septic shock. *Crit Care Med* 2002; **30**: 1250–5.
46. Hotchkiss RS, Karl IE. Sepsis – theory and therapies. *N Engl J Med* 2003; **348**: 1600–2.
47. De Jonge E. Effects of selective decontamination of digestive tract on mortality and antibiotic resistance in the intensive-care unit. *Curr Opin Crit Care* 2005; **11**: 144–9.
48. Russell JA. Management of sepsis. *N Engl J Med* 2006; **355**: 1699–713.

62

Nosocomial infection

Neil Soni

Nosocomial or hospital-acquired infections are a major problem in hospitals, affecting up to 9% of inpatients at any one time. Intensive care units (ICUs) represent 2–10% of hospital beds, but are responsible for 25% of all nosocomial blood stream and pulmonary infections. In the European Prevalence of Infection in Intensive Care (EPIC) snapshot of prevalence the infection rate in ICU was 20.62%.[1] Nosocomial infection is, at least in theory, a preventable cause of morbidity and mortality (Table 62.1).

EPIDEMIOLOGY

The prevalence of nosocomial infection is reported as being between 3 and 12% in most institutions but varies considerably between different sites within each institution.[2] The vulnerability of the patient population, the nature of interventions and cross-infection are but three of many factors. This is seen clearly if one compares the range between ophthalmology and critical care – 0–23%.[3]

The site of infection varies with location so that, whereas the urinary tract and the chest are common throughout the hospital, within the ICU surgical wound infection, pneumonia and blood stream infection are far more common (8–12%).

The impact of nosocomial infection is impressive. Ventilator-associated pneumonia (VAP) is common, has significant morbidity with increased length of stay, associated costs and a twofold increase in mortality.[4] It has been suggested that blood stream infections, surgical wound infections and nosocomial pneumonia result in 14, 12 and 13 attributable extra hospital days respectively.[5] Catheter-related blood stream infection (CR-BSI) was also associated with major morbidity although, curiously, not necessarily mortality.[6] The mortality rates directly due to these infections are hard to separate from the mortality attributed to the presenting severity of illness, which in its own right may have predisposed to infection. What is clear is that nosocomial infection is associated with increased mortality, and huge financial and resource costs.[2]

THE MECHANISMS INVOLVED IN NOSOCOMIAL INFECTION

A range of factors come together to enable nosocomial infection to occur. Some may be risk factors in their own right whereas other may simply represent an identifier of a sicker and therefore more vulnerable population (Table 62.2).

HOST

The vulnerability of a potential host will be determined by several factors:

- the acute illness or problem that required ICU admission
- the chronic health status and underlying disease. Conditions such as diabetes predispose to infective problems
- the status of their immunocompetence, which may involve medications, such as steroids
- the integrity of natural defences, such as the skin and mucous membranes. This may be disrupted by burns, surgery or by breakdown of tissues such as pressure areas. The presence of invasive devices (e.g. endotracheal tube, intravenous devices) provides a conduit past the natural defences
- antibiotics given to the patient which may encourage emergence of particular strains or resistant organisms
- blood transfusion has been suggested as a risk factor[7]

ENVIRONMENT

Local environmental pressures play their part. The combination of antibiotics, in particular multiple antibiotics, and cross-infection predisposes a vulnerable population to pseudomembranous colitis from *Clostridium difficile* toxin.[8] Epidemiological patterns, such as the prevalence of *Enterococcus faecalis* as a common pathogen in the surgical population, may be linked to widespread cephalosporin usage. Much of the multiresistance problem probably originates from antibiotic pressures.[9] Cross-infection is the biggest single problem in intensive care and transmission is by various means, but still the most common is by hands.[10]

Table 62.1 Principles of diagnosis of nosocomial infections

- Diagnosis of infection usually requires the combination of both clinical findings and the results of diagnostic tests
- Clinical diagnosis of infection from direct observation at surgery, endoscopy or other diagnostic procedure is an acceptable criterion for an infection
- It must be hospital-acquired. There must be no evidence that the infection was present or incubating at the time of hospital admission. Infection acquired in hospital, but only evident after hospital discharge, also fulfils the criteria
- Usually no specific time during or after hospitalisation is given to determine whether an infection is nosocomial or community-acquired. Each infection is examined for evidence that links it to hospitalisation (this is a matter of controversy)

Table 62.2 Risk factors for nosocomial infection

Patient
- Severity of illness
- Underlying diseases
- Nutritional state
- Immunosuppression
- Open wounds
- Invasive devices
- Multiple procedures
- Prolonged stay
- Ventilation
- Multiple or prolonged antibiotics
- Blood transfusion

Environment
- Changes in procedures or protocols
- Multiple changes in staff; new staff
- Poor aseptic practice – poor hand-washing
- Patient-to-patient: busy, crowded unit, staff shortages

The organism
- Resistance
- Resilience in terms of survival
- Formation of slime or ability to adhere
- Pathogenicity
- Prevalence

ORGANISM

The host usually lives in synergistic or symbiotic tranquillity with a huge range of organisms (Table 62.3). Antibiotics suppress many normal organisms and allow the emergence and overgrowth of a usually insignificant organism or resistant organism of the same type. For example, an intrinsic organism such as *Candida* will flourish in the presence of broad-spectrum antibiotics and this overgrowth may result in symptomatic or even invasive candidiasis. Cephalosporin use may encourage the intrinsically resistant but quiescent enterococci to emerge as a dominant and problematic organism.

Table 62.3 Common commensals that may cause infection in a vulnerable host

Site	Common commensal organisms
Skin	*Staphylococcus epidermidis*, streptococci, *Corynebacterium* (diphtheroids), *Candida*
Throat	*Streptococcus viridans*, diphtheroids
Mouth	*Streptococcus viridans, Moraxella catarrhalis, Actinomyces*, spirochaetes
Respiratory tract	*Streptococcus viridans, Moraxella*, diphtheroids, micrococci
Vagina	Lactobacilli, diphtheroids, streptococci, yeast
Intestines	*Bacteroides*, anaerobic streptococci, *Clostridium perfringens, Escherichia coli, Klebsiella, Proteus*, enterococci

Extrinsic organisms may be introduced from the environment, from other patients, from staff or from surfaces. These may be organisms which are thriving in that environment because of local pressures (e.g. antibiotics), or from poor hygiene. Examples include *Acinetobacter* and, of course, meticillin-resistant *Staphylococcus aureus* (MRSA). On admission, patients will be carrying a range of organisms that have the potential to cause problems, but during their stay they are likely to acquire a new ecology from their surroundings. In a hospital that ecology may be quite hostile, with multiresistance being common.

The individual characteristics of the organism are important. These include their resilience in the local environment, the ease of transmission and the individual pathogenicity. This clearly interacts with the vulnerability of the host, as some usually innocuous organisms, such as *Candida* or *Serratia marcescens*, will only cause problems in vulnerable hosts whereas others, such as some strains of *Staphylococcus aureus*, *Acinetobacter* or *Clostridium difficile*, may be intrinsically more virulent.

THE ORGANISMS

A vast range of organisms can cause nosocomial infection (Table 62.4). It must be emphasised that each hospital and each ICU will have its own local ecology and knowing this ecology is important. Regional, national and international surveys give indications of general trends but this does not supplant local knowledge.

Nosocomial infection is dynamic in that it is influenced by many environmental factors, the type of patient, type of surgery or illness, the antibiotic usage profile and many other variables. This dynamism is illustrated by the Gram-positive infections of the 1950s and 1960s, giving way to the Gram-negative infections of the 1970s and, while the multiresistant Gram-positive organisms are a major anxiety currently, they are already being superseded by super-resistant organisms, such as *Stenotrophomonas* and *Acinetobacter*. The ease of transmission or development of resistance is a key factor in the current explosion in multiresistance.

Table 62.4 Organisms responsible for the majority of nosocomial infections

Methicillin-resistant *Staphylococcus aureus* (MRSA)
Coagulase-negative *Staphylococcus* (CNS)
Enterococcus spp. (*E. faecalis, E. faecium*)
Pseudomonas aeruginosa
Acinetobacter baumanii
Stenotrophomonas maltophilia
Enterobacter spp.
Klebsiella spp.
Escherichia coli
Serratia marcescens
Proteus spp.
Candida spp. (*C. albicans, C. glabrata, C. krusei*)

Other organisms may be a problem in the severely immunocompromised, such as those with acquired immunodeficiency syndrome (AIDS: see Chapter 60)

The combination of sick patients and widespread use of potent antibiotics selects out problematic organisms and, as this epitomises intensive care practice, it is in ICU where multiresistance is common.

The organisms causing nosocomial infection may be endogenous or exogenous. Illness and antibiotics may both encourage the emergence and overgrowth of endogenous organisms that were normally suppressed and hence ecological change takes place in the skin, nasopharynx and gut. Alternatively the same factors influence colonisation with exogenous organisms from the environment. Cross-infection plays a significant role, as does the size of the local reservoir of exogenous organisms. The colonising organisms are well placed to invade or be introduced by invasive procedures, by devices or simply through areas of injury. Infection follows.

MULTIRESISTANT ORGANISMS

Many of the organisms that cause nosocomial infection are characterised by multiresistance. There are several mechanisms involved in resistance and in its spread. Enzymes, such as the β-lactamases, render a large array of antibiotics useless. Class 1 β-lactamase is effective against some β-lactam-containing antibiotics but extended-spectrum β-lactamases (ESBL), which incorporate enzymes, such as TEM-24, will produce cross-resistance to multiple classes of antibiotics, including fluoroquinolones and aminoglycosides. Resistance may be produced by a combination of mechanisms, such as in *Pseudomonas aeruginosa*, where the resistance is due to a combination of derepression of protein efflux systems, cephalosporinases and derepression of AmpC enzyme.

Resistance is acquired in a variety of ways. Mutation of any gene occurs at a rate of one cell in 10^7 and, if this cell is then presented with antibiotics that it can survive, it will become a dominant cell, reproducing at a rate of 10^9 overnight. An example of this might be the development of AmpC β-lactamase in *Enterobacter*, when patients are treated with third-generation cephalosporins. A similar example is the loss of porin OprD in *P. aeruginosa* in the presence of imipenem.

Table 62.5 The influence of extended-spectrum β-lactamases (ESBL) on resistance in *Klebsiella*

Antibiotics	ESBL-negative (% resistant)	ESBL-positive (% resistant)
Gentamicin	8	76
Amikacin	3	52
Ciprofloxacin	3	31
All the above	0	5

(Reproduced from Livermore DM, Yuan M. Antibiotic resistance and production of extended-spectrum beta-lactamases amongst *Klebsiella* spp. from intensive care units in Europe. *J Antimicrob Chemother* 1996; **38:** 409–24.)

The big problem, particularly with ESBL, is that they can spread by plasmid transmission which is very rapid. The enzyme production is encoded chromosomally within an organism, and can then be transferred between bacteria by plasmids. Transposons transfer genes between plasmids. Examples of this include:

1. SHV-1 plasmid β-lactamase from *Klebsiella*
2. plasmid AmpC β-lactamases from *Citrobacter*
3. aminoglycoside-modifying enzymes from aminoglycoside-producing streptomycetes

The phenomenon of induction is also seen. This is the process whereby the presence of an antibiotic appears to 'induce' or speed up the production of the relevant enzyme so that the organism rapidly becomes resistant.

Staphylococcal resistance to meticillin occurs due to an altered penicillin-binding protein, which has low affinity for all β-lactam agents. It is linked to a *MecA* gene. This gene does not develop readily and spread of meticillin resistance is by vector transmission, not de novo production of resistance[7] (Table 62.5).

SOME COMMON ORGANISMS

See Table 62.4 for organisms responsible for the majority of nosocomial infections.

Escherichia Coli

E. coli was one of the first organisms to become multiresistant. The spread of its resistance is a model of how the problem develops in different environments. Currently in Europe, about 4% of *E. coli* is resistant to ceftazidime but in Turkey this figure is 26%. The trend towards an increase in resistance seems to correspond with the use of quinolones.[11]

Enterobacter species, cloacae and Aerogenes

Part of the normal intestinal flora, these species tend to develop ESBL relatively easily, making them multiresistant to a wide range of antibiotics, including ceftazidime. The prevalence of resistance in many western ICUs is running at about 35% and rising. This organism has been implicated in cross-colonisation in ICU and the relevant enzymes, including TEM-24, impart cross-resistance to multiple classes of antibiotics. Prompt recognition and treatment are usually effective.[12]

Klebsiella

Klebsiella has become increasingly resistant with the acquisition of ESBL, and can be multiresistant. The incidence is incredibly variable between countries.

Pseudomonas

Pseudomonas are versatile opportunistic pathogens common in the critically ill; they may colonise patients with chronic lung disease. Resistance is able to develop in a range of ways and produces a very broad spectrum of resistance, making it potentially very difficult to treat and resulting in the increased popularity of combination therapy.[13] It is associated with adverse outcome in the critically ill.[14]

Stenotrophomonas Maltophilia

This is an increasingly common and troublesome environmental organism. It is often resistant to β-lactam antibiotics, quinolones and to aminoglycosides. It also produces a carbapenamase, which makes it resistant to carbapenems.

Acinetobacter Baumanii

Acinetobacter baumanii is an increasing and major problem. It survives even in dry environments and, despite its name, spreads and cross-infects readily (*a cineto*: without movement). They are multiresistant and, although they were sensitive to carbapenems, they are increasingly resistant even to these agents, presumably through gene exchange. They become rapidly resistant and the profile of resistance is unpredictable but can be extremely broad, with some organisms recently only sensitive to colistin.[15]

Coagulase-Negative Staphylococci (CNS)

CNS are low-virulence organisms, but are increasingly causing nosocomial infection. Their resilience may be in part due to the production of biofilm. Frequently meticillin-resistant, they are also resistant to multiple classes of antibiotics, but are usually sensitive to glycopeptides. As glycopeptide resistance patterns alter, newer agents, such as quinupristin, dalfopristin and linezolid, will have a role.

Staphylococcus Aureus

This is a virulent pathogen causing a wide range of infections. Meticillin resistance started in the early 1960s, and although rates between countries and ICUs vary considerably, there has been an inexorable rise in its prevalence in most countries. It is easily identified. It both colonises and infects, but is relatively easily treated with glycopeptides. More recent reports of occasional glycopeptide-resistant organisms are therefore a major source of concern. It has been a model of the failure of some infection control methods. It is being increasingly assessed in terms of suppressibility with a selective decontamination of the digestive tract (SDD)-style approach to elimination.[16]

Enterococcus Faecalis and Faecium

These organisms emerged with increased third-generation cephalosporin use. *E. faecalis* is more commonly isolated and may still be sensitive to ampicillin but more than 30% are resistant to aminoglycosides. This contrasts with *E. faecium*, which has a resistance rate of 7% to vancomycin (and rising), 53% to ampicillin and 30% to aminoglycosides. Glycopeptide resistance is increasing and vancomycin-resistant enterococcus (VRE), unheard of 10 years ago, is now being regularly identified.[17]

Tuberculosis

Not normally seen as a nosocomial infection, this has the potential to become a nosocomial problem. As numbers increase and infected patients are not recognised on admission, there is the possibility of rapid spread to both other patients and staff. In particular multiresistant tuberculosis is on the increase. At present there are occasional outbreaks but these could easily increase.

Clostridium difficile

This originally emerged as an organism that became a problem after certain antibiotics, including clindamycin. It is now clear that in the critically ill it often emerges after almost any broad-spectrum antibiotics, although usually after several courses and some considerable time. Probably as important is the observation of case clusters, indicating that cross-infection is important. The organism produces a toxin that causes pseudomembranous colitis, but paradoxically, testing for the toxin provides a rapid diagnostic pathway that can facilitate early treatment. Aggressive pseudomembranous colitis is a potentially catastrophic disease and, although it usually settles on metronidazole or vancomycin orally, not only is recurrence common but it can also progress to severe colitis and necessitates radical surgery such as colectomy.[18] Surgery carries a high mortality rate, quoted at 11% for total colectomy, and very high mortality for less aggressive surgery such as hemicolectomy in the presence of toxic megacolon.[19]

Candida Sepsis

Candida sepsis is almost always a nosocomial problem, probably endogenous in origin, and related to overgrowth secondary to antibiotic pressures. Occasionally clusters of more unusual *Candida* such as *C. glabrata* or *C. krusei* are seen in the ICU, suggesting cross-infection. The prevalence of species is defined by each unit but *C. albicans* is most common. There is some evidence to suggest that the widespread use of azoles may have infiuenced the relative increase in *C. glabrata* and *C. krusei* species. Definitive diagnosis is by blood culture but presumptive diagnosis is suggested by the triad of clinical infection, a high-risk patient and *Candida* at more than two sites. Antifungal treatment should depend on the sensitivity of the species involved.

In the next decade, three organisms will dominate nosocomial infection and one, MRSA, will provide a historical perspective. The organisms are *Stenotrophomonas*

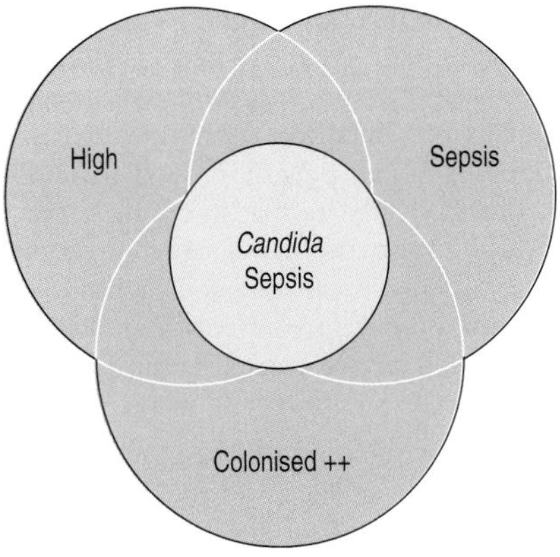

Figure 62.1 Diagnostic triad of *Candida* sepsis.

and *Acinetobacter*, which are rapidly becoming more common and less easy to treat. The third, although in relatively small numbers, relates to the rising incidence of multiresistant tuberculosis, which not only has potential but is already providing infection control challenges in the critically ill (Figure 62.1).

COLONISATION AND INFECTION

Many organisms both colonise and infect, but differentiating between colonisation and infection is difficult. In essence the presence of the organism may not indicate infection and, in complex patients with multiple colonisations and infection, determining which the culprit is may be difficult or even impossible. As a consequence, treatment is often based on probability or the weight of evidence, rather than certainty.

MRSA colonises very readily and causes infection in a significant proportion of cases but is often easily identified and treated. VRE is still relatively uncommon. It does colonise, although the incidence of overt infection appears low, at present, but is difficult to treat when it occurs. *Acinetobacter* colonises and infects very readily, may take days to identify and is difficult to treat.[20]

SITES OF INFECTION

The main sites of nosocomial infection are the chest, wounds and intravenous lines. Urinary tract infection, often quoted as common, seems to be seen rarely in the critically ill.

NOSOCOMIAL PNEUMONIA

Nosocomial pneumonia is a common problem in the critically ill, particularly in ventilated patients, with an incidence of 15–30%.[21–23]

Aetiology

There are several possible mechanisms, including aspiration from the nasopharynx, local spread or haematogenous spread of infection. Some 45% of healthy adults aspirate in their sleep. In the sick the nasopharynx colonises rapidly with a wide range of organisms, usually Gram-negatives, and aspiration is encouraged by the unconscious state, the presence of a nasogastric tube or by endotracheal intubation. Pneumonia will develop in up to 25% of colonised patients, compared with a 3% incidence in non-colonised patients. It may also be related to the colonisation of the upper gastrointestinal tract, which may in turn colonise the nasopharynx.

Factors that are likely to encourage colonisation of the pharyngeal areas with organisms include antibiotics and nasogastric tubes. Also implicated are alterations in the host defences in the pharynx, changes in the local pH, the amount of surface mucin and impairment of other local immune defence mechanisms.

Patient factors predisposing to nosocomial pneumonia include acute severity of illness; chronic illness, especially chronic lung disease; diabetes; immunosuppression; advanced age; recent surgery to thorax or abdomen; intubation; and bronchoscopy. Environmental factors include broad-spectrum and prolonged use of antibiotics; potential pathogens in the vicinity; bacterial properties such as ability to adhere to surfaces; cross-infection; 24-hour ventilator tubing changes; and foreign bodies such as nasogastric tubes. Intubated and ventilated patients have a higher rate of nosocomial infection than patients receiving non-invasive ventilation. However, this may be due to different patient populations with different underlying problems and background morbidity.[24] The role of neutralisation by H_2 antagonists and proton pump inhibitors is still debated.[25–27]

Diagnosis

The general criteria for diagnosis are general signs of infection; clinical signs of a chest infection; purulent sputum; radiological evidence, such as new pulmonary infiltrates; and positive cultures, from sputum or blood.[21,23,28,29] These produce a non-specific diagnosis. Expectorated sputum is difficult to assess, but should contain < 25 polymorphs and > 10 squamous epithelial cells per low-power field. In ICU it is more usual to provide samples from the endotracheal tube and then to use quantitative techniques. This can achieved with protected brush specimens (PBS) bronchoalveolar lavage (BAL) and protected BAL. These are difficult and time-consuming and it appears that non-bronchoscopic techniques such as blind tracheal aspirates through the endotracheal tube are both practical and reasonably effective from a clinical – if not a research – viewpoint[23,30] (Table 62.6).

The Organisms

Aerobic Gram-negatives predominate, including *Pseudomonas aeruginosa, Enterobacter* spp., *Klebsiella, Escherichia coli, Serratia marcescens* and *Proteus*; between them, these account for about 70% of infections. Staphylococci, in particular MRSA, account for a small but significant number of nosocomial pneumonias. Early-onset VAP,

Table 62.6 Principles for the diagnosis of nosocomial pneumonia

Crackles on auscultation or dullness to percussion on physical examinaion of the chest and any of the following:
• New onset of purulent sputum
• Organism isolated from blood cultures
• Isolation of pathogen from specimen obtained by transtracheal aspirate, bronchial brushing or biopsy
• Chest radiography examination shows no or progressive infiltration, consolidation, cavitation or pleural effusion
• Isolation of virus or detection of virus antigen in respiratory secretions
• Diagnostic single antibody titre (IgM) or fourfold increase in paired serum samples (IgG) for pathogen
• Histopathological evidence of pneumonia

IgM, immunoglobulin M.

between 48 hours and 5 days, may be due to community pathogens, such as methicillin-sensitive *Staphylococcus aureus*, *Streptococcus pneumoniae* and *Haemophilus infiuenzae*, as well as Gram-negative enteric bacilli (GNEB). This has been described as early endogenous infection. In contrast, later onset, after 5–7 days, involves more resistant species such as MRSA, *Pseudomonas aeruginosa*, *Acinetobacter baumannii* and *Stenotrophomonas maltophilia*.[31,32] This has been called secondary endogenous and exogenous infection.

Prevention

Prevention is by methods that reduce aspiration, cross-infection and contamination of respiratory devices.[29] Several recommended methods are:

- hand-washing
- limiting antibiotic use
- changing ventilator circuits at longer intervals – 1 week
- orotracheal, rather than nasotracheal intubation
- removing nasogastric tube
- semirecumbent position – this reduces aspiration
- avoiding muscle relaxants
- avoiding reintubation
- using non-invasive ventilation, where possible

Other more controversial methods include:

- antibiotic prophylaxis after intubation
- continuous suctioning of subglottic secretions
- early enteral nutrition: benefits of the colonisation of the gastrointestinal tract might be offset by problems with nasogastric tubes and nasopharyngeal colonisation
- the use of heat moisture exchangers
- closed suctioning: with some limited evidence it reduces VAP

Treatment

The use of inappropriate or inadequate antibiotics leads to an increased mortality, so current trends are towards initial broad-spectrum antibiotics followed by reassessment and de-escalation.[33,34] The principle is that an empirical broad-spectrum approach will cover the relevant organisms but once the specific organism is identified the antibiotics can be rationalised to focus on that organism; this is clearly harder to apply in practice than in theory. As the spectrum of resistance grows it is highly likely that it will be increasingly difficult to apply this broad-spectrum empiric treatment, especially with late-onset VAP. Surveillance of current colonisation, awareness of an individual ICU's ecology and targeted treatment will replace empiric regimens. At present, combination therapy is recommended, but there is little evidence to support it over monotherapy.[23,33,35–37]

Another area of interest is duration of treatment with antibiotics. Many regimens are traditional rather then evidence-based and may result in unnecessarily prolonged treatment. There is a trend to reducing courses. For VAP an 8-day course may be adequate.[30] There has not yet been a move towards using a clinical or bacterial response to treatment as an indicator for the duration of treatment, although it may be on the horizon.

The attributable mortality with nosocomial pneumonia is difficult to determine because patients requiring ventilation often have a high intrinsic mortality. Rates of 30% have been quoted: pneumonia accounts for 60% of deaths from nosocomial infections. In addition, nosocomial pneumonia increases length of stay by 12–23 days.[4,38,39]

WOUND INFECTION

Wound infections are common and represent 20% of all nosocomial infection. The organisms involved may be those introduced at the time or from later contamination.

RISK FACTORS

- The procedure itself and the level of contamination prior to or during surgery. In clean elective surgery the incidence should be less than 10%, but where contamination may occur (e.g. bowel surgery) it may be as high as 15%. In contaminated procedures, the rate rises to around 20%, and where infection already exists it may be 40% or higher.
- The surgeon's technical ability[40]
- Host factors: see Table 62.2
- The use of antibiotic prophylaxis
- Duration of stay in ICU

THE ORGANISMS

The organisms are frequently determined by the type of surgery and procedure. Skin commensals are common, such as staphylococci or streptococci, and are usually early infections. These are characterised by fever, pain and redness around the site. With streptococcal infection this may be quite confluent. Gram-negative organisms may also cause infection. Drainage is important.

PREVENTION

Clean theatres, good operating technique and thorough asepsis, both in the theatre and postoperatively, are important.

ANTIBIOTIC PROPHYLAXIS

This is a difficult and contentious area. The unnecessary use of broad-spectrum antibiotics should be avoided, but there are some areas of surgery where prophylaxis has a proven place. If there is no risk of infection with a clean procedure there is no place for antibiotics. If contamination is either seen or likely to occur, the use of antibiotics is to provide cover for the spillage. There may be other circumstances where the patient is particularly vulnerable to bacteraemia, such as with valve disease or where the consequences of infection would be disastrous. Effective prophylaxis requires an antibiotic:

- which covers the most likely organisms
- to be given prior to contamination
- at peak dosage at the time of contamination

A single dose should suffice, although a second dose is recommended if the procedure extends beyond 3 hours. Prolonged administration:

- increases the chance of antibiotic resistance
- unnecessarily exposes the patient to adverse effects from the drugs
- encourages colonisation with resistant organisms
- ensures that if a late infection occurs it will be with an organism resistant to the prophylaxis

In many circumstances the evidence supporting prophylaxis is minimal, and frequently the antibiotics used are inappropriate to the perceived risk. Local factors, including the local ecology, will determine specific requirements. With grafts, mesh or prostheses the morbidity from infection is so great as to justify using prophylaxis even if the evidence is marginal (Table 62.7).

Table 62.7 Surgical prophylaxis

Type of surgery	
Abdominal wall	Insertion of mesh. Staphylococcal or streptococcal cover. In the groin, Gram-negative cover may be needed
Cardiac	Protection of valves and grafts. Staphylococci may be resistant
Vascular	Protection of grafts. Staphylococci are a major consideration. If the groin is involved, it may require Gram-negative cover
Orthopaedic	Prostheses. Staphylococci are an increasing problem
Biliary upper GI	Usually Gram-negative and anaerobic cover, with an awareness of resistant enterococci
Colorectal	Protection against faecal flora. Cephalosporins and metronidazole have been popular but predispose to developing enterococci such as *Enterococcus faecalis* or *E. faecium*, which may be multiresistant
Gynaecological	Conventionally broad-spectrum involving cephalosporins or, currently, augmentin. Metronidazole is also favoured
Urological	Protection from instrumentation of the urinary tract, Gram-negative cover. Awareness of any existing infection

GI, gastrointestinal.

LINE SEPSIS

The use of intravascular devices in hospital practice is ubiquitous. There is both a significant morbidity, resulting in prolongation of hospital stay, and an attributable mortality associated with their use due to infection.[41–43]

PERIPHERAL LINES

The use of peripheral lines is commonly associated with phlebitis, which may be chemical but is frequently a precursor of infection. Usually peripheral lines should only be in situ for less than 72 hours.

ARTERIAL LINES

Curiously, arterial lines seem to become colonised and infected less frequently than other peripheral devices. Nevertheless they do become colonised and should be regularly changed. Complications include infected radial aneurysms or thrombosis.

PULMONARY ARTERY CATHETERS

The introducers are a potential source of infection, as is the part of the catheter in the introducer. They are frequently left in situ when they should have been removed earlier.

CENTRAL VENOUS CATHETERS

Colonisation of catheters is common and it is likely that this is a precursor of infection. Colonisation rates are in the order of 5–40%, determined in part by the risk factors involved (see below). Infection rates are approximately 10% of the colonised catheters.[44]

DEFINITIONS

1. Colonised catheter: growth of > 15 colony-forming units (semiquantitative) or 10^3 (quantitative) from a

Table 62.8 Risk factors for catheter infection

Host risk factors
Site: subclavian is a lower risk than internal jugular and femoral
Catheter material: antibacterial catheters may reduce infection, antiseptic catheters reduce colonisation
Number of lumens: multilumen catheters increase the infection risk[30]
Number of administrations through the lines
Dressing type: frequency of changes
Skin preparation
Experience of technique of personnel
Occurrence of bacteraemia
Tunnelling: often used for long-term access but the data are contentious[31]

proximal or distal catheter segment in the absence of accompanying clinical symptoms and signs.

2. CR-BSI: isolation of the same organism from the catheter segment (see above) as from a peripheral blood culture in a patient with signs of infection and in the absence of another source. In the absence of laboratory corroboration of infection then effervescence of infection after removal of the catheter may be taken as circumstantial evidence.

Extrinsic mechanisms associated with developing catheter sepsis include infection from the skin and insertion site; contamination from the hub and then internally spread; and contamination of drugs or fluids administered through the catheter. Bacteraemia seeding to catheter is an intrinsic mechanism.

The actual mechanics by which the organisms colonise the catheter is important. Some organisms, such as CNS, produce a polysaccharide film of 'slime' that develops on the catheter while the host's proteins such as fibronectin may also provide a matrix in which the organism can adhere, and which may provide a protective barrier against both white cells and antibiotics. Polyvinyl chloride or polythene is more prone to this film developing than some other materials such as silicone (Table 62.8).

THE ORGANISMS

The organisms involved in catheter sepsis are many and varied. There is a 25% incidence of CNS, which are increasingly recognised as pathogens. *Staphylococcus aureus* and MRSA are prevalent. There may be seeding, resulting in vertebral osteomyelitis and a variably reported incidence of endocarditis. Enterococci are increasingly seen. Occasionally fungi are found and may again be associated with seeding to the eyes or heart.

TREATMENT OF CATHETER INFECTION

The most important aspect of treatment is a high index of suspicion that leads to removal of the device if infection is present either locally or systemically.[42] Although fever and bacteraemia are likely to resolve rapidly after removal of the line, appropriate antibiotics are indicated. The recommended duration of treatment varies: 5–7 days for CNS, 10–14 days for *S. aureus*, Gram-negative organisms and fungi, and 4–6 weeks if there is evidence of endocarditis, infected thrombus or osteomyelitis, or clinical line sepsis is still present after 3 days.[42] Lines removed should be cultured. If an infection is present it is best to avoid replacing the central venous catheter if possible for a few days. In situations where it is uncertain if the line is implicated in infection, some advocate replacing a new line over a wire. If the removed catheter is subsequently shown to be infected, then it must be removed.

The situation is slightly different with Broviac or Hickman catheters. Occasionally administration of antibiotics through the catheter will eradicate the infection and save the line. Unfortunately, it is not always successful: the risk of failure should be balanced against the value of the line. Some medical catastrophes have been the consequence of persisting with infected Hickman lines.

PREVENTION

Important issues include adequate hand-washing; adequate skin disinfection; insertion under aseptic conditions; intravenous team to insert and manage lines; anchoring of lines to prevent excessive movement; closed systems with limited interruptions to the lines; application of sterile dressings to the insertion site; and daily inspection of catheter site. Replacement of intravenous administration sets at 72 hours is optimal. Stopcocks may be essential, but are portals of infection. Local antiseptics are advocated for site care, but there is little difference between gauze and transparent dressings, although efforts to reduce local humidity at the site may be important.[45–47]

Techniques of unproven benefit include antiseptic cream at insertion site; routine changes of dressings at frequent intervals; occlusive antimicrobial dressings; in-line filters; tunnelling of central venous catheters; and routine flushing of long-term central venous catheters.

METHODS OF INFECTION CONTROL

Each hospital has an infection control team that can employ techniques to reduce infection (Table 62.9).

The most important aspects of preventing nosocomial infection and facilitating infection control are simple

Table 62.9 Roles of infection control teams

Surveillance and investigation of infection outbreaks
Education of staff
Review of antibiotic utilisation
Review of antibiotic resistance patterns
Review of infection control procedures and policies

hygiene, such as hand-washing, and being aware that the problem exists. There are several ways in which the issue of nosocomial infection can be addressed. These include surveillance, screening, isolation, eradication and strategic planning.[48]

SURVEILLANCE

Routine culture of both patients and environment provides information on the organisms currently prevalent, and is a useful tool in guiding management when infection occurs. It also provides information on cross-infection rates. Using 'typing' techniques, individual organisms can be tracked, and this is of particular importance in following outbreaks.

SCREENING

This tries to prevent multiresistance by identifying patients carrying high-risk organisms. In the critically ill, to be effective it requires isolating the patient until cultures are available. It is clearly of benefit with rare or very threatening infection, such as the haemorrhagic fevers, but cumbersome and ineffectual with an organism as prevalent as MRSA. Future problems with *Acinetobacter* may need re-evaluation of its role.

ISOLATION

Although physical barriers undoubtedly reduce cross-contamination, isolation may be hazardous as it often indicates lower-intensity care. The relative risks need to be addressed.

ERADICATION

This requires the use of potent antibiotics ± antiseptics to eliminate the organism, which may be colonising rather than infecting. It exposes potent therapeutic agents and facilitates the development of resistance or the emergence of more resistant strains. It is therefore a hazardous undertaking in strategic terms.

STRATEGIC PLANNING

There are two elements. One is enforcing hygienic practice, which is simple, cheap and very effective. The other is looking towards means of reducing both nosocomial infection and the emergence of resistance. This is essentially the planned use of antibiotics.

Currently the same agents are used in agriculture, the community and in hospital, which provides vast potential for the emergence of resistance. In human practice the widespread use of potent agents in the community will impinge on hospitals. In hospitals focused antibiotic use in one area will be undermined by generalised use in another. There should be controls across the boundaries of these areas of use.

On an individual basis the approach to management must change. In the past, empiric treatment on the basis of likely organisms led to the use of very-broad-spectrum antibiotics. It is already clear that in an individual who has been in hospital for any period of time, using any antibiotic is likely to miss some resistant strains. Narrow-spectrum targeted treatment will cease to be an option and will become a necessity. Prolonged broad-spectrum antibiotic management aimed at dealing with any eventuality will be replaced by short-duration specific and effective regimens.

SELECTIVE DECONTAMINATION OF THE DIGESTIVE TRACT

SDD is based on the idea that overgrowth of colonising organisms in the gut predisposes to nosocomial infection so that reducing or eliminating the reservoir of organisms from the nasopharynx and from the gastrointestinal tract will prevent infection. To achieve this, oral non-absorbable antibiotics, such as polymyxin, tobramycin, gentamicin, neomycin and nystatin, are applied to the oropharynx and administered through nasogastric tubes. Parenteral antibiotics have been added to some regimens. Although the positive results outweigh the negative ones, the uptake of this technique has been limited.[31,49,50] Concerns over generating resistance have not been substantiated nor completely refuted.[51–53]

A new controversial but interesting application has been in attempting to eliminate multiresistant organisms such as MRSA with an MRSA-targeted regimen, which is claimed to eradicate MRSA.[16] It remains a controversial area.

USEFUL WEBSITES

http://www.cdc.gov/ncidod/dhqp/pdf/nnis/NosInf Definitions.pdf.

REFERENCES

1. Vincent JL, Bihari DJ, Suter PM *et al.* The prevalence of nosocomial infection in intensive care units in Europe. Results of the European Prevalence of Infection in Intensive Care (EPIC) Study. EPIC International Advisory Committee. *JAMA* 1995; **274**: 639–44.
2. Rosenthal VD, Guzman S, Orellano PW. Nosocomial infections in medical–surgical intensive care units in Argentina: attributable mortality and length of stay. *Am J Infect Control* 2003; **31**: 291–5.
3. Sax H, Ghugonnet S, Harbarth P *et al.* Variation in nosocomial infection prevalence according to patient setting: a hospital wide survey. *J Hosp Infect* 2001; **48**: 27–32.
4. Safdar N, Dezfulian C, Collard HR *et al.* Clinical and economic consequences of ventilator-associated pneumonia: a systematic review. *Crit Care Med* 2005; **33**: 2184–93.
5. Pittet D. Pneumonie nosocomiale: incidence, morbidité et mortalité chez le patient intube-ventilé. *Schweiz Med Wochenschr* 1994; **124**: 227–35.

6. Blot SI, Depuydt P, Annemans L *et al.* Clinical and economic outcomes in critically ill patients with nosocomial catheter-related bloodstream infections. *Clin Infect Dis* 2005; **41**: 1591–8.
7. Taylor RW, O'Brien J, Trottier SJ *et al.* Red blood cell transfusions and nosocomial infections in critically ill patients. *Crit Care Med* 2006; **34**: 2302–8; quiz 9.
8. Ortiz R, Lee K. Nosocomial infections in neurocritical care. *Curr Neurol Neurosci Rep* 2006; **6**: 525–30.
9. Edgeworth JD, Treacher DF, Eykyn SJ. A 25-year study of nosocomial bacteremia in an adult intensive care unit. *Crit Care Med* 1999; **27**: 1421–8.
10. Pittet D, Hugonnet S, Harbarth S *et al.* Effectiveness of a hospital-wide programme to improve compliance with hand hygiene. Infection Control Programme. *Lancet* 2000; **356**: 1307–12.
11. Hanberger H, Diekema D, Fluit A *et al.* Surveillance of antibiotic resistance in European ICUs. *J Hosp Infect* 2001; **48**: 161–76.
12. Blot SI, Vandewoude KH, Colardyn FA. Evaluation of outcome in critically ill patients with nosocomial *Enterobacter* bacteremia: results of a matched cohort study. *Chest* 2003; **123**: 1208–13.
13. Obritsch MD, Fish DN, MacLaren R *et al.* Nosocomial infections due to multidrug-resistant *Pseudomonas aeruginosa*: epidemiology and treatment options. *Pharmacotherapy* 2005; **25**: 1353–64.
14. Aloush V, Navon-Venezia S, Seigman-Igra Y *et al.* Multidrug-resistant *Pseudomonas aeruginosa*: risk factors and clinical impact. *Antimicrob Agents Chemother* 2006; **50**: 43–8.
15. Cisneros JM, Rodriguez-Bano J. Nosocomial bacteremia due to *Acinetobacter baumannii*: epidemiology, clinical features and treatment. *Clin Microbiol Infect* 2002; **8**: 687–93.
16. Wenisch C, Laferl H, Szell M *et al.* A holistic approach to MRSA eradication in critically ill patients with MRSA pneumonia. *Infection* 2006; **34**: 148–54.
17. Weber SG, Gold HS. *Enterococcus*: an emerging pathogen in hospitals. *Semin Respir Crit Care Med* 2003; **24**: 49–60.
18. Gerding DN. Treatment of *Clostridium difficile*-associated diarrhea and colitis. *Curr Top Microbiol Immunol* 2000; **250**: 127–39.
19. Koss K, Clark MA, Sanders DS *et al.* The outcome of surgery in fulminant *Clostridium difficile* colitis. *Colorectal Dis* 2006; **8**: 149–54.
20. Theaker C, Azadian B, Soni N. The impact of *Acinetobacter baumannii* in the intensive care unit. *Anaesthesia* 2003; **58**: 271–4.
21. Guidelines for prevention of nosocomial pneumonia. Centers for Disease Control and Prevention. *MMWR Recomm Rep* 1997; **46**: 1–79.
22. Mehta RM, Niederman MS. Nosocomial pneumonia. *Curr Opin Infect Dis* 2002; **15**: 387–94.
23. Ostendorf U, Ewig S, Torres A. Nosocomial pneumonia. *Curr Opin Infect Dis* 2006; **19**: 327–38.
24. Girou E, Brun-Buisson C, Taille S *et al.* Secular trends in nosocomial infections and mortality associated with noninvasive ventilation in patients with exacerbation of COPD and pulmonary edema. *JAMA* 2003; **290**: 2985–91.
25. Keenan SP, Heyland DK, Jacka MJ *et al.* Ventilator-associated pneumonia. Prevention, diagnosis, and therapy. *Crit Care Clin* 2002; **18**: 107–25.
26. Dodek P, Keenan S, Cook D *et al.* Evidence-based clinical practice guideline for the prevention of ventilator-associated pneumonia. *Ann Intern Med* 2004; **141**: 305–13.
27. Cook D, Heyland D, Griffith L *et al.* Risk factors for clinically important upper gastrointestinal bleeding in patients requiring mechanical ventilation. Canadian Critical Care Trials Group. *Crit Care Med* 1999; **27**: 2812–17.
28. Depuydt P, Myny D, Blot S. Nosocomial pneumonia: aetiology, diagnosis and treatment. *Curr Opin Pulm Med* 2006; **12**: 192–7.
29. Flanders SA, Collard HR, Saint S. Nosocomial pneumonia: state of the science. *Am J Infect Control* 2006; **34**: 84–93.
30. Chastre J, Luyt CE, Combes A *et al.* Use of quantitative cultures and reduced duration of antibiotic regimens for patients with ventilator-associated pneumonia to decrease resistance in the intensive care unit. *Clin Infect Dis* 2006; **43** (Suppl. 2): S75–81.
31. Silvestri L, Mannucci F, van Saene HK. Selective decontamination of the digestive tract: a life saver. *J Hosp Infect* 2000; **45**: 185–90.
32. Hospital-acquired pneumonia in adults: diagnosis, assessment of severity, initial antimicrobial therapy, and preventive strategies. A consensus statement, American Thoracic Society, November 1995. *Am J Respir Crit Care Med* 1996; **153**: 1711–25.
33. Bodmann KF. Current guidelines for the treatment of severe pneumonia and sepsis. *Chemotherapy* 2005; **51**: 227–33.
34. Porzecanski I, Bowton DL. Diagnosis and treatment of ventilator-associated pneumonia. *Chest* 2006; **130**: 597–604.
35. Costa SF, Newbaer M, Santos CR *et al.* Nosocomial pneumonia: importance of recognition of aetiological agents to define an appropriate initial empirical therapy. *Int J Antimicrob Agents* 2001; **17**: 147–50.
36. Rello J, Lorente C, Diaz E *et al.* Incidence, etiology, and outcome of nosocomial pneumonia in ICU patients requiring percutaneous tracheotomy for mechanical ventilation. *Chest* 2003; **124**: 2239–43.
37. Alvarez-Lerma F, Alvarez B, Luque P *et al.* Empiric broad-spectrum antibiotic therapy of nosocomial pneumonia in the intensive care unit: a prospective observational study. *Crit Care* 2006; **10**: R78.
38. Beyersmann J, Gastmeier P, Grundmann H *et al.* Use of multistate models to assess prolongation of intensive care unit stay due to nosocomial infection. *Infect Control Hosp Epidemiol* 2006; **27**: 493–9.
39. Hunter JD. Ventilator associated pneumonia. *Postgrad Med J* 2006; **82**: 172–8.
40. Holzheimer RG, Haupt W, Thiede A *et al.* The challenge of postoperative infections: does the surgeon make a difference? *Infect Control Hosp Epidemiol* 1997; **18**: 449–56.

41. O'Grady NP, Alexander M, Dellinger EP *et al.* Guidelines for the prevention of intravascular catheter-related infections. *Infect Control Hosp Epidemiol* 2002; **23**: 759–69.
42. Mermel LA, Farr BM, Sherertz RJ *et al.* Guidelines for the management of intravascular catheter-related infections. *J Intraven Nurs* 2001; **24**: 180–205.
43. Mermel LA. New technologies to prevent intravascular catheter-related bloodstream infections. *Emerg Infect Dis* 2001; **7**: 197–9.
44. Hannan M, Juste RN, Umasanker S *et al.* Antiseptic-bonded central venous catheters and bacterial colonisation. *Anaesthesia* 1999; **54**: 868–72.
45. Chatzinikolaou I, Raad II. Intravascular catheter-related infections: a preventable challenge in the critically ill. *Semin Respir Infect* 2000; **15**: 264–71.
46. Raad I, Hanna HA, Awad A *et al.* Optimal frequency of changing intravenous administration sets: is it safe to prolong use beyond 72 hours? *Infect Control Hosp Epidemiol* 2001; **22**: 136–9.
47. Rizzo M. Striving to eliminate catheter-related blood stream infection; a literature review of evidence-based strategies. *Semin Anesth Periop Med Pain* 2005; **24**: 4.
48. Bearman GM, Munro C, Sessler CN, Wenzel RP. Infection control and the prevention of nosocomial infections in the intensive care unit. *Semin Respir Crit Care Med* 2006; **27**: 310–24.
49. Carlet JM. Controversies in the antibiotic management of critically ill patients. *Semin Respir Crit Care Med* 2001; **22**: 51–60.
50. Zwaveling JH, Maring JK, Klompmaker IJ *et al.* Selective decontamination of the digestive tract to prevent postoperative infection: a randomized placebo-controlled trial in liver transplant patients. *Crit Care Med* 2002; **30**: 1204–9.
51. Bonten MJ, Krueger WA. Selective decontamination of the digestive tract: cumulating evidence, at last? *Semin Respir Crit Care Med* 2006; **27**: 18–22.
52. Al Naiemi N, Heddema ER, Bart A *et al.* Emergence of multidrug-resistant Gram-negative bacteria during selective decontamination of the digestive tract on an intensive care unit. *J Antimicrob Chemother* 2006; **58**: 853–6.
53. de Jonge E. Effects of selective decontamination of digestive tract on mortality and antibiotic resistance in the intensive-care unit. *Curr Opin Crit Care* 2005; **11**: 144–9.

63

Severe soft-tissue infections

Hugo Sax and Didier Pittet

The skin is the largest organ and acts as an excellent barrier against infection. It consists of the epidermis and dermis and resides on fibrous connective tissue, the superficial and deep fasciae (Figure 63.1). The fascial cleft, with nerves, arteries, veins, lymphatic and adipose tissue, lies between these fascial planes. Normal skin flora includes *Corynebacterium* spp., coagulase-negative staphylococci, *Micrococcus* spp., *Lactobacillus* and, rarely, *Staphylococcus aureus.* Colonisation by Gram-negative bacteria occurs in hospital patients; once altered, skin flora includes a higher proportion of *S. aureus* which ultimately becomes pathogenic.

These colonising microorganisms seldom cause skin and soft-tissue infections, but serious infections can occur if: there is a break in the skin because of traumatic lesion or maceration; soft tissues are ischaemic and non-viable; colonising bacteria are particularly virulent; or the patient is immunocompromised (Figure 63.2).[1–9] Conditions predisposing to infection include diabetes mellitus, cirrhosis, malnutrition, major trauma, advanced age, renal failure, steroid use, collagen vascular disease and malignancies.[1–10] Differentiation between soft-tissue infections can be difficult and one unified management approach to severe forms is appropriate.[11–13] Management decisions are further based on likely causative organism, depth of infection and clinical severity.[8]

Soft-tissue infections are usually caused by bacterial entry through skin lesions or perforation of adjacent intestinal structures. Skin lesions can on occasion be the manifestations of systemic infection; examples of this are bacteraemia by meningococci, staphylococci, *Pseudomonas aeruginosa*, *Candida* spp., and bacterial endocarditis.[3] These will not be specifically addressed here.

CLASSIFICATION

The bacteriology and subtypes of severe soft-tissue infections have not changed significantly over the last century.[8,14–16] Community-acquired meticillin-resistant *Staphylococcus aureus* (MRSA), however, can be seen as an emerging cause of severe tissue infection with a high prevalence in certain parts of the world.[17–19] The classification of soft-tissue infections can be confusing, partly because individual organisms can cause different clinical syndromes. Consequently, there are a wealth of terms often referring to the same diseases (e.g. Meleney's gangrene, haemolytic streptococcal gangrene and progressive bacterial synergistic gangrene).[14] Classification by the anatomical structure involved is more logical, but it has to be borne in mind that some conditions involve several soft-tissue levels and that some cases may evolve froma minor entity to a more severe form with more diffuse anatomical involvement (see Figure 63.1).

IMPETIGO

Impetigo,[1–3] more common in children, is a superficial skin infection caused by group A streptococci, *Staphylococcus aureus*, or both. Mild infections can be managed with topical antibiotics; more serious infections need a first-generation cephalosporin. A penicillinase-resistant penicillin is mostly chosen in severe empirical conditions (e.g. dicloxacillin).[20] Increasing resistance in streptococci and staphylococci might prohibit the use of erythromycin, which has been the alternative in the penicillin-allergic patient. For community-acquired MRSA, co-trimoxazole is an alternative.

FOLLICULITIS

This is an infection arising in hair follicles and apocrine glands.[2,3] *S. aureus* is the usual causative organism. Topical antibiotic treatment is usually all that is required. When confluent, folliculitis can evolve to furunculosis and may need surgical drainage as sole effective therapy. If accompanied by cellulitis and/or sepsis, antibiotics are added (see section on cellulitis). Repeated folliculitis raises the possibility of chronic granulomatous disease, an inherited immunodeficiency syndrome based on granulocyte malfunction.[21] Affected individuals are at risk for severe soft-tissue infections, sometimes with rare pathogens such as *Aspergillus* spp.

ERYSIPELAS

This superficial dermal infection is largely caused by group A streptococci and also by other streptococci and *Staphylococcus aureus.*[1–3,8,9] The prominent lymphatic blockade results in a painful bright red patch with a raised

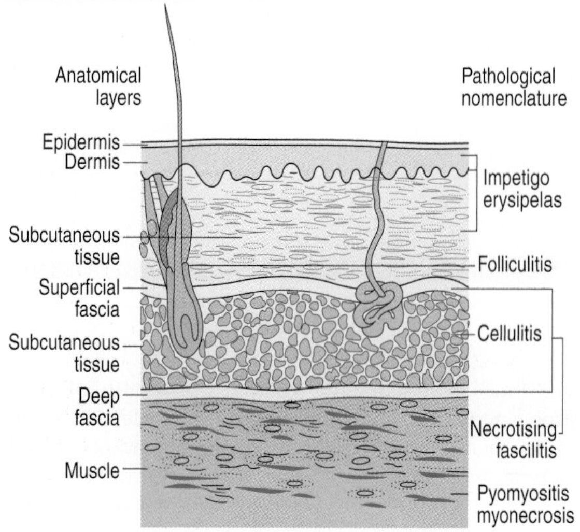

Figure 63.1 Anatomy of skin and nomenclature of skin and deep-tissue infections.

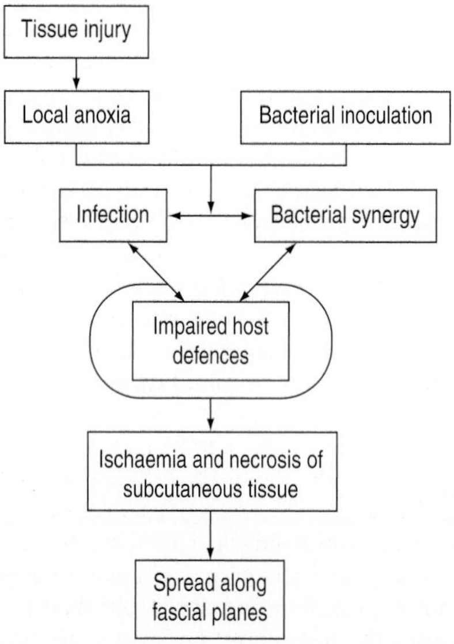

Figure 63.2 Pathogenesis of severe soft-tissue infections.

sharp border, which clearly demarcates the infection from normal surrounding skin. Fever and chills often precede the skin eruption. Predisposing conditions include ulcers, venous stasis, diabetes, alcoholism and paraparesis. High-dose penicillin is still the drug of choice in the absence of underlying disease and the possibility to observe the evolution of the lesion. Severe infections in diabetic patients require a third-generation cephalosporin, piperacillin-tazobactam or a carbapenem. If mobilisation is premature, signs recur and treatment failure may falsely be suspected. However, recurrent erysipelas does occur with persistent lymphoedema.

CELLULITIS

Cellulitis[1,2,3,5–9,22] is an acute spreading infection of the skin extending below the superficial fascia, usually involving only the upper part of the subcutaneous tissue. It can occur at any body site, but is most frequent in the lower extremities and in the face. There is less lymphatic involvement so the borders of the infection are often not well defined and differentiation between cellulitis and erysipelas is sometimes difficult. Fever, malaise and rigors are common. It is more common in patients with tissue oedema. Cellulitis is most commonly due to *Streptococcus pyogenes*, but other Gram-positive and negative organisms can also cause this condition according to location and exposure history.[9]

Typically, *S. pyogenes* cellulitis may appear hours after surgical intervention with fast progression of the erythematic zone over a large surface and can be accompanied by bacteraemia and sepsis. Many of these organisms may produce gas, hence crepitus is sometimes present (Table 63.1).

Other forms of cellulitis present with necrosis (gangrene) include anaerobic infections with *Clostridium* spp. or non-clostridial anaerobes sometimes mixed with Gram-negative pathogens that are facultative anaerobes. This latter condition may be hard to distinguish from deeper forms of infection such as necrotising fasciitis and myositis and may be crepitant. Immediate assessment by magnetic resonance imaging (MRI) and surgical exploration determines fascial and muscular involvement and allows for adequate debridement. Potent empirical therapy must include all possible pathogens because of the impossibility of deducing bacterial aetiology and depth from the initial clinical presentation. For antimicrobial therapy, see under necrotising fasciitis, below.

Periocular cellulitis is a medical emergency. It needs immediate clinical and then radiological assessment to distinguish the periorbital from the more severe orbital cellulitis. Clinical signs for the latter include visual disturbance because of optical nerve involvement. Definite diagnosis can only be established by computed tomography (CT). External facial cellulitis may involve the venous system draining into the sinus venosus and, thus, lead to thrombosis. The aetiology includes a wider range of bacteria: *Streptococcus pneumoniae, Haemophilus influenzae, Moraxella catarrhalis, Staphylococcus aureus*, group A streptococci and anaerobes.

Table 63.1 Infective causes of soft-tissue crepitus

Cellulitis	Usually anaerobic organisms, clostridial and non-clostridial
Bursitis	Gram-negative organisms
Necrotising fasciitis	Usually type I (mixed infections, Gram-negative organisms)
Myonecrosis	Clostridial organisms
Infected vascular gangrene	Any organism

A severe and fulminant form of cellulitis with hemorrhagic bullous lesions can be caused by marine bacteria of the *Vibrio* spp., mostly with a history of contact with sea-water or raw fish.[23] After fresh-water exposure of wounds[24] or application of medical leeches,[25] *Aeromonas hydrophilia* is a possible aetiology.

TREATMENT

Appropriate microbiological tests are undertaken prior to starting antibiotics. Any skin abrasion or sites that drain are swabbed for Gram stain and culture. Needle aspiration, skin biopsy and blood cultures produce only a 25% positive yield.[1] Treatment involves site elevation and high-dose oxacillin or a first-generation cephalosporin. If there is a possibility of MRSA, vancomycin is indicated instead. In severe cases, the addition of clindamycin is beneficial because of its antitoxic effect and enhanced intracellular activity.[26] If Gram-negative rods are suspected or identified (e.g. an immunocompromised patient or involvement of intestinal tract lesions), a third-generation cephalosporin should be considered. In a patient with prolonged hospitalisation or in penetrating foot infections, a cephalosporin with anti-*Pseudomonas* activity is preferred. If *Vibrio* spp. are suspected or isolated, doxycycline may be added. In the absence of controlled studies, some authors recommend ceftazidime[27,28] in addition to tetracyclines because of the high mortality of 50%.[23]

Pyoderma gangrenosum has a similar appearance, but a completely different aetiology and therapeutic management. It is a rare idiopathic, inflammatory, ulcerative disease of undetermined cause that is more frequent in patients with ulcerative colitis and rheumatoid arthritis and presents as deep ulcers with undermined borders, usually on the lower extremities or abdomen. It is often triggered by surgical intervention and only secondarily colonised with skin flora. Treatment is conservative and includes steroid medication.[29]

NECROTISING FASCIITIS

Necrotising fasciitis[1,2,3,5–8,10–13,30–35] is a deeper infection of the skin with extensive undermining of surrounding tissues. Interest in this fulminant infection has recently increased.[14,30,36] The World Health Organization reports only 160 cases since 1989, but the incidence in the USA is about 100 cases annually and recently there has been an increased incidence of group A streptococcal fasciitis in Europe.[14,30]

It usually occurs on the extremities, perineum and abdominal wall. Involvement of male genitalia is known as Fournier's gangrene.[15] Two types are described, depending on causative organisms.[33] Type I are mixed infections usually caused by Gram-positive and negative aerobe and anaerobe bacteria or *Vibrio* spp. Type II infections are caused by group A streptococci (occasionally with *Staphylococcus aureus*). Secondary infections with zygomycetes may occur.[32,34] There is no difference in the clinical course, morbidity and mortality between the two types of infection.

CLINICAL PRESENTATION

A history of minor trauma is common and necrotising fasciitis can complicate surgery and varicella infections.[30,37] Predisposing factors include cirrhosis, diabetes and other immunocompromised states. Necrotising fasciitis begins as an area of cellulitis that typically fails to improve on antibiotics and quickly spreads. Pathophysiological sequelae of sepsis result in microthrombi and impaired , leading to gangrene. Pain is a predominant feature and frequently out of keeping with other presenting symptoms and signs. Sometimes no external sign is apparent and increasing pain may even be the only initial symptom. Fever, rigors and shock are common.[30] Half of the cases of necrotising fasciitis present together with a streptococcal toxic-shock syndrome.[20] Manifestations of the systemic inflammatory response syndrome are evident and multiple-organ dysfunction develops in most cases. Bullae may form, and late lesions may resemble deep burns that are painfree because of the necrosis of nerve fibres. Reduced skin surface sensitivity and elevated creatine phosphokinase may suggest fascial involvement. Crepitus may be present (see Table 63.1). The normally adherent fascia may be easily peeled off the underlying muscle bed.

Retroperitoneal necrotising fasciitis is particularly vicious, with a high mortality due partly to the difficulty in diagnosis.[38] Abdominal or perineal trauma or sepsis is always the predisposing event. Diagnosis can only be made at laparotomy for the presenting acute abdomen. Broad-spectrum antibiotic therapy and aggressive surgery (repeated debridement of all necrotic tissue) with planned 'relook' laparotomies are strongly suggested.

Necrotising fasciitis concerning the face, eyelid or lip are rather of type II, whereas that of the neck is more often of type I and associated with a fourfold mortality compared to the facial form.[39]

MANAGEMENT

Because of rapid progression, early diagnosis and treatment are crucial for the prognosis. Two major diagnostic tools are appropriate. We recommend that a highly experienced surgeon in the treatment of necrotising fasciitis be involved as early as possible with surgical incision, probing of fascial consistency and histological diagnosis on a frozen-section specimen of doubtful fascia intraoperatively.[40] The other mainstay of diagnosis is MRI. Recently, a score has been proposed to discriminate between necrotising and non-necrotising severe soft-tissue infections based on a set of six laboratory results.[41]

A complete microbiological investigation is of the utmost importance. This includes sampling for culture by needle aspiration of any crepitant area and blood cultures. Treatment with antibiotics alone is usually inadequate. Immediate extensive surgical removal of necrotic and damaged tissues is essential.[11,12,30–32,34] Planned surgery at 24-hour intervals to debride spreading necrotic tissue is necessary until the necrotic process stops. If extremities are involved, amputation may be life-saving.

Initial antibiotic therapy includes a carbapenem or a third-generation cephalosporin plus clindamycin while awaiting Gram stain and culture results. Clindamycin 600 mg intravenously 6-hourly is added because of toxin inhibition and anaerobic activity.[26] If fungi (e.g. mucormycosis) are isolated, amphotericin B 0.5 mg/kg per day intravenously should be given for at least 2 weeks.[32,34] As in cellulitis, *Vibrio* spp. are treated with both a third-generation cephalosporin and tetracycline.[27]

Supportive care, especially organ support, is also fundamental treatment, and is discussed in other chapters. Hyperbaric oxygen therapy has no proven benefit and is likely to delay surgical intervention. Mortality from necrotising fasciitis is high, and survival appears improved when surgery is undertaken early.

PYOMYOSITIS AND MYONECROSIS

Muscles are remarkably resistant to infection so bacterial infections are rare. Pyomyositis is a focal infection usually caused by *Staphylococcus aureus*. Myonecrosis is caused by *Clostridium* spp. or various other bacteria when it evolves from cellulitis.[1,2,4–7,11,12,31,32,35,42–44] Bacteria might act synergistically and often produce various toxins (Figure 63.2).[4,32] As infection is likely to be mixed, differentiation of pyomyositis and myonecrosis is bacteriological, and only important for antibiotic choices.

PYOMYOSITIS

Pyomyositis is more common in the tropics. The causative organism in over 90% of cases is *S. aureus*, with others being *Streptococcus pyogenes, Escherichia coli* and *S. pneumoniae*. Pyomyositis often follows blunt trauma to torso, thigh or buttock muscles. Spontaneous staphylococcal muscle abscesses may occasionally occur.[2] Initial presentation is with aching muscles which feel indurated on examination. If untreated, the muscles become erythematous and boggy and are eventually destroyed. Spontaneous drainage of debris and pus does not occur. Instead, there is contiguous spread to surrounding tissues and metastatic spread to the chest (e.g. empyemas) and heart (e.g. endocarditis and pericarditis).

Investigations include needle biopsy (for Gram stain of the aspirate), ultrasound (for localised muscle oedema) and, more recently, MRI.[2] Large increases in serum creatine phosphokinase may be indicative of the degree of muscle involvement.[44] Antibiotic therapy with a penicillinase-resistant penicillin or a first-generation cephalosporin may be successful in the early stages. More often, though, the condition is not recognised early because of diagnostic difficulties and extensive surgical drainage becomes necessary for a favourable outcome.[44] Even after disfiguring muscle destruction, functional prognosis is good.

MYONECROSIS

The bacterial infection of muscles by clostridial organisms (usually *Clostridium perfringens* or *C. septicum*) has been called gas gangrene as crepitus may occur. However, other causes of skin crepitus are just as common (see Table 63.1). Predisposing causes are contaminated wounds (e.g. in trauma and septic abortions) and surgery in immunocompromised patients.

Onset is often abrupt, with involved areas being very painful and swollen. The patient presents with signs of severe sepsis. If a wound is present, there is usually a profuse serosanguineous discharge of sweet odour. Later, the skin becomes red, yellow, green or black. Bullae and crepitus may form.

A Gram stain revealing Gram-positive rods of *Clostridium* is diagnostic. Treatment of myonecrosis involves prompt, extensive surgical debridement of all infected tissue and antibiotics (i.e. high-dose penicillin plus clindamycin).[2] At surgery, the muscle is pale or brick-coloured and does not bleed. Hyperbaric oxygen has its proponents[45,46] and may be beneficial in conjunction with good supportive care. However, there is no prospective evidence to support the use of hyperbaric oxygen.[47]

SPECIAL AREAS OF SOFT-TISSUE INFECTION

NECK INFECTIONS

Since the advent of antibiotics, oropharyngeal infections are no longer major causes of neck infections.[48–50] Dental infection and regional trauma are now more common causes. Neck infections include Ludwig's angina, retropharyngeal abscesses, parapharyngeal abscesses and necrotising cervical fasciitis. Ludwig's angina is a submandibular-space infection. There is deep and tender swelling of the submandibular and submaxillary area, with swelling of the floor of the mouth and elevation of the tongue.

Causative organisms are the usual mouth commensals, Gram-negative rods and *Staphylococcus aureus*. Pain and odynophagia are almost always the presenting symptoms. Local swelling is usually present. Trismus and dental pathology are common. Systemic inflammatory signs occur in about two-thirds of patients.

Neck X-rays usually demonstrate some abnormality. CT or MRI will define anatomy and may help to decide on a course of conservative, expectant therapy.[50] Oesophagoscopy should be performed on all retropharyngeal abscesses, as foreign-body ingestion is a possible predisposing event.

Table 63.2 Pathogens and presumptive antibiotic therapy in severe soft-tissue infections*

Disease	Suspected pathogens	Initial antibiotic choice*	Remarks†
Impetigo	*Staphylococcus aureus*, group A streptococci	First-generation cephalosporin, clindamycin, oral amoxicillin/clavulanate, dicloxacillin	Check for local resistance of streptococci against clindamycin
Folliculitis	*Staphylococcus aureus, Candida* spp., *Pseudomonas aeruginosa, Pityrosporum ovale*		Local therapy usually sufficient, antibiotic treatment only with cellulitis (see cellulitis). Surgical drainage if large and fluctuant
Erysipelas	Group A streptococci (occasionally, group B, C, G or *Staphylococcus aureus*)	Penicillin G or amoxicillin still drugs of choice (if no underlying disease and possible to observe), first-generation cephalosporin	Severe infections in diabetic patients: third-generation cephalosporin, piperacilllin/tazobactam or carbapenem
Cellulitis	Group A streptococci, *Staphylococcus aureus*; rarely, various other organisms	Oxacillin, first-generation cephalosporin, clindamycin (for severe penicillin allergy)	Resistance in *Streptococcus pyogenes* and *Staphylococcus aureus* against clindamycin exists. Vancomycin in case of high likelihood of MRSA
Necrotising fasciitis	Type I: anaerobic species (*Bacteroides, Peptostreptococcus* spp.), together with facultative anaerobes, non-A streptococci, Enterobacteriaceae (*Esherichia coli, Enterobacter, Klebsiella*, etc.) Type II: group A streptococci alone or with *Staphylococcus aureus*	Carbapenem if polymicrobial, high-dose penicilline plus clindamycin if *Streptococcus* or *Clostridium*, vancomycin if MRSA	Surgical debridement absolutely essential. Empirical therapy must cover for all pathogens. Add vancomycin if MRSA likely
Pyomyositis	*Staphylococcus aureus*, group A streptococci (rarely), Gram-negative bacilli (very rarely), anaerobic bacteria other than *Clostridium*	Oxacillin, or first-generation cephalosporin	Surgical drainage essential
Myonecrosis	*Clostridium perfringens*, other clostridia	High-dose penicillin plus clindamycin	Surgical exploration and debridement crucial with open wound healing; hyperbaric oxygen debated. If extending from cellulitis/necrotising fasciitis, see those sections

MRSA, methicillin-resistant *Staphylococcus aureus*.
*Once causative pathogen(s) has(ve) been identified, antibiotic choice can be modified and spectrum narrowed.
†Be aware of local endemicity of community- or hospital-acquired MRSA. Co-trimoxazole is a good choice in most community-acquired low-grade infections; for all other cases use vancomycin.

Airway control must take top priority in any neck swelling. Antibiotics, in doses similar to necrotising fasciitis, should incorporate cover for Gram-positive cocci and Gram-negative rods. Penicillin or clindamycin plus gentamicin, or a third-generation cephalosporin plus metronidazole, are suitable. Some abscesses may be treated conservatively, especially those in children.[50] However, early surgical drainage remains the mainstay of management for large neck abscesses that impinge on airway patency, or deep infections that pursue a fulminant course.

Retrotonsillar abscess may evolve to Lemierre's syndrome, an infection with anaerobic bacteria, mostly *Fusobacterium necrophorum*, that gain access to the jugular vein and lead to metastatic infections in the liver, lung and brain. Because of possible involvement of anaerobes that produce beta-lactamase, a beta-lactamase-resisting beta-lactam antibiotic should be used.[51]

REFERENCES

1. Conly J. Soft tissue infections. In: Hall JB, Schmidt GA, Wood LDH (eds) *Principles of Critical Care.* New York: McGraw-Hill; 1992: 1325–34.
2. Canoso JJ, Barza M. Soft tissue infections. *Rheum Dis Clin North Am* 1993; **19**: 293–309.
3. Swartz MN. Cellulitis and subcutaneous tissue infections. In: Mandell GL, Bennett JE, Dolin R (eds) *Principles and Practice of Infectious Diseases*, 6th edn. New York: Elsevier Churchill Livingstone; 2004: 1172–94.
4. Pasternack M, Swartz M. Myositis. In: Mandell GL, Dolin R (eds) *Principles and Practice of Infectious Diseases*, 6th edn. New York: Elsevier Churchill Livingstone; 2004: 1194–204.
5. Ahrenholz DH. Necrotising fasciitis and other soft tissue infections. In: Rippe JM, Irwin RS, Alpert JS *et al.* (eds) *Intensive Care Medicine.* Boston: Little, Brown; 1991: 1334–42.
6. Cha JY, Releford BJ Jr, Marcarelli P. Necrotising fasciitis: a classification of necrotising soft tissue infections. *J Foot Ankle Surg* 1994; **33**: 148–55.
7. Sutherland ME, Meyer AA. Necrotising soft-tissue infections. *Surg Clin North Am* 1994; **74**: 591–607.
8. Vinh DC, Embil JM. Rapidly progressive soft tissue infections. *Lancet Infect Dis* 2005; **5**: 501–13.
9. Swartz MN. Clinical practice. Cellulitis. *N Engl J Med* 2004; **350**: 904–12.
10. Ward RG, Walsh MS. Necrotising fasciitis: 10 years' experience in a district general hospital. *Br J Surg* 1991; **78**: 488–9.
11. Kaiser RE, Cerra FB. Progressive necrotising surgical infections – a unified approach. *J Trauma* 1981; **21**: 349–55.
12. Freischlag JA, Ajalat G, Busuttil RW. Treatment of necrotising soft tissue infections. The need for a new approach. *Am J Surg* 1985; **149**: 751–5.
13. Anaya DA, Dellinger EP. Necrotising soft-tissue infection: diagnosis and management. *Clin Infect Dis* 2007; **44**: 705–10.
14. Loudon I. Necrotising fasciitis, hospital gangrene, and phagedena. *Lancet* 1994; **344**: 1416–19.
15. Fournier AJ. Clinical study of fulminating gangrene of the penis. *Semin Med* 1884; **4**: 69.
16. Meleney FL. Hemolytic streptococcus gangrene. *Arch Surg* 1924; **9**: 317–19.
17. Moran GJ, Krishnadasan A, Gorwitz RJ *et al.* Meticillin-resistant *S. aureus* infections among patients in the emergency department. *N Engl J Med* 2006; **355**: 666–74.
18. Fridkin SK, Hageman JC, Morrison M *et al.* Meticillin-resistant *Staphylococcus aureus* disease in three communities. *N Engl J Med* 2005; **352**: 1436–44.
19. Miller LG, Perdreau-Remington F, Rieg G *et al.* Necrotising fasciitis caused by community-associated meticillin-resistant *Staphylococcus aureus* in Los Angeles. *N Engl J Med* 2005; **352**: 1445–53.
20. Bisno AL, Stevens DL. Streptococcal infections of skin and soft tissues. *N Engl J Med* 1996; **334**: 240.
21. Lekstrom-Himes JA, Gallin JI. Immunodeficiency diseases caused by defects in phagocytes. *N Engl J Med* 2000; **343**: 1703–14.
22. Stevens DL. Cellulitis, pyoderma, abcesses and other skin and subcutaneous infections. In: Cohen J, Powderly WG (eds) *Infectious Diseases.* Edinburgh: Mosby; 2004: 145–55.
23. Morris JG Jr, Black RE. Cholera and other vibrioses in the United States. *N Engl J Med* 1985; **312**: 343–50.
24. Hiransuthikul N, Tantisiriwat W, Lertutsahakul K *et al.* Skin and soft-tissue infections among tsunami survivors in southern Thailand. *Clin Infect Dis* 2005; **41**: e93–6.
25. Sartor C, Limouzin-Perotti F, Legre R *et al.* Nosocomial infections with *Aeromonas hydrophila* from leeches. *Clin Infect Dis* 2002; **35**: e1–5.
26. Russell NE, Pachorek RE. Clindamycin in the treatment of streptococcal and staphylococcal toxic shock syndromes. *Ann Pharmacother* 2000; **34**: 936–9.
27. Bowdre JH, Hull JH, Cocchetto DM. Antibiotic efficacy against *Vibrio vulnificus* in the mouse: superiority of tetracycline. *J Pharmacol Exp Ther* 1983; **225**: 595–8.
28. Chuang YC, Yuan CY, Liu CY *et al. Vibrio vulnificus* infection in Taiwan: report of 28 cases and review of clinical manifestations and treatment. *Clin Infect Dis* 1992; **15**: 271–6.
29. Bennett ML, Jackson JM, Jorizzo JL *et al.* Pyoderma gangrenosum. A comparison of typical and atypical forms with an emphasis on time to remission. Case review of 86 patients from 2 institutions. *Medicine (Baltimore)* 2000; **79**: 37–46.
30. Chelsom J, Halstensen A, Haga T *et al.* Necrotising fasciitis due to group A streptococci in western Norway: incidence and clinical features. *Lancet* 1994; **344**: 1111–15.
31. Baxter CR. Surgical management of soft tissue infections. *Surg Clin North Am* 1972; **52**: 1483–99.
32. Patino JF, Castro D. Necrotising lesions of soft tissues: a review. *World J Surg* 1991; **15**: 235–9.
33. Giuliano A, Lewis F Jr, Hadley K *et al.* Bacteriology of necrotising fasciitis. *Am J Surg* 1977; **134**: 52–7.
34. Patino JF, Castro D, Valencia A *et al.* Necrotising soft tissue lesions after a volcanic cataclysm. *World J Surg* 1991; **15**: 240–7.
35. Stevens DL. Necrotising fasciitis, gas gangrene, myoxitis and myonecrosis. In: Cohen J, Powderly WG (eds) *Infectious Diseases.* Edinburgh: Mosby; 2004: 145–55.
36. Burge TS, Watson JD. Necrotising fasciitis. *Br Med J* 1994; **308**: 1453–4.
37. Wilson GJ, Talkington DF, Gruber W *et al.* Group A streptococcal necrotising fasciitis following varicella in children: case reports and review. *Clin Infect Dis* 1995; **20**: 1333–8.
38. Mokoena T, Luvuno FM, Marivate M. Surgical management of retroperitoneal necrotising fasciitis by planned repeat laparotomy and debridement. *S Afr J Surg* 1993; **31**: 65–70.

39. Banerjee AR, Murty GE, Moir AA. Cervical necrotising fasciitis: a distinct clinicopathological entity? *J Laryngol Otol* 1996; **110**: 81–6.
40. Stamenkovic I, Lew PD. Early recognition of potentially fatal necrotising fasciitis: use of frozen-section biopsy. *N Engl J Med* 1984; **310**: 1689.
41. Wong CH, Khin LW, Heng KS *et al.* The LRINEC (Laboratory Risk Indicator for Necrotising Fasciitis) score: a tool for distinguishing necrotising fasciitis from other soft tissue infections. *Crit Care Med* 2004; **32**: 1535–41.
42. Ahrenholz DH. Necrotising soft-tissue infections. *Surg Clin North Am* 1988; **68**: 199–214.
43. Stone HH, Matin JD. Synergistic necrotising cellulitis. *Ann Surg* 1972; **175**: 702–10.
44. Hird B, Byne K. Gangrenous streptococcal myositis: case report. *J Trauma* 1994; **36**: 589–91.
45. Kingston D, Seal DV. Current hypotheses on synergistic microbial gangrene. *Br J Surg* 1990; 77: 260–4.
46. Brown DR, Davis NL, Lepawsky M *et al.* A multicenter review of the treatment of major truncal necrotising infections with and without hyperbaric oxygen therapy. *Am J Surg* 1994; **167**: 485–9.
47. Heimbach D. Use of hyperbaric oxygen. *Clin Infect Dis* 1993; **17**: 239–40.
48. Sethi DS, Stanley RE. Deep neck abscesses – changing trends. *J Laryngol Otol* 1994; **108**: 138–43.
49. Linder HH. The anatomy of the fasciae of the face and neck with particular reference to the spread and treatment of intraoral infections (Ludwigs's) that have progressed into adjacent fascial spaces. *Ann Surg* 1986; **204**: 705–14.
50. Broughton RA. Nonsurgical management of deep neck infections in children. *Pediatr Infect Dis J* 1992; **11**: 14–18.
51. Sinave CP, Hardy GJ, Fardy PW. The Lemierre syndrome: suppurative thrombophlebitis of the internal jugular vein secondary to oropharyngeal infection. *Medicine (Baltimore)* 1989; **68**: 85–94.

64

Principles of antibiotic use

Jeffrey Lipman

The intensive care unit (ICU) is always the area of any hospital associated with the greatest use of antibiotics. Much of this high usage is unavoidable, but the clinician working in the ICU must realise that there is an essential consequence of this use. Antibiotic use which should eliminate susceptible organisms promotes (over)growth of other, non-susceptible organisms, especially fungi. As far as bacteria are concerned, antibiotics confer enormous selective advantage to resistant strains, and therefore these strains will congregate where their advantage is greatest, in the ICU. Resistance (and fungal overgrowth) is a direct consequence of usage, and every course of inappropriate antibiotics should be avoided to help reduce the burden of resistance.

Antibiotic stewardship[1] has been suggested as a new strategy to help limit resistance. This involves selecting an appropriate drug and optimising its dose and duration to cure an infection while minimising toxicity and conditions for selection of resistant bacterial strains. Inadequate doses of even the 'correct' antibiotic may lead to survival of initially susceptible organisms.[2,3] For the optimal use of antibiotics not only should antibiotic pharmacokinetics be understood, but there should be clear and rational principles on which each specific antibiotic prescription in the ICU is based. Also, it is probably better to have portions of the ICU population receive different classes of antibiotics at the same time.

Although this chapter will provide basic principles for most of the antibiotic classes commonly used in the ICU, some important antimicrobial agents will not be specifically addressed here, namely macrolides, clindamycin and the antifungal agents.

GENERAL PRINCIPLES[4–8]

1. All appropriate microbiological specimens, including blood cultures, should be obtained before commencing antibiotic therapy. An immediate Gram-stained report may indicate the appropriate antibiotic to use; otherwise a 'best-guess' choice is made, which is dependent on the clinical situation. This important and common clinical phenomenon involves trying to predict the infecting organism(s).
2. Blood cultures should be taken from a venepuncture site, after adequate skin antisepsis, and not from an intravenous or arterial catheter. Two separate sets of 20 ml (for adults) should be taken, the timing of which is less important.[9] Depending on what system is used, probably 10 ml should be placed into two different blood culture bottles.
3. Once a decision is made to administer antibiotics, they should be administered **without delay**.
4. The decision for empiric therapy, i.e. cover for the most 'likely' organisms causing any specific infection, must include various factors such as the site of the infecting organism (respiratory tract pathogens differ from those of abdominal infections), community versus hospital-associated infection; recent previous antibiotic prescription; ward versus ICU-acquired infection and knowledge of the organisms commonly grown in patients in any specific area. This latter point is where ward/unit surveillance becomes important.[10,11]
5. Whilst there should be an attempt to use a narrow-spectrum antibiotic whenever practicable, appropriate therapy, particularly for empirical choice for nosocomial sepsis, mandates initial broad-spectrum antibiotics, even a combination, until culture results are back,[12] at which time de-escalation should be embarked upon (see below). Inappropriate and/or delayed correct antibiotic use in the ICU has been shown to have an impact on morbidity and mortality[12,13] (Table 64.1).
6. Monotherapy with a single agent effective against the expected organisms aims to decrease the risk of drug antagonism, reaction or toxicity.[14,15] Monotherapy often costs less than multiple antibiotic usage.
7. The clinical response to treatment already given should always be considered, when bacteriological results suggest a change in antibiotics.
8. A standard 2-week course of antibiotics is unnecessary and probably harmful. There is a move to use shorter courses for pneumonia[16,17] (see Table 64.1).
9. In consultation with infectious disease specialists, additional tests such as antibiotic minimum inhibitory concentration (MIC), antibiotic assay, serum bactericidal activity and synergy tests of antibiotic combinations may be useful in serious infections (e.g. endocarditis and infections in immunocompromised

Table 64.1 New paradigm of treatment for nosocomial sepsis

Old	New
Start with penicillin	Get it right first time (broad-spectrum)
Cost-efficient low dose	Hit hard up front
Low doses = fewer side-effects	Low dose → resistance
Long courses ≥ 2 weeks	Seldom longer than 7 days

patients). Sensitivity tests should be interpreted carefully. In vitro sensitivity does not equate with clinical effectiveness; in vitro resistance generally predicts clinical ineffectiveness.

10. Consultations with the laboratory staff and infectious diseases/clinical microbiology specialists are always useful and should be mandatory in serious infections (e.g. meningococcal sepsis, meticillin-resistant staphylococci and multiresistant Enterobacteriaceae).
11. The pharmacokinetics and pharmacodynamics (e.g. penetration into relevant tissues) as well as the spectrum of activity of the antibiotic must be considered. Antibiotic pharmacokinetic principles should determine the dosage and frequency of antibiotic regimens (see below).
12. Adequate drug doses should be given. The intravenous route is preferable in critically ill patients, but other routes should be considered when appropriate (e.g. rectal metronidazole[18]).
13. Serum levels of potentially toxic antibiotics should be monitored, especially if hepatic or renal dysfunction is present.
14. Prophylactic use of antibiotics should be limited to certain situations, should cover organisms that can potentially cause infections in that specific group of patients (e.g. organisms causing skin and soft-tissue infections differ from those implicated in intra-abdominal infections) and should be given at the appropriate timing (see below).
15. General signs of infection are signs of systemic inflammation. Although bacterial infection is likely, non-bacterial infection and non-infective causes should also be considered. High procalcitonin and C-reactive protein levels may be discriminatory for infection,[19] as are interleukin-6 levels, although these are difficult to measure.
16. Antibiotic guidelines are only one aspect of infection control.[20] Hand-washing and hand hygiene in general are vital and fundamental aspects of infection control.[20] Identification and elimination of reservoirs of infection, blocking transmission of infection, barrier nursing, interrupting progression from colonisation to infection and eliminating risk factors such as invasive devices are also important.

COMMON ERRORS WHEN USING ANTIBIOTICS

1. Administration of antibiotics before microbiological specimens are obtained.
2. Inadequate quantity and poor quality of blood cultures.
3. Extended use of antibiotics after eradication of infection (e.g. a 2-week course for ventilation associated pneumonia[16])
4. Antibiotic 'surfing' (i.e. switch from one combination to another) when patient is not improving without delving into the cause of persistent inflammatory response.
5. Inadequate and delayed therapy and/or incorrect dosing of antibiotics.
6. Failure to predict adequately 'resident' microbial flora and therefore inability to choose correctly empiric antibiotics for nosocomial infections, i.e. no adequate surveillance data.
7. Failure to recognise toxic effects of antibiotics, particularly when polypharmacy is used.
8. Use of combination therapy, irrespective of infection.

SPECIFIC ISSUES

PHARMACOKINETIC PRINCIPLES

The goal of antimicrobial prescription is to achieve effective active drug concentrations (a combination of dose and duration) at the site of infection whilst avoiding, or at least minimising, toxicity.

The various antibiotic classes have different 'kill characteristics' and therefore should be dosed differently[21] (Table 64.2).

β-LACTAMS (ALL PENICILLINS AND CEPHALOSPORINS, MONOBACTAMS)[22,23]

1. Studies of β-lactam antibiotics on Gram-negative bacilli show a bactericidal activity that is relatively slow, time-dependent and maximal at relatively low

Table 64.2 Pharmacodynamic properties of selected antibiotics

Antibiotics	Aminoglycosides	Fluoroquinolones	β-lactams Carbapenems Glycopeptides?
PD kill characteristics	Concentration-dependent	Concentration-dependent with time dependence	Time-dependent
Optimal PK parameter	C_{max}:MIC	AUC:MIC	$T >$ MIC

PD, pharmacodynamic; PK, pharmacokinetic; C_{max}, peak serum concentration; MIC, minimum inhibitory concentration; AUC, area under concentration–time curve; $T >$ MIC, time above MIC.

concentrations. Bacterial killing is almost entirely related to the time that levels in tissue and plasma exceed a certain threshold. The maximum time plasma β-lactams levels should be allowed to fall below MIC is 40% of the dosing interval.

2. β-lactam antibiotics lack a significant postantibiotic effect (PAE), particularly against Gram-negative organisms, and it is not necessary to achieve very high peak plasma concentrations. PAE is the continued suppression of bacterial growth despite zero serum concentration of antibiotic. It is suggested that concentrations of any β-lactam should be maintained at about 4–5 times MIC for long periods, as maximum killing of bacteria in vitro occurs at this level. If antibiotic concentrations fall below this threshold in the in vitro models, bacterial growth is immediately resumed.
3. Thus, it is important for the efficacy of β-lactams that the dosing regime maintains adequate plasma levels for as long as possible during the dosing interval. It is not surprising, then, that dosing regimes of β-lactam antibiotics are being re-evaluated to keep plasma levels above certain thresholds of MICs of Gram-negative organisms for longer periods of the dosing interval.[24,25]

CARBAPENEMS

1. Similarly to β-lactams, the carbapenems also have time-dependent kill characteristics but have some PAE.
2. Prolonged infusions (over 3 hours) have been utilised to improve time above MIC.[25,26]
3. In vitro data suggest low concentrations may predispose to development of resistant organisms.[2]

AMINOGLYCOSIDES (THE BEST PHARMACOKINETICALLY STUDIED OF THE ANTIBIOTIC CLASSES)[22,23]

1. The above contrasts with the kill characteristic of the aminoglycosides, which is concentration-dependent. Experimentally, a high peak concentration of an aminoglycoside antibiotic provides a better, faster killing effect on standard bacterial inocula.
2. All aminoglycosides exhibit a significant PAE. The duration of this effect is variable, but the higher the previous peak, the longer the PAE. This phenomenon allows drug concentration to fall significantly below MIC of the pathogen without allowing regrowth of bacteria and hence not compromising antibacterial efficacy. The phenomenon of PAE is much more prevalent in aminoglycosides than other antibiotics and more pronounced with Gram-negative bacilli than with other bacteria.
3. These principles allow for single daily doses of aminoglycosides (also termed extended interval dosing). Combining various meta-analyses involving thousands of patients, once-daily administration was found to be more efficacious, with reduced toxicity, higher peak/MIC ratios, further prolonged PAE and reduced administration costs.
4. With renal dysfunction[27] the dose should be altered according to creatinine clearance. If $\geq$ 60 ml/min, give 5–7 mg/kg daily; if 59–40 ml/min, the same dose at an interval of 36 hours; 39–20 ml/min, increase the dosing interval to 48 hours.

QUINOLONES[22,23]

1. In contrast ciprofloxacin has a combination of both the above (concentration-dependent and time-dependent effects) as well as some PAE.
2. Although one suggested 'target' parameter for a good clinical bactericidal effect is a high peak, the most validated parameter is the area under the inhibitor curve (AUIC), i.e. AUC/MIC: values >125 translate into better clinical cures.
3. There is general concern about the emergence of resistance related to inappropriately low doses of ciprofloxacin[3] (see Table 64.1).

GLYCOPEPTIDES[22,23]

1. Vancomycin induces a PAE and a postantibiotic sub-MIC effect. These combined effects suggest that bacterial regrowth will not occur for prolonged periods following a fall in drug concentrations to levels below the MIC.
2. Continuous infusions of vancomycin may have some advantages.

Aminoglycosides and glycopeptides distribute well into fluids of the extravascular, extracellular space, and less well into tissues. This has two important implications. Firstly these agents should not be first-line agents for, nor monotherapy for, solid-organ infections (lung, kidney, liver). Secondly, in situations where extravascular fluid shifts are significant, such as in situations of 'third-space losses' of abdominal sepsis and in severe burns, the volume of distribution of these drugs is significantly affected. Hence for any serum level required a larger dose may have to be administered. The volume of distribution of the quinolones (very large) suggests that penetration is excellent into most tissues and hence these drugs are good for solid-organ infections. Similarly β-lactams as a group (including carbapenems) all have reasonable tissue penetration.

ANTIBIOTIC PROPHYLAXIS[4,6,7,28]

The main indications for prophylaxis are:

1. When surgery involves incision through an area of colonisation or normal commensal flora and a resultant potential infection has morbidity or mortality.
2. When a procedure (e.g. catheterisation, instrumentation, intubation, dental work) potentially produces a bacteraemia in the presence of an immunocompromised patient or when the potential bacteraemia occurs in the presence of an abnormal heart valve or a prosthesis.

Basic principles of choice of prophylactic regimen should include:

1. The organisms colonising the area through which the incision is made should be covered (Gram-positives if skin is breached, Gram-negatives and anaerobes if bowel is opened).
2. A similar case should be made for colonising organisms through the area breached by catheterisation or instrumentation (Gram-negatives for bladder catheterisation, Gram-positives and anaerobes for dental procedures).
3. If prevalence of a resistant organism in a specific area is high (e.g. meticillin-resistant *Staphylococcus aureus* (MRSA) in burns units), then those organisms should be covered by the prophylactic regimen.

TIMING AND DURATION OF PROPHYLAXIS

1. Optimal blood levels of antibiotic(s) are needed when the occurrence of the potential bacteraemia occurs, i.e. for surgery, optimal timing of the antibiotic should be at, or just prior to, induction of anaesthesia and skin incision.[28]
2. For prolonged procedures where bacteraemias are still a potential occurrence a second dose of antibiotic(s) may be considered.
3. There is no extra benefit of postoperative antibiotic prophylaxis.

DOSES

Comments on dosing regimens are provided below. Doses suggested below are intravenous, for a 70-kg adult with *normal* renal function. All these drugs accumulate with renal dysfunction and modified doses should be used accordingly.

1. Doses for β-lactams vary with each different drug *but* recent emphasis supports lower boluses with more frequent administration, i.e. 4-hourly versus 8-hourly or bd versus daily. Continuous infusions may become the standard of practice.[25]
2. Aminoglycosides: tobramycin and gentamicin 7 mg/kg as a loading dose on the first day, followed by 5 mg/kg per day. Amikacin 20 mg/kg as the loading dose followed by 15 mg/kg per day. These doses are the same for adults and children, neonates excluded.
3. Quinolones: ciprofloxacin *at least* 400 mg bd (up to tds).
4. Glycopeptide: vancomycin at least 2 g/day either as continuous infusion or in divided doses (40 mg/kg per day for children).
5. Carbapenems: meropenem or imipenem: 3 g/day in at least three divided doses.

SURVEILLANCE

Some type of simple laboratory-oriented surveillance which primarily collects data and resistance patterns of microbiological isolates is important. There are a few international projects,[11] but each unit should have access to its own such data as there is increasing prevalence of resistant organisms in ICUs. This is complicated even further by different units having differing resistance patterns.[10] Empiric antibiotic therapy must take these factors into account. Some form of surveillance that provides units with their own microbiological data, updatable quarterly or biannually, is therefore beneficial in helping choose empiric and prophylactic regimens that are applicable to any specific unit.[10]

MULTIRESISTANT ORGANISMS

Although this chapter is on antibiotics, the point must be made that without good, efficient and effective infection control policies in all areas treating critically ill patients, the spread of multiresistant organisms would be rampant and the control thereof useless.[20] Part of these policies should involve attention to good hand hygiene and the use of antiseptic soaps and alcohol-based hand rubs.[20] Hands are still the most documented and incriminated mode of transmission of infection. In this regard a decrement in nursing numbers has also been incriminated in outbreaks of infections, possibly due to the time it takes to wash adequately between procedures.[20]

1. Multiresistant streptococci and vancomycin-resistant enterococci (VRE), although not common in all countries, are an increasing worldwide problem, as is community-acquired MRSA.
2. The prevalence of MRSA is wider, with many ICUs having this organism almost endemic. Community-acquired MRSA is becoming a huge problem, largely because of identification and initial treatment.[29] It differs from the hospital-associated strain in that it is far less multidrug-resistant, but nevertheless it is oxacillin-resistant.
3. New agents are available for treatment of resistant Gram-positive infections.[30]
4. Antibiotic resistance is agent-specific. Often resistance is claimed to be against third-generation cephalosporins, but this is largely to ceftazidime (particularly the extended-spectrum beta-lactamases of *Klebsiella pneumoniae, Escherichia coli* and some Enterobacteriaceae).
5. Worrying Gram-negative organisms are *Klebsiella pneumoniae, Pseudomonas aeruginosa, Acinetobacter baumanii* spp. and *Stenotrophomonas maltophilia* (the latter specifically, for which trimethoprim may need to be used). A common feature of these organisms is intrinsic resistance to multiple antibiotics. *P. aeruginosa* and *Acinetobacter* complex (also named *A. baumanii*) have become particular problems. Sulbactam and polymixin B or colistin have been used for these problem organisms.[31]
6. Since the carbapenems there are no new agents for multiresistant Gram-negative organisms,[1] although tigecycline has recently been launched.

MONOTHERAPY VERSUS COMBINATION THERAPY[14,15]

1. Much of the work in this area was performed before the clinical introduction of the carbapenems, penicillin/betalactamase combinations and fourth-generation cephalosporins. It seems that newer single agents are adequate apart possibly for resistant pseudomonal infections.[12]
2. There is no clear evidence supporting the claim that combination antimicrobial therapy prevents emergence of resistance.[14]
3. However combination therapy is often suggested for endocarditis and some pseudomonal infections.[12] When combination therapy is used, preference should be given to the combination therapy of two different classes of antibiotics and then classes that act synergistically. The combination of two β-lactam antibiotics should not be used.

BROAD-SPECTRUM INITIAL COVER WITH DE-ESCALATION[32] (SEE TABLE 64.1)

In view of the morbidity and mortality of delayed appropriate therapy for nosocomial sepsis,[12,13,32] particularly pneumonias, patients with risk factors for infection with resistant pathogens should initially receive broad-spectrum antibiotics, possibly even combination therapy,[12,32] and, as soon as the pathogen and the susceptibilities are available, treatment should be simplified to a more targeted one – so-called 'de-escalation' therapy.[32] In the limited studies to date, de-escalation has led to less antibiotic usage, shorter durations of therapy, fewer episodes of secondary pneumonia and reduced mortality, without increasing the frequency of antibiotic resistance.

TIME TO ANTIBIOTICS AS A QUALITY INDICATOR

Recent data suggests that a delay of even hours of appropriate antibiotic administration increases morbidity and mortality.[33] A delay in antibiotic administration has therefore become an important negative factor in patient outcomes. Similar to the concept of "time to lysis", antibiotic administration from the time of recognition of infection may in future become a quality indicator of infection management.

REFERENCES

1. Fishman N. Antimicrobial stewardship. *Am J Med* 2006; **119**: S53–61.
2. Tam VH, Schilling AN, Neshat S *et al.* Optimization of meropenem minimum concentration/MIC ratio to suppress in vitro resistance of *Pseudomonas aeruginosa*. *Antimicrob Agents Chemother* 2005; **49**: 4920–7.
3. Zhou J, Dong Y, Zhao X *et al.* Selection of antibiotic-resistant bacterial mutants: allelic diversity among fluoroquinolone-resistant mutations. *J Infect Dis* 2000; **182**: 517–25.
4. Reese RE, Douglas RG Jnr (eds) *A Practical Approach to Infectious Diseases*. Boston: Little, Brown; 1986.
5. Lundberg GD. Making use of the microbiology laboratory. 1. Use of the laboratory. *JAMA* 1982; **247**: 857–9.
6. Sanford JP. *Guide to Antimicrobial Therapy.* West Bethesda, Maryland: Antimicrobial Therapy; 1993.
7. Mandell GL, Douglas RG, Bennett JE. *Principles and Practice of Infectious Diseases*, 4th edn. New York: Churchill Livingstone; 1994.
8. Neu HC. Antimicrobial agents: role in the prevention and control of nosocomial infections. In: Wentzel RP (ed.) *Prevention and Control of Nosocomial Infections,* 2nd edn. Baltimore: Williams & Williams; Chapter 18.
9. Weinstein MP. Current blood culture methods and systems: clinical concepts, technology, and interpretation of results. *Clin Infect Dis* 1996; **23**: 40–6.
10. Namias N, Samiian L, Nino D *et al.* Incidence and susceptibility of pathogenic bacteria vary between intensive care units within a single hospital: implications for empiric antibiotic strategies. *J Trauma* 2000; **49**: 638–45.
11. Marchese A, Schito GC. Role of global surveillance in combating bacterial resistance. *Drugs* 2001; **61**: 167–73.
12. Mutlu GM, Wunderink RG. Severe pseudomonal infections. *Curr Opin Crit Care* 2006; **12**: 458–63.
13. Kollef MH. Inadequate antimicrobial treatment: an important determinant of outcome for hospitalized patients. *Clin Infect Dis* 2000; **31** (Suppl. 4): S131–8.
14. Paul M, Benuri-Silbiger I, Soares-Weiser K *et al.* Beta lactam monotherapy versus beta lactam-aminoglycoside combination therapy for sepsis in immuno-competent patients: systematic review and meta-analysis of randomised trials. *Br Med J* 2004; **328**: 668–72.
15. Safar N, Handelsman J, Maki DG. Does combination antimicrobial therapy reduce mortality in Gram-negative bacteraemia? A meta-analysis. *Lancet Infect Dis* 2004; **4**: 519–27.
16. Chastre J, Wolff M, Fagon JY *et al.* Comparison of 8 vs 15 days of antibiotic therapy for ventilator-associated pneumonia in adults: a randomized trial. *JAMA* 2003; **290**: 2588–98.
17. Singh N, Rogers P, Atwood CW *et al.* Short-course empiric antibiotic therapy for patients with pulmonary infiltrates in the intensive care unit. A proposed solution for indiscriminate antibiotic prescription. *Am J Respir Crit Care Med* 2000; **162**: 505–11.
18. Baker EM, Aitchison JM, Crindland JS *et al.* Rectal administration of metronidazole in severely ill patients. *Br Med J* 1983; **287**: 311–14.
19. Uzzan B, Cohen R, Nicolas P *et al.* Procalcitonin as a diagnostic test for sepsis in critically ill adults and after surgery or trauma: a systematic review and meta-analysis. *Crit Care Med* 2006; **34**: 1996–2003.

20. Pittet D, Allegranzi B, Sax H *et al.* Evidence-based model for hand transmission during patient care and the role of improved practices. *Lancet Infect Dis* 2006; **6**: 641–52.
21. Craig WA. Pharmacokinetic/pharmacodynamic parameters: rationale for antibacterial dosing of mice and men. *Clin Infect Dis* 1998; **26**: 1–10.
22. Pinder M, Bellomo R, Lipman J. Pharmacological principles of antibiotic prescription in the critically ill. *Anaesth Intens Care* 2002; **30**: 134–44.
23. Roberts J, Lipman J. Antibacterial dosing in intensive care: pharmacokinetics, degree of disease and pharmacodynamics of sepsis. *Clin Pharmacokinet* 2006; **45**: 755–73.
24. Lipman J, Wallis S, Rickard C. Low cefepime levels in critically ill septic patients: pharmacokinetic modeling indicates improved troughs with revised dosing. *Antimicrob Agents Chemother* 1999; **43**: 2559–61.
25. Kasiakou SK, Lawrence KR, Choulis N *et al.* Continuous versus intermittent intravenous administration of antibacterials with time-dependent action: a systematic review of pharmacokinetic and pharmacodynamic parameters. *Drugs* 2005; **65**: 2499–511.
26. Lomaestro BM, Drusano GL. Pharmacodynamic evaluation of extending the administration time of meropenem using a Monte Carlo simulation. *Antimicrob Agents Chemother* 2005; **49**: 461–3.
27. Nicolau DP, Freeman CD, Belliveau PP *et al.* Experience with a once daily aminoglycoside program administered to 2184 adult patients. *Antimicrob Agents Chemother* 1995; **39**: 650–5.
28. Classen DC, Evans RS, Pestotnik SL *et al.* The timing of prophylactic administration of antibiotics and the risk of surgical-wound infection. *N Engl J Med* 1992; **326**: 281–6.
29. Nimmo GR, Coombs GW, Pearson JC *et al.* Meticillin-resistant *Staphylococcus aureus* in the Australian community: an evolving epidemic. *Med J Aust* 2006; **184**: 384–8.
30. Schmidt-Ioanas M, de Roux A, Lode H. New antibiotics for the treatment of severe staphylococcal infection in the critically ill patient. *Curr Opin Crit Care* 2005; **11**: 481–6.
31. Rahal JJ. Novel antibiotic combinations against infections with almost completely resistant *Pseudomonas aeruginosa* and *Acinetobacter* species. *Clin Infect Dis* 2006; **43** (Suppl. 2): S95–9.
32. Niederman MS. De-escalation therapy in ventilator-associated pneumonia. *Curr Opin Crit Care* 2006; **12**: 452–7.

65

Tropical diseases

Ramachandran Sivakumar and Michael E Pelly

Once an exotic and esoteric topic, modern travel and the quest for unusual holidays has the potential to bring tropical diseases to every ICU. This chapter covers some important diseases, which are common in the tropical belt.

MALARIA

EPIDEMIOLOGY AND PATHOGENESIS

It is estimated that four species of *Plasmodium* (*vivax*, *malariae*, *ovale* and *falciparum*) cause 300–500 million infections per year. Most of the 1–3 million deaths per year due to malaria are caused by *Plasmodium falciparum* and the majority of deaths are in children under 5 years in sub-Saharan Africa. Malaria is also widely prevalent in the Indian subcontinent and South-East Asia. It is transmitted from human to human by the bite of infected female *Anopheles* mosquitoes. After development in the liver, there is invasion of red cells by parasites, which is followed by their multiplication, and rupture of the red cells. The cycle is then repeated in red cells. In *vivax* and *ovale* infections, development to dormant forms can occur in the liver, which may lead to relapse.

CLINICAL FEATURES

UNCOMPLICATED MALARIA

Initial symptoms of malaria are non-specific and similar to a viral illness. Classic symptoms of fever, aches, and headache are usually, but not always, present. Other features such as diarrhoea, vomiting, cough, and abdominal pain, may confuse the unwary. Unusual presentations are more common in children and may be missed. Classical rigors or fevers occurring on specific days (tertian or quartan) are usually absent in early falciparum infection. Clinical signs may be unhelpful although hepatosplenomegaly may be present fairly early.

SEVERE MALARIA

Risk factors for severe malaria

- Children under 5 years in endemic regions
- Adults and children in areas of low endemicity
- Non-immune travellers to endemic areas

Definition

The diagnosis of severe malaria requires the presence of one or more of the following with no other confirmed cause occurring in a patient with asexual *Plasmodium falciparum* parasitaemia:[1]

- impaired conscious state
- multiple convulsions
- respiratory distress
- pulmonary oedema
- circulatory collapse
- abnormal bleeding
- jaundice
- haemoglobinuria
- severe anaemia

The incubation period is at least 7 days. The usual range is 9–14 days but this may be longer. Anaemia, jaundice, renal dysfunction, haemostatic abnormalities, thrombocytopenia, pulmonary oedema, shock, hypoglycaemia, and severe metabolic acidosis are common in severe malaria. Several of the above coexist or may develop in rapid succession. Cough, convulsions, and hypoglycaemia are more common in children. Jaundice is common, but hepatic failure is uncommon. The acidosis of malaria is multifactorial and probably very similar to other forms of sepsis involving tissue hypoxia, liver dysfunction, and impaired renal handling of bicarbonate.

The differential diagnosis of malaria includes:

- meningitis, typhoid fever, septicaemia
- severe influenza, dengue and other arboviral infections
- haemorrhagic fevers
- hepatitis, leptospirosis
- rickettsial diseases, e.g. scrub typhus
- relapsing fever (*Borrelia recurrentis*)
- febrile convulsions in children

Pregnancy increases the risk of development of severe malaria. During pregnancy both maternal and fetal morbidity and mortality are increased.

Poor prognostic indicators include age under 3 years, cerebral malaria, circulatory collapse and organ dysfunction. Laboratory evidence of poor prognosis includes hyperparasitaemia ($> 250\ 000/\mu l$ or $> 5\%$), peripheral schizontaemia, severe anaemia (PCV $< 15\%$ or Hb < 50 g/l), raised blood urea > 60 mg/dl and serum creatinine > 265 µmol/l (> 3.0 mg/dl), raised venous lactate (> 5 mmol/l), raised CSF lactate (> 6 mmol/l), low CSF glucose and a very high concentration of TNF-α.

Cerebral malaria

Cerebral malaria may be the most common non-traumatic encephalopathy worldwide. The term is restricted to the syndrome in which altered consciousness due to malaria could not be attributed to convulsions, sedatives, hypoglycaemia or to a non-malarial cause. It is distinguished from the postictal state if unconsciousness persists for more than 30 minutes after a convulsion.

Clinical, histopathological and laboratory studies have suggested two potential mechanisms:

- mechanical hypothesis – cytoadherence of parasitised erythrocytes
- cytotoxic hypothesis – neuronal injury by malarial toxin and excessive cytokine production.

Cerebral malaria has few specific features, but there are differences in clinical presentation between African children and non-immune adults.[2]

Clinical findings include:

- coma
- convulsions
- raised intracranial pressure
- hypoglycaemia
- acidosis
- abnormalities of tone and posture (the commonest being symmetrical pyramidal signs)
- retinopathy – retinal haemorrhages, cotton wool spots, papilloedema, retinal whitening and retinal vessel abnormalities, all of which are more common in children.

DIAGNOSIS

Microscopy of thick and thin films remains the gold standard for both the diagnosis and to follow the efficacy of treatment. In the non-immune patient there is a close association between parasite levels and complications; however, severe complications can occur in patients with low counts.

Rapid diagnostic tests (RDTs) which detect specific antigens (proteins) produced by malaria parasites are useful in diagnosis. Current tests are based on the detection of histidine-rich protein 2 (HRP2) (which is specific for *P. falciparum*), pan-specific or species-specific parasite lactate dehydrogenase (pLDH), or other pan-specific antigens such as aldolase. Many commercial assays are available. Some tests detect only one species (*P. falciparum*), while others detect one or more of the other three species. RDTs do not give information about the parasite load and their sensitivity and specificity decrease at low parasitaemia. Hence, it is important to seek microbiological advice regarding the RDTs used locally.

Polymerase chain reaction (PCR) tests based on detecting malarial DNA are more sensitive than microscopy but are expensive and do not give estimates of parasite load.

TREATMENT OF MALARIA[3]

WHO has recently issued new guidelines for the treatment of malaria.

FALCIPARUM MALARIA (TABLE 65.1)

To counter the threat of resistance of *P. falciparum* to monotherapies, and to improve treatment outcome, combinations of antimalarials are now recommended by WHO for the treatment of falciparum malaria. Antimalarial combination therapy is the simultaneous use of two or more blood schizontocidal drugs with independent modes of action. Artemisin-based combination therapy (ACT) is the recommended treatment for uncomplicated falciparum malaria.

One of the following ACTs is currently recommended: artesunate + amodiaquine, artesunate + sulfadoxine–pyrimethamine, artesunate + mefloquine, or artemether–lumefantrine. The choice of ACT in a country or region will be based on the level of resistance of the partner medicine in the combination.

Severe falciparum malaria (Table 65.2)

Two classes of drug are currently available for the parenteral treatment of severe malaria: the cinchona alkaloids (quinine and quinidine) and the artemisinin derivatives (artesunate, artemether and artemotil). Recent evidence[4,5] suggests superior efficacy of artesunate over quinine in adults. The dosage of artemisinin derivatives does not need adjustment in vital organ dysfunction.

Following initial parenteral treatment, once the patient can tolerate it, current practice is to switch to oral therapy and complete a full 7 days of treatment. In non-pregnant

Table 65.1 WHO recommendations for treatment of uncomplicated *P. falciparum* malaria

Artesunate + amodiaquine
4 mg/kg of artesunate and 10 mg base/kg of amodiaquine given once a day for 3 days
Artesunate + sulfadoxine–pyrimethamine
4 mg/kg of artesunate given once a day for 3 days and a single administration of sulfadoxine–pyrimethamine (25/1.25 mg base/kg body weight) on day 1
Artesunate + mefloquine
4 mg/kg of artesunate given once a day for 3 days and 25 mg base/kg of mefloquine, usually split over 2 or 3 days
Artemether–lumefantrine
Are available as co-formulated tablets containing 20 mg of artemether and 120 mg of lumefantrine. The recommended treatment for persons weighing more than 34 kg is 4 tablets twice a day for 3 days

Table 65.2 WHO recommendations for treatment of severe *P. falciparum* malaria

Artesunate
2.4 mg/kg i.v. or i.m. given on admission (time = 0), then at 12 hours and 24 hours, then once a day is recommended in low transmission areas or outside malaria endemic areas. If artesunate is not available, quinine i.v. should be used.
For children in high transmission areas, one of the following antimalarial medicines is recommended as there is insufficient evidence to recommend any of these antimalarial medicines over another for severe malaria:
• artesunate 2.4 mg/kg i.v. or i.m. given on admission (time = 0), then at 12 hours and 24 hours, then once a day
• artemether 3.2 mg/kg i.m. given on admission then 1.6 mg/kg body weight per day
• quinine 20 mg salt/kg on admission (i.v. infusion or divided i.m. injection), then 10 mg/kg every 8 hours; infusion rate should not exceed 5 mg salt/kg per hour

Table 65.3 WHO recommendations for treatment of *P. vivax*, *ovale* and *malariae* malaria

Uncomplicated *P. vivax* malaria
Chloroquine 25 mg base/kg divided over 3 days, combined with primaquine 0.25 mg base/kg, taken with food once daily for 14 days is the treatment of choice for chloroquine-sensitive infections. In Oceania and Southeast Asia the dose of primaquine should be 0.5 mg/kg.
Amodiaquine (30 mg base/kg divided over 3 days as 10 mg/kg single daily doses) combined with primaquine should be given for chloroquine-resistant *vivax* malaria.
Complicated *P. vivax* malaria
Treatment is the same as severe *P. falciparum* malaria.
***P. ovale* and *malariae* malaria**
Treatment is the same as uncomplicated *vivax* malaria but without primaquine for *malariae*.

adults, doxycycline (3.5 mg/kg per day) is added to quinine, artesunate or artemether and should also be given for 7 days. During pregnancy or in children, clindamycin is used instead of doxycycline.

In patients with features of severe malaria, a mixed infection with *falciparum* should be assumed even if only a benign species is identified in the film. Occasionally, severe malaria can occur with *vivax* species. If the clinical suspicion is high, a therapeutic trial of antimalarial treatment is justified, even if the film is negative.

Severe malaria leads to severe septic shock, and the principles of management are the same including resuscitation and provision of supportive treatment. These patients are at risk of acute lung injury but do need adequate fluid resuscitation. Convulsions must be actively treated. Complications should be managed as they present. The threshold for dialysis should be low. Pneumonia and bacterial septicaemia are also common, and should be recognised and treated.

Exchange blood transfusion (EBT) has been used in severe malaria. However, recent WHO guidelines[3] do not recommend EBT, and note the lack of consensus on indications, benefits and dangers involved, or on practical details such as the volume of blood that should be exchanged. Traditional indications for EBT if pathogen-free compatible blood is available are:

- parasitaemia > 30%, even in the absence of clinical complications
- parasitaemia > 10% in the presence of severe disease, especially cerebral malaria, acute renal failure, ARDS, jaundice and severe anaemia and/or poor prognostic factors (e.g. elderly patient, late stage parasites (schizonts) in the peripheral blood)
- parasitaemia > 10% and failure to respond to optimal chemotherapy after 12–24 hours

OTHER FORMS OF MALARIA

Treatment of other forms of malaria is outlined in Table 65.3.

PROGNOSIS

Data are largely derived from endemic areas where presentation with convulsions, acidosis or hypoglycaemia is associated with a poorer outcome. Mortality in an artesunate-treated severe falciparum malaria group in one trial[5] was still high (15% vs. 22% in quinine-treated patients). In cerebral malaria, mortality is around 20%. The prognosis of cerebral malaria is frequently determined by the management of other complications such as renal failure and acidosis, but neurological sequelae are increasingly recognised.

TUBERCULOSIS

EPIDEMIOLOGY

Tuberculosis continues to be a devastating disease worldwide, with an estimated 8 million new cases and 2.6–2.9 million deaths annually. Medical conditions which predispose to tuberculosis include HIV infection, silicosis, diabetes, chronic renal failure/haemodialysis, malnutrition, solid organ transplant, gastrectomy, jejunoileal bypass, injection and inhalational drug abuse, alcoholism, chronic pulmonary disease and prolonged steroid use. Social factors such as institutional living conditions (nursing homes, homeless shelters, prisons), urban dwelling and poverty are associated with an increased risk of tuberculosis.

PATHOGENESIS

Tuberculosis (TB) is usually caused by *Mycobacterium tuberculosis* and four others (*M. bovis*, *M. africanum*, *M. microti* and *M. canetti*) grouped in the Mycobacterium complex. The genus Mycobacterium consists of many different species, all of which appear similar on acid-fast staining.

Inhalation of tubercle bacilli leads to one of four possible outcomes: immediate clearance of the organism, primary or progressive primary disease, chronic or latent infection, and reactivation disease. Latent infection refers to the presence of tuberculous infection (positive tuberculin reaction) without the disease.

The majority of primary TB infections are asymptomatic; clinical pneumonia occurs in 5–10% of adults with a higher incidence in children and those suffering from HIV infection. *M. tuberculosis* microfoci that have remained dormant after primary infection may undergo reactivation resulting in secondary TB, often referred to as reactivation disease. This is responsible for 90% of TB in patients not infected with HIV.

CLINICAL SPECTRUM

The manifestations of TB are protean and TB should be considered in the differential diagnosis of all patients with fever of unknown origin, night sweats, or unexplained weight loss. Besides the lungs, it can also involve the central nervous system, peritoneum, pericardium, gastrointestinal and genitourinary tract, bone and joints, lymph nodes and skin. Occasionally it can be disseminated in the form of miliary tuberculosis.

PULMONARY TUBERCULOSIS

Typically, reactivation disease starts in the apex of one or both lungs, leading to chronic inflammation and fibrosis. Pulmonary TB is often asymptomatic initially, though cough, dyspnoea and haemoptysis are useful clues. Hilar lymphadenopathy is the most common pulmonary presentation in children. It may occasionally present very late as extensive disease in both lungs with severe lung damage including cavitation, and pneumothoraces.

Sputum, induced sputum, bronchial washings and transbronchial biopsy of infiltrates should be performed to isolate the organism. Computed tomography (CT) is more sensitive than chest radiography for detection of infiltrates, cavities, lymphadenopathy, miliary disease, bronchiectasis, bronchial stenosis, bronchopleural fistula and pleural effusion.

Tuberculous pleural effusion

Pleural TB may result in pleural effusion, pleural empyema with or without bronchopleural fistula. Thoracocentesis and pleural biopsy should be performed. Positive cultures are found in less than 25% of cases. Pleural biopsy shows granulomatous inflammation in approximately 60% of patients. However, when culture of three biopsy specimens is combined with histological examination, the diagnosis can be made in up to 90% of cases. Pleuroscopy-guided biopsies increase the yield in pleural sampling.

The pleural fluid should be examined for total protein and glucose content, WBC count and differential, and fluid pH. Raised adenosine deaminase (ADA) levels have been found to be useful in the diagnosis, with levels more than 70 U/l in pleural fluid strongly favouring tuberculous aetiology and levels less than 40 U/l making it less likely; ADA also has a good negative predictive value. However, ADA assay should not be considered as an alternative to biopsy and culture.[6] Raised γ-interferon has also been found to be useful. The clinical utility of PCR testing in tuberculous pleural effusion is limited.[7]

TUBERCULOUS MENINGITIS

Tuberculous meningitis[8] remains the most serious relevant manifestation of TB to the intensive care physician. Tuberculous meningitis results from haematogenous spread. There is a thick gelatinous exudate around the sylvian fissures, basal cisterns, brainstem and cerebellum.

The majority of patients with TB meningitis have had recent contact with TB, followed by a prodrome of vague ill-health lasting 2–8 weeks. Later, signs and symptoms of meningeal irritation appear. Cranial nerve palsies occur in 20–25% of patients and papilloedema may be present. Choroidal tubercles are rare but almost pathognomonic. Visual loss due to optic nerve involvement may occasionally be the presenting feature. There may be focal neurological deficit such as hemiplegia; extrapyramidal movements and seizures are other manifestations. As the disease progresses, cerebral dysfunction sets in and the mortality approaches 50%.

Diagnostic algorithms have been suggested but they are unlikely to provide sufficient assurance to confidently exclude other diagnoses.[9,10] The key is a high degree of clinical suspicion, especially in the critically ill. In one study, TB meningitis was considered as a diagnosis in only 36% of cases and only 6% received immediate treatment.[11]

Definitive diagnosis of TB meningitis depends upon the detection of the organism in CSF, either by smear examination or by bacterial culture. The yield from smear is variable, but generally low. Culture of the CSF for the organisms is not invariably positive. Raised ADA level is not specific.

The sensitivity and specificity of a commercial nucleic acid amplification assay for the diagnosis of TB meningitis are 56% and 98% respectively.[12] Careful bacteriology is as good as, or better than, the commercial nucleic acid amplification assays, but molecular methods may be more useful when antituberculous drugs have already been commenced. However, the diagnosis of TB meningitis cannot be excluded by these tests, even if both are negative.[8]

CT or magnetic resonance imaging (MRI) of the brain, which are sensitive but not specific, may reveal thickening and intense enhancement of meninges, especially in basilar regions. Hydrocephalus and tuberculomas may also be present. Infarcts due to either vasculitis or mechanical strangulation of the vessels by the surrounding exudates are detected in up to 40%. The radiological differential diagnosis includes cryptococcal meningitis, cytomegalovirus encephalitis, sarcoidosis, meningeal metastases and lymphoma.

TUBERCULOUS EMERGENCIES

- Massive haemoptysis
- Respiratory failure
- Pericardial tamponade
- Small intestinal obstruction
- Tuberculous meningitis
- Status epilepticus due to tuberculomas

DIAGNOSIS OF TUBERCULOSIS

Once considered, isolate the patient and sample all potential sites for acid fast staining and culture. Pleural, peritoneal, pericardial and other fluids must be cultured and analysed for differential cell count, protein, glucose and ADA. Histological examination for granulomatous infection is useful in bronchial, pleural, peritoneal and skeletal tissues. Peritoneal biopsies are best obtained via laparoscopy. Newer culture media have reduced the time for culture to 2 weeks.

Nucleic acid amplification (NAA) tests amplify target nucleic acid regions that uniquely identify the *M. tuberculosis* complex, and are available as commercial kits or in-house assays. They can be applied to clinical specimens within hours. Based on current evidence, NAA tests cannot replace conventional diagnostic approaches using microscopy and culture.

The current status of NAA tests is summarised below:

- NAA tests, in general, have high specificity and positive predictive value; they are useful in ruling in rather than ruling out TB.
- A positive NAA test in smear-positive patients can differentiate *M. tuberculosis* from non-tuberculous mycobacteria (NTM); treatment can then be started.
- The interpretation of a smear-positive/NAA-negative test is controversial.
- Treatment can be started in smear-negative/NAA-positive patients with a high clinical suspicion, particularly when prompt treatment is imperative.
- If clinical suspicion is high, TB is not excluded by both a negative smear and NAA.
- NAA results may remain positive for months. This method should be used only for initial diagnosis and not follow-up.

Serodiagnosis of tuberculosis, despite remaining a poor confirmatory tool in areas of low incidence, may be useful in exclusion of disease.

Drug susceptibility tests should be performed on initial isolates from all patients in order to identify an effective antituberculous regimen, and may have to be repeated if the patient remains culture positive after 3 months.

TREATMENT OF TUBERCULOSIS

Local guidelines are of paramount importance and advice should be sought. The commonest regimen used is isoniazid (5 mg/kg) and rifampicin (10 mg/kg) for 6 months with the addition of pyrazinamide (15–30 mg/kg) and ethambutol (5–25 mg/kg) for the first 2 months. It has been suggested that instead of ethambutol, prothionamide is preferable as a fourth drug in tuberculous meningitis. Steroids are generally recommended in tuberculous meningitis[13,14] and pericardial tuberculosis.

DRUG-RESISTANT TUBERCULOSIS

This is an increasing problem. Multidrug-resistant tuberculosis (defined as resistance to two or more of the first-line antituberculous drugs, usually isoniazid and rifampicin) can be primary (no prior antituberculous therapy) or secondary (development of resistance during or after chemotherapy).

Diagnosis depends upon collection of adequate specimens for culture prior to the initiation of antituberculous therapy. In critically ill patients, rapid diagnosis of drug resistance is of paramount importance. With the improvements in the culture methods and the availability of newer techniques, including phage-based assays, rapid identification of resistance is possible.[15] When resistance is present to two or more first-line agents, parenteral aminoglycoside (streptomycin, amikacin, etc.) and fluoroquinolones are generally added. Specialist microbiological advice should be sought.

TYPHOID FEVER

Typhoid fever is caused by *Salmonella typhi* and less commonly by paratyphi A, B and C. Even non-typhoidal salmonellae have occasionally been isolated.[16] Typhoid fever, common in South and South-East Asia, is almost exclusively caused by fecal–oral spread. In the developed world, cases are either seen in international travellers or occasionally caused by infected food.

CLINICAL FEATURES

The incubation period is 5–21 days. Typhoid presents non-specifically with fever, chills, abdominal pain and constitutional symptoms. Constipation may be more frequent than diarrhoea. Hepatosplenomegaly, erythematous macular rash (30%) and relative bradycardia may be present. Relative bradycardia is not specific for enteric fever but is a useful clue.[17]

COMPLICATIONS

- Shock
- Intestinal perforation
- Gastrointestinal haemorrhage
- Jaundice and encephalopathy[18]
- Neuropsychiatric manifestations

- Septic arthritis, pericarditis, etc.
- Obstetric complications in pregnant women

DIAGNOSIS[19]

Anaemia, leukopenia/leukocytosis and deranged liver function are common. Blood cultures are positive in up to 80% of cases, and are the investigation of choice; 10–15 ml yields higher success than smaller volumes.[20] Though culturing urine, stool, rose spots and duodenal contents is useful, bone marrow culture is the most sensitive, and its yield remains unchanged up to 5 days after commencement of treatment.[21]

Serodiagnosis using Widal tests has limited clinical value. Commercial serological tests such as Typhidot-M and Tubex, which detect IgM antibodies against different *S. typhi* antigens, have a higher sensitivity and specificity.[22] Nested PCR is very promising in the diagnosis of typhoid fever.

TREATMENT[23]

In both uncomplicated and complicated typhoid fever, the treatment of choice is the fluoroquinolones (ciprofloxacin or ofloxacin 15 mg/kg for 5–7 days in uncomplicated and 10–14 days in complicated infections). In fluoroquinolone-resistant cases, azithromycin, cefixime or ceftriaxone can be used. There is some concern in using fluoroquinolones in children as they have been shown to cause cartilage toxicity in immature animals, but this appears largely unfounded in clinical trials.[24,25]

Dexamethasone reduces mortality in severe typhoid fever: delirium, obtundation, stupor, coma, or shock.[26] Ileal perforation, which may occur late, classically in the third week of febrile illness, requires prompt surgical intervention, and segmental resection has been recommended as the procedure of choice.[27,28]

CHOLERA

Cholera is caused by enterotoxin-producing *Vibrio cholerae*.[29] The incubation period varies from 12 hours to several days. The clinical case:infection ratio is about 1:10. It starts abruptly with painless watery diarrhoea associated with vomiting and painful muscle cramps. Vomiting may be the first symptom before diarrhoea.

Stool examination shows neither leukocytes nor erythrocytes. Dark field microscopy examination may reveal rapidly motile, comma-shaped bacilli in fresh stool. Commercial assays detecting O antigen in stool samples, which take less than 5 minutes, are now available and are as sensitive and specific as stool culture. Aggressive rehydration is the mainstay of treatment; very large quantities of fluid may be needed. Adjunctive antimicrobial therapy is effective in shortening the duration of diarrhoea. Single dose doxycycline (300 mg) or single dose ciprofloxacin (1 g) is very effective, but azithromycin has recently been shown to be superior.[30]

LEPTOSPIROSIS

This is caused by *Leptospira interrogans*. It occurs due to exposure to contaminated water. The disease has an incubation period of 7–10 days with a range of 2–20 days. It has two phases: the septicaemic phase and the immune phase. Clinical features include conjunctival suffusion or haemorrhages (useful diagnostic clue), uveitis, severe muscle tenderness, non-oliguric renal failure, hypokalaemia, hepatic dysfunction, pulmonary haemorrhage, ARDS, myocarditis, rhabdomyolysis, thrombocytopenia, DIC, haemorrhage into the skin and internal organs, and digital gangrene. Weil's syndrome is characterised by hepatorenal dysfunction, bleeding diathesis and pulmonary involvement.

Diagnosis is made with isolation of the organism by culture (blood, urine, CSF) or serology using the gold standard microscopic agglutination test (MAT). Both culture and serology should be attempted if available, and local microbiological advice should be sought. Treatment is with penicillin G or ceftriaxone. In penicillin-allergic patients, doxycycline can be used.

DENGUE FEVER

EPIDEMIOLOGY AND PATHOGENESIS

It is estimated 100 million cases of dengue fever and 250 000 cases of dengue haemorrhagic fever occur each year throughout the world.[31] The causative agent is a flavivirus with four distinct serogroups, and it is transmitted by the bite of Aedes mosquitoes. Two patterns of transmission have been recognised: epidemic due to isolated introduction of dengue to a region, usually due to a single serotype, and hyperendemic, referring to the continuous circulation of multiple dengue virus serotypes.

Following a mosquito bite, viraemia begins and usually lasts up to 7 days. Infection with one of the four serotypes (primary infection) provides life-long immunity against that serotype but not against the other serotypes (secondary infection). Epidemiological studies have suggested that the risk of severe disease (dengue haemorrhagic fever/dengue shock syndrome) is significantly higher in secondary than primary infection.

CLINICAL FEATURES

The clinical presentation varies from mild febrile illness to severe haemorrhagic fever. Most infections are asymptomatic. WHO classifies dengue infection as undifferentiated fever, dengue fever (DF) and dengue haemorrhagic fever (DHF)/dengue shock syndrome (DSS).

Dengue fever has an incubation period of 3–14 days and is characterised by the sudden onset of fever, severe headache, retro-orbital pain on moving the eyes, and fatigue. It is often associated with severe myalgia and arthralgia (breakbone fever). Maculopapular rash, flushed facies and injected conjunctiva are common. Haemorrhagic manifestations can occur in DF and should not be confused with DHF.

Dengue haemorrhagic fever occurs primarily in children < 10 years and is characterised by plasma leakage syndrome and haemoconcentration (20% or greater rise in haematocrit), pleural effusion or ascites. The diagnosis is made if the following symptoms and signs are present: bleeding, a platelet count < 100000 per mm^3 and plasma leakage. Haemorrhagic manifestations without evidence of plasma leakage do not constitute DHF. The mechanism underlying the profound capillary leak in DHF but not in DF is poorly understood. It is important to watch for the onset of DHF which typically occurs 4–7 days after the onset of the disease, approximately at the time of defervescence. Decrease in platelet count and rise in haematocrit are useful clues.[32]

Dengue shock syndrome is characterised by profound hypotension and shock.

DIAGNOSIS

Dengue should be suspected in all febrile patients who live in, or have returned from, endemic areas in the preceding 2 weeks. Leukopenia, thrombocytopenia with a positive tourniquet test, and raised AST are frequently seen; the former two tests have the highest sensitivity (about 90%) for the diagnosis of early dengue.[32] A positive tourniquet test cannot differentiate DHF from DF.

IgM immunoassay allows rapid confirmation of the diagnosis. If it is negative, particularly in the first 6 days of the illness, the diagnosis should not be ruled out. Acute and convalescent sera should be analysed by haemagglutination assay or IgG immunoassay for a fourfold rise in titre. Virus isolation and reverse transcriptase PCR (RT-PCR) are available but are usually not used in the clinical setting.

TREATMENT

Supportive therapy for shock, especially appropriate and prompt fluid replacement, can reduce mortality. WHO guidelines on fluid management are available.[33] In DSS, steroids have not been shown to be useful.[34] Once capillary leakage abates, fluid overload and pulmonary oedema can become problematic.

HANTA VIRUS

Hantaviruses are rodent viruses distributed worldwide, with over 150000 cases being registered annually. There are two major clinical syndromes: hantavirus cardiopulmonary syndrome (HCPS) and haemorrhagic fever with renal syndrome (HFRS). Both are acquired by exposure to aerosols of rodent excreta.

HANTAVIRUS CARDIOPULMONARY SYNDROME

The incubation period is about 3 weeks. There are two phases: the prodromal phase is characterised by a relatively mild febrile illness, typically lasting 3–5 days, and the cardiopulmonary phase is characterised by severe, rapidly progressive respiratory failure. In the latter phase, acute pulmonary oedema due to increased capillary permeability occurs. Progress from the prodromal to cardiopulmonary phase is dramatic. In severe cases, significant myocardial depression also occurs, resulting in low cardiac output and hypotension. Acute renal failure can occur. The combination of thrombocytopenia, myelocytosis, haemoconcentration, lack of significant toxic granulation in neutrophils, and more than 10% of lymphocytes with immunoblastic morphological features is highly sensitive and specific. Enzyme-linked immunosorbent assay (ELISA) for IgM and IgG antibodies is useful in the diagnosis. Hantavirus can also be detected by tissue RT-PCR. Immunohistochemical staining of tissue reveals hantaviral antigen. Treatment is mainly supportive with intravenous fluids, inotropes, mechanical ventilation, extracorporeal membrane oxygenation and blood products. Intravenous ribavirin is probably ineffective in the treatment of HCPS in the cardiopulmonary stage.[35]

HAEMORRHAGIC FEVER WITH RENAL SYNDROME

This is characterised by fever, renal failure and haemorrhagic manifestations. The disease has five progressive stages: febrile, hypotensive, oliguric, diuretic, and convalescent. Non-specific constitutional symptoms are followed by shock, oliguria, DIC and haemorrhagic manifestations. Diagnosis is made using ELISA for IgG and IGM antibodies. Treatment is supportive, including renal support. Ribavirin has been found to be useful.[36]

ARBOVIRAL ENCEPHALITIS

Viruses transmitted to human beings by the bites of arthropods (especially mosquitoes and ticks) are major causes of encephalitis worldwide. Although different viruses can cause encephalitis, an antigenically related group of flaviviruses accounts for a major proportion of cases. These include mosquito-borne diseases such as Japanese encephalitis, West Nile virus encephalitis, St Louis encephalitis, Murray Valley encephalitis[37] and tick-borne encephalitis. Viral encephalitis is characterised by a triad of fever, headache and altered level of consciousness. Other common clinical findings include disorientation, behavioural and speech disturbances, and focal or diffuse neurological signs such as hemiparesis or seizures. The incubation period is usually 5–15 days. Other manifestations include recurrent seizures, including status epilepticus, a flaccid paralysis resembling that of poliomyelitis, and parkinsonian-type movement disorders. Flavivirus encephalitis is usually diagnosed by IgM capture ELISA.

Treatment is supportive. Interferon-α, ribavirin and intravenous immunoglobulin have all been tried with mixed success.

VIRAL HAEMORRHAGIC FEVERS (VHF)

EPIDEMIOLOGY

Lassa virus, Rift valley fever, Congo–Crimean haemorrhagic fever, haemorrhagic fever with renal syndrome, Marburg and Ebola viruses, yellow fever and dengue haemorrhagic fever are some of the most important viral haemorrhagic fevers. Increased vascular permeability is the primary defect. Petechial haemorrhages are usually associated with fever and myalgias. Later, frank mucous membrane haemorrhage may occur, with accompanying hypotension, shock and circulatory collapse. Multisystem organ failure can occur. There is a wide variation in the relative severity of the clinical presentation.

At least four of the haemorrhagic fevers – Lassa fever (LF), Ebola virus, Marburg virus and Congo–Crimean haemorrhagic fever (CCHF) – are capable of person-to-person transmission through close contact with infected blood and other body secretions. Epidemiological studies of VHF in humans indicate that, although possible, the airborne route does not readily transmit infection from person to person.

CLINICAL FEATURES

The patient will have either been in an endemic area or been in contact with someone from an endemic area. Viral haemorrhagic fevers[38] generally have an abrupt onset with an incubation period < 10 days. The incubation period can be up to 21 days. They present as acute febrile illnesses with a prodrome that often includes severe headache, dizziness, flushing, conjunctival injection, myalgia, lumbar pain and prostration. Gastrointestinal symptoms with nausea, vomiting, abdominal pain and diarrhoea may occur.

Leukopenia or leukocytosis, thrombocytopenia and elevated serum aminotransferases may be evident early in the disease; a petechial rash may appear on days 3–10. Coagulation profiles become progressively more abnormal, and overt haemorrhagic features of the disease (ecchymoses, epistaxis, gingival bleeding, melaena, haematuria, etc.) may supervene from day 5 onward, or sometimes even earlier. Multiple organ failure supervenes and death may ensue. Clinical improvement becomes apparent towards the end of the second week of illness in patients who survive.

DIAGNOSIS

A high index of suspicion is needed and VHF should be suspected in the following circumstances:

- Unexplained fever in patients who have visited areas where VHF are endemic, within 3 weeks of becoming ill. The likelihood is greater if they have camped in the bush, slept on the ground or in rural farms, or had any bites or contact with sick animals.
- Febrile medical and nursing staff in the endemic areas and laboratory workers who handle VHF viruses.
- Febrile contacts.

Tests on samples present an extreme biohazard risk. The diagnosis may be made by isolating virus from blood or body fluids, positive IgM antibody or by showing a fourfold rise in antibody titre. Detection of characteristic virions by electron microscopy establishes the diagnosis of Marburg and Ebola viruses. If needed for infection control, electron microscopy of tissues (especially liver) at autopsy is confirmatory.

TREATMENT

Therapy is essentially supportive for a severe shock state. Haemorrhage is managed by replacement of blood, platelets and clotting factors as indicated. Ribavirin is useful in treating LF and CCHF. Ribavirin may reduce mortality by 10-fold if treatment is begun within 6 days of onset. A 30 mg/kg i.v. loading dose is followed by 15 mg/kg every 6 hours for 4 days and then 7.5 mg/kg every 8 hours for another 6 days.

PRECAUTIONS

In most countries these diseases must be notified immediately. In addition to universal blood and body fluid precautions, airborne isolation, including use of goggles, high-efficiency masks, a negative pressure room with no air circulation, and positive pressure filtered air respirators have all been recommended, as is surveillance of contacts. If applicable, to prevent further mosquito transmission, patients should be isolated in well-screened rooms sprayed with residual insecticides.

REFERENCES

1. WHO. *Management of Severe Malaria. A Practical Handbook*, 2nd edn. Geneva: WHO; 2000.
2. Idro R, Jenkins NE, Newton CJRC. Pathogenesis, clinical features, and neurological outcome of cerebral malaria. *Lancet Neurol* 2005; **4**: 827–40.
3. WHO. *Guidelines for the Treatment of Malaria*. Geneva: WHO; 2006. www.who.int/malaria/docs/Treatment Guidelines2006.pdf.
4. Adjuik M, Babiker A, Garner P *et al.* Artesunate combinations for treatment of malaria: meta-analysis. *Lancet* 2004; **363**: 9–17.
5. Dondorp A, Nosten F, Stepniewska K *et al.* Artesunate versus quinine for treatment of severe falciparum malaria: a randomised trial. *Lancet* 2005; **366**: 717–25.
6. Laniado-Laborin R. Adenosine deaminase in the diagnosis of tuberculous pleural effusion: is it really an ideal test? A word of caution. *Chest* 2005; **127**: 417–18.

7. Moon JW, Chang YS, Kim SK *et al.* The clinical utility of polymerase chain reaction for the diagnosis of pleural tuberculosis. *Clin Infect Dis* 2005; **41**: 660–6.
8. Thwaites GE, Tran TH. Tuberculous meningitis: many questions, few answers. *Lancet Neurol* 2005; **4**: 160–70.
9. Kumar R, Sing SN, Kohli N. A diagnostic rule for tuberculous meningitis. *Arch Dis Child* 1999; **81**: 221–4.
10. Thwaites GE, Chau TT, Stepniewska K *et al.* Diagnosis of adult tuberculous meningitis by use of clinical and laboratory features. *Lancet* 2002; **360**: 1287–92.
11. Kent SJ, Crowe SM, Yung A *et al.* Tuberculous meningitis: a 30 year review. *Clin Infect Dis* 1993; **17**: 987–94.
12. Pai M, Flores LL, Pai N *et al.* Diagnostic accuracy of nucleic acid amplification tests for tuberculous meningitis: a systematic review and meta-analysis. *Lancet Infect Dis* 2003; **3**: 633–43.
13. Prasad K, Volmink J, Menon GR. Steroids for treating tuberculous meningitis. *Cochrane Database Syst Rev* 2000; (3): CD002244.
14. Thwaites GE, Nguyen DB, Nguyen HD *et al.* Dexamethasone for the treatment of tuberculous meningitis in adolescents and adults. *N Engl J Med* 2004; **351**: 1741–51.
15. Nahid P, Pai M, Hopewell PC. Advances in the diagnosis and treatment of tuberculosis. *Proc Am Thorac Soc* 2006; **3**: 103–10.
16. Obeogbulam SI, Oguike JU, Gugnani HC. Microbiological studies on cases diagnosed as typhoid/enteric fever in Nigeria. *J Commun Dis* 1997; **27**: 97–100.
17. Ostergaard L, Huniche B, Anderson PL. Relative bradycardia in infectious diseases. *J Infect* 1996; **33**: 185–91.
18. Kamath PS, Jalihal A, Chakraborty A. Differentiation of typhoid fever from fulminant hepatic failure in patients presenting with jaundice and encephalopathy. *Mayo Clin Proc* 2000; **75**: 462–6.
19. Bhutta ZA. Current concepts in the diagnosis and treatment of typhoid fever. *BMJ* 2006; **333**:78–82.
20. Bhan MK, Bahl R, Bhatnagar S. Typhoid and paratyphoid fever. *Lancet* 2005; **366**: 749–62.
21. Gasem MH, Dolmans WM, Isbandri BB *et al.* Culture of *Salmonella typhi* and paratyphi in blood and bone marrow in suspected typhoid fever. *Trop Geogr Med* 1995; **47**: 164–7.
22. Olsen SJ, Pruckler J, Bibb W *et al.* Evaluation of rapid diagnostic tests for typhoid fever. *J Clin Microbiol* 2004; **42**: 1885–9.
23. WHO. *The Diagnosis, Treatment, and Prevention of Typhoid Fever.* Geneva: WHO, 2003. http://www.who.int/vaccine_research/documents/en/typhoid_diagnosis.pdf .
24. Bethell DB, Hien TT, Phi LT *et al.* The effects on growth of single short courses of fluoroquinolones. *Arch Dis Child* 1996; **74**: 44–6.
25. Doherty CP, Saha SK, Cutting WA. Typhoid fever, ciprofloxacin and growth in young children. *Ann Trop Paediatr* 2000; **20**: 297–303.
26. Hoffman SL, Punjabi NH, Kumala S *et al.* Reduction of mortality in chloramphenicol-treated severe typhoid fever by high-dose dexamethasone. *N Engl J Med* 1984; **310**: 82–8.
27. Ameh EA, Dogo PM, Attah MM *et al.* Comparison of three operations for typhoid perforation. *Br J Surg* 1997; **84**: 558–9.
28. Shah AA, Wani KA, Wazir BS. The ideal treatment of the typhoid enteric perforation – resection anastomosis. *Int Surg* 1999; **84**: 35–8.
29. Sack DA, Sack RB, Nair GB *et al.* Cholera. *Lancet* 2004; **363**: 223–33.
30. Saha D, Karim MM, Khan WA *et al.* Single-dose azithromycin for the treatment of cholera in adults. *N Engl J Med* 2006; **354**: 2452–62.
31. Gubler DJ. Dengue and dengue haemorrhagic fever. *Clin Microbiol Rev* 1998; **11**: 480–96.
32. Wilder-Smith A, Schwartz E. Dengue in travelers. *N Engl J Med* 2005; **353**: 924–32.
33. WHO. *Dengue.* Geneva: WHO; 1997. http://www.who.int/csr/resources/publications/dengue/024-33.pdf.
34. Panpanich R, Sornchai P, Kanjanaratanakorn K. Corticosteroids for treating dengue shock syndrome. *Cochrane Database Syst Rev* 2006; **3**: CD003488.
35. Mertz GJ, Miedzinski L, Goade D *et al.* Placebo-controlled, double-blind trial of intravenous ribavirin for the treatment of hantavirus cardiopulmonary syndrome in North America. *Clin Infect Dis* 2004; **39**: 1307–13.
36. Huggins JW, Hsiang CM, Cosgriff TM *et al.* Prospective, double blind, concurrent, placebo-controlled clinical trial of intravenous ribavirin therapy of haemorrhagic fever with renal syndrome. *J Infect Dis* 1991; **164**: 1119–27.
37. Solomon T. Flavivirus encephalitis. *N Engl J Med* 2004; **351**: 370–8.
38. Richards GA, Murphy S, Jobson R *et al.* Unexpected Ebola virus in a tertiary setting: clinical and epidemiologic aspects. *Crit Care Med* 2000; **28**: 240–4.

Part Eleven

Severe and Multiple Trauma

66

Severe and multiple trauma

James A Judson

Trauma can be defined as physical injury from mechanical energy. It is usually categorised as blunt or penetrating. In Western countries, severe blunt trauma is common, caused by road crashes, falls and, less frequently, blows and assault. Severe penetrating trauma, usually from stabbings and gunshots, is less common except in larger cities of the USA,[1,2] South Africa and war zones. Blunt trauma is often more difficult to treat than penetrating trauma. Assessment is more difficult, because injuries are frequently internal, multiple and not obvious initially. The risk of missing serious injuries can only be lessened by a systematic approach and repeated assessments.[3–5]

ASSESSMENT AND PRIORITIES

TRIAGE

An important first step is triage – sorting patients with acute life-threatening injuries and complications from those whose lives are not in danger. The severity of total body injury is related to the number of separate injuries present, and to the severity of individual injuries. Assessment can be made either at the scene of injury or on arrival at hospital. As in any emergency, assessment, diagnosis and treatment need to be concurrent. There is limited time for detailed histories, examinations, investigations or well-considered diagnoses before starting emergency care. Most patients with severe injury can be distinguished early by the following:

- *Depressed consciousness* in the trauma patient can be related to brain injury, hypoxaemia, shock, alcohol or other ingested drugs, or precipitating neurological or cardiac events. Frequently, a combination of factors is present, and the precise extent of physical brain injury is not known initially. Initial treatment in any case is determined by the level of consciousness rather than its exact cause.
- *Breathing difficulties* are common in patients with trauma to the head, face, neck and chest. If rapid or distressed breathing is present, airway obstruction, laryngeal injury, pulmonary aspiration and lung or chest wall injury (especially pneumothorax and lung contusion) must be considered.
- *Shock* is almost always hypovolaemic from blood loss, but other types of shock occasionally occur in trauma (see below).

PRIORITIES

A trauma patient often has multiple problems requiring attention. Determining priorities is not always easy. In general, the priorities are to:

- *Support life*: the patient is kept alive with resuscitative techniques, while the various injuries and complications are attended to
- *Locate and control bleeding*, which may be varied (see below)
- *Prevent brainstem compression* and spinal cord damage
- Diagnose and treat all other injuries and complications

BASIC TREATMENT PRINCIPLES

A systematic approach to managing severe and multiple trauma is important. Effective programmes developed by the American College of Surgeons are now well established.[6] A number of basic treatment principles apply to all severe trauma patients.

EMERGENCY ASSESSMENT (PRIMARY SURVEY)

The following must be recognised and treated before anything else:

- *A – Airway obstruction*: suggested by noisy (or silent) breathing, with paradoxical chest movements and breathing distress, and inadequate airway protection from impaired gag reflexes in patients with depressed consciousness.
- *B – Breathing difficulty*: suggested by tachypnoea, abnormal pattern of breathing, cyanosis or mental confusion.
- *C – Circulatory shock*: manifested by cold peripheries with delayed capillary refill, rapid weak pulse or low blood pressure (see below).

OXYGEN AND VENTILATORY THERAPY

High-flow oxygen by mask is given to all trauma patients. However, patients with severe trauma frequently require ventilatory support. A restless uncooperative patient should be intubated under a rapid sequence induction to facilitate resuscitation.

BLOOD CROSSMATCH AND TESTS

Six units of red cells should be crossmatched urgently, but it is impossible to predict the amount of blood that will be required. Blood is concurrently sent for baseline haematological and biochemical tests, including blood ethanol level. Blood ethanol is clinically useful in assessing individual patients with depressed consciousness, quite apart from epidemiological and preventive medicine,[7] and legal considerations.

FLUID RESUSCITATION

Resuscitation fluids are given (see below). If necessary, two or three large 14- or 16-gauge i.v. cannulae are inserted in upper limb, external jugular or femoral veins.

ANALGESIA

Analgesia is easily overlooked. Opioid agents should be titrated i.v., and not given i.m. or subcutaneously. Large doses may be needed.

URINE OUTPUT

A urinary catheter is inserted unless a ruptured urethra is suspected (because of blood at the urinary meatus, severe fractured pelvis or abnormal prostate position on rectal examination), in which case a suprapubic catheter is indicated. Urine output monitoring is an important guide to resuscitation.

OTHER INJURIES

All injuries should be evaluated.

CLINICAL EVALUATION OF INJURIES (SECONDARY SURVEY)

Injuries are easily missed in an emergency, especially when one injury is obvious. A secondary, and even a tertiary, survey should be performed.[5] The back and the front of the patient should be examined. Special attention is paid to regions with external lacerations, contusions and abrasions. All body regions are examined systematically.

HEAD

Neurological observations are made. The ears and nose are inspected for cerebrospinal fluid and blood, and the scalp is examined thoroughly.

FACE

Bleeding into the airway should be excluded, and the face and jaws tested for abnormal mobility.

SPINE

A cervical spine fracture or dislocation is assumed in all patients with depressed consciousness until proved otherwise. Signs of spinal cord injury should be sought (e.g. warm dilated peripheries from loss of vasomotor tone, diaphragmatic breathing, paralysis, priapism and loss of anal tone). The thoracic and lumbar spine should be inspected and palpated.

THORAX

Fractured ribs in themselves are not usually life-threatening but haemothorax, pneumothorax, lung contusion and chest wall instability (flail chest) will require attention if present. Less common but very serious injuries can occur to the heart and great vessels (see Chapter 69).

ABDOMEN

The spleen, liver and mesenteries are often damaged. Retroperitoneal haemorrhage is common. Injuries to the pancreas, duodenum and other hollow viscera are less frequent, and may be missed until signs of peritonitis occur. Renal injury with retroperitoneal haemorrhage is suggested by haematuria and loin pain (see Chapter 71).

PELVIS

Pelvic fractures may be difficult to detect clinically, especially in the unconscious patient. Blood loss may be massive, particularly with posterior fractures involving sacroiliac dislocation. Ruptured bladder and ruptured urethra may occur with anterior fractures.

EXTREMITIES

A litre or more of blood may be lost into a fractured femur. Long bone fractures are more serious when they are open, comminuted or displaced, or if associated with nerve or arterial damage.

EXTERNAL

Contusions may be extensive and serious, especially in falls from heights, and may be overlooked if the victim's back is not examined. Road crash victims may sustain serious burns or abrasions.

SHOCK IN THE TRAUMA PATIENT

The earliest, most constant and reliable signs of shock are seen in the peripheral circulation. A patient with cold, pale peripheries has shock until proved otherwise. Tachycardia is not always present and hypotension is a late sign of shock. The commonest form of shock in trauma is hypovolaemic shock.

HYPOVOLAEMIC SHOCK

If the neck veins are empty, hypovolaemic shock should be inferred. Possible sites of blood loss causing shock are:

- *External loss*, which is obvious clinically from blood-soaked clothing and pooled blood.
- *Major fractures*, which are obvious clinically by deformity, swelling, crepitus, pain and tenderness (e.g. femurs) or seen on a plain X-ray (e.g. pelvis).
- *Pleural cavity*, detected on urgent chest X-ray. Intrapleural drains will reveal the amount and rate of blood loss.
- *Peritoneal cavity*, detected by laparotomy, diagnostic peritoneal lavage, computed tomography (CT) scan or ultrasound. Clinical examination of the abdomen can be misleading when the patient is intoxicated, has depressed consciousness or has multiple injuries. A single clinical examination is of limited value: changes over time are more important.
- *Retroperitoneum*, detected at laparotomy or by CT scan, or inferred when all the above are negative, especially in the presence of pelvic or lumbar spine fracture.

CARDIOGENIC SHOCK

If the trauma patient with shock has distended neck veins, possible causes are tension pneumothorax, concurrent myocardial infarction, cardiac tamponade or myocardial contusion.

NEUROLOGICAL SHOCK

Patients with paraplegia or tetraplegia from spinal cord injury may have low blood pressure with warm dilated peripheries accompanied by lax anal tone and by priapism in the male (see Chapter 70). This is a diagnosis of exclusion and all causes of hypovolaemic shock (see above) must be sought.

SEPTIC SHOCK

Occasionally, patients with pulmonary aspiration may develop septic shock. This is unlikely to confuse the initial trauma assessment soon after injury, but may require consideration some hours or a day or two later.

ABDOMINAL ULTRASOUND

Technological advances in ultrasound scanning and the increasing availability of FAST (focused assessment with sonography for trauma) scanning in emergency departments make this modality attractive in trauma, and it is becoming increasingly used. However:

- It is operator-dependent
- It may have an unacceptably high false-negative rate
- There is a small but important false-positive rate for intra-abdominal bleeding[8]
- It is unable to diagnose ruptured bowel
- It is not good for bleeding in the pelvis

Its main usefulness is probably in the unstable patient when it is positive, to indicate the need for laparotomy without the necessity to proceed to diagnostic peritoneal lavage (DPL).[9] FAST scans performed by enthusiastic amateurs in emergency departments without a treatment algorithm can be misleading and therefore worse than useless.

DIAGNOSTIC PERITONEAL LAVAGE

Diagnostic peritoneal lavage is indicated to diagnose intra-abdominal bleeding

- In shocked patients who are not proceeding straight to laparotomy
- In patients without shock when repeated clinical examination of the abdomen for 6 hours is not possible because of sedation or anaesthesia

Caution is needed with pregnancy, previous abdominal surgery or massive pelvic injury. Isotonic saline 1 l (or 10 ml/kg) is instilled into the peritoneal cavity, after drainage of the stomach and bladder. The presence of more than 10 ml frank blood on catheter aspiration necessitates immediate laparotomy; otherwise a lavage fluid specimen should be examined for red and white cell counts and amylase concentration. A red cell count over 100 000 per mm^3, white cell count over 500 per mm^3, or an increased amylase concentration suggests bleeding or viscus injury, and laparotomy should be undertaken immediately. These absolute figures are debatable and lower values are accepted in penetrating trauma.[6,10] Peritoneal lavages inevitably result in some false-positive laparotomies. However, in severe trauma, morbidity of a non-therapeutic laparotomy (i.e. no definitive surgery) is small compared with the dire consequences of missing significant intra-abdominal injury.[11]

CT ABDOMEN

Abdominal CT is not indicated in shock, but can be useful in the stable patient. Improved availability of CT scanning, and technological advances with reduced scanning times and better definition, is increasingly favouring CT abdomen over DPL in patients who are sufficiently stable to tolerate the procedure safely. It needs to be performed quickly and safely, with gastric and i.v. contrast, and interpreted by radiologists experienced in trauma. Visualisation of abdominal and pelvic organs and haemorrhage is excellent,[12,13] but results can be misleading and disastrous with poor technique.[4]

FLUID RESUSCITATION

FLUIDS

Almost all patients who are hypotensive or noticeably vasoconstricted will need blood transfusion. However, as cross-matched blood is not immediately available, other fluids are used first. Uncrossmatched group O Rh-negative blood is occasionally indicated in the exsanguinating patient, but in general transfusion of large quantities of blood is wasteful while bleeding is uncontrolled. The place of hypertonic fluids in trauma resuscitation is unresolved.

Isotonic saline or a balanced salt solution should be the first fluid infused. Shocked patients may need 2–3 l in the first few minutes. One litre bags or bottles and giving sets with in-line pumps should be used on all i.v. lines. If fluid resuscitation is likely to be extensive, warmed fluids and rapid infusion devices should be used. Albumin solutions (and probably other colloid resuscitation fluids) are contraindicated in trauma patients, since the SAFE study, conducted in ICU patients, showed higher mortality in patients given albumin, in the predetermined trauma subgroup, particularly in those with traumatic brain injury.[14] By 20–30 minutes crossmatched red cells should be available. Platelets and fresh frozen plasma are reserved for documented or suspected coagulopathy (i.e. dilutional coagulopathy from fluids deficient in haemostatic factors, and disseminated intravascular coagulopathy (DIC) from prolonged shock).

All resuscitation fluids have a high sodium concentration, similar to that of extracellular fluid. Glucose 5% and glucose–saline solutions are not effective resuscitation fluids. Few trauma patients actually require them in the first day.

LIMITED FLUID RESUSCITATION

In penetrating trauma, there is some evidence that extensive fluid resuscitation prior to haemostasis may be detrimental, presumably because of higher blood pressure, displacement of blood clot and dilution of coagulation factors.[15]

In blunt trauma, there is no such evidence. Furthermore, it is not appropriate to generalise the evidence from penetrating trauma to blunt trauma because these two types of trauma are quite different. In penetrating trauma, the bleeding is often from single arteries without extensive tissue injury, and complete haemostasis can often be easily achieved.

In contrast, in blunt trauma, the bleeding is often venous as well as arterial, with capillary oozing into the soft tissues which may continue for hours. It can often not be controlled, or can be only partly controlled, by operative surgery, interventional radiology or reduction and fixation of fractures. Accordingly, fluid resuscitation in the face of continuing blood loss is an important part of the treatment of circulatory shock in blunt trauma (see section on Inadequate resuscitation). Nevertheless, fluid resuscitation is not an alternative to haemostasis and must not be used as an excuse for delaying haemostasis in blunt trauma.

Furthermore, traumatic brain injury is often present in blunt trauma, which frequently involves several body regions. Hypotension is disastrous to an already injured brain, and must not be prolonged by deliberate under-resuscitation (see Chapter 67, section on Traumatic brain injury – Emergency treatment).[16–18]

URINE OUTPUT

Hourly urine output is a useful guide to resuscitation from shock. Minimal acceptable urine output is 0.5 ml/kg per hour, but 1–2 ml/kg per hour is more adequate. Furosemide has no place in initial resuscitation. Apart from adequate resuscitation, diuresis can be due to ethanol, mannitol, dopamine, nephrogenic or neurogenic diabetes insipidus, or non-oliguric renal failure. Polyuria may mask early recognition of acute renal failure.

INADEQUATE RESUSCITATION

Patients in shock have depleted interstitial fluid as well as circulating blood volume, and need trauma resuscitation fluid volumes greater than the actual volume of blood lost. With blunt injury, volume losses often continue for 24–48 hours. Prolonged shock from delayed and inadequate resuscitation leads to renal failure, acute respiratory distress syndrome (ARDS), sepsis, DIC and multiple organ dysfunction.[19,20]

PULMONARY OEDEMA

Pulmonary oedema during resuscitation may be related to fluid overload, direct lung trauma, aspiration of gastric contents, pulmonary responses to non-thoracic trauma and reactions to resuscitation fluids. They can all cause leaky capillaries and produce non-cardiogenic pulmonary oedema.

RADIOLOGY FOR TRAUMA PATIENTS

Patients with depressed consciousness, breathing difficulties or unstable circulation should be X-rayed in the emergency department, and not sent to a radiology department remote from skilled resuscitation facilities. Conversely, extensive imaging examinations of shocked patients in the emergency department are unacceptable. Only three examinations should be requested in the emergency department.

CHEST

This is the only X-ray ever justified in an unresuscitated patient. A supine film is usually sufficient. An erect film is better for showing intrapleural air or fluid, ruptured diaphragm, free abdominal gas and for defining an abnormal mediastinum, but is often impractical in shock or suspected spinal injury. It can be done later if feasible. An obvious pneumothorax does not require a chest X-ray before insertion of an intercostal drain.

LATERAL CERVICAL SPINE

This should be performed in all patients with head injury or multiple injuries because cervical spine fractures are often missed. With head or facial injuries, a cervical fracture should be assumed initially and a cervical collar applied. The lateral cervical spine X-ray can be taken later. It is only an initial screening examination for cervical spine fractures and does not 'clear' the spine.

PELVIS

Unexplained blood loss can be due to a missed pelvic fracture. A dislocated hip can be missed in multiple injuries. A pelvic X-ray is not needed in awake patients with no pelvic abnormalities.

OTHER RADIOLOGICAL INVESTIGATIONS

Other X-rays should be performed after adequate resuscitation in the radiology department, operating room or intensive care unit (ICU):

- *Skull*: plain skull X-rays do not guide immediate treatment. A CT scan of the brain is a more useful urgent investigation.
- *Extremities*: X-rays of the extremities to assess bony injuries are not urgent unless there is vascular injury. Therefore, these films should not be taken in the emergency department for diagnosis, unless the patient is going directly to the operating room for fracture fixation.
- *Spine*: X-rays of thoracic or lumbosacral spine are seldom indicated in the emergency department.
- *Abdomen*: a plain abdominal X-ray is of limited value in the initial evaluation of trauma.
- *CT abdomen*: this can be valuable to evaluate a patient who is haemodynamically sufficiently stable to tolerate the procedure safely (see above).
- *CT head*: this is vital in the treatment of traumatic brain injuries.
- *CT neck*: The most reliable way to exclude or delineate cervical spine injuries is by a CT neck scan,[4,21] which can conveniently be done when the patient is going to the CT scanner for other examinations.
- *CT thorax*: apart from diagnosis of aortic injury, CT thorax is of limited value in the trauma patient. Visualisation of thoracic structures is excellent but it seldom discovers important undiagnosed injuries which affect patient treatment.[22] If aortic injury is suspected, multislice CT is the current definitive diagnostic test. The use of aortic stent grafts for this injury, in locations where this technology is available, means that CT is not only the best diagnostic test, but necessary for preoperative planning.[23] Aortography is no longer the definitive diagnostic test for traumatic aortic rupture.
- *Urethrography* is used when urethral injury is suspected. Properly done CT abdomen may well demonstrate bladder injury, otherwise *cystography* is used.
- *Interventional radiology*: percutaneous transcatheter embolisation is therapeutic rather than diagnostic. It can provide life-saving haemostasis in massive retroperitoneal haemorrhage associated with pelvic fracture.[24] The logistics of managing such haemodynamically unstable patients in the radiology department are formidable.

THE EXSANGUINATING PATIENT

With exsanguination secondary to penetrating thoracic injury, there is a place for Emergency Room thoracotomy, but this approach has little place in blunt trauma.[25] The exsanguinating blunt trauma patient needs rapid intubation, volume resuscitation, bilateral intrapleural drains or thoracostomies, chest and pelvic X-ray, and a rapid trip to the operating room if it seems likely that the bleeding is in the thorax or abdomen.

TRAUMATIC BRAIN INJURY (SEE CHAPTER 67)

Injuries to the head region are common, but those requiring urgent cranial operations are less so. Traumatic brain injury may initially be obvious amongst multiple injuries, but may not be the most important injury. Conversely, traumatic brain injury may seem unimportant initially. Traumatic brain injury is a major determinant of outcome in critically injured patients.

EMERGENCY TREATMENT

Resuscitation measures, as in the Emergency assessment (primary survey) section above, are undertaken. Victims with one or both dilated unreactive pupils, or a rapidly deteriorating level of consciousness not due to hypoxia or shock, should be given mannitol 1 g/kg i.v. to relieve brainstem compression, until definitive diagnosis and treatment can be arranged. Mannitol should be given only if the patient has been adequately volume resuscitated as it may add to hypovolaemia. There is much interest in hypertonic saline, particularly in head trauma, and concentrated salt may eventually turn out to be a better agent than mannitol in this setting because it does not produce hypovolaemia.[26,27]

Shocked trauma patients with or without traumatic brain injuries require the same crystalloid resuscitation fluids. Treatment of shock and maintenance of cerebral perfusion are vital, as hypotension is disastrous to an already damaged brain.[16–18] Contrary to common belief, sodium-containing fluids are not inherently dangerous in traumatic brain injury. However, after adequate resuscitation, further sodium administration is usually not indicated. Excessive (free) water is potentially dangerous, as it can lead to hypo-osmolar brain swelling.[28]

NEUROLOGICAL EVALUATION

Factors such as hypoxaemia, shock, alcohol, analgesics, anaesthetic agents, muscle relaxants and other drugs depress consciousness and confound neurological signs. Clinical neurological evaluation includes the Glasgow Coma Scale (GCS)[29,30] and a search for lateralising signs.

CT scanning is indicated in all patients who will not obey verbal commands, especially if they are rendered neurologically inaccessible by sedative and relaxant agents. Lateralising motor or pupillary signs with a deteriorating level of consciousness are indications for immediate CT scanning (or, if unavailable, emergency burr holes). In an unstable patient, a laparotomy for intra-abdominal haemorrhage should take priority over a head CT scan.[31]

SEVERITY AND MORBIDITY OF TRAUMA

Severity of injury is measured by the abbreviated injury scale (AIS), updated over the years, most recently in 2005.[32–34] AIS divides the body into six regions: head and neck, face, thorax, abdomen, pelvis and extremities, and external. Specific injuries in each body region are coded on a scale of 1 (minor), 2 (moderate), 3 (serious, not life-threatening), 4 (severe, life-threatening, survival probable), 5 (critical, survival uncertain) and 6 (unsurvivable). The AIS was designed for motor vehicle injuries, but has been validated for blunt and penetrating trauma. It can provide a basis for research, education, audit and allocation of resources.

Severity of trauma is related not just to the severity of individual injuries, but also to the combined effects of multiple injuries. Multiple injuries are graded by the injury severity score (ISS), which is an empirical system based on the AIS grades for the three worst body regions.[35,36] ISS gives a score between 0 and 75 for total body injury; 16 or more indicates major trauma. Death with an ISS below 24 should be rare. Above an ISS of 25, there is a stepwise increase in mortality, with very high rates over 50.[37,38]

AIS and ISS study mostly the anatomy of injury. Other factors influence trauma mortality and morbidity, including age, pre-existing health, degree of physiological derangement, standard of prehospital and early hospital care and complications. Degree of physiological derangement can be measured by the revised trauma score,[39] which is computed from the coded values of GCS, systolic blood pressure and respiratory rate, usually at admission to the emergency department. The TRISS severity index is based on the revised trauma score, ISS, and patient age.[40] It correlates well with outcome, and has been used to compile survival norms for blunt and penetrating trauma.[37,38] Physiological scoring systems such as APACHE (acute physiology, age and chronic health evaluation) do not work well for trauma patients (see Chapter 3).[41,42] Preinjury illness (comorbidity) has a profound effect on trauma outcome.[43]

Shock influences trauma mortality and morbidity. The 'golden hour' is a catchy concept based on the observation that the longer the patient is in shock, the higher the probability of immediate or delayed complications. However, the specific timeframe of an hour has no real validity. Complications of shock include renal failure, acute respiratory distress syndrome, sepsis, liver failure and multiorgan dysfunction.[19,20,44] Acute oliguric renal failure on the first day after trauma is now rare, but non-oliguric renal failure is often seen 2–4 days later, caused by the shock and delayed or inadequate resuscitation. It is often heralded by polyuria, which is misinterpreted as a sign of adequate resuscitation.

EPIDEMIOLOGY OF INJURIES

Only a minority of victims of severe trauma reach hospital alive.[45,46] The majority of deaths are immediate (within minutes) at the scene of injury. Some deaths are early (within hours) in the emergency department or the operating room, and a few are late (after days or weeks) and occur in the ICU or ward.[47] Those in the ICU are mostly from severe head injury within a few days and, less commonly, multiorgan dysfunction later.

Of trauma admissions to hospital, only a minority have severe or multiple trauma.[48] In order of frequency, life-threatening injuries involve the head, abdomen and chest (Table 66.1), and are often multiple. The hospital services which this small number of severely injured patients use out of proportion to their numbers are major surgery, intensive care, radiography and CT scanning.[48] Major trauma outcome studies in the USA,[37] the UK[38] and Australia[49] offer valuable epidemiological data. The USA study found that the mortality of direct admissions is strongly related to serious head injury.

ORGANISATION OF TRAUMA CARE

Many of the problems of trauma care are organisational. Problems faced by health authorities are the provision of advanced care at the scene of injury, rapid

Table 66.1 Percentage of ICU trauma patients with grades of injury in different body regions

	AIS ≥ 4	AIS = 3	AIS = 1 or 2	AIS = 0
Head and neck	64	9	10	18
Face	2	11	8	79
Thorax	10	17	6	67
Abdomen	16	6	2	77
Extremities	1	33	10	56
External	0	<1	64	36

Data on 3965 adult trauma patients (excluding burns) in the DCCM, Auckland Hospital, 1988–2006. Abbreviated injury scale (AIS-80) codes:[31] 0 = no injury; 1 = minor; 2 = moderate; 3 = serious; not life-threatening; 4 = severe; life-threatening, survival probable; 5 = critical; survival uncertain; 6 = unsurvivable. In tertiary referral centres, these figures will vary with the mix of local and referred patients.[50]

transportation to hospital, policies on which hospitals should receive trauma patients, systems for rapid evaluation and decision-making in hospitals, and rapid, safe patient transfer between hospitals. If survival from major trauma is to be maximised, prehospital and hospital care must be coordinated.

Regionalisation of trauma care has become an accepted concept.[2,51] Trauma centres are designated hospitals which meet certain requirements. Main prerequisites are rapidly available experienced surgeons, anaesthetists and neurosurgeons, and a minimum number of patients seen annually for staff expertise. Regionalisation involves the concept of ambulances bypassing non-designated hospitals.[2] Helicopters are used increasingly to speed patient transportation.[52] Trauma teams are teams of surgeons and intensivists or anaesthetists who immediately attend the trauma victim on arrival at hospital.[2–4,44]

Trauma registries and databases are important tools in organising and improving trauma care. The UK major trauma outcome study[38] showed that the doctors in charge of resuscitation were often junior, delays in performing urgent operations were common, and the number of preventable deaths was significant. A hospital may not see enough trauma patients to justify a trauma team or supply adequate experience for its staff, and may not have all the facilities required by trauma patients. Transfer to a trauma hospital may be desirable, but geography and limited transport facilities may make such transfers hazardous.

In Western countries, trauma is a leading cause of death and disability under the age of 38 years.[37] Reduction of mortality and morbidity depends on public education, new legislations, on-site advanced care, rapid evacuation (see Chapter 4), hospital trauma expertise and coordination of services.[53,54]

REFERENCES

1. Trunkey DD. Trauma. *Sci Am* 1983; **249**: 20–7.
2. Trunkey DD. Overview of trauma. *Surg Clin North Am* 1982; **62**: 3–7.
3. Trunkey DD. Initial treatment of patients with extensive trauma. *N Engl J Med* 1991; **324**: 1159–263.
4. Enderson BL, Maull KI. Missed injuries: the trauma surgeon's nemesis. *Surg Clin North Am* 1991; **71**: 399–418.
5. Janjua KJ, Sugrue M, Deane SA. Prospective evaluation of early missed injuries and the role of tertiary trauma survey. *J Trauma* 1998; **44**: 1000–6.
6. Committee on Trauma, American College of Surgeons. *Advanced Trauma Life Support (ATLS) Program for Physicians*, 7th edn. Chicago: American College of Surgeons; 2004.
7. Soderstrom CA, Cowley RA. A national alcohol and trauma center survey: missed opportunities, failures of responsibility. *Arch Surg* 1987; **122**: 1067–71.
8. Shackford SR, Rogers FB, Osler TM *et al.* Focused abdominal sonogram for trauma: the learning curve of nonradiologist clinicians in detecting hemoperitoneum. *J Trauma* 1999; **46**: 553–64.
9. Branney SW, Moore EE, Cantrill SV *et al.* Ultrasound based key clinical pathway reduces the use of hospital resources for the evaluation of blunt abdominal trauma. *J Trauma* 1997; **42**: 1086–90.
10. Day AC, Rankin N, Charlesworth P. Diagnostic peritoneal lavage: integration with clinical information to improve diagnostic performance. *J Trauma* 1992; **32**: 52–7.
11. Weigelt JA, Kingman RG. Complications of negative laparotomy for trauma. *Am J Surg* 1988; **156**: 544–7.
12. Trunkey DD, Federle MP. Computed tomography in perspective [editorial]. *J Trauma* 1986; **26**: 660–1.
13. Padbani HR, Watson CJE, Clements L *et al.* Computed tomography in abdominal trauma: an audit of usage and image quality. *Br J Radiol* 1992; **65**: 397–402.
14. Finfer S, Bellomo R, Boyce N *et al.* A comparison of albumin and saline for fluid resuscitation in the intensive care unit. *N Engl J Med* 2004; **350**: 2247–56.
15. Bickell WH, Wall MJ, Pepe PE *et al.* Immediate versus delayed fluid resuscitation for hypotensive patients with penetrating torso injuries. *N Engl J Med* 1994; **331**: 1105–9.
16. Chestnut RM, Marshall LF, Klauber MR *et al.* The role of secondary brain injury in determining outcome from severe head injury. *J Trauma* 1993; **34**: 216–92.
17. Wilden JN. Rapid resuscitation in severe head injury. *Lancet* 1993; **342**: 1378.
18. Brain Trauma Foundation. *Guidelines for the Management of Severe Traumatic Brain Injury.* New York: Brain Trauma Foundation; 2007. http://www.braintrauma.org/
19. Cowley RA, Trump BF. Editors' summary: Organ dysfunction in shock. In: Cowley RA, Trump BF (eds) *Pathophysiology of Shock, Anoxia, and Ischaemia.* Baltimore, MD: Williams & Wilkins; 1982: 281–4.
20. Faist E, Baue AE, Dittmer H *et al.* Multiple organ failure in polytrauma patients. *J Trauma* 1983; **23**: 775–87.
21. Daffner RH, Sciulli RL, Rodriguez A *et al.* Imaging for evaluation of suspected cervical spine trauma: a 2-year analysis. *Injury* 2006; **37**: 652–8.
22. Paul A, Blostein PA, Hodgman CG. Computed tomography of the chest in blunt thoracic trauma: results of a prospective study. *J Trauma* 1997; **43**: 13–8.
23. Nzewi O, Slight RD, Zamvar V. Management of blunt thoracic aortic injury. *Eur J Vasc Endovasc Surg* 2006; **31**: 18–27.
24. Panetta T, Sclafani SJA, Goldstein AS *et al.* Percutaneous transcatheter embolisation for massive bleeding from pelvic fractures. *J Trauma* 1985; **26**: 1021–9.
25. Boyd M, Vanek VW, Bourguet CC. Emergency room resuscitative thoracotomy: when is it indicated? *J Trauma* 1992; **33**: 714–21.
26. Suarez JI, Qureshi AI, Bhardwaj A *et al.* Treatment of refractory intracranial hypertension with 23.4% saline. *Crit Care Med* 1998; **26**: 1118–22.

27. Prough DS, Zornow MH. Mannitol: an old friend on the skids? *Crit Care Med* 1998; **26**: 997–8.
28. Fishman RA. Effects of isotonic intravenous solutions on normal and increased intracranial pressure. *Arch Neural Psychiatry* 1953; **70**: 350–60.
29. Teasdale G, Jennett B. Assessment of coma and impaired consciousness: a practical scale. *Lancet* 1974; **2**: 81–4.
30. Jennett B, Teasdale G. Aspects of coma after severe head injury. *Lancet* 1977; **1**: 878–81.
31. Thomason M, Messick J, Rutledge R *et al.* Head CT scanning versus urgent exploration in the hypotensive blunt trauma patient. *J Trauma* 1993; **34**: 40–5.
32. American Medical Association Committee on Medical Aspects of Automotive Safety. Rating the severity of tissue damage: I – the abbreviated scale. *JAMA* 1971; **215**: 277–80.
33. Committee on Injury Scaling. The Abbreviated Injury Scale – 1980 Revision. Morton Grove, IL: American Association for Automotive Medicine; 1980.
34. Committee on Injury Scaling. The Abbreviated Injury Scale – 2005 Revision. Des Plaines, IL: American Association for Automotive Medicine; 2005.
35. Baker SP, O'Neill B, Haddon W *et al.* The injury severity score: a method for describing patients with multiple injuries and evaluating emergency care. *J Trauma* 1974; **14**: 187–96.
36. Baker SP, O'Neill B. The injury severity score: an update. *J Trauma* 1976; **16**: 882–5.
37. Champion HR, Copes WS, Sacco WJ *et al.* The major trauma outcome study: establishing national norms for trauma care. *J Trauma* 1990; **30**: 1356–65.
38. Yates DW, Woodford M, Hollis S. Preliminary analysis of the care of injured patients in 33 British hospitals: first report of the United Kingdom major trauma outcome study. *BMJ* 1992; **305**: 737–40.
39. Champion HR, Sacco WJ, Copes WS *et al.* A revision of the trauma score. *J Trauma* 1989; **29**: 623–9.
40. Boyd CR, Tolson MA, Copes WS. Evaluating trauma care: the TRISS method. *J Trauma* 1987; **27**: 370–8.
41. McAnena OJ, Moore FA, Moore EE *et al.* Invalidation of the APACHE II scoring system for patients with acute trauma. *J Trauma* 1992; **33**: 504–7.
42. Roumen RMH, Redl H, Schlag G *et al.* Scoring systems and blood lactate concentrations in relation to the development of adult respiratory distress syndrome and multiple organ failure in severely traumatized patients. *J Trauma* 1993; **35**: 349–55.
43. Sacco WJ, Copes WS, Bain LW *et al.* Effect of preinjury illness on trauma patient survival outcome. *J Trauma* 1993; **35**: 538–43.
44. Cowley RA, Dunham CM (eds). *Shock Trauma/Critical Care Manual.* Baltimore, MD: University Park Press; 1982.
45. Baker CC, Oppenheimer L, Stephens B *et al.* Epidemiology of trauma deaths. *Am J Surg* 1980; **140**: 144–50.
46. Smeeton WMI, Judson JA, Synek BJ *et al.* Deaths from trauma in Auckland: a one year study. *N Z Med J* 1987; **100**: 337–40.
47. Sauaia A, Moore FA, Moore EE *et al.* Epidemiology of trauma deaths: a reassessment. *J Trauma* 1995; **38**: 185–93.
48. Streat SJ, Donaldson ML, Judson JA. Trauma in Auckland: an overview. *N Z Med J* 1987; **100**: 441–4.
49. Cameron P, Dziukas L, Hadj A *et al.* Major trauma in Australia: a regional analysis. *J Trauma* 1995; **39**: 545–52.
50. Data updated from that published in: Gardiner JP, Judson JA, Smith GS *et al.* A decade of ICU trauma admissions in Auckland, New Zealand. *N Z Med J* 2000; **113**: 326–7.
51. Eggold R. Trauma care regionalisation: a necessity. *J Trauma* 1983; **23**: 260–2.
52. Freeark RJ. The trauma center: its hospitals, head injuries, helicopters, and heroes (1982 AAST presidential address). *J Trauma* 1983; **23**: 173–8.
53. Judson JA. Trauma management: modern concepts [editorial]. *N Z Med J* 1985; **98**: 8–9.
54. Trunkey DD. On the nature of things that go bang in the night. *Surgery* 1982; **92**: 123.

67

Severe head injury

John A Myburgh

Despite improvements in resuscitation and vital organ support, the management of patients with traumatic brain injury in the intensive care unit (ICU) presents a challenge to all members of the critical care team. As head injury is associated with a high mortality and morbidity, the benefits of intensive treatment and care may not become apparent until months or years later during rehabilitation after injury.

EPIDEMIOLOGY

Traumatic brain injury has been termed a 'silent global epidemic'. It accounts for up to 30% of all trauma-related deaths and is the leading cause of death in young males in developed countries. The impact of mechanisation in developing countries has resulted in a sharp increase in the incidence and mortality from vehicular trauma.

In addition to this high mortality, the cost of survivors in these societies in emotional, social and financial terms is substantial as the effects of the original injury may persist for many years.

AETIOLOGY

Vehicular trauma, industrial accidents, falls and assaults account for the majority of head injury, with marked variations in patterns of injury across the world. For example, in Australasia, the incidence of head injury due to vehicular trauma is decreasing due to the success of preventive strategies such as restraint devices, speed control and stricter drink-driving legislation.[1]

DEMOGRAPHICS

The numbers of patients with traumatic brain injury presenting to hospitals vary widely in accordance with hospital admission policies and capabilities. Typical figures of all-cause head injury admissions in developed countries range from 200 to 300 per 100 000 patients.

Age and gender-specific data typically show two peaks: one in the second and third decades, with a male:female ratio of 2:1; the latter in the seventh to ninth decades with a more equivalent gender ratio.

PATTERNS OF INJURY

Traumatic brain injury represents a range of injury from mild head injury that may fully recover to severe injury associated with high mortality or high levels of disability.

Injury may be either blunt or penetrating, with the latter associated with a higher mortality.

Although the majority of head injuries (70–80%) are minor, a significant proportion of these patients may have poor functional outcomes due to secondary brain insults, missed injuries and comorbidities. Of the 20–30% who constitute moderate to severe head injury, approximately 10% of these are dead on admission whilst the remainder will usually require admission to the ICU for management in the first 7–10 days.

PATHOPHYSIOLOGY

Brain injury is a heterogenous pathophysiological process. It encompasses a spectrum of injury that includes the degree of brain damage at the time of injury (primary injury) in addition to insults that occur during the post-injury phase (secondary injury). These processes are depicted in Figure 67.1.

Both primary and secondary injuries are associated with the development of variable degrees of intracranial inflammation and disruption of cerebrovascular autoregulation.

An understanding of these processes is essential in order to quantify the severity of injury, direct appropriate management strategies and interpret information from clinical monitoring systems.

PRIMARY BRAIN INJURY

The severity of primary injury is determined by the degree of neuronal damage or death at the time of impact. This is a major determinant of outcome from traumatic brain injury and, with the exception of surgically evacuable mass lesions, is usually irreversible.

Primary brain injuries include all types of injury to the brain parenchyma and vasculature. Primary injuries that are associated with adverse outcome include traumatic subarachnoid haemorrhage and non-evacuable mass lesions, particularly in critical parts of the brain such as the posterior fossa.

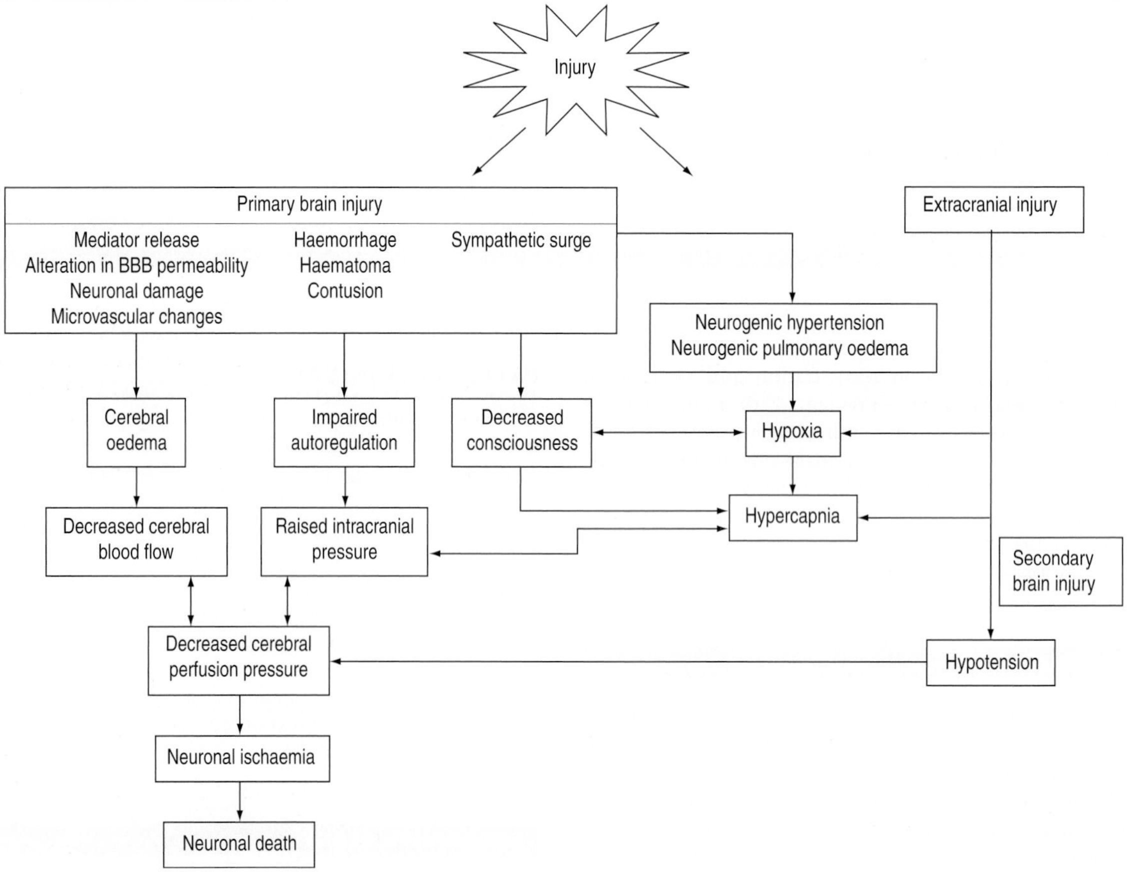

Figure 67.1 Pathophysiology of traumatic brain injury.

SECONDARY BRAIN INJURY

Secondary brain insults are characterised by a reduction in cerebral substrate utilisation, particularly oxygen (Table 67.1). Of these insults, hypotension (defined as a systolic blood pressure of < 90 mmHg), hypoxia (oxygen saturation < 90% or $Pa\text{O}_2$ < 50 mmHg), hypoglycaemia, hyperpyrexia (temperature > 39°C) and prolonged hypocapnia ($Pa\text{CO}_2$ < 30 mmHg) have been shown to independently worsen survival following traumatic brain injury.

Secondary insults may occur during initial resuscitation, transport both between and within hospitals, during anaesthesia and surgery, and subsequently in the ICU. These insults may initiate or propagate pathophysiological processes which may fatally damage neurones already rendered susceptible by the primary injury. Consequently, a vicious circle of secondary brain damage may develop with adverse outcomes.

INTRACRANIAL INFLAMMATION

As the brain is enclosed within the rigid skull and dura, small increases in intracranial volume result in sharp increases in intracranial pressure (Monro–Kelly doctrine). Consequently, the brain is a poorly compliant organ that has a limited capacity to accommodate pathological increases in intracranial pressure.

Traumatic brain injury invokes an inflammatory response characterised by the release of cytokines, free

Table 67.1 Secondary brain insults following traumatic brain injury that are associated with increased morbidity and mortality

Systemic	Intracranial
Hypoxia	Seizure
Hypotension	Delayed haematoma
Hypocapnia	Subarachnoid haemorrhage
Hypercapnia	Vasospasm
Hyperthermia	Hydrocephalus
Hypoglycaemia	Neuroinfection
Hyperglycaemia	
Hyponatraemia	
Hypernatraemia	
Hyperosmolality	
Infection	

radicals, excitatory amino acids and other mediators. The consequence of this response is disruption and alteration in the permeability of the blood–brain barrier, glial swelling and alterations in regional and global cerebral blood flow. The extent of this inflammatory process is an important determinant of intracranial pressure that may persist for some time following injury. Furthermore, alteration in blood–brain permeability may render the cerebral circulation susceptible to the effects of drugs that do not normally cross, such as osmotic diuretics and exogenous catecholamines.

CEREBRAL BLOOD FLOW AND AUTOREGULATION

Normally, cerebral blood flow is maintained at a constant rate in the presence of changing perfusion pressures by myogenic and metabolic autoregulation. These homeostatic mechanisms are impaired following head injury due to neuronal damage and intracranial inflammation. Distinct patterns of cerebral blood flow have been described following head injury that have direct clinical relevance with regard to management[2] (Figure 67.2).

THE HYPOPERFUSION PHASE

Cerebral blood flow is reduced by extrinsic and intrinsic mechanisms in the first 72 hours following injury, with resultant global and regional ischaemia. Because myogenic autoregulation is markedly impaired during this period, cerebral blood flow in the hypoperfusion phase is directly dependent on systemic blood pressure. Resultant neuronal ischaemia may result in 'cytotoxic' cerebral oedema and increased intracranial pressure.

In order to maintain cerebral perfusion, systemic blood pressure must be maintained during this phase so that cerebral perfusion pressure (defined as the difference between mean arterial pressure and intracranial pressure) is maintained between 60 and 70 mmHg.[3]

THE HYPERAEMIC PHASE

Following the initial hypoperfusion phase, autoregulatory mechanisms may start to recover with improved cerebral blood flow.

During this phase, intracranial inflammation and/or effects of medical therapies directed at maintaining adequate cerebral perfusion pressure may result in cerebral hyperaemia and increased intracranial pressure. The consequences of hyperaemia, inflammation and altered blood–brain permeability result in 'vasogenic' cerebral oedema.

This hyperaemic phase may persist for up to 7–10 days post injury and occurs in 25–30% patients. As there is restoration or increased cerebral blood flow during this phase, a range of cerebral perfusion pressure is recommended (50–70 mmHg).[4]

THE VASOSPASTIC PHASE

In a small cohort of patients (10–15%), particularly those with severe primary and secondary injuries or those with significant traumatic subarachnoid haemorrhage, a vasospastic phase characterised by typical cerebral blood flow patterns may persist. This phase represents a complex of cerebral hypoperfusion due to arterial vasospasm, posttraumatic hypometabolism and impaired autoregulation.[5]

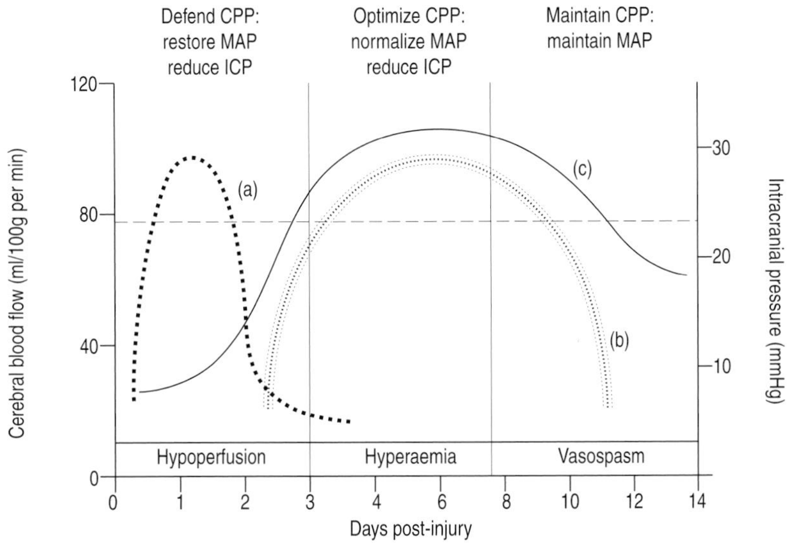

Figure 67.2 Conceptual changes in cerebral blood flow and intracranial pressure (ICP) over time following traumatic brain injury: (a) cytotoxic oedema; (b) vasogenic oedema; (c) cerebral blood flow. CPP, cerebral perfusion pressure; MAP, mean arterial pressure.

RESUSCITATION

INITIAL ASSESSMENT

The resuscitation of head-injured patients should follow the principles outlined in the Advanced Trauma Life Support (ATLS®) guidelines for the early management of severe trauma.[6]

The initial emphasis is directed at assessing and controlling the airway, ensuring adequate oxygenation and ventilation, establishing adequate intravenous access and correcting haemodynamic inadequacy. Neurological assessment and brain-specific treatment should only follow once cardiorespiratory stability has occurred. Given the direct association between hypotension and hypoxia and adverse outcomes in traumatic brain injury, this is an absolute priority.

With respect to head-injured patients, the following principles in the initial assessment apply.[7,8]

AIRWAY

All patients with severe head injury (traumatic coma), marked agitation or significant extracranial trauma require early oral endotracheal intubation.

Depending on the skill of the operator and available facilities, this should be performed using a rapid sequence induction with cricoid pressure and in-line immobilisation of the cervical spine.

All head-injured patients should be assumed to have a potential cervical spine injury, and should be immobilised in a rigid collar until that possibility is definitively excluded.

BREATHING (= VENTILATION)

Patients should be ventilated in 100% oxygen using 6–10 ml/kg tidal volumes until blood gas analysis is available.

Oxygenation should be maintained at at least 100 mmHg (13 kPa) and the ventilator adjusted to achieve a normal arterial carbon dioxide tension (35–40 mmHg; 4.5–5.0 kPa).

Non-depolarising muscle relaxants and narcotics such as fentanyl may facilitate ventilation in the immediate post-intubation period in combative patients.

Empirical hyperventilation during initial resuscitation is not indicated until adequate oxygenation, haemodynamic stability and urgent computed tomography have been achieved.[9]

CIRCULATION (= CONTROL OF SHOCK)

Prompt restoration of circulating blood volume and restoration of a euvolaemic state is critical.[10]

An emerging body of evidence recommends the use of crystalloids, specifically normal saline, for fluid resuscitation of patients with traumatic brain injury. The use of albumin for fluid resuscitation is associated with increased mortality and should be avoided.[11] Hypertonic saline may have a role as a small-volume resuscitation fluid that is useful in expanding intravascular volume, with additional beneficial effects on cerebral blood flow and reduction of cerebral oedema,[12] although there is no evidence of reduced mortality when used in the prehospital period.[13]

Early arterial monitoring for accurate measurement of mean arterial pressure and central venous catheter placement for providing a guide to volume replacement and administration of blood and drugs is essential. The placement of these lines must not delay volume resuscitation.

Inotropes, such as adrenaline (epinephrine) or noradrenaline (norepinephrine), or vasopressors such as phenylephrine or metaraminol, may be used to defend blood pressure once correction of hypovolaemia is underway or achieved.[4] This may be necessary if sedatives or narcotics are coadministered.

The use of military antishock trousers (MAST suit) in traumatic brain injury is not recommended.

DISABILITY (= NEUROLOGICAL ASSESSMENT)

Assessment of neurological function following injury is important to quantify the severity of neurotrauma and to provide prognostic information. The level of function may be influenced by associated injuries, hypoxia, hypotension and/or drug or alcohol intoxication. Similarly, recording the mechanism of injury is important, as high velocity injuries are associated with a greater degree of neuronal damage. It is important to review ambulance and emergency personnel and records in order to obtain the most accurate information.

Level of consciousness

The ATLS® recommends an initial assessment during initial resuscitation based on the response to stimulation: Awake, Verbal, Pain, Unresponsive (AVPU). This provides a rapid and practical grading of function with severe head injuries defined as those who respond to pain only or who are unresponsive.

The Glasgow Coma Scale (GCS) has an established place in the management of traumatic brain injury and is the most widely accepted and understood scale.[14] Whilst originally described as a prognostic index, it provides an overall assessment of neurological function, derived from three parameters: eye opening, verbal response and motor response (Table 67.2).

The best responses in the GCS components should be recorded following cardiorespiratory resuscitation and prior to surgical intervention in order to provide prognostic information. A GCS of 14–15 indicates a mild injury, 9–13 a moderate injury and 3–8 is classified as severe. In the severely injured, such as intubated patients or those with ocular or facial trauma, the motor response is the most useful.

Pupillary responses

Pupil size and reactivity are important when consciousness is impaired. Whilst not part of the GCS, pupillary function should always be assessed and recorded at the same time as the GCS, particularly prior to the administration of narcotics, sedatives or muscle relaxants.

Table 67.2 The Glasgow Coma Scale.[14] The best response following non-surgical resuscitation is scored

Best eyes open score		Best verbal response		Best motor response	
Spontaneously	4	Orientated, adequate	5	Obeys spoken command	6
On spoken command	3	Disorientated, confused	4	Localized pain	5
To pain	2	Inappropriate words	3	Flexion withdrawal	4
No response	1	Incomprehensible	2	Abnormal flexion	3
		No response	1	Extension	2
				No response	1
		Intubated patients:			
		Appears able to converse	5		
		Questionable ability to converse	3		
		Unresponsive	1		

In the absence of traumatic mydriasis, abnormalities of pupil size and reactivity may indicate compression of the third cranial nerve, suggesting raised intracranial pressure or impending herniation, particularly when associated with lateralising motor signs and depressed consciousness

Papilloedema is uncommon in the acute phase of head injuries.

Motor function

In addition to the motor response of the GCS, decerebrate or decorticate posturing, hemiparesis or lateralising signs, paraparesis and quadriparesis (given the high association with spinal injuries with traumatic brain injury) should be documented concurrently with the GCS and pupillary responses.

SECONDARY SURVEY

Once the initial assessment is complete and resuscitation underway, a thorough secondary survey adopting a 'top-to-toe' approach is mandatory. This is outlined in the ATLS® approach to the traumatised patient.[6]

The principles outlined in the initial assessment form the basis for prioritising interventions in the secondary survey in traumatic brain injury. Extracranial causes of hypoxia such as pulmonary contusion or haemo/pneumothorax must be excluded and promptly treated. Haemorrhage – both externally from fractures or lacerations and internally from major vascular disruption or visceral injuries – must be aggressively treated until circulatory stability is achieved. There is no place for 'permissive hypotension' in head-injured patients as has been advocated in selected cases of penetrating trauma.

Target mean arterial pressure should be estimated in the context of the patient's premorbid blood pressure. Higher pressures may be necessary in hypertensive or elderly patients. The early use of inotropes such as adrenaline or noradrenaline may be necessary to achieve this.

An approach of 'damage-control surgery' is now advocated in head-injured patients to minimise secondary insults. In the initial 24–48 hours following injury, only life- or limb-threatening injuries should be addressed, following which patients are transferred to the ICU for stabilisation and monitoring. Thereafter, semi-urgent surgery such as fixation of closed fractures or delayed plastic repairs may be done. Patients with severe head injury undergoing prolonged emergency surgery should ideally have intracranial pressure monitoring placed as soon as possible.

Routine X-rays of the chest, pelvis and cervical spine and baseline blood tests (including blood alcohol level in appropriate cases) are part of the secondary survey.

BRAIN-SPECIFIC RESUSCITATION

The place of interventions and therapies specifically directed at reducing intracranial pressure has been extensively reviewed in evidence-based guidelines for the management of severe head injury. Whilst there is little evidence for the role of some therapies such as empirical hyperventilation and osmotherapy during resuscitation, they continue to be widely used in clinical practice.

HYPERVENTILATION

Ventilation-induced reductions in $Pa\text{CO}_2$ result in marked reductions in cerebral blood flow and consequently in intracranial pressure. However, as cerebral blood flow may be reduced during the initial period following injury, further reductions in cerebral perfusion will result if hyperventilation is used during this phase (Figure 67.2).

Hyperventilation is associated with reductions in cerebral oxygenation, particularly in areas of neuronal damage, potentially exacerbating cerebral hypoxia. The combination of induced cerebral ischaemia in the damaged brain therefore offsets any theoretical benefit of reducing intracranial pressure. Consequently, empirical hyperventilation is not indicated during initial resuscitation when cerebral blood flow is compromised.

However, hyperventilation remains a potent non-surgical clinical tool of reducing intracranial pressure. In the resuscitated head-injured patient with unequivocal clinical signs of raised intracranial pressure or impending tentorial herniation (pupillary dilatation, lateralising signs or a witnessed neurological deterioration), hyperventilation is an option.

Reductions of $Pa\text{CO}_2$ to levels ≤30 mmHg (4 kPa) may be therefore considered prior to urgent imaging or surgery for evacuation of a mass lesion.[9]

OSMOTHERAPY

Osmotically active agents, such as mannitol, are widely used in the treatment of traumatic brain injury. Theoretically, mannitol is administered to increase plasma osmolality in order to cause net efflux of fluid from areas of damaged, oedematous brain, with resultant reduction in intracranial pressure. An intact blood–brain barrier is necessary for this to occur. Following intravenous administration of mannitol, an immediate plasma expanding effect that reduces haematocrit and viscosity ensues, which temporarily increases cerebral blood flow. Subsequent reductions in intracranial pressure probably result from restoration in cerebral perfusion pressure and rheological changes in cerebral blood flow, rather than specific cerebral dehydration.

Osmotherapy is associated with a number of potentially adverse effects. Mannitol exerts an osmotic effect over a narrow range of plasma osmolality (290–330 mosm/l) above which theoretically beneficial effects may be negated. Mannitol will induce an osmolal gap between measured and calculated osmolality, so that regular measurements of serum osmolality are necessary to monitor the amount administered. This gap may be further increased by alcohol that is frequently present in the acute period. Mannitol will enter the brain where the blood–brain barrier is damaged, thereby potentially increasing cerebral oedema by increasing brain osmolality. Mannitol is a potent osmotic diuretic that may compromise haemodynamic stability by inducing an inappropriate diuresis in a hypovolaemic patient. Consequently, systemic hypotension may ensue which may cause further cerebral ischaemia or subsequent organ dysfunction such as acute renal failure. This effect may be exacerbated by the concomitant administration of catecholamines in order to defend systemic blood pressure.

Given the high risk with minimal benefit during resuscitation, the routine use of mannitol is not recommended in the absence of raised intracranial pressure and in patients where cerebral blood flow is compromised.[15]

Similarly to hyperventilation, mannitol is considered as an option only in resuscitated patients with unequivocal signs of raised intracranial pressure prior to imaging or evacuation of a mass lesion. Although doses are frequently quoted as 0.25–1.0 g/kg, lower doses are equally as effective as higher doses in terms of improving cerebral perfusion and are associated with a lower incidence of side-effects.

Hypertonic saline (3% solution) exerts similar osmotic plasma expanding effects to mannitol. These solutions do not exert an osmolal gap so that serum sodium reflects serum osmolality allowing easier titration. These solutions have been advocated as 'small-volume resuscitation fluids' that may be very effective in restoring systemic and cerebral perfusion in the acute phase following injury. In addition to reducing intracranial pressure, these solutions would appear to be superior to mannitol for resuscitation.[16]

EMERGENCY SURGICAL DECOMPRESSION ('BURR HOLES')

The advent of better equipped in-field resuscitation, medical retrieval, imaging and innovations such as teleradiology and telemedicine has largely superseded the need to perform urgent craniotomy in head-injured patients. In most instances, patients are resuscitated, stabilised and imaged with CT scans prior to any surgical intervention. This may involve transfer to a specialised trauma centre. CT scanning provides accurate information and directs the surgeon to a mass lesion that needs evacuation under optimal circumstances.

In remote communities without immediate access to CT scanning, surgical evacuation may be lifesaving in patients with a clear history of an expanding mass lesion such as an extradural or subdural haematoma. These include patients with low velocity injuries to the temporal region and an associated skull fracture that have clinical signs of intracranial herniation or a witnessed deterioration.

IMAGING

X-RAYS

All head-injured patients receive the routine 'trauma series' of X-rays, namely chest, pelvis and cervical spine (lateral, anteroposterior and peg views), although the last may be superseded by high resolution CT scan of the entire cervical spine.[17]

Skull X-rays have essentially been superseded by CT scanning and their routine use in the emergency evaluation of head-injured patients has been questioned.

COMPUTED TOMOGRAPHY (CT SCAN)

CT scanning is the most informative radiological technique in the evaluation of the acute head injury and is now standard in virtually all patients following head injury. CT scanning invariably requires moving the patient to a radiological suite. This must only be done once initial assessment and resuscitation are complete and the patient is stable enough to be transported by appropriately trained and equipped personnel.

The following patients should undergo CT head scan following traumatic brain injury:

- All patients with a history of loss of consciousness or traumatic coma.
- Combative patients where clinical assessment is masked by associated alcohol, drugs or extracranial injuries. These patients may require endotracheal intubation, sedation and ventilation to facilitate completion of CT scanning.

Table 67.3 Classification of CT scan appearance following traumatic brain injury.[16] Examples are shown in Figure 67.3a

Category	Definition
Diffuse injury (DI) I	No visible intracranial pathology seen on CT scan
DI II (diffuse injury)	Cisterns are present with midline shift 0–5 mm and/or Lesion densities present No high or mixed density > 25 mm May include bony fragments and foreign bodies
DI III (swelling)	Cisterns are compressed or absent with midline shift 0–5 mm No high or mixed density > 25 mm
DI IV (shift)	Midline shift > 5 mm No high or mixed density > 25 mm
Evacuated mass lesion	Any lesion surgically evacuated
Non-evacuated mass lesion	High or mixed density lesion > 25 mm, not surgically evacuated

Technological advances in imaging now enable quick, high resolution digital images of the brain parenchyma and bony compartments. The most important role of CT scanning is prompt detection of mass lesion such as extradural or subdural haematomas. Thereafter, the degree of brain injury may be quantified by radiological criteria (Table 67.3 and Figure 67.3a).[18]

These criteria are important for:

1. providing an index of injury severity
2. providing criteria for intracranial pressure monitoring
3. comparing the progression of injuries with subsequent scans
4. providing an index for prognosis

These criteria should be recorded following each CT scan, particularly when patients are transferred to secondary or tertiary centres. Examples of typical injuries appear in Figure 67.3a and 67.3b.

The presence of traumatic subarachnoid haemorrhage should be recorded. This is an important index of severity of injury and is relevant for prognostication.[19]

CEREBRAL ANGIOGRAPHY

Cerebral angiography should be considered when a vascular injury, such as carotid artery dissection, is suspected in head-injured patients. This may be indicated by a large isodense lesion on CT scan or when the patient's clinical condition is not consistent with the CT findings (e.g. a dense hemiparesis in the absence of a mass lesion).

MAGNETIC RESONANCE IMAGING

Magnetic resonance imaging (MRI) provides accurate detail of parenchymal damage, specifically small collections and non-haemorrhagic contusions. However, the information provided is not significantly better than that obtained from CT scanning to warrant routine use of MRI in the acute phase of injury. In addition, the placement and monitoring of an acute traumatised patient in an MRI scanner poses an additional risk that is not justified by the information provided.

MRI may have an important role in prognostication at a later stage in management, particularly in mild and moderate head injury.

INTERHOSPITAL TRANSFER

All severely head-injured patients should be managed in a specialised neurotrauma centre in close collaboration with intensive care physicians and neurosurgeons.[20] This may involve intra- or interhospital transportation. This is a potentially hazardous exercise and has the potential to adversely affect outcome by causing secondary insults. Consequently, appropriately skilled and equipped personnel should only do this once resuscitation, stabilisation and initial imaging are completed.

A full primary and secondary survey and review of all documentation and investigation is required following transfer to a secondary or tertiary centre.

INTENSIVE CARE MANAGEMENT

There is no standard or uniform method of managing traumatic brain injury in the ICU. Most practices are determined by local preferences and experience, caseload and resources. The Brain Trauma Foundation of the American Association of Neurological Surgeons[21] and the European Brain Injury Consortium[22] have published evidence-based management guidelines for the management of severe brain injury. These publications provide very few standards by which to direct therapy and the majority of issues addressed are presented either as management guidelines or options.

Although management of head injury in the ICU will be considered in two sections – supportive therapy and brain-specific therapy – these occur simultaneously. The principles of management focus on the integration of all monitoring information in the context of the underlying injury so that secondary brain injury is prevented.

SUPPORTIVE THERAPY

Following initial resuscitation, good intensive care management forms the basis of head injury management and is regarded as a continuum of care. This takes priority over brain-specific therapies, which to date remain inconclusive in their efficacy.

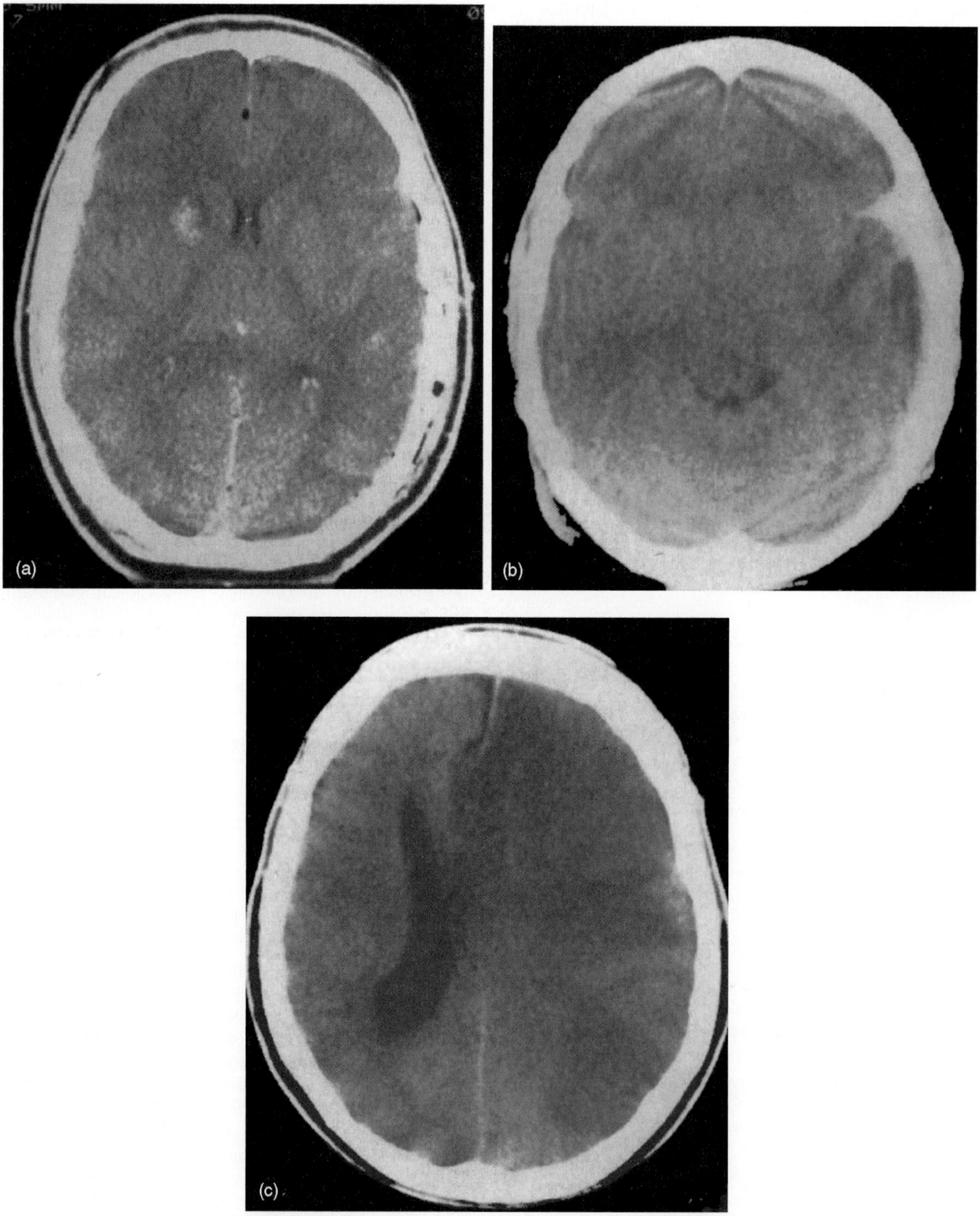

Figure 67.3a Computed tomographic classification of diffuse axonal injury (Table 67.3).[33] Panel (a) Diffuse injury II; Panel (b) Diffuse injury III; Panel (c) Diffuse injury IV.

Continued

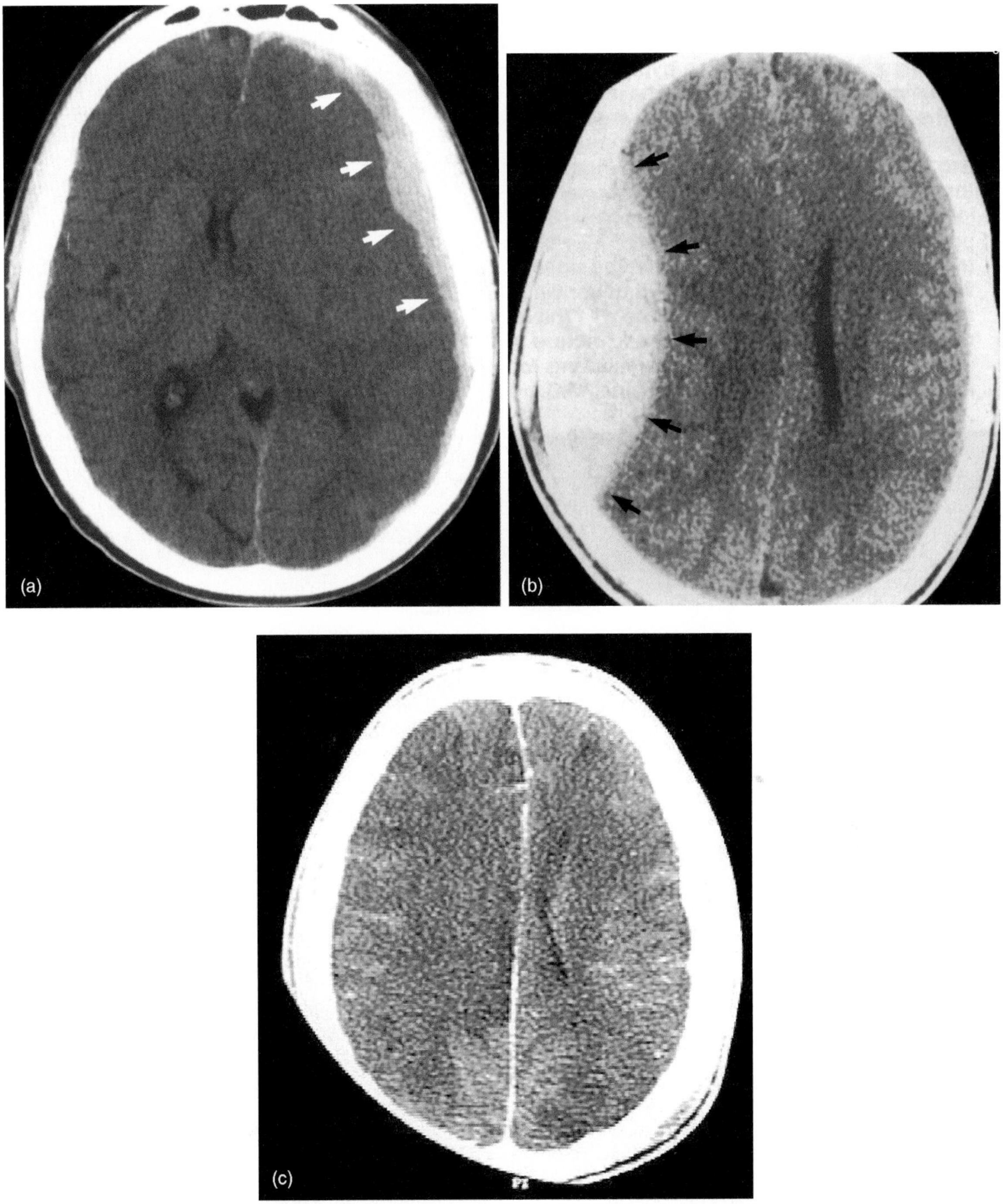

Figure 67.3b Intracranial haemorrhages. Panel (a) Acute subdural haematoma; Panel (b) Acute extradural haematoma; Panel (c) Acute traumatic subarachnoid haemorrhage.

HAEMODYNAMIC MANAGEMENT

Monitoring

Accurate measurement of systemic blood pressure is essential and should be measured via an arterial catheter referenced to the aortic root. A large artery such as the femoral artery should be considered in haemodynamically unstable patients as radial or dorsalis pedis arterial catheters may underestimate true systemic pressure in shocked patients. Given the importance of maintaining adequate systemic pressures, non-invasive measurement of blood pressure is not recommended during the acute phase of monitoring.[10]

Therapy should be titrated to mean arterial pressure in accordance with the patient's premorbid blood pressure – i.e. in older patients, higher mean arterial pressure (e.g. 80 mmHg) may be necessary.

Volume status should be assessed using clinical criteria, central venous pressure monitoring and hourly urine output.

Pulmonary artery catheterisation for the measurement of cardiac output and pulmonary artery pressures is rarely indicated in head-injured patients and is not recommended on current evidence.

Fluid management

The attainment of a euvolaemic state is essential throughout intensive care management. This is determined by standard measurements such as serum sodium and osmolality, urea and creatinine, pulse rate, right atrial and mean arterial pressure and urine output.

Resuscitative fluids depend on local preferences, as there is no evidence to recommend crystalloids over colloids.

Optimal rheology for the cerebral circulation requires a haematocrit of approximately 30%: patients should be transfused if actively bleeding or to maintain a haemoglobin between 8.5 and 10 g/l.

Maintenance fluids should be directed at maintaining a normal osmolality. As a general principle, glucose-containing solutions are not recommended; however, these may be required (i.e. as 5% dextrose in water) if patients become hyperosmolal (> 320 mosm/l).

Inotropic therapy

Inotropes such as adrenaline, noradrenaline or dopamine are frequently used to augment mean arterial pressure to attain an adequate cerebral perfusion pressure. These should only be commenced once volume resuscitation is actively underway or complete. The early use of inotropes is increasingly being advocated during resuscitation as an important strategy during the hypoperfusion phase.[4]

There are no conclusive trials to recommend one inotrope over another or combination of inotropes. Adrenaline, noradrenaline and dopamine are equally effective in augmenting cerebral perfusion pressure. The degree by which these agents directly affect the cerebral circulation following head injury is unknown, although there is some evidence suggesting that dopamine has both direct cerebrovascular and adverse neuroendocrine effects.[23,24]

Adrenaline is widely used as an initial inotropic agent in doses titrated to achieve a desired mean or cerebral perfusion pressure. Whilst effective, it may be associated with metabolic side-effects such as hyperlactataemia and hyperglycaemia, which may complicate metabolic management. For this reason, noradrenaline is currently regarded by many as the initial agent of choice for patients with traumatic brain injury.[25]

Doses may range widely and high doses may be required to attain a desired cerebral perfusion pressure, particularly if cerebral perfusion pressures are targeted for > 72 hours. It is important to prescribe inotropes in the context of the underlying injury. Lower cerebral perfusion pressure targets (i.e. 50–70 mmHg), and therefore doses of inotropes, may be necessary if patients develop cerebral hyperaemia. Titration of inotropes may require an index of cerebral blood flow such as jugular venous saturation monitoring during this phase.

Neurogenic hypertension

Neurogenic hypertension is common in the latter phases following injury (> 5 days) and is usually centrally mediated. It may be associated with ECG changes and/or supraventricular arrhythmias. It is usually self-limiting and correlates with the severity of injury. Treatment depends on the severity of the problem: β-blockers or centrally acting agents such as clonidine are usually effective; vasodilators are relatively contraindicated.

RESPIRATORY THERAPY

Monitoring

Continuous measurement of arterial oxygen saturation is essential.

Continuous measurement of end-tidal carbon dioxide is frequently performed, although the reliability is questionable and should be intermittently checked with arterial blood gases.

Monitoring of ventilatory parameters should be consistent with standard approaches and includes measurement of tidal volumes, respiratory rates, and inspiratory and expiratory airway pressures.

Ventilation

The majority of patients with severe head injury will require mechanical ventilation to ensure adequate oxygenation and to maintain an arterial carbon dioxide tension between 36 and 40 mmHg (4.8–5.3 kPa).

The principles of optimal ventilation, humidification and weaning are addressed elsewhere. Strategies such as 'permissive hypercapnia' that are advocated for selected patients with acute lung injury or acute respiratory distress syndrome do not have a role in head-injured patients due to the requirement to maintain normocapnia.

Positive end-expiratory pressure (PEEP) is recommended at low levels (5–10 cmH_2O) to maintain functional residual capacity and oxygenation. Higher levels may compromise blood pressure, particularly in hypovolaemic patients, and should be used with caution. High levels of PEEP (> 15 cmH_2O) may compromise cerebral venous return but adverse effects on intracranial pressure are uncommon.

Weaning from ventilation should commence once intracranial pathology has stabilised – resolution of cerebral oedema on CT scan, control of intracranial hypertension and adequate cerebral perfusion pressures.

Trials of extubation should be carefully considered so that subsequent hypoxic episodes do not occur, as these are potent secondary insults.

Patients with slow recovery of adequate consciousness should be considered for early tracheostomy, either percutaneously or surgically.

Neurogenic pulmonary oedema

This is a dramatic clinical syndrome that occurs in most patients with severe head injury and correlates with severity of injury. The underlying pathophysiological process is complex, but is primarily related to centrally mediated sympathetic overactivity. It is characterised by sudden onset of clinical pulmonary oedema, hypoxia, low filling pressures, poor lung compliance and bilateral lung infiltrates, usually within 2–8 hours following injury.

The process is usually self-limiting and treatment is primarily supportive, aimed at ensuring adequate oxygenation and ventilation. This usually requires endotracheal intubation and mechanical ventilation with the administration of PEEP. Ablation of sympathetic overactivity is effectively done with adequate sedation; β-blockade is usually unnecessary. Diuretics are effective but must be titrated against the volume status of the patient so that cerebral perfusion pressure is not compromised.[26]

The development of pulmonary oedema in patients with cardiac disease should be regarded as cardiogenic until proven otherwise.

Nosocomial pneumonia

Head-injured patients who require prolonged ventilation are at increased risk of nosocomial pneumonia. This is associated with secondary brain injury and an increased mortality.[27] Risk factors include barbiturate and hypothermia therapy. Diagnosis and treatment are discussed elsewhere.

SEDATION, ANALGESIA AND MUSCLE RELAXANTS

There are no standards for sedation and analgesia in head injured patients – protocols will depend on local preferences and resources. The level of sedation and analgesia required for head-injured patients depends on the degree of traumatic coma, haemodynamic stability, intracranial pressure and systemic effects of the head injury itself.

During the resuscitation phase, where cerebral hypoperfusion is common, sedation should be titrated to cause the least effect on systemic blood pressure. During this period, short-acting narcotics such as fentanyl are useful, particularly if patients have associated extracranial injuries. These agents have relatively little adverse effect on haemodynamics and have the additional benefit of tempering systemic sympathetic surges that frequently occur after injury. As narcotics affect pupillary responses, these must be documented before administration, and CT scan should be performed soon afterwards to define baseline intracranial pathology. Short-term muscle relaxants such as vecuronium are useful during this phase to control combative patients following intubation, ventilation and sedation.

During the intensive care phase, the requirements for sedation are different. Sedation should be titrated to have the patient sedated as lightly as possible to allow clinical assessment of neurological function and to facilitate mechanical ventilation. The level of sedation will depend on haemodynamic stability and the degree of intracranial pressure. Infusions of narcotics and benzodiazepines (e.g. morphine and midazolam) are useful in providing moderate to deep levels of sedation and are effective in controlling surges of intracranial pressure. However, these agents may accumulate, resulting in a delay in return of consciousness or, if used for prolonged periods, may be associated with an emergence delirium state.

The use of propofol as a sole sedating agent has become popular.[28] It provides deep levels of sedation, which is effective in controlling systemic sympathetic swings and rises in intracranial pressure. It is rapidly reversible on cessation allowing prompt assessment of neurological status and does not accumulate. In addition, pupillary responses are not directly affected. Propofol should be used with caution in haemodynamically unstable patients, as it is a potent negative inotrope. The prolonged use of propofol is associated with tachyphylaxis and significant caloric loading from the lipid vector. Concerns have been raised about myocardial depression and sudden cardiac death, particularly if large doses are administered.[29]

The routine use of muscle relaxants is not recommended either to facilitate sedation or to control raised intracranial pressure. The prolonged use of these agents is associated with adverse outcome in traumatic brain injury and prolonged use of non-depolarising muscle relaxants is associated with polyneuromyopathies.

BODY POSITION

Patients should be nursed at 30–45° head elevation to facilitate ventilation, improve oxygenation, and reduce the risk of aspiration. The head should be kept in a neutral position.[30]

PHYSIOTHERAPY

Physiotherapy has an important role to play in the removal of lung secretions, prevention of contractures and venous thrombosis. Patients with raised intracranial pressure may require boluses of sedation before chest physiotherapy to prevent acute rises in intracranial pressure.

METABOLIC MANAGEMENT

Routine measurement of biochemistry is essential with the aim of keeping all parameters within normal limits. The syndrome of inappropriate antidiuretic hormone secretion (SIADH) and diabetes insipidus may occur following head injury. Management is discussed elsewhere.

Hyperglycaemia is common following severe head injury and is usually centrally mediated and transient. Blood sugar levels should be maintained within normal limits with insulin infusions. The role of 'tight' glycaemic control (i.e. 4.0–6.0 mmol/l) in patients with traumatic brain injury has not been determined and as hypoglycaemia is a recognised secondary insult, normal blood sugar levels (i.e. 8.0–10.0 mmol/l) are recommended.

Core temperature should be routinely monitored as hyperthermia has been identified as a cause of secondary injury. However, the real incidence of hyperpyrexic secondary brain damage may be underestimated as a temperature gradient of 1–2°C between core and brain temperature has been demonstrated and efforts should be directed at maintaining core temperature at 37.5°C.

NUTRITION

The caloric needs of head-injured patients must be addressed as soon as possible following resuscitation. Early enteral feeding is recommended.[31]

Placement of a nasogastric and/or enteral feeding tubes in head-injured patients is usually via the oral route until an anterior cranial fossa (fractured cribriform plate) is excluded. Thereafter, post-pyloric tubes, via the oral, nasal or percutaneous route, are recommended as gastroparesis is common following head injury.

STRESS ULCER PROPHYLAXIS

The incidence of gastric erosions and 'stress ulceration' has markedly decreased with better resuscitation and early enteral feeding. Head-injured patients are at no more risk than other critically ill patients for developing stress ulceration.

H_2 antagonists, such as ranitidine, should be used in ventilated patients until enteral feeding is established, following which they may be ceased.

Patients with a previous history of peptic ulceration should remain on antacid therapy for the duration of the intensive care stay.

THROMBOPROPHYLAXIS

Head-injured patients, particularly those requiring prolonged ventilation and sedation, or with extracranial injuries, are at increased risk for developing thromboembolism. The use of anticoagulants such as fractionated or low molecular weight heparins is contraindicated in patients with intracranial haemorrhage. Consequently, the role of thromboprophylactic agents in head injury is difficult and there are no standards for their use.[32]

As a general rule, anticoagulants should not be used in head-injured patients with any evidence of destructive intracranial pathology or haemorrhage, until there is resolution of these processes on CT scan.

Non-pharmacological methods of thromboprophylaxis such as elastic stockings or pneumatic calf compressors are unproven, but provide a reasonable alternative. Frequent surveillance using Doppler ultrasound of the iliofemoral veins in high-risk patients, such as those with pelvic fractures, should be performed. Patients who develop deep-vein thromboses and who cannot be anticoagulated should be considered for inferior vena caval filters. The use of anticoagulants in head-injured patients with proven pulmonary embolism will depend on the relative risk to the patients' life.

ANTIBIOTICS

These should be used sparingly and in accordance with accepted microbiological principles. Prophylactic antibiotics should only be prescribed to cover insertion of intracranial pressure monitors and are not recommended for basal skull fractures.[33] Frequent cultures of leaking or draining cerebrospinal fluid should be taken and infection treated specifically.

BRAIN-SPECIFIC MONITORING

The most accurate assessment of brain function following traumatic brain injury is a full clinical neurological examination in the absence of drugs or sedatives. However, this is often not possible for the majority of head-injured patients managed in the ICU.

Ideally, neuromonitoring should provide accurate and integrated information about intracranial pressure–volume relationships (elastance), patterns and adequacy of cerebral perfusion, and an assessment of cerebral function. No such monitor exists, although each of these parameters may be monitored in various ways with variable levels of accuracy and clinical utility.

CLINICAL ASSESSMENT

Regular assessments of GCS, pupillary signs and motor responses (see above) should be made and recorded in the ICU flow chart. Concomitant sedation may influence the level of consciousness and this should be recorded. Initially, these assessments are recorded hourly, but this may change as patients become more stable.

A witnessed deterioration in GCS, especially the motor response, or the development of new lateralising signs should be regarded as life-threatening intracranial hypertension or tentorial herniation until proven otherwise.

INTRACRANIAL ELASTANCE

Intracranial pressure monitoring

The recognition that raised intracranial pressure is associated with adverse outcome led to the measurement of this parameter in order to quantify the degree of injury and to assess the response to treatments directed at reducing intracranial pressure.

The Brain Trauma Foundation guidelines recommend intracranial pressure monitoring in patients with traumatic coma (severe head injury: GCS = 8 following non-surgical resuscitation)[34] with either:

- abnormal CT scan:
  - diffuse injury II–IV (Table 67.3) or
  - high or mixed density lesions > 25 mm
- normal CT scan with two or more of the following features.
  - age > 40 years
  - unilateral or bilateral motor posturing
  - significant extracranial trauma with systolic hypotension (< 90 mmHg)

Coagulopathy is a contraindication to intracranial pressure monitoring. Measurement of intracranial pressure[35] with an intraventricular catheter is the most accurate and clinically useful method. It has the advantages of zero calibration, cerebrospinal fluid drainage for raised intracranial pressure and allows dynamic testing of pressure–volume relationships. Disadvantages include technical difficulty with insertion, particularly in patients with cerebral oedema and compression of the lateral ventricles, and an increased incidence of infection.

Solid state systems such as fibreoptic (e.g. Camino®) or strain gauge tipped catheters (e.g. Codman®) may be placed intraparenchymally or intraventricularly. These systems transduce intracranial pressure to provide high fidelity waveforms. They are small calibre and although requiring a small craniotomy (burr hole) for insertion, may be inserted at the bedside. Disadvantages include inability to perform zero calibration after insertion and baseline drift that may be clinically significant after 5 days.

Fluid-filled subdural catheters have been used for many years. However, these are no longer recommended due to the development of more accurate solid state systems. Subdural pressures do not accurately reflect global intracranial pressure, particularly in the presence of a craniectomy. Pressure readings may also be affected by local clot formation within the catheter.

Measurements are used to calculate cerebral perfusion pressure: mean arterial pressure minus intracranial pressure. For this calculation, both measurements should be referenced to the external auditory meatus (equivalent to the circle of Willis).

Intracranial pressure monitoring should be continued until the patient can be assessed clinically, intracranial pressure has stabilised (< 20–$25\ cmH_2O$) and cerebral oedema has resolved on CT scan. This occurs in the majority of patients within 7 days. Patients with refractory intracranial hypertension may require monitoring for longer periods, although this may be complicated by drift (with solid state systems), infection (with intraventricular catheters) or occlusion (subdural catheters). In this situation, intracranial pressure monitors may need to be replaced or removed and patients assessed by serial CT scan or clinically.

CEREBRAL BLOOD FLOW

Currently, there is no method of routinely measuring cerebral blood flow at the bedside. Technological advances such as mapping with labelled xenon under computed tomography and laser Doppler flowmetry provide useful imaging of regional and cerebral blood flow. However, these techniques are intermittent, labour intensive and limited to research-based units.

A number of qualitative measurement techniques are available that provide an indirect assessment of cerebral blood flow that may be useful, particularly when used in conjunction with other modalities such as intracranial pressure monitoring and CT scanning. Interpretation of these measurements must be taken within the clinical context, particularly the time course of the underlying injury (Figure 67.2).

Jugular bulb oximetry

Measurement of oxygen saturation in the jugular bulb by the retrograde placement of a fibreoptic catheter provides an indirect assessment of cerebral perfusion. Low jugular venous saturations ($< 55\%$) may be indicative of cerebral hypoperfusion due to systemic hypotension or hypocapnia. High levels of jugular venous saturation ($> 85\%$) may be indicative of cerebral hyperaemia or inadequate neuronal metabolism, such as occurs during the hyperaemic phase or during the evolution of brain death. Both low and high jugular venous saturation are associated with adverse outcomes.[36]

There are insufficient data to provide evidence-based indications for the routine use of jugular bulb oximetry. Its use is limited to experienced units when an index of cerebral blood flow is required during adjunctive therapies in patients with intracranial hypertension – for example, cerebral perfusion pressure augmentation with catecholamines, barbiturate coma, hyperventilation or hypothermia.

Transcranial Doppler

Transcranial Doppler ultrasonography with a 2 MHz pulsed Doppler probe allows non-invasive, intermittent or continuous assessment of the velocity of blood flow through large cerebral vessels. Insonation through a naturally occurring acoustic window such as the transtemporal approach allows insonation of the anterior, middle and posterior cerebral arteries, terminal internal carotid artery and anterior and posterior communicating arteries.[37]

Measured indices of flow include systolic, mean and diastolic flow velocities. Distinct patterns associated with normal, hyperaemic, vasospastic and absent flow are recognised. Derived indices such as the Gosling pulsatility index (systolic/diastolic difference divided by the mean velocity) and Lindegaard ratio (between middle cerebral artery to extracranial internal carotid artery) may assist in differentiating these flow patterns.

Despite increasing use of transcranial Doppler to diagnose posttraumatic hyperaemia and vasospasm, there are insufficient data to provide evidence-based indications for the routine use of transcranial Doppler.

Continuous measurements and trends of transcranial Doppler provide a better assessment of flow/velocity patterns than intermittent or daily measurements. The technique is operator-dependent and there may be significant variations in velocity patterns during the course of the injury. Consequently, interpretation of intermittent measurements should be made in conjunction with other variables such as CT scan appearance, intracranial pressure and, where applicable, jugular venous saturation.

CEREBRAL FUNCTION AND METABOLISM

Electroencephalography

Electroencephalography has been used for many years to assess seizure activity that may be masked by sedatives or muscle relaxants and to provide an objective estimate of the degree of electrical neuronal depression with barbiturate therapy. Whilst seizures may not be clinically apparent in a proportion of patients, and may constitute an important secondary insult, the accuracy and reliability of electroencephalography in ICUs is questionable due to outside electrical interference from monitors and ventilators.[38]

The development of bispectral index (BIS monitoring) as a measurement of depth of anaesthesia has led to the suggestion that this may be an alternative to the use of electroencephalography with barbiturate or sedative therapy in traumatic brain injury. Bispectral index has not been validated in this context and cannot be recommended as a titration end-point.[39]

Other forms of electroencephalography such as processed electroencephalography and integrated cerebral function monitors have a limited role in head-injured patients due to the amount of data generated and the need for skilled personnel to acquire and interpret the data.

Evoked potentials

Measurement of evoked potentials, assessing the integrity of sensory and motor pathways, may provide diagnostic and prognostic information; however, because of the complexity of the technique, it is not recommended for general use.[40] The reliance of one variable, such as evoked potentials, to predict outcome from traumatic brain injury is not recommended.

Neuronal function

Research developments in microprobe technology have resulted in specific electrodes that may be placed into the brain parenchyma to measure brain oxygen, pH and carbon dioxide tensions. These may be individual electrodes or combined with other sensors such as pressure monitors to form multimodal tissue monitors.

Cerebral microdialysis is a technique that measures brain extracellular fluid metabolites. Dialysate is obtained through a microdialysis catheter inserted through the same burr hole as an intracranial pressure monitor to measure concentration and fluxes of markers of intracranial inflammation (e.g. lactate, pyruvate and purines).[41]

Whilst these systems provide highly specific information about the biochemical milieu of focal areas of brain tissue, their clinical utility is limited to research centres.

BRAIN INJURY SURVEILLANCE

Serial assessment of the anatomical injury is an essential part of monitoring head injury. This is done by serial CT scanning at frequent intervals depending on the neurological status of the patient.

Any patient who develops an unexplained neurological deterioration or significant validated deviation of monitored parameters should have a CT scan so that new or delayed intracranial mass lesions are identified.

CT scans should be assessed and scored according to the classification outlined in Table 67.3. The progression or resolution of axonal injury, cerebral oedema, contusion and haemorrhages should be recorded. Other parameters such as intracranial pressure and jugular venous saturation should be interpreted in accordance with the CT scan appearance.

However, as CT scanning requires transport of the patient to a radiology suite, this should only be done by experienced personnel when the patient is stable.

BRAIN-SPECIFIC THERAPY

Treatment options directed at ameliorating brain injury are limited. Despite intensive research into defining the pathobiological processes in primary injury, studies analysing therapies designed to modulate intracranial inflammation have not been successful. These include aminosteroids, calcium channel blockade and *N*-methyl-D-aspartic acid (NMDA) antagonists.[42]

Brain-specific or 'targeted' therapy is directed at maintaining cerebral perfusion pressure and minimising intracranial pressure. Whilst there is an inherent relationship between these two principles, priorities are different depending on the time course of the underlying injury. This is important as strategies directed at one may have adverse effects in the other (Figure 67.2).

DEFENCE OF CEREBRAL PERFUSION PRESSURE

The pathophysiological principles outlined on p. 765 are important in defining strategies to optimise cerebral perfusion pressure following injury. Whilst the Brain Trauma Foundation guidelines recommend a cerebral perfusion pressure of 60–70 mmHg, this figure may not be applicable over the entire time course following injury.[3]

This requires a change from a 'set and forget' philosophy to one of 'titration against time' in order to prescribe desirable therapeutic targets.

Hypoperfusion phase (0–72 hours)

Cerebral hypoperfusion is present in the majority of patients with severe head injury (GCS = 8). During this phase, augmentation of cerebral perfusion pressure is paramount and should be done by maintaining adequate haemodynamic function.

The principles outlined above on 'Haemodynamic management' become the mainstay of defence of cerebral perfusion pressure. This phase should be regarded as an extension of resuscitation and supportive treatment. During this period, a cerebral perfusion pressure of at least 60 mmHg is recommended. In addition to reduced cerebral blood flow, intracranial pressure may be increased by mass lesions or 'cytotoxic' cerebral oedema. The latter will usually respond to restoration of cerebral perfusion pressure.

During this phase, medical therapies directed at raised intracranial pressure such as osmotherapy or hyperventilation should only be used if cerebral perfusion pressure is maintained at an appropriate level and the patient is adequately monitored.

Assessment of adequacy of the response to augmentation of cerebral perfusion pressure is made by intracranial pressure trends, CT scan appearance and, where possible, neurological assessment. If patients appear to have stabilised, sedation may be reduced with the aim of extubation.

Hyperaemic phase (3–7 days)

Approximately 25–30% of patients will develop clinical signs of cerebral hyperaemia, characterised by raised intracranial pressure, persistent cerebral oedema on CT scan and possibly confirmed by high jugular venous saturations.[43] This may be due to vasogenic cerebral oedema caused by intracranial inflammation or by catecholamine infusions often used to augment cerebral perfusion pressure.

The diagnosis of catecholamine-induced cerebral hyperaemia is difficult. This should be suspected in patients who require progressively increasing doses of catecholamines (e.g. $> 20\ \mu g/min$ of adrenaline or noradrenaline) to attain a prescribed cerebral perfusion pressure of 60 mmHg. This phenomenon is due to tachyphylaxis to prolonged catecholamine infusions and may be responsible for iatrogenically increasing intracranial pressure.

If CT appearance is unchanged, cerebral perfusion pressure targets may be lowered in order to use lower doses of inotropes. This exercise may be facilitated by jugular venous saturation monitoring or transcranial Doppler to provide an index of adequate cerebral blood flow for the lower cerebral perfusion pressure.

If patients continue to have raised intracranial pressure, strategies directed at reducing intracranial pressure should be considered.

REDUCTION OF INTRACRANIAL PRESSURE

In the absence of intracranial mass lesions, raised intracranial pressure is usually an indicator of severity of the underlying injury and represents exhausted intracranial elastance.

The most effective methods of reducing raised intracranial pressure are mechanical interventions such as removal of mass lesions, drainage of cerebrospinal fluid or decompressive craniectomy.

A number of medical strategies directed at reducing intracranial pressure have been used for many years. Despite widespread use and firmly held beliefs, there is little evidence to support the routine use of these therapies.[44]

Intracranial pressure should be maintained at $< 25\ cmH_2O$.[45] Trends of intracranial pressure are equally as important and should be assessed within the context of cerebral perfusion pressure and the methods used to defend it.

Surgical evacuation of mass lesions

The prompt detection and evacuation of mass lesions causing raised intracranial pressure is the most effective method of relieving intracranial hypertension. Although the majority of these lesions will be present immediately after injury and will be treated during the resuscitative phase, approximately 10% patients will develop delayed intracranial haematomas. These are detected by sudden unexplained rises in intracranial pressure or by CT scan surveillance.

Close liaison and coordination with neurosurgeons is essential.

Cerebrospinal fluid drainage

Drainage of cerebrospinal fluid through an intraventricular catheter is an effective method of reducing intracranial pressure. If present, these catheters should be placed 5–10 cm above the head and opened for drainage every 1–4 hours.

Decompressive craniectomy

Wide, bilateral, frontoparietal craniectomies are increasingly being advocated to reduce intracranial pressure in patients with refractory intracranial hypertension. Whilst there are numerous case series demonstrating dramatic improvements, there are no conclusive outcome-based trials to make firm recommendations.[46]

Recent experience in paediatric patients is encouraging and the role of pre-emptive decompressive craniectomy in high-risk patients is yet to be determined.[47]

Osmotherapy

The rationale and role of osmotherapy using mannitol or hypertonic solution is addressed on p. 780. The same principles during resuscitation apply during intensive care management.

Mannitol or hypertonic saline should only be used in patients with validated intracranial hypertension who are euvolaemic, haemodynamically stable, with a serum osmolality < 320 mosm/l.

There is no evidence that osmotherapy or induced dehydration improves outcome or is more effective in cytotoxic than vasogenic cerebral oedema.[15]

Hyperventilation

The role of hyperventilation during intensive care management is limited to the indications outlined on p. 780.

The routine prolonged use of hyperventilation in head-injured patients is associated with a worse outcome than patients ventilated to normocapnia. This is probably due to reductions of cerebral blood flow and secondary brain ischaemia.

Current evidence-based guidelines do not recommend the use of routine hyperventilation.[9]

Hypothermia

Induced hypothermia has been used for many years to reduce cerebral metabolism and thereby raised intracranial pressure. A sound theoretical benefit exists in experimental models where hypothermia is induced immediately following injury with prompt reduction in raised intracranial pressure. However, these benefits have not translated into improved outcomes in a number of clinical trials.[48]

Induced hypothermia (to temperatures of 30–33°C) is associated with prolonged ventilation and increased susceptibility to nosocomial infection, and may be associated with increased morbidity and mortality in head-injured patients.

Currently, hypothermia is regarded as a 'second tier' option in patients with refractory intracranial hypertension, but on current evidence, cannot be recommended.

Barbiturate coma

The role of barbiturates in traumatic brain injury is similar to hypothermia. Despite experimental evidence that barbiturates reduce cerebral metabolism and reduce intracranial pressure, no definitive studies have shown a benefit in clinical trials. Barbiturates have invariably been used in patients with refractory intracranial hypertension where a positive outcome was unlikely, making interpretation of these trials difficult.

Titration of barbiturate coma to burst suppression on an electroencephalograph is suggested as a reasonable end-point. However, this is often difficult to obtain and measure.

Barbiturates may cause hypotension and reduce cerebral blood flow, potentially exacerbating secondary insults in patients with cerebral oligaemia. Prolonged use of barbiturates will delay awakening and predispose the patient to nosocomial infection.

Barbiturates are a 'second tier' option in patients with refractory intracranial hypertension and not recommended on current evidence.[49]

Steroids

Steroids have been advocated for many years to ameliorate intracranial inflammation, thereby reducing intracranial pressure. A large international study has provided conclusive evidence that steroids may be associated with adverse outcomes in traumatic brain injury, and therefore have no place in management.[50,51]

Cerebral blood volume regulation

Following resuscitation and stabilisation, a strategy reducing cerebral perfusion pressure to > 50 mmHg using colloids, β-blockade, clonidine and dihydroergotamine may be effective in minimising secondary cerebral hyperaemia and vasogenic oedema. This strategy requires a measurement of cerebral blood flow to demonstrate adequate cerebral perfusion.[52]

CEREBRAL VASOSPASM

Posttraumatic cerebral vasospasm occurs in approximately 10–15% of patients. It is associated with a high morbidity and mortality. It is frequently present in patients with traumatic subarachnoid haemorrhage and is a marker of severity of injury.

Cerebral angiography and transcranial Doppler are frequently used to diagnose vasospasm, although false positives and negatives exist with both techniques and the true incidence of clinically significant vasospasm is uncertain.

Treatment options remain limited. Calcium antagonists, such as nimodipine, have not been shown to be effective in traumatic subarachnoid haemorrhage. Strategies that have been used in aneurysmal subarachnoid haemorrhage such as 'triple H' therapy (induced hypertension, hypervolaemia and haemodilution) or chemical angioplasty have not been evaluated in traumatic subarachnoid haemorrhage and are not recommended.[5]

SEIZURE PROPHYLAXIS

Seizures are infrequent following traumatic brain injury and usually present at the time of injury. These should be treated with anticonvulsants (e.g. diazepam, midazolam) when they occur. Subsequent prophylaxis with phenytoin is recommended only in patients with destructive parenchymal lesions on CT scan and continued for 10 days following injury. Short-term seizure prophylaxis does not prevent late onset posttraumatic epilepsy.[53]

OUTCOME AND PROGNOSIS

Patient factors that determine outcome from traumatic brain injury include severity of primary and secondary injuries, low GCS on presentation,[54] advanced age (> 60 years)[55] and comorbidities. Prediction of outcome is difficult and must be made with circumspection as significant functional improvements, particularly in young patients, may occur over time.

There are patients in whom the prognosis is clearly very poor or hopeless. A proportion of these patients will become brain dead and may be considered for organ donation. This is discussed elsewhere. In other patients, it may be appropriate to withdraw active treatment. This increasingly complex process requires time, careful consideration and consensus with all members of the health care and relatives.

Outcomes from traumatic brain injury are difficult to quantify. Whilst mortality is an easy end-point to measure, functional outcome is an equally important measurement, as the effects of traumatic brain injury on psychosocial recovery and duration of rehabilitation often take extended periods of time.

The future challenge facing the intensive care management of traumatic brain injury is to determine whether standards of practice and innovations improve mortality and functional survival. There is a responsibility to ensure that accurate outcome data are collected both at institution and regional levels. This will define the epidemiology and provide the basis for future studies.

REFERENCES

1. Myburgh JA, Cooper DJ, Finfer SR *et al.* Epidemiology and 12-month outcomes from traumatic brain injury in Australia and New Zealand. *J Trauma* 2008; **64**: 854–62.
2. Martin NA, Patwardhan RV, Alexander MJ *et al.* Characterization of cerebral hemodynamic phases following severe head trauma: hypoperfusion, hyperemia, and vasospasm. *J Neurosurg* 1997; **87**: 9–19.
3. BTF Guidelines. Brain Trauma Foundation. American Association of Neurological Surgeons. Guidelines for cerebral perfusion pressure. *J Neurotrauma* 2000; **17**: 497–506.
4. Myburgh JA. Driving cerebral perfusion pressure with pressors: how, which, when? *Crit Care Resusc* 2005; 7: 200–5.
5. Oertel M, Boscardin WJ, Obrist WD *et al.* Posttraumatic vasospasm: the epidemiology, severity, and time course of an underestimated phenomenon: a prospective study performed in 299 patients. *J Neurosurg* 2005; **103**: 812–24.
6. American College of Surgeons Committee on Trauma. *Advanced Trauma Life Support for Doctors.* Chicago IL: American College of Surgeons; 1997.
7. BTF Guidelines. The Brain Trauma Foundation. The American Association of Neurological Surgeons. Initial management. *J Neurotrauma* 2000; **17**: 463–70.
8. BTF Guidelines. Brain Trauma Foundation. American Association of Neurological Surgeons. Resuscitation of blood pressure and oxygenation. *J Neurotrauma* 2000; **17**: 471–8.
9. BTF Guidelines. Brain Trauma Foundation. American Association of Neurological Surgeons. Hyperventilation. *J Neurotrauma* 2000; **17**: 513–20.
10. BTF Guidelines. Brain Trauma Foundation. American Association of Neurological Surgeons. Hypotension. *J Neurotrauma* 2000; **17**: 591–5.
11. SAFE Study Investigators. A comparison of albumin and saline for fluid resuscitation in the intensive care unit. *N Engl J Med* 2004; **350**: 2247–56.
12. Qureshi AI, Suarez JI. Use of hypertonic saline solutions in treatment of cerebral edema and intracranial hypertension. *Crit Care Med* 2000; **28**: 3301–13.
13. Cooper DJ, Myles PS, McDermott FT *et al.* Prehospital hypertonic saline resuscitation of patients with hypotension and severe traumatic brain injury: a randomized controlled trial. *JAMA* 2004; **291**: 1350–7.
14. Teasdale G, Jennett B. Assessment of coma and impaired consciousness. A practical scale. *Lancet* 1974; **2**: 81–4.
15. BTF Guidelines. Brain Trauma Foundation. American Association of Neurological Surgeons. Mannitol. *J Neurotrauma* 2000; **17**: 521–6.
16. Doyle JA, Davis DP, Hoyt DB. The use of hypertonic saline in the treatment of traumatic brain injury. *J Trauma* 2001; **50**: 367–83.
17. Cooper DJ, Ackland HM. Clearing the cervical spine in the unconscious head injured patient. *Crit Care Resusc* 2005; 7: 181–4.
18. BTF Guidelines. Brain Trauma Foundation. American Association of Neurological Surgeons. Computed tomography scan features. *J Neurotrauma* 2000; **17**: 597–627.
19. Servadei F, Murray GD, Teasdale GM *et al.* Traumatic subarachnoid hemorrhage: demographic and clinical study of 750 patients from the European brain injury consortium survey of head injuries. *Neurosurgery* 2002; **50**: 261–7.
20. BTF Guidelines. Brain Trauma Foundation. American Association of Neurological Surgeons. Trauma systems. *J Neurotrauma* 2000; **17**: 457–62.
21. BTF Guidelines. Brain Trauma Foundation. American Association of Neurological Surgeons. Management and prognosis of severe traumatic brain injury. *J Neurotrauma* 2000; **17**: 449–554.
22. Maas AI, Dearden M, Teasdale GM *et al.* EBIC-guidelines for management of severe head injury in adults. European Brain Injury Consortium. *Acta Neurochir (Wien)* 1997; **139**: 286–94.
23. Myburgh JA, Upton RN, Grant C *et al.* A comparison of the effects of norepinephrine, epinephrine, and dopamine on cerebral blood flow and oxygen utilisation. *Acta Neurochir Suppl (Wien)* 1998; **71**: 19–21.
24. Van den Berghe G, de Zegher F. Anterior pituitary function during critical illness and dopamine treatment. *Crit Care Med* 1996; **24**: 1580–90.
25. Ract C, Vigue B. Comparison of the cerebral effects of dopamine and norepinephrine in severely head-injured patients. *Intensive Care Med* 2001; **27**: 101–6.
26. McManis P, Lee C, Morgan M *et al.* Neurogenic pulmonary oedema. *Aust N Z J Med* 2000; **30**: 514.
27. Ewig S, Torres A, El Ebiary M *et al.* Bacterial colonization patterns in mechanically ventilated patients with traumatic and medical head injury. Incidence, risk factors, and association with ventilator-associated pneumonia. *Am J Respir Crit Care Med* 1999; **159**: 188–98.
28. Kelly DF, Goodale DB, Williams J *et al.* Propofol in the treatment of moderate and severe head injury: a randomized, prospective double-blinded pilot trial. *J Neurosurg* 1999; **90**: 1042–52.
29. Cremer OL, Moons KGM, Bouman ACB *et al.* Long-term propofol infusion and cardiac failure in adult head-injured patients. *Lancet* 2001; **357**: 117–18.
30. Winkelman C. Effect of backrest position on intracranial and cerebral perfusion pressures in traumatically brain-injured adults. *Am J Crit Care* 2000; **9**: 373–80.
31. BTF Guidelines. Brain Trauma Foundation. American Association of Neurological Surgeons. Nutrition. *J Neurotrauma* 2000; **17**: 539–48.
32. Hammond FM, Meighen MJ. Venous thromboembolism in the patient with acute traumatic brain injury: screening, diagnosis, prophylaxis, and treatment issues. *J Head Trauma Rehabil* 1998; **13**: 36–50.
33. Jacobs DG, Westerband A. Antibiotic prophylaxis for intracranial pressure monitors. *J Natl Med Assoc* 1998; **90**: 417–23.

34. BTF Guidelines. Brain Trauma Foundation. American Association of Neurological Surgeons. Indications for intracranial pressure monitoring. *J Neurotrauma* 2000; **17**: 479–92.
35. BTF Guidelines. Brain Trauma Foundation. American Association of Neurological Surgeons. Recommendations for intracranial pressure monitoring technology. *J Neurotrauma* 2000; **17**: 497–506.
36. Macmillan CS, Andrews PJ, Easton VJ. Increased jugular bulb saturation is associated with poor outcome in traumatic brain injury. *J Neurol Neurosurg Psychiatry* 2001; **70**: 101–4.
37. Castillo MA. Monitoring neurologic patients in intensive care. *Curr Opin Crit Care* 2001; **7**: 49–60.
38. Procaccio F, Polo A, Lanteri P *et al.* Electrophysiologic monitoring in neurointensive care. *Curr Opin Crit Care* 2001; **7**: 74–80.
39. Myles PS, Cairo S. Artifact in the bispectral index in a patient with severe ischemic brain injury. *Anesth Analg* 2004; **98**: 706–7.
40. Carter BG, Butt W. Review of the use of somatosensory evoked potentials in the prediction of outcome after severe brain injury. *Crit Care Med* 2001; **29**: 178–86.
41. Peerdeman SM, Girbes AR, Vandertop WP. Cerebral microdialysis as a new tool for neurometabolic monitoring. *Intensive Care Med* 2000; **26**: 662–9.
42. Maas AI, Steyerberg EW, Murray GD *et al.* Why have recent trials of neuroprotective agents in head injury failed to show convincing efficacy? A pragmatic analysis and theoretical considerations. *Neurosurgery* 1999; **44**: 1286–98.
43. Marmarou A, Fatouros PP, Barzo P *et al.* Contribution of edema and cerebral blood volume to traumatic brain swelling in head-injured patients. *J Neurosurg* 2000; **93**: 183–93.
44. BTF Guidelines. Brain Trauma Foundation. American Association of Neurological Surgeons. Critical pathway for the treatment of established intracranial hypertension. *J Neurotrauma* 2000; **17**: 537–8.
45. BTF Guidelines. Brain Trauma Foundation. American Association of Neurological Surgeons. Intracranial pressure treatment threshold. *J Neurotrauma* 2000; **17**: 493–5.
46. Munch E, Horn P, Schurer L *et al.* Management of severe traumatic brain injury by decompressive craniectomy. *Neurosurgery* 2000; **47**: 315–22.
47. Taylor A, Butt W, Rosenfeld J *et al.* A randomized trial of very early decompressive craniectomy in children with traumatic brain injury and sustained intracranial hypertension. *Childs Nerv Syst* 2001; **17**: 154–62.
48. Clifton GL, Miller ER, Choi SC *et al.* Lack of effect of induction of hypothermia after acute brain injury. *N Engl J Med* 2001; **344**: 556–63.
49. BTF Guidelines. Brain Trauma Foundation. American Association of Neurological Surgeons. Use of barbiturates in the control of intracranial hypertension. *J Neurotrauma* 2000; **17**: 527–30.
50. Edwards P, Arango M, Balica L *et al.* Final results of MRC CRASH, a randomised placebo-controlled trial of intravenous corticosteroid in adults with head injury – outcomes at 6 months. *Lancet* 2005; **365**: 1957–9.
51. Roberts I, Yates D, Sandercock P *et al.* Effect of intravenous corticosteroids on death within 14 days in 10008 adults with clinically significant head injury (MRC CRASH trial): randomised placebo-controlled trial. *Lancet* 2004; **364**: 1321–8.
52. Eker C, Asgeirsson B, Grande PO *et al.* Improved outcome after severe head injury with a new therapy based on principles for brain volume regulation and preserved microcirculation. *Crit Care Med* 1998; **26**: 1881–6.
53. BTF Guidelines. Brain Trauma Foundation. American Association of Neurological Surgeons. Role of antiseizure prophylaxis following head injury. *J Neurotrauma* 2000; **17**: 549–54.
54. BTF Guidelines. Brain Trauma Foundation. American Association of Neurological Surgeons. Glasgow Coma Scale Score. *J Neurotrauma* 2000; **17**: 563–72.
55. BTF Guidelines. Brain Trauma Foundation. American Association of Neurological Surgeons. Age. *J Neurotrauma* 2000; **17**: 573–82.

68

Maxillofacial and upper-airway injuries

Cyrus Edibam

MAXILLOFACIAL INJURIES

Life-threatening haemorrhage and airway obstruction are common complications accompanying severe blunt or penetrating maxillofacial and neck injury. Injuries may be isolated or part of multisystem trauma. Up to 20% of people with facial injury will have life-threatening associated injuries: 15% with closed head injury, 3.5% with airway obstruction and 1.5% with pulmonary contusion and/or aspiration.[1–3] Urgent skilled airway management and awareness of other commonly associated injuries to the brain, cervical spine, thorax and oesophagus are paramount in preventing adverse outcomes. This chapter outlines the basic anatomy, pathology, complications and common pitfalls in the emergency management of maxillofacial, upper-airway and non-bony neck trauma.

EPIDEMIOLOGY

Maxillofacial trauma occurs most frequently in the 20–25 years age group, decreasing in frequency either side of this age group. It is three to five times more likely to occur in males than in females. Blunt injury is by far the commonest mechanism, accounting for nearly 97% of all maxillofacial injuries.[4] Motor vehicle accidents (MVAs) account for nearly three-quarters of blunt injuries, with falls, physical assault, contact sports and industrial accidents accounting for the remainder. Legislative changes and preventative measures involving drink-driving, seatbelt and airbag use have seen a reduction in the incidence of MVA-related maxillofacial injury.[5,6] In multiple trauma patients with an injury severity score (ISS) > 12, maxillofacial injury occurs in up to 17%, with a corresponding mortality rate of 13%.[4]

ANATOMICAL ASPECTS

Fractures, haemorrhage, soft-tissue damage and oedema are the commonest manifestations of blunt facial trauma. The severity of facial injury is directly related to the velocity of force applied.[7] Common fractures of facial bones are maxilla (23%), orbital region (22%), zygoma (16%), nasal bones (15%), mandible (13%), teeth (8%), alveolar ridge (2%) and temporomandibular joint (TMJ) 1%.[4]

MANDIBULAR FRACTURES

The mandible is a unique, horseshoe-shaped bone that is tubular and weakest where the cortices are thinnest; most fractures occur at vulnerable points, regardless of the point of impact.[8] Common sites are the ramus (condylar neck and angle of the mandible) and body at the level of the first or second molar. Multiple fractures are common (64%),[8] with body of mandible fractures often being accompanied by fractures of the opposite angle or neck, due to transmitted forces. Mandibular fragments are often distracted due to the action of the lower jaw muscles. Respiratory obstruction may occur after bilateral mandibular angle or body fractures due to the posterior displacement of the tongue – the 'Andy Gump' fracture.[9,10]

MIDFACIAL FRACTURES

The bones of the middle third of the face are relatively thin and poorly reinforced. Fracture dislocations occur through the bones and suture lines and the facial skeleton acts as a compressible energy-absorbing mass that gives on impact. The series of compartments (nasal cavity, paranasal sinuses and orbits) within the bony framework collapse progressively, absorbing energy and protecting the brain, spinal cord and other vital structures.[11] Multiple complex facial fractures usually result and isolated facial bone fractures are rare. Le Fort described three great lines of weakness in the facial skeleton and thus derived the Le Fort classification of fractures[12] (Figure 68.1). Le Fort fractures are perpendicular to the three main vertical buttresses of the facial skeleton – the nasomaxillary, zygomaticomaxillary and pterygomaxillary 'pillars'. Le Fort fractures rarely occur in their pure form with mixed patterns prevailing (e.g. right hemifacial Le Fort I and left hemifacial Le Fort II). Airway obstruction from posterior movement of the soft palate against the tongue and the posterior pharyngeal wall may occur. Oral secretions, blood, bone and tooth debris and pharyngeal wall haematomas may worsen airway compromise.

LE FORT I (ALSO KNOWN AS GUERIN'S FRACTURE)

This fracture involves only the maxilla at the level of the nasal fossa. It follows a horizontal plane at the level of the nose. The fracture separates the palate from the

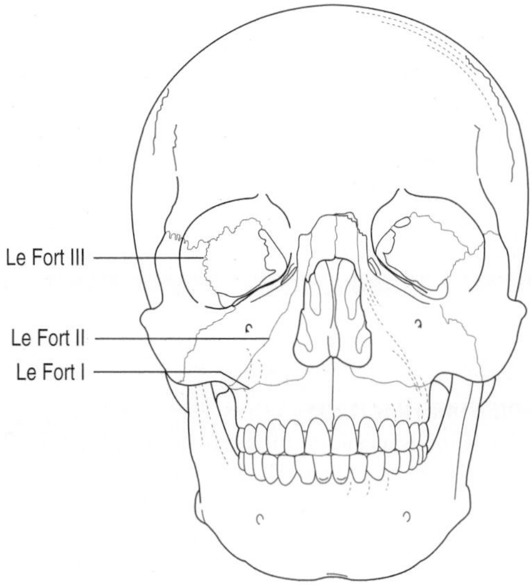

Figure 68.1 Le Fort classification of facial fractures.

remainder of the facial skeleton (i.e. palate–facial disjunction) and is usually caused by direct low-maxillary blows or by a lateral blow to the maxilla.

LE FORT II

This is the most common midface fracture.[13] The maxilla, nasal bones and medial aspect of the orbit are involved which results in a freely mobile, pyramidal-shaped portion of the maxilla (i.e. pyramidal disjunction). The fracture line extends from the lower nasal bridge through the medial wall of the orbit, and crosses the zygomaticomaxillary process. It is caused by direct blows to the mid-alveolar area, or by lateral impacts and inferior blows to the mandible when the mouth is closed.

LE FORT III

This is known as craniofacial disjunction because the fracture line runs parallel to the base of the skull, separating the midfacial skeleton from the cranium. The fracture extends through the upper nasal bridge and most of the orbit and across the zygomatic arch. It involves the ethmoid bone, and thus may transect the cribriform plate at the base of the skull.[13,14] These fractures result from superiorly directed blows to the nasal bones.[13]

TEMPOROMANDIBULAR JOINT

Mechanical TMJ impairment may result from condylar or zygomatic arch fractures and can prevent jaw opening even after muscle relaxants have been administered.[15]

ZYGOMATIC, ORBITAL AND NASAL FRACTURES

Zygomatic fractures are uncommon, but its attachments to the maxilla, frontal and temporal bones are vulnerable and may be disrupted. When the zygoma is displaced, disruption of the lateral wall and floor of the orbit may ensue. Orbital injury is commonly associated with midface trauma. The severity of injury in the orbital region varies from oedema and ecchymosis of the periosteal soft tissue to subconjunctival haemorrhage and loss of visual acuity or ocular rupture. Blinding injuries reported with facial fractures occur in 3–12% and most are secondary to globe perforation rather than optic nerve injury.[16] Orbital blowout fractures occur when pressure is directly applied to the eye, and is hydraulically transmitted via the globe to the interior bony structures. The weaker inferior wall usually fractures, causing enophthalmos, diplopia, impaired eye movement and infraorbital hypoaesthesia. Nasal fractures are common, with epistaxis and septal haematoma being the prime concerns.

SOFT-TISSUE INJURIES

Abrasions, contusions, lacerations to the tongue, palate, pharynx, cheek, eyelids, nasolacrimal duct, ear, parotid gland and facial nerve can occur. Oedema evolving over 24–48 hours can be massive and cause gross distortion of soft-tissue structures. Patency of an initially unobstructed airway may become compromised during this period.

HAEMORRHAGE

Haemorrhage following blunt maxillofacial injury is extremely common. Life-threatening bleeding is fortunately rare. Various series have reported the incidence to be between 1 and 10%.[1,17–19] Most severe haemorrhage is associated with midfacial fractures although soft-tissue lacerations alone can cause significant blood loss. Swallowing of large quantities of blood may conceal haemorrhage and predispose to aspiration.[20]

The origin of bleeding in facial trauma is complicated, as the vascular supply is derived from both the internal and external carotid arteries, with anastomoses occurring between them as well as between both halves of the face. The internal maxillary artery, especially the intraosseous branches, is the main source of bleeding in facial injury, because the artery passes within the common Le Fort fracture borders.[16] The comminuted nature of maxillary fractures makes the detection of an exact site of vessel damage nearly impossible.[16] Branches of the internal carotid artery such as the lacrimal and zygomatic branches, as well as the anterior and posterior ethmoidal arteries, may contribute to bleeding.

ASSOCIATED INJURIES

More than half of all patients with maxillofacial injuries will have other injuries and these are listed below.

Basilar skull fracture

The anterior cranial fossa is often involved in craniofacial injuries. Fractures involving the frontal bone, frontal sinus, nasoethmoid complex or fronto-orbital complex result in bone defects in the skull base and can cause dural tears with resultant leakage of cerebrospinal fluid (CSF). CSF fistulae occur in 10–30% of basilar skull fractures.[21] The clinical finding of CSF rhinorrhoea is not diagnostic for anterior cranial fossa lesions, as this represents only the site of exiting CSF. The origin may be from a temporal bone fracture, because CSF from the middle ear discharges into the nose via the Eustachian tube. A middle cranial fossa defect can produce rhinorrhoea through the sphenoid sinus. The vast majority of fistulae present within 1 week of injury. Meningitis in patients with midface fractures is uncommon, despite the fact that approximately 36% of patients sustaining Le Fort fractures with anterior cranial fossa fractures have CSF leaks.[22,23]

Pulsating exophthalmos and the presence of an orbital bruit may lead to the diagnosis of a carotido-cavernous fistula, which may develop following fractures involving the skull base and orbit.

Head and cervical spine injury

The incidence of head injury in those with maxillofacial trauma has been variably reported to be between 15% for severe head injury, increasing to 80% if all grades of head injuries are included.[1,4,24] Cervical spine injury has been reported in up to 11% of patients.

The association between maxillofacial and cervical spine injury depends on the mechanism of injury. Falls and motor vehicle accident victims are more likely to have cervical injury than sporting or personal assault victims.[25] Cervical spine fracture occurs with mandibular injury in 3%[16] and is attributed to forces exerted directly or indirectly from the facial skeleton to the neck. C1/C2 and C5–C7 are at particular risk.

Other injuries

Thoracic (9–40%) and abdominal (5–40%) trauma and limb fractures (30%) are other common coexistent injuries.[24,26] Traumatic occlusion of the internal carotid artery (ICA) is a rare complication of maxillofacial trauma occurring in less than 0.5% of patients presenting with blunt maxillofacial injury.[27,28] It is usually recognised when a patient develops an unexplained neurological deficit, most often hemiplegia, subsequent to trauma or surgery of the head, face or neck. Assessment of the carotid circulation by CT angiography is a useful investigation if carotid injury is suspected.

ASSESSMENT OF INJURY

The obvious priorities are airway management and control of haemorrhage and identifying other life-threatening injuries. These are discussed later in detail. Once the patient is stable, formal assessment of the facial injuries can proceed.

HISTORY

Evaluation of facial fractures begins with a history of the injury. The mechanism of injury is important in order to assess the likelihood of other injuries.

EXAMINATION

Physical examination includes inspection of the deformity, presence of enophthalmos, asymmetry, dental malocclusion, nasal septal deviation or haematoma, CSF rhinorrhoea and the extent of jaw opening. Other signs associated with basal skull fracture should also be noted (haemotympanum, Battle's sign, raccoon eyes). Tenderness and mobility on bimanual palpation of the alveolar process and the infraorbital rim or frontozygomatic suture indicates the presence of a complex midfacial fracture. Naso-orbito-ethmoid instability can also be established by bimanual palpation. Visual acuity (in the conscious patient), corneal integrity and pupillary reflexes as well as eye movements (failure of upward movements in orbital blowout fracture) should be assessed early and thoroughly. Facial nerve function should also be assessed if possible. The presence of a bruit over the orbit may indicate a carotido-cavernous fistula.

INVESTIGATION

Radiographic studies include a posterior–anterior, lateral oblique, stereo Water's view, stereo Caldwell's view and Panorex views. However, use of CT scanning, especially with the three-dimensional reconstructive ability, is now the preferred and most accurate method of imaging. In addition to bony distortion, fluid in the paranasal sinuses, optic nerve integrity and soft-tissue distortion, the brain, upper cervical spine and other body areas can be visualised concurrently. Other investigations such as colour Doppler ultrasound studies, CT angiography or standard angiography of the great vessels in the neck may be required in cases of possible carotid dissection or carotido-cavernous fistulae. Nasal discharge should be tested to determine the presence of a CSF fistula. Assay for β-2 transferrin is more valuable than the traditional glucose assay for CSF leak detection.[29]

AIRWAY MANAGEMENT

Airway management in maxillofacial injury is potentially complex due to multiple concurrent compromising factors (Table 68.1).

IMMEDIATE PRIORITIES

- Assess and monitor for signs of airway obstruction
- Clear airway, assist respiration
- Definitive airway intervention

As swelling and oedema are progressive in the initial hours after injury, even an unobstructed airway may become compromised. Careful close monitoring in an intensive care unit (ICU) or high-dependency unit (HDU) is essential. Maintaining the head-up position and the use of humidified oxygen may lessen the likelihood of later airway compromise. Sudden obstruction may occur with clot dislodgement and inhalation. Signs of partial obstruction include noisy breathing, stridor, intercostal, supraclavicular recession and restlessness.

Occasionally, patients may assume positions that lessen airway obstruction (e.g. sitting forward or even prone).[30] Simple measures such as suction and clearing the airway and insertion of an oropharyngeal airway may suffice.

Table 68.1 Airway problems in maxillofacial trauma

General problems	Management
Haemorrhage/debris	Suction, volume replacement
Impaired laryngoscopy	Head down
Aspiration risk from blood swallowing	Definitive control of haemorrhage (see text)
Clot inhalation/obstruction	
Teeth, bone fragments	
Oedema soft tissue haematomas	Monitor airway closely
Increases over 48 hours	Head up 30°
Mask fit can be poor	Maintain spontaneous ventilation during airway manipulation; laryngeal mask ventilation
Specific problems	
Bilateral mandibular body/angle fractures	Anterior traction on tongue or jaw, towel clip or suture through tongue and elevate
Posterior displacement of tongue	
TMJ impairment	
Mandibular condyle, zygomatic arch	Nasotracheal intubation (blind/fibreoptic) or surgical airway may be required (see text)
Mouth opening limited	
Midfacial fracture	
Mask seal poor	Anterior traction on mobile segment
Soft palate collapses against pharynx	
Basilar skull	
Nasotracheal intubation contraindicated	Avoid nasal intubation
Pneumocephalus from mask ventilation	
Cervical spine injury	Orotracheal intubation with in-line stabilisation; fibreoptic intubation; surgical airway

In midfacial injuries, anterior digital traction on the mobile mid-segment may relieve obstruction. In bilateral mandibular fractures of the angle or body, a towel clip or suture through the tongue may allow anterior traction on the unsupported tongue and relieve obstruction.

Bag and mask ventilation may be difficult due to distorted anatomy, and this should be borne in mind when a decision to intubate is made. Failure of these simple manoeuvres necessitates definitive airway management

TECHNIQUES (FIGURE 68.2)

Facilities to perform a surgical airway must be available prior to elective intubation. The chosen technique for securing the airway depends on the presence of airway obstruction and the likelihood of difficult direct laryngoscopy (extent of jaw opening, gross anatomical distortion and swelling, operator experience). In a combative patient or if urgent intubation is necessary, then a rapid sequence induction can be used if airway difficulty is not anticipated. If direct laryngoscopy is likely to be difficult or impossible, then spontaneous respiration must be maintained and intubation carried out under local anaesthesia.

Analgesia can be achieved with a combination of sprayed or nebulised lidocaine (4%) to the posterior pharynx as well as a transcricoid injection of 2–4 ml lidocaine (2%). Adjunctive superior laryngeal and glossopharyngeal nerve blocks can be used.[31,32] The orotracheal route for intubation is the route of choice in the presence of basal skull fracture.

If cervical spine injury is present or suspected, in-line stabilisation is mandatory. A variety of intubation techniques can be used – for example, direct laryngoscopy, fibreoptic guided laryngoscopy (oral/nasal), use of a light wand stylet, blind nasal and retrograde intubation techniques.[33,34] The operator should use the technique with which he/she is most comfortable. Excessive bleeding may render fibreoptic techniques useless.

Failure to intubate in the presence of airway obstruction necessitates emergency cricothyroidotomy. Tracheostomy may be required in those likely to need prolonged ventilatory support (e.g. multiple facial fractures combined with a head injury), and is best performed as a semi-elective procedure in the operating room.[16]

MANAGEMENT OF HAEMORRHAGE

Topical vasoconstrictors may not be effective with ongoing nasal haemorrhage. Anterior nasopharyngeal packs are sometimes effective at reducing blood loss. Foley catheters passed into the posterior nasopharynx with the balloons filled with air may stem blood loss, especially if anterior traction is applied.[20] Plastic or maxillofacial surgical opinion should be sought regarding operative reduction and stabilisation of fractures and direct ligation of bleeding vessels if haemorrhage is persistent. External carotid ligation and angiographic embolisation can be used as a last resort.

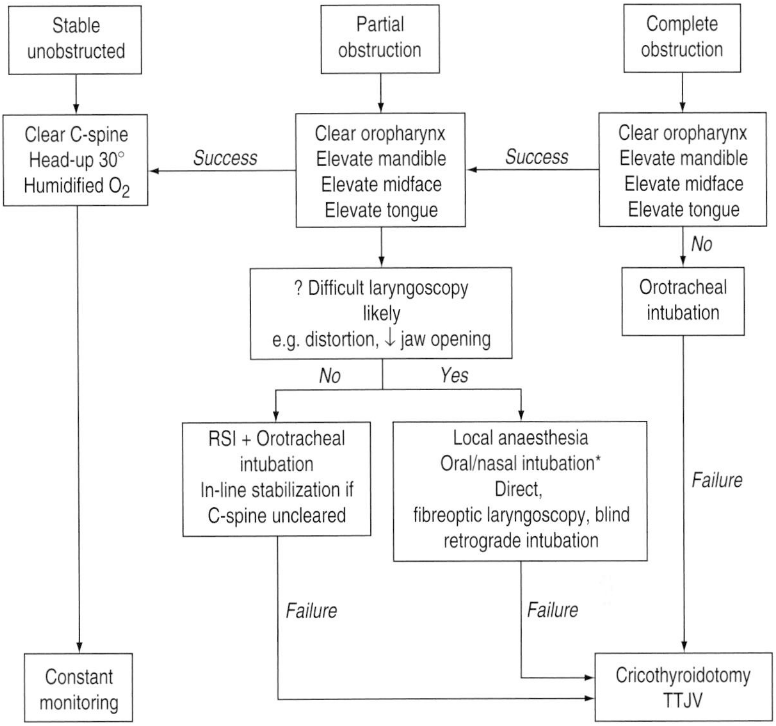

Figure 68.2 An airway management algorithm for maxillofacial trauma. C-spine, cervical spine; RSI, rapid sequence induction; TTJV, transtracheal jet ventilation. *Nasotracheal route contraindicated in basilar skull fracture.

DEFINITIVE MANAGEMENT

Definitive surgery is generally delayed 4–10 days to allow swelling to subside. The timing of surgery may be further delayed if a severe head injury coexists. Early surgery may be warranted if orbital injury with optic nerve compromise is present. The use of high dose steroids in optic nerve compression is controversial and good data do not exist regarding its efficacy.[16] Irrigation and debridement of open wounds, closure of facial lacerations and removal of foreign bodies must be undertaken as soon as is practicable, preferably within 24 hours.

The use of prophylactic antibiotics in the presence of basilar skull fracture and CSF leak is controversial and local protocols should be followed.[21] Persistent CSF leaks (> 2 weeks) or those complicated by meningitis or pneumocephalus are repaired surgically.[21] Appropriate tetanus prophylaxis must be given.

The use of modern internal fixation techniques have reduced the need for intermaxillary fixation following elective facial fracture repair, with only unstable comminuted fractures requiring this form of fixation. Submental intubation during fracture repair is now being used as an alternative to tracheostomy.[35]

INJURIES TO THE LARYNX AND TRACHEA

Direct trauma to the airway is rare, accounting for less than 1% of traumatic injury seen in most major centres.[15,36] The bony protection afforded to the airway by the sternum and mandible and death from asphyxia at the accident scene account for the rarity of the injury. Laryngotracheal injury can be classified as blunt or penetrating. Failure to recognise these injuries, their complications and specific pitfalls in airway management can lead to death.[37,38]

MECHANISM OF INJURY

BLUNT INJURY

Common causes include motor vehicle accidents where the extended neck impacts with the steering wheel or dashboard. The 'clothesline injury' occurs when a cyclist or horse rider collides with a cable or wire causing direct injury to the upper airway. Assaults and strangulation account for the remainder of blunt injuries. Direct blows are more likely to injure the cartilages of the larynx while flexion/extension injuries are most commonly associated with tracheal tears and laryngotracheal transection.[37] The larynx above the cricoid cartilage is injured in 35%, manifesting as oedema, contusions, haematomas, lacerations, avulsion and fracture dislocation, most commonly of the thyroid and arytenoid cartilages.

The cricoid cartilage itself is injured in 15%, which may cause recurrent laryngeal nerve dysfunction.[36] The cervical trachea is injured in 45%.[38] Tracheal transection most often occurs at the junction between the cricoid cartilage and trachea.[39] Oedema fluid and air dissecting within submucosal layers of the larynx and trachea may cause airway obstruction. Air in the soft tissues can cause epiglottic emphysema and narrowing of the supraglottic airway.[40] Straining, talking and coughing may worsen the oedema.

PENETRATING INJURY

Penetrating injuries usually result from stab or gunshot wounds. The anterior triangle of the neck is the most common site of entry. The cervical trachea is most commonly involved in stab wounds. The larynx is injured in about one-third of those with upper-airway injuries.[38]

ASSOCIATED INJURIES

Common associations with blunt laryngotracheal injury include cervical spine, head injury and multisystem trauma. Of those with penetrating neck trauma, major vascular injuries (carotid, jugular, subclavian, vertebral arteries) occur in 25–50%, pharyngeal or oesophageal injury in 30%, neural injury (spinal cord, brachial plexus) in 12% and apical thoracic injury in 10%.[7]

ASSESSMENT OF INJURY

Definitive investigation and management depend on the airway status and presence of associated injury. The degree of injury is not readily assessable on the basis of any one clinical symptom or sign (Table 68.2) and delayed diagnosis is common. Plain radiography (CXR, cervical spine) is performed in all cases. CT scanning demonstrates fractures of cartilages, haematomas and other injuries and is used in stable patients with laryngeal tenderness, endolaryngeal oedema and small haematomas. When obvious signs of injury are not present and there is a satisfactory airway, fibreoptic laryngotracheoscopy under local anaesthesia can demonstrate vocal cord dysfunction, integrity of the cartilaginous framework and laryngeal mucosa. Rigid laryngoscopy can be used when adequate visualisation is not achieved with the former. Pharyngo-oesophagoscopy, contrast studies, open exploration and angiography may be required to exclude aerodigestive tract and major vascular injuries.

Table 68.2 Clinical features in laryngotracheal injury

Symptoms
Respiratory distress
Hoarseness
Dysphonia
Cough
Stridor, noisy breathing
Dysphagia
Signs
Abnormal laryngeal contour
Subcutaneous emphysema
Cervical ecchymosis
Haemoptysis
Investigations
Plain radiography
Air in soft tissues
Pneumomediastinum
Pneumothorax
Cervical spine fracture
CT scan
Cartilage and soft tissue injury
Altered airway patency
Laryngoscopy
Vocal paralysis
Mucosal or cartilage disruption
Haematoma
Laceration

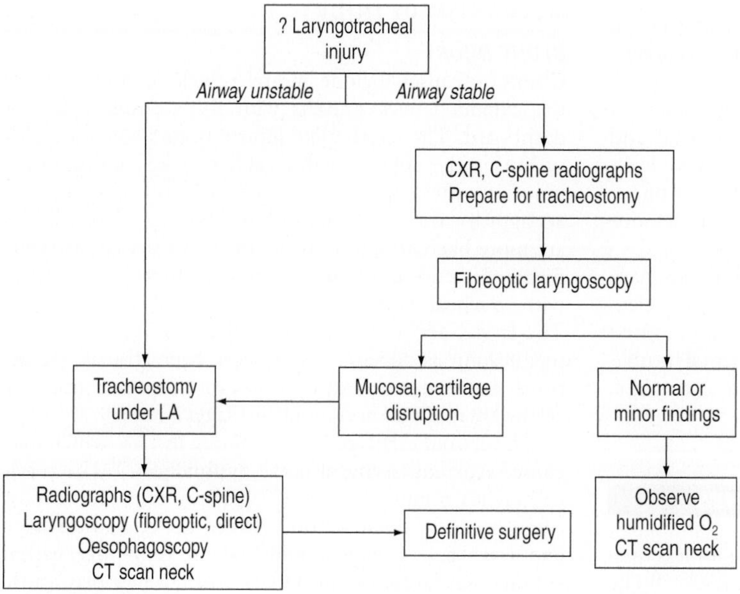

Figure 68.3 Airway assessment and management algorithm for laryngotracheal trauma. CXR, chest X-ray; C-spine, cervical spine; CT, computed tomography; LA, local anaesthesia.

AIRWAY MANAGEMENT

Major complications from airway manipulation can occur after laryngotracheal trauma. Blind intubation can lead to complete airway obstruction due to creation of false passages and mucosal disruption.[15] Cricoid pressure can lead to laryngotracheal separation and is contraindicated. Positive pressure ventilation can rapidly worsen air leaks and wherever possible the patient should maintain spontaneous respiration until a tube has been placed distal to the site of injury. Cricothyroidotomy is not recommended as it may compound laryngeal injury. Gaping airway wounds can be intubated under direct vision pending subsequent surgery.[38] The optimal mode of intubation is thus tracheostomy under local anaesthesia (Figure 68.3). Excessive movement of the cervical spine during airway manipulation should be avoided in cases of blunt trauma.

REFERENCES

1. Gwyn PP, Carraway JH, Horton CE. Facial fractures: associated injuries and complications. *Plast Reconstr Surg* 1971; **47**: 225–30.
2. Tung T, Tseng WS, Chen CT *et al.* Acute life threatening injuries in facial trauma patients. A review of 1025 patients. *J Trauma* 2000; **49**: 420–4.
3. Luce EA, Tubb TD, Moore AM. Review of 1000 major facial fractures and associated injuries. *Plast Reconstr Surg* 1979; **63**: 26–30.
4. Hogg NJ, Stewart TC, Armstrong JE *et al.* Epidemiology of maxillofacial injuries at trauma hospitals in Ontario, Canada, between 1992 and 1997. *J Trauma* 2000; **49**: 425–32.
5. Telfer MR, Jones GM, Shepherd JP. Trends in the aetiology of maxillofacial fractures in the United Kingdom (1977–1997). *Br J Oral Maxillofac Surg* 1991; **29**: 250–5.
6. Hussain KW, Wijetunge DB, Grubnic S *et al.* A comprehensive analysis of craniofacial trauma. *J Trauma* 1994; **36**: 34–7.
7. Miller RH, Duplechain JK. Penetrating wounds of the neck. *Otolaryngol Clin North Am* 1991; **24**: 15–29.
8. Halazonetis JA. The weak regions of the mandible. *Br J Oral Surg* 1968; **6**: 37–48.
9. Bavitz JB, Collicott PE. Bilateral mandibular fractures contributing to airway obstruction. *Int J Oral Maxillofac Surg* 1995; **24**: 273–5.
10. Seshul MB, Sinn DP, Gerlock AJ Jr. The Andy Gump fracture of the mandible: a cause of respiratory obstruction or distress. *J Trauma* 1978; **18**: 611–12.
11. Wenig BL. Management of panfacial fractures. *Otolaryngol Clin North Am* 1991; **24**: 93–101.
12. Le Fort R. Experimental study of fractures of the upper jaw. *Rev Chir Paris* 1901; **23**: 208–27, 360–79 (Reprinted in *Plast Reconstr Surg* 1972; **50**: 497–506).
13. Manson PN, Hoopes JE, Su CT. Structural pillars of the facial skeleton: an approach to the management of Le Fort fractures. *Plast Recontr Surg* 1980; **66**: 54–61.
14. Cruise CW, Blevins PK, Luce EA. Naso-ethmoidal-orbital fractures. *J Trauma* 1980; **20**: 551–6.
15. Crosby R. The difficult airway 2. *Anesthesiol Clin North Am* 1997; **13**: 495–749.
16. Ardekian L, Rosen D, Peled M *et al.* Life-threatening complications and irreversible damage following maxillofacial trauma. *Injury* 1998; **29**: 253–6.
17. Ardekian L, Samet N, Shoshani Y. Life threatening bleeding following maxillofacial trauma. *J Cranio-Maxillofac Surg* 1993; **21**: 336–40.
18. Thaller SR, Beal SL. Maxillofacial trauma: a potentially fatal injury. *Ann Plastic Surg* 1991; **27**: 281–90.
19. Buchanan RT, Holtmann B. Severe epistaxis in facial fractures. *Plast Reconstr Surg* 1983; **71**: 768–90.
20. Murakami WT, Davidson TM, Marshall LF. Fatal epistaxis and craniofacial trauma. *J Trauma* 1983; **23**: 57–61.
21. Marentette LJ, Valentino J. Traumatic anterior fossa cerebrospinal fluid fistulae and craniofacial considerations. *Otolaryngol Clin North Am* 1991; **24**: 151–63.
22. Maxwell JA, Goldware SI. Use of adhesive in surgical treatment of cerebrospinal fluid leaks. *J Neurosurg* 1973; **39**: 322–36.
23. Laun A. Traumatic cerebrospinal fluid fistulae in the anterior and middle cranial fossae. *Acta Neurochir* 1982; **84**: 215–22.
24. Adams C, Januszkiewicz J, Judson J. Changing patterns of severe craniomaxillofacial trauma in Auckland over eight years. *Aust N Z J Surg* 2000; **70**: 401–4.
25. Davidson JSD, Birdsell BD. Cervical spine injury in patients with skeletal trauma. *J Trauma* 1989; **29**: 1276–8.
26. Schultz RC, Oldham RJ. An overview of facial injuries. *Surg Clin North Am* 1977; **57**: 987–1010.
27. Punjabi AP, Plaisier BR, Haug RH *et al.* Diagnosis and management of blunt carotid artery injury in oral and maxillofacial surgery. *J Oral Maxillofac Surg* 1997; **55**: 1388–95.
28. Marciani RD, Israel S. Diagnosis of blunt carotid artery injuries in patients with facial trauma. *Oral Surg Oral Med Oral Pathol Oral Radiol Endod* 1997; **83**: 5–9.
29. Skedros DG, Cass SP, Hirsch BE *et al.* Beta-2 transferrin assay in clinical management of cerebral spinal fluid and perilymphatic fluid leaks. *J Otolaryngol* 1993; **22**: 341–4.
30. Neal MR, Groves J, Gell IR. Awake fibreoptic intubation in the semi-prone position following facial trauma. *Anaesthesia* 1996; **51**: 1053–4.
31. Webb AR, Fernando SS, Dalton HR *et al.* Local anaesthesia for fibreoptic bronchoscopy: transcricoid injection or the spray as you go technique. *Thorax* 1990; **45**: 474–7.
32. Gotta AW, Sullivan CA. Superior laryngeal nerve block: an aid to intubating the patient with a fractured mandible. *J Trauma* 1984; **24**: 83–5.
33. King H, Huntington C, Wooten D. Translaryngeal guided intubation in an uncooperative patient with

maxillofacial injury: a case report. *J Trauma* 1994; **36**: 885–6.
34. Verdile VP, Chang JL, Bedger R. Nasotracheal intubation using a flexible lighted stylet. *Ann Emerg Med* 1990; **19**: 506–10.
35. Chandu A, Smith ACH, Gebert R. Submental intubation: an alternative to short-term tracheostomy. *Anaesth Intensive Care* 2000; **28**: 193–5.
36. Gussack GS, Jurkovich GJ, Luterman F. Laryngotracheal trauma: a protocol approach to a rare injury. *Laryngoscope* 1986; **96**: 660–5.
37. Mathison DJ, Grillo H. Laryngotracheal trauma. *Ann Thorac Surg* 1987; **43**: 254–63.
38. Cicala RS, Kudsk KA, Butts A *et al.* Initial evaluation and management of upper airway injuries in trauma patients. *J Clin Anesth* 1991; **3**: 91–8.
39. Trone TH, Schaefer SD, Carder HM. Blunt and penetrating laryngeal trauma: a 13 year review. *Otolaryngol Head Neck Surg* 1980; **88**: 257–61.
40. Sacco JJ, Halliday DW. Submucosa epiglottic emphysema complicating bronchial rupture. *Anesthesiology* 1987; **66**: 555–7.

69

Chest injuries

Ubbo F Wiersema

CHEST INJURIES

The majority of chest injuries in Australasia result from blunt trauma due to motor vehicle crashes. Less frequent causes include falls and penetrating injuries from stab or gunshot wounds. Associated extrathoracic injuries are common. Chest injuries account for a quarter of all trauma deaths. Immediate death from blunt chest trauma is usually due to blunt rupture of the thoracic aorta, heart or major vessel. Patients who survive the immediate post-trauma period may still have life-threatening injuries that require timely intervention. Most patients can be managed with simple measures, including intercostal tube drainage, analgesia, oxygen therapy and mechanical ventilation. Thoracotomy is infrequently required.[1,2]

A systematic team approach to immediate assessment and resuscitation is important. This is followed by a detailed secondary survey and appropriate further investigations to identify all injuries and determine patient disposition.

IMMEDIATE MANAGEMENT

During the primary survey a rapid assessment of the respiratory, circulatory and neurological status of the patient is made (Table 69.1). Airway patency is ensured, oxygen administered by facemask and ventilation assessed. Obvious external bleeding is controlled. Two large bore intravenous cannulae are sited, blood samples taken for crossmatch, haematology and biochemistry tests, and intravenous fluids commenced. Intravenous opioid analgesia is given as repeated small boluses, titrated to effect. There are four critical chest injuries that should be sought during the primary survey for which immediate intervention may be life saving:

- tension pneumothorax
- open (sucking) pneumothorax
- massive haemothorax
- pericardial tamponade

In addition, the clinical features of flail chest should be sought as these will no longer be apparent if positive-pressure ventilation is instituted (see below). A chest radiograph is integral to the initial assessment and should be performed promptly. Subcostal ultrasonography of the heart as part of the focused assessment with sonography for trauma (FAST) should be performed with penetrating chest trauma, or if there is haemodynamic instability.[3] An ECG is important in the assessment for blunt cardiac injury (see below).[4]

Endotracheal intubation and mechanical ventilation are indicated for the patient with a compromised airway, severe head injury, or gross hypoventilation and/or hypoxaemia not attributable to pneumothorax. Haemodynamic instability should be anticipated (Table 69.2). Emergency cricothyroidotomy or tracheostomy is only rarely required when an airway obstruction cannot be bypassed by translaryngeal intubation. A nasogastric tube (or orogastric, if facial injuries are suspected) should be inserted to decompress the stomach after endotracheal intubation.

PNEUMOTHORAX

Pneumothorax visible on the initial chest radiograph should be treated with insertion of an intercostal tube connected to an underwater seal drainage system (Figure 69.1). A single-bottle drainage system without suction is usually adequate. Low-pressure suction (20 cmH_2O) is applied if the pneumothorax fails to fully resolve, or if there is associated haemothorax (Figure 69.2). A three-bottle system (or commercially available three-in-one system) allows more accurate control of suction (Figure 69.3). Presumptive antibiotics are not indicated.[5]

Tension pneumothorax results from progressive accumulation of air in the pleural space, leading to vena caval compression and cardiopulmonary decompensation. Clinically, tension pneumothorax is characterised by:

- tachypnoea and tachycardia
- hyperinflated chest
- contralateral tracheal deviation
- hyperresonance to percussion
- reduced breath sounds
- hypotension and jugular venous distension

If tension pneumothorax is suspected clinically an intercostal tube should be inserted immediately, prior to the chest radiograph. Needle thoracostomy with a large bore cannula inserted into the second intercostal space in the

Table 69.1 Immediate management of chest trauma

Assure patent airway, oxygenation and ventilation
Exclude or treat:
Pneumothorax
Haemothorax
Pericardial tamponade
Assess extrathoracic injuries
Provide analgesia
Reconsider endotracheal intubation and ventilation

Table 69.2 Causes of cardiovascular collapse on induction of anaesthesia and positive-pressure ventilation in chest-injured patients

Excessive anaesthetic agent
Hypovolaemia
Oesophageal intubation with hypoxaemia
Tension pneumothorax
Pericardial tamponade
Anaphylaxis
Systemic air embolism
Severe blunt cardiac injury

midclavicular line may be used to drain air more rapidly for patients in extremis. However, this is rarely necessary and may puncture the lung, fail to reach the pleural space, or kink when the needle is removed from within the cannula. Whether successful or not, needle thoracostomy must be followed by formal intercostal tube drainage.

Open pneumothorax occurs when a chest wall defect allows direct communication of a pneumothorax with the exterior, usually after penetrating trauma. Tension can develop if air can enter but not exit through the defect. Treatment involves application of an occlusive, non-adherent, square dressing sealed along three edges over the wound after sterile skin preparation. This allows air to escape but not to enter through the wound, but should be followed by intercostal tube insertion at a site not immediately adjacent to the wound.

Simple pneumothorax may develop tension at any stage, especially with positive-pressure ventilation (Table 69.2). A small pneumothorax may be missed on the initial chest radiograph. In the supine position pleural air collects anteroinferiorly and is demonstrated radiologically by a deep sulcus sign or increased radiolucency of one side of the chest compared to the other (Figure 69.4).[6]

Occult pneumothorax is defined as visible on chest CT (or upper slices of an abdominal CT) but not plain radiograph.[7] Drainage is not mandatory, but should be considered if prolonged surgery is anticipated, there is significant cardiorespiratory compromise or interhospital transport is necessary. With a conservative approach the patient should be carefully monitored for deterioration from expansion of the pneumothorax.[7]

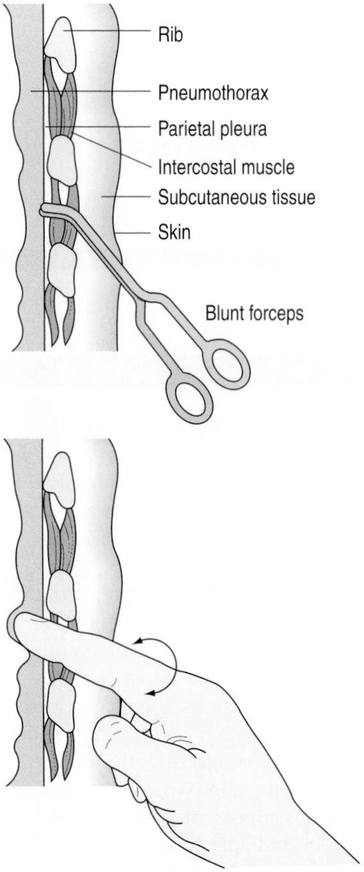

Figure 69.1 Intercostal tube insertion. After sterile preparation and drape, 1% lidocaine is infiltrated in the mid-axillary line at the level of the nipple. A 2–3 cm transverse skin incision is made. Dissection is performed by blunt forceps down to the pleura, passing just superior to the rib surface to avoid injury to neurovascular structures. A gloved finger is used to confirm separation of lung from chest wall. A large bore (32 French) intercostal tube is inserted without a trocar and directed anteriorly for pneumothorax or posteriorly for haemothorax. Curved forceps clamped to the tip of the tube can be used to guide the tube through the chest wall. The tube is immediately connected to an underwater seal drainage system (Figures 69.2 and 69.3) and checked for satisfactory drainage and tidal rise and fall in fluid level with respiration. Non-absorbable sutures are used to seal the skin incision around the tube and secure the tube. The intrathoracic position of the tube is checked with a chest radiograph.

Subcutaneous emphysema over the chest wall in a patient with blunt chest trauma is almost always associated with pneumothorax, but should raise suspicion of other injuries (Table 69.3). The pneumothorax may not be visible on the plain chest radiograph, either because it is obscured by the emphysema or because it has largely decompressed into subcutaneous tissues. An intercostal tube should be inserted.

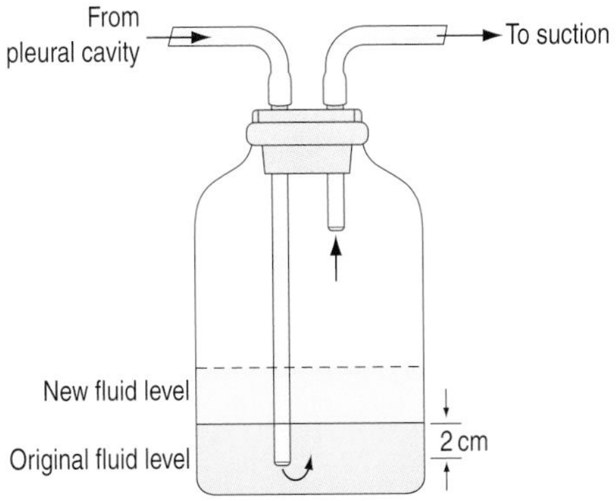

Figure 69.2 Single-bottle drainage system for haemopneumothorax. Air drainage will become more difficult if there is also fluid drainage, raising the fluid level in the bottle (dashed line) and increasing the depth of immersion of the hollow rod. This can be overcome by applying low pressure suction (20 cmH_2O). Arrows indicate direction of airflow.

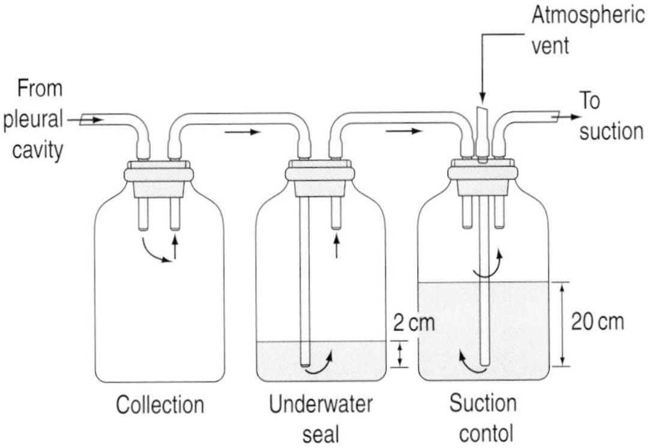

Figure 69.3 Three-bottle chest drainage system. The first bottle (connected to the intercostal tube) is a fluid collection chamber, the second functions as a one-way valve (underwater seal), and the third (connected to wall suction) limits the amount of suction applied. The level of suction is set by adjusting the depth of the atmospheric vent whilst ensuring that it bubbles continuously. Commercially available drainage systems function on the same principles as the three-bottle system. Arrows indicate direction of airflow.

If there is no associated fluid collection the chest tube can be removed once the pneumothorax is no longer visible on chest radiograph and there has been no air drained for at least 24 hours. Persistent air leak and incomplete drainage of a pneumothorax after intercostal tube insertion should prompt investigation for tracheobronchial injury. However, the depth of the tube within the pleural space and tubing connections should be checked to ensure that extraneous air is not being inadvertently entrained. Incomplete drainage with no air leak is usually due to tube malplacement.

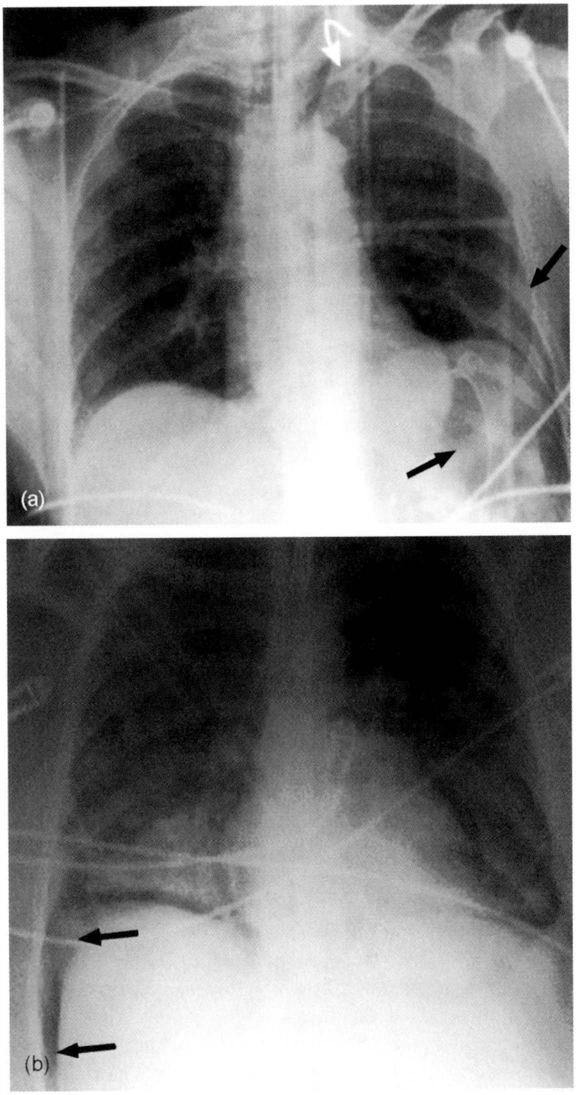

Figure 69.4 (a) Moderate-sized left pneumothorax on supine chest radiograph. The visceral pleura is visible at the lung apex (curved arrow). Hyperlucency is visible in the left lower chest (straight arrows). (b) Supine chest radiograph of right-sided deep sulcus sign (arrows). Miller LA. Chest wall, lung, and pleural space trauma. *Radiol Clin North Am* 2006; **44:** 213–224, viii.

HAEMOTHORAX

Haemothorax visible on chest radiography should be drained as completely as possible (Figure 69.1). The tube can be removed once radiographic clearance is achieved, with < 100 ml/24 hours drainage. A small haemothorax (< 300 ml) (visible on ultrasound or CT) may initially be managed conservatively, but should be drained if it enlarges.

Massive haemothorax, defined as > 1500 ml, causes life-threatening circulatory compromise from

Table 69.3 Causes of pneumothorax, subcutaneous emphysema and/or pneumomediastinum

Lung puncture
Tracheobronchial injury
Oesophageal injury
Facial or pharyngeal injury
Abdominal or retroperitoneal injury (air tracking up)

hypovolaemia and vena caval compression as well as hypoxaemia. This requires immediate tube drainage. If the amount of ongoing bleeding following initial drainage is low, the patient remains haemodynamically stable after initial resuscitation, and the blood is venous in appearance, the patient can be managed with close observation. Ongoing bleeding of > 200 ml/h, or > 600 ml over 6 hours (massive haemothorax equivalent), is an indication to proceed to thoracotomy.

PERICARDIAL TAMPONADE

Pericardial tamponade should be suspected in any patient with a gunshot wound to the chest or stab wound to the precordium. It occurs rarely with blunt trauma, but should be suspected if there is hypotension out of proportion to blood loss, and distended neck veins. Pulsus paradoxus may be detected in the spontaneously breathing patient. The differential diagnosis includes tension pneumothorax (most likely) and cardiogenic shock from severe blunt cardiac injury or delayed and inadequate resuscitation. Pericardial fluid can be detected with ultrasound (FAST scan).[3] Cardiac structures are imaged via a subcostal view using a low-frequency transducer (3.5 MHz) to provide good tissue depth penetration. Echocardiography, or operative subxiphoid window, can be used if diagnostic uncertainty remains.

Haemodynamically unstable patients should undergo thoracotomy.[8] Subxiphoid pericardiotomy can be performed in selected stable patients, but may require conversion to open thoracotomy. Needle pericardiocentesis is rarely effective in the acute setting, but may have a role in the drainage of delayed pericardial effusions following stab wounds.[8]

CARDIAC ARREST AND EMERGENCY THORACOTOMY

External cardiac massage is invariably unsuccessful in the trauma setting. Indeed, cardiac compression may cause further injury to intrathoracic structures and obstruct access to the patient for more potentially useful interventions such as (bilateral) intercostal tube insertion. For patients with witnessed loss of vital signs after penetrating chest trauma, emergency thoracotomy should be considered if suitably experienced medical personnel are available.[8] This is rarely successful for blunt trauma. The standard approach is a left-sided anterolateral thoracotomy. This allows access to the thoracic cavity for specific interventions:[8]

- Release of pericardial tamponade
- Control of intrathoracic bleeding
- Control of massive air embolism or bronchopleural fistula
- Cross-clamping of the descending aorta
- Internal cardiac massage

These temporising (damage control) measures are followed by transfer to the operating room for completion of surgery:[9]

- Definitive repair of cardiac injury
- Pulmonary tractotomy, wedge resection, or lobectomy/pneumonectomy for lung injury
- Repair or grafting of vascular injury

Postoperatively the patient is admitted to the intensive care unit (ICU) for rewarming, correction of coagulopathy and resuscitation.

SPECIFIC INJURIES

Specific chest injuries should be systematically excluded. Imaging techniques play an important role. Choice of investigation is influenced by clinical findings. The degree of haemodynamic and respiratory instability will determine whether the patient can be moved to an imaging facility. Local availability of equipment and clinician expertise may limit the options available. Extrathoracic injuries will often determine investigation and management priorities. With the advent of rapid high-resolution CT scanners, routine chest CT has become increasing popular, particularly in patients who require abdominal or head CT.[10] Endotracheal intubation and mechanical ventilation may be required to facilitate investigations (e.g. the combative trauma patient with ethanol intoxication).

BLUNT AORTIC INJURY

Blunt aortic injury usually occurs at the junction between the mobile arch and fixed descending aorta, just distal to the origin of the left subclavian artery, as a result of severe deceleration injury. Less frequently, the ascending aorta or arch vessels are injured by direct trauma. Blunt aortic injuries may be divided into:[11]

- *significant* aortic injury, with disruption of the intima and full thickness of the media. There is a high risk of rupture
- *minimal* aortic injury, with laceration limited to the intima and inner media. Radiologically this manifests as an intimal flap < 1 cm with minimal periaortic haematoma. There is a low risk of rupture

Most patients with blunt aortic injury die at the scene from complete aortic wall transection or associated

Table 69.4 Chest radiograph signs of blunt aortic injury

Signs of periaortic haematoma	Indirect signs
Widened mediastinum (> 8 cm)	Left haemothorax
Obscured aortic knuckle	Left pleural cap
Opacification of aortopulmonary window	Fractured first or second ribs
Deviation of trachea, left main bronchus or nasogastric tube	
Thickened paratracheal stripe	

injuries. Of those that reach hospital, 90% will have a significant injury.[11] Clinical signs include unequal upper limb pulses, pseudocoarctation or interscapular murmur, but these are rarely detected.[12] Aortic injury should be suspected if the mechanism of injury is suggestive of rapid deceleration, such as high speed (greater than 90 km/h) motor vehicle or motorcycle crashes, or a pedestrian hit by a vehicle.[13]

Historically, chest radiography has been the screening test (to detect mediastinal haematoma) and aortic angiography the diagnostic test for blunt aortic injury.[12,14] More recently, CT and echocardiography have been introduced for screening and diagnostic purposes:[15]

- *Chest radiograph* features of blunt aortic injury are caused by distortion of normal mediastinal contour by periaortic haemorrhage. A widened mediastinum (> 8 cm at the level of the aortic knuckle) is the principal finding (Table 69.4).[12,16] A good quality erect chest radiograph has a high sensitivity (> 90%), but low positive predictive value for aortic injury. Historically, this has resulted in a large number of negative aortograms.[12,13] Furthermore, a supine chest radiograph accentuates mediastinal width and in the acute trauma setting is often of lower quality. Measurement of left mediastinal width (> 6 cm), or left mediastinal width to mediastinal width ratio (> 0.6), may improve specificity.[16]
- *Single slice helical chest CT* may demonstrate direct signs of aortic injury. However, more commonly aortic injury manifests indirectly with periaortic haematoma, and a further diagnostic test is required.[13] Nevertheless, by differentiating periaortic haematoma from other types of mediastinal haematoma, and excluding other causes of an abnormal mediastinal contour, helical CT provides a useful screening test. Routine chest CT has thus been advocated for haemodynamically stable patients with a high-risk mechanism of injury, especially if other CT scans are planned.[13,17] *Multirow detector chest CT* (with more than 16 detectors) provides sufficient resolution in multiple planes for CT to be used as the sole diagnostic test. However, the diagnostic role of CT for branch vessel injuries remains undefined (Table 69.5).[18]
- *Transoesophageal echocardiography* is rapid and portable, making it suitable for examination of the unstable patient (who is intubated). It provides high diagnostic accuracy for aortic injury and also allows examination for blunt cardiac injury.[19,20] However, imaging of the distal aorta, proximal arch and major branches is limited. Thus, if signs of mediastinal haematoma are detected, but an aortic injury not identified, further diagnostic testing is warranted.[19] It is contraindicated if an upper-airway or oesophageal injury is suspected.
- *Aortic angiography* is relatively time consuming and requires transfer of the patient to the angiography room, making it potentially hazardous in the unstable patient. However, it is the preferred diagnostic test if branch vessel injury is suspected (Table 69.5)[18] or if uncertainty remains after other diagnostic imaging.[14] It is also necessary for endoluminal stent placement, and may be required for operative planning.

Table 69.5 Signs of aortic branch vessel injury

Supraclavicular haematoma
Pulse discrepancy in arms
Brachial plexus palsy or stroke
Widened upper mediastinum on chest radiograph

Significant aortic injury requires prompt surgical or endoluminal stent repair.[21] However, this should not take priority over other life-saving operations (e.g. craniotomy or laparotomy).[12] Surgical options include direct repair (clamp and sew) or techniques that maintain distal aortic perfusion.[14] The latter reduce the risk of postoperative paraplegia from spinal cord ischaemia, but often require systemic heparinisation, which may exacerbate bleeding from other injuries.[15] Surgery should be deferred, sometimes indefinitely, if severe associated injuries or comorbidities make the operative risk unacceptably high.[12,22] In such cases endoluminal stent repair may still be feasible.[21] Conservative management includes antihypertensive therapy (β-blockers ± vasodilators) and serial imaging to assess for expanding pseudoaneurysm that will require intervention. Minimal aortic injury may also be managed expectantly.[11,15,20]

BLUNT CARDIAC INJURY

Blunt cardiac injury results from compression of the heart between the sternum and the spine, abrupt pressure changes within cardiac chambers or deceleration shear injury. A wide spectrum of injuries has been described, but may be classified according to the clinical sequelae and need for intervention:[4]

- *Minor ECG and cardiac enzyme abnormalities*: Sinus tachycardia and premature beats are common, but usually resolve within 24 hours without intervention.
- *Complex arrhythmias*: This may cause heart failure, or persistent hypotension, and may warrant antiarrhythmic therapy.

- *Free wall rupture*: This is usually fatal, but atrial rupture may present with haemopericardium ± tamponade. Immediate drainage and repair is required.
- *Heart failure* may develop from gross myocardial injury, septal rupture (causing left-to-right shunt) or valvular injury (causing regurgitation). The latter may not manifest until weeks later. Septal rupture and severe valvular injury require surgery. Myocardial dysfunction may require inotropic support.
- *Coronary artery injury*: This is very rare and ST elevation on ECG is more likely to be due to a primary myocardial infarction.

All patients should have an ECG on admission (Figure 69.5). If this is normal and the patient is young, haemodynamically stable, and has no history of cardiac disease, the risk of significant injury is very low and no further cardiac evaluation is required. Other patients should be monitored for late sequelae of significant cardiac injury (arrhythmia or heart failure).[4] Patients who remain haemodynamically stable, with only minor ECG changes, and who have a normal troponin level at 6–8 hours post injury, have a low risk of cardiac complications.[4,23] Echocardiography is indicated for patients with hypotension unexplained by other injuries, heart failure, or persistent arrhythmias.[4] Undisplaced sternal fracture does not of itself warrant cardiac evaluation.[24]

TRACHEOBRONCHIAL INJURY

Blunt rupture of the trachea or bronchi results from crush injury or rapid deceleration with shearing of the airway between a fixed trachea and mobile lungs. The proximal right main bronchus is the most common site of injury.[25] Large injuries present with respiratory distress, subcutaneous emphysema and haemoptysis (Table 69.3).[26] The chest radiograph demonstrates pneumothorax and mediastinal emphysema. Dramatic deterioration may follow the institution of positive-pressure ventilation (Table 69.2). With smaller injuries, initial findings are often overshadowed by associated injuries with delay in diagnosis. Persistent pneumothorax with a large air leak, or recurrent

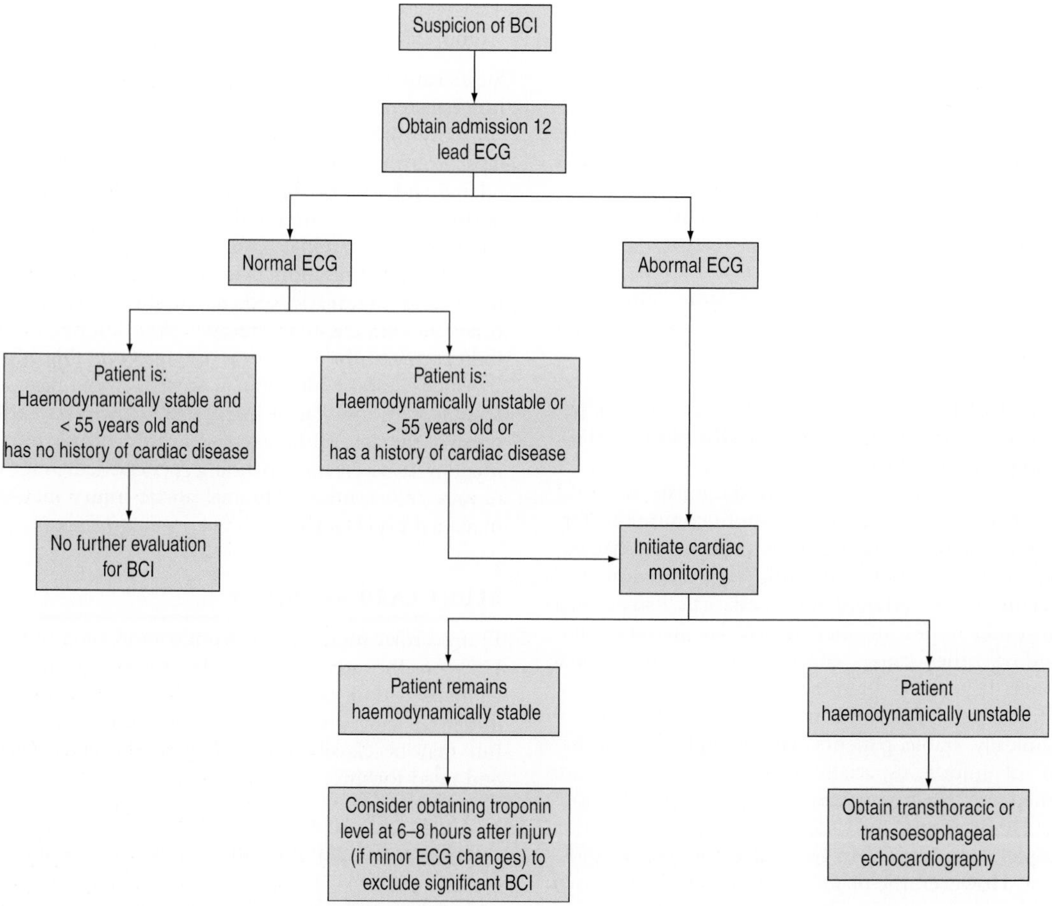

Figure 69.5 Algorithm for evaluation of patients suspected of having blunt cardiac injury (BCI). (Modified from Schultz JM, Trunkey DD. Blunt cardiac injury. *Crit Care Clin* 2004; **20**: 57–70.)

pneumothoraces and pulmonary collapse, should prompt further investigation. Flexible bronchoscopy confirms the diagnosis and identifies the level of injury. Treatment is usually primary repair, although non-operative management has been described.[27] Late complications of either approach include postobstructive pneumonia, empyema or bronchiectasis.[25]

With penetrating trauma the cervical trachea is most commonly injured. Immediate management involves tracheal intubation (preferably with flexible bronchoscopy) with the cuff positioned distal to the tear to ablate the air leak. With a large neck wound the endotracheal tube can be passed directly through the wound in emergency situations.

DIAPHRAGMATIC RUPTURE AND DIAPHRAGMATIC PARESIS

The usual mechanism of diaphragmatic rupture is gross abdominal compression from direct vehicular intrusion. The risk of rupture is higher with lateral impact collisions, but not seat belt use.[28] Associated injuries are very common.[28] Rupture of the left hemidiaphragm is more common, because the right hemidiaphragm is congenitally stronger and protected by the liver.

Symptoms (dyspnoea and chest pain) are non-specific. Rarely bowel sounds are audible on chest auscultation. Diagnostic chest radiograph findings are herniation of bowel into the thoracic cavity and nasogastric tube above the left hemidiaphragm. Indirect signs include an elevated or distorted diaphragmatic outline, or pleural effusion, but these may be obscured by adjacent pulmonary pathology, phrenic nerve injury or with positive-pressure ventilation.[29] The low diagnostic accuracy of chest radiography often results in delayed diagnosis unless further imaging is performed. Multidetector CT has high diagnostic accuracy, but magnetic resonance imaging or video thorascopy may be required if uncertainty persists.[29–31] Prompt operative repair is important to prevent bowel incarceration or perforation. The choice of surgical approach (laparotomy or thoracotomy) is dictated by associated injuries.

Traumatic phrenic nerve palsy, or postoperative diaphragmatic dysfunction, may go unrecognised whilst the patient is on mandatory positive-pressure ventilation. With the transition to spontaneous ventilation, paradoxical abdominal and chest wall movement, reduced vital capacity, and difficulty weaning from ventilatory support become evident.

OESOPHAGEAL INJURY

Rupture of the oesophagus from blunt trauma is rare. Penetrating trauma usually causes injury to the cervical portion of the oesophagus. Oesophageal injury may also result from attempted endotracheal intubation or gastric tube insertion during resuscitation of the trauma patient.[32] Clinical features include chest pain, dysphagia, pain on swallowing and subcutaneous emphysema (Table 69.3). Chest radiograph findings include pneumothorax and/or hydrothorax, mediastinal emphysema or widened mediastinum.[26] Prompt diagnosis by oesophagoscopy or gastrograffin swallow is important. Treatment is immediate surgical repair.[32] Delayed recognition or repair (more than 12 hours post injury) leads to septic shock from mediastinal contamination. Extensive irrigation and drainage are then required, but postoperative complications are common.[32]

PULMONARY INJURY

Pulmonary contusion is characterised by interstitial haemorrhage and oedema, with a secondary inflammatory reaction. Clinically, there is increased work of breathing, impaired gas exchange and sometimes haemoptysis. The chest radiograph demonstrates patchy interstitial infiltrates or consolidation not confined to anatomical segments. Gas exchange and radiographic findings may initially be unremarkable, with deterioration over the first 24–48 hours.[2,6] CT is more sensitive at detecting contusion, and quantification of lung volume affected predicts risk of acute respiratory distress syndrome (ARDS).[33] In the absence of complications (ARDS, pneumonia or aspiration), clinical and radiological recovery can be expected within 3–5 days.[6,33]

Treatment is supportive with humidified oxygen therapy, and encouragement of deep breathing and coughing in the spontaneously breathing patient. Non-invasive ventilation can be used in selected patients if gas exchange is poor. Intubation and mechanical ventilation are indicated for refractory hypoxaemia, or if intubation is required for non-pulmonary reasons. Routine corticosteroids are not indicated. Antibiotics should be reserved for superimposed pneumonia.[2]

Pulmonary laceration occurs when disruption of lung architecture, with formation of an air- or blood-filled cavity, occurs after blunt or penetrating trauma.[6] On chest radiography lacerations are often initially obscured by adjacent contusion, but typically take many weeks to resolve, and may be complicated by abscess formation or bronchopleural fistula.[6]

BONY INJURIES

Half of all rib fractures are missed on plain chest radiography, but should be suspected if there is localised tenderness over the chest wall. Good analgesia to prevent pulmonary complications from sputum retention is essential.[34] This risk may not be clinically apparent initially, but deterioration in respiratory status over the next few days should be anticipated, especially in the elderly, smokers or patients with pre-existing pulmonary disease. First and second rib fractures, scapula fracture and sternoclavicular dislocation are markers of high-energy trauma.[6]

Most sternal fractures occur in restrained occupants involved in frontal impact vehicular crashes. Associated

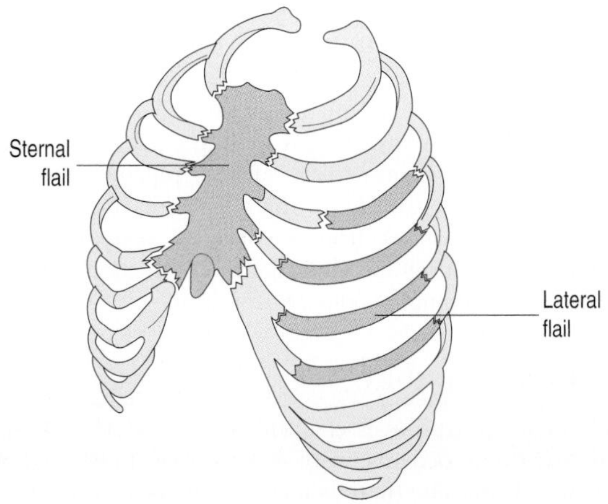

Figure 69.6 Types of flail chest. (Modified from Wanek S, Mayberry JC. Blunt thoracic trauma: flail chest, pulmonary contusion, and blast injury. *Crit Care Clin* 2004; **20**: 71–81.)

thoracolumbar spine fractures are common.[24] Blunt cardiac injury should be suspected with displaced sternal fractures.[24]

FLAIL CHEST

Fracture of at least four consecutive ribs in two or more places results in a flail segment with paradoxical movement of the chest wall during tidal breathing (Figure 69.6).[2] Associated pulmonary contusion is often present. Younger patients with no other major injuries, no pulmonary comorbidities, and good analgesia can often be managed with non-invasive ventilation or oxygen therapy alone.[35] Deteriorating gas exchange and sputum retention are indications for intubation and mechanical ventilation. Prolonged ventilatory support is often not necessary in patients whose associated injuries and comorbidities are not severe. Surgical stabilisation has been advocated for severe flail to reduce the duration of ventilation.[36]

EXTRAPLEURAL HAEMATOMA

Traumatic extrapleural haemorrhage arises when chest wall bleeding does not enter the pleural space.[37] Chest radiography shows a parietal shadow that does not cause blunting of the costophrenic angle or shift with gravity. A large haematoma should be evacuated with a chest tube or by thoracotomy.

SYSTEMIC AIR EMBOLISM

This is more frequent with penetrating injuries and is immediately life threatening. The typical presentation is circulatory collapse after institution of positive-pressure ventilation, when the pulmonary airspace pressure exceeds pulmonary venous pressure (Table 69.2). Focal neurological changes in the absence of head injury also suggest the diagnosis. Characteristic head CT findings have been described.[38]

When suspected, maintenance of spontaneous ventilation is preferred. If positive-pressure ventilation is necessary, an FiO_2 of 1.0 should be used, with ventilatory pressures and volumes reduced to a minimum. Selective lung ventilation, using a double lumen endotracheal tube or bronchial blocker, and/or high frequency ventilation, should be considered.[8] However, urgent thoracotomy, with hilar clamping or lung isolation, is usually indicated.[8] Hyperbaric oxygen therapy has been used to treat cerebral air embolism, but is often impractical.[38]

COMPLICATIONS AND ICU MANAGEMENT

On admission to ICU, rewarming, correction of coagulopathy and ongoing fluid resuscitation are often required. Pericardial tamponade and persistent air leak should be anticipated in post-thoracotomy patients.[9] A restrictive approach to fluid therapy is indicated for patients who have undergone lung surgery. However, care should be taken to ensure adequate fluid resuscitation. A judicious transfusion policy should be employed with all patients.[39]

As with other critically ill or injured patients, prophylactic measures against thromboembolism[40] and upper gastrointestinal stress ulceration should be used. Adequate nutrition is important to ameliorate the hypermetabolic and catabolic metabolic changes, reduce the incidence of sepsis, and improve outcome. Nutrition should be instituted early, preferably via the enteral route. Nasogastric feeding may be limited by gastric stasis, in which case nasojejunal feeding is usually successful.

ACUTE RESPIRATORY FAILURE AND MECHANICAL VENTILATION

Respiratory complications are common. When acute lung injury occurs early after trauma, common causes are pulmonary contusion, aspiration, massive transfusion and prolonged shock or delayed resuscitation with severe systemic inflammatory response. Aspiration with persistent lobar collapse is an indication for bronchoscopy to exclude bronchial obstruction from particulate obstruction. When lung injury develops several days later, sepsis – of either pulmonary or non-pulmonary origin – is a more likely cause.

The approach to mechanical ventilation for intubated patients follows the same principles as with other critically ill patients:

- Patients with acute lung injury/ARDS should be ventilated with a lung-protective strategy.[41] However, high PEEP and permissive hypercapnia are contraindicated if there is associated head injury.

- Patients with pneumothorax or tracheobronchial injury should be managed with low PEEP, low peak airway pressures, and early transition to spontaneous ventilation if possible.
- Patients with flail chest may benefit from the splinting effect of moderate levels of PEEP.
- Failure to wean from mechanical ventilation should raise suspicion of fluid overload, diaphragmatic injury, cardiac dysfunction or flail.

SPUTUM RETENTION

Sputum retention leads to progressive pulmonary collapse, with impaired gas exchange, increased work of breathing and increased risk of infection. Smokers, or patients with pre-existing respiratory disease, are particularly at risk. In the spontaneously breathing patient, good analgesia without excessive sedation is required to allow the patient to breathe deeply and cough adequately. In the intubated/ventilated patient, humidification, tracheal suctioning and regular position changes are important. In unintubated patients with an inadequate cough, but no other indication for ventilation, a minitracheostomy may avoid the need for conventional intubation.

ANALGESIA

Adequate analgesia is essential for deep breathing and effective coughing, which, if achieved, will reduce the likelihood that endotracheal intubation is needed for less severely injured patients. Analgesia also facilitates chest physiotherapy and early mobilisation, reducing pulmonary morbidity. The choice of analgesia depends on the severity of illness and may vary over time. Options include:[34]

- *Intravenous morphine* by frequent small boluses or continuous infusion. This is the mainstay of analgesia for severely injured patients who are intubated and ventilated. Patient-controlled analgesia (PCA) using morphine can be used for cooperative unintubated patients.
- *Thoracic epidural infusion* of combined opioid and local anaesthetic agent (e.g. fentanyl 2 μg/ml + bupivacaine 0.125% at 5–15 ml/h). This is the preferred option for unintubated patients, particularly the elderly, if four or more ribs are fractured, or if there are cardiopulmonary comorbidities. It may also be used to facilitate successful extubation of ventilated patients who still have significant analgesia requirements
- *Intercostal nerve block.* This can be used if only a few lower ribs are fractured. Either a single large bolus (20 ml of 0.5% bupivacaine) can be injected into one intercostal space, or smaller amounts can be injected at multiple levels. Repeated injections may be required.
- *Paravertebral block.* This is rarely used unless thoracic surgery is performed.
- *Non-steroidal anti-inflammatory agents.* These should only be used in fully resuscitated patients with normal renal function and no other contraindications.
- *Paracetamol* given regularly except in the presence of hepatic dysfunction.

PNEUMONIA

Sepsis is the principal cause of late death after major trauma. Breach of the skin surface barrier, devitalised tissues, and the presence of invasive drains and catheters make the trauma patient especially prone to bacterial invasion. In the chest-injured patient, pulmonary contusion, emergency intubation, shock, blood transfusion and the presence of extrathoracic injuries increase the risk of nosocomial pneumonia.[42]

Early-onset pneumonia (within the first few days of hospitalisation) may result from aspiration at the time of injury, particularly after head injury. Common pathogens are *Haemophilus influenzae*, Pneumococcus and anaerobes. Late-onset nosocomial pneumonia is more likely to be due to aerobic Gram-negative bacilli and *Staphylococcus aureus.*

The diagnosis of pneumonia is suspected if there are new or progressive infiltrates on the chest radiograph and deterioration in respiratory status. However, new infiltrates may also be caused by pulmonary contusion, pleural fluid collections, atelectasis, aspiration and pulmonary oedema. Infection is supported by the presence of purulent sputum, new fever and leukocytosis. Confirmation depends on culture of tracheal aspirate or bronchoscopic samples.[43] Antibiotic therapy should be targeted at causative organisms. Prompt empiric antibiotics should be started in unstable patients, with re-evaluation at 48–72 hours.

Preventative measures include careful hand cleansing, reduced duration of intubation and ventilation, semirecumbent position, enteral nutrition, avoidance of excessive sedation or hyperglycaemia, and avoidance of prolonged prophylactic antibiotics.[43] The role of selective decontamination of the digestive tract remains controversial.

RETAINED HAEMOTHORAX AND EMPYEMA

Haemothorax that is not adequately drained within a few days becomes clotted and unable to drain via intercostal tube. The clot becomes organised and fibrosed with progressive pleural thickening (fibrothorax). This results in loss of lung volume, impaired pulmonary compliance and increased risk of empyema formation. Retained haemothorax should be evaluated by ultrasound or CT. Small haemothoraces (< 300 ml) in clinically stable patients where the pleural cavity has not been violated may be observed. However, in the presence of respiratory compromise, suspected empyema or retained haemothorax over 500 ml, further drainage is required. This should be performed within 5–7 days, before the development of fibrothorax or empyema.

If the initial chest tube is poorly positioned or blocked, a second tube may be placed through a different skin incision, preferably under ultrasound or CT guidance. In the absence of a bleeding diathesis or empyema formation, early evacuation of retained haemothorax (within a few days of the initial haemothorax) can be attempted with intrapleural administration of a thrombolytic agent. Streptokinase 250 000 units, or urokinase 100000 units, in 100 ml saline is instilled into the intercostal tube for 4 hours each day until resolution of haemothorax with minimal further drain losses.[44] Alternatively, video-assisted thoracoscopic surgery (VATS) may be used in haemodynamically stable patients who can tolerate single lung ventilation.[30,31] Failure of these techniques, or empyema formation, requires formal thoracotomy ± decortication.

FAT EMBOLISM SYNDROME

Fat embolism invariably occurs in patients with long bone fractures.[45] Although fat embolism syndrome (with pulmonary, neurological and cutaneous sequelae) is uncommon, oxygen desaturation occurs frequently, and may be more severe and prolonged in patients with parenchymal lung injury.[46] Treatment is supportive, but early resuscitation and fracture stabilisation are important preventative measures.[45] Early (< 24 hours) intramedullary nailing is the fixation method of choice, resulting in fewer orthopaedic complications than other fixation methods, and fewer pulmonary complications than delayed surgery.[47] However, internal fixation may provoke further fat embolism, require a longer operative time, and result in more blood loss than external fixation.[47] Thus, in severely chest-injured patients, temporary stabilisation using external fixation, with intramedullary nailing several days later, is preferred.[47]

PROGNOSIS

Reported mortality rates for chest-injured patients vary greatly, reflecting the severity of chest injury and associated extrathoracic injuries. Initial physiological markers that predict adverse outcome are low Glasgow Coma Scale score, hypotension and high respiratory rate. In patients with severe blunt trauma, mortality is significantly higher with bilateral than unilateral chest injuries, and depends more on the extent of parenchymal lung injury than the extent of chest wall injury.[48] Older age correlates strongly with worse outcome, even though the elderly are more likely to suffer rib fractures than parenchymal lung injury.[48] In the elderly, the risk of death or pneumonia increases with each additional rib fractured. In younger patients, better physiological reserve means that outcome is only significantly worsened if four or more ribs are fractured.[34,49] Obese patients (BMI > 30) are likely to suffer more complications during hospitalisation than non-obese patients.[50]

REFERENCES

1. Kulshrestha P, Munshi I, Wait R. Profile of chest trauma in a level I trauma center. *J Trauma* 2004; **57**: 576–81.
2. Wanek S, Mayberry JC. Blunt thoracic trauma: flail chest, pulmonary contusion, and blast injury. *Crit Care Clin* 2004; **20**: 71–81.
3. Scalea TM, Rodriguez A, Chiu WC *et al.* Focused Assessment with Sonography for Trauma (FAST): results from an international consensus conference. *J Trauma* 1999; **46**: 466–72.
4. Schultz JM, Trunkey DD. Blunt cardiac injury. *Crit Care Clin* 2004; **20**: 57–70.
5. Maxwell RA, Campbell DJ, Fabian TC *et al.* Use of presumptive antibiotics following tube thoracostomy for traumatic hemopneumothorax in the prevention of empyema and pneumonia – a multi-center trial. *J Trauma* 2004; **57**: 742–8; discussion 748–9.
6. Miller LA. Chest wall, lung, and pleural space trauma. *Radiol Clin North Am* 2006; **44**: 213–24, viii.
7. Ball CG, Kirkpatrick AW, Laupland KB *et al.* Incidence, risk factors, and outcomes for occult pneumothoraces in victims of major trauma. *J Trauma* 2005; **59**: 917–24; discussion 924–5.
8. Hunt PA, Greaves I, Owens WA. Emergency thoracotomy in thoracic trauma – a review. *Injury* 2006; **37**: 1–19.
9. Rotondo MF, Bard MR. Damage control surgery for thoracic injuries. *Injury* 2004; **35**: 649–54.
10. Guerrero-Lopez F, Vazquez-Mata G, Alcazar-Romero PP *et al.* Evaluation of the utility of computed tomography in the initial assessment of the critical care patient with chest trauma. *Crit Care Med* 2000; **28**: 1370–5.
11. Malhotra AK, Fabian TC, Croce MA *et al.* Minimal aortic injury: a lesion associated with advancing diagnostic techniques. *J Trauma* 2001; **51**: 1042–8.
12. Nagy K, Fabian T, Rodman G *et al.* Guidelines for the diagnosis and management of blunt aortic injury: an EAST Practice Management Guidelines Work Group. *J Trauma* 2000; **48**: 1128–43.
13. Dyer DS, Moore EE, Ilke DN *et al.* Thoracic aortic injury: how predictive is mechanism and is chest computed tomography a reliable screening tool? A prospective study of 1,561 patients. *J Trauma* 2000; **48**: 673–82; discussion 682–3.
14. Fabian TC, Richardson JD, Croce MA *et al.* Prospective study of blunt aortic injury: multicenter trial of the American Association for the Surgery of Trauma. *J Trauma* 1997; **42**: 374–80; discussion 380–3.
15. Degiannis E, Boffard K. Critical decisions in trauma of the thoracic aorta. *Injury* 2002; **33**: 317–22.
16. Wong YC, Ng CJ, Wang LJ *et al.* Left mediastinal width and mediastinal width ratio are better radiographic criteria than general mediastinal width for predicting blunt aortic injury. *J Trauma* 2004; **57**: 88–94.
17. Mirvis SE. Thoracic vascular injury. *Radiol Clin North Am* 2006; **44**: 181–97, vii.

18. Holdgate A, Dunlop S. Review of branch aortic injuries in blunt chest trauma. *Emerg Med Australas* 2005; **17**: 49–56.
19. Cinnella G, Dambrosio M, Brienza N *et al.* Transesophageal echocardiography for diagnosis of traumatic aortic injury: an appraisal of the evidence. *J Trauma* 2004; **57**: 1246–55.
20. Vignon P, Martaille JF, Francois B *et al.* Transesophageal echocardiography and therapeutic management of patients sustaining blunt aortic injuries. *J Trauma* 2005; **58**: 1150–8.
21. Andrassy J, Weidenhagen R, Meimarakis G *et al.* Stent versus open surgery for acute and chronic traumatic injury of the thoracic aorta: a single-center experience. *J Trauma* 2006; **60**: 765–71; discussion 771–2.
22. Hirose H, Gill IS, Malangoni MA. Nonoperative management of traumatic aortic injury. *J Trauma* 2006; **60**: 597–601.
23. Rajan GP, Zellweger R. Cardiac troponin I as a predictor of arrhythmia and ventricular dysfunction in trauma patients with myocardial contusion. *J Trauma* 2004; **57**: 801–8; discussion 808.
24. von Garrel T, Ince A, Junge A *et al.* The sternal fracture: radiographic analysis of 200 fractures with special reference to concomitant injuries. *J Trauma* 2004; **57**: 837–44.
25. Kiser AC, O'Brien SM, Detterbeck FC. Blunt tracheobronchial injuries: treatment and outcomes. *Ann Thorac Surg* 2001; **71**: 2059–65.
26. Euathrongchit J, Thoongsuwan N, Stern EJ. Nonvascular mediastinal trauma. *Radiol Clin North Am* 2006; **44**: 251–8, viii.
27. Self ML, Mangram A, Berne JD *et al.* Nonoperative management of severe tracheobronchial injuries with positive end-expiratory pressure and low tidal volume ventilation. *J Trauma* 2005; **59**: 1072–5.
28. Reiff DA, McGwin G Jr, Metzger J *et al.* Identifying injuries and motor vehicle collision characteristics that together are suggestive of diaphragmatic rupture. *J Trauma* 2002; **53**: 1139–45.
29. Iochum S, Ludig T, Walter F *et al.* Imaging of diaphragmatic injury: a diagnostic challenge? *Radiographics* 2002; **22**(Spec No): S103–16; discussion S116–8.
30. Carrillo EH, Richardson JD. Thoracoscopy for the acutely injured patient. *Am J Surg* 2005; **190**: 234–8.
31. Lowdermilk GA, Naunheim KS. Thoracoscopic evaluation and treatment of thoracic trauma. *Surg Clin North Am* 2000; **80**: 1535–42.
32. Asensio JA, Chahwan S, Forno W *et al.* Penetrating esophageal injuries: multicenter study of the American Association for the Surgery of Trauma. *J Trauma* 2001; **50**: 289–96.
33. Miller PR, Croce MA, Bee TK *et al.* ARDS after pulmonary contusion: accurate measurement of contusion volume identifies high-risk patients. *J Trauma* 2001; **51**: 223–8; discussion 229–30.
34. Simon BJ, Cushman J, Barraco R *et al.* Pain management guidelines for blunt thoracic trauma. *J Trauma* 2005; **59**: 1256–67.
35. Gunduz M, Unlugenc H, Ozalevli M *et al.* A comparative study of continuous positive airway pressure (CPAP) and intermittent positive pressure ventilation (IPPV) in patients with flail chest. *Emerg Med J* 2005; **22**: 325–9.
36. Tanaka H, Yukioka T, Yamaguti Y *et al.* Surgical stabilization of internal pneumatic stabilization? A prospective randomized study of management of severe flail chest patients. *J Trauma* 2002; **52**: 727–32; discussion 732.
37. Rashid MA, Wikstrom T, Ortenwall P. Nomenclature, classification, and significance of traumatic extrapleural hematoma. *J Trauma* 2000; **49**: 286–90.
38. Ho AM, Ling E. Systemic air embolism after lung trauma. *Anesthesiology* 1999; **90**: 564–75.
39. Croce MA, Tolley EA, Claridge JA *et al.* Transfusions result in pulmonary morbidity and death after a moderate degree of injury. *J Trauma* 2005; **59**: 19–23; discussion 24.
40. Knudson MM, Ikossi DG. Venous thromboembolism after trauma. *Curr Opin Crit Care* 2004; **10**: 539–48.
41. Fan E, Needham DM, Stewart TE. Ventilatory management of acute lung injury and acute respiratory distress syndrome. *JAMA* 2005; **294**: 2889–96.
42. Croce MA, Tolley EA, Fabian TC. A formula for prediction of posttraumatic pneumonia based on early anatomic and physiologic parameters. *J Trauma* 2003; **54**: 724–9; discussion 729–30.
43. Guidelines for the management of adults with hospital-acquired, ventilator-associated, and healthcare-associated pneumonia. *Am J Respir Crit Care Med* 2005; **171**: 388–416.
44. Inci I, Ozcelik C, Ulku R *et al.* Intrapleural fibrinolytic treatment of traumatic clotted hemothorax. *Chest* 1998; **114**: 160–5.
45. White T, Petrisor BA, Bhandari M. Prevention of fat embolism syndrome. *Injury* 2006; **37**(Suppl 4): S59–67.
46. Wong MW, Tsui HF, Yung SH *et al.* Continuous pulse oximeter monitoring for inapparent hypoxemia after long bone fractures. *J Trauma* 2004; **56**: 356–62.
47. Pape HC, Giannoudis P, Krettek C. The timing of fracture treatment in polytrauma patients: relevance of damage control orthopedic surgery. *Am J Surg* 2002; **183**: 622–9.
48. Pape HC, Remmers D, Rice J *et al.* Appraisal of early evaluation of blunt chest trauma: development of a standardized scoring system for initial clinical decision making. *J Trauma* 2000; **49**: 496–504.
49. Brasel KJ, Guse CE, Layde P *et al.* Rib fractures: relationship with pneumonia and mortality. *Crit Care Med* 2006; **34**: 1642–6.
50. Brown CV, Neville AL, Rhee P *et al.* The impact of obesity on the outcomes of 1,153 critically injured blunt trauma patients. *J Trauma* 2005; **59**: 1048–51; discussion 1051.

70

Spinal injuries

Geoff A Gutteridge

There are few injuries that have a more devastating impact on both the patient and their family than spinal cord injuries (SCI). The physical, psychological and functional sequelae of permanent disability are immense. In addition, the economic cost to the individual and to society, with the loss of productivity and costs of hospitalisation, rehabilitation and ongoing care, are enormous.

AETIOLOGY

The incidence of SCI in developed countries is 12–53 new cases per million population per year (excluding deaths before reaching hospital).[1] There is some variation in the incidence and causes in different countries. About 80% of SCI are male, usually in the 15–35 years age group.

SCI are due mainly to motor car, motor bike and bicycle accidents (50%), falls (15–20%) and sporting injuries (10–25%).[1] Alcohol ingestion is frequently an associated factor. Work-related injuries account for 10–25%, and physical violence for 10–20% of SCI, especially from gunshot injury in the USA. Sporting and recreational injuries appear to be increasing (but with fewer now due to diving), and there is an increasing incidence of SCI in the elderly, especially from falls.[2] Ischaemic SCI is occasionally due to aortic injury or cross clamping. Pre-existing spinal pathology predisposes to SCI, including osteoarthritis, spinal canal stenosis, ankylosing spondylitis, rheumatoid arthritis and congenital abnormalities.

Fifty-five per cent of SCI are cervical (most at the C4–6 levels), with thoracic, thoracolumbar and lumbosacral injuries each being 15% of SCI. Forty-five per cent of SCI are complete and 55% incomplete. Between 20 and 60% of patients with SCI have significant associated injuries such as head and chest injuries.[1]

PATHOGENESIS

SPINAL INJURY

CERVICAL SPINE

Injury to the cervical spine has been classified several ways[3–5] relating to the mechanism of injury using the two-column concept. Differences appear to be due to the fact that compression of the anterior column is associated with distraction of the posterior column, and vice-versa. Injuries may be grouped according to the predominant mechanism of injury (Table 70.1) with these mechanisms having characteristic radiological patterns.

THORACOLUMBAR SPINE

The classification of Denis[6] using the three-column concept of the spine has been widely adopted. Major injuries are classified as in Table 70.2.

SPINAL CORD INJURY

Trauma to the spinal cord results in immediate primary and delayed secondary injury processes.

PRIMARY INJURY

Direct mechanical injury may produce focal compression, laceration or traction injury to the cord. Actual transection is unusual. Ischaemic injury may result from interference to the segmental spinal arterial supply.

SECONDARY INJURY

An understanding of secondary injury mechanisms has come from experimental SCI in animals.[1,7] Local hypoperfusion and ischaemia begin at the site of injury, extending progressively over hours from the site of injury in both directions. There is loss of spinal cord autoregulation, complicated by arterial hypotension with high SCI. Apart from ischaemia, other mechanisms may contribute to the secondary injury. These include the release of free radicals, eicosanoids, calcium, proteases, phospholipases and excitotoxic neurotransmitters (e.g. glutamate).

Petechial haemorrhages begin in the grey matter, progress over hours and may result in significant haemorrhage into the cord. There is oedema, cellular chromatolysis and vacuolation, and ultimately neuronal necrosis. Apoptosis, especially of oligodendrocytes, also occurs.[1] In the white matter vasogenic oedema, axonal degeneration and demyelination follow. Infiltration of polymorphs occurs in the haemorrhagic areas. Late coagulative necrosis and cavitation subsequently take place.

Table 70.1 Cervical spine injuries

Hyperflexion
Hyperflexion and rotation
Hyperextension
Hyperextension and rotation
Vertical compression or burst injury
Lateral flexion
Direct shearing
Penetrating
Other

Table 70.2 Major thoracolumbar spine injuries

Compression fractures
Burst fractures
Seat belt type injuries
Fracture dislocations

CLINICAL PRESENTATION

Spinal and spinal cord injuries should be suspected after severe trauma or head injuries, if there are motor or sensory symptoms or signs, or the patient reports neck or back pain.

NEUROLOGICAL ASSESSMENT

A detailed neurological examination is essential, including motor function, sensory function (spinothalamic and dorsal column) and reflexes, as well as anal motor function, sensation and reflexes. The vital capacity should be measured. This neurological examination provides the most useful information with respect to assessment of the SCI and to prognosis. However, it may be difficult to conduct on presentation due to head or other injuries, pain, alcohol or the administration of analgesic or other drugs.

In an alert patient SCI may be obvious with limb paralysis or weakness, numbness and absence of reflexes.

With a complete SCI there is muscle paralysis, with somatic and visceral sensory loss below a discrete segmental level. *Spinal shock* is usually present, with the additional features of muscle flaccidity, absence of tendon reflexes, vaso- and venodilatation, loss of bladder function and paralytic ileus. This term refers to a form of neurogenic 'shock' with temporary loss of somatic and autonomic reflex activity below the neurological level of injury. It usually lasts for 1–3 weeks before the recovery of distal reflex activity in the isolated cord segment.

TERMINOLOGY

The terminology for SCI has now been standardised.[8]

- *Tetraplegia* (preferred to quadriplegia) refers to impairment or loss of motor and/or sensory function in the cervical segments of the spinal cord due to damage of the neural elements within the spinal canal.

Table 70.3 American Spinal Injury Association (ASIA) impairment scale

A	Complete: No sensory or motor function is preserved in the sacral segments S4–S5
B	Incomplete: Sensory but not motor function is preserved below the neurological level and includes the sacral segments S4–S5
C	Incomplete: Motor function is preserved below the neurological level, and more than half of key muscles below the neurological level have a muscle grade less than 3
D	Incomplete: Motor function is preserved below the neurological level, and at least half of key muscles below the neurological level have a muscle grade greater than or equal to 3
E	Normal: Sensory and motor function is normal

- *Paraplegia* refers to impairment or loss in the thoracic, lumbar or sacral segments of the cord, as well as conus and cauda equina injuries within the spinal canal.
- *Neurological level* is reported as the most caudal cord segment with normal motor and sensory function on both sides. As differences often exist it is preferred to describe the individual motor and sensory levels on each side (as the most caudal segments with normal motor and sensory function, respectively). In this context, normal motor function refers to a motor grade of 3, with all cephalad motor levels being grade 5.
- *Skeletal level* refers to the level with the greatest vertebral damage on X-ray.
- *Complete* injury refers to the absence of motor and sensory function in the lowest sacral segment.[9] A *zone of partial preservation* exists if there is partial innervation of motor and sensory segments below the neurological level. This term is only used in complete SCI. If partial innervation of motor and sensory function is found below the neurological level *and* includes the lowest sacral segment (with anal sensation and voluntary external anal sphincter contraction) the injury is defined as *incomplete*. Grading of complete and incomplete SCI utilises the ASIA impairment scale[8] (Table 70.3).

INCOMPLETE SCI

Incomplete SCI tend to occur in characteristic syndromes.[10]

- The *central cord syndrome* is the most common, usually resulting from hyperextension injury to the neck, often in the elderly with a narrow spinal canal. There is disproportionate paralysis in the arms compared with the legs, and variable sensory loss.
- The *anterior cord syndrome* has extensive bilateral paralysis with loss of pain and temperature sensation, but preservation of sensory function in the posterior white columns.
- The *Brown–Sequard syndrome* is due to damage to one side of the spinal cord with loss of ipsilateral motor and

proprioceptive function, as well as contralateral pain and temperature sensation. It usually results from penetrating injury.

- The *conus medullaris syndrome* is due to T12/L1 injury with damage to lumbar and sacral cord segments producing extensive paralysis in the legs of both upper and lower motor neurone type.
- The *Cauda equina syndrome* results from skeletal injuries below L1 with damage to the lumbosacral nerve roots resulting in lower motor neurone paralysis, and bladder and bowel areflexia.
- Spinal cord injury without radiological abnormality (SCIWORA) occurs mainly in children, but is now very uncommon with magnetic resonance imaging (MRI).

UNCONSCIOUS OR UNCOOPERATIVE PATIENTS

The neurological examination may be difficult if the patient is unconscious or uncooperative. In this case a number of signs may be helpful in drawing attention to a SCI as in Table 70.4. Confirmation of SCI may be established by MRI or somatosensory-evoked potentials (SSEP).

SPINE

Alert patients will report neck or back pain and tenderness with spinal injuries. A palpable gap may be felt between the spinous processes of thoracolumbar vertebrae. However, a spinal injury is readily overlooked in association with head or other major injuries, or alcohol ingestion.

ASSOCIATED INJURIES

CERVICAL SPINE INJURY/TETRAPLEGIA

Overall with major trauma the incidence of cervical spine injury (CSI) is 1–3%.[11] However, 2–10% of patients with head injuries have a CSI. The more severe the head injury, the more likely is CSI to be present. Patients with head injuries should be assumed to have a CSI until proved otherwise. Of patients with a cervical SCI, 25% have some degree of head injury, with 2–3% having a severe injury.[1,12]

Table 70.4 Signs of SCI in unconscious or uncooperative patients

Response to pain above, but not below a suspected level
Flaccid areflexia in the arms and/or legs
Elbow flexion with the inability to extend suggestive of cervical SCI
Paradoxical pattern of breathing with indrawing of upper chest on inspiration (in the absence of upper respiratory tract obstruction or chest injury)
Inappropriate vasodilatation (in association with hypothermia, or in the legs but not the arms with thoracolumbar SCI)
Unexplained bradycardia, hypotension
Priapism
Loss of anal tone and reflexes

THORACOLUMBAR SPINE INJURY/PARAPLEGIA

Chest injuries are often present and are difficult to assess with the inability to take an erect chest X-ray, and the presence of a mediastinal haematoma associated with the vertebral injury. Contrast-enhanced helical CT of the chest may be used to assess other chest injuries, and to exclude an aortic injury,[13] although aortography may be preferred for this purpose.

Abdominal injuries are difficult to diagnose if there is a SCI. However, they should be suspected if there is excessive hypotension, referred shoulder pain, or free gas or fluid seen on X-ray of the spine or chest. Abdominal CT, diagnostic peritoneal lavage or ultrasound may be used to delineate these injuries.[14]

IMAGING

PLAIN X-RAYS (FIGURE 70.1)

Plain X-rays remain the primary screening method for suspected spinal injuries in symptomatic patients, except in unconscious or multitrauma patients. However, the absence of a detectable abnormality does not exclude a spinal injury. Lesions may not be seen if the views are inadequate or of poor technical quality, or the observer is inexperienced. Even without these limitations, plain X-rays of the neck frequently miss fractures and subluxations,[15,16] and a high index of suspicion should be maintained. Adequate views of the entire cervical spine from the base of the skull down to and including the C7–T1 junction should always be obtained. Abnormalities of the prevertebral soft tissues are often present and indicative of subtle injuries.[4]

With the cervical spine the three-view trauma series is standard in most hospitals (Table 70.5). This consists of lateral, anteroposterior (AP) and odontoid (open mouth) views. A five-view series with supine oblique views has been recommended as improving the diagnostic yield,[17] but other studies show no difference in the detection rate. Lateral and AP views are standard screening views for the thoracolumbar spine.

COMPUTED TOMOGRAPHY (CT) SCANNING

The sensitivity of CT scanning is much greater than plain X-rays in the detection of spinal injuries,[15] especially with the newer multidetector CT machines. CT scanning now has an essential role in the detection and evaluation of spinal injuries, as well as the exclusion of injuries with spinal clearance.[18]

Indications for CT scanning have been regarded as:

- inadequate plain X-rays
- high clinical suspicion of injury despite normal plain X-rays, e.g. ongoing or persistent neck pain or tenderness, or the development of neurological symptoms or signs
- suspicious plain X-ray findings

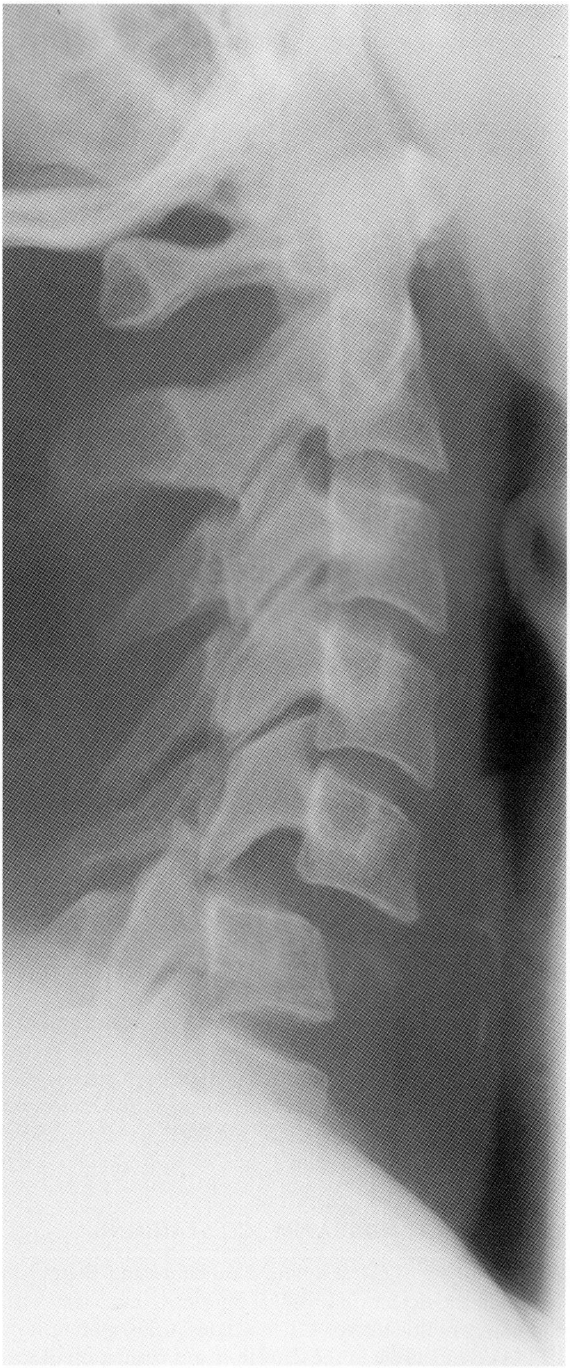

Figure 70.1 Plain lateral X-ray of the cervical spine showing a C5/6 dislocation.

- abnormal plain X-rays: further investigation of fracture, subluxation or dislocation seen on plain X-rays. Additional fractures are frequently found in the same, adjacent or distant vertebrae
- evaluation of the spinal canal

Table 70.5 Basic examination of plain X-rays of cervical spine

Must include occipital condyles to C7–T1 junction	
Lateral is the most important view and will show most injuries	
Check for:	
Alignment:	
Vertebral bodies	Anterior, posterior spinal lines
Spinous processes	
Pedicles in AP view	Lateral alignment
Laminae in oblique views	Spinolaminar line
	Posterior cervical line
Bony changes:	
Bony integrity, density, contour	
Vertebral body height	Anterior, posterior, lateral
Pedicles, laminae	
Spines, transverse processes	
Atlas, dens	
Spaces:	
Intervertebral disc spaces	
Interspinous spaces	
Predental (atlas–dens) space	
Facet joints	
Atlanto-axial, atlanto-occipital joints	
Soft tissues:	
Prevertebral soft tissue shadow	

However, CT scanning should now be undertaken in all suspected or proven spinal injuries. If patients are unconscious or have suffered severe or multiple trauma, CT scanning should be undertaken as the first line imaging, without screening plain X-rays, for the evaluation of cervical and thoracolumbar injuries.[2,19] Sagittal and coronal reconstructions should be routinely obtained. CT scanning of the spine should be coordinated with CT of other regions if needed. CT myelography has now been replaced by MRI, but may be indicated if MRI is not available or is contraindicated.

MAGNETIC RESONANCE IMAGING (MRI) (FIGURE 70.2)

MRI allows visualisation of soft tissues including ligaments, intervertebral discs and the spinal cord itself where it may show the site, extent and nature of the SCI.[4] However, it involves a prolonged study with physical isolation of the patient in a difficult environment. Nevertheless, it provides important information in evaluation of the neurological deficit, assessment of prognosis and in the planning of surgical management of SCI. MRI is urgent if there is an unexplained neurological deficit, discordance between the skeletal and neurological levels of injury or worsening neurological status.

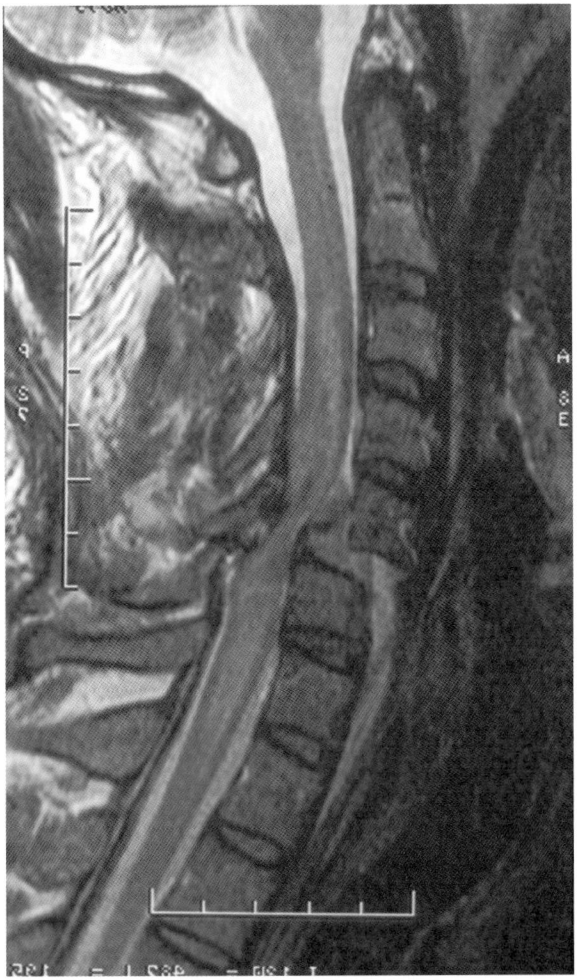

Figure 70.2 T2 weighted MRI of the same patient as in Figure 70.1 showing severe spinal cord damage.

CLEARANCE OF THE CERVICAL SPINE

Although familiarity with common injuries is desirable, in view of the severe consequences of a missed spinal injury, clearance of the spine must only be undertaken by a suitably experienced specialist after adequate imaging. Neurological deterioration with missed spinal injuries still occurs, usually as a result of insufficient imaging.[20]

The Canadian C-spine rule[21,22] now provides guidelines for the need for imaging in alert, stable trauma patients in an emergency department setting, but this would not frequently apply to patients in the intensive care unit (ICU). Clearance of the cervical spine in unconscious ICU patients remains controversial with no standardised approach.[23] The best approach would seem to be fine-cut helical multidetector CT scanning with reconstructions,[18] reserving the further use of MRI for selected cases such as those with a high-velocity mechanism of injury or high injury severity score, rather than using flexion/extension imaging to detect unstable ligamentous injuries.[16,24,25]

Early clearance of CSI is desirable to allow early removal of the cervical collar with its associated problems of pressure sores, difficult access for airway management and insertion of central venous lines, and increased intracranial pressure with head injuries.[26]

MANAGEMENT

The main principles in the early management of a spinal injury relate to the prevention of secondary injury and the provision of optimum conditions for neurological recovery. Emphasis should be on resuscitation measures and immobilisation, together with good protocols for clearance of the spine.

PREHOSPITAL MANAGEMENT

It should be assumed that all severe trauma patients have a spinal injury until proven otherwise. If a SCI is obvious, basic trauma assessment and resuscitation principles still apply.

RESPIRATION AND CIRCULATION

An adequate airway must be established by clearance of foreign material, jaw thrust and an oro- or nasopharyngeal airway if necessary. Adequate ventilation must be ensured with the provision of supplementary oxygen by facemask. Immediate endotracheal intubation and artificial ventilation may be required.

Hypotension may be due to a high SCI and will need some plasma volume expansion to correct relative hypovolaemia, but excessive volume expansion should be avoided. Hypovolaemia may also be due to other injuries.

IMMOBILISATION

If a CSI is suspected, the patient may have to be extricated from the scene of the accident. Manual stabilisation of the head in a neutral position is used with four people lifting and one controlling the head and neck. The neck is immobilised in a rigid, hard collar that should be applied without neck movement. The patient is placed supine on a rigid spine board with straps and occipital padding.[26] Sandbags should be placed on either side of the head, and the head secured with the application of broad tape across the forehead. With a suspected thoracolumbar spinal injury (TLSI) the patient is again lifted as a single unit or log rolled as necessary.

HYPOTHERMIA

Prevention of hypothermia in the field is important with SCI.

EMERGENCY MANAGEMENT

The initial management of spinal injuries follows the usual trauma triage principles with a primary survey, resuscitation and a careful secondary survey. The measures previously mentioned for establishing an adequate airway, and for providing adequate ventilation and circulation should be continued to minimise any further spinal cord insult.

After stabilisation, definitive X-rays and CT are undertaken whilst maintaining spinal immobilisation. A cervical collar does not provide rigid immobilisation and manual stabilisation is still necessary with patient transfers.[27] The prevention of hypothermia is a continuing issue in both the emergency and radiology departments. Morphine analgesia is likely to be required for pain at the spinal fracture site and/or other injury.

With SCI, a nasogastric tube should be inserted to prevent aspiration of gastric content and bowel distension from the associated ileus. A urinary catheter should also be inserted to monitor the urine output and prevent overdistension of the bladder. Attention to the skin, taking care to prevent pressure areas, is important. If high-dose corticosteroids are to be used they should be started within 8 hours from the time of SCI (see pharmacological treatment). If stable, early transport to a definitive care facility such as a multidisciplinary SCI referral centre is recommended. This approach has been shown to result in fewer complications and a reduced hospital length of stay.[2] Initially, patients (especially tetraplegics) should be admitted to the ICU for the detection and management of respiratory and cardiovascular problems.[28]

HOSPITAL/ICU MANAGEMENT

RESPIRATORY

Respiratory dysfunction

Respiratory dysfunction is a major cause of morbidity after SCI, especially in tetraplegics.[29,30]

Tetraplegia The diaphragm is innervated by the C3–5 segments. With a C5 SCI the diaphragm is intact but about 50% still need short-term mechanical ventilation (MV). With a C4 SCI there is partial loss of diaphragmatic innervation, and nearly all need short-term MV. With a C3 SCI most of the diaphragmatic innervation is lost, and all need initial MV, with about 50% requiring permanent MV.[29] Scalene muscle weakness and intercostal muscle paralysis lead to a paradoxical pattern of breathing, and abdominal muscle paralysis produces an inability to cough.

The vital capacity (VC) is markedly reduced and is usually 1.0–1.5 l on presentation. In C5–6 complete SCI the VC is decreased to 31% of predicted during the first week, and with C4 lesions to 24%.[31] It often undergoes a further decrease due to atelectasis, and sometimes from ascent of the neurological level. However, there is usually a significant increase in VC by 3–5 weeks after injury, reaching values of 44–51% of predicted by 3 months.[31] This is thought to be due to stiffening of the ligaments and joints of the rib cage, and the return of intercostal muscle tone preventing indrawing of the chest wall by the diaphragm. The VC and tidal volume are dependent on posture and surprisingly are greatest when supine due to the more cephalad position of the diaphragm.[30,32] Hypoxaemia is very common in the early phase.

Paraplegia The diaphragm is intact, but there is paralysis of the intercostal and abdominal muscles dependent on the neurological level of the SCI. The VC is reduced but is usually adequate, and there is variable impairment of the cough mechanism.

Respiratory management

The aims of respiratory management are to prevent hypoxaemia, and the development of respiratory complications and failure. Humidified oxygen should be provided by facemask. A regimen of 2-hourly postural change is instituted on a turning bed, or with log rolling, to prevent atelectasis. An intensive physiotherapy regimen is started with 4-hourly deep breathing using non-invasive ventilatory support by mouthpiece, with bronchodilators if necessary. Assisted coughing (where the physiotherapist pushes on the abdomen synchronous with glottic closure as the patient attempts to cough) may be used to clear sputum. Serial evaluation of respiratory rate, oxygenation, vital capacity and chest X-ray is necessary.

Respiratory complications

Respiratory complications are frequent and the major reason for SCI patients to be admitted to the ICU. They are dependent on the level of the SCI, the presence of underlying respiratory disease, age and associated injuries. Respiratory complications are the leading early cause of death after SCI, with most attributed to pneumonia.

These complications consist of atelectasis, sputum retention, pneumonia and acute respiratory failure (ARF). There is also the risk of aspiration of mouth secretions and gastric content, acute respiratory distress syndrome (ARDS), acute pulmonary oedema and pulmonary embolism. Indications for intubation and MV include an inability to clear secretions, progressive atelectasis or pneumonia, or frank ARF. Intubation and MV should also be undertaken for associated head or chest injuries, or if the VC falls below 12–15 ml/kg.

Endotracheal intubation with CSI The options are awake fibreoptic nasotracheal intubation or orotracheal intubation under general anaesthesia. No particular approach has been shown to be superior, and either is acceptable depending on individual circumstances. Factors determining the choice include the urgency of the situation, the skill and training of medical staff, the availability of equipment, the conscious state of the patient and the associated injuries.[11]

Awake nasotracheal intubation with topical anaesthesia allows continuous neurological assessment, but should only be attempted with an alert cooperative patient. It is contraindicated if urgent intubation is required, or if there is coagulopathy, nasal obstruction or basal skull fracture. Blind intubation often requires multiple attempts, and has a significant complication and failure rate. Fibreoptic intubation is a more acceptable technique for those with appropriate training, although desaturation during the procedure is common.

Orotracheal intubation under anaesthesia is a safe technique, despite the greater potential for neck movement, and there is no evidence to suggest that neurological outcome is worse.[11,33] Preparation should be made for a rapid sequence induction and a difficult intubation. The anterior part of the collar is removed to allow adequate mouth opening, manual stabilisation of the head is performed without traction, and cricoid pressure is applied. Intravenous atropine is given, followed by the induction agent and muscle relaxant. Suxamethonium should be avoided between 10 days and 7 months after SCI to prevent severe hyperkalaemia.[34] Rocuronium is then the preferred relaxant.

After intubation, MV is instituted using larger tidal volumes and an I:E ratio of at least 1:2. Persistent and/or recurrent atelectasis remains a problem, with the added risk of nosocomial ventilator-associated pneumonia.

Tracheostomy Once intubated, tracheostomy is usually necessary. It improves comfort and communication, and facilitates weaning from MV and discharge from the ICU. Percutaneous tracheostomy may be used after internal fixation of the cervical spine, but often the neck cannot be extended into the optimal position. Surgical tracheostomy is preferred and is ideally performed in the ICU.

Weaning from MV With high tetraplegics weaning can be very prolonged, difficult and is frequently complicated by recurrent atelectasis. Weaning is usually started after resolution of any pulmonary pathology, in the supine position and having a VC of at least 10 ml/kg. No method of weaning has been shown to be superior. Weaning is most conveniently begun by conversion to pressure support ventilation, ideally with flow triggering. Incremental reduction in the pressure support level is carried out as tolerated, before conversion to a T-piece or tracheostomy shield. Alternatively, T-piece trials may be used from the outset, but need much more psychological support to prevent patient anxiety and loss of confidence. Nearly all C4 or lower tetraplegics, and about 50% of C3 tetraplegics can be weaned from MV given time.[29] When weaned, patients may be discharged from the ICU, but tracheostomy decannulation should be delayed until it is clear that the patient is coping off MV, atelectasis does not recur, sputum production is minimal and aspiration is not occurring.

C1–3 tetraplegics who cannot be weaned are usually managed with permanent MV via a home ventilator. Some of these patients may be suitable for phrenic nerve pacing.[35] Other tetraplegics with very limited ventilatory reserve are likely to require nocturnal ventilatory support.

CARDIOVASCULAR

Cardiovascular dysfunction

With tetraplegia there is loss of supraspinal sympathetic control of the heart and peripheral vasculature, with unopposed vagal activity. In the early phase of spinal shock there is also loss of autonomic reflex activity in the isolated cord segment. These changes lead to sinus bradycardia and arterial hypotension associated with systemic vaso- and venodilatation. Similar problems are seen in paraplegia, especially with SCI above T6. Patients are sensitive to further hypotension with postural change, blood or fluid loss, and intermittent positive-pressure ventilation (IPPV).

Cardiovascular management

Monitoring should include ECG, arterial blood pressure (BP), subclavian or femoral central venous pressure (CVP) and urine output. Some plasma volume expansion is necessary to correct a degree of relative hypovolaemia. Previously mean arterial pressures (MAP) of 60–70 mmHg have been tolerated if the urine output was adequate (> 0.5 ml/kg per hour). However, animal evidence strongly suggests that hypotension after SCI contributes to secondary ischaemic injury of the cord. Clinical studies of BP elevation suggest improved neurological outcomes without adverse effects.[36] Consensus guidelines now recommend prompt correction of hypotension, and maintenance of MAP at 85–90 mmHg with vasopressors for the first 7 days after SCI.[37]

Cardiovascular complications

Venous thromboembolism Venous thromboembolism has a 40% incidence without prophylaxis, with pulmonary embolism accounting for up to 15% of deaths in the first year after SCI. Consensus guidelines[38] for prevention recommend intermittent pneumatic compression or electrical calf muscle stimulation, plus enoxaparin 30 mg twice daily or adjusted dose unfractionated heparin (to a high normal activated partial thromboplastin time) starting within 72 hours and continued for 8–12 weeks depending on risk factors. If high risk and anticoagulation fails or is contraindicated, an inferior vena caval filter should be inserted.

Bradycardia, asystole Due to disruption of sympathetic pathways and unopposed vagal activity these problems are extremely common after high SCI. With severe cervical SCI the incidence of persistent bradycardia was 100% and transient marked bradycardia (heart rate < 45 per min) 71%, with cardiac arrest occurring in 16% of patients. These arrhythmias peaked in the first week and resolved 2–6 weeks after injury.[39] Tracheal suction in the presence of hypoxia appears to be a cause of cardiac arrest preventable with atropine.

Acute pulmonary oedema This is now less common, but does occur with misguided attempts to correct hypotension with excessive volume expansion, in the absence of CVP monitoring.

Autonomic hyperreflexia This is not a problem in the early phase. It begins within 6 months of SCI after recovery from spinal shock, and is usually only significant with SCI above the T6 level.[40] In response to an afferent stimulus below the neurological level there is excessive paroxysmal autonomic reflex activity. The stimulus is often bladder or bowel distension, but may be cutaneous stimulation or surgery. The massive sympathetic efferent response causes intense vasoconstriction that produces severe hypertension, with the risk of seizures and cerebral haemorrhage. Baroreceptor-mediated bradycardia may occur with reflex vasodilatation above the neurological level in paraplegics. Treatment consists of preventing or removing the stimulus, placing the patient in an upright posture and, if necessary, short-acting i.v. antihypertensive drugs such as nitroprusside.

NEUROLOGICAL

Drug treatment strategies are aimed to reduce secondary injury mechanisms, and to allow recovery of damaged neurones. Encouraging results have been achieved with animal experiments but only minimal improvement in human SCI using corticosteroids. In the NASCIS 2 trial,[41] methylprednisolone – if started within 8 hours of SCI (30 mg/kg bolus followed by 5.4 mg/kg per hour for 23 hours) – resulted in mildly improved motor and sensory scores at 6 months and 1 year. A further trial, NASCIS 3,[42] showed some improvement in motor score and functional outcome if methylprednisolone started within 3–8 hours of SCI was given for 48 hours rather than 24 hours. However, this was associated with more sepsis and pneumonia. The administration of methylprednisolone has been widely, but not universally, accepted. Criticism of these studies has followed from reanalysis of the NASCIS data[43] and systematic review of all published studies.[44] An attempt to set guidelines[45] concluded that methylprednisolone for 24 or 48 hours was only an option for treatment of acute SCI, and that it should only be undertaken with the knowledge that evidence suggesting harmful side-effects was more consistent than suggestion of clinical benefit. No additional evidence has been forthcoming and the controversy remains.[46,47]

In human studies, GM-1 ganglioside, tirilazad, naloxone and nimodipine have shown no benefit.

Muscle spasticity is a late problem not seen in the acute phase in ICU. It develops after resolution of spinal shock.

SKELETAL

The principles of management include adequate reduction, maintenance of position, and immobilisation until stability has been achieved. There are both conservative and surgical options to management of injury to the spine.

Conservative measures for CSI include closed reduction, traction in head tongs or a halo, collars or the application of a halo-thoracic brace. For TLSI postural realignment may be used. However, some of these techniques require prolonged periods of immobilisation in bed. Mechanical turning beds facilitate this approach. Some believe that most spinal injuries, and especially TLSI, should be treated without surgery.[27]

Surgical techniques utilise open reduction and internal fixation to provide sufficient stability to allow early mobilisation. External supports such as a collar or brace may be added. Surgery is now utilised more frequently with the aim of achieving early stability and pain control, earlier mobilisation and rehabilitation, less muscle wasting, fewer hospital complications and earlier time for hospital discharge. If surgery is undertaken it is probably best performed at the earliest opportunity that other injuries and complications allow. In a multicentre study in North America, surgery was performed on 65% of acute SCI with little agreement as to timing.[48] Although claims have been made for fewer complications with earlier mobilisation and hospital discharge, there is no clear evidence in favour of surgical management.

With regard to the SCI itself, animal studies have consistently shown improved neurological outcomes with early surgical decompression of the spinal cord.[49] A recent systematic review of human studies concluded that early (< 24 hours) decompression produced better outcomes than delayed decompression or conservative treatment, especially for incomplete SCI with neurological deterioration.[50] However, there is no conclusive evidence of benefit of early decompression of the spinal cord in clinical practice, and this aspect also remains controversial.[49]

Physiotherapy measures are needed to preserve a full range of movement in paralysed joints and to prevent contractures.

TEMPERATURE

With high SCI the loss of sympathetic nerve function and an inability to shiver leads to poikilothermia. Regular temperature monitoring is needed together with an approach to prevent hypothermia.

GASTROINTESTINAL

A range of GI problems are associated with SCI. Paralytic ileus and acute gastric dilatation are frequent problems in the first few days. A nasogastric tube should be inserted immediately to protect against aspiration and respiratory impairment from abdominal distension. It may then be used for early enteral nutrition once these problems have resolved. Stress ulceration with GI bleeding has an incidence of 3–5%.[41] H_2 antagonists or proton pump inhibitors should be used for prevention. Acute acalculous cholecystitis, pancreatitis and the superior mesenteric artery syndrome are uncommon. Constipation and faecal impaction readily develop after a number of days. A preventative bowel regimen consisting of faecal softeners, suppositories and laxatives should be started early.

URINARY

After SCI there is paralysis of the bladder detrusor and urinary retention with the risk of bladder overdistension. A urethral catheter should be inserted early and placed on continuous drainage. Bladder training techniques with intermittent catheterisation are delayed until the patient is stable and has been discharged from the ICU. Bacterial colonisation of the urine is accepted while catheterised.

SKIN

Pressure sores readily develop and may cause considerable morbidity, prolonged hospitalisation and need extensive plastic surgery for closure. They must be prevented by meticulous attention to 2-hourly postural change, the use of pneumatic pressure mattresses or pillows, and to the protection of bony pressure points.

METABOLIC

Hyponatraemia has been reported to be common after complete and severe incomplete SCI.[51] Immobility after SCI leads to calcium mobilisation from bone, hypercalciuria and occasionally hypercalcaemia. Atrophy of denervated muscle, muscle wasting, weight loss and negative nitrogen balance are marked. Enteral nutrition should meet caloric needs (preferably estimated by indirect calorimetry) but nitrogen loss has to be accepted.[52]

PAIN

Pain is common after SCI. Pain may result from vertebral fractures or the gut. Neuropathic pain may occur at, or below the level of SCI. Intravenous opioids, ketamine, lidocaine and gabapentin are effective for neuropathic pain.[53]

PSYCHOLOGICAL

Prolonged supportive care is necessary for both patients and their families to deal with depression, and to help them accept and adapt to neurological disability. After intubation or tracheostomy tetraplegics have great difficulty with communication, as they are unable to write or use an alphabet board. Lip reading is utilised until a speaking tracheostomy tube can be used or a one-way speaking valve can be attached to the tracheostomy tube.

OUTCOME

After the acute care phase SCI patients undergo extensive periods of rehabilitation to maximise their functional ability before returning to the community.

NEUROLOGICAL RECOVERY

The prognosis for neurological recovery is best judged by neurological examination 72 hours post SCI. Most complete tetraplegics regain one motor level and do not recover functional lower limb movement. Incomplete SCI have much more recovery, and more than 50% of incomplete tetraplegics become ambulatory.[54,55] Significant spinal cord haemorrhage seen on MRI indicates a very low probability of motor recovery, but if < 4 mm the prognosis is better.[56]

SURVIVAL

Hospital survival after SCI is now more than 90%, with increasing life expectancy in the longer term. Long-term survival studies have shown a higher mortality risk with a higher neurological level, complete SCI, older age and earlier year of injury.[57] Most deaths are now due to respiratory and heart disease, with a decreasing proportion due to urinary complications.

REFERENCES

1. Sekhon LH, Fehlings MG. Epidemiology, demographics and pathophysiology of acute spinal cord injury. *Spine* 2001; **26**: S2–12.
2. Fisher CG, Noonan VK, Dvorak MF. Changing face of spine trauma care in North America. *Spine* 2006; **31**: S2–8.
3. Holdsworth F. Fractures, dislocations and fracture-dislocations of the spine. *J Bone Jt Surg* 1970; **52A**: 1534–51.
4. Harris JH, Mirvis SE. *The Radiology of Acute Cervical Spine Trauma*, 3rd edn. Baltimore: Williams and Wilkins; 1996: 213–44.
5. Allen BL, Ferguson RL, Lehmann TR *et al.* A mechanistic classification of closed, indirect fractures and dislocations of the lower cervical spine. *Spine* 1982; **7**: 1–27.
6. Denis F. The three column spine and its significance in the classification of acute thoracolumbar spinal injuries. *Spine* 1983; **8**: 817–31.
7. Tator CH, Fehlings MG. Review of the secondary injury theory of acute spinal cord trauma with emphasis on vascular mechanisms. *J Neurosurg* 1991; **75**: 15–26.
8. Maynard FM, Bracken MB, Creasey G *et al.* International standards for neurological and functional classification of spinal cord injury. *Spinal Cord* 1997; **35**: 266–74.
9. Waters RL, Adkins RH, Yakura JS. Definition of complete spinal cord injury. *Paraplegia* 1991; **29**: 573–81.
10. Tator CH. Classification of spinal cord injury based on neurological presentation. In: Narayan RK, Wilberger JE, Povlishock JT (eds) *Neurotrauma*. New York: McGraw-Hill; 1996: 1059–73.
11. Crosby ET. Airway management in adults after cervical spine trauma. *Anesthesiology* 2006; **104**: 1293–318.
12. Holly LT, Kelly DF, Counelis GJ *et al.* Cervical spine trauma associated with moderate and severe head injury: incidence, risk factors and injury characteristics. *J Neurosurg* 2002; **96**(3 Suppl): 285–91.
13. Lang-Lazdunski L, Pons F, Jancovici R. Update on the emergency management of chest trauma. *Curr Opin Crit Care* 1999; **5**: 488–99.
14. Schuster-Bruce M, Nolan J. Priorities in the management of blunt abdominal trauma. *Curr Opin Crit Care* 1999; **5**: 500–10.
15. Woodring JH, Lee C. Limitations of cervical radiography in the evaluation of acute cervical trauma. *J Trauma* 1993; **34**: 32–9.

16. Cooper DJ, Ackland HM. Clearing the cervical spine in unconscious head injured patients – the evidence. *Crit Care Resusc* 2005; 7: 181–4.
17. Turetsky DB, Vines FS, Clayman DA *et al.* Technique and use of supine oblique views in acute cervical spine trauma. *Ann Emerg Med* 1993; **22**: 685–9.
18. Brown CV, Antevil JL, Sise MJ *et al.* Spiral computed tomography for the diagnosis of cervical, thoracic and lumbar spine fractures: its time has come. *J Trauma* 2005; **58**: 890–5.
19. Tins BJ, Cassar-Pullicino VN. Imaging of acute cervical spinal injuries: review and outlook. *Clin Radiol* 2004; **59**: 865–80.
20. Levi AD, Hurlbert RJ, Anderson P *et al.* Neurological deterioration secondary to unrecognized spinal instability following trauma – a multicentre study. *Spine* 2006; **31**: 451–8.
21. Stiell IG, Wells GA, Vandemheen KL *et al.* The Canadian C-spine rule for radiography in alert and stable trauma patients. *JAMA* 2001; **286**: 1841–8.
22. Stiell IG, Clement CM, McKnight RD *et al.* The Canadian C-spine rule versus the NEXUS low-risk criteria in patients with trauma. *N Eng J Med* 2003; **349**: 2510–8.
23. Lien D, Jacques T, Powell K. Cervical spine clearance in Australian intensive care units. *Crit Care Resusc* 2003; **5**: 91–6.
24. Ackland HM, Cooper DJ, Malham GM *et al.* Magnetic resonance imaging for clearing the cervical spine in unconscious intensive care trauma patients. *J Trauma* 2006; **60**: 668–73.
25. Hogan GJ, Mirvis SE, Shanmuganathan K *et al.* Exclusion of unstable cervical spine injury in obtunded patients with blunt trauma: is MR imaging needed when multi-detector row CT findings are normal? *Radiology* 2005; **237**: 106–13.
26. Hadley MN. Cervical spine immobilization before admission to hospital. *Neurosurgery* 2002; **50**(Suppl): S7–15.
27. Rechtine GR. Nonoperative management and treatment of spinal injuries. *Spine* 2006; **31**: S22–7.
28. Hadley MN. Management of acute spinal cord injuries in an intensive care unit or other monitored setting. *Neurosurgery* 2002; **50**(Suppl): S51–7.
29. Mansel JK, Norman JR. Respiratory complications and management of spinal cord injuries. *Chest* 1990; **97**: 1446–52.
30. Winslow C, Rozovsky J. Effect of spinal cord injury on the respiratory system. *Am J Phys Med Rehabil* 2003; **82**: 803–14.
31. Ledsome JR, Sharp JM. Pulmonary function in acute cervical cord injury *Am Rev Respir Dis* 1981; **124**: 41–4.
32. Baydur A, Adkins RH, Milic-Emili J. Lung mechanics in individuals with spinal cord injury: effects of injury level and posture. *J Appl Physiol* 2001; **90**: 405–11.
33. Shatney CH, Brunner RD, Nguyen TQ. The safety of orotracheal intubation in patients with unstable cervical spine fracture or high spinal cord injury. *Am J Surg* 1995; **170**: 676–80.
34. Yentis SM. Suxamethonium and hyperkalaemia. *Anaesth Intensive Care* 1990; **18**: 92–101.
35. DiMarco AF. Restoration of respiratory muscle function following spinal cord injury. Review of electrical and magnetic stimulation techniques. *Respir Physiol Neurobiol* 2005; **147**: 273–87.
36. Vale FL, Burns J, Jackson AB *et al.* Combined medical and surgical treatment after acute spinal cord injury: results of a prospective pilot study to assess the merits of aggressive medical resuscitation and blood pressure management. *J Neurosurg* 1997; **87**: 239–46.
37. Hadley MN. Blood pressure management after acute spinal cord injury. *Neurosurgery* 2002; **50**(Suppl): S58–62.
38. Hadley MN. Deep venous thrombosis and thromboembolism in patients with cervical spinal cord injuries. *Neurosurgery* 2002; **50**(Suppl): S73–80.
39. Lehmann KG, Lane JG, Piepmeier JM *et al.* Cardiovascular abnormalities accompanying acute spinal cord injury in humans: incidence, time course and severity. *J Am Coll Cardiol* 1987; **10**: 46–52.
40. Colachis SC. Autonomic hyperreflexia with spinal cord injury. *J Am Paraplegia Soc* 1992; **15**: 171–86.
41. Bracken MB, Shepard MJ, Collins WF *et al.* A randomized controlled trial of methylprednisolone or naloxone in the treatment of acute spinal cord injury. *N Eng J Med* 1990; **322**: 1405–11.
42. Bracken MB, Shepard MJ, Holford TR *et al.* Administration of methylprednisolone for 24 or 48 hours or tirilazad mesylate for 48 hours in the treatment of acute spinal cord injury. *JAMA* 1997; **277**: 1597–604.
43. Hurlbert JR. Methylprednisolone for acute spinal cord injury: an inappropriate standard of care. *J Neurosurg* 2000; **93**(1 Suppl): 1–7.
44. Short DJ, El Masry WS, Jones PW. High dose methylprednisolone in the management of acute spinal cord injury – a systematic review from a clinical perspective. *Spinal Cord* 2000; **38**: 273–86.
45. Hadley MN. Pharmacological therapy after acute cervical spinal cord injury. *Neurosurgery* 2002; **50**(Suppl): S63–72.
46. Baptiste DC, Fehlings MG. Pharmacological approaches to repair of the injured spinal cord. *J Neurotrauma* 2006; **23**: 318–34.
47. Sayer FT, Kronvall E, Nilsson OG. Methylprednisolone treatment in acute spinal cord injury: the myth challenged through a structured analysis of published literature. *Spine J* 2006; **6**: 335–43.
48. Tator CH, Fehlings MG, Thorpe K *et al.* Current use and timing of spinal surgery for management of acute spinal cord injury in North America: results of a retrospective multicenter study. *J Neurosurg* 1999; **91**(1 Suppl): 12–18.
49. Fehlings MG, Perrin RG. The timing of surgical intervention in the treatment of spinal cord injury: a systematic review of recent clinical evidence. *Spine* 2006; **31**: S28–35.
50. La Rosa G, Conti A, Cardali S *et al.* Does early decompression improve neurological outcome of spinal cord injured patients? Appraisal of the literature using a

meta-analytical approach. *Spinal Cord* 2004; **42**: 503–12.

51. Peruzzi WT, Shapiro BA, Meyer PR *et al.* Hyponatremia in acute spinal cord injury. *Crit Care Med* 1994; **22**: 252–8.
52. Hadley MN. Nutritional support after spinal cord injury. *Neurosurgery* 2002; **50**(Suppl): S81–4.
53. Acute spinal cord injury. In: Australian and New Zealand College of Anaesthetists and Faculty of Pain Medicine. *Acute Pain Management: Scientific Evidence*, 2nd edn. 2005: 148–50.
54. Kirshblum SC, O'Connor KC. Levels of spinal cord injury and predictors of neurological recovery. *Phys Med Rehabil Clin N Am* 2000; **11**: 1–27.
55. Burns AS, Ditunno JF. Establishing prognosis and maximizing functional outcomes after spinal cord injury. *Spine* 2001; **26**: S137–145.
56. Boldin C, Raith J, Fankhauser F *et al.* Predicting neurological recovery in cervical spinal cord injury with postoperative MR imaging. *Spine* 2006; **31**: 554–9.
57. Frankel HL, Coll JR, Charlifue SW *et al.* Long term survival in spinal cord injury: a fifty year study. *Spinal Cord* 1998; **36**: 266–74.

71

Abdominal and pelvic injuries

Colin McArthur

Although important abdominal injuries are present in only 16–27% of hospital trauma admissions,[1] abdominal and pelvic injuries can represent up to 60% of missed diagnoses in preventable trauma deaths.[2] Most abdominal and pelvic injuries are caused by blunt trauma; penetrating aetiologies account for 6–21% of cases, depending on the society concerned.[1,3] Important considerations with abdominal and pelvic injuries are:

- potential for severe haemorrhage
- difficulties in diagnosing visceral injury
- severity of associated injuries (e.g. chest and head)
- complications, especially sepsis

MECHANISMS OF INJURY

BLUNT INJURIES

Road crashes account for most abdominal and pelvic blunt injuries. Injuries may also result from falls, assaults and industrial accidents.[1] Associated injuries are frequent, involving the thorax (most common), head and extremities. Seat belts and airbags reduce mortality in motor vehicle crashes (mainly by limiting brain injury), but are associated with more lower body injuries. Abdominal and pelvic injuries are more likely with vehicular side-on collisions, and when crashes result in a deformed steering wheel.[4]

PENETRATING INJURIES

Stab and gunshot wounds account for most penetrating injuries to the abdomen.

STAB AND LACERATION WOUNDS

Entry sites do not accurately predict the nature of deeper injury. Penetration of the thoracic cavity should be suspected with upper abdominal wounds; conversely, lower chest wounds may involve abdominal structures. Selective management of haemodynamically stable patients using investigation algorithms that accurately predict intra-abdominal injury has superseded mandatory laparotomy.[5]

GUNSHOT WOUNDS

Injuries depend on missile calibre, and its velocity and trajectory. Intra-abdominal, thoracic and multiple organ injuries and mortality are substantially greater than with stab wounds. Laparotomy should be performed in all cases with haemodynamic instability, peritonitis or a clinically unevaluable abdomen. A non-operative approach for solid organ injury[6] carries the risk of missed bowel injury.

INITIAL TREATMENT AND INVESTIGATIONS

RESUSCITATION

Ensuring adequacy of airway, ventilation and oxygenation are immediate priorities. However, circulatory resuscitation should not delay surgery for uncontrolled haemorrhage.[7] End-points for replacement of blood volume are controversial.[8] If rapid surgical haemostasis is provided in penetrating trauma, delaying or limiting fluid resuscitation before surgery may improve outcome.[9] Pneumatic antishock garments provide no benefit.[7,10]

CLINICAL ASSESSMENT

A full clinical examination (including the back) by experienced clinicians is most important. The mechanism of injury may direct attention to particular anatomical areas.[4]

- Contusions, external wounds and their relationship to underlying viscera are noted
- Abdominal distension, tenderness and peritonism are sought but auscultation for bowel sounds is not useful
- The rectum is examined for prostatic position, anal tone, blood or other evidence of injury
- Gastric aspirate and urine are inspected for blood

Isolated penetrating injuries present few diagnostic problems, but the decision to explore the abdomen can be difficult. Blunt abdominal trauma is often part of multiple injuries, and is more difficult to diagnose clinically, except when abdominal signs are obvious.

Nevertheless, in conscious patients, serial assessments can accurately identify those with significant intra-abdominal pathology. In the presence of impaired consciousness, intellectual disability or spinal, chest or pelvic injury, clinical assessment is unreliable. Other more visually spectacular injuries may also divert attention from the abdomen.

Laparotomy is indicated on clinical grounds when there is:

- shock with signs of intra-abdominal haemorrhage (e.g. peritonism or increasing distension)
- evisceration or peritonism without shock in penetrating trauma

In all other situations where clinical examination is inadequate, further investigations must be undertaken.[11]

PLAIN X-RAYS

A chest X-ray (preferably erect) is essential. It may demonstrate free intraperitoneal gas, herniation of abdominal contents through a ruptured diaphragm, or other abnormalities. Plain films of the abdomen are of no benefit. An anteroposterior pelvic X-ray is indicated for all victims of blunt trauma, except conscious patients with normal pelvis on examination.[12]

INVESTIGATIONS FOR OCCULT ABDOMINAL INJURY

ULTRASONOGRAPHY

Focused abdominal sonography for trauma (FAST) can be performed rapidly in the resuscitation room without compromising ongoing treatment. It requires significant training to achieve acceptable accuracy,[13] and although highly specific, its sensitivity of around 85%[14] is less than that of peritoneal lavage or CT in detecting free intra-abdominal fluid following either blunt[15,16] or penetrating[17] trauma. FAST can also identify pericardial fluid, but not hollow viscus injury or the nature of solid organ injury.[16] FAST may reduce the need for other investigations,[18] but the small but important false-negative rate must be considered in determining its role in abdominal assessment algorithms.

PERITONEAL LAVAGE

Diagnostic peritoneal lavage (DPL)[19] is indicated in blunt trauma when there is haemodynamic instability or uncertain clinical findings, and in penetrating trauma when peritoneal breach is suspected.

Open and closed (percutaneous guidewire) methods are both satisfactory.[20]

DPL is unjustified when an indication for laparotomy already exists. It is relatively contraindicated in pregnancy, significant obesity and previous abdominal surgery.

If required in these situations (or with pelvic fractures), the supraumbilical open method should be considered. DPL undertaken early remains reliable in the presence of pelvic fractures.[21] DPL detects intraperitoneal injury with up to 98% accuracy,[19] but its high sensitivity can result in a significant non-therapeutic laparotomy rate. Cell counts of lavage effluent are more accurate than qualitative methods, but hollow viscus injury is difficult to detect. Generally accepted criteria for a positive DPL are shown in Table 71.1.

Table 71.1 Criteria for positive diagnostic peritoneal lavage

Clinical		
Initial aspiration of > 10 ml frank blood		
Egress of lavage fluid via chest tube or urinary catheter		
Bile or vegetable material in lavage fluid		
Laboratory		
	Blunt injury	*Penetrating injury*
Red cells		
Definite	> 100 × 10⁹/l	> 20 × 10⁹/l
Indeterminate	50–100 × 10⁹/l	5–20 × 10⁹/l
White cells	> 0.5 × 10⁹/l	0.5 × 10⁹/l
Amylase	> 20 IU/l	> 20 IU/l
Alkaline phosphatase	> 10 IU/l	> 10 IU/l

COMPUTED TOMOGRAPHY (CT)

CT requires a still patient, a high-resolution scanner and experienced interpretation to match the sensitivity of peritoneal lavage. The value of enteral contrast is controversial.[22] Cuts from the top of the diaphragm to the symphysis pubis following i.v. contrast are required. CT is particularly useful to assess the retroperitoneum and pelvic fractures, and to delineate the nature of abdominal injury (thus guiding non-operative management of some solid organ injuries). It may not detect all hollow viscus trauma, but multidetector row CT is more specific and sensitive for bowel injury.[23] Magnetic resonance imaging offers no advantage over CT in evaluating acute abdominal trauma, and poses significant logistical problems.

The safety of undertaking CT in acute trauma depends on the degree of cardiorespiratory stability relative to the speed of scanning and access to resuscitation support.

CHOICE OF INVESTIGATION

- FAST is non-invasive, rapid and reasonably accurate when used by trained staff. It can screen for haemoperitoneum but negative studies should be followed by another investigation[15,16]
- DPL is invasive, takes some time and is accurate in identifying intraperitoneal bleeding or contamination, but may miss diaphragmatic injuries and does not examine the retroperitoneum. It is an alternative to FAST in unstable patients with blunt trauma, and stable patients with anterior stab wounds
- CT is non-invasive, time-consuming, accurate, and has a primary role in defining the location and magnitude of intra-abdominal injuries in stable patients with blunt trauma or penetrating trauma to the flank or back
- FAST, DPL and CT are complementary,[24] and should all be available. If CT is unavailable, DPL rather than FAST is indicated in the stable patient with blunt trauma in whom clinical examination is inadequate

LAPAROSCOPY

Diagnostic laparoscopy may be useful in the haemodynamically stable patient. It is good at visualising the diaphragm and identifying a need for laparotomy, but may miss specific organ injuries, particularly of the bowel. Laparoscopy appears best suited for the evaluation of equivocal penetrating wounds.[25]

ANGIOGRAPHY

Selective angiography and embolisation are valuable in detecting and treating the source of major haemorrhage from spleen, liver, pelvis and retroperitoneal structures.

LAPAROTOMY

Laparotomy can be regarded as both therapeutic and diagnostic. Intra-abdominal injury may be detected by means discussed above, but often only laparotomy can accurately diagnose specific injuries. In severe and multiple trauma, the morbidity of a negative laparotomy is insignificant compared to the dire consequences of not diagnosing and treating a serious injury.

Operative treatment of more severe injuries with difficult haemostasis can cause a lethal triad of hypothermia, acidosis and coagulopathy. A 'damage control' laparotomy[26] with control of haemorrhage and contamination, intraperitoneal packing, elective re-exploration and removal of packs 24–48 hours later should be performed.

- Angiography should be considered and may be required for inaccessible arterial bleeding
- Temporary prosthetic closure is often required to avoid elevated intra-abdominal pressure
- Survival is better when the decision to terminate the initial procedure is made earlier

SPECIFIC INJURIES

SPLEEN

The spleen is the organ most frequently injured by blunt trauma. Injuries vary from a small subcapsular haematoma to hilar devascularisation or shattered spleen, but are rarely fatal with good medical care.[27] Diagnosis may be delayed in mild trauma. When associated chest or neurological injuries are severe, minor splenic injury may not initially be detected unless further investigation is undertaken. Fractures of the lower left ribs are a common association. Minor trauma may cause splenic injury when the spleen is enlarged (e.g. from malaria, lymphomas and haemolytic anaemias).

Immediate splenectomy is indicated in patients with splenic avulsion, fragmentation or rupture, extensive hilar injuries, failure of haemostasis, peritoneal contamination from gastrointestinal injury or rupture of diseased spleen.[27] However, overwhelming infection by encapsulated organisms, such as Pneumococcus, can occur early or late (even years) after splenectomy in 0–2% of individuals. It is a particular risk following splenectomy in children and young adults. Polyvalent pneumococcal vaccine (Pneumovax) and haemophilus and meningococcal vaccines should be administered following splenectomy.[28]

If associated abdominal injuries have been excluded, a non-operative approach can give splenic salvage rates of over 80%. Arterial embolisation can further reduce the need for laparotomy.[29] Failure rates are higher with higher grade injuries.[28]

Other treatment alternatives include operative procedures to conserve splenic tissue (e.g. topical haemostatic agents, suture repair, absorbable mesh, partial splenectomy and splenic artery ligation). Benefits of splenectomy with autotransplantation of splenic tissue are unproven.

LIVER

The liver is the second most commonly injured organ after blunt abdominal trauma, and has been the most frequently missed injury in deaths from trauma.[2] Diagnosis is made by laparotomy in unstable patients, or CT in stable patients. Injuries range from small subcapsular haematomas to major parenchymal disruption and laceration of hepatic veins or even hepatic avulsion.

CT assessment enables most patients to be managed without operation. Patients should be haemodynamically stable, have associated major abdominal injuries excluded, and be assessed repeatedly. Follow-up CT scans can show the resolution of injury, which typically takes 2–3 months. CT-guided percutaneous drainage, endoscopic retrograde cholangiopancreaticogram (ERCP) and angioembolisation can treat the complications of a non-operative approach such as bile leak, haemobilia, necrosis, abscess and delayed haemorrhage.[28]

If surgery is required, early determination of indications for a damage control approach is important. Perihepatic packing gives best haemostasis. Angiography may identify and treat uncontrolled arterial bleeding. Early complications of liver injury relate to the effects of hypoperfusion or massive blood transfusion. Late complications are usually associated with sepsis.[30]

GASTROINTESTINAL TRACT (GIT)

Injury to the GIT is more common following penetrating than blunt trauma. The very high likelihood of bowel injury in abdominal gunshot wounds should mandate laparotomy. Laparoscopy can be used to identify those with stab wounds for laparotomy when peritoneal violation cannot be excluded. Posterior stab wounds may damage retroperitoneal structures. CT examination with contrast enema may identify colonic injury better than clinical assessment or DPL.[5]

Blunt abdominal injuries to stomach, duodenum, small intestine, colon and their mesenteries are difficult to evaluate. Physical signs may be absent initially.

FAST or DPL may provide a general indication for laparotomy, but are not accurate in diagnosing isolated bowel trauma (especially of the duodenum) because of its retroperitoneal location.

CT is a sensitive indicator of free intraperitoneal air, but signs of duodenal perforation or haematoma are subtle, even with enteral contrast. Consequently, duodenal injury is often missed. A high index of suspicion should be maintained in patients with persistent abdominal pain and tenderness.[31]

Bleeding from mesenteric vessels is often self-limiting and may not require surgical control. However, vessel damage can cause ischaemia and infarction, and may require resection of affected bowel. Uncomplicated blunt or penetrating bowel injury can usually be managed by primary repair and anastomosis rather than colostomy.[32] A faecal diversion procedure with delayed repair is indicated in significant peritoneal contamination.

PANCREAS

Blunt injuries to the pancreas require considerable force and are often associated with duodenal, liver and splenic trauma. CT is the most useful investigation. Acute hyperamylasaemia does not predict pancreatic or hollow viscus injury.[33]

Minor injuries require simple drainage and haemostasis. Severe injuries to the body and tail of the pancreas are best managed by distal pancreatectomy. Severe injuries involving the proximal pancreas and duodenum with intact ampulla and common bile duct can be treated by drainage alone if associated duodenal injury is simple to repair. Pancreaticoduodenectomy is required if there is disruption of the ampullary–biliary–pancreatic union or major devitalisation. Complications such as pancreatitis, fistula, abscess and pseudocyst are common.[34,35]

KIDNEY AND URINARY TRACT

Blunt injury to the urinary tract is more common than penetrating injury. Identification and treatment of other major injuries often take precedence. Gross haematuria should be investigated; CT is the examination of choice. Urinary extravasation may be missed unless a repeat scan 10–20 minutes after contrast injection is performed. Unless there is unexplained shock, microscopic haematuria does not require further investigation. Renovascular pedicle or ureteric injuries may not cause any haematuria. Most renal injuries resolve with expectant management. Lacerations involving the collecting system or injury to the renal pedicle usually require operative intervention, although restoration of renal function following long warm ischaemic times is unusual. If major renal injury is discovered at emergency laparotomy, intraoperative i.v. urography is prudent to ensure contralateral function and will identify urinary extravasation. Angioembolisation may be useful in controlling renal haemorrhage.[36]

Bladder rupture is commonly associated with pelvic fractures. Over 95% of patients have macroscopic haematuria. Retrograde cystography is the investigation of choice because CT has a high false-negative rate. Intraperitoneal bladder rupture requires operative repair and urinary drainage. Patients with sterile urine and extraperitoneal rupture can be managed with catheter drainage alone.[37]

Urethral trauma is caused by direct blunt injury, or occurs in association with pelvic injury. It should be suspected if there is blood at the urinary meatus, perineal injury or abnormal position of the prostate on rectal examination in the male. In the absence of these findings, cautious urethral catheterisation is appropriate. Treatment of urethral trauma is suprapubic drainage and subsequent definitive repair.

DIAPHRAGM

Diaphragmatic injury occurs in fewer than 5% of cases of blunt injury, is left-sided in 80% of cases, and is commonly associated with injuries to abdominal organs. It should also be suspected in penetrating trauma below the fifth rib. Diagnosis can be difficult, especially in the presence of positive-pressure ventilation, and may become evident only after ventilatory support is discontinued.

- Chest X-rays are commonly abnormal but often with non-specific findings
- DPL is insensitive for isolated diaphragmatic injuries
- Laparoscopy and thoracoscopy provide good views of the diaphragm

Spontaneous healing does not occur, and all defects should be repaired. The risk of associated injuries in acute cases mandates an abdominal approach.[38]

BONY PELVIS AND PERINEUM

Pelvic fractures are primarily caused by vehicular trauma or falls. Associated injuries to the bladder, urethra and intra-abdominal organs are common. Injuries may be life-threatening initially from major haemorrhage, or later from sepsis. Significant morbidity can result from damage to pelvic nerves, urethra or the structural integrity of the pelvis. Pelvic injury is suggested by pain on movement, structural instability, gross haematuria or peri-pelvic ecchymosis. Rectal examination is mandatory to identify rectal injury and prostatic position.

Radiography can confirm bony injury, but CT is required to identify associated intra-abdominal injuries (in the haemodynamically stable) and can assist in planning operative stabilisation. FAST has a significant false-negative rate with major pelvic fractures.[39]

Patients with haemodynamic instability and pelvic fractures must have intra-abdominal haemorrhage excluded. Early open supraumbilical DPL or FAST are the investigations of choice. If grossly positive, laparotomy should precede external fixation or angiography. If DPL is positive by cell count alone or FAST negative, the risk of life-threatening intra-abdominal haemorrhage is relatively low, and achieving haemostasis for pelvic bleeding becomes the priority; CT and/or laparotomy should follow if the patient is still unstable.

- Emergency measures to improve tamponade by reducing pelvic volume (pelvic binding or C-clamp) and prompt angiography and selective embolisation can significantly reduce mortality[40]
- External fixation of the pelvis can control venous and small arteriolar bleeding near fracture sites, and will also reduce the volume of an open pelvis
- Bleeding from large vessels such as the aorta, common and external iliac arteries, and common femoral artery requires surgical control

Pelvic fractures range from simple fractures of individual bones requiring bed rest alone to complex fractures. Early operative stabilisation of complex pelvic fractures is preferred in the intensive care unit (ICU), as it facilitates respiratory care, pain control and early mobilisation. Compound pelvic fractures involving the perineum, rectum or vagina require aggressive surgery (including diversion of the faecal stream) to avoid high mortality.

RETROPERITONEAL HAEMATOMA

Retroperitoneal haematoma is frequent following blunt trauma, and is commonly caused by injury to the lumbar spine, bony pelvis, bladder or kidney or, less commonly, to the pancreas, duodenum or major vascular structures. Diagnosis may be inferred by excluding other sites of major blood loss, or presumed by signs of underlying organ injury.

CT is the most useful investigation in the stable patient.

A central haematoma should be explored with proximal vascular control, because of the risk of pancreatic, duodenal or major vascular injury. A lateral or pelvic haematoma should not be explored, unless there is evidence of major arterial injury, intraperitoneal bladder rupture or colonic injury.[41]

TRAUMA IN PREGNANCY

Women injured during pregnancy pose problems of altered physiology, risk to the gravid uterus and fetus, and conflict of priorities between mother and fetus.

- High-flow oxygen must be given until maternal hypoxaemia, hypovolaemia and fetal distress have been excluded
- Reduced respiratory reserve demands earlier intervention
- Maternal compensation for blood loss is at the expense of uteroplacental blood flow
- Mothers should be positioned to avoid aortocaval compression
- Secondary survey must include a vaginal examination
- Intravenous access should be in the upper limbs
- Transfusions should be Rhesus compatible
- All Rhesus-negative mothers should receive immune globulin, because of the immunological risk of even minor fetomaternal haemorrhage[42]

Only X-rays that may significantly alter therapy should be taken (with appropriate shielding), especially if under 20 weeks' gestation.

Ultrasound is the preferred investigation as it is safe and can accurately detect free intra-abdominal fluid, confirm gestation and fetal well-being, and identify placental abnormalities. DPL is safe if performed by the open method above the fundus. CT may miss injuries due to abdominal crowding.

Retroperitoneal haemorrhage is more common in pregnant patients. Placental abruption may conceal significant blood loss. Treatment may be expectant or by caesarean section, depending on the condition of the mother and fetus. Uterine rupture is unusual and will often require hysterectomy. Rarely, perimortem caesarean section may be indicated in a dead or dying mother, to attempt to save the fetus.

Placental abruption, fetal distress and fetal loss are rare following blunt injury, but premature uterine contractions are common.

Continuous cardiotocography (indicated at viable gestations) is the most sensitive test to detect obstetric complications, but is required for only 4 hours unless abnormalities are noted.[42] Kleihauer–Betke tests to identify fetomaternal haemorrhage are not predictive of fetal or maternal morbidity.

HAEMORRHAGE

Patients with haemorrhage from abdominal and pelvic injuries can suffer the same complications of shock and massive transfusion as any patient with severe haemorrhage. Dilutional coagulopathy is common following resuscitation with fluids deficient in haemostatic factors. Patients resuscitated with crystalloids, colloids and red cells often require platelet and fresh frozen plasma transfusions. Disseminated intravascular coagulation occurs infrequently in trauma, usually when shock has been prolonged.

SEPSIS

Intra-abdominal sepsis remains an important preventable cause of death after trauma. Predisposing factors include:

- peritoneal contamination from GIT injury
- external wounds
- invasive procedures
- delayed diagnosis of hollow viscus injuries
- splenectomy
- devitalised tissue

Early diagnosis and effective lavage and drainage procedures may reduce the incidence of intra-abdominal sepsis.

Prophylactic antibiotics for 24 hours are satisfactory for penetrating injuries. Intra-abdominal sepsis should be excluded if unexplained fever and/or neutrophil leukocytosis or multiple organ failure develops. Septic shock may represent a second shock insult to the trauma patient, leading to multiorgan dysfunction.

GASTROINTESTINAL FAILURE

GIT failure in various forms, ranging from stress ulceration and delayed gastric emptying to paralytic ileus, is a frequent occurrence. Prophylaxis against stress ulceration may be indicated. Enteral nutrition is associated with a lower incidence of sepsis following trauma.[43] Feeding through a jejunostomy tube placed during surgery or radiologically in the ICU is usually feasible. Parenteral nutrition may be necessary in patients with severe bowel or retroperitoneal injuries.

RAISED INTRA-ABDOMINAL PRESSURE

Abdominal distension with raised intra-abdominal pressure may be seen in the critically injured as a consequence of haemorrhage, bowel oedema, ileus or surgical packs. This can have severe adverse effects on respiratory, cardiovascular and renal function.[44] Alleviation is by abdominal decompression using interposed synthetic mesh[45] or by leaving the abdomen open, with or without visceral packing. The abdomen is subsequently closed by staged repair as the distension resolves.

REFERENCES

1. Cameron P, Dziukas L, Hadj A *et al.* Patterns of injury from major trauma in Victoria. *Aust N Z J Surg* 1995; **65**: 848–52.
2. Anderson ID, Woodford M, de Dombal FT *et al.* Retrospective study of 1000 deaths from trauma in England and Wales. *BMJ* 1988; **296**: 1305–8.
3. Champion HR, Copes WS, Sacco WI *et al.* The Major Trauma Outcome Study: establishing norms for trauma care. *Trauma* 1990; **30**: 1356–65.
4. Yoganandan N, Pintar FA, Gennarelli TA *et al.* Patterns of abdominal injuries in frontal and side impacts. Proceedings of the Annual Conference. *Assoc Advance Automot Med* 2000; **44**: 17–36.
5. Chiu WC, Shanmuganathan K, Mirvis SE *et al.* Determining the need for laparotomy in penetrating torso trauma: a prospective study using triple contrast enhanced abdominopelvic computed tomography. *J Trauma* 2001; **51**: 860–8.
6. Demetriades D, Hadjizacharia P, Constantinou C *et al.* Selective nonoperative management of penetrating abdominal solid organ injuries. *Ann Surg* 2006; **244**: 620–8.
7. Spahn DR, Cerny V, Coats TJ *et al.* Management of bleeding following major trauma: a European guideline. *Crit Care* 2007; **11**: 414.
8. Roberts I, Evans P, Bunn F *et al.* Is the normalisation of blood pressure in bleeding trauma patients harmful? *Lancet* 2001; **357**: 385–7.
9. Bickell WH, Wall MJ, Pepe PE *et al.* Immediate versus delayed resuscitation for hypotensive patients with penetrating torso injuries. *N Engl J Med* 1994; **331**: 1105–9.
10. Mattox KL, Bickell WH, Pepe PE *et al.* Prospective MAST study in 911 patients. *J Trauma* 1989; **29**: 1104–12.
11. Prall JA, Nichols JS, Brennan R *et al.* Early definitive abdominal evaluation in the triage of unconscious normotensive blunt trauma patients. *J Trauma* 1994; **37**: 792–7.
12. Koury HI, Peschiera JL, Welling RE. Selective use of pelvic roentgenograms in blunt trauma patients. *J Trauma* 1993; **34**: 236–7.
13. Gracias VH, Frankel HL, Gupta R *et al.* Defining the learning curve for the focussed abdominal sonogram for trauma (FAST) examination: implications for credentialling. *Am Surg* 2001; **67**: 364–8.
14. Lee BC, Ormsby EL, McGahan JP *et al.* The utility of sonography for the triage of blunt abdominal trauma patients to exploratory laparotomy. *Am J Roentgenol* 2007; **188**: 415–21.
15. Hsu JM, Joseph AP, Tarlinton LJ *et al.* The accuracy of focused assessment with sonography in trauma (FAST) in blunt trauma patients: experience of an Australian major trauma service. *Injury* 2007; **38**: 71–5.
16. Griffin XL, Pullinger R. Are diagnostic peritoneal lavage or focussed abdominal sonography for trauma safe screening investigations for haemodynamically stable patients after blunt abdominal trauma? A review of the literature. *J Trauma* 2007; **62**: 779–84.
17. Udobi KF, Rodriguez A, Chiu WC *et al.* Role of ultrasonography in penetrating abdominal trauma: a prospective clinical study. *J Trauma* 2001; **50**: 475–9.
18. Ollerton JE, Sugrue M, Balogh Z *et al.* Prospective study to evaluate the influence of FAST on trauma patient management. *J Trauma* 2006; **60**: 785–91.
19. Nagy KK, Roberts RR, Joseph KT *et al.* Experience with over 2500 diagnostic peritoneal lavages. *Injury* 2000; **31**: 479–82.
20. Hodgson NF, Stewart TC, Girotti MJ. Open or closed diagnostic peritoneal lavage for abdominal trauma? A meta-analysis. *J Trauma* 2000; **48**: 1091–5.
21. Mendez C, Gubler KD, Maier RV. Diagnostic accuracy of peritoneal lavage in patients with pelvic fractures. *Arch Surg* 1994; **129**: 477–82.
22. Tsang BD, Panacek EA, Brant WE *et al.* Effect of oral contrast administration for abdominal computed tomography in the evaluation of acute blunt trauma. *Ann Emerg Med* 1997; **30**: 7–13.
23. Romano S, Scaglione M, Tortora G *et al.* MDCT in blunt intestinal trauma. *Eur J Radiol* 2006; **59**: 359–66.
24. Gonzalez RP, Ickier J, Gachassin P. Complementary roles of diagnostic peritoneal lavage in the evaluation of blunt abdominal trauma. *J Trauma* 2001; **51**: 1128–34.
25. Poole GV, Thomas KR, Hauser CJ. Laparoscopy in trauma. *Surg Clin North Am* 1996; **76**: 547–56.

26. Shapiro MB, Jenkins DH, Schwab CW *et al.* Damage control: collective review. *J Trauma* 2000; **49**: 969–78.
27. Wilson RH, Moorehead RJ. Management of splenic trauma. *Injury* 1992; **23**: 5–9.
28. Spelman D, Buttery J, Daley A *et al.* Guidelines for the prevention of sepsis in asplenic and hyposplenic patients. *Int Med J* 2008; **38**: 349–56.
29. Haan JM, Bochicchio GV, Kramer N *et al.* Nonoperative management of blunt splenic injury: a 5-year experience. *J Trauma* 2005; **58**: 492–8.
30. Lee SK, Carrillo EH. Advances and changes in the management of liver injuries. *Am Surg* 2007; **73**: 201–6.
31. Hughes TM. The diagnosis of gastrointestinal tract injuries resulting from blunt trauma. *Aust N Z J Surg* 1999; **69**: 770–7.
32. Demetriades D, Murray JA, Chan L *et al.* Penetrating colon injuries requiring resection: diversion or primary anastomosis? An AAST prospective multicenter study. *J Trauma* 2001; **50**: 765–75.
33. Boulanger BR, Milzman DP, Rosati C *et al.* The clinical significance of acute hyperamylasemia after blunt trauma. *Can J Surg* 1993; **36**: 63–9.
34. Boffard KD, Brooks AJ. Pancreatic trauma – injuries to the pancreas and pancreatic duct. *Br J Surg* 2000; **166**: 4–12.
35. Krige JE, Beningfield SJ, Nicol AJ *et al.* The management of complex pancreatic injuries. *S Afr J Surg* 2005; **43**: 92–102.
36. Santucci RA, Wessells H, Bartsch G *et al.* Evolution and management of renal injuries: consensus statement of the renal trauma subcommittee. *BJU Int* 2004; **93**: 937–54.
37. Gomez RG, Ceballos L, Corburn M *et al.* Consensus statement on bladder injuries. *BJU Int* 2004; **94**: 27–32.
38. Rosati C. Acute traumatic rupture of the diaphragm. *Chest Surg Clin North Am* 1998; **8**: 371–9.
39. Tayal VS, Neilsen A, Jones AE *et al.* Accuracy of trauma ultrasound in major pelvic injury. *J Trauma* 2006; **61**: 1453–7.
40. Bim WL, Smith WR, Moore EE *et al.* Evolution of a multidisciplinary pathway for the management of unstable patients with pelvic fractures. *Ann Surg* 2001; **233**: 843–50.
41. Feliciano DV. Management of traumatic retroperitoneal haematoma. *Ann Surg* 1990; **211**: 109–23.
42. Mattox KL, Goetzl L. Trauma in pregnancy. *Crit Care Med* 2005; **33**: S385–9.
43. Kudsk KA, Croce MA, Fabian TC *et al.* Enteral versus parenteral feeding. Effects on septic morbidity after blunt and penetrating abdominal trauma. *Ann Surg* 1992; **215**: 503–13.
44. Saggi BH, Sugerman HJ, Ivatury RR *et al.* Abdominal compartment syndrome. *J Trauma* 1998; **45**: 597–609.
45. Torrie J, Hill AA, Streat SJ. Staged abdominal repair in critical illness. *Anaesth Intensive Care* 1996; **24**: 368–74.

Part Twelve

Environmental Injuries

72

Near drowning

Cyrus Edibam

DEFINITIONS

The American Heart Association Guidelines for Resuscitation[1] suggest that the term 'submersion victim' be used to describe a person who experiences some swimming-related stress that is sufficient to require support in the field plus transportation to an emergency facility for further observation and treatment. 'Drowning' refers to death within 24 hours following a submersion event and the term 'near drowning' should no longer be used.

EPIDEMIOLOGY

Drowning causes over 400 000 deaths worldwide.[2] Of these, 4000 are reported from the USA (approximately 1.5 deaths per 100 000 population),[3] 500 from Australia[4] and 700 from the UK.[5] The incidence of non-fatal submersion events has been estimated to be 2–20 times more common than drowning.[6] More than half of all submersion events occur in children less than 5 years old, the majority being 1–2 years old.[7,8] Males predominate, with peaks at 5 and 20 years of age. Private swimming pools and natural water bodies close to home present the greatest risk to young children.[8] Other sites include bathtubs, fish tanks, buckets, toilets and washing machines. Adolescent drowning tends to occur in rivers, lakes, canals and beaches.[9] Lack of adult supervision is almost always to blame for toddler accidents; however, child abuse must also be considered. Alcohol and drug intoxication is associated with up to 40% of adolescent drowning.[10] Other risk factors include epilepsy (18%), trauma (16%) and cardiopulmonary disease (14%).[11] Hyperventilation prior to underwater swimming suppresses the physiological response to rising carbon dioxide tension, allowing hypoxia to ensue with consequent loss of consciousness and water breathing.[12]

PATHOPHYSIOLOGY

Voluntary apnoea and reflex responses occur upon submersion. The *diving response* is characterised by apnoea, marked generalised vasoconstriction and bradycardia in response to cold-water stimulus of the ophthalmic division of the trigeminal nerve. Blood is thus shunted preferentially to the brain and heart. In infants the response may be marked,[13] but only 15% of fully clothed adults show a significant response. Although the diving reflex appears to play a powerful role in oxygen conservation in animals, its role in humans is unknown but may be protective.[14]

At some point after submersion involuntary inspiration occurs which leads to aspiration of water and often vomitus. Laryngeal spasm may occur which may explain the approximate 15% incidence of *dry drowning*, where little or no fluid is found in the lungs.[15,16] Gasping then occurs and water aspiration continues. Up to 22 ml/kg of water has been estimated to be the maximal survivable inhaled water volume.[17] This is followed by a phase of secondary apnoea and loss of consciousness. Hypoxaemic death ensues if the person is not retrieved and resuscitated. Acute lung injury (ALI) – often termed *secondary drowning*, the pathophysiology of which is discussed elsewhere in the book – occurs in up to 72% of symptomatic survivors.[18] Multiple organ dysfunction and cerebral damage may become evident in those that survive to hospital.

SALT VS FRESH WATER ASPIRATION

The differences between salt and fresh water drowning should be downplayed.[1] On the basis of animal studies it was thought that hypertonic seawater aspiration would draw plasma volume into the pulmonary interstitial space, leading to hypovolaemia, hypernatraemia and haemoconcentration. Similarly, aspiration of hypotonic fresh water was thought to lead to the passage of large volumes into the blood stream, leading to hypervolaemia, dilutional hyponatraemia, haemolysis and haemoglobinuria.

Modell *et al.*[19] showed that volumes of water normally aspirated rarely translate into clinically meaningful syndromes. Orlowski and colleagues[20] showed little difference in observed cardiovascular effects in a canine model using six solutions of differing tonicity. They concluded that the cardiovascular effects seen with drowning and aspiration of water are not dependent on the tonicity of the aspirated fluid, but are the direct result of anoxia. Of 91 patients seen with severe submersion, no patient had serious electrolyte abnormalities or haemolysis. In another series, only 15% of retrieved but unresuscitatable patients had any of the expected electrolyte changes.[17] Generally, most patients with ALI/pulmonary oedema will be hypovolaemic by the time they reach hospital.[12] No clinically detectable difference in the patterns of lung injury is seen between salt and fresh water drowning; both types reduce pulmonary surfactant quantity and function.[21]

WATER CONTAMINANTS

The incidence of pneumonia complicating submersion injury may be greater than 15% in those who survive long enough.[18] Rivers, lakes and coastal waters are greater reservoirs for microbes than well-kept swimming pools. In fresh water, Gram-negative bacteria predominate along with anaerobes and *Staphylococcus* spp., fungi, algal and protozoan species. *Aeromonas* spp. are ubiquitous water-borne bacteria and can be responsible for severe pneumonia.[22]

Chemicals in polluted water (e.g. kerosene[23]), chlorine[24] and particulate matter (e.g. sand[25]) can cause severe pulmonary dysfunction.

TEMPERATURE

Victims of submersion may develop primary or secondary hypothermia. If submersion occurs in icy water (<5°C) hypothermia may develop rapidly and provide some protection against hypoxia. Surface cooling is unlikely to produce adequate protective hypothermia before hypoxia ensues.[14] Most survivors of prolonged submersion almost always involve small children in icy water and it has been postulated that protective core cooling occurs rapidly due to cold-water aspiration, ingestion and absorption, though the mechanisms remain controversial.[26]

Of more importance in cold-water submersion are the detrimental 'cold-shock' responses.[27] These responses include a 'gasp' followed by uncontrollable hyperventilation and reduction in maximal breath-hold times, vasoconstriction, tachycardia, hypertension and increased myocardial oxygen consumption. These responses may lead to motor dyscoordination and swimming failure as well as cardiac arrhythmias, hence even strong swimmers may drown quickly in icy waters.

MANAGEMENT

BASIC LIFE SUPPORT

Prompt retrieval from the water is essential as is immediate on-site resuscitation. Expired air resuscitation and external cardiac compression should be applied immediately after retrieval. If trauma is suspected, especially in diving and surfing accidents, head and spinal injuries are assumed and due caution in stabilising the cervical spine during airway manipulation and transport is required. The Heimlich manoeuvre is no longer recommended in the management of submersion injury as the volume of aspirated water removed at the time of attempt is small and the risk of gastric aspiration is great.[1] Rewarming should be commenced immediately with the use of blankets and further heat loss should be avoided. When experienced personnel arrive, bag and mask ventilation and advanced cardiac life support is initiated.

INITIAL HOSPITAL MANAGEMENT

Resuscitation continues on arrival to hospital. Endotracheal intubation and mechanical ventilation is instituted if hypoxaemia is severe despite high-flow oxygen or assisted bag and mask respiration. Ventilatory failure, characterised by increasing respiratory distress and rising carbon dioxide levels, and the presence of an impaired conscious level or severe agitation may also necessitate intubation. Insertion of a nasogastric tube to decompress the stomach should be performed if possible but may be difficult in a hypoxic agitated patient. Attempts to actively rewarm the patient are initiated as soon as possible.

ASSESSMENT

HISTORY

Attempts should be made to elucidate the time and the duration of submersion, the presence of polluted water and likely contaminants, delay in resuscitation attempts and the likelihood of alcohol ingestion, drug use, preexisting medical conditions and coexisting trauma.

EXAMINATION

A thorough secondary survey is carried out, concentrating on cardiorespiratory examination in particular, looking for signs of respiratory distress, wheeze, crepitations and peripheral circulatory insufficiency. Neurological status should also be assessed. Clinical deterioration in those with minor symptoms and signs can occur and the patient should be reassessed at frequent intervals.

INVESTIGATIONS

These depend on the clinical circumstances and could include:

- arterial blood gases/lactate level
- plasma biochemistry/serum osmolality: electrolyte abnormalities are unlikely in sea or fresh water drowning. CK should be measured as rhabdomyolysis has been reported[28]
- haematology: tests for haemolysis, e.g. total haemoglobin (tHb), free Hb and myoglobin concentrations in the plasma and urine
- toxicological assays for drug and alcohol levels should be considered
- chest X-ray, 12 lead ECG
- microbiology: tracheal aspirates or sputum for Gram stain, microscopy and culture

- trauma imaging: cervical and/or thoracolumbar spine views; CT head if head injury is suspected or the patient is comatose. Imaging of other body areas is dependent upon the clinical likelihood of injury

ADMISSION CRITERIA

Asymptomatic patients with no clinical findings on cardiorespiratory examination and a normal chest radiograph and blood gas are unlikely to develop ALI and pneumonia and thus do not require hospital admission.[18,29] All other patients should be admitted to a high-dependency area or intensive care unit for continuous monitoring and rewarming.

RESPIRATORY SUPPORT

Severe agitation or coma mandates intubation and mechanical ventilation; otherwise oxygenation is initially maintained with high-flow oxygen or continuous positive airway pressure (CPAP) by tight fitting facemask. Superimposed ventilatory failure may be managed with non-invasive inspiratory pressure assistance in addition to CPAP (often termed bilevel positive airway pressure or non-invasive pressure support). The use of intravenous and inhaled bronchodilators may reduce airflow resistance and the work of breathing. Selective pulmonary vasodilators such as inhaled nitric oxide or inhaled prostacyclin may be useful in severe refractory hypoxaemia. In severe cases, extracorporeal membrane oxygenation has been used in some centres.[30]

CARDIOVASCULAR SUPPORT

Patients with ALI are often hypovolaemic regardless of the type of water ingestion. Cautious volume expansion and the use of catecholamine infusion may improve cardiac output and blood pressure. Fluid replacement with isotonic fluids is aimed at restoring adequate end-organ perfusion without compromising respiratory function. The use of a central venous or pulmonary artery catheter may be necessary to achieve these goals. In cases where severe circulatory insufficiency or cardiac arrest is associated with severe hypothermia, cardiopulmonary bypass has been used successfully.[31]

CEREBRAL PROTECTION

Recent data show a better neurological outcome with induced hypothermia (32–34°C) after cardiac arrest due to ventricular fibrillation.[32] Although no specific data for the cerebral protective effects of hypothermia exist for patients suffering hypoxic brain injury associated with submersion, the data would suggest that comatose drowning victims should not be actively rewarmed above 34°C.

No other specific cerebral protective measures have proven efficacy in post anoxic encephalopathy associated with drowning.[33] Maintenance of an adequate cerebral perfusion pressure (mean arterial pressure >90 mmHg in adults, 60–70 mmHg in children) is the most important goal of therapy. Prevention of cerebral venous and thus intracranial hypertension can be achieved by neutral neck positioning, avoiding occlusive endotracheal tube ties and head-up positioning. Avoiding hypocapnia ($Pa\text{CO}_2$ <30 mmHg), reducing cerebral metabolic rate with sedation, preventing hypoglycaemia and hyperthermia, and the use of anticonvulsants in those with documented seizures are simple measures to prevent secondary cerebral injury.

OTHER THERAPIES

There is no role for prophylactic corticosteroid therapy in the prevention of acute lung injury after submersion.[12] Prophylactic antibiotic therapy is unproven and the decision to commence therapy is made on the degree of water contamination, need for mechanical ventilation and severity of respiratory failure in each case.[18] Baseline microbiological studies should be sent prior to commencement of therapy.

PROGNOSIS

Mortality rate for those surviving more than 24 hours was 24% in a recent large series,[18] with three quarters succumbing in the early stages after injury. Moderate to severe brain damage is reported in 33% of survivors.[8] The outcome in children is similar, with 30% having selective deficits and 3% with persistent vegetative state.[34] No difference in mortality between fresh and salt water submersion has been documented.[11] Lower core temperatures appear to be associated with a better prognosis, except if this occurs after rescue. However, hypothermia in warm water immersion and severe hypothermia (<30°C) in cold water immersion is indicative of prolonged immersion and poor outcome.[27] Table 72.1 lists some factors associated with death or severe neurological impairment. None of these predictors is infallible and survival with normal cerebral function has been noted despite the presence of some or all of these factors.[12]

Table 72.1 Predictors of death or severe neurological impairment after submersion

At site of immersion:
Immersion duration > 10 minutes[35]
Delay in commencement of CPR > 10 minutes[8]
In the emergency department
Asystole on arrival[36] or CPR duration > 25 minutes
Fixed dilated pupils[37] and Glasgow Coma Score < 5[38]
Fixed dilated pupils and arterial pH < 7.0[39]
In the ICU
No spontaneous, purposeful movements and abnormal brainstem function 24 hours after immersion
Abnormal CT scan within 36 hours of submersion

REFERENCES

1. AHA Resuscitation Guidelines. Submersion or near-drowning. *Circulation* 2000; **102**(Suppl I): I-233–6.
2. World Health Organization. The World Health Report, 2002: Reducing risks, promoting healthy life. Geneva: WHO, 2002.
3. National Center for Injury Prevention and Control. WISQARS Leading Causes of Death Reports, 1999–2000. http://webappa.cdc.gov/cgi-bin/broker.exe.
4. Pearn J. Drowning in Australia: a national appraisal with particular reference to children. *Med J Aust* 1977; **ii** :770–1.
5. Golden F St C, Rivers JF. The immersion accident. *Anaesthesia* 1975; **30**: 364–73.
6. Weinstein M, Kreiger BP. Near drowning: epidemiology, pathophysiology and initial treatment. *J Emerg Med* 1996; **14**: 461–7.
7. Centers for Disease Control. Fatal injuries to children – United States, 1986. *MMWR* 1990; **39**: 442–51.
8. Orlowski JP. Drowning, near drowning, and ice-water submersions. *Pediatr Clin North Am* 1987; **34**: 75–92.
9. Wintemute GJ. Childhood drowning and near drowning in the United States. *Am J Dis Child* 1990; **144**: 663–9.
10. Wintemute GJ, Kraus JF, Teret SP *et al.* Drowning in childhood and adolescence: a population based study. *Am J Public Health* 1987; 77: 830–2.
11. Spilzman D. Near drowning and drowning classification. A proposal to stratify mortality based on the analysis of 1831 cases. *Chest* 1997; **112**: 660–5.
12. Modell JH. Drowning. *N Engl J Med* 1993; **328**: 253–6.
13. Daly M deB, Angell-James JE, Elsner R. Role of carotid-body chemoreceptors and their reflex interactions in bradycardia and cardiac arrest. *Lancet* 1979; **1**: 764–7.
14. Gooden BA. Why some people do not drown; hypothermia versus the diving response. *Med J Aust* 1992; **152**: 629–32.
15. Karch SB. Pathology of the lung in near drowning. *Am J Emerg Med* 1986; **4**: 1.
16. Kringsholm B, Filskov A, Kock K. Autopsied cases of drowning in Denmark 1987–1989. *Forensic Sci Int* 1991; **52**: 85–92.
17. Modell JH, Davis JH. Electrolyte changes in human drowning victims. *Anesthesiology* 1969; **30**: 414–20.
18. van Berkel M, Bierens JJL, Lie RLK *et al.* Pulmonary oedema, pneumonia and mortality in submersion victims: a retrospective study in 125 patients. *Int Care Med* 1996; **22**: 101–7.
19. Modell JH, Graves SA, Ketover A. Clinical course of 91 consecutive drowning victims *Chest* 1976; **70**: 231–8.
20. Orlowski JP, Abulleil MM, Phillips JM. The hemodynamic and cardiovascular effects of near-drowning in hypotonic, isotonic, or hypertonic solutions. *Ann Emerg Med* 1989; **18**: 1044–9.
21. Sachdev R. Near drowning. *Crit Care Clin* 1999; **15**: 281–96.
22. Ender PT, Dolan MJ, Farmer JC *et al.* Near-drowning associated Aeromonas pneumonia. *J Emerg Med* 1996; **14**: 737–41.
23. Segev D, Szold O, Fireman E *et al.* Kerosene-induced severe acute respiratory failure in near-drowning. Reports on four cases and review of the literature. *Crit Care Med* 1999; **27**: 1437–40.
24. DeNicola LK, Falk JL, Swanson ME *et al.* Submersion injuries in children and adults. *Crit Care Clin* 1997; **13**: 477–502.
25. Dunagan D, Cox J, Chang MC *et al.* Sand aspiration with near drowning. Radiographic and bronchoscopic findings. *Am J Respir Crit Care Med* 1997; **156**: 292–5.
26. Conn AW, Miyassaka K, Katayama M *et al.* A canine study of cold water drowning in fresh versus saltwater. *Crit Care Med* 1995; **23**: 2023–36.
27. Golden F St C, Tipton MJ, Scott RJ. Immersion and near drowning. *Br J Anaes* 1997; **79**: 214–25.
28. Agar JW. Rhabdomyolysis and acute renal failure after near drowning in cold salt water. *Med J Aust* 1994; **161**: 686–7.
29. Causey AL, Tilelli JA, Swanson ME. Predicting discharge in uncomplicated drowning. *Am J Emerg Med* 2000; **18**: 9–11.
30. Thalmann M, Trampitsch E, Haberfellner N *et al.* Resuscitation in near-drowning with extracorporeal membrane oxygenation. *Ann Thorac Surg* 2001; **72**: 607–8.
31. Letsou GV, Kopf GS, Elefteriades JA *et al.* Is cardiopulmonary by-pass effective for treatment of hypothermic arrest due to drowning or exposure? *Arch Surg* 1992; **127**: 525–8.
32. Oddo M, Schaller MD, Feihl F *et al.* From evidence to clinical practice: effective implementation of therapeutic hypothermia to improve patient outcome after cardiac arrest. *Crit Care Med* 2006; **34**: 1865–73.
33. Bohn DJ, Biggard WJ, Smith CR *et al.* Influence of hypothermia, barbiturate therapy and intracranial pressure monitoring on morbidity and mortality after near drowning. *Crit Care Med* 1986; **14**: 529–34.
34. Pearn J. Medical aspects of drowning in children. *Ann Acad Med Singapore* 1992; **21**: 433–55.

73

Burns

David P Mackie

The last half of the twentieth century witnessed a sustained improvement in the survival of patients suffering thermal injury. Arguably, the single most important development has been the establishment of centralised burn care which made possible advances in fluid resuscitation, life support techniques and the prevention of infection. With optimal care, children and young adults with burns of more than 80% of total body surface area (TBSA) now stand a reasonable chance of survival.[1]

Improvements in survival have gradually led to a shift of emphasis in burn care towards qualitative aspects, such as rehabilitation and quality of life. The complexity of care has led to the concept of the multidisciplinary burn team, in which all aspects of care are coordinated in an integrated approach to clinical management.[1]

PATHOPHYSIOLOGY

LOCAL EFFECTS

Thermal injury produces complex local and systemic responses. The local inflammatory response results in vasodilatation and an increase in vascular permeability. The changes are immediate and combine to produce extravasation of fluid and plasma protein at the site of injury. In extensive burns, oedema becomes generalised. The greatest rate of oedema formation occurs in the first few hours, but further extravasation occurs up to 24 hours post burn.[2] The total amount of oedema formed depends on the extent of injury and the volume and rate of fluid administration. Without fluid replacement, hypovolaemic shock occurs, limiting the extent of extravasation. On the other hand, excessive fluid administration will produce excessive oedema. By 24 hours post burn, oedema formation is largely complete and vascular integrity restored.

The process of deepening of the burn wound beyond the area of heat necrosis following injury is at least partly due to microvascular stasis. Events occurring within minutes and hours of injury that contribute to stasis include microthrombus formation, neutrophil adherence, fibrin deposition and endothelial swelling. Diverse agents, including antioxidants and anti-inflammatory drugs, have been shown to attenuate this process in experimental settings, but none is yet established in clinical practice. Empirically, it is assumed that maintenance of good tissue oxygenation, avoidance of overresuscitation and prevention of wound dehydration all contribute to wound healing by preventing undue extension of necrosis in the wound bed.

CIRCULATORY EFFECTS

Circulatory effects of burn injury become significant in burns of over 15% TBSA. Changes are rapid and the magnitude is roughly proportional to the extent of burn injury. Cardiac output is reduced immediately following injury. Secretion of adrenaline (epinephrine), noradrenaline (norepinephrine), vasopressin and angiotensin cause an increase in systemic and pulmonary vascular resistance. Circulating levels of agents with myocardial depressant properties, such as interleukin-1 and TNF-α, are increased following burn injury, but developing hypovolaemia and increased blood viscosity may be equally important.[3]

Cardiac output recovers gradually during the second post-burn day, reaching supranormal levels by day 3 as the hypermetabolic response to burn injury becomes manifest. Circulatory dynamics are complicated by resorption of oedema fluid and by continuing evaporative fluid loss from the wounds. Prolonged elevation of renin/angiotensin and antidiuretic hormone (ADH) has been well documented and circulating blood volume may remain subnormal into the second week post burn.[4]

METABOLIC EFFECTS

The hypermetabolic state, which ensues from around the third post-burn day until the wounds are substantially healed, is a manifestation of the systemic inflammatory response syndrome. The state is partly sustained by evaporative and radiant heat loss through the wounds, and energy expenditure can be reduced by increasing the ambient temperature and by the use of occlusive dressings.[5,6] Other factors known to influence the metabolic rate include pain, fear and anxiety. There is also a suggestion that bacterial colonisation may aggravate hypermetabolism.[7,8] Burn patients often develop moderate pyrexia, even when all microbial cultures are negative.

PHARMACOLOGICAL EFFECTS

The pharmacokinetics and pharmacodynamics of many drugs are markedly altered in burn patients. During the first 24 hours, when the cardiac output is depressed, absorption and distribution of administered drugs are delayed. Thereafter, increased cardiac output leads to accelerated drug absorption and distribution, while oedema fluid acts as an ill-defined third space. At the same time, renal blood flow and creatinine clearance are increased, particularly in younger patients. Drugs excreted via this route, such as the quinolone and aminoglycoside antibiotics, may therefore fail to reach effective levels at conventional dosages.[9] On the other hand, toxic levels may ensue if renal failure supervenes. If possible, therefore, antibiotic administration should be guided by measurement of plasma concentrations.

Serum albumin levels are low in burn patients, and drugs bound to this protein, including some benzodiazepines, will show increased bioavailability. On the other hand, α_1-glycoprotein levels, which bind fentanyl, are increased. Detoxification via redox pathways, such as cytochrome P-450, is depressed, lengthening the half-life of drugs such as diazepam.[10] Accumulation of benzodiazepine derivatives may be increased.

The pharmacodynamics of muscle relaxants are significantly altered due to an increase in peri-junctional acetylcholine receptors.[11] Patients become relatively insensitive to non-depolarising agents, while administration of succinylcholine may give rise to excessive release of potassium, and cardiac arrest.

The burn wound is a significant route of drug absorption as well as drug loss. For example, the topical sulfonamide agent, mafenide, may cause metabolic acidosis through inhibition of renal carbonic anhydrase; deafness has been reported following the topical use of gentamicin.

CLINICAL MANAGEMENT

FIRST AID

Immediate aid comprises stopping the burn process, followed by the removal of clothing and cooling the wound, preferably with tepid, running water, for 10–20 minutes. This provides pain relief and may prevent deepening of the wound.[12] Hypothermia should be avoided. Oxygen should be given, if available, and patients with burns to head and neck should be kept in a semi-upright position. Burn injury can only be assessed properly in hospital conditions, and priority should be given to early evacuation of the victim.

GENERAL MANAGEMENT: 0–24 HOURS

On admission, a careful history should be taken of the circumstances of the injury, and to elucidate past medical history. The patient should be undressed, weighed, and carefully examined to exclude additional traumatic injury.

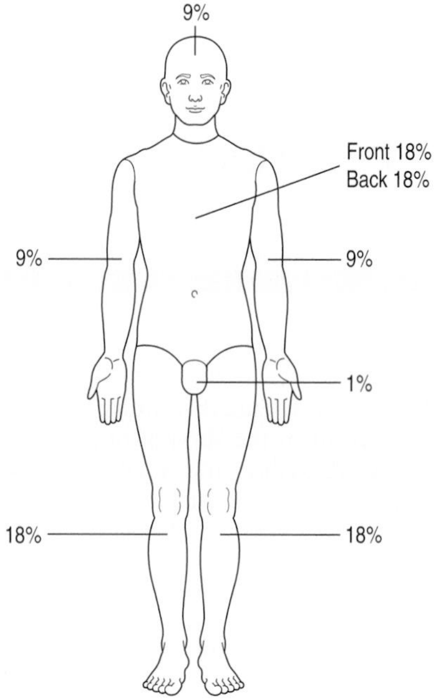

Figure 73.1 Rule of nine to estimate body surface area burns in adults.

The extent and depth of injury is assessed with the aid of printed Lund and Browder charts, or by using the 'rule of nines' (Figure 73.1). The rule of nines is modified for children (Figure 73.2). A nasogastric tube and urinary catheter should be inserted in patients requiring resuscitation therapy. Escharotomies may be required for circular burns of the trunk and limbs.

FLUID THERAPY: 0–24 HOURS

Fluid therapy is required for injuries exceeding 15% of body surface area (10% in children and the elderly), preferably via a wide-bore peripheral i.v. cannula (preferably not in a burned area). The aim is to provide sufficient salt and water to preserve normal organ function, while minimising oedema formation. Excessive fluid administration increases the risk of circulatory overload in the days following the resuscitation period. Potentially fatal complications of excessive fluid administration include the abdominal compartment syndrome in adults[13] and the occurrence of cerebral oedema in children.[14] An increasing tendency in recent years to overresuscitate burn patients has been signalled.[15,16] In contrast to other traumatic injuries, burn hypovolaemia is gradual, obligatory and predictable. Aggressive fluid administration will not restore the circulating volume[17] and in the absence of frank shock, bolus fluids should not be given.

Various resuscitation formulae have been published in the past to guide initial fluid therapy. These formulae are entirely experience-based and many are of historical interest only, but all comprise a fluid intake of 2–4 ml/kg

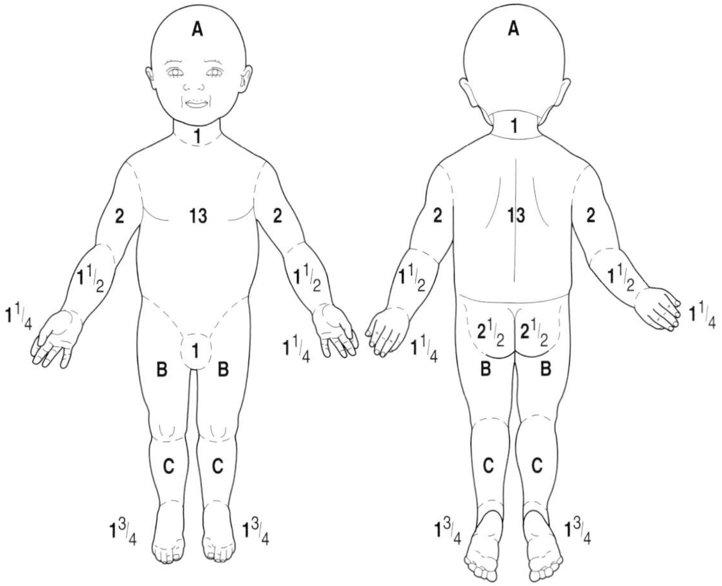

Figure 73.2 Surface area percentages by age.

Age	<1 year	1 year	5 years	10 years	15 years	Adult
Area A = ½ of head (%)	9.5	8.5	6.5	5.5	4.5	3.5
Area B = ½ of one thigh (%)	2.75	3.25	4.0	4.25	4.5	4.75
Area C = ½ of one leg (%)	2.5	2.5	2.75	3.0	3.25	3.5

body weight per % burn in 24 hours, and a sodium intake of approximately 0.5 mmol/kg per % burn.[18] These findings have led some to employ resuscitation regimens based on the administration of hypertonic sodium solutions, which require a smaller volume of fluid. However, the solute load may be excessive, requiring extra water administration in subsequent days, with an increased risk of fluid overload. The use of isotonic saline solutions is therefore preferred by those without experience of burns resuscitation.

The most widely used resuscitation formula for adults is based on the Parkland Formula, which has been adopted by major training programmes, such as the Advanced Trauma Life Support and the Emergency Medicine for Severe Burns:

> 4 ml Ringer-Lactate solution × kg body weight × % TBSA burn in the first 24 hours, of which half should to be given in the first 8 hours ***post burn*** and the other half in the next 16 hours

The formula thus incorporates a faster rate of administration if initial treatment has been delayed.

Children require extra fluid to compensate for basal needs. For children under 30 kg, the resuscitation formula of Carvajal[19] is useful:

$$\text{Fluid requirement (ml)} : 0-24 \text{ hours post burn} = (2000 \times \text{TBSA}) + (5000 \times \text{TBSAB})$$

where TBSA is the total body surface area (m^2) and TBSAB is total body surface area burned (m^2). Again half of the calculated amount is given in the first 8 hours.

These formulae are to be regarded as guidelines only. The actual amount of fluid given depends on the clinical condition and the actual amount of fluid administered can vary widely from that predicted. Adequacy of resuscitation is monitored by vital signs and a targeted urine output of 0.5–1 ml/kg per hour in adults and 1–2 ml/kg per hour in children. Other indicators include warm extremities and return of gut peristalsis. Fluid intake may be adjusted to maintain urine output at the desired range. Requirements are increased in the presence of mechanical ventilation, additional traumatic injury and dehydration (e.g. fire-fighters).

Invasive monitoring is not essential in uncomplicated burns and the results may be misleading, as central pressures are invariably low. Hypoalbuminaemia develops rapidly and may be extreme. The extent to which burn patients will tolerate hypoalbuminaemia is unknown and clinical studies into best practice are awaited. In our unit at present, albumin is given to maintain serum albumin above 15 g/l, commencing 12 hours post burn when capillary integrity has been largely restored.

Thirst is common, but unrestricted oral fluids will increase oedema formation. Controlled quantities of nutritional liquids are recommended to protect gut integrity.[20]

In patients with extensive injuries, tube feeding at a low rate can be commenced within a few hours of injury.

FLUID THERAPY AFTER 24 HOURS

During the second 24 hours, enteral nutritional intake is increased, while the total rate of fluid administration is gradually reduced. At the end of the second day, fluid intake should allow for generous urine production, while compensating for evaporative losses through the wounds.

The actual fluid loss through wounds varies widely, and depends on the type of burn and topical wound treatment. A useful formula to obtain a rough estimate for insensible fluid loss is:

$$(25 + \%\ \text{body surface burn}) \times \text{m}^2\ \text{body surface area} = \text{evaporative fluid loss (ml/h)}$$

Electrolyte disturbance is common following burn injury and requires treatment. Hypernatraemia is often a sign of hypovolaemia, confirmed if urine sodium is low. The condition is perilous, especially in the first week post burn, as oliguria and renal failure may develop unexpectedly. The amount of free water given should be increased gradually, particularly in the elderly, to avoid fluid overload. Patients who are in fluid balance may require sodium supplementation to compensate for solute loss in wound exudates.

HAEMOGLOBINUREA/MYOGLOBINUREA

Tissue injury from deep burns, particularly electrical injury, causes the release of myoglobin and haemoglobin from damaged cells. Diagnosis is made on observing discoloration of the urine, from faint pink in mild cases to almost black. Fluid administration should be increased; additional measures such as mannitol (12.5 g/l resuscitation fluid) to encourage diuresis, and bicarbonate to alkalinise the urine pH and increase the rate of pigment excretion may be considered.

PAIN THERAPY

During the first 24 hours, pain management is best achieved by incremental doses of i.v. morphine, or equivalent opiate. Thereafter, the pain suffered by burn patients may be divided into background pain, which is continuous, and procedural pain caused by interventions.[21] The recurring ordeal of dressing changes, physiotherapy exercises and surgical procedures generates apprehension and anxiety, which compound distress.

Regular pain therapy is required to counter background pain, topped up by extra analgesics prior to procedures. In recent years, the advent of slow-release oral opiate medication has greatly improved the administration of analgesia. Procedural pain is best treated with continuous i.v. morphine or fentanyl, with titrated incremental boluses as required. Patient-controlled analgesia is effective, although modification of the control button may be necessary for those with bandaged hands. Ketamine in subanaesthetic doses is extremely useful for procedural pain in children. The influence of anxiety and depression on pain perception suggests additional avenues of therapy.[22] Non-pharmacological interventions, such as hypnosis and other distraction techniques, are an effective adjunct in susceptible patients.[23] Many burn patients may develop posttraumatic distress syndrome, and the emergence of symptoms may require additional support. Above all, an attitude of reassurance and understanding by all carers is indispensable.

NUTRITION

The hypermetabolic response is roughly proportional to the extent of injury. In young adults and children with extensive burns, energy expenditure may be doubled. In addition, protein and substantial amounts of trace elements, such as zinc, copper and selenium are lost in wound exudate.[24]

There is no doubt that burn patients require additional calories and proteins, but traditional formulae for calculating requirements produce overestimates in the context of current burn care.[25] In the absence of direct metabolic measurements we currently use an empirical formula for estimating caloric intake:

$$\text{Caloric requirement} = \text{REE} + (\text{REE} \times \%\ \text{TBSA burn}/100)$$

where REE is the resting energy expenditure calculated from the Harris and Benedict equation.

Patients with extensive burns will require tube feeds, which are generally well tolerated. If gastric emptying is problematic, a post-pyloric tube is usually effective. A high-protein proprietary feed is usually adequate, but should be supplemented by extra trace elements and vitamins. The possible benefit of glutamine supplements in burns has recently been reviewed.[26] Adequacy of feeding is best assessed by monitoring body weight. Adjunctive therapy aimed at promoting anabolism includes the use of insulin to maintain normoglycaemia, the administration of oxandrolone (10 mg twice daily for adults),[27] and the use of β-blockers to control tachycardia and extensive catabolism.[28]

WOUND HEALING

Treatment of extensive, full-thickness burn wounds by early excision and grafting has been firmly linked to survival.[29] Wound excision should be completed within the first week, before bacterial colonisation and neovascular infiltration of the wound bed develop. These operations are therefore urgent. Successfully grafted wounds will heal within 5 weeks, reducing the time available for bacterial infection to develop, and shortening the period of physiological disturbance. Wounds covered with widely meshed autografts lose large amounts of fluid, unless protected by a semipermeable layer, such as allograft skin. Autograft donor sites are a further source of fluid loss.

For wounds treated conservatively, the main effort is devoted to the prevention of infection. Topical antimicrobial agents are commonly used, but may have potential side-effects (Table 73.1). These compounds change the appearance of the wound and should never be applied until expert wound inspection is complete. A number of biosynthetic materials are currently available, which are designed to improve cosmetic and functional outcome. Despite the use of antiseptic dressings or biosynthetic coverings there is still a risk of microbial infection developing and unexplained signs of sepsis may necessitate urgent wound revision.

Table 73.1 Commonly used topical antimicrobial agents

Agent	Comments
Silver sulfadiazine (SSD)	The most widely used agent with broad spectrum cover. Hypersensitivity (rarely) and transient leucopenia have been reported
Cerium nitrate 0.5%	Often added to SSD, and forms a stable eschar. It is reported to bind 'burn toxins'. Methaemoglobinaemia has been reported
Silver nitrate 0.5%	Applied as a soak, and is especially effective against *Pseudomonas*. However, it may increase sodium loss, and potentially can cause methaemoglobinaemia
Mafenide acetate 5–10%	Effective but short-lived antimicrobial, requiring repeated application. It has good penetration, and its side-effects (pain and metabolic acidosis) are less evident with 5% solution
Chlorhexidine	Aqueous solution (0.2%) or 1% gel provides broad spectrum cover, but is rapidly inactivated, and may cause local pain, and rarely causes hypersensitivity
Nitrofurazone	In polyethylene glycol (PEG) solution it is effective against *S. aureus*, but resistance develops early. Side-effects include hypersensitivity (common), hyperosmolarity, and renal failure due to PEG absorption has been reported
Povidone iodine	In PEG solution provides broad spectrum cover, but is rapidly inactivated. It prevents wound maceration. Side-effects include occasional hypersensitivity, renal dysfunction due to excessive PEG, metabolic acidosis and rarely dysfunction
Antibiotics	Have been used in solutions, creams, gels and sprays, but selection and development of resistant strains is inevitable, with a risk of systemic toxicity through absorption. Their usage is generally discouraged

PREVENTION OF WOUND INFECTION

Bacterial infection is still the most common cause of death in burns. Depression of the immune system is well documented.[30] At the same time, the burn wound presents a favourable medium for bacterial growth.

BACTERIOLOGICAL SURVEILLANCE

Routine bacteriological surveillance of burn patients (at least twice weekly) is essential. The growth of pathogens from wound swabs may reflect growing resistance to topical wound therapy, indicating a need for change. When infection is suspected, the choice of an appropriate antibiotic will be governed by prior knowledge of the colonising micro-organisms and their antibiograms. In addition, the effectiveness of prophylactic measures can only be assessed by regular monitoring of the microflora present within the burns unit.

PATIENT ISOLATION

In an effort to reduce wound colonisation and contamination from cross-infection, barrier nursing of patients with extensive injuries is mandatory. The importance of isolation measures has been stressed,[31] but a significant proportion of patients still become colonised by micro-organisms from endogenous reservoirs, which cannot be controlled by barrier nursing alone.[32,33] Positive experiences have been reported with selective decontamination of the digestive tract,[8,34] but large scale prospective trials have not been performed.

THE GASTROINTESTINAL TRACT

Loss of gut integrity following burn injury has been well demonstrated.[35] In addition to reactive damage following reperfusion of the ischaemic gut, mediators derived from the burn wound itself may also be involved.[36] Clinical strategies aimed at protecting the gastrointestinal tract include optimal fluid therapy during the first hours following injury to prevent mesenteric hypoperfusion, and the institution of early enteral nutrition, which can be safely commenced within a few hours of injury.[20] Diets enriched with glutamine may contribute to the maintenance of gut integrity.[26,37] Whatever the merits of each approach, all are secondary to the maintenance of effective hygienic policies in all aspects of patient care.

WOUND SEPSIS

Local effects include disruption of wound healing and deepening of the injury.

Systemic effects are often insidious. Prodromal signs are common and may include gastrointestinal stasis, increasing positive fluid balance, increasing insulin resistance and increasing pyrexia. As sepsis progresses, clinical deterioration becomes manifest: tachypnoea, circulatory instability, thrombocytopenia and oliguria may herald the onset of multiorgan failure. Leukocyte counts and C-reactive protein elevation are affected by the systemic inflammatory response syndrome (SIRS) and are unreliable indicators in the absence of clinical signs and symptoms. Blood cultures are indicated if sepsis is suspected.

ANTIBIOTIC THERAPY

This is chosen on the basis of bacteriological surveillance data, and should be given early, if possible. Fluid therapy in burn patients is complicated by evaporative fluid loss, which may increase if the wound surface degenerates. Supportive therapy for (multi-) organ failure should be implemented as indicated.

The causes of sepsis will persist until wound coverage is achieved and operative wound treatment should not be postponed. Although mortality is appreciable, experience has repeatedly shown that the prognosis is by no means hopeless.

INHALATION INJURY

The term inhalation injury includes three distinct types of injury which often, but not always, occur together. The presence of inhalation injury may increase resuscitation fluid requirements in patients with extensive cutaneous burns.

HEAT INJURY TO THE UPPER AIRWAY

Burns due to the inhalation of hot gases (steam excepted) rarely extend beyond the larynx. The development of mucosal and facial oedema can cause respiratory obstruction, particularly in children.

DIAGNOSIS

Facial burn, singed nasal hairs, visible burn to oropharynx, and hoarseness are typical features.

TREATMENT

If the condition is suspected, early endotracheal intubation is safest, before the procedure is rendered hazardous by oedema formation.

EFFECTS OF SMOKE ON THE RESPIRATORY SYSTEM

Many of the chemicals that are contained in smoke are highly reactive and produce damage to the tracheobronchial tree. Detachment of epithelial cells and the development of tracheobronchial oedema cause airway narrowing and cast formation. Small airway closure leads to hypoxaemia and respiratory failure. Later, bronchorrhoea and mucosal sloughing may cause atelectasis and provide a focus for infection. In the absence of a cutaneous injury the clinical course is usually benign. However, the presence of an extensive skin burn increases the likelihood of acute respiratory distress syndrome (ARDS); respiratory infection may follow.

DIAGNOSIS

There is a history of exposure in a confined space, cough, breathlessness, wheeze, stridor, hypoxaemia, and soot particles in the pharynx. Diagnosis is confirmed by bronchoscopy, which may reveal soot in the bronchial tree, mucosal injury and tracheobronchial oedema.

TREATMENT

Mild cases may be treated by high-flow oxygen administration by mask. The mainstay of treatment in severe cases is intubation and ventilatory support with positive end-expiratory pressure (PEEP) to maintain small-airway patency. Regular bronchial toilet is recommended to clear debris and to prevent respiratory infection. Endotracheal tubes may become blocked with detritus. As small-airway obstruction is common, ventilation pressures may be adversely affected. Various strategies, such as high-frequency ventilation, have been advocated to minimise the risks of barotrauma.

Prolonged respiratory assistance may be necessary. The added respiratory requirements of the hypermetabolic state combined with inevitable loss of muscle mass frequently frustrate early weaning efforts.

INHALATION OF TOXIC GASES

Of the many toxic compounds[38] in smoke (Table 73.2), carbon monoxide (CO) deserves special mention. The affinity of CO for haemoglobin is 240 times that of oxygen. The loss of oxygen transport capacity is dependent on the concentration of inhaled CO and the duration of exposure. In addition, CO binds to cytochrome systems, inhibiting cellular oxidative processes. The half-life of COHb is 4 hours when breathing air, compared with 45 minutes when breathing 100% oxygen.

DIAGNOSIS

Carbon monoxide poisoning should be suspected in all cases of exposure to combustion products in a closed space. The classic cherry red appearance of the CO victim is seldom evident; early signs may be mistaken for inebriation. Symptoms range from a throbbing headache in mild exposure (10–25% COHb) to weakness, dizziness, confusion and nausea (25–40% COHb), progressing to collapse, unconsciousness and convulsions (40–60% COHb). Death is increasingly likely at COHb concentrations of $>60\%$. Patients exposed to high levels of CO may exhibit signs of cardiac instability. Signs of cerebral irritability may persist for days or weeks following apparent recovery.

TREATMENT

Administration of the highest concentration of oxygen available, as soon as possible after exposure. Loss of consciousness is an indication for oxygen delivery via an endotracheal tube. The use of hyperbaric oxygen, if immediately available, seems logical, but additional benefit has not been proven.

HYDROGEN CYANIDE TOXICITY

Hydrogen cyanide (HCN) toxicity frequently occurs in conjunction with CO inhalation. Inhaled concentrations of 200 ppm are rapidly fatal and HCN may account for many deaths at fire accident scenes.[39] Conventional treatment is as for CO intoxication. Removal by chelating agents, such

Table 73.2 Common inhaled toxic gases

Gas	Source	Effect
Carbon monoxide	Organic matter	Tissue hypoxia, lipid peroxidation
Carbon dioxide	Organic matter	Narcosis, tachycardia, hypertension
Nitrogen dioxide	Wallpaper, wood	Bronchial irritation, dizziness, pulmonary oedema
Hydrogen chloride	Plastics	Severe mucosal irritation
Hydrogen cyanide	Wood, silk, nylons, polyurethane	Headache, coma, acidosis
Benzene	Petrol, plastics	Mucosal irritation, coma
Ammonia	Nylon	Mucosal damage, extensive lung injury
Aldehyde	Wood, cotton, paper	Mucosal irritation

as hydroxycobalamin or by the administration of sodium thiosulphate is also possible, but treatment would have to be immediate, based on a presumptive diagnosis, and is therefore not generally recommended.

FUTURE PROSPECTS

The outlook for young patients with extensive burn injuries, treated under optimal conditions, is now such that little further progress may be expected in terms of survival alone. Mortality among the elderly does, however, remain high. The major thrust of research is currently directed at improving functional and cosmetic outcome following burns. While the most visible efforts concern the development of techniques and materials to improve the quality of wound healing, advances in the field of intensive care are also relevant: strategies aimed at preventing ventilator-associated morbidity are equally applicable to burn patients, who often require prolonged ventilatory support; new insights into the inflammatory responses may improve the general condition of burn patients, increasing resistance to infection and improving tissue repair. There is growing interest in the psychological effects of thermal trauma, which includes new approaches to the management of pain and mental distress.

In the past, the establishment of burn centres has been largely opportunistic, often depending on the dedication of individual specialists. As the provision of medical services undergoes increasing scrutiny, the organisation of burn care in many countries may be subject to reorganisation. It is of the utmost importance that specialists involved in the field of burn care become actively engaged in this process, in order to guarantee continued quality of care for their population.

REFERENCES

1. Herndon DN, Blakeney PE. Teamwork for total burn care: achievements, directions and hopes. In: Herndon DN (ed) *Total Burn Care*, 2nd edn. London: WB Saunders; 2002: 11–15.
2. Demling RH, Mazess RB, Witt RM *et al.* The study of burn wound edema using dichromatic absorptiometry. *J Trauma* 1978; **18**: 124–8.
3. Cioffi WG, De Meules JE, Gamelli RL. The effects of burn injury and fluid resuscitation on cardiac function in vitro. *J Trauma* 1986; **26**: 638–43.
4. Cioffi WG, Vaughan GM, Heironimus JD *et al.* Dissassociation of blood volume and flow in regulation of salt and water balance in burn patients. *Ann Surg* 1991; **214**: 213–9.
5. Wilmore DW, Mason AD, Johnson DW *et al.* Effect of ambient temperature on heat production and heat loss in burn patients. *J Appl Physiol* 1975; **38**: 593–7.
6. Caldwell FT, Bowser GH, Crabtree JH. The effects of occlusive dressings on the energy expenditure of severely burned children. *Ann Surg* 1981; **193**: 579–91.
7. Waymack JP. Antibiotics and the post-burn hypermetabolic response. *J Trauma* 1990; **30**: S30–5.
8. Mackie DP, van Hertum WAJ, Schumburg T *et al.* Prevention of infection in burns: preliminary experience with selective decontamination of the digestive tract in patients with extensive injuries. *J Trauma* 1992; **32**: 570–5.
9. Alexander D, Richard K, Morris S *et al.* Application of newer antibiotic concepts in the use of ciprofloxacin for treatment of infections in the burn patient. *J Burn Care Rehab* 2001; **22**: S137.
10. Martyn JAJ, Greenblatt GS, Quinby WC. Diazepam kinetics following burn injury. *Anesth Analg* 1983; **62**: 293–7.
11. Martyn JAJ, Fukushima Y, Chon JY *et al.* Muscle relaxants in burns, trauma, and critical illness. *Int Anesthesiol Clin* 2006; **44**: 123–43.
12. Davies JWL. Prompt cooling of the burned area: a review of the benefits and the effector mechanisms. *Burns* 1982; **9**: 1–16.
13. Ivy ME, Atweh NA, Palmer J *et al.* Intra-abdominal hypertension and abdominal compartment syndrome in burn patients. *J Trauma* 2000; **49**: 387–91.
14. Prekop R, Bardosova G, Simko S *et al.* Brain oedema in burned children. *Acta Chir Plast* 1984; **26**: 184–92.
15. Pruitt BA Jr. Protection from excessive resuscitation: 'pushing the pendulum back'. *J Trauma* 2000; **49**: 567–8.
16. Friedrich JB, Sullivan SR, Engrav LH *et al.* Is supra-Baxter resuscitation in burns patients a new phenomenon? *Burns* 2004; **39**: 583–90.
17. Holm C, Mayr M, Tegeler J *et al.* A clinical randomised study on the effects of invasive monitoring on burn shock resuscitation. *Burns* 2004; **30**: 798–807.

18. Settle JAD. Principles of replacement fluid therapy. In: Settle JAD (ed) *Principles and Practice of Burns Management*. London: Churchill Livingstone; 1996: 217–22.
19. Carvajal HF. A physiologic approach to fluid therapy in severely burned children. *Surg Gynecol Obstet* 1980; **150**: 379–84.
20. Alexander JW, Gottschlich MM. Nutritional immunomodulation in burn patients. *Crit Care Med* 1990; **18**: S149–53.
21. Choinière M, Melzak R, Rondeau J *et al.* The pain of burns: characteristics and correlates. *J Trauma* 1989; **29**: 1531–9.
22. Taal LA, Faber AW, van Loey NEE *et al.* The abbreviated burn-specific anxiety scale: a multi-centre study. *Burns* 1999; **25**: 493–7.
23. Miller AC, Hickman LC, Lemasters GK. A distraction technique for control of burn pain. *J Burn Care Rehabil* 1992; **13**: 576–80.
24. Berger MM, Cavadini C, Chiolero R *et al.* Influence of large intakes of trace elements on recovery after burns. *Nutrition* 1994; **10**: 327–34.
25. Wolfe RR. Caloric requirements of the burned patients. *J Trauma* 1981; **21**: 712–4.
26. Windle EM. Glutamine supplementation in critical illness: evidence, recommendations, and implications for clinical practice in burn care. *J Burn Care Rehab* 2006; **27**: 764–72.
27. Wolf S, Edelman L, Kemalyan N *et al.* Effects of oxandrolone on outcome measures in the severely burned: a multicenter prospective double-blind trial. *J Burn Care Res* 2006; **27**:131–41.
28. Pereira CT, Murphy KD, Herndon DN. Altering metabolism. *J Burn Care Rehabil* 2005; **26**: 194–9.
29. Muller MJ, Ralston D, Herndon DN. Operative wound management. In: Herndon DN (ed) *Total Burn Care*, 2nd edn. London: WB Saunders; 2002: 170–82.
30. Abraham E. Physiologic stress and cellular ischemia: relationship to immunosuppression and susceptibility to sepsis. *Crit Care Med* 1991; **19**: 613–8.
31. McManus AT, Mason WF, McManus WF *et al.* A decade of reduced Gram negative infections and mortality. Abstracts, 5th European Burns Association Congress 1992: M2.
32. Burke JF, Quimby WC, Bondoc CC *et al.* The contribution of a bacterially isolated environment to the prevention of infection in seriously burned patients. *Ann Surg* 1977; **186**: 377–87.
33. Lee JJ, Marvin JA, Heimbach DM *et al.* Infection control in a burns centre. *J Burn Care Rehabil* 1990; **11**: 575–80.
34. Manson WL, Klasen HJ, Sauer EW. Selective intestinal decontamination for prevention of wound colonization in severely burned patients: a retrospective analysis. *Burns* 1992; **18**: 98–102.
35. Deitch EA. Intestinal permeability is increased in burn patients shortly after injury. *Surgery* 1990; **107**: 411–16.
36. Trop M, Schiffrin EJ, Carter EA. Effect of platelet activating factor on reticulo-endothelial system function. *Burns* 1991; **17**: 193–7.
37. Peng X, Yan H, You Z *et al.* Glutamine granule-supplemented enteral nutrition maintains immunological function in severely burned patients. *Burns* 2006; **32**: 589–93.
38. Prien T, Traber DL. Toxic smoke compounds and inhalation injury – a review. *Burns* 1988; **14**: 451–60.
39. Purser DA, Grimshaw P, Berril KR. Intoxication by cyanide in fires: a study in monkeys using polyacrylonitrile. *Arch Environmental Health* 1984; **39**: 394–400.

74

Thermal disorders

Anwar Hussein

Body temperature is normally very tightly controlled by a balance between heat production and heat loss, through a complex feedback mechanism involving the thermoregulatory centre in the hypothalamus. In the intensive care unit (ICU), fever (pyrexia) is usually due to resetting of the thermoregulatory set-point at a higher level by activation of heat-conserving mechanisms, whereas hyperthermia is due to failure of effector mechanisms to maintain body temperature at the normal set-point.

Although the pathogenesis of hyperthermia varies between different aetiologies, the complications are similar:

- metabolic acidosis
- hyperkalaemia
- rhabdomyolysis
- renal failure
- disseminated intravascular coagulation (DIC)
- liver failure
- death

THERMOREGULATION

Control of body temperature, like most complex biological systems, is maintained by a complicated system of sensors and controls. The target set-point varies by <1°C per day on a circadian basis, and by <½°C monthly in women. However, at any given time the core temperature is within a few tenths of 1°C of the set-point.

The three major components of the thermoregulatory system are:

- afferent input
- central control
- effector responses

Temperature is sensed by A-δ fibres (most cold signals) and unmyelinated C fibres (most warm signals). These sensors are distributed throughout the body but the largest contribution is from the thermal core (deep abdominal and thoracic tissues, and neuraxis).

Signals from these sensors ascend via the spinothalamic tracts in the anterior spinal cord to the thermoregulatory centre located in the preoptic region of the hypothalamus near the floor of the third ventricle. This region contains heat-sensitive neurones but also receives neural input from other thermoreceptors. The preoptic region receives afferent information from peripheral thermoreceptors, determines the thermoregulatory set-point and coordinates appropriate responses.

Temperature is then regulated by a variety of central structures that compare integrated thermal inputs from skin, neuraxis and deep tissues with reference temperatures for each thermoregulatory response.

The most important effector response in humans against extreme environments is behavioural, and outweighs autonomic changes. At extremes of age, hypothalamic temperature regulation is impaired and less effective.

Humoral mediators from the circulation act to alter temperature primarily via the organum vasculosum of the lamina terminalis (OVLT), an area of fenestrated capillaries in the hypothalamus that permits cytokine access to neuronal receptors. Cytokines appear to be the endogenous pyrogens, with interleukin-6 (IL-6) and prostaglandin-E_2 (PGE_2) being a final common pathway. In addition to elevating body temperature, several cytokines also reduce the thermoregulatory set-point, and are known as endogenous cryogens.[1]

Patients in the ICU are likely to have disturbance of both heat production and heat loss. Heat is produced as a result of metabolic activity and energy expenditure. Inflammation or infection as part of an acute phase response results in an increase in body temperature and energy expenditure. Pyrexia in turn results in an increased metabolic rate; however, reducing activity with sedation and muscle relaxation reduces energy expenditure.

Regulation of heat loss, which is the predominant effector of thermoregulation, is usually disturbed in the ICU population. Patients are usually nursed semi-naked, bed-bathed frequently, sedated and sometimes paralysed, and infused with drugs and fluids at ambient temperature. This effect is particularly pronounced during renal replacement therapy. Peripheral blood flow may be affected by vasopressors and the ability to shiver abolished by muscle relaxants. Behavioural defences may be compromised by sedative use. All of these effects play a variable part and, together with the method of temperature measurement, should be considered when evaluating fever in the ICU.

FEVER IN THE ICU

Fever is defined by a *regulated* hyperthermia, that is, it is a regulated elevation in the preoptic set-point temperature. Endogenous pyrogens as well as other mediators inhibit warm-sensitive neurones that normally facilitate heat loss and suppress heat production. This elevates the set-point temperature for all thermoregulatory responses and activates cold defences such as vasoconstriction and shivering, which decrease heat loss and increase metabolic heat production respectively. The set-point temperature returns to normal when pyrogen concentrations decrease, triggering heat loss by vasodilatation and sweating.[2]

Fever may reflect a wide variety of pathological processes including infection, inflammation, trauma, malignancy and connective tissue diseases (Table 74.1), necessitating a systematic and comprehensive diagnostic approach.[3] It is often assumed that a patient presenting with a fever should be treated, regardless of the presence or absence of other symptoms. However, the evidence that anti-fever treatments lead to an improvement in morbidity or mortality, or even patient comfort, is lacking.[4]

The development of fever in response to infection may be a protective adaptive response, and appears to be a phylogenetically preserved evolutionary response because of its survival value.[5] In mammalian models, increasing body temperature results in enhanced resistance to infection. In humans, retrospective clinical trials have shown a positive correlation between maximum temperature on the day of bacteraemia and increased survival in patients with Gram-negative bacteraemia and spontaneous bacterial peritonitis.[6] Also, septic patients with hypothermia have a poorer outcome than those who develop fever, although this causality is less clear. Both local and systemic hyperthermia has been used to facilitate cancer treatment. The protective effects of fever result from increased immune and cytokine functions.[7–10]

Temperature elevation has been shown to enhance:

- antibody production
- neutrophil and macrophage mobility and function
- cytokine production
- T-lymphocyte activity
- reduction of serum iron, which is required for bacterial growth

In addition, elevated temperatures inhibit some pathogens, such as *Streptococcus pneumoniae*.[11]

Moderate fever is a common occurrence in ICU patients, but approximately half of these are non-infectious in origin.[12–14] The presence of fever frequently results in the performance of diagnostic tests and exposes the patient to unnecessary invasive procedures and inappropriate use of antibiotics.[15]

Whilst very high fevers (> 40°C) are dangerous, it is less clear whether moderate elevation of body temperature is detrimental and, indeed, may be protective.[4] Moreover, artificially lowering the temperature of a febrile patient may mask the signs of infection and make diagnosis and monitoring more difficult. Any decision to adopt anti-fever measures, physical or pharmacological, must take into consideration the variable response by this patient population. Antipyretics may be ineffective.

Table 74.1 Causes of fever in the ICU

System	Infectious aetiology	Non-infectious aetiology
Cardiovascular	Endocarditis Catheter-related infection Pacemaker infection	Myocardial infarction Deep-vein thrombosis Pericarditis
Respiratory	Pneumonia Empyema Sinusitis	Atelectasis Chemical pneumonitis Pulmonary emboli
Alimentary	Abdominal abscess Biliary infection Peritonitis Diverticulitis Viral hepatitis Antibiotic-related colitis	Inflammatory bowel disease Acalculous cholecystitis Pancreatitis Ischaemic colitis Non-viral hepatitis Gastrointestinal haemorrhage
Renal	Pyelonephritis Urinary tract infection	
Central nervous	Meningitis Encephalitis	Cerebral haemorrhage/ infarct Seizures
Rheumatological	Septic arthritis Osteomyelitis Gout	Connective tissue disease Vasculitis
Endocrine		Adrenocortical insufficiency Alcohol and drug withdrawal Hyperthyroidism
Skin/soft tissue	Cellulitis Decubitus ulcer Wound infections	Burns Intramuscular injections Haematoma
Other	Parotitis Pharyngitis Otitis media	Drug fever Transfusion reaction Neoplasms

The usual concern about external cooling measures inducing peripheral vasoconstriction, reducing heat loss and making the pyrexia worse by shivering and hypermetabolism, may not be observed in sedated ICU patients.[16] The most likely cause for this response is the drugs used to maintain sedation.[17,18]

Pyrexia is associated with a number of deleterious physiological effects. Cardiac output, oxygen consumption, carbon dioxide production and energy expenditure are all increased, particularly in the presence of shivering. Oxygen consumption is increased on average by 10%/°C.[2] These changes are poorly tolerated by patients with limited cardiorespiratory reserve, and this group of patients would probably derive benefit from cooling measures. Other patient groups that require special consideration include those with immunosuppression, prosthetic implants and acute brain injury. Recent trials of therapeutic moderate hypothermia and traumatic brain injury indicate that hypothermia is a complicated treatment that is likely to benefit only a subgroup of patients with traumatic brain injury.[19–21]

HEAT STROKE

A diagnosis of heat stroke is suggested when hyperthermia is associated with neurological abnormalities after exposure to high ambient temperature and/or vigorous exercise. Rectal temperature is usually greater than 42°C. Two distinct forms are recognised, and the spectrum of injury includes milder forms of thermal injury often termed heat stress.

Exertional heat stroke is a consequence of prolonged, intense exercise in warm humid environments, often seen in athletes and military recruits. Classic heat stroke is commonly seen in sedentary, elderly patients with underlying illnesses during heat waves. Factors predisposing to heat stroke are listed in Table 74.2. About 80% of heat stroke deaths occur in people aged 50 years and older, because of the diminished ability of the older body to compensate for increased core temperatures. Heat stroke is estimated to be the cause of approximately 1700 deaths each year in the USA.[22] The European heat wave of 2003 was responsible for > 14 000 excess deaths within 2 weeks in France alone, of which a third were attributed to heat stroke, hyperthermia or dehydration.[23,24] A high mortality rate of > 62% was reported for this cohort, which is higher than that for leading killers in ICUs such as acute respiratory distress syndrome (ARDS) and septic shock.[25] Furthermore, there is a late mortality contributed by survivors who have sustained neurological injury. A study of former heat stroke patients suggests that susceptible individuals have a poorer physiological response to heat stress in terms of core temperature, heart rate and sweat response.

There are two autonomic responses to heat stress: sweating and active precapillary vasodilatation. Sweating is extremely effective and can dissipate up to 10 times the basal metabolic rate, provided that environmental conditions such as ambient temperature, humidity and wind speed are optimal. The resemblance between heat illness and the effects of antimuscarinic drugs, which produce a central anticholinergic syndrome, is explained by the postganglionic, cholinergic sympathetic innervation of sweat glands. Vascular responses to heat stress include vasodilatation of peripheral vascular beds and vasoconstriction of splanchnic and renal beds. During severe heat stress, blood flow through the top millimetre of skin can be equal to the entire resting cardiac output.

Table 74.2 Predisposing factors to heat stroke

Age	Elderly
Environmental	High ambient temperature and humidity Heat waves Poor ventilation
Behavioural	Lack of acclimatisation Salt and water deprivation Obesity
Underlying conditions	Infection/fever Diabetes Malnutrition Alcoholism Hyperthyroidism Impaired sweat production Healed burns Ectodermal dysplasia Impaired sweating Cardiovascular disease Fatigue Potassium deficiency
Drugs	Anticholinergics Antiparkinsonians Antihistamines Butyrophenones Phenothiazines Tricyclics Diuretics Sympathomimetics

PATHOGENESIS

The pathogenesis of multiple organ failure in heat stroke is complex. Although direct cellular damage from increased temperature constitutes the initiating insult,[26] the precise sequence of injury and responsible mediators are poorly understood. At the cellular level, thermal injury results in increased membrane permeability, which in turn stimulates membrane enzymes such as Na^+K^+-ATPase to maintain membrane integrity. This ATP-consuming enzyme activity is also responsible for nerve impulse conduction, which is markedly curtailed when ATP is depleted. This results in tissue oedema, reduced oxygen extraction and neuronal injury. High temperatures ameliorate ATP synthesis leading to fatigue.

Recent evidence suggests that the pathways for tissue injury in heat stroke share many features with that of sepsis, endotoxaemia and systemic inflammation. Increased levels of circulating endotoxin and cytokines have been identified in patients with heat stroke.[27,28] The use of anti-endotoxin antibodies in primate models of heat stroke suggests that endotoxin at least in part mediates the tissue injury associated with hyperthermia. There was also a significant correlation between plasma IL-6 concentration and the severity of heat stroke. Since this cytokine is known to modulate the hypothalamic set-point, the ramifications of such a response in an already hyperthermic patient are obvious.

Activation of coagulation factors[29] and release of endothelin and adhesion molecules[30,31] from activated or injured endothelium have also been demonstrated in heat stroke. These recent observations lead to the speculation that certain mediators that are implicated in the pathogenesis of acute organ injury are also elevated in heat stress, but become intense when heat stroke develops and are not normalised upon cooling.

CLINICAL PRESENTATION

Heat stroke induces multiple organ failure and the clinical presentation reflects this. The first clinical signs may be neurological, and include restlessness, delirium, pupillary abnormalities, seizures and coma. Brainstem reflexes may be lost in the presence of brainstem-evoked potentials. There may be focal pathology including cerebellar injury, which may remain permanent. Lumbar puncture may show increased protein, xanthochromia and lymphocytic pleocytosis.

The signs of distributive shock, with a hyperdynamic haemodynamic profile not dissimilar to that of sepsis, are present in a large number of patients. The marked hyperventilation results in respiratory alkalosis, and hypoxaemic respiratory failure may be due to cardiac failure or acute lung injury.

Dehydration follows excessive insensible losses although sweating is generally absent in the terminal stages of classic heat stroke, leaving a hot, dry skin. Hypovolaemia is a consequence of dehydration and fluid redistribution, and results in reduced organ perfusion. A severe metabolic (lactic) acidosis is present. The major biochemical abnormalities include hyperglycaemia, hypophosphataemia, and raised serum enzymes and acute phase proteins (Table 74.3). Haematological findings include leukocytosis, thrombocytopenia, and activation of coagulation and fibrinolysis.

Exertional heat stroke differs slightly in that additional findings include rhabdomyolysis and acute renal failure that is associated with hyperkalaemia, hyperphosphataemia and hypocalcaemia (Table 74.3).

Table 74.3 Biochemical differences between classic and exertional heat stroke

	Classic heat stroke	Exertional heat stoke
Arterial gases	Mixed respiratory alkalosis	Severe metabolic acidosis
Serum electrolytes	Na^+, Mg^{2+}, Ca^{2+} are usually normal Hypophosphataemia	Hyperkalaemia Hypocalcaemia Hyperphosphataemia
Blood glucose	Hyperglycaemia	Hypoglycaemia
Creatinine kinase	Moderately increased	Markedly increased
Hepatic enzymes	Markedly increased	Moderately increased
Acute phase proteins	Markedly increased	Moderately increased

MANAGEMENT

Heat stroke is a medical emergency. The principal therapeutic objectives are rapid cooling to below 40°C and support of vital organ systems. Heat is dissipated by:

- conduction (immersion in ice-cold water or packed ice)
- evaporation (repeated wetting of skin with tepid water and fanning the patient at room temperature and low humidity)

Evaporation is considerably more effective. Pharmacological treatment with antipyretic agents, or dantrolene,[32] is ineffective. Prevention of vasoconstriction and shivering by overcooling is important because of the danger of subsequent rebound hyperthermia. Core and skin temperature monitoring is useful, but measurement of rectal temperature should be avoided because it lags considerably during cooling. Cooling can be stopped when core temperature reaches below 39°C. However, despite cooling, about 25% of patients experience failure of one or more organ systems.

Fluid and electrolyte imbalance, and acid–base disturbances must be corrected cautiously with appropriate fluids tailored to the individual and guided by measurements of filling pressure, serum electrolytes and haematocrit.

The mechanism of acute renal failure is multifactorial but rhabdomyolysis is the major component. Early institution of alkaline diuresis and mannitol may obviate the need for renal replacement therapy.

Oxygen therapy and controlled ventilation may be indicated, and anticonvulsants required. Prophylactic antibiotics and steroids are not recommended. Blood glucose must be controlled aggressively. Finally, any underlying illness should be sought and treated accordingly.

OUTCOME

The largest study reported of heat stroke patients in intensive care suggests an alarmingly high mortality of > 60%,[23] although this diminishes substantially with early recognition and aggressive treatment. The incidence of permanent neurological deficit remains at 7–15%. Variables associated independently with reduced hospital survival include:

- high core temperature
- high simplified acute physiology score (SAPS) II score
- having heat stroke at home
- prolonged prothrombin time
- vasoactive therapy within 24 hours
- admission to ICU lacking air conditioning

DRUG-INDUCED HYPERTHERMIAS

In contrast to fever, the thermoregulatory set-point during hyperthermia remains unchanged at normothermic levels; however, body temperature increases in an uncontrolled fashion and overrides the ability of effector mechanisms to dissipate heat. Although a raised body temperature is not necessarily due to increased heat production but rather due to an imbalance between heat production and loss, most hyperthermias result as a consequence of net heat gain. Hyperthermia can result in dangerously high core temperatures by two mechanisms:

- excessive exogenous heat exposure
- excessive endogenous heat production

The numerous causes of hyperthermia are listed in Table 74.4. This section will review the relatively common causes of drug-induced hyperthermias, including malignant hyperthermia, neuroleptic malignant syndrome, and the sympathomimetic and anticholinergic syndromes.

Table 74.4 Causes of hyperthermia

Disorders of excessive heat production	Exertional hyperthermia Heat stroke (exertional) Malignant hyperthermia Neuroleptic malignant syndrome Lethal catatonia Thyrotoxicosis Phaeochromocytoma Salicylate intoxication Sympathomimetic drug abuse Delirium tremens Seizures Tetanus
Disorders of diminished heat dissipation	Heat stroke (classic) Dehydration Autonomic dysfunction Anticholinergic poisoning Neuroleptic malignant syndrome
Disorders of hypothalamic function	Cerebrovascular accidents Encephalitis Trauma Granulomatous diseases Neuroleptic malignant syndrome

MALIGNANT HYPERTHERMIA

Malignant hyperthermia (MH) is a rare pharmacogenetic myopathy usually manifested when a susceptible individual is exposed to anaesthetic triggering agents. It is characterised by an intense hypermetabolic state and skeletal muscle rigidity upon exposure to volatile anaesthetics and depolarising muscle relaxants. In extreme cases, body temperature may exceed 42°C and the arterial pH reach 6.8, and can be rapidly fatal. The incidence of an MH reaction during general anaesthesia varies between 1/60 000 when succinylcholine is used, and 1/250 000 when only volatile agents are used. It is more frequent in children (1/15 000), with more than 50% of cases occurring before the age of 15 years.

PATHOGENESIS

Skeletal muscle is the principal tissue involved in an MH reaction. The primary defect is thought to be in the sarcolemma, and in particular the calcium release channel also termed the ryanodine receptor (RYR1). In MH, exposure of skeletal muscle to triggering agents depolarises the muscle hypersensitively to release massive amounts of calcium ions from the sarcoplasmic reticulum (SR), thus vastly increasing its cytoplasmic concentration. It is believed that the altered kinetics of the ryanodine receptor is due to exaggerated release of calcium by small increases in cytoplasmic calcium concentration (calcium-induced calcium release), as well as a decrease in inhibitory effects of high calcium concentrations. ATP-dependent membrane pumps (Ca^{2+}-ATPase) attempt to return the calcium back to the SR, resulting in a sustained glycolytic and aerobic metabolism. Recovery of calcium by the SR is often incomplete, causing prolonged excitation–contraction coupling and leading to muscle rigidity. Muscle contractures impede blood flow and perturb nutrient supply and waste removal from this hypermetabolic reaction. Eventually, oxidative phosphorylation is uncoupled, metabolism becomes anaerobic, and a severe lactic and respiratory acidosis develops. As muscle constitutes about 40% of body mass and is a major source of body heat, increased activity results in hyperthermia.

Membrane phospholipase A_2 is also activated by calcium, leading to an increase in mitochondrial and sarcoplasmic permeability, with further loss of calcium regulation and release of intracellular contents (potassium [K^+], calcium [Ca^{2+}], creatinine kinase (CK) and myoglobin) into the circulation.

CLINICAL PRESENTATION

The earliest sign of an impending MH crisis is an unexplained rise in end-tidal CO_2 and heart rate, and not necessarily an increase in body temperature. This classic crisis of acute fulminant MH with its multiplicity of marked metabolic and muscle anomalies and sympathetic stimulation is unmistakable, but now rare. The pattern of presentation has altered since its first description in 1960, as anaesthetic techniques and succinylcholine use have changed.

The more gradual appearance of signs following exposure to triggering agents may be more difficult to diagnose as the signs may be subtle, non-specific and have variable intensity, incidence and temporal association (Table 74.5).[33] Apart from the classic crisis, other forms of MH – including smouldering, recurring, delayed and abortive – may also occur. Other conditions that may mimic MH include inadequate levels of anaesthesia or analgesia, sepsis, ischaemia or anaphylaxis. Early diagnosis is important as immediate treatment is associated with improved outcome. Masseter muscle spasm (MMS) has been associated with MH.[34] When MMS is the only presenting sign, the incidence of MH susceptibility is likely to be low. However, this incidence is increased if MMS is associated with other muscle or metabolic signs.

Halothane is the most potent of the contemporary volatile anaesthetic agents at inducing sustained contractures in isolated muscle strips from MH patients, and has formed the basis of diagnostic testing for MH for 30 years. There may be a difference amongst the volatile anaesthetics in their relative potency to trigger an MH reaction. Succinylcholine will cause an increase in the calcium concentration in the cytosol of normal muscle, and it appears that this release of calcium is exaggerated in MH muscle. Non-depolarising muscle relaxants are generally accepted to be safe in MH. A list of safe and implicated drugs is shown in Table 74.6.

Several neuromuscular and musculoskeletal abnormalities such as scoliosis, strabismus, muscular dystrophy and central core disease have been associated with MH susceptibility but definitive evidence for this association is lacking. Patients with neuroleptic malignant syndrome are not considered at risk of developing MH under general anaesthesia.

MH susceptibility has been diagnosed for the last 30 years on the basis of abnormal in vitro contractures to separate exposures to halothane and caffeine performed on freshly biopsied muscle strips. Recently, a ryanodine contracture test has been shown to be more specific and may be of additional value.

Table 74.6 Drug use in malignant hyperthermia

Contraindicated drugs	Safe drugs
Halothane	Nitrous oxide
Enflurane	Barbiturates
Isoflurane	Propofol
Desflurane	Etomidate
Sevoflurane	Ketamine
Succinylcholine	Opiates
Verapamil	Amide/ester local anaesthetics
Nifedipine	Noradrenaline (norepinephrine)
Diltiazem	Adrenaline (epinephrine)
	Dopamine
	Dobutamine

Table 74.5 Clinical features of malignant hyperthermia

Timing	Clinical signs	Changes in monitored variables	Biochemical changes
Acute	Sustained jaw rigidity after succinylcholine Tachypnoea Rapid exhaustion of soda lime Hot soda lime canister High pulse rate Irregular pulse	Increased minute ventilation Rising end-tidal CO_2 Tachycardia Ventricular ectopics Peaked T waves on ECG	Increased $Paco_2$ Decreased pH Increased $[K^+]$
Intermediate	Patient hot to touch Cyanosis Dark blood in wound Irregular pulse	Rising core body temperature Falling Spo_2 Ventricular ectopics Peaked T waves on ECG	Decreased *Pao*2 Increased $[K^+]$
Late	Generalised muscle rigidity Prolonged bleeding Dark urine Oliguria Irregular pulse Death	Ventricular ectopics Peaked T waves on ECG	Increased creatine kinase Myoglobinuria Increased $[K^+]$

Adapted from Hopkins PM. Malignant hyperthermia: advances in clinical management and diagnosis. *BJA* 2000; **85**: 118–28.

MOLECULAR GENETICS OF MH

MH is a heterogenetic disorder that is autosomal dominant with variable penetration and expression. Recent advances in molecular genetics have supported the concept for a role of the *RYR1* gene in the pathogenesis of MH. The *RYR1* gene is found at position 13.1 on chromosome 19 q and codes for the ryanodine receptor that regulates calcium transport across the calcium release channel. However, only 50% of MH families show genetic linkage to the *RYR1* gene, and more than 17 mutations at this locus have been described so far. The mutation does not always segregate with in vitro contracture testing within a family. Furthermore, *RYR1* linkage is not found in some MH families. Although all known mutations share the final common pathway of excessive calcium release from the SR, the genetic diversity of this disease precludes DNA-based diagnosis at present.

MANAGEMENT

Once a diagnosis of MH is suspected, and other diagnoses excluded, treatment should be based as follows:

- Stop all anaesthetic triggering drugs, increase fresh gas flow to purge the anaesthetic machine, and substitute a new breathing circuit. Valuable time should not be lost changing the machine and is no longer recommended. Increase ventilation to two to three times the minute volume to aid removal of CO_2.
- Abandon surgery if possible, or continue using safe drugs (Table 74.6).
- Administer intravenous dantrolene, which is the only specific therapy, at an initial dose of 2.5 mg/kg and repeat at 5–10-minute intervals until the drug reverses the metabolic derangements of MH (maximum dose 10 mg/kg). Dantrolene acts by inhibition of SR calcium release but without affecting uptake. It may be repeated at 1–2 mg/kg 4-hourly for 1–3 days and then given orally if still required.
- Arrhythmias not responsive to correction of acidosis and hyperkalaemia should be treated in the conventional manner. However, calcium antagonists are contraindicated as these drugs interact with high-dose dantrolene to cause severe hyperkalaemia and cardiovascular collapse.
- Cool the patient using simple measures such as tepid sponging, fanning and cool intravenous fluids in order to avoid vasoconstriction, which impedes heat loss. Occasionally, more aggressive cooling methods may be required.
- Frequent blood samples should be taken for analysis of blood gases, potassium, creatinine kinase, myoglobin and coagulation. Treat hyperkalaemia and acidosis early and aggressively.
- Measure urine output for impending signs of acute renal failure. Diuresis with mannitol or furosemide may be considered in addition to fluids to attempt to prevent myoglobin precipitation in renal tubules. Mannitol doses should incorporate that contained in dantrolene preparations.
- Continue monitoring closely in the post acute phase according to signs and severity. Renal protection therapy and control of coagulopathy are desirable.
- Consider alternative diagnoses if there is no response to dantrolene, e.g. other myopathies, sepsis, thyrotoxic storm, phaeochromocytoma.
- After recovery, patients and relatives should be referred to an MH screening centre.

OUTCOME

The mortality rate from MH has declined from 70% in the 1960s to less than 10% worldwide. This vast improvement is attributed to increased awareness and understanding by anaesthetists, improved monitoring techniques (especially capnography and pulse oximetry) and the availability and early use of intravenous dantrolene. Late recognition of MH may result in a poor outcome despite treatment with dantrolene.

NEUROLEPTIC MALIGNANT SYNDROME

The neuroleptic malignant syndrome (NMS) is a relatively rare but potentially fatal idiosyncratic reaction to neuroleptic drugs that is not dose related. Many features of this syndrome remain controversial as several other medical conditions generate similar symptoms, but characteristic findings include:

- encephalopathy
- muscle rigidity
- hyperthermia
- autonomic dysfunction

The incidence is estimated to vary between 0.07 and 2.2%. All ages are affected but males are disproportionately represented in some studies.

PATHOGENESIS

The pathophysiology of NMS remains unclear. Two mechanisms – a neuroleptic-induced perturbation of central thermo- and neuroregulatory mechanisms and an abnormal reaction of skeletal muscle – have been proposed.

Hypothalamic thermoregulation involves noradrenergic, serotonergic, cholinergic and central dopaminergic pathways. Neuroleptic blockade of dopamine receptors in the hypothalamus leads to disturbances in thermoregulation and heat dissipation. In addition, blockade of dopamine receptors in the basal ganglia is thought to cause muscle hypertonicity and contraction, leading to further heat production. Drugs linked to NMS appear to share the ability to antagonise dopamine receptors (primarily D_2 receptors) or to lower synaptic dopamine levels. Recent work suggests that glutaminergic excitatory amino acids may influence central dopamine activity and be more important in the development of NMS.

A common pathogenesis of NMS and MH has been suggested by virtue of similar clinical features (hyperthermia, rigidity, raised serum muscle enzymes), abnormal in vitro contracture tests and, interestingly, successful treatment with dantrolene in both. However, conflicting results have been reported regarding the prevalence of MH susceptibility among NMS patients. Neuroleptic agents induce muscle contracture in vitro; however, no difference was found in response to four neuroleptic drugs between muscle from NMS patients and normal individuals.[35]

Although biochemical studies suggest the involvement of genetic factors in the pathogenesis of NMS, the molecular basis remains elusive. There does not appear to be an association between NMS and the mutations in the *RYR1* gene associated with MH.

CLINICAL PRESENTATION

The presentation and course of NMS can be quite variable; it may take a relatively benign and self-limiting course, or it may be fulminant and fatal, although the latter is rare. NMS usually develops within 2–4 weeks of starting antipsychotic therapy but the majority of the cases develop within the first week. The main symptoms that indicate a high probability of NMS include:

- hyperthermia
- muscle rigidity
- elevated serum creatinine kinase
- autonomic instability

A predictable progression of symptoms may be identified in many patients with NMS where mental status changes and rigidity precede hyperthermia and autonomic dysfunction:[36]

- temperature elevation can be mild or severe, but is rarely greater than 42 °C as seen in heat stroke
- muscle rigidity is characterised by a 'lead pipe' increase in tone that may result in decreased chest wall compliance and hypoventilation
- extrapyramidal symptoms may also be present
- autonomic instability is demonstrated by labile hypertension (hypotension is rare), tachycardia and sweating
- altered consciousness is typically of the form of delirium and agitation that may progress to stupor and coma

Other clinical features of lesser frequency include dysarthria, dysphagia, chorea, mutism and seizures. Elevated serum creatinine kinase is now considered to be a major feature of NMS. Other non-specific laboratory abnormalities include leukocytosis, mildly elevated hepatic enzymes, and secondary electrolyte disturbances including hypocalcaemia, hypomagnesaemia and hypophosphataemia. Urine analysis often reveals proteinuria and myoglobinuria from rhabdomyolysis. The electroencephalograph (EEG) may show diffuse slowing. CT scans of the brain as well as examination of cerebrospinal fluid is usually normal in NMS.

All classes of neuroleptic medications have been implicated in NMS including butyrophenones, phenothiazines, thioxanthenes and benzamides, as well as newer drugs such as clozapine and risperidone. Haloperidol and fluphenazine are the most frequently reported agents. Other agents that block dopamine receptors or inhibit dopamine release have been associated with NMS including metoclopramide, reserpine and α-methylparatyrosine. Discontinuation of anti-parkinsonian drugs (leading to a relative decrease in dopamine levels) has also been associated with NMS.

Risk factors include organic brain disease, functional psychoses, dehydration and rapid loading of antipsychotics.

Complications include:

- acute renal failure from rhabdomyolysis
- respiratory failure from hypoventilation and aspiration pneumonia
- cardiovascular collapse
- irreversible neurological injury may result from extreme temperatures

The differential diagnosis of NMS includes all disorders that can present with a combination of hyperthermia, rigidity and encephalopathy. These include CNS infections, cerebral masses, tetanus, heat stress, MH, catatonia and drug toxicities (lithium, atropine and monoamine oxidase inhibitors).

Neuroleptic-induced heat stroke is differentiated from NMS by its faster onset, absence of extrapyramidal signs and sweating (anticholinergic properties of neuroleptics), and a history of physical exertion and exposure to a hostile environment. Like NMS, lethal catatonia can present with hyperthermia, akinesia and muscle rigidity. The importance of distinguishing the catatonias from NMS lies in the differential treatment. Benzodiazepines are usually required for the former.

SEROTONERGIC SYNDROME

Drugs that enhance serotonergic neurotransmission or lead to a relative increase in synaptic levels of serotonin can result in a toxic state that resembles features of NMS. These drugs include selective serotonin reuptake inhibitors (SSRIs), monoamine oxidase inhibitors (MAOIs) and tricyclic antidepressants (TCAs), either alone or in combination. Serotonin syndrome may complicate the administration of drugs frequently used in anaesthetic practice, including pethidine and tramadol, in combination with the above drugs. This syndrome is a toxic effect that appears to be due to hyperstimulation of 5-HT_{1A} receptors in the brain and spinal cord. This is differentiated from NMS, which is an idiosyncratic response to antipsychotics and not serotonergic drugs.

Clinical features of the serotonergic syndrome include encephalopathy, hyperreflexia, nausea and vomiting, and autonomic instability. Sweating and mild increases in temperature are evident in 50% of cases. Rhabdomyolysis, hyperkalaemia, renal failure, DIC and seizures are all rare but reported findings. The serotonergic syndrome is usually self-limited, and resolves uneventfully once the offending drug has been withdrawn. However, rarely severe forms require more aggressive supportive therapy analogous to the treatment of NMS. Specific treatments including the use of serotonin antagonists have been proposed; however, these cannot be recommended at present due to lack of well-designed studies.

MANAGEMENT

Management of mild forms of NMS may only require early recognition, withdrawal of all neuroleptic, dopamine-depleting or dopamine-antagonist medication, and general supportive therapy. Cessation of all psychotropic drugs should be considered. Rarely, severe cases require aggressive treatment of fluid/electrolyte and acid–base balance as well as cardiorespiratory function. Because acute renal failure is the most frequent complication of NMS, therapy must be directed at renal protection from myoglobin injury. The hyperthermic patient should be cooled as described previously in this chapter. Haemodialysis may be required for renal failure, but is not useful for clearing neuroleptic drugs as these are protein-bound and therefore too large to dialyse.

The benefit of adding specific pharmacotherapies in addition to supportive measures is unclear, but potential use cannot be excluded. Treatments with bromocriptine (a dopamine agonist) and dantrolene have led to a faster resolution of symptoms than with supportive therapy alone.[37] However, the place of dantrolene in the treatment of NMS is less well defined. Bromocriptine seems to be well tolerated by psychotic patients despite being a strong central dopamine agonist. The drug is effective within 24 h, with a reduction in rigidity followed by resolution of temperature and normalisation of blood pressure. Similarly, amantadine, as well as a combination of levodopa-carbidopa, has also been reported to be effective. Anticholinergic drugs have little effect on muscle rigidity or hyperthermia. Non-specific adjuncts, such as the use of benzodiazepines, have been reported to be useful in agitated patients. Electroconvulsive therapy (ECT) may be of value in selected patients, e.g. those with refractory NMS, those who remain catatonic or those with ECT-responsive psychotic symptoms.

OUTCOME

A mortality of 22% prior to 1980 has been halved since 1984. This reduction has occurred largely due to early diagnosis, supportive therapy and advances in critical care medicine, rather than a consequence of therapy with either dantrolene or dopamine agonists. Renal failure increases the mortality rate to approximately 50%; however, prognosis remains good in survivors.

SYMPATHOMIMETIC AND ANTICHOLINERGIC SYNDROMES

SYMPATHOMIMETIC POISONING

Mild to severe hyperthermia may be associated with all centrally acting sympathomimetics. These drugs produce their clinical effects by increasing synaptic concentrations of noradrenaline (norepinephrine), dopamine and serotonin.

Cocaine predominantly blocks the presynaptic uptake of noradrenaline, although neurotransmission of dopamine and serotonin is also affected. Amphetamines and related drugs augment the release of noradrenaline, dopamine and serotonin from presynaptic nerve terminals and inhibit their uptake from the synapse. Some amphetamine metabolites also inhibit monoamine oxidase.

Central thermoregulatory disturbances from sympathomimetics may arise from complex interactions of these neurotransmitters in the brainstem and hypothalamus. The syndrome of hyperthermia associated with sympathomimetic poisoning bears similarity to that of heat stroke, MH, NMS and serotonin syndrome. This may reflect the final common pathway associated with the consequences of severe hyperthermia. Sympathomimetics such as MDMA ('ecstasy') have been shown to induce marked hyperthermia through central mechanisms involving 5-HT_2 receptors, with subsequent rhabdomyolysis, DIC and multiorgan failure.[38] Hyperkinetic muscle action, motor excitability and seizures may contribute to the rise in core temperature. Furthermore, elevated levels of both cocaine and amphetamine result in peripheral vasoconstriction, thus impairing heat dissipation. Mortality appears to be related to the extent and duration of hyperthermia.

Therapy involves rapid cooling measures as outlined previously, together with support of failing organ systems. Benzodiazepines may relieve myotonic and hyperkinetic thermogenesis. However, patients who remain agitated and non-compliant should be paralysed and ventilated to permit institution of aggressive cooling measures. In moderately severe hyperthermia, dantrolene therapy has been described to improve outcome by enabling rapid muscle relaxation and control of temperature. However, the basis of its utility in this setting has not been established.

ANTICHOLINERGIC POISONING

The central and peripheral symptoms of anticholinergic syndrome result from the blockade of muscarinic acetylcholinergic receptors. Central toxicity results in:

- confusion
- tremor
- hallucinations
- myoclonus
- agitation

whereas peripheral signs of toxicity include:

- dry mucous membranes
- mydriasis
- blurred vision
- tachycardia
- urinary retention

Muscular hyperactivity from agitation, restlessness and convulsions in combination with impaired sweating may result in hyperthermia and rhabdomyolysis. Excessive temperatures can lead to multiorgan failure as described for other types of heat illness.

HYPOTHERMIA

Hypothermia is defined as a core body temperature below 35 °C. In the UK, hypothermia accounts for 1% of winter admissions, particularly amongst the elderly population. The leading causes of hypothermia in the USA are exposure due to alcoholism, drug addiction, mental illness, or accidents involving immersion in cold water. The mortality rate from accidental hypothermia varies according to its severity, but averages 21% when core temperature is decreased to 28–32°C.[39] However, a core temperature of 32 °C or less in trauma victims is associated with a mortality rate near 100%, and any hypothermia is considered a poor prognostic sign.[40,41]

Hypothermia is traditionally classified as:

- mild (temperature 32–35°C)
- moderate (temperature 28–32°C)
- severe (temperature below 28°C)

Significant hypothermia in terms of severity and duration results in multiple systemic derangements that ultimately lead to impaired tissue oxygenation. The major defence against cold stress is behavioural adaptation. However, autonomic thermoregulatory responses orchestrated by the hypothalamus are also activated to prevent heat loss and generate heat production. These include:

- peripheral vasoconstriction
- shivering
- increase in metabolism.

The four physical mechanisms of heat loss from the body surfaces are conduction, convection, radiation and evaporation.

Hypothermia may be induced deliberately for therapeutic purposes, e.g. cardiovascular surgery or neuroprotection, or it may be accidental. Primary accidental hypothermia occurs when an otherwise healthy individual experiences overwhelming cold stress, e.g. cold-water immersion. Secondary accidental hypothermia occurs despite mild environmental conditions and is due to illness or injury-induced perturbations in thermoregulation and heat production, e.g. drug intoxication or trauma.

The causes and predisposing conditions of hypothermia are listed in Table 74.7; however, the most frequent causes appear to be exposure, hypoglycaemia and the use of depressant drugs including alcohol. An impaired thermoregulatory system together with a reduced functional reserve makes the elderly more susceptible.

Administration of anaesthesia impairs the ability to maintain thermal homeostasis, decreases heat production and causes heat loss due to vasodilatation and exposure. General anaesthesia also alters the threshold for thermoregulatory vasoconstriction and shivering in the non-paralysed patient.[42]

Table 74.7 Causes and predisposing conditions of hypothermia

Age	Extremes of age
Environmental	Exposure to cold Immersion Poor living conditions
Drugs	Anaesthetic agents Phenothiazines Barbiturates Alcohol
Central nervous system disorders	Cerebrovascular accidents Trauma Spinal cord transections Brain tumours Wernicke's encephalopathy Alzheimer's and Parkinson's disease Mental illness
Endocrine dysfunction	Hypoglycaemia Diabetic ketoacidosis Hyperosmolar coma Panhypopituitarism Hypoadrenalism Hypothyroidism
Trauma	Major trauma
Debility	Severe cardiac, renal, hepatic impairment Malnutrition, sepsis
Skin disorders	Burns Exfoliative dermatitis

PATHOGENESIS AND CLINICAL PRESENTATION

Hypothermia depresses all organ functions resulting in decreased cardiac function, shock, respiratory failure, confusion, muscle rigidity, renal failure and death. The cardiovascular response in hypothermia initially comprises an increase in heart rate, cardiac output and blood pressure in response to shivering and increased metabolic demand. Peripheral vasoconstriction is due to activation of the sympathetic nervous system as well as local cutaneous reflexes, resulting in shunting of peripheral blood to the central pool. With worsening hypothermia:

- progressive cardiovascular depression leads to a reduction in tissue perfusion
- cardiac output is halved at 28°C as a result of decreased heart rate and contractility
- conduction and pacemaker activity are reduced, and there is prolongation of PR, QRS and QT intervals as well as non-specific ST-T wave changes. The characteristic J or Osborn wave may be seen when core temperature is below 33°C

- atrial fibrillation and heart block are also common below this temperature. Ventricular fibrillation and asystole can occur below 28°C and 20°C respectively. Fibrillation may occur earlier if the myocardium is diseased or stimulated, either mechanically or pharmacologically

An initial increase in respiratory rate during hypothermia is followed by progressive depression of rate, vital capacity and minute volume. The cough reflex is abolished, exposing the patient to an increased risk of aspiration pneumonia. Bronchial secretions, atelectasis and pulmonary oedema may develop. Apnoea may occur below 24°C. The oxyhaemoglobin dissociation curve is shifted to the left, resulting in reduced oxygen delivery to the tissues, but this is partially balanced by a right shift due to the underlying acidosis.

Shivering occurs in the early phase of hypothermia and is characterised by intense heat and energy production from the metabolism of stored fuels. Non-shivering thermogenesis is probably only of importance in children. Metabolic processes slow by approximately 6%/°C, and the metabolic rate is reduced by half at 28°C.[43] A mixed respiratory and metabolic acidosis results from hypoventilation and reduced tissue perfusion, leading to lactate accumulation from anaerobic metabolism. Hepatic function is depressed, affecting most enzymatic and detoxifying processes. There is a high risk of developing pancreatitis.

There is generalised cerebral depression as the metabolism of the brain declines with a fall in core temperature. This adaptation is neuroprotective and may improve the chances of survival even after prolonged hypothermic arrest. Cerebral blood flow falls as a consequence of reduced cardiac output and increased blood viscosity at a rate of 7%/°C drop in temperature.[44] Confusion can cause illogical behaviour (e.g. aggression) and paradoxical undressing. Coma, pupillary dilatation, absence of tendon reflexes and rigidity are present below 28°C. Cerebral electrical activity ceases below 20°C.

Hypothermia causes an initial increase in catecholamine and cortisol release as a result of the stress response. There is a delayed increase in serum thyroxine levels. Below 30°C, pituitary and pancreatic functions, as well as catecholamine secretion, are blunted. Blood sugar concentration is increased as a result of increased glycogenolysis and insulin resistance.

Haemoconcentration develops as a consequence of hypovolaemia as well as fluid shifts between compartments. Hypothermia increases blood viscosity by 2%/°C. Splenic sequestration results in leukopenia and thrombocytopenia. Low temperature also interferes with the intrinsic coagulation cascade. In severe hypothermia, platelet dysfunction and DIC are common.

MANAGEMENT

Once the diagnosis of hypothermia has been made, further heat loss must be prevented and rewarming started with close monitoring to avoid complications. Individual management should be modified according to aetiology and severity of hypothermia, as well as the functional reserve of the patient. Severe hypothermia, especially in the immersion victim, can mimic death, with apnoea, cardiac standstill, coma, unreactive pupils, and a silent electrocardiogram and electroencephalogram. Successful resuscitation of such patients has been reported and death should not be assumed until resuscitation has failed in an adequately warmed patient (at least 35°C).[45]

General measures begin with removal of the patient from the cold environment as rapidly as possible. Rough handling must be avoided during transport as this may precipitate fatal arrhythmias in severe hypothermia. Also, transport in the upright position must be avoided because cerebral blood flow may be compromised due to orthostatic hypotension.

Recommendation for basic and advanced life support for hypothermic patients is according to the principles of Advanced Cardiorespiratory Life Support (ACLS). Aggressive rewarming should be continued during resuscitation until the core temperature is at least 35°C. A resuscitation protocol based on core temperature and cardiac monitoring may be used.[46] If core temperature is unknown or known to be above 28°C, cardiopulmonary resuscitation (CPR) should be instituted for apparent cardiac arrest. If the patient is known to be severely hypothermic (< 28°C) but maintains sinus rhythm, chest compression may precipitate ventricular fibrillation (VF) and may be best withheld.

Vascular cannulation may be difficult in the presence of intense vasoconstriction and a central catheter is inevitably required, taking precautions to avoid myocardial stimulation.

For the same reasons, a pulmonary artery catheter should be deferred until normothermia has been re-established. Hypotension should be treated with aggressive warm fluid therapy. Lactated Ringers should be avoided because the liver may not be able to metabolise lactate to bicarbonate.

Atrial arrhythmias, bradycardia or atrioventricular block generally do not require treatment with antiarrhythmic agents unless decompensated, and resolve on rewarming.

Electrical defibrillation may not be effective at body temperature below 30°C. Indeed, VF may resolve spontaneously upon rewarming.

Sodium bicarbonate should be avoided because of paradoxical intracellular acidosis, and severe alkalosis on rewarming may induce refractory VF and left shift of the oxyhaemoglobin dissociation curve, thereby reducing tissue oxygen uptake. Progressive cardiac depression during rewarming ('recovery shock', 'afterdrop') may be due to further cooling of blood as it redistributes from the core to the relatively colder periphery.[47]

The increased metabolic demand during rewarming requires oxygen therapy. Patients in coma or respiratory failure should be intubated and ventilated with warm gases. Drug administration during hypothermia may reach toxic levels after rewarming because of functionally prolonged half-lives, and therefore should be used sparingly. Insulin treatment should be delayed until the temperature is above 30°C. It should be administered in small doses because degradation is slow and accumulation may occur with rebound hypoglycaemia as the patient is warmed.

REWARMING

Various methods of rewarming have been employed depending upon the severity of the hypothermia (Table 74.8). Careful monitoring and supportive therapy are mandatory during rewarming.

Passive warming involves removing the patient from a cold environment and allowing to rewarm spontaneously in a warm room (30°C). It is best for patients with mild hypothermia who have no circulatory compromise. Rewarming is gradual at 0.5–1.0°C/h.

Patients with moderate or severe hypothermia should be treated with active rewarming, which consists of active external rewarming or active core rewarming. Patients with moderate hypothermia and no evidence of circulatory collapse can initially be treated with active external rewarming techniques. These include use of immersion, radiant heat, forced air and electric blankets. Convective (forced air) warming at 43°C has been shown to increase body temperature by 2–3°C/hour, and is extremely effective in both preventing and treating hypothermia, as well as preventing shivering in the postoperative period.[48,49]

Active core rewarming is best used for patients with moderate to severe hypothermia. Techniques include:

- airway rewarming
- gastrointestinal
- peritoneal or pleural cavity lavage
- extacorporeal rewarming
- cardiopulmonary bypass

Active core rewarming methods are extremely rapid but invasive, and the inherent risks should be considered in the management.

Table 74.8 Rewarming methods

Passive	Warm environment >30°C (rate 0.5–1.0 °C/hour) Insulating cover (warm blanket)
Active, external	Conduction methods Warmed pads, blanket Convective methods (rate at 2–3°C/hour) Hot air blower (e.g. Bair Hugger) Radiant methods
Active, core	Humidified warm inspired gases (rate 0.5–1.5°C/hour) Warmed intravenous fluids Body cavity lavage (rate 2–3°C/hour) Gastric irrigation Pleural irrigation Peritoneal dialysis Extracorporeal methods Haemodialysis, continuous arteriovenous or venovenous rewarming (rate 5°C/hour) Cardiopulmonary bypass (rate up to 10°C/hour)

In airway rewarming, inspired gas is heated and humidified up to 40 °C, and delivered either through a facemask or an endotracheal tube. It insulates the respiratory tract and stops heat and moisture lost through breathing. The rate of rewarming is about 0.5–1.5 °C/h. Volume expansion with intravenous fluids warmed with heat exchangers or by microwave can also be used. However, this method is insufficient by itself as very large volumes would be required to achieve a significant rise in body temperature.

Peritoneal lavage with heated dialysate, and closed pleural irrigation using warm sterile saline (temperature 40–42°C) through large bore tubes may also be attempted.[50,51] These methods are equally effective in raising temperature (2–3°C/h), but impossible in patients with thoracoabdominal injuries.

Haemodialysis and continuous arteriovenous or venovenous rewarming techniques are extremely effective in raising body temperature (5 °C/h). The advantages of this technique include non-requirement of heparinisation if heparin-bonded tubing is used, rapid reversal of hypothermia, decreased total fluid requirements, decreased organ failure, decreased length of ICU stay and decreased early mortality.[52] Patients with severe cardiovascular dysfunction may not tolerate high arteriovenous fistula flows.

The best method for rewarming patients with severe hypothermia who have haemodynamic instability involves the use of cardiopulmonary bypass. Its advantages include the highest rewarming rate (up to 10°C/h), control of rewarming rate, oxygenation, fluid composition and haemodynamic support.[53] However, associated risks include heparinisation, haemolysis and air embolism.

Afterdrop is a phenomenon seen with rewarming where tissues that have been vasoconstricted and very cold start to become perfused again. Blood returning from these areas may be cold and will result in a late reduction in core temperature. This may be seen when core temperature is approaching normal and after active measures have been stopped.

OUTCOME

Poor prognostic factors include aetiology and severity of hypothermia, advanced age, comorbid states and cardiorespiratory arrest. Hypothermia associated with trauma or sepsis carries a high mortality.

REFERENCES

1. Kluger MJ. Fever: role of pyrogens and cryogens. *Physiol Rev* 1996; **71**: 93–127.
2. Lenhardt R, Kurz A, Sessler DI. Thermoregulation and hyperthermia. *Acta Anaesthesiol Scand Suppl* 1996; **40**: 34–8.
3. O'Grady WP, Barie PS, Bartlett JG *et al.* Practice guidelines for evaluating new fever in critically ill adult patients? *Clin Infect Dis* 1998; **26**: 1042–59.
4. Gozolli V, Schottker P, Suter PM *et al.* Is it worth treating fever in intensive care unit patients. *Arch Int Med* 2001; **161**: 121–3.

5. Kluger MJ, Kozak W, Conn CA *et al.* The adaptive value of fever. *Infect Dis Clin North Am* 1996; **10**: 1–20.
6. Weinstein MR, Iannini PB, Stratton CW *et al.* Spontaneous bacterial peritonitis: a review of 28 cases with emphasis on improved survival and factors influencing prognosis. *Am J Med* 1978; **64**: 592–8.
7. Azocar J, Yunis EJ, Essex M. Sensitivity of human natural killer cells to hyperthermia. *Lancet* 1982; **1**: 16–17.
8. Biggar W, Bohn DJ, Kent G *et al.* Neutrophil migration *in vitro* and *in vivo* during hyperthermia. *Infect Immunol* 1984; **46**: 857–9.
9. Jampel HD, Duff GW, Gershon RK *et al.* Fever and immunoregulation: III. Hyperthermia augments the primary in vitro humoral immune response. *J Exp Med* 1983; **157**: 1229–38.
10. van Oss CJ, Absolom DR, Moore LL *et al.* Effect of temperature on chemotaxis, phagocyte engulfment, digestion and oxygen consumption of human polymorphonuclear leucocytes. *J Reticuloendothel Soc* 1980; **27**: 561–5.
11. Styrt B, Sugarman B. Antipyresis and fever. *Arch Intern Med* 1990; **150**: 1589–97.
12. Cunha BA, Shea KW. Fever in the intensive care unit. *Infect Dis Clin North Am* 1996; **10**: 185–209.
13. Circiumaru B, Baldock G, Cohen J. A prospective of fever in the intensive care unit. *Intensive Care Med* 1999; **25**: 668–73.
14. Cunha BA. Intensive care, not intensive antibiotics. *Heart Lung* 1994; **23**: 361–2.
15. Marik PE. Fever in the ICU. *Chest* 2000; **117**: 855–69.
16. Poblette B, Romand JA, Pilchard C *et al.* Metabolic effects of intravenous propacetamol, metamizol or external cooling in critically ill febrile sedated patients. *BJA* 1997; **78**: 123–7.
17. Kurz A, Go JC, Sessler DI. Alfentanil slightly increases the sweating threshold and markedly reduces the vasoconstrictor and shivering thresholds. *Anesthesiology* 1995; **83**: 293–9.
18. Kurz A, Sessler DI, Annadata R *et al.* Midazolam minimally impairs thermoregulatory control. *Anesth Analg* 1995; **81**: 393–8.
19. Hindman BJ, Todd MM, Gelb AW *et al.* Mild hypothermia as a protective therapy during intracranial aneurysm surgery: a randomized prospective pilot trial. *Neurosurgery* 1999; **44**: 23–33.
20. Marion DW, Penrod LE, Kelsey SF *et al.* Treatment of traumatic brain injury with moderate hypothermia. *N Engl J Med* 1997; **336**: 540–6.
21. Bernard SA, Jones BM, Buist M. Experience with prolonged induced hypothermia in severe head injury. *Crit Care* 1999; **3**: 167–72.
22. Centers for Disease Control. Heat related illness and deaths: United States, 1994–95. *MMWR* 1995; **44**: 465–8.
23. Hemon D, Jorgla E. The heat wave in France in August 2003. *Rev Epidemiol Sante Publique* 2004; **52**: 3–15.
24. Kosatsky T. The 2003 European heat waves. *Eur Surveill* 2005; **10**: 1–15.
25. Missett B, De Jonghe B, Bastuji-Garin S *et al.* Mortality of patients with heatstroke admitted to intensive care units during the 2003 heat wave in France: a national multiple-center risk factor study. *Crit Care Med* 2006; **34**: 1087–92.
26. Sminia P, van der Zee J, Wondergem J *et al.* Effect of hyperthermia on the central nervous system: a review. *Int J Hyperthermia* 1994; **10**: 1–30.
27. Bouchama A, Parhar RS, El-Yazigi A *et al.* Endotoxaemia and release of TNF and IL-1α in acute heat stroke. *J Appl Physiol* 1991; **70**: 2640–4.
28. Bouchama A, Al-Sedairy S, Siddiqui S *et al.* Elevated pyrogenic cytokines in heat stroke. *Chest* 1993; **104**: 1498–502.
29. Bouchama A, Bridley F, Hammami MM *et al.* Activation of coagulation and fibrinolysis in heat stroke. *Thrombosis Haemostasis* 1996; **76**: 909–15.
30. Bouchama A, Hammami MM, Hay A *et al.* Evidence for endothelial cell activation/injury in heatstroke. *Crit Care Med* 1996; **24**: 1173–8.
31. Hammami MM, Bouchama A. Levels of soluble L-selectin and E-selectin in heatstroke and heatstress. *Chest* 1998; **114**: 949–50.
32. Bouchama A, Cafege A, deVol EB *et al.* Ineffectiveness of dantrolene sodium in the treatment of heatstroke. *Crit Care Med* 1991; **19**: 176–80.
33. Hopkins PM. Malignant hyperthermia: advances in clinical management and diagnosis. *BJA* 2000; **85**: 118–28.
34. Ramirez JA, Cheetham ED, Laurence AS. Succinylcholine, masseter spasm and later malignant hyperthermia. *Anaesthesia* 1998; **53**: 1111–16.
35. Reyford HG, Cordonnier C, Adnet P *et al.* The *in vitro* exposure of muscle strips from patients with neuroleptic malignant syndrome cannot be correlated with the clinical features. *J Neurol Sci* 1990; **98**: 527.
36. Velamoor VR, Norman R, Caroff SN *et al.* Progression of symptoms in neuroleptic malignant syndrome. *J Nerv Ment Dis* 1994; **182**: 168–13.
37. Rosenberg MR, Green M. Neuroleptic malignant syndrome: a review of response to therapy. *Arch Intern Med* 1989; **149**: 1927–31.
38. McKenna DJ, Peroutka SJ. Neurochemistry and neurotoxicity of 3,4 methylenediaoxymetamphetamine (MDMA, 'ecstasy'). *J Neurochem* 1990; **54**: 14–22.
39. Danzl D, Pozos RS, Auerbach PS *et al.* Multicentre hypothermia survey. *Ann Emerg Med* 1987; **16**: 1042–55.
40. Jurkovic GJ, Greiser WB, Luterman A *et al.* Hypothermia in trauma victims: an ominous predictor of survival. *J Trauma* 1987; **27**: 1019–24.
41. Smith CE. Focus on: Perioperative hypothermia. Trauma and hypothermia. *Curr Anaesth Crit Care* 2001; **12**: 87–95.
42. Sessler DI. Consequences and treatment of perioperative hypothermia. *Anesthesiol Clin North Am* 1994; **12**: 425–56.
43. Corneli HM. Accidental hypothermia. *J Pediatr* 1992; **120**: 671–9.
44. Morley-Forster PK. Unintentional hypothermia in the operating room. *Can Anaesth Soc J* 1986; **33**: 516–27.
45. Larach MG. Accidental hypothermia. *Lancet* 1995; **345**: 493–8.

46. Zell SC, Kurtz KJ. Severe experimental hypothermia: a resuscitation protocol. *Ann Emerg Med* 1985; **4**: 339–45.
47. Giesbrecht GG, Bristow GK. A second post-cooling afterdrop: more evidence for a convective mechanism. *J Appl Physiol* 1992; **73**: 1253–8.
48. Smith CE, Yamat RA. Avoiding hypothermia in the trauma patient. *Curr Opin Anaesthesiol* 2000; **13**: 167–74.
49. Smith CE, Patel N. Hypothermia in adult trauma patients: anaesthetic considerations. Part II. Prevention and treatment. *Am J Anesthesiol* 1997; **24**: 29–36.
50. Otto KJ, Metzler MH. Rewarming from experimental hypothermia: comparison of heated aerosol inhalation, peritoneal lavage and pleural lavage. *Crit Care Med* 1988; **16**: 869–75.
51. Brunette DD, Biros M, Mlinek EJ *et al.* Internal cardiac massage and mediastinal irrigation in hypothermic cardiac arrest. *Am J Emerg Med* 1992; **10**: 32–4.
52. Gentilello LM, Jurkovic GJ, Stark MS *et al.* Is hypothermia in the victim of major trauma protective or harmful? *Ann Surg* 1997; **226**: 439–49.
53. Walpoth BH, Walpoth-Aslan BN, Mattle HP *et al.* Outcome of survivors of accidental deep hypothermia and circulatory arrest treated with extracorporeal blood warming. *N Engl J Med* 1997; **337**: 1500–5.

75

Electrical safety and injuries

Lester A H Critchley

Patients suffering from the consequences of electrocution and associated burns occasionally require intensive care unit (ICU) management. Patients and staff in the ICU are at risk of electrocution from faulty electrical equipment. The necessity of direct patient contact with electrical equipment increases this risk, and when therapy involves an invasive contact close to the heart, microshock is an additional hazard. Faulty electrical equipment can also result in power failures, fires and explosions. The use of mobile phones and related devices nearby patient equipment can lead to malfunctioning.

PHYSICAL CONCEPTS

Electricity is produced by the movement of negatively charged electrons. A potential difference or voltage, measured in volts (V), exists between two points if the number or density of electrons is greater at one point. When these points are connected by a conductor, the potential difference will cause electrons or an electric current (I), measured in amperes (A), to flow. Resistance (R), measured in ohms (O), opposes this flow of electrons. Resistance is low in a conductor, because electrons can move freely from atom to atom. However, resistance is high in an insulator as electrons are unable to move freely. Voltage, current and resistance are related by Ohm's law:

$$V = I \times R$$

When an electric current flows through a resistance, it dissipates energy as heat. The heating effect per second, or power, is measured in Joules (J)/s or Watts (W):

$$\text{Power} = V \times I = I^2 \times R$$

When a current flows in one direction, such as produced by a battery, it is called a direct current. Electricity to homes, hospitals and factories is supplied as an alternating current which flows back and forth at a frequency, i.e. cycles per second or hertz (Hz). Voltage and frequency specifications vary worldwide. This may cause problems when electrical equipment, designed to be used in one region, is used elsewhere. Voltage specifications range from 100 V (i.e. Japan) to 240 V (i.e. Australia), with 220 V being most commonly supplied (i.e. UK, most of Europe and Asia). The frequency most commonly supplied is 50 Hz. North America is a notable exception, where the specification is 110–120 V and 60 Hz.

A current flowing in a circuit produces electric and magnetic fields, which induce currents to flow in neighbouring circuits. When this results in a current flowing between the two circuits, it is called coupling. With capacitive coupling, high frequency currents are most easily passed, and the size of the current is greatest when the circuits are close. Inductive coupling can result from the strong magnetic fields produced by heavy duty electrical equipment, such as transformers, electric motors and magnetic resonance imaging machines. The most common problem associated with coupling is electrical interference or 'noise'. Monitoring equipment is designed to 'filter' out this noise. However, in certain circumstances, such as the use of high frequency surgical diathermy and magnetic resonance, sufficient amperage can be induced to cause microshock and burns.[1,2] Smaller electromagnetic fields emitted by hand-held devices, such as mobile phones, can affect the programming of microprocessors. Cases of patient equipment malfunctions have been reported.[3]

Static electricity has no free flow of electrons. Insulated objects can become highly charged, usually by repeated rubbing. The charge is dissipated by electrons jumping onto another neighbouring object of a different potential. 'Jumping' electrons ionise and heat the air through which they pass, causing a spark which may ignite an inflammable liquid or gas. Lightning is a type of static electrical discharge. Direct currents of 12 000–200 000 A and voltages in the millions are involved; however, flow lasts only a fraction of a second.[4]

PHYSIOLOGICAL CONSIDERATIONS

For a current to flow through the body, the body must complete a circuit. Usually this involves the current flowing from its source to ground through the body. The pathophysiological effects depend on the size of the current, and this depends on the voltage and electrical resistance of the body, most of which occurs in the skin. Dry skin has a resistance in excess of 100 000 O.[5] However, skin resistance is markedly reduced (to 1000 O)[6] if the skin is wet, or if a conductive jelly has been applied. Hence, from

Ohm's law, dry skin in contact with 240 V mains supply will result in a harmless 0.24 mA current flowing through the body, whereas moist or wet skin will result in a potentially lethal 240 mA current.

ELECTROCUTION

Most cases of electrocution occur in the workplace (about 60%) or at home (about 30%), where misuse of extension cables is the main culprit.[6] Pathophysiological processes involved in true electrical injuries are poorly understood. The extent of injury depends on (i) the amount of current that passes through the body, (ii) the duration of the current, and (iii) the tissues traversed by the current (Table 75.1).

The extent of injury is most directly related to amperage. However, usually only the voltage involved is known. In general, lower voltages cause less injury, although voltages as low as 50 V have caused fatalities. An electric current passing through the body produces these main effects.

TISSUE HEAT INJURY

Currents in excess of 1 A generate sufficient heat energy to cause burns to the skin and occult thermal injury to internal tissues and organs. Blood vessels and nervous tissue appear to be particularly susceptible.[6]

DEPOLARISATION OF MUSCLE CELLS

An alternating current of 30–200 mA will cause ventricular fibrillation.[7] Currents in excess of 5 A cause sustained cardiac asystole, which is the principle used in defibrillation. Apart from ventricular fibrillation, other arrhythmias may occur. Myocardial damage is common and may result in ST and T-wave changes. Global left ventricular dysfunction may occur hours or days later, despite initial minimal ECG changes.[8,9] Myocardial infarction has also been reported.[10] Specific markers of myocardial injury, such as cardiac troponin, should be checked in all suspected cases of electrical injury to the heart.[11]

Tetanic contractions of skeletal muscle occur with currents in excess of 15–20 mA. The threshold is particularly low with alternating currents at the household frequency of 50–60 Hz. Tetanic contraction will prevent voluntary release of the source of electrocution, and violent muscle contractions may cause fractures of long bones and spinal vertebrae.[6]

Table 75.1 Origin and pathophysiological effects of different levels of electrical injury

Current (A)	Source	Effects on victim
10–100 μA	Earth leakage	Microshock (ventricular fibrillation)
300–400 μA	Faulty equipment	Tingling (harmless)
> 1 mA	Faulty equipment	Pain (withdraw)
> 10 mA	Faulty equipment	Tetany (cannot let go)
> 100 mA	Faulty equipment	Macroshock (ventricular fibrillation)
> 1 A	Faulty equipment	Burns and tissue damage
> 1000 A	High tension injury	Severe burns and loss of limbs
> 12 000 A	Lightning	Coma, severe burns and loss of limbs

VASCULAR INJURIES

Blood vessels may become thrombosed and occluded as a result of the thermal injury. Compartment syndromes are seen secondary to tissue oedema, causing tissue ischaemia and necrosis. Affected limbs may even require amputation.[12]

NEUROLOGICAL INJURIES

Neurological injuries may be central or peripheral, and immediate or late in onset. Monoparesis may occur in affected limbs, and the median nerve is particularly vulnerable.[6,13] Electrocution to the head may result in unconsciousness, paralysis of the respiratory centre, and late complications such as epilepsy, encephalopathy and parkinsonism.[6,13] Spinal cord damage resulting in para- or tetraplegia can result from a current traversing both arms.[6,13] Autonomic dysfunction may also occur, causing acute vasospasm or a late sympathetic dystrophy.[6]

RENAL FAILURE

Acute renal failure may result from the myoglobinuria and toxins produced by extensive muscle necrosis.[13]

OTHER INJURIES

Electrocution can cause the victim to fall or be thrown, and clothing to catch fire, resulting in associated injuries. High voltage injuries can rupture the eardrum.[14] Cataracts may later develop.[13]

MICROSHOCK

The above domestic/industrial electrocution is known as macroshock, when current flowing through the intact skin and body passes through the heart. In the ICU, potential microshock electrocution exists. Microshock occurs when there is a direct current path to the heart muscle. The pathway may be provided by a saline-filled

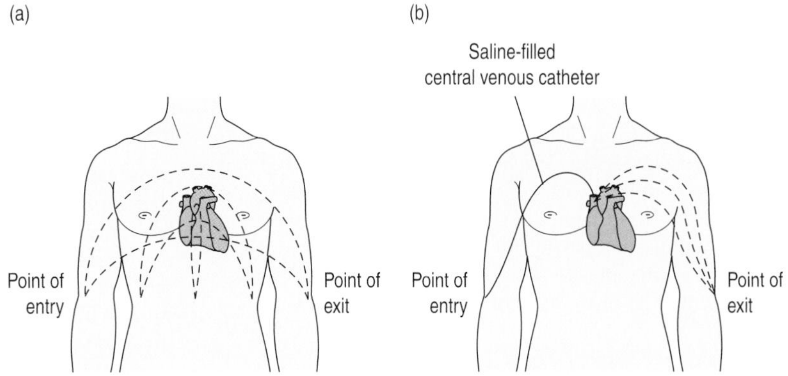

Figure 75.1 Microshock: (a) low current density at the heart; (b) high current density at the heart if there is a conducting pathway, such as a saline–filled catheter.

monitoring catheter, pulmonary artery catheter, or transvenous pacemaker wires. The current required to produce ventricular fibrillation in microshock is extremely small, in the order of 60 mA.[15] Currents of 1–2 mA are barely perceptible and produce tingling of the skin (Table 75.1). Hence a lethal microshock may be transmitted to a patient via a staff member who is unaware of the conducted current. Microshock can result from direct contact with faulty electrical equipment, stray currents from capacitive coupling or earth leakage. Such small currents are potentially lethal because a high current density is produced at the heart (Figure 75.1).

HIGH TENSION AND LIGHTNING INJURIES

High tension electricity (> 1000 V) involves voltage much greater than domestic supply, usually many thousands of volts. Tissue damage is mainly due to the generation of heat, as high amperage currents are involved. Witnesses have described tissues actually exploding.[16]

Lightning injury is a type of high tension injury. It is rare and its incidence depends upon geographic location. Victims can be thrown several feet as a result of violent muscular contractions. Electrical arcing of the air causes intense heat, resulting in superficial burns and clothes igniting. Characteristic entrance and exit site burns are seen, which have a spider-like appearance with redness and blistering. Victims are usually unconscious in the initial phase. However, many victims survive,[4] and good recovery has been reported despite initial hopeless neurological responsiveness (e.g. fixed dilated pupils).[17] Immediate death usually results from cardiorespiratory arrest; asystole is more common than ventricular fibrillation.[4]

MANAGEMENT OF ELECTRICAL INJURIES

Treatment of electrical injuries is mainly supportive and includes the following.

FIRST AID AND RESUSCITATION

It is imperative to make the immediate environment safe for rescuers. Power sources should be switched off and wet areas avoided where possible. Instinctive attempts to grab the electrocuted victim must be avoided until it is safe to do so. Cardiopulmonary resuscitation is carried out when indicated, and continued even if the prognosis seems hopeless. The neck and spine should be protected from possible fractures.

INVESTIGATIONS

Investigations are indicated to detect damaged organs. They include ECG, echocardiography, CT of the head, EEG, X-rays of the spine and long bones, haemoglobin, serum electrolytes, creatine kinase and urine myoglobin to assess muscle damage, and nerve conduction studies. Arteriograms may help in the decision to amputate a limb.[12]

HOSPITAL AND ICU MANAGEMENT

Management is directed towards treatment of burns, ischaemic and necrotic tissue, and injured organs. The principle of treating electrical burns is complete excision because of the risks of acute renal failure and sepsis. Fasciotomies and amputations may be necessary. Tetanus toxoid and antibiotics, especially penicillin, are given if indicated.

ELECTRICAL HAZARDS IN ICU

The ICU has the potential to inflict both macroshock and microshock injuries to staff and patients. Potential sources of these electrical hazards are as follows.

MAJOR ELECTRICAL FAULTS

The casing and insulated wiring of electrical equipment protect against electric shock. Faulty wiring or components, and deterioration of internal insulation, can result in the casing becoming ‘live’. Contact with live casing or wires can result in an electric current flowing through the victim to ground. The outcome largely depends on the resistance offered by the body to the current. If it is low, such as in a wet environment, sufficient current can flow to cause death.

MICROSHOCK CURRENTS

EARTH LEAKAGE CURRENTS

Within all pieces of electrical equipment, stray low amperage electrical currents exist that usually flow to earth, called earth leakage currents. They originate from current leaks across imperfect insulation of wires, capacitive and inductive coupling within the equipment, and coupling from electric and magnetic fields that exist in the working environment, such as the 50–60 Hz mains supply. Normally these currents are small and harmless, but they have the potential to cause microshock.

PACING WIRES AND CENTRAL VENOUS LINES

In certain circumstances, sufficient current to cause microshock can be passed by capacitive and inductive coupling to intracardiac pacing wires and central venous lines. Ventricular fibrillation has resulted from capacitive coupling with thermistor wires in a pulmonary artery catheter.[1]

DIFFERENT EARTH POTENTIALS

Inadequate or faulty earthing can result in separate earthing points being at different resting potentials. If contact is made between the two earthing points, sufficient current can flow to cause microshock.

STAFF–PATIENT CONTACT

Small currents capable of causing microshock can be transmitted unknowingly to a patient by a staff member who simultaneously touches faulty electrical equipment and the patient. If this current returns to earth via an intracardiac connection, a high current density will pass through the heart resulting in microshock.

INDUCTIVE CURRENTS

Inductive coupling from the strong magnetic fields produced by magnetic resonance imaging can cause overheating of wires and equipment. Severe burns have resulted from the use of pulse oximetry during magnetic resonance imaging, and specially designed wiring and probes are recommended.[2] Similar problems can exist with any intravascular device containing wires, such as a pulmonary artery catheter. More recently, problems have arisen from the interference caused by personal computers, mobile phones and related devices with patient equipment. Many hospitals have banned the use of such devices in areas where patients are treated.

OTHER RELATED HAZARDS

Electrical equipment has the potential to cause other hazards such as thermal injury, fires and power failures. Preliminary critical incident reports suggest that power failures are the most commonly encountered incidents involving electricity in the ICU. Power failures can be disastrous, as many patients' lives depend on electrically driven 'life support' equipment. Because of frequent work outside the ICU, the intensivist should also be aware of potential electrical hazards outside ICU.

ELECTRICAL SAFETY STANDARDS

Most Western countries have standards of electrical safety that apply to the use of medical equipment. For example, Australian Standards (AS 3003 and AS 3200) set minimum requirements for Australian hospitals. AS 2500 covers the safe use of electricity in patient care areas.[18] Britain and Europe follow the International Electrotechnical Commission Code[19,20] and the USA follows the National Electric Code 1993.[21] These standards have not changed significantly over the last few decades and are now easily accessible on the internet. Hospitals should establish their own committees to ensure that adequate standards are applied. However, patient care areas differ in their safety requirements and commonly used classifications are listed below. The ICU should conform to (1b) and preferably (1c).

1. (a) *Unprotected areas*, where only routine electrical safety standards are applied.
   (b) *Body protected areas*, where the level of electrical safety is sufficient to minimise the risk of macroshock when the patient is in direct contact with electrical equipment and the skin impedance is reduced or bypassed.
   (c) *Cardiac protected areas*, where the level of electrical safety is sufficient to minimise the risk of direct microshock to the heart.
2. *Wet locations*, where spillage of water and physiological solutions, such as saline and blood, frequently occurs.
3. Until recently, standards existed for the safe use of inflammable anaesthetics agents.

MEASURES TO PROTECT STAFF AND PATIENTS[22,23]

EARTHING, FUSES AND CIRCUIT BREAKERS

Earthing reduces the risk of macroshock. The casing in most electrical equipment is connected to ground by a very low resistance wire. If a fault arises, the earth wire offers a low resistance path to ground. The high amperage current that results will blow the main fuse or circuit breaker, thus warning that a fault is present. Additional protection can be achieved by connecting all the earthing points in a patient care area together by a very low resistance wire. This reduces the risk of microshock occurring from earthing points at different potentials, and is commonly used in cardiac protected areas.

POWER SUPPLY ISOLATION

MAINS ISOLATION

The power supply is isolated from earth using a mains isolation transformer. If contact is made with live faulty circuitry, the risk of electric shock is reduced because stray currents no longer preferentially flow through patient or staff member to earth. Presence of stray earth leakage currents can be detected by using a line isolation monitor. This type of system is particularly useful in wet locations where the body may offer a very low resistance to earth.

INTERNAL ISOLATION

The mains power supply is isolated from the patient connection by using transformers and photoelectric diodes. The casing is still earthed to protect against faulty circuitry. This method of protection is commonly used in ICU equipment.

EARTH LEAKAGE CIRCUIT BREAKERS

These are devices that switch off the electrical supply if small currents are detected flowing to earth. They can be used to protect against microshock. A major disadvantage is that power supply to essential life-supporting equipment is switched off.

EQUIPMENT CHECKS

The purchase of new equipment should be strictly controlled, and circuit diagrams should be provided. All new equipment should be checked for function and current leaks before use in the ICU. Preventative maintenance of equipment should be done regularly. Dated stickers should be used to show when the equipment was last checked. All faulty equipment must be removed from service, labelled appropriately, and recommissioned only after thorough checking.

RESERVE POWER SUPPLIES AND ALARMS

All essential equipment should have a reserve power supply (usually a battery) and alarms that warn of power failure. All hospitals should provide an emergency back-up power supply in case of power cuts.

PERSONNEL EDUCATION

Staff should be taught correct ways to handle electrical equipment. Equipment with frayed wires should never be used, plugs should never be tugged, trolleys should never be wheeled over power cords, and two pieces of equipment should never be handled simultaneously. Staff should also respond appropriately to alarms.

REFERENCES

1. McNulty SE, Cooper M, Staudt S. Transmitted radiofrequency current through a flow directed pulmonary artery catheter. *Anesth Analg* 1994; **78**: 587–9.
2. Peden CJ, Menon DK, Hall AS *et al.* Magnetic resonance for the anaesthetist. *Anaesthesia* 1992; **47**: 508–17.
3. Hayes DL, Carrillo RG, Findlay GK *et al.* State of the science: pacemaker and defibrillator interference from wireless communication devices. *Pacing Clin Electrophysiol* 1996; **19**: 1407–9.
4. Apfelberg DB, Masters FW, Robinson DW. Pathophysiology and treatment of lightning injuries. *J Trauma* 1974; **14**: 453–60.
5. Bruner JMR. Hazards of electrical apparatus. *Anesthesiology* 1976; **28**: 396–424.
6. Fontneau NM, Mitchell A. Miscellaneous neurologic problems in the intensive care unit. In: Irwin RS, Cerra FB, Rippe JM (eds) *Intensive Care Medicine*, 4th edn. Philadelphia: Lippincott-Raven; 1999: 2127–35.
7. Loughman J, Watson AB. Electrical safety in hospitals and proposed standards. *Med J Aust* 1971; **2**: 349–55.
8. Lewin RF, Arditti A, Sclarovsky S. Non-invasive evaluation of cardiac injury. *Br Heart J* 1983; **49**: 190–2.
9. Jensen PJ, Thomsem PEB, Bagger JP *et al.* Electrical injury causing ventricular arrhythmias. *Br Heart J* 1987; **57**: 279–83.
10. Walton AS, Harper RW, Coggins GL. Myocardial infarction after electrocution. *Med J Aust* 1988; **148**: 365–7.
11. Karras DJ, Kane DL. Serum markers in the emergency department diagnosis of acute myocardial infarction. *Emerg Med Clin North Am* 2001; **19**: 321–37.
12. Hunt JL, McManus WF, Haney WP *et al.* Vascular lesions in acute electric injuries. *J Trauma* 1974; **14**: 461–73.
13. Solem L, Fischer RP, Strate RG. The natural history of electrical injury. *J Trauma* 1977; **17**: 487–92.
14. Ogren FP, Edmunds AL. Neuro-otologic findings in the lightning-injured patient. *Semin Neurol* 1995; **15**: 256–62.
15. Watson AB, Wright JS, Loughman J. Electrical thresholds for ventricular fibrillation in man. *Med J Aust* 1973; **1**: 1179–82.
16. Burke JF, Quinby WC, Bondoc C *et al.* Patterns of high tension electric injury in children and adolescents and their management. *Am J Surg* 1977; **133**: 492–4.
17. Hanson GC, McIlwaith GR. Lightning injury: two case histories and a review of management. *Br Med J* 1973; **4**: 271–4.
18. Australian Standard 2500. *Guide to the Safe Use of Electricity in Patient Care.* Sydney: Standards Association of Australia; 1988.
19. CEI-IEC 601-1&2. *Medical Electrical Equipment*, 2nd edn. Geneva: International Electrotechnical Commission; 1988.
20. Herrmann D. A preview of IEC safety requirements for programmable electronic medical systems. *Med Dev Diag Indust* 1995; **17**: 106–11.
21. Early MW, Murray RH, Caloggero JM. *National Electrical Code Handbook*, 6th edn. Quincy: National Fire Protection Association; 1993.
22. Litt L, Ehrenwerth J. Electrical safety in the operating room: important old wine, disguised new bottles. *Anesth Analg* 1994; **78**: 417–19.
23. Ehrenwerth J. *Electrical Safety in and around the Operating Room.* ASA Refresher Course in Anesthesia. Philadelphia: JB Lippincott; 1994: 123.

76

Envenomation

James Tibballs

Envenomation by species of snakes, spiders, ticks, bees, ants, wasps, jellyfish, octopuses or cone shell snails may threaten life, while envenomation by other creatures may cause serious illness.[1] Although this chapter focuses on Australia, the principles of management are widely applicable elsewhere except for stings by scorpions which are not a significant health problem in Australia. Immediate advice on management may be obtained from the Australian Venom Research Unit (AVRU) advisory service on their 24-hour telephone number within Australia on 1300 760 451, from overseas on 61 3 8344 7753 or from their website at http://www.avru.org.

SNAKES

EPIDEMIOLOGY

Australia is habitat to a large number of venomous terrestrial and marine snakes (Families Elapidae and Hydrophiidae). The genera responsible for the majority of serious illness are Brown Snakes (*Pseudonaja*), Tiger Snakes (*Notechis*), Taipans (*Oxyuranus*), Black Snakes (*Pseudechis*) and Death Adders (*Acanthophis*).

The mean death rate in Australia from 1981 to 1999 was 2.6 per year[1] (~0.014/100 000), usually occurring because of massive envenomation, snake bite in remote locations, rapid collapse, or due to delayed or inadequate antivenom therapy. However, as many as 2000 people are bitten each year and of these at least 300 require antivenom treatment. This morbidity and mortality is far less than that observed in surrounding countries. Death and critical illness is due to (1) progressive paralysis leading to respiratory failure, (2) bleeding, or (3) renal failure occurring as a complication of rhabdomyolysis, disseminated intravascular coagulation (DIC), haemorrhage, haemolysis or to their combinations. Rapid collapse within minutes after a snake bite is due to anaphylaxis to venom or possibly due to the myocardial effects of DIC causing hypotension.

Snake bite is often 'accidental' when a snake is trodden upon or suddenly disturbed. However, many bites occur when humans deliberately interfere with snakes or handle them. The herpetologist or snake collector is at special risk. Not only do they invariably sustain bites in the course of their work[2] or hobby, but they are also at risk of developing allergic reactions to venoms and to the antivenoms used in their treatment. Contact with exotic snakes has additional problems.

SNAKE VENOMS

Venoms are complex mixtures of toxins, usually proteins, which kill the snake's prey and aid its digestion. Many are phospholipases. The main toxins cause paralysis, coagulopathy, rhabdomyolysis and haemolysis (Table 76.1). Coagulopathy may be due to a procoagulant effect by prothrombin activators (Factor Xa-like enzymes), with consumption of clotting factors, or due to a direct anticoagulant effect.

SNAKE BITE AND ENVENOMATION

Although a bite may be observed, envenomation is less common because no venom or a variable amount of venom is injected. Bites are relatively painless and may be unnoticed. This is in marked contrast to many overseas crotalid and viperid snakes, where massive local reaction and necrosis are often a major feature as a result of proteolytic enzymes. Paired fang marks are usually evident but sometimes only scratches or single puncture wounds are found. In general, Australian snake venoms do not cause extensive damage to local tissues and are usually confined to mild swelling and bruising, and continued slight bleeding from the bite site.

SYMPTOMS AND SIGNS OF ENVENOMATION

Not all possible symptoms and signs occur in a particular case: in some cases, one symptom or sign may dominate the clinical picture, and in other cases they may wax and wane (Table 76.2). These phenomena are explained by variations in toxin content of venoms of the same species in different geographical areas, and by variable absorption of different toxins.

The cause of transient hypotension soon after envenomation is obscure but it may be related to intravascular coagulation.[3,4] Prothrombin activators gain access to the circulation within a number of minutes after subcutaneous injection. There is often tachycardia and relatively minor ECG abnormalities. Other causes of hypotension such as direct cardiac toxicity remain unproven. Hypotension may be secondary to myocardial hypoxaemia.

Table 76.1 Main components of Australian snake venoms

Neurotoxins
Presynaptic and postsynaptic neuromuscular blockers present in all dangerous venomous snakes. May cause paralysis
Postsynaptic blockers readily reversed by antivenom
Presynaptic blockers are more difficult to reverse, particularly if treatment is delayed
Some presynaptic blockers are also rhabdomyolysins
Prothrombin activators
Present in many important species
Cause disseminated intravascular coagulation with consumption of clotting factors including fibrinogen
Intrinsic fibrin(ogen)lysis generates fibrin(ogen) degradation products
Significant risk of haemorrhage
Anticoagulants
Present in a relatively small number of dangerous species
Prevent blood clotting without consumption of clotting factors
Rhabdomyolysins
Some presynaptic neurotoxins also cause lysis of skeletal and cardiac muscle
Apart from loss muscle of mass, may cause myoglobinuria and renal failure
Haemolysins
Present in a few species
Rarely a serious clinical effect

Table 76.2 Progressive onset of major systemic symptoms and signs of untreated envenomation (in massive envenomation or in a child, a critical illness may develop in minutes rather than hours)

< 1 hour after bite
Headache
Nausea, vomiting, abdominal pain
Transient hypotension associated with confusion or loss of consciousness
Coagulopathy (laboratory testing)
Regional lymphadenitis
1–3 hours after bite
Paresis/paralysis of cranial nerves, e.g. ptosis, double vision, external ophthalmoplegia, dysphonia, dysphagia, myopathic facies
Haemorrhage from mucosal surfaces and needle punctures
Tachycardia, hypotension
Tachypnoea, shallow tidal volume
> 3 hours after bite
Paresis/paralysis of truncal and limb muscles
Paresis/paralysis of respiratory muscles (respiratory failure)
Peripheral circulatory failure (shock), hypoxaemia, cyanosis
Rhabdomyolysis
Dark urine (due to myoglobinuria or haemoglobin)
Renal failure

Tender or even painful regional lymph nodes are moderately common but are not per se an indication for antivenom therapy, since lymphadenitis also occurs with bites by mildly venomous snakes which do not cause serious systemic illness.

Occasionally intracranial haemorrhage occurs. In the case of untreated or massive envenomation, rhabdomyolysis may occur. This usually involves all skeletal musculature and sometimes cardiac muscle. The resultant myoglobinuria may cause renal failure. Direct nephrotoxicity has been suspected in a few cases of Brown Snake bites, but is as yet unproven.

A high intake of alcohol by adults before snake bite is common, and may make management quite difficult initially. Pre-existing treatment (e.g. warfarin therapy) or disease (e.g. gastrointestinal tract ulceration) may complicate management of coagulopathy.

SNAKE BITE IN CHILDREN

Snake bite in young children presents additional problems. It is difficult to diagnose when a bite has not been observed. The symptoms of early envenomation may pass unsuspected and the signs, particularly cranial nerve effects, are difficult to elicit. Bite marks may be difficult to distinguish from the effects of everyday minor trauma. Lastly, the onset of the syndrome of envenomation is likely to be more rapid than in adults and the severity of envenomation more acute because of the relatively higher ratio of venom to body mass. Presentation may be cardiorespiratory failure.

IDENTIFICATION OF THE SNAKE

Identification of the snake guides selection of the appropriate antivenom, and provides an insight into the expected syndrome. Administration of the wrong antivenom may endanger the victim's life because there may be very little neutralisation of venom. A venom detection kit can be used to identify the snake venom. If the snake cannot be identified, a specific antivenom, or a combination of monovalent antivenoms or polyvalent antivenom should be administered on a geographical basis (see Tables 76.3 and 76.4).

IDENTIFICATION BY VENOM DETECTION KIT TEST

The venom detection kit (VDK) is an in vitro test for detection and identification of snake venom at the bite site, in urine, blood or other tissue in cases of snake bite in Australia and Papua New Guinea. It is an enzyme immunoassay using rabbit antibodies and chromogen and peroxide solutions. A positive result will indicate the type of antivenom to be administered. It detects venom from a range of snake genera including Tiger, Brown, Black, Death Adder and Taipan. Individual species of snake cannot be identified by the test and several genera may yield a positive result in a specified well. The incidences of false-positive and false-negative tests of the kit remain unknown, but are generally regarded as low. The test is

Table 76.3 Antivenom and initial dosages when snake identified

Snake	Antivenom	Dose (units)
Common Brown Snake	Brown Snake	4000
Chappell Island Tiger Snake	Tiger Snake	12 000
Copperheads	Tiger Snake	3000–6000
Death Adders	Death Adder	6000
Dugite	Brown Snake	4000
Gwardar	Brown Snake	4000
Mulga (King Brown) Snake	Black Snake	18 000
Papuan Black Snake	Black Snake	18 000
Red-bellied Black Snake	Tiger Snake *or* Black Snake*	3000 18 000
Rough-scaled (Clarence River) Snake	Tiger Snake	3000
Sea-Snakes	Sea-Snake *or* Tiger Snake	1000 3000
Small-scaled (Fierce) Snake	Taipan	12 000
Taipans	Taipan	12 000
Tasmanian Tiger Snake	Tiger Snake	6000
Tiger Snake	Tiger Snake	3000

*Smaller protein mass Tiger Snake antivenom preferable. Antivenom units per vial: Brown Snake 1000; Tiger Snake 3000; Black Snake 18 000; Taipan 12 000; Death Adder 6000; polyvalent 40 000.
Note: (1) If the victim on presentation is critically ill, 2–3 times these amounts should be given initially; (2) additional antivenom may be required in the course of management since absorption of venom may be delayed.

Table 76.4 Antivenom and initial dosages when identity of snake uncertain

State	Antivenom	Dose (units)
Tasmania	Tiger Snake	6000
Victoria	Tiger Snake *and* Brown Snake	3000 4000
New South Wales and ACT; Queensland; South Australia; Western Australia; Northern Territory	Polyvalent	40 000
Papua New Guinea	Polyvalent	40 000

Note: (1) If the victim on presentation is critically ill, 2–3 times these amounts should be given initially; (2) additional antivenom may be required in the course of management since absorption of venom may be delayed.

very sensitive, able to detect venom in concentrations as low as 10 ng/ml, and can yield a visual qualitative result in test wells in approximately 25 minutes. On occasion, a positive test may be present but the patient is asymptomatic. A decision to administer antivenom should be made on clinical grounds. A very high concentration of venom in a sample may overwhelm the test and yield a spuriously negative result (Hook effect). If that possibility exists, a diluted sample should be re-tested.

IDENTIFICATION BY PHYSICAL CHARACTERISTICS

This can be misleading. Non-herpetologists should consult an identification guide[1] with reference to scale patterns to identify a specimen correctly if antivenom therapy is to be based on morphological characteristics alone.

IDENTIFICATION BY CLINICAL EFFECTS

The appearance of a bite site cannot be used to reliably identify the snake.

The constellation of symptoms and signs may be used to a limited degree in identification. For example, within the common genera, paralysis associated with procoagulopathy may be caused by a Tiger Snake, Taipan, Brown Snake, Rough-scaled Snake, *Hoplocephalus* spp. or Red-bellied Black Snake, but if rhabdomyolysis also occurs, a bite by a Brown Snake is improbable. Paralysis associated with anticoagulation may be caused by a Black Snake (other than a Red-bellied Black Snake), Copperhead or Death Adder, but if rhabdomyolysis occurs, a bite by a Death Adder is improbable. Paralysis with neither coagulopathy nor rhabdomyolysis may be caused by a Death Adder bite.

This information is of limited practical importance. It is essential to administer antivenom at the first opportunity when indicated, rather than wait until the full syndrome becomes apparent to enable an 'educated clinical guess' in selection of the appropriate antivenom.

MANAGEMENT OF SNAKE ENVENOMATION

The essentials of management are:

- resuscitation: mechanical ventilation and restoration of blood pressure with intravenous fluids, inotropic and vasoactive agents as needed
- application of a pressure-immobilisation first-aid bandage
- administration of antivenom
- performance of investigations

From a practical point of view, one of three clinical situations arises after snake bite. A plan of management for each of these is summarised in Figure 76.1.

- Victim presents with a critical illness
- Victim envenomated but not critically ill
- Victim bitten but does not appear envenomated

When the envenomated victim is not critically ill, more time is available to identify the snake by investigations

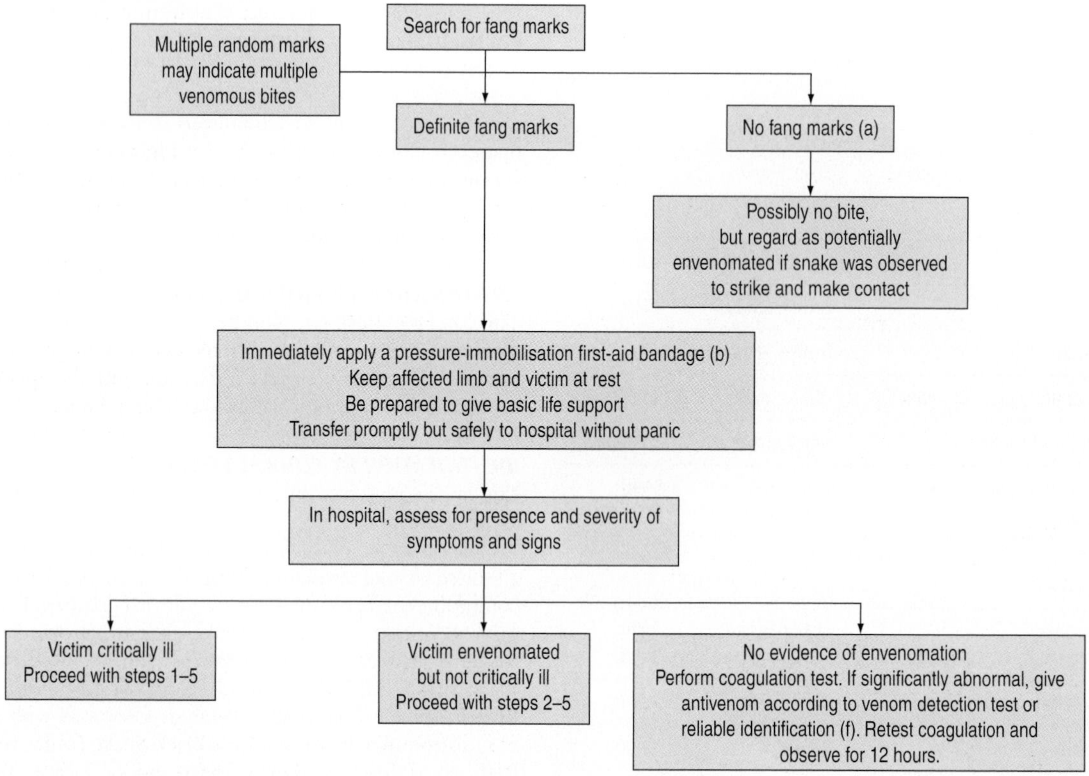

1. Resuscitate (treat hypoxaemia and shock)
   Be prepared to intubate and mechanically ventilate. Admit to intensive care.
2. Apply pressure-immobilisation bandage. Do not remove if already applied [b]
3. Give antivenom intravenously [c,d,e,f,g]
   - Give monovalent if species reliably known or appropriate antivenom indicated by venom detection test.
   - In critically ill victim, don't wait for venom detection test result or if species cannot be determined; give according to geographic location:
     Victoria – Brown and Tiger Snake
     Tasmania – Tiger Snake
     Other states and territories – polyvalent
   - Titrate antivenom against clinical and coagulation status (NOTE: Death Adders don't cause significant coagulopathy).
4. Perform investigations
   - Bite swab for venom detection. (First-aid bandage may be cut to expose bite site, and then reinforced)
   - Blood for venom detection, coagulation, type and crossmatch blood (if bleeding), fibrin degradation products, full blood examination, enzymes, electrolytes, urea, creatinine
   - Urine for venom detection, red blood cells, haemoglobin, myoglobin.
5. Examine frequently to detect slow onset of paralysis [h], coagulopathy, rhabdomyolysis and renal failure.

Dangers and mistakes in management

a. Fang marks not visible to naked eye.
b. Premature release of bandage may result in sudden systemic envenomation. Leave in situ until victim reaches full medical facilities. If clinically envenomated, remove only after antivenom given.
c. Erroneous identification of snake may cause wrong antivenom to be given. If in any doubt treat as unidentified.
d. Antivenom without premedication. Anaphylaxis is not rare and may not respond to treatment.
e. Insufficient antivenom. Titrate dose against clinical and coagulation status.
f. Blood and coagulation factors (fresh frozen plasma, cryoprecipitate) not preceded by antivenom will worsen coagulopathy.
g. Antivenom given without clinical or laboratory evidence of envenomation.
h. Delayed onset of paralysis may be missed. Victim must be examined at least hourly.

Figure 76.1 Management of snake bite.

and to administer specific monovalent antivenom. A pressure-immobilisation bandage should be applied if not already in place, and not removed until antivenom has been administered.

When the victim has been bitten, but not apparently envenomated, admission to hospital is advisable with observation and examination hourly for at least 12 hours in the case of a child but less time for an adult. The syndrome of envenomation may be very slow in onset over numerous hours with an initial period free of symptoms. A test of coagulation should always be performed. If a coagulopathy is present, specific monovalent antivenom should be administered after identification of the species or as indicated by a VDK test. If only a mild coagulopathy is present it may be acceptable to withhold antivenom in the anticipation of spontaneous resolution but coagulation should be checked at intervals and the victim maintained under surveillance until coagulation is normal.

THE PRESSURE-IMMOBILISATION TECHNIQUE OF FIRST AID

Since at least 95% of snake bites occur on the arms or legs,[1] Sutherland's first-aid pressure-immobilisation technique[5] is applicable to the majority of cases. With this technique, a crêpe (or crêpe-like) bandage is applied from the fingers or toes up the limb as far as possible, encompassing the bite site. It should be as firm as required for a sprained ankle. Additional immobilisation is applied to the entire limb by a rigid splint, with the aim of immobilising the joints either side of the bite site.

Venom is usually deposited subcutaneously. The systemic spread of venom is largely dependent on its absorption by way of the lymphatics[6] or the small blood vessels. Application of a pressure less than arterial to the bitten area when combined with immobilisation of the limb effectively delays the movement of venom to the central circulation.[5] Although it is a first-aid technique designed for use in the field, it should be part of initial management in hospital since it halts further absorption of venom. There is some experimental[1] and anecdotal[7] evidence with Death Adder bites that the technique inactivates some venom at the bite site but prolonged application has not been subjected to a controlled study.

Removal of the pressure-immobilisation bandage

Removal may precipitate a sudden elevation in blood concentration of venom and collapse of the victim. On the other hand, first aid has not been proven to inactivate venom in humans. Its removal therefore should be dictated by the circumstance. When an asymptomatic snake-bite victim reaches hospital with the recommended first-aid measures in place, these should not be disturbed until antivenom, appropriate staff and equipment have been assembled. If the victim is symptomatic and antivenom is indicated, the first-aid measures should not be removed until after antivenom has been administered, and reapplied if the victim's condition deteriorates. A swab of the bite site may be obtained by removing the splint temporarily and then cutting a window in the bandage. Thereafter the bandage should be made good and the splint reapplied.

ANTIVENOM

CSL Ltd (Parkville, Australia) produces highly purified equine monovalent antivenoms against the venoms of the main terrestrial snakes, including Tiger Snake, Brown Snake, Black Snake, Death Adder and Taipan. A polyvalent antivenom – a mixture of aliquots of all these – is also available. A sea-snake antivenom is also produced from horses immunised with Beaked Sea-Snake (*Enhydrina schistosa*) and Tiger Snake venom.

Antivenom should be administered according to the identity of the snake or, if unknown or doubtful, according to the result of a VDK test (Table 76.3). If neither of these criteria can be fulfilled, and if the situation warrants immediate antivenom therapy, the geographical location may be used a guide, since the distribution of many species is known (Table 76.4). Polyvalent antivenom should not be used when a monovalent antivenom could be used appropriately. For bites by uncommon snakes, when antivenom is indicated, polyvalent antivenom, or a monovalent antivenom as indicated by a VDK test, should be chosen.

Dose

One vial of specific antivenom neutralises in vitro the average yield on 'milking' – a process whereby venom is harvested by inducing the snake to bite through a latex membrane. If the amount of venom injected at a bite is greater than the average yield on milking, one vial of antivenom will not be adequate therapy. In severe cases of envenomation, a number of vials of antivenom will need to be administered. Absorption of venom from a bite site(s) is a continuing process.

The initial doses of antivenom are given in Tables 76.3 and 76.4. The need for subsequent doses should be guided by the clinical response. After bites by species with coagulopathic effects the victim's coagulation status is a useful guide.

The dose of antivenom required varies because the amount of venom injected cannot be determined, and snakes may bite multiple times. Victims may present late after envenomation when toxins have already become bound to target tissues and cannot be easily neutralised. Some victims in this circumstance have required mechanical ventilation for many weeks despite large amounts of appropriate antivenom. A child requires more antivenom than an adult envenomated by the same amount of venom, and a victim in poor general health will likewise require more. Finally, antivenoms are manufactured against specific species and may have less neutralising ability against different species of the same genus or against unrelated species, even when the antivenom chosen is nonetheless appropriate.

Administration

The decision to administer antivenom must be based on clinical criteria of envenomation, not restricted to the result of a VDK test. A positive VDK test establishes the diagnosis of envenomation and the choice of antivenom, but does not imply that antivenom should or should not be given.

However, if the victim is significantly envenomated, antivenom must be administered since there is no other effective treatment. Antivenom may be withheld if envenomation is so mild that spontaneous recovery may occur or the consequences of antivenom administration are likely to outweigh the benefit to be gained, e.g. in a herpetologist known to have allergy to antivenom.

Snake antivenoms must be given by the intravenous route, or in dire circumstances if a vein cannot be cannulated, by the intraosseous route in a child. The large volume of fluid and slow absorption render the intramuscular route useless in emergencies.

A test dose of antivenom to determine allergy should not be done. It is unreliable and a waste of precious time.

Premedication

Antivenom should be preceded by premedication with subcutaneous adrenaline (epinephrine), approximately 0.25 mg for an adult and 0.005–0.01 mg/kg for a child, at least 5–10 minutes before commencement of infusion. In the moribund or critically ill victim, when it is essential to administer antivenom quickly, the epinephrine may be given intramuscularly or even intravenously in smaller doses. However, in general, epinephrine is not recommended by either of those routes because of the risk of intracerebral haemorrhage due to the combination of possible hypertension and coagulopathy. Although intracerebral haemorrhage has been recorded in the past in association with premedication, all such cases were accompanied by intravenous epinephrine, none with subcutaneous epinephrine. On the other hand, the incidence of adverse reactions (8–13%) to antivenom is sufficient to warrant premedication with epinephrine, which is the only medication proven effective in reducing the incidence of antivenom-induced reactions and their severity.[8]

It is not prudent to forgo premedication and elect to treat anaphylaxis if it occurs. Iatrogenic anaphylaxis has a high mortality despite vigorous and expert resuscitation.[9] If an adverse reaction to the first vial of antivenom has not occurred, subsequent vials do not need to be preceded by epinephrine. The reaction rate to polyvalent antivenom is higher than to monovalent antivenoms and should not be used when a monovalent antivenom or combinations will suffice.

The antihistamine, promethazine, is ineffective in this setting[10] and may cause obtundation and hypotension, both of which may exacerbate and confound a state of envenomation. It is not recommended. Other drugs such as steroids and aminophylline are also not useful in preventing anaphylaxis because their actions, apart from being unproven, are too slow in onset, but steroids are useful for preventing serum sickness.

Infusion

The antivenom may be injected slowly into a running intravenous line or diluted in Hartmann's or other crystalloid solution in approximately 1 in 10 volumes in a burette and administered over 15–30 minutes if the situation is not critical. This measure reduces the risk of an anaphylactoid reaction resulting from its binding with complement. For small children, if multiple vials are required, the dilution may be less to prevent excessive fluid administration. In emergencies the antivenom may be infused quickly in high concentration.

Adverse reactions

Antivenom infusion should always be administered in a location equipped and staffed by personnel capable of managing anaphylaxis. Management of anaphylaxis is discussed in detail in Chapter 58. Intramuscular epinephrine is the key treatment in a dose of approximately 0.25–1.00 mg for adults and 10 μg/kg for children. Antivenom therapy should be discontinued temporarily and restarted when the victim's condition is stable.

Lesser degrees of immediate adverse reaction restricted to headache, chest discomfort, fine rash, arthralgia, myalgia, nausea, abdominal pain, vomiting, and pyrexia may be managed by temporary cessation of infusion and administration of steroids and antihistamine before recommencement.

A delayed hypersensitivity reaction, serum sickness, should be anticipated and patients warned of the symptoms and signs which usually appear several days to 2 weeks after antivenom administration. Severity may range from a faint rash and pyrexia to serious multisystem disease including lymphadenitis, polyarthralgia, urticaria, nephritis, neuropathy and vasculitis. The incidence of serum sickness appears to be greater with the use of multiple doses of monovalent antivenom and with polyvalent antivenom. Prophylactic treatment is a course of steroids, e.g. prednisolone 1 mg/kg per day for 5 days.

INVESTIGATIONS AND MONITORING

Tests should be performed regularly, interpreted quickly and treated promptly to counter venom effects and its complications. Serial coagulation tests and tests of renal function are especially important. Absorption of venom from the bite site is a continuing process and management must anticipate unabsorbed venom. Apart from regular monitoring of vital signs and oxygenation, the following are specifically needed.

BITE SITE

A swab for venom testing should be done. It has the highest likelihood of detecting venom provided the site has not been washed. The site may be squeezed to yield venom if it has been washed.

URINE

Test the urine for venom that may be present when venom in blood has been bound by antivenom and is therefore undetectable. Urine should also be tested for blood and protein. If the urine is pigmented a distinction should be made between haemoglobinuria and myoglobinuria, which is impossible with simple ward tests. Urine output should be recorded.

BLOOD

- Coagulation tests should include prothrombin time, activated thromboplastin time, serum fibrinogen and fibrin degradation products
- A full blood examination and blood film for haemoglobin level, evidence of haemolysis and platelet count. A mild elevation in white cell count is expected
- Electrolytes, urea, creatinine and creatine phosphokinase (isoenzymes and troponin are useful) to monitor rhabdomyolysis and possible renal compromise

ELECTROCARDIOGRAM

Sinus tachycardia, ventricular ectopy and ST segment and T-wave changes are not uncommon. These effects may be the direct result of venom toxins or from electrolyte disturbances caused by rhabdomyolysis or renal failure.

SECONDARY MANAGEMENT

COAGULATION FACTOR AND BLOOD TRANSFUSION

Although coagulopathy often resolves after several doses of antivenom it does not per se restore coagulation – it permits newly released or manufactured coagulation factors to act unopposed by venom. If coagulation is not restored after several doses of antivenom over several hours, it is prudent to administer fresh frozen plasma and to remeasure coagulation at intervals. Because regeneration of coagulation factors takes many hours, treatment of isolated coagulopathy entirely with antivenom while waiting for their regeneration exposes the patient to serious haemorrhage and implies overdosage with antivenom. Administration of coagulation factors should be preceded by antivenom to neutralise venom prothrombin activator. Platelets may be required but whole blood is rarely needed.

INTRAVENOUS FLUIDS, RHABDOMYOLYSIS AND RENAL PROTECTION

After acute resuscitation, administer intravenous fluids in sufficient volume to maintain urine output at about 40 ml/kg per day in an adult and 1–2 ml/kg per hour in a child to prevent tubular necrosis as a consequence of rhabdomyolysis. Life-threatening hyperkalaemia and hypocalcaemia may develop with rhabdomyolysis. Haemofiltration or dialysis may be required.

HEPARIN

Although this anticoagulant has prevented the action of prothrombin activators in animal models of envenomation, it does not improve established disseminated intravascular coagulation.[11] It is not recommended. Emphasis instead should be on treating the cause by neutralising venom with antivenom.

ANALGESIA AND SEDATION

Australian snake bite does not cause severe pain. However, sedation is required for the mechanically ventilated venom-paralysed victim and analgesia for rhabdomyolysis.

CARE OF THE BITE SITE

Usually no specific care is required. Occasionally the site may blister, bruise, ulcerate or necrose, particularly when a first-aid bandage has been in place for a considerable time or when the bite was by a member of the Black Snake genus, such as a Mulga Snake or Red-bellied Black Snake.

OTHER DRUGS

Antibiotics are not routinely required but should be considered as for any potentially contaminated wound. Sea-snake bites may cause Gram-negative infections. Tetanus prophylaxis should be reviewed.

SEA-SNAKE BITE

Some sea-snake venoms cause widespread damage to skeletal muscle with consequent myoglobinuria, neuromuscular paralysis or direct renal damage. Many have not been researched. The principles of treatment are essentially the same as for envenomation by terrestrial snakes. The venoms of significant species are neutralised with CSL Ltd Beaked Sea-Snake (*Enhydrina schistosa*) antivenom. If that preparation is not available, Tiger Snake or polyvalent antivenom should be used. Sea-snake bites are uncommon in Australia and no deaths have been recorded.

UNCOMMON AND EXOTIC SNAKE BITE

Zoo personnel, herpetologists and amateur collectors who catch, maintain or breed species of uncommon Australian snakes or who import or breed exotic (overseas) snakes are at risk, as are personnel in the Australian Quarantine and Inspection Service (AQIS). There are no specific antivenoms to the venoms of uncommon Australian snakes, but neutralisation is provided by polyvalent antivenom or by monovalent antivenom, as indicated by the VDK. Exotic snake antivenoms are maintained by Venom Supplies Ltd, Tanunda, South Australia (Tel: 08 8563 0001), Royal Melbourne Hospital (Tel: 03 9342 7000), Royal Adelaide Hospital (Tel: 08 8223 4000), Australian Reptile Park (Tel: 02 4340 1022) and by Taronga Zoo (Mosman, Tel: 02 9969 2777). The locations of antivenoms in Australia for treatment of bites by specific exotic snakes are maintained by AVRU at http://www.avru.org/reference/reference_avhold.html.

LONG-TERM EFFECTS OF SNAKE BITE

After appropriate treatment, recovery is expected but it may be slow, taking many weeks or months, particularly from a critical illness or after delayed presentation with neurotoxicity and rhabdomyolysis. Isolated neurological or ophthalmic signs may persist. Long-term loss of taste or smell occurs occasionally.

SPIDERS

Although several thousand species of spiders exist in Australia, only Funnel-web Spiders (genera *Atrax* and *Hadronyche*) and the Red-back Spider (*Latrodectus hasselti*) have caused death or significant systemic illness. All spiders have venom and a few, particularly the White-tailed Spider (*Lampona cylindrata*) and the Common Black House Spider (*Badumna insignis*), have caused severe local injury, although this occurs rarely.[1,12,13] Causes for ulcerated skin lesions other than spider bites should be sought.

FUNNEL-WEB SPIDERS

Many species of the Funnel-web genera *Atrax* and *Hadronyche* inhabit Queensland, New South Wales, Victoria, Tasmania and South Australia but only spiders from New South Wales and southern Queensland have caused significant illness and death. These are large dark-coloured aggressive spiders. A systematic review involving 138 cases identified 77 cases of severe envenomation with 13 deaths, but none occurred after introduction of antivenom in 1981 and the vast majority (97%) responded to antivenom therapy.[14] All deaths were attributed to the Sydney Funnel-web Spider (*A. robustus*)[1] which inhabits an area within an approximate 160 km radius of Sydney and is inclined to roam after rainfall, enter houses and seek shelter among clothes or bedding, giving a painful bite when disturbed.

Severe envenomation is also caused by the southern tree (*H. cerberea*), northern tree (*H. formidabilis*), Port Macquarie (*H.* sp. 14), Toowoomba or Darling Downs (*H. infensa*) and Blue Mountains (*H. versuta*) species. In contrast to other spiders, male Funnel-web Spiders have more potent venom than female spiders.

Bites do not always result in envenomation, but envenomation may be rapidly fatal. The early features of the envenomation syndrome include nausea, vomiting, profuse sweating, salivation and abdominal pain. Life-threatening features are usually heralded by the appearance of muscle fasciculation at the bite site, which quickly involves distant muscle groups. Hypertension, tachyarrhythmias, vasoconstriction, hypersalivation and bronchorrhoea occur. The victim may lapse into coma, develop central hypoventilation and have difficulty maintaining an airway free of secretions. Finally, respiratory failure, pulmonary oedema and severe hypotension culminate in death. The syndrome may develop within several hours but it may be more rapid. Several children have died within 90 minutes of envenomation, and one died within 15 minutes. An active component in the venom is a polypeptide which stimulates the release of acetylcholine at neuromuscular junctions and within the autonomic nervous system, and the release of catecholamines.

Treatment consists of the application of a pressure-immobilisation bandage, intravenous administration of antivenom and support of vital functions, which may include airway support, mechanical ventilation and intensive cardiovascular support.

RED-BACK SPIDER

This spider is distributed throughout Australia and is found outdoors in household gardens in suburban and rural areas. Related species and similar effects of envenomation ('Latrodectism') occur in many parts of the world. Red-back Spider bite is the most common cause for antivenom administration in Australia at 300–400 per annum. The adult female is identified easily. Its body is about 1 cm in size and has a distinct red or orange dorsal stripe over its abdomen. When disturbed, it gives a pin prick-like bite. The bite site becomes inflamed and, during the following minutes to several hours, severe pain, exacerbated by movement, commences locally and may extend up the limb or radiate elsewhere. The pain may be accompanied by profuse sweating, headache, nausea, vomiting, abdominal pain, fever, hypertension, paraesthesias and rashes. In a small percentage of cases when treatment is delayed, progressive muscle paralysis may occur over many hours, requiring mechanical ventilation. Untreated, muscle weakness, spasm and arthralgia may persist for months after the bite. Death has not occurred since the introduction of an antivenom in 1956.

If the effects of a bite are trivial and confined to the bite site, antivenom may be withheld; otherwise, antivenom should be given intramuscularly. The antivenom may be given intravenously in cases of refractory pain but the risk of anaphylaxis may be higher than by the intramuscular route which is very low ($< 0.5\%$). A premedication with promethazine is recommended and epinephrine should be at hand. In contrast to a bite from a snake or Funnel-web Spider, a bite from a Red-back Spider is not immediately life threatening. There is no proven effective first aid, but application of a cold pack or iced water may help relieve pain. Bites by *Steatoda* spp. (cupboard spiders) may cause a similar syndrome and can be treated effectively with Red-back Spider antivenom.[15]

BOX JELLYFISH

This creature, *Chironex fleckeri*, is probably the most venomous in the world. It has caused at least 63 deaths in the waters off northern Australia.[16] It has a cuboid bell up to 30 cm in diameter. Numerous tentacles arise from the corners of the bell and trail several metres. It is semitransparent and difficult to see by anyone wading or swimming in shallow water. The tentacles are lined with millions of nematocysts which, on contact with skin, discharge a threaded barb which pierces subcutaneous tissue, including small blood vessels. Contact with the tentacles causes severe pain and envenomation, from which death may occur within minutes. Death is probably due to both neurotoxic effects causing apnoea and direct cardiotoxicity, although the precise mode of action of the venom is unknown. In mechanically ventilated animals, fatal hypotension occurs rapidly on envenomation.[17] The skin which sustains the injury may heal with disfiguring scars.

First aid, which must be administered on the beach, consists of dousing the skin with acetic acid (vinegar) which inactivates undischarged nematocysts. Adherent tentacles can then be removed. Cardiopulmonary resuscitation may be required on the beach. An ovine antivenom is available but prevention is of paramount importance. Water must not be entered when this jellyfish is known to be close inshore. Wet suits, clothing and 'stinger suits' offer protection.

IRUKANDJI

Stings by the Irukandji, *Carukia barnesi*, and possibly by other jellyfish may cause a syndrome known as the Irukandji syndrome. The Irukandji is a small cubozoan jellyfish with a squarish bell a little more than 1 cm in diameter. Single tentacles trail from its corners. When submerged it is virtually impossible to see.

Its sting is mild and marked only by a small area of erythema. However, severe general illness may follow with abdominal cramps, hypertension, back pain, nausea and vomiting, limb cramps, chest tightness and marked distress.[18] Occasionally, cardiogenic pulmonary oedema has necessitated mechanical ventilation and inotropic therapy, while hypertension has caused two deaths by stroke. The mechanism is uncertain, but experimental studies in animals have shown that Irukandji extracts cause a hyperadrenergic syndrome secondary to massive release of catecholamines[19] which may explain at least in part the cause of heart failure. Pain relief is the most important feature of management in mild to moderate cases. In a series of 10 victims with 'Irukandji syndrome', intravenous magnesium salts provided pain relief and a reduction in blood pressure.[20] Antihypertensive therapy with phentolamine or a 'titratable' nitrate may be required in the initial phase of management.

AUSTRALIAN PARALYSIS TICK

This tick (*Ixodes holocyclus*) injects a toxin that causes flaccid paralysis after some 3–5 days of feeding on humans. The onset of illness resembles that of Guillain–Barré syndrome. Prompt, careful and entire removal of tick(s) is necessary, followed by a period of observation to ensure that late onset paralysis does not occur. No antitoxin is available.

BEES, WASPS AND ANTS

Anaphylactic reactions to bee and wasp stings cause approximately the same number of deaths in Australia each year as do snake bites at an average of 2.3 per annum.[20] The common European Honey Bee (*Apis mellifera*) is largely responsible. Jumper and Bull Ants (*Myrmecia* spp.) may also cause anaphylaxis. Persons who develop reactions to bites should seek immunotherapy and carry injectable epinephrine.

BLUE-RINGED OCTOPUSES

Several species of *Hapalochlaena* inhabit the Australian coastline. When handled, these octopuses bite and inject tetrodotoxin – a neurotoxin found in many different species of marine animals. It causes rapid onset of flaccid paralysis. Approximately a dozen deaths have been recorded. The required treatment is mechanical ventilation until spontaneous recovery occurs.

STINGING FISH

Numerous marine and fresh-water fish carry venom in glands attached to stinging spines. The most dangerous is the Stonefish (*Synanceia* spp.). When trodden upon, venom is injected. The immediate effect is extreme pain. Several deaths have been recorded, presumedly due to the known depressive effects of the toxins on cardiovascular and neuromuscular function, and myotoxicity. An antivenom is available. Local or regional nerve blockade may be required for pain relief. Other stinging fish, such as the freshwater Bullrout (*Notesthes robusta*) also cause excruciating pain when their spines are contacted. Immersion of the affected limb in warm-to-hot water provides pain relief.

VENOMOUS CONE SHELLS

From within their beautiful shells, many gastropod molluscs rapidly eject a venom-laden harpoon to almost instantaneously immobilise and kill prey. The numerous conotoxins, short proteins, stimulate or block neuronal and neuromuscular receptors, causing rapid death. A handful of human deaths have been recorded, when shells have been carelessly or unwittingly handled. There is no antivenom. Mechanical ventilation would be required until spontaneous recovery occurs.

REFERENCES

1. Sutherland SK, Tibballs J. *Australian Animal Toxins.* Melbourne: Oxford University Press; 2001.
2. Pearn JH, Covacevich J, Charles N *et al.* Snakebite in herpetologists. *Med J Aust* 1994; **161**: 706–8.

3. Tibballs J, Sutherland S, Kerr S. Studies on Australian snake venoms. Part I: the haemodynamic effects of Brown Snake (Pseudonaja) species in the dog. *Anaesth Intensive Care* 1989; **17**: 466–9.
4. Tibballs J. The cardiovascular, coagulation and haematological effects of Tiger Snake (*Notechis scutatus*) venom. *Anaesth Intensive Care* 1998; **26**: 529–35.
5. Sutherland SK, Coulter AR, Harris RD. Rationalization of first-aid measures for elapid snakebite. *Lancet* 1979; **1**: 183–6.
6. Howarth DM, Southee AE, Whyte IM. Lymphatic flow rates and first-aid in simulated peripheral snake or spider envenomation. *Med J Aust* 1994; **161**: 695–700.
7. Oakley J. Managing death adder bite with prolonged pressure bandaging. 6th Asia–Pacific Congress on Animal, Plant and Microbial Toxins and 11th Annual Scientific Meeting of the Australasian College of Tropical Medicine, 8–12 July 2002. Queensland, Australia: Cairns Colonial Club; 2002: 29.
8. Premawardhena AP, de Silva CE, Fonseka M *et al.* Low dose subcutaneous adrenaline to prevent acute adverse reactions to antivenom serum in people bitten by snakes: randomised, placebo controlled trial. *BMJ* 1999; **318**: 1041–3.
9. Pumphrey RS. Lessons for management of anaphylaxis from a study of fatal reactions. *Clin Exp Allergy* 2000; **30**: 1144–50.
10. Fan HW, Marcopito LF, Cardoso JL *et al.* A sequential randomised and double blind trial of promethazine prophylaxis against early anaphylactic reactions to antivenom for Bothrops snake bites. *BMJ* 1999; **318**: 1451–3.
11. Tibballs J, Sutherland SK. The efficacy of heparin in the treatment of Common Brown Snake (*Pseudonaja textilis*) envenomation. *Anaesth Intensive Care* 1992; **20**: 33–7.
12. Isbister GK, Gray MR. White-tail spider bite: a prospective study of 130 definite bites by Lampona species. *Med J Aust* 2003; **179**: 199–202.
13. Pincus SJ, Winkel KD, Hawdon GM *et al.* Acute and recurrent skin ulceration after spider bite. *Med J Aust* 1999; **171**: 99–102.
14. Isbister GK, Gray MR, Balit CR *et al.* Funnel-web spider bite: a systematic review of recorded clinical cases. *Med J Aust* 2005; **182**: 407–11.
15. Isbister GK, Gray MR. Effects of envenoming by comb-footed spiders of the genera *Steatoda* and *Achaearanea* (family Theridiidae: Araneae) in Australia. *J Toxicol Clin Toxicol* 2003; **41**: 809–19.
16. Williamson JA, Fenner PJ, Burnett JW *et al. Venomous and Poisonous Marine Animals.* Sydney: University of New South Wales Press; 1996.
17. Tibballs J, Williams D, Sutherland SK. The effects of antivenom and verapamil on the haemodynamic actions of *Chironex fleckeri* (Box jellyfish) venom. *Anaesth Intensive Care* 1998; **26**: 40–5.
18. Little M, Mulcahy RF. A year's experience of Irukandji envenomation in far north Queensland. *Med J Aust* 1998; **169**: 638–41.
19. Winkel KD, Tibballs J, Molenaar P *et al.* Cardiovascular actions of the venom from the Irukandji (*Carukia barnesi*) jellyfish: effects in human, rat and guinea-pig tissues in vitro and in pigs in vivo. *Clin Exp Pharmacol Physiol* 2005; **32**: 777–88.
20. Corkeron M, Pereira P, Makrocanis C. Early experience with magnesium administration in Irukandji syndrome. *Anaesth Intensive Care* 2004; **32**: 666–9.
21. Levick NR, Schmidt JO, Harrison J *et al.* Review of bee and wasp sting injuries in Australia and the USA. In: Austin AD, Dowton M (eds) *Hymenoptera.* Melbourne: CSIRO Publishing; 2000.

77

Blast injury and gunshot wounds: pathophysiology and principles of management

Stephen Brett

Widespread terrorist outrages in the recent past have once again served to emphasise that unpredictable events can suddenly deliver numbers of casualties to civilian hospitals, with unfamiliar patterns of injury. An understanding of the pathophysiology of blast injury, and the impact of such events on hospital function, will help medical staff make appropriate management decisions, often under difficult circumstances.[1–4]

BLAST INJURY

PHYSICS OF EXPLOSIONS[5]

An explosion is the almost instantaneous release of stored energy. The energy may come from, for example, pressurised gas, a nuclear reaction or stored chemical energy. Thus specific 'explosives' are not necessarily required. *Explosives* are materials that contain stored chemical energy that may be released rapidly. High-performance explosives release this energy by means of a chemical reaction which propagates through the explosive material faster than the speed of sound; thus the *detonation velocity* is of the order of 8 km/s compared with the speed of sound in air, 0.33 km/s.[5] This produces a supersonic shock front (blast wave) with a rapidly expanding cloud of gaseous reaction products which causes damage to structures and people in the vicinity. In effect, there is an extremely rapid increase in atmospheric pressure, 'positive overpressure', the duration of which is dependent on the magnitude of the explosive charge. This dies away exponentially and is followed by a *negative* pressure phase produced by gases forced away from the centre of the blast leaving a vacuum. Blast winds may subsequently move paradoxically towards the explosion as pressures equalise.

The blast wave carries with it energised environmental debris and device fragments. These are propelled substantial distances. In air, the blast wave intensity dies away rapidly with distance (with an inverse cube relationship) while debris travels further with the capacity to damage and injure at much greater distances. This is reversed in an underwater blast. Water propagates the blast wave effectively but 'drag' reduces the range of debris and device fragments.

In addition to the kinetic energy released, heat and light energy are also produced, and can contribute to damage and injury. For a deliberate explosion, such as that produced by a military or terrorist device, the precise characteristics depend upon a number of factors including the size and nature of the container, the environment, and the dispositions of buildings and rooms.

CLASSIFICATION OF BLAST INJURY

By convention blast injuries are classified according to which feature of the explosion was involved in wound generation.[6,7] In outline:

- *Primary injury*: caused by interaction of the blast wave and the body, particularly injuring the lungs, abdominal contents, the ears and contributing to traumatic amputation
- *Secondary injury*: produced by energised debris and weapon fragments – predominantly leading to penetrating and soft tissue injuries
- *Tertiary injury*: caused by displacement of the victim by the mass movement of air – 'blast winds'; this group includes long bone fractures and head injury
- *Quaternary injury*: this is a miscellaneous group including crush injury from falling masonry (leading to renal failure) and flash burns

EXPLOSIVE DEVICES (TABLE 77.1)

Conventional military anti-personnel devices rely on fragment generation to produce 'secondary' injuries. The device's casing is designed to produce fragments, and may contain preformed fragments or notched wire to increase the fragment load. An 81 mm mortar round contains a small quantity (~1 kg) of high explosive; the blast

Table 77.1 Types of explosive devices

Conventional munitions: e.g. grenades, aerial bombs, mortar bombs, rockets	All types of blast injury may occur, but penetrating injuries from multiple fragments predominate. Primary fragments are derived from the munition; preformed within the shell or from the casing when the munition explodes. Other materials (building debris, vehicle components) energised by the blast form secondary fragments.
Terrorist devices: typically contain a few kilograms of explosive (*NB*: Recent attacks have been larger, more sophisticated and specifically designed to maximise casualties)	Although the reported incidence of primary blast injuries varies from 1 to 76%, serious primary blast injury is uncommon and secondary and tertiary injuries predominate. Mortality is low unless the device is large, explodes in a confined space or there is structural collapse. Less than 50% of those presenting to hospital will require admission.[2]
Antipersonnel landmines: common in developing countries; indiscriminate in action	Patterns of injury: • Traumatic amputation of foot or leg, due to standing on a buried 'point detonating' mine. Mine fragments, grass, soil, parts of shoe and foot are blown upwards with substantial proximal tissue damage and contamination. • More random distribution of penetrating injuries caused by fragment mine triggered near victim by a tripwire. • Severe upper limb and facial injuries due to handling of a mine.
Enhanced-blast munitions, e.g. fuel-air or thermobaric explosives	Designed to injure by primary blast effect rather than by fragmentation. Used in recent conflict situations.

itself would only be lethal within 2–3 m, but the fragment cloud generated will seriously injure or kill within a radius of around 85 m. Improvised explosive devices (IED), built by terrorists, contain material (e.g. bolts, nails) to increase secondary injury. Larger devices, such as air-delivered free-fall bombs, missiles or artillery shells, contain sufficient explosive to produce secondary injury by throwing bricks, masonry debris and glass substantial distances. In addition, the blast may collapse physical structures such as walls and buildings.

Anti-personnel mines are broadly of two types:

- *buried mines* detonate and disrupt the foot and lower leg, blasting debris from the mine, the ground, footwear and device fragments up fascial planes towards the knee
- *above ground mines*, initiated by trip or command wires or electronic sensors, produce a preformed fragment load leading to secondary injury, with a high incidence of ocular damage

PRIMARY BLAST INJURY

A blast wave passing through an individual behaves like an acoustic wave, giving up energy at interfaces between materials of differing acoustic quality, causing damage. Air-containing organs – the lungs, the gut and the ears – are particularly vulnerable.[8,9] Massive pressure pulses, causing body wall distortion, can tear solid organs from their vascular supplies. Recent work suggests that traumatic amputation is caused by shock wave-induced stress concentrations that fracture the long bones which are subsequently removed by flailing and blast wind effects.[10] This explains why amputations are generally not through joints.[11]

Primary blast injury (PBI) is unusual amongst survivors,[12] but very common in those killed immediately.[13] The blast wave dies away rapidly with distance, but device fragments and energised debris travel and injure at greater distances. If a casualty is close enough to sustain primary injury there will be overwhelming secondary and tertiary damage. The majority of survivors from an explosion will have sustained secondary or tertiary injuries.[12] Military and terrorist devices are specifically designed to maximise casualties by the use of fragments.

Primary injury does sometimes occur and an understanding of mechanisms is useful in guiding management of such casualties. Survivors presenting with signs of one PBI (e.g. visceral perforation) must be assumed to have damage to other vulnerable regions and investigated accordingly. Casualties as close to the blast as other overwhelmingly injured fatalities must be investigated carefully for PBI. The absence of eardrum damage does not exclude PBI, as eardrum rupture depends on a number of factors, including critically the orientation of the head to the blast.

THE LUNG

Immediate effects of severe blast exposure may include apnoea and bradycardia.[9] The blast wave produces disruption of the alveolar–capillary barrier leading to intra-alveolar haemorrhage that may be massive. This occurs in regions of the chest subjected most directly to the incident blast wave (not by a pressure pulse travelling down the trachea). The wave may 'echo' around the pleural cavity, exhibiting interference effects and injuring other regions at points of stress wave concentration. Such regions include the juxtamediastinal tissue and the diaphragmatic recesses. Pulmonary contusions are produced, with associated shunt and reduction in compliance, and pulmonary fat embolism has recently been described.[14] The surface of the lung may evolve bullae, which are mechanically weak and may rupture producing pneumothoraces. These may present early

Table 77.2 Clinical features of blast lung

Symptoms	Dyspnoea Cough – dry to productive with frothy sputum; haemoptysis Chest pain or discomfort (typically retrosternal)
Signs	Cyanosis Torrential pulmonary haemorrhage Tachypnoea Reduced breath sounds, dullness to percussion Coarse crackles, wheeze Features of pneumothorax or haemopneumothorax. Subcutaneous emphysema. Retrosternal crunch (pneumomediastinum) Retinal artery air emboli

Table 77.3 Radiological evidence of blast lung

Diffuse pulmonary opacities or 'infiltrates' (typically these develop within a few hours, become maximal at 24–48 hours and resolve over 7 days)
Pneumothorax/haemopneumothorax
Interstitial (peribronchial) emphysema
Subcutaneous emphysema
Pneumomediastinum
Pneumoperitoneum (usually secondary to perforation of an abdominal viscus, but tension pneumoperitoneum has been ascribed to blast lung)

or late, perhaps triggered by mechanical ventilation. Damage to hilar structures may be produced by severe and long duration overpressures; pulmonary artery and vein injuries are usually rapidly fatal. A variety of clinical features have been described and these are summarised in Table 77.2. Radiological features are outlined in Table 77.3.

Investigations obtained may depend on availability and prioritisation if the casualty burden is high. Chest X-ray (CXR), blood gas analysis and pulse oximetry monitoring are useful. CXR will provide data concerning pneumothorax, pneumomediastinum, subcutaneous and interstitial emphysema and subdiaphragmatic air from visceral perforation. The CXR is a poor modality for quantifying extent of contusion, for which computed tomography (CT) is better.[15,16] CT may be unavailable or overwhelmed with demand. In the majority of cases CT will not provide management-altering data. The priority is close clinical observation of conventional parameters to identify the drift toward respiratory failure.

The management of significant PBI is similar to that of any other pulmonary contusion with a number of corollaries from the pathology. PBI renders the lungs prone to development of pneumothorax, and importantly, significant air emboli may be created.[17] Historically, continuous positive airway pressure (CPAP) and mechanical ventilation were regarded as so hazardous as to be treatments of last resort. This was due to fear of creating or exacerbating air embolism. Modern strategies based around modest gas exchange targets, with limited volume excursion and pressure change, has ameliorated these concerns.[18,19] A variety of non-conventional strategies including hyperbaric chambers, inhaled nitric oxide, high frequency jet ventilation and extracorporeal membrane oxygenation (ECMO) have been tried with varying success. The prognosis for pulmonary function in survivors is generally excellent.[20]

THE ABDOMEN

The hollow viscera are at risk of primary blast injury, particularly in cases of immersion blast. Isolated PBI to the gut is unusual in air blast, and generally occurs in the presence of severe secondary and tertiary injuries. At high overpressures, immediate rupture of the gut wall occurs with bleeding and spillage of intraluminal contents into the peritoneal cavity. More commonly, and at lower overpressures, haemorrhage develops within the intestinal wall, ranging from small petechiae to confluent haematomas. These lesions are characterised by varying degrees of vascular damage and thus some will progress to necrosis of the gut wall and late perforation.[21]

With large numbers of casualties, surgical triage is difficult. Data derived from a pig model provide some guidance as to those contusions at greater risk of late perforation.[22] Bowel contusions $>$ 15 mm diameter and colonic contusions $>$ 20 mm diameter were at higher risk and warranted resection; smaller lesions could be treated conservatively. Circumferential lesions and those on the antimesenteric border were also associated with greater evidence of microvascular damage and perforation risk. Subcapsular haematomas, lacerations of solid organs, testicular rupture and retroperitoneal haematomas have all been described. These result from high blast loads and are likely to present early with abdominal signs and cardiovascular instability. In some patients the indications for exploratory laparotomy are obvious; in others PBI to the abdomen represents a diagnostic challenge, since it may be clinically silent until complications are advanced.

THE EARS[23]

Damage to the ears includes sensorineural deafness, tympanic membrane rupture, injury to the ossicles and implantation cholesteatoma. These injuries are clearly not of major importance in the immediate management of the critically injured. Acute deafness may be very distressing to the victim, and impair assessment of conscious level. It may prevent gaining an accurate history of the circumstances of the blast that might assist in assessing risk of PBI. The absence of PBI to the ear has a poor negative predictive value for PBI to the lungs and gut.

TRAUMATIC AMPUTATION

Common in mine injury, traumatic amputation is unusual in blast survivors. It is common in those who are killed immediately or die quickly.[13] The amputations do not generally occur through joints.[10] That situation is seen in ejecting fast jet pilots exposed to high wind speeds

(1100 km/h). The common sites are the upper third of the tibia, and the upper or lower third of the femur. Computer modelling and evidence from isolated animal limb studies[10] demonstrate that the blast wave generates stress concentrations at particular points in long bones, causing fractures before displacement occurs. Subsequently, blast wind-induced displacement removes the limb. The implication of this is that any survivors with traumatic amputation, not obviously due to fragment damage, must be regarded as at very high risk for PBI to the lungs and gut, even if not manifest immediately, and observed accordingly.

The surgical strategy is initially one of extensive debridement leaving only viable tissue. The resulting wound is loosely packed and allowed to drain, with planned secondary inspection and soft tissue closure after a few days.[24] Bone stock is preserved with the intention that a myoplastic stump can be organised at a later date, but the surgeon must acknowledge that this may be the final stump.[25] The vascular damage which occurs under these circumstances is severe, and heroic efforts to revascularise partially amputated limbs may be counterproductive; any venous anastomosis attempted is likely to be precarious, and may jeopardise survival due to prolonged shock.

SPECIAL CIRCUMSTANCES

Under certain circumstances a relatively high incidence of PBI may be encountered, for example if casualties are protected from fatal secondary injury by personal body armour or environmental structures. Alternatively, an explosion in a confining space may produce exacerbation of the overpressure experienced by an individual, by summation of incident blast energy and that reflected from rigid surfaces. Casualties at a distance from the explosion normally considered safe (for primary effects) for a 'free field' blast, might experience an enhanced blast effect and be at risk for PBI; survivors may have a high incidence of PBI. This has been well described for terrorist bombs in buses[26] and more recently trains.[27]

Conventional military devices exert their anti-personnel effects by secondary and tertiary action. Fuel-air weapons function by delivering a cloud of fuel vapour over or around a target which, once optimally mixed with air, is then detonated. These devices have a very low integral fragment load, but have an enhanced blast effect experienced throughout the fuel cloud that may cover a wide area; the thermal output is also substantial. Originally designed to assist in mine clearance, these weapons are ideal for attacking enemy troops in trenches or built-up areas.[28] The development of these weapons was initially difficult, but most of the technical problems have been overcome, and new generations have appeared. Such devices are reported to have been deployed in recent conflicts, and are available in air-delivered, artillery, tank-mounted and shoulder-launched variants. Now fairly widely available, this class of enhanced blast effect weapon is likely to become an increasing threat. Individuals caught in the centre of the vapour cloud are unlikely to survive, but people at the margins can be predicted to have a high incidence of PBI, significant burns and injuries associated with collapse of buildings.

SECONDARY BLAST INJURY

Secondary injury can be due either to the effects of energised environmental debris, or to material integral to the explosive device itself. Environmental debris may include glass fragments or material from any vehicle used to deliver the device. Clearly a careful exposure and physical and radiological examination is required, bearing in mind that material penetrating one body cavity may travel some distance and produce damage in another. In the terrorist context, material removed, and indeed excised, and amputated tissue must be retained for forensic examination.

Surgical strategy hinges around the identification and removal of large pieces of foreign material, or those associated with, or likely to cause, neurovascular compromise.[29] Systematic removal of all minute fragments may cause more tissue destruction than might otherwise have occurred.[30,31]

Modern anti-personnel munitions (grenades, mortar rounds) are designed to incapacitate or kill by delivering high-energy small fragments into the target. Such weapons have caused the majority of wounds to military personnel in recent conflicts.[32] Preformed fragments often have a mass of 0.1–0.2 g and an initial velocity of ~1500 m/s. Because of irregular shape, velocity falls rapidly, but penetration can still occur at substantial distances. Soldiers in field conditions wear clothes contaminated with soil (and *Clostridia* spp.), and the skin is covered with faecal organisms and pyogenic *Streptococci* and *Staphylococci* spp.[33] High-energy fragments produce temporary cavities (see below) with negative intracavity pressure. Small fragments shred clothing and contaminated clothing fibres are driven or drawn into the wound. Wounds characterised by cavitation will have contamination distributed throughout a greater volume of tissue than might have been anticipated, or exhibited by lower energy wounds. The benefit of the early administration of antibiotics to prevent or retard the development of infection is well established.

Many of these wounds are to the limbs and these are small and multiple. The orthodox operative doctrine was derived from experiences in World War I where large fragments produced the majority of wounds. Newer weapons producing smaller wounds have caused a re-examination of this philosophy; selected wounds may be managed conservatively with cleansing, closed fracture management, antibiotics and observation, and criteria (Table 77.4) have been published.[34–36]

High-energy fragments can produce fractures, and can penetrate the body wall and injure the lungs or visceral structures. As the body wall is penetrated, the fragment energy is significantly reduced so that in survivors reaching hospital intracavity damage will tend to be localised.[31] Thus, mesenteric and gut perforations tend to be small and discrete. Small bowel wounds can generally be

Table 77.4 Factors to be considered in the management of small fragment wounds

Risk factors for infection[34]	Criteria where non-operative management may be appropriate[30,35,36]
Prolonged time between wounding and presentation for treatment Lack of prior wound cleansing Wound size > 1 cm Failure to comply with wound care instructions Low to medium energy transfer fractures	Entry/exit wound < 1 cm No evidence of permanent cavitation within the wound No neurovascular compromise No compartment syndrome Stable fracture pattern No signs of infection Have been treated early with dressings and antibiotics

repaired primarily; the management of large bowel wounds remains controversial. There is an increasing enthusiasm for primary resection and repair with or without proximal diversion.[37] The pursuit of small fragments, which have transited the colon into the retroperitoneal tissues, may be counterproductive.[38]

Recent reports after terrorist incidents have highlighted that biological material from fellow victims, or even suicide bombers, may penetrate casualties and present a risk of viral transmission,[39] thus vaccination or post-exposure prophylaxis should be considered.

TERTIARY BLAST INJURY

Head injuries, long bone, spinal and pelvic fractures and soft-tissue injuries can all be caused by casualties being displaced by the blast winds. Furthermore, limb flailing contributes to the pathogenesis of traumatic amputation. The management of such injuries follows conventional trauma doctrines.

QUATERNARY BLAST INJURY

This classification includes injuries not otherwise classified, and includes superficial flash burns and crush injury from collapsing buildings. Depending on the exact explosives and physical circumstances, burn injuries may impose a substantial challenge, the combination of burns plus secondary injuries posing a very substantial infection risk.[40,41]

MINES

It has been estimated that around 100 million anti-personnel mines are currently in the ground worldwide and a further 250 million are stockpiled. A mine explodes every 20 minutes, injuring or killing approximately 26 000 people per year, most commonly children and agricultural workers. Many of these people die before reaching medical assistance[42] (Table 77.5).

Table 77.5 Classification of anti-personnel mine injury[42]

	Activation	Injury pattern
Pattern 1	Mine stepped on	Severe lower limb, perineal and genital injuries
Pattern 2	Device explodes near victim: activated by other victim or an above-ground mine	Less severe lower extremity injuries; injuries to head, chest and abdomen common
Pattern 3	Handling injury	Severe facial and upper limb injury

An anti-personnel mine is designed to incapacitate and maim rather than to kill – an exception being trip- or command-wire detonated above ground mines (e.g. 'Claymore' mines). A small quantity of explosive is detonated by pressure, and device fragments, soil and footwear remnants are forced upwards. The shock wave is concentrated in the tibia which fractures; the subsequent expansion of explosive products opens up tissue planes, causing substantial damage and contamination, and often completes the traumatic amputation. Limbs not amputated at first instance often require surgical amputation due to overwhelming soft-tissue damage. Damage to the contralateral limb is likely to be less severe, but meticulous attention must be paid to avoid complications leading to a second amputation. In addition, up to 5% of casualties suffer ocular injuries, and this figure is higher for handling injuries and above ground mines. Injuries to the perineum, the external genitalia and the rectum are all common. Many patients will require laparotomy for penetrating trauma.[43,44]

The wounds are heavily contaminated with soil organisms. The surgical strategy consists of:

- initial débridement – exposing and exploring all tissue planes
- removing devitalised tissue and foreign material
- subsequent delayed closure

Primary closure of wounds[45] and heroic limb salvage for limited posterior foot injuries[46] have been reported. Complication rates are likely to be high under all but the most ideal circumstances, and the expertise and facilities required to attempt this approach safely are not available to the vast majority of those injured.

GUNSHOT WOUNDS

Small arms ammunition can be divided broadly into two types: rifle rounds, which are supersonic, and subsonic handgun or submachine gun rounds. This leads to a superficially attractive classification of gunshot wounds (GSW) into high- or low-velocity wounds. This has now been superseded with the realisation that *energy transfer* is the important factor. The kinetic energy available is governed by the equation:

$$\text{Kinetic energy} = 1/2 \times \text{mass} \times \text{velocity}^2$$

High-velocity rounds have inherently more energy available. The amount of energy transferred is governed by a variety of factors, including:

- the resistance of the tissues penetrated
- direct impact on to bone
- whether the round penetrated point first or was unstable in flight

Thus, low-velocity wounds caused by handguns (or even shotguns) at close range may cause massive tissue destruction, and occasionally high-velocity rounds may pass directly through a casualty causing very little damage.

PATHOLOGY AND MANAGEMENT OF GUNSHOT WOUNDS

The phenomenon of *temporary cavitation* is generally a feature of high-velocity rounds.[47] The bullet penetrating a casualty is preceded by a shock wave which forces tissue away from its path, producing a temporary cavity, the diameter of which is many times that of the projectile itself (Figure 77.1). The cavity is instantly under negative pressure which draws environmental debris, clothing fragments and resident skin organisms into the casualty, via the entry wound. In addition, the tissue forming the walls and margins of the cavity is damaged and devitalised,

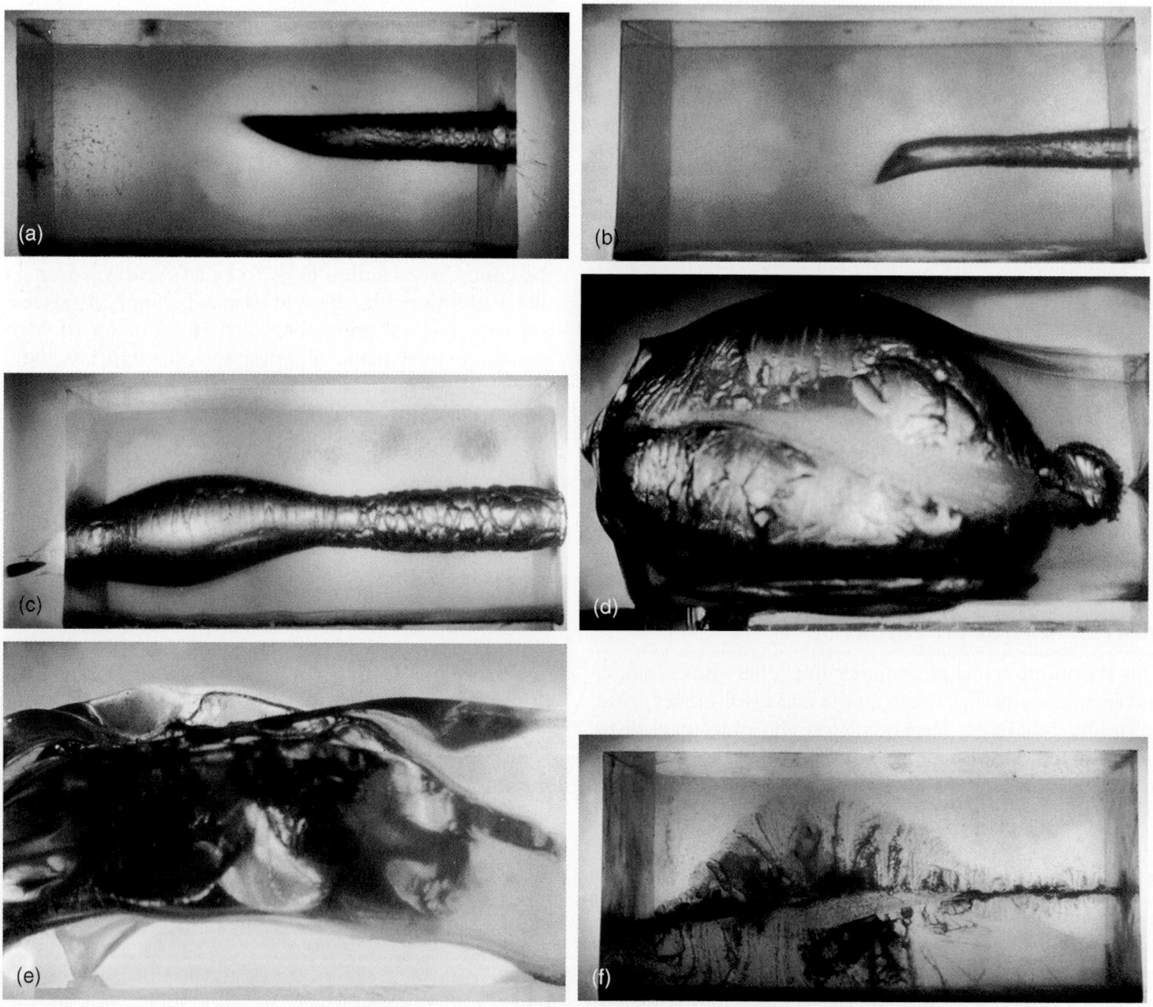

Figure 77.1 High speed camera capturing (a) a rifle round penetrating a block of ballistic gelatin; the round is fired through simulated clothing. The round yaws and tumbles shortly after penetration (b), a temporary cavity forms (c), oscillates (d) and collapses (e). Cloth fragments that have been drawn in to the 'wound' are clearly visible (f).

forming a substrate for infection with the inoculating organisms. Shock wave and cavitation effects may be responsible for fractures not directly involved with the wound track.[47–49] Skeletal muscle is fairly elastic and tolerates cavitation reasonably well, whereas organs constrained by inelastic capsules or bony structures, such as the liver and brain, fare very badly.

Rounds may yaw and tumble prior to or after impact, leading to an unpredictable path through the victim; this is a particular feature of bullets from high-velocity smaller calibre rifles, known as assault rifles. Such injuries commonly involve more than one body cavity. Thus, extensive radiological studies must be performed prior to surgical exploration if at all possible. Occasionally, minute fragments of radio-opaque bullet debris may mark the path of the wound track.[50] The presence or absence, and size of any exit wound are an imperfect guide to the magnitude of wound trauma.[47] The behaviour of bullets is unpredictable, and attempting to predict this from knowledge of the weapon and firing distance may produce a misleading treatment plan.

The severity of fractures produced by direct impact on bone is governed largely by energy transfer. High-energy weapons such as military and hunting rifles produce fractures with a high degree of comminution, whereas the majority of ballistic fractures due to handguns are minimally fragmented.[51,52]

Gunshot wounds become infected quickly due to the effects outlined above. Military surgical doctrine is for extensive wide local excision and delayed primary closure of limb wounds (Figure 77.2). This strategy evolved from conflicts during which both time of wounding to time of surgery intervals were long, and contamination with coliforms and soil organisms was likely. In civilian practice the wounding to treatment interval is usually short, and a less mutilating surgical strategy can sometimes be adopted.[53] Under certain circumstances upper limb wounds can be treated on an outpatient basis, with suitable wound cleansing, immobilisation and perhaps an antibiotic prescription.[54–56]

The majority of casualties surviving to hospital admission will require surgical exploration. The degree of debridement required will be governed by the operative findings and anatomy, rather than assumptions derived from knowledge of the weapon. Under certain circumstances, and with haemodynamically stable patients,

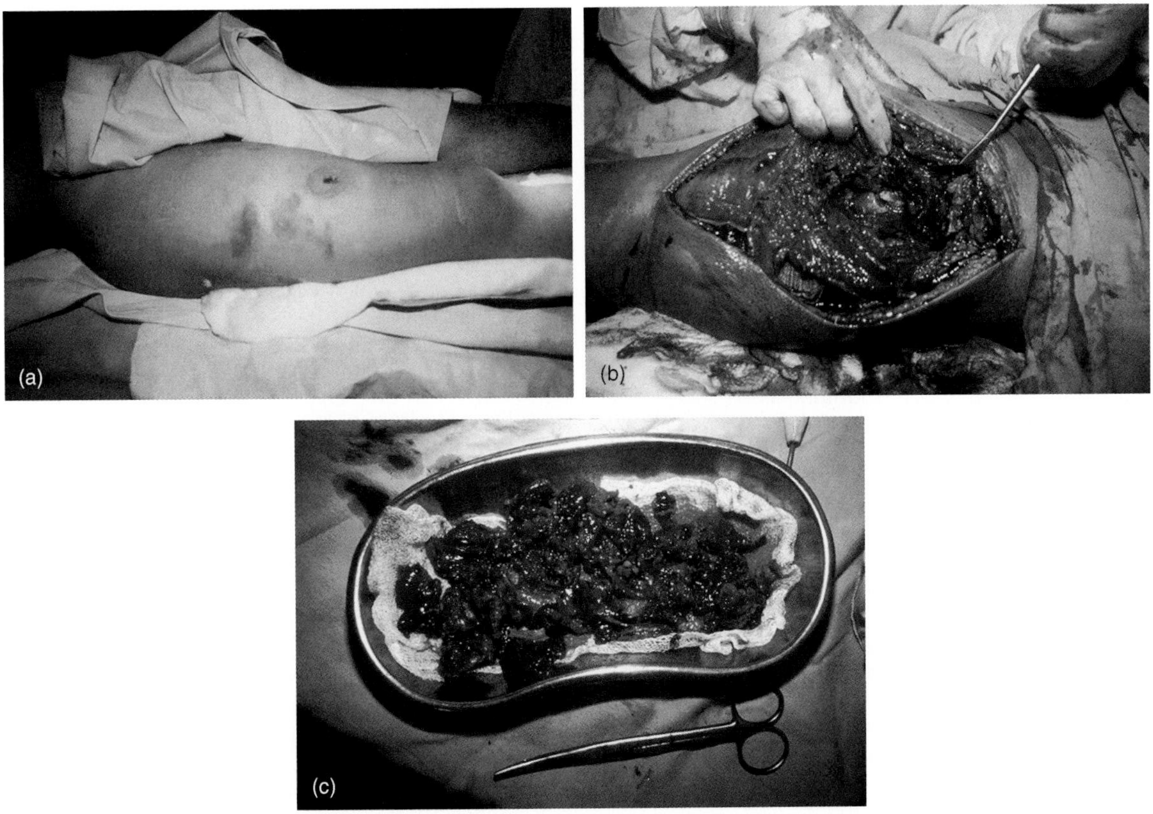

Figure 77.2 (a) Rifle wound of the thigh with small entrance wound, (b) substantial damage to muscle visible at exploration, and (c) typical mass of devitalised, contaminated tissues removed. Both Figure 77.1 and 77.2 courtesy of Professor Jim Ryan, Leonard Cheshire Professor of Conflict Recovery, University College, London.

penetrating abdominal wounds may be evaluated laparoscopically, potentially avoiding a negative laparotomy.[57,58]

ANTIBIOTIC CONSIDERATIONS

The combination of a wound, devitalised tissue and foreign material is ideal for the development of infection. Whether or not an infection develops depends on the quantity of bacteria and foreign material inoculated, and the time interval during which the bacteria can divide prior to wound irrigation, surgery or antibiotic administration.[59,60] Antibiotics can lengthen the safe period prior to establishment of infection if surgery is to be delayed.[61] The mainstay of treatment is surgery but during conflict this may not be available immediately and thus early dressing and antibiotics have an important role. As *Clostridia* spp. and β-haemolytic *Streptococci* have caused the majority of infective complications of war wounds, simple benzyl penicillin has been the most valuable first-line prophylactic and therapeutic agent, with strong evidence to support its continued use.[33,59] Ballistic fractures carry a significant risk of staphylococcal osteomyelitis and require flucloxacillin. In civilian circumstances the bacterial inoculum is orders of magnitude less. Thus, for simple limb gunshot wounds, if there is minimal inoculated material and the wound is attended to early, a far weaker argument for prophylactic use exists. The optimum duration of postoperative prophylaxis remains unclear;[59] evidence exists that even for penetrating hollow viscus injury, a short course may be adequate.[62]

SUMMARY

Detailed descriptions of the surgical management of individual injuries are beyond the scope of this book. However, with an understanding of pathophysiology it should be possible to generate an appropriate management plan. These injuries are likely to provide clinical challenges for the foreseeable future.

REFERENCES

1. Kluger Y, Peleg K, Daniel-Aharonson L *et al.* The special injury pattern in terrorist bombings. *J Am Coll Surg* 2004; **199**: 875–9.
2. Arnold JL, Halpern P, Tsai MC *et al.* Mass casualty terrorist bombings: a comparison of outcomes by bombing types. *Ann Emerg Med* 2004; **43**: 263–73.
3. Shamir MY, Rivkind A, Weissman C *et al.* Conventional terrorist bomb incidents and the intensive care unit. *Curr Opin Crit Care* 2005; **11**: 580–4.
4. Almogy G, Mintz Y, Zamir G *et al.* Suicide bombing attacks: can external signs predict internal injuries? *Ann Surg* 2006; **243**: 541–6.
5. Cullis IG. Blast waves and how they interact with structures. *J R Army Med Corps* 2001; **147**: 16–26.
6. Zuckerman S. Experimental study of blast injury to the lungs. *Lancet* 1940; **2**: 219–24.
7. Krohn PL, Whitteridge D, Zuckerman S. Physiological effects of blast. *Lancet* 1942; **1**: 252–8.
8. Horrocks CL. Blast injuries: biophysics, pathophysiology and management principles. *J R Army Med Corps* 2001; **147**: 28–40.
9. Guy RJ, Kirkman E, Watkins PE *et al.* Physiologic responses to primary blast. *J Trauma* 1998; **45**: 983–7.
10. Hull JB, Cooper GJ. Pattern and mechanism of traumatic amputation by explosive blast. *J Trauma* 1996; **40**: S198–205.
11. Hull JB, Bowyer GW, Cooper GJ *et al.* Pattern of injury in those dying from traumatic amputation caused by bomb blast. *Br J Surg* 1994; **81**: 1132–5.
12. Brismar B, Bergenwald L. The terrorist bomb explosion in Bologna, Italy, 1980: an analysis of the effects and injuries sustained. *J Trauma* 1982; **22**: 216–20.
13. Mellor SG, Cooper GJ. Analysis of 828 servicemen killed or injured by explosion in Northern Ireland 1970–84: the Hostile Action Casualty System. *Br J Surg* 1989; **76**: 1006–10.
14. Tsokos M, Paulsen F, Petri S *et al.* Histologic, immunohistochemical and ultrastructural findings in human blast lung injury. *Am J Respir Crit Care Med* 2003; **168**: 549–55.
15. Schild HH, Strunk H, Weber W *et al.* Pulmonary contusion: CT vs plain radiograms. *J Comput Assist Tomogr* 1989; **13**: 417–20.
16. Wagner RB, Jamieson PM. Pulmonary contusion. Evaluation and classification by computed tomography. *Surg Clin North Am* 1989; **69**: 31–40.
17. Keren A, Stessman J, Tzivoni D. Acute myocardial infarction caused by blast injury of the chest. *Br Heart J* 1981; **46**: 455–7.
18. Sorkine P, Szold O, Kluger Y *et al.* Permissive hypercapnia ventilation in patients with severe pulmonary blast trauma. *J Trauma* 1998; **45**: 35–8.
19. Avidan V, Hersch M, Armon Y *et al.* Blast lung injury: clinical manifestations, treatment and outcome. *Am J Surg* 2005; **190**: 945–50.
20. Hirshberg B, Oppenheim-Eden A, Pizov R *et al.* Recovery from blast lung injury: one-year follow-up. *Chest* 1999; **116**: 1683–8.
21. Cripps NPJ, Cooper GJ. Intestinal injury mechanisms after blunt abdominal impact. *Ann R Coll Surg Engl* 1997; **79**: 115–20.
22. Cripps NPJ, Cooper GJ. Risk of late perforation in intestinal contusions caused by explosive blast. *Br J Surg* 1997; **84**: 1298–303.
23. Garth RJ. Blast injury of the ear: an overview and guide to management. *Injury* 1995; **26**: 363–6.
24. Covey DC, Lurate RB, Hatton CT. Field hospital treatment of blast wounds of the musculoskeletal system during the Yugoslav civil war. *J Orthop Trauma* 2000; **14**: 278–86.
25. Coupland RM. Amputation for antipersonnel mine injuries of the leg: preservation of the tibial stump using a medial gastrocnemius myoplasty. *Ann R Coll Surg Engl* 1989; **71**: 405–8.

26. Pizov R, Oppenheim-Eden A, Matot I *et al.* Blast lung injury from an explosion on a civilian bus. *Chest* 1999; **115**: 165–72.
27. De Ceballos JP, Turegano-Fuentes F, Perez-Diaz D *et al.* 11 March 2004: The terrorist bomb explosions in Madrid, Spain – analysis of the logistics, injuries sustained and clinical management of casualties treated at the closest hospital. *Crit Care* 2005; **9**: 104–11.
28. Demonstration of fuel-air weapon available at: http://www.nawcwpns.navy.mil/clmf/faeseq.html.
29. Hill PF, Edwards DP, Bowyer GW. Small fragment wounds: biophysics, pathophysiology and principles of management. *J R Army Med Corps* 2001; **147**: 41–51.
30. Coupland RM. Hand grenade injuries among civilians. *JAMA* 1993; **270**: 624–6.
31. Bowyer GW. Management of small fragment wounds: experience from the Afghan border. *J Trauma* 1996; **40**: S170–2.
32. Patel TH, Wenner KA, Price SA *et al.* A US Army forward surgical team's experience in Operation Iraqi Freedom. *J Trauma* 2004; **57**: 201–7.
33. Mellor SG, Easmon CSF, Sanford JP. Wound contamination and antibiotics. In: Ryan JM, Rich NM, Dale RF *et al.* (eds) Ballistic Trauma. London: Edward Arnold; 1997: 61–71.
34. Ordog GJ, Sheppard GF, Wasserberger JS *et al.* Infection in minor gunshot wounds. *J Trauma* 1993; **34**: 358–65.
35. Ordog GJ, Wasserberger J, Balasubramanium S *et al.* Civilian gunshot wounds – outpatient management. *J Trauma* 1994; **36**: 106–11.
36. Bowyer GW. Management of small fragment wounds in modern warfare: a return to Hunterian principles? *Ann R Coll Surg Engl* 1997; **79**: 175–82.
37. Gonzalez RP, Falimirski ME, Holevar MR. Further evaluation of colostomy in penetrating colon injury. *Am Surg* 2000; **66**: 342–6; discussion 346–7.
38. Edwards DP, Brown D, Watkins PE. Should colon-penetrating small missiles be removed? An experimental study of retrocolic wound tracks. *J Invest Surg* 1999; **12**: 25–9.
39. Wong JM, Marsh D, Abu-Sitta G *et al.* Biological foreign body implantation in victims of the London July 7th suicide bombings. *J Trauma* 2006; **60**: 402–4.
40. Kennedy PJ, Haertsch PA, Maitz PK. The Bali burn disaster: implications and lessons learned. *J Burn Care Rehab* 2005: **26**: 125–31.
41. Silla RC, Fong J, Wright J *et al.* Infection in acute burn wounds following the Bali bombings: a comparative prospective audit. *Burns* 2006; **32**: 139–44.
42. Coupland RM, Korver A. Injuries from antipersonnel mines: the experience of the International Committee of the Red Cross. *BMJ* 1991; **303**: 1509–12.
43. Bilukha OO, Brennan M, Woodruff BA. Death and injury from landmines and unexploded ordnance in Afghanistan. *JAMA* 2003; **290**: 650–3.
44. Centers for Disease Control. Injuries associated with landmines and unexploded ordnance – Afghanistan, 1997–2002. *CDC MMWR* 2003; **52**: 859–62.
45. Atesalp AS, Erler K, Gur E *et al.* Below-knee amputations as a result of land-mine injuries: comparison of primary closure versus delayed primary closure. *J Trauma* 1999; **47**: 724–7.
46. Selmanpakoglu N, Guler M, Sengezer M *et al.* Reconstruction of foot defects due to mine explosion using muscle flaps. *Microsurgery* 1998; **18**: 182–8.
47. Cooper GJ, Ryan JM. Interaction of penetrating missiles with tissues: some common misapprehensions and implications for wound management. *Br J Surg* 1990; 77: 606–10.
48. Clasper JC, Hill PF, Watkins PE. Contamination of ballistic fractures: an in vitro model. *Injury* 2002; **33**: 157–60.
49. Hill PF, Clasper JC, Parker SJ *et al.* Early intramedullary nailing in an animal model of a heavily contaminated fracture of the tibia. *J Orthop Res* 2002; **20**: 648–53.
50. Ragsdale BD, Sohn SS. Comparison of the terminal ballistics of full metal jacket 7.62-mm M80 (NATO) and 5.56-mm M193 military bullets: a study in ordnance gelatin. *J Forensic Sci* 1988; **33**: 676–96.
51. Ragsdale BD, Josselson A. Experimental gunshot fractures. *J Trauma* 1988; **28**: S109–15.
52. Rose SC, Fujisaki CK, Moore EE. Incomplete fractures associated with penetrating trauma: etiology, appearance, and natural history. *J Trauma* 1988; **28**: 106–9.
53. Bowyer GW, Rossiter ND. Management of gunshot wounds of the limbs. *J Bone Joint Surg Br* 1997; **79**: 1031–6.
54. Knapp TP, Patzakis MJ, Lee J *et al.* Comparison of intravenous and oral antibiotic therapy in the treatment of fractures caused by low-velocity gunshots. A prospective, randomized study of infection rates. *J Bone Joint Surg Am* 1996; **78**: 1167–71.
55. Dickson K, Watson TS, Haddad C *et al.* Outpatient management of low-velocity gunshot-induced fractures. *Orthopedics* 2001; **24**: 951–4.
56. Byrne A, Curran P. Necessity breeds invention: a study of outpatient management of low velocity gunshot wounds. *Emerg Med J* 2006; **23**: 376–8.
57. Miles EJ, Dunn E, Howard D *et al.* The role of laparoscopy in penetrating abdominal trauma. *JSLS* 2004; **8**: 304–9.
58. Ahmed N, Whelan J, Brownlee J *et al.* The contribution of laparoscopy in evaluation of penetrating abdominal wounds. *J Am Coll Surg* 2005; **201**: 213–6.
59. Zimmerli W, Waldvogel FA, Vaudaux P *et al.* Pathogenesis of foreign body infection: description and characteristics of an animal model. *J Infect Dis* 1982; **146**: 487–97.
60. Simpson BW, Wilson RH, Grant RE. Antibiotic therapy in gunshot wound injuries. *Clin Orthop Relat Res* 2003; **408**: 82–5.
61. Mellor SG, Cooper GJ, Bowyer GW. Efficacy of delayed administration of benzylpenicillin in the control of infection in penetrating soft tissue injuries in war. *J Trauma* 1996; **40**: S128–34.
62. Kirton OC, O'Neill PA, Kestner M *et al.* Perioperative antibiotic use in high-risk penetrating hollow viscus injury: a prospective trial of 24 hours versus 5 days. *J Trauma* 2000; **49**: 822–32.

78

Biochemical terrorism

Munita Grover and Michael E Pelly

Biochemical terrorism is defined as the use of biological or chemical agents to intimidate, incapacitate or eradicate crops, livestock, civilian and military personnel.[1] It is well suited for attack by poorer nations against the rich, and is known as a poor man's atom bomb, or asymmetric method of attack. The large scale use of mustard and nerve gases in the Iran/Iraq war,[2] the dissemination of nerve gas sarin on the Tokyo underground,[3] and the discovery by UN inspectors in Iraq of SCUD missiles, rockets and aerial bombs primed with Botulinum and aflatoxins[4,5] have highlighted the need for planning.

CHARACTERISTICS OF BIOLOGICAL WEAPONS (TABLES 78.1 AND 78.2)

Intended target effects are due either to infection with disease-causing micro-organisms and other replicative entities, including viruses, fungi and prions, or to the toxins they elaborate. Their effects depend on the ability to multiply in the person, animal or plant attacked.[6] Sequelae depend on host factors (state of nutrition, immunocompetence) and environment (sanitation, temperature, humidity, water quality, population density).[7]

CLASSIFICATION

Although classification of biological weapons can be taxonomy based (e.g. bacterial/viral/fungal), it is also useful to examine particular features such as:

- *Infectivity*: proportion of persons exposed to a given dose that become infected. This reflects the capability of an agent to enter, survive and replicate
- *Virulence*: ratio of the number of clinical cases to the number of infected hosts. May differ for strains of the same pathogen.
- *Lethality*: ability of agent to cause death in an infected population
- *Pathogenicity*: ratio of number of clinical cases to the number of exposed persons, which reflects the capability of an agent to cause disease
- *Incubation period*: time elapsing between exposure to the agent and first signs and symptoms of disease
- *Contagiousness*: number of secondary cases following exposure to a primary case in relation to the total number exposed
- *Stability*: ability of an agent to survive the environment

Another useful classification system available is that from the Centers for Disease Control and Prevention (CDC) Atlanta:

CATEGORY A

High-priority agents include organisms that pose a risk to national security because they can be easily disseminated or transmitted from person to person. They result in high mortality rates and have the potential for major public health impact, which might cause public panic and social disruption, and require special action for public health preparedness. Examples include anthrax, botulism, plague, smallpox, tularaemia and viral haemorrhagic fevers.

CATEGORY B

Second highest priority agents include those that are moderately easy to disseminate. They result in moderate morbidity rates and low mortality rates, and require specific enhancements of CDC's diagnostic capacity and enhanced disease surveillance. Examples include brucellosis, salmonella, glanders, melioidosis, psittacosis, Q fever, ricin toxin, typhus, staphylococcal enterotoxin B and viral encephalitis.

ROUTES OF DISSEMINATION

- Inhalational exposure using sprays or aerosols: Optimal particle size for alveolar deposition is 0.6–5 microns. Particles larger than this are filtered by the nose, and smaller particles are exhaled. This can be achieved using aerosol generators mounted on stationary objects or primed onto trucks, cars, boats, cruise missiles and planes. Environmental factors such as wind velocity, cloud cover, rainfall and humidity affect the efficiency of dissemination.[7]
- Cutaneous: Via wounds and mucous membranes.
- Ingestion via food and water: Hand to mouth contact is a suitable vehicle, for example the Rajneeshee cult successfully disseminated Salmonella via salads, infecting 750 people in 1984.

Table 78.1 Potential weapons

Biological diseases	Chemical agents
Bacillus anthracis (anthrax)	Blisters/vesicants
Clostridium botulinum toxin (botulism)	Distilled mustard (HD)
Yersinia pestis (plague)	Lewsite (L)
Variola major (smallpox)	Mustard gas (H)
Francisella tularensis (tularaemia)	Nitrogen mustard (HN-2)
Viral haemorrhagic fever	Phosgene oxime (CX)
Coxiella burnetii (Q fever)	Blood
Brucella melitensis (brucellosis)	Arsine (SA)
Burkholderia mallei (glanders)	Cyanogen chloride (CK)
Ricin toxin (*Ricinus communis* – castor beans)	Hydrogen chloride
Staphylococcus enterotoxin B	Hydrogen cyanide (AC)
Niaph virus	Choking/pulmonary damage
Hantaviruses	Chlorine (CL)
	Nitrogen oxide (NO)
	Phosgene (CG)
	Nerve
	Sarin (GF)
	Soman (GD)
	Tabun (GA)
	VX
	Incapacitating
	LSD
	Cannabinoids

Table 78.2 Criteria for a successful biological weapon[6]

Assailant
Has methods to treat own forces and population
Target population
Non-immune
Little or no access to immunisation or treatment
Bioweapon
Consistently produces disease/death
Highly contagious or infective in low doses
Short and predictable incubation period
Difficult to identify in target population
Suitable for mass production, storage and weaponisation
Stable during dissemination
Low persistence after delivery

DETECTION OF A BIOTERRORIST EVENT (TABLE 78.3)

This may be obvious if large numbers of military personnel become ill with similar syndromes, but any release is likely to be a covert event. Furthermore, genetic engineering may result in altered pathogenicity, incubation periods, clinical effects and response to treatment or immunisation.

Table 78.3 Epidemiological evidence of an attack

Increasing incidence of disease in a normally healthy population
Higher incidence in subgroups, e.g. outdoor workers/shared ventilation
Increasing numbers seeking help with similar symptoms
Rise in endemic disease at an uncharacteristic time
Large numbers of rapidly fatal cases
Any patient with an uncommon disease which has bioterrorist potential
Large numbers of dying animals or fish, and unusual swarms of insects

SPECIFIC AGENTS

ANTHRAX

Anthrax[8] is an acute infectious zoonosis caused by *Bacillus anthracis*, a Gram-positive, spore-forming bacillus. The infective dose is 8000–50 000 spores and routes of transmission include inhalation, ingestion and skin contact. Person-to-person transmission does not occur for the pulmonary form but secondary cutaneous lesions may occur after direct exposure to vesicle secretions. As spraying by aircraft is a potential threat to a large city, pulmonary exposure is the most likely route in a mass casualty situation.

CLINICAL FEATURES

Pulmonary exposure[9,10]

- Incubation period is 2–60 days
- Prodrome with flu-like symptoms
- Interim improvement followed by respiratory failure, cardiovascular collapse. Widened mediastinum on CXR, due to haemorrhagic mediastinitis and lymphadenopathy
- Gram-positive bacilli on blood cultures

Cutaneous exposure

- Incubation period is 1–7 days
- Mostly head, hands and forearms
- Pruritus, erythema, oedema and maculopapular lesions progress to depressed black eschars within 2–6 days. Eschars fall off without scarring

Gastrointestinal exposure

- Incubation period is 1–7 days
- Usually follows ingestion of infected meat
- Presents with abdominal pain, cramps, haematemesis and bloody diarrhoea, followed by toxaemia and cardiovascular collapse
- Gram-positive blood cultures

Post exposure management[11]

- Universal precautions for medical personnel
- Warning to laboratory and coroners personnel regarding pathology specimens

- Contact infection control team
- Minimal handling of fomites
- Thorough decontamination with soap and water
- Disinfection of surfaces with 0.5% hypochlorite solution

TREATMENT

Most strains used for bioterrorism will produce β-lactamases, and cephalosporinases were produced by the latest cases in the USA. Appropriate antibiotics include:

- ciprofloxacin: adults 500 mg b.d. for 8 weeks; children 20–30 mg/kg per day
- doxycycline: adults 100 mg b.d. for 8 weeks; children 5 mg/kg per day
- amoxicillin: in children and pregnant patients amoxicillin 40 mg/kg per day (max 500 mg t.d.s.) is appropriate if the organism is penicillin sensitive

Immunisation with anthrax vaccine consists of three doses at 0, 2 and 4 weeks. Prophylaxis of contacts should continue for 8 weeks and include immunisation if exposure is confirmed. Preventative immunisation using an inactivated cell-free vaccine is available but presently only administered to military personnel.

BOTULISM

Botulism[5] is caused by *Clostridium botulinum*, an anaerobic Gram-positive bacillus that produces a neurotoxin. Seven forms of the toxin have been identified from A to G, but human botulism is due mainly to strains A, B and E. The neurotoxin contains a zinc protease that acts at the presynaptic terminal of the neuromuscular junction to prevent the fusion of vesicles of acetylcholine with the presynaptic membrane, therefore preventing release of acetylcholine and causing a flaccid paralysis. The LD_{50} for type A is 0.001 μg/kg.

Routes of exposure are either inhalation or ingestion, and there is an incubation period of 12–36 hours. Person-to-person transmission does not occur.

Clinical features include a responsive patient with no fever. There is a symmetric descending flaccid paralysis in a proximal to distal pattern without a sensory deficit. Cranial neuropathies (mainly bulbar) lead to diplopia, dysphagia, dysphonia and dysarthria. Respiratory dysfunction may occur due to upper-airway obstruction or muscle paralysis. The diagnosis is clinical, and confirmation is with the mouse bioassay in which mice are pretreated with antitoxin and exposed to the patient's serum. A pentavalent toxoid vaccine is available for prevention, but routine immunisation is not recommended.

TREATMENT

Patients should be monitored with frequent assessment of gag, cough reflexes, inspiratory force and vital capacity. Mechanical ventilation may be protracted, and may be punctuated by nosocomial infections requiring antibiotics.

Aminoglycosides and clindamycin are contraindicated because of their ability to increase blockade.[12] Administration of the trivalent (A, B, E) antitoxin should not be delayed while awaiting confirmation of the diagnosis. This horse serum has <9% hypersensitivity reactions, and <2% incidence of anaphylaxis. Skin testing is advisable.[13] A heptavalent antitoxin is under investigation. Passive administration of neutralising antibody minimises further damage.[14]

Treatment of children, pregnant women and immunocompromised patients should be no different; all have received equine antitoxin without short-term sequelae.

Prophylaxis of contacts involves close observation and, at the first sign of illness, treatment with antitoxin, neutralising antibody and administration of the pentavalent toxoid vaccine.

SMALLPOX

Smallpox[15] is an acute viral illness caused by variola virus (orthopoxvirus). The last documented case was in Somalia in 1977. It is transmitted from person to person via the airborne route. The infective dose is 10–100 virions, with an incubation period of 7–17 days.

In a non-immune society, the impact would be devastating[16] as the person-to-person spread would be difficult to check, and many countries have very poor health structures with overcrowding in the cities. In addition, the impact of global travel would change the epidemic and allow it to move rapidly from continent to continent.

There are two other major factors that may change the profile of a predicted epidemic: the potential use of new antiviral agents against smallpox and the HIV epidemic. Predictions are difficult.

CLINICAL FEATURES[17]

There is a flu-like prodrome with malaise, fever and headache. There is also a synchronously evolving maculopapular rash forming pustules over the head and extremities; the mouth and pharynx may also be affected. Multiorgan failure commonly complicates smallpox. Diagnosis is clinical with confirmation by identification of brick-shaped virions from vesicular fluid using electron microscopy.

PREVENTION

Routine vaccination with vaccinia virus stopped in 1972. The immune status of vaccinated individuals is unclear, but if a single dose vaccine was administered it is assumed the subject is non-immune. A preventative vaccination programme is currently under review.

TREATMENT

Vaccination within 4 days of exposure.[18] However, complications include:

- post-vaccinial encephalitis
- vaccinia gangrenosa
- eczema vaccinatum
- generalised vaccinia
- inadvertent inoculation

Five groups are considered high risk for these complications. These are pregnancy, HIV infection, chemotherapy, eczema and immune disorders.[19] In these cases, vaccinia immune globulin should be given simultaneously. Other treatments include:

- supportive care with isolation
- antibiotics for secondary bacterial infections
- cidofovir, a nucleoside DNA polymerase inhibitor, is under investigation but needs to be given i.v. and causes renal toxicity.[20]

PLAGUE

Plague[21] is an acute bacterial disease caused by the Gram-negative *Yersinia pestis*, from the enterobacter species.[22] Although usually transmitted by fleas causing bubonic and septicaemic plague, a bioterrorist event is likely to be airborne resulting in pneumonic plague. The infective dose is <100 organisms, and has an incubation period of 2–3 days. It is unlikely that spread would be person to person.

Plague presents with fever, haemoptysis, chest pain and dyspnoea. Gram-negative rods are found in mucopurulent sputum, and on Wright's, Giemsa or Wayson stain appear as bipolar rods with a safety pin appearance. The diagnosis can be confirmed on blood culture, and with fluorescent antibody testing. There is radiographic evidence of bronchopneumonia, and multi organ failure soon develops. Until 72 hours of antibiotic therapy have been completed, plague is communicable.

A formalin-killed vaccine exists but is ineffective and unavailable. Post exposure immunisation has no benefit.

TREATMENT[21]

Once the diagnosis is considered, isolation and universal precautions should be instituted. Historically, streptomycin (1 g b.d. i.m.) reduced mortality to 5%, and gentamicin (5 mg/kg per day) has also been used successfully. Tetracycline and doxycycline (100 mg b.d.) have been used, but in Madagascar 13% of strains were resistant to doxycycline. Animal studies have demonstrated efficacy of fluoroquinolones including ciprofloxacin (400 mg b.d.), ofloxacin and levofloxacin. No human trials exist so far. Chloramphenicol (25 mg/kg q.i.d.) is recommended for plague meningitis.

CHARACTERISTICS OF CHEMICAL AGENTS

The North Atlantic Treaty Organization definition of a chemical agent is a 'chemical substance which is intended for use in military operations to kill, seriously injure, or incapacitate people because of its physiological effects'.[2] In addition to physiological effects, these agents promote psychological warfare.[23]

ROUTES OF DISSEMINATION

The principal hazard is inhalation of liquid, vapour, or droplets (0.6–5 microns). Delivery may be by artillery shells, missiles or aerial bombing. In the Tokyo subway attack in 1995, terrorists left plastic bags on the subway filled with sarin after piercing them with umbrella tips. There were 3796 casualties and 12 deaths.[3]

Toxicity depends on the concentration and time of exposure, is measured in units of concentration and time (mg/min m^3), known as the Haber product.[7] Most chemical agents are designed to penetrate the skin, respiratory epithelium and cornea, unlike biological agents. Penetration is promoted by thinner, more vascular, moister, hairy skin, and by high humidity, spills and aerosols.

RICIN

Ricin is one of the most toxic biological agents known – a Category B bioterrorism agent and a Schedule number 1 chemical warfare agent. Ricin toxin can be extracted from castor beans, purified and treated to form a pellet, a white powder, or dissolved in water or weak acid to be released as a liquid. It is stable under ambient conditions. Particles of <5 microns have been used for aerosol dispersion in animal studies. Ricin particles can remain suspended in undisturbed air for several hours, and resuspension of settled ricin from disturbed surfaces also may occur.

TRANSMISSION

Ricin would need to be dispersed in particles smaller than 5 microns to be used as an effective weapon by the airborne route. It is very difficult to prepare particles of this size. Routes of exposure include inhalation, parenteral (injection) ingestion, dermal contact (exposure risk is low, except where absorption is through non-intact skin or via a solvent carrier) or ocular contact. Although ricin may adhere to skin, person-to-person transmission through casual contact has not been reported. Despite the fact that ricin may adhere to clothing or be present on surfaces, there is low potential for transmission via contact with contaminated clothing or contaminated surfaces.

RISK GROUPS

- There is worldwide distribution of castor plants. Ricin is produced when castor oil is made from castor beans, but the general public is not considered at risk for exposure
- Persons in or around castor oil processing plants. However, it would take a deliberate act to make ricin and use it as a poison
- Persons in the dispersal area of a ricin aerosol release
- Persons who are victims of parenteral injection with ricin
- Persons who ingest castor beans, or food or water contaminated with ricin
- It is not known whether certain populations are more vulnerable to the health effects of ricin exposure (e.g. children, pregnant women, the elderly, those with immunosuppression, or underlying respiratory or gastrointestinal tract disease); however, persons with pre-existing tissue irritation or damage who are exposed to ricin may sustain further injury and greater absorption of ricin toxin

PATHOGENESIS

- Ricin is a toxalbumin, a biological toxin whose mechanism of action is inhibition of protein synthesis in eukaryotic cells; cell death results from the absence of proteins
- The effects of ricin poisoning depend upon the amount of ricin exposure, the route of exposure and the person's premorbid condition
- Ingestion and mastication of three to six castor beans is the estimated fatal dose in adults. The fatal dose in children is not known, but is likely to be less
- Most cases of castor bean ingestion do not result in poisoning: ricin release requires mastication, and the degree of mastication is likely to be important in determining the extent of poisoning. Ricin is not as well absorbed through the gastrointestinal tract when compared to injection or inhalation
- Inhalation or injection of ricin would be expected to lead to a more rapid onset of symptoms of ricin poisoning and to a more rapid progression of poisoning compared to ingestion, given the same exposure amount

Data on inhalational exposure to ricin in humans are extremely limited, and systemic toxicity has not been described. Animal studies suggest that inhalation is one of the most lethal forms of ricin poisoning. Following severe ricin poisoning, damage to vital organs may be permanent or have lasting effects. No long-term effects are known to exist from ricin exposure that did not result in symptoms.

LABORATORY DIAGNOSIS

Non-specific laboratory findings in ricin poisoning include:

- metabolic acidosis
- impaired liver and renal function tests
- hematuria
- leukocytosis (two- to five-fold higher than normal value)

The presence of leukocytosis and/or abnormal liver and renal function tests may suggest ricin-associated illness in the correct clinical context but are not very specific. There are no specific clinically validated assays for detection of ricin that can be performed by the hospital/health care facility clinical laboratory, and no methods are available for the detection of ricin in biological fluids. However, tests for ricinine, an alkaloidal component of the castor bean plant, are being developed. The potential uses of tests for either ricin or ricinine in human biological samples would primarily be for purposes of confirming exposure or assessing the prevalence of exposure rather than diagnostic use.

Testing for ricin in environmental samples will most likely not be immediately available to assist in clinical decision-making. However, they may document the potential for exposure or affirm the exposure circumstances.

LABORATORY TESTING

Tests performed on ricin-suspicious samples include:

- time-resolved fluorescence immunoassay: antibody binds to ricin
- polymerase chain reaction: locates and makes copies of parts of the DNA contained in the castor bean plant. The search specifically identifies the DNA of the gene that produces the ricin protein

TREATMENT

As no antidote exists for ricin, exposure must be avoided if possible. Otherwise, all efforts must be directed to minimising exposure through decontamination. Supportive care is, in part, dictated by the route of exposure: inhalation, ingestion, skin or eye exposure, and includes measures such as ventilation, i.v. fluids, and treatment of seizure or hypotension.

SARIN

Sarin ($C_4H_{10}FO_2P$, isopropylmethylphosphofluoridate) is a colourless and odourless liquid at room temperature. It is volatile and incompatible with metals or concrete, which lead to production of hydrogen gas. Hydrolysis of sarin forms acids. It is thermally stable $<49°C$, but clings to clothing and releases slowly for 30 minutes. Toxicity is through inhibition of the enzyme acetylcholinesterase.

The route of exposure determines which clinical features (Table 78.4) appear first.[24] Post inhalation respiratory and eye symptoms appear, whereas post cutaneous exposure diaphoresis and muscle fasciculation occur. Immediate first aid is to remove the patient from the area of danger to a well-ventilated area before removal of clothing and decontamination of the skin. This can be achieved using mists of water, or dilute sodium hypochlorite. Eyes are irrigated with water or normal saline.

Table 78.4 Sarin toxicity

Mild	Rhinorrhitis Dyspnoea Miosis Blurred vision
Moderate	Diaphoresis Drooling Bronchospasm Nausea, vomiting, cramps Weakness Twitching Headache Confusion
Severe	Involuntary defecation/urination Convulsions Respiratory arrest Coma, death

Assessment follows airway, breathing and circulation. Patients with compromised airways, due either to direct effects or secondary to reduced level of consciousness, require intubation and positive-pressure ventilation. Aggressive suctioning may be needed for bronchial secretions.

TREATMENT

- Anticholinergics to antagonise the muscarinic effects, usually i.v. atropine in 2 mg doses, every 3–5 minutes, until the patient is atropinised. It may need to be continued for 24 hours at 2 mg/h^2
- Oximes to reactivate the anticholinesterase enzyme at nicotinic sites, e.g. pralidoxime mesilate 30 mg/kg by slow i.v. injection, up to 2–4 g. This should be prompt, as dealkylation of the inhibited enzyme renders it resistant to reactivation
- Prophylactic anticonvulsants to prevent seizures. Diazepam 5 mg by any route has been shown to reduce morbidity in animal studies

MUSTARD GAS

Mustard gas ($C_4H_8Cl_2S$, Bis-(2-Chloroethyl) sulphide) is a yellow oily liquid at room temperature. It has a faint garlic odour and evaporates to form a vapour that penetrates clothing. Although mortality is low, poisoning tends to incapacitate. It is a bifunctional alkylating agent that is carcinogenic (oral cavity, larynx, bronchus), and irritates skin and mucosa (Table 78.5). Mustard gas is also myelotoxic (pancytopenia) and teratogenic. Assessment is similar to sarin.[25]

TREATMENT

Patients with large burns are resuscitated as any other burn; however, fluid losses are transudates, so protein losses are less.[26] Pain control is important and frequently requires analgesics, such as morphine. Tense blisters are dressed with silver sulfadiazine. Mustard burns take at least 12 weeks to heal, but early excision and grafting does not reduce healing time.[27,28] Eye lesions usually heal in 2 weeks, and are aided by topical antibiotics and saline irrigation. Oxygen, antibiotics for secondary pneumonia, physiotherapy and ventilation are the mainstays of treatment for respiratory effects.

Table 78.5 Features of mustard gas toxicity

Eyes	Lacrimation, conjunctivitis, photophobia
Skin	Erythema, blistering, partial to full-thickness burns
Respiratory tract	Rhinorrhoea, tracheobronchitis, bronchopneumonia
Systemic	Nausea, vomiting, diarrhoea, bradycardia, hypotension

REFERENCES

1. Spencer R, Wilcox M. Agents of biological warfare. *Rev Med Microbiol* 1993; **4**: 138–43.
2. Evison D, Hinsley D, Rice P. Chemical weapons. *BMJ* 2002; **324**: 332–5.
3. KB O. Aum Shinrikyo: once and future threat? *Emerg Infect Dis* 1999; **5**: 513–16.
4. Zilinskas R. Iraq's biological weapons: the past as future? *JAMA* 1997; **278**: 418–24.
5. Arnon SS, Schechter R, Inglesby TV *et al.* Botulinum toxin as a biological weapon. Medical and Public Health Management. *JAMA* 2001; **285**: 1059–70.
6. Beeching NJ, Dance DA, Miller AR *et al.* Biological warfare and bioterrorism. *BMJ* 2002; **324**: 336–9.
7. WHO. *Health Aspects of Chemical and Biological Weapons.* Geneva: WHO; 2001: 2.
8. Inglesby TV, Henderson DA, Bartlett JG *et al.* Anthrax as a biological weapon. Concensus statement. *JAMA* 1999; **281**: 1735–45.
9. Meselson M, Guillemin J, Hugh-Jones M *et al.* The Sverdlovsk anthrax outbreak of 1979. *Science* 1994; **266**: 1202–7.
10. Swartz M. Recognition and management of anthrax – an update. *N Engl J Med* 2001; **345**: 1621–6.
11. English JF. Overview of bioterrorism readiness plan: a template for health care facilities. *Am J Infect Control* 1999; **27**: 468–9.
12. Schulze J, Toepfer M, Schroff KC *et al.* Clindamycin and nicotinic neuromuscular transmission. *Lancet* 1999; **354**: 1792–3.
13. Black R, Gunn R. Hypersensitivity reactions with botulinal antitoxin. *Am J Med* 1980; **69**: 567–70.
14. Amersdorfer P, Marks J. Phage libraries for the generation of anti-botulinum scFv antibodies. *Methods Mol Biol* 2000; **145**: 219–40.
15. Breman J, Henderson D. Poxvirus dilemmas: monkeypox, smallpox and biological terrorism. *N Engl J Med* 1998; **339**: 556–9.
16. Gani R, Leach S. Transmission potential of smallpox in contemporary populations. *Nature* 2001; **414**: 748–51.
17. Henderson DA, Inglesby TV, Bartlett JG *et al.* Smallpox as a biological weapon: medical and public health management. *JAMA* 1999; **281**: 2127–30.
18. Vaccinia vaccine: recommendations of the Immunization Practices Advisory Committee (ACIP). *MMWR Recomm Rep* 1991; **40**: 1–10.
19. Redfield RR, Wright DC, James WD *et al.* Disseminated vaccinia in a military recruit with human immunodeficiency virus. *N Engl J Med* 1987; **316**: 673–6.
20. Lalezari JP, Stagg RJ, Kuppermann BD *et al.* Intravenous cidofovir for peripheral cytomegalovirus retinitis in patients with AIDS: a randomised, controlled trial. *Ann Intern Med* 1997; **126**: 257–63.
21. Inglesby TV, Dennis DT, Henderson DA *et al.* Plague as a biological weapon: medical and public health management. *JAMA* 2000; **285**: 2763–73.
22. Perry R, Fetherston J. Yersinia pestis – aetiologic agent of plague. *Clin Microbiol Rev* 1997; **10**: 35–66.

23. Wesseley S, Hyams K, Bartholomew R. Psychological implications of chemical and biological weapons. *BMJ* 2001; **323**: 878–9.
24. Tu A. Overview of sarin terrorist attacks on Japan. *ACS Symp Ser* 2000; **745**: 304–7.
25. Newman-Taylor A, Morris A. Experience with mustard gas casualties. *Lancet* 1991; **337**: 242.
26. Mellor S, Rice P, Cooper G. Vesicant burns. *Br J Plast Surg* 1991; **44**: 434–7.
27. Eldad A, Weinberg A, Breiterman S *et al.* Early non-surgical removal of chemically injured tissue enhances wound healing in partial thickness burns. *Burns* 1998; **24**: 166–72.
28. Rice P, Brown RF, Lam DG *et al.* Dermabrasion: a novel concept in the surgical management of sulphur mustard injuries. *Burns* 2000; **26**: 34–40.

Part Thirteen

Pharmacological Considerations

79

Pharmacokinetics, pharmacodynamics and drug monitoring in critical illness

Richard N Upton, John A Myburgh and Raymond G Morris

Pharmacokinetics (PK) is the study of the absorption, distribution, metabolism and elimination (ADME) of drugs, usually by measurement of drug concentrations in blood or plasma. Pharmacodynamics (PD) is the study of the effects of a drug on the body. The pharmacokinetics of a drug is one determinant of its pharmacodynamics. Pharmacokinetic-pharmacodynamic (PK-PD) analysis seeks to summarise the behaviour of a drug in the body, to understand the sources of variability in this behaviour, and to use this knowledge to design rational, and ideally individualised, dosing regimens. The aim of this chapter is to review some basic PK and PD principles, to introduce the concepts that an intensive care physician may encounter when reading a contemporary PK-PD paper, and to consider the influence of critical illness on the pharmacokinetics and pharmacodynamics of drugs used in intensive care.

DOSE–RESPONSE RELATIONSHIPS

Most drugs exert their effects by binding to receptors[1] such as an enzyme or membrane ion channel. The binding to the receptor directly or indirectly triggers a chain of biological events leading to the observable effects of the drug. The magnitude of effect is a function of:

- the number of receptors present
- the willingness of a drug to associate with a receptor (receptor affinity)
- the presence of other compounds competing for the binding site on the receptor (agonists/antagonists)
- the concentration of the free (unbound) drug in the vicinity of the receptor

As the number of receptors present is finite, drugs have a maximum achievable effect. Classically, a plot of drug effect versus the logarithm of a wide range of doses will be described by a sigmoid-shaped dose–response curve (Figure 79.1). In practice, the range of doses used in patients is often narrower, and is confined to a smaller section of the dose–response curve.

Note that a drug effect can be plotted in individuals (e.g. mean arterial pressure vs. drug concentration) or for a population of individuals (e.g. % of patients responding to increasing doses of an antihypertensive). The shape of dose–response curves is often defined by three parameters:

- the maximum possible effect (E_{max})
- the dose at which 50% of E_{max} is achieved (the median effective dose, or ED_{50})
- a parameter controlling the steepness of the linear section of the curve (sometimes called the Hill coefficient, Figure 79.1)

Analogous curves can often be drawn for each of the adverse or toxic effects of a drug. The ratio of the median toxic dose and the median effective dose is termed the therapeutic index. The smaller the therapeutic index of a drug, the greater the potential to do harm rather than good.

Any drug should be administered with a clear understanding of the expected benefits to the patient. While it is more difficult to cause drug toxicity by administering a drug with a high therapeutic index, careless use can result in treatment failure and unnecessary cost. Drugs with a low therapeutic index should be used with considerable caution, with the assistance of titration to measured drug effects, dose nomograms or measurements of drug concentrations (therapeutic monitoring).

TITRATION

Many drugs used in intensive care have a relatively rapid onset of a directly measurable physiological effect (Table 79.1). They can therefore be used by a process of titration of dose versus effect to achieve the desired therapeutic outcome. While titration can be an empirical process, efficient titration strategies are guided by an understanding of the kinetics and dynamics of a drug. Important issues include an understanding of:

- the time required for the drug to achieve peak effect after intravenous bolus administration; multiple doses within this time period may result in 'overshoot' of effect

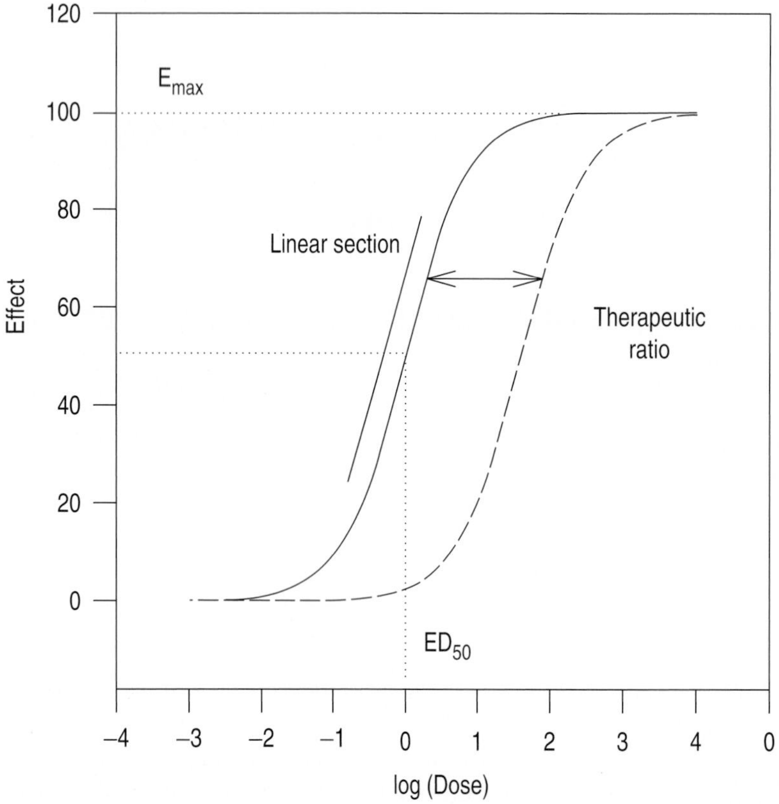

Figure 79.1 The basic concepts of dose–response curves for the therapeutic and toxic effects of a hypothetical drug. Each curve can be described by the maximum effect (E_{max}) and the dose at which half of the maximum effect is achieved (ED_{50}). The Hill coefficient (n) controls the steepness of the linear section of the curve. When this is very steep, drugs have a threshold effect and behave in an 'on or off' manner.

- potential for drug accumulation with repeated bolus doses that may manifest as a stronger, longer action for subsequent doses
- potential range of dose sizes for titration
- optimisation of initiating, increasing or decreasing the rate of an intravenous infusion
- the effects of evolving pathophysiology and tolerance
- potential kinetic and dynamic interactions with co-administered drugs

Developing this understanding requires knowledge of some fundamental pharmacokinetic and pharmacodynamic concepts.

PHARMACOKINETICS

Key pharmacokinetic concepts include volume of distribution (V) and clearance (CL). These can be applied to individual organs or to the whole body.

VOLUME OF DISTRIBUTION IN AN ORGAN

A drug administered to a patient will directly or indirectly enter the blood and be distributed by the blood circulation around the body. Drug enters the organs of the body via the afferent arterial blood supply. Any given molecule can then either diffuse into the organ or leave via the efferent venous blood (Figure 79.2). At steady state (when the arterial concentrations are constant and the net rates of diffusion into and out of the organ are equal), the total amount of drug in the organ (A) will often be a fixed ratio of the afferent arterial concentration (C). This ratio is known as an apparent volume of distribution (V):

$$V = A/C = \text{mg}/(\text{mg/l}) = \text{l} \qquad (1)$$

The process of normalising amount (e.g. mg) for concentration (e.g. mg/l) produces a constant with the units of volume (l).

A given organ is characterised by the size of defined 'physiological' spaces and its relative proportions of water, lipids and drug-binding sites (Figure 79.2). The important physiological spaces are:

- the *intravascular* space (about 3% of the total mass of the organ)
- the *interstitial* space (about one-third of total organ mass). It is separated from the intravascular space by the endothelium, which has pores of sufficient size to allow the passage of most drugs (transcapillary exchange) but not (effectively) plasma proteins
- the *intracellular* space (about two-thirds of total organ mass). It is separated from the interstitial space by the lipid barriers of the parenchymal cell membranes

Table 79.1 PK-PD summary for some commonly used drugs

Class	Family	Drug	Titrated index	PK summary	Possible changes in critical illness	Dose comment
Inotropes[2]	Catecholamines	Noradrenaline	MAP Filling pressures Indirect evidence of organ hypoperfusion	High systemic clearance (3 l/min) Low Vss (0.1 l/kg) $t_{1/2}$ = 2 minutes[3]	Clearance to one-third normal $t_{1/2}$ to three times normal[3] CO dependent kinetics?	By titration Initial infusion 3–5 µg/min, 3–10 minutes to reach constant effect
		Adrenaline		Similar to noradrenaline	Similar to noradrenaline	
	Phosphodiesterase inhibitors	Milrinone		Mainly renal clearance (0.5 l/min) Moderate Vss (0.25 l/kg) $t_{1/2}$ = 1.5–2 hours[4]	Half-life increased to 20 hours in CHF + RF[5]	Loading dose needed Difficult to titrate 12.5–50 µg/kg i.v. over 20 minutes, then 0.375–0.75 µg/kg per min
		Levosimendan		Parent $t_{1/2}$ = 1 hour Active metabolite $t_{1/2}$ = 80 hours[6]		Loading dose needed Actions persist long after last dose
Vasopressor	Catecholamines	Noradrenaline	MAP once hypovolaemia corrected	See above		See above
	Others	Phenylephrine		Low hepatic clearance (0.03 l/min) High Vss (5 l/kg) $t_{1/2}$ = 0.08 and 0.8 hours[7]	Expect variable clearance and drug interactions	Beware MAO inhibitors Short-term use Loading dose needed, 100–180 µg/min then 40–60 µg/min
		Vasopressin		Peptide High CL Low Vss $t_{1/2}$ = 8–15 minutes[8]		Used in catecholamine resistance Threshold effect – do not titrate Infusion 0.04 units/min
Antihypertensives		GTN	MAP, ICP	Variable kinetics Very high CL (> CO) Low Vss $t_{1/2}$ = 2–3 minutes[9]	Expect CO dependent kinetics	Tolerance after 24 hours Infusion 0–20 mg/hour
		Sodium nitroprusside		Variable kinetics Very high CL (> CO) Low Vss $t_{1/2}$ = 2–3 minutes[10]	Expect CO dependent kinetics	Tolerance Potential cyanide toxicity Infusion 0–20 mg/hour
		Labetalol		High hepatic clearance (1.2 l/min) Very high Vss (3–11 l/kg) $t_{1/2}$ = 3–5 hours[11]	Expect CL to depend on CO and HBF	Loading dose needed Give bolus doses slowly Infusion 25–150 mg/hour

Continued

Table 79.1 PK-PD summary for some commonly used drugs—*Continued*

Class	Family	Drug	Titrated index	PK summary	Possible changes in critical illness	Dose comment
		Metoprolol		High hepatic clearance (polymorphic) High Vss (3 l/kg) $t_{1/2} = 3–7$ hours[12]	Expect CL to depend on CO and HBF	Usually repeat bolus doses, 1–5 mg slowly up to 15 mg
Antiarrhythmics	Bradyarrhythmias	Adrenaline	ECG	See above		See above, short-term emergency use
		Atropine		High renal and hepatic clearance (1.1 l/min) High Vss (4 l/kg) $t_{1/2} = 2$ and 222 minutes[13]		Bolus 0.6 or 1.0 mg
	Supraventricular arrhythmias	Adenosine		Very high systemic clearance (CL > CO) Low Vss $t_{1/2} < 2$ minutes[14]	Expect CO dependent kinetics	Increasing i.v. bolus (3, 6, 12,18 mg) until desired effect Higher doses needed for peripheral vs. central venous lines
		Verapamil		Initial redistribution after bolus Moderate hepatic clearance (0.5 l/min) High Vss (2.5 l/kg) $t_{1/2} = 0.2$ and 4 hours[15]	Little change with renal failure	Bolus 5 mg then 10 mg 10 minutes later if needed
		Amiodarone		Variable hepatic clearance (0.1–0.7 l/min) Variable Vss (0.01–2.11 l/kg) $t_{1/2} = 3–80$ hours[16]	Animal data suggest lower clearance in biliary stasis Renal failure affected total CL but not tissue levels[17]	5 mg/kg over 30–60 minutes, then 1200 mg over remainder of 24 hours Accumulates with chronic dosing giving long recovery times
	Ventricular arrhythmias	Amiodarone		See above		See above
Respiratory		Salbutamol	Respiratory status	Local effect, only R enantiomer active Mainly renal clearance (0.7 l/min) $t_{1/2} = 2$ hours[18] Variable pulmonary bioavailability		Nebulised, MDI or infusion (0.5–1 mg/hour)
Sedatives		Propofol	Sedation-agitation score, possibly EEG Stopped daily for neurological assessment	Rapid redistribution after bolus High extrahepatic clearance (2.2 l/min) High Vss (4.5 l/kg) $t_{1/2} = 1.5$, 30 and 350 minutes[19]	CO dependent kinetics[20] Higher doses needed in hypercarbia[21]	Prolonged infusions risk hypertriglyceridaemia, Bolus doses given slowly, Infusion starts at 30 mg/hour[22]

	Midazolam		Redistribution after a bolus Active metabolite Low hepatic clearance (0.15 l/min) Moderate Vss (1.4 l/kg) $t_{1/2} = 2.5–3.5$ hours[23]	Highly variable kinetics[24] $t_{1/2}$ of parent and metabolite prolonged in illness[25] Haemodialysis removes parent, not metabolite Free fraction changes in renal failure prolong action	Active metabolite Bolus 1–5 mg Infusion 1–15 mg/hour
Anticonvulsants	Phenytoin	Seizure activity, therapeutic monitoring	Highly variable, saturable hepatic clearance Therapeutic monitoring Reduced protein binding increases the unbound concentration	Drug interactions via hepatic metabolism	Loading dose 15–20 mg/kg over 30 minutes Maintenance 300 mg/24 hours titrated to concentration
Analgesics	Morphine	Patient controlled/ feedback if possible	Active metabolites (M6G, M3G) High hepatic clearance (1.3 l/min) Moderate Vss (0.9 l/kg) $t_{1/2} = 3–4$ hours Slow, actively opposed brain penetration	Higher brain concentrations. when BBB compromised[26] Metabolites accumulate in renal failure[27] CL depends on CO and HBF Haemodialysis removes parent and metabolite	Tolerance Active M6G metabolite a problem for long infusions and renal failure Bolus 0.5–5 mg Infusion 1–10 mg/hour
	Fentanyl		Rapid redistribution after bolus Moderate hepatic clearance (0.6 l/min) High Vss (5 l/kg) $t_{1/2} = 1$, 20 and 500 minutes[28] Moderately rapid brain penetration ($t_{1/2} = 6$ minutes)	Prolonged recovery from long infusions Long half-life in critically ill[29] Expect CL to depend on CO and HBF Little effect of renal failure	Tolerance Accumulates with longer infusions (> 6 hours) giving long recovery times
Muscle relaxants	Vecuronium	Peripheral nerve stimulation if in doubt before withdrawing sedation	Low hepatic clearance (0.3 l/min) Low Vss (0.2 l/kg) $t_{1/2} = 1.2$, 14 and 62 minutes[30] Rapid blood effect equilibrium ($t_{1/2} = 3$ minutes)	Expect variable CL Active metabolite Longer action in hepatic and renal failure Duration of action increased in hypothermia	Restricted uses and always under sedation Bolus 2–8 mg

Continued

Table 79.1 PK-PD summary for some commonly used drugs—*Continued*

Class	Family	Drug	Titrated index	PK summary	Possible changes in critical illness	Dose comment
Renal		Furosemide	Urine output	Low renal and hepatic clearance (0.13 l/min) Low Vss (0.3 l/kg) $t_{1/2} = 1.25$ and 33 hours[31]	Dose adjustment in renal failure complex[31]	Possible tolerance Infusion 2.5–10 mg/hour
		Spironolactone		Kinetics of parent drug probably less relevant than that of active metabolites	Dose adjustment in renal failure complex Little effect of hepatic failure Metabolism increased with chronic dosing	Significant active metabolites Avoid or increase dose interval with renal failure or cirrhosis, 25–100 mg b.d.
Antibiotics		Many	Culture Clinical response	Wide range[32]	Drug dependent[32]	May require up to 48 hours for full effects of regimen

BBB, blood–brain barrier; CHF, congestive heart failure; CL, clearance; CO, cardiac output; GTN, glyceryl trinitrate; HBF, hepatic blood flow; ICP, intracranial pressure; MAO, monoamine oxidase; MAP, mean arterial pressure; MDI, metered dose inhaler; RF, renal failure; Vss, volume of distribution at steady state.

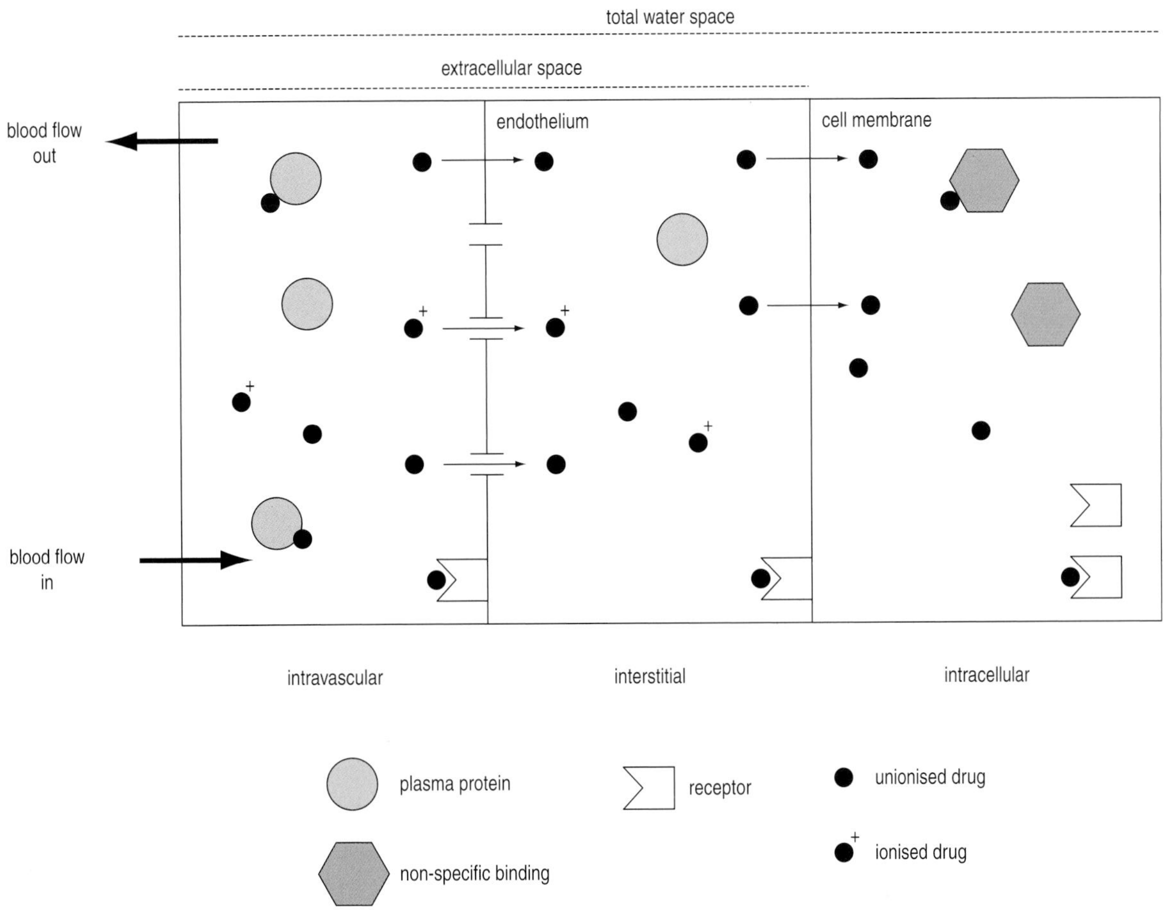

Figure 79.2 Processes governing drug entry into a tissue.

A drug may act on receptors in any of these spaces. The physicochemical properties of a drug dictate which physiological spaces are accessible to the drug. A drug can exist in blood in several forms: ionised or unionised (governed by the local pH and the pKa of the drug), and bound or unbound to plasma proteins.

- Only unbound (free) drug can diffuse into the interstitial space via capillary pores or via a paracellular route
- Only unbound, unionised drug can diffuse across cell membranes (transcellular route)

Consequently, drugs that are *highly bound* or *highly ionised* in blood generally have smaller distribution volumes in an organ. For example, the distribution volume of propofol in the brain is less than expected based on its high lipophilicity because it is highly bound in plasma. Paradoxically, highly lipophilic drugs in general do not penetrate tissues as extensively as moderately lipophilic compounds, as high lipophilicity is correlated with high binding in plasma.[33]

A distribution volume (V) provides information about how much drug is in an organ at steady state, but provides no information about how quickly steady-state concentrations in the organ would be achieved. The fastest possible rate is when diffusion across the endothelium and cell membranes is significantly faster than organ blood flow (Q). In this case, the uptake into the organ is 'flow-limited', and the half-life of organ equilibration is given by:

$$t_{1/2} = 0.693 \times V/Q \qquad (2)$$

Note that if the distribution volume of an organ is relatively large or the organ blood flow is low, the time required for an organ to completely equilibrate (at least five times $t_{1/2}$) with the blood can be quite long despite flow-limited kinetics.

When the diffusion rate across the endothelium and cell membranes is significantly less than organ blood flow (Q), the uptake into the organ is 'membrane-limited' and less affected by changes in organ blood flow. Morphine shows membrane-limited uptake into the brain.[34]

THE SPECIAL CASE OF THE BRAIN

Drug penetration into the brain is further restricted compared to that of other organs because of passive and active defence mechanisms collectively known as the blood–brain barrier (BBB). The passive component is the tight junctions of endothelial cells in the brain, which means that passage across the endothelium is solely by the transcellular route, and therefore restricted to lipophilic compounds. The active component is a range of transmembrane transporters. Some of these allow the uptake of endogenous compounds (e.g. amino acids and glucose). Of more pharmacological importance are a range of efflux transporters that actively pump drugs from the brain to the blood.[35] The clinical significance of these transporters is currently being defined, but may be particularly important for some drugs. For example, loperamide is a potent opioid, but has no central effects at normal doses because it is excluded from the brain by P-glycoprotein.[36] Similarly, the concentration of morphine in the brain is kept low by active transport. When the BBB is damaged, morphine concentrations in the brain are found to be higher.[26]

CLEARANCE IN AN ORGAN

The liver and the kidney have the special (but not exclusive) role of removing drug from the body. The liver can either transport a drug from the blood into the bile or metabolise a drug into another chemical entity (metabolite). Metabolism can be Phase I (e.g. by oxidation or reduction by enzymes of the cytochrome P-450 (CYP) family, or hydrolysis by esterases) or Phase II (e.g. conjugation with another compound to form a glucuronide or sulphate). The kidney excretes drug by filtration, and potentially active secretion, into the urine. Usually metabolites are less active than their parent compound, are more polar and more readily excreted in bile or urine.

The rate (R) that the liver or kidney can remove drug from the body is usually proportional to the concentration of drug in the blood (C) (i.e. first-order kinetics). This proportionality constant is known as drug clearance (CL):

$$CL = R/C = (\text{mg/min})/(\text{mg/l}) = 1/\text{min} \qquad (3)$$

The process of normalising rate (e.g. mg/min) for concentration (e.g. mg/l) produces a constant with the units of flow (l/min). For an organ, the clearance can be shown to be equal to the blood flow (Q) through the organ multiplied by the extraction ratio of the drug across the organ (E). If the liver, for example, completely removes all drug passing through it, then $E = 1$ and the clearance of the drug is hepatic blood flow. If half the drug is removed, $E = 0.5$ and the clearance is half the hepatic blood flow. Clearance can also be calculated for the whole body, where it represents the total rate of removal of the drug from the body.

HEPATIC DRUG CLEARANCE

There are a number of factors that affect drug metabolism by the liver, but they can be classified by the extraction ratio of the drug across the liver: high (> 0.7), intermediate or low (< 0.3).

- *High extraction drugs*: There is a relative excess of the enzymes that metabolise a drug (i.e. a high intrinsic clearance). The rate-limiting step is supply of the drug to the liver, so hepatic clearance depends on hepatic blood flow (which is proportional to cardiac output[37]) and is unaffected by changes in the amount of active enzyme (and therefore enzyme inhibition or enzyme induction) and changes in free fraction of the drug.
- *Low extraction drugs*: There is a relative shortage of the enzymes that metabolise the drug (i.e. a low intrinsic clearance) and the rate-limiting step is the activity of the enzymes themselves. Hepatic clearance is independent of hepatic blood flow but is affected by enzyme inhibition or enzyme induction, other competing drugs, and changes in free fraction of the drug (the form accessible to the enzyme).

When the concentration of some drugs is relatively high (e.g. ethyl alcohol, phenytoin, high-dose barbiturates), the metabolic pathway becomes saturated, and the drug is slowly eliminated at a fixed rate (i.e. a zero-order process). A corollary is that small increases in a dose of a drug will cause marked sustained increases in plasma concentration during zero-order kinetics compared with administration during first-order elimination kinetics.

RENAL DRUG CLEARANCE

Three processes govern the net clearance of a drug or metabolite by the kidneys: glomerular filtration, tubular secretion and tubular reabsorption. Filtration in the glomerulus normally allows the passage of the free but not protein-bound drug into the renal tubules. Therefore, drugs that are not subject to tubular secretion or reabsorption have a renal clearance that equals the glomerular filtration rate (normally 0.1 l/min). Drugs that are actively secreted into the tubules (usually charged molecules) can have higher renal clearances up to a theoretical maximum of renal blood flow (1.2 l/min). Drugs that are lipophilic and uncharged are filtered, but rapidly diffuse back across the tubule into the blood stream so that their net renal clearance is zero.

HALF-LIFE IN THE BODY

For a given drug, each organ of the body has characteristic rates of distribution (equilibration half-life) or clearance (extraction). When these complex processes are summed together, however, the sum appears to reduce to changes in blood concentrations that can be described by one, two or three exponential functions, each with an associated half-life term. Half-lives can describe the rate of decline of the blood drug concentration following a dose, or the rate of increase in concentration during an infusion. Half-life is defined as the time taken for the drug concentration in the blood to decrease (or increase) by 50%, and when only one half-life is evident it is related to distribution volume and clearance as follows:

$$t_{1/2} = 0.693 \times V/CL \qquad (4)$$

In this case, clearance and distribution volume describe the apparent behaviour of the drug in the body as a whole. This volume and clearance can be used to calculate dose regimens for this special case.

- *Intravenous bolus dose*: Shortly after a bolus dose of A mg, the initial blood concentration will be:

$$A/V \qquad (5)$$

  It will decline to 50% of this concentration in one half-life, and to 6% of this concentration in four half-lives.
- *Intravenous infusion*: For a constant rate infusion of X mg/min, the final steady-state concentration during the infusion will be:

$$X/CL \qquad (6)$$

  It will reach 50% of this concentration in one half-life, and 94% of this concentration in four half-lives.

The distribution volume can sometimes provide information about the location of a drug in the body:[38] a drug that distributes only in the *intravascular space* (e.g. one that is tightly bound to plasma proteins, such as indocyanine green) will have a distribution volume of about 0.075 l/kg; a drug that distributes into the *extracellular space* (e.g. one that is charged and cannot cross cell membrane, such as furosemide) will have a distribution volume of about 0.21 l/kg; and a drug that distributes into the *total water space* (e.g. one that is uncharged, lipophilic but does not bind to proteins, such as antipyrine) will have a distribution volume of about 0.6 l/kg. Drugs with higher distribution volumes can be assumed to be bound in blood and/or tissues.

INTERPRETING HALF-LIVES

Clinicians find the concept of half-life an attractive way to summarise the behaviour of a drug. Its simplicity is appealing, but some caution is required as a drug can have more than one half-life. For many drugs, half-lives can be found that represent initial mixing of the drug in blood, distribution, elimination and sometimes slow sequestration into tissues such as fat. The most relevant half-life(s) is the one that is dominant in determining a drug's duration of action. Thus, elimination half-life is of limited use if termination of drug effect is caused by redistribution after a bolus (e.g. propofol). The measured half-life of drug also depends on the design of the study (whether frequent early blood samples were taken), can be assay dependent (the terminal half-life of propofol has increased with newer assay methods with lower detection limits) and varies between arterial and venous blood (rapid distribution half-lives are generally more apparent in arterial blood). Finally, the half-life of a drug is not a constant – it depends on the physiological and pathophysiological state of a patient and their drug history.

PHARMACOKINETIC MODELS

It is feasible to describe the behaviour of drug in the body using the concepts of distribution volumes, clearances and half-lives. However, pharmacokineticists are often required to predict the consequences of dose changes on the concentrations and effects of a drug – this requires a mathematical representation (or model) of the behaviour of drug. A model is defined by a set of equations (representing the basic structure) and a set of parameter values for those equations (representing the behaviour of a specific drug).

There are three basic forms of pharmacokinetic models:

- *Compartmental models* are the most common and most traditional pharmacokinetic model, and assume that the body can be represented by a central compartment and possibly one or more peripheral compartments. While these models have proved serviceable in some areas of therapeutics, as they do not represent organ blood flow they therefore have some limitations in intensive care where patient physiology is labile.
- *Physiological models* represent the major organs of the body, with drug supply to and from the organs dictated by vascular anatomy and organ blood flow. While they have been developed for some important drugs, in particular for animals, they are consequently less common in the literature for humans (with some notable exceptions[23]) because they require a large amount of data for their development. They have the advantage of being able to predict the consequences of changes in both dose regimen and physiological status.
- *Recirculatory models* are an intermediate between compartment and physiological models. Recirculatory models can provide a simple conceptual framework for the important relationship between cardiac output, bolus injection rate and initial drug concentrations[39] that is lacking in compartmental models.

In a traditional pharmacokinetic analysis, the model is fitted to pooled data from a group of patients to estimate, for example, the mean clearance for the group (e.g. $CL =$ 1.8 l/min). In contrast, the population approach is a type of modelling that fits data from individual patients simultaneously.[40] It is possible to estimate not only the mean value of clearance but also its variability in the population (e.g. $CL = 1.8 \pm 0.2$ l/min). The population pharmacokinetic approach is of particular relevance to intensive care, as it can accommodate wide inter- and intra-patient variability and does not require that all patients in a study have the same dose or blood sampling schedule.

PRACTICAL APPLICATIONS

BOLUS INJECTION RATE

Dose regimens specifying an intravenous bolus injection often do not state the time over which the bolus should be administered, and often subjective and highly variable descriptions such as 'slow' are used. However, the rate of injection of a bolus is often crucial in determining the magnitude of transient toxic effects. This is because rapid injections cause disproportionately high transient 'first-pass' concentrations in arterial blood and target organs. For example, if the peak arterial concentration after 100 mg of propofol injected over 20 seconds is 60 mg/l, it will be only 10 mg/l if it is injected over 2 minutes.[39] High arterial propofol concentrations are associated with adverse haemodynamic effects.[41] Figure 79.3 shows a conceptual hydraulic model which illustrates ways that rapid injections transiently 'load' the blood and target organs with drug.

The high 'first-pass' concentrations achieved after a bolus injection are also inversely affected by cardiac output,[39] and particular caution is required in low cardiac output states. For example, if an injection of propofol over 20 seconds into a cardiac output of 5 l/min gave a peak arterial concentration of 60 mg/l, then for a cardiac output of 10 l/min the peak concentration would be 30 mg/l, and for 2 l/min it would be 150 mg/l. The conceptual hydraulic model in Figure 79.3 can also be used to develop a mental picture of how cardiac output affects bolus kinetics. There are very few drugs for which intravenous injection over less than 2 minutes is indicated.

REPEAT BOLUS OR INFUSION

Whilst drugs with relatively long half-lives and wide therapeutic indices can be given by repeat bolus administration, those with short half-lives and narrow therapeutic indices (e.g. catecholamines) can be given in a more predictable and titratable manner by infusion.

LOADING DOSES

Drugs with relatively long half-lives (due to large distribution volumes and/or low clearance) can take a considerable amount of time (five times the half-life) to reach steady state once a constant rate infusion is initiated. A loading dose (either a bolus or a short period of higher infusion rate) can decrease the time required to reach steady state by adding additional drug that can compensate for the drug initially being 'lost' from the blood into peripheral distribution volumes (see Table 79.1 for drug-specific information on loading doses).

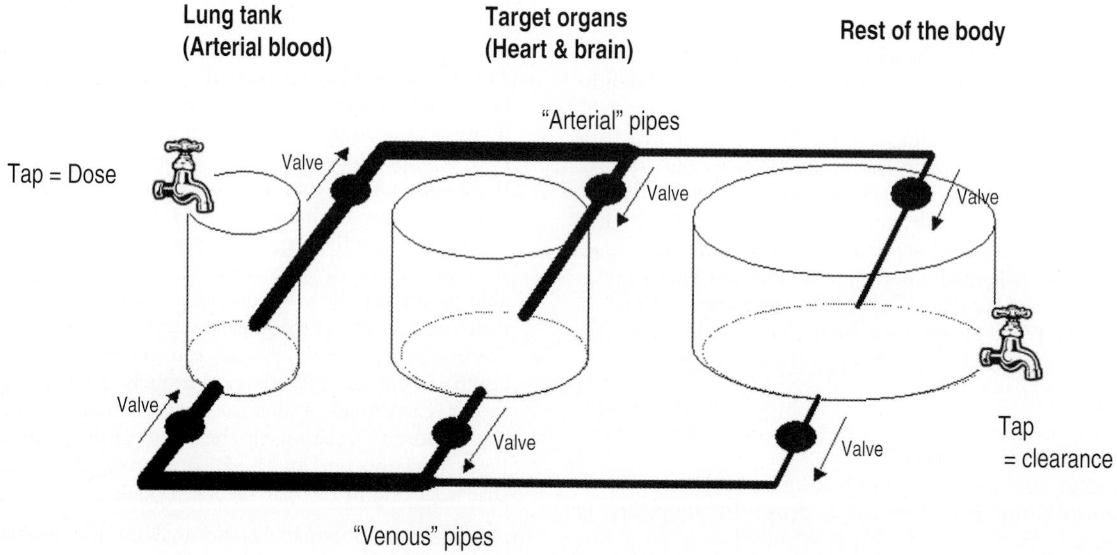

Figure 79.3 A conceptual hydraulic model of the important factors governing drug disposition after i.v. bolus administration based on recirculatory principles. This example illustrates the case where a drug acts in a well-perfused target organ such as the heart or the brain but has a large volume of distribution. Three water tanks represent drug in the lung, important target organs and the 'rest of the body'; in each tank *the height of the water is proportional to the drug concentration*. Pipes connect the tanks to represent the circulation; the diameters of the pipes are proportional to the blood flow to each organ. To impart recirculatory characteristics like the real circulation, one-way valves are fitted before and after each tank in the directions shown. Intravenous drug administration corresponds to adding to the lung tank; drug clearance is a 'leak' from the 'body' tank. The reader is asked to imagine the consequences of a rapid i.v. injection, e.g. pouring a bucket into the lung tank. It can be seen that there will be high levels of water in both the lung and target organ tank until the water has had the time to distribute into the body or be cleared; in vivo this would potentially manifest as transient toxic drug effects in the target organs. By slowing the 'injection' down and pouring more slowly, lower peak concentrations can be achieved.

MAINTENANCE DOSE

Once steady state has been achieved, it is traditionally taught that the steady-state blood concentrations are a function only of dose rate and drug clearance (Eq 6). However, intensivists should be aware that haemodynamic status can also significantly affect the steady-state blood concentration due to the key role of cardiac output (Figure 79.3) and blood flow-dependent clearance.[37] For example, administering catecholamines during a constant rate infusion of propofol could rapidly increase the cardiac output and lower the propofol concentrations in the blood and brain sufficiently to cause emergence from anaesthesia.[42] This behaviour is particularly evident for high clearance drugs.[39]

CHANGING INFUSION RATES

The immediate effect of changing the rate of drug infusion will depend on the half-life of the drug. For drugs with long half-lives (e.g. midazolam and morphine), an increase in dose requirements should be met by titrating small boluses to achieve the new state, and then increasing the infusion rate by an appropriate amount. Decreases in requirements should be met by switching off the infusion and then restarting at a lower rate after the new desired state has been reached. If severe illness causes the volume of distribution of a drug to be doubled, then its half-life will also be doubled. Severe illness may also decrease clearance of a drug; halving clearance will cause a similar doubling of half-life. Should both effects occur together, half-life will be increased fourfold, having a significant effect on the duration of action of a drug.

OFFSET TIMES

It should be appreciated that the half-life for some drugs depends on the duration of the infusion. This is particularly evident for drugs with high distribution volumes and whose bolus kinetics are governed significantly by redistribution rather than clearance (e.g. fentanyl). For short infusions, the plasma half-life after the infusion will be less than the terminal elimination half-life. However, as the duration of infusion becomes sufficient to achieve steady state, the half-life upon stopping the infusion will increase until it equals the terminal elimination half-life.[43]

ROUTES OF DRUG ADMINISTRATION

ORAL

Traditionally the enteral route has been avoided in the critically ill because alterations in gut motility, blood flow, pH, function and first-past metabolism by the liver contribute to variability in drug response. Gastric emptying is also impaired by many factors including anticholinergics, antacids, phenothiazines and opioids, inotropes (especially dopamine), traumatic brain injury and diabetes mellitus.

However, there is an increasing trend to resume premorbid oral medications as soon as possible after the intercurrent illness has resolved or vital organ function has stabilised. Furthermore, some commonly used drugs have no suitable parenteral equivalents (e.g. statins, angiotensin-converting enzyme inhibitors, angiotensin II inhibitors, aspirin, digoxin, oral anticoagulants and some antibiotics such as fusidic acid and rifampicin). Consequently, the use of the oral route is becoming more common. One confounding issue is that critically ill patients are increasingly also fed via the enteral route.[44] Enteral feeding may reduce drug availability due to absorption of drug onto enteral feed components, nasogastric tubing or by reduced absorption due to the pH of the feed. Conversely, the administered drug has the potential to block the feeding tube.

SUBCUTANEOUS AND INTRAMUSCULAR

Subcutaneous and i.m. injection may also be unpredictable because systemic transfer of drug is dependent on blood flow at the site of injection, which in turn depends on posture, activity, site of injection and degree of vasoconstriction or vasodilatation at that site.

INTRAVENOUS

The i.v. route is used for speed, convenience, reliability, titratability and lack of enteral formulations of some drugs. Intravenous apparatus including glass, plastics and rubber may absorb drugs, decreasing the dose delivered (e.g. insulin, heparin, amiodarone). When several drugs are delivered through the same i.v. line, chemical incompatibility may also occur. This may be a result of pH effects altering solubility, solvent effects (e.g. precipitation of the propylene glycol used to dissolve some preparations of diazepam when diluted excessively) and cation–anion interactions causing precipitation or formation of less active, yet soluble complexes (e.g. thiopentone or calcium in combination with most other drugs). Although precipitation can be detected by visual inspection, lack of visual changes does not mean there has not been loss of potency (e.g. heparin and dopamine, insulin and total parenteral nutrition).[45]

When infusing drugs i.v., the method of administration can alter the amount of drug delivered dramatically. Simple infusions using a drip chamber to regulate flow are not adequate when infusing inotropes, and mechanical drop counters and peristaltic pumps may be erratic, especially if drug is not adequately diluted and the flow rate is low. Syringe pumps are the most accurate, but may also be unreliable at low flow rates (1–2 ml/h). As siphoning from or flushing of i.v. lines can also result in drug overdose, it is essential that anti-reflux valves are used when more than one infusion is running into a single i.v. site.

PK-PD CHANGES IN CRITICAL ILLNESS

Critically ill patients often have multiple organ dysfunction, causing alterations in drug handling and effect in the body at all levels. The net effect of these multiple changes is difficult to predict. Frequently, the main effect is to increase inter-patient variability in response, even if typical patient response is altered little. Intra-patient variability also occurs over brief periods of time in response to changes in a patient's condition.

CIRCULATORY FAILURE

Circulatory failure causes a greater percentage of cardiac output to go to essential organs (e.g. heart and brain) and decreased blood flow to peripheral tissues (Table 79.2). The net effects are:

- Increased drug concentrations in the heart and brain (Figure 79.3)
- Decreased drug concentrations in the periphery
- Decreased renal blood flow and shunting of blood from cortical to juxtamedullary nephrons. Glomerular filtration rate and tubular excretion are decreased, decreasing extraction of drugs and metabolites
- Decreased liver blood flow. Hepatocellular function may be impaired, decreasing clearance of both highly extracted drugs due to failure of delivery to the liver, and of poorly extracted drugs due to failure of cellular metabolism

Table 79.2 Distribution of cardiac output in healthy and critically ill patients

Organ	% Body weight	% Cardiac output	Change in % of cardiac output in critical illness
Lungs	2	100	Nil
Heart	0.5	5	+++
Brain	2	14	+++
Kidneys	0.5	23	– – –
Liver/ splanchnic	10	28	– – –
Endocrine/ bone marrow	2	6	– –
Skin	6	9	– –
Muscle	50	16	– –
Fat	15	5	– –
Other	12	5	– –

In the critically ill, cardiac output may vary widely depending on therapy, and distribution will depend on the amount of peripheral vasoconstriction (e.g. from hypovolaemia) or vasodilatation (e.g. from systemic inflammatory response syndrome).

Mechanical ventilation may cause further decreases in liver blood flow by increasing intrathoracic pressure and therefore decreasing venous return.

The initial effect is a large decrease in distribution volumes and clearance of drugs. The effects are more profound on drugs that are usually rapidly distributed such as sedatives. Fluid and inotropic therapy may alter these effects over brief periods of time. With volume overload, there may be an increase in initial distribution volume but with a more prolonged distribution half-life.

HEPATIC FAILURE

Hepatic failure may increase or decrease volume of distribution and total body clearance, and increase excretion half-life of hepatically metabolised drugs. Loading doses are often not greatly affected. In the critically ill, there is usually a decrease in liver blood flow and therefore the rate at which drugs are delivered to the liver for metabolism. Flow-dependent drugs include morphine, propofol, labetalol, metoprolol and atropine (Table 79.1). Vasopressors do not usually decrease liver blood flow because of increases in cardiac output.

There is a poor correlation between derangement of conventional tests of liver function and the degree of impairment of drug metabolism. In addition, the degree of impairment may vary widely over short periods of time. In the critically ill, metabolism of some drugs will almost cease, as indicated by a lack of formation of metabolites and very high plasma concentrations (e.g. midazolam[46]).

Hepatic failure tends to decrease the amount of drug bound because of accumulation of metabolites which compete for binding sites on protein. For example, elevated concentrations of bilirubin decrease protein binding of sulphonamides, tetracyclines, penicillins and cephalosporins. A decrease in protein binding will offset increases in volume of distribution when the drug is highly protein bound, such as most penicillins and erythromycin. For drugs with low protein binding, such as aminoglycosides, a decrease in protein binding will have little effect on free plasma concentrations.

RENAL FAILURE

Renal drug clearance is reduced by renal failure, and distribution volumes will increase if there is significant fluid retention leading to increased half-lives of drugs cleared by the kidneys. Drug doses may be decreased to as little as 10% of normal. In the case of drugs that are metabolised by the liver and metabolites excreted by the kidneys, there may be accumulation of active metabolites (e.g. morphine-6-glucuronide). Renal failure usually affects glomerular function more than tubular function, so excretion of aminoglycosides which depend more on glomerular filtration are affected more than excretion of penicillins which are dependent on tubular function.

Creatinine clearance is usually a poor guide to renal function in the critically ill because there may be alterations in the rate of formation of creatinine as well as its excretion by the kidneys. Algorithms for drug dose based on creatinine clearance may be similarly unreliable, particularly in critically ill patients. Accumulation of metabolic products may cause decreases in protein binding of drugs. For example, uraemia decreases binding of penicillins, sulphonamides and cephalosporins and in the case of phenytoin excretion is increased.

Renal replacement therapy drastically alters volumes and clearances of drugs. Effects vary with the mode of dialysis, the type of membrane in use and the drugs in question. For most modern membranes little information is available, but what is known has been reviewed.[47]

SYSTEMIC INFLAMMATORY RESPONSE SYNDROME

In acute severe illness, such as sepsis and multiple organ failure, there is an increase in capillary permeability and total body water secondary to the increased capillary permeability and hypoalbuminaemia. This increases the volume of distribution of drugs, so that increased loading doses may be required to attain a satisfactory therapeutic concentration. Similar changes occur in patients with major burns, and this may be due to circulating cytokines. The volume of distribution may also change over short periods of time. When patients start to recover, serum concentrations may increase because of the decreasing volume of distribution of the drug (e.g. vancomycin[48]) as well as decrease because of resumption of normal metabolism and clearance (e.g. midazolam[46]). Circulatory, hepatic and renal failure may also add the characteristic changes already described, of decreased clearance or metabolism and accumulation of active metabolites.

CHANGES IN RECEPTORS IN ACUTE ILLNESS

Drug receptors may change in the critically ill, affecting drug response. One cause of tolerance, which is a decreased drug effect for a given dose or plasma concentration, is altered receptor function. Catecholamines show an increase in receptor numbers in response to a lack of agonist (upregulation) and a decrease in receptor numbers in response to increased concentrations of agonist (downregulation). Drug affinity for receptors is also pH dependent. Acidosis decreases the affinity of catecholamines for their receptors, and is a significant problem when there is a pH < 7.1. Hypothermia also decreases drug affinity for receptors.

Proliferation of extrajunctional acetylcholine receptors on muscle after acute injuries such as burns and denervation can lead to hyperkalaemia following the use of suxamethonium.

PROTEIN BINDING

For most drugs, it is the free (unbound) drug that can enter an organ and bind to receptors, be metabolised or be eliminated (Figure 79.2). Albumin is the dominant binding protein in plasma, and the extent of binding is related in a non-linear manner to the concentration of albumin.[49] In most cases, the number of drug-binding sites available on albumin greatly exceeds the number of drug molecules, and the free drug concentration is proportional to the total drug concentration. Most acidic drugs, including all antibiotics, bind to albumin. Basic drugs, such as phenytoin and propranolol, bind mainly to α_1-acid glycoprotein. During acute illness, α_1-acid glycoprotein concentrations increase, with increased drug binding. Lipoproteins can bind highly lipophilic drugs such as propofol. It is also important to consider the dissociation rate of the drug–protein complex.[50] When this is slow, the binding is 'restrictive' (e.g. warfarin) and free drug concentrations are very important. When dissociation is fast, the binding is 'permissive' (e.g. propranolol) and free drug concentrations are less important for processes such as hepatic clearance where rapid dissociation from protein can supply drug to liver enzymes within one pass through the liver.

Changes in protein binding in critical illness can occur due to drug interactions at the protein binding site[50] or changes in the concentrations of binding protein. However, the net effect is drug dependent, and can be negligible if the free concentration determines both drug effect and drug clearance. Changes can be significant in some contexts. Midazolam (usually 96% protein bound) increases its effect in renal failure despite increased clearance, due to reduced protein binding.[51] Similarly, the anaesthetic effect of propofol increases during haemodilution due to increases in free propofol concentration, even though the total concentration is unchanged.[52]

DRUG MONITORING

If no alternative is available, it may be necessary to use a drug with a narrow therapeutic index. When no direct clinical measure of clinical response is possible, plasma drug concentrations may be measured if there is a relationship between this concentration and pharmacological effects (efficacy and/or toxicity). Toxicity may be associated with peak drug concentration (e.g. seizures and arrhythmias from theophyllines) or with mean concentration (e.g. ototoxicity from aminoglycosides). Some drugs for which there are accepted therapeutic and/or toxic concentrations are shown in Table 79.3.

Drug assays usually measure total plasma concentration of the drug; however, it is the fraction not bound to proteins in plasma that is responsible for the pharmacological effect(s). These plasma protein levels do change during critical illness and so the unbound fraction can be different from that in relatively healthy persons, thus modifying the relationship between measured drug concentration and clinical effect. Regardless of measured concentration, evidence of clinical efficacy or toxicity

Table 79.3 Therapeutic drug monitoring in the critically ill

Drug	Therapeutic concentrations	Toxic effects and guidelines to dosage
Antiarrhythmics		
Digoxin	0.5–0.8 ng/ml in CHF patients[53]	Monitor ECG – dysrhythmia/ conduction defects
Antibiotics		
Gentamicin	Peak 5–10 μg/ml, trough < 2	Renal and ototoxicity Once daily high dose Check trough (or extended dosing interval use trough < 0.5 μg/ml)
Amikacin	Peak 8–16 μg/ml, trough < 4	As above
Vancomycin	Peak 20–40 μg/ml, trough < 10	
Anticonvulsants		
Phenytoin	10–20 mg/l	Arrhythmias Check free concentration if uraemia/low albumin
Theophyllines		
Aminophylline	10–20 mg/l	> 25 mg/l

must be monitored regularly and the drug concentration used as a part of the clinical decision process with the view to individualising the patient's dosage to optimise beneficial response(s). Given these considerations, the relatively small expense of therapeutic drug monitoring must be weighed against the risks of toxicity or treatment failure.

DRUG BY DRUG SUMMARY

Table 79.1 summarises the kinetic properties of some drugs commonly used in intensive care. The reader is referred to other chapters in this book for detailed commentary on the use of specific drugs.

ACKNOWLEDGEMENTS

Updated and modified from the chapter in the previous edition by T G Short and G C Hood. Dose regimens in Table 79.1 are modified from the ICU Handbooks of the Royal Adelaide Hospital (2003) and Waikato Hospital (2004). Dose regimens are for illustration only and local guidelines should be consulted.

REFERENCES

1. Alexander SP, Mathie A, Peters JA. Guide to receptors and channels, 2nd edn. *Br J Pharmacol* 2006; **147** (Suppl 3): S1–168.
2. Lehtonen LA, Antila S, Pentikainen PJ. Pharmacokinetics and pharmacodynamics of intravenous inotropic agents. *Clin Pharmacokinet* 2004; **43**: 187–203.
3. Beloeil H, Mazoit JX, Benhamou D *et al.* Norepinephrine kinetics and dynamics in septic shock and trauma patients. *Br J Anaesth* 2005; **95**: 782–8.
4. Hilleman DE, Forbes WP. Role of milrinone in the management of congestive heart failure. *DICP* 1989; **23**: 357–62.
5. Taniguchi T, Shibata K, Saito S *et al.* Pharmacokinetics of milrinone in patients with congestive heart failure during continuous venovenous hemofiltration. *Intensive Care Med* 2000; **26**: 1089–93.
6. Hengstmann JH, Goronzy J. Pharmacokinetics of 3H-phenylephrine in man. *Eur J Clin Pharmacol* 1982; **21**: 335–41.
7. Stroshane RM, Koss RF, Biddlecome CE *et al.* Oral and intravenous pharmacokinetics of milrinone in human volunteers. *J Pharm Sci* 1984; **73**: 1438–41.
8. Dunser MW, Wenzel V, Mayr AJ *et al.* Management of vasodilatory shock: defining the role of arginine vasopressin. *Drugs* 2003; **63**: 237–56.
9. Bogaert MG. Clinical pharmacokinetics of nitrates. *Cardiovasc Drugs Ther* 1994; **8**: 693–9.
10. Schulz V. Clinical pharmacokinetics of nitroprusside, cyanide, thiosulphate and thiocyanate. *Clin Pharmacokinet* 1984; **9**: 239–51.
11. McNeil JJ, Louis WJ. Clinical pharmacokinetics of labetalol. *Clin Pharmacokinet* 1984; **9**: 157–67.
12. Mehvar R, Brocks DR. Stereospecific pharmacokinetics and pharmacodynamics of beta-adrenergic blockers in humans. *J Pharm Pharm Sci* 2001; **4**: 185–200.
13. Ali-Melkkila T, Kanto J, Iisalo E. Pharmacokinetics and related pharmacodynamics of anticholinergic drugs. *Acta Anaesthesiol Scand* 1993; **37**: 633–42.
14. Blardi P, Laghi Pasini F, Urso R *et al.* Pharmacokinetics of exogenous adenosine in man after infusion. *Eur J Clin Pharmacol* 1993; **44**: 505–7.
15. Koike Y, Shimamura K, Shudo I *et al.* Pharmacokinetics of verapamil in man. *Res Commun Chem Pathol Pharmacol* 1979; **24**: 37–47.
16. Latini R, Tognoni G, Kates RE. Clinical pharmacokinetics of amiodarone. *Clin Pharmacokinet* 1984; **9**: 136–56.
17. Fruncillo RJ, Swanson BN, Bernhard R *et al.* Effect of renal failure or biliary stasis on the pharmacokinetics of amiodarone in the rat. *J Pharm Sci* 1986; **75**: 150–4.
18. Boulton DW, Fawcett JP. Enantioselective disposition of salbutamol in man following oral and intravenous administration. *Br J Clin Pharmacol* 1996; **41**: 35–40.
19. Schuttler J, Ihmsen H. Population pharmacokinetics of propofol: a multicenter study. *Anesthesiology* 2000; **93**: 1557–60.
20. Upton RN, Ludbrook GL. A physiologically based, recirculatory model of the kinetics and dynamics of propofol in man. *Anesthesiology* 2005; **103**: 344–52.

21. Vinayak AG, Gehlbach B, Pohlman AS *et al.* The relationship between sedative infusion requirements and permissive hypercapnia in critically ill, mechanically ventilated patients. *Crit Care Med* 2006; **34**: 1668–73.
22. Barr J, Egan TD, Sandoval NF *et al.* Propofol dosing regimens for ICU sedation based upon an integrated pharmacokinetic–pharmacodynamic model. *Anesthesiology* 2001; **95**: 324–33.
23. Bjorkman S. Prediction of drug disposition in infants and children by means of physiologically based pharmacokinetic (PBPK) modelling: theophylline and midazolam as model drugs. *Br J Clin Pharmacol* 2005; **59**: 691–704.
24. Swart EL, Zuideveld KP, de Jongh J *et al.* Comparative population pharmacokinetics of lorazepam and midazolam during long-term continuous infusion in critically ill patients. *Br J Clin Pharmacol* 2004; **57**: 135–45.
25. Boulieu R, Lehmann B, Salord F *et al.* Pharmacokinetics of midazolam and its main metabolite 1-hydroxymidazolam in intensive care patients. *Eur J Drug Metab Pharmacokinet* 1998; **23**: 255–8.
26. Ederoth P, Tunblad K, Bouw R *et al.* Blood–brain barrier transport of morphine in patients with severe brain trauma. *Br J Clin Pharmacol* 2004; **57**: 427–35.
27. Lotsch J. Opioid metabolites. *J Pain Symptom Manage* 2005; **29**: S10–24.
28. Shafer SL, Varvel JR. Pharmacokinetics, pharmacodynamics, and rational opioid selection. *Anesthesiology* 1991; **74**: 53–63.
29. Murphy EJ. Acute pain management pharmacology for the patient with concurrent renal or hepatic disease. *Anaesth Intensive Care* 2005; **33**: 311–22.
30. Caldwell JE, Heier T, Wright PM *et al.* Temperature-dependent pharmacokinetics and pharmacodynamics of vecuronium. *Anesthesiology* 2000; **92**: 84–93.
31. Vree TB, van der Ven AJ. Clinical consequences of the biphasic elimination kinetics for the diuretic effect of furosemide and its acyl glucuronide in humans. *J Pharm Pharmacol* 1999; **51**: 239–48.
32. Roberts JA, Lipman J. Antibacterial dosing in intensive care: pharmacokinetics, degree of disease and pharmacodynamics of sepsis. *Clin Pharmacokinet* 2006; **45**: 755–73.
33. van de Waterbeemd H, Smith DA, Jones BC. Lipophilicity in PK design: methyl, ethyl, futile. *J Comput Aided Mol Des* 2001; **15**: 273–86.
34. Upton RN, Ludbrook GL, Martinez AM *et al.* Cerebral and lung kinetics of morphine in conscious sheep after short intravenous infusions. *Br J Anaesth* 2003; **90**: 750–8.
35. de Boer AG, van der Sandt ICJ, Gaillard PJ. The role of drug transporters at the blood–brain barrier. *Annu Rev Pharmacol Toxicol* 2003; **43**: 629–56.
36. Sadeque AJ, Wandel C, He H *et al.* Increased drug delivery to the brain by P-glycoprotein inhibition. *Clin Pharmacol Ther* 2000; **68**: 231–7.
37. Stenson RE, Constantino RT, Harrison DC. Interrelationships of hepatic blood flow, cardiac output, and blood levels of lidocaine in man. *Circulation* 1971; **43**: 205–11.
38. Rowland M, Tozer TN. *Clinical Pharmacokinetics*, 2nd edn. Philadelphia: Lea and Febiger; 1989.
39. Upton RN. The two-compartment recirculatory model – an introduction to recirculatory pharmacokinetic concepts. *Br J Anaesth* 2004; **92**: 475–84.
40. Csajka C, Verotta D. Pharmacokinetic–pharmacodynamic modelling: history and perspectives. *J Pharmacokinet Pharmacodyn* 2006; **33**: 227–79.
41. Zheng D, Upton RN, Martinez AM *et al.* The influence of the bolus injection rate of propofol on its cardiovascular effects and peak blood concentrations in sheep. *Anesth Analg* 1998; **86**: 1109–15.
42. Myburgh JA, Upton RN, Grant C *et al.* Epinephrine, norepinephrine and dopamine infusions decrease propofol concentrations during continuous propofol infusion in an ovine model. *Intensive Care Med* 2001; **27**: 276–82.
43. Bailey JM. Context-sensitive half-times: what are they and how valuable are they in anaesthesiology? *Clin Pharmacokinet* 2002; **41**: 793–9.
44. Magnuson BL, Clifford TM, Hoskins LA *et al.* Enteral nutrition and drug administration, interactions, and complications. *Nutr Clin Pract* 2005; **20**: 618–24.
45. Florence AT, Attwood D. *Physicochemical Principles of Pharmacy*, 4th edn. London: Pharmaceutical Press; 2005.
46. Shelly MP, Mendel L, Park GR. Failure of critically ill patients to metabolise midazolam. *Anaesthesia* 1987; **42**: 619–26.
47. Bohler J, Donauer J, Keller F. Pharmacokinetic principles during continuous renal replacement therapy: drugs and dosage. *Kidney Int Suppl* 1999: S24–8.
48. Gous AG, Dance MD, Lipman J *et al.* Changes in vancomycin pharmacokinetics in critically ill infants. *Anaesth Intensive Care* 1995; **23**: 678–82.
49. Wilkinson GR. Plasma and tissue binding considerations in drug disposition. *Drug Metab Rev* 1983; **14**: 427–65.
50. Colmenarejo G. In silico prediction of drug-binding strengths to human serum albumin. *Med Res Rev* 2003; **23**: 275–301.
51. Vinik HR, Reves JG, Greenblatt DJ *et al.* The pharmacokinetics of midazolam in chronic renal failure patients. *Anesthesiology* 1983; **59**: 390–4.
52. Takizawa E, Takizawa D, Hiraoka H *et al.* Disposition and pharmacodynamics of propofol during isovolaemic haemorrhage followed by crystalloid resuscitation in humans. *Br J Clin Pharmacol* 2006; **61**: 256–61.
53. Rathore SS, Curtis JP, Wang Y *et al.* Association of serum digoxin concentration and outcomes in patients with heart failure. *JAMA* 2003; **289**: 871–8.

80

Management of acute poisoning

Duncan L A Wyncoll

Acute poisoning remains one of the commonest medical emergencies, accounting for 5–10% of hospital medical admissions. Although in the majority of cases the drug ingestion is intentional, the in-hospital mortality remains low (< 0.5%).[1] There are specific antidotes available for a small number of poisons and drugs; however, in most intoxications, basic supportive care is the main requirement and recovery will follow. This chapter is a hands-on guide to the general management of acute poisoning and drug intoxication. Larger reference books should be sourced, or internet-based information services (e.g. Toxbase – http://www.spib.axl.co.uk) referred to, if specific detail is required.

Clinical toxicology remains an experience-based specialty; consequently, many recommendations are based on a small literature of case reports, rather than controlled clinical studies. In recent years, toxicological experts have produced position statements and clinical guidelines on certain aspects of care, and these will be referenced when possible.

GENERAL PRINCIPLES

The general principles of the management of poisoned patients are diagnosis, clinical examination and resuscitation, investigations, drug manipulation, specific measures and continued supportive care. In the more acute situations, these actions often have to be carried out simultaneously.

AIRWAY AND VENTILATION

In acute poisoned patients who are unconscious, dentures should be removed and the oropharynx cleared of food and vomit. Tracheal intubation and airway protection is almost always necessary when a patient tolerates insertion of an oropharyngeal airway. Inadequate spontaneous ventilation, determined clinically or by arterial blood gas (ABG) analysis, obviously requires ventilatory support. Venous access should be established, and circulatory assessment must be made. Basic observations, including blood pressure, pulse rate, peripheral perfusion and urine output, should be recorded. There are very few tricks or traps as to the use of invasive monitoring and inotropic drugs, and the principles are similar to those covered elsewhere in this book.

CLINICAL EXAMINATION

A standard clinical examination should be carried out, looking particularly for needle marks or evidence of previous self-harm. The Glasgow Coma Scale, although designed for head-injured patients, is frequently used. However, descriptive documentation of the degree of impaired consciousness is much more valuable. When patients are unconscious and no history is available, the diagnosis depends upon excluding other common causes of coma (Table 80.1) and consideration of any circumstantial evidence. Specific attention should be paid to the temperature, pupil size, respiratory and heart rate, as these may help to restrict the list of potential toxins (Table 80.2).

INVESTIGATIONS

Important initial investigations include:

- *Urinalysis*: with a sample kept for later analysis if required (rapid reaction dipsticks are available to screen for common drugs of abuse/recreational drugs; however, their reliability is questioned by some).
- *Basic biochemistry*: many drugs are dependent on renal elimination. Significant renal insufficiency may alter management.
- *ABG analysis*: Metabolic and/or respiratory acidosis is most common. Aspirin may initially cause a respiratory alkalosis. Metabolic alkaloses are unusual.
- *Anion gap* $= ([Na^+] + [K^+]) - ([Cl^-] + [HCO_3^-])$: It is normally 10–14. Ethanol, methanol, ethylene glycol, metformin, cyanide, isoniazid or salicylates are the most frequent causes a high anion gap metabolic acidosis in clinical toxicology.
- *Osmolal gap*: this is the difference between the laboratory measured osmolality (O_m) and the calculated osmolality (O_c). $O_c = 2(Na^+ + K^+) + \text{urea} + \text{glucose}$. The osmolal gap is normally < 10. Causes of a raised osmolal gap are ethanol, methanol and ethylene glycol.
- *Chest X-ray*: inhalation of gastric contents is not uncommon.
- *Drug levels*: these are rarely helpful except in specific poisonings. They include paracetamol, salicylates, iron, digoxin and lithium.

Table 80.1 Common causes of coma other than acute poisoning

Intracranial bleeds
Subarachnoid haemorrhage
Subdural/extradural haematomas
Meningitis or encephalitis
Diabetic comas
Uraemic encephalopathy

Table 80.2 Clinical effects of the common poisons

Convulsions	Tricyclics, isoniazid, lithium, amfetamines, theophylline, carbon monoxide, phenothiazines, cocaine
Skin	
Bullae	Barbiturates, tricyclics
Sweating	Salicylates, organophosphates, amfetamines, cocaine
Pupils	
Constricted	Opioids, organophosphates
Dilated	Hypoxia, hypothermia, tricyclics, phenothiazines, anticholinergics
Temperature	
Pyrexia	Anticholinergics, tricyclics, salicylates, amfetamines, cocaine
Hypothermia	Barbiturates, alcohol, opioids
Cardiac rhythm	
Bradycardia	Digoxin, β-blockers, organophosphates
Tachycardia	Salicylates, theophylline, anticholinergics
Arrhythmias	Digoxin, phenothiazines, tricyclics, anticholinergics

GUT DECONTAMINATION

EMESIS

Ipecacuanha-induced emesis is no longer recommended for two reasons:[2] first, it is ineffective at removing significant quantities of poisons from the stomach and, second, it limits the use of activated charcoal.

GASTRIC LAVAGE

Unless performed within 1 hour of drug ingestion, it is no longer recommended.[3] The joint American and European toxicologists' statement states that if performed after this time the amount of poison removed is insignificant, and lavage may only propel unabsorbed poison into the small intestine. However, this view has recently been questioned and is based on limited data.[4] Prior intubation is essential when laryngeal competence is absent or doubtful, especially because, in the majority of overdoses, pulmonary aspiration is more lethal than the ingested drug.

To perform gastric lavage, the patient should be positioned head-down on the left side, and then a large-bore tube (36–40 Fr) with large side holes is passed into the stomach. The tube is aspirated before lavage is started, then tepid water instilled and recovered completely before continuing. The lavage is repeated until the return is clear; stomach massage or gastroscopy may assist removal of coalesced drug masses. Sodium, water and heat balance are of major importance in children. Gastric lavage is contraindicated in ingestions of corrosives, caustics and acids as oesophageal or gastric perforation may occur. Inhalation of petrol, paraffin or white spirits can cause intense pneumonitis.

ACTIVATED CHARCOAL

Activated charcoal (AC) remains the first-line treatment for most acute poisonings.[5] Owing to its large surface area and porous structure it is highly effective at adsorbing many toxins with few exceptions. Exceptions include elemental metals, pesticides, strong acids and alkalis, and cyanide. It should be given to all patients who present within 1 hour of ingestion, although it is also acceptable to administer it after 1 hour if it follows an overdose of a substance that slows gastric emptying (e.g. opioids, tricyclic antidepressants). Because of international guidelines recommending administration of AC within 1 hour, it is vital to identify rapidly those who present after a potentially serious overdose so that it can be given swiftly.[6]

Repeated doses of AC can increase the elimination of some drugs by interrupting their entero-enteric and enterohepatic circulation. Indications for repeated dose AC are shown in Table 80.3.[7] AC is given in 50 g doses for adults and 1 g/kg for children. It commonly causes vomiting; therefore consider giving an antiemetic prior to administration. Repeated doses are given at 4-hourly intervals.

WHOLE BOWEL IRRIGATION

This is a newer method of gastric decontamination that is indicated for a limited number of poisons.[8] Whole bowel irrigation involves administration of non-absorbable polyethylene glycol solution to cause a liquid stool and reduce drug absorption by physically forcing contents rapidly through the gastrointestinal tract. Polyethylene glycol preparations are still occasionally used in surgical units for 'bowel preparation' prior to surgery. It may have a

Table 80.3 Drug intoxications where multiple-dose activated charcoal may be beneficial

Carbamazepine
Theophylline
Digoxin
Quinine
Phenobarbital
Dapsone
Sustained-release preparations

role in treating large ingestions of drugs that are not absorbed by AC. Indications include large ingestions of iron or lithium, ingestion of drug-filled packets/condoms ('body packers'), and large ingestions of sustained-release or enteric-coated drugs (e.g. theophylline or calcium channel blockers). At present, efficacy is based on case reports alone.

ENHANCING DRUG ELIMINATION

In the overwhelming majority of patients who present after an overdose, gut decontamination techniques and supportive care are all that is required. In a limited number of acute poisonings it may be necessary to consider methods to enhance elimination.

URINARY ALKALINISATION

Urinary alkalinisation (previously termed *forced alkaline diuresis*) may be useful for serious poisonings with:

- salicylates
- phenobarbital (with repeated dose AC)
- chlorpropamide
- methotrexate

Intravenous sodium bicarbonate (approximately 1.26%) is infused to maintain a neutral balance and attempt to achieve a urine pH of approximately $\geq$ 7.5. The term 'urine alkalinisation' emphasises that urine pH manipulation is the prime objective of treatment; the terms 'forced alkaline diuresis' and 'alkaline diuresis' should be discontinued. According to international position statements it should be considered the treatment of choice for moderate to severe salicylate poisoning.[9] Care must be taken to ensure the potassium does not fall rapidly.

EXTRACORPOREAL TECHNIQUES

Numerous extracorporeal techniques are potentially available to aid drug removal in the poisoned patient. These include plasmapheresis, haemodialysis, haemofiltration, haemodiafiltration and haemoperfusion. There are limited data on drug clearance by these techniques in the literature and it is not possible to extrapolate from one system to the other. At present, knowledge of the principles of the methods and the kinetics of the drug involved is relied upon.

Extracorporeal techniques should only be considered when there are clinical features or markers of severe toxicity, failure to respond to full supportive care coupled with poisoning by a drug that can potentially be removed. Impairment of the normal route of elimination of the compound may also influence the decision. Use of extracorporeal techniques is probably only worthwhile if total body clearance is increased by at least 30%. Haemoperfusion is rarely performed in most intensive care units and intermittent haemodialysis is often confined to renal units. Consequently, the use of continuous haemofiltration, with or without dialysis, using filtration rates of greater than 50–100 ml/kg per hour, is likely to be as equally effective as when an extracorporeal technique is indicated.

CONTINUED SUPPORTIVE THERAPY

Self-poisoned patients do not always meet with the sympathies of the admitting medical team. Try to think of such patients as medical challenges, rather than merely instances of self-inflicted illness. Apart from specific measures that are described later, general care of the unconscious unstable patient should be continued. This includes monitoring of vital signs and provision of organ support when necessary. Attention should also be paid to fluid balance, correction of electrolytes, initiation of nutritional support, and prompt treatment of nosocomial infection.

Overall, in spite of the significant initial physiological disturbance, this group of patients usually has a good outcome.

SPECIFIC THERAPY OF SOME COMMON OR DIFFICULT OVERDOSES

This section emphasises only those features that may aid clinical diagnosis or prognosis. Treatment suggestions are always intended to support those measures described under general principles. Some new and controversial therapies are mentioned.

AMPHETAMINES (INCLUDING 'ECSTASY', MDMA)

CLINICAL FEATURES

Symptoms of mild overdose include sweating, dry mouth and anxiety. Although the majority of ecstasy patients are dehydrated, a proportion have hyponatraemia from drinking water to excess. More severe features include hypertonia, hyperreflexia, hallucinations and hypertension. Supraventricular dysrhythmias may follow with coma, convulsions and the risk of haemorrhagic stroke. A hyperthermic syndrome may develop with hyperpyrexia leading to rhabdomyolysis, metabolic acidosis, acute renal failure, disseminated intravascular coagulation (DIC) and multiple organ failure.[10]

TREATMENT

AC should be considered up to 1 hour post ingestion. Benzodiazepines are useful for agitated or psychotic patients and may have a central effect in reducing tachycardia, hypertension and hyperpyrexia. If benzodiazepines fail to control hypertension, other classes of antihypertensives should be started, such as α-blockers, labetalol or direct vasodilators. Hypertonic saline may need to be considered in severe hyponatraemia. Hyperthermia should be treated in the standard manner including administration of cold fluids. Dantrolene has been used in the treatment of ecstasy-related hyperpyrexia; however, it has been suggested that it treats the effects and not the cause, and that it may be better to direct treatment at the central mechanisms of thermoregulation.[11] Beyond this, there have been a few reports of the use of clozapine or olanzapine as a treatment for hyperpyrexia.

BARBITURATES

CLINICAL FEATURES

The central nervous, cardiovascular and respiratory systems are depressed. Cardiovascular depression is due to vasomotor centre depression and a toxic effect on myocardium and peripheral vessels. Hypotension and relative hypovolaemia may be significant.

TREATMENT

Treatment is supportive; however, repeated dose AC and urinary alkalinisation should be considered.

BENZODIAZEPINES

CLINICAL FEATURES

Overdose is common, but clinical features are not usually severe unless complicated by other CNS depressant drugs (such as alcohol), pre-existing disease or the extremes of age. Toxicity commonly produces drowsiness, dysarthria, ataxia and nystagmus; however, agitation and confusion can occur.

TREATMENT

AC can be given if patients present within 1 hour of ingestion, yet supportive treatment is usually all that is required. Flumazenil is a specific antagonist, but its brief duration of action limits its use to diagnostic purposes. Moreover, as flumazenil may cause other symptoms in patients who have ingested a cocktail of drugs (e.g. precipitation of fits in patients co-ingesting tricyclic antidepressants), its administration risks increasing morbidity and mortality.[12]

β-BLOCKERS

CLINICAL FEATURES

There is a wide variation in the individual response to β-blocker overdose. Those with cardiac disease are more at risk of complications. Hypotension and bradycardia predominate and are often refractory to standard resuscitation measures. The degree of heart block can range from a prolonged PR interval through to complete heart block and asystole. Cardiogenic shock and pulmonary oedema are not uncommon.[13]

TREATMENT

AC should be considered up to 1 hour post ingestion and multiple-dose charcoal in patients who have ingested sustained-release preparations. The role of atropine is not clear, although it is commonly used in patients who have bradycardia and hypotension. If symptomatic treatment fails, then other options such as glucagon (up to 10 mg i.v.), an adrenaline infusion or cardiac pacing are indicated. Although part of medical folklore, the evidence for glucagon is limited to animal studies.[14] It often comes as a dried powder with a phenol diluent, so if used, the glucagons powder should be dissolved in 5% dextrose, since the phenol diluent in large amounts is a myocardial depressant.

BUTYROPHENONES (INCLUDING HALOPERIDOL)

CLINICAL FEATURES

Drowsiness and extrapyramidal effects are most common. Rarely hypotension, QT prolongation, arrhythmias and convulsions develop.

TREATMENT

AC should be considered up to 1 hour post ingestion, otherwise treatment is supportive. Extrapyramidal symptoms can be treated with procyclidine or benzatropine. If ventricular arrhythmias do occur they are best treated with cardioversion; Class 1a antiarrhythmics are theoretically detrimental.

CALCIUM CHANNEL BLOCKERS

CLINICAL FEATURES

The cardiac effects of these drugs predominate in overdose, particularly hypotension and atrioventricular block, although reflex tachycardia occurs with nifedipine. Hypotension occurs due to peripheral vasodilatation and negative inotropy. Severe toxicity may occur in patients who initially appear well, when sustained-release preparations have been ingested.

TREATMENT

AC should be considered up to 1 hour post ingestion and multiple-dose charcoal in patients who have ingested sustained-release preparations. Treatment remains supportive; however i.v. calcium chloride is often given in patients who remain hypotensive despite fluid administration.[15] Atropine is often used for bradycardia, and occasionally cardiac pacing may be necessary. In persistent low cardiac output states, phosphodiesterase inhibitors, levosimendan or high-dose insulin may need to be considered.[16]

CANNABIS

CLINICAL FEATURES

Overdose is unusual following smoking of cannabis; however, high doses can produce an acute paranoid psychosis. Ataxia, nystagmus, tachycardia and confusion have been reported after ingestion in children. In adults, i.v. abuse of the crude extract may cause abdominal pain, fever, hypotension, pulmonary oedema and DIC.

TREATMENT

Treatment is supportive and most patients only have mild symptoms. AC should be considered for children who have ingested cannabis.[17]

CARBAMAZEPINE

Absorption is slow and unpredictable; moreover, maximum serum concentrations may not be achieved until 72 hours after ingestion. Carbamazepine undergoes enterohepatic recirculation and is metabolised to an active metabolite.

CLINICAL FEATURES

Nystagmus, ataxia, tremor and fits are common but, in severe overdose, fluctuating coma and severe tachycardia or bradycardia may occur. Plasma concentrations of carbamazepine and the active metabolite can be measured, but they do not correlate well with toxicity.

TREATMENT

Gastric lavage should be used if a patient presents within 1 h of a massive overdose. Multiple-dose AC is indicated in large ingestions or symptomatic patients, and may help elimination even if initiated several hours after the overdose.

CARBON MONOXIDE (CO)

Haldane first described symptoms of CO toxicity in 1919 and the mechanisms of toxicity remain unclear. Smokers may have up to 10% of their haemoglobin bound to CO (i.e. carboxyhaemoglobin, COHb) without deleterious effects. During CO poisoning, oxygen delivery to the heart and brain is increased. There is no marker that reliably detects CO poisoning. Whilst coma and/or COHb levels > 40% always indicate serious poisoning, delayed deterioration can occur in their absence. Affinity of CO for haemoglobin is approximately 240 times that of oxygen.

CLINICAL FEATURES

Neurological signs vary from mild confusion through to seizures and coma. A history of loss of consciousness should always be sought and may be the only indicator of significant poisoning. ST segment changes may be present on electrocardiogram (ECG). In the absence of respiratory depression or aspiration, $Pa\text{O}_2$ will be normal. It is essential that $Sa\text{O}_2$ is measured directly by a co-oximeter, and not calculated. Cherry-pink skin is only seen in textbooks; cyanosis is far more common.

TREATMENT

After basic resuscitative measures, high-flow oxygen (up to 100% if possible) should be administered and continued until the COHb level is less than 5%. This sometimes takes up to 24 hours. Hyperbaric oxygen (HBO), although often used, remains controversial. There have been eight randomised controlled trials of HBO versus normobaric oxygen. Unfortunately, many of these are of poor quality and it is not possible to show any statistical benefit of HBO in reducing neurological sequelae at 1 month.[18] Considering the frequently encountered logistical difficulties in transferring an unconscious patient to an HBO centre, it cannot be recommended based on the data currently available.

CHLOROQUINE

CLINICAL FEATURES

Hypotension, hypokalaemia, convulsions, ventricular arrhythmias and sudden cardiac arrest may result from severe poisoning.

TREATMENT

AC should be considered up to 1 hour post ingestion. Vasopressors may be required until hypotension is reversed, together with diazepam for agitated patients. Hypokalaemia is common and may be protective in the early stage. It is self-correcting and consequently aggressive potassium replacement is not recommended.[19]

COCAINE

CLINICAL FEATURES

Features of severe intoxication include hyperreflexia, drowsiness and convulsions.[20] Severe hypertension may cause subarachnoid or intracerebral haemorrhage, and coronary artery spasm may result in myocardial infarction or ventricular arrhythmias; fatalities generally occur early. Hyperthermia associated with rhabdomyolysis, acute renal failure and DIC may also occur.

TREATMENT

The toxic dose is variable and depends upon tolerance, presence of other drugs and route of administration, but ingestion of > 1 g is potentially fatal. Blood pressure and ECG monitoring should be instituted early and AC administered within 1 hour of ingestion. Benzodiazepines are useful for agitated or psychotic patients and may have a central effect in reducing tachycardia, hypertension and hyperpyrexia. If benzodiazepines fail to control hypertension, other classes of antihypertensives should be started, such as α-blockers, labetalol or direct vasodilators such as i.v. nitrates. The use of β-blockers is controversial and should be used with caution because of the risk of unopposed α-stimulation. Hyperthermia should be treated in the standard manner including administration of cold fluids, physical cooling measures and in the presence of convulsions, sedation, paralysis and ventilation.

CYANIDE

CLINICAL FEATURES

Severe toxicity is rapidly fatal; however, features include coma, respiratory depression, hypotension and metabolic acidosis. More moderate features include brief loss of consciousness, convulsions and vomiting. Rescuers must ensure that they do not get contaminated themselves.

TREATMENT

Inhaled amyl nitrate and 100% oxygen may well have been given at the scene, since it is present in 'cyanide antidote kits'. Following this there are a number of options:

1. Patients with severe features need dicobalt edetate 300 mg i.v. over 1 minute, followed by 50 ml dextrose 50% i.v., with a further 300 mg if there is no response.
2. Patients with moderate features should be given sodium thiosulphate 12.5 g i.v.
3. Hydroxocobalamin i.v. can also be given, but suitable preparations are not always available.
4. Patients with a metabolic acidosis should be given sodium bicarbonate.

DIGOXIN

CLINICAL FEATURES

Toxicity may result from ingestion of greater than 2–3 mg, or more commonly from taking too high a daily dose and/or a reduction in renal elimination. Any cardiac arrhythmia may occur and adverse effects may be delayed for some hours. Severe poisoning can produce hyperkalaemia and hypotension.

TREATMENT

AC should be considered up to 1 hour post ingestion and multiple-dose charcoal may be effective by interrupting enterohepatic recirculation of the drug. A digoxin serum level may be helpful although it does not equate to the total body burden. Hyper/hypokalaemia and hypomagnesaemia should be corrected. Cardiac pacing may be necessary to control symptomatic bradyarrhythmias and amiodarone may be useful for tachyarrhythmias. DC shock should be avoided if possible, but when essential must be initiated at low energy levels. Digoxin-specific antibodies are indicated in severe hyperkalaemia resistant to basic treatment, bradycardia resistant to atropine, or ventricular arrhythmias; repeated dosing is sometimes required in chronic toxicity as tissue redistribution of digoxin from deeper stores occurs.[21]

GAMMA-HYDROXYBUTYRIC ACID (GHB)

CLINICAL FEATURES

In moderate to high ingestion (> 50 mg/kg), coma, convulsions, bradycardia, hypotension and severe respiratory depression can be seen, and other CNS depressant drugs potentiate the effects. Most patients who present to hospital merely require supportive care, and even those who present in coma are often awake within 2–4 h; very few require intensive care.[22]

TREATMENT

AC can be given for ingestions of > 20 mg/kg if within 1 hour of presentation. Most patients with symptoms should be admitted and observed until symptoms resolve, which is usually fairly quickly. Benzodiazepines are the drug of choice for convulsions.

IRON

CLINICAL FEATURES

The corrosive action on gastric mucosa results in vomiting, pain, haematemesis and melaena, and gastric perforation. Severe poisoning is reflected by plasma concentrations more than 90 μmol/l in children and 145 μmol/l in adults within 4 hours of ingestion.

TREATMENT

Desferrioxamine mesylate (an iron chelator) 5 g is left in the stomach after lavage. Simultaneously, 2 g is injected i.m. and an infusion of 15 mg/kg per hour (maximum 80 mg/kg) is commenced. Treatment is continued until serum concentration and clinical status are satisfactory.

ISONIAZID

CLINICAL FEATURES

Severe toxicity is characterised by coma, respiratory depression, hypotension and convulsions, and may result from doses > 80 mg/kg. Protracted convulsions can cause rhabdomyolysis and acute renal failure.

TREATMENT

Gastric lavage followed by AC should be considered for large ingestions seen within 1 hour. Convulsions should be controlled with diazepam and pyridoxine, which is a specific antidote for isoniazid poisoning. Pyridoxine should be given prophylactically for large ingestions as early as possible, since it may prevent the development of complications.

LITHIUM

CLINICAL FEATURES

Serum lithium levels > 1.5 mmol/l are toxic, with the main feature being varied neurological symptoms and signs. Severe poisoning may result in permanent neurological damage and nephrogenic diabetes insipidus.

TREATMENT

Serum concentrations > 3.5–4.0 mmol/l or patients with signs of severe toxicity generally require extracorporeal elimination techniques. Nevertheless, the majority of patients respond to general supportive measures.

METHANOL AND ETHYLENE GLYCOL

CLINICAL FEATURES

Methanol and ethylene glycol are relatively non-toxic, but their ingestion is a medical emergency, because of their metabolism (following a latent period of 12–18 hours) to formic acid and glycolic acid respectively. These toxic metabolites account for the metabolic acidosis, ocular toxicity, renal failure and mortality that are occasionally seen. Mild features include dizziness, drowsiness and abdominal pain. When treatment is delayed, metabolic acidosis develops with drowsiness, coma and convulsions. The osmolal and the anion gap are increased.

TREATMENT

AC does not adsorb either methanol or ethylene glycol. The metabolic acidosis should be treated with sodium bicarbonate and the serum electrolytes measured. Ethanol prevents formation of the toxic metabolites and previously has been the most established treatment. However, ethanol dosing is complex, requires repeated monitoring and has adverse effects. The recent introduction of fomepizole (4-methypyrazole), although expensive, has significantly simplified the treatment of ethylene glycol and methanol poisoning, and is now strongly recommended as first-line therapy in some national guidelines.[23,24] It has been shown to be safe and effective, with minimal adverse effects,[25] and potentially prevents the need for haemodialysis in patients presenting with visual disturbances or severe acidosis.[26] If the ethylene glycol blood concentration is > 20 mg/dl or if there is a good history of ethylene glycol/methanol ingestion with an osmolal gap > 10, then patients should receive a loading dose of 15 mg/kg, followed by 10 mg/kg every 12 hours for 48 hours.

Folinic acid should also be given since it enhances the metabolism of formic acid.

MONOAMINE-OXIDASE INHIBITORS (MAOIs)

CLINICAL FEATURES

MAOIs cause an accumulation of amine neurotransmitters and are readily absorbed from the gastrointestinal tract and metabolised in the liver. Overdose results in neuromuscular excitation (muscle spasm, rigidity and opisthotonos) and sympathetic overactivity (tremor, tachycardia, hyperthermia, hypertension with fixed and dilated pupils).

TREATMENT

Management is similar to that of intoxication with amfetamines and cocaine (see above).

NON-STEROIDAL ANTI-INFLAMMATORY DRUGS (NSAIDs)

CLINICAL FEATURES

NSAIDs are commonly ingested in overdose. Fortunately, however, serious problems, other than a bad attack of gastritis, are rare. Exceptions to this rule include mefenamic acid or large ingestions of ibuprofen where self-limiting convulsions and renal failure have been reported.[27] Patients who do not develop symptoms within 4 hours are unlikely to experience delayed toxicity.

TREATMENT

AC can be given for large ingestions (> 10 tablets) that are seen within 1 hour of the overdose. Seizures should be treated with a benzodiazepine and an oral proton pump inhibitor may ease symptoms of gastrointestinal irritation.

OPIOIDS

CLINICAL FEATURES

Overdose is characterised by pinpoint pupils, drowsiness, shallow breathing and ultimately respiratory failure.

TREATMENT

AC may be effective for oral ingestions, otherwise treatment is supportive. Naloxone 0.1–0.4 mg i.v. can be given by bolus; repeat doses may be required if there is an inadequate response. Intubation and mechanical ventilation are required if respiratory failure is not rapidly reversed by naloxone.

PARACETAMOL

In normal adults, doses > 10 g may exceed the ability of hepatic glutathione to conjugate the toxic metabolite. Plasma concentrations > 200 mg/l at 4 hours or ≥ 50 mg/l at 12 hours (Figure 80.1) are usually associated with hepatic damage. Treatment should begin at lower levels for those considered to be high risk (see Table 80.4). While i.v. acetylcysteine administered more than 16 hours after ingestion may not prevent severe liver damage, it should still be given since outcome from paracetamol-induced fulminant hepatic failure is improved.[28] Although severe hepatic injury has a 10% mortality, the majority of patients recover within 1–2 weeks.

CLINICAL FEATURES

Nausea and vomiting may be the only features present in the first 24 hours.

TREATMENT

- Measure drug concentrations as described in general principles.
- Administer AC as soon as possible, even if more than 4 hours after overdose.[29]
- *N*-acetylcysteine 150 mg/kg in 200 ml 5% dextrose is infused over 15 minutes, followed by 50 mg/kg in 500 ml 5% dextrose over 4 hours and 100 mg/kg in 1 l 5% dextrose over 16 hours (total dose 300 mg/kg in 20 hours). Maximum protective effect is time-dependent. An ingestion–treatment interval of less than 10 hours gives the best results.
- In fulminant hepatic failure, the last dose (100 mg/kg in 1 l 5% dextrose over 16 hours) is repeated until the patient's INR is < 2.
- Expert opinion should be sought early on from a regional centre if liver failure is progressive since liver transplantation may become necessary.

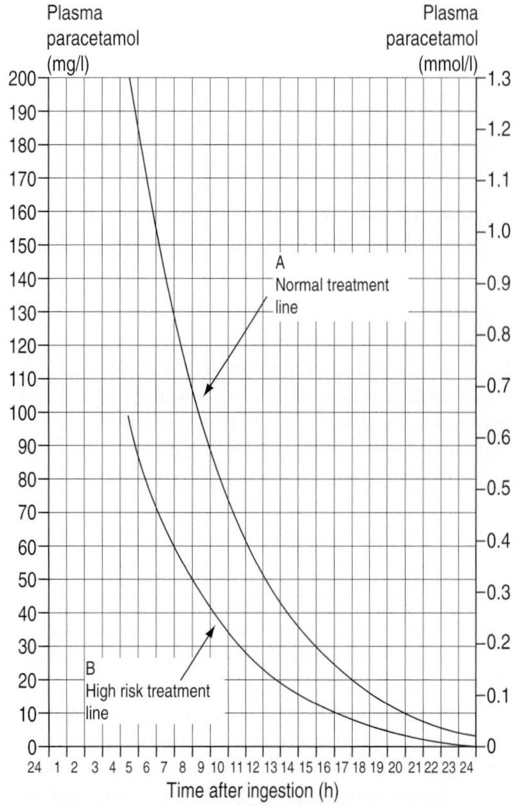

Figure 80.1 Treatment lines following paracetamol overdose in relation to time after ingestion and plasma levels. (Figure from Paracetamol Information Centre, London and the Welsh National Poisons Unit, Cardiff.)

Table 80.4 Those at high risk of liver damage following paracetamol overdose

Regular alcohol consumption
Regular use of enzyme-inducing drugs
Phenytoin, carbamazepine, phenobarbital, rifampicin
Conditions causing glutathione depletion
HIV, eating disorders, malnutrition and cystic fibrosis

PARAQUAT

In adult humans the lethal dose is 3–6 g (i.e. 15–30 ml of 20% w/v liquid concentrate). The mortality rate in patients ingesting the liquid concentrate is about 45%.[30] The lung is the primary target organ, with the injury being enhanced by oxygen. Peak concentrations are achieved between 0.5 and 2.0 hours.

CLINICAL FEATURES

Initial symptoms are gastrointestinal pain and vomiting with corrosive effects on the mouth, pharynx and oesophagus. Dyspnoea and pulmonary oedema follow within 24 hours, progressing to irreversible fibrosis and death. Cardiac, renal and hepatic dysfunctions are common.

TREATMENT

AC should be given if the patient presents within 1 hour. Other than basic measures such as antiemetics, analgesics and fluid replacement, the efficacy of specific treatment options is not established. Palliative care is probably the best approach in patients with very high plasma and urinary levels.

PHENYTOIN

CLINICAL FEATURES

Absorption is slow and unpredictable; moreover, maximum serum concentrations may not be achieved until 72 hours after ingestion. After initial nausea and vomiting, neurological symptoms develop including drowsiness, dysarthria and ataxia, and may ultimately progress to seizures. Cardiovascular toxicity is rare unless the overdose has been given i.v.

TREATMENT

Most patients require nothing more than supportive measures.

SALICYLATES (ASPIRIN)

Moderate toxicity occurs with serum concentrations 500–750 mg/l (3600–5500 μmol/l) and severe toxicity with concentrations > 750 mg/l. Serum concentrations alone do not determine prognosis. The elimination half-life increases significantly with increasing concentrations. Small reductions in pH produce large increases in non-ionised salicylate, which then penetrates tissues.

CLINICAL FEATURES

Tinnitus, deafness, diaphoresis, pyrexia, hypoglycaemia, haematemesis, hyperventilation and hypokalaemia may all occur. Coma, hyperpyrexia, pulmonary oedema and acidaemia are reported as more common in fatal cases, which present late.

TREATMENT

Multiple-dose AC may be effective but is not established. Vitamin K and glucose are used to correct hypoprothrombinaemia and hypoglycaemia. Urinary alkalinisation (see above) will decrease the amount of non-ionised drug available to enter tissues, but is hazardous and should only be used for the most severely ill patients. Extracorporeal techniques are very effective in removing salicylates and correcting acid–base disturbance. Although indications for their use are yet to be defined, they should be considered for severe cases.[31]

SELECTIVE SEROTONIN REUPTAKE INHIBITORS (SSRIs) or 5-HT Drugs

Drugs include citalopram, fluoxetine, fluvoxamine, paroxetine and sertraline. These drugs have increasingly replaced the tricyclic antidepressants and generally appear to be much safer in overdose.

CLINICAL FEATURES

Drowsiness, tachycardia and mild hypertension are the commonest features. Seizures and coma can occur, as well as a serotonin syndrome in 14% cases.[32]

TREATMENT

AC should be considered up to 1 hour post ingestion, otherwise treatment is supportive. Benzodiazepines should be used to treat agitated or hyperthermic patients. There are case reports of cyproheptadine being used to treat severe toxicity with SSRIs.[33]

THEOPHYLLINE

CLINICAL FEATURES

Acute theophylline poisoning is potentially very serious and severe poisoning carries a high mortality. Toxic effects such as agitation, tremor, nausea, vomiting and sinus tachycardia become evident at < 30 mg/l (167 μmol/l). Concentrations > 60 mg/l (333 μmol/l) in acute poisoning or > 40 mg/l (222 μmol/l) in chronic usage frequently result in seizures, malignant ventricular arrhythmias, severe hypotension and death.[34] A key feature is hypokalaemia, which predisposes to arrhythmias and rhabdomyolysis. Measuring plasma theophylline levels confirms the ingestion and may help in deciding elimination methods; in the majority of poisoned patients they do not aid management. Sustained-release preparations may result in delayed onset and prolonged toxicity.

TREATMENT

Gastric lavage is indicated for those who present early, but multiple-dose AC is highly effective. Electrolyte and acid–base disturbances should be corrected rapidly since this may be the only treatment required in many cases. Convulsions should be treated with benzodiazepines and cardiac arrhythmias with β-blockers in non-asthmatic patients. Extracorporeal elimination techniques may be indicated for severe cases. Whole bowel irrigation may be of use for sustained-release preparation overdoses.

TRICYCLIC ANTIDEPRESSANTS (TCAs)

CLINICAL FEATURES

These drugs remain the leading cause of death from overdose in patients arriving at the emergency department alive and account for up to one half of all overdose-related adult intensive care admissions.[35] Features include anticholinergic effects such as warm dry skin, tachycardia, blurred vision, dilated pupils and urinary retention. Severe features include respiratory depression, reduced conscious level, cardiac arrhythmias, fits and hypotension. Arrhythmias may be predicted by a QRS duration > 100 ms on the ECG; a QRS duration of > 160 ms increases risk of seizures.[36] All forms of rhythm and conduction disturbance have been described, and are not necessarily predicted by the ECG.[37] Amoxapine typically causes features of severe poisoning in the absence of QRS widening. Cardiac toxicity is due mainly to quinidine-like actions, slowing phase 0 depolarisation of the action potential. Other mechanisms include impaired automaticity, cholinergic blockade and inhibition of neuronal catecholamine uptake. Toxicity is worsened by acidaemia, hypotension and hyperthermia.

TREATMENT

After supportive care as outlined above, including multiple-dose AC, continuous cardiac monitoring is essential. Increasing arterial pH to ≥ 7.45 significantly reduces the available free drug and this may be the best way to avoid TCA toxicity. Mild hyperventilation and 8.4% sodium bicarbonate in 50 mmol aliquots achieves this strategy and may improve outcome.[38] Bicarbonate should probably be given in all cases of QRS prolongation (even in the absence of metabolic acidosis), malignant arrhythmias, hypotension or metabolic acidosis. If arrhythmias occur, avoid Class 1a agents; lidocaine may be best. Benzodiazepines are the drug of choice for sedation, treatment of seizures and may prevent emergence delirium.

VALPROATE

CLINICAL FEATURES

Most overdoses follow a benign course, with nausea, mild drowsiness and confusion. Coma can occur in large ingestions with cerebral oedema.

TREATMENT

Valproate levels are of little value, except to confirm the ingestion. There is poor correlation between depth of coma and free or total valproate levels. Supportive management is all that is usually required. Rapid absorption occurs and therefore gastric lavage or AC is of little benefit.

REFERENCES

1. Gunnell D, Ho D, Murray V. Medical management of deliberate drug overdose: a neglected area for suicide prevention? *Emerg Med J* 2004; **21**: 35–8.
2. American Academy of Clinical Toxicology; European Association of Poison Control Centres and Clinical Toxicologists. Position statement: ipecac syrup. *Clin Toxicol* 1997; **35**: 699–709.
3. American Academy of Clinical Toxicology; European Association of Poison Control Centres and Clinical Toxicologists. Position statement: gastric lavage. *Clin Toxicol* 1997; **35**: 711–9.
4. Eddleston M, Juszczak E, Buckley N. Does gastric lavage really push poison beyond the pylorus? A systematic review of the evidence. *Ann Emerg Med* 2003; **42**: 359–64.
5. Chyka PA, Seger D, Krenzelok EP *et al.* American Academy of Clinical Toxicology; European Association

of Poisons Centres and Clinical Toxicologists. Position paper: single-dose activated charcoal. *Clin Toxicol* 2005; **43**: 61–87.
6. Karim A, Ivatts S, Dargan P, Jones A. How feasible is it to conform to the European guidelines on administration of activated charcoal within one hour of an overdose? *Emerg Med J* 2001; **18**: 390–2.
7. American Academy of Clinical Toxicology; European Association of Poison Control Centres and Clinical Toxicologists. Position statement and practice guidelines on the use of multi-dose activated charcoal in the treatment of acute poisoning. *Clin Toxicol* 1999; **37**: 731–51.
8. American Academy of Clinical Toxicology; European Association of Poison Control Centres and Clinical Toxicologists. Position statement: whole bowel irrigation. *Clin Toxicol* 1997; **35**: 753–62.
9. Proudfoot AT, Krenzelok EP, Vale JA. Position paper on urine alkalinisation. *J Toxicol Clin Toxicol* 2004; **42**: 1–26.
10. Hall AP, Henry JA. Acute toxic effects of 'Ecstasy' (MDMA) and related compounds: overview of pathophysiology and clinical management. *Br J Anaesth* 2006; **96**: 678–85.
11. Padkin A. Treating MDMA ('Ecstasy') toxicity. *Anaesthesia* 1994; **49**: 259.
12. Seger DL. Flumazenil – treatment or toxin? *J Toxicol Clin Toxicol* 2004; **42**: 209–16.
13. Shepherd G. Treatment of poisoning caused by beta-adrenergic and calcium-channel blockers. *Am J Health Syst Pharm* 2006; **63**: 1828–35.
14. Bailey B. Glucagon in beta-blocker and calcium channel blocker overdoses: a systematic review. *J Toxicol Clin Toxicol* 2003; **41**: 595–602.
15. DeWitt CR, Waksman JC. Pharmacology, pathophysiology and management of calcium channel blocker and beta-blocker toxicity. *Toxicol Rev* 2004; **23**: 223–38.
16. Megarbane B, Karyo S, Baud FJ. The role of insulin and glucose (hyperinsulinaemia/euglycaemia) therapy in acute calcium channel antagonist and beta-blocker poisoning. *Toxicol Rev* 2004; **23**: 215–22.
17. MacNab A, Anderson E, Susak K. Ingestion of cannabis: a cause of coma in children. *Pediatr Emerg Care* 1989; **5**: 238–9.
18. Buckley NA, Isbister GK, Stokes B *et al.* Hyperbaric oxygen for carbon monoxide poisoning: a systematic review and critical analysis of the evidence. *Toxicol Rev* 2005; **24**: 75–92.
19. Jaeger A, Sauder P, Kopferschmitt J *et al.* Clinical features and management of poisoning due to antimalarial drugs. *Med Toxicol Adverse Drug Exp* 1987; **2**: 242–73.
20. Paul S, York D. Cocaine abuse: an expanding health-care problem for the 1990s. *Am J Crit Care* 1992; **1**: 109–13.
21. Bateman DN. Digoxin-specific antibody fragments: how much and when? *Toxicol Rev* 2004; **23**: 135–43.
22. Liechti ME, Kunz I, Greminger P *et al.* Clinical features of gamma-hydroxybutyrate and gamma-butyrolactone toxicity and concomitant drug and alcohol. *Drug Alcohol Depend* 2006; **81**: 323–6.
23. Barceloux DG, Krenzelok EP, Olson K *et al.* American Academy of Clinical Toxicology practice guidelines on the methanol poisoning. *J Toxicol Clin Toxicol* 1999; **37**: 537–60.
24. Barceloux DG, Bond GR, Krenzelok EP *et al.* American Academy of Clinical Toxicology practice guidelines on the methanol poisoning. *J Toxicol Clin Toxicol* 2002; **40**: 415–46.
25. Brent J, McMartin K, Phillips S *et al.* Fomepizole for the treatment of methanol poisoning. *N Engl J Med* 2001; **344**: 424–9.
26. Megarbane B, Borron SW, Trout H *et al.* Treatment of acute methanol poisoning with fomepizole. *Intensive Care Med* 2001; **27**: 1370–8.
27. Smolinske SC, Hall AH, Vandenberg SA. Toxic effects of nonsteroidal anti-inflammatory drugs in overdose. *Drug Safety* 1990; **5**: 252–74.
28. Keays R, Harrison PM, Wendon JA *et al.* Intravenous acetylcysteine in paracetamol induced fulminant hepatic failure: a prospective controlled study. *N Engl J Med* 1991; **303**: 1026–9.
29. Spiller HA, Winter ML, Klein-Schwartz W *et al.* Efficacy of activated charcoal administered more than four hours after acetaminophen overdose. *J Emerg Med* 2006; **30**: 1–5.
30. Hwang KY, Lee EY, Hong SY. Paraquat intoxication in Korea. *Arch Environ Health* 2002; **57**: 162–6.
31. Dargan PI, Wallace CI, Jones AL. An evidenced based flowchart to guide the management of acute salicylate (aspirin) overdose. *Emerg Med J* 2002; **19**: 206–9.
32. Isbister GK, Bowe SJ, Dawson A *et al.* Relative toxicity of selective serotonin reuptake inhibitors in overdose. *J Toxicol Clin Toxicol* 2004; **42**: 277–85.
33. McDaniel WW. Serotonin syndrome: early management with cyproheptadine. *Ann Phamacother* 2001; **35**: 870–3.
34. Shannon M. Predictors of major toxicity after theophylline overdose. *Ann Intern Med* 1993; **119**: 1161–7.
35. Newton EH, Shih RD, Hoffman RS. Cyclic antidepressant overdose: a review of current management strategies. *Am J Emerg Med* 1994; **12**: 376–9.
36. Boehert MT, Lovejoy FH. Value of the QRS duration versus the serum drug level in predicting seizures and ventricular arrhythmias after an acute overdose of tricyclic antidepressants. *N Eng J Med* 1985; **313**: 474–9.
37. Harrigan RA, Brady WJ. ECG abnormalities in tricyclic antidepressant ingestion. *Am J Emerg Med* 1999; **17**: 387–93.
38. Hoffman JR, Votey SR, Bayer M *et al.* Effect of hypertonic sodium bicarbonate in the treatment of moderate-to-severe cyclic antidepressant overdose. *Am J Emerg Med* 1993; **11**: 336–41.

81

Sedation, analgesia and muscle relaxation in the intensive care unit

Peter V van Heerden

Despite the widespread use of sedative and analgesic agents in the intensive care unit (ICU), the goals of sedation and analgesia are not well-established. Indications for the use of sedative agents include:

- to enable the critically ill patient to tolerate invasive and uncomfortable monitoring and treatment procedures
- to reduce oxygen consumption[1] by reducing patient arousal and activity
- to promote amnesia for events in the ICU

Sedatives may also be used as specific treatment for conditions such as epilepsy or tetanus. The delirious patient may require sedation to maintain safety of the patient and carers.

Combinations of opioids and benzodiazepines are commonly used to provide 'sedation' in the ICU. High doses of opioid analgesics may result in significant sedation in their own right and are synergistic with sedative agents such as benzodiazepines. The distinction between sedation and analgesia is therefore blurred, and makes the definition and attainment of clear sedation goals elusive.

Skilled use of analgesics in the modern ICU ensures that critically ill patients should no longer suffer pain. Pain management relies largely on the use of opioid analgesics, together with regional anaesthetic techniques. Poor management of sedation and analgesia in the critically ill patient may contribute to ongoing psychological morbidity, such as posttraumatic stress disorder.

SEDATION

Sedation of patients in the ICU is an integral part care and compassion for the critically ill patient.

Sedative agents are used in an attempt to:

- allay anxiety over the patient's own illness, the welfare of relatives or the risk of death
- ensure adequate rest
- reduce the impact of unpleasant sensations, such as thirst
- reduce the distress of invasive treatment and monitoring, such as endotracheal intubation
- blunt awareness of the environment over which the patient has very little control and in which he/she may be unable to communicate

Attention to such details as avoiding potentially distressing situations, where possible, allowing adequate access to caring visitors maintaining of adequate communication with the patient and a positive outlook by the carers will satisfy many of these goals. Small comforts, such as ice chips by mouth, a comfortable mattress or relaxation audio tapes all help this process.

LEVEL OF SEDATION

The level of sedation required will vary, depending on the indication, e.g. heavy sedation may be necessary during the control of status epilepticus, while a much lower level of sedation will be required to tolerate endotracheal intubation. Modern modes of mechanical ventilation do not demand heavy sedation in order to be comfortably tolerated. The aim of sedation should be clear to the treating team and the desired level of sedation should be determined and documented. Once sedation is instituted, the level of sedation should be regularly assessed. Protocol-based therapy reduces drug costs and enhances the quality of sedation and analgesia.[2] Failure to follow such a protocolised approach can result in significant problems, such as:[3]

- 'oversedation' with an increased risk of nosocomial pneumonia
- the need for more frequent neurological assessments including computed axial tomography (CT) scans
- prolonged stay in the ICU
- an increased incidence of psychological problems, such as posttraumatic stress disorder and depression

Level of sedation may be assessed by means of a number of measurement tools including:

- Scoring systems such as the Ramsay scale (see Table 81.1), which is a six-point scale that ranges from anxious and

Table 81.1 Ramsay scale

Level	Response
Awake levels	
1	Patient anxious and agitated or restless or both
2	Patient cooperative, orientated and tranquil
3	Patient responds to commands only
Asleep levels	
4	Brisk response to a light glabellar tap or loud auditory stimulus
5	Sluggish response to a light glabellar tap or loud auditory stimulus
6	No response to a light glabellar tap or loud auditory stimulus

agitated (level 1) to unresponsive (level 6), judged in response to a standardized stimulus (loud auditory stimulus or glabellar tap).[3] This scale has good interrater reliability and provides a numerical score, suitable for charting on the ICU observation chart and for descriptive purposes.

- Electroencephalography (EEG), which may be either 'raw' or 'processed' and is able to provide a measure of cerebral activity. This monitor is more suitable for assessing depth of anaesthesia and may be difficult to interpret in the encephalopathic patient. Newer, easy-to-use devices using integrated EEG are now appearing but their efficacy and role in the ICU have yet to be established. Use is also limited by practical considerations, such as interference due to movement artefact. To date these monitors have not enjoyed widespread use in the ICU, but may be useful for specific indications such as ensuring an isoelectric EEG trace in patients being treated for intracranial hypertension.
- Visual analogue scales, which are more suited to the assessment of pain (see below), or for use as a research tool.
- Evoked potentials.

Level of sedation may also be assessed by monitoring physiological parameters for signs of distress. A 'drug free' period every day, when sedative agents are completely withdrawn, is an excellent means of assessing level of sedation[4] – by taking note of the time for a patient to either wake up or rise to a predetermined level on the Ramsay scale.

THE IDEAL SEDATIVE

There is no ideal sedative agent. Sedatives in the future may target specific aspects of sedation, such as hypnosis, anxiolysis or amnesia, without necessarily providing the whole spectrum of sedation for each patient. Currently a good sedative would address the following:

- hypnosis/sleep
- anxiolysis
- amnesia
- be anticonvulsant
- be non-cumulative
- be independent of renal or hepatic metabolic pathways
- not produce respiratory or cardiovascular depression
- have minimal interaction with other drugs
- be of modest cost
- have a rapid onset and short offset time
- have no prolonged effects on memory
- have no long-term psychological effects

SEDATIVE AGENTS USED IN THE ICU

BENZODIAZEPINES

Benzodiazepines (BZAs), as a class, are probably the most widely used sedatives in ICUs. These agents provide hypnosis, amnesia and anxiolysis. They do not provide analgesia. BZAs are good anticonvulsant drugs and also provide some muscle relaxation. They act via BZA receptors, which are closely associated with $GABA_A$ receptors, resulting in intracellular influx of chloride when activated. These drugs may be given by mouth (PO), per rectum (PR) or intravenously (i.v.). Most commonly in the ICU they are administered by intermittent or continuous i.v. infusion, e.g. midazolam in 1 mg/ml dilution, titrated to effect.

Dosage of these agents is by titration and may vary widely depending on factors such as:

- prior exposure to BZA (increased tolerance)
- age and physiological reserve
- volume status (hypovolaemic patients are more sensitive)
- renal and hepatic dysfunction
- co-administered drugs (whether BZA is combined with an opioid)
- history of alcohol consumption (increased tolerance)

Although some BZAs (e.g. midazolam) are reported to be short-acting, water-soluble agents, there is still potential for accumulation of both parent compound and active metabolites in patients with hepatic and renal dysfunction. This may result in prolonged sedation and increased length of mechanical ventilation and ICU stay. In the critically ill, there may be extensive derangement of the pharmacokinetic profiles of BZAs. There is therefore some difficulty in predetermining suitable dosages of these agents. Typically, midazolam in doses of 0.02–0.2 mg/kg per hour may be suitable, with the level titrated to individual response. Longer acting agents, such as diazepam, may be given by intermittent i.v. injection, e.g. diazepam 5–10 mg i.v., as necessary.

BZAs are often combined with opioids in a compound 'sedative' infusion. This allows lower doses of BZA to be used, while capitalising on the opioid effects of respiratory and cough suppression, to facilitate mechanical ventilation.

Flumazenil, the specific BZA antagonist, may be used to reverse the effect of BZAs to reduce unwanted acute side-effects, such as severe hypotension or respiratory depression, or to allow acute neurological assessment of the sedated patient.

INTRAVENOUS ANAESTHETIC AGENTS

Propofol

The i.v. anaesthetic agent propofol (2,6-di-isopropylphenol) is frequently used for sedation in the ICU. It is fast acting, very effective and has a rapid offset of action (due to its rapid metabolism to inactive metabolites in the liver). These features make it very suitable for use in patients requiring short-term sedation or for anaesthesia for procedures in the ICU. Although propofol has been shown to reduce time on mechanical ventilation compared with BZA (specifically midazolam) sedation, it has not been shown to reduce time in the ICU.[5,6] Caution is required in hypovolaemic patients or those with impaired myocardial function, as severe hypotension may result. Doses for ICU sedation are generally much lower than the 6–12 mg/kg per hour required for anaesthesia. The diluent in which propofol is delivered is lipid-rich and may have to be taken into account as a source of nutrition and indeed cause of hyperlipidaemia, depending on dosage and duration of therapy. Disodium edetate, present in the propofol solution, does not appear to be harmful in patients receiving long-term infusions of propofol.[7]

There has been some recent concern about the so-called 'propofol infusion syndrome' where particularly paediatric patients, but also adults, have developed severe heart failure (preceded by metabolic acidaemia, fatty infiltration of the liver and striated muscle damage) after prolonged high-dose infusions of propofol.[8] Caution should therefore be exercised when using propofol for prolonged periods.

Thiopentone

Thiopentone is reserved for specific indications, such as management of intractable intracranial hypertension (to reduce cerebral metabolism) or for the treatment of status epilepticus. It is not commonly used as a general sedative agent. Its use is limited by its long duration of action and long terminal half-life when used for prolonged infusions.

Ketamine

Ketamine acts by blocking *N*-methyl-D-aspartic acid (NMDA) receptors. It produces a sedative state known as 'dissociative anaesthesia', with the following characteristics:

- mild sedation
- amnesia
- analgesia
- reduced motor activity

The lack of respiratory and cardiovascular depression at lower doses makes this a very safe drug for use in the ICU. Limitations to its use include hallucinations and delirium during the recovery/withdrawal phase. These may be ameliorated by BZA administration. Ketamine may be used specifically for sedation in severe asthmatics (for its bronchodilator effect), in patients following head injury (for its effect at the NMDA receptor) or in patients where analgesia is difficult (e.g. extensive burns).

Etomidate

Etomidate is no longer used for ICU sedation due to its adrenocortical suppressant (immunosuppressant) action.

MAJOR TRANQUILLIZERS

Butyrophenones (e.g. haloperidol) and phenothiazines (e.g. chlorpromazine) are very useful agents for the sedation of delirious patients in the ICU. They act via a range of receptors including dopaminergic (D_1 and D_2), α-adrenergic, histamine, serotonin and cholinergic receptors. Main actions include:

- reduced motor activity
- apathy and reduced initiative
- sedation and drowsiness
- reduced aggression
- antiemetic

Unwanted effects with these drugs are common and include:

- extrapyramidal effects (dystonia and tardive dyskinesia)
- endocrine effects (e.g. lactation)
- anticholinergic effects (e.g. blurred vision, dry mouth, urinary retention, constipation)
- hypotension
- neuroleptic malignant syndrome

The main advantage of major tranquillizers over large doses of minor tranquillizers is that they can be used to gain control in difficult situations (e.g. when delirious patients may be a risk to themselves or their carers) without a major risk of respiratory depression. These agents should not be used for long-term sedation, except where they are used for the specific treatment of psychosis. Typically, haloperidol, diluted to a 1 mg/ml solution, may be given by repeated i.v. injection in doses of 5–20 mg/hour until the delirious patient is approachable. Repeat dosages would then be titrated to allow easy arousal of the patient, with the patient otherwise calm. Haloperidol may also be given by mouth or by i.m. injection.

Olanzapine, a newer 'atypical' antipsychotic agent, is also a useful agent for the sedation of delirious patients when given in oral doses of 5–20 mg/day. It has a much lower side-effect profile than the more 'typical' antipsychotics, especially with respect to motor side-effects. Olanzapine may also be given as oral/sublingual wafers. This is a particularly useful route of administration in the uncooperative patient.

VOLATILE ANAESTHETIC AGENTS

The widespread use of volatile anaesthetic agents for sedation in the ICU has been limited by:

- the cost of prolonged administration
- the more complex set-up required for the administration of these agents (vaporizer, scavenging apparatus, etc.)
- specific side-effects, e.g. 'halothane' hepatitis, accumulation of fluoride ions and consequent renal dysfunction (enflurane and isoflurane) and inactivation of methionine synthase and bone marrow depression (nitrous oxide)

Volatile agents are useful for short periods of anaesthesia during invasive procedures in the ICU. They may be used, with effect, for longer periods for sedation (up to a few days) in acute severe asthma, due to their bronchodilatory action. Short-term administrations of Entonox (50% nitrous oxide in oxygen) are still useful for analgesia and sedation during painful procedures (e.g. removal of intercostal catheters). This may be given by demand valve (controlled by the patient) or be administered by the medical staff.

OPIOIDS

Although opioids are used primarily for their analgesic action in the ICU (see below), they also produce a degree of sedation. They therefore complement the effect of other sedatives used in the ICU, with which they are often given in combination.

DEXMEDETOMIDINE

Dexmedetomidine is a novel highly selective α_2-agonist, which has been shown to provide safe analgesia and sedation in the ICU when given as a single agent by i.v. infusion.[9]

Dosages are: loading dose of 1 μg/kg over 10 min, followed by an infusion of 0.2–0.7 μg/kg per hour.

Infusions longer than 24 hours are currently not recommended. Side-effects may be predicted from the mechanism of action and include hypotension, bradycardia, hypoxaemia and atrial fibrillation. More established α_2-agonists, such as clonidine, may be used to enhance sedation and analgesia when BZA and opioids are used as the mainstay of sedation in the ICU.

ANALGESIA

Pain management is an important priority in the care of critically ill patients.

Many patients present to the ICU with painful conditions or undergo painful procedures during their ICU stay. Pain has a number of adverse consequences:

- it produces anxiety
- it contributes to lack of sleep
- it worsens delirium
- it enhances the stress response – increases circulating catecholamine levels and oxygen consumption
- it results in respiratory embarrassment due to atelectasis and sputum retention
- it leads to immobility and venous and gut stasis

Pain management comprises a number of modalities in addition to analgesics and local and regional anaesthesia/analgesia, such as:

- a caring and supportive medical team that the patient can trust
- warm and comfortable surroundings
- attention to pressure areas (e.g. regular turning)
- the use of warm packs
- the use of simple analgesics as appropriate
- bowel and bladder care
- adequate hydration and amelioration of thirst (e.g. moistening the mouth)
- early tracheostomy where indicated to reduce the discomfort of endotracheal intubation
- splinting and early fixation of fractures.

When drug therapy is required to alleviate pain, the following groups of drugs are commonly used:

- opioid analgesics
- simple analgesics
- non-steroidal anti-inflammatory drugs (NSAIDs)
- novel agents, such as dexmedetomidine (see above) and tramadol
- local anaesthetic agents
- inhaled agents (see volatile anaesthetic agents above)
- ketamine (see above)
- ‘multimodality’ supplemental treatments such as acupuncture, acupressure, massage and transcutaneous electrical nerve stimulation (TENS)

OPIOIDS

Opioids remain the mainstay of analgesia in the ICU. This group of drugs encompasses:

- morphine and its analogues (e.g. morphine, diamorphine, codeine)
- semisynthetic and synthetic agents
  - phenylpiperidine derivatives (e.g. pethidine, fentanyl)
  - methadone derivatives (e.g. methadone, dextropropoxyphene)
  - benzomorphan derivatives (e.g. pentazocine)
  - thebaine derivatives (e.g. buprenorphine)

The effects of opioids are mediated via the three main opioid receptor subtypes μ, κ and σ. These G-protein coupled receptors inhibit adenyl cyclase and effects include:

- analgesia (supraspinal, spinal and peripheral)
- sedation
- pupillary constriction
- respiratory depression and cough suppression
- euphoria or dysphoria
- reduced gastrointestinal motility
- physical dependence

Opioids are titrated to effect by intermittent injection (usually i.v. in the ICU) or by continuous infusion, which may be nurse controlled (nurse-controlled analgesia, NCA) or controlled by the patient (patient-controlled analgesia, PCA). A suitable regimen is a 1 mg/ml dilution of morphine given by continuous i.v. infusion, titrated to patient comfort. This is often combined with a BZA (e.g. midazolam) to produce a ‘sedative/analgesic’ infusion for use in very ill patients on mechanical ventilation (see sedation above). Opioids are also administered via the subarachnoid, extradural, transdermal and intranasal routes.

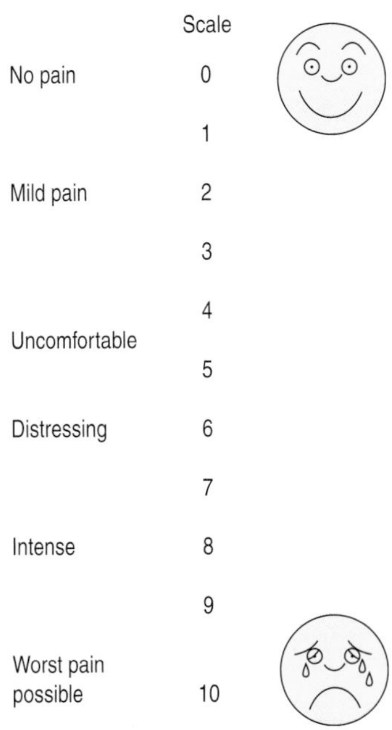
Scale
No pain 0
1
Mild pain 2
3
4
Uncomfortable
5
Distressing 6
7
Intense 8
9
Worst pain possible 10

Figure 81.1 Visual analogue score for the assessment of pain.[3]

The effect of analgesia in the clinical setting is judged by:

- patient response, if they are conscious, either verbally by describing the level of pain subjectively or by using a visual analogue score (Figure 81.1)[3] or other assessment, such as behavioural pain scales[10]
- physiological markers of distress, e.g. tachycardia, hypertension, diaphoresis, restlessness

These indicators should be assessed in the clinical context, i.e. is the pathophysiological process likely to be responsible for some, or considerable pain? Analgesia should be administered for a specific indication and to desired effect. Many factors lead to a wide variation in the experience of pain including:

- personality traits
- the previous experience of pain
- fear
- interpretation of events/disorientation/deperonalization
- age
- degree of tissue damage
- chronic disease and debility

In the critically ill, the use of opioids may be complicated by:

- wide interindividual responses to similar dosages, mandating titration of the analgesic, especially in debilitated and elderly patients
- severe hypotension following rapid administration, particularly in hypovolaemic patients. Fentanyl and sufentanil may offer advantages over morphine in terms of 'cardiostability'
- prolonged duration of action, due to accumulation of parent compound and metabolites (e.g. morphine and its major metabolites morphine-3-glucuronide and morphine-6-glucuronide) in the elderly and in patients with renal and hepatic dysfunction. Use of drugs with shorter half-lives (e.g. alfentanil) or which are less dependent on hepatic and renal pathways for metabolism and excretion (e.g. remifentanil) can reduce this problem
- constipation, requiring careful attention to detail and the judicious use of prokinetic agents (e.g. metoclopramide, erythromycin) to overcome gastric stasis and enable enteral feeding, or pruritents to aid evacuation
- the development of tolerance requiring increasing doses to achieve the same effect
- withdrawal symptoms on cessation/reduction of opioid medication. The 'abstinence syndrome' is characterized by:
  - irritability
  - tremor
  - aggression
  - fever
  - diaphoresis
  - piloerection
  - pupillary dilation
  - diarrhoea
  - insomnia

Early recognition of these symptoms of withdrawal is not always simple in the ICU patient and may be mistaken for sepsis or delirium. Treatment is by re-institution of and then slow withdrawal of the opioid, especially after prolonged periods of administration. Alternatively, symptoms may be controlled with a combination of long-acting opioid (e.g. methadone), BZA and α_2-agonists (e.g. clonidine).

A knowledge of drug-related (as opposed to class-related) side-effects is important when using opioids other than morphine, e.g. the interaction between pethidine and the older monoamine oxidase inhibitors, the potential for seizures with high dose or prolonged use of pethidine, chest wall rigidity occasionally seen with high doses of fentanyl.

The specific opioid antagonist naloxone has little role to play in the ICU, except for the treatment of severe hypotension, unwanted sedation or respiratory depression following opioid usage. Rapid reversal of opioid effect for the purpose of neurological assessment may be another valid use of naloxone.

PHARMACOKINETIC CONSIDERATIONS

The pharmacokinetics of analgesics and sedatives can be affected by such factors as:

- patient's fluid volume status
- capillary leak (changing volume of distribution)
- serum protein levels
- renal function
- hepatic function

- hepatic blood flow
- competition of combinations of drugs for carrier molecules, metabolic and excretory pathways

All of these factors make the rational choice of an appropriate drug in the appropriate dose difficult in the critically ill patient.

Use of simple analgesics or NSAIDs to treat pain will reduce the amount of opioid required.

SIMPLE ANALGESICS

Paracetamol and other simple analgesics (e.g. salicylates) are particularly effective for:

- bone and joint pain
- soft tissue pain
- perioperative pain
- inflammatory conditions
- as part of multimodal analgesia, to reduce opioid requirements

These drugs are given by mouth, via a nasogastric tube, per rectum or i.v. to supplement analgesia in the critically ill (e.g. paracetamol 1–2 g 4–6-hourly). Use is limited by the risk of hepatic dysfunction if used in high dose or for prolonged periods.

NSAIDs

The commonly used NSAIDs are carboxylic acids (e.g. indometacin, ibuprofen, mefenamic acid) or enolic acids (e.g. piroxicam). NSAIDs are useful for supplemental/multimodal analgesia in the ICU for the conditions listed for simple analgesics above. They are given by mouth, via a nasogastric tube, per rectum or by i.m. injection (e.g. indometacin 100 mg twice daily PR or ketorolac 10–15 mg 4–6-hourly i.m.) for pain and pyrexia. Side-effects include:

- renal dysfunction
- gastrointestinal haemorrhage
- increased bleeding tendency due to platelet inhibition

The newer cyclooxygenase 2 (COX-2) specific inhibitors, such as valdecoxib and its injectable precursor parecoxib, have a much lower side-effect profile than traditional NSAIDs. These drugs should be used only for short periods, due to recent evidence regarding increased cardiovascular morbidity associated with long-term use of the COX-2 inhibitors.[11]

TRAMADOL

Tramadol is a more recent addition to the analgesic range. It acts via the μ receptor, as well as by inhibiting the uptake of serotonin and noradrenaline (norepinephrine), with presynaptic stimulation of serotonin release, thereby enhancing the effects of the descending analgesia system. It is useful for moderate to severe pain in the postoperative patient in doses of 50–100 mg i.v., oral or i.m. 4–6-hourly to a maximum of 600 mg/day.

LOCAL ANAESTHETICS – REGIONAL ANAESTHESIA/ ANALGESIA

The use of local anaesthetic techniques in the critically ill patient is limited by:

- pain often emanating from multiple sources, and therefore not amenable to a single regional technique
- the requirement for 'mandatory' sedation/analgesia in order for the patient to tolerate endotracheal intubation, making a regional technique for another source of pain (e.g. laparotomy wound) superfluous
- the need to treat pain over a prolonged period, mandating either repetition of the regional block (e.g. intercostal nerve blocks for pain from an upper abdominal incision, or femoral nerve blocks for a fractured femur) or the placement of an indwelling catheter (e.g. epidural catheter). Indwelling catheters also have a defined safe duration of insertion (usually 3–4 days) before they need to be removed and replaced
- coagulopathy frequently seen in this group of patients, making procedures such as epidural injection less safe
- comorbidities (e.g. severe ischaemic heart disease) in the critically ill patient

When a regional technique is considered viable (e.g. thoracic epidural for the treatment of pain due to fractured ribs), then the following need to be considered:

- the procedure should be carried out by adequately trained personnel (usually with an anaesthesia background)
- regional techniques may be very time-consuming, requiring additional staff to properly position the patient and assist the proceduralist
- regional techniques may carry serious complication risks (e.g. subarachnoid injection of local anaesthetic or epidural haematoma during placement of epidural catheters, with serious haemodynamic, neurological and respiratory consequences)
- good preparation is paramount:
  - informed consent from patient or legal surrogate
  - recent normal coagulation profile, or correction of abnormal profile
  - the knowledge and ability to deal with complications (e.g. sudden hypotension)
  - experience with the drugs being used (typically a mixture of local anaesthetic, such as ropivacaine 0.2%, and an opioid, such as fentanyl 2 μg/ml, are used for epidural infusion)

- adequate training of nursing staff to monitor the level of block, haemodynamic parameters and for possible complications

Within the context above, the following blocks may be useful in individual patients:

- femoral nerve block for lower limb injuries (10 ml of 7.5 mg/ml ropivacaine injected intermittently 8–12-hourly into the region of the femoral nerve immediately inferior to the inguinal ligament)

- intercostal nerve blocks for thoracic and upper abdominal injuries or wounds (2–3 ml of 7.5 mg/ml ropivacaine injected into the region of appropriate intercostal nerves – usually at three or four sites unilaterally or bilaterally)
- brachial plexus or i.v. regional anaesthesia for isolated upper limb injuries or procedures (e.g. fracture manipulation)
- epidural analgesia for thoracic and abdominal pain
- intrapleural analgesia/anaesthesia, applied either via a catheter placed for this purpose or via intercostal drains previously placed for treatment of pneumothorax

MUSCLE RELAXANTS

The routine use of muscle relaxants for prolonged periods is a rare occurrence in the ICU since the advent of mechanical ventilators that provide assisted modes of ventilation (as opposed to mandatory modes used previously). Spontaneous assisted ventilation for almost all mechanically ventilated patients is now encouraged. Current indications for the use of muscle relaxants in the ICU include:

- to complement general anaesthesia for endotracheal intubation and initiation of mechanical ventilation or for short surgical procedures (e.g. tracheostomy)
- to facilitate the safe transport of patients and the acquisition of adequate radiographic images (e.g. CT or MRI)
- to facilitate mandatory mechanical ventilation when adequate sedation/analgesia alone is not adequate to achieve control, for example:
  - to increase chest wall compliance (e.g. in the severe asthmatic or to facilitate venous drainage in the patient with severe intracranial hypertension)
  - to facilitate precise control of respiratory parameters, such as airway pressure or $Pa\text{CO}_2$ (e.g. permissive hypercapnia in patients with acute respiratory distress syndrome or normocapnia in patients with impaired cerebral autoregulation)
  - to reduce $\dot{V}O_2$ in the severely hypoxaemic patient
- specific indications, such as treatment of muscle spasm in tetanus

Before muscle relaxants are used, patients should already be (or about to be commenced) on mechanical ventilation, there should be the expertise and equipment available to deal with 'difficult intubation' or accidental extubation, and patients should be sedated/anaesthetised to prevent the awareness of being paralysed while inadequately sedated. Muscle relaxants may be given by intermittent i.v. injection or by continuous i.v. infusion.

CHOICE OF MUSCLE RELAXANT

Depolarising muscle relaxants are to be used with caution in the ICU patient who has:

- multiple injuries
- renal failure
- neurological problems (e.g. paraplegia)
- burns
- been immobilised for a prolonged period of time

The risk of severe hyperkalaemia following administration of suxamethonium in these settings is high. Rocuronium, a rapid-onset, non-depolarising muscle relaxant, may be a suitable alternative.

Non-depolarising agents are the most commonly used relaxants in the ICU. Their use may be complicated by:

- Accumulation of the parent compound or active metabolites in patients with hepatic or renal insufficiency. Atracurium and cisatracurium are useful agents in these patients due to their inactivation pathways being independent of the kidney and the liver. Accumulation of the epileptogenic metabolite laudanosine may be a problem with atracurium.
- Histamine release following usually rapid injection of certain of these agents (e.g. atracurium). Vecuronium has been shown to be very 'cardiostable'.
- Protective reflexes (e.g. cough, gag, blink) are abolished and the patient is not able to move and posture him/herself. This requires increased vigilance and attention from the attendants.
- Neurological assessment of the paralysed patient is not possible and requires strict attention to detail to ensure the patient is adequately sedated while paralysed.
- Prolonged duration of action may result from:
  - patient factors, such as electrolyte disturbances (e.g. hypokalaemia, hypophosphataemia)
  - drug factors, such as myopathy associated with the use of steroidal relaxants (e.g. pancuronium, vecuronium), especially when used in conjunction with corticosteroids or aminoglycoside antibiotics.

When muscle relaxants are to be used, they should be used for a clearly defined indication, for as short a time as possible. In addition, the appropriate drug should be used and its use should be monitored regularly (e.g. train of four, post-tetanic count or double burst stimulation). Alternatively, muscle relaxants may be withheld at least once a day, until the return of muscle activity. This drug-free period may be combined with a sedation-free period every day in stable patients to allow adequate neurological assessment.

REFERENCES

1. Rhoney DH, Parker DJ. Use of sedative and analgesic agents in neurotrauma patients: effects on cerebral physiology. *Neurol Res* 2001; **23**: 237–59.
2. MacLaren R, Plamondon JM, Ramsay KB *et al.* A prospective evaluation of empiric versus protocol-based sedation and analgesia. *Pharmacotherapy* 2000; **20**: 662–72.
3. Wiener-Kronish JP. Problems with sedation and analgesia in the ICU. *Pulm Pers* 2001; **18**: 1–3.
4. Kress JP, Pohlman AS, O'Connor MF *et al.* Daily interruption of sedative infusions in critically ill patients

undergoing mechanical ventilation. *N Engl J Med* 2000; **342**: 1471–7.
5. Hall RI, Sandham D, Cardinal P *et al.* Propofol vs midazolam for ICU sedation: a Canadian multicenter randomized trial. *Chest* 2001; **119**: 1151–9.
6. Walder B, Elia N, Henzi I *et al.* A lack of evidence of superiority of propofol versus midazolam for sedation in mechanically ventilated critically ill patients: a qualitative and quantitative systemic review. *Anesth Analg* 2001; **92**: 975–83.
7. Abraham E, Papadakos PJ, Tharratt RS *et al.* Effects of propofol containing EDTA on mineral metabolism in medical patients with pulmonary dysfunction. *Intensive Care Med* 2000; **26**(Suppl 4): S422–32.
8. Bray RJ. The propofol infusion syndrome in infants and children: can we predict the risk? *Curr Opin Anaesthesiol* 2002; **15**: 339–42.
9. Nasraway SA. Use of sedative medications in the intensive care unit. *Semin Respir Crit Care Med* 2001; **22**: 165–74.
10. Aissaoui Y, Zeggwahg AA, Zekraoui A *et al.* Validation of a behavioural pain scale in critically ill, sedated and mechanically ventilated patients. *Anesth Analg* 2005; **101**: 1470–6.
11. Lee YH, Ji JD, Song GG. Adjusted indirect comparison of celecoxib versus rofecoxib on cardiovascular risk. *Rheumatol Int* 2007; **27**: 477–82.

82

Inotropes and vasopressors

John A Myburgh

The pharmacological support of the failing circulation is a fundamental part of critical care. The principal aim of these drugs is to restore inadequate systemic and regional perfusion to physiological levels.

DEFINITIONS

Inotropic agents are defined as drugs that act on the heart by increasing the velocity and force of myocardial fibre shortening. The consequent increase in contractility results in increased cardiac output and blood pressure. Characteristics of the ideal inotrope are shown in Table 82.1.

Vasopressors are drugs that have a predominantly vasoconstrictive action on the peripheral vasculature, both arterial and venous. These drugs are used primarily to increase mean arterial pressure.

The distinction between these two groups of drugs is often confusing. Many of the commonly used agents such as the catecholamines have both inotropic and variable effects on the peripheral vasculature that include venoconstriction, arteriolar vasodilatation and constriction.

Vasoregulatory agents may modulate the responsiveness of the peripheral vasculature to vasoactive drugs in pathological states such as sepsis. These agents include vasopressin and corticosteroids.

Given the overlap of pharmacodynamic effects of these drugs, the term 'vasoactive therapy' is a more appropriate description.

THE FAILING CIRCULATION

PHYSIOLOGY

Traditionally, cardiac output is discussed in terms of factors that govern cardiac function. These include preload, afterload, heart rate and rhythm, and contractility. Whilst this perspective is helpful in managing patients whose circulatory function is limited by cardiac disease, it is incomplete.

Cardiac output is controlled by the peripheral vasculature that is as energetic at returning blood to the heart as the heart is at pumping blood to the periphery[1] (Figure 82.1).

Blood is pumped down a pressure gradient that is determined by the force of myocardial ejection (contractility) and impedance to ventricular ejection (afterload). The resultant mean arterial pressure is the major 'afferent' determinant of regional perfusion pressure. Twenty per cent of the blood volume is contained in the arterial ('conducting') vessels. There is a marked drop in perfusion pressure and flow across the capillary beds to allow diffusion of substrates and oxygen. The difference between mean arterial pressure and the pressure in end capillaries ('efferent' perfusion pressure) determines regional, or organ-specific, perfusion pressure.

Blood enters the venous system and is returned to the heart via a pressure gradient determined by mean systemic pressure and right atrial pressure. The amount of blood returned to the heart determines the degree of ventricular filling prior to systole (preload), which subsequently determines stroke volume and cardiac output.

Under physiological conditions, the venous ('capacitance') system contains approximately 70% of the total blood volume which acts as a physiological reservoir ('unstressed' volume). Under conditions where circulatory demands increase, increased sympathetic tone will cause contraction of this reservoir. The resultant autotransfusion ('stressed' volume) may increase venous return by approximately 30% and subsequently cardiac output.[2,3]

Both the arterial and venous systems are integrated under complex neurohormonal influences. These include the adrenergic, renin–angiotensin–aldosterone, vasopressinergic and glucocorticoid systems in addition to local mediators such as nitric oxide, endothelin, endorphins and the eicosanoids.[4]

PATHOPHYSIOLOGY

Circulatory dysfunction or failure may be considered in terms of the major determinants of cardiac output, although there is marked interdependence between these factors.

Table 82.1 The ideal inotrope

Increases contractility
Increases mean arterial pressure
Increases cardiac output
Improves regional perfusion
No increase in myocardial oxygen consumption
Avoidance of tachycardia
Non-arrhythmogenic
Maintenance of diastolic blood pressure
Does not develop tolerance
Titratable
Rapid onset
Rapid termination of action
Compatible with other drugs
Non-toxic
Cost effective

HEART RATE FAILURE

Profound bradycardia will reduce both cardiac output and mean arterial pressure if sympathetic tone is compromised. Inotropes will increase both rate and speed of conduction, in addition to augmenting peripheral venous return, thereby restoring cardiac output and mean arterial pressure.

Tachycardia is associated with decreased left coronary artery perfusion, due to reduction of diastolic time, during which coronary perfusion occurs. This may exacerbate myocardial ischaemia in patients with coronary artery disease, particularly if mean arterial pressure, specifically diastolic blood pressure, is compromised. Therefore, drugs that shorten diastolic time or compromise coronary perfusion should be used with caution in susceptible patients.

PRELOAD FAILURE

Loss of intravascular blood volume or extracellular fluid is the most common cause of inadequate ventricular preload. This is corrected with appropriate fluids to maintain and restore a euvolaemic state. Hypovolaemia must be recognised and treated as soon as possible, preferably before vasoactive therapy is used.

There are other determinants of ventricular preload and venous return. Factors such as loss of muscle tone, positive intrathoracic pressure, loss of atrial systole (atrial fibrillation) and ablation of sympathetic tone will also compromise preload by reducing venous return. Under these circumstances, volume replacement alone may be insufficient to maintain adequate preload and vasoactive therapy may be required to increase venous return.

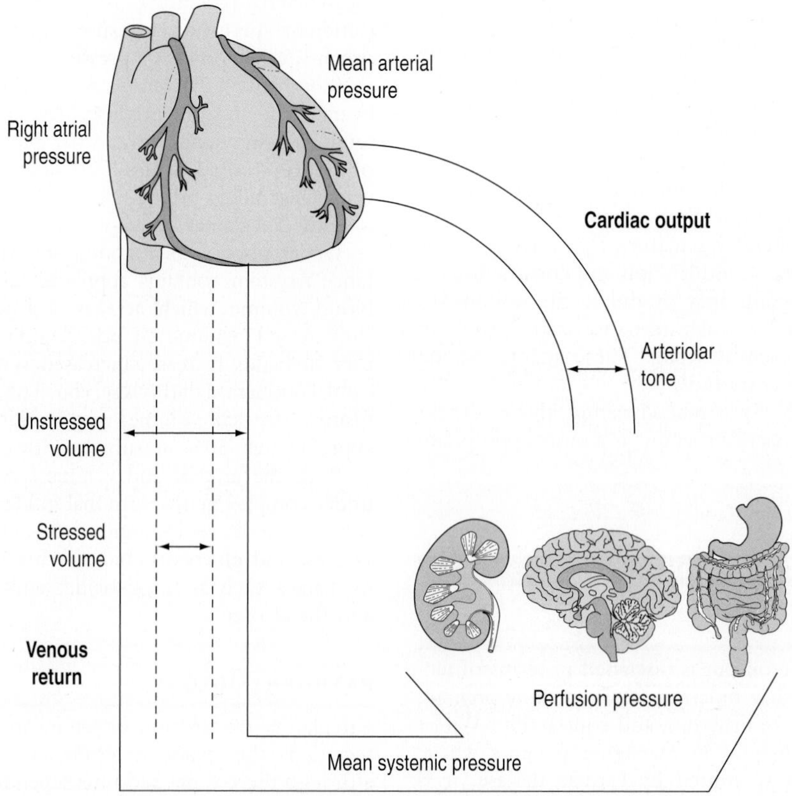

Figure 82.1 Schematic relationship of the determinants of cardiac output and venous return.

MYOCARDIAL FAILURE

Myocardial or 'pump' failure may be divided into disorders of systolic ejection (systolic dysfunction) and diastolic filling (diastolic dysfunction).

Systolic dysfunction occurs as a result of reduced effective myocardial contractility. This may be due to primary myocardial factors such as ischaemia, infarction or cardiomyopathy. Myocardial depression of both right and left ventricular function may occur in severe sepsis or following prolonged infusions of catecholamines. Increased impedance to ventricular ejection (e.g. hypertensive states) or structural abnormalities (e.g. aortic stenosis or hypertrophic obstructive cardiomyopathy) may cause systolic dysfunction.

Diastolic dysfunction is characterised by reduced ventricular compliance or increased resistance to ventricular filling during diastole. It may be due to mechanical factors such as structural abnormalities of the ventricle (e.g. restrictive cardiomyopathy) or to impaired diastolic relaxation that occurs with myocardial ischaemia or severe sepsis. This results in elevated end-diastolic pressure and pulmonary venous congestion. Episodic or 'flash' pulmonary oedema is a common clinical sign of diastolic dysfunction.[5] Tachycardias that shorten diastolic time may exacerbate diastolic failure. Diastolic dysfunction frequently accompanies systolic failure, in both acute and chronic cardiac failure, particularly in elderly patients.

In the presence of systolic dysfunction, adequate stroke volume may be maintained by an increase in left ventricular end-diastolic volume (the Frank–Starling relationship), provided diastolic function is optimal. However, if the loss of effective myocardial mass is critical, the ventricle will be unable to maintain an adequate stroke volume and cardiac output will fall. In this situation, systolic dysfunction usually requires treatment with inotropic agents in order to augment stroke volume, thereby increasing cardiac output and mean arterial pressure.

VASOREGULATORY FAILURE

Disruption or impairment of regulation of the peripheral vasculature may result in circulatory failure. This includes acute sympathetic denervation, such as high quadriplegia, epidural or total spinal anaesthesia ('spinal' shock); distributive failure such as anaphylaxis; or pathological 'vasoplegia' that occurs in severe sepsis.

These syndromes are characterised by reduced responsiveness of the peripheral circulation to endogenous or exogenous sympathetic stimulation. This results in pooling in the venous circulation due to the inability to provide a 'stressed' volume.[4]

Management of these conditions has traditionally focused on the arterial circulation with attempts to increase systemic vascular resistance, often regarded inaccurately as treatment of 'afterload failure'. This is a misnomer as the problem is predominantly impaired venous return, compounded to a lesser extent by pathological arteriolar vasodilatation.[6] Clearly, the effects of vasoregulatory failure will be exacerbated by concomitant hypovolaemia. Fluid loading to restore effective intravascular volume is essential.

Vasoactive agents may have a role in restoring vasoregulatory tone once adequate volume has been established.

CLASSIFICATION

The common ultimate cellular mechanism of action of these agents involves an influence on the release, utilisation or sequestration of intracellular calcium (Figure 82.2). These agents are divided into two main groups based on whether or not their actions depend upon increases in intracellular cyclic adenosine 3,5-monophosphate (cAMP) and are outlined in Table 82.2.

CATECHOLAMINES

Sympathomimetic amines are the most frequently used vasoactive agents in the intensive care unit (ICU) and include the naturally occurring catecholamines dopamine, noradrenaline (norepinephrine) and adrenaline (epinephrine), and the synthetic substances dobutamine, isoprenaline and dopexamine.

RECEPTOR BIOLOGY

PHYSIOLOGICAL

Agonists bind to populations of adrenergic receptors, largely divided into α and β subgroups. Further subgroups of α- (α_{1A}, α_{1B}, α_{2A}, α_{2B}, α_{2C}) and β-receptors (β_1, β_2, β_3) have been identified.[7]

Signal transduction from agonist–receptor occupation to the effector cell is modulated by conformational changes in G proteins associated with these receptors. Under the additional influence of second messengers such as nitric oxide, endothelin and eicosanoids, these conformational changes promote the release of calcium from intracellular stores and increase membrane calcium permeability. Subsequent phosphorylation of substrate proteins via protein kinases act as third messengers to trigger a cascade of events which lead to specific cardiovascular effects.

β-Receptor occupancy predominantly activates adenyl cyclase to increase the conversion of adenosine triphosphate to cAMP. α-Receptor occupancy acts independently of cAMP by activation of phospholipase C which increases inositol phosphates (IP_3 and IP_4) and diacyl glycerol.

This complex agonist–receptor–effector relationship is responsible for homeostatic mechanisms such as physiological responses to stress and autoregulation.

PATHOPHYSIOLOGICAL

The activity and function of this system is dynamic and may be markedly influenced by pathological states. This may

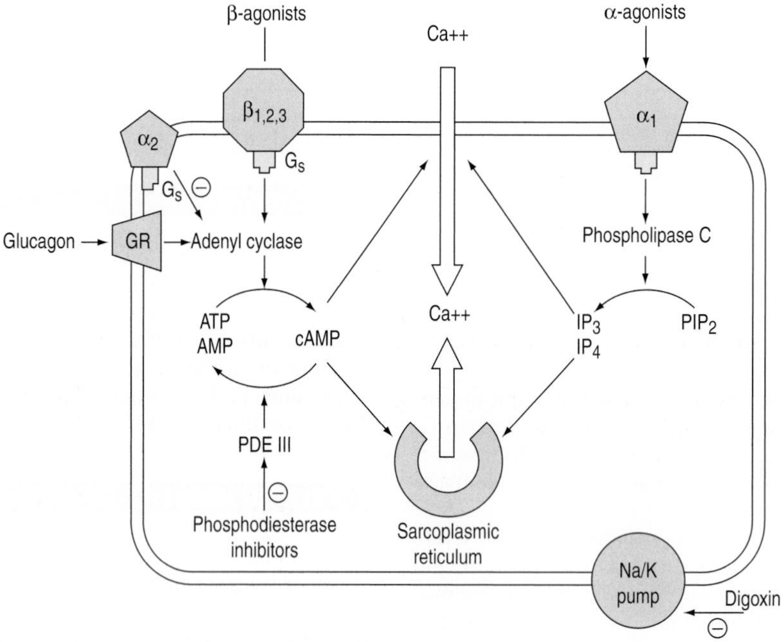

Figure 82.2 Schematic representation of the action of inotropic drugs on intracellular calcium in myocytes. AMP, adenosine monophosphate; ATP, adenosine triphosphate; cAMP, cyclic AMP; GR, glucagon receptor; Gs, G protein complex; IP, inositol phosphate 3; PDE III, phosphodiesterase III; PIP_2, phosphoinositol diphosphate.

Table 82.2 Classification of inotropes

cAMP dependent	cAMP independent
Catecholamines (β-adrenergic agonists)	Catecholamines (α-adrenergic agonists)
Adrenaline	Adrenaline
Noradrenaline	Noradrenaline
Dopamine	Dopamine
Dobutamine	Digoxin
Dopexamine	Calcium salts
Isoprenaline	Thyroid hormone
Phosphodiesterase inhibitors	
Amrinone	
Milrinone	
Enoximone	
Levosimendan	
Calcium sensitisers	
Levosimendan	
Glucagon	

result in qualitative changes in the agonist–receptor–effector organ relationship (desensitisation) where receptors no longer respond to physiological or pharmacological sympathetic stimulation to the same extent. Quantitative changes such as reduced receptor density, receptor sequestration and enzymatic uncoupling (downregulation) may also result in impaired responses.[8]

BIOSYNTHESIS

The biosynthesis and chemical structures of the naturally occurring catecholamines are shown in Figure 82.3a.

Catecholamines consist of an aromatic ring attached to a terminal amine by a carbon chain. The configuration of each drug is important for determining affinity to respective receptors.

Dopamine is hydroxylated to form noradrenaline, which is the predominant peripheral sympathetic chemotransmitter in humans, acting at all adrenergic receptors. The release of noradrenaline from sympathetic terminals is controlled by reuptake mechanisms mediated via α_2-receptors and augmented by adrenaline released from the adrenal gland at times of stress. Noradrenaline is converted to form adrenaline that is subsequently metabolised in liver and lung.

All catecholamines have very short biological half-lives (1–2 minutes) and a steady state plasma concentration is achieved within 5–10 minutes after the start of a constant infusion. This allows rapid titration of drug to a clinical end-point such as mean arterial pressure.

Adrenaline and noradrenaline infusions produce blood concentrations similar to those produced endogenously in shock states, whereas dopamine infusions produce much higher concentrations than those naturally encountered. Dopamine may exert much of its effect by being converted to noradrenaline, thus bypassing the rate-limiting (tyrosine hydroxylase) step in catecholamine synthesis.

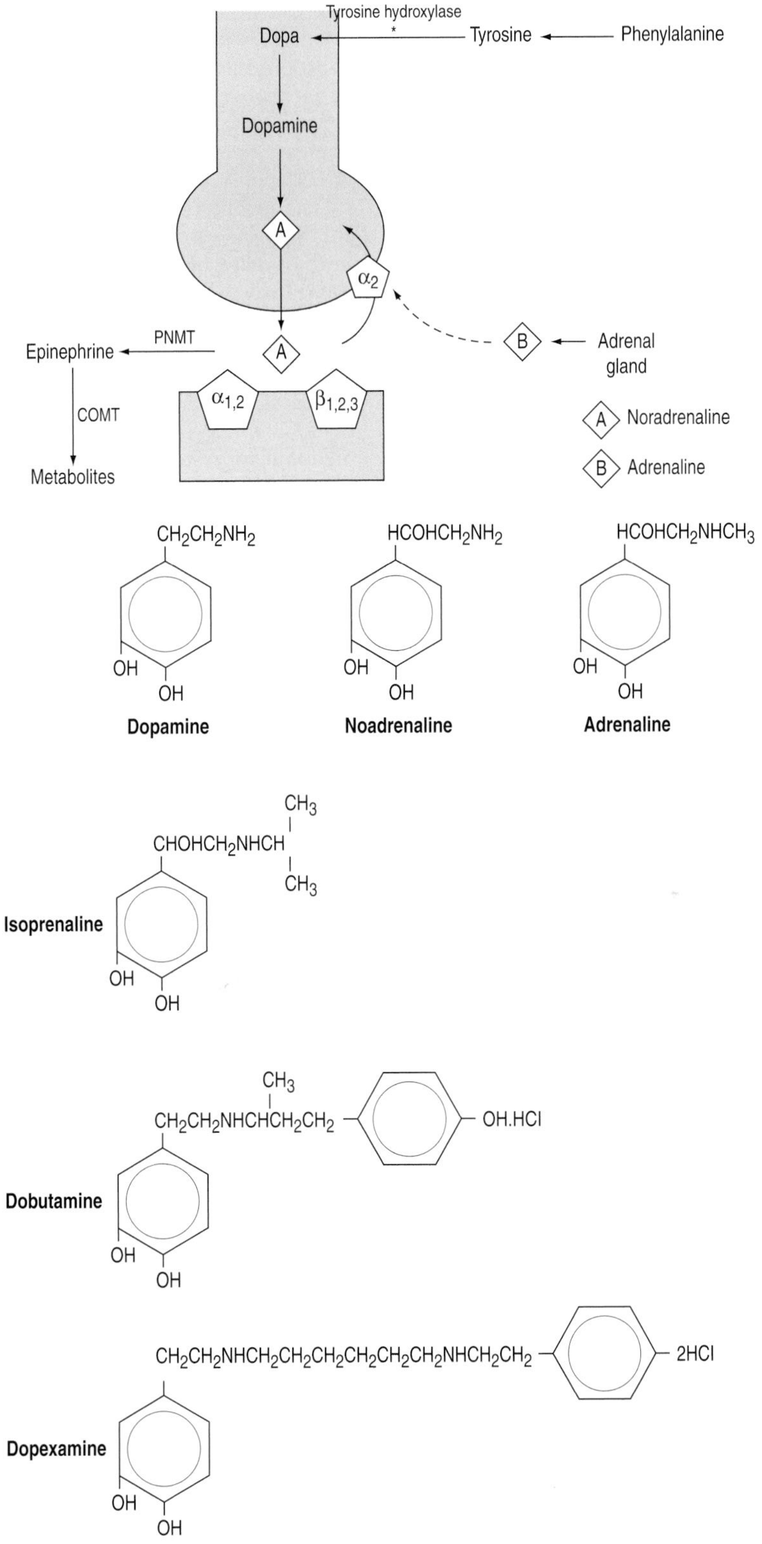

Figure 82.3 (a) Biosynthesis of catecholamines in sympathetic terminals. *Rate-limiting step by tyrosine hydroxylase. COMT, catechol-*O*-methyl transferase; PNMT, phenylethanolamine-*N*-methyltransferase. (b) Chemical structure of endogenous and synthetic catecholamines.

The synthetic catecholamines are derivatives of dopamine (Figure 82.3b). These agents are characterised by increased length of the carbon chain, which confers affinity for β-receptors. Dobutamine is a synthetic derivative of isoprenaline. These agents have relatively little affinity for α-receptors due to the configuration of the terminal amine, which differs from the endogenous catecholamines.

Adrenaline, noradrenaline and isoprenaline all have hydroxyl groups on the β-carbon atom of the side chain, and this is associated with 100-fold greater potency than dopamine or dobutamine.

SYSTEMIC EFFECTS

The systemic effects of any of these agents will vary greatly between patients and within individuals at different times. Adequacy of response is often unpredictable and depends on the aetiology of circulatory failure and systemic comorbidities. In some patients, dramatic responses to small doses may occur, whilst in others, large doses of inotropes may be required to support the failing circulation.

The classification of sympathomimetic agents into α- and β-agonists, based on the above structure/function relationships, is only a crude predictor of systemic effects.

Adrenaline, noradrenaline and dopamine are all predominantly β-agonists at low doses, with increasing α-effects becoming evident as the dose is increased.

The synthetic catecholamines are all predominantly β-agonists.

CARDIOVASCULAR

The cardiovascular effects of the catecholamines under physiological conditions are shown in Table 82.3.

Noradrenaline, adrenaline and dopamine all tend to increase stroke volume, cardiac output and mean arterial pressure, with little change in heart rate and a low incidence of dysrhythmias. The effects on the peripheral vasculature are similar, with all agents increasing venous return without significant changes in calculated systemic vascular resistance.

Isoprenaline increases cardiac output predominantly by increasing heart rate and by moderate inotropy. This occurs without a significant change in blood pressure due to predominant β_2-receptor induced veno- and vasodilatation.

The profile of dobutamine is similar to isoprenaline, although increases in heart rate are not as pronounced. Both of these agents may decrease mean arterial pressure, particularly in hypovolaemic patients, due to reduced venous return caused by venodilatation. The adverse effects of dobutamine and isoprenaline on heart rate and mean arterial pressure may compromise patients with ischaemic heart disease. However, the vasodilatory effects of dobutamine may be useful in selected patients with predominant systolic heart failure as a means of reducing afterload.

In the failing myocardium, particularly in patients with cardiac failure following cardiopulmonary bypass or septic shock, endogenous stores of noradrenaline are markedly reduced.[9] Furthermore, there may be significant desensitisation and downregulation of cardiac β-receptors. In these situations, α_1- and α_2-receptors have an important role in maintaining inotropy and peripheral vasoresponsiveness.[10] This may be expressed clinically as 'tolerance' or tachyphylaxis to catecholamines, particularly with predominantly β-agonists such as dobutamine. This phenomenon may explain the requirement for high doses of catecholamines in refractory shock states. Consequently, the role of β-agonists in patients with severe myocardial failure has been questioned.

Catecholamines have a significant effect on the venous circulation. These drugs primarily restore or maintain 'stressed volumes' of the capacitance vessels under pathological conditions, thereby maintaining or increasing cardiac output and mean arterial pressure. This is important in 'vasoplegic' states such as septic shock.[11]

Table 82.3 Cardiovascular effect of catecholamines

Agent	β_1-effects	β_2-effects	α_1-effects	α_2-effects
	+ chronotropy + dromotropy + inotropy	+ inotropy vasodilatation bronchodilatation	+ inotropy vasoconstriction	+ inotropy vasoconstriction
Noradrenaline				
Adrenaline	β-effects predominate at low dose; α-effects predominate at high dose			
Dopamine				
Dobutamine	+	+	(+)	–
Isoprenaline	+	(+)	–	–
Dopexamine	+	+	–	–

+ stimulation; (+) mild effect; – no effect.

In clinically used doses, intravenously administered catecholamines have minimal direct vasoconstrictive effects on conducting arterial vessels. Consequently, derived indices such as systemic vascular resistance do not reliably reflect the effect of catecholamines on the peripheral vasculature.

The development of peripheral gangrene in refractory septic shock has been attributed to catecholamine-induced vasoconstriction. There is little evidence to support this as the development of tissue gangrene in these situations primarily occurs as a consequence of intravascular thrombosis caused by sepsis-mediated coagulopathy.

CEREBRAL

Under physiological conditions, catecholamines do not normally cross the blood–brain barrier. Cerebral blood flow is maintained at a constant rate over a range of perfusion pressure by cerebral autoregulation. Under conditions where the integrity of the blood–brain barrier is altered, such as following traumatic brain injury and aneurysmal subarachnoid haemorrhage, or where upper and lower autoregulatory thresholds are exceeded, exogenous catecholamines may directly enter the cerebral circulation.[12]

The degree by which these agents directly affect the cerebral circulation following head injury is unknown, although there is some evidence suggesting that dopamine has a direct effect causing increased cerebral blood flow and intracranial pressure.[13]

RENAL

The kidney is an efficient autoregulator, maintaining constant glomerular filtration and renal blood flow by neurohumoral mechanisms such as the renin–angiotensin–aldosterone system. All catecholamines will increase renal blood flow to a similar extent because of increased cardiac output and mean arterial pressure with a resultant natriuresis. Catecholamine-mediated increases in renal blood flow do not affect glomerular filtration rate.

A direct natriuresis may also result from inhibition of cAMP in the renal tubules. This effect has been attributed primarily to low doses of dopamine (2 μg/kg per min), although this occurs to a similar extent with adrenaline, noradrenaline and dobutamine. The use of low dose "renal" dopamine has been shown to be ineffective in preventing renal dysfunction in susceptible patients.[14]

SPLANCHNIC

Splanchnic autoregulation is not as robust as the brain and kidney. Perfusion is more dependent on mean arterial pressure and the duality of the mesenteric and portal systems. Concerns about catecholamine-induced splanchnic vasoconstriction with mesenteric and hepatic ischaemia have not been substantiated.[15]

Dopamine and dopexamine have been promoted as selective splanchnic vasodilators, but there are no conclusive studies indicating a significant benefit over noradrenaline or adrenaline. Many studies have used gastric intramucosal pH (pHi), a surrogate measurement of splanchnic blood flow, as the primary end-point. However, as pHi remains an unvalidated measurement, the results of many of the comparative trials of the different sympathomimetics are inconclusive. All catecholamines are equally effective in increasing splanchnic perfusion by improving cardiac output and mean arterial pressure.

METABOLIC

Catecholamine-mediated β-stimulation may result in hyperglycaemia, hypokalaemia and hypophosphataemia, which may need monitoring and correcting.

Adrenaline is associated with the development of hyperlactataemia and an acidaemia, due to activation of pyruvate dehydrogenase.[16] Whilst pH may fall to levels around 7.2, the acidosis is not associated with impaired tissue perfusion or cellular dysoxia. In most patients who are haemodynamically stable, this is a self-limiting phenomenon and is not associated with adverse outcomes.[17] This may become an issue in severe sepsis with the development of a metabolic acidosis.

NON-CATECHOLAMINES

PHOSPHODIESTERASE INHIBITORS

Phosphodiesterase inhibitors are compounds that cause non-receptor mediated competitive inhibition of phosphodiesterase isoenzymes (PDE), resulting in increased levels of cAMP (Figure 82.2). Importantly, cAMP also affects diastolic heart function through the regulation of phospholamban, the regulatory subunit of the calcium pump of the sarcoplasmic reticulum. This enhances the rate of calcium re-sequestration and thereby diastolic relaxation.

For cardiovascular tissue, inhibition of isoenzyme PDE III is responsible for the therapeutic effects. Cardiac effects are characterised by positive inotropy and improved diastolic relaxation. The latter is termed lusitropy and may be beneficial in patients with reduced ventricular compliance or predominant diastolic failure.[18]

These agents also cause potent vasodilatation with reductions in preload, venous return and afterload as well as a reduction in pulmonary vascular resistance. The term 'inodilation' has been used to describe this dual haemodynamic effect.

Tolerance is not a feature. These agents may have a place in the management of patients with β-receptor downregulation by causing intrinsic inotropic stimulation and by sensitising the myocardium to β-agonists. Other speculative actions include inhibition of platelet aggregation and reduction of postischaemic reperfusion injury.

Titration pharmacokinetics of phosphodiesterase inhibitors are markedly different from catecholamines. Drug half-lives may be prolonged and excretion is predominantly renal. Hypotension may result from vasodilatation, and combined use with catecholamines (e.g. noradrenaline or adrenaline) may be necessary and complementary to maintain mean arterial pressure.

Phosphodiesterase inhibitors that have been used in clinical practice include the bipyridine derivatives amrinone and milrinone, the imidazolones enoximone and piroximone, and the calcium sensitiser levosimendan. The cardiovascular effects are similar.

The oral form of amrinone is no longer used clinically due to a high incidence of thrombocytopenia, gastrointestinal and neurological side-effects. Milrinone and enoximone are more potent agents and are currently used in clinical practice, with the latter exhibiting more inotropic effects than vasodilatation. Enoximone is more rapidly metabolised, but the metabolite is active and its cardiovascular effects persist for some hours. There is evidence that prolonged use of these agents is associated with an increased mortality in patients with severe heart failure.

Levosimendan is a dose-dependent selective phosphodiesterase inhibitor with a unique action on myocardial calcium metabolism.[19] By increasing myofilament calcium sensitivity throughout the cardiac cycle by binding to cardiac troponin C, associated conformational changes induce improved inotropic and lusitropic function. Vasodilatation is also induced through ATP-sensitive potassium channels. Calcium-sensitive actions predominate at low doses, whilst PDE-inhibition effects predominate at higher doses. The half-life of levosimendan is shorter than older PDE III inhibitors (approximately 1 hour) and it may be given by infusion. Two large trials have demonstrated improved haemodynamic function compared to dobutamine in cardiogenic shock and myocardial infarction, and improved short-term mortality,[20,21] although definitive outcome-based results in critically ill patients are awaited.

DIGOXIN

Digitalis glycosides have been used for the treatment of heart failure for 200 years and the vagotonic effects used to control the ventricular response in selected supraventricular tachyarrhythmias.

The effects of digoxin are largely mediated by an increase in intracellular calcium concentrations produced indirectly by inhibition of the $Na+/K+$ membrane pump resulting in increased myocardial contractility (Figure 82.2). The effects on impulse conduction are mediated through change in both vagal and sympathetic tone, which may also increase venous return.

Digoxin has a narrow therapeutic index, is highly protein bound and is largely excreted unchanged in the urine. Alteration in renal function may prolong the normal half-life of about 35 hours to 5 days.

The role of digoxin in acute cardiac failure is questionable. It has minimal effects as an inotrope and evaluation of its efficacy is difficult. In the presence of high levels of sympathetic activity, the positive inotropic effect is negligible and there is usually a poor response in acute myocardial failure, myocarditis, advanced cardiomyopathy, shock states and cardiac tamponade.

The potential for toxicity in the critically ill patient is increased by hypokalaemia, hypomagnesaemia, hypercalcaemia, hypoxia and acidosis. Toxicity is manifested by dysrhythmias that may assume any form including supraventricular tachyarrhythmias, bradycardia, ventricular ectopy and conduction block at any level.

Monitoring digoxin levels in critically ill patients is recommended, although interpretation of these levels is difficult. A concentration of 1–2 ng/ml represents an acceptable risk:benefit ratio, but concentrations of greater than 2 ng/ml may be associated with toxicity in some patients. However, correlation between blood concentrations, efficacy and toxic manifestations is poor. Clinical criteria remain the most reliable assessment of toxicity, but with the exception of dysrhythmias, may be difficult to elicit in ICU patients.

Drugs commonly used in the ICU, such as amiodarone, calcium channel blockers and erythromycin, demonstrate adverse drug interactions with digoxin. These may interfere with the radioimmune assay to reflect apparently increased digoxin blood concentrations. The place of digoxin in the critically ill patient is therefore limited due to unpredictable efficacy and toxicity. Careful titration of short-acting inotropes and drugs such as amiodarone for control of ventricular rate in supraventricular tachycardia in critically ill patients have largely superseded its use.

The role digoxin in chronic heart failure is well established, particularly in association with angiotensin-converting enzyme inhibitors.[22] These drugs may have a role in long-term intensive care patients with associated chronic cardiac failure. In critically ill patients, digoxin should only be administered by slow intravenous injection, as oral bioavailability varies considerably due to altered gastric motility or perfusion. A loading dose (1–1.5 mg in three or four divided doses, 4–6 hours apart) followed by a maintenance dose (0.125–0.5 mg/day) is a satisfactory regimen. Smaller doses should be used in the elderly, small patients, patients with renal, electrolyte and acid–base disturbances, and myxoedema.

Blood for assay should be taken at least 6 hours after an oral dose and 1 hour after an intravenous dose.

GLUCAGON

Glucagon is a naturally occurring polypeptide that directly stimulates adenyl cyclase via specific receptors to increase cAMP concentration in myocardial cells resulting in positive inotropy without producing myocardial excitability (Figure 82.2). Large doses are required to achieve this effect which is associated with a high incidence of metabolic side-effects.

No definitive cardiovascular role for this agent has been established apart from anecdotal reports of its use in severe β-blocker and tricyclic poisoning.

THYROID HORMONE

Thyroid hormone is required for synthesis of contractile proteins and normal myocardial contraction. It is also a regulator of the synthesis of adrenergic receptors.

Low levels of thyroid hormone have been demonstrated in brain-dead organ donors, in patients with refractory cardiogenic shock, particularly following cardiopulmonary bypass, and secondary to myxoedema. Preliminary studies suggest that treatment with thyroid hormone in these patients may reduce the need for vasoactive therapy to achieve satisfactory haemodynamics.

SELECTIVE VASOPRESSORS

Vascular responsiveness is mediated via adrenergic receptors: α-mechanisms predominantly cause vasoconstriction; β-mechanisms, specifically β_2-receptors, mediate vasodilatation (Table 82.3).

Noradrenaline, adrenaline and dopamine have variable effects on the peripheral vasculature and should not be regarded principally as vasoconstrictors or vasopressors.

There are few selective 'vasoconstrictors' that predominantly have a role in vasodilated states such as regional (epidural) anaesthesia or selected patients with acute spinal injury. Their utility in critically ill patients remains limited and they have an unproven role in patients with catecholamine-resistant septic shock and cardiopulmonary resuscitation.

PHENYLEPHRINE AND METARAMINOL

These agents are direct-acting α_2-agonists that are selective vasoconstrictors, both venous and arterial, with minimal β-activity. They have similar pharmacokinetics to catecholamines and may be given by infusion. In patients with normal sympathetic tone, these drugs may cause reflex bradycardia, particularly following bolus administration.

EPHEDRINE

Ephedrine is a synthetic, direct- and indirect-acting, non-catecholamine sympathomimetic that acts on both α- and β-receptors. Duration of action is longer than equivalent doses of adrenaline and it is generally unsuitable as an infusion.

VASOREGULATORY AGENTS

PATHOPHYSIOLOGY

In addition to adrenergic regulation, neurohumoral influences have a 'permissive' or regulatory role in maintaining vasomotor tone. These are mediated through the renin–aldosterone–angiotensin axis and local mediators such as vasopressin, corticosteroids, nitric oxide and endothelin.

The response of the whole neurohumoral system may become blunted in conditions such as severe sepsis, where qualitative and quantitative changes may occur. In this context, failure of vasomotor responsiveness may be considered as part of the multiple organ failure.

VASOPRESSIN

Specific vasopressinergic receptors (V_1, V_2) have been identified in association with sympathetic terminals. Vasopressin is a naturally occurring peptide secreted by the posterior pituitary gland. Reduced serum levels of vasopressin have been demonstrated in septic shock and following cardiopulmonary bypass, suggesting an inflammatory-mediated mechanism. Levels are maintained during cardiogenic shock.

A proportion of patients with severe septic shock requiring high levels of catecholamines to support the circulation may respond to low doses of infused vasopressin (0.04 U/hour) significantly reducing doses of infused catecholamine. This phenomenon appears to be independent of any directly attributable vasopressor effect; rather it is a supplemental 'catecholamine sparing' strategy, particularly in patients with mild to moderate shock states.[23] The impact in severe shock or on mortality has not been substantiated in a large clinical trial (VASST Study).[24]

STEROIDS

The role of steroid supplementation in circulatory failure has been studied for many years. Whilst immunosuppressive or anti-inflammatory doses have been shown to be ineffective, particularly in septic shock, replacement of 'stress response' doses (approximately 100–200 mg hydrocortisone per day) have been shown to improve vasoresponsiveness to catecholamine infusions in selected patients with refractory shock.

Patients who respond to low doses of steroids may have biochemical evidence of hypoadrenalism, although the diagnosis of this remains difficult to determine in critically ill patients.[25] Early studies of adrenal replacement therapy have suggested improvement in organ function and survival in 'non-responders' to adrenal stimulation with corticotropin.[26] although this effect has not been substantiated in a large randomised controlled trial (CORTICUS Study).[27]

CLINICAL USES

Currently, there are no definitive studies comparing the efficacy of one inotrope (or combination of inotropes) over another in terms of improving survival.

DRUG SELECTION

In most instances, individual experience and preference determine selection of inotrope(s).

On a pathobiological basis, exogenous catecholamines are essentially used to augment endogenous mechanisms that may be failing at a number of levels. In this context, vasoactive therapy should be regarded as 'cardiovascular neuroendocrine augmentation therapy'.

Noradrenaline or adrenaline may be considered as the first-line drug in most causes of circulatory failure. An emerging body of evidence confirms this statement (CATS and CAT Studies).[28]

Dopamine predominantly acts as a precursor of noradrenaline and may be used as an alternative to noradrenaline, although all of the endogenous catecholamines have similar pharmacodynamic profiles.

Prediction of the response of an individual to a catecholamine is problematic as marked inter- and intra-individual variability to the response of inotropic agents may occur.

The haemodynamic and metabolic response of an agent must be carefully monitored and evaluated. If there is not a satisfactory response, or if undesirable effects are obtained, the dose or agent should be changed.

MONITORING

Accurate monitoring of the circulation is essential in patients with circulatory failure to assess baseline parameters and the response of vasoactive drugs.

Clinical assessment of the circulation remains the cornerstone of monitoring these patients and includes frequent assessment and recording of pulse rate and rhythm, blood pressure, adequacy of peripheral perfusion, skin turgor, level of consciousness and urine output.

The majority of patients with circulatory failure managed in the ICU require haemodynamic monitoring as clinical signs may be masked or influenced by sedation, ventilation or organ failure. This should provide accurate information about the state of the circulation and be interpreted within the context of the underlying pathophysiology.

The following principles are important in patients requiring vasoactive drugs.

BLOOD PRESSURE

All patients receiving vasoactive drugs in all but trivial doses should have accurate monitoring of mean arterial pressure, ideally with an intra-arterial catheter referenced to the aortic root.

Adequacy of tissue perfusion correlates with mean arterial pressure. Accordingly, vasoactive drugs are titrated to achieve a mean arterial pressure that is commensurate with the patient's premorbid blood pressure.

Circulatory dysfunction is commonly defined as a mean arterial pressure $\leq$ 50 mmHg for 1 hour despite adequate fluid resuscitation, although this may vary between patients and will depend on the aetiology.

A large artery such as the femoral artery should be considered in haemodynamically unstable patients as radial or dorsalis pedis arterial catheters underestimate true systemic pressure in shocked patients.

The measurement of systolic and diastolic blood pressures may be inaccurate in haemodynamically unstable patients, particularly if non-invasive devices are used. These devices tend to overread in hypotensive patients and underread in hypertensive patients.

VOLUME STATUS

Right atrial pressure monitoring via a central venous catheter provides the best assessment of volume status.[29] Accuracy may be affected by tricuspid regurgitation or pulmonary hypertension.

Left atrial pressure may be measured via direct placement of a left atrial catheter, usually during cardiac surgery. Pulmonary artery occlusion pressure may be used as an indirect measurement of left atrial pressure. However, this measurement may be affected by respiratory artefact, positive airway pressure, tachycardia, hypovolaemia and poor ventricular compliance.

The response and trend to fluid loading and/or vasoactive drug provides more useful information than absolute values.

CARDIAC OUTPUT

As cardiac output is the major determinant of mean arterial pressure, adequate pressure will usually indicate adequate flow (cardiac output). This relationship depends on the adequacy of venous return and level of afterload.

In selected patients with primary myocardial failure, an assessment of cardiac output is useful to quantify baseline function and to assess the response of the heart to drug therapy. Measurement of cardiac output may be done non-invasively using transthoracic or transoesophageal echocardiography or invasively using a pulmonary catheter, ideally using a continuous cardiac output display system, although the use of these catheters have decreased substantially.

Systemic vascular resistance is frequently calculated and used as a surrogate index of afterload. However, the clinical utility of systemic vascular resistance is limited to providing a crude estimate of global vascular tone, as it does not reflect afterload, arteriolar tone or venous return. Consequently, systemic vascular resistance should not be used as a criterion for selection of vasoactive drug or as a titratable end-point.

TISSUE PERFUSION

Restoration of reduced tissue perfusion is a primary aim of inotropic therapy. This may assessed clinically by improvements in urine output, serum urea and creatinine, reversal of metabolic acidosis and reduction in serum lactate.

Global indices of oxygenation such as systemic oxygen delivery ($\dot{D}O_2$), oxygen consumption ($\dot{V}O_2$) and oxygen extraction ratio ($\dot{D}O_2/\dot{V}O_2$) have not been shown to correlate with tissue perfusion or adequacy of resuscitation. Measurement of regional tissue perfusion such as pHi (splanchnic) and jugular venous saturation (cerebral) are limited by poor specificity and are not used routinely.

DOSAGES AND DRUG ADMINISTRATION

Vasoactive drugs, such as catecholamines or vasopressors, are administered by continuous infusion through a dedicated central venous catheter using drug delivery systems such as infusion pumps or syringe drivers.

Infusion lines should be free of injection portals and clearly marked with identifying labels.

Concentrations of infusions should be standardised in accordance with individual unit protocols. Suggested infusion concentrations are shown in Table 82.4.

These infusions in ml/hour approximate μg/min. Absolute doses with regard to body weight are not relevant; rather the titrated clinical effect. Vasoactive drugs are usually prescribed as a titration against a desired mean arterial pressure.

SPECIFIC SITUATIONS

The following is a summary of the clinical uses of inotropes and vasopressors in common conditions of circulatory failure. Specific pharmacology and physiological effects are discussed above.

CARDIOPULMONARY RESUSCITATION

Adrenaline has been used for circulatory collapse at least since 1907. The International Liaison Committee on Resuscitation guidelines recommends adrenaline as first-line inotrope/vasopressor in cardiopulmonary resuscitation.[30] Doses are 1 mg intravenously every 3 minutes.

The use of 'high dose' adrenaline (5 mg), noradrenaline or phenylephrine in cardiopulmonary resuscitation has not been demonstrated to improve return of spontaneous circulation or survival.

Adrenaline is recommended as first-line therapy for 'medical pacing' for severe bradyarrhythmias that do not respond to atropine. Isoprenaline has traditionally been used for this purpose; however, its use has been superseded by adrenaline due to concerns about efficacy and lack of α-adrenergic activity.

CARDIOGENIC SHOCK

Theoretically, catecholamine infusions may confer some advantages in cardiogenic shock, particularly in association with acute myocardial infarction. In patients with systolic heart failure, adrenaline, noradrenaline, dopamine and dobutamine have been shown to cause satisfactory short-term effects. This may allow the myocardium time to recover from post ischaemic 'stunning', particularly after revascularisation. However, no increased long-term survival due to their use has been demonstrated.[31]

The role of phosphodiesterase inhibitors (e.g. milrinone) and calcium sensitisers (e.g. levosimendan) in acute heart failure has yet to be determined, but they may have a potential role in patients with diastolic heart failure. Due to their non-adrenergic mechanism of action, these agents may be useful in patients who are 'resistant' to catecholamines.

Table 82.4 Infusion concentrations of commonly used vasoactive drugs

Agent	Infusion concentration	Dose
Adrenaline	6 mg/100 ml 5% dextrose	Titrate ml/hour (= μg/min)
Noradrenaline	6 mg/100 ml 5% dextrose	Titrate ml/hour (= μg/min)
Dopamine	400 mg/100 ml 5% dextrose	Titrate ml/hour (~ μg/kg per min)
Dobutamine	500 mg/100 ml 5% dextrose	Titrate ml/hour (~ μg/kg per min)
Isoprenaline	6 mg/100 ml 5% dextrose	Titrate ml/hour (= μg/min)
Milrinone	10 mg/100 ml 5% dextrose	Loading dose: 50 μg/kg over 20 min Infusion: 0.5 μg/kg per min
Levosimendan	25 mg/100 ml 5% dextrose	Loading dose: 24 μg/kg over 10 min Infusion: 0.1 μg/kg per min
Phenylephrine	10 mg/100 ml 5% dextrose	Titrate ml/hour (= 100 μg/hour)
Metaraminol	100 mg/100 ml 5% dextrose	Titrate ml/hour (= mg/hour)
Ephedrine	300 mg/100 ml 5% dextrose	Titrate ml/hour (= 3 mg/hour)
Vasopressin	20 units/20 ml 5% dextrose	2.4 ml/hour (0.04 U/min)
Hydrocortisone	100 mg/100 ml 5% dextrose	Loading dose: 100 mg Infusion: 0.18 mg/kg per hour

SEPARATION FROM CARDIOPULMONARY BYPASS

Numerous combinations of catecholamines have been used successfully to wean patients from cardiopulmonary bypass. However, there are no definitive studies demonstrating significant benefits of one catecholamine over another. Similarly, the question whether mechanical support devices, such as intra-aortic counterpulsation, offer a significant advantage over inotropes following cardiac surgery remains unanswered.

Adrenaline, noradrenaline and/or dopamine have been found to increase cardiac output with little increase in heart rate or afterload and are often regarded as first-line drugs. At higher doses (> 40 μg/kg per min), dopamine has been shown to cause more tachycardia than adrenaline and noradrenaline. Dobutamine may be associated with vasodilatation and hypotension.

There is no conclusive evidence that the catecholamines, including noradrenaline, cause vasospasm of arterial conduits in clinically used doses.

Phosphodiesterase inhibitors, such as milrinone and levosimendan, either as sole agents or in conjunction with adrenaline or noradrenaline, have been used with success. These may have a role following mitral valve replacement in patients with pulmonary hypertension or preoperative diastolic failure.[32]

Cardiopulmonary bypass may be associated with a systemic inflammatory response syndrome characterised by a hyperdynamic, vasodilated 'low systemic vascular resistance' state.[33] Noradrenaline is frequently advocated as a 'vasopressor' agent in this context to restore mean arterial pressure that may be reduced as a consequence. This condition is usually self-limiting with a nadir 8 hours post bypass. Although catecholamines may be required to achieve appropriate target mean arterial pressure and cardiac output, caution should be applied if high doses (e.g. > 30 μg/min noradrenaline) are required. This may be associated with tachyphylaxis and potentiation of catecholamine dependency.

RIGHT VENTRICULAR FAILURE

Right ventricular infarction and major pulmonary embolism may be associated with acute right ventricular failure. Right ventricular depression may also occur in severe sepsis. Restoration of preload is critical in these conditions, as the failing right ventricle is particularly susceptible to reductions in preload.[34]

Inotropes such as noradrenaline and adrenaline are regarded as first-line drugs in these situations in order to maintain adequate mean arterial pressure so that right coronary artery perfusion, which occurs throughout the cardiac cycle, is maintained.

Concerns about pulmonary artery vasoconstriction and increased right ventricular afterload by noradrenaline and adrenaline appear to be unfounded. Consequently, the use of traditional vasodilators such as isoprenaline in acute right ventricular failure has been superseded by these drugs.

SEPTIC SHOCK

The cardiovascular effects of the sepsis syndrome and septic shock are complex and range from a hyperdynamic, vasodilated state to one of increasing myocardial failure and paralysis of the peripheral vasculature (vasoplegia).[35] The latter represents inability of the venous circulation to respond to endogenous or exogenous catecholamines with resultant venous pooling.

Consequently, it is important to establish that the patient is not hypovolaemic before using a catecholamine infusion in septic shock, as 20% of patients will respond, at least initially, to intravascular volume expansion.

An increasing body of literature now recommends the use of catecholamines as first-line agents in the treatment of septic shock. The Surviving Sepsis Campaign guidelines[36] recommend either noradrenaline or dopamine be used as the first-line choice vasopressor/inotrope. The basis for this recommendation is weak as there is no high-quality evidence to recommend one catecholamine over another. Concerns about adverse metabolic and splanchnic side-effects of adrenaline are unsubstantiated, and there is an emerging body of evidence that noradrenaline and adrenaline are equally effective in treating septic shock (CAT Study: unpublished data). Furthermore, there is evidence that dopamine may be associated with adverse outcomes, possibly due to neuroendocrine[37,38] and immunological effects, and its use is being questioned in the absence of superiority to noradrenaline or adrenaline.

The efficacy of dobutamine as a sole agent or in combination with noradrenaline in septic shock is questionable and appears to add little to the efficacy of noradrenaline or adrenaline in terms of resolution of shock or mortality (CATS and CAT Studies).[28] Furthermore, the use of dobutamine to increase or augment oxygen delivery has been proven to be ineffective in septic shock.[36]

Doses required to achieve adequate mean arterial pressure in septic shock may vary: noradrenaline or adrenaline infusions (up to 50 μg/min) may be necessary. Patients who develop marked catecholamine dependency, in the absence of other acute remediable causes such as active infection, may respond to low doses of vasopressin or 'stress response' doses of hydrocortisone, although there is marked inter-individual variation in response to these drugs (see above).

ANAPHYLAXIS

Adrenaline is the drug of choice for anaphylactic reactions and for life-threatening bronchospasm, as it blocks mediator release and specifically reverses end-organ effects (see Chapter 58).

A dose of 0.1 mg, as 1 ml of 1:10 000 solution, may be injected subcutaneously, intramuscularly or intravenously. Repeated doses or infusions of up to 100 μg/min may be required. A strong slowing pulse indicates a pressor effect and provides a useful clinical end-point for the rate of infusion. This α-agonist effect is probably also of considerable importance in anaphylaxis, as deaths are frequently due to prolonged refractory hypotension caused by acute biventricular failure. Early intravenous fluid therapy is also important.

RENAL PROTECTION

Augmentation of mean arterial pressure in order to prevent or ameliorate acute renal failure in critically ill patients is an important use of inotropes. In addition to ensuring adequate preload, catecholamines may be used to defend renal perfusion by maintaining mean arterial pressure at appropriate levels. This is important in hypertensive patients, where higher mean arterial pressure may be required to maintain renal perfusion, particularly when these patients develop intercurrent causes of circulatory failure.

'Renal' dose dopamine (2 μg/kg per min) has been advocated for many years as a renal protective agent by causing renal vasodilatation. However, this has not been substantiated in controlled clinical trials in susceptible patients[14] or as an adjunctive agent with other inotropes in septic shock. In addition, the prolonged use of low dose dopamine is associated with suppression of anterior and posterior pituitary hormonal secretion and impairment in T-cell function. Consequently, low dose dopamine is no longer recommended.

Equivalent renal protection has been demonstrated with dopamine, noradrenaline and dobutamine and it is likely that this effect relates primarily to defence of renal perfusion, rather than a specific renal effect.

CEREBRAL PERFUSION PRESSURE

Augmentation of cerebral perfusion pressure is an important strategy in patients with pathological reductions in cerebral blood flow. This is well described following traumatic brain injury and aneurysmal subarachnoid haemorrhage and is discussed elsewhere in this volume See Chapter 45 page 564. Catecholamine interactions on the cerebral vasculature are discussed above.

Noradrenaline, adrenaline, dopamine and phenylephrine have been used to augment cerebral perfusion pressure, although there is no conclusive evidence to recommend one drug over another.[13]

REFERENCES

1. Guyton AC, Lindsay AW, Kaufmann BN. Effect of mean circulatory filling pressure and other peripheral circulatory factors on cardiac output. *Am J Physiol* 1955; **180**: 463–8.
2. Jacobsohn E, Chorn R, O'Connor M. The role of the vasculature in regulating venous return and cardiac output: historical and graphical approach. *Can J Anaesth* 1997; **44**: 849–67.
3. Magder S. The classical Guyton view that mean systemic pressure, right atrial pressure, and venous resistance govern venous return is/is not correct. *J Appl Physiol* 2006; **101**: 1533.
4. Magder S, Rastepagarnah M. Role of neurosympathetic pathways in the vascular response to sepsis. *J Crit Care* 1998; **13**: 169–76.
5. Cotter G, Kaluski E, Moshkovitz Y *et al.* Pulmonary edema: new insight on pathogenesis and treatment. *Curr Opin Cardiol* 2001; **16**: 159–63.
6. Magder S, Vanelli G. Circuit factors in the high cardiac output of sepsis. *J Crit Care* 1996; **11**: 155–66.
7. Hein L. Adrenoceptors and signal transduction in neurons. *Cell Tissue Res* 2006; **326**: 541–51.
8. Lamba S, Abraham WT. Alterations in adrenergic receptor signaling in heart failure. *Heart Fail Res* 2000; **5**: 7–16.
9. Levy RJ, Deutschman CS. Evaluating myocardial depression in sepsis. *Shock* 2004; **22**: 1–10.
10. Heusch G. Alpha-adrenergic mechanisms in myocardial ischemia. *Circulation* 1990; **81**: 1–13.
11. Magder S, Rastepagarnah M. Role of neurosympathetic pathways in the vascular response to sepsis. *J Crit Care* 1998; **13**: 169–76.
12. Myburgh JA. Quantifying cerebral autoregulation in health and disease. *Crit Care Resusc* 2004; **6**: 59–67.
13. Myburgh JA. Driving cerebral perfusion pressure with pressors: how, which, when? *Crit Care Resusc* 2005; **7**: 200–5.
14. Bellomo R, Chapman M, Finfer S *et al.* Low-dose dopamine in patients with early renal dysfunction: a placebo-controlled randomised trial. Australian and New Zealand Intensive Care Society (ANZICS) Clinical Trials Group. *Lancet* 2000; **356**: 2139–43.
15. Sakka SG, Meier-Hellmann A, Reinhart K. Do fluid administration and reduction in norepinephrine dose improve global and splanchnic haemodynamics? *Br J Anaesth* 2000; **84**: 758–62.
16. Day NP, Phu NH, Bethell DP *et al.* The effects of dopamine and adrenaline infusions on acid–base balance and systemic haemodynamics in severe infection. *Lancet* 1996; **348**: 219–23.
17. Totaro RJ, Raper RF. Epinephrine-induced lactic acidosis following cardiopulmonary bypass. *Crit Care Med* 1997; **25**: 1693–9.
18. Erhardt L. An emerging role for calcium sensitisation in the treatment of heart failure. *Expert Opin Investig Drugs* 2005; **14**: 659–70.
19. Innes CA, Wagstaff AJ. Levosimendan: a review of its use in the management of acute decompensated heart failure. *Drugs* 2003; **63**: 2651–71.
20. Follath F, Cleland JG, Just H *et al.* Efficacy and safety of intravenous levosimendan compared with dobutamine in severe low-output heart failure (the LIDO study): a randomised double-blind trial. *Lancet* 2002; **360**: 196–202.
21. Moiseyev VS, Poder P, Andrejevs N *et al.* Safety and efficacy of a novel calcium sensitizer, levosimendan, in patients with left ventricular failure due to an acute myocardial infarction. A randomized, placebo-controlled, double-blind study (RUSSLAN). *Eur Heart J* 2002; **23**: 1422–32.
22. The Digitalis Investigation Group. The effect of digoxin on mortality and morbidity in patients with heart failure. *N Engl J Med* 1997; **336**: 525–33.

23. Rozenfeld V, Cheng JW. The role of vasopressin in the treatment of vasodilation in shock states. *Ann Pharmacother* 2000; **34**: 250–4.
24. Russell JA, Walley KR, Singer J, Gordon AC, Hebert PC, Cooper DJ, Holmes CL, Mehta S, Granton JT, Storms MM, Cook DJ, Presneill JJ, Ayers D for the VASST Investigators. Vasopressin versus norepinephrine infusion in patients with septic shock. *New England Journal of Medicine* 2008; **358**: 877–87.
25. Prigent H, Maxime V, Annane D. Science review: mechanisms of impaired adrenal function in sepsis and molecular actions of glucocorticoids. *Crit Care* 2004; **8**: 243–52.
26. Annane D, Sebille V, Charpentier C *et al.* Effect of treatment with low doses of hydrocortisone and fludrocortisone on mortality in patients with septic shock. *JAMA* 2002; **288**: 862–71.
27. Sprung CL, Annane D, Keh D, Moreno R, Singer M, Freivogel K, Weiss YG, Benbenishty J, Kalenka A, Forst H, Laterre P-F, Reinhart K, Cuthbertson BH, Payen D, Briegel J for the CORTICUS Study Group. *New England Journal of Medicine* 2008; **358**: 111–24.
28. Annane D, Vignon P, Renault A, Bollaert P-E, Charpentier C, Martin C, Troche G, Ricard J-D, Nitenberg G, Papazian L, Azoulay E, Bellisant E for thr CATS Study Group. *Lancet* 2007; **370**: 676–84.
29. Magder S. Central venous pressure: a useful but not so simple measurement. *Crit Care Med* 2006; **34**: 2224–7.
30. Guidelines 2000 for Cardiopulmonary Resuscitation and Emergency Cardiovascular Care. Part 6: advanced cardiovascular life support: section 6: pharmacology II: agents to optimize cardiac output and blood pressure. The American Heart Association in collaboration with the International Liaison Committee on Resuscitation. *Circulation* 2000; **102**: I129–135.
31. Mann HJ, Nolan PE Jr. Update on the management of cardiogenic shock. *Curr Opin Crit Care* 2006; **12**: 431–6.
32. Raja SG, Rayen BS. Levosimendan in cardiac surgery: current best available evidence. *Ann Thorac Surg* 2006; **81**: 1536–46.
33. Kristof AS, Magder S. Low systemic vascular resistance state in patients undergoing cardiopulmonary bypass. *Crit Care Med* 1999; **27**: 1121–7.
34. Haji SA, Movahed A. Right ventricular infarction: diagnosis and treatment. *Clin Cardiol* 2000; **23**: 473–82.
35. MacKenzie IM. The haemodynamics of human septic shock. *Anaesthesia* 2001; **56**: 130–44.
36. Dellinger RP, Vincent JL. The Surviving Sepsis Campaign sepsis change bundles and clinical practice. *Crit Care* 2005; **9**: 653–4.
37. Van den Berghe G, de Zegher F. Anterior pituitary function during critical illness and dopamine treatment. *Crit Care Med* 1996; **24**: 1580–90.
38. Sakr Y, Reinhart K, Vincent JL *et al.* Does dopamine administration in shock influence outcome? Results of the Sepsis Occurrence in Acutely Ill Patients (SOAP) Study. *Crit Care Med* 2006; **34**: 589–97.

83

Vasodilators and antihypertensives

John A Myburgh

Vasodilators are a generic group of drugs that are primarily used in the intensive care unit (ICU) for the management of acute hypertensive states and emergencies. In addition, they have an important role in the management of hypertension and cardiac failure.[1]

PHYSIOLOGY

Blood pressure is controlled by a complex physiological neurohormonal system involving all components of the cardiovascular system.[2,3] Traditionally, clinical practice has focused on the arterial circulation as the major regulator of systemic pressure. The importance of venous circulation in determining mean arterial pressure and cardiac output is discussed in Chapter 82.

The role of the peripheral vasculature, including both arteriolar and venous systems, in the regulation of blood pressure may be conceptually regarded as a balance between vasodilatation and vasoconstriction[3] (Figure 83.1).

CALCIUM FLUX

The concentration of intracellular ionised calcium is the primary determinant of vascular smooth muscle tone: increases lead to smooth muscle contraction, decreases cause relaxation. Control of calcium influx and efflux is determined by adrenergic receptor occupation and changes in membrane potential, mediated through voltage gated channels (see Chapter 82, Figure 82.2).

ENDOTHELIAL SYSTEM

The endothelium has a central role in blood pressure homeostasis by secreting substances such as nitric oxide, prostacyclin and endothelin.[3] These substances are continuously released by the endothelium and are integral in regional autoregulation.[4]

Nitric oxide is synthesised from L-arginine by nitric oxide synthases. It is released under the influence of endothelial agonists such as noradrenaline (norepinephrine), acetylcholine and substance P and in response to mechanical factors such as endothelial shear forces and pulsatile flow. Nitric oxide diffuses into underlying smooth muscle where it activates guanylate cyclase to increase cyclic guanosine monophosphate (cGMP). Subsequent phosphorylation results in relaxation of underlying smooth muscle and vasodilatation.

Prostacyclin is synthesised via the arachidonic pathway and has a minor role in the control of vascular tone.

Endothelin is an endothelium-derived vasoconstrictor peptide that is associated with increases in vascular smooth muscle intracellular calcium. It acts as endogenous ligand to regulate voltage-gated calcium channels, thereby producing vasoconstriction, usually in response to shear stresses, tissue hypoxia, angiotensin II and inflammatory mediators (e.g. interleukin-6 and nuclear factor κB).

RENIN–ANGIOTENSIN–ALDOSTERONE SYSTEM

Angiotensinogen is converted by renin to form angiotensin I, which is subsequently converted to angiotensin II by angiotensin-converting enzyme (ACE). Angiotensin II has a number of effects that are responsible for blood pressure homeostasis. These include release of aldosterone, direct activation of α-adrenergic receptors on vascular smooth muscle and a direct effect in the endothelium. These effects are directed at defending blood pressure and are integral in the stress response. Angiotensin-converting enzyme is also responsible for the inactivation of bradykinins that have predominantly vasodilatory effects, coupled to arachidonic acid synthesis and generation of prostacyclin.

ADRENERGIC SYSTEM

The sympathetic nervous system is integrally involved with all of the above systems, regulating vascular tone at central, ganglionic and local neural levels. Adrenergic stimulation of β-receptors is associated with vasodilatation; α-receptor stimulation results in vasoconstriction. The vascular effects of the catecholamines and vasopressors are discussed in Chapter 82.

Adrenergic stimulation is the predominant system in regulating venous tone.[5] This is due to endothelial differences in veins resulting in less production of nitric oxide and reduced responsiveness to angiotensin II.

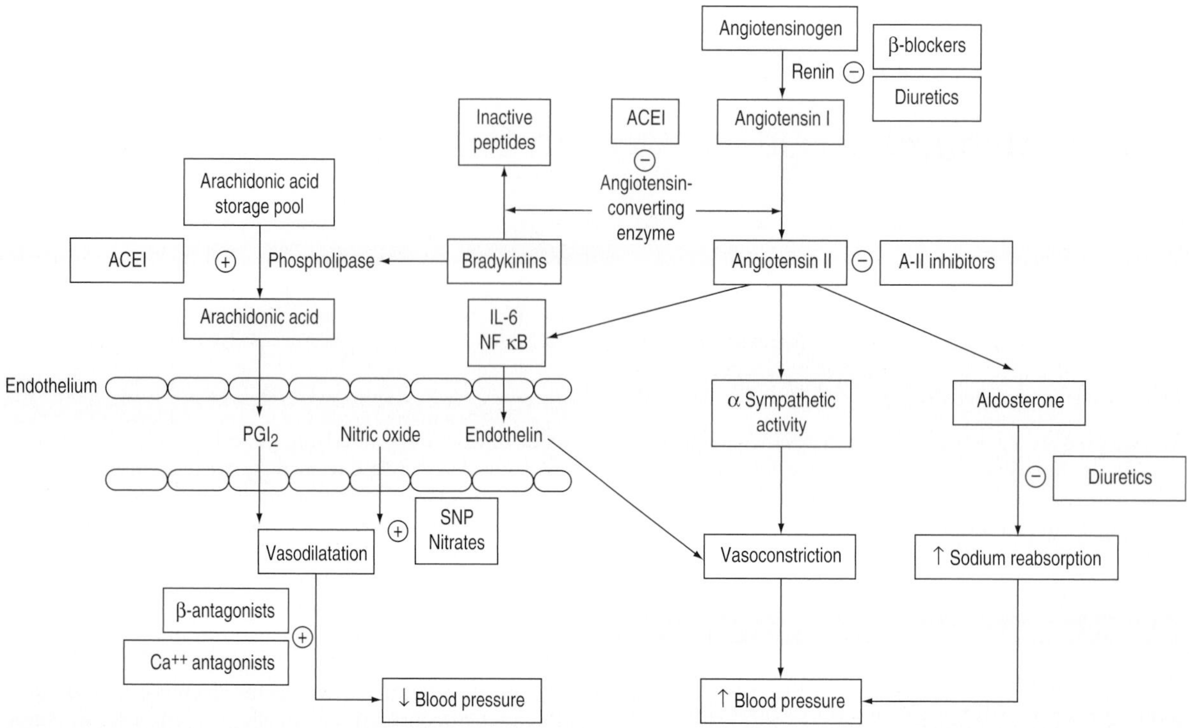

Figure 83.1 Schematic diagram of the neurohormonal factors determining vasomotor tone. Mechanism of action of vasodilators is shown by (−) for inhibition, (+) for stimulation. ACEI, angiotensin-converting enzyme inhibitors; A-II, angiotensin II; IL, interleukin; NF, nuclear factor; PGI_2, prostacyclin; SNP, sodium nitroprusside.

PATHOPHYSIOLOGY

Hypertensive states develop as a result of impaired or abnormal homeostatic processes, causing an imbalance between vasoconstrictive and vasodilatory effects.

Essential hypertension is the most common cause of hypertension and is due to abnormal neurohormonal regulation, particularly exaggerated effects of renin–angiotensin activity.

Secondary causes of hypertension include structural abnormalities such as aortic stenosis or renal artery stenosis; endocrine conditions such as phaeochromocytoma, Cushing's syndrome and pregnancy-induced hypertension; or central causes such as hypertensive encephalopathy or raised intracranial pressure.

CALCIUM ANTAGONISTS

Calcium antagonists have numerous effects on the cardiovascular system, influencing heart rate conduction, myocardial contractility and vasomotor tone. Entry of calcium through voltage-gated calcium channels is a major determinant of arteriolar, but not venous, tone.[6]

There are three major groups of arterioselective calcium antagonists: dihydropyridines (e.g. nifedipine, nimodipine, nicardipine and amlodipine), phenylalkylamines (e.g. verapamil) and benzothiazepines (e.g. diltiazem).

Magnesium is a physiological calcium antagonist, and is used therapeutically as magnesium sulphate.

NIFEDIPINE

Nifedipine is a predominant arteriolar vasodilator, with minimal effect on venous capacitance vessels and no direct depressant effect on heart rate conduction.

It may be administered intravenously, orally or sublingually, and has a rapid onset of action (2–5 minutes) and duration of action of 20–30 minutes.

Nifedipine is frequently used to treat angina pectoris, especially that due to coronary artery vasospasm. Peripheral vasodilatation results in decreased systemic blood pressure, often associated with sympathetic stimulation resulting in increased cardiac output and heart rate that may counter the negative inotropic, chronotropic and dromotropic effects of nifedipine. Nevertheless, nifedipine may be associated with profound hypotension in patients with ventricular dysfunction, aortic stenosis and/or concomitant β-blockade. For this reason, the use of sublingual nifedipine as a method of treating hypertensive emergencies is no longer recommended.[7]

Nifedipine and related drugs may cause diuretic-resistant peripheral oedema that is due to redistribution of extracellular fluid rather than sodium and water retention.

NIMODIPINE

Nimodipine is a highly lipid-soluble analogue of nifedipine. High lipid solubility facilitates entrance into the central nervous system where it causes selective cerebral arterial vasodilatation.

It may be used to attenuate cerebral arterial vasospasm following aneurysmal subarachnoid haemorrhage. Improved outcomes have been demonstrated in patients with Grade 1 and 2 subarachnoid haemorrhage.[8] Systemic hypotension may result from peripheral vasodilatation that may compromise cerebral blood flow in susceptible patients. Similarly, cerebral vasodilatation may increase intracranial pressure in patients with reduced intracranial elastance.

It may be given by intravenous infusion or enterally with equal effect.

AMLODOPINE

Amlodipine is an oral preparation that has a similar pharmacodynamic profile to nifedipine. In addition to arteriolar vasodilatory and cardiac effects, amlodipine has been shown to exert specific anti-inflammatory effects in hypertension, diabetic nephropathy and in modulating high-density lipoprotein (HDL) in patients with hypercholesterolaemia.[9] These effects have seen amlodipine increasingly being used for treatment of hypertension in high-risk patients, and may have a role in stable critically ill patients with associated comorbidities.

VERAPAMIL

The primary effect of verapamil is on the atrioventricular node and this drug is principally used as an antiarrhythmic for the treatment of supraventricular tachyarrhythmias. For this reason, concomitant therapy with β-blockers or digoxin is not recommended.

Verapamil is not as active as nifedipine in its effects on smooth muscle and therefore causes less pronounced decrease in systemic blood pressure and reflex sympathetic activity. It has a limited role as a vasodilator.[10]

DILTIAZEM

Diltiazem has a similar cardiovascular profile to verapamil, although its vasodilatory properties are intermediate between nifedipine and verapamil. Diltiazem exerts minimal cardiodepressant effects and is unlikely to potentiate β-blockers.

MAGNESIUM SULPHATE

Magnesium regulates intracellular calcium and potassium levels by activation of membrane pumps and competition with calcium for transmembrane channels. Physiological effects are widespread, affecting cardiovascular, central and peripheral nervous systems and the musculoskeletal junction.[11]

It acts as a direct arteriolar and venous vasodilator causing reductions in blood pressure. Modulation of centrally mediated and peripheral sympathetic tone results in variable effects on cardiac output and heart rate.

Consequently, it has an established role in the treatment of pre-eclampsia and eclampsia,[12] perioperative management of phaeochromocytoma[13] and treatment of autonomic dysfunction in tetanus.[14]

DIRECT-ACTING VASODILATORS

These drugs act directly on vascular smooth muscle and exert their effects predominantly by increasing the concentration of endothelial nitric oxide. These drugs are also known as nitrovasodilators.[15]

SODIUM NITROPRUSSIDE

Sodium nitroprusside is a non-selective vasodilator that causes relaxation of arterial and venous smooth muscle. It is compromised of a ferrous ion centre associated with five cyanide moieties and a nitrosyl group. The molecule is 44% cyanide by weight.

It is reconstituted from a powdered form. The solution is light-sensitive requiring protection from exposure to light by wrapping administration sets in aluminium foil. Prolonged exposure to light may be associated with an increase in release of hydrogen cyanide, although this is seldom clinically significant.

When infused intravenously, sodium nitroprusside interacts with oxyhaemoglobin, dissociating immediately to form methaemoglobin while releasing free cyanide and nitric oxide. The latter is responsible for the vasodilatory effect of sodium nitroprusside.

Onset of action is almost immediate with a transient duration, requiring continuous intravenous infusion to maintain a therapeutic effect.

Tachyphylaxis is common, particularly in younger patients. Large doses should not be used if the desired therapeutic effect is not attained, as this may be associated with toxicity.

Sodium nitroprusside produces direct venous and arterial vasodilatation, resulting in a prompt decrease in systemic blood pressure. The effect on cardiac output is variable. Decreases in right atrial pressure reflect pooling of blood in the venous system, which may decrease cardiac output. This may result in reflex tachycardia that may oppose the overall reduction in blood pressure. In patients with left ventricular failure, the effect on cardiac output will depend on initial left ventricular end-diastolic pressure. Sodium nitroprusside has unpredictable effects on calculated systemic vascular resistance. Homeostatic mechanisms in preserving cardiac output may explain tachyphylaxis to prolonged infusions.

Sodium nitroprusside may increase myocardial ischaemia in patients with coronary artery disease by causing an intracoronary steal of blood flow away from ischaemic areas by arteriolar vasodilatation. Secondary tachycardia may also exacerbate myocardial ischaemia.

Due to its non-selectivity, sodium nitroprusside has direct effects on most vascular beds. In the cerebral circulation, sodium nitroprusside is a cerebral vasodilator, leading to increases in cerebral blood flow and blood volume. This may be critical in patients with increased intracranial pressure. Rapid and profound reductions in mean arterial pressure produced by sodium nitroprusside may exceed the autoregulatory capacity of the brain to maintain adequate cerebral blood flow.

Sodium nitroprusside is a pulmonary vasodilator and may attenuate hypoxic pulmonary vasoconstriction, resulting in increased intrapulmonary shunting and decreased arterial oxygen tension. This phenomenon may be exacerbated by associated hypotension.

The prolonged use of large doses of sodium nitroprusside may be associated with toxicity related to the production and cyanide and, to a lesser extent, methaemoglobin.[16]

Free cyanide produced by the dissociation of sodium nitroprusside reacts with methaemoglobin to form cyanmethaemoglobin, or is metabolised by rhodenase in the liver and kidneys to form thiocyanate. A healthy adult can eliminate cyanide at a rate equivalent to a sodium nitroprusside infusion of 2 μg/kg per min or up to 10 μg/kg per min for 10 minutes, although there is marked inter-individual variability.

Toxicity should be considered in patients who become resistant to sodium nitroprusside despite maximum infusion rates and who develop an unexplained lactic acidosis. In high doses, cyanide may cause seizures.

Treatment of suspected cyanide toxicity is cessation of the infusion and administration of 100% oxygen. Sodium thiosulphate (150 mg/kg) converts cyanide to thiocyanate, which is excreted renally. For severe cyanide toxicity, sodium nitrate may be infused (5 mg/kg) to produce methaemoglobin and subsequently cyanmethaemoglobin. Hydroxocobalamin, which binds cyanide to produce cyanocobalamin, may also be administered (25 mg/hour to maximum of 100 mg).

GLYCERYL TRINITRATE

Glyceryl trinitrate is an organic nitrate that generates nitric oxide through a different mechanism from sodium nitroprusside.

The pharmacokinetics allows glyceryl trinitrate to be given by infusion, with a longer onset and duration of action than sodium nitroprusside. Glyceryl trinitrate may also be administered sublingually, orally or transdermally.

Tachyphylaxis is common with glyceryl trinitrate; doses should not be increased if patients no longer respond to standard doses. Glass bottles or polyethylene administration sets are required as glyceryl trinitrate is absorbed into standard polyvinylchloride sets.

The effects on the peripheral vasculature are dose dependent, acting principally on venous capacitance vessels to produce venous pooling and decreased ventricular afterload. These are important mechanisms in patients with cardiac failure.

Glyceryl trinitrate primarily dilates larger conductance vessels of the coronary circulation, resulting in increased coronary blood flow to ischaemic subendocardial areas, thereby relieving angina pectoris. This is in contrast to sodium nitroprusside that may cause a coronary steal phenomenon.

Reductions in blood pressure are more dependent on blood volume than sodium nitroprusside. Precipitous falls in blood pressure may occur in hypovolaemic patients with small doses of glyceryl trinitrate. In euvolaemic patients, reflex tachycardia is not as pronounced as with sodium nitroprusside. At higher doses, arteriolar vasodilatation occurs without significant changes in calculated systemic vascular resistance.

Glyceryl trinitrate is a cerebral vasodilator and should be used with caution in patients with reduced intracranial elastance. Headache due to this mechanism is a common side-effect in conscious patients.

ISOSORBIDE DINITRATE

Isosorbide dinitrate is the most commonly administered oral nitrate for the prophylaxis of angina pectoris. It has a physiological effect that lasts up to 6 hours in doses of 60–120 mg. The mechanism of action is the same as glyceryl trinitrate. Hypotension may follow acute administration, but tolerance to this develops with chronic therapy.[17]

HYDRALAZINE

Hydralazine is a potent, arterioselective, direct-acting vasodilator that acts via stimulation of cGMP and inhibition of smooth muscle myosin light chain kinase.

Following intravenous administration, hydralazine has a rapid onset of action, usually within 5–10 minutes. It may also be administered intramuscularly or orally. The drug is partially metabolised by acetylation, for which there is marked inter-individual variability (35% population are slow acetylators). Whilst this does not have much clinical significance regarding the antihypertensive effects, it is important with respect to toxicity.[17]

Hydralazine causes predominantly arteriolar vasodilatation that is widespread but not uniform. It is associated with direct and reflex sympathetic activity, so that cardiac output and heart rate are increased. Prolonged use of hydralazine stimulates renin release and is associated with sodium and water retention. Consequently, hydralazine is frequently administered with β-blockers and/or diuretics.

Chronic use of hydralazine may be associated with immunological side-effects including a lupus syndrome, vasculitis, haemolytic anaemia and rapidly progressive glomerulonephritis.

DIAZOXIDE

Diazoxide is chemically related to the thiazide diuretics and is a potent, non-selective, direct-acting vasodilator. The mechanism of action is unclear, but it is a predominantly arteriolar vasodilator.[18] Diazoxide is administered intravenously or intramuscularly. It has a rapid onset (3–5 minutes) and prolonged duration of action (1–2 hours), often with precipitous reductions in blood pressure. Diazoxide has similar cardiovascular effects to hydralazine and is associated with significant reflex sympathetic stimulation, resulting in increased cardiac output and heart rate.

It is a useful drug in accelerated hypertension associated with acute renal failure such as glomerulonephritis and has been used in severe pregnancy-induced hypertension and eclampsia. Stimulation of catecholamine release prohibits the use of diazoxide in patients with phaeochromocytoma.

It is associated with metabolic side-effects such as hyperglycaemia and sodium and water retention.

α-ADRENERGIC ANTAGONISTS

Several groups of compounds act as α-adrenergic blockers with variable affinity for populations of α-receptors. Physiology and pathophysiology may influence the responsiveness of the drug receptor–effector relationship. Receptor pathobiology is discussed in Chapter 82. Consequently, there may be marked inter- and intra-individual variability in the patient's response to these drugs.

There are six main groups of α-receptor antagonists: imidazolines (e.g. phentolamine), haloalkylamines (e.g. phenoxybenzamine), prazosin, β-adrenergic antagonists with a receptor antagonism (labetalol, carvedilol), phenothiazines (chlorpromazine) and buyrophenones (haloperidol).

PHENTOLAMINE

Phentolamine is a non-selective, competitive antagonist at α_1- and α_2-receptors. At low doses, phentolamine causes prejunctional inhibition of noradrenaline release (via α_2-receptor inhibition). At higher doses, more complete α-receptor blockade is achieved, with enhancement of effects of β-agonists due to increased local concentration of noradrenaline produced by α_2-blockade (see Chapter 82, Figure 82.3a).

Phentolamine is administered intravenously and may be given intermittently or by infusion. Onset is rapid (within 2 minutes), with a duration of action of 10–15 minutes.

Arteriolar and venous vasodilatation reduces systemic blood pressure, without significant changes in calculated systemic vascular resistance. Effects on cardiac output are variable, and there is modest reflex sympathetic stimulation without significant increases in heart rate.

PHENOXYBENZAMINE

Phenoxybenzamine is a non-selective, non-competitive, α_1- and α_2-receptor antagonist. Blockade is also produced on histamine, serotonin and acetylcholine muscarinic receptors. Reuptake of noradrenaline is blocked, thereby potentiating the effects of β-agonists.

Phenoxybenzamine is usually administered orally, but may also be given intravenously. It has a long onset of action and prolonged duration of action (3–4 days). It causes a gradual reduction in systemic blood pressure, without rapid reflex sympathetic activity.

Prolonged use is associated with increased β-adrenergic effects, predominantly increased heart rate, for which combination therapy with β-blockade is used. Phenoxybenzamine is primarily used in the management of phaeochromocytoma, either preoperatively or long term in inoperable patients. It may also be used to control autonomic hyperreflexia in patients with spinal cord transection.[19]

PRAZOSIN

Prazosin is a relatively arterioselective, competitive, α_1-receptor antagonist. It acts postjunctionally and therefore does not inhibit reuptake of noradrenaline. Consequently, it produces less tachycardia for a given reduction in systemic blood pressure.

It is administered orally and usually used for essential or renovascular (hyper-reninaemia) hypertension. It is frequently used in combination with β-blockers and diuretics, particularly in patients with renal dysfunction.

LABETALOL

Labetalol is specific competitive antagonist at α_1-, β_1- and β_2-adrenergic receptors. β-Blockade effects predominate, with a blockade potency approximately 10% of prazosin. Labetalol has partial agonist effects on β_2-receptors. The ratio of α_1:β-receptor blockade is 1:4.

It is administered intravenously, has a rapid onset of action (5–10 minutes) with a duration of 2–6 hours. It may be given by infusion.

Systemic blood pressure and cardiac output are reduced by a combination of negative inotropy, arterial and venous vasodilatation. Reflex tachycardia is attenuated by β-blockade.

Side-effects such as bronchospasm and hyperkalaemia relate predominantly to β-blockade.

CARVEDILOL

Carvedilol is a non-selective β-blocker with α_1-antagonist activity. Most of the vasodilator activity relates to α_1-antagonism, although at high concentrations it also blocks calcium entry. The ratio of α_1:β-receptor blockade is 1:10.

It is administered orally; no intravenous preparation is available.

Recent studies have demonstrated slowing of progression of congestive cardiac failure and improved mortality, particularly when used in conjunction with ACE inhibitors in patients with mild to moderate cardiac failure.[20,21] It may also be used in patients who cannot be treated with ACE inhibitors.

HALOPERIDOL AND CHLORPROMAZINE

These drugs act as competitive α-receptor antagonists causing non-selective vasodilatation and blockade of noradrenaline reuptake.

These drugs are primarily used as major tranquillisers or antipsychotics; their effect on the peripheral vasculature should be regarded as a side-effect, rather than a specific therapeutic action.

Reduction of systemic blood pressure is variable and may be precipitous, particularly in hypovolaemic patients with high sympathetic drive. These drugs may be useful in neurogenic hypertension, and are not regarded as first-line vasodilators.

SYMPATHOMIMETICS

The peripheral vascular effects of β-adrenergic agonists such as adrenaline (epinephrine), noradrenaline, dopamine and the synthetic catecholamines dobutamine and isoprenaline are discussed in Chapter 82.

At low doses, adrenaline, noradrenaline and dopamine are predominantly β-agonists and cause both arterial and venous vasodilatation which may cause reductions in mean arterial pressure.

Dobutamine and isoprenaline are predominantly β-agonists and may cause decreases in mean arterial pressure, particularly in hypovolaemic patients or those with increased sympathetic drive. These agents may have a role in reducing left ventricular afterload in patients with systolic heart failure.

ANGIOTENSIN-CONVERTING ENZYME INHIBITORS

Angiotensin converting enzyme (ACE) inhibition has become a cornerstone in the management of patients with hypertension, cardiac failure and ischaemic heart disease.[22,23] These drugs act by non-selective, competitive, irreversible inhibition to the angiotensin I binding site.

There are a very large number of ACE inhibitors on the market with very high penetration into the ambulant patient population. These drugs are administered orally; there are no routinely used parenteral preparations. Consequently, many critically ill patients admitted to the ICU may be taking ACE inhibitors. As a general rule, ACE inhibitors are stopped in most critically ill patients until vital organ (specifically renal) function is stabilised and the patient can take orally or enterally. Thereafter, doses are gradually increased over time with close monitoring of renal function.

PREPARATIONS

Captopril is the prototype and is still widely used. It is administered orally in increasing doses and intervals to a maximum dose of 50 mg 8 hourly. It may be administered sublingually in acute hypertension (5–25 mg), with an onset of action in 20–30 minutes, duration of 4 hours. There are no significant differences in the cardiovascular effects between captopril and other preparations. It is contraindicated in patients with bilateral renal artery stenosis and should be avoided in pregnancy.

Enalapril is a pro-drug, effective by hepatic metabolism to enalaprilat, producing a slower and more controlled action. It is administered orally in 5 mg increments to a total of 20 mg twice daily.

Lisinopril has the advantage of single daily dosing and may be useful in stable critically ill patients.

CARDIOVASCULAR EFFECTS

The cardiovascular effects of ACE inhibition are widespread, with effects that influence the peripheral vasculature, cardiac performance, and salt and water homeostasis. Consequently, ACE inhibitors are not principally regarded as vasodilators, although they have both direct and indirect effects on the peripheral vasculature.

Increased production of endothelial vasodilators such as prostacyclin and decreased production of endothelin by angiotensin result in generalised venous and arteriolar vasodilatation. This occurs in the absence of reflex sympathetic activity or changes in heart rate, due to the modulation of adrenergic stimulation. Systemic blood pressure is reduced without changes in cardiac output or heart rate.

ACE inhibition is associated with improved myocardial performance following acute myocardial infarction due to left ventricular remodelling and improvement in neurohumoral activation. These drugs have been shown to improve survival following myocardial infarction in patients with left ventricular dysfunction.[24]

'First-dose hypotension' is described in patients receiving ACE inhibitors for the first time. This may occur particularly in patients who are salt and water depleted, or those who develop sensitivity to the drug. Drug sensitivity may also present as a sudden decrease in renal function following commencement of the drug (see below).

RENOVASCULAR EFFECTS

ACE inhibitors may cause renal failure, particularly in patients with renovascular disease, hyperreninaemic hypertension and acute renal dysfunction. The renal effects of ACE inhibitors may be potentiated by diuretics, non-steroidal anti-inflammatory agents and β-blockers.

As a rule in intensive care patients, ACE inhibitors are started in suitable patients once renal function has stabilised and the patient no longer requires inotropic support.

SIDE-EFFECTS AND TOXICITY

In addition to renal dysfunction, ACE inhibitors may be associated with a number of side-effects. The most common of these is cough, which is due to the increased production of kinins.[25]

Severe angioneurotic oedema causing upper-airway obstruction may occur with all ACE inhibitors, although this is less common with enalapril and lisinopril. This is due to increased activation of bradykinins. ACE inhibitors are contraindicated in patients with a history of hereditary or idiopathic angioneurotic oedema.[26]

Neutropenia and agranulocytosis are uncommon but potentially lethal side-effects in susceptible patients.

ANGIOTENSIN RECEPTOR BLOCKERS

These are a newer class of antihypertensive drugs that cause irreversible, selective blockade of angiotensin II at AT_1 receptors.[27,28]

Losartan is the prototype, which has been followed by newer compounds such as irbesartan, valsartan and telmasartan. These drugs are oral preparations; there is no parenteral form.

The cardiovascular profile of angiotensin receptor blockers is similar to the ACE inhibitors, although definitive studies on long-term survival following acute myocardial infarction or in patients with cardiac failure have yet to be done.

The selective blockade of angiotensin II offers several possible advantages over ACE inhibitors. These drugs are long acting and may be given once daily; onset of action is slow, thereby avoiding first-dose hypotension; side-effects such as cough and angioneurotic oedema are less common.[29]

CENTRALLY ACTING AGENTS

These agents modulate adrenergic stimulation at central nervous system and spinal cord level.

The vasomotor centre of the medulla mainly controls sympathetic pressor influences, although other brainstem, midbrain and spinal centres have a role.

Most central responses are mediated through α_2-adrenergic receptors, which modulate the release and reuptake of noradrenaline, with subsequent effects on the peripheral vasculature and cardiac function.

CLONIDINE

Clonidine is a centrally acting α_2-agonist which stimulates inhibitory neurones in the vasomotor centre. This results in a reduction in sympathetic outflow from the central nervous system and is associated with negative inotropy and reduction in heart rate. Systemic blood pressure is reduced by this mechanism, with associated arteriolar and venous vasodilatation. Clonidine has centrally acting analgesic properties, which make it a suitable drug in patients with postoperative hypertension.

Peripherally, it stimulates prejunctional α_2-receptors, thereby decreasing noradrenaline release, but may also have an effect at postjunctional α_1-receptors causing vasoconstriction. This may present as rebound hypertension following initial reduction of blood pressure, as there is variable duration of the central and peripheral effects.

Clonidine is administered by intravenous injection; it cannot be given by infusion. It has a rapid onset of action (5–10 minutes) and duration of action of 20–30 minutes. It has both central and peripheral effects.

METHYLDOPA

Methyldopa has been used in the treatment of hypertension for 30 years. It acts as a centrally acting 'false' transmitter following metabolism to methylnoradrenaline and subsequent stimulation of α_2-receptors, although the precise mechanism is not clear.

It has no direct effect on cardiac or renal function. Cardiac output is maintained without changes in heart rate. Consequently, it may arrest or improve hypertensive nephropathy. It has a limited role in hypertensive emergencies, but is useful in accelerated essential, renovascular and pregnancy-induced hypertension.

It is administered orally in doses of 250 mg to 2 g per day. An intravenous preparation is available.

OTHER ANTIHYPERTENSIVE AGENTS

β-ADRENERGIC ANTAGONISTS

β-Blockers have been used for the treatment of hypertension for over 30 years and have an increasingly important role in the management of cardiac failure.[30–32]

In addition to decreasing heart rate and contractility, β-blockers have other neurohumoral effects that affect vascular tone. These relate to inhibition of renin release from juxtaglomerular cells (Figure 83.1) and prejunctional inhibition of noradrenaline that result in reduction in vascular tone and blood pressure. A central effect of β-blockers has also been proposed.

The mode of action has been described in terms of selectivity to blockade of β-adrenergic receptors – β_1 and/or β_2. While this is an appropriate pharmacological distinction, the clinical activity of these drugs is not as predictable due to mixed populations of β_1- and β_2-receptors in most organs and variable receptor responsiveness in physiological and pathophysiological conditions. Consequently, there is marked inter-individual variability in the response to these drugs. In high enough doses, whether intentionally or due to toxicity, all β-blockers will cause generalised antagonism with resultant therapeutic and toxic effects.

Lipid-soluble β-blockers include propranolol and metoprolol that are predominantly excreted by the liver; atenolol and sotalol are predominantly renally excreted, warranting caution with these drugs in patients with renal dysfunction.

β-Blockers may be given orally or intravenously. As there is significant first-pass metabolism, doses for oral and intravenous administration are markedly different.

Esmolol is an intravenous β-blocker that is rapidly metabolised by red cell esterases. Its rapid onset of action and short duration allow infusion of drug, making it a useful drug in patients with acute hypertensive states associated with tachycardia. Labetalol and carvedilol are discussed above.

β-Blockers are frequently used as adjuncts to vasodilators in the treatment of hypertensive emergencies and states, particularly where reflex tachycardia and sympathetic stimulation occurs (e.g. hydralazine, nifedipine and prazosin).

Side-effects and toxicity of β-blockers include bradycardia (which may be profound), hypotension, bronchoconstriction, aggravation of peripheral vascular ischaemia, hyperkalaemia and masking of the sympathetic response to hypoglycaemia.

DIURETICS

As with β-blockers, diuretics have an established place in the management of hypertension. In addition to their effects on salt and water excretion and inhibition of aldosterone, direct vasodilatory effects are associated with diuretics such as furosemide and the thiazides.

These drugs have a rapid venodilatory action, which may be due to inhibition of a noradrenaline-activated chloride channel on veins. Reductions of blood pressure and right atrial pressure may occur following low doses, and may present before an associated diuresis.

All diuretics should be used with caution in patients with renal dysfunction and avoided until a euvolaemic state is achieved.

DRUG SELECTION

The clinical use of vasodilators in intensive care is different from their use in ambulatory patients. In the critically ill patient, these drugs are primarily used to control acute rises in mean arterial pressure associated with sympathetic stimulation, or as specific treatment of hypertensive emergencies.[33]

The ideal vasodilator is therefore one that has a rapid and predictable onset of action, allows titration to achieve a desired systemic blood pressure, does not compromise cardiac output, does not cause significant reflex tachycardia and is non-toxic.

The selection of drug to treat hypertensive states will depend on the predominant cause of hypertension and the mechanism of action in the homeostatic pathway outlined in Figure 83.1.

There are no large studies investigating optimum therapy in patients presenting with hypertensive emergencies. These conditions occur in a heterogenous group of patients and drug selection is essentially determined by the underlying pathophysiology, personal preference and experience.[33]

MONITORING

The principles of haemodynamic monitoring in patients receiving vasoactive drugs is outlined in Chapter 82.

Patients with severe hypertension or those receiving infusions or doses of potent vasodilators such as sodium nitroprusside, glyceryl trinitrate, diazoxide or nifedipine should be monitored via an intra-arterial catheter.

The use of non-invasive measurement devices are not recommended in patients with hypertensive emergencies.

As peripheral vasodilators have significant effects on both the arterial and venous systems, measurement of volume status is important. In the majority of patients, establishing a euvolaemic state is essential before commencing a vasodilator.

DOSAGES AND DRUG ADMINISTRATION

Vasodilators administered via infusion are delivered through a dedicated central venous catheter using infusion pumps or syringe drivers and titrated to achieve a target mean arterial pressure.

Infusion lines should be free of injection portals and clearly marked with identifying labels.

Concentrations of infusions should be standardised in accordance with individual unit protocols. Suggested infusion concentrations and common drug doses are shown in Table 83.1.

SPECIFIC SITUATIONS

The following is a summary of the clinical uses of the above drugs in hypertensive states commonly encountered in the ICU. Specific pharmacology and physiological effects are discussed above.

ACUTE HYPERTENSION

The most common cause of hypertension in intensive care patients is pain or agitation, particularly in postoperative patients. It is important that patients have adequate analgesia and sedation before antihypertensives or vasodilators are used.

Other common causes of hypertension include hypothermia, urinary retention, positional discomfort and omission of pre-admission antihypertensives, particularly β-blockers.

Table 83.1 Dose and infusion concentrations of commonly used vasodilators and antihypertensives in intensive care

Agent	Infusion/Dose	Caution
Sodium nitroprusside	50 mg/250 ml 5% Dextrose; range 3–40 ml/hour	Cyanide toxicity (> total dose 0.5 mg/kg per 24 hours) Photodegradation Raised intracranial pressure Rebound hypotension Shunt and oxygen desaturation
Glyceryl trinitrate	30 mg/100 ml 5% Dextrose; range 2–25 ml/hour	Drug binding to polyvinylchloride Tachyphylaxis Raised intracranial pressure
Hydralazine	10–20 mg i.v. bolus 20–40 mg 6–8-hourly	Tachycardia Myocardial ischaemia
Diazoxide	50–100 mg i.v. boluses 15–30 mg/min infusion	Precipitous hypotension Hyperglycaemia
Trimetaphan	1–4 mg/min infusion	Mydriasis, ileus Bradycardia
Phentolamine	1–10 mg i.v. boluses 5–30 mg/hour infusion	Tachycardia
Phenoxybenzamine	Oral: 10 mg/day until postural hypotension i.v.: 1 mg/kg per day	Idiosyncratic hypotension
Prazosin	2–10 mg/day, 8-hourly	
Nifedipine	5–10 mg oral/sublingual	Precipitous hypotension
Amlodipine	5–10 mg oral b.d.	Caution in renal impairment
Captopril	6.25–50 mg orally, 8-hourly Acute hypertension: 6.5–25 mg sublingually p.r.n.	Caution in renovascular hypertension and renal failure Pregnancy Angioneurotic oedema
Enalapril	5–20 mg 8-hourly	
Enalaprilat	0.625–5 mg bolus	Caution in renal failure and hypovolaemia
Losartan	25–100 mg/day	Caution in renal failure
Clonidine	25 μg to 150 mg i.v. bolus	Acute, perioperative centrally mediated hypertension May cause rebound hypertension with chronic use
Atenolol	1–10 mg i.v. boluses 25–100 mg oral b.d.	Caution in poor left ventricular function, asthma Hyperkalaemia Potentiated in renal failure
Metoprolol		As for atenolol, safe in renal failure
Esmolol	Loading dose 0.5 mg/kg 10–40 mg/hour infusion	
Labetalol	20–80 mg i.v. boluses 0.5–4 mg/min infusion	
Magnesium sulphate	40–60 mg/kg loading (or 6 g) 2–4 g/hour infusion	Maintain serum magnesium > 1.5–2 mmol/l

The majority of instances of acute hypertension in the ICU will respond to simple measures addressing the above.[34]

Sustained hypertension may be treated acutely with incremental doses or infusions of short-acting drugs such as glyceryl trinitrate, sodium nitroprusside, phentolamine, hydralazine, nifedipine or clonidine. Infusions of vasodilators may be required if hypertension persists, or if the patient in unable to take longer acting oral agents such as prazosin or amlodipine. Hypertension associated with tachycardia may be treated with β-blockers.

HYPERTENSIVE ENCEPHALOPATHY

Hypertensive encephalopathy is defined as an acute organic brain syndrome occurring as a result of failure of cerebrovascular autoregulation. There may be differences in the degree of hypertension that cause encephalopathy. It may present as confusion, visual disturbances, blindness, seizures or stroke. If not adequately treated, hypertensive encephalopathy may result in intracerebral haemorrhage, coma or death.[35]

Hypertensive encephalopathy may occur in patients with untreated or undertreated hypertension or in association with other diseases such as renal disease (e.g. glomerulonephritis, renovascular disease), thrombotic thrombocytopenic purpura, immunosuppressive therapy, collagen vascular diseases or eclampsia. Consequently, drug treatment will depend on the context in which it occurs.

The aim of drug therapy in these patients is to reduce blood pressure in a controlled, predictable and safe way. Acutely, short-acting, titratable parenteral drugs are suitable in emergency situations. Sodium nitroprusside can be used safely in most circumstances. Although sodium nitroprusside may increase intracranial pressure, associated reductions in mean arterial pressure offset this effect. Phentolamine is equally effective. Esmolol may be useful as an adjunctive agent.[36]

Other agents that are useful in controlling severe hypertension include hydralazine, diazoxide, nifedipine, clonidine and ACE inhibitors (although these must be used cautiously in patients with associated renal dysfunction). Combination therapy is usually required, although this should be done with caution to minimise additive effects with resultant hypotension.

Patients with hypertensive emergencies are frequently hypovolaemic due to excessive sympathetic stimulation. In the absence of left ventricular failure, judicious fluid replacement may reduce blood pressure and improve renal function, thereby minimising precipitous hypotension that may result following administration of some drugs. Diuretics are generally avoided in these conditions unless there is evidence of left ventricular failure.[36]

ACUTE STROKE

Acute stroke syndromes frequently occur in the setting of severe hypertension. The reduction of mean arterial pressure must be balanced by the maintenance of adequate cerebral perfusion pressure and cerebral blood flow. Ischaemic or infarcted brain is vulnerable to critical reductions in cerebral blood flow, while excessive mean arterial pressure may increase the risk of cerebral haemorrhage.[37]

Acutely, blood pressure should be maintained in a normal range until intracranial pathology has been identified by CT scan. Aggressive reduction in blood pressure is not recommended in patients with ischaemic stroke, whilst hypertension in patients with aneurysmal subarachnoid haemorrhage or intracranial haemorrhage may be managed by drugs outlined above.

AORTIC DISSECTION

Aortic dissection is the most dramatic and most rapidly fatal complication of severe hypertension. Blood pressure should be decreased as rapidly as possible to normal or slightly hypotensive levels. Titrations are usually made to achieve systolic blood pressures of 100–110 mmHg or mean arterial pressure of 55–65 mmHg. This will depend on the patient's premorbid blood pressure and the accuracy of blood pressure measurement. It is important to maintain blood pressure at levels compatible with adequate cerebral and renal perfusion.[38]

This is best achieved initially by a combination of β-blockers (e.g. esmolol, labetalol or atenolol), then in combination with vasodilators such as sodium nitroprusside or glyceryl trinitrate. Tachycardia must be avoided as this is a significant determinant of aortic shear force that may exacerbate the dissection.

Aortic dissection distal to the left subclavian artery is managed conservatively with antihypertensive therapy. Proximal dissections are managed surgically after acute control of blood pressure.

ACUTE MYOCARDIAL ISCHAEMIA

Myocardial ischaemia in the absence of obstructive coronary atherosclerosis may be precipitated by severe hypertension. This occurs by increased left ventricular wall stress, reduced preload, tachycardia and increased myocardial metabolic demand. Severe ischaemia may result in acute left ventricular failure.

Intravenous glyceryl trinitrate is useful in this situation and may be used in combination with β-blockers such as esmolol, labetalol or carvedilol.

ACE inhibitors may be used in the acute situation and may be required for longer term treatment.

PHAEOCHROMOCYTOMA

Tumours of the adrenal medulla secrete catecholamines that result in initial paroxysmal, then sustained, severe hypertension. They may present to the ICU as a hypertensive emergency or perioperatively for surgical ablation.[39]

Acute hypertensive crises associated with phaeochromocytoma are managed with incremental doses or infusions of phentolamine. Untreated patients may be significantly hypovolaemic and may require judicious volume replacement. β-Blockers should not be used in the acute stage as these will potentiate unopposed α-adrenergic stimulation.

Phenoxybenzamine forms the mainstay of treatment and preparation for surgery. This is commenced in 20–30 mg increments and continued until blood pressure is controlled. Excessive β-adrenergic effects are treated with β-blockers after sufficient α-blockade with phenoxybenzamine.[19]

Magnesium sulphate is useful in the perioperative management of phaeochromocytoma. It is given by infusion at 2–4 g/hour.[13]

RENAL FAILURE

Renal insufficiency may be a cause or consequence of a hypertensive emergency. Patients on haemodialysis (particularly those receiving erythropoietin therapy) and renal transplant patients (especially those receiving ciclosporin or corticosteroids) commonly present with severe hypertension. In patients with new onset renal failure accompanying severe hypertension, blood pressure must be controlled without potentiating renal dysfunction. Drugs such as calcium antagonists, phentolamine or prazosin may preserve renal blood flow and are appropriate in these patients. ACE inhibitors and diuretics should be used with caution until renal function has stabilised or improved.

Patients in the recovery phase of acute renal failure are usually hypertensive. This is a normal physiological response and should not be treated unless there is associated myocardial or cerebral ischaemia.[40]

PRE-ECLAMPSIA AND ECLAMPSIA

In addition to delivery of the baby and placenta, parenteral magnesium sulphate is the treatment of choice to prevent the evolution of pre-eclampsia to eclampsia (seizures and deteriorating encephalopathy[12]). Other parenteral drugs that have been used for many years for pregnancy-induced hypertensive states include hydralazine, phentolamine, diazoxide and labetalol.[41]

ACE inhibitors and angiotensin receptor blockers are contraindicated in pregnancy. This is discussed in Chapter 55.

DRUG INTERACTIONS

Severe rebound hypertension may result following abrupt cessation of antihypertensive treatment. Drugs associated with this discontinuation syndrome include clonidine, methyldopa, β-blockers, guanethidine and diuretics. The degree of rebound depends on the rapidity of drug withdrawal, dosage, renovascular and cardiac function. Antihypertensives should be reintroduced according the status of the patient and the degree of hypertension managed accordingly.

Interaction with monoamine oxidase inhibitors and drugs such as indirect sympathomimetics, narcotics and tyramine-containing foods may result in a hypertensive emergency. This is best managed acutely with α- and/or β-blockers.

REFERENCES

1. Erdmann E. The management of heart failure – an overview. *Basic Res Cardiol* 2000; **95**(Suppl 1): I3–7.
2. Cohn JN. Left ventricle and arteries: structure, function, hormones, and disease. *Hypertension* 2001; **37**: 346–9.
3. Spieker LE, Flammer AJ, Luscher TF. The vascular endothelium in hypertension. *Handb Exp Pharmacol* 2006; **176**: 249–83.
4. Egan K, FitzGerald GA. Eicosanoids and the vascular endothelium. *Handb Exp Pharmacol* 2006; **176**: 189–211.
5. Magder S, De Varennes B. Clinical death and the measurement of stressed vascular volume. *Crit Care Med* 1998; **26**: 1061–4.
6. Schulman IH, Zachariah M, Raij L. Calcium channel blockers, endothelial dysfunction, and combination therapy. *Aging Clin Exp Res* 2005; **17**: 40–5.
7. Varon J, Marik PE. The diagnosis and management of hypertensive crises. *Chest* 2000; **118**: 214–27.
8. Rinkel GJ, Feigin VL, Algra A *et al.* Calcium antagonists for aneurysmal subarachnoid haemorrhage. *Cochrane Database Syst Rev* 2005; CD000277.
9. Zanchetti A, Julius S, Kjeldsen S *et al.* Outcomes in subgroups of hypertensive patients treated with regimens based on valsartan and amlodipine: an analysis of findings from the VALUE trial. *J Hypertens* 2006; **24**: 2163–8.
10. De Cicco M, Macor F, Robieux I *et al.* Pharmacokinetic and pharmacodynamic effects of high-dose continuous intravenous verapamil infusion: clinical experience in the intensive care unit. *Crit Care Med* 1999; **27**: 332–9.
11. Saris NE, Mervaala E, Karppanen H *et al.* Magnesium. An update on physiological, clinical and analytical aspects. *Clin Chim Acta* 2000; **294**: 1–26.
12. Altman D, Carroli G, Duley L *et al.* Do women with pre-eclampsia, and their babies, benefit from magnesium sulphate? The Magpie Trial: a randomised placebo-controlled trial. *Lancet* 2002; **359**: 1877–90.
13. James MF, Cronje L. Pheochromocytoma crisis: the use of magnesium sulfate. *Anesth Analg* 2004; **99**: 680–6.
14. Thwaites CL, Yen LM, Loan HT *et al.* Magnesium sulphate for treatment of severe tetanus: a randomised controlled trial. *Lancet* 2006; **368**: 1436–43.
15. Vassalle C, Domenici C, Lubrano V *et al.* Interaction between nitric oxide and cyclooxygenase pathways in endothelial cells. *J Vasc Res* 2003; **40**: 491–9.
16. Alaniz C, Watts B. Monitoring cyanide toxicity in patients receiving nitroprusside therapy. *Ann Pharmacother* 2005; **39**: 388–9.
17. Ferdinand KC. Isosorbide dinitrate and hydralazine hydrochloride: a review of efficacy and safety. *Expert Rev Cardiovasc Ther* 2005; **3**: 993–1001.

18. Frank G. Diazoxide and trimethaphan used? *Chest* 2001; **119**: 316.
19. Prys-Roberts C. Phaeochromocytoma – recent progress in its management. *Br J Anaesth* 2000; **85**: 44–57.
20. Packer M, Coats AJ, Fowler MB *et al.* Effect of carvedilol on survival in severe chronic heart failure. *N Engl J Med* 2001; **344**: 1651–8.
21. Kopecky SL. Effect of beta blockers, particularly carvedilol, on reducing the risk of events after acute myocardial infarction. *Am J Cardiol* 2006; **98**: 1115–9.
22. Stone PH. Review: ACE inhibitors reduce mortality and cardiovascular endpoints in stable coronary artery disease. *ACP J Club* 2006; **145**: 32.
23. Remuzzi G, Ruggenenti P. Overview of randomised trials of ACE inhibitors. *Lancet* 2006; **368**: 555–6.
24. Nickenig G, Ostergren J, Struijker-Boudier H. Clinical evidence for the cardiovascular benefits of angiotensin receptor blockers. *J Renin Angiotensin Aldosterone Syst* 2006; 7(Suppl 1): S1–7.
25. Dicpinigaitis PV. Angiotensin-converting enzyme inhibitor-induced cough: ACCP evidence-based clinical practice guidelines. *Chest* 2006; **129**: S169–73.
26. Beltrami L, Zingale LC, Carugo S *et al.* Angiotensin-converting enzyme inhibitor-related angioedema: how to deal with it. *Expert Opin Drug Saf* 2006; **5**: 643–9.
27. See S. Angiotensin II receptor blockers for the treatment of hypertension. *Expert Opin Pharmacother* 2001; **2**: 1795–804.
28. Bhatia V, Bhatia R, Mathew B. Angiotensin receptor blockers in congestive heart failure: evidence, concerns, and controversies. *Cardiol Rev* 2005; **13**: 297–303.
29. Cooper ME, Webb RL, de Gasparo M. Angiotensin receptor blockers and the kidney: possible advantages over ACE inhibition? *Cardiovasc Drug Rev* 2001; **19**: 75–86.
30. Krum H. Guidelines for management of patients with chronic heart failure in Australia. *Med J Aust* 2001; **174**: 459–66.
31. Packer M. Current role of beta-adrenergic blockers in the management of chronic heart failure. *Am J Med* 2001; **110**(Suppl 7A): S81–94.
32. Gheorghiade M, Eichhorn EJ. Practical aspects of using beta-adrenergic blockade in systolic heart failure. *Am J Med* 2001; **110**(Suppl 7A): S68–73.
33. Moser M, Izzo JL Jr, Bisognano J. Hypertensive emergencies. *J Clin Hypertens* (Greenwich) 2006; **8**: 275–81.
34. Slama M, Modeliar SS. Hypertension in the intensive care unit. *Curr Opin Cardiol* 2006; **21**: 279–87.
35. Mabie WC. Management of acute severe hypertension and encephalopathy. *Clin Obstet Gynecol* 1999; **42**: 519–31.
36. Vaughan CJ, Delanty N. Hypertensive emergencies. *Lancet* 2000; **356**: 411–7.
37. Sokol SI, Kapoor JR, Foody JM. Blood pressure reduction in the primary and secondary prevention of stroke. *Curr Vasc Pharmacol* 2006; **4**: 155–60.
38. Ahmad F, Cheshire N, Hamady M. Acute aortic syndrome: pathology and therapeutic strategies. *Postgrad Med J* 2006; **82**: 305–12.
39. Graham GW, Unger BP, Coursin DB. Perioperative management of selected endocrine disorders. *Int Anesthesiol Clin* 2000; **38**: 31–67.
40. Palmer BF. Impaired renal autoregulation: implications for the genesis of hypertension and hypertension-induced renal injury. *Am J Med Sci* 2001; **321**: 388–400.
41. Watson D. The detection, investigation and management of hypertension in pregnancy. *Aust N Z J Obstet Gynaecol* 2000; **40**: 361.

Part Fourteen

Metabolic Homeostasis

84

Acid–base balance and disorders

Thomas J Morgan

THEORETICAL CONSIDERATIONS

The structural integrity of intracellular enzymes is essential for survival. Proton activity at enzymatic sites of action in cytosol and organelles must be tightly controlled. In critical illness, with survival under threat, direct monitoring of any intracellular site remains an impractical ideal. Clinicians are obliged to track extracellular data, usually from tests on arterial blood, knowing that plasma pH exceeds intracellular pH by 0.6 pH units on average.

WATER DISSOCIATION AND ACID–BASE

Stewart reminded us of the central role of water in aqueous acid–base equilibria.[1] Mammals are approximately 60% water. It follows that the behaviour of water is fundamental to our understanding of acid–base physiology. Water (simplistically) dissociates as follows:

$$H_2O \leftrightarrow H^+ + OH^-$$

By the Law of Mass Action, at any equilibrium $[H^+][OH^-] = Kw\,[H_2O]$, where Kw is the temperature-dependent dissociation constant. Water is a vast proton reservoir, its concentration several orders of magnitude greater than that of its two dissociation products (55.5 M vs. 160 nM at 37°C). When conditions favour proton release, for example with increased temperature, water dissociates and pH falls. With conditions less favourable, protons return to their source, and pH rises.

An advantage of its numeric predominance is that $[H_2O]$ can be combined with Kw to form a new constant, K′w. The equilibrium equation then simplifies to:

$$[H^+][OH^-] = K'w \qquad \textit{Equation 84.1}$$

pH AND ACID–BASE NEUTRALITY

The negative logarithm of the proton concentration, or more exactly proton 'activity', is termed pH. In aqueous solutions, neutrality occurs when $[H^+] = [OH^-]$, so that $([H^+])^2 = K'w$. Thus neutral pH = 0.5 pK′w. At 37°C, neutral pH is 6.8, which is the normal mean intracellular pH in health. The pH of the surrounding extracellular fluid, usually > 7.3, is relatively alkaline.

THE PaCO$_2$/PH RELATIONSHIP – THE ACID–BASE 'WINDOW' FOR CLINICIANS

About 15 moles of CO_2 are generated daily by aerobic metabolism. CO_2 travels along a partial pressure gradient from its intracellular source (PCO$_2$ > 50 mmHg) to the atmosphere (PCO$_2$ = 0.3 mmHg). The primary exit point is the lungs, with transit facilitated by a large, perpetually refreshed blood–air interface. En route, CO_2 equilibrates with all aqueous environments. The PCO$_2$ in any body fluid is thus an equilibrium value, determined by the interplay between regional CO_2 production, regional blood flow, alveolar perfusion and alveolar ventilation.

Clinicians use the relationship between arterial PCO$_2$ (PaCO$_2$) and arterial pH as the acid–base assessment platform. This is appropriate, because the PaCO$_2$/pH curve is a fundamental physiological property (Figure 84.1). Several factors determine the shape and position of this curve.

THE PaCO$_2$/pH RELATIONSHIP IS DEFINED BY SEVERAL SIMULTANEOUS EQUATIONS

In body fluids, pH is a function of water dissociation modified by CO_2, other weak acids and certain electrolytes. All equilibria obey the Laws of Mass Action and Mass Conservation, and must achieve overall electrical neutrality. Non-diffusible ions exert electrochemical forces across membranes, known as Gibbs Donnan effects, which influence the final acid–base result.

Therefore apart from Equation 1, several other equations must be satisfied simultaneously at any equilibrium. They relate to:

1. The interaction of carbon dioxide with water:

$$CO_2 + H_2O \leftrightarrow H_2CO_3 \leftrightarrow H^+ + HCO_3^-$$

By applying the Law of Mass Action and substituting [dissolved CO_2] for $[H_2CO_3]$, the following expression can be derived:

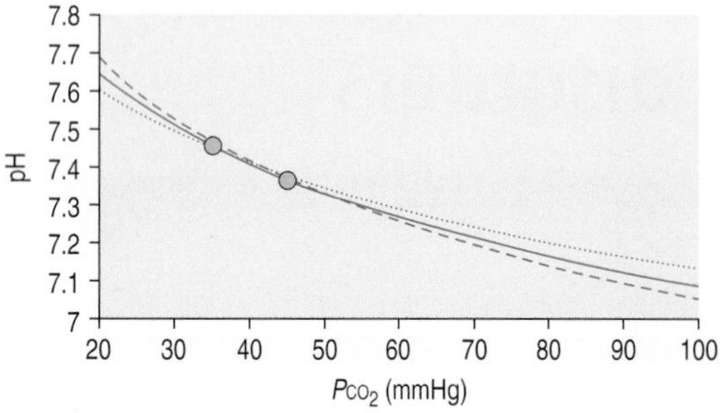

Figure 84.1 Pco_2/pH relationships. The solid line shows the normal in vivo $Paco_2$/pH relationship. The normal $Paco_2$ range is between the filled circles. To the left of the circles there is an increasing acute respiratory alkalosis, and to the right an increasing acute respiratory acidosis. The interrupted curve represents the normal in vitro whole blood relationship, and the dotted curve is the same relationship for separated plasma. A point of commonality exists at $Pco_2 = 40$ mmHg.

$$pH = 6.1 + \log_{10}([HCO_3^-]/\alpha PCO_2) \quad \textit{Equation 84.2}$$

This is the Henderson–Hasselbalch equation, where α is the plasma CO_2 solubility coefficient (0.03), and 6.1 is the pKa, the negative logarithm of the dissociation constant. The Henderson–Hasselbalch equation generates the plasma $[HCO_3^-]$ in blood gas readouts.

2. Bicarbonate dissociation to carbonate. At equilibration:

$$[H^+][CO_3^{2-}] = Keq[HCO_3^-] \quad \textit{Equation 84.3}$$

3. Non-volatile weak acid dissociation. Fluid compartments have varying concentrations of non-CO_2 generating (non-volatile) molecules with weak acid properties. In other words, their overall negative charge alters in parallel with pH. In plasma, they consist mainly of albumin and to a lesser extent inorganic phosphate. In red cells haemoglobin predominates. Much smaller concentrations of non-volatile weak acid also appear in interstitial fluid, primarily as phosphate. For convenience, Stewart modelled all non-volatile weak acids in each compartment as having a single anionic form (A^-) and a single conjugate base form (HA).

$$HA \leftrightarrow H^+ + A^-$$

By applying the Law of Mass Action:

$$[H^+][A^-] = Keq[HA] \quad \textit{Equation 84.4}$$

4. Conservation of mass. Stewart termed the total concentration of non-volatile weak acids in any compartment 'A_{TOT}', where $A_{TOT} = [HA] + [A^-]$. A_{TOT} is an imposed mass constant. It does not vary with pH. A change in pH merely signals a shift in the balance between HA and A^-.

5. Electrical neutrality, linked to Stewart's concepts of strong ions and strong ion difference. Certain elements such as Na^+, K^+, Ca^{++}, Mg^{++} and Cl^- exist as completely ionised entities in body fluids. At physiological pH this includes anions with pKa values of 4 or less, for example sulphate, lactate, and β-hydroxybutyrate. Stewart described compounds exhibiting this property as 'strong ions'. In body fluids there is a surfeit of strong cations, referred to by Stewart as the strong ion difference (SID). In other words, SID = [strong cations] – [strong anions]. Being a 'charge' space, SID is expressed in mEq/l. SID calculated from measured strong ions in normal plasma is 42 mEq/l.

   Hence, by the Law of Electrical Neutrality:

$$SID + [H^+] - [HCO_3^-] - [CO_3^{2-}] - [A^-] - [OH^-] = 0 \quad \textit{Equation 84.5}$$

6. Gibbs Donnan forces. These alter equilibria across semipermeable membranes, with electrical gradients balanced against concentration gradients. The plasma compartment (volume 3 l), the erythrocyte compartment (volume 2 l) and the interstitial space (volume 13.5 l) each contains different concentrations of non-diffusible anions, mainly albumin or haemoglobin. Erythrocytes, which harbour most of these trapped negative charges, attract diffusible cations (such as Na^+, K^+) from adjacent compartments while repelling diffusible anions (primarily Cl^-). However, several cations are continually redistributed against the Donnan forces by energy-dependent transmembrane pumps, to prevent cell swelling and haemolysis. Importantly, chloride, the major anion, remains fully susceptible to the Donnan effects.

The trapped anions have weak acid properties. Any pH shift alters their negative charge, driving further ionic redistributions, particularly chloride, between compartments. The net effect is that plasma SID goes up and down with $PaCO_2$ (Figure 84.2), the origin of the so-called Hamburger effect. Importantly, ionic shifts are confined within the total extracellular space, so that extracellular SID does not alter with PCO_2. This is fortuitous for clinicians, forming the basis of the CO_2 invariance of standard base excess (see below).

At any equilibrium, Equations 1–5 plus the Donnan equilibria must be satisfied simultaneously. In such a system, pH and HCO_3^-, as well as CO_3^{2-}, A^- and OH^-, cannot be altered directly, only via any of three independent variables imposed on the system but not altered directly by the system. These are SID (total extracellular SID, immune to Gibbs Donnan forces), extracellular A_{TOT}, and $Paco_2$, which is externally regulated by alveolar ventilation. Hence, in arterial blood, pH is defined by $Paco_2$, extracellular SID and extracellular A_{TOT}.

Thus it can be seen that for any individual the $Paco_2$/pH relationship is a unique acid–base 'signature' (Figure 84.1) and ultimately a complex function of extracellular SID and A_{TOT}.

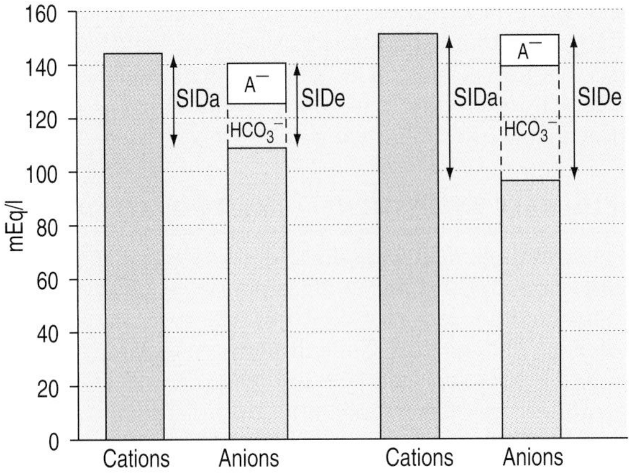

Figure 84.2 Gamblegrams of plasma strong and weak ions (in vitro data from CO_2 equilibrated normal blood). On the left, $P_{CO_2} < 20$ mmHg; on the right, the same blood with $P_{CO_2} >$ 200 mmHg. The transition from hypocapnia to hypercapnia increases SIDa, with ionic redistribution between red cells and plasma due to altered Gibbs Donnan forces. There are almost identical increases in SIDe ($[A^-] + [HCO_3^-]$), also known as 'buffer base', although $[A^-]$ actually falls. Note that the SIG, which is SIDa minus SIDe, remains close to zero.

WEAK IONS AND BUFFER BASE

SID is a charge space. Weak ions, which arise from variably dissociating conjugate bases, occupy this space. These include H^+, OH^-, HCO_3^-, CO_3^{2-} and A^-. Their total net charge must always equal SID. However, HCO_3^- and A^-, together known as the 'buffer base' anions, take up virtually the entire space on their own (Figure 84.2) since the other ions are measured in either micromoles/l or, in the case of protons, nanomoles/l. SID therefore not only dictates the buffer base concentration but is also numerically identical to it. In other words, SID = $[HCO_3^-] + [A^-]$. This fact, plus Figge's linear approximations[2] for calculating A^-, allows us to simplify Stewart's equations in plasma, reducing them to three without sacrificing accuracy.[3]

$$[A^-] = [\text{Alb}] \times (0.123 \times \text{pH} - 0.631) + [\text{Pi}] \times (0.309 \times \text{pH} - 0.469)$$

$$[HCO_3^-] = 0.0301' P_{CO_2}' 10^{(\text{pH}-6.1)}$$

$$\text{SIDe} = [HCO_3^-] + [A^-]$$

[Alb] is albumin concentration expressed in g/l. [Pi] is phosphate concentration in mmol/l. P_{CO_2} is in mmHg. SIDe is effective SID, also known as 'buffer base' (Figure 84.2).

SID calculated from measured plasma concentrations of strong ions is termed the 'apparent' SID, or SIDa (Figure 84.2). Discrepancies between SIDe and SIDa imply the presence of unmeasured ions in plasma (see below).

ISOLATED CHANGES IN SID AND A_{TOT}

At any given Pa_{CO_2}, a falling SID or a rising A_{TOT} reduce pH, moving the equilibrium towards a metabolic acidosis. Conversely, a rising SID or a falling A_{TOT} create a metabolic alkalosis. Many argue that SID and A_{TOT} act individually and should therefore be regarded as independent metabolic acid–base variables. By this argument we could have a strong ion acidosis or alkalosis combined with either a hyperalbuminaemic (high A_{TOT}) acidosis or a hypoalbuminaemic (low A_{TOT}) alkalosis.[4] However, SID and A_{TOT} do appear to be linked, with the SID set-point adjusting to A_{TOT}. In particular, SID seems to fall in hypoalbuminaemia, presumably by renal chloride adjustment.[5,6]

HOW ACID–BASE DISTURBANCES AFFECT THE PA_{CO_2}/PH RELATIONSHIP

Acute respiratory disturbances move data points along the prevailing Pa_{CO_2}/pH curve, to the left in respiratory alkalosis, and to the right in respiratory acidosis (Figure 84.1). In contrast, metabolic disturbances (altered extracellular SID and/or A_{TOT}) shift the entire curve up or down (Figure 84.3). A down-shifted curve means that the pH at any given Pa_{CO_2} is lower than normal, which – depending on the Pa_{CO_2} – represents either a primary metabolic acidosis or else metabolic compensation for a respiratory alkalosis. With an up-shifted curve, the pH at any given Pa_{CO_2} is higher than normal, signifying either a primary metabolic alkalosis or else compensation for a respiratory acidosis.

TEMPERATURE CORRECTION OF BLOOD GAS DATA – 'ALPHA-STAT' VERSUS 'PH-STAT' APPROACHES

Blood gas analysers operate at 37°C. Their software can convert pH and gas tensions to values corresponding to the patient core temperature for interpretation and action. This is the 'pH-stat' approach. The alternative is

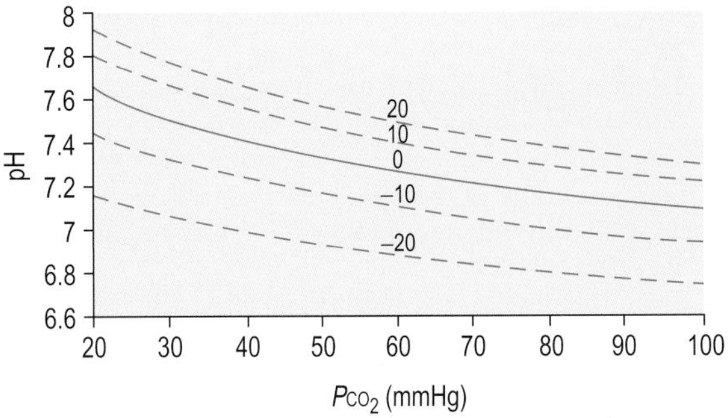

Figure 84.3 Pa_{CO_2}/pH curve shifts and associated SBE values (mEq/l). Alterations in metabolic acid–base status shift the curve down (SBE increasingly negative) or up (SBE increasingly positive).

to act on values as measured at 37°C – the 'alpha-stat' approach.

'Alpha' is the ratio of protonated imidazole to total imidazole on the histidine moieties in protein molecules. At 37°C, under normal acid–base conditions, the mean intracellular pH is 6.8 (the neutral pH at 37°C). Alpha is then approximately 0.55. Maintaining alpha close to 0.55 preserves enzyme structure and function, and is thus a fundamental goal.

'Alpha-stat' logic is best illustrated by considering blood in a blood gas syringe. When placed on ice, the $P\text{CO}_2$ falls as its solubility coefficient increases. Water dissociation is reduced, due to the hypocapnia and to the temperature-induced decrease in K′w. Consequently, there is a progressive alkalaemia, which on rewarming in the blood gas analyser reverts immediately. Throughout these phenomena, alpha stays constant. The reason is that the fall of the imidazole pKa with temperature is about half the fall in pK′w.

Hence, a simple way to keep alpha at 0.55 in hypothermia is to maintain uncorrected $P\text{aCO}_2$ and pH measurements in their 37°C reference ranges.[7,8] This mimics the hypothermic physiology of ectothermic (cold-blooded) animals. Similar arguments apply in fever, the more common intensive care unit (ICU) scenario. Many intensivists follow the alpha-stat approach, whatever the core temperature.

Those who favour the pH-stat approach argue that it is more consistent with the physiology of hibernating endothermic mammals, and that it allows better maintenance of cerebral perfusion in hypothermia.[9] This approach was used during an influential trial of mild hypothermia following out-of-hospital cardiac arrest.[10]

RENAL PARTICIPATION IN ACID–BASE

In the absence of renal function, there is a progressive metabolic acidosis. About 60 mEq of strong anions, particularly sulphate, but also hippurate and others, are produced daily as metabolic end-products. These accumulate in renal failure, reducing extracellular SID. So does free water, which brings sodium concentrations closer to chloride, again reducing SID. Hyperphosphataemia contributes by increasing A_{TOT}, although in acute renal failure this is commonly offset by coexistent hypoalbuminaemia.[11]

Traditionally, renal acid–base homeostasis is described in terms of resorption of filtered bicarbonate primarily in the proximal tubule, and excretion of fixed acids through titration of urinary buffers, particularly phosphate, and through excretion of ammonium, primarily in the distal tubule.[12]

From the physical chemical perspective, the traditional analysis of renal acid–base homeostasis is misleading, since it is based on H^+ or HCO_3^- 'balances'. H^+ and HCO_3^- are dependent variables, responsive exclusively to $P\text{CO}_2$, SID and A_{TOT}, and not subject to 'in versus out' balance sheets. The physical chemical explanation is simple. The kidneys regulate extracellular SID via urinary SID, the principal tool being tubular NH_4^+ acting as an adjustable cationic partner for tubular Cl^- and other urinary strong anions.[13] The kidneys also modify A_{TOT} via phosphate excretion, which is a totally different concept from that of 'titratable acidity'.

ACID–BASE ASSESSMENT – THE TWO 'SCHOOLS'

By convention, acid–base disorders are divided into respiratory ($P\text{aCO}_2$) and metabolic (non-$P\text{aCO}_2$). $P\text{aCO}_2$ is the undisputed index of respiratory acid–base status. Two 'schools', Boston and Copenhagen, separated by a large ocean,[14] have formed around the identification and quantification of metabolic acid–base disturbances. Both succeed as navigation systems, if used correctly.

Stewart's concepts neither invalidate nor supplant the traditional approaches,[15–17] but rather help us to understand their physiological basis, evaluate their relative merits, and extend their utility.[18] SID by itself is not a reliable measure of metabolic acid–base status, for three reasons:

- Plasma SID, the only SID measurable by clinicians, is subject to Donnan effects, which means it varies with $P\text{aCO}_2$ (the only SID that does not is total extracellular SID).
- In any compartment, SIDa and at times SIDe can be quite inaccurate reflections of the true SID. For example, unmeasured strong anions give SIDa positive bias, and unmeasured weak anions such as infused gelatin give SIDe negative bias.
- SID on its own is only half the story, since metabolic acid–base status is a function of the interplay between SID and A_{TOT}. In a healthy individual a plasma SID of 42 mEq/l may be normal, but in the presence of hypoalbuminemia (reduced A_{TOT}) it represents a metabolic alkalosis. Hence there is little point in attempting to track SID clinically.

For a pure metabolic index to succeed, it must integrate the effects of extracellular SID and A_{TOT}, irrespective of the $P\text{aCO}_2$. The best of these (in the author's opinion) is standard base excess, the flagship of the Copenhagen school. However, Boston school devotees can navigate quite successfully using empiric plasma bicarbonate-based 'rules of thumb'.

BASE EXCESS AND STANDARD BASE EXCESS

In 1960, Siggaard-Andersen introduced 'base excess' (BE).[19] BE was defined as zero when pH = 7.4, $P\text{CO}_2$ = 40 mmHg (both at 37 °C). If pH ≠ 7.4 or $P\text{CO}_2$ ≠ 40 mmHg, BE was defined as the concentration of titratable hydrogen ion required to return the pH to 7.4 while maintaining $P\text{CO}_2$ at 40 mmHg.

In the lead-up, Astrup, Siggaard-Andersen, Engel and others had equilibrated the blood of Danish volunteers with known CO_2 tensions at varying haemoglobin concentrations, after first adding known amounts of acid or base. The data were then used to create an 'alignment nomogram' which allowed the determination of BE from simultaneous measurements of pH, $P\text{CO}_2$ and haemoglobin concentration.

Seventeen years later, Siggaard-Andersen published the Van Slyke equation for calculating BE.[20] It was derived from known physical chemical relationships, and was claimed to match the empiric nomogram. The Van Slyke equation computes ($\Delta[\text{HCO}_3^-] + \Delta[\text{A}^-]$) – in other words, the deviation from normal of the buffer base concentration in whole blood. From the Stewart perspective, buffer base and SID are interchangeable terms. Hence Stewart would describe BE as the abnormality in whole blood SID at the prevailing A_{TOT}.

It became clear that BE loses its CO_2 invariance in vivo, where Gibbs Donnan forces drive ions between intravascular and interstitial compartments. As a result, a primary change in $Pa\text{CO}_2$ shifts BE in the opposite direction. The solution was to calculate BE at a haemoglobin concentration of approximately 50 g/l, replicating the mean extracellular haemoglobin concentration and thus more closely modelling the extracellular environment.[21] This is standard base excess (SBE).

As a metabolic acid–base index, SBE is close to ideal, being both quantitative and demonstrably independent of $Pa\text{CO}_2$.[22] A useful formula is:

$$\text{SBE} = 0.93 \times ([\text{HCO}_3^-] + 14.84 \times (\text{pH} - 7.4) - 24.4)$$

with SBE and $[\text{HCO}_3^-]$ values in mEq/l. This formula can be further refined to allow for changes in plasma A_{TOT} due to variations in albumin and phosphate.[23] However, because haemoglobin is the predominant weak acid, the end result is very similar.

A typical SBE reference range (in mEq/l) is −3.0 to +3.0. If SBE < -3.0 mEq/l, there is a down-shifted $Pa\text{CO}_2$/pH curve. This could represent either a primary metabolic acidosis or else compensation for a primary respiratory alkalosis, depending on the $Pa\text{CO}_2$ and the pH (see below). SBE quantifies the increase in extracellular SID (in mEq/l) needed to shift the curve back to the normal position without changing A_{TOT} (Figure 84.3). In terms of the original BE definition, this is roughly the required dose of sodium bicarbonate in mmol per litre of extracellular fluid. Similarly, if SBE is > 3.0 mEq/l, there is an up-shifted curve, either a metabolic alkalosis or compensation for a respiratory acidosis. The SBE is the decrease in extracellular SID needed to shift the curve back to the normal position at the prevailing A_{TOT}. Conceptually, it approximates the dose of HCl required per litre of extracellular fluid. SBE is thus 'extracellular SID excess' or 'SIDex'.[24]

THE BICARBONATE-BASED APPROACH TO METABOLIC ACID–BASE – THE BOSTON 'RULES OF THUMB'

Boston 'school' devotees calculate the plasma $[\text{HCO}_3^-]$ from the measured pH and $Pa\text{CO}_2$, and match this value with the $[\text{HCO}_3^-]$ deemed appropriate for the measured $Pa\text{CO}_2$, using empiric 'rules of thumb' derived from clinical and experimental data (Table 84.1).[25] An offset denotes a metabolic acid–base disturbance.

The Boston method is largely qualitative, since by focusing on plasma bicarbonate alone it ignores the A^- component of the buffer base (SIDe) concentration (Figure 84.2). The Boston rules of thumb can only tell us whether the $Pa\text{CO}_2$/pH curve is shifted up or down. Unlike SBE, they cannot tell us how much.

Table 84.1 Compensation – mechanisms and rules

Disorder	Compensation	Simple rules	Boston rules
Uncompensated respiratory acidosis and alkalosis	Nil	SBE −3.0 to +3.0	Respiratory acidosis: $\text{HCO}_3^- = 24 + 0.1 \times (Pa\text{CO}_2 - 40)$ Respiratory alkalosis: $\text{HCO}_3^- = 24 + 0.2 \times (Pa\text{CO}_2 - 40)$
Compensated respiratory acidosis and alkalosis	Respiratory acidosis: extracellular SID increased by decreasing urinary SID Respiratory alkalosis: extracellular SID decreased by increasing urinary SID	pH is normal or $\text{SBE} = 0.4 \times (Pa\text{CO}_2 - 40)$	Respiratory acidosis: $\text{HCO}_3^- = 24 + 0.35 \times (Pa\text{CO}_2 - 40)$ Respiratory alkalosis: $\text{HCO}_3^- = 24 + 0.5 \times (Pa\text{CO}_2 - 40)$
Metabolic acidosis	Hyperventilation reduces $Pa\text{CO}_2$	$Pa\text{CO}_2$ = last 2 digits of pH or $Pa\text{CO}_2 = 40 + \text{SBE}$ ($Pa\text{CO}_2$ rarely < 10 mmHg)	$Pa\text{CO}_2 = 1.5 \times (\text{HCO}_3^- + 8)$
Metabolic alkalosis	Hypoventilation increases $Pa\text{CO}_2$	$Pa\text{CO}_2$ = last 2 digits of pH or $Pa\text{CO}_2 = 40 + \text{SBE}$ ($Pa\text{CO}_2$ rarely > 60 mmHg)	$Pa\text{CO}_2 = 0.6 \times (\text{HCO}_3^- - 24)$

SBE, standard base excess; SID, strong ion difference.

ACID–BASE DISORDERS – CLASSIFICATION

PRIMARY ACID–BASE DISORDERS

Primary acid–base disorders dictate the direction of the pH disturbance. They are designated by the suffix 'osis', and can be either respiratory ($Pa\text{CO}_2$) or metabolic. Hence we can have a respiratory or metabolic acidosis or alkalosis. The final pH abnormality (if any) is designated by the suffix 'aemia'. In acidaemia, plasma pH is < 7.35; in alkalaemia, plasma pH is > 7.45. The pH in opposing primary acid–base disturbances can be normal.

COMPENSATION AND ITS EFFECT ON pH

Compensation is a counterresponse to a primary acid–base disorder. It reduces the severity of the pH disturbance. When the primary disturbance is respiratory ($Pa\text{CO}_2$), the compensation is metabolic (renal alteration of SID); if the primary disturbance is metabolic (abnormal SID relative to the prevailing A_{TOT}), the compensation is respiratory ($Pa\text{CO}_2$).

Metabolic compensation

In respiratory acid–base disturbances, the kidneys adjust extracellular SID by regulating urinary SID, primarily via urinary chloride. In prolonged hypocapnia, there is a compensatory fall in extracellular SID, achieved by increasing urinary SID. In sustained hypercapnia, the kidneys decrease urinary SID and thereby increase extracellular SID. Renal compensation for chronic respiratory acid–base disturbances takes time, but is ultimately very effective. Over the $Pa\text{CO}_2$ range 25–80 mmHg, which encompasses most chronic respiratory disturbances, full compensation will normalise the arterial pH.[22,26,27] However, this can take up to 5 days.

Respiratory compensation

By contrast, respiratory compensation for metabolic disturbances is much faster, but less effective. A normal pH is *never* regained. Metabolic acid–base disturbances activate feedback loops linked to alveolar ventilation, forcing $Pa\text{CO}_2$ in the direction that reduces the pH perturbation. The loops are driven by CSF and plasma pH acting on the central and peripheral chemoreceptors respectively. In severe metabolic acidosis, minute ventilation often increases more than eightfold, the resultant hypocapnia blunting the acidaemia. In contrast, metabolic alkalosis suppresses minute ventilation, the hypercapnia reducing the pH rise.

In both cases the full response evolves over 12–24 hours, at first driven entirely by the peripheral chemoreceptors. The central chemoreceptors dampen the initial response, since SID equilibration between plasma and CSF is gradual, whereas $P\text{CO}_2$ equilibration is immediate.

A normal pH combined with an abnormal $Pa\text{CO}_2$ can mean one of two things. Either there are two primary opposing acid–base disorders, one respiratory and one metabolic, or else there is a fully compensated respiratory acid–base disturbance. A 'normal' $Pa\text{CO}_2$ combined with an abnormal pH always represents two primary acid–base disturbances (see Table 84.1).

ACID–BASE 'SCANNING TOOLS'

ELECTRICAL GAPS (TABLE 84.2)[28]

Accumulating strong anions reduce SID, causing metabolic acidosis. Other than chloride and now increasingly L-lactate, strong anions are not routinely measured. However, they can be especially injurious, creating a need for rapid detection and early intervention. Critical care practitioners use electrical 'gaps' as early warning systems.

Table 84.2 Factors affecting the anion gap (AG), the albumin-corrected anion gap (AGc) and the strong ion gap (SIG)

Factor	AG	AGc	SIG
[Pi] ↑	Increased	Increased	No effect
[Pi] ↓	Decreased	Decreased	No effect
pH ↑	Increased	Increased	No effect
pH ↓	Decreased	Decreased	No effect
$[Ca^{++}]$ and $[Mg^{++}]$ ↑	Decreased	Decreased	No effect
$[Ca^{++}]$ and $[Mg^{++}]$ ↓	Increased	Increased	No effect
[Alb] ↑	Increased	No effect	No effect
[Alb] ↓	Decreased	No effect	No effect
L-Lactate	Increased	Increased	No effect
Unmeasured strong anions (e.g. D-lactate, ketoacids, salicylate)	Increased	Increased	Increased
Unmeasured weak anions (polygelinate, myeloma IgA bands)	Increased	Increased	Increased
Unmeasured strong cations (lithium)	Decreased	Decreased	Decreased
Unmeasured weak cations (THAMH+, myeloma IgG bands)	Decreased	Decreased	Decreased
Chloride overestimation (bromism, hyperlipidemia, high bicarbonate)	Decreased	Decreased	Decreased
Sodium underestimation (hypernatraemia)	Decreased	Decreased	Decreased

Anion gap (AG)

The plasma AG is calculated (in mEq/l) as $[Na^+] + [K^+] - [Cl^-] - [HCO_3^-]$, although $[K^+]$ is omitted in many laboratories. A typical reference range is 7–17 mEq/l. The AG quantifies [unmeasured anions] – [unmeasured cations], both strong and weak. The AG is increased by unmeasured anions, and reduced by unmeasured cations. In health, most of the AG consists of A^-, the negative charge on albumin and phosphate. The AG is altered by A_{TOT} fluctuations, which affect A^- directly, and by severe pH disturbances, which act via the A^- component (Table 84.2). When used for its primary purpose, which is scanning for unmeasured strong anions, AG sensitivity and specificity are low.

Albumin-corrected anion gap (AGc)[4]

The AGc was devised to correct for variations in plasma [albumin]. It is calculated as AG + 0.25 × (40 – [albumin]), assuming a normal plasma [albumin] of 40 g/l. By attributing a fixed negative charge to albumin, and making no adjustment for pH, error remains. This is minor, except in severe alkalaemia.

Strong ion gap (SIG)

The SIG concept was proposed by Jones in 1990,[29] and progressed by others.[2,30] It is calculated as SIDa – SIDe, where SIDa = $[Na^+] + [K^+] + [Ca^{++}] + [Mg^{++}] - [Cl^-]$ – [L-lactate], and SIDe = $[A^-] + [HCO_3^-]$. The unmeasured ions creating the 'gap' can be either strong or weak, but the term 'strong ion gap' has persisted.

In the absence of measurement error, the SIG should be zero unless there are unmeasured ions, the list of which is smaller than with AG and AGc (Table 84.2).[28] SIG is under evaluation as a scanning tool. Its signal is subject to the summated variability of multiple analytes. In many centres, the normal SIG is 4 mEq/l or more, the positive bias presumably due to locally adopted measurement technologies and variations in analytic reference standards. A refinement, 'net unmeasured ions' (NUI), has been successfully incorporated into an acid–base diagnostic module and linked to a laboratory information system.[31]

THE OSMOLAL GAP

The osmolal gap scans for unmeasured osmotically active molecules. It is calculated as measured osmolality – (1.86 × $([Na^+] + [K^+])$ + [urea] + [glucose]). The normal osmolal gap is < 10 mosm/kg. If there is an unexplained high AGc, a simultaneously raised osmolal gap suggests poisoning by methanol or ethylene glycol. However, a number of other molecules elevate the osmolal gap. These include other alcohols, mannitol and glycine, acetone and glycerol in ketoacidosis, and unknown solutes in lactic acidosis and renal failure.

PRACTICAL CONSIDERATIONS

THE DIAGNOSTIC SEQUENCE

At the outset, the clinician examining a set of blood gases should ignore derived variables such as bicarbonate or standard base excess. Most (frequently all) of the important information can be gleaned from the measured variables, $Pa\text{CO}_2$ and pH.

PRIMARY SURVEY

1. Take a history and perform a clinical examination.
2. Scan for primary disorders by matching the $Pa\text{CO}_2$ and pH combination with one of nine possible scenarios (Table 84.3).

SECONDARY SURVEY

1. Apply 'rules of thumb' (Table 84.1) where applicable. This step assesses compensation for any primary acid–base disturbances.
2. Note absent or inappropriate respiratory compensation in primary metabolic acid–base disorders, and identify this as a separate acid–base disturbance. For example, in diabetic ketoacidosis, if the arterial pH = 7.20 and the $Pa\text{CO}_2$ = 20 mmHg, the patient has a metabolic acidosis with normal respiratory compensation (Table 84.1). If, however, the pH = 7.20 with a $Pa\text{CO}_2$ = 32 mmHg, the metabolic acidosis has an accompanying respiratory acidosis (despite the hypocapnia). This is a greater cause for concern, signalling imminent respiratory decompensation. Conversely, if at this pH, $Pa\text{CO}_2$ = 12 mmHg, there is an accompanying respiratory alkalosis.
3. Calculate the AG or preferably the AGc. If either is elevated, unmeasured anions are likely. If low or negative, suspect laboratory error, but consider lithium intoxication, IgG myeloma and others (Table 84.2).

Table 84.3 Acid–base status – primary survey

pH	$Pa\text{CO}_2$ (mmHg)	Primary process(es)
7.35–7.45	35–45	None
7.35–7.45	> 45	1. Chronic respiratory acidosis or 2. Respiratory acidosis, metabolic alkalosis
7.35–7.45	< 35	1. Chronic respiratory alkalosis 2. Respiratory alkalosis, metabolic acidosis
< 7.35	< 35	Metabolic acidosis
< 7.35	> 45	Respiratory acidosis
< 7.35	35–45	Respiratory acidosis, metabolic acidosis
> 7.45	> 45	Metabolic alkalosis
> 7.45	< 35	Respiratory alkalosis
> 7.45	35–45	Respiratory alkalosis, metabolic alkalosis

4. Compare any AGc elevation with the SBE or [HCO_3^-]. An elevated AGc should be accompanied by a similar reduction in SBE or [HCO_3^-]. If not, there are dual disorders. For example, if AGc = 20 mEq/l and SBE = −15 mEq/l, the metabolic acidosis is due to a combination of an unmeasured anion and a narrowed difference between chloride and sodium (a combined normal and raised anion gap metabolic acidosis). If AGc = 20 mEq/l and the SBE = 0 mEq/l, there is a combined metabolic alkalosis and anion gap metabolic acidosis.
5. If there is no obvious cause for an elevated AGc, perform specific assays (e.g. L-lactate, β-hydroxybutyrate, D-lactate, salicylate). A concurrently raised osmolal gap suggests methanol or ethylene glycol toxicity. Urinary organic anions may reveal pyroglutamate.[32]

CLINICAL ACID–BASE DISORDERS

METABOLIC ACIDOSIS

In metabolic acidosis, the extracellular SID is low relative to A_{TOT}. This can represent a narrowing of the difference between [Na^+] and [Cl^-] (normal AGc, Table 84.4), or an accumulation of other anions (elevated AGc, Table 84.4). Although a normal AGc acidosis is often hyperchloraemic, the absolute [Cl^-] is not important, just its value relative to [Na^+].

Clinical features

Clinical features are those of acidaemia itself (Table 84.5), combined with specific toxicities of individual anions. These include blindness and cerebral oedema (formate),[33] crystalluria, renal failure and hypocalcaemia (oxalate),[34] and tinnitus, hyperventilation and fever due to uncoupling of oxidative phosphorylation (salicylate).[35]

Table 84.4 Causes of metabolic acidosis

Normal AGc	Raised AGc
Saline infusions	L-Lactate acidosis
Organic anion excretion	Ketoacidosis
Ketoacidosis	β-Hydroxybutyrate, acetoacetate
Glue sniffing (hippurate, benzoate)	Renal failure
Loss high SID enteric fluid	Sulphate, hippurate, urate, other organic anions
Small intestinal, pancreatic, biliary	Phosphate accumulation increases A_{TOT}
Urinary/enteric diversions	Ethylene glycol poisoning
High urinary SID	Glycolate, oxalate
Renal tubular acidosis	Methanol poisoning
High urinary SID	Formate
Post hypocapnia	Pyroglutamic acidosis
High urinary SID	Pyroglutamate
TPN and NH_4Cl administration	Toluene (glue sniffing)
	Hippurate, benzoate
	Short bowel syndrome
	D-lactate

AGc, albumin-corrected anion gap; SID, strong ion difference; TPN, total parenteral nutrition.

Table 84.5 Adverse effects of metabolic acidosis

Reduced myocardial contractility, tachy- and bradydysrhythmias, systemic arteriolar dilatation, venoconstriction, centralization of blood volume
Pulmonary vasoconstriction, hyperventilation, respiratory muscle failure
Reduced splanchnic and renal blood flow
Increased metabolic rate, catabolism, reduced ATP synthesis, reduced 2,3-DPG synthesis
Confusion, drowsiness
Increased inducible nitric oxide synthase (iNOS) expression, proinflammatory cytokine release
Hyperglycaemia, hyperkalaemia
Cell membrane pump dysfunction
Bone loss, muscle wasting

The adverse effects of acidaemia (Table 84.5) are more prominent at pH < 7.2. Acidaemia also has potential benefits. For example, the Bohr effect increases tissue oxygen availability, although this is rapidly counteracted by reduced 2,3-diphosphoglycerate concentrations. Lowering pH is protective in a number of experimental hypoxic stress models.[36,37] During mild acidaemia therefore, the net result of harm versus benefit can be debated.

Infusion-related acidosis[38,39]

Large volumes of intravenous saline cause a normal AGc metabolic acidosis. The SBE rarely falls below −10 mEq/l. With appropriate respiratory compensation, the pH will frequently remain above 7.3. An unresolved question is whether this is severe enough to cause harm.

Infusion-related acidosis is driven by the 'effective' SID of the crystalloid. Rapid infusion alters plasma SID towards the effective crystalloid SID, but also causes a metabolic alkalosis by diluting A_{TOT}. The SID of saline is zero (equal concentrations of the strong cation Na^+ and the strong anion Cl^-). At such a low SID, rapid infusion reduces extracellular SID precipitously, outstripping the metabolic alkalosis of A_{TOT} dilution.

To balance saline, some Cl^- must be replaced with HCO_3^-, or else with strong anions which undergo metabolic 'disappearance', such as lactate, gluconate or acetate. Enough chloride must be replaced to balance the fall in extracellular SID against the A_{TOT} dilution effect. Experimentally this value is 24 mEq/l.[38]

Renal tubular acidosis (RTA)

In RTA, urinary SID is inappropriately high in the setting of a low extracellular SID. The disturbance is in renal tubular Cl^- handling, either from reduced ammonium production proximally (Type 4) or distally (Type 1), or

Table 84.6 Types of renal tubular acidosis

	Type 1	Type 2	Type 4
Mechanism	Impaired distal NH_4^+ secretion	Increased proximal chloride resorption	Hyperkalaemic suppression of proximal tubular NH_4^+ production
Some causes	Idiopathic, hypercalciuric, amphotericin B, lithium carbonate, rheumatoid arthritis, Sjögren's disease, systemic lupus erythematosus, cirrhosis, renal transplant rejection, obstructive uropathy, primary hyperparathyroidism, hyperglobulinaemia	*With other proximal tubular defects = Fanconi syndrome*: Genetic, light chain nephropathy, acetazolamide, heavy metals, aminoglycosides, valproate, chemotherapy, renal transplantation, amyloidosis, paroxysmal nocturnal haemoglobinuria	*Reduced aldosterone secretion or sensitivity*: Hyporeninaemia, adrenal insufficiency, ACE inhibitors, NSAIDs, cyclosporin, heparin, amiloride, spironolactone, triamterene, pentamidine, diabetes, obstructive uropathy, interstitial nephropathies, renal transplant rejection, analgesic nephropathy
SBE	Can be < -15 mEq/l	–6 to -15 mEq/l	A -6 to -8 mEq/l
Plasma $[K^+]$	Usually low	Low	High
Urine pH post furosemide	> 5.5	< 5.5 (Bicarbonaturia with $NaHCO_3^-$ infusion)	Usually < 5.5
Urinary AG	Positive	Negative	Positive
Urinary NH_4^+	Reduced	Normal or high	Usually reduced

AG, anion gap; SBE, standard base excess.

increased proximal tubular chloride resorption (Type 2). Causes are legion (Table 84.6).

Apart from treating underlying causes and preventing hypercalciuria, management in Types 1 and 2 RTA is based on administering sodium bicarbonate or citrate to correct extracellular SID, and preventing and treating hypokalaemia using potassium citrate (not chloride). In Type 4 RTA, inciting agents are ceased where relevant, and adrenal insufficiency treated with mineralocorticoid replacement. Alkali supplements and furosemide are occasionally necessary.[12]

Lactic acidosis

This is discussed in Chapter 15.

Management of metabolic acidosis

Management is directed at the underlying cause. When instituting mechanical ventilation, a sudden reduction in minute volume can be lethal. For example, a patient with an arterial pH of 6.9 and $Pa\text{CO}_2$ of 10 mmHg is hyperventilating maximally. If the $Pa\text{CO}_2$ is allowed to return to 'normal' (40 mmHg) on instituting mechanical ventilation, the arterial pH will immediately fall to 6.7. If the $Pa\text{CO}_2$ is inadvertently allowed to rise to 60 mmHg, the pH will be 6.6.

Administration of buffers – sodium bicarbonate, 'carbicarb' and sodium lactate

In lactic acidosis and organic acidoses in general, it is difficult to justify the administration of buffers (see Chapter 15).[40] However, infusing $NaHCO_3$ to correct a severe normal AGc acidosis may be appropriate. Other conditions where $NaHCO_3$ administration is often indicated include severe hyperkalaemia, methanol and ethylene glycol poisoning, and tricyclic and salicylate overdose. A $NaHCO_3$ dose of 1 mmol/kg increases SBE approximately 3 mEq/l.

When administering $NaHCO_3$, the aim is to increase SID. The active agent is therefore sodium, not bicarbonate. The only reason NaOH is not used is its alkalinity (pH 14). However, two problems arise from the high CO_2 content (CO_{2TOT}) of $NaHCO_3$ (approximately 1028 mmol/l in a 1 M solution): one is the need for CO_2 impermeable storage; the other is the potential to create paradoxical intracellular respiratory acidosis, which can be demonstrated in vitro by adding $NaHCO_3$ to cultured cells.[41]

One approach is to reduce CO_{2TOT}, the trade-off being a rise in pH. In carbicarb (CO_{2TOT} = 750 mmol/l, $P\text{CO}_2$ = 2 mmHg, pH = 9.8), half the monovalent bicarbonate becomes divalent carbonate. Its use is still under evaluation. In Europe, sodium lactate (0.167 M, pH 6.9) is an alternative. The role of lactate is not to generate bicarbonate, but to undergo metabolic 'disappearance', leaving sodium to increase the SID.

Adding a weak base (B_{TOT}) will also shift the $Pa\text{CO}_2$/pH curve upward. THAM (tris-hydroxymethyl aminomethane, or tris buffer) is a weak base with a pKa of 7.7 at 37 °C. $THAM\text{-}H^+$ allows buffer base and thus SBE to increase without changing extracellular SID or A_{TOT}. THAM is CO_2 consuming, with good cell penetration, and causes an immediate intracellular metabolic and respiratory alkalosis.

Presumably in CSF this phenomenon is behind its propensity to cause sudden apnoea. THAM accumulates in renal failure. Other problems include hyperosmolality, coagulation and potassium disturbances, and hypoglycaemia. The use of THAM requires further evaluation.

Finally, it should be recognised that to cause an appreciable increase in P_{aCO_2}, $NaHCO_3$ has to be administered very rapidly (e.g. over 5 minutes).[42] Even then the rise is transient, and usually less than 10 mmHg. With slow administration, over 30–60 minutes, $NaHCO_3$ should have minimal effects on CO_2 production and intravascular P_{CO_2}. The exception is when pulmonary perfusion is massively reduced, such as in cardiac arrest.

Other potential adverse effects of buffer administration include a sudden increase in haemoglobin–oxygen affinity, the production of a hyperosmolar state, reduced $[Ca^{++}]$ and $[Mg^{++}]$, and rebound alkalosis on resolution of an organic acidosis.

METABOLIC ALKALOSIS

In metabolic alkalosis, extracellular SID is high relative to A_{TOT}. Metabolic alkalosis has been described as the most common acid–base disturbance. With modern definitions it is more often seen as part of a 'mixed' disorder.

Causes (Table 84.7)

Metabolic alkalosis can be precipitated by:

- low urinary SID
- loss of low SID enteric fluid
- gain of high SID fluid

Table 84.7 Metabolic alkalosis – causes

Low urinary SID	Enteric losses of low SID fluid	Gain of high SID fluid
Loop or thiazide diuretics Post hypercapnia Corticosteroids Cushing's syndrome Primary mineralocorticoid excess Carbenoxolone Glycyrrhetinic acid (liquorice) Hypercalcaemia Milk-alkali syndrome Magnesium deficiency Bartter's and Gitelman's syndromes	Pyloric stenosis, vomiting, nasogastric suction Villous adenoma Laxative abuse	$NaHCO_3$ administration Sodium citrate (plasma exchange, > 8 units stored blood) Renal replacement fluids with high SID (> 35 mEq/l) Milk-alkali syndrome

SID, strong ion difference.

Clinical features

A high plasma pH (> 7.55) has a number of adverse effects (Table 84.8). Mortality in critical illness escalates as the pH rises above 7.55, although how much is causation versus association is unclear.

Table 84.8 Severe metabolic alkalosis – multisystem effects

Central nervous system
Vasospasm
Seizures
Confusion, drowsiness
Neuromuscular
Weakness, tetany, muscle cramps
Cardiovascular
Arrhythmias – supraventricular and ventricular
Decreased contractility
Respiratory
Decreased alveolar ventilation
Atelectasis, hypoxaemia
Metabolic
Hyperlactaemia
Low [Pi], $[Ca^{++}]$, $[Mg^{++}]$ and $[K^{+}]$
Haemoglobin–oxygen affinity
Initially increased (until counteracted by increased 2,3-DPG)

Treatment

The first step is to remove the cause. Measures can then be instituted to accelerate the reduction in extracellular SID. They include:

- Correcting effective volume depletion (reduced skin turgor, postural hypotension, high urea:creatinine ratio, urinary $[Cl^-] < 20$ mmol/l). Albumin preparations simultaneously increase A_{TOT} and reduce SID, and are thus likely to be more effective than saline.[43]
- Administering KCl to correct potassium depletion. The vital component here is the chloride. Simplistically, potassium (strong cation) enters the depleted intracellular compartment in excess of chloride (strong anion), increasing extracellular SID. This explanation ignores associated Gibbs Donnan phenomena.
- Acetazolamide therapy to increase urinary SID (requires adequate renal function).
- Administration of HCl, which has a negative SID.[44,45] Minute ventilation, hypercapnia and oxygenation generally (but not invariably) improve. For full correction the calculated HCl requirement (in mmol) is 0.3 × SBE × Wt (kg). HCl can be infused over 24 hours

as a 0.2 M solution in dextrose through a central venous catheter. Regular checks of SBE (every 4 hours) are advisable. HCl can also be given indirectly, as NH_4Cl, or arginine or lysine hydrochloride. All require hepatic deamination.
- Renal replacement therapy.

Metabolic alkalosis in the setting of effective volume depletion has been termed 'saline responsive', in the sense that saline overcomes the alkalinising renal hypovolaemic response (low urinary SID). In fact, all metabolic alkaloses will respond if sufficient saline can be administered safely (see Infusion-related acidosis).

As with metabolic acidosis, care is required when instituting mechanical ventilation. Unless minute volume settings are reduced, it is possible to precipitate extreme alkalaemia.

RESPIRATORY ACIDOSIS

Causes (Table 84.9)

The risk is increased when CO_2 production is high and when ventilation is inefficient (large alveolar or apparatus dead space, respiratory muscle disadvantage due to hyperinflation).

Clinical features

These include the effects of acidaemia (Table 84.5). However, acute hypercapnia has important central nervous effects, including confusion, drowsiness, asterixis, fitting and raised intracranial pressure. Hypercapnia also activates the sympathetic–adrenal and renin–angiotensin systems, reducing renal blood flow, glomerular filtration rate and urine output.

Treatment

Management is directed at the underlying cause. Mechanical ventilation, either non-invasive or invasive, may be required.

RESPIRATORY ALKALOSIS

Causes

Respiratory alkalosis arises in a number of clinical scenarios (Table 84.10).

Clinical features

With the exception of the complications of hypoventilation, all the multisystem effects of alkalaemia apply.

Treatment

Management should be directed towards the underlying cause.

Table 84.9 Some causes of respiratory acidosis

Mechanism/ affected site	Acute	Chronic
Respiratory centre suppression	Sedative and narcotic drugs, CNS injury, CNS infection, brainstem vasculitis or infarction	Obesity hypoventilation syndrome
Airway obstruction	Inhalational injury, Ludwig's angina, laryngeal trauma	Obstructive sleep apnoea, vocal cord paresis, subglottic and tracheal stenosis
Mechanical ventilation	Permissive hypercapnia	
Neural/ neuromuscular	Spinal cord injury, Guillain–Barré syndrome, myasthenia gravis, muscle relaxants, envenomation, acute poliomyelitis, critical illness weakness syndromes	Phrenic nerve damage, paraneoplastic syndromes, post-polio syndrome
Muscle	Myopathy, low [K^+], high [Mg^+], low [Pi], diaphragmatic injury, shock	Muscular dystrophies, motor neurone disease
Decreased chest wall compliance	Abdominal distension, burns, pneumothorax, large pleural effusions	Obesity, kyphoscoliosis, ankylosing spondylitis
Loss of chest wall integrity/geometry	Flail segment	Thoracoplasty
Increased small airways resistance	Asthma, bronchiolitis	Chronic obstructive pulmonary disease
Deceased lung compliance	Acute lung injury, pneumonia, pulmonary oedema, vasculitis, haemorrhage	Pulmonary fibrosis

Table 84.10 Conditions predisposing to respiratory alkalosis

Acute	Chronic
Hypoxaemia	Pregnancy
Hepatic failure	High altitude
Sepsis	Chronic lung disease
Asthma	Neurotrauma
Pulmonary embolism	Chronic liver dysfunction
Pneumonia, acute lung injury	
CNS disorders – stroke, infection, trauma	
Drugs – salicylates, selective serotonin reuptake inhibitors	
Opiate and benzodiazepine withdrawal	
Mechanical hyperventilation – intentional or inadvertent	
Pain, anxiety, psychosis	

REFERENCES

1. Stewart PA. How to understand acid–base. In: Stewart PA (ed) *A Quantitative Acid–Base Primer for Biology and Medicine*. New York: Elsevier: 1981.
2. Figge J, Mydosh T, Fencl V. Serum proteins and acid–base equilibria: a follow-up. *J Lab Clin Med* 1992; **120**: 713–9.
3. Anstey CM. Comparison of three strong ion models used for quantifying the acid–base status of human plasma with special emphasis on the plasma weak acids. *J Appl Physiol* 2005; **98**: 2119–25.
4. Fencl V, Jabor A, Kazda A *et al.* Diagnosis of metabolic acid–base disturbances in critically ill patients. *Am J Respir Crit Care Med* 2000; **162**: 2246–51.
5. Wilkes P. Hypoproteinemia, strong-ion difference, and acid–base status in critically ill patients. *J Appl Physiol* 1998; **84**: 1740–8.
6. Wooten EW. Analytic calculation of physiological acid–base parameters in plasma. *J Appl Physiol* 1999; **86**: 326–34.
7. Patel RL, Turtle MR, Chambers DJ *et al.* Alpha-stat acid–base regulation improves neuropsychologic outcome in patients undergoing coronary artery bypass grafting. *J Thorac Cardiovasc Surg* 1996; **111**: 1267–79.
8. Stephan H, Weyland A, Kazmaier S *et al.* Acid–base management during hypothermic cardiopulmonary bypass does not affect cerebral metabolism but does affect blood flow and neurological outcome. *Br J Anaesth* 1992; **69**: 51–7.
9. Sakamotot T, Kurosawa H, Shin'oka T *et al.* The influence of pH strategy on cerebral and collateral circulation during hypothermic cardiopulmonary bypass in cyanotic patients with heart disease: results of a randomised trial and real-time monitoring. *J Thorac Cardiovasc Surg* 2004; **127**: 12–19.
10. Bernard SA, Gray TW, Buist MD *et al.* Treatment of comatose survivors of out-of-hospital cardiac arrest with induced hypothermia. *N Engl J Med* 2002; **346**: 557–63.
11. Rocktäschel J, Morimatsu H, Uchino S *et al.* Impact of continuous veno-venous haemofiltration on acid–base balance. *Int J Artif Organs* 2003; **26**: 19–25.
12. Soriano JR. Renal tubular acidosis; the clinical entity. *J Am Soc Nephrol* 2002; **13**: 2160–70.
13. Kellum JA. Determinants of plasma acid–base balance. *Crit Care Clin* 2005; **21**: 329–46.
14. Severinghaus JW. Siggaard-Andersen and the 'Great Trans-Atlantic Acid-Base Debate'. *Scand J Clin Lab Invest* 1993; **214**(Suppl): 99–104.
15. Gluck SJ. Acid–base. *Lancet* 1998; **352**: 474–9.
16. McNamara J, Worthley LI. Acid–base balance: part I. Physiology. *Crit Care Resusc* 2001; **3**: 181–7.
17. McNamara J, Worthley LI. Acid–base balance: part II. Pathophysiology. *Crit Care Resusc* 2001; **3**: 188–201.
18. Kellum JA. Clinical review: reunification of acid–base physiology. *Crit Care* 2005; **9**: 500–7.
19. Siggaard-Andersen O, Engel K. A micro method for determination of pH, carbon dioxide tension, base excess and standard bicarbonate in capillary blood. *Scand J Clin Lab Invest* 1960; **12**: 172–6.
20. Siggaard-Andersen O. The Van Slyke equation. *Scand J Clin Lab Invest* 1977; **37**(Suppl 146): 15–20.
21. Siggaard-Andersen O, Fogh-Andersen N. Base excess or buffer base (strong ion difference) as measure of a non-respiratory acid–base disturbance. *Acta Anesth Scand* 1995; **39**(Suppl 107): 123–8.
22. Schlichtig R, Grogono AW, Severinghaus JW. Human $PaCO_2$ and standard base excess compensation for acid–base imbalance. *Crit Care Med* 1998; **26**: 1173–9.
23. Wooten EW. Calculation of physiological acid–base parameters in multicompartment systems with application to human blood. *J Appl Physiol* 2003; **95**: 2333–44.
24. Schlichtig R, Grogono AW, Severinghaus JW. Current status of acid–base quantitation in physiology and medicine. *Int Anesthesiol Clin* 1998; **16**: 211–33.
25. Narins RB, Emmett M. Simple and mixed acid–base disorders: a practical approach. *Medicine* 1980; **59**: 161–87.
26. Martinu T, Menzies D, Dial S. Re-evaluation of acid–base prediction rules in patients with chronic respiratory acidosis. *Can Respir J* 2003; **10**: 311–15.
27. Lim VS, Katz AI, Lindheimer MD. Acid–base regulation in pregnancy. *Am J Physiol* 1976; **231**: 1764–70.
28. Morgan TJ. What exactly is the strong ion gap, and does anybody care? *Crit Care Resusc* 2004; **6**: 155–9.
29. Jones NL. A quantitative physicochemical approach to acid–base physiology. *Clin Biochem* 1990; **23**: 189–95.
30. Kellum JA, Kramer DJ, Pinsky MR. Strong ion gap: a methodology for exploring unexplained anions. *J Crit Care* 1995; **10**: 51–5.
31. Lloyd P, Freeborn R. Using quantitative acid–base analysis in the ICU. *Crit Care Resusc* 2006; **8**: 19–30.
32. Dempsey GA, Lyall HJ, Corke CF *et al.* Pyroglutamic acidemia: a cause of high anion gap metabolic acidosis. *Crit Care Med* 2000; **28**: 1803–7.
33. Gonda A, Gault H, Churchill D *et al.* Hemodialysis for methanol intoxication. *Am J Med* 1978; **64**: 749–57.

34. Peterson CD, Collins AJ, Himes MJ *et al.* Ethylene glycol poisoning. *N Engl J Med* 1981; **304**: 21–3.
35. Chapman BJ, Proudfoot AT. Adult salicylate poisoning: deaths and outcome in patients with high plasma salicylate concentrations. *Q J Med* 1989; **72**: 699–707.
36. Bonventre JV, Cheung JY. Effects of metabolic acidosis on viability of cells exposed to anoxia. *Am J Physiol* 1985; **249**: C149–59.
37. Heijnen BH, Elkhaloufi Y, Straatsburg IH *et al.* Influence of acidosis on liver ischemia and reperfusion injury in an in vivo rat model. *J Appl Physiol* 2002; **93**: 319–23.
38. Morgan TJ, Venkatesh B, Hall J. Crystalloid strong ion difference determines metabolic acid–base change during acute normovolaemic haemodilution. *Intensive Care Med* 2004; **30**: 1432–7.
39. Morgan TJ. The meaning of acid–base abnormalities in ICU Part III: Effects of fluid administration. *Crit Care* 2005; **9**: 204–11.
40. Levraut J, Grimaud D. Treatment of metabolic acidosis. *Curr Opin Crit Care* 2003; **9**: 260–5.
41. Levraut J, Giunti C, Ciebiera JP *et al.* Initial effect of sodium bicarbonate on intracellular pH depends on the extracellular nonbicarbonate buffering capacity. *Crit Care Med* 2001; **29**: 1033–9.
42. Levraut J, Garcia P, Giunti C *et al.* The increase in CO_2 production induced by $NaHCO_3$ depends on blood albumin and hemoglobin concentrations. *Intensive Care Med* 2000; **26**: 558–64.
43. Bellomo R, Morimatsu H, French C *et al.* The effects of saline or albumin resuscitation on acid–base status and serum electrolytes. *Crit Care Med* 2006; **34**: 2891–7.
44. Worthley LI. Intravenous hydrochloric acid in patients with metabolic alkalosis and hypercapnia. *Arch Surg* 1986; **121**: 1195–8.
45. Brimioulle S, Berre J, Dufaye P *et al.* Hydrochloric acid infusion for treatment of metabolic alkalosis associated with respiratory acidosis. *Crit Care Med* 1989; **17**: 232–6.

85

Fluid and electrolyte therapy

Anthony Delaney and Simon Finfer

The management of patients' fluid and electrolyte status requires an understanding of body fluid compartments as well as an understanding of water and electrolyte metabolism. These principles will be considered along with the commonly encountered fluid and electrolyte disturbances. Recent evidence for the use of fluid therapy in a number of common clinical scenarios will also be presented.

FLUID COMPARTMENTS (TABLE 85.1, FIGURE 85.1)

TOTAL BODY WATER

In humans, water contributes approximately 60% of body weight, with organs varying in water content (Table 85.2). The variation of the percentage of total body weight as water, between individuals, is largely governed by the amount of adipose tissue. The average water content as a percentage of total body weight is 60% for males and 50% for females. Total body water as a percentage of total body weight decreases with age, due to a progressive loss of muscle mass, causing bone and connective tissue to assume a greater percentage of total body weight[1–3] (Table 85.3).

Total body water is commonly divided into two volumes, the extracellular fluid (ECF) volume and the intracellular fluid (ICF) volume.[2] Sodium balance regulates the ECF volume, whereas water balance regulates the ICF volume. Sodium excretion is normally regulated by various hormonal and physical ECF volume sensors, whereas water balance is normally regulated by hypothalamic osmolar sensors.[4]

EXTRACELLULAR FLUID

ECF is defined as all body water external to the cell, and is commonly subdivided into plasma and interstitial fluid volumes. The ECF is normally 40% of total body water and 25% of total body weight. With acute or chronic illness, ICF volume is reduced, and ECF volume is increased and may even exceed the ICF volume. The ECF volume can be divided into the plasma volume, the extracellular fluid volume, and the interstitial volume.

INTRACELLULAR FLUID

ICF is defined as all the body water within cells and, unlike the ECF compartment, is an inhomogeneous, multicompartmental entity, with different pH and ionic composition depending upon the organ or tissue being considered. The ICF volume is often determined by inference from the difference in measurements of the total body water and ECF spaces. This estimation suffers from the inaccuracies inherent in both ECF and total body water measurements. In general, the ICF is considered to be 60% of total body water and 35% of total body weight.

TRANSCELLULAR FLUID

Fluids in this compartment have a common characteristic of being formed by transport activity of cells. The fluid is extracellular in nature and will be considered as part of the interstitial volume. It may vary from 1 to 10 l, with larger volumes occurring in diseased states (e.g. bowel obstruction or cirrhosis with ascites), and is formed at the expense of the remaining interstitial and plasma volumes.

WATER METABOLISM

Water balance is maintained by altering the intake and excretion of water. Intake is controlled by thirst, whereas excretion is controlled by the renal action of antidiuretic hormone (ADH). In health, plasma osmolalities of about 280 mOsm/kg suppress plasma ADH to concentrations low enough to permit maximum urinary dilution.[5] Above this value, an increase in ECF tonicity of about 1–2% or a decrease in total body water of 1–2 l, causes the posterior pituitary to release ADH, which acts upon the distal nephron to increase water reabsorption. Maximum plasma ADH concentrations are reached at an osmolality of 295 mOsm/kg.[5] The osmotic stimulation also changes thirst sensation and, in the conscious ambulant individual, initiates water repletion (drinking), which is more important in preventing dehydration than ADH secretion and action. Thus, in health, the upper limit of the body osmolality (and therefore serum sodium) is determined by the osmotic threshold for thirst, whereas the lower limit is determined by the osmotic threshold for ADH release.[6]

Table 85.1 Body fluid compartments

Fluid compartment	Volume (ml/kg)	% Total body weight
Plasma volume	45	4.5
Blood volume	75	7.5
Interstitial volume	200	20
Extracellular fluid volume	250	25
Intracellular fluid volume	350	35
Total body fluid volume	600	60

Table 85.2 Water content of various tissues

Tissue	% Water content
Brain	84
Kidney	83
Skeletal muscle	76
Skin	72
Liver	68
Bone	22
Adipose tissue	10

Increase in osmolality caused by permeant solutes (e.g. urea) does not stimulate ADH release. ADH may also be released in response to hypovolaemia and hypotension, via stimulation of low and high pressure baroreceptors. ADH release is extremely marked when more than 30% of the intravascular volume is lost. ADH may also be stimulated by pain and nausea, which are thought to act through the baroreceptor pathways.[4] ADH release may also be stimulated by a variety of pharmacological agents (Table 85.4). Renal response to ADH depends upon an intact distal nephron and collecting duct, and a hypertonic medullary interstitium. The capacity to conserve or excrete water also depends upon the osmolar load presented to the distal nephron.[4]

WATER REQUIREMENTS

Water is needed to eliminate the daily solute load, and to replace daily insensible fluid loss (Table 85.5). With a normal daily excretion of 600 mOsm solute, maximal and minimal secretions of ADH will cause urine osmolality to vary from 1200 to 30 mOsm/kg respectively, and the urine output to vary from 500 ml to 20 l/day respectively. Skin and lung water losses vary, and may range from 500 ml to 8 l/day depending on physical activity, ambient temperature and humidity.

DISORDERS OF OSMOLALITY

TONICITY

Osmolality is a measure of the number of osmol/kg water. The osmolality of the ECF is due largely to sodium salts. Clinical effects of hyperosmolality, due to excess solute, depend upon whether the solute distributes evenly throughout the total body water (e.g. permeant solutes of alcohol or urea) or distributes in the ECF only (e.g. impermeant solutes of mannitol or glucose). With impermeant solutes, hyperosmolality is associated with a shift of fluid from the ICF to the ECF compartment. Hyperosmolality due to increased impermeant solutes is known

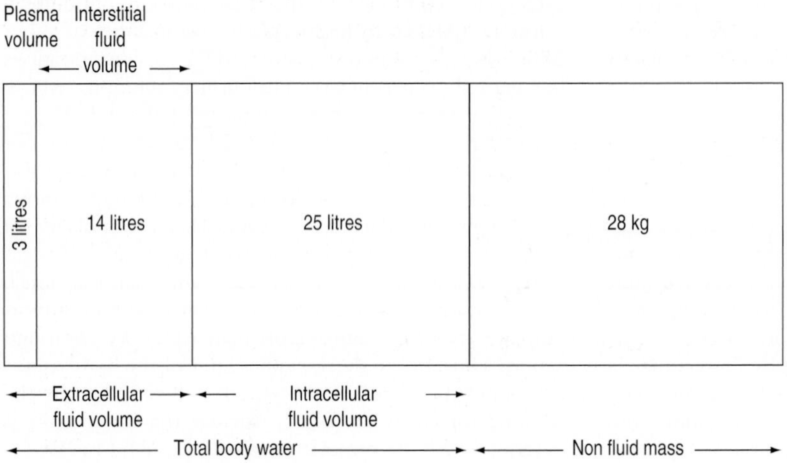

Figure 85.1 Body fluid compartments.

Table 85.3 Water content as a percentage of total body weight

Age (years)	Males (%)	Females (%)
10–15	60	57
15–40	60	50
40–60	55	47
> 60	50	45

Table 85.4 Drugs affecting ADH secretion

Stimulate	Inhibit
Nicotine	Ethanol
Narcotics	Narcotic antagonists
Vincristine	Phenytoin
Barbiturates	
Cyclophosphamide	
Chlorpropamide	
Clofibrate	
Carbamazepine	
Amitriptylline	

as hypertonicity. This condition may also be associated with a reduction in the serum sodium concentration (see below).

WATER EXCESS

In a 70-kg man, for every 1 l excess water, ECF increases by 400 ml and ICF increases by 600 ml, on average. The osmolality also decreases by 6–7 mOsm/kg and the serum sodium falls by 3.0–3.5 mmol/l.

WATER DEFICIENCY

In a 70-kg man, for every 1 l water loss, 600 ml is lost from the ICF and 400 ml from the ECF. The osmolality also increases by 7–8 mOsm/kg and the serum sodium rises by 3.5–4.0 mmol/l.

ELECTROLYTES

Chemical compounds in solution may either:

- Remain intact (i.e. undissociated), in which case they are called non-electrolytes (e.g. glucose, urea)
- Dissociate to form ions, in which case they are called electrolytes. Ions carry an electrical charge (e.g. Na^+, Cl^-). Ions with a positive charge are attracted to a negative electrode or cathode, and hence are called 'cations'. Conversely, ions with a negative charge travel towards a positive electrode or anode and are called 'anions'. Each body water compartment contains electrolytes with different composition and concentration (Table 85.6)

SODIUM

Sodium is the principal cation of the ECF and accounts for 86% of the ECF osmolality. In a 70-kg man, total body sodium content is 4000 mmol (58 mmol/kg) and is divided into a number of compartments (Table 85.7). ECF concentration of sodium varies between 134 and 146 mmol/l. The intracellular sodium concentration varies between different tissues, and ranges from 3 to 20 mmol/l.

The standard Western society dietary sodium intake is about 150 mmol/day, but the daily intake of sodium varies widely, with urinary losses ranging from < 1 to > 240 mmol/day.[7] Sodium balance is influenced by renal hormonal and ECF physical characteristics. The complete renal adjustment to an altered sodium load usually requires 3–4 days before balance is restored.

HYPONATRAEMIA

Hyponatraemia is defined as a serum sodium less than 135 mmol/l and may be classified as isotonic, hypertonic or hypotonic, depending upon the measured serum osmolality (Table 85.8).

Table 85.5 Daily fluid balance (for a 70-kg man at rest in a temperate climate)

	Input (ml)			Output (ml)	
	Seen	Unseen		Seen	Unseen
Drink	1000	–	Urine	1000	–
Food	–	650	Skin	–	500
Water of oxidation	–	350	Lungs	–	400
			Faeces	–	100
Total	1000	1000	Total	1000	1000

Table 85.6 Electrolyte composition of body fluid compartments

Electrolyte	ICF (mmol/l)	ECF (mmol/l)	
		Plasma	Interstitial
Sodium	10	140	145
Potassium	155	3.7	3.8
Chloride	3	102	115
Bicarbonate	10	28	30
Calcium (ionized)	< 0.01	1.2	1.2
Magnesium	10	0.8	0.8
Phosphate	105	1.1	1.0

Table 85.7 The sodium compartments in a 70-kg man

	Total (mmol)	(mmol/kg)
Total body sodium	4000	58
Non-exchangeable bone sodium	1200	17
Exchangeable sodium	2800	40
Intracellular sodium	250	3
Extracellular sodium	2400	35
Exchangeable bone sodium	150	2

Table 85.8 Common causes of hyponatraemia

1. **Spurious result**
   - Isotonic
     - Hyperlipidaemia
     - Hyperproteinaemia
   - Hypertonic
     - Hyperglycaemia
     - Mannitol, glycerol, glycine or sorbitol excess
2. **Water retention**
   - Renal failure
   - Hepatic failure
   - Cardiac failure
   - Syndrome of inappropriate ADH secretion
   - Drugs
   - Psychogenic polydipsia
3. **Water retention and salt depletion**
   - Postoperative, post trauma or patients with excess fluid losses given inappropriate fluid replacement
   - Adrenocortical failure
   - Diuretic excess

Isotonic hyponatraemia

Plasma normally contains 93% water and 7% solids (5.5% proteins, 1% salts and 0.5% lipids). If the solid phase is elevated significantly (e.g. in hyperlipidaemia or hyperproteinaemia), any device which dilutes a specific amount of plasma for analysis will give falsely lower values for all measured compounds. This effect produces 'factitious hyponatraemia' and is associated with a normal measured serum osmolality.[8] Measurement of plasma sodium by an ion-selective electrode is not affected by the volume of plasma 'solids' and therefore 'pseudohyponatraemia' will not occur with this method.[8]

Hypertonic hyponatraemia

In patients who have hypertonicity due to increased amounts of impermeant solutes (e.g. glucose, mannitol, glycerol or sorbitol), a shift of water from the ICF to the ECF occurs to provide osmotic equilibration, thus diluting the ECF sodium. Such resultant hyponatraemia is often associated with an increased measured osmolality. For example, in the presence of hyperglycaemia, for every 3 mmol/l rise in glucose, the serum sodium decreases by 1 mmol/l.[9]

Hypotonic hyponatraemia

Hyponatraemia is almost always caused by an excess of total body water, due to excessive hypotonic or water-generating i.v. fluids (e.g. 1.5% glycine, 0.45% saline or 5% glucose) or excessive ingestion of water, particularly in the presence of high circulating ADH concentrations. It may rarely be caused by loss of exchangeable sodium or potassium. In the latter circumstances, a loss of approximately 40 mmol of sodium or potassium, without a change in total body water content, is required to lower the serum sodium by 1 mmol/l. As hyponatraemia may be associated with an alteration in both total body water and total body sodium, the ECF may be increased (hypervolaemia), decreased (hypovolaemia) or exhibit no change (isovolaemia).[5]

In health, a fluid intake up to 15–20 l may be tolerated before water is retained and hyponatraemia occurs. In psychogenic polydipsia, if the water intake exceeds the renal capacity to form dilute urine, water retention and hyponatraemia will occur. With this disorder, the plasma osmolality exceeds urine osmolality. In circumstances where ADH is increased (e.g. hypovolaemia, hypotension, pain or nausea), or where renal response to ADH is altered (i.e. in renal, hepatic, pituitary, adrenal or thyroid failure), water retention occurs with lower intakes of fluid.

Transurethral resection of prostate (TURP) syndrome

Clinical features The TURP syndrome consists of hyponatraemia, cardiovascular disturbances (hypertension, hypotension, bradycardia), an altered state of consciousness (agitation, confusion, nausea, vomiting, myoclonic and generalised seizures) and, when using glycine solutions, transient visual disturbances of blurred vision, blindness and fixed dilated pupils, following TURP. It has also been described following endometrial ablation.[10] It may occur within 15 minutes or be delayed for up to 24 hours postoperatively,[11] and is usually caused by an excess absorption of the irrigating fluid which contains 1.5% glycine with an osmolality of 200 mosm/kg. Hyponatraemic syndromes have also been described when irrigating solutions containing 3% mannitol or 3% sorbitol have been used. Symptomatology usually occurs when > 1 l of 1.5% glycine or > 2–3 l of 3% mannitol or sorbitol are absorbed.[12]

The excess absorption of irrigating fluid causes an increase in total body water (which is often associated with only a small decrease in plasma osmolality), hyponatraemia (as glycine, sorbitol or mannitol reduces the sodium component of ECF osmolality) and an increase in the osmolar gap.[12,13] When glycine is used, other features include hyperglycinaemia (up to 20 mmol/l; normal plasma glycine concentrations range from 0.15 to 0.3 mmol/l), hyperserinaemia (as serine is a major metabolite of glycine), hyperammonaemia (following deamination of glycine and serine), metabolic acidosis and hypocalcaemia (due to the glycine metabolites glyoxylic acid and oxalate). Because glycine is an inhibitory neurotransmitter, and as it passes freely into the intracellular compartment when glycine solutions are used, hyperglycinaemia may be more important in the pathophysiology of this disorder than a reduction in body fluid osmolality and cerebral oedema.[14]

Treatment Treatment is largely supportive with the management of any reduction in plasma osmolality being based on the measured plasma osmolality and not the plasma sodium. If the measured osmolality is > 260 mOsm/kg and mild neurological abnormalities exist, and if the patient is haemodynamically stable with normal renal function, close observation and reassurance (e.g. the visual disturbances are reversible and will last for less than 24 hours) are usually all that is needed. If the patient is hypotensive and bradycardic with severe and unresolving neurological abnormalities, haemodialysis may be warranted. Hypertonic saline is only used if the measured osmolality is < 260 mOsm/kg and severe non-visual neurological abnormalities exist.[15]

Syndrome of inappropriate ADH secretion (SIADH)

This syndrome is a form of hyponatraemia in which there is an increased concentration of ADH inappropriate to any osmotic or volume stimuli that normally affect ADH secretion.[16] Diagnostic criteria and common causes are listed in Tables 85.9 and 85.10, respectively.

Table 85.9 Criteria for the diagnosis of syndrome of inappropriate antidiuretic hormone (SIADH)

Hypotonic hyponatraemia
Urine osmolality greater than plasma osmolality
Urine sodium excretion greater than 20 mmol/l
Normal renal, hepatic, cardiac, pituitary, adrenal and thyroid function
Absence of hypotension, hypovolaemia, oedema and drugs affecting ADH secretion
Correction by water restriction

Table 85.10 Aetiologies of syndrome of inappropriate antidiuretic hormone (SIADH)

Ectopic ADH production by tumours
Small cell bronchogenic carcinoma
Adenocarcinoma of the pancreas or duodenum
Leukaemia
Lymphoma
Thymoma
Central nervous system disorders
Cerebral trauma
Brain tumour (primary or secondary)
Meningitis or encephalitis
Brain abscess
Subarachnoid haemorrhage
Acute intermittent porphyria
Guillain–Barré syndrome
Systemic lupus erythematosus
Pulmonary diseases
Viral, fungal and bacterial pneumonias
Tuberculosis
Lung abscess

Clinical features While cerebral manifestations are usually absent when the sodium concentration exceeds 125 mmol/l, progressive symptomatology of headache, nausea, confusion, disorientation, coma and seizures are often observed when plasma sodium is below 120 mmol/l.[17]

Treatment Initial treatment should be fluid restriction with close monitoring of serum sodium. If serum sodium concentration is not increasing with fluid restriction, judicious administration of sodium as intravenous normal or hypertonic saline may be required. As the true duration and rapidity of onset of hyponatraemia is often unclear, the presence and severity of symptoms may be used as the trigger for active correction of hyponatraemia.[17] The evidence base available to guide therapy is limited and there is consequently no consensus on the optimum rate at which to correct the serum sodium concentration. The major concern is to avoid neurological damage from untreated seizures or cerebral oedema and from myelinolysis.[17] In the absence of good evidence, recommended rates at which to increase the sodium concentration vary from 0.5 to 2 mmol/l per hour. Unless the treating clinician feels that more rapid correction is indicated, it seems prudent to correct the serum sodium concentration at a slower rather than a faster rate.

Cerebral salt wasting

Cerebral salt wasting (CSW) is a syndrome occurring in patients with a cerebral lesion and an excess renal loss of sodium and chloride.[18] The exact aetiology of the syndrome remains unclear. Although hyponatraemia is not necessary for the diagnosis, the syndrome is commonly associated with hyponatraemia.[19] The diagnosis of CSW is suspected in patients with a cerebral lesion, such as subarachnoid haemorrhage, traumatic brain injury or a cerebral tumour, when there is an elevated urine output, with elevated urinary sodium in the absence of a physiological cause for increased sodium excretion.[19] The syndrome can be differentiated from the SIADH, as patients with CSW will have evidence of ECF depletion (e.g. negative fluid balance, tachycardia, increased haematocrit, increased urea, low central venous pressure) as opposed to the SIADH where ECF volume will be normal or slightly expanded.[20] Treatment of patients involves exclusion of other causes of hyponatraemia and increased urine output, replacement of sodium and fluid losses, and possibly fludrocortisone.[21]

Hypertonic saline

Hypertonic saline, most commonly as 3% saline, is used as a therapy for patients with symptomatic hyponatraemia. Due to the osmolarity (1000 mosm/l) of 3% saline , it must be given through a central line, and care must be taken to avoid the known complications of its use. Complications reported with hypertonic saline therapy include congestive cardiac failure and central pontine and extrapontine myelinolysis (osmotic demyelination syndrome).[22,23] Careful haemodynamic and electrolyte monitoring throughout saline administration is required. There is still no uniform agreement that osmotic demyelination is produced by a rapid correction of hyponatraemia.

While hypertonic saline has been proposed as a therapy for raised intracranial pressure in a number of clinical settings,[24] its use remains controversial.[25] In a recent methodologically sound (adequate allocation concealment, blinded and using intention to treat analysis) randomised clinical trial, which included 229 patients with severe traumatic brain injury, resuscitation with 250 ml of 7.5% saline was not associated with improved mortality or functional outcomes compared to Hartmann's solution.[26]

Vasopressin receptor antagonists

V_2 receptor antagonists, such as lixivaptan, tolvaptan and OPC-31260, have recently been developed. These agents come from a novel class of non-peptide agents that bind to V_2 receptors in the distal tubule of the kidney and prevent vasopressin-mediated aquaporin mobilisation, and thus promote an aquaresis.[27] These agents have been trialled as therapeutic options for the treatment of hyponatraemia in a number of clinical settings including hyponatraemia associated with cardiac failure, cirrhosis and SIADH.[27,28] At present the role of V_2 receptor antagonists in the management of hyponatraemia in the critically ill remains uncertain.

HYPERNATRAEMIA

Hypernatraemia, defined as a serum sodium greater than 145 mmol/l, is always associated with hyperosmolality and may be caused by excessive administration of sodium salts (bicarbonate or chloride), water depletion or excess sodium and loss of water (Table 85.11).

Table 85.11 Causes of hypernatraemia

Water depletion
Extrarenal loss
Exposure
GIT losses (often with excess saline replacement)
Renal loss
Osmotic diuresis – urea, mannitol, glycosuria
Diabetes insipidus
Neurogenic
Post traumatic, fat embolism
Metastatic tumours, craniopharyngioma, pinealoma, cysts
Meningitis, encephalitis
Granulomas (TB, sarcoid)
Guillain–Barré syndrome
Idiopathic
Nephrogenic
Congenital
Hypercalcaemia, hypokalaemia
Lithium
Pyelonephritis
Medullary sponge kidney
Polycystic kidney
Post obstructive uropathy
Multiple myeloma, amyloid, sarcoid
Salt gain
Hypertonic, saline or sodium bicarbonate

Excessive ingestion of sodium salts is rare but intravenous infusion of large volumes of sodium-containing fluids is common in the management of hospitalised patients. Hypernatraemia often occurs in the recovery phase of acute illness when spontaneous diuresis or diuretic therapy results in more rapid clearance of free water than sodium. Pure water depletion is uncommon, unless water restriction is applied to a patient who is unconscious or unable to obtain or ingest water, as the thirst response normally corrects water depletion. If it occurs, the serum sodium concentration increases, in association with loss of both ECF and ICF.

Clinical features

Hypernatraemia usually produces symptoms if the serum sodium exceeds 155–160 mmol/l (i.e. osmolality > 330 mOsm/kg). The clinical features include increased temperature, restlessness, irritability, drowsiness, lethargy, confusion and coma.[29] Convulsions are uncommon. The diminished ECF volume may reduce cardiac output, thereby reducing renal perfusion, leading to pre-renal renal failure.

Treatment

For pure water depletion, this consists of water administration. If i.v. fluid is required, 5% glucose or hypotonic saline solutions (0.45% saline) are often used, as sterile water infusion causes haemolysis. In rare cases, i.v. sterile water may be used, by administering through a central venous catheter.[30] Since rapid rehydration may give rise to cerebral oedema, the change in serum sodium should be no greater than 0.5 mmol/l per hour.[29]

POTASSIUM

Potassium is the principal intracellular cation and accordingly (along with its anion) fulfils the role of the ICF osmotic provider. It also plays a major role in the functioning of excitable tissues (e.g. muscle and nerve). As the cell membrane is 20-fold more permeable to potassium than sodium ions, potassium is largely responsible for the resting membrane potential. Potassium also influences carbohydrate metabolism and glycogen and protein synthesis.

Total body potassium is 45–50 mmol/kg in the male (3500 mmol/70 kg) and 35–40 mmol/kg (2500 mmol/65 kg) in the female; 95% of the total body potassium is exchangeable. As ECF potassium ranges from 3.1 to 4.2 mmol/l, the total ECF potassium ranges from 55 to 70 mmol. About 90% of the total body potassium is intracellular: 8% resides in bone, 2% in ECF water and 70% in skeletal muscle. With increasing age (and decreasing muscle mass), total body potassium decreases.

FACTORS AFFECTING POTASSIUM METABOLISM

The potassium content of cells is regulated by a cell wall pump-leak mechanism. Cellular uptake is by the Na^+/K^+ pump which is driven by Na^+/K^+ ATPase. Movement of potassium out of the cell is governed by passive forces (i.e. cell membrane permeability and chemical and electrical gradients to the potassium ion).

Acidosis promotes a shift of potassium from the ICF to the ECF, whereas alkalosis promotes the reverse shift. Hyperkalaemia stimulates insulin release, which promotes a shift of potassium from the ECF to the ICF, an effect independent of the movement of glucose. β_2-adrenergic agonists promote cellular uptake of potassium by a cyclic AMP-dependent activation of the Na^+/K^+ pump, whereas α-adrenergic agonists cause a shift of potassium from the ICF to the ECF.[31] Aldosterone increases the renal excretion of potassium; glucocorticoids are also kaliuretic, an effect which may be independent of the mineralocorticoid receptor.

Normally, mechanisms to reduce the ECF potassium concentration (by increasing renal excretion and shifting potassium from the ECF to the ICF) are very effective. However, mechanisms to retain potassium in the presence of potassium depletion are less efficient, particularly when compared to those of sodium conservation. Even with severe potassium depletion, urinary loss of potassium continues at a rate of 10–20 mmol/day. Metabolic alkalosis also enhances renal potassium loss, by encouraging distal nephron Na^+/K^+, rather than Na^+/K^+ exchange.

HYPOKALAEMIA

Hypokalaemia is defined as a serum potassium of less than 3.5 mmol/l (or plasma potassium less than 3.0 mmol/l). It may be due to decreased oral intake, increased renal or

Table 85.12 Causes of hypokalaemia

Inadequate dietary intake (urine $K^+ < 20$ mmol/l)
Abnormal body losses
Gastrointestinal (urine $K^+ < 20$ mmol/l)
Vomiting, nasogastric aspiration
Diarrhoea, fistula loss
Villous adenoma of the colon
Laxative abuse
Renal (urine $K^+ > 20$ mmol/l)
Conn's syndrome
Cushing's syndrome
Bartter's syndrome
Ectopic ACTH syndrome
Small cell carcinoma of the lung
Pancreatic carcinoma
Carcinoma of the thymus
Drugs
Diuretics
Corticosteroids
Carbapenems, amphotericin B, gentamicin
Cisplatin
Renal tubular acidosis
Magnesium deficiency
Compartmental shift
Alkalosis
Insulin
Na^+/K^+ ATPase stimulation
Sympathomimetic agents with β_2 effect
Methylxanthines
Barium poisoning
Hypothermia
Toluene intoxication
Hypokalaemic periodic paralysis
Delayed following blood transfusion (see Chapter 88)

gastrointestinal loss, or movement of potassium from the ECF to the ICF (Table 85.12).

Clinical features

These include weakness, hypotonicity, depression, constipation, ileus, ventilatory failure, ventricular tachycardias (characteristically torsades de pointes), atrial tachycardias, and even coma.[32] With prolonged and severe potassium deficiency, rhabdomyolysis and thirst and polyuria, due to the development of renal diabetes insipidus, may occur. The ECG changes are relatively non-specific, and include prolongation of the PR interval, T-wave inversion and prominent U-waves.

Treatment

Intravenous or oral potassium chloride will correct hypokalaemia, particularly if it is associated with metabolic alkalosis. If the patient has renal tubular acidosis and hypokalaemia, potassium acetate or citrate may be preferred to potassium chloride. Intravenous administration of potassium should normally not exceed 40 mmol/hour, and plasma potassium should be monitored at 1–4-hourly

Table 85.13 Causes of hyperkalaemia

Collection abnormalities
Delay in separating RBC
Specimen haemolysis
Thrombocythemia
Excessive intake
Transiently following blood transfusion (see Chapter 88)
Exogenous (i.e. i.v. or oral KCl, massive blood transfusion)
Endogenous (i.e. tissue damage)
Burns, trauma
Rhabdomyolysis
Tumour lysis
Decrease in renal excretion
Drugs
Spironolactone, triamterine, ameloride
indomethacin
Captopril, enalapril
Renal failure
Addison's disease
Hyporeninaemic hypoaldosteronism
Compartmental shift
Acidosis
Insulin deficiency
Digoxin overdosage
Succinylcholine
Arginine hydrochloride
Hyperkalaemic periodic paralysis
Fluoride poisoning

intervals.[33] In patients with acute myocardial infarction and hypokalaemia, some recommend i.v. potassium to maintain the serum potassium at 4.0 mmol/l.[34] The plasma concentration should be monitored closely.

HYPERKALAEMIA

Hyperkalaemia is defined as a serum potassium greater than 5.0 mmol/l or plasma potassium greater than 4.5 mmol/l. It may be artifactual (from sampling errors such as in vitro haemolysis); true hyperkalaemia may be due to excessive intake, severe tissue damage, decreased excretion or body fluid compartment shift (Table 85.13).

Clinical features

These include tingling, paraesthesia, weakness, flaccid paralysis, hypotension and bradycardia. The characteristic ECG effects include peaking of the T-waves, flattening of the P-wave, prolongation of the PR interval (until sinus arrest with nodal rhythm occurs), widening of the QRS complex, and the development of a deep S-wave. Finally, a sine wave ECG pattern which deteriorates to asystole may occur at serum potassium levels of 7 mmol/l or greater.

Treatment

This is directed at the underlying cause, and may include dialysis. Rapid management of life-threatening hyperkalaemia may be achieved by:[35]

- Calcium chloride 5–10 ml i.v. of 10% (3.4–6.8 mmol, which is used to reduce the cardiac effects of hyperkalaemia)
- Sodium bicarbonate, 50–100 mmol i.v.
- Glucose, 50 g i.v. with 20 units of soluble insulin
- Oral and rectal resonium A, 50 g
- Diuresis with furosemide, 40–80 mg i.v.

CALCIUM

Almost all (99%) of the body calcium (30 mmol or 1000 g or 1.5% body weight) is present in bone. A small but significant quantity of ionised calcium exists in the ECF, and is important for many cellular activities, including secretion, neuromuscular impulse formation, contractile functions and clotting. Normal daily intake of calcium is 15–20 mmol, although only 40% is absorbed. The average daily urinary loss is 2.5–7.5 mmol. The total ECF calcium of 40 mmol (2.20–2.55 mmol/l) exists in three forms: 40% (1.0 mmol/l) is bound to protein (largely albumin), 47% is ionised (1.15 mmol/l) and 13% is complexed (0.3 mmol/l) with citrate, sulphate and phosphate. The ionised form is the physiologically important form, and may be acutely reduced in alkalosis which causes a greater amount of the serum calcium to be bound to protein.[36] While the serum ionised calcium can be measured, total serum calcium is usually measured, which can vary with the serum albumin concentrations. A correction factor can be used to offset the effect of serum albumin on serum calcium. This is 0.02 mmol/l for every 1 g/l increase in serum albumin (up to a value of 40 g/l), added to the measured calcium concentration. For example, if measured serum calcium is 1.82 mmol/l, and serum albumin is 25 g/l, corrected serum calcium $= 1.82 + [(40–25) \times 0.02]$ mmol/l $= 2.12$ mmol/l. It has been suggested that ionised calcium, where available, is a better indicator of calcium status in the critically ill.[37]

HYPOCALCAEMIA

Common causes of hypocalcaemia include hypoparathyroidism and pseudohypoparathyroidism, septic shock, acute pancreatitis and rhabdomyolysis.[38] Clinical features of a reduced serum ionised calcium include tetany, cramps, mental changes and decrease in cardiac output. Symptomatic hypocalcaemia should be treated with i.v. calcium, either as calcium chloride or calcium gluconate. It should be remembered that 1 ml of calcium chloride has three times as much elemental calcium as 1 ml of calcium gluconate, and so the former is the preferred formulation in acute situations. Calcium should be administered via a central vein when practical due to the risk of tissue damage if extravasated.[38]

HYPERCALCAEMIA

The clinical features of hypercalcaemia include nausea, vomiting, pancreatitis, polyuria, polydipsia, muscular weakness, mental disturbance and ectopic calcification. Some of the common causes of hypercalcaemia include endocrine diseases such as hyperparathyroidism and thyrotoxicosis, renal failure, malignancy, thiazide diuretics and prolonged immobilisation.[38]

Severe hypercalcaemia (> 3.3 mmol/l) or more moderate symptomatic hypercalcaemia will require specific therapy. A cause for the elevated calcium concentration should be sought, and specific treatment may be warranted. General measures include restoration of intravascular volume with normal saline, followed by the use of a loop diuretic such as furosemide to promote calcium excretion. The use of bisphosphonates, such as pamidronate (30–90 mg by i.v. infusion), is recommended for severe cases.[39] Other therapies to consider include steroids, calcitonin and mithramycin.

MAGNESIUM

Magnesium is primarily an intracellular ion which acts as a metallo-coenzyme in numerous phosphate transfer reactions. It has a critical role in the transfer, storage and utilisation of energy.

In humans, the total body magnesium content is 1000 mmol, and the plasma concentrations range from 0.70 to 0.95 mmol/l. The daily oral intake is 8–20 mmol (40% of which is absorbed) and the urinary loss, which is the major source of excretion of magnesium, varies from 2.5 to 8 mmol/day.[40]

HYPOMAGNESAEMIA

Hypomagnesaemia is caused by decreased intake or increased loss (Table 85.14). Clinical features include neurological signs of confusion, irritability, delirium tremors, convulsions and tachyarrhythmias. Hypomagnesaemia is often associated with resistant hypokalaemia and hypocalcaemia. Treatment consists of i.v. magnesium sulphate as a bolus of 10 mmol, administered over 5 minutes, followed by 20–60 mmol/day.

Table 85.14 Causes of magnesium deficiency

Gastrointestinal disorders
Malabsorption syndromes
GIT fistulas
Short-bowel syndrome
Prolonged nasogastric suction
Diarrhoea
Pancreatitis
Parenteral nutrition
Alcoholism
Endocrine disorders
Hyperparathyroidism
Hyperthyroidism
Conn's syndrome
Diabetes mellitus
Hyperaldosteronism
Renal diseases
Renal tubular acidosis
Diuretic phase of acute tubular necrosis
Drugs
Aminoglycosides
Carbenicillin, ticarcillin
Amphotericin B
Diuretics
Cis-platinum
Cyclosporin

HYPERMAGNESAEMIA

Hypermagnesaemia is often caused by excessive administration of magnesium salts or conventional doses of magnesium in the presence of renal failure. Clinical features include drowsiness, hyporeflexia and coma, vasodilatation and hypotension, and conduction defects of sinoatrial and atrioventricular nodal block and asystole may occur. Treatment is directed towards increasing excretion of the ion, which may require dialysis. Intravenous calcium chloride may be used for rapidly treating the cardiac conduction defects.[40]

MAGNESIUM THERAPY

There are increasing reports of the use of magnesium as a therapy for a variety of conditions. A randomised control trial of over 10 000 women with pre-eclampsia demonstrated the efficacy of magnesium in the prevention of eclampsia,[41] and it is also a recommended treatment for established eclampsia. It has been used to treat atrial fibrillation, to achieve both rate control and reversion to sinus rhythm in a number of settings, including post cardiac surgery, and in the emergency department.[42,43] Magnesium, given either intravenously or nebulised, may be beneficial for patients with acute severe asthma.[44,45] There are also preliminary trials to suggest that magnesium may prevent delayed cerebral ischaemia due to vasospasm in patients with subarachnoid haemorrhage.[46]

PHOSPHATE

While most of the body phosphate exists in bone, 15% is found in the soft tissues as ATP, red blood cell 2,3-DPG, and other cellular structural proteins, including phospholipids, nucleic acids and phosphoproteins. Phosphate also acts as a cellular and urinary buffer.[40]

HYPOPHOSPHATAEMIA

Hypophosphataemia may be caused by a decreased intake, increased excretion or intracellular redistribution (Table 85.15). While hypophosphataemia may be

Table 85.15 Causes of hypophosphataemia

Hyperparathyroidism
Vitamin D deficiency
Vitamin D resistant rickets
Renal tubular acidosis
Alkalosis
Parenteral nutrition
Alcoholism
Refeeding syndrome

symptom-free, clinical features have been described which include paraesthesia, muscle weakness, seizures, coma, rhabdomyolysis and cardiac failure. Hypophosphataemia may be a prominent feature of the refeeding syndrome when it may be accompanied by other electrolyte disturbances such as hypokalaemia and hypomagnesaemia. Treatment consists of close monitoring and replacement as oral or i.v. sodium or potassium phosphate, 50–100 mmol/24 hours.

HYPERPHOSPHATAEMIA

Hyperphosphataemia is usually caused by an increased intake or decreased excretion (Table 85.16). Clinical features include ectopic calcification of nephrocalcinosis, nephrolithiasis and band keratopathy. Treatment may require haemodialysis; otherwise oral aluminium hydroxide and even hypertonic glucose solutions to shift ECF phosphate into the ICF can be used.

FLUID AND ELECTROLYTE REPLACEMENT THERAPY

GENERAL PRINCIPLES

In critical illness many of the body's normal homeostatic mechanisms are deranged and basic life-preserving senses such as hunger and thirst may be abolished by disease processes or by treatments such as the use of sedation. As a result, the survival of critically ill patients depends on the administration of appropriate volumes of fluids, and appropriate quantities of electrolytes and nutrition by their medical and nursing attendants. Basal requirements for water, electrolytes and nutrients are discussed in Chapter 87. In addition to basal requirements, many critically ill patients have abnormal fluid and electrolyte losses that must be replaced; examples are discussed below.

Table 85.16 Causes of hyperphosphataemia

Rhabdomyolysis
Renal failure (acute or chronic)
Vitamin D toxicity
Acidosis
Tumour lysis
Hypoparathyroidism
Pseudohypoparathyroidism
Diphosphonate therapy
Excess i.v. administration

GASTROINTESTINAL LOSSES

The daily volumes and composition of gastrointestinal tract (GIT) secretions in mmol/l are shown in Table 85.17. Clinical effects of fluid loss from the GIT are largely determined by the volume and composition of the fluid, and therapy is usually directed at replacing the losses. Gastric fluid loss (e.g. from vomiting and nasogastric suction) results in water, sodium, hydrogen ion, potassium and chloride depletion. Hence, metabolic alkalosis, hypokalaemia, hypotension and dehydration develop if the saline and potassium chloride losses are not correctly replaced.

Pancreatic and biliary fluid losses (e.g. pancreatic or biliary fistula)

These may result in hyperchloraemic acidosis with hypokalaemia, hypotension and dehydration if the losses of bicarbonate, potassium and saline are not correctly replaced.

Intestinal losses (e.g. fistula or ileostomy losses, diarrhoea and ileus)

These result in hypokalaemia, hypotension and dehydration if the saline and potassium losses are not replaced.

RESUSCITATION FLUIDS

Systemic hypotension is a common feature of acute critical illness and first-line treatment is usually the administration of intravenous resuscitation fluid. The fluids available to clinicians to maintain or expand intravascular volume are crystalloids, colloids and blood products; the properties of colloid solutions and blood products are discussed in Chapter 89.

Whether the choice of resuscitation fluid influences patients' outcomes has been the subject of long-running debate. The debate has been fuelled by the conflicting

Table 85.17 Daily volume and electrolyte composition of GIT secretions

Electrolytes (mmol/l)	Vol (l)	H^+	Na^+	K^+	Cl^-	HCO_3^-
Saliva	0.5–1.0	0	30	20	10–35	0–15
Stomach	1.0–2.5	0–120	60	10	100–120	0
Bile	0.5	0	140	5–10	100	40–70
Pancreatic	0.75	0	140	5–10	70	40–70
Small and large gut	2.0–4.0	0	110	5–10	100	25

and inconclusive results of a number of meta-analyses.[47–50] At present, the published data do not provide unequivocal support for either side of the debate. The only adequately powered trial to date, the Saline versus Albumin Fluid Evaluation Study, found that saline and albumin produced comparable outcomes in a heterogeneous population of adult patients.[51] Whether specific fluids are beneficial or harmful in more highly selected subpopulations of critically ill patients is not yet clear. A number of investigator-initiated trials are currently underway and are expected to report their results in the next few years. These trials may provide clinicians with the data needed to make rational fluid choices.

REFERENCES

1. Edelman IS, Leibman J. Anatomy of body water and electrolytes. *Am J Med* 1959; **27**: 25–77.
2. Gamble J. *Chemical Anatomy, Physiology and Pathology of Extracellular Fluid*. Cambridge, MA: Harvard University Press; 1954.
3. Moore FD, Olesen KH, McMurray JD. *Body Composition in Health and Disease*. Philadelphia: WB Saunders; 1963.
4. Bie P. Osmoreceptors, vasopressin, and control of renal water excretion. *Physiol Rev* 1980; **60**: 961–1048.
5. Humes HD. Disorders of water metabolism. In: Kokko JP, Tannen RL (eds) *Fluid and Electrolytes*. Philadelphia: WB Saunders; 1986: 118–49.
6. Phillips PJ. Water metabolism. *Anaesth Intensive Care* 1977; **5**: 295–304.
7. Intersalt Cooperative Research Group. Intersalt: an international study of electrolyte excretion and blood pressure. Results for 24 hour urinary sodium and potassium excretion. *BMJ* 1988; **297**: 319–28.
8. Weisberg LS. Pseudohyponatremia: a reappraisal. *Am J Med* 1989; **86**: 315–8.
9. Katz MA. Hyperglycemia-induced hyponatremia – calculation of expected serum sodium depression. *N Engl J Med* 1973; **289**: 843–4.
10. Arieff AI, Ayus JC. Endometrial ablation complicated by fatal hyponatremic encephalopathy. *JAMA* 1993; **270**: 1230–2.
11. Gravenstein D. Transurethral resection of the prostate (TURP) syndrome: a review of the pathophysiology and management. *Anesth Analg* 1997; **84**: 438–46.
12. Hahn RG. Fluid and electrolyte dynamics during development of the TURP syndrome. *Br J Urol* 1990; **66**: 79–84.
13. Ghanem AN, Ward JP. Osmotic and metabolic sequelae of volumetric overload in relation to the TURP syndrome. *Br J Urol* 1990; **66**: 71–8.
14. Jensen V. The TURP syndrome. *Can J Anaesth* 1991; **38**: 90–6.
15. Agarwal R, Emmett M. The post-transurethral resection of prostate syndrome: therapeutic proposals. *Am J Kidney Dis* 1994; **24**: 108–11.
16. Bartter FC, Schwartz WB. The syndrome of inappropriate secretion of antidiuretic hormone. *Am J Med* 1967; **42**: 790–806.
17. Reynolds RM, Padfield PL, Seckl JR. Disorders of sodium balance. *BMJ* 2006, **332**: 702–5.
18. Cort JH. Cerebral salt wasting. *Lancet* 1954; **266**: 752–4.
19. Singh S, Bohn D, Carlotti AP *et al.* Cerebral salt wasting: truths, fallacies, theories, and challenges. *Crit Care Med* 2002; **30**: 2575–9.
20. Rabinstein AA, Wijdicks EF. Hyponatremia in critically ill neurological patients. *Neurologist* 2003; **9**: 290–300.
21. Hasan D, Lindsay KW, Wijdicks EF *et al.* Effect of fludrocortisone acetate in patients with subarachnoid hemorrhage. *Stroke* 1989; **20**: 1156–61.
22. Sterns RH, Riggs JE, Schochet SS Jr. Osmotic demyelination syndrome following correction of hyponatremia. *N Engl J Med* 1986; **314**: 1535–42.
23. Martin RJ. Central pontine and extrapontine myelinolysis: the osmotic demyelination syndromes. *J Neurol Neurosurg Psychiatry* 2004; **75**(Suppl 3): iii, 22–8.
24. Bhardwaj A, Ulatowski JA. Hypertonic saline solutions in brain injury. *Curr Opin Crit Care* 2004; **10**: 126–31.
25. White H, Cook D, Venkatesh B. The use of hypertonic saline for treating intracranial hypertension after traumatic brain injury. *Anesth Analg* 2006; **102**: 1836–46.
26. Cooper DJ, Myles PS, McDermott FT *et al.* Prehospital hypertonic saline resuscitation of patients with hypotension and severe traumatic brain injury: a randomized controlled trial. *JAMA* 2004; **291**: 1350–7.
27. Yeates KE, Morton AR. Vasopressin antagonists: role in the management of hyponatremia. *Am J Nephrol* 2006; **26**: 348–55.
28. Palm C, Pistrosch F, Herbrig K *et al.* Vasopressin antagonists as aquaretic agents for the treatment of hyponatremia. *Am J Med* 2006; **119**(7 Suppl 1): S87–92.
29. Adrogue HJ, Madias NE. Hypernatremia. *N Engl J Med* 2000; **342**: 1493–9.
30. Worthley LI. Hyperosmolar coma treated with intravenous sterile water. A study of three cases. *Arch Intern Med* 1986; **146**: 945–7.
31. Sterns RH, Cox M, Feig PU *et al.* Internal potassium balance and the control of the plasma potassium concentration. *Medicine (Baltimore)* 1981; **60**: 339–54.
32. Phelan DM, Worthley LI. Hypokalaemic coma. *Intensive Care Med* 1985; **11**: 257–8.
33. Stockigt JR. Potassium metabolism. *Anaesth Intensive Care* 1977; **5**: 317–25.
34. American Heart Association Guidelines for Cardiopulmonary Resuscitation and Emergency Cardiovascular Care. Part 8: Stabilization of the patient with acute coronary syndromes. *Circulation* 2005; **112**(24 Suppl): IV-89–110.
35. American Heart Association Guidelines for Cardiopulmonary Resuscitation and Emergency Cardiovascular Care. Part 10.1: Life-threatening electrolyte abnormalities. *Circulation* 2005; **112**(24 Suppl): IV-121–5.
36. Thomas DW. Calcium, phosphorus and magnesium turnover. *Anaesth Intensive Care* 1977; **5**: 361–71.
37. Slomp J, van der Voort PH, Gerritsen RT *et al.* Albumin-adjusted calcium is not suitable for diagnosis of

hyper- and hypocalcemia in the critically ill. *Crit Care Med* 2003; **31**: 1389–93.

38. Bushinsky DA, Monk RD. Electrolyte quintet: calcium. *Lancet* 1998; **352**: 306–11.
39. Ariyan CE, Sosa JA. Assessment and management of patients with abnormal calcium. *Crit Care Med* 2004; **32**(4 Suppl): S146–54.
40. Weisinger JR, Bellorin-Font E. Magnesium and phosphorus. *Lancet* 1998; **352**: 391–6.
41. Altman D, Carroli G, Duley L *et al.* Do women with pre-eclampsia, and their babies, benefit from magnesium sulphate? The Magpie Trial: a randomised placebo-controlled trial. *Lancet* 2002; **359**: 1877–90.
42. Davey MJ, Teubner D. A randomized controlled trial of magnesium sulfate, in addition to usual care, for rate control in atrial fibrillation. *Ann Emerg Med* 2005; **45**: 347–53.
43. Henyan NN, Gillespie EL, White CM *et al.* Impact of intravenous magnesium on post-cardiothoracic surgery atrial fibrillation and length of hospital stay: a meta-analysis. *Ann Thorac Surg* 2005; **80**: 2402–6.
44. Rowe BH, Bretzlaff JA, Bourdon C *et al.* Intravenous magnesium sulfate treatment for acute asthma in the emergency department: a systematic review of the literature. *Ann Emerg Med* 2000; **36**: 181–90.
45. Hughes R, Goldkorn A, Masoli M *et al.* Use of isotonic nebulised magnesium sulphate as an adjuvant to salbutamol in treatment of severe asthma in adults: randomised placebo-controlled trial. *Lancet* 2003; **361**: 2114–17.
46. van den Bergh WM, Algra A, van Kooten F *et al.* Magnesium sulfate in aneurysmal subarachnoid hemorrhage: a randomized controlled trial. *Stroke* 2005; **36**: 1011–15.
47. Cochrane Injuries Group Albumin Reviewers. Human albumin administration in critically ill patients: systematic review of randomised controlled trials. *BMJ* 1998; **317**: 235–40.
48. Vincent JL, Navickis RJ, Wilkes MM. Morbidity in hospitalized patients receiving human albumin: a meta-analysis of randomized, controlled trials. *Crit Care Med* 2004; **32**: 2029–38.
49. The Albumin Reviewers. Human albumin solution for resuscitation and volume expansion in critically ill patients. *Cochrane Database Syst Rev* 2004; (4): CD001208, pub2.
50. Roberts I, Alderson P, Bunn F *et al.* Colloids versus crystalloids for fluid resuscitation in critically ill patients. *Cochrane Database Syst Rev* 2004; CD000567.
51. The SAFE Study Investigators. A comparison of albumin and saline for fluid resuscitation in the intensive care unit. *N Engl J Med* 2004; **350**: 2247–56.

86

Metabolic response to injury and infection

Ian K S Tan

Injury and infection evoke in the host a hypermetabolic inflammatory response and a compensatory hypometabolic hypoimmune response. The magnitude of the response is proportional to the extent of injury. Additional components of illness, such as ischaemia and reperfusion or resuscitation, nutritional status, surgical procedures, transfusions, drugs and anaesthetic techniques, genetic polymorphisms and concurrent diseases, impact on the response. Some components of the metabolic response, or the failure to regulate the response, are destructive, and its modulation may improve patient survival.[1]

MEDIATORS OF THE METABOLIC RESPONSE

Following directed adhesion to endothelium and migration into tissue, neutrophils undergo an oxidative burst, producing a large variety of free radicals (species with one or more unpaired electrons) and reactive oxygen species (ROS), overwhelming natural scavenging and antioxidant defences, such as superoxide dismutase and glutathione peroxidase. These free radicals and ROS directly damage cells. Proteases, arachidonic acid metabolites (leukotrienes, thromboxanes and prostaglandins) and adhesion molecules are produced, amplifying the inflammatory cascade. Inducible nitric oxide synthase is activated, and nitric oxide is produced. Tissue macrophages become primed and activated.

CYTOKINES

Cytokines are soluble, non-antibody, regulatory proteins released from the activated immunocytes, and are responsible primarily for the inflammatory and counter-inflammatory response. Injury and infection cause cytokine release from activated leukocytes, endothelial cells and fibroblasts. T-helper type 1 (TH1) lymphocytes primarily impact cell-mediated immunity and secrete tumour necrosis factor-α (TNF-α), interleukin-2 (IL-2) and interferon-γ (IFN-γ), while TH2 lymphocytes impact antibody-mediated immunity and secrete IL-4 and IL-10. The TH1/TH2 cytokine profile determines the immunostimulatory/immunosuppressive balance. Cytokines generally exert their effects in a paracrine fashion, but in severe injury and infection, they enter the circulation and act as hormones. The following are major cytokines involved in the response to stress:

- TNF-α is a necessary and sufficient proximal mediator. After endotoxin challenge, TNF-α concentrations peak before other mediators. TNF-α administration reproduces all features of septic shock, including hypermetabolism, fever, anorexia, hyperglycaemia, decreased lipogenesis, marked protein catabolism and lactic acidosis. TNF-α activates the hypothalamic–pituitary–adrenal (HPA) axis. Soluble TNF-α receptors, a natural antagonist to TNF-α, also increase; this may be a regulatory response which contributes to later immunosuppression.
- IL-1β (endogenous pyrogen) produces much the same metabolic effects as TNF-α, and the combined effect of the two cytokines is greater than the effect of either alone. IL-1β is a potent inducer of the HPA axis as well as central and peripheral noradrenergic neurons. IL-6 is the main mediator of the acute phase response. Similar to TNF-α and IL-1β, IL-6 levels correlate with severity of illness and outcome. IL-8 induces neutrophil adhesion, chemotaxis and enzyme release. IL-2 generation is decreased. Anti-inflammatory cytokine (IL-4, IL-10, transforming growth factor-β) and antagonist (IL-1 receptor antagonist) levels increase. IL-4 activates B lymphocytes.
- Colony-stimulating factors stimulate the proliferation of haemopoietic cells, superoxide and cytokine production by neutrophils and macrophages. Disproportionate monocytopoiesis over granulocytopoiesis occurs. Erythropoietin production is suppressed.
- IFN-γ stimulates fibroproliferation, upregulates TNF receptors and induces TNF synthesis. IFN-γ production is synergistically induced by IL-12 and IL-18. IFN-α/β secretion is induced in viral infections and is proinflammatory.
- High mobility group box 1 (HMGB1) is a late pro-inflammatory mediator. It induces the expression of adhesion molecules in endothelial cells, increases enterocyte permeability, and further release of pro-inflammatory cytokines from leukocytes.
- Counter-inflammatory cytokines accumulate at the site of injury. Prostaglandin E_2 inhibits further synthesis of inflammatory cytokines, and spermine inhibits

their release. Transforming growth factor-β inhibits monocyte activation.

NEUROENDOCRINE MEDIATORS

Cytokine release from the site of injury or infection triggers vagal afferent impulses to the dorsal vagal complex (DVC) in the medulla oblongata. Synaptic connections with the rostroventral medulla and locus ceruleus, and the hypothalamic nuclei, activate the sympathetic nervous system and the HPA axis respectively.[2] High circulating cytokine levels may also cross the blood–brain barrier, or affect neurons at circumventricular organs lacking a blood–brain barrier, such as the area postrema. In general, a biphasic response is observed following injury and infection: an initial neuroendocrine 'storm' followed by a decrease. The following are some neuroendocrine mediators involved in the response to stress:

- *Reflex vagal efferent nerves* secrete acetylcholine, which by binding to α_7 subunits of the nicotinic receptor, suppresses proinflammatory cytokine synthesis from immunocytes.
- *Reflex sympathetic efferents* increase catecholamine levels, causing tachycardia and calorigenesis with increased oxygen consumption. Blood flow redistribution occurs depending on tissue receptor balance. Glycogenolysis, gluconeogenesis and lipolysis are stimulated. Activation of β_2-adrenergic receptors decreases synthesis of proinflammatory cytokines and increases the synthesis of anti-inflammatory cytokines. However, α_2-adrenoreceptor activation may increase TNF production.
- *HPA axis* activation results in high adrenocorticotropin hormone (ACTH) and cortisol levels, driving gluconeogenesis, proteolysis and lipolysis. Primarily by suppressing the nuclear factor (NF)-κB pathway, cortisol attenuates damage from excessive proinflammatory cytokine synthesis, while activating synthesis of anti-inflammatory IL-4 and IL-10. With prolonged critical illness, ACTH levels fall, but cortisol remains elevated with persistent loss of diurnal variation in secretion. Corticosteroid-binding globulin levels fall, and free cortisol levels may be increased. TNF decreases glucocorticoid response, and peripheral glucocorticoid resistance may vary between tissues.
- *Growth hormone* (GH) levels increase acutely with increased pulsatile frequency, but concomitant peripheral GH resistance occurs initially with low levels of GH-binding protein (GHBP) and insulin-like growth factor (IGF-1). Levels of the inversely regulated IGF-binding protein (IGFBP-1) increase, which correlates with mortality. Subsequently, loss of hypothalamic stimulation, as well as decreased ghrelin (a potent growth hormone secretagogue) levels, causes greatly reduced GH burst amplitudes, but peripheral GH sensitivity recovers.[3]
- *The thyroid axis* behaves in a similar fashion, with transient increases in thyrotropin (TSH) and thyroxine (T_4) levels, and reduced conversion of T_4 to tri-iodothyronine (T_3). Chronically, reduced thyrotrophin-releasing hormone (TRH) secretion leads to low/normal levels and pulsatility in TSH, low T_4 levels and further falls in T_3 levels, termed the 'sick euthyroid syndrome'.
- *Prolactin* (PRL) levels increase transiently, followed by reduced pulsatile amplitudes. As T-lymphocyte function is prolactin-dependent, this contributes to late loss of immune competence.
- *Luteinising hormone* (LH) levels increase transiently, followed by reduced pulsatile amplitudes. Low testosterone and high estradiol levels occur.[4] Dehydroepiandrosterone levels are low. Estrogens inhibit proinflammatory cytokine production.
- *α-Melanocyte stimulating hormone* (α-MSH) levels increase, leading to immunosuppression via inhibition of the NF-κB pathway.
- *Insulin and glucagon* levels are increased but the insulin levels are inappropriately low for the level of hyperglycaemia. Insulin resistance is characterised by impaired glycogen synthesis. The increased glucagon: insulin ratio augments gluconeogenesis. Insulin has anti-inflammatory properties by inhibiting the NF-κB pathway, and prevents mitochondrial ultrastructural abnormalities, possibly by inhibiting hyperglycaemia-induced production of superoxide. Leptin levels increase acutely, then decrease.
- *Procalcitonin* levels increase and remain high, and its level correlates with severity of illness, so that procalcitonin has become a useful marker of systemic infection and a guide to therapy. Calcitonin levels, however, are variable and not necessarily elevated. Of the other members of the calcitonin superfamily, calcitonin gene-related peptide (CGRP) and adrenomedullin levels greatly increase; they are anti-inflammatory and contribute to vasodilatation.
- *The renin–angiotensin–aldosterone axis* is activated, causing fluid retention. Subsequently, aldosterone levels fall while renin remains elevated.
- *Arginine vasopressin* (AVP) levels increase initially, then return to normal or low levels despite persistent shock, in part due to depletion of stored hormone. Downregulation of V_1 receptors (which mediate AVP's vasoconstricting effect) occurs in sepsis.
- *Vasoactive intestinal peptide* secretion is induced, probably by nitric oxide, inhibiting production of proinflammatory cytokines and stimulating secretion of IL-10.

THE METABOLIC RESPONSE

The metabolic response to injury and infection begins with the activation of receptors throughout the body by the above mediators. These receptors include toll-like receptors (TLR)-2 and TLR-4, and the receptor for advanced glycation end products (RAGE). Subsequent intracellular activation of the NF-κB pathway leads to gene induction and production of mRNA for the synthesis of proinflammatory cytokines. Catecholamines can initiate rapid functional changes via protein phosphorylation, which does not require gene induction. Behavioural effects such as anorexia, possibly due to elevated leptin levels, also affect the metabolic response. The metabolic effects may be described at three levels.

CELLULAR METABOLIC EVENTS

Intracellularly, heat shock protein (HSP) synthesis is induced. Many HSPs are also expressed constitutively. HSPs act as 'chaperones', assisting in the assembly, disassembly, stabilisation and internal transport of other intracellular proteins. HSPs facilitate translocation of the glucocorticoid-receptor complex from the cytosol to the nucleus, and inhibit NF-κB activity. HSPs have cellular protective roles in sepsis and ischaemia-reperfusion.[5]

Mitochondrial dysfunction limits cell metabolism and may be responsible for the ensuing multiorgan dysfunction of severe injury and infection. Electron transport chain complexes are inhibited by excessive nitric oxide and peroxynitrite generated during sepsis.[6] Additionally, poly (ADP-ribose) polymerase-1 (PARP-1) is activated, reducing cell nicotinamide adenine dinucleotide (NADH) content, a substrate for ATP generation. The reduced ATP production may have functional consequences, such as diaphragmatic dysfunction.[7] It has been hypothesised that this 'metabolic shutdown' is an adaptive response similar to hibernation.[8]

Apoptosis, or programmed cell death, may finally be induced when death receptors are engaged by their ligands, or by mitochondrial-mediated pathways.[9] Death receptors include Fas and TNF receptor type I (TNFRI), and this pathway activates caspase. The mitochondrial pathway, mediated in part by glycogen synthase kinase-3β activation, causes activation of caspase. Caspases 8 and 9 activate caspase 3, which commits the cell to death. TNF-α, IL-10, cortisol and nitric oxide all induce apoptosis. Apoptosis further augments immunosuppression. It is probable that bioenergetic failure and the apoptotic death of immune cells are the major causes of death in late sepsis.

INTERMEDIARY METABOLISM

Protein metabolism: IL-1, TNF, related cytokines and hormonal changes trigger an extreme protein catabolism. Glutamine, alanine and other amino acids are mobilised from skeletal muscle and taken up by hepatocytes and gut mucosa. Glutamine depletion may occur. Increased ureagenesis and nitrogen loss occurs. Levels of branch chained amino acids (leucine, isoleucine, valine) fall with peripheral oxidation. The fraction of energy expenditure derived from glucose is reduced, while that derived from amino acid oxidation in the Krebs cycle is increased.

Carbohydrate metabolism: hyperglycaemia results from glycogenolysis, accelerated gluconeogenesis and peripheral insulin resistance. Lactate production increases from peripheral tissue, areas of injury and the white cell mass, and serves as substrate for gluconeogenesis in hepatocytes. In the terminal phase of severe illness, hypoglycaemia may occur.

Fat metabolism: lipolysis is increased with increased turnover of triglycerides and fatty acids, and plasma free fatty acid levels are high. TNF, IL-1 and IL-6 decrease lipoprotein lipase activity, contributing to hypertriglyceridaemia. Both high- and low-density lipoprotein (HDL and LDL) cholesterol levels are low. Ketosis is suppressed, indicating that fat is not a major calorie source. Glycerol generated from lipolysis further contributes to gluconeogenesis. The action of cyclooxygenase and lipoxygenase on arachidonic acid (a tissue phospholipid) produces inflammatory leukotrienes, thromboxanes and prostaglandin E_2.

Electrolyte and micronutrient metabolism: salt and water retention occurs, with hyponatraemia, masking the loss of lean tissue. Protein loss is accompanied by potassium, magnesium and phosphate loss. Serum hypocalcaemia with increased intracellular calcium commonly occurs. Zn redistributes to liver and bone marrow. Zn deficiency is associated with impaired IL-2 production and wound healing. Selenium levels are low and correlate with mortality. Selenium is required by glutathione peroxidases and thioredoxin reductases to prevent oxidative damage. Fe levels decrease.

SYSTEMIC PROTEIN SYSTEM RESPONSES

The acute phase response is a systemic response to injury characterised by redirection of hepatic protein synthesis and haematological alterations. Production of proteins involved in defence is increased (protease inhibitors, fibrinogen, C-reactive protein, haptoglobulin, complement C3), while synthesis of serum transport and binding molecules is reduced (albumin, transferrin). Serum levels of acute phase reactants such as C-reactive protein can be used for diagnostic, monitoring and prognostic purposes.

Complement cascade triggering produces the membrane attack complex, chemoattractants (C3a, C5a), vasoactive anaphylatoxins (C3a, C4a, C5a), opsonins (C3b), stimulation of neutrophil and monocyte oxidative burst (C3b) and neutrophil adherence to endothelium (C5a).

TNF-α induces the expression of tissue factor on leukocyte and endothelial cell surfaces, triggering the coagulation cascade. Depletion of endogenous anticoagulants such as antithrombin, protein C, and tissue factor pathway inhibitor (TFPI) occurs. In turn, activated coagulation factors amplify inflammation.

FACTORS AFFECTING THE METABOLIC RESPONSE

ENERGY BALANCE AND OXYGEN DELIVERY

Hypermetabolism increases oxygen demand and consumption. Capillary permeability increases, causing reduced intravascular filling, and inadequate oxygen delivery can lead to anaerobic metabolism and inadequate production of high-energy phosphates. In adequately resuscitated patients, aerobic glycolysis with lactate production rather than anaerobic glycolysis is characteristic of the metabolic response to stress.[10] Subsequent cell swelling from injury and resuscitation activates phospholipase A_2, augmenting the inflammatory cascade.[11]

SURGICAL PROCEDURES AND ANAESTHETIC TECHNIQUES

Total afferent neuronal blockade (somatic and autonomic block) (e.g. by epidural anaesthesia), and minimally invasive surgery, both of which greatly attenuate the metabolic changes of surgical injury, have been associated with reduced morbidity.[12,13] Improved analgesia, avoidance of endotracheal intubation and maintenance of consciousness may also contribute to the effect.

STARVATION AND NUTRITION

Starvation alone produces adaptive hypometabolism with the use of fat as the primary fuel, sparing protein. In contrast, injury and infection result in hypermetabolism with prominent protein catabolism. Starvation in combination with the metabolic changes of stress produces a hypoalbuminaemic malnourished state. Malnutrition clearly contributes to morbidity and mortality. However, current forms of nutrition do not adequately reduce protein catabolism or promote protein synthesis, so that a positive energy balance often results in fat and fluid gain instead.[14]

DRUGS AND DISEASE

Adverse effects of steroids include increased infection rates and myopathy (particularly in conjunction with the use of neuromuscular blocking drugs). Commonly used intensive care unit (ICU) drugs such as the catecholamines, dopamine, corticosteroids, theophylline, calcium-channel blockers, antibiotics and blood transfusions all have immunomodulatory effects. Diseases such as diabetes will clearly impact on the metabolic response to stress. Apart from concurrent disease, the inciting organism may itself modulate its host response by affecting cytokine mediators, their production, secretion and elimination, or by interacting with their receptors.[15]

GENETIC POLYMORPHISMS

From epidemiological studies, a large genetic influence on the outcome of sepsis can be found.[16] Unfortunately, studies on specific genetic polymorphisms involving mediators of the metabolic response have generally been underpowered, and the evidence is conflicting.

SECONDARY INSULTS

Secondary insults, such as device-related sepsis, the use of bioincompatible membranes for renal support, mechanical ventilator-induced lung injury, pain and hypothermia, will increase the severity and duration of the metabolic response.

VALUE OF THE METABOLIC RESPONSE

The cytokines and neuroendocrine mediators reprioritise metabolic processes, increasing the supply of substrates to active tissues involved in defence against injury. Inflammation localises the area of injury. Cardiovascular changes divert blood flow to inflamed areas and vital organs, while salt and water retention maintains overall perfusion. Sympathectomised and adrenalectomised animals fare poorly when stressed. Etomidate, which blocks cortisol synthesis, was associated with increased mortality when used for ICU sedation.[17]

Disadvantages of the metabolic response include increased oxygen consumption and myocardial work, which is detrimental to patients with marginal cardiovascular reserves. The redistribution of blood flow away from the 'non-vital' gut organ may result in translocation of bacteria and endotoxin into the circulation. High catecholamine levels are arrhythmogenic to the compromised heart. Systemic inflammation can result in systemic tissue destruction. Hyperglycaemia is associated with an increased incidence of infection.

MODULATING THE METABOLIC RESPONSE

Modulation of the metabolic response in order to accelerate recovery and improve morbidity and mortality is an expanding area of research. Large multicentre trials have failed to show consistent benefits with therapies targeted at specific cytokine components of the metabolic response to infection. This has led to the development of therapies providing non-specific suppression or elimination of circulating mediators, or monitoring the state of 'immunologic dissonance' in order to provide individualised therapy.

Antioxidants show promise in improving survival. The substitution of omega-3 fatty acids for omega-6 fatty acids in inflammatory mediators modulates the metabolic response. Clinically, enteral nutrition with eicosapentaenoic acid (EPA or fish oil), γ-linolenic acid (GLA or borage oil) and antioxidant vitamins[18] has been shown to reduce mortality. Selenium prevents excessive oxidative damage, but was not shown to reduce mortality when supplemented in pharmacological doses, and a larger trial is needed.[19] Ethyl pyruvate is another promising antioxidant able to directly neutralise peroxides and peroxynitrite non-enzymatically. Statins decrease the activation of the NF-κB pathway, and inhibit superoxide production. Experimentally, statins have been shown to prolong survival time in sepsis,[20] but randomised controlled trials in humans are required.[21]

Protein catabolism leading to loss of muscle has functional consequences such as respiratory muscle weakness. A 25% body weight loss in the presence of injury may be fatal. Wound healing and multiple facets of host defence are impaired, increasing the risk of nosocomial infection. Parenteral glutamine supplementation has been reported to reduce mortality.[22] Of the anabolic agents (GH, IGF-1 and testosterone derivatives), GH has received the most attention in the setting of critical illness. GH increased mortality in a heterogeneous group of critically ill patients.[23] It is possible that patient selection, unmasking of glutamine deficiency and high GH doses (mean 0.1 mg/kg per day) resulted in the adverse outcome. Combined GH, IGF-1 and glutamine-supplemented parenteral nutrition has been shown to produce net protein gain.[24]

'Intensive insulin therapy' to attain a glucose of 4.4–6.1 mmol resulted in significant prevention of acute renal failure, and shortened time to weaning from mechanical ventilatory support.[25] The mortality benefit shown in a previous trial could not be corroborated. Frequent hypoglycaemia may accompany the technique and further studies are underway.

A meta-analysis of steroid usage in septic shock found that high-dose steroids given over a short time increased mortality, while lower doses of hydrocortisone for 5–7 days and subsequently tapered resulted in improvement in survival and shock reversal.[26] In the largest trial, the benefit was found only in patients who had a less than 9 μg/dl increase in cortisol after 250 μg tetracosactrin intravenously.[27] Given the difficulties in free cortisol kinetics and definition of 'relative adrenal insufficiency' in the critically ill, this finding requires external validation.

The extracellular fluid is the aqueous medium within which the mediators of the metabolic response function, so that blood purification may modulate the intensity of the metabolic response and hence influence outcome. A randomised trial of 425 ICU patients with acute renal failure to ultrafiltration doses of 20 ml/hour per kg, 35 ml/hour per kg and 45 ml/hour per kg by continuous veno-venous haemofiltration resulted in survival at 15 days after treatment discontinuation of 41%, 57% and 58% respectively.[28] Extension of the above approach leads to the inference that high volume haemofiltration (i.e. intensive plasma water exchange) may further improve survival.[29]

In an initial trial, activated protein C (APC) was found to reduce 28-day mortality in patients with severe sepsis. Longer term follow-up did not reveal an overall improvement in survival, although the study was not powered to detect this end-point.[30] In less severely ill patients, APC did not influence outcome, and increased the rates of serious bleeding.[31] APC is not indicated in paediatric severe sepsis.

The most logical approach is to monitor the host response so as to provide individualised therapy. Although IFN-γ did not reduce infection or mortality in burns patients,[32] it is hypothesised that monitoring HLA-DR expression may be used to identify immunosuppressed patients who may benefit most from IFN-γ.[33]

REFERENCES

1. Russell JA. Management of sepsis. *N Engl J Med* 2006; **355**: 1699–713.
2. Webster JI, Tonelli L, Sternberg EM. Neuroendocrine regulation of immunity. *Annu Rev Immunol* 2002; **20**: 125–63.
3. Van den Berghe G, de Zegher F, Bouillon R. Acute and prolonged critical illness as different neuroendocrine paradigms. *J Clin Endocrinol Metab* 1998; **83**: 1827–34.
4. Van den Berghe G, Baxter RC, Weekers F *et al.* A paradoxical gender dissociation within the growth hormone/insulin-like growth factor I axis during protracted critical illness. *J Clin Endocrinol Metab* 2000; **85**: 183–92.
5. Bruemmer-Smith S, Stubber F, Schroeder S. Protective functions of intracellular heat-shock protein (HSP) 70-expression in patients with severe sepsis. *Intensive Care Med* 2001; **27**: 1835–41.
6. Boulos M, Astiz ME, Barua RS *et al.* Impaired mitochondrial function induced by serum from septic shock patients is attenuated by inhibition of nitric oxide synthase and poly(ADP-ribose) synthase. *Crit Care Med* 2003; **31**: 353–8.
7. Callahan LA, Supinski GS. Sepsis induces diaphragm electron transport chain dysfunction and protein depletion. *Am J Respir Crit Care Med* 2005; **172**: 861–8.
8. Singer M, De Santis V, Vitale D *et al.* Multiorgan failure is an adaptive, endocrine mediated, metabolic response to overwhelming systemic inflammation. *Lancet* 2004; **364**: 545–8.
9. Hotchkiss RS, Osmon SB, Chang KC *et al.* Accelerated lymphocyte death in sepsis occurs by both the death receptor and mitochondrial pathways. *J Immunol* 2005; **174**: 5110–8.
10. Levy B, Gibot S, Franck P *et al.* Relation between muscle Na^+/K^+ ATPase activity and raised lactate concentrations in septic shock: a prospective study. *Lancet* 2005; **365**: 871–5.
11. Cotton B, Guy J, Morris J *et al.* The cellular, metabolic, and systemic consequences of aggressive fluid resuscitation strategies. *Shock* 2006; **26**: 115–21.
12. Rodgers A, Walker N, Schug S *et al.* Reduction of postoperative mortality and morbidity with epidural or spinal anaesthesia: results from overview of randomised trials. *BMJ* 2000; **321**: 1493–7.
13. Lacy AM, Garcia-Valdecasas JC, Delgado S *et al.* Laparoscopy-assisted colectomy versus open colectomy for treatment of non-metastatic colon cancer: a randomised trial. *Lancet* 2002; **359**: 2224–9.
14. Hart DW, Wolf SE, Herndon DN *et al.* Energy expenditure and caloric balance after burn. Increased feeding leads to fat rather than lean mass accretion. *Ann Surg* 2002; **235**: 152–61.
15. Wilson M, Seymour R, Henderson B. Bacterial perturbation of cytokine networks. *Infect Immunol* 1998; **66**: 2401–9.
16. Sørensen T, Nielsen G, Andersen P *et al.* Genetic and environmental influences on premature death in adult adoptees. *N Engl J Med* 1988; **318**: 727–32.

17. Watt I, Ledingham IM. Mortality amongst multiple trauma patients admitted to an intensive therapy unit. *Anaesthesia* 1984; **39**: 973–81.
18. Pontes-Arruda A, Aragao A, Albuquerque J. Effects of enteral feeding with eicosapentaenoic acid, γ-linolenic acid, and antioxidants in mechanically ventilated patients with severe sepsis and septic shock. *Crit Care Med* 2006; **34**: 2325–33.
19. Angstwurm M, Engelmann L, Zimmermann T *et al.* Selenium in Intensive Care (SIC) study. Results of a prospective randomized, placebo-controlled, multiple-center study in patients with severe systemic inflammatory response syndrome, sepsis, and septic shock. *Crit Care Med* 2007; **35**: 118–26.
20. Merx M, Liehn E, Graf J *et al.* Statin treatment after onset of sepsis in a murine model improves survival. *Circulation* 2005; **112**: 117–24.
21. Majumdar S, McAlister F, Eurich D *et al.* Statins and outcomes in patients admitted to hospital with community acquired pneumonia: population based prospective cohort study. *BMJ* 2006; 333; 999.
22. Novak F, Heyland DK, Avenell A *et al.* Glutamine supplementation in serious illness: a systematic review of the evidence. *Crit Care Med* 2002; **30**: 2022–9.
23. Takala J, Ruokonen E, Webster N *et al.* Increased mortality associated with growth hormone treatment in critically ill adults. *N Engl J Med* 1999; **341**: 785–92.
24. Carroll P, Jackson N, Russell-Jones D *et al.* Combined growth hormone/insulin-like growth factor I in addition to glutamine-supplemented TPN results in net protein anabolism in critical illness.*Am J Physiol Endocrinol Metab* 2004; **286**: 151–7.
25. Van den Berghe G, Wilmer A, Hermans G *et al.* Intensive insulin therapy in the medical ICU. *N Engl J Med* 2006; **354**: 449–61.
26. Minneci P, Deans K, Banks S *et al.* Meta-analysis: the effect of steroids on survival and shock during sepsis depends on the dose. *Ann Intern Med* 2004; **141**: 47–56.
27. Annane D, Sebille V, Charpentier C *et al.* Effect of treatment with low doses of hydrocortisone and fludrocortisone on mortality in patients with septic shock. *JAMA* 2002; **288**: 862–71.
28. Ronco C, Bellomo R, Homel P *et al.* Effects of different doses in continuous veno-venous haemofiltration on outcomes of acute renal failure: a prospective randomised trial. *Lancet* 2000; **355**: 26–30.
29. Ratanarat R, Brendolan A, Piccinni P *et al.* Pulse high-volume haemofiltration for treatment of severe sepsis: effects on hemodynamics and survival. *Critical Care* 2005; **9**: R294–302.
30. Angus D, Laterre P, Helterbrand J *et al.* The effect of drotrecogin alfa (activated) on long term survival after severe sepsis. *Crit Care Med* 2006; **32**: 2199–206.
31. Abraham E, Laterre P, Garg R *et al.* Drotrecogin alfa (activated) for adults with severe sepsis and a low risk of death. *N Engl J Med* 2005; **353**: 1332–41.
32. Wasserman D, Ioannovich JD, Hinzmann RD *et al.* Interferon-gamma in the prevention of severe burns-related infections: a European phase III clinical trial. *Crit Care Med* 1998; **26**: 434–9.
33. Docke WD, Hoflich C, Davis K *et al.* Monitoring temporary immunodepression by flow cytometric measurement of monocytic HLA-DR expression: a multicenter standardized study. *Clin Chem* 2005; **51**: 2341–7.

87

Enteral and parenteral nutrition

Richard Leonard

It is standard practice to provide nutritional support to critically ill patients, in order to

- treat existing malnutrition
- minimise wasting of lean body mass

However, despite the universality of this practice, the evidence underlying it is often conflicting and of disappointingly poor quality.[1] The failings in the evidence seem to extend to some of the resulting debates, in which certainty appears inversely proportional to justification.[2] Inevitably, these difficulties have led many to seek clarity in meta-analysis; perhaps equally inevitably,[3] they have usually been disappointed. On so basic a question as the relative merits of enteral and parenteral routes of feeding, the two most recent meta-analyses have produced conflicting results.[4,5] Instead of choosing on which trials to base patient care, it seems the clinician must now decide which meta-analysis to believe.

The problem persists with the publication of numerous clinical practice guidelines,[6–11] which differ in important areas, although one at least has been used in a cluster randomised trial showing a 10% reduction in mortality that just failed to reach statistical significance in those intensive care units (ICUs) randomised to use the guideline – the ACCEPT study.[6] While such validation does not mean that each component of the ACCEPT guideline (Figure 87.1) is optimal, it does at least provide some support.

NUTRITIONAL ASSESSMENT

Objective assessment of nutritional status is difficult in ICU, because disease processes confound methods used in the general population. Anthropometric measures such as triceps skin-fold thickness and mid-arm circumference may be obscured by oedema. Voluntary handgrip strength, a test of functional capacity, is impractical in unconscious patients. Laboratory measures, including transferrin, pre-albumin and albumin levels, lymphocyte counts and skin-prick test reactivity, are abnormal in critical illness. Clinical evaluation – the so-called Subjective Global Assessment – is better than objective measurement at predicting morbidity.[12] Historical features of malnutrition include weight loss, poor diet, gastrointestinal symptoms, reduced functional capacity and a diagnosis associated with poor intake. Physical signs include loss of subcutaneous fat, muscle wasting, peripheral oedema and ascites.

While laboratory measures are of little value in assessing nutritional status in critically ill patients, intensivists are increasingly involved in preoperative assessment of patients undergoing major surgery. In these patients the serum albumin and operative site were closely associated with the risk of postoperative complications.[13] This raises the possibility that outcomes may be improved by treating preoperative malnutrition identified by a simple screening test.

PATIENT SELECTION AND TIMING OF SUPPORT

There are reasonable grounds to believe that it is better to provide nutritional support to critically ill patients than not to do so. This belief is based on the close association between malnutrition, negative nitrogen and calorie balance and poor outcome, and the inevitability of death if starvation continues for long enough. In otherwise healthy humans this takes several weeks to occur. There is also some direct evidence from small studies of parenteral nutrition in patients with severe head injuries[14] and of jejunal feeding in those operated on for severe pancreatitis,[15] in which the control groups received little or no nutritional support. Both studies showed decreased mortality in the groups receiving adequate nutrition.

Two questions arise from this, relating to the important problem of when nutritional support should start:

- How long is it safe to leave a critically ill patient without nutrition? In other words, which patients need to be fed artificially because they will be starved for too long, and which can safely wait until they are able to eat?
- If the patient will clearly exceed whatever period is deemed reasonable, is it better to begin feeding immediately? In other words, when should we start to feed?

Quite good evidence now supports the early institution of nutritional support, and the trend is both to tolerate

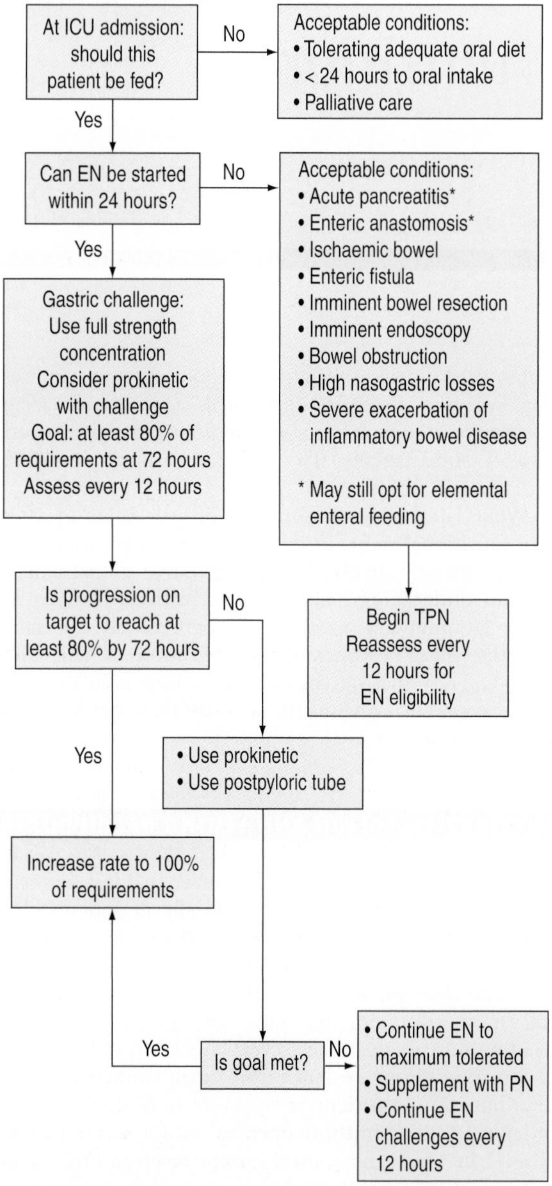

Figure 87.1 Algorithm for nutritional support used in the ACCEPT trial.[6] EN, enteral nutrition, PN, parenteral nutrition.

much shorter periods without nutrition and to begin feeding more rapidly after initial resuscitation.

In 1997, recommendations from a conference sponsored by the US National Institutes of Health, the American Society for Parenteral and Enteral Nutrition and the American Society for Clinical Nutrition suggested that nutritional support be started in any critically ill patient unlikely to regain oral intake within 7–10 days.[10] The basis for this was that at a typical nitrogen loss of 20–40 g/day dangerous depletion of lean tissue may occur after 14 days of starvation. Others have suggested a maximum acceptable delay of 7 days. A meta-analysis comparing early (first 48 hours after admission to ICU) with late enteral feeding revealed a reduction in infectious complications.[16] Two subsequent meta-analyses comparing early enteral feeding with no artificial nutritional support, and early parenteral feeding with delayed enteral feeding, both found a reduction in mortality with early support.[17] Finally, early institution of enteral feeding was an important component of the ACCEPT study guideline.[6] Patients in this study received nutritional support if they were thought unlikely to tolerate oral intake in the next 24 hours, and the goal was to start feeding within 24 hours of admission to ICU. The weight of evidence is presently in favour of this more aggressive approach.[18]

NUTRITIONAL REQUIREMENTS OF THE CRITICALLY ILL

ENERGY

Some muscle wasting and nitrogen loss are unavoidable in critical illness, despite adequate energy and protein provision.[19] This fact, coupled with the realisation that caloric requirements had previously been overestimated, has led to downward revision of intake, a process which may still be ongoing. In 1997, the American College of Chest Physicians (ACCP) published guidelines recommending a daily energy intake of 25 kcal/kg,[9] and this has remained the standard target energy intake for critically ill patients. More recently, concerns have been raised that this may be excessive. An observational study found lower mortality in those patients who received 9–18 kcal/kg/day than in those with higher and lower intakes.[20] However, meaningful benefits of hypocaloric feeding have yet to be demonstrated in prospective trials. It is, moreover, extremely important to realise that enterally fed patients frequently fail to achieve their target intake, and that significant underfeeding is certainly associated with worse outcomes.[20–22]

Attempts have also been made to tailor the energy provided to critically ill patients to their individual needs. Two methods are commonly used, indirect calorimetry and predictive equations.

Indirect calorimetry is the gold standard, and its use is becoming easier with the availability of devices designed for ICU patients. It permits measurement of the resting energy expenditure (REE). This value excludes the energy cost of physical activity, which increases later in the course of an ICU admission.[23] Calorimetry reveals deviations from values predicted by equations, such that two thirds of patients in one study were being either under- or overfed.[24] On the other hand, it could not be shown that outcomes are improved by the use of calorimetry.[25] Moreover, there are no clear data to relate measured REE to total energy expenditure in the individual patient. As a result, many units do not use calorimetry; in those that do, a target energy provision of 1.3 × measured REE is usual.[22]

There are a large number of equations claiming to predict basal metabolic rate (BMR) on the basis of weight, sex and age. The best known is the Harris–Benedict equation, which dates back more than 80 years. Schofield's equations were derived anew in the 1980s.[26] Correction factors exist to convert predictions of BMR into estimated energy expenditure by adjusting for such variables as diagnosis, pyrexia and activity. In the past these correction factors have been excessive and may have contributed to overfeeding; a more conservative approach is now advocated. The recommendations of the British Association for Parenteral and Enteral Nutrition are:[27]

1. Determine BMR from Schofield equations (Table 87.1)
2. Adjust BMR for stress (Table 87.2)
3. Add a combined factor for activity and diet-induced thermogenesis
   bed-bound, immobile +10%
   bed-bound, mobile/sitting +20%
   mobile around ward +25%

Despite the popularity of measurements or estimates of energy expenditure it is not clear that their routine use improves outcome. Many clinicians dispense with both and simply aim to deliver the ACCP's recommended target of 25 kcal/kg per day.

Table 87.1 Basal metabolic rate in kcal/day by age and gender[26]

Age	Female	Male
15–18	13.3 W + 690	17.6 W + 656
18–30	14.8 W + 485	15.0 W + 690
30–60	8.1 W + 842	11.4 W + 870
> 60	9.0 W + 656	11.7 W + 585

W = weight in kg.

Table 87.2 Stress adjustment in the calculation of basal metabolic rate[27]

Partial starvation (>10% weight loss)	Subtract 0–15%
Mild infection, inflammatory bowel disease, postoperative	Add 0–13%
Moderate infection, multiple long bone fractures	Add 10–30%
Severe sepsis, multiple trauma (ventilated)	Add 25–50%
Burns 10–90%	Add 10–70%

PROTEIN

Assessment of nitrogen balance by measuring urinary urea nitrogen is too variable to be useful in estimating protein requirements in ICU.[28] As there is an upper limit to the amount of dietary protein that can be used for synthesis,[29] there is no benefit from replacing nitrogen lost in excess of this. A daily nitrogen provision of 0.15–0.2 g/kg per day is therefore recommended for the ICU population; this is equivalent to 1–1.25 g protein/kg per day. Severely hypercatabolic individuals, such as those with major burns, are given up to 0.3 g nitrogen/kg per day, or nearly 2 g protein/kg per day.[27]

MICRONUTRIENTS

Critical illness increases the requirements for vitamins A, E, K, thiamine (B_1), B_3, B_6, vitamin C and pantothenic and folic acids.[30] Thiamine, folic acid and vitamin K are particularly vulnerable to deficiency during total parenteral nutrition (TPN). Renal replacement therapy can cause loss of water-soluble vitamins and trace elements. Deficiencies of selenium, zinc, manganese and copper have been described in critical illness, in addition to the more familiar iron-deficient state. Subclinical deficiencies in critically ill patients are thought to cause immune deficiency and reduced resistance to oxidative stress. Suggested requirements for micronutrients in critically ill patients vary between authors and depending on route of administration; the most comprehensive guidance[30] is reproduced in Tables 87.3 and 87.4. More recent but broadly similar recommendations for some compounds are also available.[31]

Commercial preparations of both enteral and parenteral feeding solutions contain standard amounts of micronutrients. Supplementation of intake of certain antioxidant vitamins and trace elements above these levels is discussed below.

WATER AND ELECTROLYTES

Water and electrolyte requirements vary widely depending on the patient's condition; typical basal intakes are shown in Table 87.5.

ROUTE OF NUTRITION

When possible patients should be fed enterally. The advantages over the parenteral route are:

- lower cost
- greater simplicity
- possibly fewer infective complications

These appear to be the only advantages of the enteral route. Despite the fervour with which some pursue the debate,[2] there is little basis for the widespread belief that the enteral route provides a clear benefit in terms

Table 87.3 Vitamin requirements in critical illness[30]

Vitamin	Function	Dose
Vitamin A	Cell growth, night vision	10000–25000 IU
Vitamin D	Calcium metabolism	400–1000 IU
Vitamin E	Membrane antioxidant	400–1000 IU
β-Carotene*	Antioxidant	50 mg
Vitamin K	Activation of clotting factors	1.5 μg/kg per day
Thiamine (vitamin B_1)	Oxidative decarboxylation	10 mg
Riboflavin (vitamin B_2)	Oxidative phosphorylation	10 mg
Niacin (vitamin B_3)	Part of NAD, redox reactions	200 mg
Pantothenic acid	Part of coenzyme A	100 mg
Biotin	Carboxylase activity	5 mg
Pyridoxine (vitamin B_6)	Decarboxylase activity	20 mg
Folic acid	Haematopoiesis	2 mg
Vitamin B_{12}	Haematopoiesis	20 μg
Vitamin C	Antioxidant, collagen synthesis	2000 mg

*Not strictly a vitamin.

Table 87.4 Trace element requirements in critical illness[30]

Element	Function	Dose
Selenium	Antioxidant, fat metabolism	100 μg
Zinc	Energy metabolism, protein synthesis, epithelial growth	50 mg
Copper	Collagen cross-linking, ceruloplasmin	2–3 mg
Manganese	Neural function, fatty acid synthesis	25–50 mg
Chromium	Insulin activity	200 mg
Cobalt	B_{12} synthesis	
Iodine	Thyroid hormones	
Iron	Haematopoiesis, oxidative phosphorylation	10 mg
Molybdenum	Purine and pyridine metabolism	0.2–0.5 mg

Table 87.5 Water and electrolyte requirements/kg per day

Water	30 ml
Sodium	1–2 mmol
Potassium	0.7–1 mmol
Magnesium	0.1 mmol
Calcium	0.1 mmol
Phosphorus	0.4 mmol

of outcome, and that the advantages of enteral feeding are unassailable.

Two hypotheses are commonly advanced in support of the putative superiority of enteral feeding. First, it appears that the lipid contained within TPN is immunosuppressive. Intravenous lipid is known to suppress neutrophil and reticuloendothelial system function, and a comparison of TPN with and without lipid in critically ill trauma patients showed a lower complication rate in those not receiving lipid.[32] Second, enteral feeding may protect against infective complications. Absence of complex nutrients from the intestinal lumen is followed in rats by villus atrophy and reduced cell mass of the gut-associated lymphoid tissue (GALT). Starved humans show these changes to a much lesser extent. Lymphocytes produced in the GALT are redistributed to the respiratory tract, and contribute heavily to mucosal immunity. In mice, this contribution is lost during TPN.

The possibility that multiple organ failure may be driven by translocation of bacteria or endotoxin across an impaired mucosal barrier has been extensively investigated in animals. While it is known that TPN is associated with increased gut permeability to macromolecules in humans, this does not seem to result in translocation.[33] Although translocation does occur following surgery, and seems to be associated with sepsis;[34] a causal relation with multiple organ failure is unproven. In fact, a reduction in septic morbidity has only been found in certain groups, primarily abdominal trauma victims,[35,36] in whom parenteral nutrition was associated with a higher incidence of abdominal abscess and pneumonia. A third study found no difference.[37] In head-injured patients there is one trial showing no effect and one each supporting either route; however in the study favouring TPN the enteral nutrition group were grossly underfed.[14,38,39]

None of these studies is less than 15 years old, and the techniques of both enteral and parenteral feeding have changed a great deal in that time. Reductions in septic complications have also been found using enteral feeding in pancreatitis.[40] In contrast, no benefit was found in sepsis, though enteral feeding was instituted late.[41] A review of 31 clinical trials comparing enteral with parenteral feeding found no consistent difference.[42]

More recent systematic analyses have, as mentioned earlier, produced conflicting results. One found a reduction in infectious complications with enteral feeding, but no difference in mortality.[5] The most recent and most robust meta-analysis considered only high-quality trials using an intention-to-treat principle. It showed a clear reduction in mortality in patients fed parenterally.[4]

The same authors performed a prospectively defined subgroup analysis comparing early enteral with parenteral feeding, which showed no difference in mortality. Another recent meta-analysis of this question reached the same conclusion.[43] On this basis, as in the ACCEPT study, the authors recommended early use of the enteral route, with rapid recourse to parenteral nutrition if this was not possible.[6,17] At present it appears that timing of nutritional support matters as much as the route used.

A well-powered randomised study comparing early parenteral with enteral feeding will soon start.[18] However, in view of the practical and financial advantages of enteral feeding, it will probably need to find a significant mortality difference in favour of the parenteral route if it is to change the present preference for enteral feeding.

ENTERAL NUTRITION

ACCESS

Nasal tubes are preferred to oral, except in patients with a basal skull fracture, in whom there is a risk of cranial penetration. A large-bore (12–14 Fr) nasogastric tube is usually used at first. Once feeding is established and gastric residual volumes no longer need to be checked this can be replaced with a more comfortable fine-bore tube. A stylet is needed to assist in passage of fine-bore tubes. The position of all tubes must be checked on X-ray before feeding is started, as misplacement is not uncommon and intrapulmonary delivery of feed is potentially fatal.

Nasojejunal tubes are beneficial if impaired gastric emptying is refractory to prokinetic agents[6] (see below) or in pancreatitis. Spontaneous passage through the pylorus following blind placement is not reliable, but may be increased by the administration of single doses of 200 mg erythromycin or 20 mg metoclopramide.[44] However endoscopic or fluoroscopic assistance is needed for truly reliable transpyloric tube placement, although new developments in tube technology may soon obviate the logistic difficulties these methods entail. Unsurprisingly, two meta-analyses of various inconclusive studies have produced conflicting results on the question of whether nasojejunal feeding reduces the risk of aspiration or ventilator-associated pneumonia.[7,45] At present, the uncertain quality of the evidence concerning their benefits, coupled with the cost and logistic difficulty of placing them, precludes the routine use of nasojejunal tubes for all patients.

An alternative method of access in those needing long-term enteral feeding is percutaneous gastrostomy, which is usually performed endoscopically. Percutaneous jejunal access can be obtained either via a gastrostomy or by direct placement during incidental laparotomy.

REGIMEN

Slowly building up the rate of feeding is not proven to avoid diarrhoea or high gastric residual volumes. Head-injured patients fed with target intake from the outset have fewer infective complications.[46] Nonetheless, it is presently common practice to start delivering around 30 ml/hour and build up to the target intake depending on tolerance, as judged by gastric residual volumes. These are assessed by aspiration of the tube every 4 hours. Gastric residual volumes over 150 ml on two successive occasions have been associated with an increased incidence of ventilator-associated pneumonia;[47] contrastingly, others have found no link between high residual volumes and the risk of aspiration.[48] Nevertheless, if the residual volume is consistently greater than 200 ml, treatment with prokinetic agents (metoclopramide 10 mg every 8 hours or erythromycin 250 mg every 12 hours intravenously) appears to increase tolerance of feeding, though there is no discernible effect on mortality or morbidity.[44] In refractory cases a nasojejunal tube often permits successful enteral feeding, because small bowel function is resumed quicker than gastric emptying. A nasogastric tube is still needed to drain the stomach. Diarrhoea, abdominal distension, nausea and vomiting may suggest intolerance, despite low gastric volumes. Absence of bowel sounds is common in ventilated patients and should not be taken to indicate ileus.

Fine-bore tubes should not be aspirated as this causes them to block. Various folk remedies have been tried for unblocking tubes, including instillation of Coca-Cola™ fruit juice and pancreatic enzyme supplements. The instillates should be left in situ for an hour or more.

COMPOSITION

Commercially available enteral feeding solutions vary widely in composition. Polymeric feeds contain intact proteins (derived from whey, meat, soy isolates and caseinates) and carbohydrates in the form of oligo- and polysaccharides. These require pancreatic enzymes for absorption.

Elemental feeds with defined nitrogen sources (amino acids or peptides) are not of benefit when used routinely, but may enable feeding when small bowel absorption is impaired, for instance in pancreatic insufficiency or following prolonged starvation. Lipids are usually provided by vegetable oils consisting mostly of long-chain triglycerides, but some also contain more easily absorbed medium-chain triglycerides. The proportion of non-protein calories provided as carbohydrate is usually two thirds.

Electrolyte composition varies widely, with sodium- and potassium-restricted formulations available. Vitamins and trace elements are usually added by the manufacturers so that daily requirements are present in a volume containing roughly 2000 kcal. The possible benefits of providing additional doses of some of these substances to critically ill patients are considered below.

COMPLICATIONS

Enteral feeding is an independent risk factor for ventilator-associated pneumonia.[49] Sinusitis due to nasogastric intubation may necessitate changing to an orogastric tube. Fine-bore tubes are vulnerable to misplacement in the trachea or to perforation of the pharynx, oesophagus, stomach or bowel. Percutaneous endoscopic gastrostomy is associated with a high 30-day all-cause mortality in acutely ill patients, in whom it may be best avoided.[50] Other complications include insertion site infection, serious abdominal wall infection and peritonitis. Surgically placed jejunostomies can cause similar problems, and may also obstruct the bowel.

Diarrhoea is common in ICU patients, particularly those being fed enterally. It is often multifactorial and causes considerable distress and morbidity, particularly when the patient is repeatedly soiled with watery stool. Common causes include antibiotic therapy, *Clostridium difficile* infection, faecal impaction and a non-specific effect of critical illness. Malabsorption, lactose intolerance, prokinetic agents, magnesium, aminophylline, quinidine and medications containing sorbitol (e.g. paracetamol syrup and cimetidine) are occasional culprits. Rate of administration of enteral feed also plays a role. Faecal impaction, medication-induced diarrhoea and *C. difficile* infection must be excluded or treated, while malabsorption may respond to elemental diet. Slowing the rate of feeding sometimes helps; diluting the formula does not.

Metabolic complications include electrolyte abnormalities and hyperglycaemia. Severely malnourished patients are at risk of refeeding syndrome (see below) if nutritional support is begun too rapidly.

PARENTERAL NUTRITION

Parenteral nutritional support is indicated when adequate enteral intake cannot be established within an acceptable time. In some cases, absolute gastrointestinal failure is obvious, while in others it only becomes apparent after considerable efforts to feed enterally have failed. As discussed above, there is increasing evidence that if enteral feeding cannot be established early, then the parenteral route should be used until it can. Nevertheless, the aim in all patients fed intravenously should be to revert to enteral feeding as this becomes possible.

Parenteral feeding solutions may be prepared from their component parts under sterile conditions. Ready-made solutions also exist, but any necessary additions must be made in the same way.

In ICU patients the daily requirements are infused continuously over 24 hours. Careful biochemical and clinical monitoring is important, particularly at the outset (Table 87.6).

Table 87.6 Minimum monitoring during total parenteral nutrition. Less stable patients may require more intensive surveillance

Nursing	Temperature Pulse Blood pressure Respiratory rate Fluid balance Blood sugar (4 hourly when commencing feed)
Daily (at least)	Review of fluid balance Review of nutrient intake Blood sugar Urea, electrolytes and creatinine
Weekly (at least)	Full blood picture Coagulation screen Liver function tests Magnesium, calcium and phosphate Weight
As indicated	Zinc Uric acid

ACCESS

The major concern with central venous access for TPN is prevention of infection. The following considerations apply:[51]

- *insertion site*: subclavian lines have lower infection rates than internal jugular or femoral lines
- *tunnelling* may reduce infection rates in internal jugular lines but apparently not in short-term subclavian lines. It is not recommended for routine use
- *expertise* of operator and adequacy of ICU *nurse staffing levels* affect infection rate
- *skin preparation*: 2% chlorhexidine in alcohol is the most effective
- *sterile technique*: maximal sterile barrier procedures (mask, cap, gown, gloves, and large drape) are known to reduce catheter-related bacteraemia rates sixfold. There is a bewildering resistance to use of these precautions outside ICUs
- *dressings*: permeable polyurethane transparent dressings are superior to impermeable
- *antimicrobial catheters*: catheters coated with either chlorhexidine and silver sulfadiazine or rifampicin and minocycline are several times less likely to cause bacteraemia than standard polyurethane catheters.

The duration of the anti-infective effect appears to be longer with the antibiotic-coated catheters (2 weeks versus 1 week)

- *scheduled exchange* has not been proven to reduce catheter-related sepsis
- *guide-wire exchange* is associated with increased bacteraemia rates, which in routine use outweigh the reduced mechanical complications

In practice, pre-existing central access is used in the first instance. If a multilumen catheter is used, one lumen should be dedicated to administration of TPN and not used for any other purpose. Three-way taps should be avoided and infusion set changes carried out daily under sterile conditions. For long-term TPN (more than 2 months) specialised catheters with a tunnelled cuff or a subcutaneous port are recommended.

COMPOSITION

ENERGY

Energy is provided by a combination of carbohydrate and lipid. The optimal balance between the two is unknown; often 30–40% of non-protein energy is given as lipid. Alternatively, glucose may be relied upon for almost all the energy, with lipid being infused once or twice a week to provide essential fatty acids.

Glucose is the preferred carbohydrate and is infused as a concentrated solution. Exceeding the body's capacity to metabolise glucose (4 mg/kg per min in the septic patient) can lead to hyperglycaemia, lipogenesis and excess CO_2 production. Endogenous insulin secretion increases to control blood sugar levels. However, many patients require additional insulin, particularly diabetics. This may be infused separately, but when requirements are stable it is more safely added to the TPN solution. Persistent hyperglycaemia is better addressed by reducing the glucose infusion rate than by large doses of insulin.

Lipid provides essential fatty acids (linoleic and linolenic acids) and a more concentrated energy source than glucose. It may thus avoid the complications of excess glucose administration. However, there are concerns of immunosuppression from lipid infusion, as discussed above. Current lipid preparations consist of soybean oil emulsified with glycerol and egg phosphatides.

NITROGEN

Nitrogen is supplied as crystalline solutions of L-amino acids. Commercially available preparations vary in their provision of conditionally essential amino acids. Glutamine, tyrosine and cysteine are absent from many because of instability.

MICRONUTRIENTS

Vitamin and trace element preparations are added to TPN solutions in appropriate amounts. Thiamine, folic acid and vitamin K are particularly vulnerable to depletion and additional doses may be necessary.

ELECTROLYTES

Amino acid preparations contain varying quantities of electrolytes; additional amounts may need to be added to the solution.

COMPLICATIONS

Parenteral nutrition has the potential for severe complications.

- *Catheter-related sepsis* is addressed above. Other complications of central venous cannulation are discussed elsewhere
- *Electrolyte abnormalities* include hypophosphataemia, hypokalaemia and hypomagnesaemia, especially in the first 24–48 hours
- *Hyperchloraemic metabolic acidosis* may result from amino acid solutions with a high chloride content. Replacing some chloride with acetate in the TPN solution will resolve this where necessary
- *Rebound hypoglycaemia* may occur when TPN is discontinued suddenly. TPN should be weaned over a minimum of 12 hours. If it cannot be continued, an infusion of 10% dextrose should be started and blood sugars closely monitored
- *Refeeding syndrome* may occur when normal intake is resumed after a period of starvation. It is associated with profound hypophosphataemia, and possibly hypokalaemia and hypomagnesaemia. With the restoration of glucose as a substrate, insulin levels rise and cause cellular uptake of these ions. Depletion of ATP and 2,3-DPG results in tissue hypoxia and failure of cellular energy metabolism. This may manifest as cardiac and respiratory failure, with paraesthesiae and seizures also reported. Thiamine deficiency may also play a part
- *Liver dysfunction* is common during TPN. Causes include hepatic steatosis, intrahepatic cholestasis and biliary sludging from gallbladder inactivity. The problems necessitating TPN in the first place may also cause liver dysfunction
- *Deficiencies* of trace elements and vitamins (especially thiamine, folic acid and vitamin K) may occur

NUTRITION AND SPECIFIC DISEASES

ACUTE RENAL FAILURE

The advent of continuous renal replacement therapy means that dietary fluid and protein restriction is rarely necessary in ICU. Use of specialised lipid or amino acid formulations in TPN is not supported by evidence, and in general normal nutritional support is appropriate in acute renal failure.

LIVER DISEASE[10,52]

Energy requirements in ICU patients are not altered by the presence of chronic liver disease. Lipolysis is increased, so lipid must be used with caution to avoid hypertriglyceridaemia (not more than 1 g/kg per day). Protein restriction may be required in chronic hepatic encephalopathy; starting with 0.5 g/kg per day, the dose may be cautiously increased towards a normal intake. Hepatic encephalopathy may in part be due to depletion of branched-chain amino acids (BCAAs) permitting increased cerebral uptake of aromatic amino acids, which produce inhibitory neurotransmitters. In protein-intolerant patients the use of feeds enriched with BCAAs may permit greater protein intake without worsening encephalopathy. Their routine use is not indicated.[17] Thiamine and fat-soluble vitamin deficiencies are common in patients with chronic liver disease.

Fulminant hepatic failure reduces gluconeogenesis; hypoglycaemia is a common problem necessitating glucose infusion. Lipid is well tolerated. Energy and protein requirements are similar to those above. BCAAs have not been shown to be superior to standard amino-acid solutions.

RESPIRATORY FAILURE

Oxidation of fat produces less carbon dioxide than glucose. There have been attempts to use this to assist in weaning from mechanical ventilation by providing 50% of energy intake as lipid, with mixed results. Avoidance of overfeeding is much more important.

ACUTE PANCREATITIS

Until recently, TPN was a cornerstone of the management of severe acute pancreatitis to minimise pancreatic stimulation. This has changed with the publication of studies showing jejunal feeding to be safe, effective and associated with reductions in infective complications compared with TPN.[40] Elemental feeds and pancreatic enzyme supplements are logical if malabsorption is a problem. Despite the shift towards enteral feeding of patients with pancreatitis, some can only be fed intravenously.

OBESITY

The possibility that obese patients specifically may benefit from hypocaloric feeding was assessed by comparing 40 obese patients fed target intakes of <20 or 25–30 kcal/kg per day.[53] Other than a reduction in ICU stay, no benefit was shown. At present there is insufficient evidence to justify feeding obese patients differently from others.

ADJUNCTIVE NUTRITION

Certain substances have been used as adjuncts to feeding solutions, in attempts to modulate the metabolic and immune responses to critical illness. While this is an area of much promise, in general no conclusive benefit has yet been shown in unselected critically ill patients. The situation has been complicated by a tendency to study several compounds simultaneously, at arbitrary doses and in heterogeneous populations, then to perform retrospective subgroup analysis in order to demonstrate an effect. The evidence would be a great deal clearer if supplements with an established therapeutic window were evaluated individually. Such interventions are at least as much matters of pharmacology as of nutrition, and should be investigated as such.

GLUTAMINE

Glutamine serves as an oxidative fuel and nucleotide precursor for enterocytes and immune cells, mainly lymphocytes, neutrophils and macrophages. It also appears to regulate the expression of many genes related to signal transduction and to cellular metabolism and repair. During catabolic illness glutamine is released in large quantities from skeletal muscle, in order to supply this need. In these circumstances it may become 'conditionally essential' and is vulnerable to depletion, with potentially adverse effects on gut barrier and immune function, which may in turn impair the ability to survive a sustained period of critical illness once glutamine stores are depleted.

The evidence on glutamine supplementation in critical illness is as contradictory as in other areas of nutritional support. Reductions in infectious complications and length of ICU stay were shown in small early studies of enterally fed trauma and burns patients, but a much larger study in unselected ICU patients found no effect on any outcome.[54] TPN solutions have historically contained no glutamine because of problems with stability and solubility. These are now being overcome by use of dipeptides, but clinical studies of intravenous glutamine supplementation during TPN have also been conflicting. One early trial in ICU patients requiring TPN showed a reduction in late mortality which only became apparent after 20 days, and which persisted at 6 months.[55] There are suggestions from meta-analysts that there is now a demonstrable mortality benefit from higher doses of parenteral glutamine;[56] this awaits confirmation in a prospective trial. In the meantime, it seems that the patients most likely to benefit are those requiring TPN for more than 10 days.[55]

SELENIUM

Selenium is crucial to the regulation of glutathione peroxidase, the major scavenging system for oxygen free radicals. Low plasma selenium levels are common in ICU patients, and a number of small studies have shown potential benefits, again mostly when larger doses are given intravenously. A very recent large randomised trial of selenium 1000 μg intravenously for 14 days has shown a reduction in mortality when patients breaching trial protocols were excluded, but the intention-to-treat analysis did not reach statistical significance.[57] Parenteral selenium supplementation may well soon be proven to be beneficial in unselected ICU patients.

ANTIOXIDANT VITAMINS

Vitamins A, C and E are also involved in systemic defence against oxidant stress, and have been studied in various combinations and doses, with and without selenium. Of the trials not using selenium, only one has shown a reduction in deaths using large enteral doses of vitamins C and E; the control group, however, had a very high mortality rate.[58] It is hard to recommend routine supplementation with antioxidant vitamins on present evidence.

ARGININE AND IMMUNONUTRITION

Arginine is a non-essential amino acid which acts as a precursor of nitric oxide, polyamines (important in lymphocyte maturation) and nucleotides. Animal studies suggest enhanced cell-mediated immunity and survival when arginine is supplemented. Several commercially available enteral feeding solutions combine omega-3 fatty acids, arginine, nucleotides and in one case glutamine to produce so-called immune-enhancing diets. They have been assessed in a number of trials, few of them in patient groups likely to be admitted to ICU outside North America. Meta-analysis has suggested reductions in hospital stay and infections, but not in mortality.[59,60] Subgroup analysis revealed an increase in mortality when arginine supplementation was given to septic patients;[60] interim safety assessment of a randomised controlled trial[61] led to its early cessation when this finding was replicated in the subgroup of patients with sepsis, though this may have been a chance effect.[17]

At present it appears that such diets should not be used in septic patients. While there are suggestions of benefit in other groups, notably patients undergoing major surgery or suffering a burn injury, there is little basis for their general use in ICU patients unless it is justified by future adequately powered prospective trials comparing their individual components with meaningful controls.

REFERENCES

1. Doig GS, Simpson F, Delaney A. A review of the true methodological quality of nutritional support trials conducted in the critically ill: time for improvement. *Anesth Analg* 2005; **100**: 527–33.
2. Marik PE, Pinsky M. Death by parenteral nutrition. *Intensive Care Med* 2003; **29**: 867–9.
3. LeLorier J, Gregoire G, Benhaddad A *et al.* Discrepancies between meta-analyses and subsequent large randomized, controlled trials. *N Engl J Med* 1997; **337**: 536–42.
4. Simpson F, Doig GS. Parenteral vs. enteral nutrition in the critically ill patient: a meta-analysis of trials using the intention to treat principle. *Intensive Care Med* 2005; **31**: 12–23.
5. Gramlich L, Kichian K, Pinilla J *et al.* Does enteral nutrition compared to parenteral nutrition result in better outcomes in critically ill adult patients? A systematic review of the literature. *Nutrition* 2004; **20**: 843–8.
6. Martin CM, Doig GS, Heyland DK *et al.* Multicentre, cluster-randomized clinical trial of algorithms for critical-care enteral and parenteral therapy (ACCEPT). *CMAJ* 2004; **170**: 197–204.
7. Heyland DK, Dhaliwal R, Drover JW *et al.* Canadian clinical practice guidelines for nutrition support in mechanically ventilated, critically ill adult patients. *J Parenter Enteral Nutr* 2003; **27**: 355–73.
8. Jacobs DG, Jacobs DO, Kudsk KA *et al.* Practice management guidelines for nutritional support of the trauma patient. *J Trauma* 2004; **57**: 660–78.
9. Cerra FB, Benitez MR, Blackburn GL *et al.* Applied nutrition in ICU patients. A consensus statement of the American College of Chest Physicians. *Chest* 1997; **111**: 769–78.
10. Klein S, Kinney J, Jeejeebhoy K *et al.* Nutrition support in clinical practice: review of published data and recommendations for future research directions. Summary of a conference sponsored by the National Institutes of Health, American Society for Parenteral and Enteral Nutrition, and American Society for Clinical Nutrition. *Am J Clin Nutr* 1997; **66**: 683–706.
11. Kreymann KG, Berger MM, Deutz NE *et al.* ESPEN guidelines on enteral nutrition: intensive care. *Clin Nutr* 2006; **25**: 210–23.
12. Baker JP, Detsky AS, Wesson DE *et al.* Nutritional assessment: a comparison of clinical judgement and objective measurements. *N Engl J Med* 1982; **306**: 969–72.
13. Kudsk KA, Tolley EA, DeWitt RC *et al.* Preoperative albumin and surgical site identify surgical risk for major postoperative complications. *J Parenter Enteral Nutr* 2003; **27**: 1–19.
14. Rapp RP, Young B, Twyman D *et al.* The favorable effect of early parenteral feeding on survival in head-injured patients. *J Neurosurg* 1983; **58**: 906–12.
15. Pupelis G, Selga G, Austrums E *et al.* Jejunal feeding, even when instituted late, improves outcomes in patients with severe pancreatitis and peritonitis. *Nutrition* 2001; **17**: 91–4.
16. Marik PE, Zaloga GP. Early enteral nutrition in acutely ill patients: a systematic review. *Crit Care Med* 2001; **29**: 2264–70.
17. Doig G, Simpson F. Evidence-based guidelines for nutritional support of the critically ill: results of a bi-national guideline development conference. Sydney: EvidenceBased.net; 2005.
18. Doig GS, Simpson F. Early enteral nutrition in the critically ill: do we need more evidence or better evidence? *Curr Opin Crit Care* 2006; **12**: 126–30.
19. Streat SJ, Beddoe AH, Hill GL. Aggressive nutritional support does not prevent protein loss despite fat gain in septic intensive care patients. *J Trauma* 1987; **27**: 262–6.
20. Krishnan JA, Parce PB, Martinez A *et al.* Caloric intake in medical ICU patients: consistency of care with guidelines and relationship to clinical outcomes. *Chest* 2003; **124**: 297–305.
21. Rubinson L, Diette GB, Song X *et al.* Low caloric intake is associated with nosocomial bloodstream

infections in patients in the medical intensive care unit. *Crit Care Med* 2004; **32**: 350–7.
22. Villet S, Chiolero RL, Bollmann MD *et al.* Negative impact of hypocaloric feeding and energy balance on clinical outcome in ICU patients. *Clin Nutr* 2005; **24**: 502–9.
23. Plank LD, Hill GL. Sequential metabolic changes following induction of systemic inflammatory response in patients with severe sepsis or major blunt trauma. *World J Surg* 2000; **24**: 630–8.
24. Makk LJ, McClave SA, Creech PW *et al.* Clinical application of the metabolic cart to the delivery of total parenteral nutrition. *Crit Care Med* 1990; **18**: 1320–7.
25. Saffle JR, Larson CM, Sullivan J. A randomized trial of indirect calorimetry-based feedings in thermal injury. *J Trauma* 1990; **30**: 776–82.
26. Schofield W. Predicting basal metabolic rate; new standards and review of previous work. *Hum Nutr Clin Nutr* 1985; **39C** 5–41.
27. Working Party of the British Association for Parenteral and Enteral Nutrition. *Current Perspectives on Enteral Nutrition in Adults.* Maidenhead: BAPEN; 1999.
28. Konstantinides FN, Konstantinides NN, Li JC *et al.* Urinary urea nitrogen: too insensitive for calculating nitrogen balance studies in surgical clinical nutrition. *J Parenter Enteral Nutr* 1991; **15**: 189–93.
29. Larsson J, Lennmarken C, Martensson J *et al.* Nitrogen requirements in severely injured patients. *Br J Surg* 1990; **77**: 413–6.
30. Demling RH, DeBiasse MA. Micronutrients in critical illness. *Crit Care Clin* 1995; **11**: 651–73.
31. Shenkin A. Micronutrients in the severely-injured patient. *Proc Nutr Soc* 2000; **59**: 451–6.
32. Battistella FD, Widergren JT, Anderson JT *et al.* A prospective, randomized trial of intravenous fat emulsion administration in trauma victims requiring total parenteral nutrition. *J Trauma* 1997; **43**: 52–8.
33. Sedman PC, MacFie J, Palmer MD *et al.* Preoperative total parenteral nutrition is not associated with mucosal atrophy or bacterial translocation in humans. *Br J Surg* 1995; **82**: 1663–7.
34. MacFie J, O'Boyle C, Mitchell CJ *et al.* Gut origin of sepsis: a prospective study investigating associations between bacterial translocation, gastric microflora, and septic morbidity. *Gut* 1999; **45**: 223–8.
35. Moore FA, Moore EE, Jones TN *et al.* TEN versus TPN following major abdominal trauma – reduced septic morbidity. *J Trauma* 1989; **29**: 916–22.
36. Kudsk KA, Croce MA, Fabian TC *et al.* Enteral versus parenteral feeding. Effects on septic morbidity after blunt and penetrating abdominal trauma. *Ann Surg* 1992; **215**: 503–11.
37. Adams S, Dellinger EP, Wertz MJ *et al.* Enteral versus parenteral nutritional support following laparotomy for trauma: a randomized prospective trial. *J Trauma* 1986; **26**: 882–91.
38. Grahm TW, Zadrozny DB, Harrington T. The benefits of early jejunal hyperalimentation in the head-injured patient. *Neurosurgery* 1989; **25**: 729–35.
39. Young B, Ott L, Twyman D *et al.* The effect of nutritional support on outcome from severe head injury. *J Neurosurg* 1987; **67**: 668–76.
40. Marik PE, Zaloga GP. Meta-analysis of parenteral nutrition versus enteral nutrition in patients with acute pancreatitis. *BMJ* 2004; **328**: 1407.
41. Cerra FB, McPherson JP, Konstantinides FN *et al.* Enteral nutrition does not prevent multiple organ failure syndrome (MOFS) after sepsis. *Surgery* 1988; **104**: 727–33.
42. Lipman TO. Grains or veins: is enteral nutrition really better than parenteral nutrition? A look at the evidence. *J Parenter Enteral Nutr* 1998; **22**: 167–82.
43. Peter JV, Moran JL, Phillips-Hughes J. A metaanalysis of treatment outcomes of early enteral versus early parenteral nutrition in hospitalized patients. *Crit Care Med* 2005; **33**: 213–20.
44. Booth CM, Heyland DK, Paterson WG. Gastrointestinal promotility drugs in the critical care setting: a systematic review of the evidence. *Crit Care Med* 2002; **30**: 1429–35.
45. Marik PE, Zaloga GP. Gastric versus post-pyloric feeding: a systematic review. *Crit Care* 2003; **7**: R46–51.
46. Taylor SJ, Fettes SB, Jewkes C *et al.* Prospective, randomized, controlled trial to determine the effect of early enhanced enteral nutrition on clinical outcome in mechanically ventilated patients suffering head injury. *Crit Care Med* 1999; **27**: 2525–31.
47. Mentec H, Dupont H, Bocchetti M *et al.* Upper digestive intolerance during enteral nutrition in critically ill patients: frequency, risk factors, and complications. *Crit Care Med* 2001; **29**: 1955–61.
48. McClave SA, Lukan JK, Stefater JA *et al.* Poor validity of residual volumes as a marker for risk of aspiration in critically ill patients. *Crit Care Med* 2005; **33**: 324–30.
49. Drakulovic MB, Torres A, Bauer TT *et al.* Supine body position as a risk factor for nosocomial pneumonia in mechanically ventilated patients: a randomised trial. *Lancet* 1999; **354**: 1851–8.
50. Abuksis G, Mor M, Plaut S *et al.* Outcome of percutaneous endoscopic gastrostomy (PEG): comparison of two policies in a 4-year experience. *Clin Nutr* 2004; **23**: 341–6.
51. Fraenkel DJ, Rickard C, Lipman J. Can we achieve consensus on central venous catheter-related infections? *Anaesth Intensive Care* 2000; **28**: 475–90.
52. Mizock BA. Nutritional support in hepatic encephalopathy. *Nutrition* 1999; **15**: 220–8.
53. Dickerson RN, Boschert KJ, Kudsk KA *et al.* Hypocaloric enteral tube feeding in critically ill obese patients. *Nutrition* 2002; **18**: 241–6.
54. Hall JC, Dobb G, Hall J *et al.* A prospective randomized trial of enteral glutamine in critical illness. *Intensive Care Med* 2003; **29**: 1710–6.
55. Griffiths RD, Jones C, Palmer TE. Six-month outcome of critically ill patients given glutamine-supplemented parenteral nutrition. *Nutrition* 1997; **13**: 295–302.
56. Heyland DK. Critical care nutrition. Kingston, Ontario: Critical Care Nutrition; 2006. http://www.criticalcarenutrition.com

57. Angstwurm MW, Engelmann L, Zimmermann T *et al.* Selenium in Intensive Care (SIC): results of a prospective randomized, placebo-controlled, multiple-center study in patients with severe systemic inflammatory response syndrome, sepsis, and septic shock. *Crit Care Med* 2007; **35**: 118–26.
58. Crimi E, Liguori A, Condorelli M *et al.* The beneficial effects of antioxidant supplementation in enteral feeding in critically ill patients: a prospective, randomized, double-blind, placebo-controlled trial. *Anesth Analg* 2004; **99**: 857–63.
59. Heys SD, Walker LG, Smith I *et al.* Enteral nutritional supplementation with key nutrients in patients with critical illness and cancer: a meta-analysis of randomized controlled clinical trials. *Ann Surg* 1999; **229**: 467–77.
60. Heyland DK, Novak F, Drover JW *et al.* Should immunonutrition become routine in critically ill patients? A systematic review of the evidence. *JAMA* 2001; **286**: 944–53.
61. Bertolini G, Iapichino G, Radrizzani D *et al.* Early enteral immunonutrition in patients with severe sepsis: results of an interim analysis of a randomized multicentre clinical trial. *Intensive Care Med* 2003; **29**: 834–40.

Part Fifteen

Haematological Management

88

Blood transfusion

James P Isbister

Blood component therapy has a central therapeutic role in clinical medicine, but blood banking and transfusion medicine has tended to focus on the blood component supply rather than the demand/patient perspective. The clinical focus should naturally be on 'what is best for the patient?' not, 'what is best for the blood supply?'

Demand for blood components continues to increase. Reasons include the greater burden of chronic disease due to ageing of the population, increasing severity of illness of intensive care unit (ICU) patients and both a widening range of clinical indications for blood components and newer blood-intensive surgical procedures. This is tempered by greater focus on appropriate use.

When prescribing blood component therapy, the clinical problem and patient's needs must be accurately identified and clearly understood. Often therapy is required for haematological deficiencies until the basic disease process can be corrected (e.g. surgical control for acute haemorrhage, or support for bone marrow suppression until the marrow recovers). Therapy may be aimed at controlling the effects of a deficiency or preventing secondary problems. Alternatively, the indication is passive immunotherapy (e.g. Rhesus prophylaxis) or high-dosage intravenous immunoglobulin as immunomodulatory therapy.

In recent years the role of blood transfusion in a wide range of clinical settings is being critically reassessed. Careful risk assessment and the use of blood conservation techniques have made 'bloodless' surgery possible in most elective surgical settings. Added to the uncertainty about the indications and benefits of allogeneic blood transfusion is the accumulating evidence that blood transfusion is an independent risk factor for poorer clinical outcomes. Clearly many transfusions are both indicated and lifesaving, but it is appropriate that there is greater focus on transfusion alternatives, techniques to minimise exposure and closer attention to the quality and immediate efficacy of blood components.

Traditionally, transfusion has been regarded as the 'default' decision when there is clinical uncertainty. The benefits of transfusion have been assumed with little or no evidence to support the assumption and patients are thereby unnecessarily exposed to potential morbidity or even mortality. Given that the decision-making process for using blood component therapy can be difficult, that indications may be controversial or when there is no evidence for potential benefit, there are good common sense and scientifically evidence-based reasons to adopt a non-transfusion default position.[1,2] If allogeneic blood component therapy can be avoided, the potential hazards cease to be an issue.

Both evidence-based transfusion medicine and the fact that blood is altruistically donated should ensure that blood is seen as a valuable and unique natural resource that should be conserved and managed appropriately. It should only be used as therapy when there is evidence for potential benefit, when alternatives have been considered and potential harm has been minimised. Potential hazards must be balanced against benefits and wherever possible the benefits and risks should be explained to the patient/relatives.

In considering the use of allogeneic blood transfusion the following questions need to be addressed:

- What is the timeframe of the decision-making process?
- Is it an elective decision?
- What is the haemopoietic defect?
- What is the most appropriate therapy for the patient?
- Are there alternatives to allogeneic transfusion?
- What component is indicated and where should it be obtained?
- How should the component be administered and monitored?
- What are the potential hazards of the blood component therapy?
- Can the risk of adverse effects be avoided or minimised?
- What is the cost of the haemotherapy?
- Is the patient fully informed of the medical decisions?

Safe and effective transfusion requires attention to the following details (Figure 88.1):

- Clearly defined indication and benefits of blood components
- Accurate patient identification for blood group compatibility
- Identification and careful management of high-risk patients
- Appropriate handling, administration and monitoring

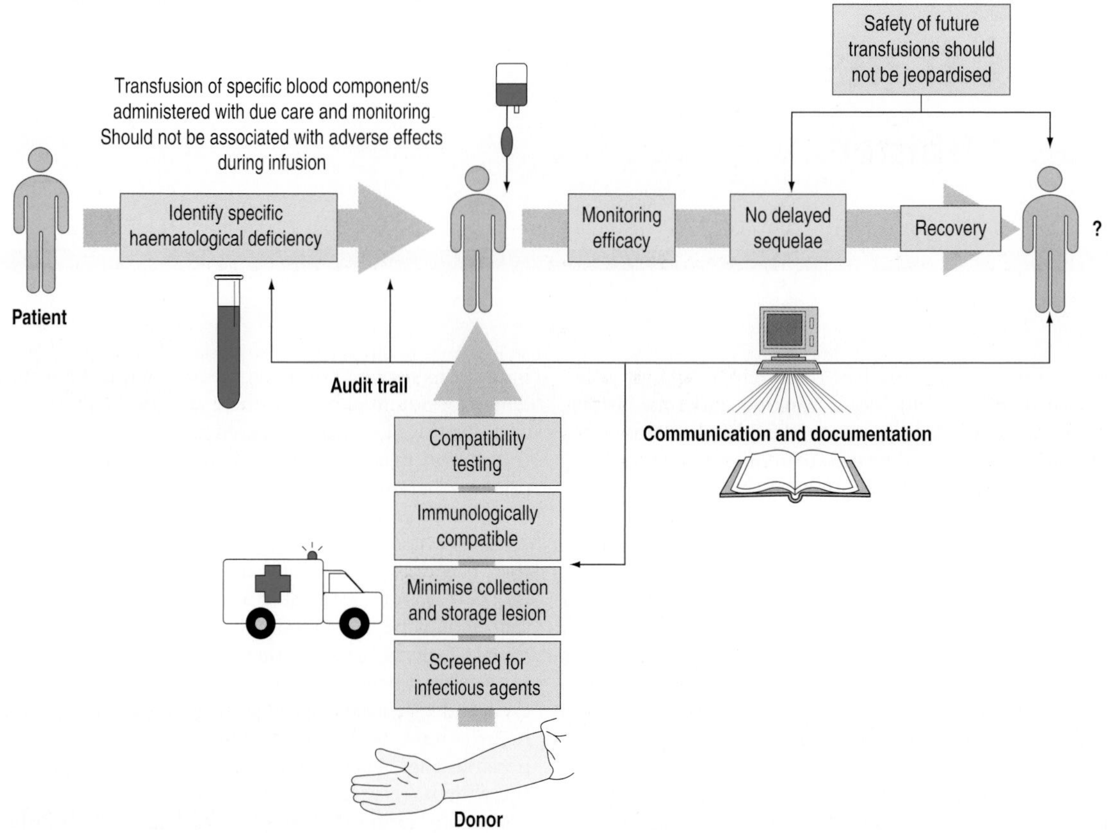

Figure 88.1 What is a safe transfusion?

- Provision of adequate amounts and quality of component(s)
- Communication of benefits and risk to the patient/relatives
- The infusion should not be associated with preventable ill effects
- Awareness of possible transfusion-related complications
- Early diagnosis and prompt action in relation to adverse events of transfusion
- Accurate documentation
- Input into quality assurance programmes

BLOOD STORAGE AND THE STORAGE LESIONS

Blood is altered from the moment of collection and the 'lesions' of collection – anticoagulation, separation, cooling, preservation and storage – compound and progressively increase until the date of expiry.[3] The extent of these changes is determined by collection technique, the specific blood component, the preservative medium, the container, storage time and storage conditions. The threshold storage time for blood components has generally been arbitrarily determined by in vitro studies and assessment of in vivo survival. In the case of red cell concentrates, greater than 75% of transfused cells should survive post transfusion.

Storage results in quantitative and/or qualitative deficiencies in blood components, which may reduce the immediate efficacy of a transfusion. In parallel with these storage changes is an accumulation of degenerate material (e.g. microaggregates and procoagulant material), release of vasoactive agents, cytokine generation and haemolysis.[4] Many of the changes occurring during storage are related to the presence of leukocytes and can be minimised by prestorage leukoreduction.[5] Red cells undergo a change from their biconcave disc shape to spiky spherocytes (echinocytes) and in so doing lose their flexibility. There are also changes in the red cell membrane resulting in an increased tendency to adhere to endothelial cell surfaces in the microcirculation, especially if there is activation of endothelial cells, for example in the presence of the systemic inflammatory response (e.g. with shock or sepsis).[6] There is evidence that the immediate post-transfusion function of stored red cells and haemoglobin in delivering oxygen to the microcirculation and unloading is questionable, and several hours are required for red cell oxygen carriage and delivery to return to normal.[7,8] It is important to differentiate between the storage

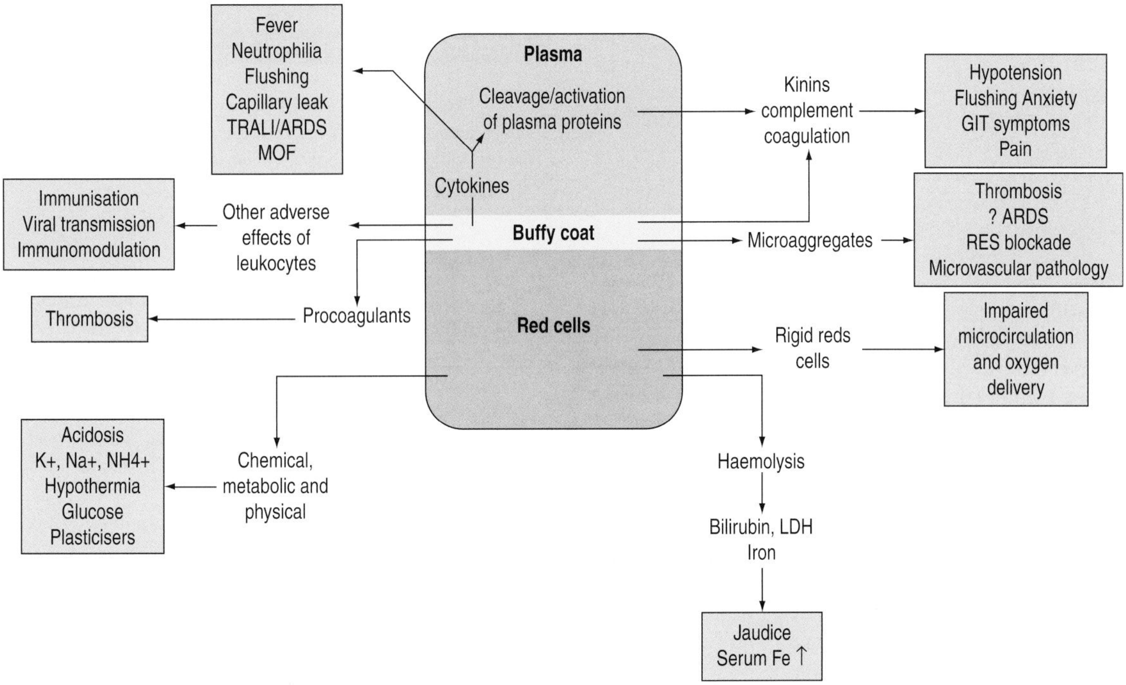

Figure 88.2 The storage lesions. ARDS, adult respiratory distress syndrome; GIT, gastrointestinal tract; MOF, multiorgan failure; RES, reticuloendothelial system; TRALI, transfusion-related acute lung injury.

lesion being responsible for failure to achieve clinical/laboratory end-points due to reduced survival and/or qualitative defects in cellular function and the 'toxic' effects of blood storage (Figure 88.2).

The use of blood filters has been an acknowledgement of the existence of the blood storage lesion and its possible clinical significance. The 170 μm blood-giving filters were first introduced into transfusion medicine to stop the occlusion of blood-giving sets. Ironically, there was little concern that the fibrin clots may harm the patient but fortunately the lung is one of nature's remarkable filters. Adult respiratory distress syndrome (ARDS) and the Vietnam War increased interest in unfiltered microaggregates accumulating during storage. Both logic and animal data suggested their implication in ARDS and that microfilters to remove microparticles 20–40 μm in size may be protective. This proved difficult to confirm but microaggregate filters do not adequately address the problem of the storage lesion and its clinical significance. Using pre-storage leukodepletion filters, and preventing the development of the storage lesion in both blood and platelets from its inception, is more logical and scientific. Universal pre-storage leukoreduction is now standard practice in many countries, although it was primarily introduced as a precautionary measure against the possible transmission of variant Creutzfeldt–Jakob disease (vCJD) and not to address the numerous other indications for the removal of leukocytes.[9]

The clinical significance of blood storage lesions is still controversial. Further studies are needed to assess their relevance in conditions such as ARDS, multiorgan failure (MOF), vasoactive reactions and alterations in laboratory parameters.[7,10,11] It is assumed that blood components have been appropriately collected, processed, stored, transported and transfused, but despite much greater attention to standard operating procedures and regulation generally, the quality of the final product cannot be guaranteed.[12] The 'assumed' quality of labile cellular blood products is based on research data and monitoring of standard operating procedures. There is rarely detailed individual product assessment prior to transfusion.[8] It is accepted that the adverse effects of storage increase with time and an arbitrary 'cut off' is mandated on the basis of research studies.

In relation to the possible clinical significance of the storage lesion, the following should be considered:

- Quantitative and qualitative deficiency of blood component
  - Failure to achieve anticipated end-points due to reduced quantity and/or quality of the blood product
  - Exposure to excessive numbers of donors in achieving efficacy
- Physical characteristics
  - Hypothermia
  - Chemical characteristics
  - Citrate toxicity
  - Acid–base imbalance
  - Glucose

- Contamination
  - Bacterial resulting in endotoxaemia or septicaemia
  - Plasticisers
- Accumulation of 'toxic' or degenerate products
  - Role of the storage lesion in transfusion-related immunomodulation
  - Role of cytokines
  - Role of reticuloendothelial system blockade
  - Accentuation of free radical pathophysiology due to free iron
- Effects of transfusion on laboratory parameters (e.g. elevations in bilirubin, neutrophils, serum iron and lactic dehydrogenase) which may lead to incorrect interpretation
- Large volume transfusions (proportional to storage age) as a risk factor for MOF and ARDS
- Early hyperkalaemia, late hypokalaemia
- Activation and consumption of the haemostatic factors with possible contribution to disseminated intravascular coagulation (DIC) and venous thromboembolism
- Non haemolytic, non-febrile transfusion reactions
- Hypotension and circulatory instability due to vasoactive substance (kinins, histamine)

THE ROLE OF LEUKOCYTES AS A 'CONTAMINANT' IN LABILE STORED BLOOD AND THE ROLE OF PRE-STORAGE LEUKODEPLETION

There are several difficulties assessing potential adverse effects of leukocytes as they may be responsible for a wide range of blood component quality and safety issues.[9] The presence of leukocytes has been shown to be responsible for specific adverse outcomes in some patients (e.g. non-haemolytic febrile transfusion reaction, platelet refractoriness and transfusion-associated graft-versus-host disease, TAGVHD), but this is the minority. In the larger context the overall available evidence, in the absence of adequate large randomised clinical trials, suggests that universal pre-storage leukodepletion may reduce transfusion-related morbidity and mortality as well as generating cost savings.[13] Leukodepletion of red cell and platelet concentrates minimises the clinical consequences of the immunomodulatory effects of allogeneic transfusion. Hence it may decrease the incidence of recurrence of some cancers, of postoperative infections, of blood stream infections and reduce ICU and hospital length of stay. In many patients transfusion-related acute lung injury (TRALI) is a multifactorial disorder and in 'at risk' patients non-leukodepleted blood may be a risk factor. Patients in whom there is activation of the systemic inflammatory response syndrome (SIRS) are at risk of developing the multiorgan failure syndrome.[5,14] Patients at particular risk include those with trauma, burns, critical bleeding, shock, sepsis and those undergoing cardiopulmonary bypass.[15–19] The quality and function of pre-storage leukodepleted red cell concentrates is better maintained on storage, ensuring better post-transfusion efficacy and survival.[6,20]

CLINICAL GUIDELINES FOR BLOOD COMPONENT THERAPY

The following is a brief summary of the clinical guidelines for the use of commonly used blood components. The use of specific concentrates or recombinant products is beyond the scope of this book.

RED CELL TRANSFUSIONS

What constitutes appropriate use of red cell transfusions in acute medicine is contentious because of the difficulties in identifying the benefits of red cell transfusion in many circumstances.[21] Pursuit of the lowest safe haematocrit continues to receive considerable attention, but pushing any aspect of a system to its limits risks 'sailing too close to the wind' which may be appropriate in some situations, but potentially hazardous in others.[22,23]

In an otherwise stable patient, the transfusion of red cell concentrates is likely to be inappropriate when the hemoglobin level is > 100 g/l. On the other hand, their use may be appropriate when haemoglobin is in the range 70–100 g/l if there are other defects in the oxygen transport system, such as cardiorespiratory dysfunction. The decision to transfuse should be supported by the need to relieve clinical signs and symptoms of impaired oxygen transport and prevent morbidity and mortality. The transfusion of red cell concentrates is likely to be appropriate when hemoglobin is < 70 g/l and the anaemia is not reversible with specific therapy in the short term, but lower levels may be acceptable in patients who are asymptomatic, especially in the younger age group.

PLATELET TRANSFUSIONS

Platelet transfusion therapy may benefit patients with platelet deficiency or dysfunction. The following are the indications for platelet transfusions:[24]

PROPHYLAXIS

- Bone marrow failure when the platelet count is $< 10 \times 10^9$/l without associated risk factors for bleeding or $< 20 \times 10^9$/l in the presence of additional risk factors
- To maintain the platelet count at $> 50 \times 10^9$/l in patients undergoing surgery or invasive procedures
- In qualitative platelet function disorders, depending on clinical features and setting (platelet count is not a reliable indicator for transfusion)

BLEEDING PATIENT

- In any haemorrhaging patient in whom thrombocytopenia secondary to marrow failure is considered a contributory factor
- When the platelet count is $< 50 \times 10^9$/l in the context of massive haemorrhage/transfusion and $<100 \times 10^9$/l in the presence of diffuse microvascular bleeding

The transfusion of platelet concentrates is not generally considered appropriate:

- when thrombocytopenia is due to immune-mediated destruction
- in thrombotic thrombocytopenic purpura and haemolytic uraemic syndrome
- in uncomplicated cardiac bypass surgery

FRESH FROZEN PLASMA

There are few specific indications for fresh frozen plasma, but its use may be appropriate:[25]

- for replacement of single factor deficiencies where a specific or combined factor concentrate is not available
- for treatment of the multiple coagulation deficiencies associated with acute DIC
- for treatment of inherited deficiencies of coagulation inhibitors in patients undergoing high-risk procedures where a specific factor concentrate is unavailable
- in the presence of bleeding and abnormal coagulation parameters following massive transfusion or cardiac bypass surgery or in patients with liver disease
- for immediate reversal of warfarin-induced anticoagulation in the presence of potentially life-threatening bleeding when prothrombin concentrates (PCC) are not available[26–28] (see Chapter 91)

The use of fresh frozen plasma is generally not considered appropriate in cases of:

- hypovolaemia
- plasma exchange procedures unless post exchange invasive procedures are planned
- treatment of immunodeficiency states

CRYOPRECIPITATE

Cryoprecipitate is prepared from freshly collected plasma and contains factor VIII, fibrinogen, von Willebrand factor, factor XIII and fibronectin. Cryoprecipitate was originally developed for treatment of haemophilia due to factor VIII deficiency, but is now prescribed to treat congenital or acquired hypofibrinogenaemia, usually in the context of liver disease, trauma, DIC, hyperfibrinolysis or massive transfusion.

IMMUNOGLOBULIN

Normal human immunoglobulin is available in intramuscular and intravenous forms for the treatment or prevention of infection in patients with proven hypogammaglobulinaemia.[29] Intravenous immunoglobulin G has been recommended as adjunctive therapy in patients with fulminant sepsis syndrome, especially those with toxic shock syndrome caused by group A streptococci.[30]

Intravenous immunoglobulin therapy also has a role in therapy of some autoimmune disorders, such as idiopathic thrombocytopenic purpura, autoimmune polyneuropathy and others (see Chapter 90).

FACTOR CONCENTRATES

There is an increasing number of plasma protein concentrates available for clinical use. Some are prepared from donor plasma and some by recombinant technology. Factor VIII and factor IX concentrates have an established role in the management of haemophilia, but others are in the process of establishing their clinical efficacy and indications. Antithrombin III (ATIII) concentrates are available for thrombophilia due to ATIII deficiency and are increasingly recommended in other disorders where ATIII may be depleted (e.g. DIC, MOF).[31] Recombinant human activated protein C has antithrombotic, anti-inflammatory and profibrinolytic properties but its role in the treatment of patients with severe sepsis remains controversial.[32]

Of recent interest is the use of the recombinant activated haemostatic proteins and inhibitors. Recombinant activated factor VII (rFVIIa) was developed for the management of haemophilic patients with coagulation factor inhibitors. rFVIIa is now being widely used 'off label' for controlling haemorrhage in the non-haemophilic setting and there is considerable controversy as to its benefits and risks.[33] There are an increasing number of case reports and series reporting on the use of rFVIIa in critical life-threatening haemorrhage. Patients with uncontrolled critical bleeding and coagulopathy, despite large transfusions and surgical intervention, have significant mortality rates and rFVIIa in these clinical situations is used as salvage therapy. rFVIIa is now being studied in controlled trials where there is critical bleeding in various clinical settings. rFVIIa initiates the extrinsic coagulation pathway when complexed to tissue factors at sites of injury and on activated platelet surfaces. It potentially has a role in a wide range of haemostatic disorders (e.g. massive blood transfusion, liver disease, uraemia, severe thrombocytopenia and platelet disorders).[34]

POTENTIAL ADVERSE EFFECTS OF ALLOGENEIC TRANSFUSION

The pathophysiology of blood transfusion reactions can broadly be divided into five categories (Figure 88.3):

- Reactions may occur due to *immunological differences* between the donor and recipient, resulting in varying degrees of blood component incompatibility. In general, in order for a reaction to occur, the recipient needs to have been previously immunised to a cellular or plasma antigen.[35]
- A wide range of *infectious agents* may be transmitted by homologous blood component therapy.

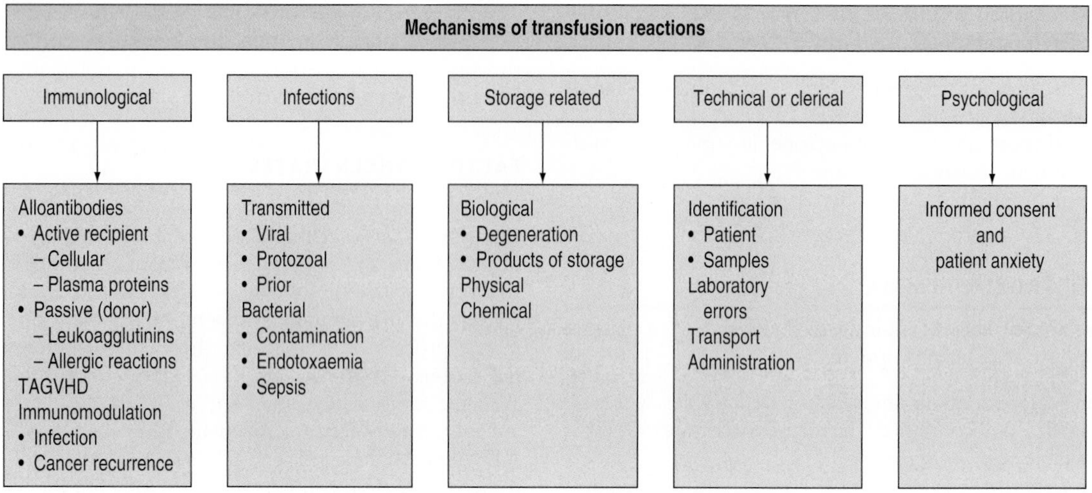

Figure 88.3 Possible mechanisms of adverse effects to blood transfusion. TAGVHD, transfusion-associated graft-versus-host disease.

- *Alterations in blood products due to preservation and storage* may result in quantitative and/or qualitative deficiencies in the blood components which will reduce transfusion efficacy and expose the patient to potentially adverse consequences from storage accumulants in the component.
- *Technical or clerical errors* that may result in adverse events in all the above categories.
- *Psychological* – informed consent issues and patient anxiety compatibility.

In terms of causation of an adverse clinical event, the possible role of blood transfusion can be classified into three categories on the basis of probability (Figure 88.4):

- *Definite – unifactorial – transfusion caused*: The well-understood and reported hazards of transfusion (i.e. immunological, technical, infectious) are generally unifactorial with a 1:1 causal relationship between the blood component transfused (usually a specific individual unit) and the adverse consequence for the patient. ABO blood group incompatibility, transfusion-related infection transmission, TAGVHD and TRALI due to donor leukoagglutinins are examples in this category.
- *Probable – oligofactorial – transfusion related*: Some adverse consequences of transfusion result from interaction with other insults, pathophysiology or host factors, but the contribution of the transfusion can usually be specifically identified. Fever, allergic reactions, hypotensive reactions, pulmonary oedema, some cases of TRALI, hyperbilirubinaemia and cytomegalovirus (CMV) transmission are examples in this category.
- *Possible – multifactorial – transfusion associated*: Transfusion may be a contributor to a complication or poor clinical outcome. In these circumstances it may be difficult to implicate transfusion directly in an individual case, nor is it necessarily the major factor. Transfusion-induced immunomodulation (TRIM) and the clinical consequences of storage lesions fall into this category. The role of transfusion being associated with adverse consequences has been established in observational studies, but causation cannot be confidently concluded. Accumulating evidence, in the absence of randomised clinical trials, supports causation, thus demanding a more precautionary approach to allogeneic blood

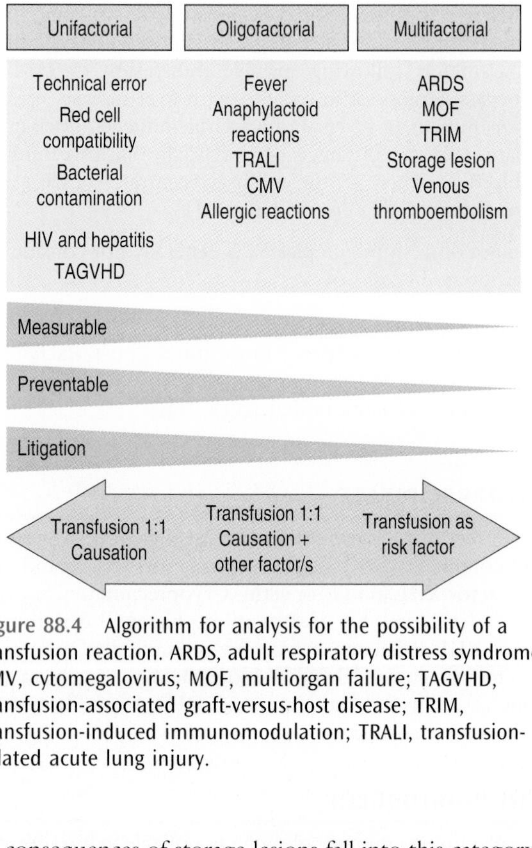

Figure 88.4 Algorithm for analysis for the possibility of a transfusion reaction. ARDS, adult respiratory distress syndrome; CMV, cytomegalovirus; MOF, multiorgan failure; TAGVHD, transfusion-associated graft-versus-host disease; TRIM, transfusion-induced immunomodulation; TRALI, transfusion-related acute lung injury.

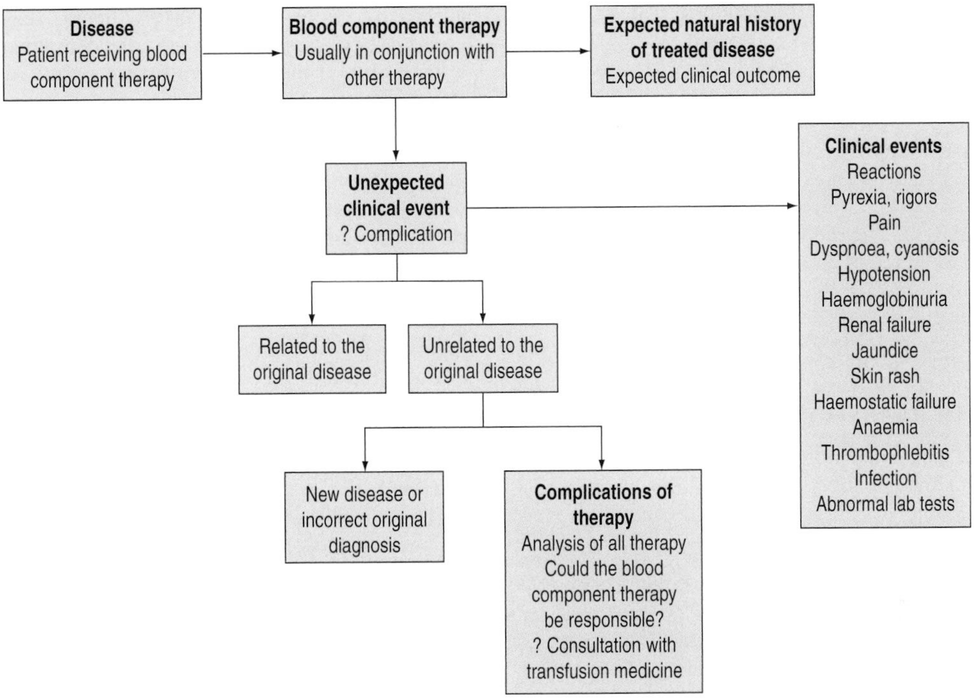

Figure 88.5 Adverse reactions to blood component therapy may just be one of the contributory factors in the differential diagnosis of any unexpected clinical presentation.

transfusion, examination of alternatives to transfusion and implementation of methods to improve the quality of transfused blood components (especially red cell and platelet concentrates). Universal pre-storage leukodepletion is currently the most important and effective strategy for minimising the clinical impact of TRIM and the blood storage lesions.

Adverse reactions to blood component therapy may present in a wide range of 'guises' and transfusion must always be considered in the differential diagnosis of any unexpected clinical presentation or indeed as a contributory factor to a clinical picture that may have several contributory factors (Figure 88.5).

PYREXIA

Mild febrile reactions are not usually a matter of concern, but rigors and temperatures above 38°C should not be ignored. The majority of febrile reactions are now considered to be an immunological reaction against one or more of the transfused cellular or plasma components, usually leukocytes.

TRANSFUSION-RELATED INFECTIONS

HEPATITIS

Post-transfusion hepatitis is a potential complication of allogeneic transfusion; donor selection, serological and nucleic acid tests ensure exclusion of infective donors. Hepatitis B and C are now almost totally preventable transfusion-transmitted diseases.

HUMAN IMMUNODEFICIENCY VIRUS

Donor selection, antibody screening and nucleic acid testing of blood donors has almost eliminated transfusion-associated HIV infection.

MONONUCLEOSIS SYNDROMES

The development of swinging pyrexia with varying degrees of peripheral blood atypical mononucleosis, 7–10 days following transfusion, can cause diagnostic confusion. Abnormalities in liver function are common. CMV infection is the commonest cause of this syndrome.

OTHER TRANSFUSION-TRANSMISSIBLE INFECTIONS

There is an increasing range of agents that have the potential to be transmitted by blood transfusion, the most recent one of concern being vCJD. The reader is referred to reviews for further information.[36,37]

BACTERIAL CONTAMINATION

Bacterial contamination of stored blood has always been recognised as a potential cause of fulminant endotoxic shock. Although a rare complication, continuing reports of its occurrence, especially in relation to platelet concentrate transfusion, have increased awareness.[38,39] The clinical features of transfusion-related bacterial sepsis in the non-anaesthetised patient include rigors, fever, tachycardia and vascular collapse, with prominent nausea, vomiting and diarrhoea. Anaesthetised patients may have a delayed onset of symptoms (fever, tachycardia, hypotension and cyanosis), followed by DIC, renal failure and sometimes ARDS. The requirement to store platelet concentrates at room temperature increases the risks of bacterial contamination. Pre-release bacterial testing is being more widely advocated as a measure to minimise the problem.

HAEMOLYTIC TRANSFUSION REACTIONS

Most severe acute haemolytic transfusion reactions are due to ABO incompatibility, have an identifiable cause and are avoidable, in contrast to delayed haemolytic reactions which are immune in nature and usually cannot be prevented.

INITIAL SYMPTOMS AND SIGNS

The classic symptoms and signs of an acute haemolytic transfusion reaction, typical of ABO incompatibility, include apprehension, flushing, pain (e.g. at infusion site, headache, chest, lumbosacral and abdominal), nausea, vomiting, rigors, hypotension and circulatory collapse.

HAEMOSTATIC FAILURE

Haemorrhagic diathesis due to DIC may be a feature, resulting in severe generalised haemostatic failure, with haemorrhage and oozing from multiple sites.[40] As the responsible transfusion is likely to have been administered for haemorrhage, increasing severity of local bleeding may be the first clue to an incompatible transfusion, especially if the patient is unconscious or anaesthetised in the operating room.

OLIGURIA AND RENAL IMPAIRMENT

Renal impairment may complicate a haemolytic transfusion reaction and its prevention or the appropriate management of established renal failure is important. If circulating volume and urinary output are rapidly restored, established renal failure is unlikely to occur. Death from acute renal failure directly caused by an incompatible blood transfusion is preventable, and there are usually other poor prognostic factors.

ANAEMIA AND JAUNDICE

A severe haemolytic transfusion reaction may be suspected from the development of jaundice or anaemia.

ALLERGIC AND ANAPHYLACTOID REACTIONS

Non-cellular blood (plasma and plasma derivatives) components are rarely considered to be a major cause for adverse reactions to transfusion therapy. However, the complexity of plasma and its various components and the effects from component processing results in a broader spectrum of potential adverse effects than frequently recognised. The antigenic heterogeneity of plasma proteins and the presence of antibodies make the non-cellular components of blood responsible for a range of adverse effects, many of which remain poorly understood and commonly pass unrecognised in clinical practice.[41]

There has been debate over the years as to the classification of allergic reactions to blood components. Clinical severity may range from minor urticarial reactions or flushing through to fulminant cardiorespiratory collapse and death. Some of these reactions are probably true anaphylaxis, but in others, mechanisms have been less clear and the term anaphylactoid has been used. To avoid implying the mechanism of the reaction, the term immediate generalised reaction has been used.

The clinical syndromes of immediate reactions have been classified as follows:

- Grade I
  - skin manifestations
- Grade II
  - mild to moderate hypotension
  - gastrointestinal disturbances (nausea)
  - respiratory distress
- Grade III
  - severe hypotension, shock
  - bronchospasm
- Grade IV
  - cardiac and/or respiratory arrest

PLASMA AND PLASMA COMPONENTS MAY CAUSE ADVERSE EFFECTS BY SEVERAL PATHOPHYSIOLOGICAL MECHANISMS

Immunological reactions to normal components of plasma may occur in two ways:

- Plasma proteins being antigenic to the recipient; they may contain epitopes on their molecules different from those on the recipient's functionally identical plasma proteins (e.g. anti-IgA antibodies)
- Antibodies in the donor plasma reacting with cellular components of the recipient's blood cells or plasma proteins

Physicochemical characteristics and contaminants of donor plasma, such as temperature, chemical additives, medications and micro-organisms may be responsible for recipient reactions.

The preparation techniques and storage conditions of blood and blood products may potentially cause adverse reaction through:

- *accumulation of metabolites* or cellular release products
- *plasma activation*, i.e. activation of some of the proteolytic systems. Importantly, the complement and

kinin/kininogen systems may generate vasoactive substances and anaphylatoxins which may be responsible for reactions. Some apparently allergic reactions to blood products may be due to vasoactive substances in the infusion. Subjective sensations may be missed in an unconscious patient. Hypotension occurring during rapid infusion of a hypovolaemic patient is likely to be interpreted as further volume loss, particularly with some plasma protein fractions that have been reported as consistently producing a transient fall in blood pressure, and a situation fraught with risk of overload can be produced

- *histamine generation*: histamine levels increase in some stored blood components and levels may be correlated with non-febrile, non-haemolytic transfusion reactions. Histamine release may be stimulated in the patient by plasma components, synthetic colloids and various medications
- *generation of cytokines* during storage may be responsible for non-haemolytic transfusion reactions
- *chemical additives*: there are various chemical additives (ethylene oxide, formaldehyde, drugs, latex) which may be responsible for immunological or non-immunological recipient reactions.

TRANSFUSION-ASSOCIATED GRAFT-VERSUS-HOST DISEASE (TAGVHD)

Graft-versus-host disease, classically observed in relationship to allogeneic bone marrow transplantation, may occur following a blood transfusion due to the infusion of immunocompetent lymphocytes precipitating an immunological reaction against the host tissues of the recipient.[42] It is most commonly observed in immunocompromised patients, but may also be seen in recipients of directed blood donation from first-degree relatives, and occasionally where donor and recipient are not related, due to homozygosity for HLA haplotypes for which the recipient is heterozygous. The syndrome usually occurs 3–30 days post allogeneic transfusion with fever, liver function test abnormalities, profuse watery diarrhoea, erythematous skin rash and progressive pancytopenia.

TRANSFUSION-RELATED ACUTE LUNG INJURY (TRALI)

TRALI is receiving a great deal of attention as a potentially serious complication of blood transfusion.[43–46] In the classic plasma neutrophil antibody-mediated form of the disease symptoms usually arise within hours of a blood transfusion.[47] In contrast to most patients with ARDS, recovery usually occurs within 48 hours. The underlying pathophysiology of 'classic' TRALI is due to the presence of leukoagglutinins in donor plasma. When complement is activated, C5a promotes neutrophil aggregation and sequestration in the microcirculation of the lung, causing endothelial damage leading to an interstitial oedema and acute respiratory failure. This classic form of transfusion-related acute lung injury has been recognised for over five decades, but was thought to be a rare complication of allogeneic plasma transfusion. As leukoagglutinins occur typically in plasma from multiparous females there is a move to using male donor only fresh frozen plasma.

It is now accepted that there has been underrecognition and underdiagnosis of TRALI, partly due to a lack of clinical awareness, but also to a broader understanding of mechanisms by which blood transfusion may cause or be a contributory factor to lung injury.[48,49] The term TRALI is now being expanded to include cases in which transfusion is identified as an independent risk factor predisposing patients to lung injury.[50,51] The reader is referred to recent reviews addressing the expanding area of concern in which transfusion, per se, is being identified as an independent risk factor for poor clinical poor outcomes, of which TRALI is only one.

TRANSFUSION-RELATED IMMUNOMODULATION (TRIM)

There is evidence that allogeneic blood transfusion is immunosuppressive in the recipient that has implications in relation to resistance to infection and the likelihood of cancer recurrence.[52–54] Donor leukocytes probably play the most important role in this immunomodulation. TRIM, along with the clinical effects of the blood storage lesion, is probably the mechanism by which allogeneic blood transfusion is responsible for poorer clinical outcomes discussed in the next section.

ALLOGENEIC TRANSFUSION AS AN INDEPENDENT RISK FACTOR FOR POORER CLINICAL OUTCOMES

Over the last decade experimental and clinical studies have identified blood transfusion as an independent risk factor for morbidity and mortality as well as increased admission rates to ICUs, increased length of hospital stay and additional costs.[18,19,55–57] Blood transfusion being implicated as part of the problem rather than optimal therapy has been a surprise to many clinicians, health administrators and patients, as it has always been assumed that blood transfusion can only be of benefit to the bleeding or anaemic patient. This long-standing belief is now being effectively challenged and currently the debate on the management of the acutely haemorrhaging or anaemic patient has moved significantly from a paradigm with a focus on transfusion to one in which the urgent control of critical bleeding is the paramount priority, with avoidance and/or minimisation of blood transfusion. There is thus increasing evidence that transfusion-related immunomodulation (TRIM) and the transfusion effects of storage lesions are responsible for poorer clinical outcomes in a range of clinical settings.[18,19,55,58–63]

However, it is not possible to categorically conclude causation and that pre-storage leukoreduction will eliminate or minimise the risk. While the case for causation is strengthened, it is important to be aware that there is minimal evidence for the efficacy or appropriateness of many transfusions, and there is evidence that restrictive red cell transfusion policies do not jeopardise clinical outcomes; indeed, the reverse may be the case.[64,65] Thus, until these issues are resolved, a precautionary approach should be adopted, with the modus operandi being to avoid or minimise allogeneic transfusion and use appropriate patient blood conservation techniques.[66] An additional association with transfusion is the higher incidence of venous thromboembolism if patients are transfused.[67]

CRITICAL HAEMORRHAGE AND MASSIVE BLOOD TRANSFUSION

There is a reappraisal of clinical practice guidelines for the use of blood components in the bleeding patient.[21,68] The guidelines are no longer for the management of massive blood transfusion, but rather for the management of critical bleeding and avoiding getting into the massive transfusion coagulopathy quagmire in which the patient can spiral down into the 'triad of death' – coagulopathy, acidosis and hypothermia.

This reappraisal of management of patients with acute haemorrhage is resulting in the challenging of long-standing dogmas. There is greater tolerance of hypotension until haemorrhage is controlled, and lower haemoglobin levels are tolerated with closer attention to the clinical context of the anaemia and its impact on systemic and local oxygen delivery, especially if there are any compromises in cardiorespiratory function. More attention and research is being directed toward the role of clear fluids and the importance of plasma viscosity, colloid oncotic pressure and functional capillary density.[69] The search for safe and effective haemoglobin-based oxygen carriers continues.[70–72]

If blood loss has been massive or there are defects in the haemostatic system, specific component therapy may be indicated. Advances in patient retrieval, resuscitation protocols, techniques for rapid and real-time diagnosis, trauma teams and early 'damage control' surgery have improved the management of acutely haemorrhaging patients. Patients are now surviving with larger volumes of blood transfusion, but sepsis, acute lung injury and multiorgan failure remain major challenges, and blood transfusion is increasingly being recognised as a two-edged sword and probably a contributory factor to these complications in which microcirculatory dysfunction is recognised as central in the pathophysiology. As already discussed, the evidence that the immediate post-transfusion ability of stored red cells and haemoglobin to deliver and unload oxygen to microcirculation may be impaired is resulting in stored red cell concentrates not being automatically the first therapy for acutely enhancing oxygen delivery. Indeed, recent animal data indicate that the immediate clinical benefit of transfused red cells in treating hypovolaemic shock relates to reconstitution of the macrocirculation, with adverse effects on the functional capillary density in the microcirculation.[73]

In previously healthy patients who have suffered an acute blood loss of less than 25% of their blood volume, restoring volume is more important than replacing oxygen-carrying capacity. Plasma volume expanders may preclude the necessity for allogeneic transfusion, especially if bleeding can be controlled. Clear fluids also allow time for transfusion compatibility testing. In the context of acute bleeding and hypovolaemic shock, the haemoglobin level is not the primary indicator for determining the need for allogeneic red cell transfusion. A normal human may survive a 30% deficit in blood volume without fluid replacement, in contrast to an 80% loss of red cell mass if normovolaemia is maintained. Minimisation of allogeneic blood transfusion is important and haemodilution with tolerance of anaemia is now accepted clinical practice. However, there are limits to haemodilution, not only from the oxygen-carrying capacity perspective. Marked reduction in blood viscosity is counterproductive as reactive peripheral vasoconstriction to maintain total peripheral resistance results in reduction in functional capillary density in the microcirculation. The role of clear fluids and the importance of plasma viscosity, colloid oncotic pressure, electrolyte composition and functional capillary density is the subject of current research.[74]

A protocol approach to blood component therapy is generally not recommended, as each patient should be treated individually. However, this remains a controversial issue with advocates for 'blind', up-front component therapy with red cell and haemostatic components, especially fresh frozen plasma and cryoprecipitate or fibrinogen concentrates. With better understanding of coagulopathy in the critical haemorrhage setting and the importance of hypofibrinogenaemia and hyperfibrinolysis there is a reanalysis of the approach to blood component therapy.[75] In an elective situation in which normovolaemia is generally maintained from the outset, defects can be predicted and appropriate blood components prescribed, a protocol approach may be justified. This should be done in close consultation with the haematologist and hospital transfusion service.

Failure of haemostasis is common in critically bleeding patients and may be complex and multifactorial in pathogenesis.[76,77] The importance of avoiding acidosis and hypothermia cannot be overemphasised as the triad of coagulopathy, acidosis and hypothermia has an extremely poor prognosis. Coagulopathy associated with critical haemorrhage is related to other aspects of the pathophysiology of the clinical setting. The assumption that there is a 'generic coagulopathy' vaguely referred to as DIC is incorrect and can result in inappropriate therapeutic decisions. The reader is referred to an expanding literature on this topic where it will be seen that there can be no standard approach to therapy.[77] This author is increasingly convinced that the pathophysiology of coagulopathy, when occurring in the context of critical haemorrhage, should be viewed as related to the primary insult/initiating event, and that a 'secondary' coagulopathy (e.g. massive stored blood transfusion, haemodilution, hypothermia, continuing tissue hypoxia, etc.) may compound the problem in the resuscitated patient. The primary mechanisms of coagulopathy relating to the initiating event may relate to trauma, hypoxia, pregnancy, microbial infection, envenomation or iatrogenic (antithrombotic) agents. In all circumstances there is activation or inhibition of some aspect of the haemostatic system, and therapy is better informed if the varied mechanisms are understood. Frequently, complex tests are required for definitive diagnosis, but the urgency of the situation cannot always await the results, and therapy may be initiated on clinical evidence with minimal laboratory information.

Many trauma patients have coagulopathy at presentation that is more related to hypovolaemic shock and not consumption or dilution. Recent evidence indicates that excessive activation of the protein C system and hypofibrinogenaemia secondary to secondary hyperfibrinolysis are important.[78] Except for severe abnormalities, haemostatic laboratory parameters correlate poorly with clinical evidence of haemostatic failure. In the massively transfused patient thrombocytopenia and impaired platelet function are the most consistent significant haematological abnormalities, correction of which may be associated with control of microvascular bleeding. Coagulation deficiency from massive blood loss is initially confined to factors V and VIII. Activated partial thromboplastin time (APTT), prothrombin time (PT) and fibrinogen assay should be performed, but the urgency of the situation does not usually allow for other specific factor assays.

A problem with the standard screen tests of coagulation function is that they do not give information about the actual formation of the haemostatic plug, its size, structure or stability. For this reason there is increasing interest in global tests of haemostatic plug formation and stability such as thromboelastography, thrombin generation tests and clot waveform analysis in which changes in light transmission in routine APTT are measured.[79] Fresh frozen plasma should be infused if the test results are abnormal, including cryoprecipitate or fibrinogen concentrates if the fibrinogen level is < 1 g/l. A case can be made for prophylactic fresh frozen plasma in infusions in patients with massive blood loss which has been replaced with red cell concentrates and plasma substitutes.

With ongoing bleeding with associated microvascular oozing various approaches may be taken. Having ensured that all identifiable haemostatic defects have been corrected, questions arise as to the role of fresh blood and, more recently, recombinant activated factor VII (rFVIIa).[80] The use of freshly collected whole blood remains controversial and is an 'emotive' subject needing some comment. The provision of fresh whole blood can present logistic, ethical and safety problems needing consideration. Many transfusion medicine specialists categorically state that there is never an indication for fresh whole blood. Such dogma can be difficult to defend in the clinical setting of the massive haemorrhage and transfusion syndrome where pathophysiology remains poorly understood and specific blood component therapy may be ineffective.

The following statements reasonably summarise the current status of fresh blood transfusion:

- Fresh blood provides immediately functioning oxygen-carrying capacity, volume and haemostatic factors in the one product
- The number of allogeneic donors to whom a patient is exposed can be reduced
- Problems associated with infusion of massive volumes of stored blood can be minimised/avoided
- The risk of transfusion-related viral infections is possibly higher than fully tested and stored blood
- The benefit in controlling haemorrhage probably relates to the presence of immediately functioning platelets

SPECIFIC HAZARDS OF MASSIVE BLOOD TRANSFUSION

Massive blood transfusion may be defined in several ways:

- replacement of the circulating volume in 24 hours
- > 4 units of blood in 1 hour with continuing blood loss
- loss of 50% of circulating blood volume within 3 hours

Any patient receiving massive blood component therapy is likely to be seriously ill and have multiple problems. Many adverse effects must be considered in conjunction with the injuries and multiorgan dysfunction. It is not always possible to define the complications caused or aggravated by massive blood transfusion.

CITRATE TOXICITY

A patient responds to citrate infusion by the removal of citrate and mobilisation of ionised calcium. Citrate is metabolised by the Krebs cycle in all nucleated cells, especially the liver. A marked elevation in the citrate concentration is seen with transfusion exceeding 500 ml in 5 minutes; the level rapidly falls when the infusion is slowed. Citrate metabolism is impaired by hypotension, hypovolaemia, hypothermia and liver disease. Toxicity may also be potentiated by alkalosis, hyperkalaemia, hypothermia and cardiac disease. The clinical significance of a minor depression of ionised calcium remains ill-defined, and it is accepted that a warm, well-perfused adult patient with normal liver function can tolerate a unit of blood each 5 minutes without requiring calcium. The rate of transfusion is more significant than the total volume transfused. Common practice is to administer 10% calcium gluconate 1.0 g i.v. following each 5 units of blood or fresh frozen plasma. Such a practice remains controversial as there is increasing concern regarding calcium homeostasis and cell function in acutely ill patients.

ACID–BASE AND ELECTROLYTE DISTURBANCES

Acid–base

Stored bank blood contains an appreciable acid load and is often used in a situation of pre-existing or continuing metabolic acidosis. The acidity of stored blood is mainly due to the citric acid of the anticoagulant and the lactic acid generated during storage. Their intermediary metabolites are rapidly metabolised with adequate tissue perfusion, resulting in a metabolic alkalosis. Hence the routine use of sodium bicarbonate is usually unnecessary and is generally contraindicated. Alkali further shifts the oxygen dissociation curve to the left, provides a large additional sodium load, and depresses the return of ionised calcium to normal following citrate infusion. Acid–base estimations should be performed and corrected in the context of the clinical situation. With continuing hypoperfusion, however, metabolism of citrate and lactate will be depressed, lactic acid production will continue, and there may be an indication for i.v. bicarbonate and calcium to correct acidosis and low ionised calcium.

Serum potassium

Although controversial, it is unlikely that the high serum potassium levels in stored blood have pathological effects in adults, except in the presence of acute renal failure. However, hypokalaemia may be a problem 24 hours after transfusion as the transfused cells correct their electrolyte composition and potassium returns into the cells. Thus, although initial acidosis and hyperkalaemia may be an immediate problem with massive blood transfusion, the net result of successful resuscitation is likely to be delayed hypokalaemia and alkalosis. With CPD (citrate–phosphate–dextrose) blood, the acid load and red cell storage lesion is less. Constant monitoring of the acid–base and electrolyte status is essential in such fluctuating clinical situations.

Serum sodium

The sodium content of whole blood and fresh frozen plasma is higher than the normal blood level due to the sodium citrate. This should be remembered when large volumes of plasma are being infused into patients who have disordered salt and water handling (e.g. renal, liver or cardiac disease).

HYPOTHERMIA

Blood warmed from 4°C to 37°C requires 1255 kJ (300 kcal), the equivalent heat produced by 1 hour of muscular work, with an oxygen requirement of 62 l. Hypothermia impairs the metabolism of citrate and lactate, shifts the oxygen dissociation curve to the left, increases intracellular potassium release, impairs red cell deformability, delays drug metabolism, masks clinical signs, increases the incidence of arrhythmias, reduces cardiac output and impairs haemostatic function. Thus a thermostatically controlled blood-warming device should be routinely used when any transfusion episode requires the rapid infusion of more than 2 units of blood.

HYPERBILIRUBINAEMIA

Jaundice is common following massive blood transfusion as a significant amount of transfused stored blood may not survive, resulting in varying degrees of hyperbilirubinaemia. During hypovolaemia and shock, liver function may be impaired, particularly in the presence of sepsis or multiorgan failure. An important rate-limiting step in bilirubin transport is the energy-requiring process of transporting conjugated bilirubin from the hepatocyte to the biliary canaliculus. Thus, although an increased load of bilirubin from destroyed transfused red cells may be conjugated, there may be delayed excretion, leading to a conjugated hyperbilirubinaemia. This 'paradoxical' conjugated hyperbilirubinaemia may be misinterpreted, leading to unnecessary investigations. The effect of resorbing haematoma and the possibility of an occult haemolytic transfusion reaction should also be considered.

BASIC IMMUNOHAEMATOLOGY

Red cell serology is a highly specialised area of knowledge and it is not possible to expect clinicians to have more than a basic working knowledge essential for patient safety. The following is a summary of core knowledge for the clinician.

SALINE AGGLUTINATION

Safe red cell transfusion has revolved around this traditional serological technique. A saline suspension of red cells is mixed with serum and observed for agglutination. Saline agglutination is used for ABO blood grouping and is one of the techniques for compatibility testing of donor blood.

THE DIRECT AND INDIRECT ANTIGLOBULIN TEST

In red cell serology, the antiglobulin test (Coombs test) is used to detect IgG immunoglobulins or complement components. The direct antiglobulin test (DAT) detects immunoglobulin or complement components present on the surface of the red cells circulating in the patient. The result is positive in autoimmune haemolytic anaemia and haemolytic disease of the newborn and during a haemolytic transfusion reaction. The indirect antiglobulin test (IAT) detects the presence of non-agglutinating antibodies in the patient's plasma, usually IgG type. Antibody screening for atypical antibodies and pretransfusion compatibility testing are the main applications of the IAT.

REGULAR AND IRREGULAR (ATYPICAL) ANTIBODIES

The regular alloantibodies (isoagglutinins) of the ABO system are naturally occurring agglutinins present in all ABO types (except AB), depending on the ABO group. Group O people have anti-A and anti-B isoagglutinins, group A have anti-B and Group B have anti-A. Group A cells are the cause of the commonest and most dangerous ABO incompatible haemolytic reactions. Atypical antibodies are not normally present in the plasma, but may be found in some people as naturally occurring antibodies or as immune antibodies. Immune antibodies result from previous exposure due to blood transfusion or pregnancy. Naturally occurring antibodies more frequently react by saline agglutination and, although they may be stimulated by transfusion, are usually of minimal clinical significance. In contrast, many of the immune atypical antibodies are of major clinical significance and their recognition is the raison d'être for pretransfusion compatibility testing and antenatal antibody screening. Most of the clinically significant immune atypical antibodies are detected by the IAT.

Blood group antigens vary widely in their frequency and immunogenicity. The D antigen of the Rhesus blood group system is common and highly immunogenic. Thus, when a Rh-negative (i.e. D-negative) patient is exposed to D-positive blood there is a high likelihood of forming an anti-D antibody. It is for this reason that the D antigen is taken into account when providing blood for transfusion, in contrast to the numerous other red cell antigens that are less common or less immunogenic. Beyond the Rh (D), and sometimes the Kell (K) blood group antigens, it is not practical, or necessary, to take notice of other blood group antigens unless an atypical antibody is detected during antibody screening procedures.

THE ANTIBODY SCREEN

On receipt of a blood sample by the transfusion service the red cells are ABO and Rh D typed and the serum is screened for atypical antibodies. This screen consists of testing the patient's serum with group O screening cells. The screening panel consists of red cells obtained usually from two group O donors containing all common red cell antigens occurring with a frequency of greater than approximately 2% in the community. If an atypical antibody is detected on the antibody screen, further serological investigations are carried out to identify the specificity of the antibody. These investigations are time consuming and when possible should be carried out electively.

THE CROSSMATCH (COMPATIBILITY TEST)

The crossmatch is the final compatibility test between the donor cells and the patient's serum. The crossmatch test tends to be overemphasised to the detriment of the antibody screen. With sophisticated knowledge of serology the emphasis in the supply of compatible blood is now concentrated on the steps prior to the final compatibility crossmatch.

THE TYPE AND SCREEN SYSTEM

As precompatibility testing has assumed the major role in the selection of blood for transfusion, there has been a rethinking of policies relating to the supply of blood for elective transfusions. Whenever elective surgery is planned for a patient who is likely to require blood transfusion, the transfusion service must receive a clotted blood sample well before the anticipated time of surgery. The precompatibility testing should be carried out during the routine working hours when facilities are geared for large workloads and enough staff is available to handle all contingencies.

THE PROVISION OF BLOOD IN EMERGENCIES

When quick clinical and laboratory decisions are made under conditions of stress it is frequently difficult for all involved personnel to appreciate the difficulties of others. The decision to give uncrossmatched, partially crossmatched or wait for crossmatched compatible blood is not easy, and certain basic serological considerations may clarify for the clinician some of the problems faced by the serologist. Depending upon the degree of urgency and the extent of previous knowledge about the patient's red cell serology, blood can be provided with varying degrees of safety. However, it should be emphasised that when a patient is exsanguinating and likely to die, the giving of ABO compatible uncrossmatched blood, especially if the antibody screen is negative, is safe and appropriate therapy.

UNIVERSAL DONOR GROUP O BLOOD

Group O blood under normal circumstances will be ABO compatible with all recipients. The transfusions should be given as red cell concentrates screened for high titre A or B haemolysins and only used in extreme emergencies. If the recipient is in the childbearing age every attempt should be made to give Rh-D negative blood until the patient's blood group is known.

ABO GROUP SPECIFIC BLOOD

Transfusion of blood of the correct ABO type circumvents the isoagglutinin problems alluded to above. Simple as this approach may seem, its safety is dependent on meticulous attention to grouping. Previous blood group information, such as a 'bracelet' group or 'unofficial' group written in the patient's records may be incorrect, and there may be considerable risk if blood is administered on the basis of this information.

SALINE-COMPATIBLE BLOOD

The administration of saline-compatible blood is, for practical purposes, the administration of ABO group specific blood.

REFERENCES

1. Isbister JP. Decision making in perioperative transfusion. *Transfus Apher Sci* 2002; **27**: 19–28.
2. Isbister JP. Clinicians as gatekeepers: what is the best route to optimal blood use? *Dev Biol (Basel)* 2007; **127**: 9–14.

3. Scott KL, Lecak J, Acker JP. Biopreservation of red blood cells: past, present, and future. *Transfus Med Rev* 2005; **19**: 127–42.
4. Anniss AM, Glenister KM, Killian JJ *et al.* Proteomic analysis of supernatants of stored red blood cell products. *Transfusion* 2005; **45**: 1426–33.
5. Sparrow RL, Patton KA. Supernatant from stored red blood cell primes inflammatory cells: influence of prestorage white cell reduction. *Transfusion* 2004; **44**: 722–30.
6. Anniss AM, Sparrow RL. Storage duration and white blood cell content of red blood cell (RBC) products increases adhesion of stored RBCs to endothelium under flow conditions. *Transfusion* 2006; **46**: 1561–7.
7. Tinmouth A, Fergusson D, Yee IC *et al.* Clinical consequences of red cell storage in the critically ill. *Transfusion* 2006; **46**: 2014–27.
8. Elfath MD. Is it time to focus on preserving the functionality of red blood cells during storage? *Transfusion* 2006; **46**: 1469–70.
9. Blajchman MA. The clinical benefits of the leukoreduction of blood products. *J Trauma* 2006; **60**(6 Suppl): S83–90.
10. Basran S, Frumento RJ, Cohen A *et al.* The association between duration of storage of transfused red blood cells and morbidity and mortality after reoperative cardiac surgery. *Anesth Analg* 2006; **103**: 15–20.
11. Ho J, Sibbald WJ, Chin-Yee IH. Effects of storage on efficacy of red cell transfusion: when is it not safe? *Crit Care Med* 2003; **31**(12 Suppl): S687–97.
12. Hogman CF, Meryman HT. Red blood cells intended for transfusion: quality criteria revisited. *Transfusion* 2006; **46**: 137–42.
13. van Hilten JA, van de Watering LM, van Bockel JH *et al.* Effects of transfusion with red cells filtered to remove leucocytes: randomised controlled trial in patients undergoing major surgery. *BMJ* 2004; **328**: 1281.
14. Despotis GJ, Zhang L, Lublin DM. Transfusion risks and transfusion-related pro-inflammatory responses. *Hematol Oncol Clin North Am* 2007; **21**: 147–61.
15. Jeschke MG, Herndon DN. Blood transfusion in burns: benefit or risk? *Crit Care Med* 2006; **34**: 1822–3.
16. Blumberg N, Fine L, Gettings KF *et al.* Decreased sepsis related to indwelling venous access devices coincident with implementation of universal leukoreduction of blood transfusions. *Transfusion* 2005; **45**: 1632–9.
17. Hebert PC, Fergusson D, Blajchman MA *et al.* Clinical outcomes following institution of the Canadian universal leukoreduction program for red blood cell transfusions. *JAMA* 2003; **289**: 1941–9.
18. Palmieri TL, Caruso DM, Foster KN *et al.* Effect of blood transfusion on outcome after major burn injury: a multicenter study. *Crit Care Med* 2006; **34**: 1602–7.
19. Malone DL, Dunne J, Tracy JK *et al.* Blood transfusion, independent of shock severity, is associated with worse outcome in trauma. *J Trauma* 2003; **54**: 898–905; discussion 907.
20. Sparrow RL, Healey G, Patton KA *et al.* Red blood cell age determines the impact of storage and leukocyte burden on cell adhesion molecules, glycophorin A and the release of annexin V. *Transfus Apher Sci* 2006; **34**: 15–23.
21. Spiess BD. Red cell transfusions and guidelines: a work in progress. *Hematol Oncol Clin North Am* 2007; **21**: 185–200.
22. Carson JL, Ferreira G. Transfusion triggers: how low can we go? *Vox Sang* 2004; **87**(Suppl 2): 218–21.
23. Vallet B, Adamczyk S, Barreau O *et al.* Physiologic transfusion triggers. *Best Pract Res Clin Anaesthesiol* 2007; **21**: 173–81.
24. Guidelines for the use of platelet transfusions. *Br J Haematol* 2003; **122**: 10–23.
25. Stanworth SJ, Brunskill SJ, Hyde CJ *et al.* Appraisal of the evidence for the clinical use of FFP and plasma fractions. *Best Pract Res Clin Haematol* 2006; **19**: 67–82.
26. Lankiewicz MW, Hays J, Friedman KD *et al.* Urgent reversal of warfarin with prothrombin complex concentrate. *J Thromb Haemost* 2006; **4**: 967–70.
27. Baker RI, Coughlin PB, Gallus AS *et al.* Warfarin reversal: consensus guidelines, on behalf of the Australasian Society of Thrombosis and Haemostasis. *Med J Aust* 2004; **181**: 492–7.
28. Schulman S, Bijsterveld NR. Anticoagulants and their reversal. *Transfus Med Rev* 2007; **21**: 37–48.
29. Looney RJ, Huggins J. Use of intravenous immunoglobulin G (IVIG). *Best Pract Res Clin Haematol* 2006; **19**: 3–25.
30. Norrby-Teglund A, Muller MP, McGeer A *et al.* Successful management of severe group A streptococcal soft tissue infections using an aggressive medical regimen including intravenous polyspecific immunoglobulin together with a conservative surgical approach. *Scand J Infect Dis* 2005; **37**: 166–72.
31. Wiedermann CJ, Hoffmann JN, Juers M *et al.* High-dose antithrombin III in the treatment of severe sepsis in patients with a high risk of death: efficacy and safety. *Crit Care Med* 2006; **34**: 285–92.
32. Gardlund B. Activated protein C (Xigris) treatment in sepsis: a drug in trouble. *Acta Anaesthesiol Scand* 2006; **50**: 907–10.
33. Mittal S, Watson HG. A critical appraisal of the use of recombinant factor VIIa in acquired bleeding conditions. *Br J Haematol* 2006; **133**: 355–63.
34. Mathew P, Simon TL, Hunt KE *et al.* How we manage requests for recombinant factor VIIa (NovoSeven). *Transfusion* 2007; **47**: 8–14.
35. Brand A. Immunological aspects of blood transfusions. *Transpl Immunol* 2002; **10**: 183–90.
36. Stramer SL. Current risks of transfusion-transmitted agents: a review. *Arch Pathol Lab Med* 2007; **131**: 702–7.
37. Alter HJ, Stramer SL, Dodd RY. Emerging infectious diseases that threaten the blood supply. *Semin Hematol* 2007; **44**: 32–41.

38. Rao PL, Strausbaugh LJ, Liedtke LA *et al.* Bacterial infections associated with blood transfusion: experience and perspective of infectious diseases consultants. *Transfusion* 2007; **47**: 1206–11.
39. Palavecino E, Yomtovian R. Risk and prevention of transfusion-related sepsis. *Curr Opin Hematol* 2003; **10**: 434–9.
40. Davenport RD. Pathophysiology of hemolytic transfusion reactions. *Semin Hematol* 2005; **42**: 165–8.
41. Gilstad CW. Anaphylactic transfusion reactions. *Curr Opin Hematol* 2003; **10**: 419–23.
42. Oto OA, Paydas S, Baslamisli F *et al.* Transfusion-associated graft-versus-host disease. *Eur J Intern Med* 2006; **17**: 151–6.
43. Swanson K, Dwyre DM, Krochmal J *et al.* Transfusion-related acute lung injury (TRALI): current clinical and pathophysiologic considerations. *Lung* 2006; **184**: 177–85.
44. Popovsky MA. Pulmonary consequences of transfusion: TRALI and TACO. *Transfus Apher Sci* 2006; **34**: 243–4.
45. Goldman M, Webert KE, Arnold DM *et al.* Proceedings of a consensus conference: towards an understanding of TRALI. *Transfus Med Rev* 2005; **19**: 2–31.
46. Nathens AB. Massive transfusion as a risk factor for acute lung injury: association or causation? *Crit Care Med* 2006; **34**(5 Suppl): S14–150.
47. Curtis BR, McFarland JG. Mechanisms of transfusion-related acute lung injury (TRALI): anti-leukocyte antibodies. *Crit Care Med* 2006; **34**(5 Suppl): S118–123.
48. Silliman CC, McLaughlin NJ. Transfusion-related acute lung injury. *Blood Rev* 2006; **20**: 139–59.
49. Silverboard H, Aisiku I, Martin GS *et al.* The role of acute blood transfusion in the development of acute respiratory distress syndrome in patients with severe trauma. *J Trauma* 2005; **59**: 717–23.
50. Croce MA, Tolley EA, Claridge JA *et al.* Transfusions result in pulmonary morbidity and death after a moderate degree of injury. *J Trauma* 2005; **59**: 19–23; discussion 24.
51. Gong MN, Thompson BT, Williams P *et al.* Clinical predictors of and mortality in acute respiratory distress syndrome: potential role of red cell transfusion. *Crit Care Med* 2005; **33**: 1191–8.
52. Blajchman MA. Transfusion immunomodulation or TRIM: what does it mean clinically? *Hematology* 2005; **10**(Suppl 1): 208–14.
53. Blumberg N. Deleterious clinical effects of transfusion immunomodulation: proven beyond a reasonable doubt. *Transfusion* 2005; **45**(Suppl 2): S33–40.
54. Raghavan M, Marik PE. Anemia, allogenic blood transfusion, and immunomodulation in the critically ill. *Chest* 2005; **127**: 295–307.
55. Chang H, Hall GA, Geerts WH *et al.* Allogeneic red blood cell transfusion is an independent risk factor for the development of postoperative bacterial infection. *Vox Sang* 2000; **78**: 13–18.
56. Strumper-Groves D. Perioperative blood transfusion and outcome. *Curr Opin Anaesthesiol* 2006; **19**: 198–206.
57. Dutton RP, Lefering R, Lynn M. Database predictors of transfusion and mortality. *J Trauma* 2006; **60**(6 Suppl): S70–77.
58. Robinson WP 3rd, Ahn J, Stiffler A *et al.* Blood transfusion is an independent predictor of increased mortality in nonoperatively managed blunt hepatic and splenic injuries. *J Trauma* 2005; **58**: 437–45.
59. Miller PR, Croce MA, Kilgo PD *et al.* Acute respiratory distress syndrome in blunt trauma: identification of independent risk factors. *Am Surg* 2002; **68**: 845–50; discussion 850–1.
60. Moore FA, Moore EE, Sauaia A. Blood transfusion. An independent risk factor for postinjury multiple organ failure. *Arch Surg* 1997; **132**: 620–4; discussion 624–5.
61. Taylor RW, O'Brien J, Trottier SJ *et al.* Red blood cell transfusions and nosocomial infections in critically ill patients. *Crit Care Med* 2006; **34**: 2302–8.
62. Koch CG, Li L, Duncan AI *et al.* Morbidity and mortality risk associated with red blood cell and blood-component transfusion in isolated coronary artery bypass grafting. *Crit Care Med* 2006; **34**: 1608–16.
63. Koch CG, Li L, Duncan AI *et al.* Transfusion in coronary artery bypass grafting is associated with reduced long-term survival. *Ann Thorac Surg* 2006; **81**: 1650–7.
64. Hebert PC, Wells G, Blajchman MA *et al.* A multicenter, randomized, controlled clinical trial of transfusion requirements in critical care. Transfusion Requirements in Critical Care Investigators, Canadian Critical Care Trials Group. *N Engl J Med* 1999; **340**: 409–17.
65. Kwan P, Gomez M, Cartotto R. Safe and successful restriction of transfusion in burn patients. *J Burn Care Res* 2006; **27**: 826–34.
66. McIntyre L, Hebert PC, Wells G *et al.* Is a restrictive transfusion strategy safe for resuscitated and critically ill trauma patients? *J Trauma* 2004; **57**: 563–8; discussion 568.
67. Nilsson KR, Berenholtz SM, Garrett-Mayer E *et al.* Association between venous thromboembolism and perioperative allogeneic transfusion. *Arch Surg* 2007; **142**: 126–32; discussion 133.
68. Practice guidelines for perioperative blood transfusion and adjuvant therapies: an updated report by the American Society of Anesthesiologists Task Force on Perioperative Blood Transfusion and Adjuvant Therapies. *Anesthesiology* 2006; **105**: 198–208.
69. Tsai AG, Cabrales P, Intaglietta M. Blood viscosity: a factor in tissue survival? *Crit Care Med* 2005; **33**: 1662–3.
70. Thyes C, Spahn DR. Current status of artificial O_2 carriers. *Anesthesiol Clin North Am* 2005; **23**: 373–89, viii.
71. Winslow RM. Targeted O_2 delivery by low-p50 hemoglobin: a new basis for hemoglobin-based oxygen carriers. *Artif Cells Blood Substit Immobil Biotechnol* 2005; **33**: 1–12.
72. Tsai AG, Cabrales P, Intaglietta M. Oxygen-carrying blood substitutes: a microvascular perspective. *Expert Opin Biol Ther* 2004; **4**: 1147–57.

73. Tsai AG, Cabrales P, Intaglietta M. Microvascular perfusion upon exchange transfusion with stored red blood cells in normovolemic anemic conditions. *Transfusion* 2004; **44**: 1626–34.
74. Wettstein R, Erni D, Intaglietta M *et al.* Rapid restoration of microcirculatory blood flow with hyperviscous and hyperoncotic solutions lowers the transfusion trigger in resuscitation from hemorrhagic shock. *Shock* 2006; **25**: 641–6.
75. Fries D, Haas T, Klingler A *et al.* Efficacy of fibrinogen and prothrombin complex concentrate used to reverse dilutional coagulopathy – a porcine model. *Br J Anaesth* 2006; **97**: 460–7.
76. Tieu BH, Holcomb JB, Schreiber MA. Coagulopathy: its pathophysiology and treatment in the injured patient. *World J Surg* 2007; **31**: 1055–65.
77. Levy JH. Massive transfusion coagulopathy. *Semin Hematol* 2006; **43**(1 Suppl 1): S59–63.
78. Brohi K, Cohen MJ, Ganter MT *et al.* Acute traumatic coagulopathy: initiated by hypoperfusion: modulated through the protein C pathway? *Ann Surg* 2007; **245**: 812–18.
79. Zwaginga JJ, Sakariassen KS, Nash G *et al.* Flow-based assays for global assessment of hemostasis. Part 2: current methods and considerations for the future. *J Thromb Haemost* 2006; **4**: 2716–17.
80. Hedner U. Mechanism of action of factor VIIa in the treatment of coagulopathies. *Semin Thromb Hemost* 2006; **32**(Suppl 1): 77–85.

89

Colloids and blood products

Michael Mythen

Colloids are plasma expanders used to expand the blood volume. Hydrostatic and osmotic forces dictate movement of fluid between the different compartments of the body across semipermeable membranes (Starling's forces).

The osmotic pressure generated by a solute is proportional to the number of molecules or ions of solute and independent of solute molecular size.

Colloid osmotic pressure (COP) is the osmotic pressure exerted by the macromolecules (the colloid molecules).[1,2] This can be measured using a membrane transducer system in which the membrane is freely permeable to small ions and water but largely impermeable to the colloid molecules.[3] The membrane pore size and the molecular size distribution of the colloid being studied will dictate the measured value (see Figures 89.2 and 89.3).[2,3] Capillary walls are made up of endothelial cells, which are freely permeable to small ions such as Na^+ and Cl^-, but are relatively impermeable to larger molecules such as colloids (Figure 89.3). A colloid is a homogeneous non-crystalline substance consisting of large molecules or ultramicroscopic particles of one substance dispersed through a second substance – the particles do not settle and cannot be separated out by ordinary filtering or centrifuging like those of a suspension such as blood.[2]

In practical terms, it is a fluid that when infused into the intravascular space should expand the blood volume by the volume infused.[3,4] Crystalloids have larger volumes of distribution dependent on their composition (Figure 89.1 and Table 89.1). Colloids or plasma substitutes have molecular weights (MW) >35 kDa, and infusion results in an initial increase in blood osmotic pressure. The ideal properties of a colloid are:

- stable with a long shelf life
- pyrogen, antigen and toxin free
- free from risk of disease transmission
- plasma volume expanding effect lasts for several hours
- metabolism and excretion do not adversely effect the recipient
- no direct adverse effects, e.g. causing a coagulopathy

COLLOID SOLUTIONS

There are two major groups of colloids – plasma derivatives or semisynthetics.[5] Plasma derivatives include human albumin solutions, plasma protein fraction, fresh frozen plasma and immunoglobulin solutions. Three principal types of semisynthetic colloid molecule are commonly used in intravenous solutions – gelatins, dextrans and hydroxyethyl starches. All colloids are presented dissolved in a crystalloid solution. Isotonic saline is still the most commonly used carrier solution but isotonic glucose, hypertonic saline and isotonic balanced electrolyte solutions are also used.

Colloids often do not consist of uniform sized molecules. Human albumin solution contains more than 95% albumin with a uniform molecular size. This is described as monodisperse. Conversely, all the semisynthetic colloids have a distribution of molecular sizes and are described as polydisperse.[1,2] The size–weight relationship is relatively constant although some colloids can have equivalent MW with different molecular size – succinylated and urea-linked gelatins have almost identical molecular weights but the succinylated product undergoes conformational change due to an increase in negative charge and is physically larger.[2,3]

HUMAN ALBUMIN SOLUTION

Human albumin is thought of as an ideal colloid and is commonly the reference solution against which other colloids are judged. Human albumin is a naturally occurring monodisperse colloid. Solutions (5% and 20%) are prepared from human plasma and heat treated to ensure that neither hepatitis nor HIV can be transmitted. It has a relatively short (~1 year) shelf life at room temperature, but a 5-year shelf life at 2–8°C. Human albumin 5% is used for the treatment of hypovolaemia in a wide variety of clinical conditions. Concentrated salt-poor 20% human albumin is used for the treatment of hypoalbuminaemia in the presence of salt and water overload (e.g. hepatic failure with ascites). Albumin has putative advantages that include limiting free radical-mediated damage but the importance of a normal serum albumin level remains uncertain.[6–8]

Human-derived colloid has a number of significant disadvantages. These are expensive products and concerns have been raised about transmission of infectious agents, such as new variant Creutzfeldt–Jakob disease (nvCJD)

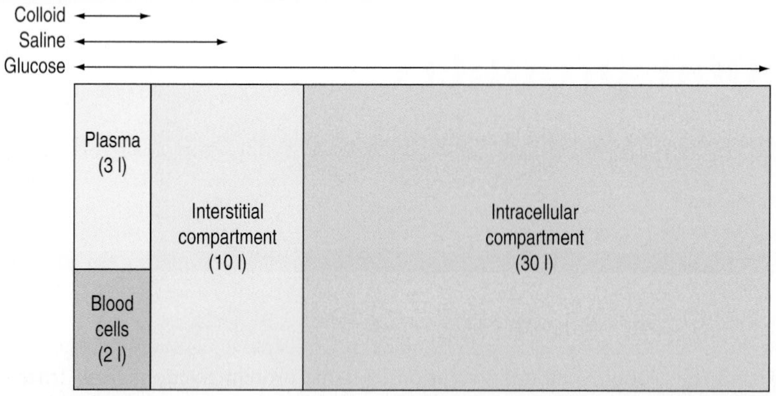

Figure 89.1 Simplified theoretical volumes of distribution of infused isotonic solutions of an ideal colloid, saline and glucose. (Reproduced with permission from Grocott MPW, Mythen MG. Fluid therapy. In: Goldhill DR, Strunin L (eds) *Clinical Anaesthesiology*. London: Baillière Tindall; 1999: 363–81.)

Table 89.1 Comparison of contents, osmolarity and pH of crystalloid solutions for intravenous administration

Solution	Osmolar (mosmol/l)	Ph	Na^+ (mmol/l)	Cl^- (mmol/l)	K^+ (mmol/l)	Ca^{2+} (mmol/l)	Glucose (mg/l)	HCO_3^- (mol/l)	Lactate (mmol/l)
Glucose 5%	252	3.5–6.5	–	–	–	–	50	–	–
Glucose 25%	1260	3.5–6.5	–	–	–	–	250	–	–
Glucose 50%	2520	3.5–6.5	–	–	–	–	500	–	–
Saline 0.9%	300	5.0	154.0	154.0	–	–	–	–	–
Glucose-saline	282	3.5–6.5	30.0	30.0	–	–	40	–	–
Ringer's	309	5.0–7.5	147.0	156.0	4.0	2.2	–	–	–
C. Na lactate*	278	5.0–7.0	131.0	111.0	5.0	2.0	–	–	29.0
Plasmalyte B	298.5	5.5	140	98	5	–	–	50	–

*Compound sodium lactate: Hartmann's solution or Ringer's lactate solution.
Reproduced with permission from Grocott MPW, Mythen MG. Fluid therapy. In: Goldhill DR, Strunin L (eds) *Clinical Anaesthesiology*. London: Baillière Tindall; 1999: 363–81.

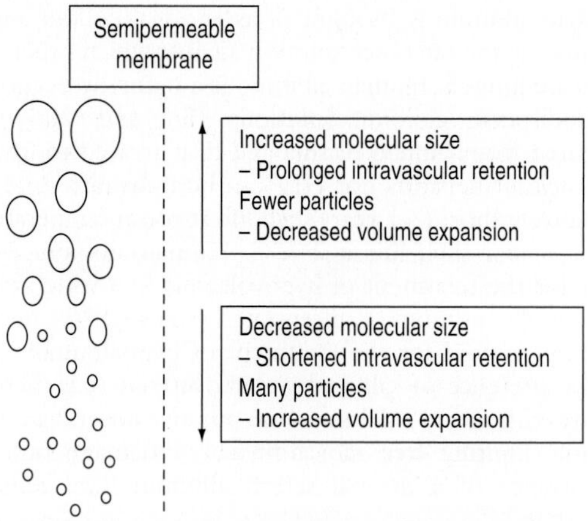

Figure 89.2 Polydispersity of colloid molecular size. (Reproduced with permission from Grocott MPW, Mythen MG. Fluid therapy. In: Goldhill DR, Strunin L (eds) *Clinical Anaesthesiology*. London: Baillière Tindall; 1999: 363–81.)

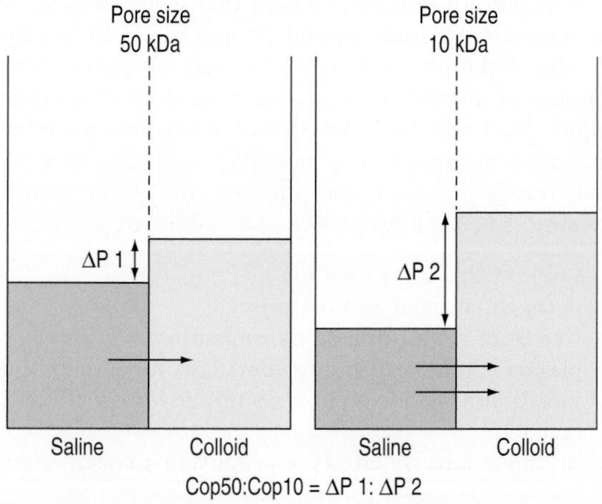

Figure 89.3 Schematic of technique for measurement of the COP50:COP10 ratio. (Reproduced with permission from Grocott MPW, Mythen MG. Fluid therapy. In: Goldhill DR, Strunin L (eds) *Clinical Anaesthesiology*. London: Baillière Tindall; 1999: 363–81.)

associated with bovine spongiform encephalopathy (BSE), that are not removed by currently available techniques. Concerns have also been raised by the conclusions of a highly controversial meta-analysis suggesting that the use of human albumin solution may be associated with increased mortality in the critically ill. These conclusions were probably unjustified,[8,9] but there is certainly no evidence that the use of human albumin has any advantages over less expensive semisynthetic alternatives[10,11] or indeed crystalloids. However, the latter applies to all colloids.[12–14]

GELATINS

Gelatins are prepared by hydrolysis of bovine collagen.[15] The commonly available preparations are succinylated gelatin (Gelofusine) and urea-linked gelatin–polygeline (Haemaccel).[1,2] Because of the significant calcium content of Haemaccel, citrated blood should not be infused through a giving set that has been previously used for this product; however, this does not apply to SAGM (saline–adenine–glucose–mannitol) blood. Gelatins are relatively inexpensive and stable, with long shelf lives. The gelatins' plasma volume expanding effect only lasts about 90–120 minutes.[3,4] They are mainly eliminated by renal excretion.

Incidence of reactions to gelatins are acceptable (<0.5%) and range from mild skin rash and pyrexia to life-threatening anaphylaxis. The reactions appear to be related to histamine release, which is probably the result of a direct effect of gelatin on mast cells. The gelatins appear to have the least impact on haemostasis and it is not clear whether they have any impact over and above simple haemodilution of clotting factors. A specific safety issue has arisen with bovine-derived gelatin products since the advent of sporadic cases of nvCJD associated with exposure to tissue infected with BSE. The gelatin used in the commercially available products in the UK, for example, is sourced from the US (which is regarded as BSE free) or from certified BSE free herds in France. The UK Spongiform Encephalopathy Advisory Committee concluded that gelatin was safe to use in this context.

DEXTRANS

Dextrans are polysaccharides biosynthesised commercially from sucrose by the bacterium *Leuconostoc mesenteroides* using the enzyme dextran sucrase.[1,2] This produces a high molecular weight dextran that is then cleaved by acid hydrolysis and separated by repeated ethanol fractionation to produce a final product with a relatively narrow molecular weight range. The products in current clinical use are described by their MW, Dextran 40 and Dextran 70 having MWs of 40 000 and 70 000 Da, respectively.

Dextran preparations are stable at room temperature and have long shelf lives. Dextran 70 is used as a plasma substitute for the treatment of hypovolaemia and has an intravascular volume-expanding effect that lasts at least 6 hours. Dextran 40 is used for its effects on microcirculatory flow and blood coagulation in some types of surgery (e.g. vascular, neuro and plastic surgery). The beneficial effects on outcome when Dextran 40 is used as an 'anti-sludging agent' remain controversial. Dextran 40 should not be used as a plasma substitute for the treatment of hypovolaemia as although it produces an immediate plasma volume expansion as a result of its small molecular weight it may obstruct renal tubules and produce renal failure.[5]

Dextrans can precipitate true anaphylactic reactions, as anti-dextran antibodies may be present due to synthesis of dextrans by lactobacilli that occur naturally as gut commensals. Dextran infusion, particularly of the high molecular weight products, can also precipitate anaphylactoid reactions. The risk of true anaphylactic reactions can be decreased about 10-fold by pretreatment with monovalent hapten-dextran. The dextrans are also associated with significant haemostatic derangements. These include:

- simple haemodilution of clotting factors
- reduction in factor VIII activity
- increase in plasminogen activation
- increase in fibrinolysis
- reduction in clot strength
- impairment of platelet function

Red cell aggregation is also reduced with the lower molecular weight dextrans. In patients whose haemostatic function is normal prior to infusion, a maximum dose of 1.5 g/kg is often recommended to avoid risk of bleeding complications. The anticoagulant effects of dextrans can be utilised perioperatively as a prophylaxis against thromboembolism.[1,2,5]

HYDROXYETHYL STARCHES

Hydroxyethyl starches (HES) are produced by hydroxyethyl substitution of amylopectin, a D-glucose polymer, obtained from sorghum or maize.[1,2] The pattern of hydroxyethyl substitution on glucose moieties influences the susceptibility to hydrolysis by non-specific amylases in the blood. A high C2 to C6 substitution ratio and a high overall degree of substitution (the proportion of glucose moieties that have been substituted) both protect against enzymatic breakdown and prolong the effective activity of HES as a plasma volume expander. The different HES products are commonly described by their weight-averaged molecular weight (MWw, number of molecules at each weight times the particle weight divided by the total weight of all the molecules). They are also described by their degree of substitution.[1,2–5] Hetastarches (C2/C6 ratio 0.6–0.7), pentastarches (C2/C6 ratio ≈0.5) and tetrastarches (C2/C6 ratio ≈0.4). Starch usage varies between countries.

In the USA, the only starches available for clinical use are high molecular weight (>450 kDa) hetastarches presented in either normal saline or a lactate-buffered, glucose-containing, balanced electrolyte solution (Hextend).[16,17] There is a move towards the use of the non-saline based starch as the administration of high volumes of normal saline to humans has been associated with clinically significant acid–base disturbances.[18–21] In particular, normal saline infusion has been shown to cause a hyperchloraemic metabolic acidosis; however, the pathogenesis and significance of this phenomenon remains controversial.[18–22] Colloids presented in balanced electrolyte solutions are becoming available outside the USA. In Europe, the trend over the past 5 years has been towards the use of lower molecular weight (130 kDa) tetrastarches presented in saline and more recently in balanced electrolyte solutions.[23] Starch preparations are stable at room temperature and have long shelf lives. The duration of intravascular retention is proportional to molecular weight[3,4,24] but is > 6 hours even for the 130 kDa tetrastarches.

HES products are associated with an acceptable incidence of adverse events including anaphylactoid reactions. Tissue deposition may result in intractable itching if large volumes of HES are infused over several days.[25] Whether the administration of large volumes of HES may cause some renal dysfunction remains controversial.[26] HES products can cause a coagulopathy.[27,28] In particular, HES products cause a reduction in factor VIII (FVIII) levels and impair platelet function causing a von Willebrand-like syndrome. These effects are greater with high molecular weight HES molecules infused at larger volumes. The effects of the high molecular weight starches on coagulation seemed to be lessened in the reformulated balanced electrolyte alternative cited above.[16]

THE ROLE OF HYPERTONIC SOLUTIONS

In recent years hypertonic (600–1800 mosmol) crystalloid and colloid solutions have been introduced for certain clinical indications.[29–33] The theoretical advantage of these solutions is that a small volume of administered fluid will provide a significant plasma volume expansion. The high osmolarity of these solutions draws tissue fluid into the intravascular space and thus should minimise tissue oedema for a given plasma volume increment. Hypertonic crystalloids and colloids presented in a hypertonic saline carrier have been shown to achieve adequate resuscitation in a number of clinical settings. A smaller volume of hypertonic solution is normally required to achieve similar plasma volume expansion. In particular, these solutions are thought to result in reduced cerebral oedema in those patients at risk of this complication and indeed these solutions may have a place in treating refractory cerebral oedema.[31–33] Outside the perioperative arena they are finding use in the management of burns patients and in prehospital resuscitation of trauma victims. They are limited at present to single dose administrations.

BLOOD SUBSTITUTES – PERFLUROCARBON AND HAEMOGLOBIN THERAPEUTICS

In future, the use of artificial or semisynthetic oxygen-carrying solutions will become increasingly common.[34] A number of products have been and are currently under evaluation: perflurocarbon, modified human haemoglobin (Hb), modified bovine Hb and recombinant Hb solutions. These products not only function as oxygen carriers but are also capable of sustained plasma volume expansion. Unlike Hb present in intact red cells, these products often have a linear O_2Hb dissociation profile and the effects of this on O_2 uptake in the lungs and release in the tissues are not yet clearly defined. Additionally, they may have specific pharmacological effects – for example, with stroma-free haemoglobin nitric oxide scavenging resulting in vasoconstriction is well recognised. A modified bovine haemoglobin solution (Hemopure) has been licensed for clinical use in South Africa since 2001 but is still not approved for use elsewhere in the world.

PLASMA DERIVATIVES

FRESH FROZEN PLASMA

Fresh frozen plasma (FFP) contains normal plasma levels of all the clotting factors, albumin and immunoglobulin. A unit is typically 200–250 ml and has a FVIII level of at least 0.7 IU/ml (i.e. 70% of normal levels) and about 0.5 g of fibrinogen. It is kept at a temperature of −50°C in order to preserve coagulant levels. FFP is indicated for the replacement of multiple clotting factor deficiencies (e.g. liver disease, coumarin anticoagulant overdose and coagulopathy associated with massive blood transfusion).[35–37] An initial dose of 12–15 ml/kg (four packs for a 70-kg adult) is appropriate. Although it is effective, FFP should not be used as a plasma volume expander solely for the treatment of hypovolaemia.

CRYOPRECIPITATE

Cryoprecipitate is usually supplied as a pool of six or so single donor units in one pack. It is prepared from FFP by using a freeze thaw method, collection of the precipitate and then resuspending it in about 20 ml of plasma. It contains about 50% of the coagulant factor activity of the original unit (e.g. fibrinogen 250 mg, FVIII 100 IU). Cryoprecipitate is stored at −30°C and remains stable for up to a year.[35] It is indicated in the treatment of coagulation defects, including massive haemorrhage and DIC if there is microvascular bleeding associated with a fibrinogen level < 0.5 g/l and as an alternative to FVIII concentrate in the treatment of inherited deficiencies of von Willebrand factor, FVIII and FXIII.[36,37] For an adult, transfusion of 3–4 g of fibrinogen (about 16 packs) should raise the fibrinogen level by 1 g/l.

FACTOR VIII

Factor VIII concentrate is prepared from large pools of donor plasma. One freeze-dried vial contains about 300 FVIII units.[35] The concentrates are heat or chemically treated to inactivate HIV-1. It is stable for 2 years when stored at 4°C. Further purification of the concentrate by chromatography results in high-purity FVIII and the relative merits of high- and intermediate-purity products are being investigated.

Recombinant FVIII is being used increasingly commonly in many parts of the world. Indications are the treatment of haemophilia A and von Willebrand's disease.[38] A dose of about 10–15 U/kg may be given, depending on the severity of bleeding and repeated 12 hourly, as required.

FACTOR IX

Factor IX concentrate (prothrombin concentrate) contains factors II, VII, IX and X in varying amounts, and is prepared from pools of plasma.[35] It is available as a freeze-dried preparation, and is reconstituted with water immediately before use. Factor IX concentrate of intermediate purity is used to treat haemophilia B and to correct bleeding disorders due to an overdose of coumarin anticoagulants in patients who cannot tolerate large volumes of FFP.[35] Purified factor IX concentrates are now available and are 100 times purer than the traditional concentrate, with 75% of total protein being factor IX.

OTHER PLASMA CONCENTRATES

Activated factor VII concentrate can be used in patients with inhibitors to factor VIII or IX, as it bypasses the requirement for these factors.[35] Activated factor VII has also been used in the treatment of severe life-threatening haemorrhage but this remains controversial.[39] Other concentrates, such as antithrombin III, C1 esterase inhibitor, and proteins C and S, are available for treating deficient patients at times of risk, such as surgery. Most of these concentrates have been used experimentally with varying success for the treatment of DIC and septic shock.

Recombinant versions of most plasma factors are either clinically available or in development and will probably become the standard of care. Recombinant activated protein C has been shown to be beneficial in a large human study for the treatment of septic shock[40] (see Chapter 11).

IMMUNOGLOBULINS (GAMMAGLOBULINS)

Normal human immunoglobulin preparation is made from plasma pools obtained from normal blood donors. It contains antibodies to hepatitis A, measles, mumps, varicella, polio and prevalent bacteria.[35] Immunoglobulins are indicated in the prevention or treatment of patients with hypogammaglobulinaemia, and may have a role in the treatment of autoimmune diseases, such as thrombocytopenic purpura and myasthenia gravis. Specific immunoglobulins are available for a range of infectious agents including tetanus, hepatitis B, rubella, measles, rabies and varicella zoster. They are made from donor plasma known to contain high levels of the specific IgG antibodies and are used for prophylaxis and treatment in patients who have not been actively immunised. Rhesus-D immunoglobulin is prepared from plasma containing high levels of anti Rh-D antibodies and it prevents sensitisation of Rh-negative mothers to Rh-D positive cells that may enter their circulation. The principal use of Rh-D immunoglobulin is in the prevention of haemolytic disease of the newborn.[41]

REFERENCES

1. Grocott MPW, Mythen MG. Fluid therapy. In: Goldhill DR, Strunin L (eds) *Clinical Anaesthesiology.* London: Baillière Tindall; 1999: 363–81.
2. Vercueil A, Grocott MP, Mythen MG. Physiology, pharmacology, and rationale for colloid administration for the maintenance of effective hemodynamic stability in critically ill patients. *Transfus Med Rev* 2005; **19**: 93–109.
3. Webb AR, Barclay SA, Bennett ED. In vitro colloid osmotic pressure of commonly used plasma expanders and substitutes: a study of the diffusibility of colloid molecules. *Intensive Care Med* 1989; **15**: 116–20.
4. Lamke LO, Liljedahl SO. Plasma volume changes after infusion of various plasma expanders. *Resuscitation* 1976; **5**: 93–102.
5. Boldt J, Suttner S. Plasma substitutes. *Minerva Anestesiol* 2005; **71**: 741–58.
6. Halliwell B. Albumin – an important extracellular antioxidant? *Biochem Pharmacol* 1988; **37**: 569–71.
7. Vincent JL, Navickis RJ, Wilkes MM. Morbidity in hospitalized patients receiving human albumin: a meta-analysis of randomized, controlled trials. *Crit Care Med* 2004; **32**: 2029–38.
8. Cochrane Injuries Group Albumin Reviewers. Human albumin administration in critically ill patients: systematic review of randomised controlled trials. *BMJ* 1998; **317**: 235–40.
9. Bunn F, Alderson P, Hawkins V. Colloid solutions for fluid resuscitation (Cochrane Review). *The Cochrane Library* 2000; **4**.
10. Stockwell M, Soni N, Riley B. Colloid solutions in the critically ill. A randomized comparison of albumin and polygeline. 1. Outcome and duration of stay in the intensive care unit. *Anaesthesia* 1992; **47**: 3–6.
11. Stockwell M, Scott A, Riley B *et al.* Colloid solutions in the critically ill. A randomised comparison of albumin and polygeline. 2. Serum albumin concentration and incidences of pulmonary oedema and acute renal failure. *Anaesthesia* 1992; **47**: 7–9.
12. Finfer S, Bellomo R, Boyce N *et al.* A comparison of albumin and saline for fluid resuscitation in the intensive care unit. *N Engl J Med* 2004; **350**: 2247–56.

13. Schierhout G, Roberts I. Fluid resuscitation with colloid or crystalloid solutions in critically ill patients: a systematic review of randomised trials. *BMJ* 1998; **316**: 961–4.
14. Choi P, Yip G, Quinonez L *et al.* Crystalloids vs colloids in fluid resuscitation: a systematic review. *Crit Care Med* 1999; **27**: 200–10.
15. Davies MJ. Polygeline. *Dev Biol Stand* 1987; **67**: 129–31.
16. Gan TJ, Bennett-Guerrero E, Phillips-Bute B *et al.* Hextend, a physiological balanced plasma expander for large volume use in major surgery: a randomized phase III clinical trial. *Anesth Analg* 1999; **88**: 992–8.
17. Waters JH, Gottlieb A, Schoenwald P *et al.* Normal saline versus lactated Ringer's solution for intraoperative fluid management in patients undergoing abdominal aortic aneurysm repair: an outcome study. *Anesth Analg* 2001; **93**: 817–22.
18. Reid F, Lobo DN, Williams RN *et al.* (Ab)normal saline and physiological Hartmann's solution: a randomized double-blind crossover study. *Clin Sci (Lond)* 2003; **104**: 17–24.
19. Brill SA, Stewart TR, Brundage SI *et al.* Base deficit does not predict mortality when secondary to hyperchloremic acidosis. *Shock* 1999; **17**: 459–62.
20. Williams EL, Hildebrand KL, McCormick SA *et al.* The effect of intravenous lactated Ringer's solution versus 0.9% sodium chloride solution on serum osmolality in human volunteers. *Anesth Analg* 1999; **88**: 999–1003.
21. Wilkes NJ, Woolf R, Stephens R *et al.* The effects of balanced versus saline based intravenous solutions on acid base status and gastric mucosal perfusion in elderly surgical patients. *Anesth Analg* 2001; **93**: 811–16.
22. Ho AM, Karmakar MK, Contardi LH *et al.* Excessive use of normal saline in managing traumatized patients in shock: a preventable contributor to acidosis. *J Trauma* 2001; **51**: 173–7.
23. Boldt J, Wolf M, Mengistu A. A new plasma-adapted hydroxyethylstarch preparation: in vitro coagulation studies using thrombelastography and whole blood aggregometry. *Anesth Analg* 2007; **104**: 425–30.
24. James MF, Latoo MY, Mythen MG *et al.* Plasma volume changes associated with two hydroxyethyl starch colloids following acute hypovolaemia in volunteers. *Anaesthesia* 2004; **59**: 738–42.
25. Morgan PW, Berridge JC. Giving long persistent starch as volume replacement can cause pruritus after cardiac surgery. *Br J Anaesth* 2000; **85**: 696–9.
26. Zander R, Boldt J, Engelmann L *et al.* [The design of the VISEP trial : Critical appraisal.] *Anaesthesist* 2007; **56**: 71–7.
27. Treib J, Baron JF. Hydroxethyl starch: effects on hemostasis. *Ann Fr Anesth Reanim* 1998; **17**: 72–81.
28. Roche AM, James MF, Bennett-Guerrero E *et al.* A head-to-head comparison of the in vitro coagulation effects of saline-based and balanced electrolyte crystalloid and colloid intravenous fluids. *Anesth Analg* 2006; **102**: 1274–9.
29. Wade CE, Grady JJ, Kramer GC. Efficacy of hypertonic saline dextran fluid resuscitation for patients with hypotension from penetrating trauma. *J Trauma* 2003; **54**(5 Suppl): S144S1448.
30. Oi Y, Aneman A, Svensson M *et al.* Hypertonic saline-dextran improves intestinal perfusion and survival in porcine endotoxin shock. *Crit Care Med* 2000; **28**: 2843–50.
31. Simma B, Burger R, Falk M *et al.* A prospective, randomized, and controlled study of fluid management in children with severe head injury: lactated Ringer's solution versus hypertonic saline. *Crit Care Med* 1998; **26**: 1265–70.
32. Dubick MA, Bruttig SP, Wade CE. Issues of concern regarding the use of hypertonic/hyperoncotic fluid resuscitation of hemorrhagic hypotension. *Shock* 2006; **25**: 321–8.
33. Shackford SR, Bourguignon PR, Wald SL *et al.* Hypertonic saline resuscitation of patients with head injury: a prospective, randomized clinical trial. *J Trauma* 1998; **44**: 50–8.
34. Farrar D, Grocott M. Intravenous artificial oxygen carriers. *Hosp Med* 2003; **64**: 352–6.
35. McClelland DBL (ed) *Handbook of Transfusion Medicine*. London: HMSO; 1989.
36. Mammen EF. Disseminated intravascular coagulation (DIC). *Clin Lab Sci* 2000; **13**: 239–45.
37. Mythen MG, Machin SJ. Derangements of blood coagulation. In: Hanson GC (ed) *Critical Care of the Surgical Patient*. London: Chapman and Hall; 1997: 185–94.
38. Hambleton J. Advances in the treatment of von Willebrand disease. *Semin Hematol* 2001; **38**: 7–10.
39. Moscardo F, Perez F, de la Rubia J *et al.* Successful treatment of severe intra-abdominal bleeding associated with disseminated intravascular coagulation using recombinant activated VII. *Br J Haematol* 2001; **114**: 174–6.
40. Bernard GR, Vincent JL, Laterre PF *et al.* Efficacy and safety of recombinant human activated protein C for severe sepsis *N Engl J Med* 2001; **344**: 699–709.
41. Greenough A. The role of immunoglobulins in neonatal rhesus haemolytic disease. *BioDrugs* 2001; **15**: 533–41.

90

Therapeutic plasma exchange and intravenous immunoglobulin immunomodulatory therapy

James P Isbister

Bloodletting to remove 'evil humours' has a long history of over 2000 years. Although not based on logic in the past, the removal of 'noxious' agents from the blood remains the rationale, but now there is scientific understanding of the pathophysiology of the diseases treated by plasma exchange.[1] Exchange transfusions revolutionised the management of haemolytic disease in the newborn, and paved the way for therapeutic plasmapheresis and plasma exchange – the removal of plasma, with replacement by albumin-electrolyte solutions or fresh frozen plasma.

Plasma exchange was initially used in the management of hyperviscosity associated with malignant paraproteinaemia, but is now also used in the treatment of a wide range of autoimmune disorders (now > 100). Nevertheless, plasma exchange is expensive and not risk-free, and debate continues on its therapeutic role in many diseases.

For the past two decades, intravenous immunoglobulin (IVIG) has increasingly been used as an immunomodulatory agent beyond its original primary use as replacement therapy in patients with humoral immune deficiency. The use of this agent will also be referred to in this chapter as it is now being used in many disorders in which plasma exchange is effective, but the convenience and safety of IVIG therapy is preferred as an alternative. However, the underlying principles in managing autoimmune diseases in which IVIG is used are similar to those of therapeutic plasma exchange. The mechanism of action of IVIG as an immunomodulatory agent remains controversial and it is likely, as fine plasma exchange, that there is more than one mechanism in play. Therapeutic efficacy of IVIG has been established in controlled trials for a range of diseases including idiopathic thrombocytopenic purpura, Kawasaki disease, Guillain–Barré syndrome, dermatomyositis, and others. There is compelling evidence that IVIG can modulate immune reactions of T-cells, B-cells and macrophages, not only interfering with antibody production and degradation, but also modulating the complement cascade and cytokine networks.

RATIONALE FOR PLASMA EXCHANGE

Theoretically, plasma exchange should be effective to treat any disorder in which there is a pathogenic circulating factor responsible for the disease. However, this premise is probably too simplistic, and other mechanisms may contribute to its beneficial effects (Table 90.1). It is a non-specific procedure, which brings about numerous, potentially undesirable, alterations in the plasma's *milieu interieur.*

PATHOPHYSIOLOGY OF AUTOIMMUNE DISEASE

Autoimmune disease originates from the breakdown of immunoregulation (i.e. immune tolerance), allowing the immune system to become autoaggressive. Autoimmune diseases having underlying humoral mechanisms result from either a circulating autoantibody against a self-antigen (alone or in combination with an environmental antigen) or circulating immune complexes (which may be deposited in the microcirculation of various organs, resulting in end-organ damage). Cellular and tissue damage is affected by the autoantibody or immune complexes activating the cellular and humoral components of the inflammatory response. The circulating proteolytic systems involved include the complement, coagulation, fibrinolytic and kinin systems. On the cellular side, neutrophils and macrophages are involved, with eosinophils and basophils also playing a part.

The varied clinical manifestations of autoimmune disorders relate more to the cell, tissue or organ involved, rather than the pathophysiological process. However, basic pathophysiological mechanisms by which autoimmune diseases occur need to be understood in order to standardise treatment. Although some cells of the host defence system, in particular the macrophages and lymphocytes, may have special differentiation appropriate to individual organs, their basic functional processes are not all that dissimilar between different organs.

Table 90.1 Rationale for plasma exchange

Removal of circulating toxic factor antibodies
Monoclonal antibodies
Autoantibodies
Alloantibodies, immune complexes, chemicals, drugs
Depletion of the mediators of inflammation
Replacement of deficient plasma factor(s)
Potentiation of drug action
Enhanced reticuloendothelial function
Altered immunoregulation
Potentiating effects of plasma exchange on other modes of therapy

In general, autoimmune disease can be an acute, self-limiting ('one hit') disorder, intermittent or a chronic perpetuating disorder. Acute autoimmune disease may have an identifiable trigger, such as an infection, followed by a 10-day to 3-week gap until the pathogenic humoral or cellular factors appear in the circulating blood. At this point, end-organ damage commences, and clinical features of the disease appear.

The course of the disease will be determined by several factors:

- biological function and importance of the system involved
- extent of damage
- replaceability or otherwise of the cells under attack
- time course of the damaging insult

The extent of damage is a product of the:

- characteristics of the antibodies or lymphocytes involved (e.g. antibody affinity, complement fixing capabilities and titre)
- function of other components of the host defence system (e.g. neutrophils, platelets, proteolytic systems and reticuloendothelial system)
- presence of other aggravating factors (e.g. infection, hormonal responses and circulatory responses)

The kinetics of the end-cell involved in the immunological damage is relevant in determining the final outcome of the disease. Ultimate recovery of organ function after 'burn out' of a self-limiting autoimmune disease, or control of a chronic autoimmune disease, is determined by the ability of the cell to replace and restore function to normal.

Cells are broadly divided into three kinetic characteristics:

- *Continuous replicators*: these cells are continuously replaced in the normal state. They are readily replaced when damaged, and if the immunological insult is removed or controlled, full replacement of the end-cells occurs. This is typically seen with the haemopoietic system, the cells lining the gut and skin cells.
- *Discontinuous replicators*: these are cells that are not being constantly replaced in the normal state, but when damaged, cell division is initiated and replacement occurs. This is seen with hepatocytes, renal tubular cells and the neuronal Schwann cells.
- *Non-replicating cells*: when damaged, these cells are irreplaceably destroyed with permanent loss of function. This is seen with neuronal cells, muscle cells and renal glomeruli.

The clinical features and final outcome of any autoimmune disease can thus be seen to be determined by many different factors, including the ability of the end-organ to repair following removal or control of the immunological insult. In many self-limiting autoimmune diseases, if the end-cell is a continuous or intermittent replicator, full recovery can be expected, as long as appropriate support to end-organ function and life support is given during the acute phase of the illness. Examples are acute tubular necrosis, acute demyelination, acute hepatic failure and some forms of marrow aplasia. However, in disorders with non-replicating cells such as acute glomerulonephritis, therapy must be aimed at removing the immunological insult or dampening its damaging affects as soon as possible, so as to minimise irreparable damage to the end-cells and thus long-term organ function. Immunological mediators may also produce disease without direct destruction of end-cells. This occurs when autoantibodies develop against cell receptors, with blocking or destruction of the receptor as is typically seen in myasthenia gravis and thyrotoxicosis.

Therapy in acute and chronic autoimmune disease aims to minimise irreparable end-organ damage and support patients during the acute illness. This therapy may include:

- non-specific therapy to suppress the effector mechanisms, e.g. corticosteroids, antiplatelet therapy, non-steroidal anti-inflammatory drugs, anticoagulation and depletion of humoral effector mechanisms by plasma exchange or defibrination
- therapy to reduce the circulating levels of a humoral factor is achieved with plasma exchange or immunoabsorption technique
- specific or broad-spectrum immunosuppressive agents to suppress or block the immune response, e.g. corticosteroids, cytotoxic agents, antilymphocyte globulin, high-dose intravenous gammaglobulin therapy
- therapy directed at altering reticuloendothelial function, which may then have effects on autoantibody and immune complex clearance, or clearance of circulating damaged cells
- intravenous immunoglobulin immunomodulatory therapy

As most disorders are multifactorial, it is unlikely that a single form of therapy will be successful. A multipronged approach to therapy needs to be planned following an analysis of the basic underlying pathophysiology. The stage of the disease is also important (Figure 90.1). Clearly, plasma exchange will have a different response when autoantibody production is rising rapidly, compared with a stage when

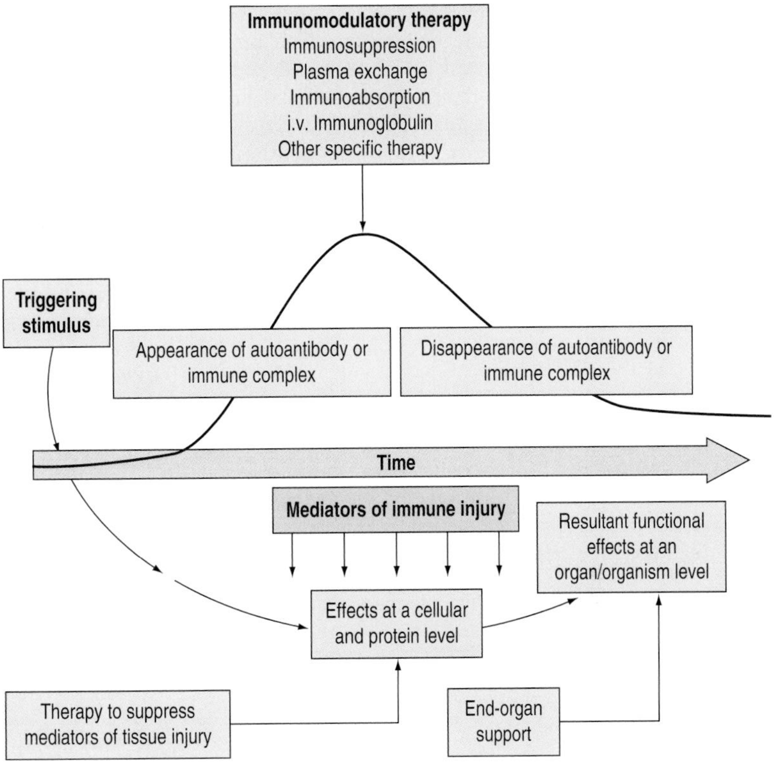

Figure 90.1 The therapy of 'one hit' autoimmune disease.

autoantibody has ceased production. Also, immunoregulation is a complex process, and therapies may interfere at different points in the immune mechanisms.

In some circumstances, specific and directed therapy may attack the most relevant link in the pathophysiological chain, but overall multiple approaches to therapy may be required. In general, plasma exchange is a temporising procedure and concomitant immunosuppressive therapy is required to maintain control. Plasma exchange for autoimmune disease should generally be regarded as a first step in immunomodulatory therapy, and restricted to acute or fulminant situations in which autoantibodies or immune complexes are responsible for life-threatening or end-organ damaging complications. There are some situations in which the humoral factor may be only transient ('one antigen hit' disorders), and no follow-up immunosuppression is required (e.g. acute postinfectious polyneuritis). Increasing monoclonal antibody therapy with rituximab (an anti-CD20 antibody) is finding a role in the longer term management of autoimmune diseases.[2,3]

The availability and recognition of the immunomodulatory effects of intravenous immunoglobulin has resulted in an exponential increase in its use in immune and inflammatory disorders, with its availability being one of the main drivers of the supply of human-derived plasma products. In most of the immune and inflammatory disorders in which plasma exchange has been used, intravenous immunoglobulin has been used. The mechanisms of action of intravenous immunoglobulin remain controversial. Intravenous immunoglobulin, fractionated from normal human plasma, was introduced as a replacement therapy for humoral immunodeficiency disorders, but is now widely used for a range of autoimmune and inflammatory diseases. Progress is being made in understanding the complex mechanisms by which IVIG has immunomodulatory actions. The mechanisms of action of IVIG involve modulation of expression and function of immunoglobulin Fc receptors, interference with activation of the complement system and the cytokine and immunoglobulin idiotype networks, and regulation of cell growth. There is also evidence for effects on activation, differentiation and effector functions of dendritic cells and T and B lymphocytes.[4]

TECHNICAL CONSIDERATIONS

Cell separators available for plasma exchange therapy are broadly divided into two groups:[5]

- machines which use centrifugation for the separation and are also suitable for specific separation and removal of blood components (e.g. plasmapheresis, thrombopheresis and leukopheresis)
- machines which separate by membrane filtration and can only be used for separation of plasma components

Either of these techniques for plasma exchange can be combined with immunoabsorption techniques, in which immunoglobulins are specifically or non-specifically removed.[6]

As plasma is removed, it is replaced volume for volume with a solution of adequate colloid activity (e.g. 5% albumin) and appropriate electrolyte composition. Although the levels of other plasma proteins are reduced by plasma exchange, there are rarely clinically significant effects. However, if extremely large volumes are exchanged, or exchanges are done frequently, it may be necessary to replace some plasma proteins. In patients with coagulation factor deficiencies or immunodeficiency, fresh frozen plasma is usually required.

INDICATIONS (TABLE 90.2)

Plasma exchange is most beneficial for immunoproliferative and autoimmune diseases. In some conditions with unclear pathophysiology, beneficial effects of plasma exchange may be due to infusion of a deficient component in the replacement plasma, rather than removal of a circulating factor.

Table 90.2 Acute diseases in which plasma exchange may be beneficial*

Immunoproliferative diseases with monoclonal immunoglobulins
Hyperviscosity syndrome
Cryoglobulinaemia
Renal failure in multiple myeloma
Autoimmune diseases due to autoantibodies or immune complexes
Goodpasture's syndrome
Myasthenia gravis
Guillain–Barré syndrome
Chronic inflammatory demyelinating polyneuropathy (CIDP)
Stiff-man syndrome
Systemic lupus erythematosus
Fulminant antiphospholipid syndrome
Thrombotic thrombocytopenic purpura
Haemolytic uraemic syndrome
Rapidly progressive glomerulonephritis
Coagulation inhibitors
Autoimmune haemolytic anaemia
Pemphigus
Paraneoplastic syndromes
Conditions in which replacement of plasma may be beneficial $\pm$ removal of toxins
Disseminated intravascular coagulation
Multiorgan dysfunction syndrome
Overwhelming sepsis syndromes (e.g. meningococcaemia)
Conditions in which the mechanisms are unknown
Reye's syndrome
Removal of protein-bound or large molecular weight toxins
Paraquat poisoning
Envenomation?

*This is an incomplete list and only includes disorders that are relatively common or in which plasma exchange has a definitive role to play.

MONOCLONAL ANTIBODIES ASSOCIATED WITH IMMUNOPROLIFERATIVE DISEASES

Monoclonal immunoglobulins are a classic feature of multiple myeloma and Waldenström's macroglobulinaemia, but may also be associated with other lymphoproliferative disorders. These monoclonal proteins may be associated with numerous clinical effects, many of which may be reversed by plasma exchange.

HYPERVISCOSITY SYNDROME

Characteristic clinical features of hyperviscosity in association with monoclonal proteins include visual disturbance, neurological dysfunction and hypervolaemia, all of which can be rapidly relieved by plasma exchange.[7]

HAEMOSTATIC DISTURBANCES

Monoclonal proteins may impair haemostasis by adversely affecting platelet function or by inhibitory effects on coagulation factors. Plasma exchange is usually effective in controlling haemorrhage and may also be helpful in preparing patients for surgery.

RENAL FAILURE

The development of renal failure in the course of multiple myeloma is generally regarded as a sign of poor prognosis. In most cases, the renal failure is multifactorial in origin, but some of these factors may be reversible by plasma exchange. Patients presenting acutely with hyperviscosity, dehydration and hypercalcaemia may show recovery of renal function following adequate hydration, alkaline diuresis and plasma exchange.

IMMUNOLOGICAL DISEASES

DISEASES MEDIATED BY SPECIFIC AUTOANTIBODIES

Goodpasture's syndrome

Circulating antiglomerular basement membrane antibodies can be demonstrated in most cases of Goodpasture's syndrome. The disease classically has a fulminant presentation with rapidly progressive renal failure and life-threatening pulmonary haemorrhage. Early diagnosis and intensive plasma exchange may be necessary to preserve renal function and control pulmonary haemorrhage. Patients who are already in anuric renal failure rarely show improvement in renal function.[8]

Myasthenia gravis

Removal of the acetylcholine receptor autoantibody is associated with clinical improvement in the majority of patients with this disorder. The beneficial effects of plasma exchange are usually transient, and the procedure should normally be used in conjunction with other forms of therapy (see Chapter 49). The major role for plasma exchange is usually in myasthenic crisis, in patients whose condition is resistant to other forms of therapy, and prior to surgery. Therapy can be monitored by acetylcholine receptor autoantibody assays and respiratory function tests. Patients undergoing plasma exchange may transiently deteriorate during the procedure, due to a combination of the physical exertion and removal of medication from the circulation, and adequate ventilatory support should be available. IVIG may also be use in myasthenia gravis.[9–11]

Stiff-man syndrome

Stiff-man syndrome (STS) is a rare neurological disorder characterised by involuntary axial and proximal limb rigidity and continuous motor unit activity on electromyography. Autoantibodies to glutamic acid decarboxylase are usually demonstrable. Although plasma exchange is successful in STS, those who are autoantibody negative are less likely to respond.[12,13]

Autoimmune haematological disorders

Haemostatic failure due to autoantibodies directed against coagulation factors may present a major management problem. Antibodies directed against factor VIII are the commonest, occurring spontaneously or in association with replacement therapy in haemophiliacs. First-line therapy in patients with coagulation factor inhibitors usually requires activated factor VII therapy with recombinant FVIIa or appropriate prothrombin concentrates.[14]

IMMUNE COMPLEX DISEASE

Rapidly progressive glomerulonephritis

Immune complex-induced rapidly progressive glomerulonephritis may occur by itself or be associated with several systemic disorders (e.g. systemic lupus erythematosus, polyarteritis nodosa and Wagener's granulomatosis).[15–17] Plasma exchange may result in improvement in renal function even in patients who present with anuria. The decomplementing and defibrinating effects of plasma exchange may be partly responsible for clinical improvement. The therapeutic role of plasma exchange in rapidly progressive glomerulonephritis is difficult to assess, but most experienced physicians feel that the procedure leads to a more rapid and complete recovery of renal function in fulminant, rapidly deteriorating cases. However, the ultimate prognosis of the disease depends on adequate immunosuppression to inhibit immune complex formation, or spontaneous disappearance of the inciting antigen.

Systemic lupus erythematosus (SLE)

Plasma exchange has a role in acute life-threatening or organ-damaging relapses of SLE. Rapid deterioration in renal function, cerebritis and acute fulminant lupus pneumonitis are clinical situations in which plasma exchange should be considered.[18]

Cryoglobulinaemia

The various forms of cryoglobulinaemia may be associated with vasculitis or hyperviscosity. In some cases, there may be an acute fulminant presentation with cutaneous vasculitis, renal failure and neurological impairment. In this situation, plasma exchange should be considered an urgent definitive form of therapy.

OTHER IMMUNE-MEDIATED DISEASES

Renal transplant rejection

Humoral mechanisms appear to play a part in hyperacute renal allograft rejection. Plasma exchange ± IVIG may be useful in tiding patients over episodes of acute graft rejection, but results of clinical trials have been conflicting.[19,20] General opinion is that plasma exchange helps in a limited number of patients who cannot be currently preselected by any clinical or laboratory criteria.

Thrombotic thrombocytopenic purpura

Thrombotic thrombocytopenic purpura (TTP) is a potentially fulminant and life-threatening disorder characterised by platelet microthrombi in small vessels, resulting in microangiopathy. The clinical syndrome is manifest by the pentad of thrombocytopenia, microangiopathic haemolytic anaemia, fever, renal dysfunction and neurological abnormalities. Abdominal symptoms, hepatic dysfunction and pulmonary abnormalities may also occur. With the appropriate clinical features, thrombocytopenia and a microangiopathic blood film, diagnosis is established.

TTP has been linked to a severe deficiency in ADAMTS13 with metalloprotease activity, with its target cleavage sequence in von Willebrand factor (vWF). The presence of an autoantibody inhibitor to this vWF reducing metalloproteinase has been documented in patients with both acute TTP and those with chronic relapsing forms. In normal plasma, vWF undergoes proteolysis by a specific protease, and deficiency of this cleaving protease reduces or abolishes the plasma clearance of ultralarge vWF multimers, resulting in intravascular aggregation of platelets, particularly at sites of intravascular shear stress. The inhibitor to the metalloproteinase has been demonstrated to be an IgG autoantibody.

There is a primary idiopathic form of the disease that usually has an acute presentation and probably has an underlying autoimmune mechanism. This form may be associated with a variety of prodromal infections (viral or bacterial). Bacterial cytotoxins, produced by *Shigella dysenteriae* type 1 and certain *Escherichia coli* serotypes, have been related to TTP and haemolytic uraemic syndrome (HUS), probably by initiating damage to vascular endothelial cells, possibly via cytokine mechanisms. TTP may be associated with various drugs (cytotoxic agents), toxins and bites. Cytomegalovirus (CMV), human immunodeficiency virus (HIV) and herpes viruses have also been implicated. Chemotherapy-associated TTP/HUS is being increasingly recognised and may be associated with a range of cytotoxic medications. Severe microangiopathy resembling TTP has also been reported as a complication of acute graft-versus-host disease in patients receiving ciclosporin prophylaxis following allogeneic bone marrow transplant.

TTP used to be a fatal disease in 90% of patients, but dramatic improvement in its outcome has occurred over the past two decades with the development of effective therapy. Plasma exchange has become the cornerstone of the treatment with fresh frozen plasma replacement.[21,22] Cryoprecipitate-poor plasma (depleted in vWF) may offer advantages over whole fresh frozen plasma. It is now possible to achieve remissions in the majority of patients and cures are now common, though unfortunately relapse may occur. The clinical course at relapse is usually milder than the disease at presentation and less aggressive therapy may be needed.

Haemolytic uraemic syndrome (HUS)

This syndrome has many similarities to TTP, but renal involvement in contrast to cerebral in TTP is the hallmark in association with microangiopathy and thrombocytopenia.[23] The prognosis and approach to management of HUS is similar to TTP. It usually occurs in children (related to bacterial or viral infections), but may rarely be seen in adults, in whom the disease may take a more chronic and sinister course. In adult cases medications are commonly implicated.

Inflammatory demyelinating neuropathies and the Guillain–Barré syndrome (GBS)

This acute self-limiting disease in which an acute demyelinating neuropathy occurs (usually following a viral infection) commonly results in admission to the intensive care unit (ICU) (see Chapter 49). There is demyelination due to postinfectious autoimmunity, with both cellular and humoral arms of the immune system attacking myelin. There is now wide experience in the use of plasma exchange and IVIG therapy in GBS, with controlled trials substantiating its benefits of shortening of the illness and complications. Therapy should be instituted early.[11,24] As GBS also responds to high-dose IVIG there is debate as to which should be the first line of therapy. Decisions are usually made on the basis of local logistics and economics as the therapies are comparable in relationship to efficacy and safety.[25] In some cases the onset of recovery after therapy may be delayed, probably due to time for remyelination to occur. Some patients show rapid improvement after plasma exchange, suggesting the presence of neuronal blocking factors. Chronic inflammatory demyelinating peripheral neuropathy (CIPD) is related to GBS, and plasma exchange and/or IVIG have important roles in treatment, in many cases requiring long-term therapy.

COMPLICATIONS

Plasma exchange is a relatively safe procedure, but close supervision by experienced physicians and apheresis operators is essential. A sound understanding of the haemodynamic, biochemical, haematological and immunological effects of plasma exchange is of paramount importance. Potential complications of plasma exchange include fluid imbalance, reactions to replacement fluids, vasovagal reactions, pyrogenic reactions, hypothermia, embolism (air or microaggregates), hypocalcaemia, anaemia, thrombocytopenia, haemostatic disturbances, hepatitis, hypogammaglobulinaemia, and altered pharmacokinetics of drugs. Prevention and treatment of most of these complications are usually obvious, but specific mention should be made of the following.

CIRCULATORY EFFECTS

Any extracorporeal procedure is likely to lead to problems of circulatory instability. Intravascular volume changes, vasovagal reactions, medications and infusion fluids may all alone, or in combination, be responsible for circulatory problems. If there are no associated oxygen transport defects, the patient will usually be able to compensate. However, if there are pre-existing defects (e.g. altered blood volume, vascular disease or renal failure), close monitoring is essential. A strict fluid and electrolyte balance should be kept at all times, both during the plasma exchange and as a daily tally.

PLASMA ONCOTIC PRESSURE

Most patients compensate for minor fluctuations in plasma oncotic pressure (COP). Patients who have oedema or local factors predisposing to interstitial fluid accumulation (e.g. raised intracranial pressure, interstitial pulmonary oedema, deep-venous thrombosis and renal impairment) need close attention.

INFECTION

Many patients who are undergoing plasma exchange are already immunosuppressed, either due to their disease or secondary to drug therapy. In patients requiring recurrent and frequent plasma exchange, attempts should be made to maintain serum immunoglobulin levels. When fresh frozen plasma is not used as replacement fluid, the bactericidal and opsonic activities of blood are probably impaired, and it is probably advantageous to infuse at least 2 units of fresh frozen plasma at the conclusion of the procedure. At the completion of a course of plasma exchange consideration may need to be given to a dose of intravenous gammaglobulin.

HAEMOSTASIS

Plasma exchange causes perturbations in the haemostatic system which may result in either bleeding or thrombosis. The significance of these alterations will depend largely on the volume and frequency of exchange, pre-existing defects in the system, anticoagulation, other risk factors for thrombosis, replacement fluids and invasive procedures.

REACTIONS TO REPLACEMENT FLUIDS

The rapid infusion of any blood component may be associated with allergic or vasomotor reactions. Plasma exchange is a rather unique situation in which blood or blood products and plasma substitutes are being infused at resuscitation rates into normovolaemic, normotensive patients.

EFFECTS OF INTRAVASCULAR PROTEINS

If plasma protein fractions or albumin are being used for replacement fluids, not only will coagulation and complement components be depleted, but various transport and binding proteins in the circulation will be significantly reduced. These may have significant effects on drug activity and elimination (e.g. antithrombin III levels may have effects on heparin activity). The effects of corticosteroids may be potentiated after plasma exchange owing to a reduction in binding proteins.

REFERENCES

1. Isbister JP. Plasma exchange: a selective form of blood-letting. *Med J Aust* 1979; **2**: 167–73.
2. Scheinberg M, Hamerschlak N, Kutner JM *et al.* Rituximab in refractory autoimmune diseases: Brazilian experience with 29 patients (2002–2004). *Clin Exp Rheumatol* 2006; **24**: 65–9.
3. Virgolini L, Marzocchi V. Rituximab in autoimmune diseases. *Biomed Pharmacother* 2004; **58**: 299–309.
4. Negi VS, Elluru S, Siberil S *et al.* Intravenous immunoglobulin: an update on the clinical use and mechanisms of action. *J Clin Immunol* 2007; **27**: 233–45.
5. Stegmayr BG. A survey of blood purification techniques. *Transfus Apher Sci* 2005; **32**: 209–20.
6. Ullrich H, Kuehnl P. New trends in specific immunoadsorption. *Transfus Apher Sci* 2004; **30**: 223–31.
7. Mehta J, Singhal S. Hyperviscosity syndrome in plasma cell dyscrasias. *Semin Thromb Hemost* 2003; **29**: 467–71.
8. Shah MK, Hugghins SY. Characteristics and outcomes of patients with Goodpasture's syndrome. *Southern Med J* 2002; **95**: 1411–8.
9. Zhu KY, Feferman T, Maiti PK *et al.* Intravenous immunoglobulin suppresses experimental myasthenia gravis: immunological mechanisms. *J Immunol* 2006; **176**: 187–97.
10. Gajdos P, Chevret S, Toyka K. Intravenous immunoglobulin for myasthenia gravis. *Cochrane Database Syst Rev* 2006(2): CD002277.
11. Green DM. Weakness in the ICU: Guillain–Barré syndrome, myasthenia gravis, and critical illness polyneuropathy/myopathy. *Neurologist* 2005; **11**: 338–47.
12. Shariatmadar S, Noto TA. Plasma exchange in stiff-man syndrome. *Ther Apher* 2001; **5**: 64–7.
13. Cantiniaux S, Azulay JP, Boucraut J *et al.* [Stiff man syndrome: clinical forms, treatment and clinical course]. *Rev Neurol (Paris)* 2006; **162**: 832–9.
14. Abshire T, Kenet G. Recombinant factor VIIa: review of efficacy, dosing regimens and safety in patients with congenital and acquired factor VIII or IX inhibitors. *J Thromb Haemost* 2004; **2**: 899–909.
15. Stegmayr BG, Almroth G, Berlin G *et al.* Plasma exchange or immunoadsorption in patients with rapidly progressive crescentic glomerulonephritis. A Swedish multi-center study. *Int J Artif Organs* 1999; **22**: 81–7.
16. Rahman T, Harper L. Plasmapheresis in nephrology: an update. *Curr Opin Nephrol Hypertens* 2006; **15**: 603–9.
17. Jayne DR, Gaskin G, Rasmussen N *et al.* Randomized trial of plasma exchange or high-dosage methylprednisolone as adjunctive therapy for severe renal vasculitis. *J Am Soc Nephrol* 2007; **18**: 2180–8.
18. Pagnoux C, Korach JM, Guillevin L. Indications for plasma exchange in systemic lupus erythematosus in 2005. *Lupus* 2005; **14**: 871–7.
19. Lehrich RW, Rocha PN, Reinsmoen N *et al.* Intravenous immunoglobulin and plasmapheresis in acute humoral rejection: experience in renal allograft transplantation. *Hum Immunol* 2005; **66**: 350–8.
20. Rocha PN, Butterly DW, Greenberg A *et al.* Beneficial effect of plasmapheresis and intravenous immunoglobulin on renal allograft survival of patients with acute humoral rejection. *Transplantation* 2003; **75**: 1490–5.
21. Brunskill SJ, Tusold A, Benjamin S *et al.* A systematic review of randomized controlled trials for plasma exchange in the treatment of thrombotic thrombocytopenic purpura. *Transfus Med* 2007; **17**: 17–35.
22. Ozkalemkas F, Ali R, Ozkocaman V *et al.* Therapeutic plasma exchange plus corticosteroid for the treatment of the thrombotic thrombocytopenic purpura: a single institutional experience in the southern Marmara region of Turkey. *Transfus Apher Sci* 2007; **36**: 109–15.
23. Amirlak I, Amirlak B. Haemolytic uraemic syndrome: an overview. *Nephrology* 2006; **11**: 213–18.
24. Raphael JC, Chevret S, Hughes RA *et al.* Plasma exchange for Guillain–Barré syndrome. *Cochrane Database Syst Rev* 2002(2): CD001798.
25. Tsai CP, Wang KC, Liu CY *et al.* Pharmacoeconomics of therapy for Guillain–Barré syndrome: plasma exchange and intravenous immunoglobulin. *J Clin Neurosci* 2007; **14**: 625–9.

91

Haemostatic failure

James P Isbister

Failure of haemostasis is common in critically ill patients and may be complex and multifactorial in pathogenesis. As haemostatic failure may complicate a wide range of medical, surgical and obstetric disorders, definitive diagnosis and specific therapy can significantly impact on outcome. Frequently, complex tests are required for definitive diagnosis, but the urgency of the situation cannot always wait for the results, and therapy may be initiated on clinical evidence with minimal laboratory information. Consultation with a clinical haematologist is strongly recommended.

NORMAL HAEMOSTASIS

The haemostatic system is a delicately controlled component of the host defence system, the role of which is to initiate haemostasis where and when required and in adequate, but not in excessive, amounts. The system closely interacts with other components of the host defence system, including the acute stress responses, inflammation, healing and immune functions. There has been a paradigm shift in our understanding of the haemostatic system from one of interacting humoral factors to an integrated cell-based system.[1,2] In view of the increasing range of focused therapies available that act on the haemostatic system to modulate its activity, it is important that core aspects of the structure and function of the system are summarised.

The conversion of blood from its fluid to solid state is an increasingly understood physiological process. The triad of vascular constriction, platelet plugging and fibrin clot formation forms haemostatic plugs and provides the framework on which haemostasis operates (Figure 91.1) and sets the scene for healing to occur. Thrombin is the potent proteolytic enzyme of the coagulation sequence converting fibrinogen to fibrin-soluble monomers, which subsequently polymerise to form the fibrin clot. Fibrinogen is the bulk protein of the coagulation system and fibrin is the end-product of this cascade of proteolytic activity, in which precursor coagulation proteins are activated to potent proteolytic enzymes, with the aid of cofactors, to produce active precursors further down the coagulation 'amplifier'. The polymerised fibrin is further acted on by factor XIII to form a stable fibrin clot. The process of thrombin generation in small amounts initially occurs in relationship to tissue factor-bearing cells and the process is subsequently transferred to the activated platelet surface where amplification occurs.

Following injury, vascular constriction reduces bleeding, and allows time to initiate haemostasis. With large volume haemorrhage, resulting systemic hypotension is an important physiological mechanism to minimise blood loss and facilitate stabilisation of the haemostatic plug. Controlled or 'tolerated' hypotension is now accepted as an important aspect of managing critical haemorrhage.[3,4] This vascular constriction is further accentuated by vasoconstrictors released in association with platelet plug formation. Vascular endothelial cells play an active part by synthesising substances which act at the membrane surface and/or interact with platelets and the coagulation system (e.g. prostacyclin, antithrombin III, plasminogen activator, von Willebrand factor, thrombomodulin, heparin cofactor II and nitric oxide).[5] Following the initial vascular reactions, successful haemostasis depends on adequate numbers of functioning platelets, coagulation cascade function, and poorly understood contributions from red cells and leukocytes.

The coagulation system is triggered via the extrinsic pathway, by which damaged tissues expose tissue factor (TF). Tissue factor is a membrane-bound protein present in cells surrounding the vascular bed. Factor VII and VIIa (a small amount circulates normally in the blood) are bound to TF activating factor X. Factor Xa interacts with the cofactor Va to form prothrombinase complexes with the generation of a small amount of thrombin on the cell surface. Factor IX is also activated by the TF/VIIa complex; it does not play a significant role in the initiation phase of coagulation, but diffuses across to platelets in the vicinity that have adhered in proximity to the site of the TF-bearing cells binding to a specific platelet surface receptor and interacting with cofactor factor VIIIa, leading to activation of factor X directly on the platelet surface. The concept of the intrinsic and extrinsic systems is more of historical and laboratory significance as it is now clear that such a division is artificial, but the concept still has value in performing and assessing haemostatic laboratory tests.

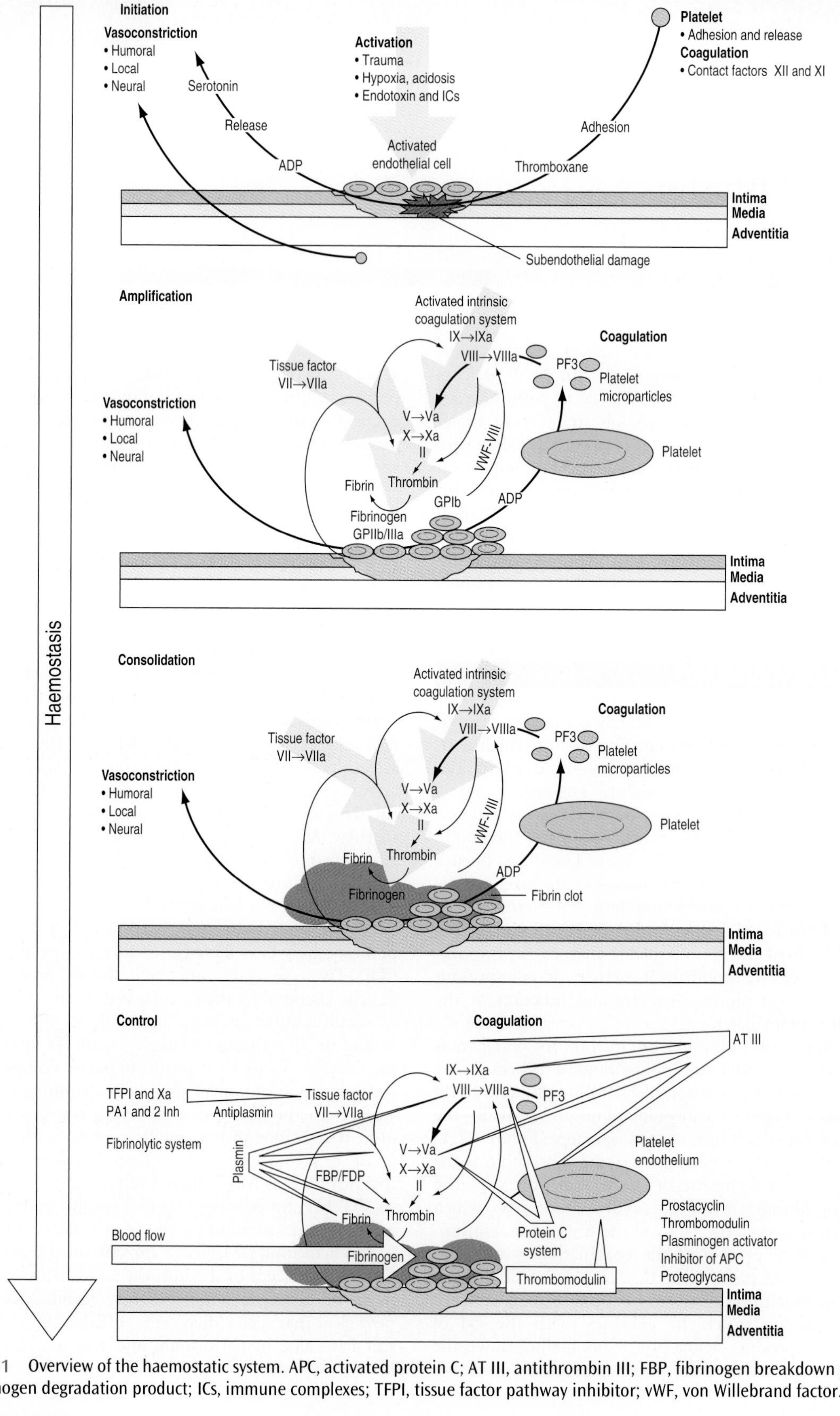

Figure 91.1 Overview of the haemostatic system. APC, activated protein C; AT III, antithrombin III; FBP, fibrinogen breakdown product; FDP, fibrinogen degradation product; ICs, immune complexes; TFPI, tissue factor pathway inhibitor; vWF, von Willebrand factor.

Von Willebrand factor (vWF) is a multimeric glycoprotein that plays a central role in haemostasis by mediating adhesion of platelets to the exposed subendothelium and linking the primary vascular/platelet phase with coagulation by being the carrier protein for coagulant factor VIII which dissociates from vWF to form a complex on the activated platelet surface with IXa (tenase complex) to activate factor X to Xa. Further vWF is released from Weibel–Palade bodies in nearby endothelial cells and platelet α-granules. Platelets interact with vWF via their surface glycoprotein Ib-IX-V complexes. This slows their motion along the subendothelium, allowing receptor interaction leading to platelet binding to collagen. Adhesion to collagen is facilitated by the GPIa-IIa receptor. GPIIb-IIIa can then bind vWF, fibrinogen, fibronectin, vitronectin and thrombospondin, providing further important sites of anchorage for the spreading platelet. The initiation phase of platelet plug formation leads to the development of a platelet monolayer over the injured subendothelium. With the concomitant activation of the coagulation cascade there is local generation of thrombin. Thrombin is a potent platelet agonist via the protease-activated receptor (PAR) to produce a haemostatic plug. Further extension occurs by platelet recruitment by platelet agonists, such as thrombin and mediators, adenosine 5-diphosphate (ADP) and thromboxane A2 released directly from platelets. P-selectin is expressed during activation and also plays a role in platelet-to-platelet cohesion.

Parallel to and within the coagulation system are complex feedback mechanisms to ensure fine-tuning and protection against inappropriate and excessive activation.[6–8] There are several inhibitory proteins, including antithrombin III, thrombomodulin, proteins C and S, tissue factor pathway inhibitor as well as the fibrinolytic system, which are all important in controlling the degree and site of fibrin formation. Indeed, thrombin itself acts as either a procoagulant or an anticoagulant depending on context. Massive activation, as may be seen in trauma and severe infections, can precipitate systemic activation, but in general, the system is well controlled and activity is localised to the area of the stimulus. Perturbations in this complex defence system can produce a wide range of clinical disorders from excessive arterial or venous thrombosis, microvascular obstruction and atheroma to haemostatic failure.

SYSTEMIC HAEMOSTATIC ASSESSMENT

There may be clinical features suggesting local or generalised failure of the haemostatic system (Figure 91.2). Clinical history is important, especially with respect to previous bleeding problems, family history, comorbid medical conditions and medications. The nature of surgery or an invasive intervention may have haemostatic issues that need specific consideration.

TESTS OF THE HAEMOSTATIC SYSTEM

Tests of whole blood clotting time and clot observation do not generally have a role in assessing haemostasis. However, in emergency settings, while waiting for laboratory results, observation of blood collected into a glass tube and maintained at 37°C for clot formation, size, retraction and possible lysis may provide crude information of a possible coagulopathy. The thromboelastogram is a more accurate and controlled procedure for 'holistic' assessment of the haemostatic system at the bedside, but requires close attention to technique and quality control. In most clinical settings, laboratory haemostatic screening tests are readily available, with near-patient testing techniques continuing to improve. A full blood count, prothrombin time (PT), activated partial thromboplastin time (APTT), fibrinogen level, D-Dimer ± thrombin clotting time (TCT) provide a broad screen for most clinically significant haemostatic disorders[9–11] (Figure 91.3). Based on these results, and following consultation with a haematologist, further specific tests of haemostasis may be performed (e.g. mixing studies, factor assays, platelet function tests and test of fibrinolytic function). In broad terms:

- PT tests the integrity of the extrinsic system
- APTT the intrinsic system
- TCT fibrinogen conversion
- D-Dimer assay measures the breakdown products from lysis of fibrin

The haemostatic system optimally functions at 37°C and laboratory coagulation tests are performed at 37°C. Hypothermia may severely impair a patient's systemic and local haemostasis despite the system being structurally intact and laboratory tests normal.

The laboratory investigation of a patient with a potential haemostatic defect depends on the degree of urgency. It may be necessary to administer blood component therapy without a definitive haemostatic defect being established. In elective settings, the defect can be accurately identified, problems pre-empted and specific blood component therapy administered prophylactically or therapeutically. A detailed clinical history and screening laboratory investigations prior to elective procedures will often avert undiagnosed emergency haemostatic crises.

There are several important principles in the collection of blood samples for haemostatic investigations. Most samples are collected into citrated tubes and the amount of anticoagulant in the tube is related to the intended amount of blood to be collected into the tube. It is important that the correct amount of blood is added to the tube and gently mixed. Attention to venepuncture technique is crucial and rapid transfer of the sample to the laboratory is important. Contamination of the sample with tissue factor due to traumatic venepuncture will activate the sample and invalidate results. Collection from vascular access lines may result in diluted or heparin-contaminated samples. Incorrect

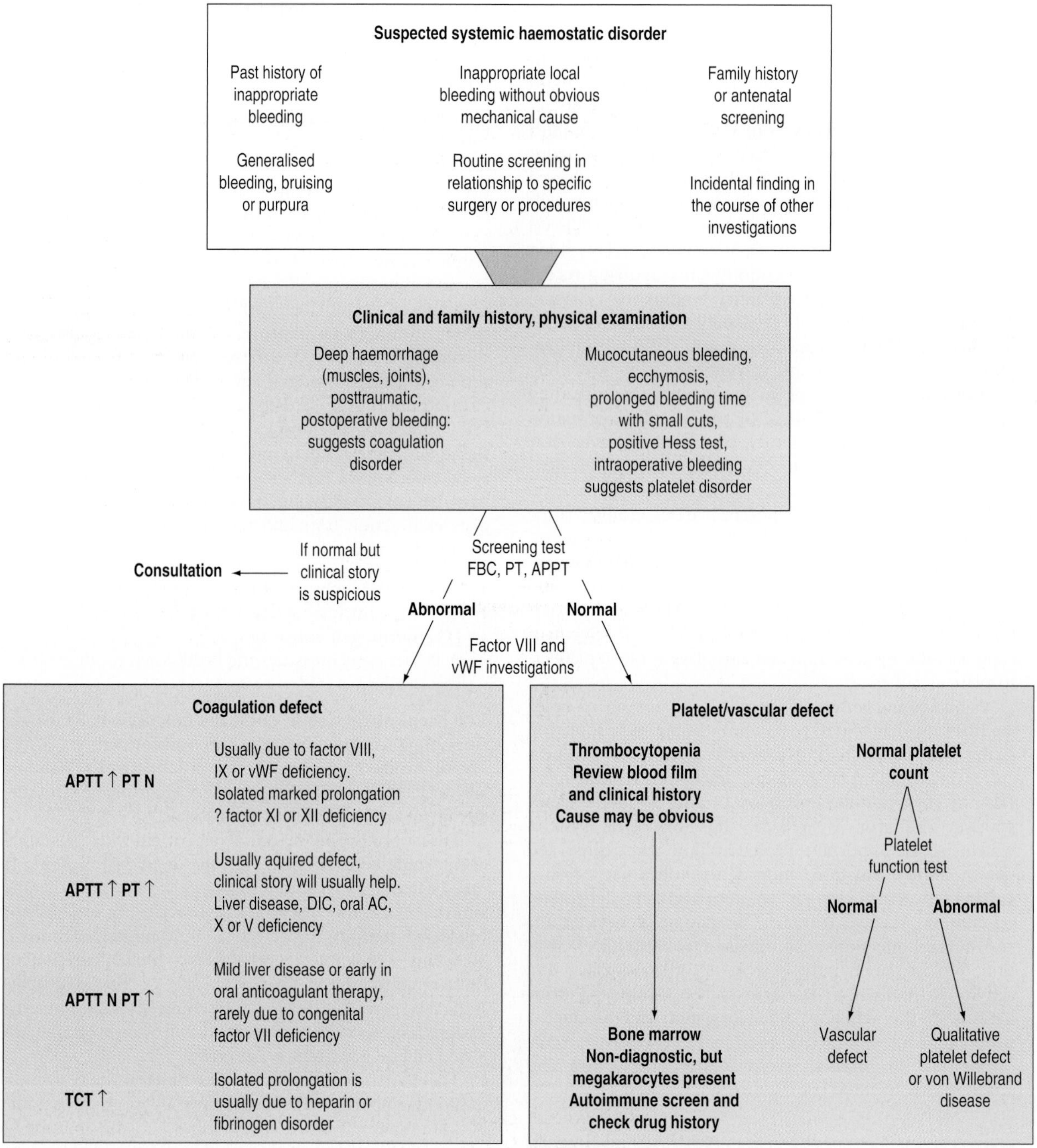

Figure 91.2 Coagulation tests.

laboratory results may be more dangerous to a patient than no results at all.

PLATELET COUNT (PC) (NORMAL 150–400 × 10^9/l)

The counting of platelets is performed as part of the full blood count by automated cell counters. It is not possible to perform accurate platelet counts on 'fingerprick' blood.

BLEEDING TIME (BT) (NORMAL 3–9 MINUTES)

The bleeding time is progressively prolonged when the platelet count falls below 75–100 × 10^9/l assuming platelet function is normal. It is also prolonged when platelet function is defective, in capillary/vascular disease and in some coagulation defects. The bleeding time is an invasive and operator-dependent test. It is not good for

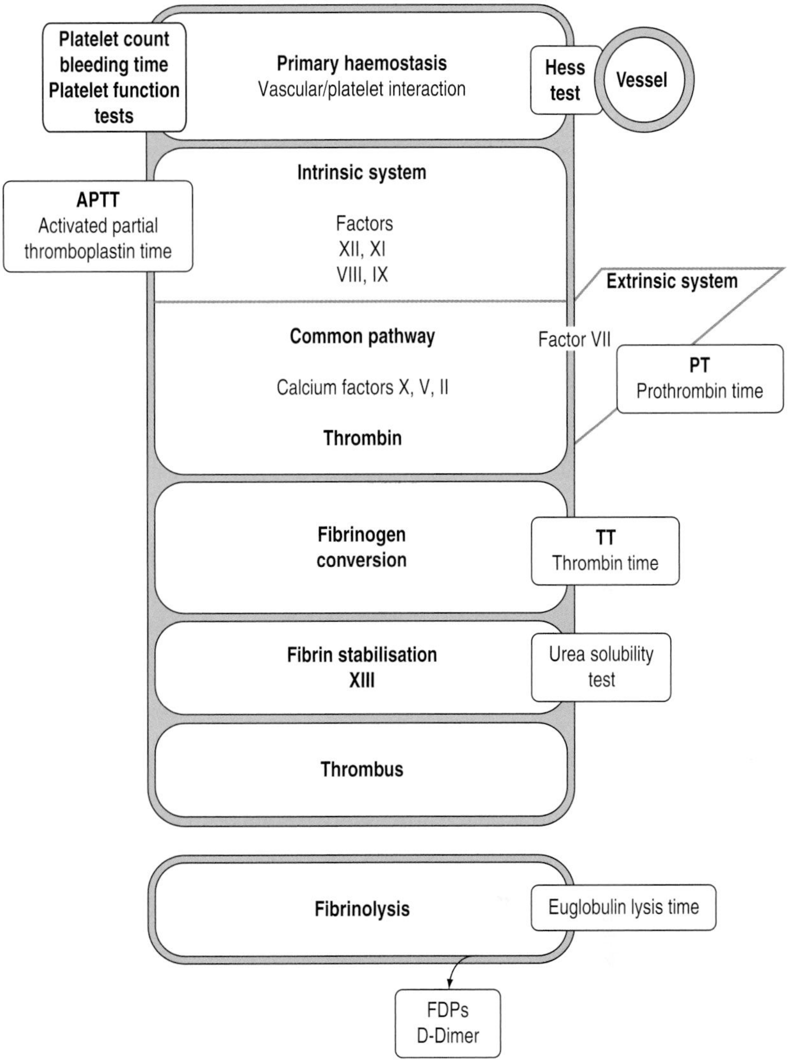

Figure 91.3 Investigations for a suspected haemostatic defect. FDPs, fibrinogen degradation products.

screening unselected patients and has generally been replaced by the platelet function analyser, PFA-100(R).

PROTHROMBIN TIME (PT) (NORMAL RANGE < 3 SECONDS ABOVE THE CONTROL)

The PT is a test of the extrinsic coagulation and prolongation may be caused by factor VII deficiency, liver disease, vitamin K deficiency or oral anticoagulant therapy. The PT is also expressed as the international normalised ratio (INR), especially when used for anticoagulant control.

ACTIVATED PARTIAL THROMBOPLASTIN TIME (APTT) (< 6 SECONDS ABOVE CONTROL)

The APTT is a test of the intrinsic coagulation system and the result must be interpreted with caution as there may be significant variation in sensitivity and specificity of the test between laboratories. In unselected patients there is poor correlation between the APTT prolongation and the presence of haemostatic failure or the likelihood of a patient bleeding. In the context of a patient suspected of having a systemic haemostatic defect, an isolated prolongation of the APTT may represent deficiency or an inhibitor of factor VIII or IX. If there is a marked isolated prolongation there may be a deficiency in the contact phase of the coagulation cascade and there is poor correlation with a bleeding tendency. Prolongation of APTT and PT may be due to deficiencies of factors X, V or II. A lupus anticoagulant may prolong the APTT and represent a prothrombotic state.

THROMBIN CLOTTING TIME (TCT) (NORMAL < 2 SECONDS LONGER THAN CONTROL)

This is a test of the final conversion of fibrinogen to fibrin. Prolongation of TCT is due to hypofibrinogenaemia, dysfibrinogenaemia, heparin, and fibrin degradation products.

D-DIMER (NORMAL < 0.25 ng/L)

The D-Dimer assay measures cleavage fragments resulting from the proteolytic action of plasmin of fibrin. Elevation of D-Dimer may be seen in the postoperative state, trauma, renal impairment, sepsis and venous thrombosis. High levels of D-Dimer suggest excessive fibrinolysis, as seen in disseminated intravascular coagulation. The test is specific for fibrinolysis and not primary fibrinogenolysis.

SPECIFIC COAGULATION FACTOR ASSAYS

Fibrinogen is the commonest routinely measured coagulation factor in patients suspected of systemic haemostatic failure. Fibrinogen concentration can be measured using clottable protein methods, end-point detection techniques or immunochemical tests. The method of Clauss is the most common fibrinogen assay used. Other assays are usually performed in the investigation for specific defects, usually after consultation with a haematologist.

EUGLOBULIN LYSIS TIME (ELT) (NORMAL RANGE > 90 MINUTES)

This test mainly reflects the presence of plasminogen activators. A shortened time is indicative of systemic fibrinolytic activation.

PLATELET FUNCTION TESTS

Platelet function tests are used for the diagnosis of platelet disorders.[12,13] In recent years there has been increasing interest in the use of platelet function tests to monitor antiplatelet therapy. Unfortunately, platelet function testing is poorly standardised and good quality control is commonly lacking. The diagnostic utility of some of the newer simpler assays of platelet function have been evaluated in a range of clinical settings, but their value remains controversial.

A popular technology is the platelet function analyser (PFA-100) in which citrated whole blood is placed in a disposable cartridge containing a membrane coated with collagen/adrenaline or collagen/ADP into which a microscopic aperture has been cut. With high shear rates contact of blood with the membrane causes platelets to aggregate and occlude the aperture. The time to occlude the aperture is recorded as the end-point and referred to as the closure time.[14] The technique is simple and rapid, but subject to a number of variables such as the platelet count, haematocrit, ABO blood group and plasma vWF levels. A normal result has a high negative predictive value and is increasingly becoming popular as a screening test for platelet dysfunction; however, false positive and negative results may occur. The test is more sensitive than the bleeding time which is now generally regarded as an obsolete test. .

THROMBOELASTOGRAM (TEG)

Thrombelastography was originally described 50 years ago, but failed to establish a role in routine laboratory haemostasis testing. Improvements in the technology, especially standardisation and computerisation, have now made the TEG a valuable tool for monitoring haemostasis as a holistic dynamic process supplementing the long-standing conventional coagulation screens. The TEG measures the viscoelastic properties of blood as it clots under low shear conditions. The patterns of changes in shear elasticity provide information about the kinetics of clot formation, growth, strength and stability of the formed clot. The TEG is increasing being used as a point of care test, providing 'real time' information about a patient's haemostatic function.[15]

CONGENITAL HAEMOSTATIC DEFECTS

Congenital bleeding disorders are relatively uncommon and are usually confined to a single defect. It is important to identify the defect so that specific replacement therapy can be given preoperatively or to arrest a particular episode of bleeding.

THE HAEMOPHILIAS

HAEMOPHILIA A (CLASSIC HAEMOPHILIA)

Haemophilia A is an X-linked disorder due to a deficiency of factor VIII. The mainstay of haemophilia treatment is coagulation factor replacement.[16,17] Coagulation factor concentrates or recombinant factor VIII are given to prevent bleeding and to control existing haemorrhage. The dose of clotting factor is calculated on the basis that one unit of coagulation factor is that amount present in 1 ml of pooled normal plasma. An individual with a plasma volume of 3000 ml would have 3000 U of the clotting factor in the circulation. If such person was a haemophiliac with <1% factor VIII level in the plasma, a dose of 3000 U of factor VIII would be required to raise the plasma level to 100% of normal.

Experience has demonstrated that doses of 15–20 U/kg body weight will control most haemarthroses, but doses of up to 30 U/kg are required for muscle haematomas or for the prevention of dental bleeding. Raising clotting factor levels to 100% of normal is indicated for severe bleeding (e.g. intracranial or intra-abdominal haemorrhage), but there is considerable patient variation in response to specific doses, and empirical 'dose-finding' may be necessary. Measurement of factor VIII levels following replacement therapy is helpful. A factor VIII concentration of 25%, usually achieved with a dose of 15 U/kg, controls joint bleeding, whereas a level of 50%, generally obtained with a dose of 30 U/kg, prevents bleeding following tooth extraction. Clotting factor is given when a haemophiliac undergoes invasive procedures, including minor invasions such as arterial blood gas sampling.

The half-life of factor VIII in the circulation is approximately 12 hours. On this basis, doses are repeated 12-hourly if it is necessary to maintain a specific plasma concentration of the factor. Clotting factor assays are performed near the end of this 12-hour period in order to confirm that adequate levels for haemostasis are being achieved. Concentrate may also be given by continuous infusion.

HAEMOPHILIA B (CHRISTMAS DISEASE)

Haemophilia B due to factor IX deficiency is less common than classic haemophilia. The general principles of management are similar, with factor IX concentrates or recombinant products being used.

VON WILLEBRAND'S DISEASE

Von Willebrand's disease (vWD), the commonest of the hereditary haemostatic disorders, with a prevalence of approximately 100 symptomatic persons per million, is due to a quantitative or qualitative defect in von Willebrand factor (vWF). Patients with defective vWD may have mucocutaneous bleeding consistent with platelet dysfunction, or spontaneous deep tissue bleeding similar to that of haemophiliacs.

Classification of vWD is complex and controversial. Therapy may be determined by the specific subtype and expert haematological consultation is important.[18,19] Clinical heterogeneity is reflected in the classification of subtypes corresponding to specific pathophysiological mechanisms.

In most cases desmopressin (DDAVP) is effective therapy, but replacement therapy may be needed for the rarer severe subtypes. DDAVP induces a haemostatic state via release of factor VIII and vWF; 0.3 μg/kg is infused slowly over 30 minutes immediately prior to surgery or to establish haemostasis in the bleeding patient. Antifibrinolytic agents may also be useful when not contraindicated as a thrombotic risk. If replacement therapy is indicated, cryoprecipitate or factor VIII concentrates containing vWF should be administered.

CONGENITAL PLATELET DISORDERS

Congenital platelet disorders are rare, the commonest severe disorder being Glanzmann's thrombaesthenia.[20] Platelet transfusions may be required for acute bleeds or in relation to elective surgery; DDAVP ± antifibrinolytic therapy and recombinant factor VIIa may all have a role.

ACQUIRED HAEMOSTATIC DISORDERS

The acquired disorders of coagulation are usually more complex and multifactorial than the hereditary disorders. A unified approach is essential for the successful management of these potentially life-threatening situations, and transfusion therapy cannot be isolated from other treatment.

CRITICAL HAEMORRHAGE AND MASSIVE BLOOD TRANSFUSION

The nature and management of haemostatic defects secondary to acute and/or massive blood loss and transfusion remains poorly understood.[21] The coagulopathy of trauma is characterised by non-surgical bleeding from mucosal lesions, serosal surfaces, wounds and vascular access sites. Hypothermia, acidosis and haemodilution are commonly present, occasionally with features of disseminated intravascular coagulation (DIC). DIC typically occurs acutely after trauma when brain, fat, amniotic fluid or other potent thromboplastins enter the circulation. It may occur less acutely when endothelial inflammation or failure reduces clearing of activated coagulation factors. The coagulopathy of trauma should be anticipated in massive transfusion situations and there is increasing support for early treatment with plasma, which may prevent or delay its onset.

Further aggravation of the complications of massive blood transfusion can be avoided or minimised if correctable defects in the haemostatic system are identified (Table 91.1). The relative importance of the different potential mechanisms responsible for haemostatic failure is difficult to determine, but the identification of correctable defects will avoid or minimise complications. Haemostatic failure correlates poorly with the volume of transfusion or components administered, but better with the nature of the insult, degree of hypovolaemia, and time to resuscitation. Trauma patients with major coagulopathy and microvascular haemorrhage usually have abnormal laboratory parameters prior to massive blood transfusion. Except for severe abnormalities, haemostatic laboratory parameters correlate poorly with clinical evidence of haemostatic failure. Thrombocytopenia and impaired platelet function are probably the most consistent significant haematological abnormalities, correction of which may be associated with control of microvascular bleeding.

Coagulation deficiency from massive blood loss is initially confined to factors V and VIII. APTT, PT and fibrinogen assay should be performed, but the urgency of the situation does not usually allow for other specific factor assays, and fresh frozen plasma (FFP), cryoprecipitate or factor concentrates should be infused if the test results are abnormal. Correction of hypofibrinogenaemia is probably more important than thought previously.[22]

Table 91.1 Possible factors contributing to haemostatic failure following massive blood transfusion

Pre-existing haemostatic defect
Loss of coagulation factors, platelets and inhibitors
Dilution of coagulation factors, platelets and inhibitors
Impaired synthesis due to effects of shock on liver and bone marrow function
Effects of trauma: disseminated intravascular coagulation (DIC) and fibrinolysis
Effects of blood storage lesion: depletion of coagulation factors and platelets, aggravation or precipitation of DIC
Depletion of modulators of haemostasis (e.g. antithrombin III, fibronectin and protein C)
Incompatible transfusion reaction: DIC
Hypothermia
? Citrate toxicity

Table 91.2 Potential problems with stored blood components

Failure to correct deficiency
Inadequate correction of deficiency
Blockade of reticuloendothelial system (microaggregates, coagulation)
Microvascular pathophysiology (ARDS, MSOF)
Accentuation of free radical pathology (leukocytes, iron)
Activation and consumption of the haemostatic system
Hyperkalaemia, hypocalcaemia, hypothermia
Vasoactive effects (hypotension)
Hyperbilirubinaemia

A case can be made for prophylactic FFP in infusions in patients with massive blood loss which has been replaced with red cell concentrates and plasma substitutes. Hypothermia must be avoided, recognised and treated rapidly.[23] Potential problems associated with large volume stored blood replacement are summarised in Table 91.2.

With ongoing bleeding with associated microvascular oozing, various approaches may be taken. Having ensured that all identifiable haemostatic defects have been corrected, questions arise as to the roles of fresh blood and, more recently, recombinant activated factor VII (rFVIIa).[24] The use of freshly collected whole blood remains controversial and is an 'emotive' subject needing some comment.[25,26] The provision of fresh whole blood can present logistic, ethical and safety problems needing consideration. Many transfusion medicine specialists categorically state that there is never an indication for fresh whole blood. Such dogma can be difficult to defend in the clinical setting of the massive haemorrhage and transfusion syndrome where pathophysiology remains poorly understood and specific blood component therapy may be ineffective. The current author, from his own experience and on the basis of current evidence, feels that the following statements reasonably summarise the current status of fresh blood transfusion:

- Fresh blood provides immediately functioning oxygen-carrying capacity, volume and haemostatic factors in the one product
- The number of allogeneic donors to whom a patient is exposed can be reduced
- Problems associated with infusion of massive volumes of stored blood can be minimised/avoided
- The risk of transfusion-related viral infections is potentially higher than fully tested and stored blood
- The benefit in controlling haemorrhage probably relates to the presence of immediately functioning platelets

HAEMOSTATIC FAILURE ASSOCIATED WITH LIVER DISEASE

The liver is the production site of nearly all the factors involved in the formation and control of coagulation (Table 91.3). Bleeding in association with liver disease can be difficult to manage. There may be a combination of excessive consumption of coagulation factors and impaired synthesis of both clotting factors and coagulation inhibitor proteins. Excessive activation of fibrinolysis may occur and defective clearing of activated clotting factors compounds the problem. Moreover, the effects of massive blood loss, shock and transfusion must also complicate the problem.

Table 91.3 Haemostatic disturbances in liver disease

Deficiency of vitamin K-dependent clotting factors II, VII, IX, X
Deficiency of fibrinogen and factor V
Dysfibrinogenaemia
Disseminated intravascular coagulation
Excessive fibrinolytic activity
Circulating anticoagulants
Platelet abnormalities

Haemostatic defects due to deficient vitamin K-dependent coagulation factors (in patients with predominantly cholestatic liver disease) may be rapidly reversed with vitamin K therapy, and blood transfusion may not be required. If the abnormality is not reversed by vitamin K, hepatocellular damage is likely to be present and FFP is appropriate replacement therapy.[27] When an elective procedure is planned, prophylactic FFP is appropriate. Low fibrinogen levels in liver disease usually indicate advanced disease and are associated with a poor prognosis, or the presence of DIC. Cryoprecipitate is generally the most readily available form of fibrinogen if concentrates are not available.

DISSEMINATED INTRAVASCULAR COAGULATION[28]

Disseminated intravascular coagulation (DIC) is a pathophysiological process and not a disease in itself. Clinical manifestations of DIC relate to occlusion of the microvessels during the obstructive phase of the syndrome and haemorrhage secondary to consumption of plasma and cellular components of the haemostatic system.[29]

Perpetuation of the process may be due to continuation of the stimulus and/or consumption of the natural inhibitors of haemostasis. DIC thus results, due to inappropriate, excessive and uncontrolled activation of the haemostatic process. This may initially occur with adequate compensation when defects may only be demonstrable in laboratory tests. If the initiating disorder is severe enough, the clinical syndrome of uncontrolled acute DIC will result with a systemic bleeding state, usually with associated end-organ failure. A compensatory secondary fibrinolysis occurs, which in some cases may accentuate the bleeding.

PATHOPHYSIOLOGY

DIC is characterised by the consumption of clotting factors and platelets within the circulation, resulting in varying degrees of microvascular obstruction due to fibrin deposition (Figure 91.4). When significant platelet and coagulation factor consumption occurs, bleeding may become a major feature.

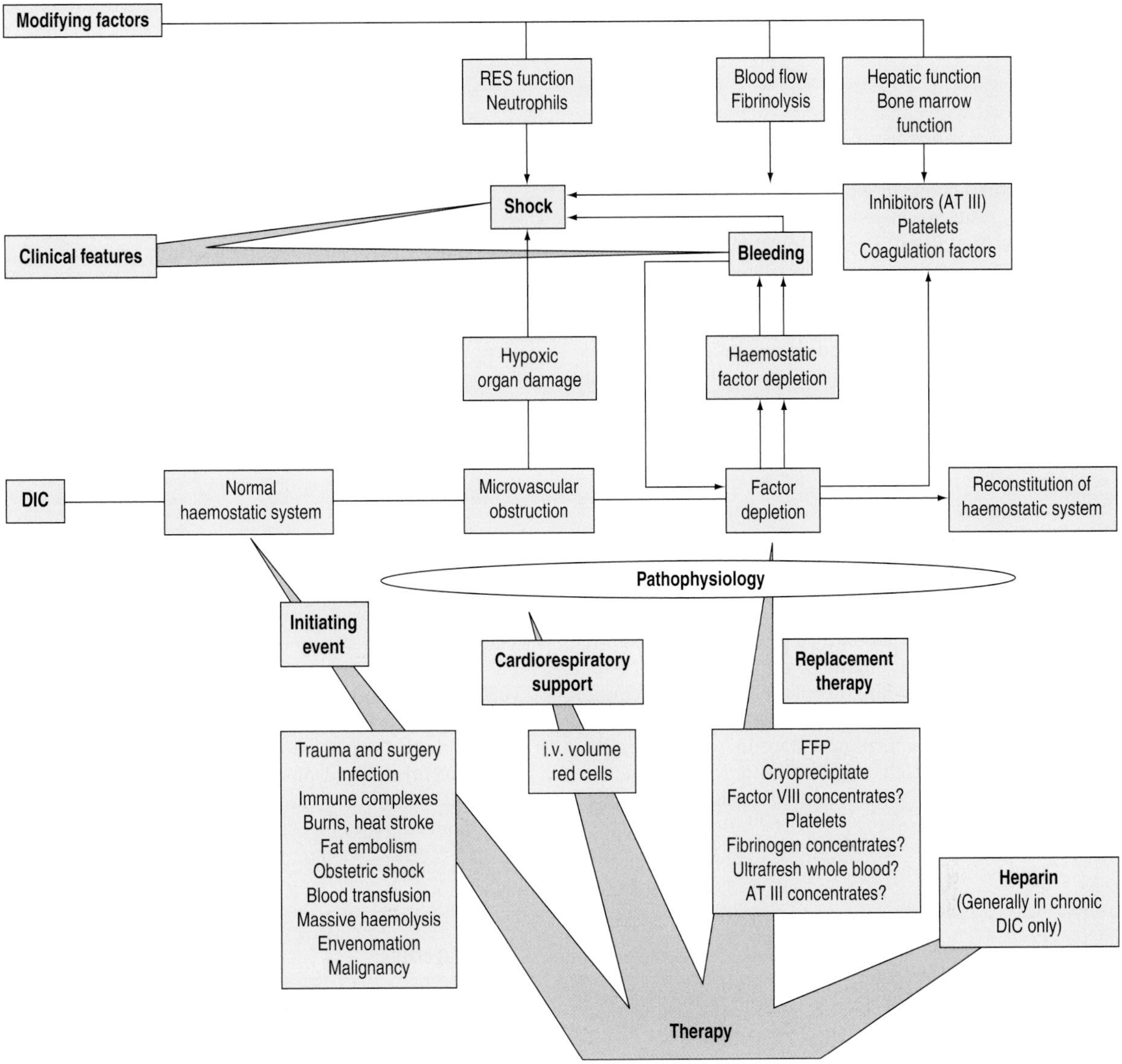

Figure 91.4 The pathophysiology and management of disseminated intravascular coagulation (DIC). AT III, antithrombin III; FFP, fresh frozen plasma; RES, reticuloendothelial system.

Mechanisms which may inappropriately activate the haemostatic system include:

- Activation of the coagulation sequence by release of tissue thromboplastins into the systemic circulation, e.g. following extensive tissue trauma, during surgery, malignancy and during an acute intravascular haemolysis.
- Vessel wall endothelial injury causing platelet activation followed by activation of the haemostatic system, predominantly via the intrinsic pathway (e.g. Gram-negative sepsis from endotoxin release, viral infections, extensive burns, prolonged hypotension, hypoxia or acidosis).
- Induction of platelet activation (e.g. septicaemia, viraemia, antigen–antibody complexes and platelet activation).

CLINICAL FEATURES

The clinical presentation of DIC varies, with patients showing thrombotic, haemorrhagic or mixed manifestations in various organ systems. The major clinical problem and presenting feature of acute DIC is bleeding. This may manifest as generalised bruising or bleeding at sites of therapeutic or traumatic invasion (venepuncture sites and surgical wounds). DIC may occur in association with a wide range of clinical disorders (see Table 91.5). When DIC occurs in acutely ill patients with multisystem organ failure the prognosis is poor. DIC may, in some patients, be an agonal event and should not be treated.

LABORATORY FINDINGS

Results of tests may be variable and difficult to interpret. Significant DIC can be present despite normal standard coagulation tests (i.e. PT, APTT and TCT). The key tests in diagnosis are those that provide evidence for excessive conversion of fibrinogen to fibrin within the circulation and its subsequent lysis. Platelet–fibrin clots create a mesh in the microcirculation in which passing red cells may be traumatised, resulting in red cell fragmentation and haemolysis. The blood film may demonstrate fragmentation of the red cells (microangiopathic haemolytic anaemia), but this is more commonly seen in chronic DIC, especially in association with malignancy.

The diagnosis is usually based on a combination of the appropriate clinical picture with a supportive pattern of laboratory tests of the haemostatic system[27] (Table 91.4). Thrombocytopenia and hypofibrinogenaemia with prolongation of the APTT, PT and TCT in conjunction with an elevation of fibrin degradation products (D-Dimer test) are supportive evidence for the diagnosis. The D-Dimer test is specific for fibrin breakdown versus primary fibrinogenolysis. More specialised test such as elevation of fibrinopeptide A and reduced levels of antithrombin III add further weight to the diagnosis.

In chronic DIC the laboratory findings are different from those in acute DIC. Many of the usual tests of haemostasis are normal or near normal. The platelet count may be normal, as may many of the haemostatic factors. However, this is a compensated state in which there is increased turnover of each of the haemostatic components. D-Dimer is elevated in this setting and a microangiopathic red cell picture is seen on the peripheral blood film.

DISORDERS ASSOCIATED WITH DIC

DIC may occur in association with a wide range of clinical disorders (Table 91.5).

THERAPY

The management of DIC remains controversial, but removal or treatment of the initiating cause is important in conjunction with general resuscitation. The early recognition of DIC and initiation of management may allow the patient to survive hours or days, granting sufficient time for definitive diagnosis and treatment of the inciting disorder. Blood component therapy should be given to the haemorrhaging patient, but the use of heparin should only be considered in selected cases.

- Fresh frozen plasma (FFP) contains all the coagulation factors and the main inhibitors, antithrombin III and protein C, in near-normal quantities and should be used if haemorrhage is occurring.[30,31]
- Cryoprecipitate contains all the components of the factor VIII complex, as well as fibrinogen, factor XIII and fibronectin in concentrated form. Between 5 and 10 units should be infused in conjunction with the fresh frozen plasma.
- Platelet transfusion may be indicated in the presence of life-threatening haemorrhage; however, this is a controversial subject and the patients tend to be resistant if the initiating cause of the DIC has not been controlled.
- It is likely that replacement therapy with antithrombin III concentrates and possibly other inhibitors of haemostasis will find a greater role in therapy.[30] Successful treatment of the bleeding phase of DIC probably

Table 91.4 Laboratory test for the diagnosis of disseminated intravascular coagulation

Analysis	Early	Late
Platelet count	↓	↓↓
Activated partial thromboplastin time (APTT)	↑	↑↑
Prothrombin time (PT)	↑	↑
Thrombin clotting time (TCT)	↑	↑
Fibrin degradation products (D-Dimer assay)	↑	↑↑
Hypofibrinogen	↓	↓↓
Other coagulation factors II, VII, VIII, X	↓	↓↓
Coagulation inhibitors: antithrombin III, protein C	↓	↓↓↓
Blood film	Usually normal in early stages	Fragmented red cells + in subacute or chronic cases
Supplementary and research tests: prothrombin fragment 1+2, thrombin–antithrombin complex (TAT complex), procalcitonin (PCT), plasmin–antiplasmin complexes (PAP complex)	↑	↑

Table 91.5 Conditions associated with disseminated intravascular coagulation

Infection
Bacterial sepsis
Viral haemorrhagic fevers
Protozoal (malaria)
Trauma
Extensive tissue injury
Head injury
Fat embolism
Malignancy
Carcinoma
Leukaemia (especially promyelocytic)
Immunological disorders
Transplantation rejection
Incompatible haemolytic blood transfusion reactions
Severe allergic reaction
Drug reactions
Extracorporeal circulations
Snake bite envenomation
Vascular disorders
Giant haemangioma
Aortic aneurysm
Pregnancy associated
Septic abortion
Abruptio placentae
Eclampsia
Amniotic fluid embolism
Placenta praevia
Burns
Hyperthermia
Liver disease and acute hepatic necrosis

depends to a variable degree on the patient being able to 'switch off' the coagulation system. Correction of depleted coagulation inhibitor levels, reticuloendothelial blockade and impaired or excessive fibrinolysis may be important.

- In general, heparin should only be used after initial adequate replacement therapy has failed to control bleeding. The decision to use heparin should not be undertaken lightly, or without due consultation. Small doses should be used initially (e.g. 50–100 units/kg body weight followed by 10–15 units/kg per hour), adjusted according to the clinical and laboratory response. Heparin is especially valuable in certain specific clinical situations, including acute promyelocytic leukaemia, the early stages of amniotic fluid embolism and immediately following a severe incompatible blood transfusion.

Management of sudden massive obstetric haemorrhage is similar to other cases of DIC except that the onset is more likely to be fulminant and unexpected and associated with greater depletion of coagulation factors, especially fibrinogen, due to marked fibrinolysis. Fresh blood is possibly warranted in some of these cases where bleeding does not stop quickly. Once the uterus has been emptied and contracted, the haemostatic failure quickly resolves. There is increasing interest in a possible role for rFVIIa in this setting.

OUTCOME

Factors which may affect the outcome of DIC include:

- the nature of the initiating event
- the host factors (e.g. state of reticuloendothelial system, levels of inhibitors of coagulation and fibrinolytic activity, hepatic synthetic function)
- the extent of end-organ damage sustained during the thrombotic phase and from shock caused during the haemorrhagic phase

ANTITHROMBOTIC THERAPY

The availability of an increasing variety of antithrombotic agents, and wider clinical use of antithrombotic therapy generally, has inevitably resulted in an increase in iatrogenic bleeding in patients presenting with other medical conditions (e.g. trauma, surgery and invasive procedures) and intensivists must be aware of the methods for rapid reversal of therapy.[32,33] Bleeding problems in patients on well-controlled anticoagulation are usually due to surgery, trauma or a local lesion (e.g. peptic ulceration). Otherwise, bleeding is due to over-anticoagulation, sometimes as a result of drug interactions. Elective surgery in this group of patients needs careful planning if haemorrhagic and thrombotic complications are to be avoided. Patients on antithrombotic therapy involved in traumatic events are a challenge in whom there is the risk of progression of the original insult, increased risk of posttraumatic complications, and mortality.

ORAL ANTICOAGULANT AGENTS

Oral anticoagulant agents induce a controlled deficiency of the vitamin K-dependent clotting factors (II, VII, IX and X), the anticoagulant action being measured by prolongation of PT (INR). The indications for reversing vitamin K antagonists depend on the clinical situation and the indication for therapy. Reversal of over-anticoagulation depends on the degree of overactivity and on the presence, or not, of haemorrhage. In most cases vigorous intervention is unnecessary and the oral anticoagulation can be temporarily ceased. Short-term reversal or temporary reversal is achieved by administration of FFP. Prothrombin complex concentrate will effectively and rapidly reverse the anticoagulant effects of warfarin, including protein C correction, and have a role in anticoagulant overdose. Previous concerns about coagulation activation do not appear to be a problem with current products.

Long-term reversal requires vitamin K, but care must be taken not to give an excessive dose if it is planned that the patient needs to return to oral anticoagulation in the long term. For most surgical interventions or invasive procedures an INR of 1.5 or less is accepted as safe. This can usually be achieved by temporarily ceasing medication.

HEPARINS

With the wide clinical use of fractionated low molecular weight (LMW) heparins, this subject has become more complex. Heparins act by potentiating the action of antithrombin III, a natural coagulation inhibitor. Unfractionated heparin acts in neutralising both thrombin and factor Xa, in contrast to the LMW heparins which predominantly neutralise factor Xa. The anticoagulant effect of unfractionated heparin is usually measured by prolongation of the APTT. LMW heparins do not prolong the APTT, are generally administered on weight basis and are not routinely monitored by a laboratory test. When monitoring is required, the anti-Xa assay is used.

ANTIPLATELET AGENTS

Antiplatelet agents are being used increasingly for prophylaxis and therapy of arterial disease, and many of the non-steroidal anti-inflammatory agents are also platelet-inhibitory drugs. Aspirin has an irreversible effect on platelet function and platelet function tests may show abnormalities for up to 10 days after medication. Most of the other non-steroidal anti-inflammatory drugs have a reversible effect lasting a matter of hours or occasionally days. Perioperative bleeding is usually mild, but occasionally may be serious, depending on the surgery, and in some situations a platelet transfusion may be necessary. In other cases, the patient may already have a mild haemostatic defect (e.g. von Willebrand's disease) and aspirin may have a synergistic effect, leading to major haemostatic failure.

Agents such as clopidogrel act as inhibitors of platelet aggregation by selectively inhibiting the binding of ADP to its platelet receptor by irreversibly modifying the platelet ADP receptor and, as a result, ADP-mediated activation of the GPIIb/IIIa complex. As with aspirin, platelets exposed to clopidogrel are affected for their lifespan and recovery of normal platelet function occurs as new platelets are produced.

REVERSAL OF ANTITHROMBOTIC AGENTS

Life-threatening bleeding in patients on warfarin requires urgent reversal and this is best achieved with prothrombin concentrate (PCC) administration in conjunction with FFP depending on the factor VII level of the PCC.[34–36] The advantages of PCC over FFP include more timely correction, absence of volume overload and potentially better restoration of the vitamin K-dependent coagulation factors. Vitamin K_1 is essential for sustained reversal, but the dose should be determined on the basis of whether temporary reversal is indicated. When there is an indication to continue warfarin therapy, vitamin K_1 should be administered in a dose that will lower or maintain the INR to a safe, but not subtherapeutic, range and will not cause resistance once warfarin is reinstated.

Immediate reversal of heparin activity can be achieved with protamine sulphate. Although formulas have been quoted for the reversal of heparin (e.g. 1 mg protamine sulphate will neutralise 100 units of heparin), it is better to titrate the dose using APTT after an initial empirical dose of 50 mg. Protamine sulphate should be injected slowly by the intravenous route. Protamine is not without risk, as it may itself impair coagulation and be associated with anaphylactoid reactions. It is not possible to reverse the effects of LMW heparins, and rFVIIa may have role in critical bleeding settings.

Antiplatelet agents, particularly acetylsalicylic acid, clopidogrel and GPIIb/IIIa inhibitors, now have a central role in preventing arterial thrombosis. Clinicians are now regularly confronted by balancing the haemorrhagic risks associated with these agents, especially in the perisurgical setting, against the thrombotic risks associated with their discontinuation. It is generally agreed that continuing acetylsalicylic acid during vascular surgery procedures and in most other settings in which the bleeding risk is likely to be low is acceptable. It is generally recommended that clopidogrel be ceased 5 days before surgery to allow regeneration of half the platelet pool. Although withdrawal of the competitive GPIIb/IIIa inhibitors at the beginning of surgery will decrease the risk of bleeding, it should be emphasised that thrombotic events in patients waiting for urgent myocardial revascularisation are a significant risk and acceptance of perioperative bleeding risk may take priority. Patient blood management techniques to minimise blood loss and transfusion should be used.[37] Platelet concentrate transfusions may be indicated in the acute setting.

NEWER ANTITHROMBOTIC AGENTS

Limitations of the currently available antithrombotic agents continue to stimulate research into new anticoagulants with improved pharmacological activity and safety.[38]

Targets of action include:

- the factor VIIa/tissue factor pathway inhibition – recombinant nematode anticoagulant peptide c2 and tissue factor pathway inhibitor
- factor Xa inhibitors – fondaparinux, idraparinux, razaxaban
- factor Va and VIIIa pathway inhibition with recombinant activated protein C, soluble thrombomodulin
- thrombin inhibitors – hirudin, bivalirudin, argatroban, ximelagatran, dabigatran

Independent of their mode of action, these agents all have the potential to cause bleeding complications.

Reversal agents do not exist for the majority of these newer agents. Recombinant activated factor VIIa may have a role in controlling bleeding, but more experience will be needed with the use of these newer agents and their bleeding risks.

ACQUIRED INHIBITORS OF COAGULATION

Major haemostatic failure may be seen with rare inhibitors of coagulation factors. Autoantibodies against factors VIII (commonest), IX, X, V and vWF have been reported. A coordinated approach to haemotherapy is essential if bleeding is to be arrested. The patients are relatively resistant to factor replacement therapy and removal of the offending autoantibody by plasma exchange and replacement with FFP ± factor concentrates is indicated. Recombinant activated factor VII may have a role yet to be defined.

PRIMARY FIBRINOLYSIS

This rare acquired disorder of haemostasis is in reality primary fibrinogenolysis because circulating plasmin is responsible for an uncontrolled proteolytic attack on the coagulation system (particularly factor VIII and fibrinogen). The disorder may complicate specific types of surgery (e.g. neurosurgery, pulmonary and prostate) or malignancy. Rapid recognition of this potentially devastating failure of haemostasis is essential if appropriate antifibrinolytic and blood component therapy (FFP and cryoprecipitate) is to be effective. With streptokinase and tissue plasminogen activator therapy of arterial and venous disease, problems of excess lysis may occur.

EXTRACORPOREAL CIRCULATION CARDIAC SURGERY

A range of haemostatic disturbances may be associated with extracorporeal circulation, most commonly cardiopulmonary bypass, and the clinician must constantly balance the risks of bleeding versus thrombosis.[39] The abnormalities are generally directly related to the time on bypass and are more likely to be seen in multiple valve replacements or re-operations. Fresh blood components have generally been advocated in cardiac bypass surgery to ensure optimal oxygen delivery and function of the haemostatic components of blood. Haemostatic failure usually becomes apparent in the operating room or soon after and appropriate laboratory investigations should be performed to allow logical therapy. It is pointless infusing large volumes of plasma products or platelets if heparin has not been adequately reversed. Increased fibrinolytic activity may in some cases also contribute to bleeding.

A predictable thrombocytopenia occurs after extracorporeal blood circulation. The postoperative platelet count in the majority of cardiac bypass patients is seldom below 100 000/μl, but platelet functional defects may contribute to bleeding and occasionally platelet concentrates are indicated. Increasingly, rFVIIa is being used to control bleeding associated with cardiac surgery. More evidence is required before definitive recommendations can be made.[40]

THROMBOCYTOPENIA AND QUALITATIVE PLATELET DEFECTS

IDIOPATHIC THROMBOCYTOPENIC PURPURA (ITP)

ITP is an autoimmune disorder where autoantibodies (IgG) are directed against the platelets, which are subsequently destroyed by the monocyte–macrophage system, predominantly in the spleen. ITP is typically a disease of children and young adults. The acute form is more commonly identifiable as postinfectious, and recovery over weeks to months is the usual natural history. The course of the chronic form is variable and may spontaneously recover, but more commonly needs specific intervention.

Therapy of ITP remains controversial.[41] Corticosteroids should generally be regarded as short-term therapy. In adults, the majority of patients respond with a rise in the platelet count. After an initial high dose (50–75 mg) of prednisolone a day until response occurs, the dose is gradually reduced. There is little evidence that corticosteroids will raise the platelet count in acute disease. However, their short-term role in reducing the incidence of bleeding, which is highest in the first weeks, may be important. High dose i.v. immunoglobulin is effective in most patients and is specifically indicated in fulminant acute disease, preoperatively and in pregnancy.

THROMBOTIC THROMBOCYTOPENIC PURPURA

Thrombotic thrombocytopenic purpura (TTP) is a disorder in which platelet aggregates form within the microvasculature, resulting in tissue ischaemia and infarction. Red blood cell fragmentation occurs, resulting in haemolysis, and the systemic platelet clumping leads to thrombocytopenia. This condition and its management are discussed in more detail in Chapter 90.

DRUG-INDUCED THROMBOCYTOPENIA

The clinical presentation of drug-induced thrombocytopenia may be as variable as ITP. Some may have a dramatic and fulminant presentation with marked haemostatic failure. Drugs with a particular reputation for inducing thrombocytopenia include quinine (also in bitter drinks), quinidine, antituberculous drugs, heparin, sedormid, thiazide diuretics, penicillins, sulphonamides, rifampicin and anticonvulsants.

Heparin-induced thrombocytopenia and thrombosis syndrome (HITTS) is an important and potentially life-threatening complication of heparin therapy.[42–44] An immune reaction occurs to heparin after 7–10 days of therapy, at which time the patient's platelets aggregate and thrombocytopenia develops; this reactivity can be demonstrated by a variety of laboratory tests. In contrast to other causes of drug-induced thrombocytopenia, there may be arterial, microvascular or venous thrombosis associated with the platelet aggregation. The best way to avoid this potentially devastating complication is to keep heparin therapy as brief as possible, and be always alert to the diagnostic possibility. The incidence is less with the use of LMW heparins, and if cross-reactivity is not demonstrated in the heparin antibody test, LMW heparins or heparinoids may have a part to play in therapy.

Quinine-induced immune thrombocytopenia with haemolytic uraemic syndrome (HUS) can be a severe drug reaction, characterised by the onset of chills, sweating, nausea and vomiting, abdominal pain, oliguria and petechial rash following quinine or quinidine exposure. Quinine-dependent platelet-reactive antibodies can usually be identified. Plasma exchange in conjunction with renal dialysis has been found to be a beneficial adjunct to therapy.

SEPSIS

Platelets play an important role in the inflammatory response and a reactive thrombocytosis is usually seen in infection. However, if there is overwhelming sepsis, associated DIC or marrow suppressive influences, thrombocytopenia may be seen. The combination of sepsis, shock, DIC, alcoholism and nutritional deficiency are common factors contributing to thrombocytopenia in critically ill patients.

QUALITATIVE PLATELET DEFECTS

The effects of aspirin and other antiplatelet agents are discussed above. Haemostatic failure is a common manifestation of renal failure. Its mechanism is not fully elucidated, but the defect can be substantially corrected by dialysis. Prolongation of the bleeding time, defects in aggregation responses, diminished adhesion and reduced platelet factor 3 availability have all been demonstrated. A relationship between the degree of anaemia and prolongation of bleeding is usually demonstrable; increasing the haemoglobin level reduces the bleeding time. Patients with the myelodysplastic syndrome may not only have thrombocytopenia, but also a qualitative platelet function defect. They are thus at high risk of bleeding in relation to any surgery or invasive procedure. β-Lactam antibiotics may also be responsible for a platelet function defect.

REFERENCES

1. Hoffman M, Monroe DM. Coagulation 2006: a modern view of hemostasis. *Hematol Oncol Clin North Am* 2007; **21**: 1–11.
2. Roberts HR, Hoffman M, Monroe DM. A cell-based model of thrombin generation. *Semin Thromb Hemost* 2006; **32**(Suppl 1): 32–8.
3. Duggan JM. Review article: transfusion in gastrointestinal haemorrhage – if, when and how much? *Aliment Pharmacol Ther* 2001; **15**: 1109–13.
4. Bickell WH, Wall MJ Jr, Pepe PE *et al.* Immediate versus delayed fluid resuscitation for hypotensive patients with penetrating torso injuries. *N Engl J Med* 1994; **331**: 1105–9.
5. Verhamme P, Hoylaerts MF. The pivotal role of the endothelium in haemostasis and thrombosis. *Acta Clin Belg* 2006; **61**: 213–19.
6. Tanaka KA, Levy JH. Regulation of thrombin activity – pharmacologic and structural aspects. *Hematol Oncol Clin North Am* 2007; **21**: 33–50.
7. Dahlback B. Blood coagulation and its regulation by anticoagulant pathways: genetic pathogenesis of bleeding and thrombotic diseases. *J Intern Med* 2005; **257**: 209–23.
8. Macias WL, Yan SB, Williams MD *et al.* New insights into the protein C pathway: potential implications for the biological activities of drotrecogin alfa (activated). *Crit Care* 2005; **9**(Suppl 4): –S3–45.
9. Adams M, Ward C, Thom J *et al.* Emerging technologies in hemostasis diagnostics: a report from the Australasian Society of Thrombosis and Haemostasis Emerging Technologies Group. *Semin Thromb Hemost* 2007; **33**: 226–34.
10. Rochon AG, Shore-Lesserson L. Coagulation monitoring. *Anesthesiol Clin* 2006; **24**: 839–56.
11. Soliman DE, Broadman LM. Coagulation defects. *Anesthesiol Clin* 2006; **24**: 549–78, vii.
12. Hayward CP, Eikelboom J. Platelet function testing: quality assurance. *Semin Thromb Hemost* 2007; **33**: 273–82.
13. Cardigan R, Turner C, Harrison P. Current methods of assessing platelet function: relevance to transfusion medicine. *Vox Sang* 2005; **88**: 153–63.
14. Karger R, Donner-Banzhoff N, Muller HH *et al.* Diagnostic performance of the platelet function analyzer (PFA-100(R)) for the detection of disorders of primary haemostasis in patients with a bleeding history: a systematic review and meta-analysis. *Platelets* 2007; **18**: 249–60.
15. Traverso CI, Caprini JA, Arcelus JI. The normal thromboelastogram and its interpretation. *Semin Thromb Hemost* 1995; **21**(Suppl 4): 7–13.
16. Bolton-Maggs PH, Pasi KJ. Haemophilias A and B. *Lancet* 2003; **361**: 1801–9.
17. Bolton-Maggs PH, Stobart K, Smyth RL. Evidence-based treatment of haemophilia. *Haemophilia* 2004; **10**(Suppl 4): 20–4.
18. Mannucci PM. Treatment of von Willebrand's disease. *N Engl J Med* 2004; **351**: 683–94.
19. Laffan M, Brown SA, Collins P *et al.* The diagnosis of von Willebrand disease: a guideline from the UK Haemophilia Centre Doctors' Organization. *Haemophilia* 2004; **10**: 199–217.
20. Hayward CP, Rao AK, Cattaneo M. Congenital platelet disorders: overview of their mechanisms, diagnostic evaluation and treatment. *Haemophilia* 2006; **12** (Suppl 3): 128–36.
21. Hardy JF, de Moerloose P, Samama CM. Massive transfusion and coagulopathy: pathophysiology and implications for clinical management. *Can J Anaesth* 2006; **53**(6 Suppl): –S4–58.
22. Fries D, Innerhofer P, Reif C *et al.* The effect of fibrinogen substitution on reversal of dilutional coagulopathy: an in vitro model. *Anesth Analg* 2006; **102**: 347–51.
23. Ketchum L, Hess JR, Hiippala S. Indications for early fresh frozen plasma, cryoprecipitate, and platelet transfusion in trauma. *J Trauma* 2006; **60**(6 Suppl): –S–8.
24. Levy JH, Fingerhut A, Brott T *et al.* Recombinant factor VIIa in patients with coagulopathy secondary to anticoagulant therapy, cirrhosis, or severe traumatic injury: review of safety profile. *Transfusion* 2006; **46**: 919–33.
25. Kauvar DS, Holcomb JB, Norris GC *et al.* Fresh whole blood transfusion: a controversial military practice. *J Trauma* 2006; **61**: 181–4.
26. Repine TB, Perkins JG, Kauvar DS *et al.* The use of fresh whole blood in massive transfusion. *J Trauma* 2006; **606** Suppl: –S5–69.

27. Ramsey G. Treating coagulopathy in liver disease with plasma transfusions or recombinant factor VIIa: an evidence-based review. *Best Pract Res Clin Haematol* 2006; **19**: 113–26.
28. Toh CH, Hoots WK. The scoring system of the Scientific and Standardisation Committee on Disseminated Intravascular Coagulation of the International Society on Thrombosis and Haemostasis: a 5-year overview. *J Thromb Haemost* 2007; **5**: 604–6.
29. Levi M. Current understanding of disseminated intravascular coagulation. *Br J Haematol* 2004; **124**: 567–76.
30. Wiedermann CJ, Kaneider NC. A systematic review of antithrombin concentrate use in patients with disseminated intravascular coagulation of severe sepsis. *Blood Coagul Fibrinolysis* 2006; **17**: 521–6.
31. Levi M, de Jonge E, van der Poll T. Plasma and plasma components in the management of disseminated intravascular coagulation. *Best Pract Res Clin Haematol* 2006; **19**: 127–42.
32. Pengo V, Pegoraro C, Iliceto S. New trends in anticoagulant therapy. *Isr Med Assoc J* 2004; **6**: 479–81.
33. Kessler CM. Current and future challenges of antithrombotic agents and anticoagulants: strategies for reversal of hemorrhagic complications. *Semin Hematol* 2004; **41**(1 Suppl 1): 44–50.
34. Lankiewicz MW, Hays J, Friedman KD *et al.* Urgent reversal of warfarin with prothrombin complex concentrate. *J Thromb Haemost* 2006; **4**: 967–70.
35. Baker RI, Coughlin PB, Gallus AS *et al.* Warfarin reversal: consensus guidelines, on behalf of the Australasian Society of Thrombosis and Haemostasis. *Med J Aust* 2004; **181**: 492–7.
36. Schulman S, Bijsterveld NR. Anticoagulants and their reversal. *Transfus Med Rev* 2007; **21**: 37–48.
37. Ferraris VA, Ferraris SP, Saha SP *et al.* Perioperative blood transfusion and blood conservation in cardiac surgery: the Society of Thoracic Surgeons and The Society of Cardiovascular Anesthesiologists clinical practice guideline. *Ann Thorac Surg* 2007; **83** (5 Suppl): –S2–86.
38. Von Heymann C, Schoenfeld H, Sander M *et al.* New antithrombotics – pharmacologic profile and implications for anesthesia and surgery. *Trans Altern Trans Med* 2006; **8**: 164–74.
39. Vincentelli A, Jude B, Belisle S. Antithrombotic therapy in cardiac surgery. *Can J Anaesth* 2006; **53** (6 Suppl): –S89–102.
40. Walsham J, Fraser JF, Mullany D *et al.* The use of recombinant activated factor VII for refractory bleeding post complex cardiothoracic surgery. *Anaesth Intensive Care* 2006; **34**: 13–20.
41. Cines DB, McMillan R. Management of adult idiopathic thrombocytopenic purpura. *Annu Rev Med* 2005; **56**: 425–42.
42. Cines DB, Rauova L, Arepally G *et al.* Heparin-induced thrombocytopenia: an autoimmune disorder regulated through dynamic autoantigen assembly/disassembly. *J Clin Apher* 2007; **22**: 31–6.
43. Levy JH, Hursting MJ. Heparin-induced thrombocytopenia, a prothrombotic disease. *Hematol Oncol Clin North Am* 2007; **21**: 65–88.
44. Selleng K, Warkentin TE, Greinacher A. Heparin-induced thrombocytopenia in intensive care patients. *Crit Care Med* 2007; **35**: 1165–76.

92

Haematological malignancies

James P Isbister

The treatment of haematological malignancy has been an evolving success story. In recent years, the prognosis for patients with acute leukaemia has changed from death within 1–3 months without effective therapy to long-term survival and cure in many cases.[1,2] In some diseases the potential for regular cure of patients has been realised, including Hodgkin's disease, childhood acute lymphoblastic leukaemia, some high-grade lymphomas and some adult leukaemias.[3] These advances have predominantly resulted from the introduction of a wide range of cytotoxic chemotherapeutic regimens which permit obliteration of the disease in conjunction with comprehensive supportive therapy. In some cases, 'supralethal' therapy is necessary, with bone marrow transplantation (autologous or allogeneic) being used as marrow 'rescue' therapy. The development of 'engineered' highly specific and targeted drugs is offering further promise (e.g. monoclonal antibodies, tyrosine kinase inhibitors for chronic myeloid leukaemia).[1]

It is important that clinicians not regularly involved in the care of these patients do not take a nihilistic approach to management of patients with haematological malignancy. If patients can be adequately supported and complications treated during the severe neutropenic stage of chemotherapy, clinical improvement may occur rapidly following marrow recovery. However, in patients requiring prolonged ventilatory support and/or dialysis, the prognosis is poor and intensive supportive therapy can usually only be justified if marrow recovery is imminent and there is a reasonable anticipated life expectancy if the crisis can be survived.

CLASSIFICATION AND PATHOPHYSIOLOGY

The heterogeneous nature of the haemopoietic and lymphoid cells, their individual kinetic characteristics and the disseminated nature of haemopoietic and lymphoid tissue explains the complexity of haematological malignancy. The numerous confusing classification systems advocated to 'clarify' understanding have in many cases increased the confusion for the non-expert. In broad terms, the haematological malignancies with origins in the marrow are classified as leukaemia or multiple myeloma, and those arising in the peripheral lymphoid tissues as Hodgkin's and non-Hodgkin's lymphomas (nodal and extranodal).

The leukaemias are divided into acute and chronic, generally according to the time span of their clinical course. In general, a leukaemia that is blastic in appearance behaves in an acute and malignant manner with a rapidly fatal outcome without therapy. This is in contrast to the chronic leukaemias in which the cells are more differentiated ('benign'), with the disease following a more indolent course. Leukaemias are classified on the basis of their cell of origin with broad division into those of myeloid origin (i.e. of haemopoietic marrow origin) and those of lymphoid origin (i.e. arising from the cells of the immune system).

Most patients with acute myeloid leukaemia present with features of bone marrow failure. Acute promyelocytic leukaemia is a unique subtype of acute myeloid leukaemia which may typically present with disseminated intravascular coagulation (DIC) requiring expert haematological management.[4] Acute lymphoblastic leukaemia is the commonest encountered in children. The lymphomas are a complex and heterogeneous group of malignancies ranging from highly malignant disorders through to low-grade indolent disease not requiring therapy.

The myelodysplastic syndromes are a group of disorders in which the main feature is bone marrow dysplasia. They are a heterogeneous group of potentially malignant haematological disorders which may be the harbingers of more classic leukaemic states or may behave as slowly evolving marrow failure syndromes. They usually occur in the elderly, have an insidious onset and may have a variety of clinical manifestations.

Dysplasia may affect any of the haemopoietic elements, with the patient presenting with a range of peripheral blood abnormalities, most commonly including anaemia, thrombocytopenia and neutropenia. Diagnosis, classification, understanding of pathophysiology and therapy have undergone enormous changes in recent years and the non-specialist can be excused for feeling confused.[5,6] There is a rising prevalence and incidence of the myelodysplastic syndromes. Epidemiological data indicate that they are more common than initially thought and probably on the increase, especially due to the ageing population and their occurrence as a late complication of cytotoxic chemotherapy.

Awareness of these relatively common disorders is important as undiagnosed patients with relatively normal blood counts may present de novo with life-threatening infection or haemorrhage in a postoperative or trauma setting.

COMPLICATIONS OF HAEMATOLOGICAL MALIGNANCY AND ITS THERAPY

METABOLIC DISTURBANCES

At presentation, haematological malignancy may be associated with a range of metabolic derangements.[7] Hyperuricaemia and hypercalcaemia are well-recognised complications which may be associated with renal failure.[8] The tumour lysis syndrome is a rarer complication which may occur spontaneously or shortly after the initiation of therapy.[9,10] There is sudden liberation of intracellular contents in quantities that overwhelm the excretory capacity of the kidneys, resulting in hyperkalaemia, hyperphosphataemia, hypocalcaemia and occasionally lactic acidosis. Pre-empting the development of this syndrome usually allows control of the metabolic effects, especially with the maintenance of high intravenous fluid intake, alkalinising the urine and administration of allopurinol. More recently, intravenous rasburicase – a recombinant uricolytic agent which, in contrast to allopurinol, acts on existing uric acid concentrations – is being used for the management of anticancer therapy-induced hyperuricaemia.[11] Rasburicase is contraindicated in patients with methaemoglobinaemia and glucose-6-phosphate dehydrogenase deficiency.

Multiple myeloma may be complicated by renal insufficiency, hypercalcaemia, hyperviscosity and hyperuricaemia. Most of these can be managed conventionally; however, with large amounts of monoclonal protein, fluid management can be difficult due to the hypervolaemia with or without hyperviscosity and plasma exchange may be indicated (see Chapter 90).

COAGULOPATHIES

A range of haemostatic disturbances may occur in association with haematological malignancy and its therapy. Most of these are considered in general terms in Chapter 91 which outlines the general principles of diagnosis and management.

ACUTE RESPIRATORY DISTRESS SYNDROME

Acute (or adult) respiratory distress syndrome (ARDS) remains a potentially lethal complication of autoaggressive inflammation. As most of the mediators (cytokines, neutrophils and endothelial adherence molecules) initiating the disease process are haemopoietic in origin it is not surprising that ARDS may occur in haemopoietic malignancies. However, ARDS is relatively uncommon in the neutropenic septic patient, probably due to the fact that the neutrophil under normal circumstances is one of the central mediators of this syndrome. ARDS and interstitial pneumonitis may be a problem due to hyperleukocytosis, transfusion-related acute lung injury (TRALI; see Chapter 88), cytomegalovirus (CMV) infection, DIC, post marrow transplantation, and sometimes in relation to chemotherapy and radiotherapy. The use of all-trans retinoic acid (ATRA) may be associated with the development of a potentially lethal ARDS/pulmonary leukostasis syndrome (retinoic acid syndrome), usually in association with a rising leukocyte count.[12] In all the settings mentioned, early recognition of the symptom complex of fever and dyspnoea (with or without pulmonary infiltrates) is important and therapy with high-dose corticosteroids decreases morbidity and mortality.

SIDE-EFFECTS OF CHEMOTHERAPY

The wide range of cytotoxic chemotherapeutic agents used in the management of haematological malignancy may be responsible for a plethora of toxicities other than bone marrow suppression. The haematologists will be aware of these and should communicate necessary information to the intensive care unit (ICU) staff.

BONE MARROW FAILURE

Most of the acute leukaemias present with clinical and laboratory features of marrow failure with anaemia, bleeding or infection. If not a problem at presentation, marrow failure is almost universal during remission induction and subsequent chemotherapy.

Neutropenia

Neutropenia should be considered in the following terms:

- Absolute neutrophil count, the rate of fall, the nadir and duration.
- Duration of the neutropenia is a critical factor determining the management and outcome. Patients with profound prolonged neutropenia of $< 0.1 \times 10^9$/l granulocytes for > 10 days require special attention and they may require different initial therapy.

For practical purposes neutropenia has been divided into the following groups:

- Neutropenia $< 0.5 \times 10^9$/l
- Neutropenia between 0.5 and 1.0×10^9/l and potentially falling
- Neutropenia 0.5–1.0×10^9/l and stable or rising
- Profound prolonged neutropenia

Figure 92.1 illustrates the numerous interacting factors to be considered when managing patients with neutropenia in association with haematological malignancy and its therapy. Table 92.1 lists the organisms which may be associated with various defects in the host defence system.

PRINCIPLES OF MANAGEMENT OF HAEMATOLOGICAL MALIGNANCIES

ICU ADMISSION

Patients with haematological malignancy may be critically ill from their disease or therapy, for brief or long

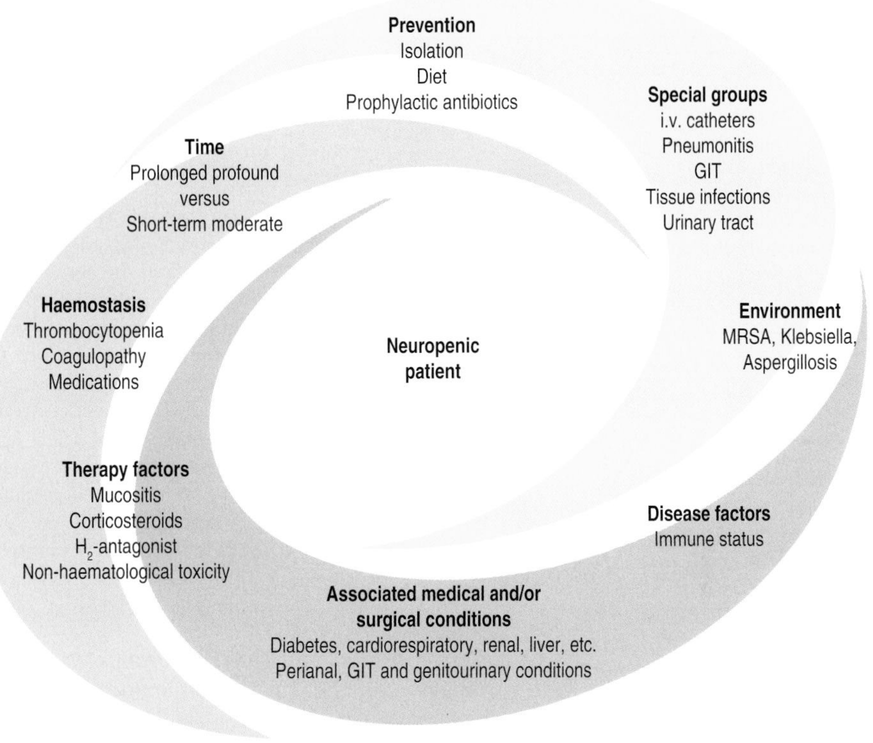

Figure 92.1 The neutropenic patient. GIT, gastrointestinal tract; MRSA, meticillin-resistant *Staphylococcus aureus*.

periods. At times during therapy they may require intensive supportive therapy and can develop a range of life-threatening complications. Rarely, it is necessary to admit critically ill patients with haematological disorders to the ICU. Under normal circumstances, admission of such patients is to be avoided as they have severely impaired host defences and poor tolerance for invasive procedures. However, mechanical ventilation may be required for severe respiratory infections or pneumonitis. Such patients may present specific problems for the ICU staff. Most patients have severe marrow failure requiring intensive transfusion support. Severe neutropenia is the main, and most life-threatening, defect in the host defence system. Nutrition can be a challenge in these patients due to a multitude of factors. The anorexia, nausea and vomiting with chemotherapy, oral mucositis, hypermetabolism, malabsorption and diarrhoea are only some of the factors mitigating against maintaining an adequate nutritional state, and parenteral nutrition may be needed if the period of therapy is prolonged.

There must be good communication between the ICU staff and clear policies on admission and treatment. If the patient's ultimate prognosis is poor, extraordinary invasive measures cannot be justified. A palliative approach will be instituted if the patient does not respond to treatment within a specific period of time. However, if the haematological malignancy has a high likelihood of cure or long-term good-quality survival, more strenuous and extended intensive care support can be justified.

INFECTION PREVENTION

Prevention of infection is extremely important and meticulous attention to sterility with invasive procedures (e.g. i.v. line insertions) is essential. Infection may be endogenously or exogenously acquired. Most patients when they are admitted to hospital become colonised with the hospital flora. The major sources of infecting organisms, however, are the patients themselves (e.g. from the oropharynx, the gastrointestinal tract, i.v. line sites, lung and local lesions).

All ICUs must demand strict adherence to infection control guidelines. The most effective procedure is hand-washing by all health care workers involved in the care of the immunocompromised patient.

Other preventive measures include sterile techniques for invasive procedures by experienced staff, maintaining a clean environment, cooked patient meals, and limited use of prophylactic antibiotics. Needless to say, excessive use of antibiotics is a major factor in the emergence of resistant strains and the susceptibility to colonisation with hospital-acquired organisms. Many would argue that the efficacy of empirical therapy in the neutropenic patient

Table 92.1 Organisms associated with immune deficiency states

Neutropenia	
Bacteria	
	Gram-negative bacilli
	Escherichia coli
	Pseudomonas aeruginosa
	Klebsiella pneumoniae
	Acinetobacter
	Gram-positive cocci
	Staphylococcus epidermidis
	Staphylococcus aureus
	Streptococci viridans group
Fungal	
	Candida
	Aspergillus
	Mucormycosis
Cellular immune dysfunction	
Bacteria	
	Listeria monocytogenes
	Salmonella
	Mycobacterium
	Nocardia asteroides
	Legionella
Fungi	
	Cryptococcus neoformans
	Histoplasma capsulatum
	Coccidioides immitis
Viruses	
	Varicella zoster
	Cytomegalovirus
	Herpes simplex
Protozoa	
	Pneumocystis jiroveci
	Toxoplasma gondii
	Cryptosporidium
Humoral immune dysfunction	
Bacteria	
	Streptococcus pneumoniae
	Haemophilus influenzae

is such that prophylaxis may be unnecessary. Reverse barrier nursing is instituted in order to minimise exposure to exogenous infection. This can be difficult in a critical care setting and will not prevent infections of endogenous origin.

INVASIVE PROCEDURES

Invasive procedures should be kept to a minimum and, when performed, appropriate steps should be taken to minimise bleeding and the risk of infection. Endotracheal intubation should be avoided or minimised if at all possible. Biopsy procedures, arterial access, and other invasive procedures should be well planned and discussed with the haematologists.

BLOOD COMPONENT THERAPY

During the period of marrow suppression red cell concentrates may need to be administered to maintain oxygen-carrying capacity at a satisfactory level. There is much debate as to the appropriate trigger for red cell transfusion. The decision is essentially a clinical one that takes into account the numerous comorbidities that may occur in these patients, such as cardiorespiratory compromise, thrombocytopenia and physical activity. In general, a fixed haemoglobin level trigger is no longer appropriate. In some patients a higher oxygen delivery may be necessary (i.e. acute respiratory failure) and a higher haemoglobin level may be required (> 120 g/l). Maintenance of a higher haemoglobin may avoid the requirement for intubation and assisted ventilation.

Regular platelet concentrates are required. In the presence of sepsis platelets are consumed rapidly and transfusions may be necessary on a daily basis, otherwise every second day is usually adequate. The patient should be examined daily for evidence of haemostatic failure (e.g. purpura, ecchymoses, mouth, fundoscopy). Granulocyte transfusion may have a role in patients with proven unresponsive bacterial sepsis.[13]

ANTIMICROBIAL THERAPY

The febrile neutropenic patient

After resistance of the malignant cell to therapy, infection is the commonest cause of death in patients with haematological malignancy. Patients usually tolerate neutropenia without developing infection until the count is $< 1.0 \times 10^9$/l and it is not until the neutrophil count falls to $< 0.2 \times 10^9$/l that spontaneous overwhelming sepsis becomes a major potentially life-threatening problem. These patients must be watched closely for infection and treated early if necessary. When the neutrophil count is $< 0.5 \times 10^9$/l any temperature above 38°C should be regarded as representing serious sepsis until proven otherwise. High-risk patients include those with pneumonitis, severe mucositis, an infected i.v. catheter and evidence of local sepsis. In patients with haematological malignancy and in allogeneic marrow transplant patients there may be pre-existing immunodeficiency.

The role of prophylactic antibiotic therapy has been controversial due to concerns related to the development of antibiotic resistant micro-organisms, but there is evidence to support their use.[14,15] Early empirical antibiotic therapy, without microbiological proof of cause, may be life-saving.[16] With most patients fever resolves, especially if marrow function returns in the short term. Ultimate proof of infection is frequently not established. Patients with agranulocytosis will not show the typical features of inflammation. For example, lung consolidation may not occur, cellulitis or sputum may not be clinically obvious, and urinary tract symptoms may be minimal. The role of steroids in suppressing temperature and clinical features of inflammation must also be considered. Non-infectious fever should be borne in mind (e.g. malignancy or drugs).

The presence of rigors, hypotension and shock may point more towards Gram-negative sepsis. The value of combination therapy with a β-lactam antibiotic in combination with an aminoglycoside has been demonstrated in patients with prolonged and severe neutropenia with Gram-negative septicaemia. Gram-negative sepsis is potentially rapidly fatal in the neutropenic patient, but is less common than in the past as the less virulent Gram-positive organisms now predominate. This may be related to several factors including the increased use of permanent indwelling intravenous devices, mucositis, H_2 antagonists and the use of quinolones as antibiotic prophylaxis. However, both streptococcal and staphylococcal sepsis can be severe and empiric use of vancomycin in high-risk patients is justified. *Staphylococcus epidermidis* is an indolent form of sepsis and time is usually available for adjustment of therapy, with most patients recovering.

The choice of empirical antibiotic therapy

Empirical antibiotic therapy should be aggressive with cover against Gram-negative sepsis as this is potentially lethal for the neutropenic patient.[17] Anaerobic cover may need to be included when there is any problem with the gastrointestinal tract (e.g. intra-abdominal or perianal problems). This is not usually necessary when problems are confined to the mouth.

The nature and site of infection is determined by a range of factors including:

- the host defence defect
- time course of neutropenia
- local microbiological ecology
- antibiotic usage (e.g. prophylaxis)
- haemostasis
- presence of indwelling lines (i.v., endotracheal, urinary)
- type of chemotherapy
- nature of disease
- patient factors (e.g. hepatic, renal, respiratory or other factors)

Antibiotic regimens

Empirical antimicrobial regimens for neutropenic patients remain a constant changing and controversial issue.[17,18] Initial empirical antibiotic therapy should cover *Pseudomonas aeruginosa, Escherichia coli, Klebsiella* species, *Streptococcus viridans, Staphylococci* (coagulase negative and coagulase positive) depending on clinical circumstances. Other organisms should be covered after the results of cultures have been assessed or it is known that a specific organism is present in the ward (e.g. *Streptococcus viridans*) or on surveillance cultures. Coverage against *Staphylococcus epidermidis* is not necessary until bacteraemia is demonstrated.

Single-drug therapy Single-agent therapy with a third-generation cephalosporin (e.g. cefotaxime, ceftriaxone, ceftazidime, cefepime) may be adequate therapy in low-risk patients, i.e. neutrophil count $> 0.5 \times 10^9$/l and expected to stay above 0.5×10^9/l or neutropenia expected to last less than 7 days. The carbapenems (e.g. imipenem and meropenem) are alternative choices to third-generation cephalosporins, having good *Pseudomonas* cover, and can also be used as monotherapy in low-risk individuals.

Two-drug therapy Two-drug therapy with an added aminoglycoside (gentamicin, tobramycin, amikacin, netilmicin) is recommended as standard initial empirical regimen in patients with prolonged and profound neutropenia and no additional risk factors.

Three-drug therapy Three-drug therapy with a glycopeptide (vancomycin, teicoplanin) added to the aminoglycoside and cephalosporin is indicated for patients who are particularly likely to be infected with coagulase-negative staphylococci, meticillin-resistant *Staphylococcus aureus, Corynebacterium* species and penicillin-resistant *Streptococcus viridans* (e.g. infected indwelling central venous catheter, pneumonitis, rash and severe mucositis).

Daily clinical assessment and review of microbiological results is essential. Antibiotic therapy is modified according to microbiological results. If no helpful microbiological information is forthcoming in the case of single- or two-drug therapy, the antibiotic regimen should be re-evaluated at 48 hours and if there has been no response, a glycopeptide added. If the fever has resolved and the cultures are negative, the aminoglycoside may be ceased.

Multiresistant Gram-negative organisms occasionally cause problems (e.g. some species of *Acinetobacter*) and need treatment with amikacin. Vancomycin-resistant *Enterococcus* is also occasionally seen although it may only be a 'commensal' rather than actual cause of infection. Therapy with a new antibiotic of the oxazolidinone class, such as linezolid, may be necessary.

With patients on three-drug therapy, antibiotic reassessment at 72 hours is appropriate. If there is no response, further investigation such as a CT chest and bronchoalveolar lavage may be indicated. Depending on the clinical state of the patient the introduction of antifungal therapy should be considered. Fungal infections are an increasing problem in patients with profound prolonged neutropenia.[19] There is an increasing range of antifungals available, including voriconazole and the echinocandins (caspofungin, micafungin). Standard amphotericin is now rarely used. Prophylaxis with new azoles such as posaconazole may reduce the incidence of *Aspergillus* as fluconazole has with *Candida* infection. The use of potent anti-*Aspergillus* agents seems to be resulting in the emergence of breakthrough fungal infections with *Mucormycosis, Scedosporium* and *Fusarium*. These are uncommon fungal infections which were only rarely seen previously.

Haemopoietic growth factors, immunotherapy and granulocyte transfusions

Genetically engineered haemopoietic growth factors are now widely used to minimise the degree and time of neutropenia. Granulocyte and granulocyte-macrophage colony-stimulating factors are glycoproteins which stimulate the proliferation and maturation of bone marrow progenitor cells, and increase the number and function of these committed cell populations. Treatment reduces the duration and severity of neutropenia in patients receiving chemotherapy and after haemopoietic stem cell transplantation.[20] Growth factors do not prevent neutropenia, but do shorten its duration, and their use has been associated with fewer infectious febrile episodes. Intravenous immunoglobulin should be infused in patients with hypogammaglobulinaemia. Granulocyte transfusion may have a role if bacterial-proven sepsis is not resolving or there is evidence of spreading local bacterial infection.

Patient subgroups

Indwelling intravenous catheters Indwelling intravenous silastic catheters provide a nidus for both infectious and non-infectious complications. The incidence of catheter-associated infections varies. Indwelling i.v. catheters present an increased risk of infection for both neutropenic and non-neutropenic patients. Coagulase-negative staphylococci are the most common cause of catheter-associated bacteraemia, but *Staphylococcus aureus, Bacillus* species, *Corynebacteria* and Gram-negative organisms (especially species of *Acinetobacter* and *Pseudomonas*) can also cause catheter infections and *Candida* infection can be catheter related. Exit-site infections and infections along the subcutaneous tunnel of the catheter can be caused by aerobic bacteria, *Mycobacteria* and fungi.

If bacteraemia is thought to be catheter related, it may be possible to avoid removal of the catheter, particularly if the infection is caused by coagulase-negative staphylococci. Even patients with Gram-negative infections can often be successfully treated with antibiotics infused through the catheter. In patients with multiple-lumen catheters, the administration of antibiotics should be rotated through all the lumens, as infection may be restricted to only one. However, removal of the catheter is usually necessary for bacteria (e.g. species of bacillus) that may not be eradicated even though sensitive to antibiotics and with candidaemia in which there is a high incidence of dissemination. Patients with tunnel infections usually require catheter removal.

Lung infiltrates Lung infiltrates in febrile patients with neutropenia represent a high risk of treatment failure. Prolonged neutropenia has a significantly adverse effect on the outcome of infection. Incorporation of systemic antifungal agents into first-line therapy, particularly in selected high-risk subgroups, may improve the outcome. Involvement of a respiratory physician with experience in managing immunocompromised patients is important. Pulmonary investigations such as fine-cut chest CT, bronchoscopy, bronchoalveolar lavage ± transbronchial biopsy may be required. Pulmonary haemorrhage can be a sudden and life-threatening cause of pulmonary infiltration and respiratory insufficiency. This usually occurs in severe thrombocytopenia associated with infection, and in patients who have become resistant to platelet transfusions.

HAEMOPOIETIC STEM CELL TRANSPLANTATION

Haemopoietic stem cell transplantation therapy is increasingly establishing a role in the treatment of a wide range of malignant and non-malignant disorders.[21] Allogeneic haemopoietic stem cell transplantation has been used as an adjunct to the treatment of acute leukaemia with an impressive success rate, which is translating into long-term survival and cure. This success is now being extended to the management of a wider range of haematological malignancies and some solid tumours. Haemopoietic stem cells can be obtained from either marrow aspiration or from the peripheral blood by apheresis using a blood cell separator following stimulation of the marrow with haemopoietic growth factors ± cytotoxic chemotherapy. Allogeneic transplantation brings with it a range of potentially serious and potentially fatal complications related to graft-versus-host disease (GVHD).[22] It does, however, have the advantage of using normal stem cells which need not be stored and a limited degree of GVHD may have a beneficial anti-tumour effect. Autologous stem cell transplantation is of particular advantage when relatively normal bone marrow can be obtained, in which case GVHD is not a problem.

The principles for the use of bone marrow transplantation in the management of malignancy include the following:

- The tumour must be responsive to chemotherapy and/or radiotherapy.
- The dose limitation of the chemotherapeutic agents used relate to marrow toxicity and not other end-organs.
- There should be a source of uncontaminated, or minimally contaminated, haemopoietic stem cells.
- Appropriate haemopoietic supportive therapy must be available during the marrow aplastic period.
- High-quality clinical and laboratory facilities must be available for the collection and preservation of haemopoietic stem cells.
- An integrated team of medical and nursing and scientific staff is essential.
- The preparation of a well-documented clinical protocol and effective implementation, with appropriate monitoring, is essential for success. The general management of the patient during the procedure is similar to the management of other patients receiving high-dose chemotherapy who will have prolonged neutropenic periods.

COMPLICATIONS OF HAEMOPOIETIC CELL TRANSPLANTATION

Respiratory failure in haemopoietic cell transplant patients

Respiratory failure is the commonest cause of death in patients undergoing bone marrow transplantation. Both CMV-induced interstitial pneumonia and the idiopathic pneumonia syndrome rarely occur in the early cytopenic phase post transplantation. Haematological reconstitution with donor-type cells seems to be a prerequisite to the development of these pulmonary complications, suggesting a key role of immunological reactions. While CMV pneumonia can be effectively treated or prevented by ganciclovir, the idiopathic syndrome is usually fatal. Due to improved prophylaxis and therapy, lethal interstitial pneumonia due to *Pneumocystis jiroveci* (formerly *P. carinii*), *herpes simplex, varicella zoster* or *Toxoplasma gondii*, as well as lethal pneumonia caused by bacteria or *Candida* species, is generally less common. However, *Aspergillus* species have emerged as frequent causative pathogens. Prolonged granulocytopenia and prolonged medication with corticosteroids are major risk factors for pulmonary aspergillosis, which is commonly fatal, but prophylaxis may be achieved by sterile air supply during the hospital stay and by prophylactic inhalation of amphotericin B. Pulmonary haemorrhage, diagnosed by bronchoalveolar lavage, may develop due to the toxicity of the conditioning regimen, or may be secondary to infectious pneumonia of various kinds. Congestive heart failure might give rise to the development of pulmonary oedema. Patients with hepatic veno-occlusive disease have a high risk of subsequent pulmonary complications.

Graft-versus-host disease (GVHD)

GVHD is a major complication of allogeneic haemopoietic stem cell transplantation, especially with the increasing use of unrelated and mismatched donors.[22] The target of the immune response in GVHD has long been regarded to be histocompatibility antigens possessed by the host, but not the donor. However, it is now recognised that self-antigens have been documented in GVHD, confirming that it is more complex than simple alloreactivity. Cytokines play a central role in mediating many of the manifestations of GVHD.

Nearly all patients with GVHD have a rash. Other features include liver and gastrointestinal dysfunction. Initial therapy for low-grade disease is systemic corticosteroids. Treatment for more severe disease may include a range of therapies, including ciclosporin, antithymocyte globulin, tacrolimus, methotrexate, PUVA and thalidomide.

Veno-occlusive disease of the liver

Veno-occlusive disease can be a major complication of haemopoietic stem cell transplantation, predominantly seen in allogeneic transplants, and is a major contributor to mortality.[23] The disorder is due to thrombotic occlusion in the small hepatic vessels, probably as a result of endothelial damage associated with high-dose chemotherapy. The problem manifests as weight gain, oedema, ascites, tender hepatomegaly, jaundice and may proceed to liver failure. Prophylaxis with low-dose heparin or prostaglandins may be useful. Treatment is predominantly supportive with fluid management a critical aspect. Treatment with tissue plasminogen activator and antithrombin III concentrates has been successful.

REFERENCES

1. Smith M, Barnett M, Bassan R *et al.* Adult acute myeloid leukaemia. *Crit Rev Oncol Hematol* 2004; **50**: 197–222.
2. Bassan R, Gatta G, Tondini C *et al.* Adult acute lymphoblastic leukaemia. *Crit Rev Oncol Hematol* 2004; **50**: 223–61.
3. Kuppers R, Yahalom J, Josting A. Advances in biology, diagnostics, and treatment of Hodgkin's disease. *Biol Blood Marrow Transplant* 2006; **12**(1 Suppl 1): 66–76.
4. Arbuthnot C, Wilde JT. Haemostatic problems in acute promyelocytic leukaemia. *Blood Rev* 2006; **20**: 289–297.
5. Vardiman JW. Hematopathological concepts and controversies in the diagnosis and classification of myelodysplastic syndromes. Hematology/the Education Program of the American Society of Hematology. Washington, DC: American Society of Hematology; 2006: 199–204.
6. Schiffer CA. Clinical issues in the management of patients with myelodysplasia. Hematology/the Education Program of the American Society of Hematology. Washington, DC: American Society of Hematology; 2006: 205–10.
7. Filippatos TD, Milionis HJ, Elisaf MS. Alterations in electrolyte equilibrium in patients with acute leukemia. *Eur J Haematol* 2005; **75**: 449–60.
8. Jibrin IM, Lawrence GD, Miller CB. Hypercalcemia of malignancy in hospitalized patients. *Hosp Physician* 2006; **42**: 29–35. http://www.turner-white.com/memberfile.php?PubCode=hp_nov06_malig.pdf.
9. Rampello E, Fricia T, Malaguarnera M. The management of tumor lysis syndrome. *Nature Clin Pract* 2006; **3**: 438–47.
10. Cairo MS, Bishop M. Tumour lysis syndrome: new therapeutic strategies and classification. *Br J Haematol* 2004; **127**: 3–11.
11. Oldfield V, Perry CM. Spotlight on rasburicase in anticancer therapy-induced hyperuricemia. *BioDrugs* 2006; **20**: 197–9.
12. Tallman MS, Andersen JW, Schiffer CA *et al.* Clinical description of 44 patients with acute promyelocytic leukemia who developed the retinoic acid syndrome. *Blood* 2000; **95**: 90–5.
13. Price TH. Granulocyte transfusion: current status. *Semin Hematol* 2007; **44**: 15–23.
14. Craig M, Cumpston AD, Hobbs GR *et al.* The clinical impact of antibacterial prophylaxis and cycling antibiotics for febrile neutropenia in a hematological malignancy and transplantation unit. *Bone Marrow Transplant* 2007; **39**: 477–82.
15. Hart S. Review: antibiotic prophylaxis reduces mortality in patients with neutropenia. *Evid Based Nurs* 2006; **9**: 50.
16. Rolston KV. Management of infections in the neutropenic patient. *Ann Rev Med* 2004; **55**: 519–26.
17. Bal AM, Gould IM. Empirical antimicrobial treatment for chemotherapy-induced febrile neutropenia. *Int J Antimicrob Agents* 2007; **29**: 501–9.

18. Paul M, Yahav D, Fraser A *et al.* Empirical antibiotic monotherapy for febrile neutropenia: systematic review and meta-analysis of randomized controlled trials. *J Antimicrob Chemother* 2006; **57**: 176–89.
19. Bow EJ. Of yeasts and hyphae: a hematologist's approach to antifungal therapy. Hematology/the Education Program of the American Society of Hematology. Washington, DC: American Society of Hematology; 2006: 361–7.
20. Crawford J. Update on neutropenia and myeloid growth factors. *J Support Oncol* 2007; **5**(4 Suppl 2): 27–46.
21. Ljungman P, Urbano-Ispizua A, Cavazzana-Calvo M *et al.* Allogeneic and autologous transplantation for haematological diseases, solid tumours and immune disorders: definitions and current practice in Europe. *Bone Marrow Transplant* 2006; **37**: 439–49.
22. Bacigalupo A. Management of acute graft-versus-host disease. *Br J Haematol* 2007; **137**: 87–98.
23. MacQuillan GC, Mutimer D. Fulminant liver failure due to severe veno-occlusive disease after haematopoietic cell transplantation: a depressing experience. *QJM* 2004; **97**: 581–9.

Part Sixteen

Transplants

93

Organ donation

Stephen J Streat

Intensivists often have responsibility for the care of organ transplant recipients and have seen the benefits they obtain from transplantation. Clinical results continue to improve, despite increasing recipient case complexity and increasing use of organs from extended-criteria deceased donors, and this success continues to drive demand for transplantation.[1] At the same time, deaths from road trauma (once the most common cause of death in deceased-donor organ donation) continue to fall in many countries as a result of both primary prevention and better treatment of traumatic brain injury. Decompressive craniectomy in particular is effective in controlling refractory intracranial hypertension[2] (and thereby reducing brain death), although whether outcomes are improved overall await the results of two ongoing clinical trials. Similarly, population-based studies have shown falls in the incidence and mortality of subarachnoid haemorrhage[3] and perhaps also intracerebral haemorrhage. Treatments for some other conditions which uncommonly contribute to deceased-donor donation (e.g. hypoxic–ischaemic encephalopathy, meningitis) have also improved.

With the exception of the USA, many countries are now experiencing a fall in brain dead organ donation. Transplant numbers have been maintained, or only modestly increased, by other strategies, including donation after cardiac death (DCD, formerly called non-heart beating donation), live donors (including altruistic donors) and the use of split livers for two recipients. There is considerable pressure on intensivists and others to provide a solution to the 'organ donor shortage', but less consideration given to restricting access to waiting lists. Despite widespread condemnation of the practice, desperate recipients from wealthy countries take part in 'transplant tourism'[4,5] in Asia (particularly in China, including organs from executed prisoners), Africa and South America. The internet has facilitated a form of altruistic but directed live donation which also is potentially vulnerable to commercial exploitation (e.g. http://www.matchingdonors.com). Slow progress continues in alternative approaches to end-stage organ failure, including artificial organs, xenotransplantation and the engineering of organs and tissues from stem cells, but none is yet available for routine clinical use.

RESPONSIBILITIES OF THE INTENSIVIST

Most intensivists are supportive of deceased-donor organ donation.[6] Those who are not should make arrangements with other intensivist colleagues for the care of potential organ donors and discussions with their families.[7] Intensivists' responsibilities include the care of dying patients and of their families in the intensive care unit – the location of organ donation itself. Intensivists therefore must either define and take responsibility for good practice in organ donation, or accept that these processes will be taken over by others with the objective of 'transforming the greatest possible number of cadavers into real donors'.[8] This personal epiphany[9,10] is not yet widely shared in intensive care medicine.

Intensivists must ensure that the processes involved in deceased-donor organ donation, now including DCD, continue to be publicly seen to be of the highest standard. These processes include the care of the dying patient and their family, determination of death, identification of the potential for organ donation to occur, offering the opportunity for organ donation to the family, maintenance of physiological stability after brain death throughout the time until organ retrieval, withdrawal of treatment and determination of death in DCD, and aftercare for the family of the deceased, irrespective of whether organ donation took place

CARE OF THE DYING PATIENT AND THEIR FAMILY

Intensivists are familiar with the care of the dying patient, including the need to avoid suffering and maintain patient dignity. The respect of the intensive care unit (ICU) staff for the humanity of the dying person is expressed in the 'patient comfort care' provided by the nursing staff, the continued involvement and attentiveness of the medical staff, and in evident compassion of all staff for the family.[11]

On behalf of all the treating team, an intensivist should establish rapport during an early meeting (e.g. the morning after admission) with the family of every intensive care patient. This is particularly important for families of patients at high risk of death or disability with whom there will often need to be several 'bad news' meetings over several days. Family meetings should be attended by whomsoever the family defines itself to include, by the intensivist, and by a member of the nursing staff supporting the family (preferably the 'bedside nurse' looking after the patient). If the family wishes, the meeting might include a chaplain, social worker or cultural health worker. The 'support' role should be kept separate from the 'bearer of bad news' role. Family meetings should be held in a separate private room large enough to accommodate all the participants, away from the bedside and protected from interruption. With evident compassion[11] the intensivist should convey an accurate account of the sequence of events, a realistic prognosis (in as much as this is possible) and the immediate treatment plan. Some families find CT or other visual information helpful. There must be enough time to answer any questions that the family may have. At the end of the meeting the intensivist should ascertain that the family understands what has been said[11] and agrees with the immediate plan. Ensuring that all team members give the family congruent messages is an essential part of maintaining the trust of the family in the ICU team. Ideally, one intensivist should speak with the family but where this is impractical it is vital that there be detailed and explicit discussions between one intensivist and another before the next family meeting. A relationship of mutual understanding and trust will enable the ICU team and the family to work together through difficult and painful issues, including withdrawal of intensive therapies,[12] death of the patient and consideration of organ donation.

Many patients who develop apparent loss of brainstem function do so despite continuance of all available surgical and medical therapy. In these circumstances, brain-oriented intensive therapies (including sedatives, opioids, neuromuscular blockers, hypothermia and osmotherapy) should be withheld pending formal assessment of brain death. In order to meet the preconditions for brain death assessment,[7] extracranial homeostasis must be maintained, and these conditions also preserve the possibility of organ donation in the future.

Withdrawal of intensive therapies is common practice in Australasian ICUs.[12–14] In the setting of severe brain damage this first involves assembling definitive prognostic information. Although neurophysiology and imaging provide important supportive information, a sedative-free clinical assessment of CNS function is an essential aspect of prognostication. During the period of sedative-free CNS assessment, some patients will suffer apparent loss of brainstem function. If brain death does not occur, but devastating brain damage has clearly occurred, those treating the patient (e.g. intensivists, neurosurgeons and others) should achieve a consensus view of prognosis and a recommended treatment plan, which might include withdrawal of intensive treatments (e.g. artificial airway, ventilatory or inotropic support, further neurosurgery). The intensivist should then discuss the prognosis and recommended plan with the family and facilitate a consensus. Withdrawal of treatment may subsequently occur, either because death is seen to be imminent and inevitable or because the likely survival outcome would not be in accord with the patient's previously expressed wishes or inferred best interests. Such a decision to limit or withdraw treatment is guided by the principles of non-malfeasance and respect for autonomy.[15] It is appropriate to withdraw all intensive therapies from such patients, while continuing to provide 'comfort care' to the patient and support to the family.[15]

The possibility of future organ donation must have no influence on a decision to limit or withdraw specific brain-oriented therapies. A minority of patients having intensive treatments withdrawn will die within a short period of time (i.e. under 1 hour) and it is in such circumstances that DCD is possible. Some families of dying patients volunteer the view that they (and/or the patient) would wish for organ donation to take place, if that is possible. Such views are commonly conveyed prior to the determination of brain death in patients who seem very likely to become or may already be brain dead, but can also be made when the patient retains brainstem function, and sometimes even prior to a decision that intensive treatments will be withdrawn. They should be sensitively acknowledged by the intensivist, and assurances given that the intensivist will revisit this issue without prompting with the family if and when the clinical circumstances are appropriate. However, the possibility of DCD must not be raised by the treating team prior to a consensus decision of the family and treating team that treatment will be withdrawn.

IDENTIFICATION OF THE POTENTIAL FOR ORGAN DONATION TO OCCUR

Most ICUs admit patients with very severe brain damage whose probability of recovery is low. The rationale for this practice is to identify any (small) subgroup of patients with reversible conditions and provide them with the necessary treatment to facilitate their recovery. There are, however, more extreme situations when the chance of recovery is thought so remote that admission of the patient to ICU would not ordinarily occur. Some intensivists advocate admitting these patients to ICU solely to allow for the future possibility that organ donation may occur, sometimes with accompanying explicit discussion and agreement of the family to such a plan.[16] Although it seems likely[16] that such an utilitarian approach might increase the number of organs available for transplant, ethical,[17] legal[18] and clinical[17] objections to the practice have all been raised.

Organ donation is possible in most situations where brain death has been confirmed. The absolute general contraindications to organ donation are few and present in a small minority of brain-dead patients. They include situations where there is an unacceptably high risk of transmission of malignancy or infection to the recipient, or where the function of the possible donor organs is

Table 93.1 Information likely to be required by transplant teams

Age, sex, weight, approximate height
Medical and social history (including comorbidity, surgery, medication, alcohol, smoking, illicit drug use, tattoos, body piercing, sexual history and allergies)
Detailed clinical history of fatal illness (including history of cardiac arrest, periods of hypotension or hypoxia, evidence of aspiration or sepsis)
Current clinical status (including physiological parameters and the extent of ventilatory and inotropic support)
Current investigations (including blood group, arterial blood gases, chest X-ray, ECG, serum urea, creatinine, electrolytes, glucose, bilirubin, transaminases, alkaline phosphatase and gamma-glutamyl transpeptidase, prothrombin ratio, activated partial thromboplastin time, haemoglobin, white cell count, platelets and all microbiology results)
Other investigations may be required later (e.g. echocardiogram or bronchoscopy)

likely to be unacceptably poor. Most extracerebral malignancies and certain infections (e.g. HIV) are likely to remain absolute contraindications but other donor factors (e.g. advanced age, recent bacterial sepsis,[19] treated HSV encephalitis, positive HCV[20] or HBV[20] serology, some 'apparently cured' malignancies) are no longer absolute contraindications. Intensivists should discuss the specific issue with the appropriate agency (donor coordinator or organ procurement organisation) rather than decide that organ donation is contraindicated on medical grounds. Similarly, the organ-specific contraindications to organ donation have reduced in recent years as the outcomes of recipients transplanted with donor organs formerly rejected have been found to be acceptable.[21] Finally, all contraindications vary somewhat between transplant centres and continue to change in a more permissive direction. Intensivists should discuss these organ-specific issues with the donor coordinator or appropriate agency before deciding that any particular organ is unsuitable for possible donation and subsequent transplantation. In most jurisdictions an appropriate authority (e.g. a coroner or medical examiner) may legally interdict organ donation under certain circumstances (e.g. homicide) and this issue must also be clarified with the donor coordinator. The donor coordinator will clarify with the transplant teams whether any organ donation is possible and whether particular organs may not be suitable, and the intensivist should ensure that the information (Table 93.1) necessary for these decisions is provided.

DETERMINATION OF BRAIN DEATH

This is a clinical responsibility of the intensivist and must be carried out according to appropriate codes of practice or clinical guidelines (see Chapter 46). The determination of brain death[7,22,23] involves several stages:

1. establishing the presence of a condition known to produce severe and irreversible structural brain damage
2. exclusion of possible confounding factors
3. determination by two independent clinical examinations that there is profound unresponsive coma and persistent absence of brainstem function

The examination and determination of brain death is facilitated by a proforma and should be documented in the medical record. When clinical examination is confounded (e.g. by barbiturate coma), then absent cerebral blood flow must instead be demonstrated by reliable imaging.[7]

The intensivist should convey the fact of brain death and its medical and legal implications to the family. It can be difficult to accept brain death as death, given the life-like appearance of the skin, the rise and fall of the chest and the warmth of the hands that are preserved by ventilatory and circulatory support.[24] Some family members appreciate an offer to view the (second) clinical examination for brain death (taking care to explain beforehand the possibility of spinal reflexes), or the cerebral blood flow study when clinical examination is confounded. This may help them to understand and accept the final awful implication of this diagnosis. Intensivists should be open to offering these options.

In the absence of organ donation, it is appropriate to remove ventilatory support at a time that allows for family needs.

DONATION AFTER CARDIAC DEATH

Donation after cardiac death (DCD), previously known as non-heart-beating donation, is increasing in many countries but is not yet practised worldwide. Kootstra and colleagues from Maastricht have long been advocates for DCD, and described four categories of 'non-heart-beating' donors; this terminology remains in common use.

- Category I: those who are dead on arrival
- Category II: those in whom cardiopulmonary resuscitation is ceased
- Category III: those in whom cardiac arrest is expected to soon occur
- Category IV: those who have cardiac arrest while brain dead

In all but Category III the situation is 'uncontrolled'.[25]

DCD practice varies considerably worldwide. Category II donors are most common in the Dutch experience but donation does occur from all categories. Almost all DCD donors in the UK, USA, Canada and Australasia are Category III (and a very few are Category IV). By contrast, in Spain, although withdrawal of treatment in ICU is far less common than in Holland or the UK,[26,27] and Category III donors are rare, immediate postmortem organ preservation measures (including cardiopulmonary bypass) can be implemented with prior consent and most DCD donors are Category I and II.[28]

Recent advocates for DCD commonly assert that 'all organ donation occurred this way' before brain death was accepted as legal death. Although organs were removed after circulatory arrest, there are differences which are not discussed and which negate the assertion that the processes are identical. Although brain death was not accepted as legal death, the syndrome had been recognised many years earlier (e.g. absent cerebral blood flow[29] was reported in 1956 and the clinical syndrome[30] in 1959). The final awful meaning of the brain death syndrome ('apnoea, fixed dilated pupils, polyuria, hyperglycaemia and spontaneous hypothermia'[31]) was understood by intensivists and nephrologists and conveyed to families at that time, prior to a discussion of organ donation (PB Doak, RV Trubuhovich, personal communications). Organ donation was not discussed with the family if some brainstem function (usually only a tracheal reflex) was known to be present. Apnoea at hypercarbia was not specifically tested for but the shared expectation of the family and the treating team was that the patient would not breathe after withdrawal of ventilatory support (although a few did, for a short time and inadequately). Cardiac arrest usually occurred in 15–20 minutes, at which point death was declared and the kidneys were removed.

In contrast to organ donation after brain death, in (Category III) DCD the patient is known not to be brain dead at the time of organ donation discussion, may well breathe after extubation and may not die in the timeframe where organ donation is possible. These differences have ethical and clinical consequences for intensivists which are discussed below.

Delayed graft function is more common (~40% vs. ~20%) in recipients of DCD kidney grafts,[32] but long-term recipient outcomes are equivalent to those who receive a graft from a brain-dead donor.[33] Both graft and patient survival after DCD liver grafts are lower than after grafts from brain-dead donors (e.g. 5-year graft survival 52% vs. 66%, 5-year patient survival 65% vs. 72%),[34,35] probably reflecting both intolerance of the liver to more than 15 minutes of warm ischaemia and impaired small vessel washout of the biliary system. Less viscous preservation solutions may ameliorate this latter problem. Patient survival is less impacted than graft survival but at the expense of an increased frequency of retransplantation. Recipient and graft outcomes after pancreas transplantation with grafts from DCD donors are similar to those from brain-dead donors.[36] Although successful lung and even heart transplantation from DCD donors is being reported, experience so far is insufficient to characterise the long-term recipient outcomes.

Following the Institute of Medicine report[37] in 1997 there has been an explosion of publications on the legal, ethical and medical issues raised by DCD[25,38,39] and more recently several national guidelines or recommendations have been produced which address these issues.[35,40,41] Recommendations for Australasia have been developed by the Australian and New Zealand Intensive Care Society.[7]

There are many potentially contentious issues, including ensuring that there has been a consensus decision to withdraw treatment before the family are presented with the option of possible organ donation after death, estimating the probability of death soon after withdrawal of treatment, use of agents (e.g. heparin) and procedures (e.g. instrumentation) prior to death that are for 'organ benefit only', location of withdrawal of treatment (ICU or operating room), presence of the family after withdrawal of treatment, use of opioids and sedatives after withdrawal of treatment, separation of clinical responsibility for end-of-life care (including opioids, sedatives and determination of death) from responsibility for organ procurement, timing of organ removal after death, abandoning the procedure (but continuing comfort care) if the patient does not die within a predetermined time (usually 1 hour) after withdrawal of treatment, ensuring that the family are fully informed and supported throughout the process, ensuring that all participating personnel are familiar with, and accepting of, DCD procedures and ensuring that appropriate protocols which explicitly address all of these issues are in place in each participating hospital. DCD should only take place in the context of such protocol wherein broad clinical, ethical and societal consensus has been achieved after wide consultation. Where this has been done, DCD has been viewed favourably by both families and hospital staff, has compensated for the fall in brain-dead donors in Holland and the UK, and has modestly increased the number of organs (particularly kidneys) available for transplant in the USA.

OFFERING THE OPPORTUNITY FOR ORGAN DONATION TO THE FAMILY

Organ donation (from deceased donors) is an activity that takes place at the end of life, usually involving an intensive care unit. It is separate from transplantation which is concerned with the care of patients with end-stage organ failure who may receive donated organs. Appreciating this distinction is fundamental to an understanding of important issues that are often ignored or dismissed in transplant-oriented publications. Organ donation fundamentally modifies human rituals at the time of death, even of death in the ICU. Organ retrieval is an invasive procedure carried out in the operating room. Although it is done respectfully and with identical surgical processes to those used on living people, it is nevertheless viewed by some[42] as 'mutilating'. Discussion of organ donation is an emotionally intense activity involving a newly bereaved family and a health professional, and requires very clear and sensitive communication. This discussion takes place when family members are experiencing the death of their family member. They must consider the issue amidst their intense grief – there is no other time. Knowledge of transplantation varies widely in the community and there is even less knowledge of organ donation processes. Some families may not previously have known that organ donation and transplantation occur! Similarly, discussion of organ donation and willingness to be part of it vary widely in the community. There is greater support of 'organ donation in principle' than either individual willingness to donate or willingness to agree to donation on behalf of a family member. Discussion of organ donation among families is promoted as a way of increasing organ donation rates and it may do so. However, some family members hold strong views against organ donation based on spiritual, religious or cultural beliefs.[42]

There are several utilitarian attitudes about organ donation including the notion that organ donation is the only possible positive outcome that can occur in the setting of brain death,[43] that it is appropriate to refer to dead or dying persons in a utilitarian way as sources of organs for transplant,[44] that for many families organ donation can assist with easing the pain of loss, and that fulfilling the previously expressed wishes of the donor should be the primary or indeed the only[45] consideration. In some jurisdictions these wishes have indeed been defined to be legally sufficient for organs to be retrieved, and are often assumed to be a means of increasing the organ donation rate[46] by excluding the family from the opportunity to prohibit organ donation and 'returning control to the individual'. This assumption may well be erroneous.[47,48] Although many countries (including Australia) have defined the status of an individual's wishes about organ donation after their death to constitute legally sufficient 'consent', it is contentious whether the word itself is appropriate in this context[10] as the person is dead at the time that the issue becomes 'live' and further, it is unlikely that any current 'register-based' record of such wishes would meet standards for informed consent[49] in a personal health care context.[50]

Implicit in a 'transplant-oriented' moral economy[51] is the judgement that for a family to agree to organ donation is both desirable and of greater moral value ('the right thing to do') than the contrary decision, particularly if organ donation was the previously expressed wish of the dead person. This judgement implicitly denies the legitimacy of the close human relationship between the family and the deceased to determine what should happen to their loved one after death,[52] but is now explicitly acknowledged, practised and advocated by many USA organ procurement organisations (S Gunderson, personal communication). Even in countries that legally allow the previously expressed wishes of the deceased to determine whether organ donation may take place, usual practice continues to both involve the family and not to proceed against family objection – accepting that the impact on the deceased's family is the most important factor determining consent practice.[53] However, in many countries this has resulted in the evolution, exposition and advocacy of strategies 'to overcome family objections'. The likely injurious effect of such 'strategies' on family bereavement[54] is not considered or reported by those who advocate for it, and whose sole measure of 'quality' or 'success' in organ donation practice is the proportion of situations in which donation occurs.

Intensivists should be aware of their own views on these matters, and indeed the views of others that might discuss organ donation with family members. Whilst intensivists most often initiate discussion of organ donation with families in Australasia, this is increasingly unusual elsewhere. Whoever undertakes this discussion should be skilled in communication with grieving people. In Australasian clinical practice, the intensivist has already established a relationship with the family, involving mutual trust and respect, in prior family meetings during the patient's final illness. This relationship naturally allows the intensivist to initiate and facilitate discussion of organ donation. Defining the discussion as 'offering the option of organ donation' rather than 'obtaining consent' (or even 'persuasion'[55]) is not coercive in language and enables the intensivist to provide complete and unbiased information, support the family in their decision-making and thank them for their consideration, whatever the decision about organ donation might be.

The intensivist must ensure that the fact of death (in the situation of brain death) is understood. When (Category III) DCD is a possibility, there must be prior consensus agreement by the family and the treating team that treatment must be withdrawn before the option of possible organ donation is raised by the intensivist. The patient is clearly not dead at this time, although death is certainly anticipated to be imminent. This imminent death should also be understood by the family before the option of DCD is offered.

In either situation there must be sufficient time for the intensivist to inform the family of the option of organ donation and what it entails, to answer any questions and if necessary to facilitate decision-making by the family. The discussion may take into account previously expressed wishes, previous family discussions, values and beliefs of the patient and of family members. This discussion must not be coercive. Language that is potentially coercive (e.g. 'fulfilling the deceased's wishes', 'doing what he would have wanted', 'something good may come of this') can redefine the situation in terms of the family coming to fulfil the intensivist's wishes and should be avoided. Finally, some language is particularly insensitive from the perspective of grieving families and should be avoided (e.g. the use of the term 'harvest' rather than 'organ retrieval' to describe the process of organ retrieval, or 'the body' rather than the person's name to describe the brain-dead person). The intensivist should facilitate the family spending time at the bedside prior to organ retrieval if they wish. Some investigations (e.g. echocardiography or bronchoscopy) may be performed during this time and the family should be informed about these. The intensivist should ensure that the family is offered the opportunity to spend time with the deceased after organ retrieval.

MAINTENANCE OF EXTRACEREBRAL PHYSIOLOGICAL STABILITY IN BRAIN DEATH

Immediately prior to brain death there is usually a period of hypertension, tachycardia and occasionally dysrhythmia, mediated by both autonomic activity and catecholamine secretion. Pulmonary oedema, biventricular dysfunction and myocardial injury may develop but there is debate about the implications of these for subsequent cardiac graft function.[56] If treatment of this adrenergic phenomenon is thought essential, then a short-acting β-blocker (e.g. esmolol) or only 'moderating' doses of a conventional β-blocker should be used. Cardiac arrest can rarely occur during this phase, usually due to tachydysrhythmia, but is often reversible. Hypertension is soon followed by hypotension, associated with marked reduction in sympathetic activity and catecholamine secretion. Hypotension may be profound in the presence of simultaneous hypovolaemia or cardiac dysfunction and can lead to cardiac arrest or loss of donor organ viability, and should be promptly treated by volume expansion and inotropic support.

Diabetes insipidus due to loss of ADH production soon follows in most but not all brain-dead persons and is manifest by brisk hypo-osmolar polyuria, which untreated will quickly lead to hyperosmolality and later to hypovolaemia. Other hormone abnormalities occur but do not have serious implications in the short term. Associated with the loss of cerebral blood flow there is loss of cerebral metabolism and a fall of around 25% in oxygen consumption and carbon dioxide production.[57] This leads to a fall in the necessary ventilatory minute volume necessary for normocarbia. The fall in resting energy expenditure (heat production) together with loss of vasomotor tone and the possibility of shivering-induced thermogenesis exacerbate the risk of hypothermia developing.

Spontaneous movements and spinal motor reflexes commonly persist in brain death.[58] These rarely include bizarre movements[22,59] which are often reproducible. Family members may be offered the opportunity to view the (perhaps second) clinical examination for brain death and should be warned about the possibility of these responses (which may not have occurred at the first examination) and given a prior explanation of them. These movements and sympathetic circulatory responses can also occur during organ retrieval in the operating room. The use of use of neuromuscular blockade and opioids is recommended in the operating room[60] although catecholamine responses are not suppressed by opioids in this situation.[61]

SUGGESTED STRATEGIES FOR MAINTAINING PHYSIOLOGICAL STABILITY

The onset of brain death is usually heralded by rises in intracranial pressure (if measured) and signs of progressive loss of brainstem function (coma, pupillary dilatation) and these features should initiate preparation for specific support strategies. This preparation should include ensuring that central venous access for inotropic support (and perhaps pressure measurement), intravenous access for rapid volume expansion and a source of external heat (e.g. a warming blanket) are all available.

VENTILATORY MANAGEMENT

The aims of ventilatory management are to maintain good oxygenation and normocarbia, minimise circulatory depression and maintain, if possible, sufficiently good lung function to allow for future lung donation to occur. The use of moderate tidal volumes (10–12 ml/kg) and addition of a low level of positive end-expiratory pressure (PEEP) (5 cmH_2O) may prevent atelectasis. Originally a Pao_2 of more than 350 mmHg on 100% oxygen and 5 cmH_2O PEEP was thought a necessary criterion for lung donation but Pao_2/Fio_2 ratios of 300 or 250 have been found to be acceptable.[62] Peak airway pressures above 30 cmH_2O should be avoided if possible. Usual pulmonary care including changes of position and sterile endotracheal suctioning must continue. When pulmonary dysfunction is severe, higher levels of PEEP may be required to prevent airway frothing or provide adequate oxygenation. The determination of apnoea during brain-death testing in such patients may require a period of mechanical hypoventilation prior to apnoea and continuation of continuous positive airway pressure (CPAP) during apnoea in such patients if serious hypoxaemia and circulatory depression are to be avoided.

CIRCULATORY MANAGEMENT

The aims of circulatory management are to maintain adequate organ perfusion and arterial pressure without producing fluid overload or excessive vasoconstriction, and without prejudicing future cardiac donation. Reasonable initial haemodynamic goals include normotension (a mean arterial pressure over 70 mmHg), heart rate of 100 beats per minute or less, and central venous pressure of 8 mmHg. Some inotropic support is almost always given (e.g. 92% of the 227 donors in 2006 in Australia and New Zealand[63]). Having established normotension with an inotrope infusion, the haemodynamic response to a controlled volume challenge should be assessed.

The choice of inotrope is the subject of more controversy than evidence. Dobutamine is not recommended. Noradrenaline (norepinephrine), usually less than 500 μg/hour, is preferred in Australasia (85% of 208 donors in 2006 who received inotrope infusions[63]) without apparent harm to organ function in recipients. Dopamine may exacerbate tubular polyuria and is not commonly used in Australasia (8% of 208 donors in 2006 who received inotrope). Adrenaline (epinephrine) may have specific benefit on renal blood flow in brain death[64] but may also increase glycaemia and thereby osmotic diuresis. Catecholamine infusion may reduce the upregulation of organ immunogenicity that occurs in brain death and lower the incidence of acute rejection in subsequent recipients of kidney grafts.[65] Although levels of thyroid hormones fall after brain death, this is probably the 'sick euthyroid syndrome' and replacement of thyroid hormone does not improve the circulation after brain death.[66–68]

Corticosteroids are often given just prior to organ removal from brain-dead donors and commonly recommended (on the basis of retrospective analyses) to increase the number of organs, particularly thoracic organs[69] that are retrieved and transplanted. Although steroids improve haemodynamics in an experimental model,[70] an early randomised human study[71] did not show any benefit in kidney graft outcomes. There are no other trials of steroids alone in human brain death and a single small trial of the combination of steroid and tri-iodothyronine (T_3) similarly did not show beneficial circulatory effects.[72]

Vasopressin infusion, at least in low doses, reduces the amount of catecholamine required to support arterial pressure[73] without apparent detriment to subsequently transplanted organs. Whether this translates into improved outcome is uncertain. Following reports using retrospective analysis with multiple logistic regression,[74,75] many authors now advocate the use of so-called 'hormonal resuscitation' (combined use of T_3, steroid and vasopressin), although these authors of papers themselves cautioned that their results 'are based on a retrospective analysis and the finding should be confirmed in future prospective randomised clinical studies'.[75]

Control of excessive polyuria will minimise the risks of developing hyperosmolality,[76] hypovolaemia or hyperglycaemia secondary to infusion of large amounts of dextrose-containing fluids. Synthetic desmopressin (1-D amino-8 D arginine vasopressin) is commonly given to control diabetes insipidus and appears safe and effective.[62,77]

Control of diabetes insipidus is an essential aspect of rational fluid therapy, and hypovolaemia should be corrected with resuscitation fluids. Haemoconcentration occurs early after experimental brain death. Crystalloid infusion has been reported to worsen pulmonary function in brain death and somewhat larger volumes will be required than if colloid is used.[78] At least moderate anaemia is well tolerated in brain death but red cells may be given if needed to maintain packed cell volume around 0.25 pending organ retrieval. Free water should be given as necessary (1–2 ml/kg per hour as 5% dextrose) to maintain serum osmolality in the range of 280–310 mosm/kg, corresponding to serum sodium below 155 mmol/l. Severe hyperosmolality (probably a marker of inadequate donor care) is associated with poor graft function in subsequent liver recipients.[76] Failure to control diabetes insipidus will lead to increased requirements of free water to control serum osmolality. If 5% dextrose is used for this then hyperglycaemia and osmotic diuresis may result.

METABOLIC MANAGEMENT

Oxygen consumption, carbon dioxide production, heat production and glucose oxidation all fall in brain death due to the loss of cerebral metabolic activity.[57] Hypothermia may easily develop in association with vasoparesis, loss of shivering, exposure to room temperature, warm polyuria and infusion of room temperature intravenous fluids. Core temperature should be kept above the 35°C required to confirm brain death.[7,22] Keeping the ambient temperature high (24°C) and using infusion fluid warmers, heated humidifiers and external warming systems may be required. Low-dose insulin infusion is occasionally required to prevent hyperglycaemia. Serum potassium should be kept above 3.5 mmol/l but potassium replacement should be given with caution as hyperkalaemia is not uncommon after brain death. Correction of hypophosphataemia does not improve haemodynamics in brain death.[79]

AFTERCARE OF THE DONOR FAMILY

Routine aftercare is increasingly recommended[80] for all families of patients who die in ICUs. Aftercare programs are well received[11] and have the potential to improve the care of subsequent families by revealing areas of inadequate or inappropriate communication.

There may be issues specific to organ donation that need to be addressed, sometimes by way of a family meeting with an intensivist at some later stage. Most organ donation agencies provide donor families with ongoing emotional support (which may extend over many years), provide them with limited anonymous information about recipients, and accept and facilitate limited anonymous communication (i.e. by letter) between recipients and donor families by mutual consent; direct contact is not recommended.

REFERENCES

1. Groth CG, Brent LB, Calne RY *et al.* Historic landmarks in clinical transplantation: conclusions from the consensus conference at the University of California, Los Angeles. *World J Surg* 2000; **24**: 834–43.
2. Aarabi B, Hesdorffer DC, Ahn ES *et al.* Outcome following decompressive craniectomy for malignant swelling due to severe head injury. *J Neurosurg* 2006; **104**: 469–79.
3. Stegmayr B, Eriksson M, Asplund K. Declining mortality from subarachnoid hemorrhage: changes in incidence and case fatality from 1985 through 2000. *Stroke* 2004; **35**: 2059–63.
4. Canales MT, Kasiske BL, Rosenberg ME. Transplant tourism: outcomes of United States residents who undergo kidney transplantation overseas. *Transplantation* 2006; **82**: 1658–61.
5. Bass D. Kidneys for cash and egg safaris – can we allow 'transplant tourism' to flourish in South Africa? *S Afr Med J* 2005; **95**: 42–4.
6. Pearson IY, Zurynski Y. A survey of personal and professional attitudes of intensivists to organ donation and transplantation. *Anaesth Intensive Care* 1995; **23**: 68–74.
7. Australian and New Zealand Intensive Care Society. *Statement on Death and Organ Donation*, 3rd edn. Melbourne: ANZICS; 2008.

8. Manyalich M, Cabrer C, Valero R *et al.* Transplant procurement management: a model for organ and tissue shortage. *Transplant Proc* 2003; **35**: 2533–8.
9. Streat S, Silvester W. Organ donation in Australia and New Zealand – ICU perspectives. *Crit Care Resusc* 2001; **3**: 48–51.
10. Streat S. Moral assumptions and the process of organ donation in the intensive care unit. *Crit Care* 2004; **8**: 382–8.
11. Cuthbertson SJ, Margetts MA, Streat SJ. Bereavement follow-up after critical illness. *Crit Care Med* 2000; **28**: 1196–201.
12. Streat S. When do we stop? *Crit Care Resusc* 2005; **7**: 227–32.
13. Ho KM, Liang J, Hughes T *et al.* Withholding and withdrawal of therapy in patients with acute renal injury: a retrospective cohort study. *Anaesth Intensive Care* 2003; **31**: 509–13.
14. Yaguchi A, Truog RD, Curtis JR *et al.* International differences in end-of-life attitudes in the intensive care unit: results of a survey. *Arch Intern Med* 2005; **165**: 1970–5.
15. Henig NR, Faul JL, Raffin TA. Biomedical ethics and the withdrawal of advanced life support. *Annu Rev Med* 2001; **52**: 79–92.
16. Riad H, Nicholls A, Neuberger J *et al.* Elective ventilation of potential organ donors. *BMJ* 1995; **310**: 714–8.
17. Manara A, Jewkes C. Intensive care units have good reasons not to do it. *BMJ* 1995; **311**: 121–2.
18. F versus West Berkshire Health Authority. 1989: 2 All ER 545–551, HL.
19. Freeman RB, Giatras I, Falagas ME *et al.* Outcome of transplantation of organs procured from bacteremic donors. *Transplantation* 1999; **68**: 1107–11.
20. The Transplantation Society of Australia and New Zealand. Organ allocation protocols. Sydney: TSANZ; 2002. http://www.tsanz.com.au/organallocationprotocols/index.asp.
21. Ojo AO, Hanson JA, Meier-Kriesche H *et al.* Survival in recipients of marginal cadaveric donor kidneys compared with other recipients and wait-listed transplant candidates. *J Am Soc Nephrol* 2001; **12**: 589–97.
22. Wijdicks EF. The diagnosis of brain death. *N Engl J Med* 2001; **344**: 1215–21.
23. Capron AM. Brain death – well settled yet still unresolved. *N Engl J Med* 2001; **344**: 1244–6.
24. Whetstine LM. Bench-to-bedside review. When is dead really dead – on the legitimacy of using neurologic criteria to determine death. *Crit Care* 2007; **11**: 208.
25. Kootstra G, Kievit J, Nederstigt A. Organ donors: heartbeating and non-heartbeating. *World J Surg* 2002; **26**: 181–4.
26. Esteban A, Gordo F, Solsona JF *et al.* Withdrawing and withholding life support in the intensive care unit: a Spanish prospective multi-centre observational study. *Intensive Care Med* 2001; **27**: 1744–9.
27. Sprung CL, Cohen SL, Sjokvist P *et al.* Ethicus Study Group. End-of-life practices in European intensive care units: the Ethicus Study. *JAMA* 2003; **290**: 790–7.
28. Sanchez-Fructuoso AI, de Miguel Marques M, Prats D *et al.* Non-heart-beating donors: experience from the Hospital Clinico of Madrid. *J Nephrol* 2003; **16**: 387–92.
29. Löfstedt S, von Reis G. [Intracranial lesions with abolished passage of x-ray contrast through the internal carotid arteries]. *Opusc Med* 1956; **1**: 199–202.
30. Wertheimer P, Jouvet M, Descites J. Apropos du diagnostic de la mort du système nerveux dans les comas avec arrêt respiratoire traités par respiration artficielle. *Presse Med* 1959; **67**: 87–8.
31. Spence M. *5th Annual Report of the Acute Respiratory Unit, Auckland Hospital 1965–66.* Auckland Hospital Board 1966.
32. Locke JE, Segev DL, Warren DS *et al.* Outcomes of kidneys from donors after cardiac death: implications for allocation and preservation. *Am J Transplant* 2007; **7**: 1797–807.
33. Metcalfe MS, Butterworth PC, White SA *et al.* A case-control comparison of the results of renal transplantation from heart-beating and non-heart-beating donors. *Transplantation* 2001; **71**: 1556–9.
34. Lee KW, Simpkins CE, Montgomery RA *et al.* Factors affecting graft survival after liver transplantation from donation after cardiac death donors. *Transplantation* 2006; **82**: 1683–8. Erratum in: *Transplantation* 2007; **83**: 521.
35. Bernat JL, D'Alessandro AM, Port FK *et al.* Report of a national conference on donation after cardiac death. *Am J Transplant* 2006; **6**: 281–91.
36. Salvalaggio PR, Davies DB, Fernandez LA *et al.* Outcomes of pancreas transplantation in the United States using cardiac-death donors. *Am J Transplant* 2006; **6**: 1059–65.
37. Institute of Medicine, National Academy of Sciences. *Non-heart-beating Organ Transplantation: Medical and Ethical Issues in Procurement.* Washington, DC: National Academy Press, 1997.
38. Vanrenterghem Y. Cautious approach to use of non-heart-beating donors. *Lancet* 2000; **356**: 528.
39. Daar AS. Non-heart-beating donation: ten evidence-based ethical recommendations. *Transplant Proc* 2004; **36**: 1885–7.
40. Ridley S, Bonner S, Bray K *et al.* Intensive Care Society's Working Group on Organ and Tissue Donation. UK guidance for non-heart-beating donation. *Br J Anaesth* 2005; **95**: 592–5.
41. Shemie SD, Baker AJ, Knoll G *et al.* National recommendations for donation after cardiocirculatory death in Canada: donation after cardiocirculatory death in Canada. *CMAJ* 2006; **175**: S1.
42. Chapman JR, Hibberd AD, McCosker C *et al.* Obtaining consent for organ donation in nine NSW metropolitan hospitals. *Anaesth Intensive Care* 1995; **23**: 81–7.
43. Murphy L. Donation – a difficult but most important discussion. *Mich Health Hosp* 1999; **35**: 20–1.
44. Fisher J. An expedient and ethical alternative to xenotransplantation. *Med Health Care Philos* 1999; **2**: 31–9.
45. May T, Aulisio MP, DeVita MA. Patients, families, and organ donation: who should decide? *Milbank Q* 2000; **78**: 323–36, 152.

46. Spital A. Mandated choice for organ donation: time to give it a try. *Ann Intern Med* 1996; **125**: 66–9.
47. Lawlor M, Kerridge I, Ankeny R *et al.* Public education and organ donation: untested assumptions and unexpected consequences. *J Law Med* 2007; **14**: 360–6.
48. Lawlor M, Billson FA. Registering wishes about organ donation may decrease the number of donors. *Med J Aust* 2007; **186**: 156.
49. Woien S, Rady MY, Verheijde JL *et al.* Organ procurement organizations Internet enrolment for organ donation: abandoning informed consent. *BMC Med Ethics* 2006; 7: E14.
50. New Zealand Health and Disability Commissioner. *Code of Health and Disability Services Consumers Rights.* Wellington: Health and Disability Commissioner; 1996. http://www.hdc.org.nz/files/hdc/code-leaflet.pdf.
51. Cassell J. *Life and Death in Intensive Care.* Philadelphia: Temple University Press; 2005.
52. Klassen AC, Klassen DK. Who are the donors in organ donation? The family's perspective in mandated choice. *Ann Intern Med* 1996; **125**: 70–3.
53. Wendler D, Dickert N. The consent process for cadaveric organ procurement: how does it work? How can it be improved? *JAMA* 2001; **285**: 329–33.
54. Kesselring A, Kainz M, Kiss A. Traumatic memories of relatives regarding brain death: request for organ donation and interactions with professionals in the ICU. *Am J Transplant* 2007; 7: 211–7.
55. Siminoff LA, Gordon N, Hewlett J *et al.* Factors influencing families' consent for donation of solid organs for transplantation. *JAMA* 2001; **286**: 71–7.
56. Deibert E, Aiyagari V, Diringer MN. Reversible left ventricular dysfunction associated with raised troponin I after subarachnoid haemorrhage does not preclude successful heart transplantation. *Heart* 2000; **84**: 205–7.
57. Bitzani M, Matamis D, Nalbandi V *et al.* Resting energy expenditure in brain death. *Intensive Care Med* 1999; **25**: 970–6.
58. Saposnik G, Bueri JA, Maurino J *et al.* Spontaneous and reflex movements in brain death. *Neurology* 2000; **54**: 221–3.
59. Ropper AH. Unusual spontaneous movements in brain-dead patients. *Neurology* 1984; **34**: 1089–92.
60. Young PJ, Matta BF. Anaesthesia for organ donation in the brainstem dead – why bother? *Anaesthesia* 2000; **54**: 105–6.
61. Fitzgerald RD, Hieber C, Schweitzer E *et al.* Intraoperative catecholamine release in brain-dead organ donors is not suppressed by administration of fentanyl. *Eur J Anaesthesiol* 2003; **20**: 952–6.
62. Gabbay E, Williams TJ, Griffiths AP *et al.* Maximizing the utilization of donor organs offered for lung transplantation. *Am J Respir Crit Care Med* 1999; **160**: 265–71.
63. Excell L, Hee K, Russ GR (eds) ANZOD *Registry Report 2007.* Adelaide: Australia and New Zealand Organ Donation Registry; 2007. http://www.anzdata.org.au.
64. Ueno T, Zhi-Li C, Itoh T. Unique circulatory responses to exogenous catecholamines after brain death. *Transplantation* 2000; **70**: 436–40.
65. Schnuelle P, Lorenz D, Mueller A *et al.* Donor catecholamine use reduces acute allograft rejection and improves graft survival after cadaveric renal transplantation. *Kidney Int* 1999; **56**: 738–46.
66. Goarin JP, Cohen S, Riou B *et al.* The effects of triiodothyronine on hemodynamic status and cardiac function in potential heart donors. *Anesth Analg* 1996; **83**: 41–7.
67. Perez-Blanco A, Caturla-Such J, Canovas-Robles J *et al.* Efficiency of triiodothyronine treatment on organ donor hemodynamic management and adenine nucleotide concentration. *Intensive Care Med* 2005; **31**: 943–8.
68. Randell TT, Hockerstedt KA. Triiodothyronine treatment is not indicated in brain-dead multiorgan donors: a controlled study. *Transplant Proc* 1993; **25**: 1552–3.
69. Follette DM, Rudich SM, Babcock WD. Improved oxygenation and increased lung donor recovery with high-dose steroid administration after brain death. *J Heart Lung Transplant* 1998; **17**: 423–9.
70. Lyons JM, Pearl JM, McLean KM *et al.* Glucocorticoid administration reduces cardiac dysfunction after brain death in pigs. *J Heart Lung Transplant* 2005; **24**: 2249–54.
71. Chatterjee SN, Terasaki PI, Fine S *et al.* Pretreatment of cadaver donors with methylprednisolone in human renal allografts. *Surg Gynecol Obstet* 1977; **145**: 729–32.
72. Mariot J, Jacob F, Voltz C *et al.* Value of hormonal treatment with triiodothyronine and cortisone in brain dead patients. *Ann Fr Anesth Reanim* 1991; **10**: 321–8.
73. Chen JM, Cullinane S, Spanier TB *et al.* Vasopressin deficiency and pressor hypersensitivity in hemodynamically unstable organ donors. *Circulation* 1999; **100**: II244–6.
74. Rosendale JD, Kauffman HM, McBride MA *et al.* Aggressive pharmacologic donor management results in more transplanted organs. *Transplantation* 2003; **75**: 482–7.
75. Rosendale JD, Kauffman HM, McBride MA *et al.* Hormonal resuscitation yields more transplanted hearts, with improved early function. *Transplantation* 2003; **75**: 1336–41.
76. Totsuka E, Dodson F, Urakami A *et al.* Influence of high donor serum sodium levels on early postoperative graft function in human liver transplantation: effect of correction of donor hypernatremia. *Liver Transpl Surg* 1999; **5**: 421–8.
77. Guesde R, Barrou B, Leblanc I *et al.* Administration of desmopressin in brain-dead donors and renal function in kidney recipients. *Lancet* 1998; **352**: 1178–81.
78. Randell T, Orko R, Hockerstedt K. Peroperative fluid management of the brain-dead multiorgan donor. *Acta Anaesthesiol Scand* 1990; **34**: 592–5.
79. Riou B, Kalfon P, Arock M *et al.* Cardiovascular consequences of severe hypophosphataemia in brain-dead patients. *Br J Anaesth* 1995; **74**: 424–9.
80. Campbell ML, Thill M. Bereavement follow-up to families after death in the intensive care unit. *Crit Care Med* 2000; **28**: 1252–3.

94

Liver transplantation

Elizabeth Sizer and Julia Wendon

Liver transplantation has revolutionised the care of patients, with both acute and chronic end-stage liver disease becoming the treatment of choice in the absence of contraindications. It has become an almost routine procedure, with the majority of patients having a short postoperative intensive care unit (ICU) stay and 1-year survival > 90%.[1–4] Indications have widened, and contraindications decreased. As a consequence, the number of patients awaiting transplantation continues to outstrip cadaveric donor rates; waiting times lengthen, hence patients become critically ill before receiving a transplant, increasing risk and perioperative complications, and impairing long-term outcome.[5] Innovative strategies have evolved as possible solutions to the lack of cadaveric donor organs, including widening the donor pool to include previously unsuitable donors (so called marginal donors), paediatric and adult living-related donation, reduced size and splitting techniques and the use of 'non-heart beating donation'.

PATIENT SELECTION

There are currently relatively few absolute contraindications to liver transplantation and no specific age limitation. Guidelines are available in regard to hepatocellular carcinoma and liver transplant. Such patients increasingly, if not inevitably, require disease-modifying treatments, (transarterial chemoembolisation and radio frequency ablation) whilst waiting for a suitable cadaveric donor.

Portopulmonary and hepatopulmonary syndromes are now an active indication for transplantation as opposed to a contraindication.[6] Such patients are likely to have a more complex postoperative course, especially if graft function is borderline or they develop sepsis. Monitoring of patients whilst on the waiting list is essential to ensure that their disease does not progress such that transplantation is no longer a feasible option. Patients must have the required cardiorespiratory reserve to tolerate the procedure. Much work has gone into the development of prognostic tools to allow accurate prediction of the need and timing for transplantation, and increasingly the model used is the model for end-stage liver disease (MELD) system. This system was initially developed for predicting survival following transjugular intrahepatic portosystemic stent (TIPS) shunt but has been shown to be equally useful in predicting survival in those awaiting liver transplantation. Once multiorgan failure has developed in a debilitated patient awaiting transplantation, survival rates decrease to 20–30% and these patients often require weeks to months of postoperative hospitalisation.[2,7]

PERIOPERATIVE ASPECTS

OPERATIVE TECHNIQUE

Orthotopic liver transplantation (OLT) involves recipient hepatectomy, revascularisation of the donor graft and biliary reconstruction.

Two main techniques are used in adult liver transplantation – those with vena cava preservation ('piggyback technique') and those using portal bypass (either internal, temporary portocaval shunt or external, veno-venous bypass). The advantages of the piggyback technique include haemodynamic stability during the anhepatic phase, without large volume fluid administration, and the negation of the need for veno-venous bypass with its associated risks and complications. Decreased transfusion requirements, shorter anhepatic time and shorter total operating time are also observed. There is no observed difference in renal function between the two techniques.[8–10] The donor hepatic artery is directly anastomosed, utilising an 'end-to-end' technique, or a conduit is constructed. Portal venous anastomosis must also be undertaken. In most patients this is an end-to-end anastomosis; however, portal venous thrombosis is no longer a contraindication to transplantation. These patients may under go a re-cannulisation procedure or require a jump graft technique. Such conduits and grafts are normally fashioned from donor vessels.

It is imperative that all those caring for the patients are aware of the surgical technique undertaken, as complications may vary. The radiologist must be aware of the technique used to allow appropriate interpretation of subsequent investigations and vascular imaging. This applies not just to the vascular anastomosis but also to the presence of a full graft, reduced size graft, right or left split graft or indeed an auxiliary graft. The biliary anastomosis is normally also undertaken as an end-to-end procedure, the donor bile duct being directly joined to the recipient duct. It is no longer standard for this to be undertaken over a T-tube, but this may be required where there is marked discrepancy between donor and recipient duct size. Some conditions (e.g. extrahepatic biliary atresia, primary sclerosing cholangitis) may preclude end-to-end anastomosis and formation of choledochojejunostomy may be required.

Split-liver grafts allow one liver to provide an organ for two recipients. Initially comprised of a child receiving the left lateral segment and an adult the remaining liver, nowadays two adults may receive grafts from one liver if the anatomy and size match allow. Such splits may be less than ideal when the recipient has a high MELD score, as is increasingly the case with the prioritisation of sick patients awaiting liver grafts. Such grafts are at increased risk of postoperative complications such as bile leaks from the cut surface and haematoma/collections at the cut surface.[3,11]

Auxiliary liver transplantation is a technique that involves subtotal recipient hepatectomy and implantation of a reduced size graft. It is a technically difficult procedure, as both portal and arterial supplies have to be constructed de novo. In addition, a duplicate biliary drainage system needs to be constructed. Hepatic venous outflow is anastomosed as usual. In acute liver failure, it has significant potential, since regeneration of the native liver may obviate the need for donor function, potentially allowing withdrawal of immunosuppression. It also has application in the treatment of some hereditary metabolic disorders where adequate metabolic function may be achieved with an auxiliary graft. The major advantage is withdrawal of immunosuppressive therapy if the patent develops severe complications, or when applicable gene therapy becomes available. The disadvantage of auxiliary transplantation in the face of acute liver failure is that the postoperative course is frequently more complicated; reasons are multifactorial, and can be due to the continued presence of a regenerating native liver or due to a smaller donor graft attempting to cope with a critical illness.

Non-heart beating transplantation (NHBD) has emerged in recent times as a potential way of increasing organs for transplantation.[12,13] The success in renal transplantation has lead to exploration of its application in the fields of liver, pancreas and lung retrieval. Most retrievals are undertaken in the context of controlled NHBD, i.e. in the context of planned withdrawal of care. Warm ischaemia can be accurately assessed and cold ischaemia minimised. Early experience with NHBD was associated with inferior survival for patients and grafts but recent experience suggests that survival is approaching that for heart beating donation. There are, however, continuing concerns over biliary and vascular complications. Prolonged cold ischaemia is associated with poor graft function and biliary complications, as are warm ischaemia times of greater than 30 minutes.[14] With regard to postoperative care, an understanding of the pre- and perioperative factors is essential in anticipating potential complications, initiation of monitoring and proactive management.

Living donor-related transplantation (LDLT) is now a routine undertaking in paediatric liver transplantation. It is becoming increasingly utilised in adult liver transplantation although its application in countries with good cadaveric donor pools is less established. Adult LDRT using right lobe grafts is an effective procedure with good survival outcomes but is associated with significant complications. From a postoperative perspective the intensive care team may be responsible for the management of both the donor and the recipient. Morbidity rates for donors are significantly higher with use of a right lobe donation compared with a left lobe graft. Mortality for donors has been reported. Survival rates now reported for living related recipients are good, with rates of 80% at 12 months.[15,16]

Adequate function of undersized transplanted liver grafts is essential to successful outcome. Primary graft non-function is relatively rare and one of the main areas of concern is that of the so-called 'small for size syndrome'.[15,17] This was first recognised in the post transplant setting but also occurs following liver resection. It is still an area under discussion but the clinical entity is that of hyperbilirubinaemia, graft dysfunction, ascites, and portal hypertension with associated end-organ dysfunction/failure. The clinical picture is that of portal hyperaemia, with portal flow passing into a small liver remnant/graft with associated pathophysiological consequences, and at a histological level there is evidence of arteriolar constriction. In some patients consideration should also be given to the potential compounder of hepatic venous outflow limitation.[18,19] Other factors that predispose to the syndrome are an inappropriate graft weight to recipient and steatotic grafts. In regard of management of this syndrome most trials have focused on optimising venous outflow and limiting/preventing portal hyperaemia and limiting portal hypertension.[15,20] Animal studies have also examined the role intrahepatic vasodilators with good effect. Management of the syndrome remains controversial but its early consideration allows the clinical team time to consider therapeutic options and interventions.

BLOOD LOSS AND COAGULOPATHY

Orthotopic liver transplantation may be associated with massive blood loss. The causes of this are multifactorial and include preoperative coagulation disorders secondary to end-stage liver disease, portal hypertension, surgical technique, adhesions related to previous surgery and intraoperative changes in haemostasis. Activation of the fibrinolytic system, especially during the anhepatic and post-reperfusion phases, occurs in some recipients. Platelet dysfunction, both quantitative and qualitative, is also common. The consequences of massive bleeding and replacement are significant, not only in terms of postoperative morbidity and mortality, but also intraoperatively, when issues such as acute hypovolaemia, reduced ionised calcium due to citrate intoxication, hyperkalaemia, acidosis and hypothermia become important. Transfusion-related acute lung injury (TRALI) is a potentially devastating complication. It is believed to result from neutrophil antibodies preformed in donor serum. The immunosuppressive effects of large volume blood transfusions are well recognised and pertinent in a group of patients who are already functionally immunosuppressed. In addition to these immediate problems is the risk of transmission of, as yet, unidentified viral infections.

Much effort has gone into reducing the amount of exogenous blood products required intraoperatively. This includes the use of cell salvage techniques with autologous transfusion, near patient testing of haemostasis, utilising both laboratory-based tests and thromboelastography. The appropriate use of antifibrinolytic drugs such as aprotinin and tranexamic acid may then be considered. These therapies appear to reduce intraoperative blood loss and transfusion requirements and possibly reduce the reperfusion injury sustained without increasing the incidence of thromboembolic complications or renal impairment.

Although it is assumed that all patients with liver disease are subject to an increased risk of bleeding there are some subgroups that are prothrombotic. Patients with preoperative portal or hepatic venous thrombosis appear to carry a higher incidence of prothrombotic mutations than the general population, and patients with primary biliary cirrhosis and primary sclerosing cholangitis are frequently prothrombotic. Such patients may require anticoagulation in the early postoperative period. Other patient groups such as those with Budd–Chiari syndrome may have a recognised prothrombotic condition with a resultant early requirement for anticoagulation.

POST-REPERFUSION SYNDROME

The post-reperfusion syndrome is a poorly understood phenomenon that occurs after reperfusion of the portal vein through the donor graft. It is characterised by hypotension, bradycardia, vasodilatation, pulmonary hypertension, hyperkalaemia and in some cases cardiac arrest. The aetiology is unclear, but a sudden increase in venous return, release of vasoactive substances, and cold potassium-rich preservation fluids are potentially implicated. The syndrome usually resolves within the first 5 minutes of reperfusion with appropriate fluid loading and electrolyte management. However, in approximately 30% of patients it lasts for significantly longer, necessitating the use of inotropes and/or vasopressors. The post-reperfusion syndrome seems more common in organs with longer preservation times and may well be associated with initial poor graft function.

POSTOPERATIVE CARE

The postoperative care of the recipient depends to some extent on preoperative comorbidity, the presence of any of the immediate complications listed above, recipient stability during the procedure and lastly the pretransplant cause of liver failure.

Straightforward recipients who return to the ICU in a stable condition with good graft function may be woken up and weaned immediately. The tracheal tube and some of the invasive monitoring lines should be removed as soon as no longer required to reduce the risk of infection and encourage mobility. Close monitoring of all physiological systems is important in the early postoperative period (Tables 94.1 and 94.2).

EARLY COMPLICATIONS

As with all postoperative surgical intensive care admissions some complications are applicable to all patients. These include haemorrhagic and pulmonary complications of any prolonged procedure in addition to specific complications pertinent to liver transplantation. These can be subdivided into technical complications, conditions and complications associated with pre-existing liver disease, and complications associated with immunosuppressive agents, graft function and massive transfusion.

CARDIOVASCULAR

End-stage liver disease is characterised by a hyperdynamic circulation, with low systemic vascular resistance, high cardiac index and a relatively reduced circulating volume. The majority of patients can be managed with adequate volume loading with or without vasopressor inotropes to maintain adequate perfusion pressures. However, in some patients this state may compensate for degrees of cardiomyopathy (which may be difficult to detect with non-invasive preoperative investigation).[21–23] The massive increase in the volume of liver transplants performed in the last decade has revealed cardiac failure as an important cause of morbidity and mortality in the transplant recipient. So-called cirrhotic cardiomyopathy, quite independent of the effects of alcohol, may be multifactorial in nature, possibly due to overproduction of nitric oxide, abnormal β-adrenoceptor structure and/or function, or the presence of some as yet unidentified myocardial depressant factor. Whatever the cause, OLT can impose severe stresses on the cardiovascular system: haemorrhage, third-space loss, impaired venous return due to caval clamping, hypocalcaemia and acidosis all impair myocardial contractility. Reperfusion can also be a time of profound circulatory instability, as discussed above. In addition, the impaired exercise tolerance of the pretransplant recipient may have limited the clinical importance of coronary ischaemia which becomes pertinent in the posttransplant period.

Haemodynamic changes after OLT are also common; hypertension with an increased systemic vascular resistance is frequent and may be due to the restoration of normal liver function and portal pressure, as well as the hypertensive effect of the calcineurin immunosuppressants. The increased afterload in the early posttransplant period may unmask cardiac dysfunction. Management of

Table 94.1 Routine investigation of posttransplant patient in the ICU

	FBC	LFTs	Coagulation	Drug levels	Cultures	Ultrasound
Day 1	√	√	√		As indicated	Routine ultrasound including hepatic artery, hepatic veins and portal vein flow between D1 and D5 unless clinically indicated at other time
Day 2	√	√	√	√		
Day 3	√	√	√	√		

Table 94.2 Monitoring of graft function in ICU

	Parameter	Comment
General	Liver perfusion	Characteristics at surgery
	Bile production	Quality ± volume if T-tube in situ
	Haemodynamics	Stabilisation, with cessation of vasopressor requirements
Coagulation	INR/Prothrombin time (hours)	8-hourly for the first 24 hours, thereafter daily unless indicated. The fall in PT is more important than the actual value. FFP should be withheld to assess graft function although platelet support should be provided as usual
Biochemistry	Glucose	Hypoglycaemia is an ominous sign. 4-hourly measurement in the first 24 hours. Euglycaemia or hyperglycaemia requiring insulin infusion is the norm
	Arterial blood gases and lactate	4–6-hourly depending on ventilatory requirement. Hyperlactataemia and acid–base disturbance should rapidly resolve. Other causes of base deficit such as renal tubular acidosis and hyperchloraemia should be excluded and managed appropriately
	AST	Should fall steadily (50% fall each day). The first measurement may reflect washout and thus the next may be higher. Daily measurements. The initial measurement reflects the degree of preservation injury.
	Bilirubin	Early increases may reflect absorption of haematoma and do not reflect graft function. Haemolysis should be considered if the graft is not blood group matched, termed passenger lymphocyte syndrome
	ALP/GGT	Usually normal; increases may reflect biliary complications or cholestasis of sepsis

myocardial dysfunction post OLT is largely empirical; diuretics, afterload reduction and positive-pressure ventilation may all be required. In the longer term, control of cardiovascular risk factors is required and many of these patients may over the years return to the intensive care environs with other system failures and considerable burdens of hypertension, coronary ischaemia, diabetes, hyperlipidaemia and renal dysfunction.

PULMONARY

Pulmonary complications are common and occur in 40–80% of recipients. The presence of preoperative impairment (e.g. pleural effusions, hypoxaemia, pulmonary hypertension or the hepatopulmonary syndrome) is strongly associated with postoperative complications. Specific conditions related to liver transplantation include right hemidiaphragm palsy as a result of phrenic nerve damage, which can occur if suprahepatic caval clamping is used intraoperatively. The commonest postoperative problems are pleural effusions, ongoing shunting secondary to the hepatopulmonary syndrome, atelectasis and, over subsequent days, infection. De novo acute lung injury and the acute respiratory distress syndrome are relatively uncommon at this stage. Other complications such as TRALI and pulmonary oedema are almost certainly underrecognised and underreported.

Specific management of portopulmonary syndrome may be required in the postoperative period if right-sided pressures are elevated, to ensure that liver congestion and graft dysfunction do not ensue.[6,24,25] Control of pulmonary pressures may require a variety of therapeutic options, with the treatment options being similar to those utilised in primary pulmonary hypertension. Concern about potential hepatotoxicity needs to be balanced against the need to control right-sided pressures and provide optimal graft function. Similarly, hepatopulmonary syndrome may take a variable time to resolve and hypoxia during this period will require management and recognition.

Respiratory complications are also seen in patients with poor muscle bulk and subsequent weakness. Similarly, the presence of osteoporosis in the pretransplant patient is frequently associated with postoperative pain and poor cough. The role of adequate analgesia is important, as in all patients, in promoting mobilisation and adequate respiratory function. In general, the management of a protracted respiratory wean follows conventional lines.

NEUROLOGICAL

The quoted incidence of central nervous system (CNS) complications varies widely from 10 to 40% in the published series. Most neurological complications occur within the first month of transplant. The commonest causes relate to persistent encephalopathy post transplant in a patient with pre-existing encephalopathy.[26,27] The causes are multiple, including hepatic, metabolic, infectious, vascular and pharmacological. A patient with acute liver failure will remain encephalopathic in the immediate posttransplant period, and is at risk for intracranial hypertension for 48 hours following transplantation, or longer in the face of graft dysfunction. De novo hepatic encephalopathy may develop in patients with severe graft dysfunction and/or primary graft non-function; again the patient is at risk of cerebral oedema. The effects of sepsis, rejection (and its treatment with high-dose steroids), drug therapy (especially the sedatives and analgesics used in the ICU setting) and the presence of renal failure may all contribute to the presence of altered conscious level. The calcineurin inhibitors are particularly associated with seizures and altered conscious level. All such patients will require brain imaging to further define the aetiology of their impaired neurology.

Other possible neurological complications are those of intracerebral haemorrhage. Such bleeds may relate to arteriovenous malformations, may be spontaneous or may be a complication of intracranial pressure monitoring, particularly in patients with acute liver failure. CNS infection normally presents later than the immediate postoperative period but should always be considered, especially in those patients with a prolonged and complicated postoperative course. All possible infecting agents, including bacterial, viral, fungal and opportunistic, should be considered. Central pontine myelinolysis is a rare but potentially devastating complication associated with rapid sodium shifts. Modern technology and the use of haemofiltration techniques allow tight control of sodium shifts in the majority of patients, and this has become a rare neurological complication.

RENAL DYSFUNCTION

Despite intraoperative efforts, renal dysfunction can be exacerbated and acute renal dysfunction is a relatively common complication, with an incidence of between 12 and 50%[28–30] and a multifactorial aetiology. Risk factors include the presence of pretransplant comorbidity (e.g. hypertension, diabetes mellitus, hepatorenal syndrome), severity of underlying liver disease, intraoperative instability, blood product requirement, drug toxicity and graft dysfunction. Mortality in those who require renal replacement is high, and graft survival is lower. To avoid exacerbation of existing renal impairment, agents with inherent nephrotoxicity, such as the calcineurin inhibitors, may be omitted or their dose significantly reduced in the early pretransplant period. There must be a balance between the risk of rejection and that of side-effects of drug therapies. Mycophenolate mofetil, a cytotoxic immunosuppressant, may be substituted in the posttransplant course to limit or mitigate against renal dysfunction, and increasingly agents such as interleukin-2 (IL-2) blockers are utilised to decrease renal dysfunction.[31]

Hepatorenal syndrome is a reversible entity following establishment of normal liver function post transplantation. There are considerable data in the literature to suggest that such patients do well with no prolongation of care or increase in mortality. Some data suggest that combined renal and liver transplant is associated with improved outcome. Patients with significant intrinsic renal dysfunction, as compared to those with functional hepatorenal dysfunction, may be offered combined liver–kidney transplantation.[32,33] Interestingly, the risk of acute rejection for combined liver–kidney grafts is as for liver transplantation as compared to the higher rate of rejection that is seen for sole renal transplant.

Intra-abdominal hypertension should always be considered in the posttransplant setting as a potential contributor to not only renal dysfunction but also cardiorespiratory dysfunction. Early consideration should be given to laparostomy in patients with elevated intra-abdominal pressures and associated organ dysfunction.[34,35]

PRIMARY NON-FUNCTION (PNF)/INITIAL POOR FUNCTION

This is a spectrum occurring in 2–23% of cases, which at worst requires urgent retransplantation. It is characterised by poor graft function from the time of reperfusion, with hyperlactataemia, coagulopathy, metabolic acidosis, hypoglycaemia, hyperkalaemia and a rapid elevation in aminotransferase concentrations, accompanied by a systemic inflammatory response.

A major reason for the initial graft dysfunction is ischaemic injury to the graft, which depends on the type of preservation fluid used, and the duration of cold and warm ischaemia time. The aetiology of primary non-function remains unclear.[36]

Vasodilator prostaglandins and antioxidants may have a role in 'rescue therapy', but controlled data are lacking.

SURGICAL PROBLEMS

Anastomotic thromboses are uncommon complications of liver transplantation, but can cause significant morbidity, which may require further invasive procedures and even urgent retransplantation. Hepatic artery thrombosis occurring in the early postoperative period is associated with a similar picture to PNF. Small vessel calibre is a risk factor, and is more prevalent in the paediatric recipient where it has also been associated with prothrombotic states such as protein C deficiency. Ultrasound is the first-line screening test and is undertaken both routinely in the immediate postoperative period and if there is a sudden rise in transaminase measurements. If the vessel is not visualised, the patient should proceed to CT angiography. If diagnosed quickly, emergency intervention can be undertaken to re-establish arterial flow; however, emergency retransplantation may be required.

Venous complications such as portal thrombosis are even more uncommon, and are usually associated with intraoperative technical difficulty, recurrence of preoperative disease or undiagnosed thrombophilia. Portal thrombosis is normally associated with portal hypertension and massive ascites, but may also be associated with graft dysfunction, especially in the paediatric population. CT scanning will interrogate the vessels and also provide information on graft perfusion: regional ischemia may be identified that may have presented as a transaminitis. Treatment is dependent on the severity of the injury but ranges from diuretics to angioplasty, surgical reconstruction or ultimately retransplantation. Regional ischaemia and areas of poor perfusion should be actively sought in patients with a transaminitis and especially in those who had received a reduced size or split-liver graft.

Biliary complications post liver transplant are relatively common. The bile duct normally receives two-thirds of its arterial supply from the gastroduodenal artery and one-third from the hepatic artery. Post transplant, the only supply is from the hepatic artery, making it vulnerable to ischaemic injury whether that be at the time of retrieval, reperfusion or postoperatively. The resulting complication depends on the type of biliary anastomosis and the timing of the insult. Strictures are more commonly observed than leaks. Management of biliary complications is in the first instance endoscopic, with stent placement and/or balloon dilatation. In patients with a T-tube in situ, cholangiography may be undertaken by that route. Open reconstruction in the early postoperative period is uncommon (Tables 94.3, 94.4 and 94.5). Bile leaks may also be seen in the postoperative period from the cut surface of a split graft. Bile leaks are associated with an increased risk of infection and potentially of pseudoaneurysm formation.

ACUTE REJECTION

Acute cellular rejection becomes a risk from approximately 5–7 days post transplant; the clinical signs of rejection are non-specific and include fever, deterioration in graft function, and a rapid rise in serum aminotransferase concentration. Liver biopsy is the only reliable diagnostic tool; however, biopsy may be relatively contraindicated due to coagulopathy. In some circumstances transjugular biopsy offers a solution to this problem. The normal management regime for an episode of acute rejection is that of pulsed methylprednisolone, 1 g for 3 days. The differential diagnosis may be that of sepsis, or problems with vascular integrity; there are some data to suggest that procalcitonin may be of use in the differentiation (Table 94.6).

SEPSIS AND FEVER

Transplant recipients are uniquely vulnerable to bacterial infection: preoperative colonisation, prolonged and technically difficult surgery, large wounds, urinary catheterisation and the frequent need for central venous access postoperatively all combine to make them at vastly increased risk. However, compared with a decade ago, the overall incidence is reduced, probably due to improved and patient-tailored immunosuppressive regimens. Sepsis remains an important and life-long complication of liver transplantation, which may require readmission to intensive care.[37,38]

The epidemiology of pathogens is evolving; the incidence of Gram-positive bacterial infection (enterococci and staphylococci) is now more common than Gram-negative sepsis. More concerning is the emergence of multiple antibiotic-resistant bacteria, in particular meticillin-resistant *Staphylococcus aureus* (MRSA), vancomycin-resistant enterococci (VRE) and extended-spectrum β-lactamase (ESBL)

Table 94.3 Technical complications of OLT

Complication	Comment
Abdominal bleeding	
Anastomosis	Immediate
Graft surface (if cut down)	Immediate
General ooze secondary to coagulopathy	Immediate
Pseudo-aneurysm formation	Can present early or late and is usually associated with intra-abdominal sepsis and biliary leaks
Vascular complications	
Hepatic artery thrombosis	Early and late
Portal vein thrombosis	Early and late; there may also be a stenosis of the portal vein rather than thrombosis
Inferior vena caval obstruction	May be infra-, supra- or retrohepatic in site
Biliary complications	
Biliary leak	Usually early
Biliary stricture	Usually late
Papillary dysfunction	Late
Roux-en-Y dysfunction	Usually late

Table 94.4 Biochemical and clinical features of technical problems

Complication	Features	Investigation	Management
Hepatic artery thrombosis	Early: rapid rise in transaminase, coagulopathy, graft failure Differential diagnosis: hyperacute rejection, primary graft non/dysfunction	Ultrasound, angiogram	Thrombectomy, retransplantation
	Late: biliary complications, strictures, sepsis, liver abscess	Ultrasound, angiogram	Angioplasty
Portal vein thrombosis	Early: rapid deterioration in graft function, acute liver failure, ascites, variceal bleeding Late: mildly abnormal LFTs, portal hypertension, varices	Ultrasound, CT, angiography, MRA Investigation as for acute portal vein thrombosis	Thrombectomy, retransplantation, conservative management

Table 94.5 Differential diagnosis of graft dysfunction in ICU

Primary non-function
Preservation injury
Rejection – hyperacute/acute
Vascular complications
Biliary complications
Drug-induced liver dysfunction
Infection – viral, bacterial, fungal
Recurrent disease (normally late)

producing Gram-negative organisms. Mortality associated with infection caused by these multiply resistant organisms is significantly greater compared with other organisms.

A decline in the incidence of both *Pneumocystis jiroveci* (formerly *P. carinii*) and cytomegalovirus infection is probably a result of both modulating immunosuppressive regimens and more effective prophylaxis. Patients should be screened for viral infections, including herpes simplex virus (HSV) and cytomegalovirus (CMV) utilising polymerase chain reaction (PCR) techniques. Opportunistic fungal infection still remains problematic, especially in the context of environmental risk factors[39,40] (Table 94.7).

FEVER

In transplant recipients, 76% of febrile episodes have a documented infectious aetiology, but acute rejection needs to be considered in the differential diagnosis. In the ICU transplant recipient the aetiology is even more likely to be infectious – often nosocomial and bacterial. In one study, pneumonia, catheter-related bacteraemia and the biliary tree were the three most common sources in the ICU population (41%). Viral infections accounted for 9% of febrile episodes, fungal infections 3% and endocarditis 3%. As mentioned above, the epidemiology of pathogens is changing and it is important to have thorough knowledge of local problem pathogens on which to base meaningful antibiotic policy.

These data have implications for the threshold to investigate febrile episodes, suspect bacterial infection and commence appropriate empirical antibiotic therapy. However, it should also be appreciated that immunosuppressed recipients do not always produce a febrile response to infection.

Table 94.6 Management of rejection in intensive care

	Comment	Characteristics	Liver biopsy	Differential diagnosis	Treatment options
Hyperacute rejection	Rare in OLT 1–10 days post transplant	Rapid deterioration in graft function: AST > 1000, Coagulopathy, acidosis	Haemorrhagic necrosis	Primary non-function/ delayed function Hepatic artery thrombosis	Retransplantation Rarely: OKT3, Cyclophosphamide, plasmapheresis (unproven)
Acute rejection	30–70% Occurs at mean of 7–9 days	Often clinically silent apart from fever and RUQ pain High AST and bilirubin Coagulation and acid–base undisturbed	Portal inflammation Endothelitis Bile duct damage	Sepsis Vascular Viral	Methylprednisolone 1 g daily for 3 days

In those who do not respond: Consider diagnosis; if correct, consider tacrolimus if induction agent is cyclosporin A, OKT3 or MMF/sirolimus if other new agents.

Table 94.7 Infection in the intensive care unit

Aetiology	Bacterial	Viral	Fungal	Protozoal
	Wound Nosocomial pneumonia Line sepsis UTI Liver Biliary	HSV CMV EBV Varicella	Candida Aspergilla PCP Cryptococcus	Toxoplasmosis Strongyloides
Timing	Any time	HSV in first few weeks CMV 3–10 weeks EBV from 4 weeks Varicella later All may be earlier in ALF or retransplantation	Usually after 4 weeks	After 3 weeks

MANAGEMENT OF CMV INFECTION AFTER LIVER TRANSPLANTATION

CMV infection is rarely associated with symptomatic illness in healthy hosts, but is a major cause of morbidity and mortality in transplant recipients; it is the single most common opportunistic infection after solid organ transplantation. In the absence of antiviral prophylaxis the overall incidence of CMV infection after OLT ranges from 23 to 85%, with approximately 50% of those developing clinical disease.

CMV infection most commonly occurs in the first 3 months after OLT, with a peak incidence in the third and fourth week. Infection may be asymptomatic or it may cause a spectrum of illness including fever, thrombocytopenia, neutropenia, pneumonia and hepatitis. The indirect effects of infection probably contribute more to the adverse effects on graft function than direct effects. CMV infection further immunosuppresses the recipient, leading to increased opportunistic fungal infection and also increased risk of Epstein–Barr virus (EBV) infection which can go on to be associated with posttransplant lymphoproliferative disease (PTLD). CMV infection is also implicated in increased rejection, although this is controversial. In those patients who proceed to transplant who are already receiving immunosuppressive agents, or in those with acute liver failure, CMV disease may present earlier in the clinical course.

The risk of CMV infection post transplant is dependent on the serological status of both the donor and recipient; the highest risk is associated with donor positive/recipient negative. Proven prophylactic strategies in the high-risk groups include long-term intravenous (i.v.) or oral (po) ganciclovir. Currently, 3 months of ganciclovir remains the gold standard in the treatment of CMV disease. In many patients, therapy will commence i.v. and then convert to oral to facilitate discharge from hospital and rehabilitation. There is no evidence to support specific immunoglobulin in addition, but it is frequently added in the management of CMV pneumonitis.

The monitoring of posttransplant patients in the intensive care and ward environment should allow for HSV, CMV and EBV PCR; treatment options can then be tailored to individual patient needs.

MANAGEMENT OF VIRAL HEPATITIS

Hepatitis C (HCV) related cirrhosis is the commonest indication for transplantation in both Europe and the USA. Post transplant, HCV viraemia is universal. Recurrent liver disease, with a more accelerated and aggressive course, is often observed; indeed, 20% are cirrhotic at 5 years post transplant.[41] Those with histological evidence of recurrence also have a greater incidence of acute rejection. Immunosuppression, especially with steroids, directly increases the HCV RNA serum load. Most transplant programmes therefore convert to single- or double-agent immunosuppression regimens as soon as possible post transplant.[42] Yet to be fully elucidated is the role of antiviral therapy (interferon and ribavirin) in both the pre- and post-transplant period. Provisional data are optimistic, although it requires considerable workload and supportive drug therapy. It would not normally be undertaken in the intensive care setting. Theoretically, early antiviral therapy is attractive as viral load is low, immunosuppressive therapy has just started and acute rejection necessitating pulsed steroids is relatively common. However, risk of infection and thrombocytopenia often contraindicates antiviral therapy in the early postoperative period.

Initial results of transplantation for hepatitis B infection (HBV) were discouraging, largely due to recurrent disease with rapid and fatal progression. Passive immunoprophylaxis with hepatitis B immune globulin (HBIG) during and after transplant and the use of antiviral agents pretransplant to suppress viral replication dramatically reduce reinfection rate. However, such therapy must be continued indefinitely following transplant to prevent disease recurrence. In respect of modulation of immunosuppression regimens, the comments made with respect to HCV are similarly applicable.

IMMUNOSUPPRESSION

As the field of transplantation evolves, new immunosuppressive regimens and drugs become available. For all combinations, however, there is a balance to be struck between the optimal prevention of rejection and the toxicity and unwanted effects of the drugs. The incidence of acute rejection rises at about 1 week after OLT; it resembles a delayed-type hypersensitivity reaction, and immunosuppressive agents are highly effective at treating it. Chronic rejection occurs over months to years and is characterised by the 'vanishing bile-duct' syndrome, pathological mechanisms are poorly understood and immunosuppressant agents are largely ineffective.[31] Currently, calcineurin inhibitors such as ciclosporin and tacrolimus, along with steroids, form the mainstay drugs after liver transplantation, certainly in the early stages. They have revolutionised the outcome of solid-organ transplantation, but both drugs are limited by their side-effects, predominantly nephro- and neurotoxicity, necessitating drug level monitoring.

These manifestations of toxicity can be difficult in the management of posttransplant immunosuppression in patients who exhibited encephalopathy or renal dysfunction pretransplant; the use of agents without renotoxic profiles may be considered in this context. It is usual to have an induction regimen beginning in the perioperative period; this usually involves a calcineurin inhibitor and steroids, which are administered in a high-dose taper regime. With time after transplantation, the level of immunosuppression required decreases and drug doses may be reduced further. Cytotoxic drugs such as azathioprine or mycophenolate mofetil (MMF) may also allow further reduction of steroids and calcineurin inhibitors. The long-term effects of immunosuppression have to be considered but are less pertinent in the immediate postoperative period.

Another variation in the regimen is the introduction of antilymphocyte antibodies (ALA) for 10–14 days in order to delay the introduction of calcineurin inhibitors: this may be desirable in patients with impaired renal function. ALA interferes with lymphocyte function in several ways: enhanced removal of activated lymphocytes by the reticuloendothelial system, downregulation of lymphocyte-binding cell surface receptors, with decreased lymphocyte activation and proliferation.

Recently, several monoclonal antibodies have been introduced. They bind to IL-2 receptors, which are only present on activated T-cells, and hence they have a more specific mode of action. The role of such agents, especially in those with renal dysfunction, is gaining greater recognition.

Sirolimus is a novel immunosuppressant that has been used extensively in renal transplantation and more recently in liver transplant recipients in whom the calcineurin inhibitors are contraindicated.[31] It resembles tacrolimus structurally, and binds to the same protein, but whereas ciclosporin and tacrolimus act by inhibiting IL-2 gene transcription, sirolimus acts by blocking post-receptor signal transduction and IL-2 dependent proliferation. In addition to its immunosuppressive actions, sirolimus is also an antifungal and antiproliferative agent. Sirolimus lacks neuro- and nephrotoxicity. However, it can raise the intracellular concentrations of cyclosporin A and tacrolimus, indirectly potentiating their toxicity. Hyperlipidaemia has also been noted although this may be a reflection of the often higher dose steroid regimens used in combination with sirolimus. Because of its antiproliferative effects, sirolimus can also cause thrombocytopenia, neutropenia and anaemia; there have also been concerns about its effects on wound healing. Sirolimus also requires therapeutic drug level monitoring, not only because serum concentrations have a high level of intra- and interindividual variability, but also because there are significant interactions with drugs that use the cytochrome P-450 3A system.

All immunosuppressive regimens should be tailored to individual patient needs and a balance struck between side-effects (short and long term) and risk of rejection.

READMISSION TO ICU/LATE COMPLICATIONS

The cause of readmission to ICU after liver transplantation varies in relation to time after transplantation. Approximately 20% of recipients require readmission, and this correlates with actuarial reduced patient and graft survival. In the period immediately after transplantation, cardiorespiratory failure is the commonest reason for readmission, due to both fluid overload and infection. Indeed, an abnormal predischarge chest X-ray is predictive of readmission as is high central venous pressure and tachypnoea. Other predictors of readmission are age, pretransplant synthetic function, bilirubin, amount of intraoperative blood products and renal dysfunction. Graft dysfunction, severe sepsis and postoperative care of surgical complications are other important causes of readmission. Bleeding and biliary anastomotic leaks represent the commonest surgical causes for readmission.

LIVER TRANSPLANTATION FOR ACUTE LIVER FAILURE

Acute liver failure is a syndrome associated with an acute onset coagulopathy, jaundice and encephalopathy; the causes are many and the syndrome is notable for its high morbidity and mortality. The acceptance of emergency liver transplantation in selected cases has revolutionised the clinical course, but outcome is sometimes disappointingly poor, often due to the rapid development of uncontrollable cerebral oedema, sepsis and multiorgan failure. There is also a short window of opportunity in listing these patients; despite highest priority listing they may receive 'marginal' organs or even ABO blood group incompatible organs. Early determination of prognosis and appropriate listing for transplant are clearly important. The King's College Hospital prognostic criteria for non-survival among patients with acute liver failure is a tool used to identify those at high risk while sparing those in whom spontaneous recovery will otherwise occur. It has been validated both in Europe and the USA (Table 94.8). Several advances in the supportive management of these patients have occurred since the original criteria were developed but their prognostic value holds true.

Table 94.8 King's College Hospital prognostic criteria for non-survival among patients with acute liver failure

Paracetamol induced	Non-paracetamol induced
pH < 7.3 (irrespective of grade of encephalopathy), following volume resuscitation and > 24 hours post ingestion *or* PT > 100 seconds (INR > 6.5) *and* creatinine > 300 μmol/l in patients with grade III–IV encephalopathy, occurring within a 24-hour timeframe	PT > 100 seconds (INR > 6.5) irrespective of grade of encephalopathy *or* pH < 7.3 following volume resuscitation *or* any three of the following variables (in association with encephalopathy): Age < 10 years or > 40 years Aetiology: non-A, non-B or drug induced Jaundice to encephalopathy > 7 days PT > 50 seconds (INR > 3.5) Serum bilirubin > 300 μmol/l

EXTRACORPOREAL HEPATIC SUPPORT

The liver has metabolic, excretory and synthetic functions, all of which need to be maintained in a patient who has liver failure until either an organ becomes available or regeneration takes place. The major components of a bioartificial liver include hepatocytes able to perform some of the functions of normal liver, a delivery system to bring blood to and from the patient, and a membrane designed to allow adequate exchange between blood and hepatocytes.

Clinical trials are in progress to evaluate the place for these devices and there has been some success with using them as a bridge to transplantation, and in acute liver failure in particular an improvement in neurological status and reduced cerebral oedema.[43] Still to be elucidated is the timescale on which these devices can be used and whether they can bridge the gap to regeneration, thus sparing the patient from transplantation.

PAEDIATRIC LIVER TRANSPLANTATION

OLT is the treatment of choice for children with end-stage liver disease. Cholestatic disorders make up the largest indication for transplantation, with extrahepatic biliary atresia plus or minus previous Kasai porto-enterostomy accounting for over 50% of paediatric transplants. Metabolic diseases and primary hepatic tumours are also common indications. As in adult recipients, multisystem effects of end-stage liver disease are common, and the occurrence of liver disease as part of a congenital syndrome (e.g. Alagille's) may warrant invasive preoperative evaluation of extrahepatic manifestation. Patient and graft survival have improved over the last decade such that 5-year patient survival is over 80%. Scarce availability of paediatric donors has driven innovations such as reduced size grafts, split-liver techniques and living donor programmes which have all contributed to expand the pool of available donors and reduce the mortality for those children waiting for suitable organs.

One of the biggest problems associated with paediatric transplantation is the relatively high incidence of vascular complications such as hepatic artery thrombosis, portal vein thrombosis and venous outflow obstruction. Risk factors for these conditions include fulminant hepatic failure, long operation time, donor/recipient age and weight discrepancies, young recipient age, low recipient weight and arterial reconstruction techniques. In order to minimise these often devastating complications, strategies to minimise the risk include delayed primary closure of the abdominal wall, maintaining the haematocrit at 22–25% to ensure laminar flow, and avoidance of platelets and blood components combined with considered use of anticoagulants.

Associated cardiac, pulmonary or renal abnormalities observed in some paediatric syndromes with liver disease may require particular attention and management such as the pulmonary stenosis seen in association with Alagille's.

HEPATOPULMONARY SYNDROMES

Changes in the cardiovascular system associated with chronic liver disease may contribute to the spectrum of cardiopulmonary disease associated with chronic liver disease and portal hypertension. A hyperdynamic state with high cardiac output, long-standing portal hypertension with the development of collateral flows, together with an imbalance of vasoactive mediators either synthesised or metabolised by the liver, may lead to characteristic changes in both flow and pressure through the pulmonary vasculature. This may be associated with hypoxia and orthodeoxia. Two ends of the spectrum are hepatopulmonary syndrome (HPS) and portopulmonary hypertension (PPH). The two conditions are rare but important, as they have vastly different impacts on risk associated with liver transplantation and long-term outcome (Table 94.9). The role of agents used in the management of primary pulmonary hypertension is yet to be examined in a controlled manner in liver disease but data thus far suggest benefit.

Diagnostic criteria for both conditions are summarised in the table.

Table 94.9 Diagnostic criteria for hepatopulmonary syndrome and portopulmonary hypertension

Hepatopulmonary syndrome	Portopulmonary hypertension
Chronic liver disease (± cirrhosis)	Portal hypertension
Arterial hypoxaemia	Mean pulmonary artery pressure > 25 mmHg
Pao_2 < 75 mmHg (10 kPa) or A–ao_2 gradient > 20 mmHg	Pulmonary artery occlusion pressure < 15 mmHg
Intrapulmonary vascular dilatation	Pulmonary vascular resistance > 120 dynes/s per cm^{-5}

HEPATOPULMONARY SYNDROME

It can be seen from Table 94.9 that hypoxia is a characteristic finding in this condition. It results from intrapulmonary vascular dilatation at the pre- and postcapillary level, leading to decreased ventilation/perfusion ratios; more uncommonly, anatomical shunt is present with atrioventricular communication. One of the postulated mechanisms of this vasodilatation is overactivity of pulmonary vasculature nitric oxide synthetase; pretransplant patients have raised levels of exhaled nitric oxide that decrease post transplant with resolution of the syndrome. Medical treatment of the syndrome has been disappointing; indeed, most transplant centres agree that the syndrome is an indication for transplantation in itself, as resolution is reported in up to 80% after transplantation.

Risk stratification based on severity is important, as vastly increased peritransplant mortality is associated with severe hypoxia and high levels of vascular shunt. Mortality overall is 16% at 90 days and 38% at 1 year. Refractory hypoxia is the indirect cause of death, which may be due to multiorgan failure, intracerebral haemorrhage and sepsis due to bile leaks. Resolution of the syndrome can take months, lending support to the theory that it is vascular remodelling rather than just acute reversal of vasodilatation that reverses hypoxia.[25,44]

PORTOPULMONARY HYPERTENSION

Up to 20% of pretransplant patients have pulmonary hypertension; this probably constitutes increased flow through the pulmonary vasculature and is not associated with increased resistance. These patients do well after transplantation. A much more ominous syndrome is the presence of pulmonary hypertension with high pulmonary vascular resistance (seen in < 4%). The aetiology of this syndrome is complex but it is characterised by a hyperdynamic high flow state with excess central volume and non-embolic pulmonary vasoconstriction. The pathological changes associated with this syndrome match those associated with primary pulmonary hypertension except that cardiac output is high in this group.

In comparison to HPS, there are several differences in terms of response to medical treatment and outcome after transplantation. The response to epoprostenol, a PGI_2 analogue, is encouraging. Decreases in pulmonary artery pressure but more importantly transpulmonary gradient (TPG) have been noted, although at least 3 months' treatment seems necessary, suggesting remodelling rather than vasodilatation is the important mechanism. A limiting factor in the treatment may also be progressive thrombocytopenia and splenomegaly. Another difference is the perioperative risk and posttransplant prognosis, Resolution is not associated with transplantation and progression can be a feature. Perioperatively, the higher the mean pulmonary artery pressure (MPAP), pulmonary vascular resistance (PVR) and TPG the greater the risk of death, usually due to acute right ventricular decompensation. If the MPAP is >35 mmHg or the PVR is >250 dyne/s per cm, mortality reaches 40%. If MPAP is >50 mm Hg some have even suggested delisting or even intraoperative cancellation as the mortality may be as high as 100%.[24]

REFERENCES

1. Roberts MS, Angus DC, Bryce CL *et al.* Survival after liver transplantation in the United States: a disease-specific analysis of the UNOS database. *Liver Transpl* 2004; **10**: 886–97.
2. Habib S, Berk B, Chang CC *et al.* MELD and prediction of post-liver transplantation survival. *Liver Transpl* 2006; **12**: 440–7.
3. Futagawa Y, Terasaki PI. An analysis of the OPTN/UNOS Liver Transplant Registry. *Clin Transpl* 2004: 315–29.
4. Burroughs AK, Sabin CA, Rolles K *et al.* 3-month and 12-month mortality after first liver transplant in adults in Europe: predictive models for outcome. *Lancet* 2006; **367**: 225–32.
5. Fink MA, Berry SR, Gow PJ *et al.* Risk factors for liver transplantation waiting list mortality. *J Gastroenterol Hepatol* 2007; **22**: 119–24.
6. Krowka MJ. Hepatopulmonary syndrome and portopulmonary hypertension: implications for liver transplantation. *Clin Chest Med* 2005; **26**: 587–97.
7. Fusai G, Dhaliwal P, Rolando N *et al.* Incidence and risk factors for the development of prolonged and severe intrahepatic cholestasis after liver transplantation. *Liver Transpl* 2006; **12**: 1626–33.
8. Reddy KS, Johnston TD, Putnam LA *et al.* Piggyback technique and selective use of veno-venous bypass in adult orthotopic liver transplantation. *Clin Transplant* 2000; **14**: 370–4.
9. Parrilla P, Sanchez-Bueno F, Figueras J *et al.* Analysis of the complications of the piggy-back technique in 1112 liver transplants. *Transplant Proc* 1999; **31**: 2388–9.
10. Cabezuelo JB, Ramirez P, Acosta F *et al.* Does the standard vs piggyback surgical technique affect the development of early acute renal failure after orthotopic liver transplantation? *Transplant Proc* 2003; **35**: 1913–4.

11. Heaton N. Small-for-size liver syndrome after auxiliary and split liver transplantation: donor selection. *Liver Transpl* 2003; **9**: S26–8.
12. Monbaliu D, Van Gelder F, Troisi R *et al.* Liver transplantation using non-heart-beating donors: Belgian experience. *Transplant Proc* 2007; **39**: 1481–4.
13. Muiesan P, Girlanda R, Jassem W *et al.* Single-center experience with liver transplantation from controlled non-heartbeating donors: a viable source of grafts. *Ann Surg* 2005; **242**: 732–8.
14. Deshpande R, Heaton N. Can non-heart-beating donors replace cadaveric heart-beating liver donors? *J Hepatol* 2006; **45**: 499–503.
15. Chan SC, Fan ST, Lo CM *et al.* Effect of side and size of graft on surgical outcomes of adult-to-adult live donor liver transplantation. *Liver Transpl* 2007; **13**: 91–8.
16. Polido WT Jr, Lee KH, Tay KH *et al.* Adult living donor liver transplantation in Singapore: the Asian centre for liver diseases and transplantation experience. *Ann Acad Med Singapore* 2007; **36**: 623–30.
17. Tucker ON, Heaton N. The 'small for size' liver syndrome. *Curr Opin Crit Care* 2005; **11**: 150–5.
18. Chan SC, Lo CM, Liu CL *et al.* Tailoring donor hepatectomy per segment 4 venous drainage in right lobe live donor liver transplantation. *Liver Transpl* 2004; **10**: 755–62.
19. Cheaito A, Craig B, Abouljoud M *et al.* Sonographic differences in venous return between piggyback versus caval interposition in adult liver transplantations. *Transplant Proc* 2006; **38**: 3588–90.
20. Chan SC, Fan ST, Lo CM *et al.* Toward current standards of donor right hepatectomy for adult-to-adult live donor liver transplantation through the experience of 200 cases. *Ann Surg* 2007; **245**: 110–17.
21. Cirrhotic cardiomyopathy: multiple reviews. *Liver Transpl* 2007; **13**: 1060–1.
22. Lee RF, Glenn TK, Lee SS. Cardiac dysfunction in cirrhosis. *Best Pract Res Clin Gastroenterol* 2007; **21**: 125–40.
23. Milani A, Zaccaria R, Bombardieri G *et al.* Cirrhotic cardiomyopathy. *Dig Liver Dis* 2007; **39**: 507–15.
24. Krowka MJ. Evolving dilemmas and management of portopulmonary hypertension. *Semin Liver Dis* 2006; **26**: 265–72.
25. Krowka MJ, Plevak D. The distinct concepts and implications of hepatopulmonary syndrome and portopulmonary hypertension. *Crit Care Med* 2005; **33**: 470.
26. Dhar R, Young GB, Marotta P. Perioperative neurological complications after liver transplantation are best predicted by pre-transplant hepatic encephalopathy. *Neurocrit Care* 2008; **8**: 253–8.
27. Saner F, Gu Y, Minouchehr S *et al.* Neurological complications after cadaveric and living donor liver transplantation. *J Neurol* 2006; **253**: 612–17.
28. Farmer DG, Venick RS, McDiarmid SV *et al.* Predictors of outcomes after pediatric liver transplantation: an analysis of more than 800 cases performed at a single institution. *J Am Coll Surg* 2007; **204**: 904–14; discussion 914–6.
29. Gonwa TA, McBride MA, Anderson K *et al.* Continued influence of preoperative renal function on outcome of orthotopic liver transplant (OLTX) in the US: where will MELD lead us? *Am J Transplant* 2006; **6**: 2651–9.
30. O'Riordan A, Wong V, McQuillan R *et al.* Acute renal disease, as defined by the RIFLE criteria, post-liver transplantation. *Am J Transplant* 2007; **7**: 168–76.
31. Perry I, Neuberger J. Immunosuppression: towards a logical approach in liver transplantation. *Clin Exp Immunol* 2005; **139**: 2–10.
32. Ruiz R, Barri YM, Jennings LW *et al.* Hepatorenal syndrome: a proposal for kidney after liver transplantation (KALT). *Liver Transpl* 2007; **13**: 838–43.
33. Ruiz R, Kunitake H, Wilkinson AH *et al.* Long-term analysis of combined liver and kidney transplantation at a single center. *Arch Surg* 2006; **141**: 735–41; discussion 741–2.
34. Biancofiore G, Bindi L, Romanelli AM *et al.* Renal failure and abdominal hypertension after liver transplantation: determination of critical intra-abdominal pressure. *Liver Transpl* 2002; **8**: 1175–81.
35. Biancofiore G, Bindi ML, Romanelli AM *et al.* Postoperative intra-abdominal pressure and renal function after liver transplantation. *Arch Surg* 2003; **138**: 703–6.
36. Fischer-Frohlich CL, Lauchart W. Expanded criteria liver donors (ECD): effect of cumulative risks. *Ann Transplant* 2006; **11**: 38–42.
37. Philpott-Howard J, Burroughs A, Fisher N *et al.* Piperacillin-tazobactam versus ciprofloxacin plus amoxicillin in the treatment of infective episodes after liver transplantation. *J Antimicrob Chemother* 2003; **52**: 993–1000.
38. Safdar N, Said A, Lucey MR. The role of selective digestive decontamination for reducing infection in patients undergoing liver transplantation: a systematic review and meta-analysis. *Liver Transpl* 2004; **10**: 817–27.
39. Cruciani M, Mengoli C, Malena M *et al.* Antifungal prophylaxis in liver transplant patients: a systematic review and meta-analysis. *Liver Transpl* 2006; **12**: 850–8.
40. Limaye AP, Bakthavatsalam R, Kim HW *et al.* Impact of cytomegalovirus in organ transplant recipients in the era of antiviral prophylaxis. *Transplantation* 2006; **81**: 1645–52.
41. Gringeri E, Vitale A, Brolese A *et al.* Hepatitis C virus-related cirrhosis as a significant mortality factor in intention-to-treat analysis in liver transplantation. *Transplant Proc* 2007; **39**: 1901–3.
42. Llado L, Xiol X, Figueras J *et al.* Immunosuppression without steroids in liver transplantation is safe and reduces infection and metabolic complications: results from a prospective multicenter randomized study. *J Hepatol* 2006; **44**: 710–6.
43. Wai CT, Lim SG, Aung MO *et al.* MARS: a futile tool in centres without active liver transplant support. *Liver Int* 2007; **27**: 69–75.
44. Schiffer E, Majno P, Mentha G *et al.* Hepatopulmonary syndrome increases the postoperative mortality rate following liver transplantation: a prospective study in 90 patients. *Am J Transplant* 2006; **6**: 1430–7.

95

Heart and lung transplantation

Cliff J Morgan

The first successful cardiac transplantation was performed at Groote Schuur, South Africa in 1967 and was followed by operations in other pioneer cardiac centres worldwide. However, it was not until the introduction of ciclosporin (cyclosporine) in 1979 that consistently improved long-term survival was achieved. To date, more than 70 000 cardiac transplantations have been performed in over 200 centres. Further improvements in immunosuppression therapy, surgical technique, detection and treatment of rejection, and general improvements in anaesthesia and postoperative care contributed to the sustained improvements, especially in centres concentrating experience and expertise above a critical mass. Typical survival figures following cardiac transplantation are in the order of 80% survival at 1 year, 70% after 5 years and 50% at 10 years.

The first successful heart and lung transplantation was performed in Stanford, USA in 1981 and was followed by successful heart–lung, single-lung and double-lung transplantations, mostly at the same centres that had led the way in cardiac transplantation.

With cardiac and lung transplantation accepted as standard treatment for a range of end-stage cardiopulmonary diseases, a large number of recipients may potentially develop critical illness, unrelated or directly related to their original condition. Around 40% of cardiac transplant recipients are readmitted to hospital within 1 year, at least a third requiring admission to intensive care units (ICUs).[1] Many of these patients present to the ICUs of non-transplant centres, especially as the number of centres performing transplantation is apparently falling. Therefore, all critical care practitioners need to be aware of the principles of management of the transplant recipient.

CARDIAC TRANSPLANTATION

The main issue with cardiac transplantation revolves around donor availability (Table 95.1). The numbers of potential recipients who fulfil internationally accepted criteria[2] (Table 95.2) vastly outnumber the available donors, so the great majority of patients with severe end-stage heart failure inevitably die before a suitable donor heart becomes available.

The cardiac equivalent of dialysis, for the maintenance of the potential renal transplant recipient until an organ is available, is simply not feasible. However, there has been progress in the medical and surgical management of severe heart failure, some of which are highly specialised treatments with limited availability and some more routine and commonplace (Table 95.3). The use of inotropic drugs such as β-agonists (e.g. dobutamine), catecholamines (e.g. epinephrine) and phosphodiesterase inhibitors (e.g. milrinone) to support the failing heart and circulation is widely practised, as is the use of intra-aortic balloon pump (IABP) counterpulsation. These treatment options are, of course, highly invasive but may be used as rescue therapy in a patient with severe or end-stage cardiac failure who may be waiting for a transplant but in whom some event such as infection of worsening myocardial ischaemia has resulted in a catastrophic deterioration. The response of the failing heart to β-agonists may be disappointing because of the tendency to β-receptor downregulation from chronic overstimulation. In these cases the phosphodiesterase inhibitor drugs such as milrinone and enoximone may have greater and more sustained potency because of their intracellular site of action.

Some patients who have been deemed inoperable in conventional terms may still benefit from cardiac surgical interventions, though in the setting of severe chronic cardiac failure the risk of death, serious morbidity and prolonged postoperative critical illness may be considered prohibitive. Sometimes a degree of reversible myocardial ischaemia may be demonstrated by thallium scanning and guide subsequent coronary artery bypass grafting. In some cases, the degree of secondary mitral valve regurgitation caused by dilatation of the left ventricle may become a haemodynamically significant lesion of itself and reconstruction of the mitral valve or remodelling of the left ventricle may prove beneficial. In extreme cases of cardiac decompensation and where other organ functions are maintained (an unusual combination) the use of mechanical assistance[4] to support the heart and buy time for a donor heart to become available ('bridge to transplant') or to provide support while a severe but temporary process (such as some viral myocarditis episodes) subsides ('bridge to recovery') may be undertaken in

Table 95.1 Illustration of the disparity between transplant operations and numbers of patients on the UK transplant registry

Organ transplanted	UK recent annual total	UK registered potential recipients
Heart	50–60	90–100
Lung	50	275
Heart and lung	5	20

Source: www.uktransplant.org.uk.

Table 95.2 Criteria to select cardiac transplant recipients

Clinical
Heart failure survival score (HFSS),[3] high risk
NYHA class III/IV heart failure refractory to maximal medical treatment
Severely limiting angina not suitable for revascularisation – surgical or medical
Recurrent symptomatic ventricular arrhythmias refractory to medical, surgical or electrophysiological treatments
Physiological
Peak oxygen consumption less than 10 ml/kg per min after reaching anaerobic threshold
Exclusion criteria
Age greater than 65 years
Transpulmonary gradient (mean PAP – mean PAOP) > 15 mmHg (2.0 kPa) or PVR > 5.0 Wood Units despite standardised reversibility testing with nitrates or inhaled nitric oxide
Insulin-dependent diabetes mellitus with end-organ dysfunction
Severe psychiatric disturbance or intellectual retardation
Current alcohol or drug abuse
Morbid obesity
Concurrent malignancy
Severe hepatic or renal disease, unrelated to cardiac disease (unless being considered for combined organ transplant)
Immunodeficiency disease
Active systemic infection

NYHA, New York Heart Association; PAOP, pulmonary artery occlusion pressure (or 'wedge' pressure); PAP, pulmonary artery pressure; PVR, pulmonary vascular resistance.

highly specialised centres. The logical conclusion is to develop permanent mechanical support devices obviating the need for transplantation but this goal appears to be a long way in the future. The cost of such therapy in both financial and human terms has to be considered in the context of general health economics. These episodes are still at best pioneering, extremely invasive, draining on the resources of critical care, blood transfusion and pharmacy, and of limited outcome benefits. On the other hand, it can be argued that earlier use of potent mechanical assistance at a stage that other organs have yet to be irretrievably damaged should be more widely attempted and, by inference, outside the major cardiac specialist centres.

DONORS AND RECIPIENTS

Most countries have seen a progressive gradual decline in the numbers of cardiac transplantations performed as a result of decreasing donor availability. Measures to optimise the donor pool for all solid organ transplants and care of potential donors are discussed elsewhere. Donor selection criteria are summarised in Table 95.4.

Matching of a potential cardiac donor with a recipient is determined by weight within 80–120% of each other, ABO blood group compatibility and negative lymphocyte crossmatch. HLA tissue type comparisons are only available after the event generally and are of prognostic and theoretical interest only.

THE TRANSPLANT PROCEDURE

The care of the cardiac transplant recipient is multifaceted and should take the following principles into account:

- General preparation of a patient (and relatives) who has suffered severe chronic illness and has been under the shadow of impending death
- Perioperative care for major cardiac surgery
- Management of specific early postoperative complications, e.g. control of rejection, containment of side-effects of immunosuppression and prompt treatment of infection
- Reintegration of the patient into society

The anaesthetic and perioperative care of these patients is not materially different from any major cardiac surgery and the important principles are well described in the literature.[11–13] However, the coordination of the timing of surgery with the arrival of the donor heart, management of the excised donor graft and the immunosuppression protocol are all crucial factors. Organ preservation after harvesting from the donor is especially important and the main factor appears to be limiting the total ischaemic time to less than 4 hours (6 hours at the extreme). The recipient may have to be called in from home and may have a full stomach. The recipient may be elated or extremely anxious, or both.

Details of perioperative care will vary from centre to centre, e.g. the timing of components of the immunosuppression regimen, exact choice of antibiotics for prophylaxis and whether or not the right internal jugular vein has to be left virgin by the anaesthetic and postoperative team so that endomyocardial biopsies may be more conveniently performed. The striking difference of the cardiac transplant recipient compared to other postoperative cardiac surgical patients is the consequences of the grafted donor heart having no nervous control. It is denervated at excision from the donor and reinnervation in the recipient does not occur.

Table 95.3 Non-transplant or bridge to transplant treatment of severe cardiac failure

Treatment modality	Notes	Applicability
Angiotensin-converting enzyme (ACE) inhibitors	Reduce cardiac work and improve output – beware exacerbation of renal failure	Ward setting to establish, then as outpatient
β-Blockers[5,6]	Improve β-receptor numbers and function	Ward setting to establish, then as outpatient
Inotropic support	Rescue therapy – rescue and restabilisation sometimes possible – requires central vascular access	CCU or ICU
Intra-aortic balloon pump counterpulsation	Rescue therapy combined with inotropes – may restabilise and thus temporary but invasive	CCU or ICU
Antiarrhythmic treatments – implantable defibrillators and advanced pacing, e.g. resynchronisation[7]	Where recurrent or severe arrhythmias threaten life or cause general destabilisations	Cardiac centre with facilities for electrophysiology
Surgical interventions	Routine (e.g. coronary artery bypass) or complex (e.g. anterior ventricular remodelling, mitral reconstruction where severe mitral regurgitation complicates cardiomyopathy)	Specialised cardiac centre
Ventricular assist devices (VAD)[8]	Short- and medium-term mechanical support for the failed heart – extremely invasive – usually holding stage or bridge to transplant	Specialised cardiac centre
Totally implanted artificial heart[9,10]	Longer term version of VAD – ultimately may be instead of transplant	Specialised cardiac centre, then possibly home

CCU, coronary care unit; ICU, intensive care unit.

Table 95.4 General criteria to select cardiac transplant donors

Age under 60 years
Brain death criteria fulfilled
Family consent obtained
Absence of infection
Absence of chest trauma
Absence of prolonged cardiac arrest
Minimal inotropic support
Viral markers (hepatitis B, C and HIV) negative
No malignancy (except primary cerebral tumour)

PHYSIOLOGY AND PHARMACOLOGY OF THE DENERVATED HEART (TABLE 95.5)

At surgery, the sinoatrial (SA) node of the recipient is retained but does not activate the grafted heart across the suture line. The donor heart has its own SA node but this is not innervated. It may be possible to discern two discrete P waves on the electrocardiogram (ECG). The donor SA node controls the graft heart rate. In the absence of autonomic innervation, only drugs or manoeuvres that act directly on the heart will have an effect. For example, the Valsalva manoeuvre or carotid sinus massage will not affect heart rate, but drugs such as adrenaline (epinephrine), noradrenaline (norepinephrine) and isoprenaline (isoproterenol) exert a positive inotropic and chronotropic effect and β-adrenergic blockers will depress myocardial function. Quinidine and digoxin will influence conductivity through their direct effects only.

The denervated heart retains its intrinsic control mechanisms,[14] e.g. a normal Frank–Starling response to volume loading, normal conductivity and intact α- and β-adrenergic receptors, possibly with enhanced responsiveness.

The coronary arteries retain their vasodilatory responsiveness to nitrates and metabolic demands. They can develop atherosclerosis in the long term, but the patient experiences no anginal pain with ischaemia or infarction because of the denervation.

Denervation results most importantly in an atypical response to exercise, hypovolaemia and hypotension. Any increase in cardiac output from increased heart rate or contractility depends on an increasing venous return and circulating catecholamines, and the response may be delayed. During exercise, muscle contraction increases venous return and the increased circulating catecholamines

Table 95.5 The pharmacology of the denervated heart

Drug	Effect on recipient	Mechanism
Digoxin	Normal increase in contractility; minimal effect on AV node	Direct myocardial effect; denervation
Adenosine	Fourfold increase in sinus and AV node blocking effect	Denervation supersensitivity
Atropine	None	Denervation
Epinephrine	Increased contractility and chronotropy	Denervation supersensitivity
Norepinephrine	Increased contractility and chronotropy	Denervation supersensitivity
Isoprenaline	Normal chronotropic effect	
Glyceryl trinitrate	No reflex tachycardia	Baroreflex disruption
Quinidine	No vagolytic effect	Denervation
Verapamil	AV block	Direct effect
Nifedipine	No reflex tachycardia	Denervation
β-Blockers	Increased antagonistic effect	Denervation
Pancuronium	No tachycardia	Denervation
Neostigmine, succinylcholine	No bradycardia	Denervation

increase the heart rate. This is a gradual response and, as exercise ceases, the heart rate and cardiac output slowly fall as the catecholamine and the response levels decrease.[15] In pathological states, the transplanted heart is especially dependent on adequate filling volumes, and attention to preload is critical.

The denervated heart is also sensitive to extremes of heart rate; arrhythmias are unusual but may cause serious haemodynamic problems. Cardiac arrhythmias can be atrial, junctional or ventricular, and may be a sign of rejection. These may resolve if the rejection is adequately treated. Occasionally, antiarrhythmic drugs that act directly on the conduction system (e.g. quinidine, disopyramide and procainamide) or electrical cardioversion are required. Verapamil and nifedipine have enhanced effects in the transplanted heart. Hypotension and bradycardia may be profound because of the absence of the normal cardiac sympathetic-mediated response to vasodilatation. Adenosine used for supraventricular tachycardias may induce asystole and cause profound hypotension in the transplanted heart. Amiodarone has been used successfully for ventricular and atrial arrhythmias, but its mild negative inotropy and vasodilatation can cause hypotension. Lidocaine is normally effective in the treatment of ventricular arrhythmias.

POSTOPERATIVE CARE

In the majority of cases the immediate postoperative course is uneventful and very similar to 'routine' cardiopulmonary bypass surgery requiring sternotomy with similar duration of postoperative ventilation and ICU length of stay, with hospital discharge being at around 10–14 days if all goes well. All the usual principles of care apply with the additional concerns regarding denervation, immunosuppression, infection, and detection and treatment of rejection.

The transplanted heart may have suffered from ischaemic damage before successful reperfusion in the recipient and may require inotropic, chronotropic or even temporary mechanical support. The severity of recipient pulmonary vascular disease may have been underestimated and even modest elevations of pulmonary vascular resistance combined with a degree of graft right ventricular myocardial dysfunction may prove troublesome or result in haemodynamic instability or catastrophic low cardiac output states. It may be necessary therefore to tide the patient over this temporary setback with a combination of various therapeutic options selected on the basis of careful clinical examination and investigation (Table 95.6). Most complex situations are assisted by or absolutely require the use of echocardiography.

IMMUNOSUPPRESSION

The details of the immunosuppression regimen will differ between transplant centres but the principles are the same.[16] Immunosuppression is induced just prior to transplantation and then maintained permanently with a combination of drugs aimed at maximal effect and minimal toxicity. Episodes of suspected or proven rejection prompt additional temporary treatment.

Since the early 1980s the regime used by most centres has been triple therapy with ciclosporin, azathioprine and corticosteroids. The initial introduction of ciclosporin in 1979 was a major step, but the drug has significant

Table 95.6 Possible support options for postoperative care of the complicated cardiac transplant recipient

Treatment	Directed at	Based on
Inotropic support, e.g. milrinone or epinephrine	Poor contractility of LV, RV or both LV and RV	Elevated filling pressures, low cardiac output, echocardiography (TTE or TOE)
Pressor support, e.g. norepinephrine	Low systemic arterial blood pressure despite adequate filling pressures and supported contractility	Arterial pressure monitoring, cardiac output and TTE or TOE
Heart rate support with chronotropic drugs (e.g. isoprenaline or milrinone) or pacing	Low intrinsic grafted heart rate	Heart rate less than 90 in the first 48 hours usually symptomatic and indication for support
Mechanical support, e.g. IABP	Poor LV function not responsive to other measures	Elevated LAP, low cardiac output, poor response to drugs, TTE or TOE
Temporary ventricular assistance – RVAD, LVAD or BiVAD	Very poor RV, LV or biventricular function	As above, no response to less invasive measures and where recovery or retransplantation may be an option
Inhaled nitric oxide	RV failure combined with reversible elevation of PVR	Filling pressures, PAP, TTE or TOE
Resternotomy	Catastrophic states where excessive bleeding or tamponade is suspected	Combination of observations but particularly TOE

IABP, intra-aortic balloon pump counterpulsation; LAP, left atrial pressure (direct or indirect); LV, left ventricle; PAP, pulmonary arterial pressure; PVR, pulmonary vascular resistance; RV, right ventricle; RVAD, LVAD, BiVAD, right, left or biventricular assist device support; TOE, transoesophageal echocardiography; TTE, transthoracic echocardiography.

problems; in addition to renal and hepatic toxicity, there is uncertain gut absorption and bioavailability (at best only 30%) which can be exacerbated by many commonly prescribed drugs.[17] Alterations in gut function may seriously reduce plasma levels to the point at which rejection may occur. Drug interactions may result in toxic levels. Plasma levels of the drug should be monitored frequently, especially in the early perioperative phase and during any complicating illness. When the gut cannot be relied upon the intravenous formulation may be used with one-third of the oral dose given by intravenous injection over 2–6 hours. Modified formulations of the drug have allegedly improved bioavailability and stability of plasma levels.[18]

Ciclosporin works through interleukin-2 (IL-2) inhibition in T lymphocytes so its action is fairly specific. Tacrolimus is an alternative to ciclosporin and has similar potency, toxicity and monitoring requirements. Azathioprine is the other commonly used drug. It has a much broader T and B lymphocyte depression effect so marrow suppression is not surprisingly a major potential side-effect. The intravenous alternative to the commonly used oral preparation is highly irritant and when the oral route is not available it is usually best omitted or an alternative used. Mycophenolate is often substituted for azathioprine. It has a much more specific effect through suppression of purine synthesis in lymphocytes, and achieves lower incidence of rejection, but at the expense of greater risk of infections.[19] Corticosteroids are very important at induction and for treatment of rejection episodes but otherwise the dose is tapered to minimise all the usual steroid side-effects.

Immunological treatment with antithymocyte globulin (ATG) derived from various species was traditionally reserved for the treatment of rejection episodes but newer monoclonal ATG-type drugs[20] may prove more effective and less allergenic. Newer approaches with the promise of greater specificity and lower toxicity include agents such as daclizumab[21] which appears to reduce episodes of rejection, but so far no convincing evidence of improved survival. The complexity of these issues makes it vital that all relevant treatment decisions are made by, or discussed with, the relevant transplant centre.

REJECTION

One or more episodes of rejection are experienced by the majority of recipients within the first 3 months after transplantation. The risk is subsequently negligible in successful grafts. The diagnosis may be suggested on clinical grounds but the gold standard remains histological examination of an endomyocardial biopsy. In some centres biopsies are performed on a routine basis, as well as when rejection is suspected. The right internal jugular vein is the preferred vascular access site for performing the biopsy so this should be considered when selecting line sites for general critical care purposes. The clinical indications or suggestions of rejection are very non-specific and include dyspnoea, weight gain, malaise, atrial arrhythmias, low voltage ECG and echocardiographic evidence of declining cardiac function. The biopsy is graded according to an internationally accepted system, but some centres have moved to a more algorithm-based approach to the patient where clinical features and monitoring of the immune response help to determine the frequency of biopsies.[22,23]

OTHER COMPLICATIONS

The other main complications include infection, malignancy and graft atherosclerosis or cardiac allograft vasculopathy (CAV).

Infection

Opportunistic infections (commonly lung) account for many of the complications and for a significant proportion of readmissions. A recent study reported that 45% of infections were bacterial and less than 10% fungal; however, the associated mortalities were 40% for fungal and less than 10% for bacterial infections.[24] Opinions vary as to the current significance of cytomegalovirus (CMV) infection. Some centres believe that CMV is a problem of the past because of better matching of CMV status, and more effective and potent prophylaxis and treatment with ganciclovir when indicated.[25] However, there is still significant risk of severe acute viral illness,[26] and a possible link between acute viraemic episodes and subsequent damage to the graft and CAV.[27]

Malignancy

The transplant recipient has a hundredfold increased risk of new malignancy (around 1–2% per year) compared to age-matched controls. The majority are skin tumours (with substantially increased susceptibility to solar radiation) and lymphomas but any neoplasm may occur. Malignancy is one of the leading causes of death or late readmission to hospital and the risk of subsequent malignancy is a significant and complex factor in the selection of optimum immunosuppression.[28]

Cardiac allograft vasculopathy (CAV)

This is the main cause of death in the long term after heart transplantation and is a multifactorial process resulting in diffuse obliterative coronary atherosclerosis.[29] The diffuse nature of the lesions makes revascularisation by angioplasty and stent, or by surgical bypass, difficult. Perhaps improvements in the control of rejection, management of CMV and drugs such as statins, calcium channel blockers and specific growth regulatory factors such as hepatocyte growth factor[30] may help.

HEART–LUNG TRANSPLANTATION

The first heart–lung transplant (HLT) was performed in Stanford in 1981. HLT was then performed for both parenchymal lung disease and pulmonary hypertension. With the advent of single- or double-lung transplantations, there is overlap between indications for these procedures. The present indications for HLT are primary pulmonary hypertension, Eisenmenger's syndrome, end-stage suppurative pulmonary disease or end-stage bilateral lung disease associated with significant cardiac failure, generally right ventricular failure.

Table 95.7 Heart–lung transplantation: donor selection criteria

Age and ABO blood group compatibility as per heart donors
Close size match of donor to recipient to avoid lung restriction (donor lung too big) or persistent residual space between lung and chest wall (donor lung too small)
Donor Pa_{O_2} > 100 mmHg (13.3 kPa) on Fi_{O_2} = 0.3 or > 300 mmHg (39.9 kPa) on Fi_{O_2} = 1.0
Normal chest X-ray

SELECTION CRITERIA (TABLE 95.7)

These are similar to those for heart transplantation, except that an elevated pulmonary vascular resistance tips clinical judgement towards HLT. Exclusion criteria for recipients are also similar but probably should include a stricter age limit (i.e. 45 years), high-dose corticosteroid therapy (relative contraindication), active bronchopulmonary fungal disease, and prior sternotomy, thoracotomy or mediastinal irradiation.

THE TRANSPLANT PROCEDURE

Heart–lung transplantation is by any definition a massive procedure. The combination of cardiopulmonary bypass with full anticoagulation and significant likelihood of pleural adhesions tethering the explanted lungs to the chest wall make for a substantial risk of major intraoperative haemorrhage and this may continue into the postoperative phase. Preservation of nerves such as the vagus, phrenic and recurrent laryngeal may be difficult and result in significant morbidity when unsuccessful.

POSTOPERATIVE CARE

This is similar to that for cardiac transplant patients, with some differences. The patient is without a bronchial arterial supply or pulmonary innervation. Lymphatic drainage of the lungs is lost. Thus patients are kept in a negative fluid balance in the early postoperative period. Active physiotherapy is required, sometimes with bronchoscopic toilet to clear secretions, as denervation prevents reflex coughing of secretions below the anastomosis (usually at around five tracheal rings above the carina). Once secretions reach the native trachea, coughing may result. Immunosuppression is given as for cardiac transplantation. Antibiotic prophylaxis will depend on local policies and results of cultures of recipient and donor sputum or secretions. Rejection is more likely to manifest first in the lungs rather than the heart graft so rejection surveillance includes frequent reassessment of pulmonary status, possibly with transbronchial biopsies.

COMPLICATIONS

Bleeding may occur due to extensive dissection and systemic pulmonary collaterals in congenital heart disease. Other early complications include tracheal anastomotic dehiscence, acute reperfusion lung injury (i.e. pulmonary oedema) due to long ischaemic times and infection. Heart–lung recipients have three times as many infections as heart recipients, and this contributes significantly to their higher mortality rate. Infection is the major cause of mortality in the first 6 months, and rejection thereafter.

IMMUNOSUPPRESSION

This is very similar to that used in heart transplantation, and also similar in single- and double-lung transplantation.

SINGLE- OR DOUBLE-LUNG TRANSPLANTATION

Early attempts at single-lung transplantation (SLT) yielded only short-term survival.[31] However, subsequent successes by the Toronto Group encouraged the development of double-lung transplantation,[32] initially by the en bloc method with tracheal anastomosis. The extensive dissection required in the recipient and the high incidence of anastomotic problems encouraged development of bilateral sequential lung transplantation (BSLT), which has found wide favour.[33] SLT is indicated for non-suppurative lung disease in a patient who does not have cardiac disease (e.g. emphysema from smoking or α_1-antitrypsin deficiency, or fibrosing alveolitis). Whilst these conditions can also be managed by BLST, SLT provides satisfactory results and makes more efficient use of a limited donor pool. BSLT is indicated for suppurative and/or bilateral lung disease (e.g. cystic fibrosis and bilateral bronchiectasis). The merits of BSLT or HLT for these conditions are controversial. With HLT, the recipient's heart may be used in a 'domino' procedure as a donor heart for a second recipient.[34] Either BLST or a domino HLT allows the most efficient use of donor organs. Lung transplantation can be combined with kidney or liver transplantation.

Recipients are accepted for lung transplantation up to age 55 years. It is usually possible to perform SLT without cardiopulmonary bypass (CPB). The requirement for CPB is higher in BSLT (approximately 5–10%) because the first lung transplanted (usually the right) must immediately provide ventilation and gas exchange whilst the other side is transplanted. CPB increases the amount of operative blood loss and the volume of colloid required in the postoperative period. The incidence of non-cardiogenic pulmonary oedema is also increased.

PHYSIOLOGY OF THE DENERVATED LUNGS

The lungs appear to remain permanently denervated. There is evidence that the bronchial artery circulation and lymphatic system regenerate after several weeks. Control of respiration is not affected by the loss of pulmonary afferent nerves. Regulation of breathing is through chest wall afferents. Patients regain spontaneous breathing early, and are usually able to be weaned off ventilation and extubated within 48 hours.

Patients who were dependent on their hypoxic drive may take time to achieve normocarbia. Arterial blood gases otherwise tend to remain normal. On exercise, minute volume, tidal volume and respiratory rate are able to increase appropriately. Bronchomotor tone is retained. The cough response is lost below the anastomosis.

POSTOPERATIVE CARE

Patients require a period of postoperative ventilation for reasons similar to all major pulmonary surgery. However, there are additional concerns regarding the temporary lung injury which almost inevitably results from the procedure, and the worry that this injury may be compounded by infection, overgenerous fluid therapy, pulmonary oxygen toxicity and barotrauma or 'volutrauma' from injudicious ventilator settings. Some degree of impaired gas transfer or widened alveolar to arterial oxygen tension gradient $(A–a)DO_2$ is very common and may further widen as a result of the following complications.

IMPLANTATION RESPONSE

This manifests within a few hours. Infiltrates in the transplanted lung or lungs appear on chest X-ray, and the lungs may appear to be oedematous with increased peribronchial cuffing. In severe cases, a picture suggestive of severe acute respiratory distress syndrome is seen with widespread loss of translucency. There is an association between ischaemic time and the severity of the response. Management is supportive with fluid restriction if tolerated.

HYPERACUTE REJECTION

This is fortunately rare. It usually results in acute graft failure with a very poor prognosis for recovery of function. Management requires continued respiratory support and consideration of retransplantation.

EARLY REJECTION

Episodes of rejection of the transplanted lung occur in almost all recipients in the first 3 months, but may occur very early in some recipients. Deterioration in PaO_2 and pulmonary infiltrates after 48–72 hours should favour a suspicion of rejection rather than implantation response. It may be difficult to distinguish between early rejection and bacterial infection. Bronchoscopic washings may be helpful and transbronchial biopsy is essential in doubtful cases. In suspicious cases, a course of pulsed steroids is appropriate with concurrent antibiotics.

SPUTUM RETENTION

Effective analgesia, aggressive physiotherapy and early mobilisation are essential to minimise this problem. Secretions below the anastomoses do not elicit a cough reflex and voluntary coughing is important.

PULMONARY INFECTION

Early pulmonary bacterial infection is common, and infection with other micro-organisms can occur later. Initially, bronchitis is more common than pneumonia. Patients with resident micro-organisms are given prophylactic antibiotics. Samples of the donor's pulmonary secretions are taken at the time of lung harvesting and may be useful in guiding the selection of antibiotics.

ANASTOMOTIC PROBLEMS

Ischaemic anastomotic ulceration is usually superficial, but occasionally deeper tissue loss eventually produces bronchial or tracheal stenosis requiring dilatation and/or stent insertion in the early months. Anastomotic dehiscence is rare but often fatal. It may be preceded by fungal invasion of the anastomosis. Fibreoptic bronchoscopy to inspect the anastomoses and remove residual secretions is performed at the conclusion of surgery or after return to the ICU. This is repeated as indicated.

LONG-TERM COMPLICATIONS

Obliterative bronchiolitis[35] which may be a manifestation of chronic rejection may eventually lead to graft failure. Recurrent infections with *Pseudomonas* or methicillin-resistant *Staphylococcus* can be serious. After the first 6 weeks, infection with CMV, any fungus, protozoan or virus presents potential hazards. Chronic renal failure due to ciclosporin therapy may persist, but is not usually a major problem unless other complications occur. Most patients have a good quality of life with few complications. The improvement in quality of life after lung transplantation may be more important as a marker of success than bald survival figures.[36]

RESULTS OF CARDIOPULMONARY TRANSPLANTATION

A very good source of information on the results of intrathoracic transplantation can be found at www.ishlt.org and in more traditional publications[37] such as the recent summary of results of transplantation in the UK.[38] These figures indicate that survival is considerably better after heart transplantation than heart–lung or lung. Almost 90% of heart recipients are alive at 3 months as compared to around 75% of heart–lung and lung recipients. Around 70% of heart recipients are still alive after 5 years; 50% or less of heart–lung and lung recipients survive this long. While these figures are quite impressive and could improve with current trends in immunosuppression and general care, the main issue remains the gross disparity between the number of patients with end-stage cardiopulmonary disease and the ever-shrinking supply of donor organs. This is all the more reason to ensure that those patients who have got as far as to benefit from such a rare and precious opportunity receive high standards of medical care throughout their remaining life.

REFERENCES

1. Brann WM, Bennett LE, Kekck BM *et al.* Morbidity, functional status, and immunosuppressive therapy after heart transplantation: an analysis of the Joint International Society for Heart and Lung Transplantation/ United Network for Organ Sharing Thoracic Registry. *J Heart Lung Transplant* 1998; **17**: 374–82.
2. Hunt SA. 24th Bethesda conference: cardiac transplantation. *J Am Coll Cardiol* 1993; **22**(Suppl 1): 1–64.
3. Aaronson KD, Schwartz JS, Chen TMC *et al.* Development and prospective validation of a clinical index to predict survival in ambulatory patients referred for cardiac transplant evaluation. *Circulation* 1997; **95**: 2660–7.
4. Glenn E, Hill DJ. Advances in mechanical bridge to heart transplantation. *Curr Opin Organ Transplant* 2000; **5**: 126–39.
5. Barnett DB. Beta blockers in heart failure: a therapeutic paradox. *Lancet* 1994; **343**: 557–8.
6. Packer M, Coats AJ, Fowler MB *et al.* Carvedilol prospective randomized cumulative survival study group. Effect of carvedilol on survival in severe chronic heart failure. *N Engl J Med* 2001; **344**: 1651–8.
7. Wasson S, Voelker DJ, Vesom P *et al.* Cardiac resynchronization therapy for CHF. *Postgrad Med* 2006; **119**: 25–9.
8. Rose EA, Gelinjns AC, Moskowitz AJ *et al.* for the REMATCH Study Group. Long-term use of a left ventricular assist device for end-stage heart failure. *N Engl J Med* 2001; **345**: 1435–43.
9. Pennington DG, Oaks TE, Lohmann DP. Permanent ventricular assist device support versus cardiac transplantation. *Ann Thorac Surg* 1999; **68**: 729–33.
10. Stevenson LW, Shekar P. Ventricular assist devices for durable support. *Circulation* 2005; **112**: 111–15.
11. Clark NJ, Martin RD. Anesthetic considerations for patients undergoing cardiac transplantation. *J Cardiothorac Anaesth* 1988; **2**: 519–42.
12. Stein KL, Darby JM, Grenvic A. Intensive care of the cardiac transplant recipient. *J Cardiothorac Anesth* 1988; **2**: 543–53.
13. Cooper DKC, Lidsky NM. Immediate postoperative care and potential complication. In: Cooper DKC, Miller LW, Patterson GA (eds) *The Transplantation and Replacement of Thoracic Organs.* Dordrecht: Kluwer; 1996: 221–8.
14. Borow KM, Neumann A, Arensman FW *et al.* Cardiac and peripheral vascular responses to adrenoreceptor stimulation and blockade after cardiac transplantation. *J Am Coll Cardiol* 1989; **14**: 1229–38.
15. Pope SE, Stinson EB, Daughters CT *et al.* Exercise response of the denervated heart in long term cardiac transplant recipients. *Am J Cardiol* 1980; **46**: 213–8.
16. Hosenpud JD. Immunosuppression in cardiac transplantation. *N Engl J Med* 2005; **352**: 2749–50.

17. Aziz T, El-Gamel A, Keevil B *et al.* Clinical impact of Neoral in thoracic organ transplantation. *Transplant Proc* 1998; **30**: 1900–3.
18. Cooney GF, Jeevanandam V, Choudhury S *et al.* Comparative bioavailability of Neoral and Sandimmune in cardiac transplant recipients over 1 year. *Transplant Proc* 1998; **30**: 1892–4.
19. Kabashigawa J, Miller L, Renlund D *et al.* A randomized controlled trial of mycophenolate mofetil in heart transplant recipients. Mycophenolate Mofetil Investigators. *Transplantation* 1998; **66**: 507–15.
20. Beniaminovitz A, Itescu S, Lietz K *et al.* Prevention of rejection in cardiac transplantation by blockade of the interleukin-2 receptor with a monoclonal antibody. *N Engl J Med* 2000; **342**: 613–9.
21. Hershberger RE, Startling RC, Eisen HJ *et al.* Daclizumab to prevent rejection after cardiac transplantation. *N Engl J Med* 2005; **352**: 2705–13.
22. Billingham ME, Cary NRB, Hammond ME *et al.* A working group for the standardisation of nomenclature in the diagnosis of heart and lung rejection; Heart Study Group. *J Heart Lung Transplant* 1990; **9**: 587–93.
23. Itescu S, Tung TC, Burke EM *et al.* An immunological algorithm to predict risk of high-grade rejection in cardiac transplant recipients. *Lancet* 1998; **352**: 263–70.
24. Aziz T, El-Gamel A, Krysiak P *et al.* Risk factors for early mortality, acute rejection, and factors affecting first-year survival after heart transplantation. *Transplant Proc* 1998; **30**: 1912–4.
25. Vuylsteke A, Wallwork J. The heart-transplanted patient in the intensive care unit: last news before the millennium. *Curr Opin Critical Care* 1999; **5**: 422–6.
26. Singh N. Infections in solid organ transplant recipients. *Curr Opin Infect Dis.* 1998; **11**: 411–7.
27. Valantine HA. Cytomegalovirus infection and allograft injury. *Curr Opin Organ Transplant* 2001; **6**: 305–9.
28. O'Neill JO, Edwards LB, Taylor DO. Mycophenolate mofetil and risk of developing malignancy after orthotopic heart transplantation: analysis of the transplant registry of the International Society for Heart and Lung Transplantation. *J Heart Lung Transplant* 2006; **25**: 1186–91.
29. Ramzy D, Rao V, Brahm J *et al.* Cardiac allograft vasculopathy: a review. *Can J Surg* 2005; **48**: 319–27.
30. Yamaura K, Ito K, Tsukioka K *et al.* Suppression of acute and chronic rejection by hepatocyte growth factor in a murine model of cardiac transplantation – induction of tolerance and prevention of cardiac allograft vasculopathy. *Circulation* 2004; **110**: 1650–7.
31. Derom F, Barbier F, Ringoir S *et al.* Ten-month survival after lung homotransplantation in man. *J Thorac Cardiovasc Surg* 1971; **61**: 835–46.
32. Toronto Lung Transplant Group. Unilateral lung transplantation for pulmonary fibrosis. *N Engl J Med* 1986; **314**: 1140–5.
33. Kaiser LR, Pasque MK, Trulock EP *et al.* Bilateral sequential lung transplantation: the procedure of choice for double lung replacement. *Ann Thorac Surg* 1991; **52**: 438–46.
34. Yacoub MH, Banner NR, Khaghani A *et al.* Heart–lung transplantation for cystic fibrosis and subsequent domino heart transplantation. *J Heart Transplant* 1990; **9**: 459–66.
35. de Hoyos AL, Patterson GA, Maurer JR *et al.* Pulmonary transplantation. Early and late results. *J Thorac Cardiovasc Surg* 1992; **103**: 295–306.
36. Anyanwu AC, McGuire A, Rogers CA *et al.* Assessment of quality of life in lung transplantation using a simple generic tool. *Thorax* 2001; **56**: 218–22.
37. ISHLT. The registry of the International Society for Heart and Lung Transplantation: Twenty third annual report. *J Heart Lung Transplant* 2006; **25**: 869–911.
38. Anyanwu AC, Rogers CA, Murday AJ *et al.* Intrathoracic organ transplantation in the United Kingdom 1995 to 1999; results from the UK cardiothoracic transplant audit. *Heart* 2002; **87**: 449–54.

Part Seventeen

Paediatric Intensive Care

96

The critically ill child

Alan W Duncan

The chapters on paediatric intensive care are intended to help intensivists outside specialised paediatric centres manage common paediatric emergencies. They should be read in conjunction with relevant adult chapters, as there are areas of common interest. Some common neonatal emergencies are also presented.

The differences between neonates and infants from adults render them susceptible to critical illness and alter their response to disease processes. Nevertheless, there are also similarities and many aspects of organ monitoring and support in adult intensive care units (ICUs) have been successfully modified for use in children and are applicable to even the smallest infants.

The major differences between paediatric and adult patients are described below.

ADAPTATION

Dramatic physiological adaptation takes place as the fetus adjusts to extrauterine life. Many changes are incomplete until some time after birth and, until then, reversion to fetal physiology may occur. Classically, this applies to the cardiorespiratory events at birth and the subsequent development of a transitional pattern of circulation (see below).

GROWTH AND DEVELOPMENT

There is progressive growth and development of all organ systems throughout childhood. 'Small-body technology' has evolved to cope with the technical aspects of paediatric critical care. Some aspects of growth are non-linear and contribute to the reduced cardiorespiratory reserve of the infant. Physiological differences that influence disease processes and their management are discussed in respective chapters in this section.

MATURATION

At birth, the immaturity of many systems and biochemical processes alters the response to pathophysiological stress and drugs. Thermoregulation, immune function and renal function are immature at birth, even in the full-term infant. Such immaturity is magnified in the premature infant; for example, surfactant deficiency in the lung causing hyaline membrane disease and liver glucuronyl transferase deficiency causing jaundice.

DIVERSE PATHOPHYSIOLOGICAL STATES

Developmental anomalies, inborn errors of metabolism, susceptibility to infection and various accidents and trauma provide a wide spectrum of paediatric critical illnesses. The response to these illnesses is modified by various aspects of adaptation, growth and development and maturation.

PAEDIATRIC INTENSIVE CARE

The development of separate paediatric ICUs recognised the unique problems and requirements of critically ill children. The paediatric ICU (PICU) should not be seen in isolation, but as part of a tertiary paediatric centre, with well-defined prehospital care, emergency medical services and retrieval teams. Minimum standards should be adopted. In general, a PICU should provide:

- a specialist trained in paediatric intensive care available at short notice
- a range of paediatric subspecialty support
- immediately available junior medical staff with advanced life support skills
- nursing staff with experience in paediatric intensive care
- allied health professionals and ancillary support staff
- specialised advanced life support equipment for children ranging in age from neonates to adolescents
- 24-hour laboratory, radiological and pharmacy services
- purpose-built PICU, recognising the special physical and emotional needs of critically ill children and their families
- a programme for teaching, continuing education, research and quality assurance

Neonatal ICUs have their own particular requirements.

CARDIORESPIRATORY EVENTS AT BIRTH

During intrauterine life, 60% of blood returning to the right atrium passes directly through the foramen ovale into the left ventricle and ascending aorta. As most of this blood is from the umbilical arteries, the heart and brain are perfused with better-oxygenated blood. Pulmonary vascular resistance (PVR) is high and most of the blood reaching the right ventricle passes through the ductus arteriosus to the descending aorta. Only 10% of right ventricle output passes to the lungs which, although non-functional, require a blood supply for nutrition, growth and development of the lung vasculature.

At birth, closure of the umbilical vessels increases systemic vascular resistance (SVR) and lung expansion leads to the dramatic fall in PVR. Pulmonary blood flow increases, leading to a rise in left atrial pressure and functional closure of the foramen ovale. The ductus arteriosus subsequently constricts and eventually thromboses.

Following the dramatic fall in PVR at birth, there is a gradual regression in muscularisation of the pulmonary arterioles over the following weeks to months. This regression is prevented if high pulmonary blood flow occurs, due to congenital heart lesions (e.g. ventricular septal defect, large patent ductus arteriosus and truncus arteriosus) or lesions associated with persistent hypoxaemia (e.g. transposition of great vessels). With these lesions, progression to irreversible pulmonary vascular disease may occur at an early age.

TRANSITIONAL CIRCULATION

Haemodynamic adaptation at birth may be delayed or reversed by a number of factors. Persistent pulmonary hypertension and patency of the fetal channels result in right-to-left shunting through the foramen ovale and ductus arteriosus (termed persistent fetal circulation or more correctly transitional circulation). A vicious cycle may develop, with increasing hypoxaemia and acidosis, increased PVR and further shunting. Unless the underlying disturbance is treated and the pulmonary hypertension is corrected, progression to death is likely. Pulmonary circulation pathophysiology is probably related to abnormalities of endogenous nitric oxide production and manipulation of this agent is proving useful in therapy.

CAUSES OF TRANSITIONAL CIRCULATION

A 'fetal' pattern may persist due to:

- low lung volume states (e.g. hyaline membrane disease and perinatal asphyxia)
- pulmonary hypoplasia (e.g. diaphragmatic hernia and Potter's syndrome)
- meconium aspiration syndrome
- chronic placental insufficiency
- perinatal hypoxia and acidosis from any cause
- sepsis (e.g. group B streptococcal infection)
- hyperviscosity syndrome

CLINICAL FEATURES

Hypoxaemia disproportional to the degree of respiratory distress is typical of transitional circulation and suggests the possibility of congenital cyanotic heart disease. In cases without significant lung disease, echocardiography may be necessary to exclude a structural cardiac lesion. Severe respiratory distress is present in cases secondary to pulmonary disease. Differential cyanosis (i.e. increased cyanosis affecting the lower limbs when compared with the head, neck and right arm) may be seen with the right-to-left shunting at ductal level. This may be confirmed by simultaneous pre- and postductal arterial blood sampling, transcutaneous $P\text{O}_2$ monitoring or oximetry.

TREATMENT

It is important to treat the underlying cause (e.g. surfactant therapy for hyaline membrane disease) in addition to therapy to reduce PVR. The main steps employed are:

- maintenance of high inspired oxygen. Alveolar oxygen tension is an important determinant of pulmonary arteriolar resistance. Sudden reductions in inspired oxygen may increase shunting through fetal channels (so-called flip-flop phenomenon)
- correction of low lung volume states with continuous positive airway pressure (CPAP) or positive-pressure ventilation with positive end-expiratory pressure (PEEP)
- correction of both metabolic and respiratory acidosis
- deliberate hyperventilation using muscle relaxants to lower $P_a\text{CO}_2$ and generate a respiratory alkalosis. This manoeuvre is limited by lung immaturity and risk of barotrauma. Rapid rates of ventilation (> 60 breaths/min) may prove beneficial
- maintenance of systemic arterial pressure with volume expanders and inotropic agents to reduce the pressure gradient favouring ductal shunting
- isovolaemic haemodilution with colloid, if indicated, to reduce hyperviscosity
- administration of pulmonary vasodilators, e.g. inhaled nitric oxide[1]

Many centres successfully employ extracorporeal membrane oxygenation (ECMO) in this situation.

THERMOREGULATION IN THE NEWBORN

Human body temperature is maintained within narrow limits. This is achieved most easily in the thermoneutral zone – the range of ambient temperature within which the metabolic rate is at a minimum. Once ambient temperature is outside the thermoneutral zone, heat production (shivering or non-shivering thermogenesis) or evaporative heat loss processes are required to maintain body temperature within normal limits. Regulatory mechanisms are less effective in the neonate (there is no shivering or sweating), who is otherwise disadvantaged by a high surface area to body weight ratio and lack of subcutaneous tissue.

The thermoneutral zone is higher in premature infants and falls with increasing postnatal age. Oxygen consumption is minimal, with an environmental or abdominal skin temperature of 36.5 °C. Oxidation of brown fat found in the interscapular and perirenal areas (non-shivering thermogenesis) is the major source of heat production when 'cold-stressed'.

Alteration of body temperature above or below normal leads to increased or decreased metabolism respectively. Attempts by the body to maintain body temperature within normal limits are associated with increased metabolism and cardiorespiratory demands. Radiation is a major source of heat loss in the neonate and is effectively minimised by double-walled incubators or by servo-controlled radiant heaters. The latter allows better access to critically ill babies for monitoring and procedures. Cold stress per se increases neonatal mortality. In the presence of respiratory or cardiac disease, it may lead to decompensation.

IMMUNOLOGY OF THE INFANT

The immunological system consists of:

- non-specific mechanisms, including phagocytosis and the inflammatory response
- specific immune responses, consisting of cell-mediated (T-cell) and humoral (B-cell) systems (see Chapter 59). These two components are intimately related and both may be abnormal in the newborn infant

The inflammatory response of the newborn is attenuated. Febrile response to infection may be lacking and both cellular (chemotaxis and phagocytosis) and humoral (complement activity and opsonisation) responses may be impaired. Cell-mediated immunity is completely absent in infants born without thymic function (DiGeorge syndrome). In the normal newborn, however, T-cell function appears to be quite well developed. Rejection of skin allografts is slower in the newborn but this seems to be related mainly to the attenuated inflammatory response.

The B-cell system, responsible for antibody production, is immature at birth. The neonate has passive immunity against some infections because of transplacental transfer of maternal antibodies. Natural immunity is acquired as a result of immunoglobulin A (IgA) in breast milk and protects against some acquired gastrointestinal infections. Overall, the immaturity and inexperience of the immune system result in a markedly increased susceptibility to infection in the first 6 months of life.

RESUSCITATION OF THE NEWBORN

Some newborn infants fail to adapt from fetal to extrauterine life and require immediate cardiopulmonary and cerebral resuscitation. The Apgar scoring system (Table 96.1) scored after 1 minute, remains the most widely accepted method of assessment. The best Apgar score is 10 and the worst is 0. There is an inverse relationship between the Apgar score and the degree of hypoxia and acidosis. It has been suggested that the 5-minute score is a guide to ultimate prognosis but this is questioned. Collection of sequential scores must not delay the institution of resuscitation.

BIRTH ASPHYXIA

The causes of birth asphyxia may be:

- placental failure – acute or chronic (e.g. toxaemia, diabetes and antepartum haemorrhage)
- drug depression due to maternal analgesics or sedatives administered immediately prior to delivery
- obstetric complications (e.g. difficult forceps, breech, caesarean section and prolapsed cord)
- fetal conditions (e.g. multiple births and prematurity)
- postnatal problems (e.g. respiratory distress immediately after birth from any cause)

MANAGEMENT

The principles of resuscitation are identical to those employed in other situations. Resuscitation must be started immediately after delivery. Although some cerebral insult may have occurred in utero or intrapartum, secondary insults from postpartum asphyxia must be avoided.

Babies suffering mild asphyxia immediately before birth with Apgar scores between 5 and 7 usually respond to stimulation and gentle suction to the nose, mouth

Table 96.1 Apgar scoring system

Score	0	1	2
Heart rate	Absent	< 100 beats/min	> 100 beats/min
Respiratory effort	Absent	Weak cry	Strong cry
Muscle tone	Limp	Some flexion	Active motion
Reflex irritability (in response to catheter in nose)	No response	Grimace	Grimace and cough or sneeze
Colour	Blue, pale	Body pink, extremities blue	Pink

and pharynx although oxygen therapy is occasionally required. Babies with moderate asphyxia (Apgar 3–4) usually respond to bag-and-mask ventilation with oxygen. Acid–base status should be determined and sodium bicarbonate administered to restore pH > 7.25. Severely asphyxiated infants (Apgar 0–2) need urgent cardiopulmonary resuscitation (CPR). After airway suction, bag-and-mask ventilation should be followed by rapid orotracheal intubation and positive-pressure ventilation with oxygen. Fear of complications of oxygen therapy must not mitigate against the administration of 100% oxygen at this stage. If the liquor contains thick meconium, it is vital that the pharynx and trachea be suctioned prior to the onset of respiration or application of positive pressure. Meconium aspiration syndrome is a preventable condition that is often difficult to manage.

Venous access via umbilical or peripheral veins must be established immediately and followed by the administration of 1–2 mmol/kg of sodium bicarbonate. Subsequent buffer therapy should be based on arterial acid–base status if available. Rapid or excessive infusions of hypertonic solutions (e.g. sodium bicarbonate or hypertonic dextrose) or volume expanders may precipitate intracranial haemorrhage, particularly in premature infants.

Asphyxiated infants are usually volume-depleted at birth and blood pressure should be immediately restored with colloids (10 ml/kg in the first instance). External cardiac massage and additional drug therapy (see below) should be employed, if necessary, to restore cardiac rhythm. Postresuscitative care to maintain cerebral perfusion pressure, correct abnormal serum biochemistry and control seizures is required to prevent secondary cerebral insults. Myocardial dysfunction may occur secondary to asphyxia. Dopamine or dobutamine (5–10 μg/kg per min) may prove useful.

The orotracheal tube should be changed to nasotracheal to enable secure fixation once a degree of stability is attained. Radiological confirmation of tube position should be made as soon as possible. The trachea is very short in the newborn and endobronchial intubation is a particular risk.

Approximate nose to mid-trachea (T2) distances are:

- 28 weeks' gestation: 7 cm
- 33 weeks' gestation: 9 cm
- term infant: 10.5 cm

CARDIORESPIRATORY ARREST IN CHILDREN

The vast majority of children lack intrinsic myocardial disease and when cardiac arrest occurs, it is usually the end result of hypoxaemia and acidosis. The most common predisposing causes are rapidly progressive upper-airway obstruction, near drowning, sudden infant death syndrome, pneumonia, sepsis, gastroenteritis and major trauma. Such children invariably arrest in asystole and this should be assumed if an electrocardiogram (ECG) is not immediately available.

Ventricular fibrillation (VF) may be anticipated in the following situations:

- congenital heart disease
- cardiomyopathies
- myocarditis
- poisoning (e.g. tricyclic antidepressant ingestion)
- hereditary prolongation of QT interval (Romano–Ward syndrome)

The International Liaison Committee on Resuscitation (ILCOR) has developed a consensus statement detailing the science underpinning paediatric and neonatal basic and advanced life support.[2] The management of paediatric cardiopulmonary resuscitation is discussed in detail elsewhere in this volume.

VASCULAR ACCESS

Venous access may be difficult, particularly in the collapsed, hypovolaemic or hypothermic child. The external jugular vein may be prominent when usual sites are inaccessible. Cannulation of central veins, apart from via the femoral and external jugular veins, is hazardous even in ideal situations and should not be attempted during cardiac arrest in small children and babies. Two may be considered: intraosseous access or endotracheal instillation.

INTRAOSSEOUS ACCESS[3]

This involves infusion into bone marrow – a non-collapsible venous system in direct communication with the circulation. In dog experiments, drugs infused in this way reach the central circulation as rapidly as those injected into a central vein. The effect of equal doses of adrenaline (epinephrine) given by intraosseous and i.v. routes is identical in shocked dogs. The technique is simple and quick to learn.

Intraosseous infusion has been successfully used in CPR.[4]

Potential complications include:

- osteomyelitis: conventional venous access should be established after resuscitation
- compartment syndromes requiring limb amputation: these have resulted from needle misplacement in muscle or administration of fluids into muscle through another bone perforation[5]

Careful placement is essential, and close observation of the limb and early removal once alternative access is achieved are recommended.

ENDOTRACHEAL INSTILLATION

Endotracheal instillation is, at best, a poor substitute for the above methods. Do not use bicarbonate and calcium as they will cause direct lung damage and cannot be administered by this route.

Epinephrine, lidocaine and atropine may be diluted in saline (newborn 1 ml, infants and preschool children 3 ml, older children 5 ml) and delivered into the bronchi through a catheter passed down the endotracheal tube.

PAEDIATRIC MONITORING

Technology has allowed most aspects of adult monitoring to be applied to neonatal and paediatric practice. The ideal paediatric haemodynamic and respiratory monitoring system should:

- be non-invasive, painless and readily interfaced with the child
- constitute minimal risk to the child
- provide specific data relevant to the child's status that are reproducible and readily understood
- respond rapidly to changes in status
- provide continuous visual and/or auditory display of data
- have appropriate alarms
- have facilities for recording data
- be inexpensive and require low maintenance

ARTERIAL CANNULATION AND PRESSURE MONITORING

Arterial cannulation is routine practice in paediatric intensive care, even in infants weighing < 1 kg. It is indicated in all critically ill infants for continuous blood pressure monitoring and accurate blood gas sampling. In the neonate, difficult 'stabs' may lead to significant errors in $Pa\text{O}_2$ and $Pa\text{CO}_2$. Umbilical arterial catheters are commonly used in newborn infants, although users must be aware of the potential vaso-occlusive complications (e.g. lower limb ischaemia, renal thrombosis, necrotising enterocolitis and rarely, paraplegia).

Peripheral arteries used include radial, ulnar, brachial, femoral, posterior tibial and dorsalis pedis. Radial and ulnar or posterior tibial and dorsalis pedis vessels must never be cannulated sequentially in the same limb. The safety of brachial and femoral cannulation lies in the presence of rich collateral vessels around the elbow and hip joints. Arterial lines are kept patent by continuous flushing with 1–2 ml/hour of heparinised normal saline (5 units heparin/ml flushing solution) or 5% dextrose. Complications include distal ischaemia, infection, retrograde embolisation and haemorrhage. Retrograde embolisation occurring with flushing is a particular risk in the small infant, depending on the length and volume of the vessel and volume and speed of injection. In a 1.5 kg infant, as little as 0.5 ml of fluid injected rapidly into the right radial artery will reach the cerebral circulation. Haemorrhage from accidental disconnection can be significant because of the relatively small blood volume. Meticulous fixation is therefore required.

CENTRAL VENOUS CANNULATION AND PRESSURE MONITORING

All routes of central venous cannulation are applicable to infants and children and must be within the skills of paediatric intensivists. The femoral route is sometimes the safest in emergency situations. Catheters utilising the Seldinger technique have greatly increased successful placement. Ultrasonography is useful to determine the exact location of veins. Multilumen catheters are recommended when infusing multiple drugs and for parental nutrition. Complications including catheter-related sepsis are the same as in adults. This risk can be reduced by adherence to a bundle of measures.[6] The need for prolonged venous access may warrant regular catheter changes, or surgical implantation of a central venous device (e.g. Infusaport, Broviac or Hickman catheter). Umbilical venous cannulation and passage of the catheter through the sinus venosus to the right atrium is useful in neonatal emergencies.

PULMONARY ARTERY PRESSURE MONITORING

Pulmonary artery (PA) pressure monitoring using flow-directed 4 and 5 FG catheters is feasible even in neonates; however, it is invasive, technically more difficult and has greater risks than in the adult. It is rarely required in the neonate, as the pulmonary circulation and response to therapy can usually be gauged indirectly from the magnitude of right-to-left shunting. Systemic levels of PA pressure are usually found in neonates with severe lung disease.

The major indication for PA pressure monitoring is following surgery for congenital heart disease (e.g. repair of ventricular septal defect with pulmonary hypertension, truncus arteriosus and obstructed total anomalous pulmonary venous drainage). A catheter is inserted directly into the PA or via the right ventricular outflow tract at the time of surgery. It is most useful in guiding weaning from mechanical ventilation.

LEFT ATRIAL PRESSURE MONITORING

Left atrial pressure monitoring is often useful after open heart surgery for congenital heart disease, and is achieved by means of a catheter placed directly in the left atrium during surgery.

CARDIAC OUTPUT MEASUREMENT

Cardiac output determination can be performed in small children by dye dilution, thermodilution or Doppler techniques. Unfortunately, errors have been substantial, and the first two techniques are invasive, intermittent and only repeatable within finite limits. Interpretation of results is made difficult or impossible in the presence of intracardiac shunts or valvular incompetence. The dye curve may, in fact, be useful in demonstrating residual intracardiac shunts. Calculation of derived variables is only as accurate as the flow measurement.

A recently developed system (PiCCO, Pulsion Medical Systems AG, Munich, Germany) provides continuous cardiac monitoring even in small infants. Cardiac output is determined both intermittently by transpulmonary thermodilution[7] and continuously through arterial pulse contour analysis.[8] The system also derives cardiac preload volume, an index of left ventricular contractility, and an estimate of intrathoracic blood volume and extravascular lung water.

TEMPERATURE MONITORING

Temperature monitoring is important in neonatal and paediatric intensive care. Prevention of cold stress requires accurate measurement of core and skin temperature. Core–toe–ambient temperature gradients provide a sensitive, albeit indirect index of cardiac output and peripheral perfusion and are useful in managing fever. Toe temperature normally lies between core temperature (tympanic or oesophageal) and ambient temperature. The toe–core temperature gradient increases with low cardiac output or vasoconstriction from any cause. Toe temperature is a useful guide to the efficacy of vasodilator therapy.

PULSE OXIMETRY

Pulse oximetry provides continuous non-invasive measurement of arteriolar saturation ($Sa\text{O}_2$) and provides a rapid indication of hypoxaemia. Accurate information is given:

- when the oxyhaemoglobin dissociation curve is shifted to the left (e.g. fetal haemoglobin and alkalosis) or to the right (e.g. sickle-cell disease and acidosis)
- in the presence of carboxyhaemoglobin (functional saturation is accurate)
- with moderately severe desaturation (e.g. cyanotic heart disease)
- with anaemia (haemoglobin concentrations above 5 g/dl)
- when skin is pigmented

Errors occur with extreme hypoperfusion, excessive movement and rapidly changing ambient light. A range of sensors is now available to monitor children of all ages.

TRANSCUTANEOUS $P\text{O}_2$ AND $P\text{CO}_2$ MONITORING

Oxygen and carbon dioxide diffuse through well-perfused skin from the superficial capillary network and can be measured using modified polarographic and glass electrodes respectively. The electrodes are heated to 43–45°C to arterialise the capillary blood and maximise capillary blood flow. Under optimal conditions, there is good correlation between arterial and transcutaneous gas tensions. Hence continuous monitoring of blood gas tensions is possible in a non-invasive way. The $Ptc\text{O}_2$–$Pa\text{O}_2$ gradient and the output of the heating element have been used as indices of microcirculation. The accuracy of these devices is mainly confined to the neonatal period.

DRUG INFUSIONS

All drugs used in cardiovascular and respiratory support are administered according to body weight; accurate delivery is crucial. Accurate drug infusions require accurate devices, of which syringe pumps are the most useful. Potentially lethal errors in calculating drug dilutions are minimised by the use of dose/dilution/infusion rate guidelines (Table 96.2).[9]

PAIN RELIEF AND SEDATION IN CHILDREN

Management of pain and agitation in children has received inadequate attention and has tended to be underestimated and underrated. Infants and children are often unable or unwilling to complain of pain. In the past, some believed that the neonate could not perceive pain. It is now clear that even neonates possess all the anatomical and neurochemical systems necessary for pain perception and exhibit physiological and behavioural responses to pain.[10] Stress responses associated with pain and agitation may increase morbidity and mortality in critically ill patients. Analgesia can be provided by narcotic infusions, local blocks and regional techniques in children of all ages. Painful procedures in the ICU must always be accompanied by appropriate analgesia. The addition of sedative agents such as benzodiazepines can reduce agitation, minimise harmful stress responses and result in narcotic sparing.

NEONATAL AND PAEDIATRIC EMERGENCY TRANSPORT

Care of critically ill neonates and children necessitates the use of specialised retrieval services linked to neonatal and paediatric ICUs. Retrieval services should offer facilities for specialist consultation in addition to secondary transport. Careful audit of such services is necessary to improve patient outcome.[11] The aim of retrieval services is to extend the intensive care facility to peripheral hospitals, allowing stabilisation by experienced personnel prior to rapid transport to a regional centre in the most appropriate vehicle (see Chapter 4). Special considerations such as thermoregulation and oxygen monitoring must be provided for in neonatal transport. Well-designed neonatal emergency transport services have resulted in significant reductions in morbidity and mortality.

Table 96.2 Calculation of drug infusion dilutions

1. Select desired drug dosage to be delivered in µg/kg per min
2. Select infusion rate of syringe pump in ml/h (from centre of table)
3. Calculate number of milligrams of drug to be mixed in 50-ml syringe e.g.: 10-kg child, 0.1–2 µg/kg per min, infusion 1–20 ml/h: put 0.3 ml/kg (= 3 mg) in 50 ml

	0.15 mg/kg in 50 ml	0.3 mg/kg in 50 ml	0.6 mg/kg in 50 ml	1.5 mg/kg in 50 ml	3 mg/kg in 50 ml	6 mg/kg in 50 ml	15 mg/kg in 50 ml	30 mg/kg in 50 ml	60 mg/kg in 50 ml
µg/kg per min									
0.05	1	ml/h							
0.1	2	1	ml/h						
0.2	4	2	1						
0.3	6	3	1.5						
0.4	8	4	2	ml/h					
0.5	10	5		1					
0.6	12	6	3						
0.7	14	7							
0.8	16	8	4						
0.9	18	9			ml/h				
1	20	10	5	2	1				
1.5		15		3	1.5	ml/h			
2		20	10	4	2	1			
3				6	3	1.5			
4			20	8	4	2	ml/h		
5				10	5		1		
6				12	6	3			
7				14	7				
8				16	8	4			
9				18	9			ml/h	
10				20	10	5	2	1	
12					14	7			
14					14	7			
15					15		3	1.5	ml/h
20					20	10	4	2	1
25							5		
30						15	6	3	1.5
40						20	8	4	2
50							10	5	
100							20	10	5
150								15	
200								20	10

Noradrenaline

Dopamine Dobutamine Salbutamol

Morphine

Lidocaine

Nitroglycerine

Thiopental

Adreanaline

Ketamine

Nitropusside
Max. hours of infusion
10
8
7
7
6

OUTCOME OF PAEDIATRIC INTENSIVE CARE

Depending on admission criteria, mortality in paediatric ICUs ranges from 5 to 15%. If patients with pre-existing severe disabilities are excluded, the majority of survivors have a normal or near-normal life expectancy. A number of scoring systems have been developed or modified for paediatric application to predict ICU mortality. These scoring systems allow comparison between different ICUs, internal audits, stratification of patients for research purposes and analysis of cost benefit. The paediatric risk of mortality (PRISM) score[12,13] and the paediatric index of mortality (PIM) score[14] are applicable to a wide range of critically ill infants and children. Although PRISM performs marginally better, PIM is easier to collect and hence less prone to errors in data collection. PIM also has the advantage that it predicts mortality based on admission parameters whereas PRISM is based on the worst variables in the first 24hours. As many paediatric ICU deaths occur in the first 24hours, PRISM is often recording the dying process rather than predicting it. Specialised scores have been developed for specific problems, e.g. the modified injury severity scale (MISS) and paediatric trauma score (PTS) for paediatric trauma, and the modified Glasgow Coma Scale (GCS) for neurological insults. Numerous scoring systems have been developed for meningococcaemia, the best validated being the Glasgow meningococcal septicaemia prognostic score (GMSPS).[15]

Compared with adult intensive care, children with equivalent therapeutic intervention scores (TISS) have a lower in-hospital and 1-month mortality.[16] In addition, non-survivors do not consume a disproportionate amount of resources. While multiple organ failure increases mortality, the prognosis is considerably better than for adults.[17] There is evidence that mortality is lower in specialist paediatric ICUs,[18] and that paediatric ICUs with a larger workload have better outcomes than those looking after fewer children.[19] General hospitals should therefore have facilities for urgent resuscitation of children prior to early transport to a specialised paediatric ICU. Unless unavoidable, critically ill children, particularly those requiring mechanical intervention, should not be cared for in an adult ICU for longer than 24 hours. The American Academy of Pediatrics, the Society of Critical Care Medicine, the British Paediatric Association and the Australian National Health and Medical Research Council have all stated that children should receive intensive care in specialist paediatric units.

REFERENCES

1. Kinsella JP, Neish SR, Dunbar ID *et al.* Clinical responses to prolonged treatment of persistent pulmonary hypertension of the newborn with low doses of inhaled nitric oxide. *J Pediatr* 1993; **123**: 103–8.
2. The International Liaison Committee on Resuscitation. The International Liaison Committee on Resuscitation (ILCOR) Consensus on Science with treatment recommendations for pediatric and neonatal patients: pediatric basic and advanced life support. *Pediatrics* 2006; **117**: 955–77.
3. Rosetti VA, Thompson BM, Miller J *et al.* Intraosseous infusion: an alternative route of pediatric intravascular access. *Ann Emerg Med* 1985; **14**: 885–8.
4. Saccheti AD, Linkenheimer R, Liberman M *et al.* Intraosseous drug administration: successful resuscitation from asystole. *Pediatr Emerg Care* 1989; **5**: 97–8.
5. Moscati R, Moore GP. Compartment syndrome with resultant amputation following intraosseous infusion. *Am J Emerg Med* 1990; **8**: 470–1.
6. Bernholtz SM, Pronovost PJ, Lipsett PA *et al.* Eliminating catheter-related bloodstream infection in the intensive care unit. *Crit Care Med* 2004; **32**: 2014–20.
7. McLuckie A, Murdoch IA, Marsh MJ *et al.* A comparison of pulmonary and femoral artery thermodilution cardiac indices in paediatric intensive care patients. *Acta Paediatr* 1996; **85**: 336–8.
8. Goedje O, Hoeke K, Lichtwarek-Aschoff M *et al.* Continuous cardiac output by femoral arterial thermodilution calibrated pulse contour analysis: comparison with pulmonary arterial thermodilution. *Crit Care Med* 1999; **27**: 2407–12.
9. Shann F. Continuous drug infusions in children: a table for simplifying calculations. *Crit Care Med* 1983; **11**: 462–3.
10. Anand KJS, Hickey PR. Pain and its effects in the human neonate and fetus. *N Engl J Med* 1987; **317**: 1321–9.
11. Henning R, McNamara V. Difficulties encountered in transport of the critically ill child. *Pediatr Emerg Care* 1991; **7**: 133–7.
12. Pollack MM, Ruttimann UE, Getson PR. Pediatric risk of mortality (PRISM) score. *Crit Care Med* 1988; **16**: 1110–6.
13. Pollack MM, Patel KM, Ruttimann UE. PRISM III: an updated pediatric risk of mortality score. *Crit Care Med* 1996; **24**: 743–52.
14. Shann F, Pearson G, Slater A *et al.* Paediatric index of mortality (PIM): a mortality prediction model for children in intensive care. *Intensive Care Med* 1997; **23**: 201–7.
15. Thompson APJ, Sills JA, Hart A. Validation of the Glasgow meningococcal septicaemia prognostic score: a 10 year retrospective survey. *Crit Care Med* 1991; **19**: 26–30.
16. Yeh TS, Pollack MM, Holbrook PR *et al.* Assessment of pediatric intensive care – application of the Therapeutic Intervention Scoring System. *Crit Care Med* 1982; **10**: 497–500.
17. Wilkinson JD, Pollack MM, Ruttimann UE *et al.* Outcome of pediatric patients with multiple organ system failure. *Crit Care Med* 1986; **14**: 271–4.
18. Pollack MM, Alexander SR, Clarke N *et al.* Improved outcomes from tertiary center pediatric intensive care: a statewide comparison of tertiary and nontertiary care facilities. *Crit Care Med* 1991; **19**: 150–9.
19. Pearson G, Shann F, Barry P *et al.* Should paediatric intensive care be centralized? Trent versus Victoria. *Lancet* 1997; **349**: 1214–7.

97

Upper respiratory tract obstruction in children

Alan W Duncan

Upper respiratory tract obstruction (URTO) is a common cause of respiratory failure in infants and children. This reflects the frequency of upper respiratory tract abnormalities and disorders, the presence of narrow airways and the structural inefficiencies of the lung and chest wall. The majority of children with critical airway obstruction are otherwise healthy, and expert management results in a normal life expectancy. Poor management can lead to cardiopulmonary arrest and hypoxic cerebral damage.

ANATOMICAL DIFFERENCES AND CLINICAL RELEVANCE

Differences in the anatomy and function of the airway are important considerations in airway maintenance, laryngoscopy and intubation. In the newborn, the nose contributes approximately 42% of total airways resistance, which is considerably less than the adult's 63%. Thus, infants are obligatory nose-breathers. The epiglottis is longer, U-shaped and floppy, and may need to be lifted with a straight-bladed laryngoscope for visualisation of the larynx and intubation. The larynx is higher in the neck (C3–4) in the neonate, and has an anterior inclination.[1] It descends over the first 3 years of life, and again at puberty, to ultimately lie opposite C6. The length of the trachea varies from 3.2 to 7.0 cm in babies weighing less than 6 kg. Accurate positioning of the tracheal tubes is required to prevent accidental extubation or endobronchial intubation. The narrowest part of the airway until puberty is the cricoid ring. This part of the airway is most vulnerable to trauma and swelling. The narrow cricoid ring also dictates tube size, and allows use of uncuffed tubes in infants and children.

PATHOPHYSIOLOGY

Although the ratio of airway diameter to body weight is relatively large in the infant, in absolute terms airway diameter is small, and a minimal reduction causes a devastating increase in airway resistance. For example, the diameter of the newborn's cricoid ring is 5 mm. A 50% reduction in radius will result in turbulent flow, and increases the pressure (and work) required to maintain breathing 32-fold.[2]

Symptoms and signs vary with the level of obstruction, the aetiology and the age of the child. Airway obstruction may be extrathoracic, intrathoracic or a combination. Extrathoracic obstruction is more pronounced during inspiration and is characterised by inspiratory stridor and prolongation of inspiration. Intrathoracic obstruction affecting either large or small airways is more pronounced during expiration and is characterised by expiratory stridor, prolonged expiration, wheeze and air trapping. Biphasic stridor is characteristic of mid tracheal lesions. These features mirror the intrapleural and airway pressure changes of the respiratory cycle (Figure 97.1). Retraction of the chest wall, an important sign of respiratory distress, reflects the negative intrapleural pressures generated combined with the compliance of the chest wall. Large negative intrapleural pressures are also transmitted to the interstitium of the lung, and may result in pulmonary oedema.[3,4] Cor pulmonale may develop secondary to chronic obstruction, hypoxia and pulmonary hypertension.[5,6]

CLINICAL PRESENTATION

Stridor is noisy breathing due to turbulent air flow. It is the cardinal feature of URTO. Parents complain that their child has noisy breathing and of 'sucking the chest in'. The pitch and timing of stridor provide information about the degree and level of obstruction.

Voice sounds may also be informative. Nasal obstruction results in hyponasality. Oropharyngeal obstruction may cause a 'hot potato' voice. Supraglottic obstruction is characterised by a muffled voice. Children with glottic lesions may be hoarse or aphonic.

Retraction of the chest wall develops as obstruction progresses. Retraction is less prominent in older children, as the chest wall is more stable. As obstruction worsens, the work of breathing increases and the accessory muscles become active. The alae nasi (vestigial muscles of ventilation) begin

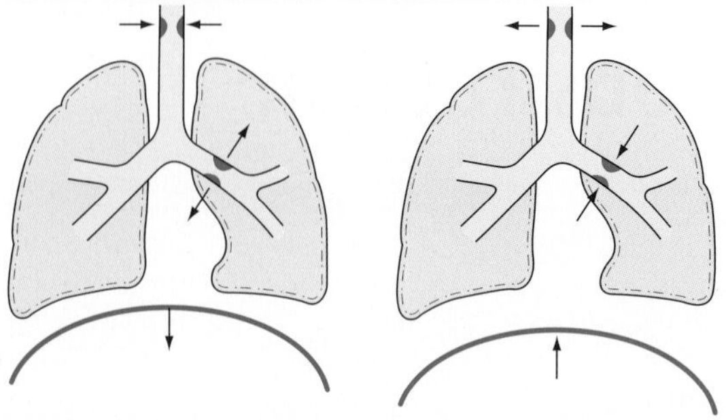

Figure 97.1 Dynamics of (a) extrathoracic and (b) intrathoracic airways obstruction.

to flare. Fever increases minute volume and magnifies any degree of obstruction. Whereas infants and older children can maintain an increased work of breathing, premature infants and neonates rapidly fatigue, and may develop apnoeic episodes.[7,8]

Auscultation over the neck and larynx may identify the site of obstruction. A foreign body in the airway may produce a mechanical or slapping sound. Decreased or absent breath sounds may occur with greater degrees of obstruction. Chronic URTO is a cause of failure to thrive, chest deformity (pectus excavatum) and cor pulmonale.[5,6] Some infants present with recurrent chest infections. Abnormal posturing (head retraction) may also be a feature, particularly in infants.

Initially, the child with airway obstruction exhibits tachypnoea and tachycardia. If obstruction is severe and persistent, exhaustion eventually occurs, and the child exhibits decreased respiratory effort, decreased stridor and breath sounds, restlessness, cyanosis, pallor and eventually bradycardia.

AETIOLOGY

A classification of the causes of URTO is presented in Table 97.1. The neonatal causes are predominantly due to congenital structural lesions. Acute inflammatory lesions, foreign bodies and trauma predominate in older infants and children.

DIAGNOSIS

The cause of URTO can often be determined from the history and clinical features. Radiographic examination of the upper and lower airways with anteroposterior and lateral views may show soft-tissue swelling or the presence of foreign bodies.[9] Air shadows may indicate fixed stenotic or compressive lesions. In children with significant respiratory distress, these investigations should be undertaken in the intensive care unit (ICU) rather than the radiology department.

Previously, barium swallow and aortography have been used to confirm the diagnosis of vascular compression of the trachea. Computed tomography (CT) has assumed importance in the assessment of fixed lesions such as intrinsic stenosis and extrinsic compression. Echocardiography, magnetic resonance imaging (MRI) and CT with contrast are useful to assess vascular anomalies.[10] Tracheobronchography may provide excellent anatomical delineation of the proximal tracheobronchial tree and allow dynamic assessment of airway calibre.

Direct visualisation of the airway may be necessary, and may also prove therapeutic (e.g. removal of a foreign body). Nasoscopy, flexible fibreoptic and rigid laryngoscopy and bronchoscopy all have a place in assessing the

Table 97.1 Causes of upper airway obstruction in children

Level	Newborn	Older infant and child
Nasal	Choanal atresia	
Oropharyngeal	Facial malformations (e.g. Pierre Robin syndrome, Treacher Collins syndrome) Macroglossia Cystic hygroma Vallecular cyst	Macroglossia/postglossectomy Angioedema Retropharyngeal abscess Tonsillar and adenoidal hypertrophy Obstructive sleep apnoea
Laryngeal	Infantile larynx Bilateral vocal cord palsy Congenital subglottic stenosis Subglottic haemangioma Laryngeal web Laryngeal cysts	Acute laryngotracheobronchitis (croup) Bacterial tracheitis Acute epiglottitis Postintubation oedema and stenosis Laryngeal papillomata Laryngeal foreign body Inhalation burns Caustic ingestion External trauma
Tracheal	Tracheomalacia Vascular ring	Foreign body Anterior mediastinal tumours (e.g. lymphoma)

paediatric airway. Investigation of the child's airway should only be undertaken in specialised centres by experienced endoscopists, radiologists and anaesthetists.

Blood gas determination is rarely useful in assessment or monitoring of URTO. An exception to this is in very young infants where hypercapnic respiratory failure may occur early and insidiously in URTO. It is dangerous practice to await respiratory failure before intervention. Mild hypoxaemia only may be present until fatigue, hypoventilation, cyanosis and hypercapnia occur. Pulse oximetry may provide useful warning information. An oxygen saturation less than 90% in a patient with pure URTO (without lung disease) is a reason for concern.

SPECIFIC AIRWAY OBSTRUCTION

EPIGLOTTITIS

Epiglottitis is a life-threatening supraglottic lesion which, prior to vaccination, was caused almost exclusively by *Haemophilus influenzae* type b. The prevalence of epiglottitis has fallen dramatically with the uptake of *H. influenzae* vaccination. It still occurs due to failure to vaccinate or vaccine failure. Occasional cases are caused by *Streptococcus, Staphylococcus, Pneumococcus* and *Meningococcus*, as well as by viruses. Non-infective causes include corrosive ingestion and thermal injury.

The diagnosis is usually obvious from history and clinical features. There is an acute onset of high fever, toxaemia and noisy breathing. The child adopts a characteristic posture, preferring to sit with mouth open, drooling saliva. The tongue is often proptosed and immobile. Cough is usually absent. These features are the legacy of an intensely painful pharynx. Due to the accompanying septicaemia, the severity of illness often appears out of proportion to the degree of airway obstruction. Typically, a low-pitched inspiratory stridor is present, accompanied by a characteristic expiratory snore. Atypical cases with cough and without fever may obscure the diagnosis.

Sudden total obstruction is not infrequent, and may be precipitated by examination of the pharynx, by placing the child in the supine position or stressful procedures (e.g. cannula insertion). When the diagnosis is in doubt, a lateral X-ray of the neck in the sitting position should be taken in the emergency department or ICU, provided that staff capable of securing the airway remain in attendance. Examination of the pharynx must not be undertaken unless personnel and facilities are available for immediate intubation.

MANAGEMENT

PARENTERAL ANTIBIOTICS

Third-generation cephalosporins are the preferred antibiotics because of emerging resistance to ampicillin and, to a lesser extent, chloramphenicol. Appropriate regimens include cefotaxime 200 mg/kg per day i.v. for 5 days, or ceftriaxone 100 mg/kg i.v. statim followed by 50 mg/kg i.v. after 24 hours. Co-trimoxazole is usually an effective enteral antibiotic if more prolonged therapy is required.

RELIEF OF AIRWAY OBSTRUCTION

All but the mildest cases require insertion of an artificial airway under anaesthesia (see below). Nasotracheal intubation is the optimal management,[11] although, depending on the available personnel, tracheostomy is a satisfactory alternative. Anaesthesia for relief of airway obstruction is described below. A tube of size appropriate for age is chosen (see Chapter 104). Extubation can be undertaken when fever subsides and the child no longer appears toxic. Most cases can be extubated in less than 18 hours. Only those complicated by pulmonary oedema, pneumonia or cerebral hypoxia (from delayed therapy) will require intubation for longer than 24 hours. It is not necessary to re-examine the larynx prior to extubation. Nebulised adrenaline (epinephrine) is of no benefit in this condition and may aggravate the situation.[12] Pulmonary oedema, when it occurs, is due to airway obstruction, septicaemia and increased lung capillary permeability.[3,13,14] It is managed according to conventional principles.

PROPHYLAXIS

Most invasive infections due to *H. influenzae* occur in children under 5 years of age. The risk of infection in close contacts is about 500-fold higher than in the general population. It is thus recommended that all members (including adults) of any household with *H. influenzae* type b infection and with another child under 4 years should be given prophylactic antibiotics. An accepted regimen is oral rifampicin 20 mg/kg per day (maximum 600 mg) for 4 days. An alternative is a single dose of ceftriaxone 100 mg/kg i.m. or i.v.

CROUP

Croup or acute laryngotracheobronchitis is due to inflammation and oedema of the glottic and subglottic regions. The narrowest part of the child's upper airway is the subglottic region, the point at which critical narrowing occurs. Retained secretions due to the bronchitic component may compound the obstruction. Croup is uncommon in children under 6 months of age, and an underlying structural lesion such as subglottic stenosis or haemangioma with superimposed infection should be suspected. Endoscopy is warranted if the child has a prior history of stridor or if symptoms persist beyond the acute episode.

Three subgroups are recognised: viral croup, spasmodic croup and bacterial tracheitis.

VIRAL CROUP

Viral croup, most commonly due to parainfluenza virus, respiratory syncytial virus and rhinovirus, is characterised by a coryzal prodrome, low-grade fever, harsh barking

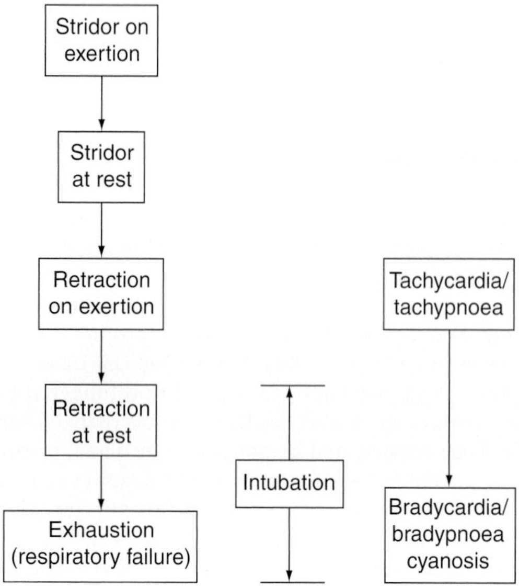

Figure 97.2 Features of progressive upper-airway obstruction.

(croupy) cough and hoarse voice. Progression of airway obstruction in severe cases is shown in Figure 97.2.

SPASMODIC CROUP

Spasmodic or recurrent croup occurs in children with an allergic predisposition.[15,16] It usually develops suddenly, often at night, and without prodromal symptoms. Endoscopy reveals pale, watery oedema of the subglottic mucosa. Such children probably represent part of the asthma spectrum, and wheeze, due to small airway flow limitation, may be a feature.

BACTERIAL TRACHEITIS

Bacterial tracheitis is uncommon but should be suspected in children exhibiting the usual features of croup, but accompanied by high fever, leukocytosis and copious purulent secretions.[17] There is a greater risk of sudden, severe obstruction from purulent secretions. *Staphylococcus aureus* is usually the cause, although *H. influenzae* and group A *Streptococcus* have also been isolated in some cases.

MANAGEMENT

Minimal disturbance is important, as restlessness will increase minute ventilation, oxygen consumption and signs of obstruction.

Adequate hydration: oral fluid intake must be encouraged to avoid dehydration. Nasogastric feeding is contraindicated, and i.v. fluids may occasionally be necessary. Overhydration must also be avoided. Hyponatraemia and convulsions due to inappropriate antidiuretic hormone secretion have been observed with prolonged, severe airway obstruction.

Oxygen therapy may mask signs of respiratory failure, but should be given to treat hypoxaemia. Its use can be guided by pulse oximetry (i.e. keep $Sa\text{O}_2 > 90\%$). Oxygen administration may further stress the young child. The need for oxygen therapy is often an indication that the child is progressing towards intubation.

Corticosteroids have dramatically reduced the need for intubation in children with croup. They are effective in both viral and spasmodic croup.[18,19] Steroids will also shorten the duration of intubation and increase the success rate of extubation.[20,21] The dose of dexamethasone is 0.6 mg/kg statim (maximum dose 10 mg) followed, if necessary, by 0.15 mg/kg 6-hourly. In very distressed children, it is best administered i.m. or i.v. to ensure absorption. Inhaled steroids are also effective in milder cases.[22]

Humidification of inspired gases was the mainstay of supportive care for decades. Controlled studies showing efficacy are lacking. A study by Bourchier *et al.* failed to demonstrate benefit and its use has been abandoned in many centres.[23]

Nebulised adrenaline will usually provide temporary relief of acute obstruction.[24] Historically, racemic adrenaline (2.25% solution, i.e. 1:88 L-adrenaline), developed for use in asthma, was employed. Indications for adrenaline nebulisation are:

- acute laryngotracheobronchitis, where relief usually lasts 1–2 hours, but may be longer if it facilitates secretions to be expelled. It is debatable whether the natural history of the disease is altered. It is an effective temporising measure until steroids have time to work. If given prior to induction, it will facilitate inhalational anaesthesia for intubation
- spasmodic croup, where one or two inhalations may produce lasting relief of airway obstruction
- post endoscopy or intubation oedema, where the benefit is often dramatic
- during transport, where administration may render the child safe for interhospital transfer without intubation

The empirical dose of racemic adrenaline is 0.05 ml/kg diluted to 2 ml with saline and nebulised with oxygen. The same dose of a strong preparation (1%) of the L-isomer can also be used. The same mass of L-adrenaline is also provided by 0.5 ml/kg (max 5 ml) of the standard 1:1000 solution of adrenaline, and this is equally effective. Antibiotics are indicated only for bacterial tracheitis where anti-staphylococcal cover is recommended.

Mechanical relief of airway obstruction: this requirement has been greatly reduced by early use of steroids. Increasing tachycardia, tachypnoea and restlessness indicate the need for tracheal intubation. An $Sa\text{O}_2$ persistently less than 90% is another reason for concern. It is important not to wait for the development of bradycardia, bradypnoea, cyanosis, exhaustion and respiratory failure. Blood gases are not a useful guide for intubation.

Table 97.2 Nasotracheal tube size in croup

Age	Size
Less than 6 months	3.0 mm
6 months to 2 years	3.5 mm
2–5 years	4.0 mm
Over 5 years	4.5 mm

Nasotracheal intubation is preferred. An orotracheal tube, size (inner diameter) 1 mm less than that predicted by age (Table 97.2) is first inserted under anaesthesia (see below). A stylet through the tube is recommended to overcome the resistance of the subglottic region. The tube is changed to a nasotracheal tube immediately after clearance of secretions.

Extubation can be performed when the child is afebrile, secretions have diminished and a leak is audible around the tube with coughing or application of positive pressure (25 cmH_2O or less). The duration of intubation averages 5 days. Children under 1 year have a higher incidence of requiring intubation and a longer duration of intubation. Reintubation may be required in some cases. Endoscopy should be performed in cases that require repeated intubation to exclude underlying lesions and subglottic injury. Tracheostomy is a suitable alternative for some situations, although complications are more significant.

OTHER SUPRAGLOTTIC LESIONS

Retropharyngeal abscess, tonsillitis, peritonsillar abscess, infectious mononucleosis and Ludwig's angina may all mimic epiglottitis. Local features will usually indicate the diagnosis. A retropharyngeal abscess can be detected by palpation and is obvious on a lateral X-ray of the neck. Airway relief, antibiotics, drainage and, rarely, neck incision form the basis of treatment for these disorders. A nasopharyngeal tube will provide relief of obstruction in most supraglottic lesions. In an emergency situation, placement of a laryngeal mask airway may be life-saving. Tonsillectomy, although best performed electively, is occasionally indicated in the acute phase of tonsillar obstruction. Steroids appear to be effective in reducing cervical lymphadenopathy and tonsillar enlargement in cases of infectious mononucleosis and the response is rapid.

TONSILLAR AND ADENOIDAL AIRWAY OBSTRUCTION

The contemporary conservative surgical approach to tonsillectomy and adenoidectomy has led to an increased incidence of hypertrophy and untreated chronic upper-airway obstruction.[25] Such children may present with severe, acute exacerbations due to intercurrent infection (e.g. tonsillitis). They may present in a toxic state with drooling, thereby mimicking acute epiglottitis. Obstruction is most marked during sleep. In the most severe cases, it may be necessary to relieve the obstruction with a nasotracheal tube or a nasopharyngeal tube positioned beyond the tonsillar bed. Tonsillectomy and adenoidectomy are generally contraindicated in the acute phase, because of increased risk of bleeding, but are performed when infection has settled.

OBSTRUCTIVE SLEEP APNOEA SYNDROME

Obstructive sleep apnoea (OSA) syndrome is characterised by intermittent upper-airway obstruction during sleep, with heavy snoring, stertorous breathing and an abnormal, irregular respiratory pattern.[26] Frequent episodes of chest-wall motion with inadequate airflow (hypopnoea) or absent airflow (obstructive apnoea) are a feature. These episodes are most frequent during rapid eye movement sleep. They are accompanied by variable degrees of oxygen desaturation. OSA may be associated with enlarged tonsils and adenoids, a large uvula or long soft palate, macroglossia, retrognathia or various neurological disorders. Obesity is a common finding.

If OSA is severe and protracted, cardiac and pulmonary decompensation may occur. Chronic hypoxia and hypercarbia lead to pulmonary hypertension and cor pulmonale.[5,6] There may also be evidence of left ventricular failure and pulmonary oedema. Urgency of treatment is dictated by the mode of presentation. Critically ill children may require immediate relief of airway obstruction (nasopharyngeal or nasotracheal tube), oxygen therapy and diuretics. Antibiotics are indicated if there is bacterial superinfection. Surgical intervention is required after stabilisation. Tonsillectomy and adenoidectomy are often dramatically beneficial. They are best removed even when not grossly enlarged. Postoperative observation in a paediatric ICU or high-dependency unit is required for those with severe OSA. Other surgical procedures, such as uvulopalatopharyngoplasty or tracheostomy, may be required when this fails. The use of nocturnal continuous positive airway pressure (CPAP) is an option in long-standing, refractory conditions, e.g. neurological disorders. It is often not feasible because it is difficult to interface CPAP masks in young and uncooperative children.

PIERRE ROBIN SYNDROME

This sequence consists of a posterior cleft palate, retrognathia and relative macroglossia. It is the cause of airway obstruction, feeding difficulties and failure to thrive in the newborn. Differential growth eventually reduces the significance of the deformity. Acute airway obstruction may be relieved by nursing the infant in the prone position, by passage of a nasopharyngeal tube or insertion of a laryngeal mask airway.[27] Occasionally, nasotracheal intubation or tracheostomy is required. Tongue–lip anastomosis has been used in the past but is now rarely performed.

CYSTIC HYGROMA

Although often conspicuous at birth, cystic hygroma is a relatively rare cause of upper-airway obstruction in infancy. The tumours consist of masses of dilated lymphatic channels. They usually occur in the neck and may involve tissues of the tongue and larynx. Occasionally, extension into the mediastinum occurs. Airway obstruction may be due to infection or haemorrhage into the lesion. Surgical excision has been the mainstay of treatment, although complete removal is difficult and recurrence is common. Treatment using sclerosing therapy is now used. Compounds used include bleomycin emulsion or OK 432.[28,29] OK 432 is produced by lyophilisation of cultures of a low virulent strain of group A *Streptococcus pyogenes* (human origin). In severe cases, long-term tracheostomy is required.

INHALATION BURNS

Inhalational injury should be suspected with burns occurring in a closed space, and when facial burns, singed nasal hairs and oropharyngeal carbonaceous material are present. Respiratory complications are the major cause of mortality in children who are burnt. Direct airway burns or inhalation of products of combustion may lead to rapidly progressive oedema. The situation may be compounded by small airway and lung injury and by the need to provide adequate analgesia. Early intubation is strongly recommended prior to an emergency situation developing. Tracheal tube fixation is critical and may be problematic with extensive facial burns; it may require suturing of the tube to the nasal septum.

SUBGLOTTIC STENOSIS

Neonates with congenital subglottic stenosis may present with severe obstruction requiring intubation at birth. Other infants present with persistent stridor or recurrent croup due to superimposed infection. Subglottic stenosis may also occur as a complication of prolonged or traumatic intubation, the result of tube pressure, mucosal ischaemia and healing by fibrosis. Prolonged intubation or tracheostomy may be required. Surgical techniques such as the cricoid split procedure or laryngotracheoplasty may be required to enlarge the airway.

SUBGLOTTIC HAEMANGIOMA

Haemangiomata are common in infancy and occur in many parts of the body. Subglottic lesions often present in the second or third month of life and owe their importance to the anatomical location. Stridor is usually both inspiratory and expiratory. A hoarse cry is indicative of vocal cord involvement. Obstruction may be severe and is aggravated by crying, struggling or superimposed infection. Cutaneous haemangiomata are seen in 50% and, if present, provide a clue to diagnosis. Definitive diagnosis rests on endoscopy. The natural history is of spontaneous resolution between the first and second years of life. Meanwhile, tracheostomy or periods of intubation may be indicated to cover episodes of obstruction. Encouraging results are being obtained with laser surgery. Intralesional injection of steroids may be of benefit.

FOREIGN BODY OR CHOKING

A foreign body must be suspected in any acute obstruction occurring in an infant or child between 6 months and 2 years of age. Older children with neurological impairment are also at risk. A foreign body lodged in the pharynx results in gagging, respiratory distress and facial congestion. Laryngeal impaction usually produces stridor, a distressing cough and aphonia. Sudden total obstruction may occur. Symptoms usually develop while the child is playing or eating.

The technique for removal of a pharyngolaryngeal foreign body without equipment in infants and children is controversial and difficult. The American Academy of Paediatrics has made recommendations to cover various ages.[30] Gravity should be utilised by placing the child prone, straddled over the arm with the head down and a hand supporting the jaw. Four back blows between the shoulder blades should be administered. If this fails, chest thrusts or finger sweep across the pharynx should be attempted. There is some risk that the latter manoeuvre may impact the foreign body in the larynx. Abdominal thrusts (the Heimlich manoeuvre) are not recommended in infants but may be useful in children older than 1 year. Expired air resuscitation should be attempted in an emergency, although the risk of gastric distension is great. The best method of removal is extraction under direct vision using a laryngoscope, forceps, suction or a finger.

Tracheal or bronchial foreign bodies produce persistent cough and wheeze, and recurrent pneumonia. A foreign body lodged in the upper oesophagus may compress the trachea and present with either acute or, more commonly, persistent stridor. Radiopaque materials are easily shown radiologically, but both anteroposterior and lateral views may be necessary. Barium studies may prove useful for non-radiopaque material in the oesophagus. Treatment is removal at bronchoscopy or oesophagoscopy.

ANTERIOR MEDIASTINAL TUMOURS

Anterior mediastinal tumours, such as lymphoma, may compress the trachea or bronchi, causing symptoms such as dry cough, stridor or wheeze. Airway compression may become severe enough to cause hyperinflation or atelectasis. Pleural effusions are common and may add to the respiratory distress. This is a high-risk situation. Symptoms may be aggravated by the supine position, especially during anaesthesia for a biopsy procedure. This is likely in patients with superior vena caval syndrome. Postural symptoms or findings on flow–volume loops may allude to this risk. Echocardiography may also provide evidence of cardiac compression which increases the risks associated with anaesthesia. Sudden complete obstruction that cannot be bypassed by a standard tracheal tube has been described. The use of armoured tubes or a rigid bronchoscope may be required. Consideration should be given to leaving the tracheal tube in situ postoperatively until corticosteroids and chemotherapy reduce the tumour mass.

ANAESTHESIA FOR RELIEF OF AIRWAY OBSTRUCTION

Inhalational induction and anaesthesia with oxygen and halothane or sevoflurane is the preferred technique for intubation. The use of muscle relaxants is hazardous if the ability to maintain a patent airway is doubtful.

Important points are:

- A prepared induction should be undertaken with efficient suction apparatus, a range of tracheal tubes, suitable stylets and bougies. Preparations must be made to intubate without deep anaesthesia if sudden obstruction occurs.
- Inhalational anaesthesia is slow in upper-airway obstruction, particularly when accompanied by lower airway or lung disease.
- Induction in the sitting position is advocated with epiglottitis. The child is laid flat after induction and prior to intubation.
- CPAP or assisted ventilation will reduce obstruction (minimise the dynamic component) and hasten induction. Care must be taken not to distend the stomach.
- Laryngoscopy is performed, and the child intubated, only when adequate depth of anaesthesia is achieved (e.g. approximately 8–10 minutes of 4% halothane in oxygen). Others recommend 6–8% sevoflurane.
- Orotracheal intubation is quickest and safest, and should be performed initially. After good tracheal toilet, the tube is changed to a nasotracheal one. Muscle relaxants may be used at this point if the operator is confident of the ability to intubate and/or ventilate.

CARE OF NASOTRACHEAL TUBE

Successful management of URTO in children requires optimal care of the nasotracheal tube. Such children must always be nursed in an ICU with adequate nursing ratios. The nasotracheal tube must be positioned at the level of the clavicular heads (T2) on an anteroposterior chest X-ray. Length of the tube from 1 to 6 years of age (in cm measured at the nose) is given by age in years + 13 cm. A meticulous technique of fixation must be employed to prevent accidental extubation.

Adequate humidification is difficult in the active child. Nevertheless, it is important to prevent obstruction of narrow tubes by inspissated secretions. Lightweight heat and moisture exchangers (HME) are very useful (e.g. Thermovent, Gibeck, and Humidvent, Portex). The HME should be changed every 24 hours to reduce contamination and increased resistance. Oxygen supplementation can be provided, if necessary. Some children will tolerate connection of a humidified T-piece.

Effective bagging and tracheal toilet is vital, and should be repeated until the airway is clear. Instillation of saline (0.5–1.0 ml) prior to suction may be necessary to remove secretions. Light sedation is used to improve tolerance of the tracheal tube and to reduce the risk of self-extubation. Midazolam, 0.1–0.2 mg/kg statim, followed by continuous infusion (0.05–0.2 mg/kg per hour) is effective. Arm restraints may also be advisable, particularly in very young children. In some restless young children, it may be safer to use heavy sedation and mechanical ventilation. Signs of obstruction are usually relieved by intubation. Mild retraction may persist in children with high fever and increased minute ventilation in the presence of a smaller than predicted tube. Fibreoptic bronchoscopy can be performed to confirm patency. The tracheal tube must be changed or removed if there is doubt about its patency.

Nasogastric tube feeding should be commenced in children who require intubation longer than 24 hours.

TRACHEOSTOMY

Tracheostomy remains a life-saving procedure and must be undertaken if tracheal intubation is impossible, or if appropriate equipment and personnel to facilitate intubation are unavailable. For chronic airway problems, it is more comfortable, allows better nasopharyngeal toilet and permits the child to leave the ICU and eventually return home. It is best performed under endotracheal anaesthesia with the neck extended. When intubation is impossible, the tracheostomy can be performed under anaesthesia via a laryngeal mask airway. A longitudinal slit is made through the second and third tracheal rings without removal of cartilage. Stay sutures in the tracheal wall lateral to the incision aid recannulation if accidental dislodgement occurs prior to formation of a well-defined tract (after 4 days). A postoperative chest X-ray should be obtained to check the position of the tip of the tracheostomy tube and to exclude pneumothorax or other complications.

Care of a newly created tracheostomy is similar to that of an endotracheal tube, with the additional problem of some discomfort and the likelihood of fresh blood in the airway. The first tracheostomy tube change is undertaken once a tract has been established, usually between 5 and 7 days.

CRICOTHYROTOMY

A wide-bore plastic i.v. cannula (14- or 16-gauge) passed into the trachea via the cricothyroid membrane may be life-saving if alternative procedures are unavailable. This should be performed with the neck extended as for tracheostomy. A system of connection to a low-pressure oxygen supply must be planned in advance. One method is to attach the hub of the cannula to the sleeve of a plastic 2–3 ml syringe (without plunger) to an adaptor from a 7.5 mm outer diameter tracheal tube, and then to a breathing circuit (e.g. Jackson Rees modification of Ayres T-piece). Jet ventilation has also been performed through a narrow cannula in this situation.

REFERENCES

1. Westhorpe RN. The position of the larynx in children and its relationship to the ease of intubation. *Anaesth Intensive Care* 1987; **15**: 384–8.
2. Badgwell JM, McLeod ME, Friedberg J. Airway obstruction in infants and children. *Can J Anaesth* 1987; **34**: 90–8.
3. Sofer S, Bar-Ziv J, Scharf SM. Pulmonary edema following relief of upper airway obstruction. *Chest* 1984; **86**: 401–3.
4. Stalcup SA, Mellins RB. Mechanical forces producing pulmonary edema in acute asthma. *N Engl J Med* 1977; **297**: 592–6.
5. Cox MA, Schiebler GL, Taylor WJ *et al.* Reversible pulmonary hypertension in a child with respiratory obstruction and cor pulmonale. *J Pediatr* 1965; **67**: 192–7.
6. Luke MJ, Mehrizi A, Folger GM *et al.* Chronic nasopharyngeal obstruction as a cause of cardiomegaly, cor pulmonale, and pulmonary oedema. *Paediatrics* 1966; **37**: 762–8.
7. Keens TG, Bryan AC, Levinson H *et al.* Development pattern of muscle fibre types in human ventilatory muscles. *J Appl Physiol Respir Environ Exercise Physiol* 1978; **44**: 909–13.
8. Muller NL, Bryan AC. Chest wall mechanics and respiratory muscles in infants. *Pediatr Clin North Am* 1979; **26**: 503–16.
9. Kushner DC, Harris GBC. Obstructing lesions of the larynx and trachea in infants and children. *Radiol Clin North Am* 1978; **16**: 181–94.
10. Siegel MJ, Nadel SN, Glazer HS *et al.* Mediastinal lesions in children. Comparison of CT and MR. *Radiology* 1986; **160**: 241–4.
11. Butt W, Shann F, Walker C *et al.* Acute epiglottitis: a different approach to management. *Crit Care Med* 1988; **16**: 43–7.
12. Kissoon N, Mitchell I. Adverse effects of racemic epinephrine in epiglottitis. *Pediatr Emerg Care* 1985; **1**: 143–4.
13. Soliman MG, Richer P. Epiglottitis and pulmonary oedema in children. *Can Anaesth Soc J* 1978; **25**: 270–5.
14. Travis KW, Todres DI, Shannon DC. Pulmonary edema associated with croup and epiglottitis. *Pediatrics* 1978; **59**: 695–8.
15. Zach M, Erben E, Olinsky A. Croup, recurrent croup, allergy and airways hyper-reactivity. *Arch Dis Child* 1981; **56**: 336–41.
16. Zach MS, Schnall RP, Landau LI. Upper and lower airway hyper-reactivity in recurrent croup. *Am Rev Respir Dis* 1980; **121**: 979–83.
17. Jones R, Santos JI, Overall JC. Bacterial tracheitis. *JAMA* 1979; **242**: 721–6.
18. Super DM, Cartelli NA, Brooks LJ *et al.* A prospective randomized double-blind study to evaluate the effect of dexamethasone in acute laryngo-tracheitis. *J Pediatr* 1989; **115**: 323–9.
19. Koren G, Frand M, Barzilay Z *et al.* Corticosteroid treatment of laryngotracheitis in spasmodic croup in children. *Am J Dis Child* 1983; **137**: 941–4.
20. Tibballs J, Shann FA, Landau FI. Placebo controlled trial of prednisolone in children intubated for croup. *Lancet* 1992; **340**: 745–8.
21. Freezer N, Butt W, Phelan P. Steroids in croup: do they increase the incidence of successful extubation? *Anaesth Intensive Care* 1990; **18**: 224–8.
22. Klassen TP, Feldman ME, Watters LK *et al.* Nebulized budesonide for children with mild to moderate croup. *N Engl J Med* 1994; **331**: 285–9.
23. Bourchier D, Dawson KP, Fergusson DM. Humidification in viral croup: a controlled trial. *Aust Paediatr* 1984; **20**: 289–91.
24. Jordan WS, Graves CL, Elwyn RA. New therapy for postintubation laryngeal edema and tracheitis in children. *JAMA* 1970; **212**: 585–8.
25. Check WA. Does drop in tonsillectomies and adenoidectomies pose new issue of adeno-tonsillar hypertrophy? *JAMA* 1982; **247**: 1229–30.
26. Guilleminault C, Tilkian A, Dement WA. The sleep apnea syndromes. *Ann Rev Med* 1976; **27**: 465–84.
27. Heaf DP, Helms PJ, Dinwiddie MB *et al.* Nasopharyngeal airways in Pierre Robin syndrome. *J Pediatr* 1982; **100**: 698–703.
28. Tanaka K, Inomata Y, Utsunomiya H *et al.* Sclerosing therapy with bleomycin emulsion for lymphangioma in children. *Pediatr Surg Int* 1990; **5**: 270–3.
29. Samuel M, McCarthy L, Boddy SA. Efficacy and safety of OK-432 sclerotherapy for giant cystic hygroma in a newborn. *Fetal Diagnosis Ther* 2000; **15**: 93–6.
30. American Academy of Pediatrics Committee on Accident and Poison Prevention. First aid for the choking child. *Pediatrics* 1988; **81**: 740–2.

98

Acute respiratory failure in children

Alan W Duncan

Established or imminent respiratory failure is the commonest reason for admission to neonatal and paediatric intensive care units (ICUs). A number of structural and functional factors contribute to the high incidence of respiratory failure, particularly in the first year of life. In addition, respiratory failure is frequently a consequence of pathology primarily affecting other organ systems, e.g. congenital heart disease or central nervous system (CNS) disease.

PREDISPOSING FACTORS

Respiratory function must equate with metabolic demands. Oxygen consumption in the infant is approximately 7 ml/kg per min (compared with 3–4 ml/kg per min in the older child and adult). Fever, illness and restlessness dramatically increase demands; during periods of apnoea or respiratory depression, $Pa\text{CO}_2$ rises at twice the rate of older children and adults. Respiratory reserve is reduced in infants and neonates due to the following factors.

STRUCTURAL IMMATURITY OF THE THORACIC CAGE[1]

The ribs are short and horizontal and the bucket motion that increases the anteroposterior and lateral dimensions of the thorax is minimal. Thus, the infant is dependent on diaphragmatic displacement of abdominal contents to increase the length and volume of the thorax. Rib cage structure and function alter between 12 and 18 months, as the child develops the erect posture. The consequence is that any impairment of diaphragmatic function (e.g. phrenic nerve palsy, abdominal distension) may precipitate respiratory failure.

The chest wall is soft and provides a poor fulcrum for respiratory effort. Retraction of bony structures and soft tissues, a prominent sign of respiratory distress, occurs with reduced lung compliance and increased airway resistance. Infant intrapleural pressure is −1 to −2 cmH_2O (−0.1 to −0.2 kPa) compared with −5 to −10 cmH_2O (−0.5 to −1.0 kPa) in the adult. This is due to the higher compliance of the chest wall (which tends to collapse in) and lower elastic recoil of the lung. The result is an increased tendency to airway closure, atelectasis and intrapulmonary shunting.

In the neonate, the diaphragm and intercostal muscles have a lower percentage of type 1 (slow twitch and high oxidative) muscle fibres and therefore fatigue more readily. Diaphragmatic muscle mass is relatively reduced. Intercostal muscle activity is inhibited during rapid eye movement sleep, further reducing ventilatory efficiency. Increased respiratory work is poorly sustained in the face of increased load and may culminate in exhaustion and apnoea.[2]

INFANT AIRWAYS

Although relatively large compared with the adult, airways of infants in absolute terms are small and more prone to obstruction. Trachea and bronchiole diameters of a 3 kg neonate are one-third and one-half respectively of those of a 60-kg adult. However, any degree of oedema or airway mucus will have a more profound effect on airway resistance in the infant.

LUNG STRUCTURE

Although the number of alveoli in the infant lung is proportionate to body size, the diffusion area is relatively small. The alveolar surface area is approximately 2.8 m^2 at birth, 32 m^2 at 8 years and 75 m^2 in the adult. Alveolar number and surface area may be reduced by in utero or early postnatal insults, including ventilator-induced injury. The infant lung also lacks the anatomical channels that allow ‘collateral ventilation’, putting the infant at greater risk of atelectasis, emphysematous changes and ventilation/perfusion abnormalities. The interalveolar pores of Kohn appear between the first and second years of life, while Lambert’s channels provide communication between bronchi and adjacent alveoli beginning at 6 years.

INCREASED SUSCEPTIBILITY TO INFECTION

The immaturity and inexperience of the immune system (cellular and humoral) result in a markedly increased susceptibility to infection in the first 6 months of life. The neonate’s T-cells are unable to produce certain cytokines which compromises the interaction between T-cells and B-cells. There is greater reactivity of T-suppressor cells to T-helper cells. Complement activation is impaired in premature and full-term neonates. The neonate's phagocytes have diminished motility, adherence and chemotaxis but bacterial killing by polymorphonuclear leukocytes is intact. In addition, there are many immune deficiency syndromes that may first reveal themselves early in postnatal life.

IMMATURITY OF LUNG FUNCTION

Premature infants in particular may have surfactant deficiency, resulting in alveolar instability, atelectasis, intrapulmonary shunting and reduced lung compliance.

IMMATURITY OF RESPIRATORY CONTROL

Inadequate respiratory drive from immaturity of the respiratory centre is a factor leading to apnoeic spells, particularly in premature infants. Opioid analgesics are associated with greater respiratory depression in young infants.

CONGENITAL ABNORMALITIES

Congenital defects of the respiratory system (lower airways, lungs, chest wall, diaphragm) or associated organs (e.g. heart, great vessels) often present with respiratory failure shortly after birth.

PERINATAL ASPHYXIA OR INJURIES

Asphyxia or intracranial haemorrhage associated with birth may result in seizures and respiratory depression.

CLINICAL PRESENTATION

Respiratory distress is manifested by tachypnoea, distortion of the chest wall (i.e. sternal and rib retraction, recession of intercostal, subcostal and suprasternal spaces) and use of accessory muscles (e.g. flaring of alae nasi and use of neck muscles).

In young infants, lethargy, pallor, apnoea, bradycardia and hypotension may be the first signs of hypoxia. The physiological anaemia of infancy may delay recognition of cyanosis, and major signs are those of CNS and cardiovascular depression. Increased work of breathing, marked by tachypnoea and chest-wall retraction, is poorly sustained; bradypnoea and apnoea are evidence of respiratory fatigue. Expiratory 'grunting' is a sign of respiratory distress that represents an attempt to maintain a positive expiratory airway pressure to prevent airway closure and alveolar collapse, the equivalent of pursed-lip breathing in the adult.

The older child with acute hypoxia, like the adult, demonstrates tachycardia, hypertension, mental confusion and restlessness prior to CNS and cardiovascular depression. Sweating occurs with CO_2 retention – a feature lacking in the newborn.

In the newborn, the effects of hypoxia and acidosis may be compounded by the development of pulmonary hypertension and reversion to a transitional circulation, with right-to-left shunting through a patent ductus arteriosus and foramen ovale. If untreated, increasing hypoxaemia, progressive acidosis and death may occur.

Conventional clinical examination of the chest should be performed. It is, however, of limited value in the neonate, as breath sounds may be transmitted uniformly through the chest, even in the presence of tension pneumothorax, lobar collapse or endobronchial intubation. The chest X-ray is an essential part of the assessment.

AETIOLOGY

Acute respiratory failure may result from upper or lower airway obstruction, alveolar disease, pulmonary compression, neuromuscular disease or injury (Table 98.1). Upper respiratory tract obstruction is discussed in Chapter 97.

TRACHEOMALACIA, TRACHEAL STENOSIS AND VASCULAR COMPRESSION

Instability of the tracheal wall (tracheomalacia) is most commonly associated with oesophageal atresia, tracheo-oesophageal fistula and various vascular anomalies. The most common causes of vascular compression are a double aortic arch and the complex of a right-sided aortic arch, left ductus arteriosus and an aberrant left subclavian artery. These produce a true vascular ring, with encirclement of the trachea and oesophagus. Anterior tracheal compression may also be due to an anomalous innominate artery. Lower tracheomalacia or tracheal stenosis may occur in association with an anomalous left pulmonary artery (pulmonary artery sling). The problem may extend to the major bronchi (bronchomalacia). Tracheomalacia and bronchomalacia also occur as isolated airway anomalies. In this situation, the severity of dynamic airway obstruction is aggravated by any condition that results in reduced lung compliance.

Division of the vascular ring and ligation or repositioning of the aberrant vessel, while removing the cause of the obstruction, do not immediately re-establish normal airway dimensions or stability. Although severity of symptoms may be alleviated by surgery, problems may persist for some years. Tracheomalacia may sometimes be stabilised by a prolonged period of nasotracheal intubation or tracheostomy with continuous positive airway pressure (CPAP). Tracheopexy, which suspends the anterior tracheal wall from the posterior sternal surface and great vessels, is occasionally useful. A slide tracheoplasty may be required to correct tracheal stenosis associated with

Table 98.1 Causes of respiratory insufficiency in infancy and childhood

Site	Neonate	Older infant and child
Upper airway obstruction		
	See Chapter 103	
Lower airway obstruction		
Tracheal	Tracheomalacia	Foreign body
	Vascular anomalies	
	Tracheal stenosis	Mediastinal tumour
Bronchial	Bronchomalacia	Foreign body
Bronchiolar	Meconium aspiration	
	Congenital cystic adenomatoid malformation	Acute viral bronchiolitis
	Lobar emphysema	
Disorders of lung function		
	Aspiration syndromes	Pneumonia
		Cystic fibrosis
	Hyaline membrane disease	
	Bronchopulmonary dysplasia	Aspiration syndromes
	Perinatal pneumonia	
	Massive pulmonary haemorrhage	Congenital heart disease
	Pulmonary oedema	Near-drowning
	Pulmonary hypoplasia	Trauma
	Diaphragmatic hernia	Burns
		Acute respiratory distress syndrome
Pulmonary compression		
	Diaphragmatic hernia	Pneumothorax
	Pneumothorax	Pleural effusion
	Repaired exomphalos or gastroschisis	Empyema
Neurological and muscular disorders		
	Diaphragmatic palsy	Poisoning
	Birth asphyxia	Meningitis
	Convulsions	Encephalitis
	Apnoea of prematurity	Status epilepticus
		Trauma
		Guillain–Barré syndrome
		Envenomation

complete tracheal rings.[3] A range of stenting devices have also been developed for complex airways and employed with mixed success.

MECONIUM ASPIRATION SYNDROME

Meconium aspiration is seen in 0.3% of live births, and is most common in term or postterm infants. There is usually a history of fetal distress in labour, or prolonged and complicated delivery. Asphyxia during labour results in the expulsion of meconium into the liquor. With the first few breaths, material in the upper airway (i.e. amniotic fluid, meconium, vernix and squames) is inhaled, obstructing small airways and producing atelectasis and obstructive emphysema. Meconium also causes a chemical pneumonitis and surfactant abnormalities. During recovery, the aspirated material is absorbed and phagocytosed.

Clinical signs include tachypnoea, retraction and cyanosis. The chest may become hyperexpanded and pneumomediastinum or pneumothorax is a frequent complication. Pulmonary hypertension and persistent fetal circulation are common.

The chest X-ray confirms the diagnosis, with coarse mottling and streakiness radiating from the hila. Lungs are overexpanded, with flattened diaphragms and an increase in the chest anteroposterior diameter. The condition is largely preventable if the airway can be aspirated rapidly and completely following delivery of the head and before the first breath.

Most of these infants require oxygen therapy. Severely affected infants require controlled mechanical ventilation (CMV), which may be difficult because of the high pressures required, the non-uniformity of ventilation, and danger of pneumothorax. Improved outcomes are now achieved using surfactant (may cause transient deterioration), inhaled nitric oxide and high-frequency oscillation.[4] Extracorporeal membrane oxygenation (ECMO) is also effective in those centres that have the facility, although its use has declined since the introduction of the above therapies. Cerebral effects of severe intrapartum asphyxia contribute to overall morbidity and mortality.

CONGENITAL CYSTIC ADENOMATOID MALFORMATION

Congenital cystic adenomatoid malformation (CCAM) of the lung results from abnormal mesenchymal proliferation and failure of maturation of bronchiolar structures early in gestation. The result is multiple lung cysts, usually within a single lobe. CCAM is often diagnosed on antenatal ultrasound. Other cases present with respiratory distress due to obstruction whilst others present with infection in the cysts and recurrent lobar pneumonia. Some cases are diagnosed incidentally on chest radiographs taken for another reason. Some cases are associated with renal dysplasia. Even asymptomatic infants are at risk of cyst expansion or infection and lobectomy is the treatment of choice for all cases.

LOBAR EMPHYSEMA

Congenital lobar emphysema is characterised by overdistension of a pulmonary lobe caused by air trapping. Most cases present in the first month of life, with tachypnoea, wheezing, grunting and cough. Signs include hyperresonance, decreased air entry and deviation of the trachea and heart away from the affected lobe. There may be asymmetry of the chest due to bulging of the affected hemithorax. Cyanosis may be associated with periods of increased respiratory distress. There may be associated cardiovascular abnormalities, rib cage abnormalities or renal dysplasia.

Radiologically, the affected lobe is overdistended with compression and deviation of the surrounding structures. The pathogenesis is unknown in over 50%, 25% have localised bronchial cartilaginous dysplasia, and the remainder have obstruction of a lobar bronchus from a mucous plug, redundant mucosa, aberrant vessels or localised stenosis. Lobectomy is the definitive surgical treatment. Care must be taken with positive airway pressure because of the risk of further overdistension.

ASPIRATION PNEUMONIA

In the newborn, aspiration may result from pharyngeal incoordination or lack of protective reflexes, due to prematurity, birth asphyxia or intracranial haemorrhage. It is particularly likely to occur with abnormalities of the alimentary tract, such as oesophageal atresia, tracheo-oesophageal fistula and oesophageal reflux. Large and small airway obstruction and pneumonia may occur.

HYALINE MEMBRANE DISEASE

This is due to deficiency of lung surfactant. Predisposing factors are prematurity, maternal diabetes and intranatal asphyxia. Postnatal hypoxia and acidosis also inhibit surfactant production. Lack of surfactant results in alveolar instability, atelectasis, intrapulmonary shunting and increased work of breathing.

Clinical signs appear shortly after birth and consist of tachypnoea, chest-wall retraction, expiratory grunting and a progressive increase in oxygen requirements. The chest X-ray reveals a reticulogranular pattern (ground-glass appearance) with air bronchograms. In uncomplicated cases, the disease is self-limiting and resolves in 4–5 days. Respiratory failure may require increasing inspired oxygen concentrations (F_{IO_2}), CPAP, intermittent mandatory ventilation (IMV) or CMV. CPAP is known to improve oxygenation, the pattern and regularity of respiration, retard the progression of the disease and reduce morbidity, particularly with early application in the extremely preterm infant. In infants with persistent pulmonary hypertension, transitional circulation and requiring high airway pressures, the use of inhaled nitric oxide and high-frequency oscillatory ventilation are beneficial.

Instillation of surfactant into the trachea has been shown to improve oxygenation and compliance (despite some initial deterioration) and reduce the risk of pneumothorax, early mortality and morbidity.[5–8] Two types of surfactant are used: synthetic (Exosurf), and bovine (Survanta) or porcine (Curosurf).

BRONCHOPULMONARY DYSPLASIA

Bronchopulmonary dysplasia (BPD), or chronic lung disease, may occur in survivors of neonatal lung disease. Its occurrence correlates with lung immaturity, high airway pressures and barotrauma. The lung architecture is abnormal with widespread fibrosis and cystic changes. There is often a reactive component to the airway disease that may be responsive to bronchodilator and anti-inflammatory therapy, such as steroids. It is a cause of chronic respiratory failure in infancy, and in severe cases progresses to cor pulmonale and death in the first 2 years of life. Prolonged low-flow home oxygen therapy may be necessary to reduce the risk of pulmonary hypertension. Superimposed bacterial and viral infection may exacerbate chronic respiratory failure and lead to further lung injury.

PNEUMONIA

Perinatal pneumonia may occur as a result of transplacental spread of a maternal infection, prolonged rupture of membranes, passage through an infected birth canal or cross-infection in the nursery. The immunoparetic state of the newborn and the need for invasive procedures increase the risk.

Clinical and radiological features may be indistinguishable from hyaline membrane disease. Antibiotics (e.g. penicillin and gentamicin) should be given until negative cultures exclude the diagnosis. The most common organisms include group B haemolytic *Streptococcus, Escherichia coli, Pseudomonas aeruginosa, Klebsiella pneumoniae* and *Staphylococcus aureus.* Group B haemolytic streptococcal infection is frequently associated with septic shock and persistent fetal circulation. Failure to suspect group B haemolytic streptococcal infections (and hence treat promptly with penicillin) will result in poor outcome. Multiresistant staphylococcal and Gram-negative bacillary infections must be suspected in longer-stay patients in neonatal ICUs.

Most pneumonia in infants and young children is of viral origin. Viruses commonly implicated are respiratory syncytial virus (RSV), influenza A1, A2 and B, and parainfluenza types 1 and 3. Adenovirus and rhinovirus are less common causes. The spectrum of illness is wide. Many infants and children have cough, fever and tachypnoea, with X-ray evidence of patchy consolidation, all of which resolve rapidly. Occasionally, infants develop life-threatening respiratory illness with extensive pneumonic changes and marked necrosis. Permanent lung damage with bronchiolitis obliterans and pulmonary fibrosis may occasionally complicate severe adenoviral pneumonia in particular.

Bacterial pneumonia also occurs. Pneumococcal pneumonia is common and usually responds dramatically to appropriate antibiotic therapy. Staphylococcal pneumonia is relatively uncommon, but may result in life-threatening respiratory failure, and is often associated with complications (e.g. empyema, pneumatocele, tension pneumothorax and suppuration in other organs). Aspiration of an effusion may be useful for diagnostic purposes. Parapneumonic effusions (empyema) may require tube thoracostomy or video-assisted thoracoscopic drainage. Resolution of the effusion can be enhanced by the instillation of thrombolytic agents such as urokinase or tissue plasminogen activator.[9] In severe cases with bronchopleural fistula, surgical resection of the necrotic area offers the best chance of survival.

Pneumonia due to *Haemophilus influenzae* may also occur and be associated with epiglottitis, meningitis, pericarditis or middle-ear disease. The prevalence of *H. influenzae* infection has reduced dramatically since the introduction of HiB immunisation.

Gram-negative pneumonia is seen mostly in infants with debilitating conditions who are hospitalised for prolonged periods. It is a particular risk for patients in ICUs with endotracheal or tracheostomy tubes. Other opportunistic infections, such as *Pneumocystis jiroveci* (formerly *P. carinii*), *Candida albicans, Aspergillus* and cytomegalovirus, may occur in immune deficiency states.

MASSIVE PULMONARY HAEMORRHAGE

This usually presents as acute cardiorespiratory collapse, accompanied by outpouring of bloodstained fluid from the trachea, mouth and nose. It is seen in association with severe birth asphyxia, hyaline membrane disease, congenital heart disease, erythroblastosis fetalis, coagulopathy and sepsis. Hypoxia is often a precipitating factor. The condition in the newborn is believed to represent haemorrhagic pulmonary oedema due to acute left ventricular failure. Treatment is that of the underlying condition with oxygenation, CMV and correction of any coagulation disturbance.

PULMONARY OEDEMA

Pulmonary oedema in the newborn period is due mostly to congenital heart disease, especially coarctation of the aorta, patent ductus arteriosus, critical aortic stenosis and, rarely, obstructed total anomalous pulmonary venous drainage.

Pulmonary oedema due to circulatory overload may also occur in erythroblastosis fetalis, the placental transfusion syndrome, or as a result of inappropriate fluid therapy. Myocarditis is a further cause seen throughout infancy and childhood. Prolonged supraventricular tachycardia may result in ventricular dysfunction and biventricular failure, including pulmonary oedema.

In the newborn period, pulmonary oedema manifests as respiratory distress and feeding difficulty and specific features of congenital heart lesions may be evident. There is a spectrum of severity, from tachypnoea with a widened alveolar–arterial oxygen gradient to life-threatening respiratory failure requiring urgent support. Chest X-ray usually shows an enlarged heart (except in total anomalous pulmonary venous drainage) and a ground-glass appearance fanning out from the hilar regions.

PULMONARY HYPOPLASIA

This is seen most often in association with congenital diaphragmatic hernia, but bilateral pulmonary hypoplasia may also occur in association with renal agenesis or dysgenesis (Potter's syndrome), in babies with severe Rhesus isoimmunisation, and in the presence of chronic amniotic fluid leak. It may also present as an isolated malformation. Unilateral hypoplasia can occur as an isolated anomaly or in association with cardiovascular defects.

DIAPHRAGMATIC HERNIA

Congenital diaphragmatic hernia (most commonly left-sided) results in respiratory failure, partly due to lung compression but mainly related to the associated pulmonary hypoplasia (both ipsilateral and contralateral). The degree of pulmonary hypoplasia is most severe in infants with absence of the diaphragm. The disturbance of pulmonary function ranges from mild to severe. In severe cases, life-threatening respiratory distress is present from birth, with cyanosis, intercostal retraction, mediastinal displacement, and poor or absent breath sounds on the affected side. The abdomen is usually scaphoid, due to much of its usual contents being in the chest. Chest X-ray shows loops of bowel in the affected hemithorax, with pulmonary compression and mediastinal displacement to the contralateral side.

Neonates presenting in the first 4 hours of life have major degrees of lung hypoplasia and have a mortality of 40% despite maximal supportive therapy. Those presenting after 4 hours of age should all survive. CMV may be complicated by tension pneumothorax and bronchopleural fistula on either side. Pulmonary hypertension with persistent fetal circulation and difficulties of CMV present major challenges. Many centres use ECMO or high-frequency ventilation in these infants. Nitric oxide is a useful pulmonary vasodilator in this condition.[4] Prolonged ventilatory support is often required but the outlook for survivors is excellent.

PNEUMOTHORAX

Spontaneous pneumothorax may occur during the birth process in normal newborns, or secondary to hyaline membrane disease or meconium aspiration. Tension pneumothorax is particularly likely to occur when CMV is required in the presence of lung immaturity, lung hypoplasia, non-uniform lung disease (e.g. staphylococcal pneumonia) and diseases characterised by air trapping (e.g. meconium aspiration, bronchiolitis and asthma).

Tension pneumothorax should be suspected with any sudden deterioration of an infant on a ventilator. Classic clinical signs are evident in older children, but are of limited value in neonates. Circulatory embarrassment may be profound and rapidly progressive. Abdominal distension due to depression of the diaphragm and congestion of intra-abdominal organs, and unilateral chest hyperexpansion are useful signs. Transillumination of the thorax using a bright light source is a sensitive guide in newborn infants. A chest X-ray is mandatory, but should be preceded by needle aspiration or drainage if the infant's condition is critical. Pre-existing pulmonary interstitial emphysema in one lung may also point to the likely side of the pneumothorax.

REPAIRED EXOMPHALOS OR GASTROSCHISIS

Complete repair of abdominal wall defects may cause marked elevation of intra-abdominal pressure when the intestines are then enclosed in a poorly developed peritoneal cavity. The diaphragm is elevated, compressing the lungs. In addition, compression of the inferior vena cava may lead to peripheral oedema, reduced cardiac output and oliguria (abdominal compartment syndrome). The associated paralytic ileus may further increase intra-abdominal pressure.

Disturbed lung function with inadequate gas exchange may require postoperative ventilation for several days. With large defects, it may be necessary to house the abdominal contents in a prosthesis to allow gradual reduction into the abdominal cavity.

DIAPHRAGMATIC PALSY

Phrenic nerve palsy is a relatively common complication of cardiothoracic surgery. It occasionally occurs as a congenital abnormality, or may result from birth trauma. Paralysis and paradoxical movement of the affected diaphragm lead to reduced lung and tidal volumes, hypoxaemia and increased work of breathing. A chest X-ray taken without positive airway pressure reveals the elevated hemidiaphragm (positive pressure may mask the radiological diagnosis). Screening with ultrasound or fluoroscopy confirms the paradoxical movement.

Paralysis of the hemidiaphragm may cause respiratory failure in infants, particularly if associated with another disorder affecting lung function. Problems are greatest in children under 3 years, due to the poor stability of the chest wall. CPAP may be an effective method of increasing lung volume, stabilising the rib cage and reducing paradoxical movement. Surgical plication of the diaphragm is usually effective in cases that fail to resolve with conservative management.

BIRTH ASPHYXIA

Birth asphyxia may result from placental failure, obstetric difficulties or maternal sedation. The resulting central respiratory depression, convulsions, intracerebral haemorrhage, meconium aspiration and transitional circulation contribute to respiratory failure. The Apgar score at 1 minute is an objective means of evaluating the degree of asphyxia; the score at 5 minutes is a guide to prognosis. Delayed spontaneous respiration (> 5 minutes) is also a poor prognostic sign. Further postnatal hypoxaemia, hypercapnia and brain ischaemia must be avoided. Severely asphyxiated infants need CMV after delivery, with correction of acidosis and hypovolaemia; inotropic drugs may be needed to maintain cerebral blood flow. It is important to prevent hypoglycaemia and control convulsions. A recent randomised control trial has shown improved cerebral outcomes with the use of early topical hypothermia, although the benefit is probably restricted to infants with less severe degrees of hypoxic–ischaemic encephalopathy.[10]

CONVULSIONS

Convulsions in the newborn are most frequent in the first 3 days of life. They are commonly due to birth asphyxia, trauma, intracranial haemorrhage and metabolic abnormalities such as hypoglycaemia or hypocalcaemia and meningitis. Seizures in older children commonly occur with fever, idiopathic epilepsy, CNS infection, poisoning, trauma and metabolic disturbances (e.g. hypoglycaemia, hyponatraemia and hypocalcaemia).

Generalised seizures may cause respiratory failure from airway obstruction, aspiration, apnoea or central respiratory depression. During grand mal seizures, ventilation may be inadequate, and oxygen consumption and CO_2 production may be increased by associated muscle activity. Anticonvulsant drugs may further depress respiration.

Initial management consists of ensuring a clear airway, adequate oxygenation and ventilation, and administering anticonvulsants. Oxygen should be given, because cerebral and total body oxygen consumption is increased, and it is difficult to assess adequacy of ventilation. Urgent control of seizures is important, as protracted seizures (longer than 1 hour) cause cerebral oedema and may result in permanent neurological sequelae, even if hypoxaemia is avoided. The underlying cause must then be determined and treated.

APNOEA OF PREMATURITY

Recurrent apnoeic episodes (> 20 seconds) are common in premature infants, and relate to immaturity of the brainstem, hypoxia, altered chemoreceptor responsiveness, diaphragmatic fatigue and the active (rapid eye movement) sleep state. Underlying causes such as hyaline membrane disease, hypoglycaemia, aspiration, sepsis, anaemia and intracranial haemorrhage should be sought. Mild episodes revert either spontaneously or with tactile stimulation. Severe episodes may require bag-and-mask ventilation. Apnoeic episodes may be reduced or prevented by theophylline or caffeine (central respiratory stimulants) or CPAP. IMV is necessary in some cases.

Many premature infants also suffer obstructive or mixed (central and obstructive) apnoea, both disorders of respiratory and airway musculature control. The infant airway collapses easily, and this is aggravated by neck flexion. Ex-premature infants may develop recurrent apnoea with intercurrent infection or following general anaesthesia and surgical procedures. This risk may persist until a postconceptual age of 46 weeks, and demands close monitoring.[11] The risk may be greater in infants with a history of apnoeic episodes, bronchopulmonary dysplasia, anaemia or neurological disease. This is transient and remarkably responsive to theophylline or caffeine loading. Ongoing maintenance therapy is often unnecessary.

STATUS ASTHMATICUS

Asthma is the commonest reason for admission to most paediatric hospitals. Asthma is an inflammatory disease affecting the airways. Airway obstruction is due to mucosal oedema, mucus plugging and bronchiolar muscle spasm. Under 2 years of age, bronchiolar muscle is poorly developed, and muscle spasm is probably of less importance, with poor response to bronchodilator therapy.

Clinical and radiological features and management of asthma in small children are similar to that in adults (see Chapter 35). Blood gas estimation is indicated for any child with acute severe asthma, if pulsus paradoxus greater than 20 mmHg (2.6 kPa) is present, or if the child fails to respond to optimal drug therapy. Hypoxaemia due to intrapulmonary shunt and $\{\dot{V}\}/\{\dot{Q}\}$ mismatching is the usual finding, and is the main cause of morbidity and mortality. High inspired oxygen therapy is therefore important. Hypocapnia in response to hypoxic drive is the rule; normocapnia or a rising $Pa\text{CO}_2$ are signs of worsening asthma or fatigue and require increased medical therapy or mechanical ventilation.

Nebulised and/or i.v. β_2-sympathomimetic amines, i.v. aminophylline and corticosteroids form the mainstay of drug therapy; maximal therapy should be introduced early. Salbutamol is nebulised with oxygen as 0.05 mg/kg of 0.5% solution diluted to 4 ml with sterile water, given 2–4-hourly initially, or more frequently in severe cases. A greater and more sustained response may be achieved by more frequent or continuous salbutamol nebulisation.[12] Inhaled ipratropium may have additional benefit, even in patients receiving maximal therapy with β_2-sympathomimetic amines.

Some centres abandoned the use of aminophylline because of its narrow therapeutic range and because of the belief that it did not add benefit to maximal therapy with salbutamol. There is evidence, however, that aminophylline does have a place in the management of severe acute asthma in children that is unresponsive to initial treatment.[13] Aminophylline is also known to possess anti-inflammatory properties. A loading dose of 5–10 mg/kg aminophylline over 1 hour produces serum levels in the therapeutic range; lower loading doses may be employed to reduce the occurrence of nausea and vomiting. Children under 9 years have increased metabolism, and require higher doses of theophylline (0.85 mg/kg per hour, equivalent to an aminophylline infusion of 1.1 mg/kg per hour). Serum concentrations should be measured (therapeutic range is 60–110 μmol/l).

Continuous infusion of salbutamol has been shown to reduce the need for CMV. It should be added when $Pa\text{CO}_2$ is rising or is greater than 60 mmHg (8 kPa), as an infusion of 5–10 μg/kg per min for 1 hour and then reduced to 1–2 μg/kg per min. An adrenaline (epinephrine) or isoprenaline infusion (0.05–2 μg/kg per min) may be useful in refractory cases.

Lactic acidosis may occur as a result of hypoxaemia and increased work of breathing. Adrenaline by infusion is also associated with lactic acidosis. Cautious bicarbonate therapy is recommended to improve cardiovascular function and bronchomotor responsiveness to theophylline and sympathomimetic agents. Isoprenaline and theophylline may both override pulmonary hypoxic vasoconstrictor responses and thereby increase intrapulmonary shunt and worsen hypoxaemia. Salbutamol is believed to be preferable in this respect.

Particular attention should be paid to fluid balance. Dehydration may lead to inspissation of secretions, but the risks of inappropriate antidiuretic hormone (ADH) secretion and pulmonary oedema must be noted.[14,15]

With aggressive medical therapy, the need for CMV should be rare. Its use should be based predominantly on clinical features rather than solely on blood gas analysis. It should not, however, be withheld out of fear of difficulties. CMV may worsen air trapping and lead to hypotension or pneumothorax. Controlled hypoventilation (permissive hypercapnia) with a long expiratory time is advocated to minimise airway pressures and air trapping. A trial of positive end-expiratory pressure (PEEP) may be justified to reduce intrinsic (auto) PEEP and air trapping, although evidence in adults suggests that PEEP may be associated with increased air trapping.[16]

ACUTE VIRAL BRONCHIOLITIS

Most cases of bronchiolitis occur in the first 6 months of life and are caused by RSV. Other viruses now identified as causing bronchiolitis include rhinovirus and human metapneumovirus. Cough, low-grade fever, tachypnoea and wheeze are the cardinal signs. Some infants, particularly ex-premature, develop apnoeic episodes. The chest is hyperinflated with rib retraction and widespread crepitations. Clinical features are due to small airways obstruction from oedema and exudate.

Management consists of minimal handling and oxygen therapy. If respiratory distress is marked, feeds should be withheld and fluids administered i.v. Progression of the disease leads to exhaustion and respiratory failure in 1–2% of cases. CPAP and/or aminophylline therapies are reported to reduce the work of breathing, lower $Pa\text{CO}_2$ and eliminate recurrent apnoea. Nebulised adrenaline may also be beneficial.[17] CMV is required in some cases, particularly when the disease occurs in association with congenital heart or chronic lung disease. High airway pressures may be required, increasing the risk of pneumothorax. The antiviral agent ribavirin is difficult to administer and has not been shown to improve outcome. Bacterial coinfection is common, and justifies the use of broad-spectrum antibiotics in severe cases.[18]

RESPIRATORY FAILURE SECONDARY TO CONGENITAL HEART DISEASE

Infants with congenital heart disease may develop respiratory failure for a number of reasons.

TYPE OF CARDIAC LESION

Congenital heart lesions producing acute respiratory failure fall into four main groups.

1. *Left heart obstruction* (e.g. critical aortic stenosis, interrupted aortic arch and coarctation of aorta). In this group, left ventricular failure leads to pulmonary oedema, reduced pulmonary compliance and respiratory failure.
2. *Large left-to-right shunts* (e.g. ventricular septal defect and patent ductus arteriosus). Respiratory failure in this group with excessive pulmonary blood flow results from volume overloading of the left ventricle, with pulmonary oedema, small airways obstruction, bronchial compression or intercurrent infection. Correction of the defect is associated with improved lung mechanics.[19]
3. *Hypoxaemic lesions*, where:
   (a) there is obstruction to pulmonary blood flow (e.g. tetralogy of Fallot and critical pulmonary stenosis)
   (b) the pulmonary and systemic circuits are in parallel (e.g. transposition of the great vessels)

(c) there is complete mixing of systemic and pulmonary venous blood (e.g. single ventricle and truncus arteriosus).

In lesions associated with reduced pulmonary blood flow, lung compliance is high. High-pressure ventilation may further impede pulmonary blood flow, leading to increased hypoxaemia and, occasionally, CO_2 retention. Hypoxaemic lesions associated with increased pulmonary blood flow have problems of reduced lung compliance and air trapping (due to small airways disease and bronchial compression) in addition to hypoxaemia (due to mixing).

4. Vascular lesions associated with compression or stenosis of large airways (e.g. vascular rings and anomalous left pulmonary artery).

INTERCURRENT INFECTION

Recurrent pneumonia and bronchiolitis are common in infants with congenital heart disease, particularly those associated with increased pulmonary blood flow.

POSTOPERATIVE

Respiratory failure may occur following repair of cardiac lesions due to low cardiac output state and pulmonary oedema, acute respiratory distress syndrome (ARDS), lobar collapse, pleural effusions, pneumonia, phrenic nerve palsy, respiratory depressant drugs, abdominal distension and ascites.

NEAR DROWNING

Respiratory failure after near drowning may result from aspiration pneumonitis or CNS depression from hypoxic–ischaemic encephalopathy. Acute gastric dilatation (associated with the immersion or resuscitation) is common and may be a contributing factor. Pulmonary oedema may be secondary to water and particulate matter inhaled, or to chemical pneumonitis from aspiration of gastric contents. Secondary infection occasionally leads to necrotising pneumonia. Prophylactic antibiotics are not of proven benefit, but there are occasional reports of fulminant ARDS associated with infection after immersion. Broad spectrum antibiotic therapy should be administered early if there is significant pulmonary disease. Ongoing therapy should be guided by culture of tracheal aspirate.

Patients with both fresh- and salt-water drowning are usually hypovolaemic, hypoxic and acidotic at the time of admission. Oxygen therapy is mandatory, even in so-called 'dry drowning'. Resuscitation usually requires volume expansion, correction of acidosis and inotropic support. Immersion hypothermia may afford some protection to the brain. Complete rewarming should not be undertaken until circulatory resuscitation is achieved. Resuscitation attempts should be sustained in the presence of severe hypothermia; in warmer climates, however, severe hypothermia implies a longer period of immersion and carries a very poor prognosis. In such circumstances it may be appropriate to cease resuscitative efforts prior to rewarming. CMV usually produces a dramatic improvement in gas exchange.

TRAUMA

Respiratory failure may follow trauma to the brain, spinal cord, chest or abdomen. High spinal cord injuries may be difficult to detect in the presence of severe brain injury. Presence of rhythmic flaring of the alae nasi without accompanying respiratory excursion is a useful sign (Duncan's sign). As the chest wall is compliant, severe pulmonary contusion can occur from blunt trauma with minimal chest-wall injury. Fractured ribs, haemothorax and pneumothorax may all precipitate respiratory failure. The diagnosis of a ruptured diaphragm is often delayed as the clinical signs are easily confused with a tension pneumothorax. CMV will effectively displace abdominal contents from the thorax and improve gas exchange prior to surgery. The chest X-ray is a mandatory investigation during resuscitation.

Acute gastric dilatation is almost invariable in the traumatised child, may mimic an acute abdomen and may exacerbate respiratory failure. Emergency decompression with a wide-bore gastric tube improves cardiorespiratory function and reduces the risk of aspiration.

ACUTE RESPIRATORY DISTRESS SYNDROME

Acute respiratory distress syndrome (ARDS) may occur in children of all ages from a variety of direct and indirect lung insults. ARDS is characterised by respiratory distress or failure, diffuse pulmonary infiltrates, reduced pulmonary compliance and hypoxaemia in the presence of a known precipitating cause and in the absence of left ventricular failure. In children, common causes include shock from any cause, pneumonia, sepsis, near drowning, aspiration and pulmonary contusion.

POISONING

Accidental poisoning is a common but preventable cause of respiratory failure, particularly in the first 4 years of life. Deliberate overdose is seen in children beyond 8 years. Tricyclic antidepressants, antihistamines, anticonvulsants and attention deficit hyperactivity disorder (ADHD) medications (clonidine, methylphenidate, dexamfetamine) are now the commonest CNS-affecting drugs ingested. Convulsions may aggravate the situation.

MENINGITIS AND ENCEPHALITIS

Meningitis is common in the early years of life. After the neonatal period, the usual causative organisms are *Haemophilus influenzae, Neisseria meningitidis* and *Streptococcus pneumoniae*. Immunisation has markedly reduced the incidence in developed countries. Rapid diagnosis and appropriate antibiotic therapy form the cornerstone of treatment. Respiratory failure is mainly associated with uncontrolled convulsions, altered conscious state or raised intracranial pressure (ICP).

Encephalitis may also cause unconsciousness and raised ICP. Associated problems are upper airway obstruction, pulmonary aspiration and central respiratory depression. In many cases of encephalitis, a causative organism is not found although viral or postinfective causes are suspected. The antiviral agent, aciclovir, should be administered until herpes encephalitis is excluded. Hyperpyrexia, convulsions and cerebral oedema may complicate encephalitis.

GUILLAIN–BARRÉ SYNDROME

This is the most common polyneuritis in childhood. Ascending paralysis may involve the intercostal muscles, the diaphragm and bulbar muscles. The onset may be rapid, with respiratory failure occurring within 48 hours. Intervention is based on clinical assessment of cough reflex and bulbar function, a measured vital capacity < 15 ml/kg, and evidence of hypoxaemia ($Sa\text{O}_2 < 90\%$). Hypoxaemia occurs relatively early due to reduced functional residual capacity, atelectasis and intrapulmonary shunting. An elevated $Pa\text{CO}_2$ is a late feature, suggesting a vital capacity in the tidal range, i.e. < 5–7 ml/kg. CMV is usually necessary if intubation is required. Unless rapid recovery is anticipated, early tracheostomy is advocated for patient comfort, to allow speech and to facilitate mobilisation. The condition is often improved by the early use of i.v. immunoglobulin therapy or plasmapheresis. Immunoglobulin is easier to deliver and probably safer. Other complications relate to autonomic involvement (arrhythmias, blood pressure lability) and ileus. Muscle pain may require analgesic relief.

Transverse myelitis may present in a similar manner and the principles of management are the same. Nerve conduction studies and MRI may be necessary to distinguish between the two conditions. Immunoglobulin therapy and plasmapheresis, however, are not effective. There are some reports of benefit from steroid therapy.

ENVENOMATION

Some animal venoms, such as those of some snakes, ticks and blue-ringed octopus, are neurotoxic and may cause muscle weakness and respiratory insufficiency. The Sydney funnel-web spider causes widespread acetylcholine release and symptoms similar to anticholinesterase poisoning. These symptoms include intense salivation, lacrimation, sweating, laryngeal and muscle spasm and pulmonary oedema. Paralysis due to tetrodotoxin may rapidly follow puffer-fish ingestion. In Australia and many other countries, specific antivenom therapy is available for most potentially lethal envenomations. Supportive therapy is required until antivenom is administered and recovery occurs.

MANAGEMENT OF ACUTE RESPIRATORY FAILURE

In some cases, definitive treatment of the underlying cause will lead to resolution of respiratory failure (e.g. relief of upper airway obstruction or reversal of drug depression). Where this is not possible, mechanical ventilatory support is required until the underlying process has resolved.

GENERAL MEASURES

GENERAL NURSING CARE

Critically ill children require a nurse:patient ratio of 1:1 and it important that the nurses are skilled in the care of a ventilated child. This is one of the important differences between a paediatric intensive care unit and a general unit that only occasionally looks after children.

THERMAL ENVIRONMENT

Maintenance of body temperature is of major importance. The immature newborn is particularly vulnerable to cold stress, which increases metabolism, rapidly depletes carbohydrate stores and causes cardiorespiratory deterioration. In a normal newborn, oxygen consumption may rise threefold on exposure to environmental temperatures of 20–25°C. Conditions are optimal when the abdominal skin temperature is 36–36.5°C.

The most satisfactory devices to maintain temperature homeostasis are servo-controlled infrared-heated open cots. These allow for observation of and access to the exposed infant. In an incubator, the environmental temperature is less stable and access is difficult. Double-glazed incubators reduce radiant heat loss. Older infants and children can be nursed in standard cots and beds.

POSTURE

Neonates are best nursed prone with the hips and knees flexed and the head turned regularly. This posture may abolish apnoeic episodes in premature infants. It also decreases gastric emptying time, making aspiration of vomitus less likely. However, if the neonate is unstable and interventions are likely, the supine position is preferred. Older infants and young children are usually nursed in the position they find most comfortable although, as in adults, there is evidence that gas exchange is improved by prone positioning in at least some ventilated children.

PHYSIOTHERAPY

The role of conventional chest physiotherapy with posturing, percussion and vibration in the paediatric ICU setting is unproven. Physiotherapy must be applied cautiously in children with cardiovascular instability or raised ICP. Chest compression and vibration in the newborn may result in rib fractures and possibly intracranial haemorrhage. Physiotherapy may cause a significant fall in $Pa\text{O}_2$. $F\text{iO}_2$ should be increased in anticipation (caution is required in premature infants who are at risk of retinopathy of prematurity). In infants, periodic gentle pharyngeal suction removes pharyngeal secretions and may stimulate coughing. Effective bagging, tracheal suction and positioning are the most useful techniques in the intubated patient.

FLUID THERAPY

Oral feeding should be suspended with severe respiratory distress, because of the difficulty in oxygen administration and the risk of abdominal distension, vomiting and aspiration. Nasogastric feeding may be cautiously employed in infants with mild to moderate respiratory distress.

Lung and airway disease is often associated with increased secretion of ADH, leading to fluid retention. Increased airway pressure (e.g. CMV and CPAP) may also increase ADH secretion. Efficient humidification via a tracheal or tracheostomy tube prevents insensible water loss from the airway, and diminishes fluid requirements. Most patients with acute lung disease benefit from some degree of fluid restriction. Fluid balance and biochemical status must be monitored carefully. In prolonged respiratory failure, it is essential to minimise wasting of the respiratory muscles and to provide energy for increased work of breathing. High-calorie oral or nasogastric feeding may be tolerated. Parenteral nutrition is particularly useful when fluid restriction is necessary, and should be commenced early if prolonged interruption to enteral feeding is likely.

MONITORING AND ASSESSMENT

Repeated clinical observation by skilled staff is necessary to detect early signs of hypoxia, increasing respiratory distress, or onset of fatigue. Deterioration may represent a progression of disease state, development of fatigue or the presence of complications. Monitoring of cardiorespiratory parameters and respiratory therapy is imperative for optimal respiratory care.

PULSE OXIMETRY

Pulse oximetry provides essential information about the state of oxygenation (i.e. $Sa\text{O}_2$) on a continuous basis. It is applicable to children of all sizes and can obviate the need for arterial cannulation in some cases. It forms part of a minimum standard for monitoring critically ill infants and children. Surprising degrees of desaturation, undetectable clinically, may be identified and treated.

BLOOD GASES

Measurement of blood gases and acid–base status is essential in cardiorespiratory assessment. Arterial blood is obtained from an indwelling cannula or by direct puncture of peripheral arteries. The latter may be distressing to the child. Results from difficult collections may not accurately reflect the true blood gas status. Topical anaesthesia using EMLA cream should be considered for non-urgent percutaneous sampling.

Peripheral arterial cannulation is routine practice in paediatric intensive care, even in infants weighing less than 1 kg. It allows continuous blood pressure monitoring and reduces sampling errors. The radial, ulnar, brachial, femoral, posterior tibial and dorsalis pedis arteries are suitable. Radial artery cannulation by cut-down should be considered when the percutaneous method fails. Radial and ulnar or posterior tibial and dorsalis pedis vessels must not be cannulated in the same limb, even at different times, because of the danger of distal limb ischaemia. The safety of brachial and femoral cannulation lies in the collateral vessels around the elbow and hip joints. Complications of arterial cannulation include distal ischaemia, infection, haemorrhage and retrograde embolisation when the cannula is flushed. Central venous blood gases provide information on the adequacy of cardiac output (mixed venous oxygen saturation) as well as trends in $P\text{CO}_2$.

In the neonate with acute respiratory failure, a preductal vessel, such as the right radial artery, is preferred. Preductal sampling is important in premature infants, because it indicates the $Pa\text{O}_2$ of blood perfusing the retina. Knowledge of the $F\text{iO}_2$ is essential to interpret information from all forms of oxygen monitoring.

CAPNOGRAPHY

Measurement of the end-tidal $P\text{CO}_2$ in the intubated patient provides a continuous guide to the adequacy of alveolar ventilation. In severe lung disease, the value does not reflect arterial $P\text{CO}_2$ (due to a wide alveolar–arterial gradient). It may still provide valuable trend information, and is also an additional means of warning of sudden reductions in cardiac output.

CHEST X-RAY

Clinical examination of the thorax may be misleading in the small infant and serial chest X-rays form a vital part of assessment. Anteroposterior supine films usually provide the necessary information. Lateral or decubitus views may be useful to localise lung pathology, or to confirm air or fluid collections. Examination should look for focal or generalised lung disease, pleural effusions, evidence of barotrauma, the size and shape of cardiac contour and the position of invasive devices. The tracheal tube should be level with the second thoracic vertebra or the ends of the clavicles, and take account of the neck posture. A change from extension to flexion may advance the endotracheal tube by 1 cm in the term neonate. As the trachea in the neonate is only 4 cm long, accurate placement is critical. Multiple chest X-rays may be required with rapidly changing clinical situations.

TRANSILLUMINATION

Transillumination of the thorax with a cold fibreoptic light source is a useful technique to detect pneumothorax in newborn infants. Transillumination occurs on the side of pneumothorax, but does not quantify the amount of air present. Bilateral pneumothoraces may cause confusion. In severe pulmonary interstitial emphysema, increased transillumination may be seen. A chest X-ray should be performed to confirm the pneumothorax when time permits.

VITAL CAPACITY AND MAXIMUM INSPIRATORY FORCE

In diseases such as Guillain–Barré syndrome, measurements of vital capacity and maximum inspiratory force are useful in older cooperative children. A vital capacity < 15 ml/kg or an inability to generate a maximum inspiratory force of less than -25 cmH_2O (-2.5 kPa) is an indication for intubation and assisted ventilation. These parameters are also useful to guide weaning and extubation or decannulation.

SPECIFIC MEASURES

OXYGEN THERAPY

Mode of administration is guided by patient size and required FiO_2. Neonates requiring less than 40% oxygen can be nursed in an incubator. Plastic headboxes are used to deliver higher concentrations to neonates and infants.

Older children tolerate appropriately sized facemasks but FiO_2 is rarely known. Masks incorporating a reservoir bag will deliver high concentrations in young children. Restless children do not tolerate facemasks and oxygen delivery may become intermittent. Once positioned, nasal cannulae are usually well tolerated. A single catheter in the postnasal space (1–2 l/min) is also an effective method of delivery. With nasal cannulae, FiO_2 depends on flow rate, size of the nasopharynx, the presence or absence of mouth-breathing and peak inspiratory flow rate. Using a single nasal cannula, a flow rate of 150 ml/kg per min provides FiO_2 about 0.5 in children under 2 years.[20] Effective humidification is difficult with nasal cannulae, and drying of mucosa and secretions may be a problem.

Therapeutic procedures, physiotherapy and handling may all increase oxygen consumption and lead to hypoxaemia and deterioration. Timing of these manoeuvres is important and a prior increase in FiO_2 may be justified.

COMPLICATIONS OF OXYGEN THERAPY IN NEONATES

RETINOPATHY OF PREMATURITY

Retinal vessels of premature infants are susceptible to the vasoconstrictive effects of high arterial oxygen tension. Visual impairment is due to retinal fibroproliferative changes or to subsequent retinal detachment. While the absolute safe maximal level and duration of hyperoxia are unknown, maintenance of a PaO_2 between 50 and 80 mmHg (6.6 and 10.6 kPa) is recommended.

BRONCHOPULMONARY DYSPLASIA

The development of chronic pulmonary insufficiency in mechanically ventilated neonates correlates best with lung immaturity, peak inspiratory pressures and other evidence of barotrauma or volutrauma. Pulmonary oxygen toxicity is probably a contributory factor. Chronic hypoxaemia, on the other hand, is a factor in the development of cor pulmonale.

INTUBATION

Tracheal intubation relieves airway obstruction, and allows accurate control of inspired oxygen, application of positive airway pressure and tracheal toilet. Nasotracheal intubation is preferred, as it allows better fixation. Implant-tested polyvinyl chloride tubes may be left in place indefinitely. For long-term use, however, tracheostomy is indicated. Disadvantages of nasotracheal intubation include bypassing nasal humidifying mechanisms, sinusitis, increased airway resistance, risk of subglottic stenosis, impaired cough reflex, loss of physiological PEEP and impaired pulmonary defence mechanisms. In neonates, the risk of laryngeal injury correlates with duration of intubation and repeated intubation trauma. The correct tracheal tube size permits a small leak when a positive pressure of less than 25 cmH_2O (2.5 kPa) is applied. Exceptions to the rule are:

- neonates: for unknown reasons, absence of leak rarely results in complications
- croup, where a smaller tube than predicted for age is passed, and subsequent development of a leak indicates resolution of subglottic oedema and is an indication for extubation
- mechanical ventilation in the presence of poorly compliant lungs, where an airtight seal may be required for effective ventilation – a risk of subglottic stenosis occurs. Alternatively, cuffed endotracheal tubes are increasingly used in children

MECHANICAL VENTILATORY SUPPORT

MECHANICAL VENTILATION

Paediatric ventilators are discussed elsewhere in this volume. The risks of barotrauma, volutrauma and oxygen toxicity demand that specific ventilator settings be prescribed for rate, peak inspiratory pressure, PEEP, CPAP, flow rate, inspiratory time, minute volume and inspired oxygen. If pulmonary function progressively deteriorates, a stepwise increase of each setting should be considered. The least harmful alternative should be undertaken first (e.g. increasing FiO_2 is probably a safer alternative than increasing PEEP). Unless contraindicated, a PEEP of 3–5 cmH_2O (0.3–0.5 kPa) is recommended in all ventilated infants to prevent airway closure. In the presence of reduced cerebral compliance, PEEP may be associated with increased intracranial pressure. Oxygenation is a priority, however, and other means of maintaining cerebral perfusion pressure should be employed if PEEP is required. Removing or reducing PEEP must be considered if there is evidence of barotrauma. Increased PEEP demands a similar increase in peak inspiratory pressure if the same tidal volume is to be maintained. Mean airway pressure is the main determinant of oxygenation. It is dependent on rate, peak inspiratory pressure, flow rate, inspiratory time and PEEP.

In general, slow ventilatory rates (e.g. neonates 30 breaths/min, infants under 12 months 25 breaths/min, children 16–20 breaths/min) and an inspiratory time of about 1 second provide optimal gas exchange. Infants under 1 kg may benefit from faster ventilatory rates and shorter inspiratory times. Short inspiratory times may, however, be associated with loss of lung volume and increased intrapulmonary shunting. Strategies to recruit alveoli are important with many lung diseases, particularly after disconnection for suction and other procedures.

CONTINUOUS POSITIVE AIRWAY PRESSURE

Continuous positive airway pressure (CPAP) applies a constant pressure gradient to the spontaneously breathing patient via a special circuit. The T-piece system requires a fresh gas flow of two to three times the predicted minute ventilation to prevent rebreathing. For CPAP to be well sustained, either the flow rate must exceed peak inspiratory flow or a reservoir bag must be incorporated into the system.

Nasotracheal intubation is the safest and most efficient method of applying CPAP, although masks, nasal cannulae or a nasopharyngeal tube may be used. These latter techniques rely on neonates being obligatory nose breathers; positive pressure is lost during crying or mouth breathing, and abdominal distension may occur. Blood gas sampling during mouth breathing may lead to errors in oxygen therapy. The stomach should be decompressed continuously with a nasogastric tube.

Benefits of CPAP include the following:

- CPAP increases functional residual capacity (FRC), recruits alveoli, promotes alveolar stability and reduces intrapulmonary shunt. An increased $Pa\text{O}_2$ results and allows a reduction in $Fi\text{O}_2$.
- CPAP promotes the stability of large and small airways. This splinting effect is useful in airway obstruction, bronchomalacia and tracheomalacia. CPAP has also been recommended in croup, bronchiolitis and even asthma.
- In neonates, CPAP may abolish or reduce apnoeic episodes and improve the rhythmicity of spontaneous breathing. Physiological amounts of CPAP (2–5 cmH_2O, 0.2–0.5 kPa) should be applied to intubated children whenever practical to prevent airway closure.

Because of the resistance of the endotracheal tube and respiratory circuit, the use of low levels of pressure support ventilation (PSV) is often more effective in minimising the work of breathing.

CPAP may reduce cardiac output or cause barotrauma. Increased ADH secretion and fluid retention are also seen, although the exact mechanism is disputed. If CPAP results in hyperinflation it may also increase pulmonary vascular resistance and right ventricular afterload. This effect is often balanced by the beneficial effect of CPAP in preventing atelectasis, optimising lung volume and thereby reducing pulmonary vascular resistance. It is often difficult to interface CPAP and other non-invasive respiratory techniques to non-sedated infants and children without causing excessive restlessness.

SEDATION AND ANALGESIA

Sedation and analgesia should be used to reduce restlessness and discomfort, and to minimise the work of breathing (see Chapter 100). In the brain injured, sedation prevents coughing, straining, unwanted autonomic responses and increases in intracranial pressure. Heavy sedation (with or without muscle relaxants) is recommended, provided supervision and monitoring facilities are adequate.

COMPLICATIONS

Complications of mechanical ventilatory support include:

- *Reduced cardiac output*: circulatory effects of increased airway pressure may be less marked in young children.[21] Nevertheless, volume expansion (e.g. with 10–20 ml/kg of colloid) may be required at the start of CMV, particularly if muscle relaxants are employed
- *Barotrauma, volutrauma* may present as:

  (a) *pulmonary interstitial emphysema* (PIE) with gas in the lung interstitium, outside the alveoli. This is most common in premature infants, although protective lung ventilation strategies have probably reduced the incidence. PIE is deleterious to gas exchange and is not readily amenable to drainage. It may produce intrapulmonary tension and mediastinal shift. Unfortunately, the initiating factor, positive pressure, may need to be increased further to restore gas exchange. It is a forerunner of pneumothorax. Management is to limit or remove positive pressure as early as possible. High-frequency oscillatory ventilation may be advantageous. Occasionally, decompression of the lung by needling or via thoracotomy may be required
  (b) *pneumothorax*
  (c) *pneumomediastinum*
  (d) *tension pneumopericardium* occasionally occurs in neonates on ventilation and may require decompression by pericardiocentesis or limited sternotomy and drainage
  (e) *pneumoperitoneum*, where a differential diagnosis from ruptured viscus may be difficult. Occasionally, drainage is required to reduce intra-abdominal tension and respiratory embarrassment.

Mechanical ventilation must be approached cautiously if air leak is a particular risk (e.g. in immature lungs and diseases characterised by air trapping). Permissive hypercapnia can often be tolerated, provided that oxygenation, perfusion and acid–base balance are acceptable.

WEANING

The risks of prolonged ventilation (ventilator-induced lung injury, ventilator-associated pneumonia, airway injury, cost) must be balanced against the risk of premature weaning and extubation. Particular risks such as those associated with pulmonary hypertension, myocardial dysfunction and the difficult airway should be considered. Weaning commences when the underlying process necessitating ventilation has resolved sufficiently, the cardiovascular system is stable and the child is awake and has sufficient respiratory drive. It is unlikely to be successful if an F_{IO_2} over 0.5 or peak airway measures greater than 25 cmH_2O (2.5 kPa) are required. PEEP should be reduced to 5 cmH_2O (0.5 kPa) or less prior to intubation. The rate of weaning is determined by the underlying pathology and the expected response.

Progression through IMV and PSV or CPAP is usually advised. Attention to the status of all organ systems must be meticulous, and some degree of fluid restriction is usually indicated. Other forms of circulatory support such as inotropic agents and vasodilators should be maintained during the weaning period. Increased work of breathing places additional demands on the cardiovascular system and may divert blood flow from other vital organs. The patient should be fasted and the abdomen decompressed prior to extubation. A period of fasting before and after long-term intubation is recommended (e.g. up to 24 hours in some cases), to allow for return of laryngeal competence.

HIGH-FREQUENCY OSCILLATORY VENTILATION

High-frequency ventilation (HFV) refers to ventilation at respiratory rates between 4 and 15 Hz, with tidal volumes close to or less than anatomical dead space. Methods of HFV most commonly used are high-frequency jet ventilation, high-frequency flow interruption and high-frequency oscillatory ventilation (HFOV). Most interest has centred on HFOV (10–15 Hz), with tidal volumes well below anatomical dead space. All three can produce adequate oxygenation and CO_2 removal in infants, children and adults with restrictive lung disease, often using lower peak and mean airway pressures than in CMV. In HFOV CO_2 removal is very efficient and occurs by a combination of accelerated diffusion and cardiogenic mixing. Oxygenation is maintained by keeping mean airway pressure above the critical opening pressure for the alveoli. High volume cycling is avoided, thereby limiting further lung injury as a result of repeated sheer stress.

Animal studies using HFOV and an 'open lung strategy' have convincingly demonstrated less of the histological changes of ARDS and less barotrauma.[22,23] Although a multicentre trial of HFOV in preterm infants failed to show benefit, a number of single centre randomised or rescue studies have demonstrated less barotrauma in very low birth weight infants, a decreased incidence of chronic lung disease (BPD) and reduced requirement for ECMO.[24,25] The combined use of HFOV and nitric oxide therapy has led to reduced use of ECMO in many centres. HFOV has an important role in the management of severe pulmonary air leak syndromes.

REFERENCES

1. Muller NL, Bryan AC. Chest wall mechanics and respiratory muscles in infants. *Pediatr Clin North Am* 1979; **26**: 503–26.
2. Keens TG, Bryan AC, Levison H *et al.* Developmental pattern of muscle fibre types in human ventilatory muscles. *J Appl Physiol Respir Environ Exercise Physiol* 1978; **44**: 909–13.
3. Kyocyildirim E, Kanani M, Roebuck D *et al.* Long-segment tracheal stenosis: slide tracheoplasty and a multidisciplinary approach improve outcomes and reduce costs. *J Thorac Cardiovasc Surg* 2004; **128**: 876–82.
4. Kinsella JP, Neish SR, Dunbar ID *et al.* Clinical responses to prolonged treatment of persistent pulmonary hypertension of the newborn with low doses of inhaled nitric oxide. *J Pediatr* 1993; **123**: 103–8.
5. Bose C, Corbet A, Bose G *et al.* Improved outcome at 28 days of age for very low birth weight infants treated with a single dose of a synthetic surfactant. *J Pediatr* 1990; **117**: 947–53.
6. Long W, Corbet A, Cotton R *et al.* A controlled trial of synthetic surfactant in infants weighing 1250 g or more with respiratory distress syndrome. *N Engl J Med* 1991; **325**: 1696–703.
7. Stevenson D, Walther F, Long W *et al.* Controlled trial of a single dose of synthetic surfactant at birth in premature infants weighing 500–699 grams. *J Pediatr* 1992; **120**: S3–12.
8. Jobe A. Pulmonary surfactant therapy. *N Engl J Med* 1993; **328**; 861–8.
9. Park CS, Chung WM, Lim MK *et al.* Transcatheter instillation into loculated pleural effusion: analysis of treatment effect. *Am J Roentgenol* 1996; **167**: 649–52.
10. Gluckman PD, Wyatt JS, Azzopardi D *et al.* Selective head cooling with mild systemic hypothermia after neonatal encephalopathy: multicentre randomised trial. *Lancet* 2005; **365**: 663–70.
11. Sims C, Johnson CM. Postoperative apnoea in infants. *Anaesth Intensive Care* 1994; **22**: 40–5.
12. Robertson CF, Smith F, Beck R *et al.* Response to frequent low doses of nebulized salbutamol in acute asthma. *J Pediatr* 1985; **106**: 672–4.
13. Yung M, South M. Randomised controlled trial of aminophylline for severe acute asthma. *Arch Dis Child* 1998; **79**: 405–10.
14. Baker JW, Yerger SY, Segar WE. Elevated plasma antidiuretic hormone levels in status asthmaticus. *Mayo Clin Proc* 1976; **51**: 31–4.

15. Stalcup SA, Mellins RB. Mechanical forces producing pulmonary edema in acute asthma. *N Engl J Med* 1977; **297**: 592–6.
16. Tuxen DV. Detrimental effects of positive end-expiratory pressure during controlled mechanical ventilation of patients with severe airflow limitation. *Am Rev Resp Dis* 1989; **140**: 5–9.
17. Sanchez I, De Koster J, Powell RE *et al.* Effect of racemic epinephrine and salbutamol on clinical score and pulmonary mechanics in infants with bronchiolitis. *J Pediatr* 1993; **122**: 145–51.
18. Korppi M, Leinonen M, Koskela M *et al.* Bacterial coinfection in children hospitalized with respiratory syncytial virus infections. *Pediatr Infect Dis J* 1989; **8**: 687–92.
19. Lanteri CJ, Kano S, Duncan AW *et al.* Changes in respiratory mechanics in children undergoing cardiopulmonary bypass. *Am J Respir Crit Care Med* 1996; **152**: 1893–900.
20. Shann F, Gatchalian S, Hutchinson R. Nasopharyngeal oxygen in children. *Lancet* 1988; **1**: 1238–40.
21. Clough JB, Duncan AW, Sly PD. The effect of sustained positive airway pressure on derived cardiac output in children. *Anaesth Intensive Care* 1994; **22**: 30–4.
22. Hamilton PP, Onayemi A, Smyth JA *et al.* Comparison of conventional and high-frequency ventilation: oxygenation and lung pathology. *J Appl Physiol* 1983; **55**: 131–8.
23. DeLemos RA, Coalson JJ, Gerstmann DR *et al.* Ventilation management of infant baboons with hyaline membrane disease: the use of high-frequency ventilation. *Pediatr Res* 1987; **21**: 594–602.
24. Clark RH, Yoder BA, Sell MS. Prospective, randomised comparison of high-frequency oscillation and conventional ventilation in candidates for extracorporeal membrane oxygenation. *J Pediatr* 1994; **124**: 447–54.
25. Clark RH, Gerstmann DR, Null DM *et al.* Prospective randomised comparison of high-frequency oscillatory and conventional ventilation in respiratory distress syndrome. *Pediatrics* 1992; **89**: 5–12.

99

Paediatric fluid and electrolyte therapy

Frank A Shann

Children need a much higher intake of water and electrolytes per kilogram of body weight than adults; this makes children more susceptible to dehydration if they have abnormal losses of water or a reduced intake. On the other hand, an inability to excrete a water load, due to immature kidneys (in neonates) or high levels of antidiuretic hormone (ADH), means that children can easily be given too much water intravenously. There are good reviews of fluid and electrolyte therapy in paediatric and neonatal intensive care.[1–5]

WATER

The full-term neonate is 80% water; this figure falls to about 60% by 12 months of age, and then remains almost constant throughout childhood. The intravenous (i.v.) fluid requirements for children in hospital are shown in Tables 99.1 and 99.2. The widely used formula for an active child shown in Table 99.1 was published in 1957,[6] and some of the measurements of energy expenditure were made almost 100 years ago. The formula is a compromise between the requirements of a fully active child and the much lower requirements at basal metabolic rate – for example, the estimate of 100 ml/kg per day for an active 10-kg child in hospital is double the 50 ml/kg per day needed for a sick child at basal state (Table 99.1).[6,7]

Table 99.3 shows that very ill children in intensive care often need much less water than the 'standard' amounts that are often given. For example, if a 15-kg child ('standard' maintenance fluid of 50 ml/hour,[6] Table 99.2) sustains a head injury and has evidence of high levels of ADH (maintenance fluid × 0.7),[8] is ventilated with humidified gas (maintenance × 0.75),[9] is paralysed (basal state, maintenance × 0.7),[6] and is maintained at a rectal temperature of 36°C (maintenance – 12%),[1] then his actual full maintenance fluid requirement is (50 × 0.7 × 0.75 × 0.7) – 12% = 16 ml/hour. Even less water should be given initially if the child is overhydrated.

In very small children, all fluid administered has to be taken into account, including the volume of drugs (bicarbonate, dextrose and antibiotics) and 'flushes' used to clear i.v. lines (after blood sampling or administration of drugs).

The estimates of water requirements in Tables 99.1–99.3 are only approximate, and water balance must be monitored closely in any child in intensive care. Unfortunately, regular, accurate weighing of very sick children is often impractical, and hydration has to be assessed using:

- the serum sodium concentration
- skin turgor
- urine output (minimum 0.5–1.0 ml/kg per hour)
- central venous pressure

In a child with oliguria following a severe ischaemic or hypoxic insult (such as birth asphyxia, near drowning or cardiac arrest), it may be helpful to measure the urine sodium concentration.[10] In oliguria due to acute tubular necrosis, where restriction of fluid intake may be necessary, the urine sodium is usually more than 40 mmol/l. In oliguria due to hypovolaemia, the urine sodium is usually less than 20 mmol/l.

SODIUM[11,12]

Sodium is predominantly an extracellular ion, so total body sodium is well represented by the serum concentration. It must be interpreted in the context of both total hydration and the relative amounts of water and sodium. Acute changes in serum sodium are usually due to changes in body water rather than changes in body sodium.

In the first 1–2 days of life, small preterm babies often have poor urine output and high transcutaneous fluid losses. They are therefore prone to hypernatraemia and hyperkalaemia, and such infants should usually be given 5% or 10% dextrose without sodium or potassium. From 2 days of age, 2–4 mmol/kg per day of sodium and potassium will usually be sufficient, but much higher intakes of sodium are needed in some preterm neonates due to their impaired renal conservation of sodium.

Hyponatraemia may be due to:[11]

- increased body water due to excessive water intake, especially in the presence of high levels of ADH (CNS disease, intermittent positive-pressure ventilation (IPPV), lung disease, vomiting, stress)
- low body sodium due to diuretic therapy, poor renal conservation of sodium, or a low sodium intake (e.g. breast milk)

Table 99.1 Approximate intravenous fluid requirements for children (ml/kg per day)

Active child in hospital	
< 10 kg	100 ml/kg per day
10–20 kg	1000 ml + (50 ml/kg per day for each kg over 10 kg)
> 20 kg	1500 ml + (20 ml/kg per day for each kg over 20 kg)
Sick, but not intubated	
< 10 kg	50 ml/kg per day
10–20 kg	500 ml + (30 ml/kg per day for each kg over 10 kg)
> 20 kg	800 ml + (20 ml/kg per day for each kg over 20 kg)
Intubated, with humidified inspired gases	
< 10 kg	35 ml/kg per day
10–20 kg	350 ml + (20 ml/kg per day for each kg over 10 kg)
> 20 kg	550 ml + (12.5 ml/kg per day for each kg over 20 kg)

Table 99.3 Modifications to the fluid intakes for active children shown in Table 99.2

Decrease	Adjustment
Humidified inspired air	× 0.75
Basal state (e.g. paralysed)	× 0.7
High ADH (IPPV, brain injury)	× 0.7
Hypothermia	− 12% per °C
High room humidity	× 0.7
Renal failure	× 0.3 (+ urine output)
Increase	
Full activity + oral feeds	× 1.5
Fever	+ 12% per °C
Room temperature > 31°C	+ 30% per °C
Hyperventilation	× 1.2
Neonate preterm (1–1.5 kg)	× 1.2
radiant heater	× 1.5
phototherapy	× 1.5
Burns first day	+ 4% per 1% area burnt
subsequently	+ 2% per 1% area burnt

ADH, antidiuretic hormone; IPPV, intermittent positive pressure ventilation.

Acute hyponatraemia causes cerebral oedema, with a grave risk of cerebral herniation and death or severe brain damage.[13] Hyponatraemia due to sodium deficit should be corrected by careful administration of sodium (Table 99.4). However, hyponatraemia is usually due to water excess rather than sodium deficiency, and this should be treated with restriction of water intake. If symptomatic, it can be corrected by careful administration of 3% sodium at 0.5 ml/kg per hour (Table 99.4), and furosemide 0.5 mg/kg i.v. if there are high ADH levels. Hyponatraemia must be corrected slowly: the serum sodium should increase by no more than 8 mmol/l each 24 hours, and even less in patients with long-standing hyponatraemia.[11]

Hypernatraemia may be due to:[12]

- reduced body water (dehydration) from a large insensible fluid loss (caused by radiant heaters or phototherapy), diarrhoea, osmotic diuresis (caused by glycosuria) or inadequate fluid intake
- increased body sodium from administration of large amounts of sodium (e.g. sodium bicarbonate) or salt poisoning

With hypernatraemic dehydration, shock should be treated with boluses of 10 ml/kg of 0.9% saline. The water deficit should then be corrected very slowly using 0.9% saline so that the serum sodium falls no faster than 0.5 mmol/l per hour to prevent cerebral oedema.[12] If salt ingestion causes severe acute hypernatraemia without dehydration, peritoneal dialysis or haemofiltration may be indicated.

POTASSIUM[14]

Potassium is predominantly an intracellular ion, so total body potassium is poorly represented by the serum concentration. The concentration of potassium in the serum depends on pH as well as the total body potassium (which is usually about 50 mmol/kg). A child may have hypokalaemia without a deficit of total body potassium in the presence of alkalosis and, conversely, there may be a large deficit of potassium without hypokalaemia in the presence of acidosis. Potassium should rarely be infused at more than 0.3 mmol/kg per hour, and it should not normally be given to a patient with severe oliguria or anuria.

Table 99.2 Approximate intravenous fluid requirements for children (ml per hour)

	Weight in kg											
	3	5	7	10	15	20	25	30	40	50	60	70
Active	12	20	30	40	50	60	65	70	80	90	95	100
Sick	6	10	14	20	25	30	35	40	45	55	60	70
Intubated	4	7	10	14	17	21	25	28	32	40	45	50

Table 99.4 Doses and formulae in paediatric fluid and electrolyte therapy

Albumin 20%	undiluted: 2–4 ml/kg 5% in 5% dextrose or saline: 10–20 ml/kg
Bicarbonate (number of mmol of deficit)	under 5 kg: base excess × wt(kg) × 0.5 (give half of this) over 5 kg: base excess × wt(kg) × 0.3 (give half of this)
Blood volume	85 ml/kg in neonate 70 ml/kg in older children
Calcium	chloride 10% (0.7 mmol/ml Ca^{++}): maximum 0.2 ml/kg i.v. stat, requirement 1.5 ml/kg per day gluconate 10% (0.22 mmol/ml Ca^{++}): maximum 0.5 ml/kg i.v. stat, requirement 5 ml/kg per day
Dextrose	for hypoglycaemia: 1 ml/kg 50% dextrose i.v. in neonate: 4 mg/kg per min (2.4 ml/kg per hour 10% dextrose) day 1, increasing to 8 mg/kg per min (up to 12 mg/kg per min with hypoglycaemia) for hyperkalaemia: 0.1 U/kg insulin and 2 ml/kg 50% dextrose i.v. stat
Magnesium	chloride 0.48 g/5 ml (1 mmol/ml Mg^{++}): 0.4 mmol (0.4 ml)/kg per dose slow i.v. 12-hourly sulphate 50% (2 mmol/ml Mg^{++}): 0.4 mmol (0.2 ml)/kg per dose slow i.v. 12-hourly
Mannitol	0.25–0.5 g/kg per dose i.v. (1–2 ml/kg of 25%) 2-hourly, provided serum osmolality < 330 mosm/kg
Packed cells	10 ml/kg raises Hb 3 g%, 1 ml/kg raises PCV 1%.
Potassium	maximum 0.3 mmol/kg per hour, requirement 2–4 mmol/kg per day, 1 g KCl = 13.3 mmol K^+. Hyperkalaemia: see dextrose
Sodium	depletion: 3% saline at 0.5 ml/kg per hour (maximum Na rise 8 mmol/l in 24 hours); requirement 2–6 mmol/kg per day, 1 g NaCl = 17.1 mmol/Na^+
Urine	minimum acceptable is 0.5–1.0 ml/kg per hour

PCV, packed cell volume.

CALCIUM, MAGNESIUM AND PHOSPHATE

Hypocalcaemia in children occurs in:

- sick neonates in the first two days of life
- infants of diabetic mothers
- exchange transfusion with citrated blood (a temporary effect)
- magnesium deficiency
- infants fed cows' milk (which has a high phosphate content)

Hypocalcaemia and hypomagnesaemia cause jitters, tetany, cardiac arrhythmias and convulsions. The doses of calcium and magnesium are given in Table 99.4. The normal intravenous maintenance requirements in infants are 1 mmol/kg per day of calcium and 0.3 mmol/kg per day of magnesium.

STANDARD PAEDIATRIC MAINTENANCE FLUIDS

'Maintenance solution' is an unfortunate term, since these solutions do not provide maintenance calorie or protein requirements (see Parenteral nutrition, below). Until recently, it was common practice to give children a hypotonic maintenance solution of approximately 0.2% saline in 4% dextrose in generous amounts, based on the water requirements of an active child.[6] This policy resulted in a high incidence of hyponatraemia – and far too many children developed cerebral oedema that resulted in death or severe brain damage.[13,15–18]

Several factors have contributed to the high incidence of hyponatraemia in children.

- The amount of dehydration present is often overestimated,[19] and rapid administration of an excessive amount of fluid will cause hyponatraemia, even if 0.9% saline is given, because the increase in intravascular volume will cause the production of urine containing more than 154 mmol/l of sodium (the amount present in 0.9% saline).[20]
- The formula that is widely used to calculate maintenance water requirements is based on the needs of active children, and prescribes too much fluid for a sick child (Table 99.1).[13]
- Many sick children have increased secretion of antidiuretic hormone even in the absence of hypovolaemia,[21,22] so they are unable to excrete the excess water when they are given large amounts of fluid.
- Some sick children lose substantial amounts of sodium in their urine, perhaps due in part to the excretion of ketones as sodium salts.[18]

There is general agreement that an isotonic fluid such as 0.9% saline should be used to correct hypovolaemia, but there has been spirited debate about whether hypotonic 0.2% saline or isotonic 0.9% saline should be used for maintenance.[5,23,24] The supporters of using 0.2% saline argue that it is logical and safe providing the volume of fluid given is never in excess of actual requirements,[25–27] but there is limited empirical evidence to support this theory.[27] The supporters of using 0.9% saline for initial maintenance therapy in sick children (with careful monitoring of the serum sodium) argue that, in practice, this has been preferable,[13,15–18] because it is difficult to ensure that no excess fluid is administered, and there is a lower risk of hyponatraemia and cerebral oedema if any excess fluid that is given is isotonic. It is especially important to use isotonic fluid during and after surgery, and whenever there is a high risk of cerebral oedema (e.g. amongst children with diabetic ketoacidosis or brain injury).[5,15–18,23,24]

Ill children with clear signs of hypovolaemia should be treated with 5–10 ml/kg boluses of 0.9% saline until the intravascular volume has been restored, and then given 0.9% saline (with potassium and dextrose as required) in the volumes shown in Tables 99.1 and 99.2 (or calculated from Table 99.3). The serum sodium concentration should be monitored carefully. If the serum sodium is less than 138 mmol/l and falling, then less 0.9% saline should be infused. If the serum sodium is more than 142 mmol/l and rising, then 0.45% or 0.2% saline should be infused with a cautious increase in the rate.

Great care should be taken to avoid hypoglycaemia in children. Hypoglycaemia is particularly dangerous in young infants,[28] while hyperglycaemia is probably less dangerous in children than it is in adults in intensive care.[29]

The key messages are:

- correct hypovolaemia using 10 ml/kg boluses of 0.9% saline
- most sick children need far less maintenance fluid than previously thought (Table 99.2)
- use isotonic maintenance fluid for the first few days of treatment with careful monitoring of the serum sodium
- avoid hypoglycaemia

DEHYDRATION AND SHOCK

Weight loss is the best guide to the degree of dehydration, if a recent weight is known. Many of the commonly used clinical signs of dehydration in children are inaccurate, and this leads to dehydration being diagnosed when it is not present, and to overestimation of the degree of dehydration.[19] The clinical signs of mild to moderate dehydration become apparent with only 3–4% dehydration in children.[19] The most reliable signs are:[30]

- decreased peripheral perfusion (as shown by pallor or reduced capillary return)
- deep breathing
- decreased skin turgor

In children with shock, intravenous access may be difficult. In these circumstances, parenteral fluid can be given rapidly into the bone marrow, which is an intravascular compartment.[31] The usual sites chosen are the junction of the upper and middle third of the tibia (0–12 months of age), the medial malleolus (1–5 years) and the iliac crest (over 5 years). A 0.9 mm (20 gauge) lumbar puncture needle or an intraosseous needle can be used; the needle is held perpendicular to the bone and pushed in *gently* with a rotary motion about its long axis – a slight decrease in resistance will be felt as the needle enters the medulla. In infants with a patent anterior fontanelle, the superior sagittal sinus is an excellent way to gain intravenous access in an emergency.[32]

Shock should be treated with an initial bolus of 10 ml/kg of 0.9% saline, followed by further boluses of 10 ml/kg until the intravascular volume has been restored.[33] After shock has been corrected with a rapid infusion of fluid, the remainder of the deficit is replaced over the next 48–72 hours, while giving maintenance requirements using 0.9% saline with dextrose and potassium chloride. Thus, a 5-kg child with 10% dehydration from diarrhoea (500 ml deficit) might receive 100 ml (20 ml/kg) of isotonic saline rapidly to restore the circulation, leaving a 400 ml deficit to be replaced over 48 hours. If the maintenance requirement is 250 ml/day (Table 99.1), then the child should be given a further 450 ml of 0.9% saline per day for the next 2 days (approximately 20 ml/hour) in addition to the initial 100 ml. Further abnormal fluid losses should be replaced with an appropriate fluid (see Table 99.5).

With hypernatraemic dehydration, shock should be treated as above, with rapid infusion of 10–20 ml/kg of isotonic saline. The remaining deficit should then be replaced *slowly* with 0.9% saline so that the serum sodium falls no faster than 0.5 mmol/l per hour to prevent cerebral oedema.[12]

In dehydration due to pyloric stenosis there is a deficit of water, hydrogen ion, chloride and potassium. Hypovolaemia should be treated by rapid infusion of 10–20 ml/kg of 0.9% saline, then 0.9% saline in 5% dextrose with 40 mmol/l of potassium chloride should be given at 50 ml/kg per day with careful monitoring of the serum electrolytes and blood glucose.

OEDEMA

Oedema is common in children in intensive care units. It may be due to:

- excess water intake, often with high levels of ADH (from CNS disease, IPPV or lung disease)
- capillary leak (due to the effects of hypoxia, ischaemia, acidosis or sepsis)
- hypoalbuminaemia
- heart failure or renal failure

Table 99.5 Composition of some body fluids in children

Fluid	Na^+ mmol/l	K^+ mmol/l	Cl^- mmol/l	HCO_3^- mmol/l	Other
Gastric fluid	20–80	10–20	100–150	0	H^+ 30–120
Bile	140–160	3–15	80–120	15–30	
Pancreatic fluid	120–160	5–15	75–135	10–45	Basal state
Jejunal fluid	130–150	5–10	100–130	10–20	
Ileal fluid	50–150	3–15	20–120	30–50	
Diarrhoeal fluid	10–90	10–80	10–110	20–70	
Sweat					
Normal	10–30	3–10	10–35	0	
Cystic fibrosis	50–130	5–25	50–110	0	
Burn exudate	140	5	110	20	Protein 30–50 g/l
Saliva	10–25	20–35	10–30	2–10	Unstimulated

Several possible causes are often present in one child, and it can be difficult to decide which is the most important. Children with oedema and high levels of ADH will have a serum osmolality less than 270 mmol/kg (with hyponatraemia) and a urine osmolality greater than 270 mmol/kg; the appropriate treatment is fluid restriction. On the other hand, in children with oedema due to capillary leak, fluid restriction and attempts to remove water (diuretics, dialysis) are unlikely to cure the oedema, and often cause hypovolaemia; in fact, large amounts of fluid (e.g. blood and normal saline) may be needed to preserve the intravascular volume in these children – the oedema will only disappear when the capillary damage resolves.

CRYSTALLOID OR COLLOID

There have been many reviews of the contentious issue of the relative merits of crystalloid or colloid fluids in critically ill patients. A widely quoted review concluded that, compared to crystalloids, albumin increased mortality by 6% (95% CI, 3–9%).[34] However, a subsequent large study in 6997 adults in Australia found no significant difference in overall mortality between normal saline and 4% albumin;[35] the mortality with albumin tended to be lower in sepsis and higher in trauma, but the differences just failed to reach statistical significance in both subgroups. The current Cochrane analysis is heavily influenced by the large Australian study, and it concludes that there is no evidence that albumin reduces mortality when compared with cheaper alternatives such as saline.[36]

There have been very few studies comparing crystalloid to colloid fluids in children, so most of the evidence comes from studies in adults. The use of albumin in paediatric and neonatal intensive care has been reviewed.[37,38] The meta-analyses do not suggest that colloid is better than crystalloid, and colloid is more expensive and carries a small risk of transmitting infection. Until more evidence is available, it seems sensible to use crystalloid as routine, but give concentrated albumin to children with severe hypoalbuminaemia (perhaps if their serum albumin is less than 25 g/l), unless the low albumin is caused by chronic malnutrition, when albumin should *not* be given.[39]

PARENTERAL NUTRITION[40–42]

'Maintenance solution' is an unfortunate medical term, particularly when small children are concerned – a solution of 5% dextrose with sodium and potassium chloride provides maintenance amounts of water, sodium, potassium and chloride, but little or no calories, protein, trace elements or vitamins. For example, 100 ml/kg per day of 5% dextrose provides 20 cal/kg per day (84 kJ/kg per day), which is only 20% of the requirement of a normal infant (let alone a child with increased calorie requirements). It has been estimated that, although an adult has the energy reserve to survive for about a year on 3 litres of 10% dextrose a day, a small preterm infant will survive only 11 days on 75 ml/kg per day of 10% dextrose.[43]

Many children in intensive care units are unable to absorb adequate amounts of food from the gut, and their nutritional reserves are small, so they often need parenteral nutrition. However, parenteral nutrition is difficult to administer and dangerous in small children – such patients should be referred to a specialist paediatric unit as soon as possible.

The usual requirements for amino acids, dextrose and fat in parenteral nutrition in children are shown in Table 99.6. The amino acid solution can be mixed with dextrose in the Pharmacy Department to make a 'nutrient solution'. A standard nutrient solution might provide 4 mmol/kg per day of sodium, 3 mmol/kg per day of potassium, and 7.5 mmol/

Table 99.6 Approximate requirements in paediatric parenteral nutrition

	Total fluid ml/kg per day*	Amino acids (g/kg per day) Day			Dextrose (g/kg per day) Day			Lipid (g/kg per day) Day				Total calories (kcal) needed (1 kcal = 4.2 kJ)
		1	2	3+	1	2	3+	1	2	3	4+	
Neonates	100	1.5	2	2	10	10–15	15–20	1	2	2	2–3	100/kg
Under 10 kg	100	1.5	2	2	10	10	15–20	1	2	2	2–3	100/kg
10–15 kg	90	1	1.5	2	5	10	15	1	1.5	2	2–3	1000 + (50/kg over 10 kg)
15–20 kg	80	1	1.5	1.5–2	5	10	10–15	1	1	1.5	2–3	1000 + (50/kg over 10 kg)
20–30 kg	65	1	1	1–2	5	10	10–15	1	1	1	1–2	1500 + (20/kg over 20 kg)
30–50 kg	50	1	1	1–2	5	5–10	10	1	1	1	1–2	1500 + (20/kg over 20 kg)

*1 ml/kg per day of fluid is needed for each kcal/kg per day; for adjustments to requirements, see Table 99.3 [Total kcal/kg per day equals g/kg per day of (amino acids × 4) + (dextrose × 4) + (lipid × 10)].
Calorie requirement of an active child in hospital.

day of calcium and phosphate (with up to 12 mmol/l for neonates). The standard solution should also contain 4 mmol/l of magnesium, 0.2 μmol/kg per day of manganese, 3 μmol/kg per day of zinc, 0.5 μmol/kg per day of copper, 0.04 μmol/kg per day of iodide, 0.005 μmol/kg per day of chromium, 20 μg/l of hydroxycobalamin, 2 mg/l of phytomenadione, 1 mg/l of folic acid, and a multivitamin preparation. For short-term nutrition, the solution need not provide fluoride, iron or vitamins A, D and E, but a paediatric multivitamin preparation should be given to children on long-term parenteral nutrition. Fat can be given as a 20% emulsion, either through a separate i.v. line or alternating with the nutrient solution. Nutrient solutions for paediatric use contain high concentrations of calcium, magnesium and phosphorus, and they should not be mixed with the fat emulsion, even in a Y-connection placed just before the cannula.

In a child on parenteral nutrition, it is important that abnormal fluid losses (Table 99.5) be replaced with an appropriate solution (in addition to the nutrient solution), and that parenteral nutrition always be introduced and withdrawn slowly. A dislodged i.v. cannula should be replaced immediately in a child on parenteral nutrition to prevent rebound hypoglycaemia. If nutrient solution is not available at any time, it should be replaced with an infusion of a similar amount of dextrose (e.g. 20% dextrose with 40 mmol/l of sodium chloride and 20 mmol/l of potassium chloride).

Children receiving parenteral nutrition are liable to develop:

- hyperglycaemia (with glycosuria and dehydration)
- hypoglycaemia
- sepsis
- extravasation of solutions with necrosis of tissue
- thrombocytopenia
- hypoproteinaemia
- electrolyte imbalance
- acidosis
- anaemia
- hyperlipaemia
- uraemia
- cholestatic jaundice

Frequent, careful monitoring is essential (Table 99.7). Initially, monitoring may need to be more frequent than suggested in Table 99.7, particularly in preterm babies. Monitoring can be less frequent once a child is stabilised on parenteral nutrition.

Table 99.7 Monitoring in paediatric parenteral nutrition

Daily: inspect i.v. site, electrolytes, acid–base, serum triglyceride (reduce lipid infusion rate if triglyceride is greater than 2–2.5 mmol/l)
Twice weekly: haemoglobin (transfuse if anaemia develops), platelets, proteins
Weekly: creatinine, magnesium, calcium, phosphate, bilirubin, aspartate aminotransferase
Blood glucose 8-hourly until the dextrose intake is stable
Test urine for glucose 8-hourly (reduce dextrose intake if more than trace)
Weigh frequently (daily if possible)

REFERENCES

1. Winters RW (ed) *The Body Fluids in Pediatrics*. Boston: Little Brown; 1973.
2. Finberg L, Kravath RE, Hellerstein S. *Water and Electrolytes in Pediatrics: Physiology, Pathophysiology and Treatment*, 2nd edn. Philadelphia: Saunders; 1993.
3. Greenbaum LA. Pathophysiology of body fluids and fluid therapy. In: Behrman RE, Kliegman RM, Jenson HB (eds) *Nelson: Textbook of Pediatrics*, 3rd edn. Philadelphia: Saunders; 2004: 191–252.
4. Dell KM, Davis ID. Fluid and electrolyte management. In: Martin RJ, Fanaroff AA, Walsh MC (eds) *Fanaroff and Martin's Neonatal–Perinatal Medicine*, 8th edn. Philadelphia: Mosby; 2005: 695–712.
5. Paut O, Lacroix F. Recent developments in the perioperative fluid management for the paediatric patient. *Curr Opin Anaesthesiol* 2006; **19**: 268–77.
6. Holliday MA, Segar WE. The maintenance need for water in parenteral fluid therapy. *Pediatrics* 1957; **19**: 823–32.
7. Talbot FB. Basal metabolism standards for children. *Am J Dis Child* 1938; **55**: 455–9.
8. Bouzarth WF, Shenkin HA. Is 'cerebral hyponatraemia' iatrogenic? *Lancet* 1982; **1**: 1061–62.
9. Sousulski R, Polin RA, Baumgart S. Respiratory water loss and heat balance in intubated infants receiving humidified air. *J Pediatr* 1983; **103**: 307–10.
10. Harrington JT, Cohen JJ. Measurement of urinary electrolytes – indications and limitations. *N Engl J Med* 1975; **293**: 1241–3.
11. Androgué HJ, Madias NE. Hyponatremia. *N Engl J Med* 2000; **342**: 1581–9.
12. Androgué HJ, Madias NE. Hypernatremia. *N Engl J Med* 2000; **342**: 1493–9.
13. Choong K, Kho ME, Menon K *et al.* Hypotonic versus isotonic saline in hospitalized children: a systematic review. *Arch Dis Child* 2006; **91**: 828–35.
14. Gennari FJ. Hypokalemia. *N Engl J Med* 1998; **339**: 451–8.
15. Taylor D, Durward A. Pouring salt on troubled waters. *Arch Dis Child* 2004; **89**: 411–4.
16. Hoorn EJ, Geary D, Robb M *et al.* Acute hyponatremia related to intravenous fluid administration in hospitalized children: an observational study. *Pediatrics* 2004; **113**: 1279–84.
17. Moritz ML, Ayus JC. Preventing neurological complications from dysnatremias in children. *Pediatr Nephrol* 2005; **20**: 1687–700.
18. Neville KA, Verge CF, Rosenberg AR *et al.* Isotonic is better than hypotonic saline for intravenous rehydration of children with gastroenteritis: a prospective randomized study. *Arch Dis Child* 2006; **91**: 226–32.
19. Mackenzie A, Barnes G, Shann F. Clinical signs of dehydration in children. *Lancet* 1989; **1**: 605–7.
20. Steele A, Gowrishankar M, Abrahamson S *et al.* Postoperative hyponatremia despite near-isotonic saline infusion: a phenomenon of desalination. *Ann Intern Med* 1997; **126**: 20–5.
21. Gerigk M, Gnehm HE, Rascher W. Arginine vasopressin and renin in acutely ill children: implications for fluid therapy. *Acta Paediatr* 1996; **85**: 550–3.
22. Neville KA, Verge CF, O'Meara MW *et al.* High antidiuretic hormone levels and hyponatremia in children with gastroenteritis. *Pediatrics* 2005; **116**: 1401–7.
23. Cunliffe M, Potter F. Four and a fifth and all that. *Br J Anaesth* 2006; **97**: 274–7.
24. Sterns RH, Silver SM. Salt and water: read the package insert. *Q J Med* 2003; **96**: 549–52.
25. Holliday MA, Friedman AL, Segar WE *et al.* Acute hospital-induced hyponatremia in children: a physiological approach. *J Pediatr* 2004; **145**: 584–7.
26. Hatherill M. Rubbing salt in the wound. *Arch Dis Child* 2004; **89**: 414–8.
27. Sanchez-Bayle M, Alonso-Ojembarrena A, Cano-Fernandez J. Intravenous rehydration of children with gastroenteritis: which solution is better? *Arch Dis Child* 2006; **91**: 716.
28. Kinnala A, Rikalainen H, Lapinleimu H *et al.* Cerebral magnetic resonance imaging and ultrasonography findings after neonatal hypoglycemia. *Pediatrics* 1999; **103**: 724–9.
29. de Ferranti S, Gauvreau K, Hickey PR *et al.* Intraoperative hyperglycemia during infant cardiac surgery is not associated with adverse neurodevelopmental outcomes at 1, 4, and 8 years. *Anesthesiology* 2004; **100**: 1345–52.
30. Steiner MJ, De Walt DA, Byerley JS. Is this child dehydrated? *JAMA* 2004; **291**: 2746–54.
31. Spivey WH. Intraosseous infusions. *J Pediatr* 1987; **111**: 639–43.
32. Shann F. Cannulation of superior sagittal sinus. *Lancet* 2002; **359**: 1700.
33. Scheinkestel CD, Tuxen DV, Cade JF *et al.* Fluid management of shock in critically ill patients. *Med J Aust* 1989; **150**: 508–17.
34. Roberts E. Human albumin administration in critically ill patients: systematic review of randomised controlled trials. *BMJ* 1998; **317**: 235–40.
35. The SAFE Study Investigators. A comparison of albumin and saline for fluid resuscitation in the intensive care unit. *N Engl J Med* 2004; **350**: 2247–56.
36. Alderson P, Bunn F, Li Wan Po A *et al.* Human albumin solution for resuscitation and volume expansion in critically ill patients. *Cochrane Database Syst Rev* 2004; Issue 4, Art No CD0001208.
37. Bohn D, Carcillo JA (eds) The use of albumin in pediatric and neonatal critical care. *Pediatr Crit Care Med* 2001; **2**(Suppl 1): S1–S39.
38. Uhing MR. The albumin controversy. *Clin Perinatol* 2004; **31**: 475–88.
39. World Health Organization. *Management of the Child with a Serious Infection or Severe Malnutrition*. WHO/FCH/CAH/00.1. Geneva: WHO; 2000.

40. Baker RD, Baker SS, Davis AM. *Pediatric Parenteral Nutrition*. New York: Aspen; 1997.
41. Shulman RJ, Phillips S. Parenteral nutrition in infants and children. *J Pediatr Gastroenterol Nutr* 2003; **36**: 587–607.
42. Poindexter BB, Leitch CA, Denne SC. Parenteral nutrition. In: Martin RJ, Fanaroff AA, Walsh MC (eds) *Fanaroff and Martin's Neonatal–Perinatal Medicine*, 8th edn. Philadelphia: Mosby; 2005: 679–93.
43. Heird WC, Driscoll JM, Schullinger JN *et al*. Intravenous alimentation in pediatric patients. *J Pediatr* 1972; **80**: 351–72.

100

Sedation and analgesia in children

Geoff Knight

All children, including preterm infants, feel and remember pain and discomfort.[1] Provision of adequate sedation and analgesia should therefore be a priority in the management of all critically ill children.

INDICATIONS AND BENEFITS

Pain in the paediatric intensive care unit (PICU) may be surgical in origin or due to the underlying illness or to procedures (e.g. central venous catheterisation, lumbar puncture and removal of drains). Sedation is frequently necessary to allow a child to tolerate an endotracheal tube and mechanical ventilation. It may also be needed to allow sleep in a brightly lit, noisy environment. As young children are unlikely to cooperate during investigations, such as an echocardiogram or computed tomographic (CT) scan, sedation is often necessary to prevent excessive movement.

In addition to its humane benefits, sedation and analgesia can suppress non-advantageous physiological responses to noxious stimuli. Analgesic suppression of the marked postsurgery stress response has been associated with significant improvements in postoperative morbidity and mortality.[2–4]

ASSESSMENT

Adequacy of pain relief and sedation is dependent on an accurate assessment of the degree of discomfort. This is particularly difficult in the critically ill child who may be preverbal, developmentally delayed, intubated and/or paralysed, or simply uncooperative. Thorough assessment requires careful and frequent consideration of a number of factors. These include the nature of the noxious stimulus, variations in physiological parameters (e.g. heart rate and blood pressure) and interpretation of subjective clues (e.g. facial expressions and posture). Parental interpretations are reliable and should be included in the overall assessment.

Pain and sedation assessment tools should also be utilised. Neonates and infants are particularly difficult to assess and validated assessment tools, including the Premature Infant Pain Profile (PIPP) and CRIES scale, are helpful objective measures of pain in this group.[5] The Multidimensional Assessment of Pain Scale (MAPS) has recently been validated as a tool for assessing postoperative pain in preverbal children.[6] Established tools such as the Face, Legs, Activity, Cry and Consolability (FLACC) Scale have been modified to enhance the pain assessment of children with cognitive impairment.[7] The COMFORT and the modified COMFORT 'Behavior' are validated observer reported sedation scales for children 1–3 years.[8] In older children, self-reporting measurement scales can be used but these require a degree of patient cooperation.

The most challenging group of patients to manage optimally are those receiving muscle paralysis. Attempts to enhance the limited clinical parameters available for interpretation with an objective measure have centred on the bispectral index (BIS). Validation studies in the paediatric intensive care environment are limited and highlight the probable inaccuracy of current methods of assessing sedation in paralysed patients.[9] In general it is preferable to err on the side of over- rather than under-sedation in the paralysed patient.

APPROACH TO MANAGEMENT

The management of discomfort, anxiety and pain should be multifaceted. Recently published consensus guidelines from the United Kingdom Paediatric Intensive Care Society present a detailed analysis of the evidence for assessment and management strategies.[10]

Management can and should, whenever possible, begin prior to the child's admission to intensive care. Orientation to the unit should be accompanied by a clear, age-appropriate explanation of the planned procedure or operation and the expected postoperative course. Parental presence during this phase and at other critical times is also important to help allay anxiety and fear. Close attention should also be paid throughout a child's admission to potentially distressing physiological factors, such as hunger and urinary retention. In addition to these supportive measures, many paediatric patients require a pharmacological form of analgesia or sedation.

Table 100.1 Single dose and infusion rates of sedative and analgesic drugs*

Drug	Bolus dose	Infusion rate
Morphine	0.1–0.2 mg/kg i.v.	10–40 μg/kg per hour
Fentanyl	1–2 μg/kg i.v.	1–10 μg/kg per hour
Remifentanil	0.1–0.5 μg/kg i.v.	0.1–0.5 μg/kg per min
Midazolam	0.1–0.2 mg/kg i.v. 0.5 mg/kg (oral)	50–200 μg/kg per hour
Ketamine	1–2 mg/kg i.v.	10–20 μg/kg per min (sedation) 4 μg/kg per min (analgesia)
Propofol	1–3 mg/kg i.v.	< 4 mg/kg per hour (short term)
Clonidine	1–2 μg/kg i.v. 4 μg/kg (oral)	0.1–2 μg/kg per hour
Dexmedetomidine	0.5–1 μg/kg i.v.	0.2–1.0 μg/kg per hour

Note: Some infusion rates are described per minute and others per hour.

Sedation and analgesia should be tailored to the patient's particular requirements. It is vital that there be continuous assessment and frequent adjustment of regimes so that optimal levels of sedation and adequate analgesia are delivered at all times. This requires a clear understanding by medical and nursing staff of the aims of management and of the pharmacology of the agents being administered. Relief of pain should be achieved with analgesic agents and care must be taken to avoid the overadministration of sedative agents when the patient's primary need is for pain relief (Table 100.1). While emphasis should be on optimal comfort, consideration should also be given to minimising side-effects. A single drug may be effective but often a combination of medications and a combination of delivery methods (e.g. i.v./oral, i.v./epidural) will be useful and may avoid the side-effects of high doses of a single agent. A recent trend towards analgesia-based sedation, as an approach to managing the ventilated adult patient, has shown benefits when compared to hypnotic-based regimes.[11]

PAEDIATRIC PHARMACOLOGICAL CONSIDERATIONS

Differences in drug handling between children and adults should be considered. Drug distribution, rates of drug metabolism and relative organ blood flows differ in children, particularly in young infants. These differences may result in greater concentrations of free drug and differing volumes of distribution. Neonates have relatively larger total body water, extracellular fluid volume, blood volume and cardiac output and significantly less body fat than adults. Their blood–brain barrier is less efficient and allows more ready entry of some drugs to the brain. Mixed-function oxidases mature quickly to adult levels by 6 months of age, and acetylation and glucuronidation mechanisms mature by about 3 months. Renal blood flow and glomerular filtration rate are low in the immediate neonatal period. However, both increase significantly in the first 2–3 days and reach adult values by around 5 months. Tubular secretory capacity reaches adult levels by 6 months of age. In general therefore, drug metabolism and clearance are relatively mature by 6 months of age but great care is required when dealing with the neonate and young infant.

NON-OPIOID AGENTS

MIDAZOLAM

Midazolam is water soluble, and has a rapid onset of action. Metabolism occurs in the liver and by 6 months of age is comparable to that of an adult. The standard i.v. sedative dose is 0.1–0.2 mg/kg and this is effective for uncomfortable procedures, such as echocardiography and cardioversion. The oral route (0.5 mg/kg) may also be useful though there is a 15-minute delay to onset of sedation. Nasal administration (0.2 mg/kg) can be useful in children who do not have established i.v. access and in whom oral agents are not appropriate. Although midazolam may be effective as the sole sedative agent for ventilated patients, higher doses, and often additional agents, are commonly required in young children (1–4 years).[12] 50–200 μg/kg per hour, in combination with an opioid (morphine 10–40 μg/kg per hour), is usually effective in facilitating mechanical ventilation. Dose-related respiratory depression occurs and hypotension can be significant in hypovolaemic patients and in those with depressed myocardial function. During continuous infusion, accumulation can occur, particularly in young infants (under 6 months) and in patients with liver dysfunction. The use of midazolam in neonatal intensive care is controversial as there are concerns regarding its safety and effectiveness as a long-term sedative in the newborn.[13]

KETAMINE

Ketamine is a dissociative anaesthetic agent with sedative, analgesic and amnesic properties. Biotransformation occurs by the microsomal enzyme system. Thus, there is little metabolism in the newborn and clearance is less and elimination half-life greater in infants than in older children and adults.[14] Ketamine's usefulness in preterm infants, to a postconceptual age of 51 weeks, is limited because of an increased risk of postanaesthetic apnoea. An initial i.v. dose of 1–2 mg/kg is usually adequate to induce deep sedation. Cardiovascular disturbance is minimal and ketamine is therefore particularly useful as the induction agent in status asthmaticus and in patients with a compromised haemodynamic state, such as tamponade. Prolonged sedation for ventilated children can be achieved with a continuous infusion of 10–15 μg/kg per min and analgesia can be provided by an infusion of 4 μg/kg per min. Concomitant use of an antisialogogue, such as glycopyrrolate, helps control the often seen increase in respiratory tract secretions. The unpleasant emergent phenomena, seen frequently in adults, probably occur less often in children. The traditional practice of concurrently administering a benzodiazepine with the aim of minimising these effects has minimal demonstrable benefit.[15]

PROPOFOL

Propofol is a rapidly acting hypnotic agent that is widely used in paediatric anaesthesia and intensive care for short- and longer-term sedation.[16,17] Although it has no analgesic properties its short half-life makes it an attractive agent for sedation. The half-life decreases with age, probably due to development of metabolising capacity and increasing hepatic flow.[18] Sedation can be achieved in the spontaneously breathing patient, with an induction dose of 1 mg/kg, followed by intermittent smaller doses: 2–3 mg/kg per hour has delivered uncomplicated satisfactory sedation to ventilated children.[19] However, propofol should be used with caution for sedation in the PICU because of the reported association between high dose (> 4 mg/kg per hour), prolonged (> 29 hours) infusions and a clinical syndrome (propofol infusion syndrome) consisting of metabolic acidosis, lipaemia, cardiac failure, arrhythmias and death.[20] The pathogenesis of this syndrome remains unclear, although it has been postulated that a disturbance of mitochondrial function leading to disordered hepatic lipid regulation underlies the disorder.[21] Lipaemia may be an early indicator of developing problems and successful use of haemodialysis in the early phase is the only therapy described.[22] There are sufficient concerns to limit the use of propofol in the PICU to short-term sedation in the stable ventilated child. Administration of propofol in the presence of shock, hypoxaemia or acute liver dysfunction, or for long-term, high-dose sedation cannot be recommended. It should be noted that the manufacturers advise against the use of propofol for sedation of children during intensive care.

THIOPENTAL

Thiopental is useful as an anaesthetic induction agent in critically ill children, although its hypotensive effects limit its use in shocked patients. The standard dose is 5 mg/kg, and this should be reduced to 2–3 mg/kg when hypotension is a risk. Thiopental is useful in the management of refractory status epilepticus and may have a role in difficult cases of raised intracranial pressure. In such cases, it is administered by continuous infusion (1–5 mg/kg per hour). Accumulation can lead to prolonged sedation.

CHLORAL HYDRATE

Chloral is an effective oral hypnotic and sedative agent with no analgesic effect. The hypnotic dose is 50 mg/kg and appropriate sedation may be achieved with lower doses. Gastric irritation can be a problem in some children. Toxic doses produce depression of respiration and cardiac contractility. Despite the disadvantage of delayed onset, chloral can be useful given prior to procedures, or as a supplemental sedative agent in the ventilated child and it can effectively induce nocturnal sleep. On a cautionary note, there is some evidence that it may not be suitable in acutely wheezing infants.[23]

CLONIDINE AND DEXMEDETOMIDINE

Clonidine is an α_2-adrenoreceptor agonist with significant neurological, neuroendocrine and cardiovascular effects that result in sedation, analgesia and reduced sympathetic outflow. It is rapidly absorbed after oral administration and has a half-life of 9–12 hours. Metabolism is via the liver and kidney and approximately 50% is excreted unchanged in the urine. A single oral dose (4 μg/kg) can provide both preoperative sedation and postoperative analgesia following moderately painful surgery.[24] An i.v. infusion (0.1–2 μg/kg per hour) in combination with midazolam (50 μg/kg per hour) has been shown to produce effective sedation in ventilated children without haemodynamic disturbance.[25] Clonidine can also have a role in the management of the autonomic storms seen following severe traumatic brain injury and in the management of opioid withdrawal.

Dexmedetomidine is a selective α_2-agonist that has many of the properties of clonidine and may produce less respiratory depression. It is metabolised in the liver and, in adults, has an elimination half-life of 2 hours. It has provided satisfactory sedation and analgesia with minimal respiratory or haemodynamic disturbance in postoperative ventilated and spontaneously breathing adult patients. Respiratory stability during infusion has been sufficient to allow successful extubation of patients who had previously failed because of agitation.[26] Use is approved and recommended by the manufacturer for the sedation of adult patients for up to 24 hours. In the paediatric population studies are limited. 0.5–1 μg/kg followed by an infusion of 0.5–1 μg/kg per hour has provided adequate sedation for non-invasive procedures.[27] 1 μg/kg followed by 0.1–2 μg/kg per hour, added to an opioid/benzodiazepine regime, has also been shown to improve patient comfort without significant respiratory depression.[28] As with clonidine, bradycardia has been seen during continuous infusion.[25,29]

OPIOID ANALGESICS

MORPHINE

Morphine is frequently used to provide analgesia and as part of a sedative regime for children on mechanical ventilation. Marked variation in pharmacokinetics in the neonatal period has been demonstrated, but infants over 1 month of age eliminate morphine efficiently and should not be more sensitive to respiratory depression than adults. Clearance and half-life (2 hours) are at adult values by 6 months of age.[30] The active metabolite is renally excreted and can therefore accumulate in renal failure. The standard i.v. dose is 0.1–0.2 mg/kg and an infusion rate of 20–40 μg/kg per hour provides safe postoperative pain relief in spontaneously breathing patients. With careful titration of dose to effect, higher rates can be administered, particularly to the child on mechanical ventilation. Patient-controlled analgesia devices delivering fixed doses of opioid, with or without a background infusion, can be used successfully by the majority of school-aged children and may occasionally be appropriate in intensive care. Histamine-related side-effects, in particular nasal itch, may warrant a change of opioid and fentanyl is an alternative.

FENTANYL AND ALFENTANIL

Fentanyl has theoretical advantages over morphine in certain situations because of its rapid onset and its systemic and pulmonary hemodynamic stability. Termination of the effects of a single dose is by redistribution. Clearance is more rapid in neonates and infants compared to adults and does not change with time during continuous infusion. However, after prolonged infusion, unchanged fentanyl is returned to the circulation from peripheral compartments, resulting in a prolonged terminal elimination half-life of approximately 21 hours.[31] The effective dose for painful procedures is 1–2 μg/kg. Fentanyl is useful as an anaesthetic agent in patients with labile pulmonary vasculature, as it can blunt changes in pulmonary vascular resistance seen with stimulation.[4] However, it does not prevent the increase in pulmonary vascular pressure caused by hypoxia.[32] Infusions of 1–5 μg/kg per hour produce effective sedation in neonates on mechanical ventilation; 1–10 μg/kg per hour is required for analgesia in older children. Tolerance, noted in both neonates and older children, can develop rapidly.[33] Fentanyl's short duration of action makes it suitable for use in epidural regimens.

Alfentanil, because of its shorter duration of action, may have advantages for analgesia or sedation for very short procedures.

REMIFENTANIL

Remifentanil is a synthetic opioid with potent analgesic properties, rapid onset of action, and, following initial redistribution, a short half-life of around 8 minutes. Metabolism occurs via non-specific esterases and is therefore relatively independent of renal and hepatic mechanisms. The short duration of action allows rapid emergence from general anaesthesia, thereby facilitating extubation or assessment of the patient's neurological state.[34] Postoperative pain needs to be managed with an alternative analgesic regime and an opioid should be administered prior to discontinuing remifentanil.

Infusions of 0.1–0.5 μg/kg per min have produced satisfactory analgesia and sedation in ventilated adult patients and there is evidence that ventilation times are shorter and weaning from ventilation more rapid in comparison to standard sedation regimes.[11,35] Although remifentanil is widely used in paediatric anaesthesia there are few data available on its use in children in intensive care. Uncomplicated and successful use in the induction and sedation of a ventilated preterm neonate has been described.[36] As metabolism is relatively independent of renal and hepatic mechanisms, remifentanil could be considered for use in patients with liver and/or renal impairment who do not have continuing pain and in whom rapid termination of sedation is required.

PARACETAMOL AND NON-STEROIDAL ANTI-INFLAMMATORY DRUGS

The addition to an analgesic regime of either paracetamol or a non-steroidal anti-inflammatory drug (NSAID) should be considered provided there are no contraindications.

Paracetamol is useful for mild to moderate pain and is an effective supplement to opioids for more severe pain. Enteral preparations, though useful, are prone to erratic absorption. The intravenous preparation Perfalgan is a more useful drug in the intensive care setting and has been shown to reduce opioid requirements in adults with few side-effects following orthopaedic surgery.[37] Data in children and neonates are limited. The recommended initial i.v. dose is 15 mg/kg (30 mg/kg p.o. or rectal) and the total daily i.v. dose should be limited to 60 mg/kg (90 mg/kg p.o.). Lower i.v. doses (7.5 mg/kg 6-hourly) are recommended for neonates. Contraindications to paracetamol include liver dysfunction and care must be taken to avoid liver injury in all children.

NSAIDs should also be considered as supplemental analgesics. Care should be taken, however, regarding the risk of bleeding, particularly in the postoperative period and in the highly stressed patient in whom gastric bleeding is more likely. Ketorolac (0.6 mg/kg) can be given i.v. and therefore has the potential to reduce the dose of opioid required in the immediate postoperative period when enteral medications are not appropriate.

INHALED AGENTS

NITROUS OXIDE

Nitrous oxide is a potent analgesic agent. It is useful in intensive care during short painful procedures such as removal of surgical drains. A mixture of 50% nitrous oxide with oxygen provides analgesia in awake and cooperative patients. It is unsuitable for repeated or continuous use because of toxicity and administration to younger children may cause distress because of the need for application of a mask.

ISOFLURANE

Isoflurane has been used for long-term sedation in intensive care in adults. As elimination is independent of hepatic and renal mechanisms, there are theoretical advantages in many critically ill patients. However, an association between isoflurane sedation and neurological abnormalities has been reported in children.[38] These abnormalities, although reversible, were a considerable clinical problem and make this technique unsuitable.

DRUG WITHDRAWAL SYNDROMES

Opioid withdrawal is a recognised problem and symptoms include poor feeding, tremors, agitation, poor sleeping, tachycardia, diarrhoea, sweating, increased muscle tone, dystonic posturing and seizures. It occurs particularly following prolonged high-dose infusions. The risk of withdrawal following a fentanyl infusion is associated with the duration of infusion and the total dose. Infusion for > 5 days or a total dose > 1.5 mg/kg was associated with greater than 50% incidence.[39]

Benzodiazepine withdrawal (agitation, anxiety, sweating, tremor) is also seen and the risk following a midazolam infusion is associated with a total dose > 60 mg/kg.[40] Careful attention to weaning an infusion in high-risk patients can minimise withdrawal symptoms. Longer-term pharmacological management is occasionally required and is best managed by administering the agent from which the patient is withdrawing. Methadone, benzodiazepines and clonidine have been used via i.v., oral and subcutaneous routes.[41] Recent evidence suggests that short-term (5-day) opioid weaning programmes can be successful.[42] Although withdrawal can be a significant problem, adequate sedation or analgesia should not be withheld because of fears of the development of drug dependence.

LOCAL ANAESTHESIA

Local anaesthesia can produce effective analgesia without systemic effects and therefore has significant advantages in many patients, particularly the postoperative group. In the intensive care setting, it can be used as the sole method of providing analgesia or in combination with i.v. agents. The risk of toxicity is related both to the dose and to the rapidity of absorption, which is dependent on local blood flow. Metabolism of the amide local anaesthetics (lidocaine, bupivacaine) is via the cytochrome P-450 system and their half-life is longer in infants less than 6 months of age. Unbound drug does not produce analgesia but is potentially toxic as infants have lower levels of the binding protein α-glycoprotein.[43] The use of local anaesthesia in infancy therefore requires careful assessment and close monitoring.

EMLA

EMLA, an emulsion of lidocaine and prilocaine, is effective in reducing the pain associated with percutaneous procedures.[44] It needs to be applied to the skin 60 minutes beforehand and thus is unsuitable for urgent procedures. Systemic absorption of the prilocaine component and subsequent methaemoglobinaemia can occur. Neonates, because of their relative deficiency of methaemoglobin reductase, are particularly at risk and EMLA should be used with caution in this group.

LOCAL INFILTRATION

Optimal analgesia for some painful procedures is possible, particularly in older children, with careful local infiltration and minimal sedation. The total dose of local anaesthetic agent infiltrated must be monitored and maximum doses not exceeded. The total dose of lidocaine should not exceed 4 mg/kg (7 mg/kg if combined with adrenaline).

NERVE BLOCKS

Femoral nerve blockade is a simple technique that produces effective analgesia in cases of femoral shaft fracture. A single injection is effective for approximately 3 hours and longer term analgesia can be provided by a continuous infusion of bupivacaine (0.125%) at 0.2–0.3 ml/kg per hour through a fine catheter placed adjacent to the femoral nerve.[45] As this technique can decrease opioid requirements, it is particularly useful in trauma patients who have suffered a coexistent head injury.

Intercostal nerve blocks may be useful after thoracotomies and liver transplants in children.[46] A single dose of 0.125% bupivacaine (maximum single dose 2 mg/kg) can produce up to 8 hours of analgesia. The dose must be carefully limited, because the relatively high blood flow to the area increases the risk of toxicity. Continuous infusions via an intercostal catheter can provide ongoing pain relief. These require careful monitoring in the PICU, particularly regarding maximal dose. There is a risk of pneumothorax with this technique and it should therefore be avoided when there is significant coexistent lung disease.

EPIDURAL ANALGESIA

Caudal, lumbar and thoracic epidural anaesthesia can provide effective control of postoperative pain in children.[47,48] The procedures must be performed by skilled experienced staff who clearly understand the risks and benefits. A complication rate of 1.5 per 1000 has been reported, with dural puncture and intravascular injection seen most commonly.[49] Other risks include cord injury, epidural infection and excessive motor blockade. Infants under 6 months are at highest risk because of their size and immature metabolism.

Many epidural catheter insertions are performed in the operating theatre and general anaesthesia is a prerequisite in most paediatric patients. PICU care may subsequently be required because of the nature of the surgery (e.g. thoracotomy, liver transplant) or because of underlying patient factors (e.g. neurological disorders, morbid obesity, age). Epidurals have been used in paediatric cardiac surgery without clear benefit over conventional postoperative analgesia.[50] Particular indications for commencing epidural analgesia in the PICU include burns in a suitable distribution (e.g. abdomen and lower limbs) and blunt chest trauma with rib fractures. Contraindications include shock, hypovolaemia, meningitis, coagulopathy and local skin infection.

Bupivacaine is the most commonly used local anaesthetic. A single dose should not exceed 2.5 mg/kg and the maximum infusion rate is 0.4 mg/kg per hour (0.2 mg/kg per hour in infants). Opioids (morphine and fentanyl) may be added and have a synergistic effect, thereby allowing less local anaesthetic agent to be used. Epidural opioids can cause sedation and respiratory depression.

REFERENCES

1. Anand KJS, Hickey PR. Pain in the foetus and neonate. *N Engl J Med* 1987; **317**: 1321–9.
2. Anand KJS, Ward-Platt MP. Neonatal and paediatric responses to anaesthesia and operation. *Int Anesthesiol Clin* 1988; **26**: 218–25.
3. Anand KJS, Hickey PR. Halothane-morphine compared with high dose sufentanil for anaesthesia and postoperative analgesia in neonatal cardiac surgery. *N Engl J Med* 1992; **326**: 1–19.
4. Hickey P, Hansen DD, Wessell DL *et al.* Blunting of stress response in the pulmonary vasculature of infants by fentanil. *Anesth Analg* 1985; **64**: 1137–42.
5. McNair C, Ballantyne M, Dionne K *et al.* Postoperative pain assessment in the neonatal intensive care unit. *Arch Dis Child Fetal Neonatal Ed* 2004; **89**: F53–541.
6. Ramelet AS, Rees N, McDonald *et al.* Development and preliminary psychometric testing of the Multidimensional Assessment of Pain Scale: MAPS. *Paediatr Anaesth* 2007; **17**: 333–40.
7. Malviya S, Voepel-Lewis T, Burke C *et al.* The revised FLACC observational pain tool: improved reliability and validity for pain assessment in children with cognitive impairment. *Paediatr Anaesth* 2006; **16**: 258–65.
8. Ista E, van Dijk M, Tibboel D *et al.* Assessment of sedation in pediatric intensive care patients can be improved by using the COMFORT 'behavior' scale. *Pediatr Crit Care Med* 2005; **6**: 58–63.
9. Aneja R, Heard AM, Fletcher JE *et al.* Sedation monitoring of children by the Bispectral Index in the paediatric intensive care unit. *Pediatr Crit Care Med* 2003; **4**: 60–4.
10. Playfor S, Jenkins I, Boyles C *et al.* Consensus guidelines on sedation and analgesia in critically ill children. *Intensive Care Med* 2006; **32**: 1125–36.
11. Park G, Lane M, Rogers S *et al.* A comparison of hypnotic and analgesic based sedation in a general intensive care unit. *Br J Anaesth* 2007; **98**: 76–82.
12. Gast-Bakker DH, ven der Werff SD, Sibarani-Ponsen R *et al.* Age is of influence on midazolam requirements in a paediatric intensive care unit. *Acta Paediatr* 2007; **96**: 414–7.
13. Ng E, Taddio A, Ohisson A. Intravenous midazolam infusion for sedation of infants in the neonatal intensive care unit. *Cochrane Database Syst Rev* 2003; CD002052.
14. Chang T, Glazko T. Biotransformation and metabolism of ketamine. *Int Anesthesiol Clin* 1974; **12**: 157–77.
15. Sherwin TS, Green SM, Khan A *et al.* Does adjunctive midazolam reduce recovery agitation after ketamine sedation for pediatric procedures? A randomised, double blind, placebo controlled trial. *Ann Emerg Med* 2000; **35**: 229–38.
16. Playfor SD, Venketash K. Current patterns of propofol use in the United Kingdom and North America. *Paediatr Anaesth* 2004; **14**: 501–4.
17. Festa M, Bowra J, Schell D. Use of propofol in Australian and New Zealand paediatric intensive care units. *Anaesth Intensive Care* 2002; **30**: 786–93.
18. Jones RDM, Chan K, Andrew LJ. Pharmacokinetics of propofol in children. *Br J Anaesth* 1990; **65**: 661–7.
19. Cornfield DN, Tegtmeyer K, Nelson MD *et al.* Continuous propofol infusion in 142 critically ill children. *Pediatrics* 2002; **110**: 1177–81.
20. Bray RJ. Propofol infusion syndrome in children. *Paediatr Anaesth* 1998; **8**: 491–9.
21. Ahlen K, Buckley CJ, Goodale DB *et al.* The 'propofol infusion syndrome': the facts, their interpretation and implications for care. *Eur J Anaesthesiol* 2006; **23**: 990–8.
22. Cray SH, Robinson BH, Cox PN. Lactic acidaemia and bradyarrhythmia in a child sedated with propofol. *Crit Care Med* 1998; **26**: 2087–92.
23. Mallol J, Sly PD. Effect of chloral hydrate on arterial oxygen saturation in wheezy infants. *Pediatr Pulmonol* 1988; **5**: 96–9.
24. Reimer EJ, Dunn GS, Montgomery CJ *et al.* The effectiveness of clonidine as an analgesic in paediatric adenotonsillectomy. *Can J Anaesth* 1998; **45**: 1162–7.
25. Ambrose C, Sale S, Howells R *et al.* Intravenous clonidine infusion in critically ill children: dose dependent

sedative effects and cardiovascular stability. *Br J Anaesth* 2000; **84**: 794–6.

26. Siobal MS, Kallet RH, Kivett VA *et al.* Use of dexmedetomidine to facilitate extubation in surgical intensive care unit patients who failed previous weaning attempts following prolonged mechanical ventilation: a pilot study. *Respir Care* 2006; **51**: 492–6.
27. Berkenbosch JW, Wankum PC, Tobias JD. Prospective evaluation of dexmedetomidine for non-invasive procedural sedation in children. *Pediatr Crit Care Med* 2005; **6**: 435–9.
28. Walker J, Maccallum M, Fischer C *et al.* Sedation using dexmedetomidine in pediatric burn patients. *J Burn Care Res* 2006; **27**: 206–10.
29. Chrystosomou C, Di Filippo S, Manrique AM *et al.* Use of dexmedetomidine in children after cardiac and thoracic surgery. *Pediatr Crit Care* 2006; **7**: 126–31.
30. McRori TI, Lynn AM, Nespecca MK *et al.* The maturation of morphine clearance and metabolism. *Am J Dis Child* 1992; **146**: 972–6.
31. Katz R, Kelly WH. Pharmacokinetics of continuous infusions of fentanyl in critically ill children. *Crit Care Med* 1993; **21**: 995–1000.
32. Vacanti JP, Crone PK, Murphy JP *et al.* The pulmonary haemodynamic response to perioperative anaesthesia in the treatment of high-risk infants with congenital diaphragmatic hernia. *J Pediatr Surg* 1984; **19**: 672–9.
33. Arnold JH, Truog RD, Scavone JM *et al.* Changes in the pharmacodynamic response to fentanyl in neonates during continuous infusion. *J Pediatr* 1991; **119**: 639–43.
34. Friesen RH, Veit AS, Archibald DJ *et al.* A comparison of remifentanil and fentanyl for fast track paediatric cardiac anaesthesia. *Paediatr Anaesth* 2003; **13**: 122–5.
35. Breen D, Karabinis A, Malbrain M *et al.* Decreased duration of mechanical ventilation when comparing analgesia based sedation using remifentanil with standard hypnotic-based sedation for up to 10 days in intensive care unit patients: a randomised trial. *Crit Care* 2005; **9**: R200–10.
36. Pereira E, Silva Y, Gomez RS *et al.* Remifentanil for sedation and analgesia in a pre-term neonate with respiratory distress syndrome. *Paediatr Anaesth* 2005; **15**: 993–6.
37. Sinatra RS, Jahr JS, Reynolds LW *et al.* Efficacy and safety of single and repeated administration of 1 gram intravenous acetaminophen injection (paracetamol) for pain management after major orthopedic surgery. *Anesthesiology* 2005; **102**: 822–31.
38. Kelsall AWR, Ross-Russell R, Herrick MJ. Reversible neurological dysfunction following isoflurane sedation in pediatric intensive care. *Crit Care Med* 1994; **22**: 1032–4.
39. Katz R, Kelly WH, Hsi A. Prospective study on the occurrence of withdrawal in critically ill children who receive fentanyl by continuous infusion. *Crit Care Med* 1994; **22**: 763–7.
40. Fonsmark L, Rasmussen YH, Carl P. Occurrence of withdrawal in critically ill sedated children. *Crit Care Med* 1999; **27**: 196–9.
41. Tobias JD. Tolerance, withdrawal and physical dependency after long-term sedation and analgesia of children in the paediatric intensive care unit. *Crit Care Med* 2000; **28**: 2122–32.
42. Berens RJ, Meyer MT, Mikhailov TA *et al.* A prospective evaluation of opioid weaning in opioid-dependent pediatric critical care patients. *Pediatr Anaesth* 2006; **102**: 1045–50.
43. Wilder RT. Local anesthetics for the pediatric patient. *Pediatr Clin North Am* 2000; **47**: 545–58.
44. Sims C. Thickly and thinly applied lignocaine–prilocaine cream prior to venepuncture in children. *Anaesth Intensive Care* 1991; **19**: 343–5.
45. Johnson CM. Continuous femoral nerve blockade for analgesia in children with femoral nerve fractures. *Anaesth Intensive Care* 1994; **22**: 281–3.
46. Shelly MP, Park GR. Intercostal nerve blockade for children. *Anaesthesia* 1987; **42**: 541–5.
47. Dalens B. Lumbar epidural anaesthesia. In: Dalens B (ed) Regional Anesthesia in Infants, Children and Adolescents. Baltimore: Williams and Wilkins; 1995: 207–48.
48. Dalens B, Khandwala R. Thoracic and cervical epidural anesthesia. In: Dalens B (ed) *Regional Anesthesia in Infants, Children and Adolescents.* Baltimore: Williams and Wilkins; 1995: 249–60.
49. Giaufre E, Dalens B, Gombert A. Epidemiology and morbidity of regional anaesthesia in children: a one year survey of the French-language Society of Pediatric Anesthesiologists. *Anesth Analg* 1996; **83**: 897–900.
50. Biche T, Roue JC, Schlegel S *et al.* Epidural sufentanil during paediatric cardiac surgery: effects on metabolic response and post-operative outcome. *Paediatr Anaesth* 2000; **10**: 609–17.

101

Shock and cardiac disease in children

Robert D Henning

Most cases of shock in childhood are caused by hypovolaemia (Table 101.1) or sepsis. The causes, clinical course, management and complications of shock differ from those in adults: severe diarrhoeal disease and congenital abnormalities are common in childhood but abdominal sepsis, pancreatitis and obstructive vascular disease are uncommon.

The following factors affect the epidemiology of shock in children:

SMALLER BODY FLUID COMPARTMENTS

A small volume of blood or diarrhoeal fluid loss, or of fluid leakage into the extravascular space may represent a large percentage loss of blood or extracellular fluid (ECF) volume in a small child (Table 101.2).

IMMATURE IMMUNE SYSTEM IN INFANTS AND TODDLERS[2]

The innate host defences of the small child are immature: the skin and the respiratory and gut mucosae are more permeable to bacteria and their toxins, and secretory IgA levels remain low throughout childhood. There is increased susceptibility to severe bacteraemias due to:

- low IgM and IgG levels
- deficient neutrophil adhesion, migration and respiratory burst activity, combined with lower levels of complement (especially C3, C9 and factor B)
- low cytokine production by monocytes

Antibody response to bacterial polysaccharide capsular antigens (e.g. *Streptococcus pneumoniae, Haemophilus* spp. and *Neisseria meningitidis*) remains poor in the preschool years. Low IgG concentrations, immunological naivety and reduced natural killer (NK) cell activity predispose young children to frequent viral infections, and the newborn to severe herpes simplex infection.[3]

Reduced cytokine production, especially in the immunologically naive, may alter the features and duration of the shock syndrome, including the ability to develop a fever, and causes deficiency in most T-cell functions, including cytotoxicity and augmentation of B-cell differentiation.[4]

MICROBIOLOGY

In the newborn, septic shock is most often caused by *Staphylococcus aureus*, group B β-haemolytic streptococci, Enterobacteriaceae, *Listeria monocytogenes*, enteroviruses (e.g. Echo or Coxsackie viruses) or herpes simplex virus.

Later in childhood, *Strep. pneumoniae, N. meningitidis, Haemophilus influenzae, Staph. aureus* and Enterobacteriaceae cause most cases of septic shock. Although severe sepsis due to *H. influenzae* type b (Hib) and *N. meningitidis* group C has been almost completely eradicated among immunised children, cases of severe sepsis involving these organisms still occur in non-immunised children, and cases of sepsis due to other serotypes are seen in immunised children.

In immunodeficient children, *Staph. aureus*, Enterobacteriaceae, *Pseudomonas* spp., *Candida albicans*, fungi and viruses such as cytomegalovirus and varicella frequently cause septic shock.

SEVERE CONGENITAL ABNORMALITIES

Children with congenital heart, lung or neurological diseases, multiple congenital abnormalities, inborn errors of metabolism and the inherited immunodeficiency syndromes are prone to develop cardiogenic, hypovolaemic or septic shock, especially in the first 2–3 years of life.

OTHER CHILDHOOD CONDITIONS THAT PREDISPOSE TO SEVERE SEPSIS

These include:

- cancer and its chemotherapy
- organ transplantation (especially bone marrow)
- multiple trauma
- burns
- prolonged paediatric intensive care unit (PICU) stay
- the presence of implanted therapeutic devices including intravascular catheters

Table 101.1 Causes of hypovolaemic shock in childhood

Bleeding
Revealed (external or into the gastrointestinal tract)
Concealed (scalp, intracranial, trunk or limbs)
Water and electrolyte loss
Bowel
Renal
Skin
Plasma loss (capillary leak)
Water deprivation (absolute or relative to losses)

Table 101.2 Body fluid compartments during childhood (ml/kg)[1]

	Total body water	Extracellular fluid	Intracellular fluid	Blood
Preterm newborn	800	550	300	95
Birth	750	450	300	85
1 year	700	350	350	80
5 years	650	250	400	75
Adult	600	200	400	70

PATHOPHYSIOLOGY

The pathophysiology of shock is described in Chapter 11 which should be read in conjunction with this chapter. The following aspects of a child's physiology affect the response to insults.

IMMATURE CARDIOVASCULAR SYSTEM[5,6]

LESS CAPABLE OF DEVELOPING CONTRACTILE FORCE

The immature myocardium has more loose connective tissue than the adult, but fewer sarcomeres per gram of tissue. The arrangement of myofibrils in the myocyte, and of myocytes in the myocardium, is less parallel than in the adult. Intracellular desmin fibrils which link the contractile elements are more randomly arranged in the infant heart. Less efficient calcium uptake, storage and release from sarcoplasmic reticulum (SR) and a higher density of cell membrane Na/Ca exchangers mean that excitation–contraction coupling is more dependent on trans-sarcolemmal Ca^{++} flux, and on ECF Ca^{++} concentration than the adult.

LESS DIASTOLIC COMPLIANCE THAN THE ADULT HEART

- Limited calcium uptake and storage into SR, more slow skeletal troponin I and more β-tropomyosin relative to α-tropomyosin mean slower diastolic relaxation of the ventricles.
- Greater myocardial collagen content and immaturity of the cytoskeleton and intercellular matrix increase the diastolic elastic recoil of the infant ventricular wall.
- Increases in end-diastolic volume of either ventricle cause greater reduction of compliance of the opposite ventricle than in the adult: when right ventricle (RV) afterload rises acutely, the consequent increase in RV end-diastolic volume distorts the left ventricle (LV) and impairs LV filling and emptying more than in the adult.

MORE TOLERANT OF HYPOXAEMIA

Although the infant heart has fewer mitochondria per gram of tissue, and a lower oxidative capacity, it has a lower oxygen demand per gram, larger glycogen reserves and a higher capacity for anaerobic glycolysis.[7] Glucose is the major myocardial energy source (rather than long chain fatty acids as in older children) and hypoglycaemia causes severe myocardial depression.

IMMATURE AUTONOMIC INNERVATION

Parasympathetic innervation of the heart is more complete than sympathetic in infants, and the infant response to severe stress (e.g. hypoxia) tends to be bradycardia rather than tachycardia.

The infant myocardium has fewer β-receptors, more α-receptors, and is more sensitive to noradrenaline (norepinephrine) than the adult. Stimulation of myocardial α-receptors in the infant is more likely to cause tachycardia than bradycardia.[8]

HIGH PULMONARY VASCULAR RESISTANCE[8]

In the fetus, the small pulmonary arteries are narrow, the pulmonary vascular resistance is high, and pulmonary blood flow is less than one-tenth of systemic flow. A thick layer of smooth muscle, which extends further out into the vascular tree than in the adult, is highly sensitive to hypoxia, hypercarbia, acidaemia, sepsis and central neural stimuli such as pain.

At birth, after the first breaths are taken, the smooth muscle cells gradually relax and become more fusiform in shape. Pulmonary vascular resistance falls immediately, then gradually declines to adult levels by 6–8 weeks of age, and smooth muscle bulk falls to adult levels by 3–4 months.[9] In the presence of lung disease, high pulmonary venous pressures (e.g. due to aortic stenosis or stenosis of the pulmonary veins) or large left-to-right shunts (e.g. ventricular septal defect (VSD) or truncus arteriosus), the high pulmonary vascular resistance and the extensive and bulky vascular smooth muscle fail to decline normally. The infant is then vulnerable to episodes of acute right heart failure whenever the pulmonary vascular resistance increases abruptly.

CLINICAL PRESENTATION OF SHOCK IN CHILDHOOD

HYPOVOLAEMIC SHOCK (SEE TABLE 101.1)

The child may have a history of fluid or blood loss, reduced fluid intake or bowel-related illness. Signs of dehydration (see Chapter 99), external bleeding or haematoma may be present. The presence of hypovolaemic shock implies a blood volume deficit greater than 30 ml/kg.

Signs of homeostatic compensation, such as tachycardia (Table 101.3), narrow pulse pressure, cool mottled limbs and slow capillary refill usually precede the onset of hypotension, which tends to occur late (after loss of 15–20% of blood volume) and precipitously in young children. In severe shock of any cause, signs of multiple organ hypoperfusion (e.g. oliguria of less than 0.5 ml/kg per hour, lethargy or coma, hypothermia, tachypnoea and increasing lactic or other metabolic acidosis) are found. Bleeding due to disseminated intravascular coagulation and liver dysfunction may occur in the first 6 hours.

In early shock, these changes are reversible by plasma volume expansion with boluses of 20 ml/kg 0.9% saline or blood, repeated as necessary. Failure to respond to two such boluses with a decrease in heart rate and capillary refill time (normal < 2 seconds after 5 seconds' pressure over the sternum) indicates refractory shock requiring more aggressive treatment (see below).

Table 101.3 Normal blood pressure, heart rate and respiratory rate in childhood[10]

Age	Blood pressure (mmHg (kPa))	Heart rate (beats/min) (2nd–98th centile)	Respiratory rate (breaths/min)
Birth	75/40 (10.0/5.3)	125 (94–155)	50
1 year	95/60 (12.6/8.0)	120 (108–168)	35
2 years	96/60 (12.8/8.0)	110 (90–152)	25
6 years	98/60 (13.0/8.0)	110 (64–133)	16
10 years	110/70 (14.6/9.3)	90 (63–130)	16
14 years	118/75 (15.7/10.0)	80 (61–120)	16

Table 101.4 Investigation of shock in children

All shocked children
- Arterial blood gases
- Plasma electrolytes, urea, creatinine, glucose, liver function tests, lactate
- Haemoglobin, platelet count, total and differential white cell count
- Coagulation screen including fibrin degradation products
- Blood group (hold serum)

If the cause of shock is unknown
- Exclude sepsis:
  - Several sets of blood cultures, percutaneous and via vascular catheters
  - Culture and Gram stain pus
  - Urine cultures from mid-stream sample or suprapubic aspirate of urine
  - Urine, stool and nasopharyngeal aspirate for virology
  - CSF bacterial and viral culture plus PCR for specific organisms
- Urine bacterial antigens
- To exclude cardiogenic shock: echocardiography, ECG, cardiac catheter
- Drug screen: urine, gastric aspirate, blood
- Metabolic screen: urinary amino acids and organic acids, plasma ammonia and glucose
- Short Synacthen test

CSF, cerebrospinal fluid; ECG, electrocardiogram; PCR, polymerase chain reaction.

Investigations (see Table 101.4) include:

- daily weighing and comparison with pre-illness weight
- close monitoring of fluid balance
- stool culture and examination for occult blood
- imaging of body cavities by CT or ultrasound for evidence of fluid or blood accumulation
- repeated full blood examination and coagulation screen
- plasma urea and electrolytes
- serum and urine osmolality

CARDIOGENIC SHOCK

Tachycardia, hypotension, low volume pulses and signs of homeostatic compensation and poor organ perfusion (see above) are usually present. Cardiomegaly, muffled heart sounds and a gallop rhythm may be found. New murmurs may appear (e.g. mitral systolic murmur due to left ventricular dilatation with consequent mitral regurgitation, or aortic diastolic murmur due to endocarditis). Chest rales, tachypnoea and wheezing indicate left heart failure, while in right heart failure, oedema appears first in the eyelids and dorsum of hands and feet. Hepatomegaly develops rapidly in children, and is a more reliable sign of right heart failure than a raised jugular venous pressure (JVP) which may be hard to detect in infants.

Table 101.5 Causes of cardiogenic shock in childhood

Structural congenital heart disease (qv)
Post cardiac surgery
Arrhythmia (qv)
Myocardial hypoxia/ischaemia
Cardiomyopathy
Congenital
Metabolic
Infective
Hypertrophic
Endocardial fibroelastosis
Valvular heart disease
Congenital
Infective
Rheumatic
Traumatic
Sepsis
Drug intoxication
Cardiac tamponade
Constrictive pericarditis
Trauma to myocardium or coronary arteries

Combinations of signs specific to individual congenital heart lesions are described below. Such signs when present (e.g. absent femoral pulses in aortic coarctation, or skull, liver or renal bruits of arteriovenous fistulae) may indicate the cause of the shock (Table 101.5), while diagnostically useful murmurs are not always present.

Investigations (see Table 101.4) should include:

- chest X-ray to assess heart size and lung vascularity and oedema, and to exclude pneumothorax
- electrocardiogram (ECG)
- echocardiography
- in some cases, CT or MR angiography or cardiac catheterisation

SEPTIC SHOCK

Septic infants usually present with a hypodynamic circulation, low cardiac output and cool extremities. Early septic shock in older children may be hypodynamic, or may be similar to that in adults, in which tachycardia, tachypnoea and hypotension are accompanied by warm extremities, wide pulse pressure and increased cardiac output. Lethargy or stupor, oliguria and Kussmaul breathing characteristic of metabolic acidosis indicate inadequate tissue oxygenation.

Severely septic children are often hypothermic rather than febrile.

As shock progresses, myocardial depression by endotoxin, tumour necrosis factor-α (TNF-α) and interleukin-1β (IL-1β) (see Chapter 11) decreases the cardiac output earlier than is the case in adults, as the less compliant infant ventricle cannot dilate to sustain the stroke volume in the face of a reduced ejection fraction.[11,12] Furthermore, the rapid and severe capillary leak that is characteristic of paediatric sepsis leads to hypovolaemia in the underresuscitated child, further reducing preload and cardiac output. For this reason, septic children often respond well to aggressive fluid resuscitation ($>$ 60 ml/kg in the first hour). Peripheral oedema caused by leakage of proteinaceous fluid from injured capillary endothelia exacerbates cellular hypoxia by increasing the diffusion distance for oxygen between capillaries and cells.

MULTIPLE ORGAN FAILURE IN SHOCKED CHILDREN

Shock of any cause leads to multiple organ failure, the clinical course and outcome of which differ from those in shocked adults:

- Myocardial depression, reduced ventricular diastolic compliance[13] and low cardiac output. Clinically important arrhythmias rarely occur.
- Acute lung injury can occur in a shocked child of any age, including the newborn. Respiratory muscle fatigue due to impaired muscle blood flow and oxygenation further reduces gas exchange.
- Acute renal failure occurs frequently, is usually reversible within 50 days, may require haemodiafiltration or peritoneal dialysis, and is rarely a significant contributor to mortality in shocked children.
- Disseminated intravascular coagulation occurs very commonly, due to activation of the coagulation pathway, increased production of plasminogen activator inhibitor-1 and reduced levels of proteins C and S, antithrombin III and thrombomodulin.[14] This contributes to failure of other organs, and combines with impaired liver function and clotting factor dilution by fluid resuscitation to cause bleeding from puncture sites and sometimes from the upper gastrointestinal tract.
- Bone marrow failure, with anaemia, granulocytopenia and thrombocytopenia, implies severe shock and is associated with a poor outcome, especially in sepsis.
- Gastrointestinal failure with paralytic ileus is often present. Significant upper gastrointestinal bleeding occurs less commonly in shocked children than in adults. The source is usually generalised oozing from gastric mucosa which responds to proton pump inhibitors and replacement of platelets and clotting factors.
- Plasma concentrations of liver enzymes and bilirubin are often raised but return to normal over a few days in survivors.
- Acalculous cholecystitis due to splanchnic ischaemia is sometimes found in older children.
- Encephalopathy with stupor or coma occurs commonly. The appearance of seizures suggests some complication of sepsis, such as glucose or electrolyte abnormality, meningitis, septic embolus or intracranial bleeding.

DISTRIBUTIVE SHOCK

The main features are hypotension, vasodilatation and hypovolaemia due to plasma leakage from capillaries. The child's extremities are warm and pink, the blood

Table 101.6 Causes of distributive shock in childhood

Sepsis
Anaphylaxis
Drugs
Neurogenic: spinal cord injury

pressure is low and the pulse pressure is wide. There is tachycardia, oliguria and stupor. Other evidence of anaphylaxis (wheezing, urticaria, swollen face or tongue), spinal cord injury (bradycardia, quadriparesis, lax anal sphincter) or drug intoxication (history, tablets, coma out of proportion to shock) may be present (Table 101.6).

INVESTIGATION

See Table 101.4.

MANAGEMENT

The child's airway, breathing (see Chapter 98) and circulation should be secured during the initial assessment. The priorities in management of the circulation are to achieve:

1. adequate perfusion of the brain and heart
2. adequate perfusion of kidneys, liver and gut
3. adequate perfusion of muscle and other tissues

ADEQUATE PERFUSION OF THE BRAIN AND HEART

This requires systolic and diastolic blood pressures of 80% of normal for age (see Table 101.3), achieved by aggressive early blood volume expansion and by pressor drugs. The conscious state is the best index of adequate brain perfusion, while improved coronary perfusion is shown by rising blood pressure with falling central venous pressure.

Preload

Intravenous fluid is given in boluses of 20 ml/kg 0.9% saline or 10 ml/kg blood or colloid, repeated every 5–10 minutes until blood pressure, heart rate and skin vasoconstriction (capillary refill time: normal < 2 seconds after 5 seconds' pressure over the sternum) and indices of organ perfusion (i.e. urine output, conscious state, blood pH and lactate) improve. Heart and liver size and increases in central venous pressure (CVP) are used to assess hypervolaemia. If more than 40 ml/kg crystalloid is given:

- consider starting an infusion of a pressor drug (sepsis and other distributive shock) or an inotrope (see below)
- monitor central venous pressure
- insert an arterial cannula for blood pressure and biochemical monitoring

Pulmonary artery catheterisation for measurement of wedge pressure and cardiac output is rarely justified in children: evidence that it improves outcome is lacking,[15] and side-effects occur commonly.[16] Non-invasive monitoring of left and right ventricular preload by transthoracic echocardiography may be more useful than atrial pressure measurement, in that it removes the confounding factors of diastolic compliance and atrioventricular (AV) valve dysfunction, but it is subjective and operator dependent.[17]

Systemic vascular resistance

In septic or hypovolaemic shock, infusion of noradrenaline (0.05–2.0 μg/kg per min) should be started (via an intraosseous cannula when no central venous cannula is in place) if volume expansion does not achieve 80% of normal systolic blood pressure for age within 10 minutes. In septic shock, vasopressin (0.0003–0.0006 U/kg per min), the action of which does not depend on downregulated α_1-receptors, may be used to reduce the dose of noradrenaline required. Vasopressin deficiency occurs commonly in septic shock[18] and in irreversible shock of other causes.[19]

Contractility

If the blood pressure then remains low despite CVP = 12 mmHg or 'adequate' LV filling on transthoracic echo, an inotrope such as adrenaline (0.05–2.0 μg/kg per min), dobutamine or dopamine (5–15 μg/kg per min) should be added. Dobutamine and dopamine downregulate β-adrenergic receptors, and dopamine depletes myocardial noradrenaline stores, so the dose of these drugs should be minimised as soon as possible. β-Agonists increase oxygen consumption (and therefore oxygen demand) by increasing free fatty acid cycling and by increasing glycogenolysis and glycolysis.[20] Dopamine suppresses prolactin, thyroid-stimulating hormone and growth hormone secretion in infants and children.[21]

In infants with cardiogenic shock, infusion of 10% calcium gluconate (0.2–0.5 ml/hour) can increase blood pressure and cardiac output. Serum ionised calcium should be monitored.

ADEQUATE PERFUSION OF KIDNEYS, LIVER AND GUT

Bowel and liver ischaemia in a shocked child impairs detoxification of drugs and toxic metabolites and may increase the risk of bacteraemia and endotoxaemia of bowel origin.[22] Hypovolaemia and low cardiac output must be corrected by blood volume expansion and inotropic drugs such as dobutamine. Vasoconstricting drugs (vasopressin, noradrenaline and dopamine doses > 5 μg/kg per min) should be reduced or stopped once heart and brain perfusion are secured.

Urine output > 0.5 ml/kg per hour and a normal (or falling) plasma creatinine concentration are the best indices of adequate renal perfusion. Monitoring of splanchnic perfusion remains unreliable. Gastric pH and gastric–arterial $P\text{CO}_2$ difference correlate somewhat with outcome in septic children (though not as well as plasma lactate)[23] and are not consistently improved by measures to restore bowel perfusion.[24] Oesophageal–arterial $P\text{CO}_2$ difference[25] and near-infrared spectroscopy of the liver[26] may offer more accurate monitoring of the adequacy of splanchnic blood flow.

ADEQUATE PERFUSION OF MUSCLE AND OTHER TISSUES

Further volume expansion and infusion of vasodilators such as milrinone may be needed to improve circulation to these tissues in shock states where myocardial depression is prominent, provided an adequate blood pressure (80% normal for age; see Table 101.3) can be sustained. Maintaining a supranormal cardiac output and oxygen delivery has not been shown to improve survival in paediatric shock, although the ability to do so may predict survival.

In the absence of a pulmonary artery catheter, the adequacy of upper or lower body blood flow is conventionally assessed by monitoring changes in central venous saturation[27] and plasma lactate, though the oxygen excess factor Ω ($Sao_2/(Sao_2 - Svo_2)$) has been used in children with intracardiac shunts.[28]

Afterload reduction in cardiogenic shock

Vasoconstrictors and blood transfusion (to achieve a haemoglobin concentration of 120 g/l) may be required at first to ensure adequate coronary and cerebral perfusion pressure. When blood pressure is adequate (see Table 101.3), the cardiac output may be improved by afterload reduction. Short-acting drugs such as milrinone or sodium nitroprusside (SNP) are preferable.

Inhaled nitric oxide (NO) 1–10 ppm via the ventilator circuit may improve RV output in children with cardiogenic shock due to pulmonary hypertension (primary or after cardiac surgery or in persistent pulmonary hypertension of the newborn). Sildenafil and bosentan have been shown to reduce pulmonary vascular resistance and to permit weaning from NO in this group of children.[29]

Infusion of vasodilators such as nitroglycerin, prostacyclin (PGI_2) and SNP reduces systemic as well as pulmonary vascular resistance. These drugs are easier to administer than NO, but are less effective pulmonary vasodilators, and they (and sildenafil and bosentan) often cause systemic hypotension.

After appropriate samples are taken for investigations (see Table 101.4), possible sepsis is treated aggressively with appropriate antibiotics (Table 101.7), replacement of invasive lines and drainage of collections of pus.

Supportive measures

Early mechanical ventilation secures adequate oxygenation and pH of arterial blood. It also reduces the work of breathing and muscle oxygen demand, diverting the limited cardiac output away from muscles to vital organs. Airway pressures and tidal volumes should be limited to the minimum needed, as impaired venous return from positive-pressure ventilation will exacerbate hypotension.

Other measures include administration of platelets and fresh frozen plasma in consumptive coagulopathy, early commencement of renal support with haemodiafiltration or peritoneal dialysis in established acute renal failure and the use of H_2 antagonists or proton pump inhibitors to prevent upper gastrointestinal bleeding.

Table 101.7 Initial antibiotic therapy in children with septic shock

Up to 8 weeks of age	
	Flucloxacillin 50 mg/kg i.v. 6-hourly *plus*
	Gentamicin 6 mg/kg i.v. per day *plus*
	Cefotaxime 50 mg/kg i.v. 6-hourly
Older child	
	Flucloxacillin 50 mg/kg i.v. 6-hourly
	Gentamicin 6 mg/kg i.v. per day

Controversial measures

- *Stress dose of hydrocortisone (4 mg/kg per day for ~5 days)*: Reduced 28-day all-cause mortality and ICU and hospital mortality in septic shock.[30]
- *Granulocyte–macrophage colony-stimulating factor*: A randomised trial found that it reduced mortality in severely ill septic, neutropenic newborns.[31]
- *Intravenous pooled polyclonal immunoglobulin (IVIG)*: Some evidence of reduced mortality from controlled trials in severe sepsis.[32]
- *Recombinant bactericidal permeability-increasing protein ($rBPI_{21}$)*: Trend to improved functional outcome in a small trial in children with severe meningococcal sepsis.[33]
- *Granulocyte transfusions for severe sepsis with neutropenia*: Trend to improved outcome when combined with IVIG in a controlled trial in septic newborns.[34]
- *High-dose steroids after antibiotics started*: Pre-1992 trials showed no benefit.[30]
- *Monoclonal anti-endotoxin, anticytokine antibodies or IL-1 receptor antagonists*: No evidence of efficacy in controlled trials.[32]
- *Activated protein C*: No evidence of improved outcome in a controlled trial in severely septic children.[35]
- *Tri-iodothyronine (T_3)*: No convincing evidence of improved outcome in trials in children with low cardiac output after cardiac surgery despite evidence that T_3 is deficient in these patients.[36]
- *Circulatory support with extracorporeal membrane oxygenation (ECMO)*: ECMO has been employed in children moribund with septic shock, with some survivors, but there is no convincing evidence of its efficacy.[37]
- *Close control of blood glucose using insulin infusion.* There is no evidence in children that it improves outcome. Infants are very vulnerable to hypoglycaemia and are sensitive to low insulin doses. Blood glucose should be monitored frequently in shocked children.

HEART FAILURE IN CHILDREN

In cardiac failure, the cardiac output is insufficient to meet the metabolic needs of the tissues without development of abnormally high ventricular end-diastolic volumes.[38]

Table 101.8 shows the main causes of heart failure in children. In many cases, several factors combine to produce heart failure (e.g. sepsis plus valve regurgitation and amiodarone).

- *Preload* may be:
  - excessive: volume loading, e.g. systemic arteriovenous malformation, large ventricular septal defect, aortopulmonary window, AV valve regurgitation or excessive fluid administration
  - inadequate: e.g. mitral stenosis, pericardial tamponade, hypertrophic cardiomyopathy or congenital hypoplasia of the left or right ventricle. Ventricular diastolic compliance may be reduced by ischaemia, postoperative myocardial oedema, sepsis, heart transplant rejection or cardiomyopathy (infiltrative or hypertrophic).
- *Excessive afterload* (ventricular systolic wall tension) may be caused by pulmonary valve stenosis or pulmonary hypertension (right ventricle); by aortic valve stenosis, aortic coarctation or hypoplasia or systemic hypertension (left ventricle); or by ventricular dilatation.

(Laplace's Law: $T = P \times R/2H$, where T is systolic wall tension, P is ventricular pressure during systole, R is ventricular radius and H is ventricular wall thickness.)

- *Inadequate contractility*: e.g. due to myocarditis, sepsis or ischaemia.
- *Heart rate* may be:
  - too fast (e.g. in supraventricular tachycardia or atrial flutter, ventricular filling time is inadequate and myocardial work is excessive).
  - too slow (e.g. complete heart block).

PRESENTING SIGNS

In childhood, heart failure may present with growth failure. Feeding is slow and may cause sweating and dyspnoea. Useful signs are tachypnoea, cardiomegaly, hepatomegaly, gallop rhythm, tachycardia and cool, mottled extremities. There may be clinical and X-ray signs of lung congestion, oedema and air trapping (due to airway compression by distended blood vessels and airway mucosal oedema: seen in large left-to-right shunts such as VSD). In infants, the JVP is a difficult sign to elicit. The liver enlarges rapidly as the right atrial pressure increases, and oedema is often non-pitting, and located in the eyelids and the dorsum of the hands and feet.[39]

INVESTIGATIONS

After a detailed history and clinical examination, investigations include:

- *chest X-ray:* for heart size, shape, position and lung vascularity
- *electrocardiogram (ECG)* and, if necessary, Holter monitoring

Table 101.8 Common causes of heart failure from infancy to adolescence

Heart failure presenting at birth
Birth asphyxia
Sepsis
Severe anaemia
Obstructive left-sided lesions presenting after closure of the ductus arteriosus (e.g. coarctation, aortic stenosis, interrupted aortic arch, hypoplastic left heart syndrome)
Aortopulmonary window, truncus arteriosus
Systemic AV fistula (e.g. liver, brain, kidney)
Congenital cardiomyopathy
Arrhythmia: congenital SVT or heart block
Persistent pulmonary hypertension of the newborn
Heart failure presenting in the first 8 weeks of life
Large left-to-right shunts (e.g. VSD, PDA, total anomalous pulmonary venous drainage) cause heart failure as pulmonary vascular resistance and the haematocrit decrease
Infiltrative cardiomyopathy
Anomalous origin of the left coronary artery from the pulmonary artery
Hypothyroidism
Heart failure presenting later in childhood
Congenital heart disease
Subaortic stenosis
VSD with or without aortic regurgitation
Systemic AV valve regurgitation
Pulmonary atresia and VSD with large aortopulmonary collaterals
Congenital heart disease post operation
Fontan procedure
Obstructed prosthetic valve
Post ventriculotomy (e.g. Fallot's tetralogy)
Coronary artery injury
Imperfect myocardial preservation during bypass
Valve regurgitation after aortic or pulmonary valvotomy
Large Blalock–Taussig shunt
Cardiomyopathy
Infective, infiltrative, neuromuscular disease
Asphyxia (e.g. near-drowning, smoke inhalation)
Ischaemia (e.g. Kawasaki disease)
Toxic: acute (e.g. eucalyptus oil, carbamazepine, verapamil, flecainide)
Toxic: chronic (e.g. anthracycline)
Metabolic (e.g. LCAD deficiency)
Heart transplant rejection
Valvular (e.g. postrheumatic, infective endocarditis, trauma)
Arrhythmia (e.g. SVT, complete heart block)
Severe polycythaemia or anaemia (haematocrit > 70% or < 15%)
Cor pulmonale (e.g. bronchopulmonary dysplasia, severe scoliosis)
Acute hypertension (e.g. glomerulonephritis, haemolytic–uraemic syndrome)

AV, arteriovenous; LCAD, long-chain acyl-CoA dehydrogenase; PDA, patent ductus arteriosus; SVT, supraventricular tachycardia; VSD, ventricular septal defect.

- *echocardiography* (usually transthoracic; less often transoesophageal): for structural abnormality; valve stenosis, regurgitation and structure; chamber size and filling; wall thickness; pericardial fluid and estimates of ventricular systolic and diastolic function; left-to-right and right-to-left shunts, and pulmonary artery pressure
- *cardiac catheterisation* when indicated to quantify shunts, measure pressures and elucidate anatomy.

Plus other investigations as indicated:

- CT angiography to demonstrate 3-dimensional extracardiac structures
- MR angiography
- blood gases; chromosomal analyses; viral culture of stool, blood and throat swabs; urine screen for amino- and ketoacids, and myocardial biopsy.

MANAGEMENT [40,41]

The development of heart failure in infancy is an emergency requiring urgent hospitalisation. Management priorities include the following:

- *Correct precipitating factors* (e.g. fever, infection, anaemia or hypertension).
- *Diagnose and correct the underlying cause* (e.g. correct an aortic coarctation; repair or replace a regurgitant valve; treat an arrhythmia or infection; correct anaemia).
- *Support the systemic and pulmonary circulations* and reduce systemic and pulmonary venous congestion:
  - Give oxygen by mask or nasal prongs.
  - Give diuretics such as furosemide and spironolactone to reduce ventricular preload and venous congestion. Spironolactone has been shown to reduce mortality in adults with cardiac failure by inhibiting ventricular remodelling and improving diastolic compliance. Addition of a sulphonamide diuretic such as metolazone or hydrochlorothiazide has been shown to produce a diuresis in children with oliguria resistant to furosemide after cardiac surgery.[42] Restriction of fluid and salt intake, head elevation and venodilator drugs such as nitroglycerin (GTN) 1–10 μg/kg per min may be required. Preload reduction may depress the cardiac output in acute correctable lesions which obstruct ventricular inflow (e.g. cardiac tamponade).
  - Reduce left ventricular afterload by infusion of milrinone (0.25–0.75 μg/kg per min) or sodium nitroprusside (0.5–5.0 μg/kg per min). Angiotensin-converting enzyme (ACE) inhibitors may be added carefully when the child's heart is capable of increasing its output to sustain an adequate blood pressure. ACE inhibitors reduce mortality in early and late heart failure by improving ventricular performance and inhibiting myocardial remodelling. Vasodilators must be used cautiously in obstructive left-sided lesions to avoid myocardial ischaemia (due to reduced aortic diastolic pressure in the presence of ventricular wall hypertrophy. Vasodilators exacerbate volume loading in VSD or aortopulmonary shunts.
  - Reduce right ventricular afterload in intubated children with nitric oxide (NO) (0.5–10.0 ppm). In non-ventilated children, and to permit weaning of nitric oxide, sildenafil (0.3 mg/kg 6-hourly enterally) or infusion of prostacyclin (PGI_2 5–15 ng/kg per min) may be used.[29,43]
  - Increase contractility acutely with i.v. infusion of dobutamine (2–10 μg/kg per min) or adrenaline (0.02–0.5 μg/kg per min). β-adrenergic agonists increase oxygen consumption, myocardial work and ventricular diastolic stiffness, and may provoke tachyarrhythmias. They should therefore be used in the lowest effective dose.
  - Levosimendan infusion (12.5 μg/kg over 10 minutes, then 0.2 μg/kg per min for 24 hours) has been shown to improve haemodynamics and 31-day survival compared with dobutamine in adults with severe heart failure, even when combined with β-blockers.[44] It offers improvement in contractility without increasing myocardial oxygen consumption or downregulating β-receptors.
  - Consider careful use of β-blockers when diastolic dysfunction is prominent and when the child's circulation is sufficiently stable for β-agonists to be withdrawn. If the child tolerates infusion of a short-acting drug such as esmolol (50 μg/kg per min gradually increased to 200 μg/kg per min), a longer-acting agent such as carvedilol may be substituted.[45]
- *Mechanical ventilation* improves myocardial performance by improving gas exchange and reducing acidaemia, work of breathing and left ventricular afterload.[46] When pulmonary hypertension is the main cause of heart failure, intubation and mechanical ventilation can improve RV output by improving gas exchange and allowing NO to be given, but a short inspiratory time and low positive end-expiratory pressure (PEEP; 4–5 cmH_2O) are used to avoid further raising pulmonary vascular resistance.
- *Sedation and muscle relaxants* reduce metabolic rate and the cardiac output needed to meet metabolic demands. In a child with severe heart failure, commencing an inotrope such as dobutamine 10 μg/kg per min via peripheral cannula if necessary, 30 minutes before intubation reduces the risk of severe hypotension during intubation.
- *Ventricular assist devices* (*VAD*) can maintain life for weeks to months in very severe but reversible cardiac failure pending ventricular recovery or heart transplantation. When severe respiratory failure complicates severe heart failure, ECMO may be needed. Aortic balloon counterpulsation is less feasible and much less often helpful in small children than in adults.

CONGENITAL HEART DISEASE

Children critically ill with congenital heart disease (CHD) often require urgent resuscitation before a definitive structural diagnosis is made. The appropriate management then depends on the mode of presentation. A paediatric cardiologist should be consulted immediately about all such children. Management of acute postoperative deterioration depends on the underlying condition, nature of surgery and cause of deterioration.

Congenital heart disease in children may present in the following ways.

SHOCK IN THE FIRST FEW DAYS OF LIFE[47]

The commonest CHD causes are obstructive lesions of the left heart, including coarctation of the aorta with or without VSD, aortic stenosis and hypoplastic left heart syndrome (HLHS). Differential diagnosis includes cardiomyopathy, systemic arteriovenous malformation (AVM), septicaemia, inborn error of metabolism, anaemia, congenital heart block and supraventricular tachycardia (SVT).

In left-sided obstructive lesions, shock develops as the ductus arteriosus closes. All pulses (especially the femoral pulses in the case of coarctation) are decreased or absent. Tachycardia, tachypnoea, oliguria, cool mottled extremities, metabolic acidosis, hepatomegaly, cardiomegaly and pulmonary oedema are often present. Murmurs are often absent.

Emergency management[48] consists of prostaglandin E_1 infusion (start at 10 ng/kg per min and increase to 25 if necessary) to provide aortic blood flow from the pulmonary artery by opening the ductus arteriosus, dopamine infusion, $NaHCO_3$ 1 mmol/kg i.v. over 1 hour to correct metabolic acidosis, and mechanical ventilation (to reduce work of breathing, maintain normocarbia and prevent apnoea due to the PGE_1). Hypocarbia and a high FiO_2 should be avoided as they reduce pulmonary vascular resistance and divert blood flow to the lungs, thereby reducing systemic blood flow. Normoglycaemia and normocalcaemia should be maintained.

ACYANOTIC HEART FAILURE

IN THE FIRST WEEK OF LIFE [47]

Coarctation, aortic stenosis, cardiomyopathy (including obstructive cardiomyopathy in an infant of a diabetic mother) and endocardial fibroelastosis, anaemia, septicaemia, overtransfusion and systemic AVM can present as heart failure. Signs include poor feeding, tachycardia, tachypnoea, sweating, hepatomegaly, cardiomegaly, gallop rhythm, alar flaring, wheezing and expiratory grunt. Femoral pulses may be absent in coarctation and bruits are audible in skull, liver or kidneys in AVM. An aortic flow murmur may be present in anaemia or AVM.

Emergency management includes oxygen, diuretics and fluid restriction (to 50% of maintenance requirements; see Chapter 99). In severe failure, mechanical ventilation and inotropic drug infusion (see above) are started, and the child is transferred to a paediatric cardiac centre. When femoral pulses are absent or if aortic stenosis is suspected, i.v. infusion of PGE_1 (5–25 ng/kg per min) is started.

AFTER 2–8 WEEKS OF AGE

Systolic murmurs and signs of heart failure appear in infants with left-to-right shunts (such as VSD, patent ductus arteriosus (PDA), aortopulmonary window and AV septal defect) due to the physiological decreases in haemoglobin concentration and pulmonary vascular resistance at this time.

Emergency management includes diuretics and oxygen given via nasal prongs. Transfusion (to haemoglobin 13–14 g/dl) may reduce left-to-right shunt. If these measures fail to control heart failure, surgery is often needed, preceded if necessary by mechanical ventilation and inotropic drug infusion (see above).

CYANOSIS

PaO_2 greater than 150 mmHg (20 kPa) breathing 100% oxygen almost completely rules out cyanotic CHD. Most cyanotic CHDs have a PaO_2 less than 60 mmHg (8 kPa). A chest X-ray should be obtained urgently. Cyanosis due to CHD occurs when:

- pulmonary blood flow is reduced (e.g. pulmonary atresia)
- pulmonary and systemic circulations are not in series but are separate (e.g. transposition of the great arteries)
- saturated and unsaturated blood mix in the heart (e.g. anomalous pulmonary venous drainage)

CYANOSIS WITH PULMONARY OLIGAEMIA ON CHEST X-RAY

This is usually caused by stenosis at, below or above the pulmonary valve, or by tetralogy of Fallot. Deep cyanosis is present, often without murmurs or with a pulmonary ejection murmur. Tachypnoea may be present. Chest X-ray shows paucity of lung vessels and concavity in the pulmonary artery segment of the left heart border.

Emergency management[47,49]

In the newborn PGE_1 infusion (5–25 ng/kg per min) is used to open the ductus arteriosus and increase pulmonary blood flow. FiO_2 of 0.5 gives a small increase in oxygen delivery, and $NaHCO_3$ is used to correct a metabolic acidosis. Gentle assisted ventilation is needed if PGE_1 causes apnoea. The lungs are very compliant and airway pressures above 12–15 cmH_2O further reduce lung blood flow. The haemoglobin concentration should be kept at 120–150 g/l by transfusion if necessary. The child needs urgent echocardiographic diagnosis and most need a Blalock–Taussig shunt.

Beyond 1 month of age If the PaO_2 is less than 30 mmHg (4.0 kPa), or if cyanotic spells occur in a child with tetralogy of Fallot despite plasma volume expansion and oral β-blockers, an urgent Blalock–Taussig shunt is needed. Urgent treatment of Fallot spells consist of high Fio_2, knee–chest (older child) or legs raised (infant) position, 0.9% saline infusion 20 ml/kg and i.v. morphine 0.1 mg/kg. If these measures fail, then esmolol (0.5 mg/kg i.v. then infusion of 50–200 μg/kg per min) may be needed to reduce subpulmonary obstruction in Fallot's tetralogy. Inotropic drugs and vasodilators should be avoided.

CYANOSIS WITH PULMONARY PLETHORA OR OEDEMA IN THE NEWBORN[47]

The commonest cardiac causes are transposition of the great arteries (TGA), single ventricle, HLHS, truncus arteriosus and total anomalous pulmonary venous drainage (TAPVD). Signs include tachypnoea, tachycardia, cardiomegaly and hepatomegaly. A murmur may be present. Differential diagnosis includes lung disease such as hyaline membrane disease and neonatal pneumonia, group B streptococcal sepsis and persistent pulmonary hypertension of the newborn.

Emergency management

Acidaemia should be corrected and Fio_2 should be high. If heart failure is present, mechanical ventilation and dobutamine infusion are used. PGE_1 infusion (5–25 ng/kg per min) is used in all cases except when a small heart accompanies cyanosis and pulmonary oedema. These signs suggest TAPVD with obstruction of the pulmonary veins, in which case PGE_1 will exacerbate the pulmonary oedema. Assessment at a paediatric cardiac centre is needed urgently. A child with TGA needs balloon atrial septostomy and the other lesions need urgent surgery.

ARRHYTHMIAS IN CHILDREN[50]

SINUS BRADYCARDIA (SEE TABLE 101.3: 2ND–98TH CENTILE OF NORMAL HEART RATE FOR AGE)

Predisposing conditions include normal sleep, hypoxaemia, acidosis, hypotension, high intracranial pressure, cervical spinal cord injury, tracheal suction and drugs such as β-blockers, amiodarone and digoxin.

MANAGEMENT

No treatment is needed for asymptomatic bradycardia unless it is extreme. Correct any reversible cause. If the sinoatrial node is damaged, atropine (20 μg/kg) or isoprenaline infusion (0.1–0.5 μg/kg per min) or temporary transoesophageal or (in an older child) transvenous pacing may be used.

BRADYCARDIA–TACHYCARDIA (SICK SINUS) SYNDROME[51]

The usual form is severe sinus bradycardia with junctional escape rhythm. It can cause syncope and even sudden death. Predisposing conditions include:

- congenital atrial anomalies (e.g. Ebstein's anomaly and AV septal defects)
- extensive atrial surgery (e.g. Fontan and Senning operations)
- viral myocarditis
- congenital sinus node dysfunction

MANAGEMENT

Atrial pacing then treat tachyarrhythmias on their merits.

ATRIOVENTRICULAR BLOCK[52] (TABLE 101.9)

Often asymptomatic, but may present with fatigue, syncope or cardiac failure.

MANAGEMENT

- *Acquired complete heart block* should be paced, regardless of symptoms, as escape rhythms are unreliable.
- *Symptomatic second or third degree AV block* requires i.v. atropine, isoprenaline infusion (0.1–0.5 μg/kg per min) and, if necessary, external cardiac massage until pacing is established. Temporary transoesophageal or (in an older child) transvenous pacing may precede insertion of a permanent pacemaker.
- *Congenital in infants*: temporary, then permanent pacing if the heart rate is < 55 beats/min, regardless of symptoms.
- *Congenital in an older child*: temporary, then permanent pacing if the heart rate is < 50 beats/min or if symptomatic, or if there are ventricular escape beats or ventricular dysfunction.

SUPRAVENTRICULAR TACHYCARDIA (SVT)

RE-ENTRANT SVT

In younger children, an accessory AV pathway is usually present, which may conduct antegrade (pre-excitation, e.g. Wolff-Parkinson-White (WPW)) or retrograde (no pre-excitation; normal QRS). These AV re-entrant tachycardias may be episodic (e.g. precipitated by an extrasystole or a junctional escape beat) or may be permanent. The latter may be associated with heart failure in infants.

In older children and adolescents, a re-entrant pathway may exist in the peri-AV node area, and is sometimes

Table 101.9 Causes of atrioventricular block

Normal variant in newborn, adolescents, athletes
Structural heart abnormalities (atrioventricular septal defects or left atrial isomerism)
Post cardiac surgery (e.g. repair of ventricular septal defect or Fallot's tetralogy, Konno procedure)
Maternal antibodies
Cardiomyopathies, myocarditis (including rheumatic) and muscular dystrophies
Drugs (e.g. carbamazepine overdose)

associated with congenital heart lesions such as Ebstein's anomaly, tricuspid atresia and AV canal defects, as well as post cardiac surgery, myocarditis, drugs, sepsis, acidosis and catecholamine administration.

Management

Infants

- *If shocked:*
  - Give O_2 by mask
  - Sedation: i.v. midazolam (0.05–0.1 mg/kg i.v.)
  - Synchronised DC cardioversion 1 joule/kg
- *If stable*:
  - Vagal stimulation: induce gag reflex or apply ice water to the whole face for ~30 seconds. Do not use eyeball pressure.
  - Overdrive atrial pacing via transoesophageal or epicardial leads
  - Adenosine by rapid i.v. bolus 0.05 mg/kg (max 3 mg) increasing by 0.05 mg/kg (max 3 mg) every 2 minutes to a maximum of 0.25 mg/kg (max 12 mg)
  - Synchronised DC cardioversion 1 joule/kg. Record ECG during reversion to sinus rhythm, as pre-excitation may only be revealed at that time
  - Consider amiodarone or (provided WPW is absent) digoxin
  - Avoid verapamil which causes shock and cardiac arrest in infants

Older children

- As above.
- Verapamil (0.1 mg/kg i.v. over 30 minutes) or atenolol (0.05 mg/kg i.v. every 5 minutes until response, maximum of 2.5 mg or four doses, then 0.1 mg/kg every 12–24 hours) may also be used.

JUNCTIONAL ECTOPIC TACHYCARDIA (JET)[50,52]

Atrioventricular dissociation and ventricular rate 160–290 beats/min with narrow QRS complexes are seen on ECG. JET usually follows cardiac surgery, especially when myocardial function is poor and when surgery involves the AV node or its blood supply (e.g. Fontan operation or repair of VSD or AV septal defect). Postoperative JET can be fatal, but is usually self-limiting after 12–72 hours.

Management

- Reduce β-adrenergic stimulation: use low-dose noradrenaline or vasopressin to maintain blood pressure. Avoid the use of pancuronium as a muscle relaxant.
- Induce hypothermia to 34–35 °C for 2–3 days with 12-hourly brief normothermia to allow assessment.
- Amiodarone infusion: 25 μg/kg per min for 4 hours, then 5–5 μg/kg per min (max 1.2 g/24 hours).
- Consider procainamide (400 μg/kg per min for 25 minutes, then 20–80 μg/kg per min) or propafenone (2 mg/kg over 2 hours i.v., then 4 μg/kg per min): beware of hypotension.

JET is usually resistant to vagal manoeuvres, adenosine and overdrive pacing.

VENTRICULAR ECTOPIC BEATS AND VENTRICULAR TACHYCARDIA

Ventricular tachycardia (VT)[51] is uncommon in childhood, but may present as syncope, poor feeding (in infants) or heart failure. The rate is 120–300 beats/min. The QRS axis is different from that of the underlying sinus rhythm. QRS duration is usually (but not always) prolonged (> 0.08 seconds). Supraventricular tachycardia with aberrant conduction is rare in children: more than 90% of wide-complex tachycardias in children are VT. Fusion or capture beats, AV dissociation and new bundle branch block also favour the diagnosis of VT.

Predisposing conditions include congenital heart lesions and their surgery (e.g. aortic and subaortic stenosis, with hypertrophy of the left ventricular wall), myocardial ischaemia, mitral valve prolapse, myocarditis, cardiomyopathy, the hereditary long QT syndromes, blunt chest trauma, hypokalaemia or hypomagnesaemia and drug toxicity (including digoxin, cocaine, phenothiazines and tricyclic antidepressants).

MANAGEMENT[50]

Synchronised DC cardioversion should be used for any child with haemodynamic compromise due to VT.

Occasionally, i.v. lidocaine (1 mg/kg) or procainamide (see above) are used to convert VT to sinus rhythm when the cardiac output is adequate. These drugs or amiodarone (see above) are also used to prevent reversion to VT after DC cardioversion. In these circumstances, serum K^+ should be kept above 4.5 mmol/l, and serum Mg^{++} above 1.0 mmol/l.

REFERENCES

1. Friis-Hansen B. Body water compartments in children: changes during growth and related changes in body composition. *Pediatrics* 1961; **28**: 169–81.
2. Lawton AR, Crowe JE. Ontogeny of immunity. In: Stiehm ER, Ochs HD, Winkelstein JA (eds) *Immunologic Disorders in Infants and Children*, 5th edn. Philadelphia: Saunders; 2004: 3–19.
3. Roberton DM. The child who is immunodeficient. In: Robinson MJ, Roberton DM (eds) *Practical Paediatrics*, 4th edn. Edinburgh: Churchill Livingstone; 1998: 3–19.
4. Lewis DB, Wilson CB. Developmental immunology and role of host defences in neonatal susceptibility to infection. In: Remington JS, Klein JO (eds) *Infectious Diseases of the Fetus and Newborn Infant*, 4th edn. Philadelphia: WB Saunders; 1995: 20–98.
5. Epstein D, Wetzel RC. Cardiovascular physiology and shock. In: Nichols DG, Ungeleider RM, Spevak PJ *et al.* (eds) *Critical Heart Disease in Infants and Children*, 2nd edn. Philadelphia: Mosby; 2006: 17–72.

6. Mahony L. Development of myocardial structure and function. In: Allen HD, Gutgesell HP, Clark EB *et al.* (eds) *Moss and Adams' Heart Disease in Infants, Children and Adolescents*, 6th edn. Philadelphia: Lippincott, Williams and Wilkins; 2001: 24–40.
7. Williams CE, Mallard C, Tan W *et al.* Pathophysiology of perinatal asphyxia. *Clin Perinatol* 1993; **20**: 305–25.
8. Anderson PAW, Kleinman CS, Lister G *et al.* Cardiovascular function during development and the response to hypoxia. In: Polin RA, Fox WW, Abman SH (eds) *Fetal and Neonatal Physiology*, 3rd edn. Philadelphia: Saunders; 2004: 635–69.
9. Martin LD, Nyhan D, Wetzel RC. Regulation of pulmonary vascular resistance and blood flow. In: Nichols DG, Ungeleider RM, Spevak PJ *et al.* (eds) *Critical Heart Disease in Infants and Children*, 2nd edn. Philadelphia: Mosby; 2006: 73–112.
10. Davignon A, Rautaharju P, Boisselle E *et al.* Normal ECG standards for infants and children. *Pediatr Cardiol* 1980; **1**: 123–52.
11. Carcillo JA. The failing cardiovascular system in sepsis. In: Chang AC, Towbin JA (eds) *Heart Failure in Children and Young Adults*. Philadelphia: Saunders; 2006: 416–27.
12. Kumar A, Haery C, Parrillo JE. Myocardial dysfunction in septic shock. *Crit Care Clin* 2000; **16**: 251–87.
13. Poelaert J, Declerck C, Vogelaers D *et al.* Left ventricular systolic and diastolic function in septic shock. *Intensive Care Med* 1997; **23**: 553–60.
14. Vincent JL. New therapeutic implications of anticoagulation mediator replacement in sepsis and acute respiratory distress syndrome. *Crit Care Med* 2000; **28**(Suppl 9): S83–5.
15. Tibby SM, Murdoch IA. Measurement of cardiac output and tissue perfusion. *Curr Opin Pediatr* 2002; **14**: 303–9.
16. Thompson AE. Pulmonary artery catheterization in children. *New Horizons* 1997; **5**: 244–50.
17. Levy RJ, Deutschman CS. Evaluating myocardial depression in sepsis. *Shock* 2004; **22**: 1–10.
18. Holmes CL, Patel BM, Russell JA *et al.* Physiology of vasopressin relevant to management of septic shock. *Chest* 2001; **120**: 989–1002.
19. Robin JK, Oliver JA, Landry DW. Vasopressin deficiency in the syndrome of irreversible shock. *J Trauma* 2003; **54**: S149–54.
20. Romijn JA, Coyle EF, Sidossis LS *et al.* Regulation of endogenous fat and carbohydrate metabolism in relation to exercise intensity and duration. *Am J Physiol* 1993; **265**(3 Pt 1): E380–91.
21. Van den Berghe G, de Zegher F, Lauwers P. Dopamine suppresses pituitary function in infants and children. *Crit Care Med* 1994; **22**: 1747–53.
22. Lichtman SM. Bacterial translocation in humans. *J Pediatr Gastroenterol Nutr* 2001; **33**: 1–10.
23. Duke TD, Butt W, South M. Predictors of mortality and multiple organ failure in children with sepsis. *Intensive Care Med* 1997; **23**: 684–92.
24. Marshall JC. An intensivist's dilemma: support of the splanchnic circulation in critical illness [comment]. *Crit Care Med* 1998; **26**: 1637–8.
25. Totapally BR, Fakioglu H, Torbati D *et al.* Esophageal capnometry during hemorrhagic shock and after resuscitation in rats. *Crit Care* 2003; 7: 79–84.
26. Schulz G, Weiss M, Bauersfeld U *et al.* Liver tissue oxygenation as measured by near-infrared spectroscopy in the critically ill child in correlation with central venous oxygen saturation. *Intensive Care Med* 2002; **28**: 184–9.
27. Marx G, Reinhart K. Venous oximetry. *Curr Opin Crit Care* 2006; **12**: 263–8.
28. Charpie JR, Dekeon MK, Goldberg CS *et al.* Postoperative hemodynamics after Norwood palliation for hypoplastic left heart syndrome. *Am J Cardiol* 2001; **87**: 198–202.
29. Beghetti M. Current treatment options in children with pulmonary arterial hypertension and experiences with oral bosentan. *Eur J Clin Invest* 2006; **3**: 16–24.
30. Annane D, Bellissant E, Bollaert PE *et al.* Corticosteroids for treating severe sepsis and septic shock. *Cochrane Database Syst Rev* 2004; Issue 1. Art. No. CD002243. http://www.mrw.interscience.wiley.com/cochrane/clsysrev/articles/CD002243/frame.html.
31. Bilgin K, Yarami A, Haspolat K *et al.* A randomized trial of granulocyte–macrophage colony-stimulating factor in neonates with sepsis and neutropenia [see comment]. *Pediatrics* 2001; **107**(1): 36–41.
32. Alejandria MM, Lansang MA, Dans LF *et al.* Intravenous immunoglobulin for treating sepsis and septic shock. *Cochrane Database Syst Rev* 2002; Issue 1. Art. No. CD001090. http://www.mrw.interscience.wiley.com/cochrane/clsysrev/articles/CD001090/frame.html.
33. Levin M, Quint PA, Goldstein B *et al.* Recombinant bactericidal/permeability-increasing protein (rBPI21) as adjunctive treatment for children with severe meningococcal sepsis: a randomised trial. *Lancet* 2000; **356**: 961–7.
34. Mohan P, Brocklehurst P. Granulocyte transfusions for neonates with confirmed or suspected sepsis and neutropaenia. *Cochrane Database Syst Rev* 2003; Issue 4. Art. No. CD003956. http://www.mrw.interscience.wiley.com/cochrane/clsysrev/articles/CD003956/frame.html.
35. Giroir B, Goldstein B, Nadel S *et al.* The efficacy of drotrecogin alfa (activated) for the treatment of pediatric severe sepsis. *Crit Care Med* 2006; **33**: A152.
36. Dimmick S, Badawi N, Randell T. Thyroid hormone supplementation for the prevention of morbidity and mortality in infants undergoing cardiac surgery. *Cochrane Database Syst Rev* 2004; Issue 3. Art. No. CD004220. http://www.mrw.interscience.wiley.com/cochrane/clsysrev/articles/CD004220/frame.html.
37. Leclerc FMD, Leteurtre SMD, Cremer RMD *et al.* Do new strategies in meningococcemia produce better outcomes? *Crit Care Med* 2000; **28**(9 Suppl): S60–3.

38. Braunwald E. Heart failure. In: Braunwald E, Fauci AS, Kasper DL *et al.* (eds) *Harrison's Principles of Internal Medicine*, 15th edn. New York: McGraw Hill; 2001: 1318–29.
39. Altman CA, Kung G. Clinical recognition of congestive heart failure in children. In: Chang AC, Towbin JA (eds) *Heart Failure in Children and Young Adults.* Philadelphia: Saunders; 2006: 201–10.
40. Chang AC, Towbin JA (eds) *Heart Failure in Children and Young Adults.* Philadelphia: Saunders; 2006.
41. Kay JD, Colan SD, Graham Jr TP. Congestive heart failure in pediatric patients. *Am Heart J* 2001; **142**: 923–8.
42. Dickerson HA, Chang AC. Diuretics. In: Chang AC, Towbin JA (eds) *Heart Failure in Children and Young Adults.* Philadelphia: Saunders; 2006.
43. Kageyama K, Shime N, Hirose M *et al.* Factors contributing to successful discontinuation from inhaled nitric oxide therapy in pediatric patients after congenital cardiac surgery. *Pediatr Crit Care Med* 2004; **5**: 351–5.
44. De Luca L, Colucci WS, Nieminen MS *et al.* Evidence-based use of levosimendan in different clinical settings. *Eur Heart J* 2006; **27**: 1908–20.
45. Packer M, Fowler MB, Roecker EB *et al.* Effect of carvedilol on the morbidity of patients with severe chronic heart failure: results of the carvedilol prospective randomized cumulative survival (COPERNICUS) study. *Circulation* 2002; **106**: 2194–9.
46. Dent CL, Nelson DP. Low cardiac output in the intensive care setting. In: Chang AC, Towbin JA (eds) *Heart Failure in Children and Young Adults.* Philadelphia: Saunders; 2006.
47. Penny DJ, Shekerdemian LS. Management of the neonate with symptomatic congenital heart disease. *Arch Dis Child Fetal Neonatal Ed* 2001; **84**: F141–45.
48. Lang P, Fyler DC. Hypoplastic left heart syndrome, mitral atresia and aortic atresia. In: Keane JF, Lock JE, Fyler DC (eds) *Nadas' Pediatric Cardiology*, 2nd edn. Philadelphia: Saunders; 2006.
49. Breitbart RE, Fyler DC. Tetralogy of Fallot. In: Keane JF, Lock JE, Fyler DC (eds) *Nadas' Pediatric Cardiology*, 2nd edn. Philadelphia: Saunders; 2006.
50. Fish FA, Benson DWJ. Disorders of cardiac conduction and rhythm. In: Allen HD, Gutgesell HP, Clark EB *et al.* (eds) *Moss and Adams' Heart Disease in Infants, Children and Adolescents*, 6th edn. Philadelphia: Lippincott Williams and Wilkins; 2001: 482–533.
51. Vetter V. Arrhythmias. In: Moller JH, Hoffman JIE (eds) *Pediatric Cardiovascular Medicine.* New York: Churchill Livingstone; 2000: 833–83.
52. Kanter RJ, Carboni MP, Silka MJ. Pediatric arrhythmias. In: Nichols DG, Ungerleider RM, Spevak PJ *et al.* (eds) *Critical Heart Disease in Infants and Children*, 2nd edn. Philadelphia: Mosby; 2006: 207–41.

102

Neurological emergencies in children

Anthony J Slater

Neurological emergencies are the most common life-threatening emergencies in children. In developed societies after the first year of life, the leading cause of death in childhood is injury, particularly traumatic brain injury. There is a range of conditions affecting the brain, spinal cord and peripheral nervous system that require prompt recognition, resuscitation and definitive management. The pathophysiology, clinical features, treatment and outcome of these acute neurological emergencies are influenced by several important differences between adults and children. These differences include response to injury, developmental maturity and capacity for growth and recovery.

PATHOPHYSIOLOGY OF BRAIN INJURIES IN CHILDREN

Brain injuries are usually caused by a primary event (e.g. trauma, ischaemia, infection or metabolic disturbance) and are frequently accompanied by secondary injuries including oedema, altered cerebrovascular autoregulation, tissue hypoxia or other cytotoxic events. It is unlikely that therapy administered after the event will influence the outcome of the primary injury. However, appropriate resuscitation and treatment and the avoidance of iatrogenic complications may prevent or reduce the impact of secondary injuries.

Features of brain injury particular to the paediatric patient are described below.

DIFFUSE CEREBRAL SWELLING

Diffuse brain swelling in the absence of oedema is a frequent early finding in paediatric brain injury, and is due to generalised cerebral vasodilatation. It often resolves in 1–2 days if there is no other significant brain injury. With more severe primary traumatic injury, diffuse cerebral swelling may be accompanied by areas of contusion, multifocal petechial haemorrhage and vasogenic oedema that progress over several days.

CEREBRAL BLOOD FLOW AND METABOLISM

The cerebral perfusion pressure (CPP) represents the difference between mean arterial pressure (MAP) and intracranial pressure (ICP).

$$CPP = MAP - ICP$$

If autoregulation is disturbed as part of the illness, CPP becomes the major determinant of cerebral blood flow, particularly in areas with more severe damage. The ideal CPP in childhood is not known. The normal range of MAP varies with age from 40 mmHg in a term neonate to 90 mmHg in an adult. The target CPP is usually adjusted with age, taking into consideration the normal blood pressure for age. For example, for an adolescent patient, therapy may be directed at maintaining a CPP of 70 mmHg, while for a child aged 5 years, the aim may be to maintain a CPP of 50 mmHg.

In conditions where vasogenic oedema occurs, arterial hypertension may increase vascular shift of fluid and worsen brain swelling. However, treatment aimed at lowering arterial pressure (e.g. with vasodilators) may interfere with homeostatic mechanisms and should be used cautiously.

The brain comprises up to 12% of body weight in infancy compared with 2–3% in adulthood. Cerebral oxygen and glucose consumption is therefore proportionately greater in childhood while glycogen stores are readily depleted. As hypoglycaemia occurs commonly in severe illnesses such as sepsis, blood glucose should be monitored regularly.

HYPOVOLAEMIA

Children have small blood volumes and commonly develop hypovolaemia from scalp bleeding or intracranial haemorrhage. For example, hypovolaemia will develop in a 5-kg infant (blood volume 400 ml) following blood loss of only 100 ml. Hypovolaemia should be treated aggressively with fluid boluses of 20 ml/kg to ensure adequate cerebral perfusion.

RELATIVE GROWTH

The child's short stature and proportionately large head confer a number of risks. The toddler's head is at the level of the front of a motor vehicle and isolated head injury is subsequently common following pedestrian injury in this age group. The neck muscles are relatively weak in infancy and they support a large head. This renders the brain prone to deceleration injury in motor vehicle crashes and in cases of domestic violence. Injury inflicted by shaking an infant by the shoulders snaps the head to and fro, leading to compression of brain tissue and rupture of delicate bridging veins.

BONE DEVELOPMENT

The skull bones in the first year of life are thin with open sutures and open fontanelles. Beyond 2 years, the skull sutures close and the cranial vault thickens. In young children there tends to be less bony protection from high impact trauma, while the non-rigid skull may expand to partially decompress expanding lesions.[1]

UNDIAGNOSED COMA

An ordered approach to diagnosis and treatment is required for a child with depressed conscious state of unknown origin. This approach must consider common life-threatening and rare treatable diseases (Table 102.1).

INITIAL MANAGEMENT

Management should always begin with rapid assessment of the adequacy of airway, ventilation and circulation. If inadequacies are detected, interventions aimed at correcting them should occur immediately. Once venous access is obtained, blood should be drawn for routine tests including immediate measurement of blood glucose. If hypoglycaemia is demonstrated 2 ml/kg of 25% glucose or 5 ml/kg of 10% glucose should be given intravenously as the neurological sequelae of unrecognised hypoglycaemia can be profound.

Concurrent with the initial assessment and resuscitation, relevant details of the present and past history should be obtained. A detailed neurological and general physical examination should be performed. It is important to document accurately the conscious state so that changes over time, particularly deterioration, can be easily recognised. The Glasgow Coma Scale (GCS) is appropriate for this purpose. The responses of children change with development and therefore the GCS requires modification for paediatric use (Table 102.2). After completing the clinical assessment, the likely diagnosis is often apparent and appropriate investigation and treatment can commence. Multiple factors may compound to produce coma. For example, a child with severe gastroenteritis may have hyperthermia, hyponatraemic dehydration, metabolic acidosis and hypovolaemic shock.

Table 102.1 Causes of coma in children

Structural	Metabolic
Trauma	Post-ictal state
Accidental	Infection
Inflicted	Meningitis
Hydrocephalus	Encephalitis
Haemorrhage	Drugs and toxins
AVM	Hypoxia–ischaemia
Aneurysms	Circulatory shock
Tumour	Biochemical
Tumour	Hypoglycaemia
Cerebral abscess	Electrolyte disorders
	Sodium/water
	Calcium
	Acid–base disturbance
	Hyperthermia
	Hepatic failure
	Haemolytic–uraemic syndrome
	Inborn errors of metabolism
	Reye's syndrome

CONTROLLED VENTILATION

Indications for ventilating a comatose child are:

- upper-airway obstruction or loss of airway reflexes
- apnoea, respiratory failure
- rapidly worsening coma
- signs of progressive elevation of ICP (i.e. bradycardia, hypertension, abnormal pupillary light reflexes and localising signs)

Once ventilation is initiated the stomach should be drained with a gastric tube and blood pressure checked every 5 minutes. Raised ICP should be considered in any case of rapidly progressive coma. Intracranial hypertension should be managed with moderate hyperventilation and intravenous mannitol (0.25 g/kg). Hypertonic saline given as 0.5 ml/kg of 20% solution (3.4 mmol/ml) can also rapidly reduce ICP.[2] Once stability is achieved, adequate sedation and analgesia is required. Muscle relaxants may be necessary to facilitate ventilation and prevent straining; however, their use precludes further neurological assessment and therefore, if long-acting muscle relaxants are continued, ICP monitoring is advisable. Hyperventilation is a short-term manoeuvre and following the early resuscitation phase, gradual return to a low-normal $Pa\text{CO}_2$ should be the aim. This is best achieved with end tidal CO_2 and ICP monitoring. Particular attention should be paid to restoring intravascular volume and maintaining an adequate CPP.

CRANIAL COMPUTED TOMOGRAPHY (CT)

A CT scan is required in comatose children with localising signs and in those in whom the diagnosis is not clear. A CT should also be performed if the conscious state is abnormal and there is a history of trauma. Even if the general condition does not warrant controlled ventilation, a CT is often best performed under general anaesthesia. Unwanted movement will cause poor-quality images and sedation alone may place the child at risk of hypoventilation or aspiration.

LUMBAR PUNCTURE

Lumbar puncture (LP) should be performed when there is reasonable suspicion of meningitis or encephalitis. The risks and contraindications to LP are discussed under bacterial meningitis.

Table 102.2 Glasgow Coma Scale for children

Glasgow Coma Scale (4–15 years)		Child's Glasgow Coma Scale (< 4 years)	
Response	**Score**	**Response**	**Score**
Eye opening		Eye opening	
Spontaneously	4	Spontaneously	4
To verbal stimuli	3	To verbal stimuli	3
To pain	2	To pain	2
No response to pain	1	No response to pain	1
Best motor response		Best motor response	
Obeys verbal command	6	Spontaneous or obeys verbal command	6
Localises to pain	5	Localises to pain or withdraws to touch	5
Withdraws from pain	4	Withdraws from pain	4
Abnormal flexion to pain (decorticate)	3	Abnormal flexion to pain (decorticate)	3
Abnormal extension to pain (decerebrate)	2	Abnormal extension to pain (decerebrate)	2
No response to pain	1	No response to pain	1
Best verbal response		Best verbal response	
Orientated and converses	5	Alert, babbles, coos, words to usual ability	5
Disorientated and converses	4	Less than usual words, spontaneous irritable cry	4
Inappropriate words	3	Cries only to pain	3
Incomprehensible sounds	2	Moans to pain	2
No response to pain	1	No response to pain	1

ADDITIONAL INVESTIGATIONS

Additional investigations include arterial blood gas analysis, serum electrolytes, glucose, urea and creatinine, liver function tests, serum ammonia, serum and CSF lactate and pyruvate, and urine analysis. Appropriate screening of blood and urine will exclude common poisons and drug intoxications.

SPECIFIC TREATMENT

The clinical signs and results of investigations generally guide treatment. If hypoglycaemia occurs, after initial correction, care should be taken to ensure that it does not recur by the administration of appropriate glucose containing i.v. fluid and regular blood glucose monitoring. Herpes simplex encephalitis can present in many ways and is not excluded by the absence of CSF pleocytosis. Aciclovir therapy should therefore be considered in any patient in whom herpes cannot be confidently excluded.

STATUS EPILEPTICUS

Convulsive status epilepticus (CSE) is usually defined as a continuous convulsion lasting 30 minutes or longer or repeated convulsions lasting 30 minutes or longer without recovery of consciousness between convulsions.[3] The common causes of CSE in children are:

- prolonged febrile convulsion
- epilepsy associated with first presentation, anticonvulsant withdrawal or intercurrent illness, often with fever
- central nervous system infection (i.e. meningitis or encephalitis)
- metabolic disturbance (e.g. hypoglycaemia, hyponatraemia, hypocalcaemia)
- trauma, including inflicted injury

PATHOPHYSIOLOGY

Many physiological changes occur during prolonged seizures. There is an initial phase of compensation lasting less than 30 minutes. Following a period of transition there is a phase of decompensation commencing between 30 and 60 minutes and evolving over hours. Physiological changes during the compensated phase include tachycardia, hypertension, increased catecholamine release and increased cardiac output. Changes within the brain include increased cerebral blood flow and increased cerebral utilisation of glucose and oxygen. After 30–60 minutes the mechanisms for homeostatic compensation fail. During the decompensated phase there may be falling blood pressure and cardiac output, hypoglycaemia, hypoxia, acidosis, electrolyte disturbance and rhabdomyolysis. The cerebral physiology is characterised by failing autoregulation and reduced cerebral blood flow and oxygen and glucose utilisation. Over hours a deficit in brain energy develops and this is associated with the development of brain damage.[4]

EXCITATORY AMINO ACIDS AND BRAIN INJURY

Mesial temporal sclerosis is the most common acquired brain lesion following CSE. There is evidence that the accumulation of a number of excitatory and inhibitory amino acids have a role in the pathophysiology of neuronal injury. In particular, glutamate accumulation and stimulation of NMDA receptors (*N*-methyl-D-aspartate) leads to an influx of intracellular calcium, which triggers a number of cytotoxic events and ultimately cell death.[5]

MANAGEMENT

The initial management is as for other neurological emergencies with attention to airway and oxygenation. Most seizures in childhood cease spontaneously in a short time, but if they persist for 5 minutes or continue after presentation to an emergency department, they should be stopped to avoid metabolic and ischaemic neuronal damage. Hypoglycaemia should be excluded or detected early. If intravenous access cannot be obtained rapidly, drugs can be administered intramuscularly, intranasally, rectally or via the intraosseous (i.o.) route. If benzodiazepines are administered within 20 minutes of a seizure commencing, the rate of seizure control is higher than if they are administered after 30 minutes.[6] This justifies early prehospital administration of benzodiazepines to children with active seizures at the time of ambulance arrival.[7] Specific drug treatment includes the following.

BENZODIAZEPINES

Diazepam, midazolam and lorazepam are the most useful agents.

Diazepam is given initially as 0.2 mg/kg i.v./i.o., and repeated up to 0.5 mg/kg. If venous access cannot be secured, it can be given per rectum. The recommended rectal dose is higher than the intravenous dose (0.5 mg/kg p.r.). Excessive sedation and respiratory depression occur with larger doses and must be dealt with effectively.

Lorazepam (0.05–0.1 mg/kg i.v.) may have advantages over diazepam as it is as effective, has a longer half-life, and causes less respiratory depression.[8,9]

Midazolam and clonazepam are also effective. When i.v. access is not available, intramuscular or intranasal administration of midazolam is an alternative to rectal diazepam.[10–12] In children presenting to an emergency department still convulsing, 0.2 mg/kg i.m. of midazolam has been reported to control 83% of seizures within 5 minutes of administration and 93% of seizures within 10 minutes.[13] Midazolam has also been used by constant i.v. infusion (1–8 μg/kg per min) to control refractory CSE in children.[14–16]

PHENYTOIN

Phenytoin should be commenced if benzodiazepines are not effective. It is given as 20 mg/kg i.v. over 30 minutes, which is followed by a maintenance dose (4 mg/kg 8-hourly past the neonatal period). It causes minimal sedation or respiratory depression, but is not suitable in neonates and in patients who are already on maintenance doses. As it is given slowly, phenytoin will not have rapid effects and if generalised CSE persists, consideration should be given to the use of thiopental (see below). Fosphenytoin, a prodrug of phenytoin, can be administered i.m. or i.v., but has a less irritant effect when given i.v.[17] Its place in the management of CSE in children is not yet clear.[18]

PHENOBARBITAL

When phenytoin is contraindicated, phenobarbital (20 mg/kg i.v. over 30 minutes) should be given. Respiratory depression and hypotension occur, particularly after benzodiazepines. Further doses can be safely administered to the ventilated child who has ongoing seizures.

THIOPENTAL

If seizures are prolonged and are not controlled by benzodiazepines, thiopental 2–5 mg/kg slowly i.v., then 1–5 mg/kg per hour by continuous infusion into a central vein can be given. Appropriately skilled staff and suitable equipment are necessary as thiopental necessitates endotracheal intubation and mechanical ventilation, and possibly inotropic drugs to counter its myocardial depressant effects. Blood concentrations need to be monitored during prolonged use. Whenever muscle relaxants are used they should be short acting to ensure ongoing seizure activity is not masked. Seizures are only controlled by anaesthetic doses of thiopental.

PARALDEHYDE

In many centres rectal paraldehyde (0.4 ml/kg mixed with an equal quantity of olive oil) is frequently used in the management of CSE.[18] One advantage of paraldehyde is that, like diazepam, it can be administered rectally if i.v. access is difficult to obtain.

OTHER MANAGEMENT

The patient must be protected from self-injury during seizures. Severe respiratory and metabolic acidosis are common and are best managed by rapid control of the seizure and maintenance of adequate ventilation and oxygenation. Once seizures are controlled, the cause should be sought. A detailed history is invaluable. A CT scan should reveal structural lesions. An LP should be deferred if the child is unconscious after a seizure. However, if the conscious state improves and there are no signs of raised ICP (see below), an LP will confirm or exclude meningitis. When the diagnosis remains unclear, viral encephalitis (e.g. herpes, enterovirus), metabolic encephalopathy, poisoning and inflicted injury should be considered.

OUTCOME

The outcome of CSE is dependent on the aetiology. Neurologically normal children in whom CSE is precipitated by fever are considered to have a good prognosis with mortality reported between 0 and 2%.[19] The incidence of neurological deficits or cognitive impairment in this group is also very low.[5] In acute symptomatic CSE (where CSE is a symptom of an acute neurological process such as infection or trauma), mortality is 12–16% and the incidence of new neurological dysfunction is more than 20%.[19] In this setting, however, it is very difficult to tease out the extent to which prolonged seizures contribute to neurological sequelae.

BACTERIAL MENINGITIS

PATHOPHYSIOLOGY

Bacterial meningitis (BM) usually occurs following haematogenous spread of organisms carried in the nasopharynx. In childhood the common bacteria causing BM are *Streptococcus pneumoniae*, *Neisseria meningitidis* and *Haemophilus influenzae* type b (Hib). Group B *Streptococcus*, *Escherichia coli* and *Listeria monocytogenes* are the most common causative organisms of neonatal BM. Occasionally, meningitis occurs as a complication of other pathology such as base of skull fracture, chronic middle ear infection or infection of a congenital dermoid sinus.

In the early stages of the disease cerebral hyperaemia occurs. This can be followed by cerebral ischaemia, which may occur by several different mechanisms. Local vasculitis of vessels transversing the subarachnoid space can progress to arterial thrombosis and focal infarction. Other vascular abnormalities including vasospasm and sagittal sinus thrombosis can also occur. Cerebral oedema is relatively common in meningitis and is caused by a combination of vasogenic, cytotoxic and hydrostatic factors. If cerebral oedema is severe, raised ICP and impaired cerebral perfusion can occur, leading to global cerebral ischaemia.

CLINICAL FEATURES

In children the typical features of BM are fever, headache, photophobia, neck stiffness and vomiting. The history may extend over several days; however, in fulminant cases the time from first symptom to coma and death may only be a few hours. Neonates and young infants do not present with the typical localised symptoms and signs. Instead, they present with generalised signs of illness including lethargy, poor feeding and pallor. Generalised or focal convulsions or apnoea may be present at presentation. Tuberculous meningitis usually presents with a more insidious onset of symptoms and may be associated with focal neurological signs.

Complications occur commonly in BM. During the early phase, meningitis may be associated with septic shock and disseminated intravascular coagulation (DIC). Fluid and electrolyte abnormalities are relatively common, particularly hyponatraemia and hypoglycaemia. Focal and generalised convulsions are relatively common and may progress to status epilepticus. During the recovery phase subdural effusions or hydrocephalus may occur.

INVESTIGATIONS

Lumbar puncture for CSF microscopy, culture and bacterial antigen testing is required for definitive diagnosis of BM and to guide antibiotic therapy. While an LP can be performed safely in the majority of children with BM, LP may precipitate brainstem herniation if raised ICP is present.[20] Identifying children at risk of this complication is difficult, so it is generally recommended that empiric antibiotic therapy be commenced and LP deferred if any of the following clinical features are present:

- depressed conscious state
- decorticate or decerebrate posturing
- focal neurological signs
- other signs of raised ICP

A normal CT scan does not exclude the possibility of elevated ICP.[20] Therefore, the decision to defer an LP should be based on clinical rather than radiological signs. In addition to signs of increased ICP, other indications for deferring the LP include cardiorespiratory instability and severe coagulopathy.

If LP is deferred, alternative methods of establishing a bacterial diagnosis include blood culture and bacterial antigen testing in urine and polymerase chain reaction (PCR) testing of blood.[21,22]

MANAGEMENT

RESUSCITATION

Severely ill patients require rapid resuscitation. Comatose patients require intubation and ventilation to prevent airway obstruction and hypoventilation. Hypovolaemia should be treated rapidly with boluses of fluid. Patients with septic shock will also require inotropic support.

CEREBRAL RESUSCITATION

General principles of supporting brain injury apply to BM. These include optimising cerebral oxygen delivery, controlling intracranial pressure and preventing cerebral metabolic stress. The role of ICP monitoring is controversial. There is some anecdotal evidence to support the use of ICP monitoring in a small number of selected cases. Unfortunately, there are no large studies that assess the benefit or harm of ICP monitoring and ICP targeted therapy in BM.

ANTIBIOTIC THERAPY

Empiric broad-spectrum antibiotics should be selected based on likely pathogens and local resistance patterns. A common protocol for BM is to use ampicillin plus cefotaxime for the first month of life and to use a third-generation cephalosporin (cefotaxime or ceftriaxone) after the first month.[23] In regions where penicillin and cephalosporin-resistant *Pneumococcus* occurs, vancomycin should be added to the initial empiric antibiotics until the causative organism is identified and the antibiotic sensitivities are known. When cephalosporin-resistant pneumococci are found to be the causative organism in meningitis, both a third-generation cephalosporin and vancomycin should be continued as vancomycin penetrates into CSF poorly and therefore should not be used as a single antibiotic. The addition of rifampicin should be considered.[24]

ADJUVANT THERAPY

Although a number of adjuvant therapies have been investigated experimentally, the only one that is commonly used clinically is dexamethasone. If dexamethasone is used it should ideally be given before the first dose of antibiotics and continued for 48 hours (0.4 mg/kg 12-hourly).[25] There is evidence that dexamethasone reduces the incidence of neurological sequelae and sensineural deafness; however, the beneficial effects are greatest in Hib meningitis.[26,27] Now that immunisation has changed the epidemiology and antibiotic-resistant pneumococcal strains are more common, it is possible that the relationship between risk and benefit of dexamethasone therapy has changed. However, current recommendations support the use of dexamethasone for children more than 6 weeks of age with bacterial meningitis.[24,28]

FLUID THERAPY

Although there is consensus that hypovolaemia should be treated rapidly and aggressively, fluid therapy after the initial resuscitation is controversial. It is important to consider both the tonicity of i.v. fluids as well as the rate of fluid administration. Although dextrose saline solutions with low sodium content (0.18–0.3% saline) are isotonic with plasma when first administered, as the dextrose crosses the blood–brain barrier or is metabolised, the net effect is that the cerebral circulation is exposed to hypotonic fluids, which potentially exacerbates cerebral oedema. Therefore, the i.v. fluid used in BM should be 0.45% or 0.9% saline in 5% dextrose.[29,30]

Restriction of maintenance fluids in BM has been commonly practised. Hyponatraemia is common and if it is assumed that this is secondary to the syndrome of inappropriate antidiuretic hormone secretion (SIADH) then fluid restriction is logical. Recent evidence, however, suggests that ADH is appropriately elevated in response to hypovolaemia[31] and that hyponatraemic patients with BM tend to be more dehydrated than normonatraemic patients.[32] Compared to fluid restriction, fluid therapy aimed at providing maintenance plus the fluid deficit has been reported to result in a more rapid correction of sodium and ADH.[31,33]

Although these studies suggest fluid restriction may not benefit all children with BM, it is important that fluid is restricted in patients with BM and true SIADH, as maintenance fluid therapy in these patients will cause the serum sodium to fall further. This complication is potentially life threatening, with the progressive fall in sodium precipitating seizures and worsening cerebral oedema. Therefore, serum sodium should be monitored closely during the first 24–48 hours of therapy in all patients with BM.

CHEMOPROPHYLAXIS FOR CONTACTS

Prophylaxis is required for every household member in cases of meningococcal infection and in cases of Hib infection when there is another child in the household under 5 years who is unimmunised. Rifampicin (10 mg/kg to a maximum of 600 mg b.d.) for 2 days in meningococcal disease or 4 days in Hib disease is appropriate. Neonates require 10 mg/kg per day. Pregnant women can be effectively managed with a single intramuscular dose of ceftriaxone (250 mg). Ciprofloxacin (15 mg/kg to a maximum of 750 mg) is also effective and has the advantage of single dose therapy.[34]

OUTCOME

Bacterial meningitis is associated with significant mortality and morbidity. Overall mortality for BM in childhood is 5–10%; however, in children requiring mechanical ventilation a mortality rate of 30% has been reported, with major neurosequelae occurring in 33% of survivors.[35]

PREVENTION

Immunisation has significantly reduced the incidence of Hib meningitis in developed countries,[36,37] while initial trials of heptavalent pneumococcal vaccine have shown a reduction in invasive pneumococcal infection in children.[38] Meningococcal serogroup C conjugate vaccines have reduced the incidence of severe meningococcal disease in infants in the UK and Australia.[39,40]

ENCEPHALITIS

Common causes of encephalitis include enteroviruses, mycoplasma, cytomegalovirus, herpes, Epstein–Barr and respiratory viruses (adenovirus and parainfluenzae). The most significant causes worldwide are the insect-transmitted arbovirus encephalitides including Australian, Japanese B and St Louis. These can cause profound coma and are associated with significant incidence of residual neurological deficit.

Presenting symptoms of encephalitis include seizures, focal neurological deficits in the setting of an acute febrile illness, confusion and coma. Meningeal irritation may not be obvious. CSF analysis may show a pleocytosis and in the early phase this can consist predominantly of neutrophils. As mentioned, herpes is the most important diagnosis to make, because it is treatable. Electroencephalography (EEG), CT and magnetic resonance imaging (MRI) are helpful in making the diagnosis. MRI is more sensitive than CT for detecting signs of encephalitis, particularly during the early stages of the illness. PCR on CSF may also aid rapid diagnosis.[41,42] Aciclovir used early improves outcome and should be commenced when the diagnosis is suspected.

The enteroviruses are important causes of encephalitis in children. In addition, they cause other acute neurological illnesses including acute flaccid paralysis due to transverse myelitis and Guillain–Barré syndrome.[43] Pleconaril is a promising new antiviral agent that appears to have clinical benefit in enteroviral infections, including CNS disease.[44] Outcome of viral encephalitis is worse in infancy than in older age groups.[45]

NON-TRAUMATIC INTRACRANIAL HAEMORRHAGE

Non-traumatic intracranial haemorrhage (ICH) is uncommon in children. Arteriovenous malformations (AVM) are a more common cause of haemorrhage in children than aneurysms[46] (Table 102.3). The presenting features are similar to those seen in adults, and include sudden severe headache, altered conscious state and seizures. Diagnosis can usually be made by CT scan. Raised ICP, if present, is managed in the usual manner. A mass lesion or acute obstructive hydrocephalus requires neurosurgical assessment.

Following diagnosis of ICH further investigations may be required to clarify the underlying cause. These include coagulation profile and platelet count. Angiographic images can be obtained with CT, MRA (magnetic resonance angiography) or digital subtraction. In some cases definitive cerebral angiography may be required to define the underlying vascular malformation or tumour. Definitive surgery or endovascular treatment of an AVM can be planned once the underlying lesion has been defined. A period of close observation is required as children may be at greater risk of rebleeding from an AVM than adults.[47] The efficacy of therapies (e.g. calcium channel blockers) used to prevent vasospasm in adults has not been studied in children with aneurysmal haemorrhage. Sequelae of ICH include hemiparesis, aphasia, seizures and hydrocephalus.

HYPOXIC–ISCHAEMIC ENCEPHALOPATHY

AETIOLOGY

The most common causes of hypoxic–ischaemic encephalopathy outside the neonatal period are:

- near-miss sudden infant death syndrome
- immersion
- accidents, including drug ingestion and strangulation
- inflicted injury

Table 102.3 Aetiology of spontaneous intracranial haemorrhage in children

Vascular malformations
Arteriovenous malformation
Capillary telangiectasia
Cavernous malformation
Venous malformation
Aneurysm
'Berry'
Mycotic
Posttraumatic
Coagulopathy
Thrombocytopenia
Haemophilia
Anticoagulant therapy
Tumours
Gliomas
Hypertension

PATHOLOGY

The brain depends on an uninterrupted supply of oxygen and glucose to produce, via aerobic glycolysis, sufficient high-energy adenosine triphosphate (ATP) to maintain neuronal membrane and synthetic function. Under anoxic conditions anaerobic glycolysis occurs which produces lactic acid but less ATP (by 18 times). As there are virtually no stores of ATP, rapid neuronal failure ensues. If ischaemia accompanies hypoxia, there is associated failure of both substrate delivery and metabolic waste removal, which amplifies the cellular insult. Ischaemia produces coma in less than 10 seconds and cerebral damage in as little as 2 minutes.

Following restoration of cerebral blood flow there is a period of relative hyperaemia followed by relative hypoperfusion. Animal studies suggest that the blood flow during this phase of postischaemic hypoperfusion is determined by the metabolic needs of the brain.[48] Cytotoxic cerebral oedema may subsequently develop, but significant elevation of ICP is unusual unless ischaemia and damage are profound.

MANAGEMENT

The principles of therapy are similar to those for other brain injuries. It is mandatory to provide rapid cardiopulmonary resuscitation (CPR) and prevent secondary insults. In cases of out-of-hospital cardiac arrest, full resuscitation must be attempted while the history is sought. Postresuscitation care is important for optimising outcome. Comatose patients with hyper- or hypotonia and a Glasgow Coma Scale score (GCS) < 8 are probably best managed by mechanical ventilation, sedation and paralysis for at least 1–2 days although benefits are not proven. Ventilation should be targeted at normocapnia, and hyperventilation avoided due to the risk of further cerebral ischaemia.[49] Haemodynamic disturbance may develop because of primary cardiac dysfunction or hypovolaemia secondary to fluid loss from capillary leak syndrome. Circulating volume should be restored and inotropic agents considered to improve the state of the circulation. The dose and choice of vasoactive agent should be individualised based on haemodynamic monitoring.

Following cardiac arrest children are usually hypothermic. Fever commonly develops during the subsequent hours and is associated with worse outcome:[50] fever should therefore be anticipated and prevented. Further to preventing fever, there is evidence that therapeutic hypothermia of 32–34°C improves outcome. There are two trials in adults following cardiac arrest[51,52] and two trials in newborns following birth asphyxia[53,54] demonstrating improved neurological outcome if hypothermia is used for between 12 and 72 hours. Although there are no paediatric trials, therapeutic hypothermia should be considered as a treatment option in children who are comatose following hypoxic–ischaemic events. Hyperglycaemia has been associated with a worse prognosis and, although it may simply be a marker of injury severity, active treatment has been advocated. The role of ICP measurement is limited as intracranial hypertension usually only occurs in the setting of severe injury and poor outcome.[55]

PROGNOSIS

The major determinants of recovery are:

- ischaemic time
- cerebral metabolic rate
- quality of resuscitation.

In immersion injuries in young children, full recovery may be possible despite prolonged ischaemia if sufficient rapid cerebral cooling has occurred. In these cases the onset of ischaemia may be delayed by bradycardia with preferential cerebral flow (the 'diving reflex'). In general, survival from out-of-hospital cardiac arrest is unlikely, even with expert CPR, if asystole is present on arrival at hospital.[56] The rare exception is the hypothermic child who presents following immersion; prolonged CPR may be justified in selected cases when profound hypothermia was induced rapidly. If cardiac output is present on arrival at hospital, with either flexion or extension to pain, recovery is likely. Normothermic patients, who present apnoeic, flaccid and unresponsive to pain, are likely to die or have serious neurological deficits. This group is also prone to further deterioration several days after the insult, with progression of cerebral oedema.[55] Coma persisting for more than 24 hours is a predictor of poor prognosis and minimal long-term improvement is likely in this group.[57] Residual neurological deficits present at the end of the first week are less likely to improve following ischaemic injury than following traumatic brain injury.

A number of ancillary tests have been investigated as predictors of neurological outcome. Somatosensory-evoked potentials (SEPs) performed at the bedside are the most useful aid to prediction. One report of 109 children with severe brain injury concluded that, with appropriate patient selection, the positive predictive value for poor outcome of bilaterally absent SEPs is 100% (95% CI, 92–100%).[58]

GUILLAIN–BARRÉ SYNDROME

CLINICAL FEATURES

Guillain–Barré syndrome (GBS) is the most common cause of acute motor paralysis in children. Although most patients develop typical ascending, symmetrical areflexic weakness, GBS may present insidiously with apparent lethargy or loss of motor milestones in the young child. There may also be rapid progression and admission criteria to the intensive care unit (ICU) include respiratory failure, bulbar palsy, severe autonomic disturbance or rapidly progressive weakness. Sensory loss is usually minimal and transient. Pain in the back and legs, possibly neurogenic in origin, is common and may be the presenting feature.[59] This pain may be severe and is often difficult to control. Papilloedema and encephalopathy occasionally occur.[60] The complications of deep venous thrombosis and thromboembolism are not common problems in young children but may occur in adolescents.

INVESTIGATIONS

An LP should be done ideally before treatment with intravenous immunoglobulin (IVIG) is commenced. CSF typically shows a white cell count $< 10 \times 10^6$, while CSF protein is usually raised but may be normal during the first week of illness. Nerve conduction studies may be normal if performed early. Neurophysiological criteria have been used to classify GBS subtypes according to either demyelinating or axonal and whether or not both sensory and motor nerves are involved.[61] Anti-ganglioside antibodies are raised in some but not all patients.[62]

If there is uncertainty about the clinical diagnosis, brain and spinal cord imaging, as well as screening for infection, should be considered.

MANAGEMENT

Adequate respiratory care is the basis of minimising morbidity and mortality in GBS. Up to one-third of patients require ventilatory support and, ideally, mechanical ventilation should be undertaken electively. Early indications are increased work of breathing, fatigue, poor cough and progressive bulbar palsy. Hypercarbia is a late sign and should be avoided. In children that are old enough to cooperate, forced vital capacity (FVC) should be monitored during the progressive phase of the illness. Mechanical ventilation should be considered if FVC falls below 15–20 ml/kg. Careful frequent clinical assessment is necessary. Once mechanically ventilated, many patients require some degree of hyperventilation to prevent 'air hunger'. Although nasotracheal intubation is satisfactory initially, a tracheostomy should be performed if recovery is delayed. This will improve comfort and allow speech via pressure-generated ventilation and an air leak around the tracheostomy tube. Successful weaning is unlikely unless vital capacity exceeds 12 ml/kg and maximum negative inspiratory force is at least 20 cmH_2O (2 kPa).

Autonomic dysfunction is an important cause of morbidity and mortality in children with GBS. Airway manipulation or induction of anaesthesia, particularly in the presence of hypoxia, may provoke serious cardiac arrhythmias. Fluctuating blood pressure, urinary retention and gut dysfunction also occur.

Plasma exchange (PE) and IVIG are effective therapies. The indications for either are rapid progression and respiratory insufficiency or weakness to the point of being unable to walk unassisted. The strongest evidence for these therapies is from adult trials.[63–65] Although large trials adequately powered to separately test the efficacy of PE and IVIG in children have not been performed, a number of small retrospective studies have described local experiences with these immune therapies in children with mixed results.[66–70] As IVIG has significant potential technical advantages over PE, IVIG is generally the first-line therapy in children. Indications for IVIG are based on the degree of functional impairment and time from onset of symptoms. The indications are not influenced by the clinical or neurophysiological subtype or the results of antibody screening. There is no evidence to support sequential treatment using both PE and IVIG.[71]

Pain is a common feature of GBS and may have a neuropathic basis. Paracetamol and non-steroidal anti-inflammatory drugs are useful, while drugs to treat neuropathic pain (including gabapentin, carbamazepine and amitriptyline) may also be beneficial.

The problems of long-term ventilation in a conscious patient, compounded by emotional immaturity, speech failure, fear of procedures and family disruption, make the management of a child with GBS and their family particularly challenging. A sensitive team approach is essential.

PROGNOSIS

The prognosis in acute GBS may be better for children than adults. Full recovery is likely if the time from maximal deficit to onset of recovery is less than 18 days. Complete recovery, despite a longer plateau phase, has been reported, however.[72] Good recovery can occur in patients who have required ventilation and the need for ventilation may not be a poor prognostic factor in children.[66] Those presenting with a subacute course are at risk of relapses and permanent motor deficits.

METABOLIC ENCEPHALOPATHY

Approximately 0.1% of babies have an inborn error of metabolism. Acute encephalopathy is one of the many ways neurometabolic diseases present in childhood.[73,74] In general, acute presentations occur in the neonatal period and early infancy. Symptoms are often vague and include lethargy, poor feeding and vomiting. Older infants and children more commonly present with a chronic encephalopathy, with features that may include seizures, long-tract signs, visual impairment and loss of milestones.

APPROACH TO DIAGNOSIS

A careful history and examination may elicit clues to a possible metabolic problem. Family history and history of drug exposure are extremely important. Valproate, in particular, has been associated with a Reye-like illness. The following readily available investigations are useful to allow a broad categorisation and direct further detailed investigations: blood gas analysis, blood sugar, serum ammonia, serum lactate, urine metabolic screen and urine ketones. While lactic acidosis and hypoglycaemia can occur in a number of disease states, including sepsis, persisting abnormalities require further investigation. This is best done in collaboration with a metabolic disease specialist or a clinical biochemist.

Lactic acidosis can be further assessed with measurement of lactate:pyruvate ratio and urine biochemical analysis may provide further diagnostic information (Table 102.4).

Table 102.4 Biochemical markers of metabolic disorders

Biochemical marker	Disorder
Hypoglycaemia	Organic acidurias Methylmalonic/propionic acidaemia Reye's syndrome Fat oxidation defects MCAD
Ketoacidosis	Diabetes mellitus Organic acidurias
Lactic acidosis	Mitochondrial encephalomyopathies Respiratory chain disorders Pyruvate carboxylase deficiency
Hyperammonaemia (2–3 × normal)	Reye's syndrome Urea cycle defects Fat oxidation defects MCAD Organic acidurias

MCAD, medium-chain acyl CoA dehydrogenase.

ASSESSMENT

Metabolic coma can be staged using Lovejoy's classification for Reye's syndrome (Table 102.5).[75]

MANAGEMENT

Initial management is largely supportive. Metabolic derangements such as acidosis and hypoglycaemia should be corrected. Acute intracranial hypertension should be managed with mechanical ventilation while the role of ICP monitoring is controversial. Hyperammonaemia should be managed with limited protein intake initially. In certain circumstances increasing ammonia metabolism using agents such as arginine and sodium benzoate is helpful. In some settings providing calories intravenously in the form of glucose and fat may help limit the extent of catabolism and thereby help to curtail the metabolic crisis. Dialysis is used to control severe hyperammonaemia

Table 102.5 Staging in metabolic encephalopathy

Stage	Coma	Pain response	Reflexes
1	Lethargy	Normal	Normal
2	Combative	Variable	Pupils sluggish
3	Coma	Decorticate	Pupils sluggish
4	Coma	Decerebrate	Pupils sluggish, abnormal oculocephalic
5	Coma	Flaccid	No pupil response, absent oculocephalic

Adapted from NIH, modification of Lovejoy.[75]

and acidosis. Continuous venovenous haemodiafiltration is considered more effective than peritoneal dialysis.[76]

REYE'S SYNDROME AND REYE-LIKE ILLNESS

Reye's syndrome is a rare disorder, occurring almost exclusively in children. It is characterised by an acute encephalopathy with brain swelling and fatty degeneration of viscera, especially the liver. Typically the patient presents with intractable vomiting followed by progressive encephalopathy. There is an association with aspirin use and a preceding varicella infection. Diagnosis can be made when a compatible history accompanies hyperammonaemia and elevation of serum hepatocellular enzymes to at least twice normal, but with a normal bilirubin concentration. Hypoglycaemia occurs in patients under 2 years. Management consists of correction of hypoglycaemia, neurological monitoring and management of raised ICP.

A wide range of conditions has been described that closely mimic typical Reye's syndrome. Ten percent of cases originally described as being Reye's syndrome were subsequently found to be due to an inherited metabolic disorder.[77] A careful approach is mandatory to ensure detection of inherited disorders.

The introduction of neonatal screening programmes using tandem mass spectrometry will see many inherited metabolic diseases diagnosed in the neonatal period, often prior to the onset of symptoms. This technology is particularly useful for detecting fatty acid oxidation defects (e.g. medium-chain acyl CoA dehydrogenase deficiency, or MCAD) and disorders of amino acid metabolism (e.g. methylmalonic acidaemia).[78]

SPINAL INJURY

INCIDENCE

Paediatric spinal trauma is relatively rare, comprising < 5% of all spinal injuries. Approximately 5% of children with severe head trauma will have a cervical spine injury. However, a high proportion of children who die following motor vehicle trauma, particularly those who suffer immediate cardiorespiratory arrest, or who die before arrival at hospital, have disruption of the spinal cord above C3, particularly at the cervicomedullary junction.[79,80]

AETIOLOGY

The commonest causes of paediatric spinal trauma are motor vehicle crashes, either as a pedestrian or passenger, falls and diving injuries. Sports-related injuries are uncommon.

PATHOPHYSIOLOGY

The patterns of spinal injury in children differ from those seen in adults in many ways. Spinal cord injury without radiographic abnormality (SCIWORA) occurs almost exclusively in children (20–60% of spinal cord injuries). It is associated with a high incidence of complete neurological deficit. Spinal injury in the first decade occurs most commonly in the first two cervical segments, with atlanto-axial rotatory subluxation, bony or ligamentous injuries, or SCIWORA and severe cord injury. Although not as common as upper cervical injuries, lower cervical injuries below C4 do occur in young children,[81] while injury may occur at more than one level. Atlanto-axial rotatory subluxation is rarely associated with neurological deficit and ligamentous injury is more likely than high cervical fractures to be associated with permanent neurological deficit.[82] As the bony spine matures, the pattern of injury becomes more adult-like with lower cervical and thoracic injuries seen in the second decade.[83,84]

CLINICAL FEATURES

The immediate effects of spinal cord damage are similar at any age. Frequently an associated head injury can render clinical assessment extremely difficult; confirmation of cord injury is sometimes delayed. Clues to the diagnosis in the unconscious patient include:

- flaccidity, immobility and areflexia below the level of the lesion
- hypoventilation with paradoxical chest movement; this occurs if intercostal muscles are paralysed and the phrenic nerves are intact (in the absence of airway obstruction)

- apnoea with rhythmic flaring of the alae nasi (Duncan's sign), seen when the lesion is above C3
- hypotension with inappropriate bradycardia and cutaneous vasodilatation below the level of injury, due to absent spinal sympathetic outflow
- priapism, which occurs frequently

There may be visible or palpable evidence of trauma to the spine and surrounding soft tissues, including retropharyngeal or retrolaryngeal haematomas. Spinal shock is common with temporary complete loss of function. As this resolves after 3–5 days, reflexes progressively return, usually starting with bulbocavernosus and anal reflexes. Incomplete lesions, including the Brown–Sequard cord hemisection, and anterior and central cord syndromes may become apparent at this stage.

INVESTIGATIONS

Resuscitation, including emergency intubation, should not be delayed to perform X-rays. The entire spinal column should, however, be X-rayed subsequently to demonstrate the presence of subluxation, fractures or dislocations. MRI is useful in both the acute setting and in assessment at later stages, and is now accepted as the standard for identifying haemorrhage, contusion or compression of the cord. CT produces better definition of bony injuries, and may also show cord involvement by haematomas, bone fragments and foreign bodies. SCIWORA was defined in an era before MRI was routinely available. In the majority of children with SCIWORA, MRI will also be normal; however, if intramedullary lesions are demonstrated with MRI, permanent neurological deficits are more likely.[85,86] Somatosensory-evoked potentials may be useful to evaluate the integrity of the spinal cord, particularly in the comatose patient.

MANAGEMENT

Achieving control of airway, ventilation and circulation is always of first priority. If tracheal intubation is indicated, and if stability of the neck is unknown, skilled assistance is necessary to immobilise the head and neck and prevent flexion or extension. Because of the sympathectomised state in high cord injuries, a relatively low blood pressure can be expected even after hypovolaemia is corrected. Significant hypotension becomes more likely the higher the lesion and the younger the patient. Haemodynamic support with a vasoconstrictor such as noradrenaline (norepinephrine) is useful if hypotension is problematic following restoration of intravascular volume. As up to 20% of patients will have multiple trauma, many will require major surgical procedures, during which the spinal cord must remain protected. If muscle relaxants are required 2–3 days following the injury, suxamethonium, which may cause fatal hyperkalaemia, should be avoided.

The use of steroids is controversial and there are no studies specific to children. Two randomised controlled trials in adults demonstrated that high-dose methylprednisolone administered within 8 hours of the injury (30 mg/kg initially followed by 5.4 mg/kg per hour for the following 24–48 hours) improved outcome.[87,88] These studies have significant limitations and the results have not been universally accepted.[89–91]

As with brain injuries, preventing secondary injury is vital. Adequate perfusion of the cord should be ensured, as autoregulation of blood flow is lost after trauma. Immobilisation can be maintained by skull tongs with axial traction or external bracing. Operative intervention is controversial with little evidence of neurological improvement from decompressive surgery. Laminectomy and decompression in children with complete cord injuries carry significant mortality.

The incidence of venous thromboembolism after spinal injury in adolescents approaches that in adults and therefore patients in this age group should receive standard prophylaxis. Venous thromboembolism is rare in prepubertal children (approximately 1%), and the risk–benefit ratio of routine prophylaxis in this age group is unknown.[92] There should be early consultation with a specialised spinal injuries unit. Optimal rehabilitation requires a team of orthopaedic and neurosurgeons, rehabilitation specialists, nurses, physiotherapists, occupational therapists, psychiatrists, social workers and schoolteachers.

PROGNOSIS

The prognosis of all spinal injuries in children may be better than in adults. In one series of 113 children with spinal column injuries, 55 (48%) had no neurological deficit, and 38 (34%) had an incomplete deficit. Of these, 23 (20%) made a complete recovery and 11 (10%) improved.[79] The remaining 20 (18%) children had a complete cord injury and, of these, 4 improved and 3 died. In a smaller series, 44% had neurological deficits, SCIWORA was seen in 21% and 11% of injuries were immediate, complete and permanent. Of the 18 children with SCIWORA, 4 had a permanent, complete deficit.[82]

REFERENCES

1. Mann KS, Chan KH, Yue CP. Skull fractures in children: their assessment in relation to developmental skull changes and acute intracranial hematomas. *Childs Nerv Syst* 1986; **2**: 258–61.
2. Suarez JI, Qureshi A, Bhardwaj A *et al.* Treatment of refractory intracranial hypertension with 23.4% saline. *Crit Care Med* 1998; **26**: 1118–22.
3. Hanhan UA, Fiallos MR, Orlowski JP. Status epilepticus. *Pediatr Clin North Am* 2001; **48**: 683–94.
4. Lothman E. The biochemical basis and pathophysiology of status epilepticus. *Neurology* 1990; **40**(S2): 13–23.
5. Scott RC, Surtees RAH, Neville BGR. Status epilepticus: pathophysiology, epidemiology, and outcomes. *Arch Dis Child* 1998; **79**: 73–7.

6. Lewena S, Young S. When benzodiazepines fail: how effective is second line therapy for status epilepticus in children? *Emerg Med Australas* 2006; **18**: 45–50.
7. Dieckmann RA. Is the time overdue for an international reporting standard for convulsive paediatric status epilepticus? *Emerg Med Australas* 2006; **18**: 1–3.
8. Chiulli DA, Terndrup TE, Kanter RK. The influence of diazepam or lorazepam on the frequency of endotracheal intubation in childhood status epilepticus. *J Emerg Med* 1991; **9**: 13–7.
9. Appleton RE, Sweeney A, Choonara I *et al.* Lorazepam vs. diazepam in the treatment of epileptic seizures and status epilepticus. *Dev Med Child Neurol* 1995; **37**: 682–8.
10. Chamberlain JM, Altieri MA, Futterman C *et al.* A prospective, randomized study comparing intramuscular midazolam with intravenous diazepam for the treatment of seizures in children. *Pediatr Emerg Care* 1997; **13**: 92–4.
11. Mahmoudian T, Zadeh MM. Comparison of intranasal midazolam with intravenous diazepam for treating acute seizures in children. *Epilepsy Behav* 2004; **5**: 253–5.
12. McIntyre J, Robertson S, Norris E *et al.* Safety and efficacy of buccal midazolam versus rectal diazepam for emergency treatment of seizures in children: a randomised controlled trial. *Lancet* 2005; **366**: 205–10.
13. Lahat E, Aladjem M, Eshel G *et al.* Midazolam in treatment of epileptic seizures. *Pediatr Neurol* 1992; **8**: 215–6.
14. Rivera R, Segnini M, Baltodano A *et al.* Midazolam in the treatment of status epilepticus in children. *Crit Care Med* 1993; **21**: 991–4.
15. Koul RL, Raj Aithala G, Chacko A *et al.* Continuous midazolam infusion as treatment of status epilepticus. *Arch Dis Child* 1997; **76**: 445–8.
16. Yoshikawa H, Yamazaki S, Abe T *et al.* Midazolam as a first-line agent for status epilepticus in children. *Brain Dev* 2000; **22**: 239–42.
17. Wheless JW. Paediatric use of intravenous and intramuscular phenytoin: lessons learned. *J Child Neurol* 1998; **13**: S11–4.
18. Appleton R, Choonara I, Martland T *et al.* The Status Epilepticus Working Party. The treatment of convulsive status epilepticus in children. *Arch Dis Child* 2000; **83**: 415–9.
19. Raspall-Chaure M, Chin RF, Neville BG *et al.* Outcome of paediatric convulsive status epilepticus: a systematic review. *Lancet Neurol* 2006; **5**: 769–79.
20. Rennick G, Shann F, de Campo J. Cerebral herniation during bacterial meningitis in children. *BMJ* 1993; **306**: 953–5.
21. Seward RJ, Towner KJ. Evaluation of a PCR-immunoassay technique for detection of *Neisseria meningitidis* in cerebrospinal fluid and peripheral blood. *J Med Microbiol* 2000; **49**: 451–6.
22. Newcombe J, Cartwright K, Palmer WH *et al.* PCR of peripheral blood for diagnosis of meningococcal disease. *J Clin Microbiol* 1996; **34**: 1637–40.
23. Feigin RD, Pearlman E. Bacterial meningitis beyond the neonatal period. In: Feigin RD, Cherry JD (eds) *Textbook of Pediatric Infectious Diseases.* Philadelphia: WB Saunders; 1998: 400–29.
24. Chavez-Bueno S, McCracken GH. Bacterial meningitis in children. *Pediatr Clin North Am* 2005; **52**: 795–810.
25. Odio CM, Faingezicht I, Paris M *et al.* The beneficial effects of early dexamethasone administration in infants and children with bacterial meningitis. *N Engl J Med* 1991; **324**: 1525–31.
26. McCracken GH, Label MH. Dexamethasone treatment for bacterial meningitis in infants and children. *Am J Dis Child* 1989; **143**: 287–9.
27. Schaad UB, Lips U, Gnehm HE *et al.* Dexamethasone therapy for bacterial meningitis. *Lancet* 1993; **342**: 457–61.
28. McIntyre PB, Berkey CS, King SM *et al.* Dexamethasone as adjunctive therapy in bacterial meningitis. A meta-analysis of randomised clinical trial since 1988. *JAMA* 1997; **278**: 925–31.
29. Duke T, Molyneux EM. Intravenous fluids for seriously ill children: time to reconsider. *Lancet* 2003; **362**: 1320–3.
30. Duke T. Fluid management of bacterial meningitis in developing countries. *Arch Dis Child* 1998; **79**: 181–5.
31. Powell KR, Sugarman LI, Eskenazi AE *et al.* Normalisation of plasma arginine vasopressin concentrations when children with meningitis are given maintenance plus replacement fluid therapy. *J Pediatr* 1990; **117**: 515–22.
32. Bianchetti MG, Thyssen HR, Laux-End R *et al.* Evidence for fluid volume depletion in hyponatraemic patients with bacterial meningitis. *Acta Paediatr* 1996; **85**: 1163–6.
33. Singhi SC, Singhi PD, Srinivas B *et al.* Fluid restriction does not improve the outcome of acute meningitis. *Pediatr Infect Dis* 1995; **14**: 495–503.
34. Cuevas LE, Kazembe P, Mughogho GK *et al.* Eradication of nasopharyngeal carriage of *Neisseria meningitidis* in children and adults in rural Africa: a comparison of ciprofloxacin and rifampicin. *J Infect Dis* 1995; **171**: 728–31.
35. Madagame ET, Havens PL, Bresnahan JM *et al.* Survival and functional outcome of children requiring mechanical ventilation during therapy for acute bacterial meningitis. *Crit Care Med* 1995; **23**: 1279–83.
36. McIntyre PB, Chey T, Smith WT. The impact of vaccination against invasive *Haemophilus influenzae* type b disease in the Sydney region. *Med J Aust* 1995; **162**: 245–8.
37. Adams WG, Deaver KA, Cochi SL *et al.* Decline of childhood *Haemophilus influenzae* type b (Hib) disease in the Hib vaccine era. *JAMA* 1993; **269**: 221–6.
38. Whitney CG, Farley MM, Hadler J *et al.* Decline in invasive pneumococcal disease after the introduction of protein–polysaccharide conjugate vaccine. *N Engl J Med* 2003; **348**: 1737–46.
39. Balmer P, Borrow R, Miller E. Impact of meningococcal C conjugate vaccine in the UK. *J Med Microbiol* 2002; **51**: 717–22.
40. Booy R, Jelfs J, El Bashir H *et al.* Impact of meningococcal C conjugate vaccine use in Australia. *Med J Aust* 2007; **186**: 108–9.

41. Aurelius E, Johansson B, Skoldenberg B *et al.* Rapid diagnosis of herpes simplex virus encephalitis by nested polymerase chain reaction assay of cerebrospinal fluid. *Lancet* 1991; **337**: 189–92.
42. Troendle-Atkins J, Demmler GJ, Buffone GJ. Rapid diagnosis of herpes simplex encephalitis by using polymerase chain reaction. *J Paediatr* 1993; **123**: 376–80.
43. McMinn P, Stratov I, Nagarajan L *et al.* Neurological manifestations of enterovirus 71 infection in children during an outbreak of hand, foot, and mouth disease in Western Australia. *Clin Infect Dis* 2001; **32**: 236–42.
44. Rotbart HA, Webster AD. Treatment of potentially life-threatening enterovirus infections with Pleconaril. *Clin Infect Dis* 2001; **32**: 228–35.
45. Koskiniemi M, Vaheri A. Effect of measles, mumps, rubella vaccination on pattern of encephalitis in children. *Lancet* 1989; **1**: 31–4.
46. Al-Jarallah A, Al-Rifai MT, Riela AR *et al.* Nontraumatic brain hemorrhage in children: etiology and presentation. *J Child Neurol* 2000; **15**: 284–9.
47. Stein BM, Wolpert SM. Arteriovenous malformation of the brain II: current concepts and treatment. *Arch Neurol* 1980; **37**: 69–75.
48. Michenfelder JD, Milde JH. Post-ischaemic canine cerebral blood flow appears to be determined by cerebral metabolic needs. *J Cereb Blood Flow Metab* 1990; **10**: 71–6.
49. International Liaison Committee on Resuscitation. International consensus on cardiopulmonary resuscitation and emergency cardiovascular care science with treatment recommendations. Part 6: Paediatric basic and advanced life support. *Resuscitation* 2005; **67**: 271–91.
50. Zeiner A, Holzer M, Sterz F *et al.* Hyperthermia after cardiac arrest is associated with an unfavorable neurologic outcome. *Arch Intern Med* 2001; **161**: 2007–12.
51. Bernard SA, Gray TW, Buist MD *et al.* Treatment of comatose survivors of out-of-hospital cardiac arrest with induced hypothermia. *N Engl J Med* 2002; **346**: 557–63.
52. Hypothermia after Cardiac Arrest Study Group. Mild therapeutic hypothermia to improve the neurologic outcome after cardiac arrest. *N Engl J Med* 2002; **346**: 549–56.
53. Shankaran S, Laptook AR, Ehrenkranz RA *et al.* Whole-body hypothermia for neonates with hypoxic–ischemic encephalopathy. *N Engl J Med* 2005; **353**: 1574–84.
54. Gluckman PD, Wyatt JS, Azzopardi D *et al.* Selective head cooling with mild systemic hypothermia after neonatal encephalopathy: multicentre randomised trial. *Lancet* 2005; **365**: 663–70.
55. Sarnaik AP, Preston G, Lieh-Lai M *et al.* Intracranial perfusion pressure in near-drowning. *Crit Care Med* 1985; **13**: 224–7.
56. Schindler MB, Cox PN, Jarvis A *et al.* Factors influencing outcome from out of hospital paediatric cardiopulmonary arrest. *Anaesth Intensive Care* 1995; **23**: 381–2.
57. Kriel RL, Krach LE, Luxenberg MG *et al.* Outcome of severe anoxic/ischaemic brain injury in children. *Paediatr Neurol* 1994; **10**: 207–12.
58. Beca J, Cox PN, Taylor MJ *et al.* Somatosensory evoked potentials for prediction of outcome in acute severe brain injury. *J Pediatr* 1995; **126**: 44–9.
59. Manners PJ, Murray KJ. Guillain–Barré syndrome presenting with severe musculoskeletal pain. *Acta Paediatr* 1992; **81**: 1049–51.
60. Cole GF, Matthew DJ. Prognosis in severe Guillain–Barré syndrome. *Arch Dis Child* 1987; **62**: 288–91.
61. Hadden RD, Cornblath DR, Hughes RA *et al.* Electrophysiological classification of Guillain–Barré syndrome: clinical associations and outcome. *Ann Neurol* 1998; **44**: 780–8.
62. Pritchard J. What's new in Guillain–Barré syndrome? *Pract Neurol* 2006; **6**: 208–17.
63. Van der Meche FGA, Schmitz PIM, Dutch Guillain–Barré Study Group. A randomised trial comparing intravenous immune globulin and plasma exchange in Guillain–Barré syndrome. *N Engl J Med* 1992; **326**: 1123–9.
64. Hughes RAC, Raphaël J-C, Swan AV *et al.* Intravenous immunoglobulin for Guillain–Barré syndrome. *Cochrane Database Syst Rev* 2006; Issue 1. Art. No. CD002063.
65. Raphaël JC, Chevret S, Hughes RAC *et al.* Plasma exchange for Guillain–Barré syndrome. *Cochrane Database Syst Rev* 2002; Issue 2. Art. No. CD001798.
66. Jansen PW, Perkin RM, Ashwal S. Guillain–Barré syndrome in childhood: natural course and efficacy of plasmapheresis. *Pediatr Neurol* 1993; **9**: 16–20.
67. Lamont PJ, Johnston HM, Berdoukas VA. Plasmapheresis in children with Guillain–Barré syndrome. *Neurology* 1991; **41**: 1928–31.
68. Shahar E, Leiderman M. Outcome of severe Guillain–Barré syndrome in children: comparison between untreated cases versus gamma-globulin therapy. *Clin Neuropharmacol* 2003; **26**: 84–7.
69. Ortiz-Corredor F, Pena-Preciado M. Use of immunoglobulin in severe childhood Guillain–Barré syndrome. *Acta Neurol Scand* 2007; **115**: 289–93.
70. Vajsar J, Sloane A, Wood E *et al.* Plasmapheresis vs intravenous immunoglobulin treatment in childhood Guillain–Barré syndrome. *Arch Pediatr Adolesc Med* 1994; **148**: 1210–12.
71. Hughes RA, Wijdicks EF, Barohn R *et al.* Practice parameter: immunotherapy for Guillain–Barré syndrome: report of the Quality Standards Subcommittee of the American Academy of Neurology. *Neurology* 2003; **61**: 736–40.
72. Briscoe DM, McMeniman LB, O'Donohoe NV. Prognosis in Guillain–Barré syndrome. *Arch Dis Child* 1987; **62**: 733–5.
73. Neville BGR. Paediatric neurology. In: Walton J (ed) *Brain's Diseases of the Nervous System.* Oxford: Oxford Medical Publications; 1993: 453–77.
74. Chaves-Carballo E. Detection of inherited neurometabolic disorders. A practical clinical approach. *Pediatr Clin North Am* 1992; **39**: 801–19.

75. National Institutes of Health Conference on Reye's Syndrome. Diagnosis and treatment of Reye's syndrome. *JAMA* 1981; **246**: 2441.
76. Schaffer F, Straube, Oh J *et al.* Dialysis in neonates with inborn errors of metabolism. *Nephrol Dial Transplant* 1999; **14**: 918–19.
77. Green A, Hall S. Investigation of metabolic disorders resembling Reye's syndrome. *Arch Dis Child* 1992; **67**: 1313–17.
78. Andresen BS, Dobrowolski SF, O'Reilly L *et al.* Medium-chain acyl CoA dehydrogenase deficiency (MCAD) mutations identified by MS/MS-based screening of newborns differ from those observed in patients with clinical symptoms: identification and characterization of a new, prevalent mutation that results in mild MCAD deficiency. *Am J Hum Genet* 2001; **68**: 1408–18.
79. Hadley MN, Zabramski MD, Browner CM *et al.* Paediatric spinal trauma. Review of 122 cases of spinal cord and vertebral column injuries. *J Neurosurg* 1988; **68**: 18–24.
80. Swan PK, Bohn DJ, Sides CA *et al.* Cervical spine damage associated with severe head injury in the paediatric patient: implications for airway management. *Anaesth Intensive Care* 1987; **15**: 115–6.
81. Givens TG, Polley KA, Smith GF *et al.* Pediatric cervical spine injury: a three year experience. *J Trauma* 1996; **41**: 310–14.
82. Ruge JR, Sinson GP, McLone DG *et al.* Pediatric spinal injury: the very young. *J Neurosurg* 1988; **68**: 25–30.
83. Birney TJ, Hanley EN. Traumatic cervical spine injuries in childhood and adolescence. *Spine* 1989; **14**: 1277–82.
84. McCall T, Fassett D, Brockmeyer D. Cervical spine trauma in children: a review. *Neurosurg Focus* 2006; **20**: E5.
85. Dare AO, Dias MS, Li V. Magnetic resonance imaging correlation in pediatric spinal cord injury without radiographic abnormality. *J Neurosurg* 2002; **97**(S1): 33–9.
86. Liao CC, Lui TN, Chen LR *et al.* Spinal cord injury without radiological abnormality in preschool-aged children: correlation of magnetic resonance imaging findings with neurological outcomes. *J Neurosurg* 2005; **103**: 17–23.
87. Bracken MB, Shepard MJ, Collins WF *et al.* A randomized controlled trial of methylprednisolone or naloxone in the treatment of acute spinal cord injury: result of the Second National Acute Spinal Cord Injury Study. *N Engl J Med* 1990; **322**: 1405–11.
88. Bracken MB, Shepard MJ, Holford TR *et al.* Administration of methylprednisolone for 24 or 48 hours or tirilazad mesylate for 48 hours in the treatment of acute spinal cord injury: results of the third National Acute Spinal Cord Injury randomized controlled trial. *JAMA* 1997; **277**: 1597–604.
89. Short DJ, El Masry WS, Jones PW. High-dose methylprednisone in the management of acute spinal cord injury – a systematic review from a clinical perspective. *Spinal Cord* 2000; **38**: 273–86.
90. Hurlbert RJ. The role of steroids in acute spinal cord injury: an evidence-based analysis. *Spine* 2001; **26**: S39–46.
91. Sayer FT, Kronvall E, Nilsson OG. Methylprednisolone treatment in acute spinal cord injury: the myth challenged through a structured analysis of published literature. *Spine J* 2006; **6**: 335–43.
92. Jones T, Ugalde V, Franks P *et al.* Venous thromboembolism after spinal cord injury: incidence, time course, and associated risk factors in 16,240 adults and children. *Arch Phys Med Rehabil* 2005; **86**: 2240–7.

103

Paediatric trauma

Neil T Matthews

The management of paediatric trauma is different from adults. Paediatric patients presenting with trauma have mechanisms of injury, clinical symptoms and examination findings which differ from adults, and differ across the range of their ages. Trauma is by far the leading cause of death in children over 1 year old, and the third leading cause less than 1 year after congenital abnormalities and sudden infant death syndrome.[1] Causes of trauma and patterns of injury are determined by age-related behaviour, with falls and assaults more common in younger children, and motor vehicle accidents more common in older children. Injury patterns differ, with impact forces dissipated over a smaller target, severe organ damage resulting without bony fracture because bones are not ossified, and greater potential for hypothermia. In general, blunt trauma with multiorgan injury is most likely.

As with adults, there are three peak mortality periods after injury:

- *minutes* at the scene, from airway obstruction, bleeding and fatal primary brain injury
- *hours* during resuscitation and transport from airway obstruction, aspiration, haemorrhage and the head injury
- *days to weeks* later from head injury or complications

The mainstay of early management is optimising the ABC of resuscitation as outlined in other chapters. Importantly, vascular access can be difficult, and expertise in intraosseous needle insertion is essential.[2]

PREVENTION STRATEGIES

Paediatric trauma requires resources and separate systems to successfully reduce mortality and morbidity.[3] New emphasis has seen the development of prevention strategies (Table 103.1), including:

- injury surveillance, prevention research, legislation and public safety campaigns
- education programmes directed at care-givers
- nationally coordinated approaches to trauma care

HEAD INJURY

Significant head injury occurs in 75% of children admitted with blunt trauma,[5] and 70% of these result in death. Causes of injury are determined by behaviour patterns, which change with age and are commonly due to falls and assaults in infants, and motor vehicle accidents (including bicycle-related injuries) in older children.

ASSESSMENT

The Glasgow Coma Scale (GCS) requires different interpretation in children, because scores tend to be more subjective and prone to misinterpretation. When using the original GCS described for adults, children under 5 years are unable to score normally for verbal and motor responses. Normal aggregate scores for age are:

- 9 at 6 months
- 11 at 12 months
- 13–14 at 5 years.

This has led to attempts to modify the scale by either changing the scoring assessment signs, or by reducing the total score (i.e. eliminating some response categories).[6] The latter does not allow for comparison of outcome data.

An example of a commonly used scale modified for infants is shown in Table 103.2. However, difficulties remain as regards the accuracy and reproducibility of GCS for infants. Clinical assessment must prioritise the signs and symptoms of cerebral oedema or raised intracranial pressure (ICP) (Table 103.3).

MANAGEMENT

The aims of therapy are to minimise secondary effects on the primary brain injury by maintaining adequate cerebral blood flow and oxygen supply, and preventing secondary ischaemic injury and herniation from raised ICP.

Table 103.1 Prevention strategies[4]

Paediatric injuries	Preventative strategies
MVA – occupant	Child car seat Seatbelt restraints Car design Airbags
MVA – pedestrian	Safety programmes in schools
Bicycle	Helmet Separate sidewalks
Playground	Equipment structural design Soft surfaces
Drowning	Surround pool fencing
Burns	Smoke detectors Water tap regulators Flammable fabric legislation
Poisoning	Preventative packaging
Violence	Hand gun legislation Crisis resolution counselling

- Deterioration in level of consciousness and the appearance of signs of herniation must be rapidly recognised.
- Airway, oxygenation and respiration should be optimised and intubation performed when the airway is compromised.
- Controlled ventilation with muscle relaxation and sedation should be instituted in the presence of hypoventilation, seizures and signs of raised ICP (see Table 103.3).
- Hypotension significantly increases mortality in children and the systemic circulation must be maintained.

Table 103.3 Signs of raised intracranial pressure

Depressed level of consciousness
Changes in respiratory pattern, blood pressure and pulse rate
Increased head circumference (less than 18 months of age)
Full or bulging fontanelle
Motor weakness
Cranial nerve palsies
Decorticate or decerebrate posturing
Vomiting
Headache
Papilloedema (late)

- Management of blood pressure is difficult because the exact ranges of cerebral autoregulation are unknown in children.[7] Hypotension is most likely from blood loss (especially from scalp lacerations) and not brain injury. Fluid management needs to balance the need for volume resuscitation with the attempt to avoid hypovolaemia.
- Hypotonic and glucose-containing solutions should be avoided because of the association with poor outcomes.[8]
- Studies on the effectiveness of induced hypothermia in paediatric trauma are ongoing.
- Hyperthermia should be avoided with a servo-controlled cooling blanket and adjustment of humidifier temperature because each 1°C temperature rise increases cerebral metabolic rate by 5%.[9]
- Cerebral venous return should be optimised by neutral head positioning. Cerebral perfusion pressure may be best with the bed flat.[10]
- Treatment of seizures with phenytoin (20 mg/kg i.v.) provides less central nervous system depression than barbiturates or benzodiazepines. Monitoring for seizures to guard against resulting increases in cerebral blood flow and oxygen consumption is difficult in the

Table 103.2 Glasgow Coma Scale modified for infants

Glasgow Coma Scale			Glasgow Coma Scale modified for infants		
Activity	Best response	Scale	Activity	Best response	Scale
Eye opening	Spontaneous	4	Eye opening	Spontaneous	4
	To speech	3		To speech	3
	To pain	2		To pain	2
	None	1		None	1
Verbal	Orientated	5	Verbal	Coos, babbles	5
	Confused	4		Irritable, cries	4
	Inappropriate words	3		Cries to pain	3
	Non-specific sounds	2		Moans to pain	2
	None	1		None	1
Motor	Obeys commands	6	Motor	Spontaneous activity	6
	Localises pain	5		Withdraws to touch	5
	Withdraws to pain	4		Withdraws to pain	4
	Abnormal flexion	3		Flexion to pain	3
	Extensor response	2		Extension to pain	2
	None	1		None	1

paralysed patient. Systems for continuous electroencephalogram monitoring are complex to interpret at the bedside and provide limited information. Post-traumatic seizures are more common under 2 years of age,[11] but their long-term incidence is not reduced by acute prophylaxis.[12]

- Continuous measurement of jugular venous oxygen saturation (Sjo_2) via fibreoptic reflection oximetry can identify global cerebral hypoperfusion and ischaemia.[13] However, its use in children is subject to technical difficulties, mainly related to catheter position. Its use is not clinically routine in paediatrics.

DIAGNOSTIC INVESTIGATIONS

Supportive investigations can be performed while emergency assessment and therapy proceed. These include pH and acid–base, serum glucose, osmolality, electrolytes, calcium, magnesium and phosphate, complete blood profile and blood crossmatch.

X-rays of skull and cervical spine (anteroposterior, lateral and C1–C2 views), chest and pelvis are needed. Ultrasound of the skull, where the fontanelle is open, measures ventricular size, and can detect intracranial haemorrhage. It is useful for repeated assessment in the unstable patient.

A cranial computed tomography (CT) scan in stable patients excludes surgically treatable lesions, assesses the size of cerebrospinal fluid (CSF) spaces, including the basal cisterns, detects herniation and shift, and shows the presence of hyperaemia, oedema, intracerebral haematomas, contusions and fractures. A normal CT scan does not exclude raised ICP. Intracranial blood collections are less common than in adults.[5] The following are poor prognostic signs:

- subdural haemorrhage (as an indication of severe trauma and damage to underlying brain tissue)
- ablated basal cisterns and midline shift
- lack of or reversal of grey/white differentiation

CEREBRAL PERFUSION PRESSURE

Maintenance of cerebral perfusion pressure (CPP) in children is important and has significant implications, but the minimal required CPP in children has not been determined. CPP depends on the difference between mean systemic blood pressure and ICP and these values vary with age. In particular, blood pressure assumes great importance in the younger age group, where physiological systolic pressures are lower:

- 85 mmHg (11.3 kPa) at 6 months
- 95 mmHg (12.6 kPa) at 2 years
- 100 mmHg (13.3 kPa) at 7 years[14]

Normal ICP is also lower,[15] being normally less than 5 mmHg (0.67 kPa) at 2 years and less than 10 mmHg (1.3 kPa) at 5 years. Thus, in younger age groups, relative hypotension has a more profound effect on CPP and outcome,[16] and hypotension may be the main cause of cerebral ischaemia. For adolescents, therapy should aim to sustain CPP at 60–70 mmHg (8.0–9.3 kPa), while maintaining normal blood volume and adequate blood pressure (with pressor agents if required). A CPP less than 40 mmHg (5.3 kPa) reduces the likelihood of intact survival. Younger patients should have therapeutic targets adjusted to age-related realistic end-points.

INTRACRANIAL PRESSURE

Mechanisms of raised ICP in childhood trauma are listed in Table 103.4. If ICP remains persistently raised and uncompensated, cerebral ischaemia and herniation result. This herniation can be cingulate, uncal (temporal lobe), cerebellar tonsillar, upward cerebellar (posterior fossa hypertension) or transcalvarian (through vault defects). Signs of herniation are as for raised ICP (Table 103.3).

MEASUREMENT OF INTRACRANIAL PRESSURE

Measurement of ICP is indicated when intracranial hypertension is likely or potential (e.g. GCS 8 or less), or where signs are hidden by muscle relaxation. Technically, measurement in children can be more difficult. Subdural catheters and intracranial transducers require careful placement in children. Ventricular catheters allow removal of CSF, but are difficult to insert when ventricles are small, and readings are difficult to interpret when ventricles collapse. Strain-gauge technology will allows easier and more meaningful measurement of ICP (including intracerebral pressure).

REDUCTION OF RAISED INTRACRANIAL PRESSURE

Several mechanisms allow physiological compensation for raised ICP in children (Table 103.5). In the child under

Table 103.4 Mechanisms of raised intracranial pressure

Increased intracranial blood volume
Intracranial bleeding (epidural, subdural, subarachnoid, intracerebral)
Cerebral hyperaemia (in the first 1–2 days post injury[17])
Increased cerebral blood flow (increased $Paco_2$, decreased Pao_2, and convulsions)
Cerebral oedema (after day 2[18])
Hydrocephalus from intraventricular blood

Table 103.5 Physiological compensatory mechanisms for raised intracranial pressure in children

Displacement of CSF to distensible spinal subarachnoid space
Compression of intracranial venous system
Increased CSF reabsorption
Reduced CSF production
Stretching of dura, unfused skull bones and skin (less than 18 months of age)

18 months of age, a gradual increase in intracranial volume is achieved by an increase in head circumference. Measurement of the circumference is important, because compensation can delay recognition of clinical signs and diagnosis in emerging intracranial pathology. The important factor in the rate of change in compliance and ICP is the elasticity of the dura, which is dependent on the rate of change in intracranial volume.

Hyperventilation is effective in lowering raised ICP. However, excessive hyperventilation may cause cerebral ischaemia, and $Pa\text{CO}_2$ should be maintained between 35 and 40 mmHg (4.7–5.3 kPa). Weaning from hyperventilation should be slow, to minimise rebound rises in ICP.[19] Fluid restriction is helpful, provided circulating blood volume is maintained.

Mannitol (0.25–0.50 g/kg i.v. slowly) reduces raised ICP by increasing the osmotic gradient across the intact blood–brain barrier and reducing cerebral oedema. Its effects may also be due to reduced blood viscosity and induced cerebral vasoconstriction. Serum osmolality should be monitored to avoid hyperosmolar states.

Furosemide (1 mg/kg) reduces cerebral water and CSF production, but excessive diuresis from mannitol or furosemide may compromise the circulation. The use of hypertonic saline in children (3%) reduces ICP and appears to be more beneficial in resuscitation. CSF drainage is possible if a ventricular drain is in situ. Controlled hypothermia reduces raised ICP in patients with refractory intracranial hypertension, but improvement in outcomes is uncertain. Surgical decompression or removal of cerebral contusion in the face of intractably raised ICP in head trauma is advocated,[5] with improved results in unremitting focal oedema.

SPINAL CORD INJURY

Spinal cord injury is rare in children. Anatomical differences in children under 8 years render their spines more mobile and subject to stress with flexible ligaments and joint capsules, less muscular support, and horizontal facet joints. In addition, the relatively large head mass increases momentum, with the fulcrum of mobility at C2–C3 as opposed to C4–C5 in the adult. Thus paediatric cervical spine injuries tend to be above C4. The use of seat belts has led to an increase in lumbar spinal cord injury in children.[20]

ASSESSMENT

Clinical assessment can be difficult, as can the interpretation of radiological investigations because of normal variation and age-dependent ossification changes. Spinal cord injury without obvious radiological abnormality (SCIWORA) occurs in 10–20% of all paediatric spinal cord injuries.[21] Sensory-evoked potentials can be a valuable adjunct to diagnosis. Spinal cord injury can only be dismissed after imaging assessments (which may include magnetic resonance imaging in the non-acute setting) and careful and repeated examination of the lucid patient.

MANAGEMENT

From the time of injury, the spine should be assumed to be unstable until proved otherwise. Immobilisation, which at times is difficult, is necessary from the time of injury in the presence of:

- signs or symptoms suggesting neurological spinal deficit
- a history of loss of consciousness
- altered mental status
- history of a high-speed accident or significant fall (including diving)
- significant head or chest trauma

Immobilisation should continue until appropriate assessment can be made, looking for abnormal peripheral neurological signs and spinal distraction pain in the presence of normal imaging.

It is often difficult to decide whether the spinal-injured child is initially best cared for in a paediatric ICU or a specialised spinal unit. This decision will be ultimately determined on the age of the child and the stability of the spine. Certainly, infants should not be managed in adult spinal units, whereas for older children, expertise in spinal care may be more important. However, once spinal column stability and surgical fixation have been achieved, children are best managed in paediatric facilities for ongoing management and rehabilitation.[22] Ongoing care is complex, and requires a multidisciplinary approach. Attention to pressure areas, bladder and bowel care and training, nutrition and prevention of contractures is essential. Symptoms of hypercalcaemia (e.g. vomiting, anorexia, nausea and malaise) can be distressing and difficult to control. Depression is common in adolescents. With high spinal cord injury, chin-operated battery-powered wheelchairs, portable ventilators and computer-activated environment control devices allow for relative independence and a functional lifestyle.

THORACIC TRAUMA

Despite a low incidence in children, thoracic trauma is usually associated with multiorgan injury and high mortality.[23] The mechanism of injury is almost entirely related to motor vehicle accidents, with penetrating trauma being uncommon. The child's small size and more elastic chest wall allow transmission of more kinetic energy to intrathoracic structures, with a high incidence of pulmonary contusions without rib fractures or flail chest.

As for adults, life-threatening injuries which require immediate intervention are upper-airway obstruction, tension pneumothorax, open pneumothorax, flail chest, pericardial tamponade and massive haemothorax (see Chapter 69). Potentially life-threatening injuries are airway rupture, pulmonary contusion, ruptured aorta, diaphragmatic rupture, oesophageal perforation and myocardial contusion. Contrast CT scan and angiography are the methods of choice in diagnosing aortic rupture in children.

ABDOMINAL TRAUMA

Abdominal trauma is usually associated with blunt injury[24] and recognition maybe difficult in the presence of multisystem injury. Mortality is relatively high and missed abdominal trauma is the leading cause of preventable morbidity and mortality.[25] The abdominal wall and thoracic cage of children provide less protection to intra-abdominal organs. Also, the liver and spleen are relatively large and more exposed below the rib cage. Forces need not be excessive to cause rupture of internal organs. Absence of bruising does not exclude injury while bruising means severe injury is likely. Lap seat belt injuries are an important cause of abdominal injury in restrained children.

Improvements in radiological imaging techniques have allowed blunt abdominal trauma to be managed conservatively in children.[26] This approach requires appropriate monitoring and supervision in a paediatric intensive care setting, with an awareness of the need for urgent intervention, i.e. laparotomy (Table 103.6).

- Ultrasonography is an important screening tool for detecting free fluid[27] and confirming intra-abdominal bleeding.
- CT scan assessment with intraluminal and i.v. contrast is indicated with clinical suspicion of abdominal injury or when physical examination is unreliable. It allows for examination of solid organs and renal tract, and detection of intraperitoneal blood and free air.
- Diagnostic peritoneal lavage is less important, and is only indicated when the source of continued bleeding is undetermined, when an urgent procedure is required for a non-abdominal injury or when a prolonged observation period is anticipated and ultrasonography or CT scan is not available.

NON-ACCIDENTAL INJURY

Non-accidental injuries to children are seen in younger age groups, and include physical assault, sexual and emotional abuse and neglect (especially inadequate supervision and deprivation of nutrition and medical care). Injuries resulting from intentional assault can be difficult to diagnose, unless a high index of awareness is maintained.

With regard to the history, suspicion should be raised when:

- the cause of the injury cannot be explained
- there is discrepancy between the volunteered history and the sustained injury, especially when the child's stage of development is taken into account
- there is a history of repeated injuries
- it is alleged that the injury is self-sustained; or
- there is a delay in seeking care

Physical examination should be thorough, to establish a pattern of injury.[29] Multiple bruises in differing stages of development can be separately estimated for age. Patterns for burns are typical for forced immersion in hot water (with sparing of the groin area) and from cigarettes. Suspicion should be raised where cerebral trauma is associated with retinal haemorrhages, subdural haematomas or fractures. Findings of retinal haemorrhages on ophthalmological examination increases suspicion for inflicted injury but do not confirm the diagnosis.[30] The most common intracranial pathology is subdural and subarachnoid haemorrhage, which account for the higher morbidity and mortality. A whole-body X-ray series and bone scan will detect fractures in differing stages of healing from multiple assaults.

Whenever non-accidental injury is suspected or diagnosed, a multidisciplinary approach is required by a specialised child protection unit to deal with medical and legal issues, and with the counselling. Urgent intervention may be necessary where the safety of other siblings is threatened.

Table 103.6 Indications for laparotomy in paediatric abdominal trauma[28]

Profound hypovolaemia
Persistent haemorrhage
Haemodynamic instability after replacement 40 ml/kg
Penetrating injury
Gastrointestinal perforation
Signs of peritonism
Pancreatic injury

TRANSPORT

The outcome of trauma in remote locations is optimal when advice, prehospital stabilisation and transport are provided by teams based in tertiary paediatric ICUs.[31] Secondary insults occur more frequently when paediatric-trained personnel are not used for transport.[32] A referral and retrieval infrastructure which links a tertiary centre to outlying areas within the region is necessary. Local health care providers must have sufficient skills to stabilise any critically ill child adequately. The transport team must offer a level of care during the stabilisation and transport phases that is equivalent to that of the receiving paediatric ICU.

It is important for regional hospitals not used to routinely caring for paediatric trauma patients to recognise and acknowledge their individual abilities and limitations. A relationship with a tertiary PICU is essential to allow appropriate and timely communication regarding advice on clinical care, prehospital stabilisation and safe transport for individual patients.

BRAIN DEATH

Determination of brain death in children has different implications.[33] Isoelectric EEGs have been reported in neonates with partially preserved clinical brain function, and cerebral death can occur without marked increase in ICP, allowing partial cerebral blood flow in the presence of brain death criteria and electrocerebral silence. In addition, partial brain recovery has been demonstrated after prolonged periods of clinical unresponsiveness. So for determination of brain death, consideration needs to be given to longer observation periods, more frequent use of confirmatory tests, and an emphasis on the history and clinical findings.

The American Academy of Pediatrics has set longer observation times which include the requirement for two separate EEGs or one EEG and a cerebral radionucleotide angiogram. These longer observation times depend on the child's age, namely:

- over 1 year of age – 12 hours' observation
- ages 1 month to 12 months – 24 hours' observation
- ages 7 days to 2 months – 48 hours' observation
- under 7 days of age – no recommendation

The Australian and New Zealand Intensive Care Society recommendations on brain death and organ donation only make reference to the under 2 months age group when 'determination of brain death may be more difficult and different time periods may be required'.[34] Importantly, there is a lack of evidence for any required observation periods, so that cerebral blood flow imaging may be required in the neonate and infant. The most important factors when determining brain death are in knowing the cause of coma, and being certain of its irreversibility. Time must be allowed for relatives to come to terms with the diagnosis, and there is a responsibility to discuss organ donation. Having relatives watch the physical examination for brain death testing is helpful.

ORGAN DONATION

During the process of brain death determination and consideration of organ donation, there are significant emotional implications for both the care-givers and the relatives:

- There is a critical time when the hopelessness of the child's outcome becomes apparent and consideration is about to be given for the declaration of brain death.
- The treatment plan previously focused on cerebral resuscitation, and intensive care staff reach a pivotal decision point when treatment is deemed unsuccessful.
- If organ donation is to be considered, then some therapies must be withdrawn to allow for an assessment of cerebral function.

This moment can be a very stressful time for the professional care-givers involved, because they need to shift from a cerebral resuscitation paradigm to withdrawal of support to allow for declaration of brain death, and then institute protocols aimed at organ resuscitation for possible organ donation.

Parents and relatives have to deal with:

- their child being taken from them unexpectedly
- the death being surrounded by tragic circumstances
- intensive medical therapy and critical decisions concerning interventions
- discussions on withdrawal of support
- confronting the issue that their child who outwardly looks no different is clinically dead; and
- subliminal conflicts of blame and guilt which can lead to conflict within family relationships

Success in asking for paediatric organs from parents is associated with:

- knowing the certainty of death
- a willingness to do good for others
- previous discussion of organ donation within the family unit; and
- a knowledge of the patient's wishes before death

Factors inhibiting a willingness to donate by parents include:

- an uncertainty in the parents understanding the diagnosis
- insufficient information and counselling from health professionals; and
- a fear of mutilation

WITHDRAWAL OF SUPPORT

The emotion surrounding a child's impending death can be overwhelming for both relatives and intensive care staff. Children are involved in sudden and catastrophic events that at times seem unreasonable and unfair. For parents, the grieving process begins before or during the intensive care admission, and intensive care staff are intimately involved in helping parents and relatives through this process. The death of any child is a tragedy, and communication between staff is important to ensure appropriate emotional support. Intensive care staff need to understand that withdrawal of therapy can be appropriate. Ensuring the process has dignity and helping relatives through their grieving process are important facets of the intensive care commitment.[35]

REFERENCES

1. Krug EG, Sharma GK, Lozana R. The global burden of injuries. *Am J Public Health* 2000; **90**: 523–6.
2. Smith R, Davis N, Bouamra O *et al.* The utilisation of intraosseous infusion in the resuscitation of paediatric major trauma patients. *Injury* 2005; **36**: 1034–8.

3. Potoka DA, Schall LC, Gardner M *et al.* Impact of pediatric trauma centres on mortality in a statewide system. *J Trauma* 2000; **49**: 237–45.
4. Maconochie I. Accident prevention. *Arch Dis Child* 2003; **88**: 275–7.
5. Lam WH, Mackersie A. Paediatric head injury: incidence, aetiology and management. *Paediatr Anaesth* 1999; **9**: 377–85.
6. Simpson D, Reilly P. Paediatric coma scale. *Lancet* 1982; **2**: 450.
7. Kokoska ER, Smith GS, Pittman T. Early hypotension worsens neurological outcome in pediatric patients with moderately severe head trauma. *J Pediatr Surg* 1998; **33**: 333–8.
8. Michaud LJ, Rivara FP, Longstreth WT *et al.* Elevated initial blood glucose levels and poor outcome following severe brain injuries in children. *J Trauma* 1991; **31**: 1362–6.
9. Ross AK. Pediatric trauma. *Anesthesiol Clin North America* 2001; **19**: 309–37.
10. Feldman Z, Kanter MJ, Robertson CS *et al.* Effect of head elevation on intracranial pressure, cerebral perfusion pressure, and cerebral blood flow in head-injured patients. *J Neurosurg* 1992; **76**: 207–11.
11. Hahn YS, Chyung C, Barthel MJ *et al.* Head injuries in children under 36 months of age. Demography and outcome. *Childs Nerv Syst* 1988; **4**: 34–40.
12. Temkin NR, Dikmen SS, Winn HR. Management of head injury. Posttraumatic seizures. *Neurosurg Clin N Am* 1991; **2**: 425–35.
13. Dearden NM, Midgley S. Technical considerations in continuous jugular venous oxygen saturation measurement. *Acta Neurochir Suppl (Wien)* 1993; **59**: 91–7.
14. Horan MJ. Report of the second task force on blood pressure in children. *Pediatrics* 1987; **79**: 1–25.
15. Welch K. The intracranial pressure in infants. *J Neurosurg* 1980; **52**: 693–9.
16. Raju TN, Vidyasagar D, Papazafiratou C. Cerebral perfusion pressure and abnormal intracranial waveforms: their relation to outcome in birth asphyxia. *Crit Care Med* 1981; **9**: 449–53.
17. Bruce DA, Alavi A, Bilaniuk L *et al.* Diffuse cerebral swelling following head injuries in children: the syndrome of 'malignant brain edema'. *J Neurosurg* 1981; **54**: 170–8.
18. Snoek JW, Minderhoud JM, Wilmink JT. Delayed deterioration following mild head injury in children. *Brain* 1984; **107**: 15–36.
19. Havill JH. Prolonged hyperventilation and intracranial pressure. *Crit Care Med* 1984; **12**: 72–4.
20. Newman KD, Bowman LM, Eichelberger MR. The lap belt complex: intestinal lumbar spin injury in children. *J Trauma* 1990; **30**: 1140–4.
21. Slack SE, Clancy MJ. Clearing the cervical spine of paediatric trauma patients. *Emerg Med J* 2004; **21**: 189–93.
22. Sherwin ED, O'Shanick GJ. The trauma of paediatric and adolescent brain injury: issues and implications for rehabilitation specialists. *Brain Inj* 2000; **3**: 267–84.
23. Peclet MH, Newman KD, Eichelberer MR *et al.* Thoracic trauma in children: an indicator of increased mortality. *J Pediatr Surg* 1990; **25**: 961–6.
24. Cooper A, Barlow B, DiScala C *et al.* Mortality and truncal injury: the pediatric perspective. *J Pediatr Surg* 1994; **29**: 33–8.
25. Holmes JF, Sokolove PE, Brant WE *et al.* Identification of children with intra-abdominal injuries after blunt trauma. *Ann Emerg Med* 2002; **5**: 500–9.
26. Erin S, Shandling B, Simpson J *et al.* Nonoperative management of traumatised spleen in children. *J Pediatr Surg* 1978; **13**: 117–9.
27. Akgur FM, Aktug T, Olguner M *et al.* Prospective study investigating routine use of ultrasonography as the initial diagnostic modality for the evaluation of children sustaining blunt abdominal trauma. *J Trauma* 1997; **42**: 626–8.
28. Rance CH, Singh SJ, Kimble R. Blunt abdominal trauma in children. *J Paediatr Child Health* 2000; **36**: 2–6.
29. Vandeven AM, Newton AW. Update on child physical abuse, sexual abuse, and prevention. *Curr Opin Pediatr* 2006; **18**: 201–5.
30. Bechtel K, Stoessel K, Leventhal JM *et al.* Characteristics that distinguish accidental from abusive injury in hospitalised young children with head trauma. *Pediatrics* 2004; **114**: 165–8.
31. Pearson G, Shann F, Barry P *et al.* Should paediatric intensive care be centralised? Trent versus Victoria. *Lancet* 1997; **349**: 1213–7.
32. McNab JM. Optimal escort for interhospital transport of pediatric emergencies. *J Trauma* 1991; **31**: 205–9.
33. Fishman MA. Validity of brain death criteria in infants. *Pediatrics* 1995; **96**: 513–5.
34. Australian and New Zealand Intensive Care Society. *Recommendations Concerning Brain Death and Organ Donation*, 2nd edn. Melbourne: ANZICS; 1998.
35. Matthews NT. Issues of withdrawal of therapy and brain death in paediatric intensive care. *Crit Care Resusc* 1999; **1**: 7–12.

104

Equipment for paediatric intensive care

James Tibballs

This chapter discusses equipment and its performance required in paediatric and neonatal intensive care. How to use equipment is not discussed. Examples of equipment are given, but exhaustive lists are not intended. Only essential equipment is considered.

Not discussed includes equipment for aerosol therapy, anaesthesia, bronchoscopy, cardiovascular monitoring, cardiac output measurement, echocardiography, ultrasonography, electroencephalographic monitoring, extracorporeal membrane oxygenation, ventricular assistance, home mechanical ventilation, hyperbaric treatment, negative pressure ventilation, nitric oxide therapy, phrenic nerve pacing, mechanical devices for treatment of shock, suction devices and tracheostomy–cricothyrotomy.

All equipment should be purchased, used and maintained in accordance with recognised local standards and manufacturers' instructions. Medical and nursing staff should read the manuals accompanying all items of equipment and receive instruction on safe use.

Numerous items including laryngoscopes, resuscitation bags and ventilator circuits are available as disposable items in response to a market demand for infection safety and reduction of sterilisation costs. The user should subject such items to measures of quality control.

AIRWAY MANAGEMENT

ENDOTRACHEAL TUBES

TUBE TYPES

Polyvinyl chloride or silastic tubes are suitable for long-term intubation. There is little difference in the safety of uncuffed and cuffed tubes provided correct sizes are used and cuff pressures are regulated. The cuff should be inflated with the minimum volume of air necessary to maintain a seal, and checked every 4–8 hours. Recording of pressure in the cuff is desirable. Nonetheless, cuffs reduce effective tube diameter, which would otherwise be available for gas flow. High-volume low-pressure cuffed tubes may be used after puberty when the cricoid region of the trachea has enlarged and is no longer a narrow region at special risk. In circumstances of poor lung compliance, high airway resistance or foreseeable difficulties changing a tube (e.g. as in facial burns), it may be preferable to use a cuffed tube from the outset.

The curve of the tube should be of the Magill type – curved but neither preformed nor of variable diameter. Preformed tubes (e.g. Rae and Childs) make suction difficult and automatically stipulate length in relation to diameter and circumference. Tubes of non-uniform diameter (e.g. Cole and Oxford) may damage the vocal cords, and do not prevent endobronchial intubation.

- Radio-opacity is necessary for correct positioning.
- All tubes should have length markings and a Murphy eye, i.e. a side aperture at the distal end, allowing gas to flow if the tip abuts against the tracheal wall.

TUBE SIZE

A selection of sizes, one larger and one smaller than the anticipated size, should be available at intubation. Tube sizes according to body weight and age are given in Table 104.1 and 104.2. A rough guide for internal diameter size in the child is age (in years)/4 + 4 mm.

Correct selection of size is necessary to avoid pressure-induced ischaemia/ulceration of tracheal mucosa and to limit aspiration around the tube. The correct size should allow not only a small leak on application of moderate inflation pressure (25 cmH_2O, 2.5 kPa) but also enable adequate pulmonary inflation and expiration. When lung compliance is poor, it is permissible to use a cuffless tube without a leak or a cuffed tube to achieve lung inflation.

PLACEMENT

Oral or nasal tubes may be used. Orally placed tubes are preferred in acute resuscitation and when only a short duration of intubation is required, e.g. for anaesthesia during insertion of a central venous cannula. Nasal placement of tubes is preferred in the setting where spontaneous or mechanical ventilation is required for prolonged periods.

Nasal tubes are more comfortable and manageable for the awake patient and are more easily secured to the face, but pose risks, which include sinus infection and necrosis of the alae nasi. Oral tubes are difficult to fix, uncomfortable and are easily occluded by biting by conscious/semiconscious patients.

Table 104.1 Orotracheal and nasotracheal tube lengths for premature neonates

Birth weight (g)	Gestation (weeks)	Oral depth (cm)	Nasal depth (cm)
750	24–25	5–5.5	6.5
1000	27	5.5	7
1500	30–31	6	8
1750	31–32	6.5	8.5
2000	33	7	9
2250	34–35	7–7.5	9.5
2500	35–36	7.5	9.5–10
2750	36–37	8	10.5
3000	37–38	8–8.5	10.5
3500	40	9	11–11.5

ETT sizes: BW <1 kg, 2.5 mm; 1–3.5 kg, 3.0 mm; >3.5 kg, 3.5 mm.

Table 104.2 Endotracheal tube sizes (internal diameter) and orotracheal and nasotracheal depths for infants and children

Body weight/ age	Size (mm)	Oral depth (cm)	Nasal depth (cm)
Newly-born 3.5 kg	3.0	9	11–11.5
1–6 months	3.5	9.5–11	12–13
6–12 months	4.0	11.5–12	13–14
2–3 years	4.5	13–13	15–16
4–5 years	5.0	14–14	17–18
6–7 years	5.5	15–15.5	19
8–9 years	6.0	16–16	20
10–11 years	6.5	17–17	21
12–13 years	7.0	18–18	22
14–16 years	7.5	19	23

TUBE LENGTH (DEPTH)

The endotracheal tube tip should be located in the mid-trachea so that the risks of accidental extubation and endobronchial intubation are minimised. Correct positioning of the tube should always be checked by auscultation in the axillae, by chest X-ray immediately after intubation and daily thereafter.[1] At intubation, visualisation of the depth of the tube passed through the cords should be a guide only, since the tube advances when the head is released from extension as the laryngoscope is removed.[2]

The lengths (depths) at which orotracheal and nasotracheal tubes can be chosen initially on the basis of weight or gestation in premature neonates are given in Table 104.1, and on the basis of age for infants and children in Table 104.2. The lengths are at the lips for oral tubes and at the exit from the nose for nasal tubes. For oral tubes, a guide to correct depth for 2 years and over is given by the formula: (age in years/2 + 12 cm), while for nasal tubes the formula is: (age in years/2 + 15 cm). The depth of insertion of any tube should be documented or marked on the tube.

LARYNGOSCOPES

The adult curved Macintosh blade is suitable for all paediatric patients except neonates and infants, in whom a straight blade is needed to displace the relatively large epiglottis anteriorly from the laryngeal inlet. A straight flat blade, e.g. Miller (size 0 or 1) or Seward blade, or a straight blade with a medial flange (Magill, Robertshaw, Oxford or Wisconsin) is equally suitable for this purpose. The latter blades displace the tongue medially and give a better view of the larynx, but leave less room for instrumentation with a sucker, introducer or forceps.

SUCTION CATHETERS

Sizes 5, 6, 8, 10 and 12 FG should be available. The suction catheter should be large enough to remove secretions but not too large to occlude the endotracheal/tracheostomy tube lumen (Table 104.3). Many suitable types are available – differing in number and location of suction ports (end and side ports are needed) and whether the tip is angled or straight. Angled tips facilitate entry into the left main bronchus. Satin-finish types with smooth port edges are needed. Single use suction catheters may be reused up to 24 hours without adding to the risk of pneumonia.[3] Closed suction systems permit suction without disconnection from ventilator as may be indicated during nitric oxide therapy, severe lung disease or frequent suction.

Table 104.3 Recommended suction catheters

Internal diameter (mm) of ETT or tracheostomy	Recommended suction catheter (FG)
2.5	5
3.0	6
3.5–5.5	8
6.0–6.5	10
7.0 and larger	12

ETT, endotracheal tube.

OROPHARYNGEAL AIRWAYS

A range of Guedel airways (sizes 000, 00, 0, 1, 2 and 3) constructed of polyvinyl chloride with a metal insert should be available: an airway that is too small may be occluded by the surface of the tongue or displace the tongue backwards to obstruct the airway; an airway that is too large may enter the oesophagus. The correct size, when placed alongside the cheek, extends from the centre of the lips to the angle of the mandible. Nasopharyngeal airways are available for the older child, but any size can be constructed from an endotracheal tube. A guide to length is from the tip of the nose to the tragus of the ear.

LARYNGEAL MASK AIRWAYS

Sizes are available to suit body weight (kg) of newborns, infants and children:

- size 1 — < 5 kg
- size 1½ — 5–10 kg
- size 2 — 10–20 kg
- size 2½ — 20–30 kg
- size 3 — 30–50 kg
- size 4 — 50–70 kg
- size 5 — 70–100 kg
- size 6 — > 100 kg

They have complementary roles in paediatric intensive care practice which are as airways under anaesthesia, a limited role during cardiopulmonary resuscitation (CPR) and as emergency relief of upper-airway obstruction.

MECHANICAL VENTILATION

RESUSCITATOR 'BAGGING' CIRCUITS

Manual pulmonary inflation is often necessary via a mask or endotracheal/tracheostomy tube. Two types of device are available: flow-inflated and self-inflated bags.

FLOW-INFLATED BAGS

These are exemplified by Jackson-Rees modified Ayre's T-piece. Gas flow must exceed 220 ml/kg per min for children and 3 l/min for infants to prevent rebreathing during manual ventilation. It is possible to control precisely the concentration of inspired oxygen, which is an advantage, especially for the premature neonate at risk of oxygen-induced retrolental fibroplasia. However, considerable experience is necessary to provide adequate ventilation without barotrauma in the intubated infant. The circuit has neither a valve nor any pressure-relief device. A pressure gauge should be incorporated in the circuit to help prevent barotrauma.

SELF-INFLATED BAGS

These bags are designed to give positive-pressure ventilation attached to either a mask or endotracheal/tracheostomy tube. Rebreathing is prevented by one-way duck-bill valves, spring disk/ball valves or diaphragm/leaf valves.

The Laerdal bag series (infant, child, adult) typify these devices. A pressure-relief valve (infant and child size) opens at 35 cmH_2O (3.5 kPa). A pressure monitor can be incorporated in the circuit. Supplemental oxygen is added to the ventilation bag, with or without attachment of a reservoir bag, whose movement may serve as a visual monitor of tidal volume during spontaneous ventilation when intubated. However, the valve may offer too much resistance for spontaneous ventilation and they should not be used to provide supplemental oxygen to a spontaneously breathing patient via a mask placed loosely over the face.

With Laerdal and Partner bags, negligible amounts of oxygen (0.1–0.3 l/min) issue from the patient valve when 5–15 l/min of oxygen is introduced into bags unconnected to patients.[4] The valve is unlikely to open unless the mask is sealed well on the face. The delivered oxygen concentration is dependent on the flow rate of oxygen, use of the reservoir bag, and the state of the pressure relief valve (whether open or closed).

- With use of the reservoir bag and oxygen flow greater than the minute ventilation, 100% oxygen is delivered.
- Without the reservoir bag the delivered gas is only 50% oxygen, despite oxygen flow rate at twice minute ventilation.
- At an oxygen flow rate of 10 l/min to the infant resuscitator bag, the delivered gas is 85–100% oxygen without the use of the reservoir bag.

Other self-inflated bags include the Combibag, Ambu, AirViva and Hudson RCI.

MASKS

Masks should facilitate an airtight seal on the face with minimal dead space.

- For neonates, Rendell-Baker Soucek masks (sizes 0 and 1) or Bennett masks (sizes 1 and 2) are suitable.
- For infants and small children, the larger Rendell-Baker Soucek masks (sizes 2 and 3) or small masks with inflatable rims, such as CIG (sizes 2 and 3) or MIE (sizes 0 and 1), are suitable.
- For older children, masks with inflatable rims are preferred.

Masks with rims created by infolding of the body are more difficult to use.

MECHANICAL VENTILATORS

CONVENTIONAL VENTILATORS

Some ventilators are designed specifically for neonates and infants. A few adult ventilators are also satisfactory. In addition to general requirements of ventilators, the paediatric ventilator should have:

- low circuit volume, compliance and resistance
- minimal dead space within the ventilator and circuit

- rapid response time for gas flow during spontaneous respiratory effort
- a lightweight circuit
- inspiratory time adjustment independent of the inspiratory/expiratory ratio
- capability for a ventilation rate up to 60 breaths/min (excluding capability for high-frequency ventilation)
- variable gas flow at least up to 2–3 l/kg per min
- electronic display of inspiratory pressure wave
- accurate measurement of low tidal volume

A generic classification of ventilators, their operational characteristics and their modes of ventilation has been proposed.[5] It is described here briefly to enable functional description and comparison of some ventilators.

Ventilators may be operationally classified as pressure, volume, flow or time controllers. These are the independent or control variables. Since only one variable can be controlled at a given time, i.e. predetermined, the remaining features of the waveform are dependent variables. If pressure, volume or flow is not predetermined, the ventilator is presumed to be a time controller in which only the timing of the inspiratory and expiratory phases is controlled.

- *Pressure controller*: the pressure waveform does not change when resistance or compliance changes, but volume waveform will.
- *Volume and flow controllers*: the volume waveform does not change when resistance and compliance change but the pressure waveform changes. In a volume controller the volume is measured and used in control whereas it is not in a flow controller. In a flow controller it is flow that is used.
- *Time controller*: both pressure and volume waveforms change when resistance and compliance change.

These concepts allow understanding of any mode of ventilation and interpretation of bedside pulmonary mechanics, i.e. resistance, compliance, time constants, etc. The manner of controlling the independent variable may be an open-loop system, in which no feedback occurs during inspiration to achieve the target goal, or a closed-loop or feedback or servo-controlled system in which the independent variable is modified according to progress during inspiration.

During inspiration, dual control may be used and may be altered from one independent variable to another. For example, in the VAPS mode (volume assured pressure support mode) of the Bird VIP Gold ventilator, control is switched from pressure to flow control if a preset tidal volume has not been achieved. In another example using the Pmax feature of the Drager Evita 4, if in flow control a pressure limit has been reached, control is passed to pressure while the tidal volume is monitored and the inspiratory time increased until the preset tidal volume has been achieved.

PHASE VARIABLES

The manner of initiation of inspiration (triggering), sustaining inspiration (limit variables), initiation of expiration (cycling) and sustaining expiration are the phase variables. Initiation of inspiration, or triggering, may be dictated by machine or patient. Usual triggers are the elapse of time or generation of pressure or flow by the patient. Flow triggering during spontaneous ventilation is more energy efficient and better tolerated than other variables, particularly when the flow sensor is located at the endotracheal tube. Mandatory breaths are all those triggered by a preset frequency or minimum minute ventilation, or terminated by a preset frequency or tidal volume. Spontaneous breaths are those initiated by the patient and terminated by lung mechanics or ventilatory drive. The quantification of the inspiratory phase is by time, pressure or volume. Initiation of expiration (termination of inspiration) or cycling is achieved by elapse of time, pressure, volume or flow. Expiration is usually sustained by pressure alone.

Modes of ventilation may be described on the following generic basis. It is derived from the controller variables. It should not be assumed that a manufacturer's mode terminology accurately defines its functional attributes or is intuitively obvious. Terminology is not necessarily interchangeable between different manufacturers. Although some new modes are genuine inventions, another purpose appears to be differentiation of product from competition. The capabilities of any ventilator can be defined by the following:

- The controller variable (pressure, volume, dual)
- The pattern of mandatory breaths versus spontaneous breaths
  - CMV is continuous mandatory ventilation (conventional IPPV)
  - SIMV is synchronised intermittent mandatory ventilation
  - CSV is continuous spontaneous ventilation.
- The phase variable for mandatory breaths, especially trigger and cycle variables
- Whether spontaneous breaths are assisted

If conditional variables exist, these act to change the pattern of ventilation – for example, to give a sigh breath based on elapse of time, or switching from patient-triggered breaths to machine-triggered breaths in the SIMV mode or mandatory minute ventilation modes.

Volume/flow-control modes are suitable for conditions in which lung compliance and resistance are variable. In these circumstances, the peak inspiratory pressure attained is a valuable observation. However, when a pressure limit is imposed, such information is lost. A mode consisting of flow control, time triggering, pressure limitation and time cycling is commonly used because of the relative ease of operation. However, relatively small leaks may severely compromise tidal volume, mean airway pressure and oxygenation. Large leaks may also delay attainment of preset pressure until late in the inspiratory cycle. Thus, it is helpful to display the volume and pressure waveforms. Some ventilators do, however, provide leak compensation (e.g. Bird VIP Gold). Gas flow should be set above 2 l/kg per min to achieve the preset pressure early in the inspiratory period. This flow rate is also suitable for peak inspiratory flow rate during spontaneous respiratory effort with intermittent mandatory ventilation.

Pressure in the circuit should be monitored in close proximity to the endotracheal tube. Changes in endotracheal tube resistance from encrustation or kinking have a major adverse effect on tidal volume.[6]

Neonates and infants have small tidal volumes (5–50 ml), and are therefore prone to alveolar hypoventilation when variable air leaks occur around the endotracheal tube and from the ventilator–humidifier circuit. Moreover, the internal compliance and compressible volume of the circuit may exceed the tidal volume. Small tidal volumes are difficult to set and maintain when the lung compliance and resistance are abnormal.[7]

Most neonatal intensive care units (ICUs) use pressure-control modes which in hyaline membrane disease achieves adequate oxygenation with minimal barotrauma.[8] The pressure-control mode is more appropriate than the volume-control mode for neonates and infants 0.5–5.0 kg body weight. Ventilators, which are pressure controllers, deliver a variable flow dependent on lung and airway characteristics.

Improvements in ventilatory management of newborns are observed with a new generation of ventilators, which utilise changes in airway pressure, airway gas flow or abdominal movement to trigger inspiration, and which have ultrashort trigger delays.[9] Previously, ventilators were unable to cope with the very short inspiratory times (mean 0.31, SD 0.06 seconds) of newborns with respiratory distress syndrome.[10] Patient-triggered ventilation (PTV) permits synchronous ventilation with better gas exchange, prevents the patient fighting the ventilator and reduces the need for neuromuscular paralysis.[11,12] Some ventilators suitable for paediatric use are the Bear Cub 2001, Bear Cub 750vs, Bird T Bird, Bird VIP Gold, Drager Babylog 8000 (plus), Drager Evita 4, Evita XL, Infant star 950, Sechrist IV-100B, Sechrist IV-200 SAVI, Siemens Servo 900C, Siemens Servo 300, Siemens Servo-*i*, Viasys Avea, and SLE 5000.

HIGH-FREQUENCY VENTILATORS

These provide ventilation at at least four times normal rate and may be classified into five types:[5]

- high-frequency positive-pressure ventilation (HF-PPV)
- high-frequency jet ventilation (HFJV)
- high-frequency flow interruption (HFFI)
- high-frequency oscillation (HFO)
- high-frequency percussive ventilation (HFPV)

High-frequency oscillatory ventilation (HFO) at 15 Hz has been shown to achieve better gas exchange with less barotrauma than conventional mechanical ventilation in infants with respiratory distress.[13,14] Examples of high-frequency oscillators are the Sensor Medics and 3100A and 3100B (adult) and the Humming series models, of which the latest is Atom Humming V. The latter also offers a synchronised intermittent mandatory ventilation mode. An example of a high-frequency jet ventilator is the Bunnell Life Pulse jet ventilator which is used in conjunction with a conventional ventilator to provide positive end-expiratory pressure (PEEP) and humidified gas for spontaneous ventilation. An example of a high-frequency positive-pressure ventilator is the Nellcor Puritan-Bennett Infant Star 950, which operates as a flow interrupter.

TRANSPORT VENTILATORS

Although 'hand-bagging' may be used during transport from the field to hospital, between hospitals and within hospitals, it is highly desirable to utilise a purpose-designed transport ventilator to ensure consistent ventilation and cardiorespiratory stability. Ventilation by machine also enables personnel to attend to other tasks. Whether pneumatic or electronically powered, it must be compact, light, rugged, easy to operate and yet provide a standard and mode of ventilation required by a wide variety of patient illnesses and equivalent to that required by any patient in the ICU. Electrically powered ventilators should have both mains and battery power.

The ventilator should be capable of providing SIMV with time or flow cycling and flow or pressure-triggering, non-invasive ventilation, continuous positive airway pressure (CPAP) and PEEP, and provide 21–100% oxygen. Controls for rate, inspiratory time, flow, tidal volume and pressure should be independent. It should be unaffected by altitude and be operable in an MRI environment. It should incorporate alarms for low and high pressure, apnoea and disconnection. All these aims are difficult if not impossible to fulfil. Examples of ventilators are Drager Oxylog 2000, Pulmonetic Systems LTV1000 and Newport HTSO.

NON-INVASIVE VENTILATION (NIV)

The application of ventilation 'BiPAP' (bilevel positive airways pressure) or CPAP by means other than intubation (NIV) has become an essential part of paediatric intensive care practice. Although a proprietary name (Respironics), 'BiPAP' has become synonymous with non-invasive ventilation. It is distinct from BIPAP (biphasic positive airway pressure), a mode available in some conventional ventilators in which spontaneous ventilation is permitted during all phases of mechanical ventilation. CPAP or BiPAP may be given by an interface of a nasal, oronasal (full face) mask with harnesses with or without a chin strap (headgear). Other interface devices such as mini-masks, nasal pillows, nasal cushions, mouthpiece/lipseal and helmets are less common in paediatrics.

CPAP is commonly used to relieve upper-airway obstruction or improve oxygenation in lung disease. BiPAP is commonly used to provide ventilation in chronic hypoventilatory states such as congenital central hypoventilation syndrome, neuromuscular diseases, pretransplantation cystic fibrosis and in acute conditions such as asthma, pneumonia and pulmonary oedema. Both CPAP and BiPAP are used before resorting to invasive ventilation and after extubation. Although stand-alone, BiPAP machines are primarily intended for use in adult patients with obstructive sleep apnoea and are not generally intended for use as life support. Consequently, many machines are not licensed to provide ventilation via endotracheal tube or tracheostomy but this capability is a distinct advantage and may be provided as an optional mode in mechanical ventilators.

The defining characteristics of BiPAP are the automatic breath-by-breath compensation for air leaks and the ability to trigger and cycle by flow or time in synchronisation with patient effort. The devices can be set to provide a spontaneous (assisted) mode, timed (mandatory) mode or a combined mode. When the inspiratory positive airway pressure (IPAP) is set the same as the expiratory positive airway pressure (EPAP), CPAP is provided. Examples of CPAP machines are Tranquility (Healthdyne) and CPAP S6 series (Resmed). Examples of BiPAP machines are the BiPAP S/T, S/T-D, S/T-D 30, Harmony and Synchrony series (Respironics), the KnightStar 335 (Nellcor-Puritan-Bennett) but not suitable for children < 30 kg, and the Sullivan VPAP II and VPAP II ST (Resmed).

OXYGEN THERAPY AND MONITORING

OXYGEN CATHETERS

Sizes 6, 8 and 10 FG should be available and placed in the same nostril as the nasogastric tube, to limit airway resistance. Size 6 FG is suitable for neonates, 8 FG for infants and small children and 10 FG for older children. It should be appreciated that oxygen catheters placed in the nasopharynx provide a small amount of PEEP, and indeed may be used for that purpose.[15] Nasal cannulae (two-pronged) are not recommended. Excessive flow may cause gastric distension. Flow rate for infants should be regulated by a low-flow meter, graduated 0–2.5 l/min.

OXYGEN MASKS

Masks may not be well tolerated by the infant or small child; oxygen catheters are preferable.

HEAD BOXES AND INCUBATORS

A clear perspex head box is the best way of administering a high concentration of oxygen to the unintubated neonate and infant. Precise oxygen therapy is possible but rebreathing, heat loss and desiccation are potential problems. To avoid rebreathing, a large flow rate (10–12 l/min) of fresh gas with predetermined oxygen content should be introduced. The practice of introducing a low flow rate of 100% oxygen into a head box (to gain a lesser concentration) may cause rebreathing and hypercarbia. If 100% oxygen is the only compressed gas available, lesser concentrations of oxygen may be attained without rebreathing by using a flow of 100% oxygen and a Venturi device. The relatively large capacity of an incubator precludes the attainment of a high concentration of oxygen, but limited oxygen therapy, up to 60%, can be achieved.

OXYGEN ANALYSERS

These are essential to regulate oxygen therapy via incubator or head box. The devices utilise either a polarographic electrode or galvanic cell (microfuel cell) as oxygen sensor. The polarographic types require a source of power (battery or mains), are more expensive to buy but cheaper to run, and have a faster response time.[13,16] An incorporated alarm is recommended. The sensing electrode should be placed close to the patient's head.

An oxygen analyser capable of monitoring deliberate hypoxic gas mixtures (e.g. OX60+, Parker Healthcare Pty Ltd) is required if nitrogen is to be used – for example, to increase pulmonary vascular resistance in management of post-Norwood repair of hypoplastic left heart syndrome.

TRANSCUTANEOUS GAS ANALYSERS

Transcutaneous gas tensions in paediatric patients equate well with arterial gas tensions. However, $Pa\text{O}_2$ is underestimated by $Ptc\text{O}_2$ during mild hyperoxaemia in neonates.[17] Transcutaneous gas values are dependent on both arterial gas tensions and on blood flow. During normovolaemia with adequate flow, $Ptc\text{O}_2$ reflects $Pa\text{O}_2$ and $Ptc\text{CO}_2$ reflects $Pa\text{CO}_2$. However, during circulatory failure, a reduction in $Ptc\text{O}_2$ reflects a reduction in flow, provided $Pa\text{O}_2$ is normal.[18] Likewise, during circulatory failure, $Ptc\text{CO}_2$ exceeds $Pa\text{CO}_2$ and is flow dependent.[19] Typical transcutaneous dual function single electrodes are Hewlett Packard Virida tcO_2/tcCO_2, Sensormedics FasTrac SaO_2/CO_2 monitor.

Continuous pulse oximetry ($Sp\text{O}_2$) has evolved to be an integral part of monitoring in neonatal and paediatric intensive care. Transcutaneous pulse oximetry is more convenient than transcutaneous partial pressure measurement. Each patient should have a pulse oximeter. The value of pulse oximetry is detection of hypoxaemia, not hyperoxaemia. They cannot be used accurately to titrate oxygen therapy, which requires blood or transcutaneous partial pressure measurement. The accuracy of pulse oximetry at low $Sa\text{O}_2$ (< 75%) is poor.[20] Numerous devices are available.

BLOOD GAS ANALYSERS

In many neonatal and paediatric conditions, frequent blood gas analysis is essential for optimal management. A blood gas analyser utilising small volumes (< 0.2 ml) is essential. The instrument should be located within or near the ICU, so that tests can be performed and the results known without delay. Hand-held bedside devices are available, e.g. i-Stat.

APNOEA MONITORS

Infant apnoea is often due to upper-airway obstruction, seizures or gastro-oesophageal reflux,[21] although it may be idiopathic and is commonly associated with prematurity. Short apnoeic spells (< 15 seconds) are normal during sleep and feeding. Significant apnoea is associated with bradycardia, cyanosis and hypotonia. The detection and treatment of apnoea in intensive care are dependent on cardiovascular monitoring and constant nursing observation. In the home or ward, where observation is less than that available in the ICU, apnoea may be detected by the use of a pressure sensor in a pad or mattress under the infant, or by impedance pneumography, in which diaphragmatic movement causes a change in resistance between two electrodes on the skin. Apnoea of central origin is detected early by these devices but obstructive apnoea, resulting in paradoxical respiratory effort, is detected late. Some devices incorporate electrocardiogram monitoring and rely upon bradycardia as evidence of hypoxaemia, which is a useful but late sign in obstructive apnoea, when both hypoxaemia and movement of the diaphragm are present. False-positive alarms are not uncommon.

THERMOREGULATION

RADIANT HEATERS AND INCUBATORS

Adequate temperature regulation is essential in neonates and infants to avoid cold stress and to maintain a thermoneutral environment.[22] Numerous heaters and incubators are available with special features for transport, resuscitation, intensive care and regular ward nursing. Open-type radiant heaters (e.g. Drager Babytherm 8000 OC, Air Shields Vickers IICS-90, Datex Ohmeda Infant Warmers series) are more suitable for use in intensive care. The ideal radiant heater should incorporate:

- servo-controlled overhead heating device with alarm for overheating
- open tilt bed of adequate area
- clear perspex removable/hinged sides
- adequate illumination
- adjustable height
- facility for X-ray examinations
- facility for phototherapy

Additional features may include facilities for bottled oxygen and air, positive pressure, resuscitation and suction equipment.

Incubators are less suitable for use in intensive care because of limited access, but are better for transportation. Heating is via a conductive mattress. Double-walled infant incubators (e.g. Air-Shields Isolette C2000) reduce heat loss, attain preset temperature rapidly, do not produce excessive air currents or sound levels, and do not permit carbon dioxide accumulation.[23] Oxygen therapy and mechanical ventilation are possible with both types of unit, but are technically easier with all open-cot radiant heaters.

CONVECTION AND CONDUCTION THERMOREGULATORS

Mattresses with circulating fluid and air-inflated blankets are essential for maintaining preset body temperatures as might be required for therapeutic hypothermia (after cardiac arrest or head injury) or restoration of normothermia after hypothermic or hyperthermic injuries.

HUMIDIFIERS

Adequate humidification of ventilator circuits is of utmost importance in the paediatric patient. Unless adequately humidified, the relatively narrow endotracheal and tracheostomy tubes are prone to encrustation and blockage. Insensible water and heat loss are also prevented with adequate humidification. High-flow heated humidifiers provide near 100% humidification (44 mg H_2O/l gas, 47 mmHg) at body temperature and are preferred. They are easily adapted for use into ventilator circuits, face and tracheostomy masks, T-piece circuits and oxygen head boxes. When used in ventilator circuits, it is important to realise that they contribute to internal compliance and a compressible volume, which produce errors in both volume-preset and pressure-preset ventilators. Ideally, the compliance should not exceed 1.0 ml/cmH_2O for infants less than 10 kg body weight.[24]

Several methods exist to maintain the water level including an airlock system, parallel-fill system, float-system and a pinch-clamp system.[5] Systems that automatically maintain a constant level are preferred for the aforementioned reasons. Incorporation of servo-control is also important. A thermistor probe incorporated into the proximal inspiratory circuit and heating of the inspiratory limb ensure that gas is delivered to the patient at body temperature. However, because some heat loss may occur along the inspiratory limb and much more along the expiratory limb (which is not heated), significant condensation (rain-out) occurs. A water trap must be incorporated to gather 'rain-out' and the circuit, particularly the expiratory limb, positioned in a dependent manner to prevent aspiration by the patient. Such water, although potentially contaminated by airway bacteria, does not pose nosocomial infection risk and may be allowed to drain into the humidifier where high temperature inhibits bacterial growth. Circuits may be changed infrequently. Examples of servo-controlled heated humidifiers are Puritan-Bennett Cascade II and Fisher and Paykel MR600, 700, 720, 850 series.

Condenser-type humidifiers or 'artificial noses' have a role in intensive care. They are passive humidifiers capturing exhaled water vapour and heat, permitting their reuse on inhalation (heat and moisture exchangers, HME). Numerous devices exist, some incorporating filters and/or hydroscopic materials leading to subclassifications of heat and moisture exchanging filter (HMEF), hydroscopic heat and moisture exchanger (HHME) and hydroscopic heat and moisture exchanging filter (HHMEF). They are often added to tracheostomy or endotracheal tubes of spontaneously breathing patients or inserted into the inspiratory limb of a ventilator circuit for short periods, e.g. for transport. They cannot replace full humidification. HMEs provide approximately one-quarter to one-third relative humidity whereas HHME/HHMEFs provide approximately one-half to three-quarters relative humidity.[5] Problems with these devices include deterioration of performance with time, resistance and dead space. The appropriate size for the patient (adult, paediatric, neonatal) must be used. They are not suitable for use if the patient is hypothermic, has thick or bloody secretions or requires frequent changes. They should never be used in conjunction with heated water humidifiers because of potential circuit blockage. They should not be moistened and the addition of oxygen, although sanctioned by some manufacturers, will compromise performance.

Unheated humidifiers of the passover, bubble, bubble diffuser and jet types are inefficient and have limited applicability in the intensive care setting. Other types of humidifiers such as jet nebulisers and ultrasonic nebulisers have little role in intensive care.

MISCELLANEOUS EQUIPMENT

INFUSION DEVICES

Numerous electromechanical devices have been developed to overcome the deficiencies of gravity-fed i.v. infusion sets. They enable constant and accurate infusion of predetermined volumes. These devices have wide clinical application and are used to control the administration of potent drugs, hormones and parenteral nutrition. Performance and application are variable.[25,26]

VOLUMETRIC PUMPS

These regulate flow rate by delivering a premeasured bolus under pressure. In some the delivery is not smooth. They utilise disposable closed cassettes. The risk of air pumping is minimal and alarms indicate infusion failure. High (up to 999 ml/hour) and low flow rates (1 ml/hour) are possible. Examples are IVAC Neo-mate 565, Alaris Medical Systems Gemini PC-1, PC-2, Abbott Lifecare 5000 'Plum' Pump, and B/Braun Infusomat fm.

SYRINGE PUMPS AND DRIVERS

These are suitable for infusion of potent drugs in concentrated form at very low rates (down to 0.1 ml/hour). They are mains electricity and/or battery powered. The latter are suitable for use during transport and miniaturised models are suitable for ambulant use. These devices are suitable for i.v., intra-arterial, intramuscular, subcutaneous infusion or enterogastric feeding, being particularly suitable for use in neonates and infants. They are not suited to infusion of large volumes and offer no safeguard against extravasation unless an overpressure alarm is incorporated. Generally, the pumps utilise specified syringes unless recalibrated. Some syringe brands do not run smoothly. At low flows (< 1 ml/hour) infusion line compliance contributes to irregular drug delivery associated with vertical displacement of the pump.[27]

Examples of syringe infusion pumps are B/Braun Perfusor, Graseby 3100, IVAC Alaris P3000, P6000, and Alaris asena GH.

INDIRECT MEASUREMENT OF BLOOD PRESSURE

Measurement of blood pressure in the critically ill neonate and infant is important in cardiovascular monitoring. Continuous direct intra-arterial measurement is preferred in cardiovascular instability, but adequate monitoring can be achieved with Doppler ultrasonography (e.g. Roche Arteriosonde) or with microprocessor analysis of oscillometric signals (e.g. Critikon Dinamap, Nippon-Colin, Ohio NIMP, Narco Scientific and Vita-Stat, Kenz BPM). The latter devices provide time-automated analysis of systolic, diastolic and mean blood pressure, as well as heart rate at specified intervals. Some portable monitoring devices provide additional data, such as invasive pressure measurement, electrocardiogram, heart rate, pulse oximetry, capnography, respiratory rate and temperature (e.g. Nellcor Propaq, Datascope Passport, Schiller Argus TM-7, S & W Diascope, BCI 6100).

Continuous non-invasive measurement of blood pressure may be measured with the Ohmeda Finapres non-invasive blood pressure monitor. Blood pressure measured with these non-invasive devices correlates well with simultaneous measurement by direct intra-arterial measurement in neonates,[28] infants and children.[29] Generally, systolic pressure is underestimated by only 2–4 mmHg (0.3–0.5 kPa), while the diastolic pressure is overestimated by a similar amount. Venostasis and radial nerve compression are occasional complications.[30]

NASOGASTRIC TUBES

These are mandatory in all intubated and/or ventilated patients as aids to prevent aspiration, and are a useful means of providing nutrition and medication. A range of sizes should be available: 5–6 FG for neonates; 8 FG for infants; 10 FG for small children and 12 FG for larger children.

PLASMAPHERESIS/HAEMOFILTRATION

Generally, the techniques described in dialytic therapy are applicable to infants and children. Although separate veins – or an artery and a vein – may be cannulated, it is common to perform these procedures via a double lumen catheter inserted into a large vein (femoral, jugular, subclavian), i.e. to perform continuous venovenous haemo/diafiltration (CVVH, CVVHD), plasmafiltration or haemoperfusion. In infants (0–1 year), this requires a 6.5 FR catheter to achieve blood flow of 25–40 ml/

min, small children (1–8 years) an 8.5 FR catheter to achieve 30–60 ml/min and in large children (> 8 years) an 11 FR catheter to achieve 50–100 ml/min via a blood pump (e.g. Gambro MPM 10, Kimal ultra or Infomed HF400). Typically, the filtration rate is approximately one-third of the blood flow while the size of the molecules appearing in the filtrate is determined by filter size. To remove molecules up to 30 000 Daltons, Gambro FH 22, 55, 66, 77 or 88 is used. To remove molecules up to 3 million Daltons, Gambro PF1000 or PF2000 is used.

DEFIBRILLATION

DC shock machines should be able to give shocks as low as 1 or 2 joules with gradations up to adult doses, with a preference for a biphasic waveform.

REFERENCES

1. Greenbaum DM, Marshall KE. The value of routine daily chest X-rays in intubated patients in the medical intensive care unit. *Crit Care Med* 1982; **10**: 29–30.
2. Bosman YK, Foster PA. Endotracheal intubation and head posture in infants. *South Afr Med J* 1977; **52**: 71–8.
3. Scoble MK, Copnell B, Taylor A *et al.* Effect of reusing suction catheters on the occurrence of pneumonia in children. *Heart Lung* 2001; **30**: 225–33.
4. Carter BG, Fairbank B, Tibballs J *et al.* Oxygen delivery using self-inflating resuscitation bags. *Pediatr Crit Care Med* 2005; **6**: 125–8.
5. Branson RD, Hess DR, Chatburn RL. *Respiratory Care Equipment.* Philadelphia: Lippincott Williams and Wilkins; 1999.
6. Abrahams N, Fisk GC, Vonwiller JB *et al.* Evaluation of infant ventilators. *Anaesth Intensive Care* 1975; **3**: 6–11.
7. Simbruner G, Gregory GA. Performance of neonatal ventilators: the effects of changes in resistance and compliance. *Crit Care Med* 1981; **9**: 509–14.
8. Reynolds EOR, Taghizadeh A. Improved prognosis of infants mechanically ventilated for hyaline membrane disease. *Arch Dis Child* 1974; **49**: 505.
9. Greenough A, Milner AD. Respiratory support using patient triggered ventilation in the neonatal period. *Arch Dis Child* 1992; **67**: 69–71.
10. South M, Morley CJ. Respiratory timing in intubated neonates with respiratory distress syndrome. *Arch Dis Child* 1992; **67**: 446–8.
11. Hird MF, Greenough A. Patient triggered ventilation using a flow triggered system. *Arch Dis Child* 1991; **66**: 1140–2.
12. Cleary JP, Bernstein G, Mannino FL *et al.* Improved oxygenation during synchronized intermittent mandatory ventilation in neonates with respiratory distress syndrome: a randomized, crossover study. *J Pediatr* 1995; **126**: 407–11.
13. Ogawa Y, Miyasaka K, Kawano T *et al.* A multicenter randomized trial of high frequency oscillatory ventilation as compared with conventional mechanical ventilation in preterm infants with respiratory failure. *Early Human Dev* 1993; **32**: 1–10.
14. HiFO study group. Randomized study of high-frequency oscillatory ventilation in infants with severe respiratory distress syndrome. *J Pediatr* 1993; **122**: 609–19.
15. Shann F, Gatachalian S, Hutchinson R. Nasopharyngeal oxygen in children. *Lancet* 1988; **2**: 1238–40.
16. Cole AGH. Small oxygen analysers. *Br J Hosp Med* 1983; **29**: 469–71.
17. Martin RJ, Robertson SS, Hopple MM. Relationship between transcutaneous and arterial oxygen tension in sick neonates during mild hyperoxaemia. *Crit Care Med* 1982; **10**: 670–2.
18. Tremper KK, Shoemaker WC, Shippy CR *et al.* Transcutaneous oxygen monitoring of critically ill adults with and without low flow shock. *Crit Care Med* 1981; **9**: 706–9.
19. Tremper KK, Shoemaker WC, Shippy CR *et al.* Transcutaneous PCO_2 monitoring on adult patients in the ICU and operating room. *Crit Care Med* 1981; **9**: 752–5.
20. Carter BG, Carlin JB, Tibballs J *et al.* Accuracy of two pulse oximeters at low arterial hemoglobin–oxygen saturation. *Crit Care Med* 1998; **26**: 1128–33.
21. Brown LW. Home monitoring of the high-risk infant. *Clin Pediatr* 1984; **11**: 85–100.
22. Hull D, Chellappah G. On keeping babies warm. In: Chiswick ML (ed) *Recent Advances in Perinatal Medicine.* Edinburgh: Churchill Livingstone; 1983: 153–68.
23. Bell EF, Rios GR. Performance characteristics of two double-walled infant incubators. *Crit Care Med* 1983; **11**: 663–7.
24. Holbrook PR, Taylor G, Pollak MM *et al.* Adult respiratory distress syndrome in children. *Pediatr Clin North Am* 1980; **27**: 677–85.
25. Shyam VSR, Tinker J. Recent developments in infusion devices. *Br J Hosp Med* 1981; **25**: 69–75.
26. Dickenson JR. Syringe pumps. *Br J Hosp Med* 1983; **29**: 187–91.
27. Weiss M, Banziger O, Neff T *et al.* Influence of infusion line compliance on drug delivery rate during acute line loop formation. *Intensive Care Med* 2000; **26**: 776–9.
28. Lui K, Doyle PE, Buchanan N. Oscillometric and intra-arterial blood pressure measurements in the neonates: evaluation and comparison of methods. *Aust Paediatr J* 1982; **18**: 32–4.
29. Savage JM, Dillon MJ, Taylor JFN. Clinical evaluation and comparison of the infrasonde, arteriosonde and mercury sphygmomanometer in measurements of blood pressure in children. *Arch Dis Child* 1979; **54**: 184–9.
30. Showman A, Betts EK. Hazard of automatic noninvasive blood pressure monitoring. *Anesthesiology* 1981; **55**: 717–19.

105

Paediatric poisoning

James Tibballs

EPIDEMIOLOGY

The peak incidence of poisoning in childhood is among 1–4 year olds. It usually occurs in the home when the child ingests a single prescribed or over-the-counter medication or a household product. Approximately 3500 young children are admitted to hospital each year in Australia.[1] This mode of poisoning is called 'accidental' – erroneously because it is usually the result of inadequate supervision or improper storage of poisons. The mortality is very low and if hospitalisation is required, it is usually brief (1–3 days). In this circumstance, care must be taken to ensure that whatever treatment is applied, it does not impose additional risk.

Occasionally, poisoning in childhood is either truly accidental as in ingestion of a decanted chemical, or is part of a syndrome of child abuse (Munchausen syndrome by proxy), or is iatrogenic as when a parent mistakes medications at home or when medical or nursing staff make errors in drug administration in hospital. Medication errors occur in approximately 5% of paediatric inpatient medication.[2] Self-poisoning in older children is usually with the intention to manipulate their psychosocial environment or to commit suicide, or is the result of substance abuse. All circumstances of poisoning require remedial action.

DIAGNOSIS

Commonly, the diagnosis of poisoning in paediatric practice is self-evident and supported by a history detailed by parents or guardians. Although a single poison is usually involved, the possibility of several or multiple poisons should be considered. Occasionally the diagnosis is unknown on presentation. Any child who presents with unexplained obtundation, fitting, hypoventilation, hypotension or has a metabolic derangement should have the diagnosis excluded.

A knowledge of important poisons is indispensable. A number of poisons or classes of poison are potentially fatal to a small child if taken as a single tablet or a teaspoonful. These include opiates (methadone, buprenorphine, lomotil), camphor, quinine derivatives, cyclic antidepressants, clonidine, sulphonylureas, salicylates and calcium channel blockers.[3]

OPTIONS FOR TREATMENT

The treatment should be determined by the poison, severity of poisoning as judged by the observed and expected effects of the poison, by the amount ingested, by the interval between ingestion and presentation and by the existence or otherwise of an antidote.

The range of treatment options is to: discharge home, observe for a short duration in the emergency department or ward, provide intensive nursing care or to treat medically. The task is to match the intensity of treatment to the severity of the poisoning, thereby avoiding under- and overtreatment.

PRINCIPLES OF MANAGEMENT

The four basic principles in management of poisoning are:

- support vital functions
- confirm the diagnosis
- remove the poison from the body
- administer an antidote. Few poisons have antidotes (Table 105.1).

Individual poisons may require specific measures. Consult toxicology texts[4–6] for details.

The vast majority of poisoning in childhood is by ingestion. The correct choice of a gastrointestinal decontamination technique is crucial to uncomplicated recovery. The choices are induced emesis, gastric lavage, activated charcoal, whole-bowel irrigation or a combination of these techniques. The efficacy, indications, contraindications and disadvantages and complications of these techniques are discussed below. A general plan of management is presented in Figure 105.1.

A crucial point in management is initial recognition that the patient is in a state of either 'full-consciousness' or 'less-than-full consciousness'. Traditionally, management has been dependent on a judgement of whether the gag reflex is present or absent, but in practice this is rarely tested. Since aspiration pneumonitis is a common feature of poisoning management, particularly among (but not confined to) CNS obtunded patients, it is prudent to regard all obtunded patients as having incompetent pharyngeal reflexes.

Table 105.1 Antidotes to some serious poisons

Poison	Antidotes	Comments
Amfetamines	Esmolol i.v. 500 μg/kg over 1 min, then 25–200 μg/kg per min Labetalol i.v. 0.15–0.3 mg/kg or phentolamine i.v. 0.05–0.1 mg/kg every 10 minutes	Treatment for tachyarrhythmia Treatment for hypertension
Benzodiazepines	Flumazenil i.v. 3–10 μg/kg, repeat 1 minute, then 3–10 μ/kg per hour	Specific receptor antagonist. Beware convulsions
β-Blockers	Glucagon i.v. 7 μg/kg, then 2–7 μg/kg per min Isoprenaline i.v. 0.05–3 μg/kg per min Noradrenaline i.v. 0.05–1 μg/kg per min	Stimulates non-catecholamine cAMP (preferred antidote) Beware β_2 hypotension Antagonises at receptors
Calcium channel blocker	Calcium chloride i.v. 10%, 0.2 ml/kg	Antagonises at receptors
Carbon monoxide	Oxygen 100%	Decreases carboxyhaemoglobin. May need hyperbaric oxygen
Cyanide	Dicobalt edetate i.v. 4–7.5 mg/kg Hydroxocobalamin (vitamin B_{12}) i.v. 70 mg/kg Amyl nitrite 0.2 ml perles by inhalation until sodium nitrite 3% i.v. 0.13–0.33 ml/kg over 4 min, then sodium thiosulphate 25% i.v. 1.65 ml/kg (max 50 ml) at 3–5 minutes	Give 50 ml 50% glucose after dose Beware anaphylaxis, hypertension Beware hypotension. Nitrites form methaemoglobin–cyanide complex. Beware excess methaemoglobin >20%. Thiosulphate forms non-toxic thiocyanate from methaemoglobin–cyanide
Digoxin	Magnesium sulphate i.v. 25–50 mg/kg (0.1–0.2 mmol/kg) Digoxin Fab i.v: acute – 10 vials per 25 tablets (0.25 mg each), 10 vials per 5 mg elixir; steady state: vials, serum digoxin(ng/ml) × BW(kg)/100	Antagonises digoxin at sarcolemma Binds digoxin
Ergotamine	Sodium nitroprusside infusion 0.5–5.0 μg/kg per min Heparin i.v. 100 units/kg then 10–30 units/kg per hour	Treats vasoconstriction. Monitor BP continuously Monitor partial thromboplastin time
Lead	Dimercaprol (BAL) i.m. 75 mg/m² 4-hourly, six doses, then i.v. $CaNa_2$ edetate (EDTA) 1500 mg/m² over 5 days if blood level >3.38 μmol/l If asymptomatic and blood level 2.65–3.3 μmol/l, infuse $CaNa_2$EDTA 1000 mg/m² per day 5 days or oral succimer 350 mg/m² 8-hourly 5 days, then 12-hourly 14 days	Chelating agents
Heparin	Protamine 1 mg/100 units heparin	Direct neutralisation
Iron	Desferrioxamine 15 mg/kg per hour 12–24 hours if serum iron >90 μmol/l (500 μg/dl) or >63 μmol/l (350 μg/dl) and symptomatic	Give slowly, beware anaphylaxis
Methanol, ethylene glycol, glycol ethers	Ethanol i.v. loading dose 10 ml/kg 10% diluted in glucose 5%, then 0.15 ml/kg per hour to maintain blood level 0.1% (100 mg/dl) Fomepizole (4-methylpyrazole) 15 mg/kg over 30 minutes, then 10 mg/kg 12-hourly, four doses. (Not available in Australia)	Competes with poison for alcohol dehydrogenase Inhibits alcohol dehydrogenase
Methaemoglobinaemia	Methylene blue i.v. 1–2 mg/kg over several minutes	Reduces methaemoglobin to haemoglobin
Opiates	Naloxone i.v. 0.01–0.1 mg/kg, then 0.01 mg/kg per hour as needed	Direct receptor antagonist

Continued

Table 105.1 Antidotes to some serious poisons—*Continued*

Poison	Antidotes	Comments
Organophosphates and carbamates	Atropine i.v. 20–50 μg/kg every 15 minutes until secretions dry Pralidoxime i.v. 25 mg/kg over 15–30 minutes then 10–20 mg/kg per hour for 18 hours or more. Not for carbamates	Blocks muscarinic effects Reactivates cholinesterase
Paracetamol	*N*-acetylcysteine i.v. 150 mg/kg in dextrose 5% over 60 minutes then 10 mg/kg per hour for 20–72 hours OR oral 140 mg/kg then 17 doses of 70 mg/kg 4-hourly (total 1330 mg/kg over 68 hours)	Restores glutathione inhibiting metabolites. Give if serum paracetamol exceeds 1500 μmol/l at 2 hours, 1000 at 4 hours, 500 at 8 hours, 200 at 12 hours, 80 at 16 hours, 40 at 20 hours. Beware anaphylaxis
Phenothiazine dystonia	Benzatropine i.v or i.m. 0.01–0.03 mg/kg	Blocks dopamine reuptake
Potassium	Calcium chloride 10% i.v. 0.2 ml/kg Sodium bicarbonate i.v. 1 mmol/kg Glucose i.v. 0.5 g/kg plus insulin i.v. 0.05 units/kg Salbutamol aerosol 0.25 mg/kg Resonium oral or rectal 0.5–1 g/kg	Antagonises cardiac effects Decreases serum potassium (slight effect). Beware hypocalcaemia Decreases serum potassium (rapid marked effect). Monitor serum glucose Decreases serum potassium (rapid marked effect) Absorbs potassium (slow effect)
Sulphonyl ureas	Glucose Octreotide 1–2 μg/kg 8-hourly	Inhibits insulin release
Tricyclic antidepressants	Sodium bicarbonate i.v. 1 mmol/kg to maintain blood pH >7.45	Reduces cardiotoxicity

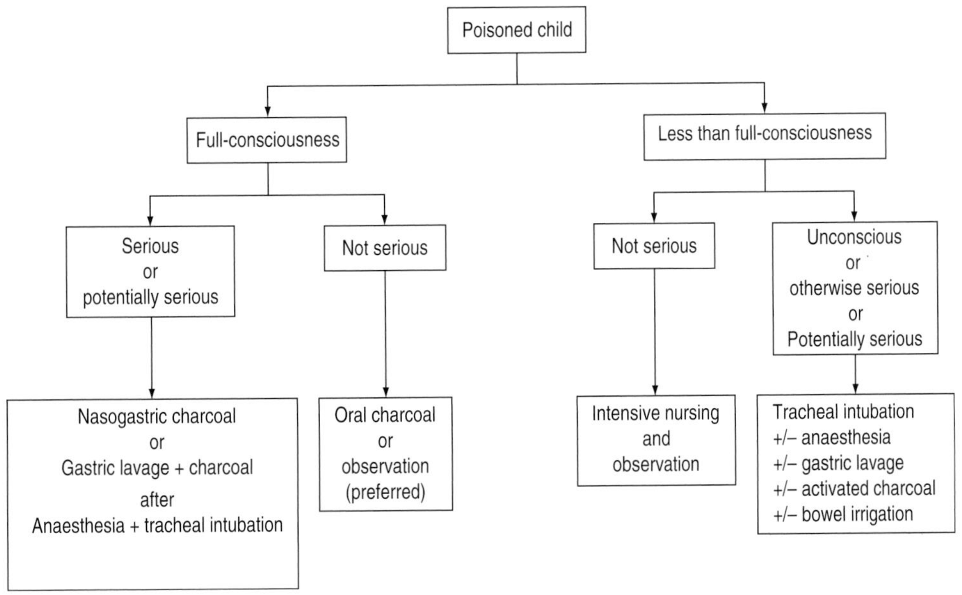

Figure 105.1 General management of the poisoned child.

The decision to attempt removal of a poison should always be made with due reference to two facts:

- The vast majority of childhood poisonings recover with merely supportive care or no treatment at all
- Aspiration pneumonitis is more serious than most poisonings

Occasionally, removal from the circulation by charcoal haemoperfusion, plasmafiltration or haemofiltration is indicated.

INDUCED EMESIS

Induced emesis is quickly disappearing from hospital practice and should not be performed routinely in this setting.[7] It does not improve outcome and may reduce effectiveness of the alternative treatments of activated charcoal, oral antidotes and whole-bowel irrigation.

Specific contraindications include actual or impending loss of full consciousness or ingestion of corrosives or hydrocarbons.[7]

Syrup of Ipecacuanha has superseded other more injurious substances as emetic agents. It contains alkaloids, mainly emetine and cephaeline, which induce emesis by stimulation of the chemoreceptor trigger zone of the medulla and by irritation of the gastric mucosa.

The efficacy of ipecacuanha (ipecac) is limited and decreases with time from ingestion. Although it causes vomiting in a high percentage (93–100%) of children within 25 minutes, the percentage of stomach contents ejected is small (28%) even when administered immediately after ingestion.[8] Moreover, solids are retained in the stomach or may even be propelled into the duodenum.[9]

In experimental drug ingestions, approximately 50–83% of ingested experimental drug is removed if ipecac is given after 5 minutes,[10] but falling to 2–44% if given at 30 or 60 minutes.[11–15] In paediatric paracetamol poisoning, the 4-hour postingestion serum level was approximately 50% of controls if ipecac-induced vomiting occurred within 60 minutes of ingestion, but no benefit was derived if emesis occurred beyond 90 minutes after ingestion.[16] Similarly, serum levels of paracetamol were reduced approximately 50% if ipecac was administered at home, inducing emesis at a mean of 26 minutes after ingestion, compared with ipecac administered at a medical facility at a mean of 83 minutes.[17]

In adults, ipecac is even less useful and has to be given immediately to have quantifiable effects.[18]

Induced emesis appears superior to gastric lavage but inferior to activated charcoal. In children poisoned with salicylate, emesis retrieved twice as much compared with gastric lavage.[19] In adult volunteers ipecac-induced vomiting, occurring at an average of 19 minutes after ingestion, removed 54% of a tracer compared with 30% with gastric lavage performed at the equivalent times after ingestion.[20–22]

The use of ipecac has potential complications:

- time-related lack of efficacy
- protracted vomiting (17%)
- diarrhoea (13%)
- lethargy (12%)[23]

More serious, but rare complications include:

- gastric, oesophageal or brain haemorrhage
- pneumomediastinum
- aspiration pneumonitis may occur, even in the fully conscious
- delayed onset of vomiting which is a threat if loss of consciousness subsequently occurs
- abuse in bulimia which may cause cardiotoxicity as well as the sequelae associated with repetitive vomiting

Critics claim that induced emesis merely creates work, delays discharge from the emergency department,[24] increases complications[24] and does not benefit the patient who presents more than 1 hour after ingestion.[25] Importantly, ipecac did not alter the clinical outcome of patients who presented awake and alert to the emergency department.[26]

Induced emesis has been largely abandoned by emergency departments but its use in the home is safe and is associated with fewer paediatric emergency department attendances.[27] Its use at home is still recommended by authoritative paediatric health organisations in the USA[28] and by approximately half of poison centre staff.[29] Although ipecac was recommended inappropriately in 20% of cases to poisons information centres, it caused little morbidity.[30]

CONCLUSION

In hospital, it has no practical role. Even when a child presents very early after significant poisoning, oral or nasogastric charcoal is preferred. Whenever induced emesis is used the child must be fully conscious on administration and expected to be fully conscious when vomiting occurs.

GASTRIC LAVAGE

Its place in the management of the poisoned victim has also been curtailed. It is an invasive technique with questionable efficacy. Moreover, it is potentially harmful and should be reserved for the child who presents soon after life-threatening poisoning such as ingestion of iron or colchicine.

It involves passage of a large bore oro- or nasogastric tube into the stomach and the repeated instillation of fluid, usually water but some authorities advocate normal or half-normal saline. The oral route is preferred because of less potential for traumatic injury but an oropharyngeal airway may be needed to prevent tube occlusion by chomping. A smaller tube may be used if the poison is a liquid. Traditionally, the child should be placed in the left lateral position to limit stomach emptying but volume of intragastric contents rather than body position determines gastric emptying.[31]

Experimental studies with therapeutic substances in volunteers, or with liquid medicines or substances instilled into the stomachs of overdose victims, reported that gastric lavage retrieved 90% at 5 minutes,[32] 45% at 10 minutes[21] and 30% at 19 minutes[20] and reduced absorption or bioavailability by 20–32% at 1 hour after ingestion.[11,33] When gastric lavage was performed 5 minutes after ingestion of tablet drugs, it failed to prevent absorption, presumedly because the tablets had not disintegrated.[34] In true overdose situations, gastric lavage within 4 hours of admission reduced serum paracetamol levels by 39%.[35]

Efficacy of gastric lavage, even with large bore tubes, is poor because tablets are not removed and lavage encourages propulsion into the duodenum.[8] In symptomatic patients, gastric lavage alone compared with gastric lavage and activated charcoal increased pneumonic aspiration and did not alter the duration of intubation or the stay in the emergency department or the intensive care unit (ICU),[36] and was not beneficial unless performed within 1 hour of ingestion.[26] A prospective randomised trial of gastric lavage in acute overdose,[37] although criticised on methodological grounds,[37,38] suggested that it made no difference to outcome of obtunded patients when preceding activated charcoal.

CONTRAINDICATIONS

- Less-than-full consciousness patient (unless already intubated) because of the risk of aspiration pneumonitis – which is not negligible even during full consciousness[36]
- After ingestion of corrosives because of the risk of perforation
- After ingestion of hydrocarbons or petrochemicals because of the risk of pneumonitis

COMPLICATIONS

- Aspiration pneumonitis
- Water intoxication
- Minor trauma to oropharynx (gastro-oesophageal perforation occurs rarely)
- Intrabronchial instillation of lavage fluid

As expected, infants and children never cooperate fully for gastric lavage, thus increasing risks of complications and the degree of psychological trauma.

If lavage is indicated, i.e. for life-threatening poisoning, rapid sequence induction of anaesthesia with intubation is advised. The largest possible lubricated tube of diameter similar to an appropriate sized endotracheal tube should be used and correct placement in the stomach confirmed. Small volumes (1–2 ml/kg) of warm tap water may be used to lavage until clear. However, most water should be retrieved to avoid hyponatraemia.

ACTIVATED CHARCOAL

Charcoal is a substance which adsorbs many drugs and is regarded as a 'universal antidote'. It is advocated as the sole treatment in most poisonings although it is overused for minor poisonings. For many poisons no data exist regarding efficacy.

Treatment of charcoal with chemicals and heat increases its surface area to approximately 950 m^2/g in so-called low surface area activated charcoal and to 2000 m^2/g in superactivated charcoal. The latter adsorbs paracetamol better[38] and is more palatable.[39,40] Activated charcoal is not pleasant to drink and was associated with vomiting in 20% of poisoned children.[41]

It is superior to induced emesis and gastric lavage in treatment of symptomatic poisoned patients.[22,26,36] Its efficacy diminishes with time after ingestion. Activated charcoal reduces absorption of ingested experimental drugs in volunteers by 85–100% when administered 5 minutes after ingestion,[10,34,42] by 40–75% at 30 minutes[9] and by 30–50% at 60 minutes.[14,42] At a mean time of 98 minutes (SD 44) or more than 2 hours after poisoning, it was not effective at all.[43,44]

Studies have suggested that charcoal alone is as effective as when combined with either emesis or with lavage.[37,38] Furthermore, combined methods have a higher incidence of aspiration, 8.5% versus none.[34] Activated charcoal failed to show a benefit in asymptomatic poisoned patients.

Repeated doses of activated charcoal enhance elimination of some drugs by increasing adsorption and by achieving postabsorption elimination by interrupting enterohepatic circulation and by removing drug from the gastrointestinal mucosa ('gastrointestinal dialysis'). Although there are multiple reports in experimental and clinical practice (Table 105.2), there is no hard evidence to show that this therapy reduces mortality or morbidity. Only in life-threatening poisoning by carbamazepine, dapsone, phenobarbital, quinine or theophylline should multiple-dose activated charcoal be considered.[45]

A suitable single dose is 1–2 g/kg. A multiple-dose regimen for children is 1–2 g/kg stat followed by 0.25–0.5 g/kg 4–6-hourly. An alternative is 0.25–0.5 g/kg hourly for 12–24 hours.[46]

CONTRAINDICATIONS

- If ileus is present
- A less-than-fully conscious patient unless already intubated
- Substances not adsorbed – for example, strong corrosive acids and alkalis, cyanide, metals (iron, lithium, mercury, lead), alcohols, glycols, petroleum distillates (not all) and essential oils[4–6]

Table 105.2 Elimination and lack of elimination of drugs by multiple dose activated charcoal[45]

Elimination increased in experimental and clinical studies	Elimination increased in volunteer studies	Elimination not increased in experimental or clinical studies
Carbamazepine	Amitriptyline	Astemizole
Dapsone	Dextropropoxyphene	Chlorpropamide
Phenobarbital	Digitoxin	Doxepin
Quinine	Digoxin	Imipramine
Theophylline	Disopyramide	Meprobamate
	Nadolol	Methotrexate
	Phenylbutazone	Phenytoin
	Phenytoin	Sodium valproate
	Piroxicam	Tobramycin
	Sotalol	Vancomycin

See text for details.

COMPLICATIONS

Aspiration of charcoal causes severe and often fatal pneumonitis, bronchiolitis obliterans and adult respiratory distress syndrome. Intratracheal instillation of activated charcoal causes a significant increase in lung microvascular permeability and arterial blood gas derangements.[47]

Constipation is common after charcoal but bowel obstruction is fortunately rare. The addition of a laxative (e.g. sorbitol or magnesium sulphate) is not recommended because although transit time through the gut is decreased, efficacy of the charcoal is reduced and life-threatening fluid and electrolyte imbalance may occur.[48]

WHOLE-BOWEL IRRIGATION

Irrigation of the bowel with an iso-osmolar solution of polyethylene glycol and electrolytes is effective in reducing absorption of experimental drug by 24–67% at 1 hour after ingestion[49,50] and up to 73% at 4 hours after ingestion.[51] However, it has not been shown conclusively to improve the outcome of poisoned patients. The technique has limited applications to sustained-release or enteric-coated drugs and remains a theoretical option for ingestions of iron, lead, zinc (substances not adsorbed by activated charcoal), packets of illicit drugs[52] and for lithium.[53] Whole-bowel irrigation may be useful in delayed presentations when poisons have progressed beyond the stomach.

Irrigation solutions are adsorbed by activated charcoal and cause desorption of drug – necessitating prior administration of charcoal if a combined technique is used.[54] However, whole-bowel irrigation did not add to the benefits of activated charcoal in an experimental model of sustained-release theophylline poisoning.[55]

A suitable regimen is approximately 30 ml/kg per hour for 4–8 hours until rectal effluent is clear. A regimen of 25 ml/kg per hour has been used safely for 5 days (total 44.3 litres),[56] but a total of 3 litres performed as well as 8 litres in a simulated poisoning.[57]

CONTRAINDICATIONS

Risk of aspiration during:

- less-than-full consciousness
- bowel obstruction or ileus

PLAN OF MANAGEMENT

A general plan of management is suggested in Figure 105.1, but each case of poisoning mandates a specific plan of management according to circumstances. The primary determinant is the state of consciousness which relates to the risk of aspiration. Apart from that, the timing of presentation in relation to the severity of poisoning and the existence or otherwise of an effective antidote dictate if removal should be attempted, and by what means.

POISONING BY SPECIFIC SUBSTANCES

Like adults, children are poisoned regularly by therapeutic prescription or over-the-counter therapeutic drugs and substances. The poisons probably reflect their availability in the home. In a survey, the most common agents responsible for hospital admission were benzodiazepines, anticonvulsants, anti-parkinsonism drugs, paracetamol, major tranquillisers, antidepressants and cardiovascular drugs.[58] The inquisitive nature of young children, however, may lead to poisoning by substances not normally regarded as dangerous – a few of these and others which have notably different management from similar poisoning in adults are considered here, briefly.

BUTTON OR DISC BATTERIES

Ingestion may cause electrolytic injury and potentially corrosive, toxic or pressure injury. There are many types of batteries that contain a variety of substances: the most important are lithium, mercury and potassium hydroxide.

Impaction in the oesophagus is the most significant situation; this can result in oesophageal perforation and tracheo-oesophageal fistula or aorto-oesophageal fistula. An impacted battery must be removed endoscopically as soon as possible. Lithium batteries are large and impact readily and they have higher voltages than other types. Electrolysis commences as soon as the battery surfaces are immersed in oesophageal fluid. The consequence is local and surrounding tissue destruction, including the trachea.[59] Strong alkali is produced at the cathode and strong acid is produced at the anode. Mercury batteries are more likely to fragment[60] but mercury poisoning is very uncommon.

Sufficient follow-up is necessary to exclude oesophageal and tracheal damage and to ensure that a battery in the stomach or distal bowel is eliminated.

PETROLEUM DISTILLATES

Numerous by-products of petroleum distillation are utilised in industrial and domestic purposes. Ingestion of these hydrocarbons may cause CNS toxicity (comprising obtundation and convulsion), gastrointestinal irritation, occasional hepatorenal toxicity, and pneumonitis.

Pneumonitis is the most significant and it may occur during ingestion or subsequent vomiting. Although variable, these substances have low surface tensions which enable their rapid dispersement throughout contiguous mucosal surfaces which include the respiratory tree. Prime examples are petrol, kerosene, lighter fluid, lamp oil and mineral spirits. Any child who ingests a distillate must be assessed for pneumonitis and this should include clinical examination, a chest X-ray and at least a non-invasive measurement of oxygenation such as pulse oximetry. Although most children who ingest petroleum distillates do not develop pneumonitis, the onset of this complication may be within 30 minutes[61] and progress rapidly to severe lung disease. An adequate period of observation (6 hours) is necessary to exclude this complication. There is a poor correlation between the amount ingested and the severity of pulmonary toxicity.

Deliberate inhalation of volatile hydrocarbons such as petrol or aerosolised paint has the additional toxicity on myocardial tissue, including fatal tachydysrhythmia, possibly due to sensitisation to endogenous catecholamines. The deliberate inhalation of paint fumes, usually via a plastic bag, is called 'chroming'.

ESSENTIAL OILS

The oils from certain plants contain mixtures of terpenes, alcohols, aldehydes, ketones and esters, which are used domestically for various purposes. The well-known oils are eucalyptus, turpentine, citronella, cloves, melaleuca, peppermint, wintergreen and lavender. In general, small amounts cause depression of conscious state, irritation of gastrointestinal tract, liver dysfunction and pneumonitis if inhaled. Each has different toxicity. For example, as little as 5 ml of eucalyptus oil[62] or 15 ml of turpentine may cause depression of conscious state.

Emesis should not be induced and gastric lavage performed only if airway protection is required.

LEAD

Children are more susceptible to lead poisoning after ingestion than are adults, possibly because of better absorption.

Acute poisoning usually occurs after ingestion of a lead salt or metallic foreign body or a lead-containing product, such as paint or traditional remedy or cosmetic. Acute poisoning by a salt may cause life-supporting cardiovascular collapse, and encephalopathy.

Chronic poisoning can occur with ingestion of lead-contaminated water, or by inhalation of leaded petrol fumes or contaminated house dust. Chronic poisoning causes multiorgan dysfunction including neuromuscular dysfunction and encephalopathy.

Treatment consists of gastric decontamination in the case of recent ingestion of lead salts. The use of chelating agents may be indicated. In the case of ingestion of a lead foreign body, serial X-rays should be taken to ensure elimination, otherwise surgical removal is indicated. In the case of multiple embedded gunshot pellets and in all cases of chronic poisoning, serum lead levels should be measured to guide chelation therapy (see Table 105.1).

PARACETAMOL

This is the most common drug ingested by children in an accidental, iatrogenic or deliberate overdose situation. Overdose has the potential for hepatic failure and, less commonly, renal failure. The onset of toxicity is delayed – up to several days. Consequently, the need for acute gastric decontamination is uncommon, but would be justifiable for acute large dose presentations. The toxicity in part is caused by the hepatic metabolite of the drug (*N*-acetyl-*p*-benzoquinoneimine) which accumulates when endogenous glutathione, which normally facilitates conversion of *N*-acetyl-*p*-benzoquinoneimine to non-toxic substances, becomes exhausted. Adequate supply of glutathione is ensured by administration of the antidote, *N*-acetylcysteine, a glutathione precursor which can be administered intravenously or orally (see Table 105.1).

The time of presentation after ingestion, as well as the dose, determines the management. If presentation is within 1 hour of ingestion, effective gastric removal or administration of activated charcoal may be all that is required pending a serum paracetamol level. In contrast, if presentation is several hours after ingestion, administration of the antidote, according to serum paracetamol level, takes precedence and although it may be administered orally or intravenously, the intravenous route is preferred.[63] Near-simultaneous administration of activated charcoal may be of some benefit but it may also cause vomiting or desorption, thus decreasing the effectiveness of the antidote. If presentation is many hours after the poisoning, activated charcoal would not be indicated, so the antidote could be administered orally if necessary according to serum paracetamol levels. In all cases, evidence of liver dysfunction mandates administration of the antidote.

The threshold single toxic dose of paracetamol indicating *N*-acetylcysteine administration is generally regarded as 150 mg/kg, although it has been suggested that a single dose less than 200 mg/kg in children less than 6 years of age may be safely managed at home.[64] However, in situations of repeated sub-150 mg/kg doses hepatotoxicity has a high mortality among children[65] and in adults.[66] Unfortunately, toxic overdosing by chronic administration is not uncommon even in paediatric institutions.[67]

No sufficient data exist on which to firmly base a decision to administer *N*-acetylcysteine to children. Time-related serum levels of paracetamol should be measured and reference made to a guideline to administer the antidote (see Table 105.1) as derived from single toxic dose adult data.[68] The serum paracetamol level indicating antidote has been predicted as > 225 mg/l (1500 μmol/l) at 2 hours after ingestion of a single overdose of elixir in children 1–5 years of age.[43] If serum levels of paracetamol cannot be obtained and > 150 mg/kg has been ingested as a single dose or liver dysfunction is present after chronic poisoning, the antidote should be given.

Adverse reactions to *N*-acetylcysteine (approximately 8%) respond to an antihistamine[69] and its temporary cessation.

IRON

Small quantities of elemental iron (> 20 mg/kg) are toxic to children. This dose may be reached by ingestion of few iron tablets. The initial effects are gastrointestinal, which may include gastric erosion, followed sometimes by an interval before cardiovascular failure occurs at 6–24 hours and then followed by multiorgan failure (including encephalopathy) and hepatic and renal failure up to some 48 hours after ingestion. In addition to general supportive measures, specific management should include abdominal X-ray to determine if unabsorbed tablets are present, in which case gastric lavage or whole-bowel irrigation may be useful. Activated charcoal is useless. Chelation therapy with desferrioxamine (see Table 105.1) should be guided by serum iron level and clinical status.

CAUSTIC SUBSTANCES

In a study of 743 children,[70] the incidence of oesophageal burns caused by ingestion of automatic machine dishwashing detergents was 59%, caustic soda 55% and drain cleaners 55%. All are strongly alkaline and are corrosive. Dishwasher detergents are presented as liquids, powders or tablet blocks and are commonly accessed in an open dishwasher.[71] Pharyngeal and oesophageal irritation, burns or corrosion may occur. There may be simultaneous ocular and dermal toxicity. Any child presenting with a history of ingestion of a caustic substance, irrespective of clinical signs, should be considered for oesophagoscopy and follow-up since the correlation between symptoms and signs and oesophageal burns is poor[70] and significant oesophageal damage may occur in the absence of more proximal injury.[72]

REFERENCES

1. Cripps R, Steel D. Childhood poisoning in Australia. Australian Government, Australian Institute of Health and Welfare. http://www.nisu.flinders.edu.au/pubs/reports/2006/injcat90.php.
2. Kaushal R, Bates DW, Landrigan C *et al.* Medication errors and adverse drug events in paediatric inpatients. *JAMA* 2001; **285**: 2114–20.
3. Michael JB, Sztajnkrycer MD. Deadly pediatric poisons: nine common agents that kill at low doses. *Emerg Med Clin North Am* 2004; **22**: 1019–50.
4. Haddad LM, Shannon MW, Winchester JF. *Clinical Management of Poisoning and Drug Overdose*, 3rd edn. Philadelphia: WB Saunders; 1998.
5. Ellenhorn MJ, Schonwald S, Ordog G *et al. Ellenhorn's Medical Toxicology*, 2nd edn. Baltimore: Williams and Wilkins; 1997.
6. Bates N, Edwards N, Roper J *et al. Paediatric Toxicology.* London: Macmillan; 1997.
7. Krenzelok EP, McGuigan M, Lheur P. Position statement: ipecac syrup. American Academy of Clinical Toxicology; European Associations of Poisons Centres and Clinical Toxicologists. *J Toxicol Clin Toxicol* 1997; **35**: 699–709.
8. Corby DG, Decker WJ, Moran MJ *et al.* Clinical comparisons of pharmacologic emetics in children. *Pediatrics* 1968; **4**: 361–4.
9. Saetta JP, March S, Gaunt ME *et al.* Gastric emptying procedures in the self-poisoned patient: are we forcing gastric content beyond the pylorus? *J Roy Soc Med* 1991; **84**: 274–6.
10. Neuvonen PJ, Vartiainen M, Tokola O. Comparison of activated charcoal and ipecac syrup in prevention of drug absorption. *Eur J Clin Pharmacol* 1983; **24**: 557–62.
11. Tenenbein M, Cohen S, Sitar DS. Efficacy of ipecac-induced emesis, orogastric lavage, and activated charcoal for acute drug overdose. *Ann Emerg Med* 1987; **16**: 838–41.
12. Curtis RA, Barone J, Giacona N. Efficacy of ipecac and activated charcoal/cathartic. Prevention of salicylate absorption in a simulated overdose. *Arch Intern Med* 1984; **144**: 48–52.
13. Danel V, Henry JA, Glucksman E. Activated charcoal, emesis, and gastric lavage in aspirin overdose. *BMJ* 1988; **296**: 1507.
14. McNamara RM, Aaron CK, Gemborys M *et al.* Efficacy of charcoal cathartic versus ipecac in reducing serum acetaminophen in a simulated overdose. *Ann Emerg Med* 1989; **18**: 934–8.

15. Vasquez TE, Evans DG, Ashburn WL. Efficacy of syrup of ipecac-induced emesis for emptying gastric contents. *Clin Nucl Med* 1988; **13**: 638–9.
16. Bond GR, Requa RK, Krenzelok EP *et al.* Influence of time until emesis on the efficacy of decontamination using acetaminophen as a marker in a pediatric population. *Ann Emerg Med* 1993; **22**: 1403–7.
17. Amitai Y, Mitchell AA, McGuigan MA *et al.* Ipecac-induced emesis and reduction of plasma concentrations of drugs following accidental overdose in children. *Pediatrics* 1987; **80**: 364–7.
18. Saincher A, Sitar DS, Tenenbein M. Efficacy of ipecac during the first hour after drug ingestion in human volunteers. *J Toxicol Clin Toxicol* 1997; **35**: 609–15.
19. Boxer L, Anderson FP, Rowe MD. Comparison of ipecac-induced emesis with gastric lavage in the treatment of acute salicylate ingestion. *Ped Pharmacol Ther* 1969; **74**: 800–3.
20. Young WF Jr, Bivins HG. Evaluation of gastric emptying using radionuclides: gastric lavage versus ipecac-induced emesis. *Ann Emerg Med* 1993; **22**: 1423–7.
21. Tandberg D, Diven BG, McLeod JW. Ipecac-induced emesis versus gastric lavage: a controlled study in normal adults. *Am J Emerg Med* 1986; **4**: 205–9.
22. Albertson TE, Derlet RW, Foulke GE *et al.* Superiority of activated charcoal alone with ipecac and activated charcoal in the treatment of acute toxic ingestions. *Ann Emerg Med* 1989; **18**: 56–9.
23. Czajka PA, Russell SL. Nonemetic effects of ipecac syrup. *Pediatrics* 1985; **75**: 1101–4.
24. Kornberg AE, Dolgin J. Pediatric ingestions: charcoal alone versus ipecac and charcoal. *Ann Emerg Med* 1991; **20**: 648–51.
25. Foulke GE, Albertson TE, Derlet RW. Use of ipecac increases emergency department stays and patient complication rates. *Ann Emerg Med* 1990; **17**: 402.
26. Kulig K, Bar-Or D, Cantrill SV *et al.* Management of acutely poisoned patients without gastric emptying. *Ann Emerg Med* 1985; **14**: 562–7.
27. Bond GR. Home use of syrup of ipecac is associated with a reduction in pediatric emergency department visits. *Ann Emerg Med* 1995; **25**: 338–43.
28. Manoguerra AS, Cobaugh DJ, Guidelines for the Management of Poisoning Consensus Panel. Guidelines on the use of ipecac syrup in the out-of-hospital management of ingested poisons. *Clin Toxicol* 2005; **43**: 1–10.
29. Marchbanks B, Lockman P, Shum S *et al.* Trends in ipecac use: a survey of poison center staff. *Vet Hum Toxicol* 1999; **41**: 47–9.
30. Wrenn K, Rodewald L, Dockstader L. Potential misuse of ipecac. *Ann Emerg Med* 1993; **22**: 1408–12.
31. Doran S, Jones KL, Andrews JM *et al.* Effects of meal volume and posture on gastric emptying of solids and appetite. *Am J Physiol* 1998; **275**: R1712–8.
32. Auerbach PS, Osterich J, Braun O *et al.* Efficacy of gastric emptying: gastric lavage versus emesis induced with ipecac. *Ann Emerg Med* 1986; **15**: 692–8.
33. Grierson R, Green R, Sitar DS *et al.* Gastric lavage for liquid poisons. *Ann Emerg Med* 2000; **35**: 435–9.
34. Lapatto-Reiniluoto O, Kivisto KT, Neuvonen PJ. Gastric decontamination performed 5 min after ingestion of temazepam, verapamil and moclobemide: charcoal is superior to lavage. *Br J Clin Pharmacol* 2000; **49**: 274–8.
35. Underhill TJ, Greene MK, Dove AF. A comparison of the efficacy of gastric lavage, ipecacuanha and activated charcoal in the emergency management of paracetamol overdose. *Arch Emerg Med* 1990; **7**: 148–54.
36. Merigian KS, Woodard M, Hedges JR *et al.* Prospective evaluation of gastric emptying in the self-poisoned patient. *Am J Emerg Med* 1990; **8**: 479–83.
37. Pond SM, Lewis-Driver DJ, Williams GM *et al.* Gastric emptying in acute overdose: a prospective randomised controlled trial. *Med J Aust* 1995; **163**: 345–9.
38. Whyte IM, Buckley NA. Progress in clinical toxicology: from case reports to toxicoepidemiology. *Med J Aust* 1995; **163**: 340–1.
39. Roberts JR, Gracely EJ, Schoffstall JM. Advantage of high-surface-area charcoal for gastrointestinal decontamination in a human acetaminophen ingestion model. *Acad Emerg Med* 1997; **4**: 167–74.
40. Fischer TF, Singer AJ. Comparison of the palatabilities of standard and superactivated charcoal in toxic ingestions: a randomized trial. *Acad Emerg Med* 1999; **6**: 895–9.
41. Osterhoudt KC, Durbin K, Alpern ER *et al.* Risk factors for emesis after therapeutic use of activated charcoal in acutely poisoned children. *Pediatrics* 2004; **113**: 806–10.
42. Neuvonen PJ, Elonen E. Effect of activated charcoal on absorption and elimination of phenobarbitone, carbamazepine and phenylbutazone in man. *Eur J Clin Pharmacol* 1980; **17**: 51–7.
43. Anderson BJ, Holford NHG, Armishaw JC *et al.* Predicting concentrations in children presenting with acetaminophen overdose. *J Pediatr* 1999; **135**: 290–5.
44. Yeates PJ, Thomas SH. Effectiveness of delayed activated charcoal administration in simulated paracetamol (acetaminophen) overdose. *Br J Clin Pharmacol* 2000; **49**: 11–14.
45. Anonymous. Position statement and practice guidelines on the use of multi-dose activated charcoal in the treatment of acute poisoning. American Academy of Clinical Toxicology; European Association of Poisons Centres and Clinical Toxicologists. *J Toxicol Clin Toxicol* 1999; **37**: 731–51.
46. Ohning BL, Reed MD, Blumer JL. Continuous nasogastric administration of activated charcoal for the treatment of theophylline intoxication. *Ped Pharmacol* 1986; **5**: 241–5.
47. Arnold TC, Willis BH, Xiao F *et al.* Aspiration of activated charcoal elicits an increase in lung microvascular permeability. *J Toxicol Clin Toxicol* 1999; **37**: 9–16.
48. Palatnick W, Tenenbein M. Activated charcoal in the treatment of drug overdose. *Drug Safety* 1992; **7**: 3–17.

49. Smith SW, Ling LJ, Halstenson CE. Whole bowel irrigation as a treatment for acute lithium overdose. *Ann Emerg Med* 1991; **29**: 536–9.
50. Tenenbein M, Cohen S, Sitar DS. Whole bowel irrigation as a decontamination procedure after acute drug overdose. *Arch Intern Med* 1987; **147**: 905–7.
51. Kirshenbaum LA, Mathews SC, Sitar DS *et al.* Whole-bowel irrigation versus activated charcoal in sorbitol for the ingestion of modified-release pharmaceuticals. *Clin Pharmacol Ther* 1989; **46**: 264–71.
52. Tenenbein M. Position statement: whole bowel irrigation. American Academy of Clinical Toxicology; European Association of Poisons Centres and Clinical Toxicologists. *J Toxicol Clin Toxicol* 1997; **35**: 753–62.
53. Scharman EJ. Methods used to decrease lithium absorption or enhance elimination. *J Toxicol Clin Toxicol* 1997; **35**: 601–8.
54. Makosiej FJ, Hoffman RS, Howland MA *et al.* An in vitro evaluation of cocaine hydrochloride adsorption by activated charcoal and desorption upon addition of polyethylene glycol electrolyte lavage solution. *J Toxicol Clin Toxicol* 1993; **31**: 381–95.
55. Burkhart KK, Wuerz RC, Donovan JW. Whole bowel irrigation as adjunctive treatment for sustained-release theophylline overdose. *Ann Emerg Med* 1992; **21**: 1316–20.
56. Kaczorowski JM, Wax PM. Five days of whole-bowel irrigation in a case of pediatric iron ingestion. *Ann Emerg Med* 1996; **27**: 258–63.
57. Olsen KM, Gurley BJ, Davis GA *et al.* Comparison of fluid volumes with whole bowel irrigation in a simulated overdose of ibuprofen. *Ann Pharmacother* 1995; **29**: 246–50.
58. Hoy JL, Day LM, Tibballs J *et al.* Unintentional poisoning hospitalizations among young children in Victoria. *Inj Prev* 1999; **5**: 31–5.
59. Tibballs J, Wall R, Velandy Koottayi S *et al.* Tracheo-oesophageal fistula caused by electrolysis of a button battery impacted in the oesophagus. *J Paediatr Child Health* 2002; **38**: 201–3.
60. Litovitz T, Schmitz BF. Ingestion of cylindrical and button batteries: an analysis of 2382 cases. *Pediatrics* 1992; **89**: 747–57.
61. Anas N, Namasonthi V, Ginsburg CM Criteria for hospitalizing children who have ingested products containing hydrocarbons. *JAMA* 1981; **246**: 840–3.
62. Tibballs J. Clinical effects and management of eucalyptus oil ingestion in infants and young children. *Med J Aust* 1995; **163**: 177–80.
63. Buckley NA, Whyte IM, O'Connell DL *et al.* Oral or intravenous N-acetylcysteine: which is the treatment of choice for acetaminophen (paracetamol) poisoning? *J Toxicol Clin Toxicol* 1999; **37**: 759–67.
64. Bond GR, Krenzelok EP, Normann SA *et al.* Acetaminophen ingestion in childhood – cost and relative risk of alternative referral strategies. *J Toxicol Clin Toxicol* 1994; **32**: 513–25.
65. Heubi JE, Barbacci MB, Zimmerman HJ. Therapeutic misadventures with acetaminophen: hepatotoxicity after multiple doses in children. *J Pediatr* 1998; **132**: 22–7.
66. Schiodt FV, Rochling FA, Casey DL *et al.* Acetaminophen toxicity in an urban county hospital. *N Engl J Med* 1997; **337**: 1112–17.
67. Hynson JJ, South M. Childhood hepatotoxicity with paracetamol doses less than 150 mg/kg per day. *Med J Aust* 1999; **171**: 497.
68. Smilkstein MJ, Bronstein AC, Linden C *et al.* Acetaminophen overdose: a 48 hour intravenous N-acetylcysteine treatment protocol. *Ann Emerg Med* 1991; **20**: 1058–63.
69. Schmidt LE, Dalhoff K. Risk factors in the development of adverse reactions to N-acetylcysteine in patients with paracetamol poisoning. *Br J Pharmacol* 2001; **51**: 87–91.
70. Bautista Casasnovas A, Estevez Martinez E, Varela Cives R *et al.* A retrospective analysis of ingestion of caustic substances by children. Ten-year statistics in Galicia. *Eur J Pediatr* 1997; **156**: 410–14.
71. Cornish LS, Parsons BJ, Dobbin MD. Automatic dishwasher detergent poisoning: opportunities for prevention. *Aust N Z J Public Health* 1996; **20**: 278–83.
72. Krenzelok EP, Clinton JE. Caustic esophageal and gastric erosion without evidence of oral burns following detergent ingestion. *JACEP* 1979; **8**: 194–6.

106

Paediatric cardiopulmonary resuscitation

James Tibballs

This chapter concerns basic and advanced cardiopulmonary resuscitation (CPR) for infants and children (Figure 106.1). The essentials of resuscitation of the 'newly-born' (at birth) infant are also provided (Figure 106.2). The recommendations are based on guidelines published by several authoritative resuscitation organisations[1–3] which are in turn derived from an extensive evaluation of the science of resuscitation conducted by the International Liaison Committee on Resuscitation.[4]

This chapter is intended primarily for use by medical and nursing personnel in hospital (health carers). To add ability to knowledge, it is advisable to undertake a specialised paediatric cardiopulmonary resuscitation course, such as the Advanced Paediatric Life Support (APLS) or Paediatric Advanced Life Support (PALS) courses. This chapter should be regarded as an addendum to Chapters 17 (Adult cardiopulmonary resuscitation), 96 (The critically ill child) and 104 (Equipment for paediatric intensive care).

Distinctions within the term paediatric are based on combinations of physiology, physical size and age. Some aspects of CPR are different for the 'newly-born', infant, small (younger) child and large (older) child. 'Newly-born' refers to the infant at birth or within several hours of birth. 'Infant' refers to an infant outside the 'newly-born' period up to the age of 12 months. Other terms, such as newborn or neonate, do not enable that distinction. 'Small/young child' refers to a child of preschool and early primary school from the age of 1–8 years. 'Large/older child' refers to a child of late primary school from the age of 9 up to 14 years. Children older than 14 years may be treated as adults but they do not have the same propensity for ventricular fibrillation as do adults.

EPIDEMIOLOGY

The causes of cardiopulmonary arrest (CPA) in infants and children are many but include any cause of hypoxaemia or hypotension or both. Common causes are trauma (motor vehicle accidents, near-drowning, falls, burns, gunshot), drug overdose and poisoning, respiratory illness (asthma, upper-airway obstruction, parenchymal diseases), postoperative (especially cardiac), septicaemia and sudden infant death syndrome. As many as 10% of newly-born infants require some form of resuscitation for varied conditions of which birth asphyxia is the most common.

BASIC LIFE SUPPORT

ASSESSMENT OF AIRWAY AND BREATHING

On determining that the patient is not responsive to tactile and auditory stimulation, not breathing normally and not moving, airway opening manoeuvres and assessment of breathing should be performed. Assessment of the patient's airway and breathing can be performed effectively in either the supine or lateral position.

Obvious causes of airway obstruction in the pharynx should be removed. Fluids such as vomitus or blood should be aspirated with a Yankauer sucker. Solid or semi-solid objects, such as food particles or foreign objects, should be removed with an instrument, e.g. Magill's forceps. Since the most common cause of airway obstruction in an obtunded state is the tongue, first-aid manoeuvres to elevate it should be performed. The manoeuvres are backward head tilt, chin lift and jaw thrust. Head tilt and chin lift are often combined. If neck injury is present or suspected, neither the head tilt nor the chin lift manoeuvre should be used. Following establishment of an airway, the presence or absence of adequate breathing is assessed by inspection of movement of the chest and abdomen, and by listening and feeling for escape of exhaled air from the mouth and nose (look, listen and feel). If adequate breathing is occurring the patient should be placed on the side in a coma position.

RESCUE BREATHING (EXPIRED AIR RESUSCITATION)

If inadequate breathing is present, rescue breathing (expired air resuscitation) or bag-valve-mask ventilation should be commenced immediately. There is no evidence to dictate the number of initial breaths. However, at least two breaths are recommended by all resuscitation organisations, with some stating up to five. While maintaining the airway, slow breaths over 1–1.5 seconds should be given with enough air to achieve adequate chest inflation. In children of all sizes, a mouth-to-mouth technique is possible by pinching the nostrils closed. In newly-born

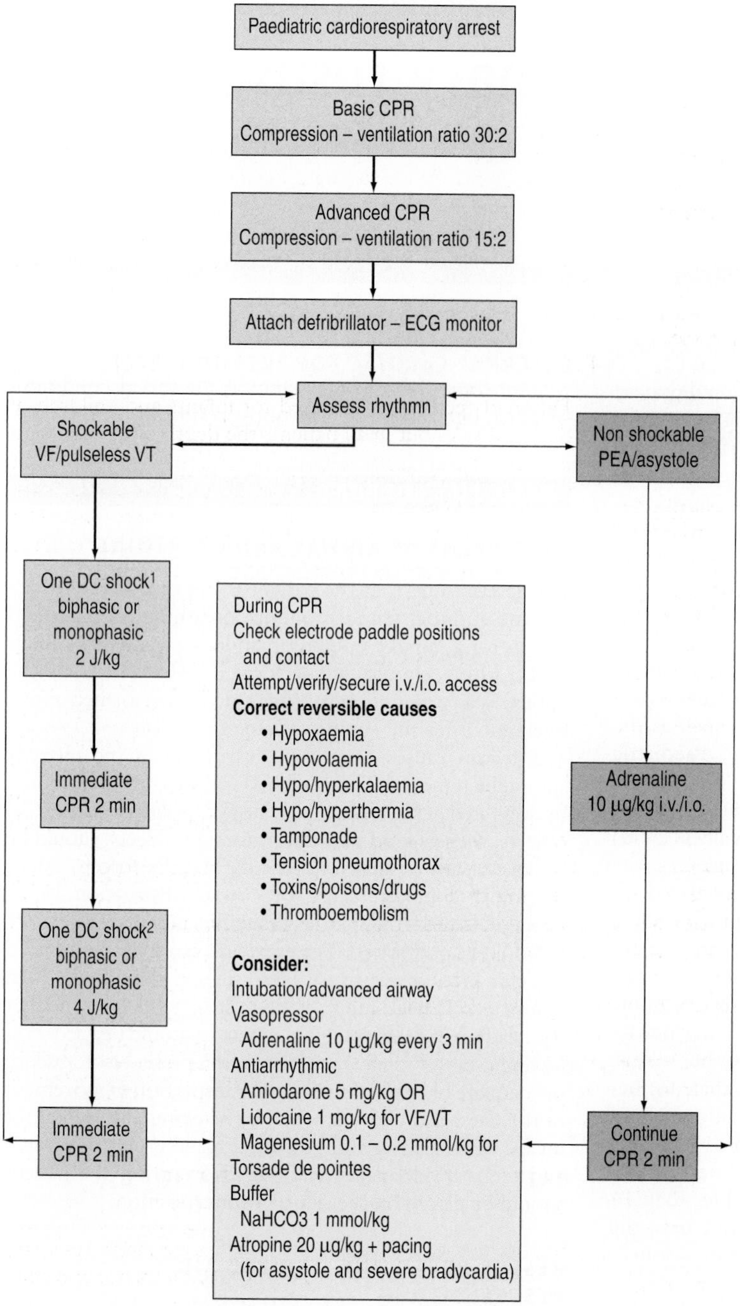

[1] For witnessed arrest, give up to three stacked shocks (2, 4, 4 J/kg) at first defibrillation attempt.

[2] If further shocks are needed these should be single shocks 4 J/Kg.

Figure 106.1 Paediatric resuscitation. PEA, pulseless electrical activity; VF, ventricular fibrillation; VT, ventricular tachycardia. (Reproduced with permission from the Australian Resuscitation Council, Melbourne.)

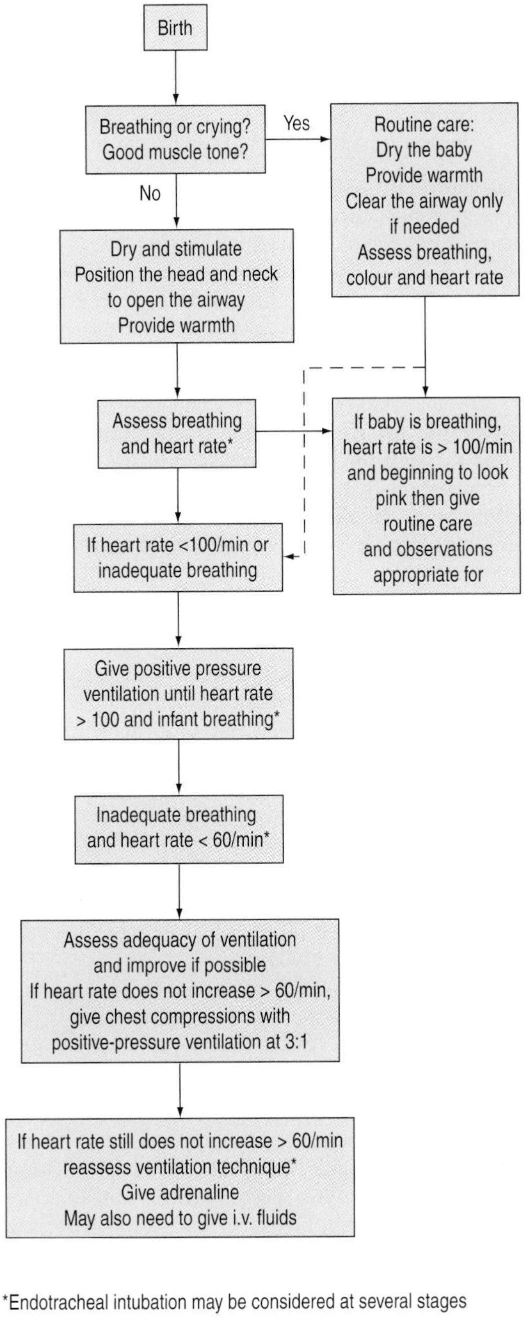

Figure 106.2 Newly-born infant resuscitation. (Reproduced with permission from the Australian Resuscitation Council, Melbourne.)

and infants, a mouth-to-mouth-and-nose technique is recommended, but if the rescuer has a small mouth, a mouth-to-nose technique is an alternative. Lack of chest rise may signify obstruction of the airway requiring repositioning of the head and neck.

ASSESSMENT OF SIGNS OF LIFE OR CIRCULATION

If 'signs of life' or 'signs of circulation' are absent (unresponsiveness, inadequate breathing, lack of movement) or a pulse cannot be detected within 10 seconds or is inadequate (<60 beats/min) external cardiac compression (ECC) should be commenced. Although the pulse check has been discarded in guidelines for lay-person CPR, because of their inability to reliably check the pulse, it has been retained in guidelines for health care personnel. Palpation of any major pulse (carotid, brachial, femoral) is appropriate.

EXTERNAL CARDIAC COMPRESSION (ECC)

Different techniques are used for infants and children of different sizes but in all patients the depth of compression is one-third the depth of their chest. For newly-born infants and infants, two techniques are in common use. In the 'two-finger technique', the middle and forefinger are used. This technique is taught to lay-persons and is also the preferred technique by a single health care rescuer. With the 'two-thumb technique', the hands encircle the thorax, approaching the chest from either above or below, and the thumbs are placed either opposite, alongside or atop one another. With this technique, the rescuer must take care to avoid restriction of the patient's chest during inflation. With premature newly-borns and small infants, the rescuer's encircling fingers may reach and stabilise the vertebral column, without limiting chest inflation. With both techniques, the sternum is compressed above the xiphoid or about one finger breadth below the internipple line.

Either a single hand or both hands may be used for infants and children as determined by the relationship between the size of the patient's chest and the hands of the rescuer. For young children, ECC can be performed with the heel of one hand. For older children, a bimanual technique as per adults may be used. In all ages, the 'centre of the chest' – which corresponds to the lower sternum – is compressed. Approximately 50% of each cycle should be compression.

RATES OF COMPRESSION AND RATIO OF COMPRESSION TO VENTILATION

In hospitals where there are usually two (or more) rescuers, the ratio of compressions to ventilation for infants and children should be 15:2. After every 15 compressions, a pause should allow delivery of two ventilations whenever expired air resuscitation or any type of mask ventilation is given. ECC can be given during the second exhalation. The aim should be to achieve about five cycles per minute, i.e. about 75 compressions and 10 breaths. If circulation returns, but respiration remains inadequate, the number of ventilations should be higher but care should be taken to avoid hypocarbia which results in cerebral ischaemia. A health care rescuer, when alone, may use the lay-person ratio of 30:2, aiming to achieve about five cycles in 2 minutes, i.e. about 75 compressions and 5 breaths per minute.

For infants and children, compressions should be delivered at a rate of 100/min, i.e. one compression every 0.6 seconds or approximately two per second. This does not mean that 100 actual compressions are given each minute. When ventilation is interposed between compressions, the actual compressions delivered will be less than 100 each minute.

If the airway has been secured, e.g. by intubation, strict coordination of compression and ventilation is not crucial: ventilation can be given against resistance imposed by chest compression. In this case about 100 compressions/minute will be achieved but ventilation should be limited to about 10–12 per minute and wherever possible guided by arterial blood gas analysis.

For newly-born infants the total number of recommended 'events' per minute is 120, with the aim of achieving 90 compressions and 30 inflations each minute, i.e. in a ratio of 3:1.

ADVANCED LIFE SUPPORT

As soon as practicable, mechanical ventilation with added oxygen should be commenced with either a bag-valve-mask or via endotracheal intubation. Although intubation is preferred (see below), valuable time should not be wasted in numerous unsuccessful attempts. Initial effective bag-valve-mask ventilation is a necessary prerequisite for successful paediatric CPR. Bags of appropriate sizes should be available for infants, small children and large children. A bag of ~500 ml volume should be available for newly-born infants. Insertion of an oropharyngeal (Guedel) airway may be necessary to facilitate bag-valve-mask ventilation. Access to the circulation and display of the electrocardiograph should also be achieved as soon as possible. Thereafter treatment should be guided by the cardiac rhythm. Underlying causes of CPA should be sought and treated.

AIRWAY MANAGEMENT

If attending personnel are skilled, the trachea should be intubated as soon as practicable. This establishes and maintains an airway, facilitates mechanical ventilation with 100% oxygen, minimises the risk of pulmonary aspiration, enables suctioning of the trachea and provides a route for the administration of selected drugs. If difficulty is experienced at initial intubation, oxygenation should be established with bag-valve-mask ventilation before a reattempt at intubation. Initial intubation should be via the oral route, not via the nasal route.

Intubation via the oral route:

- is invariably quicker than via the nasal route
- is less likely to cause trauma and haemorrhage
- enables the endotracheal tube to be more easily exchanged if the first choice is inappropriate

On the other hand, a tube placed nasally:

- can be better affixed to the face and so is less likely to enter a bronchus or be subject to inadvertent extubation
- is preferred for transport and long-term management

A nasogastric tube should be inserted after intubation to relieve possible gaseous distension of the stomach sustained during bag-valve-mask ventilation.

Correct placement of the endotracheal tube in the trachea must be confirmed. In the hurried conditions of emergency intubation at cardiopulmonary arrest, it is not difficult to mistakenly intubate the oesophagus or to intubate a bronchus. There is no substitute for:

- visualising the passage of the tip of the endotracheal tube through the vocal cords at intubation
- confirmation of bilateral pulmonary air entry by auscultation in the axillae
- continuous observation of rise and fall of the chest on ventilation

It is recommended that correct placement of the endotracheal tube be confirmed by capnography or colorimetric CO_2 detection after initial placement with the realisation that CO_2 excretion can only occur with effective pulmonary blood flow. This implies that CO_2 detection cannot be expected unless spontaneous cardiac output returns or unless external cardiac compression is effective. Oxygenation should be confirmed with use of a pulse oximeter or measurement of arterial gas tension.

Tube size

- 2.5 mm tube is used for a premature newborn <1 kg
- 3.0 mm for infants 1–3.5 kg
- 3.5 mm for infants >3.5 kg and up to age 6 months
- 4 mm for infants 7 months to 1 year
- For children over 1 year, the size is approximately determined by the formula: size (mm) = age (years)/4 + 4.

Tubes larger and smaller should be available. The correct size should allow a small leak on application of moderate pressure but also enable adequate pulmonary inflation.

The tube is inserted a specific depth to avoid accidental extubation or endobronchial intubation. Assessment of the depth of insertion at laryngoscopy is not reliable because this is performed with the neck extended. When the laryngoscope is removed the head assumes a position of neutrality or flexion and the tube depth increases.

The appropriate depth of insertion measured from the centre of the lips for an oral tube is:

- 9.5 cm for a term newborn
- 11.5 cm for a 6-month-old infant
- 12 cm for a 1 year old

An alternative formula for oral tube depth of insertion is: depth (cm) = size (mm) ×3. After 1 year the depth is given by the formula: depth (cm) = age (years)/2 + 12.

The appropriate depth of insertion for a nasal tube in this age group is: depth (cm) = age (years)/2 + 15. On a chest X-ray taken with the head in neutral position, the tip of the tube should be at the interclavicular line.

A laryngeal mask airway (LMA) may be used to establish an airway in the setting of CPA. However, its role in provision of mechanical ventilation remains uncertain. Like bag-valve-mask ventilation, it does not protect the airway from aspiration. Although insertion of an LMA is easier to learn than endotracheal intubation, training should not replace mastery of bag-valve-mask ventilation. An LMA is not suitable for long-term use or during transport when endotracheal intubation is preferred.

ELECTROCARDIOGRAPH

The electrocardiograph (ECG) should be displayed with either leads or paddles. Drug therapy or immediate direct current (DC) shock is administered according to the existing rhythm.

ACCESS TO THE CIRCULATION

According to the skills of the personnel, access to the circulation via a peripheral or central vein should be attempted immediately. Any site is acceptable. Visible or palpable peripheral veins are to be found on the dorsum of the hand, wrist, forearm, cubital fossa, chest wall, foot and ankle. In infants, scalp veins are accessible and the umbilical vein can be used up to about 1 week after birth. The external jugulars are usually distended at CPR but cannulation may be impeded by performance of intubation. Cannulation of femoral, subclavian or internal jugulars are options but difficult or hazardous in this situation. Surgical cutdown onto a long saphenous, saphenofemoral junction or basilic is a valuable skill sometimes required in traumatic exsanguination. Any pre-existing functioning line can be used provided it does not contain any drug or electrolyte precipitating the CPA.

INTRAOSSEOUS INJECTION

If intravenous (i.v.) access cannot be achieved rapidly, say within 60 seconds, intraosseous (i.o.) access should be obtained. This route has been used for patients of all ages and provides rapid, safe and reliable access to the circulation. It serves as an adequate route for any parenteral drug and fluid administration.

A metal needle with a trocar (e.g. disposable intraosseous needle; Cook, Illinois, USA) is preferable although a short lumbar puncture type of needle with an inner trocar may suffice. Although many sites have been used for bone marrow injection, the easiest to identify is the anteromedial surface of the upper or lower tibia, especially in children less than 6 years. The site of the former is a few centimetres below the anterior tuberosity and the latter a few centimetres above the medial malleolus. The handle of the device needle is held in the palm of the hand while the fingers grip the shaft about a centimetre from the tip. It is inserted perpendicular to the bone surface and a rotary action is used to traverse the cortex. Sudden loss of resistance signifies entry to bone marrow. Correct positioning of the needle is confirmed by aspiration of bone marrow (which may be used for biochemical and haematological purposes) but that is not always possible. Bone injection guns (Wais Med Ltd), which fire a needle a preset distance according to the size of the patient, enable easy i.o. injection for infants, children and adults.

Volume expanders need to be given by syringe to achieve rapid restoration of circulating volume and rapid access of drugs to the central circulation. This is best achieved using a 10-ml syringe with a three-way tap in the i.v. tubing so that the i.o. needle does not become dislodged inadvertently.

Care should be exercised to avoid complications, particularly cutaneous extravasation, compartment syndrome of the leg and osteomyelitis. Contraindications include local trauma and infection.

ENDOTRACHEAL ADMINISTRATION OF DRUGS

Lipid-soluble drugs – adrenaline (epinephrine), atropine, lidocaine and naloxone – may be administered via the endotracheal tube if neither i.v. nor i.o. access is possible. Although the optimal doses of these drugs by this route are not known, work in animal models suggests doses should be 10 times the i.v. doses. The drugs should be diluted in normal saline up to 2 ml for infants, 5 ml for small children and 10 ml for large children. It is acceptable and simplest to squirt the drugs from the syringe (after removing the needle) directly into the endotracheal tube and disperse them throughout the respiratory tree with bagging.

Neither sodium bicarbonate nor calcium salts should be administered via the tracheal route because they injure the airways.

DC SHOCK

Defibrillators should have paediatric paddles of cross-sectional area 12–20 cm^2 for use in children <10 kg body weight. For others, adult-sized paddles (50–80 cm^2) are satisfactory provided the paddles do not contact each other. Selectable energy levels should enable delivery of doses 0.5–4 J/kg. The closest level to the dose should be selected. One paddle is placed over the mid-axilla opposite the xiphoid or nipple, the other to the right of the upper sternum below the clavicle. Conductive gel (confined to the area beneath the paddles) or gel pads and firm pressure are needed to deliver optimum energy to the heart without causing skin burns. The doses for monophasic and biphasic shock are the same.

In the treatment of refractory arrhythmias, equipment failure should be excluded. An anteroposterior position of the paddles (one over the cardiac apex, one over the left scapula) may be efficacious in refractory arrhythmia. Dextrocardia may be present with congenital heart disease and the position of the paddles should be altered accordingly.

Monophasic and biphasic automated external defibrillators (AEDs) with attenuated energy doses (approximately 50 J or less) may be used for children 1–8 years of age (approximately 10–25 kg). Adult energy doses of 150–200 J may be used in children older than 8 years of age or 25 kg body weight. AEDs are not recommended for use in infants since they cannot reliably distinguish ventricular fibrillation from tachycardia and hence pose a risk of harmful DC shock.

Rescuers should be cognisant of the risk of inadvertent shock to themselves and colleagues during operation of defibrillators. They should ensure that they have no physical contact with the patient directly or indirectly at the time of electrical discharge. Paddles should be charged only when already placed on the chest of the patient. If the need to give DC shock abates while the paddles are charged, they should be disarmed before replacing them in their cradles.

TREATMENT OF SPECIFIC ARRHYTHMIAS

The following discussion of specific arrhythmias assumes that mechanical ventilation with oxygen and external cardiac compression has been commenced. The treatment of pulseless arrhythmias is summarised in Figure 106.1.

Reversible causes of arrhythmias should be sought and treated during resuscitation. For example:

- hypoxaemia or hypotension causing bradycardia may respond to ventilation
- calcium channel blockade toxicity may be treated with calcium i.v. or i.o. (chloride 10% 0.2 ml/kg, gluconate 10% 0.7 ml/kg)
- hyperkalaemia may be antagonised with a calcium salt then the level lowered with insulin (0.05 U/kg) + dextrose (0.5 g/kg), salbutamol, sodium bicarbonate, hyperventilation or combinations

All drugs should be flushed into the circulation with a small bolus of isotonic fluid. To prevent their inactivation, drugs should not be mixed in the syringe or in infusion lines.

ASYSTOLE AND BRADYCARDIA

Asystole and hypotensive bradycardia (<60 beats/min) should be treated with adrenaline 10 μg/kg i.v. or i.o. If these routes are not available, adrenaline 100 μg/kg should be administered via endotracheal tube (ETT).

Unresponsive asystole should be treated with similar doses of adrenaline (10 μg/kg i.v., i.o.; 100 μg/kg ETT) every 3–5 minutes. Higher doses, up to 200 μg/kg i.v. or i.o., may be indicated in special circumstances (e.g. β-blocker toxicity) but should not be used routinely as they have not altered outcome and predispose to complications (postarrest myocardial dysfunction, hypertension, tachycardia). In newly-born infants, the initial bolus dose is 100–300 μg/kg.

Recurrent bradycardia or asystole may require an infusion of adrenaline at 0.05–3 μg/kg per min: doses <0.3 μg/kg per min are predominantly β-adrenergic; doses >0.3 μg/kg per min are predominantly α-adrenergic. Infuse into a secure large vein. If sinus rhythm cannot be restored, sodium bicarbonate 1 mmol/kg i.v. or i.o. may be helpful but do not allow mixing with adrenaline since catecholamines are inactivated in alkaline solution.

Sinus bradycardia, sinus arrest with slow junctional or idioventricular rhythm, and atrioventricular block are the most common preterminal arrhythmias in paediatric practice. Untreated, bradycardia progresses to asystole.

Bradycardia caused by vagal stimulation should be managed with cessation of the stimulus and/or atropine 20 μg/kg i.v. or i.o. (minimum dose 100 μg) but persistent vagal-mediated bradycardia should be treated with adrenaline 10 μg/kg i.v. or i.o.

If facilities are available, bradycardia may be treated with pacing (oesophageal, transcutaneous, transvenous, epicardial) if sinus node dysfunction or heart block exists, but it is not helpful in asystole.

VENTRICULAR FIBRILLATION AND PULSELESS VENTRICULAR TACHYCARDIA

The initial dose for ventricular fibrillation (VF) or pulseless ventricular tachycardia (VT) is a single unsynchronised shock at 2 J/kg followed by immediate resumption of ECC. If VF or VT persists, subsequent single shocks of 4 J/kg are given, each separated by 2 minutes of ECC.

The witnessed (monitored) onset of VF or pulseless VT should be treated with unsynchronised DC shock initially at 2 J/kg, progressing to 4 J/kg in a stack (salvo) of three shocks. Rescuers should maintain the paddles on the chest and be prepared to deliver a series of three shocks in quick succession, pausing only to verify the rhythm. A precordial thump may be given before DC shock but its efficacy has not been proven.

Failure to revert to sinus rhythm should be treated with adrenaline 10 μg/kg i.v. or i.o. or 100 μg/kg ETT and another shock at 4 J/kg after an interval of ECC. Persistent (refractory) or recurrent VF or VT may also be treated with antiarrhythmics (amiodarone, lidocaine, magnesium) interspersed with single DC shocks. Irrespective of other drug therapy, adrenaline should be administered every 3–5 minutes. The dose of lidocaine is 1 mg/kg i.v. or i.o. bolus followed by an infusion if successful at 20–50 μg/kg per min. The dose of amiodarone is 5 mg/kg i.v. or i.o. as a bolus which may be repeated to maximum of 15 mg/kg. Magnesium, 25–50 mg/kg (0.1–0.2 mmol/kg) is indicated for polymorphic VT (torsade de pointes). The alternative to adrenaline as a vasopressor, vasopressin, has not been adequately investigated for use during CPR for children.

PULSATILE VENTRICULAR TACHYCARDIA

Haemodynamically stable VT may be treated with an antiarrhythmic agent such as amiodarone (5 mg/kg i.v. over 20–60 minutes) or procainamide (15 mg/kg i.v. over 30–60 minutes). Both drugs prolong QT interval and should not be given together. If torsade de pointes is present, magnesium (25–50 mg/kg, 0.1–0.2 mmol/kg i.v.) may be used. If cardioversion is needed, it should be synchronised at 0.5–2 J/kg under sedation/anaesthesia.

ELECTROMECHANICAL DISSOCIATION AND PULSELESS ELECTRICAL ACTIVITY

A normal ECG complex without pulse or circulation iscalled electromechanical dissociation (EMD). If untreated, the ECG initially deteriorates to an abnormal but still recognisable state when it is called pulseless electrical activity (PEA). Both conditions should be treated as for asystole and their causes ascertained and treated.

SUPRAVENTRICULAR TACHYCARDIA

Supraventricular tachycardia (SVT) is the most common spontaneous arrhythmia in childhood and infancy. It may cause life-threatening hypotension. It is usually re-entrant with a rate of 220–300/min in infants, less in children. The QRS complex is usually narrow (<0.08 seconds) making it difficult sometimes to discern from sinus tachycardia (ST). However, whereas ST is a part of other features of illness, SVT is a singular entity, and whereas the rate in ST is variable with activity or stimulation, it is uniform in SVT. In both rhythms, a P wave may be discernible. SVT with aberrant conduction (wide QRS) may resemble VT.

If haemodynamically stable (adequate perfusion and blood pressure), initial treatment of SVT should be vagal stimulation. For infants and young children, application to the face of a plastic bag filled with iced-water is often effective. Older children may be treated with carotid sinus massage or perform a Valsalva (e.g. blowing through a narrow straw). If unsuccessful, give adenosine 100 μg/kg i.v. by rapid bolus (maximum dose 6 mg), doubling once to 200 μg/kg. If unsuccessful, give synchronised DC shock (cardioversion) commencing with 0.5 J/kg, progressing if unsuccessful to 2 J/kg under sedation/anaesthesia. If SVT is accompanied by haemodynamic instability (i.e. hypotension), proceed to cardioversion (synchronised 0.5–2 J/kg) immediately although vagal stimulation or adenosine (i.v. or i.o.) may be used provided they do not delay cardioversion. Verapamil should not be used to treat SVT in infants and should be avoided in children because it induces hypotension and cardiac depression.

POST RESUSCITATION CARE

Supportive therapy should be provided until there is recovery of function of vital organs. This may require provision of oxygen therapy, mechanical ventilation, inotropic/vasopressor infusion, renal support, parenteral nutrition and other therapy for several days or longer. Recovery of infants and children is usually slow because cardiorespiratory arrest is often secondary to prolonged global ischaemia or hypoxaemia which implies that other organs sustain damage before cardiorespiratory arrest.

Particular care should be taken to ensure adequate cerebral perfusion with well-oxygenated blood. Hyperventilation is not useful for this purpose. Therapeutic hypothermia post resuscitation (33–36 °C) up to 3 days may improve neurological outcome. Inadvertently hypothermic patients, provided temperature is above 33 °C, should not be actively warmed but hyperthermia should be aggressively treated. During deliberate hypothermia shivering should be prevented with sedation and/or neuromuscular blockade, seizures should be actively sought and treated with anticonvulsant and the cause of the CPA should be investigated and treated appropriately, e.g. sepsis or drug overdose.

Complications of CPR should be sought, especially if secondary deterioration occurs. A chest X-ray should be obtained to check the position of the endotracheal tube, to exclude pneumothorax, lung collapse, contusion or aspiration, and to check the cardiac silhouette although an echocardiographic examination is preferable to specifically check contractility and to exclude a pericardial effusion. Measurement of haemoglobin, pH, gas tensions, electrolytes and glucose is important.

CESSATION OF CARDIOPULMONARY RESUSCITATION

Long-term outcome from paediatric CPR is poor, but better if arrest is respiratory alone or if CPA occurs in hospital. The decision to cease CPR should be based on a number of factors including the duration of resuscitation, response to treatment, pre-arrest status of the patient, remediable factors, likely outcome if ultimately successful, opinions of personnel familiar with the patient and, whenever appropriate, the wishes of the parents. In general, unless hypothermia or drug toxicity exists, survival to normality is most unlikely if there has been a failure to respond to full competent CPR after 30 minutes and several doses of adrenaline. In the newly-born infant, discontinuation of treatment is appropriate if CPR does not establish a spontaneous circulation within 10–15 minutes. Family members should be kept informed, allowed to be present or asked if they want to be present during resuscitation.

POST RESUSCITATION STAFF MANAGEMENT

Unfortunately, CPA occurring in hospital is often unexpected – for example, when a moribund patient arrives unannounced in the emergency department, a patient's condition deteriorates rapidly on the ward or when a mishap occurs under anaesthesia. These situations test the readiness, training, abilities and skills of individuals and the organisation of the institution. It is prudent to monitor performance with a view to improvement and not ignore the psychological impact which such events have on individuals. Sensitive debriefing sessions should be encouraged.

REFERENCES

1. Australian Resuscitation Council, Melbourne. Guidelines 12.1–12.7, 13.1–13.10. http://www.resus.org.au.
2. American Heart Association. Pediatric advanced life support. *Circulation* 2005; **112**: 167–87.
3. European Resuscitation Council Guidelines for Resuscitation 2005. Section 6. Paediatric life support. *Resuscitation* 2005; **67**(Suppl 1): S97–133.
4. International Liaison Committee on Resuscitation. Consensus on resuscitation science and treatment recommendations. Part 6. Paediatric basic and advanced life support. *Resuscitation* 2005; **67**: 271–91.

Appendix 1

Normal biochemical values

I BLOOD CHEMISTRY

S = serum
P = plasma
HWB = heparin whole blood

		0.5–1.4 g/l
α_1-Acid glycoprotein (S)		Supine – 140–530 pmol/l
Aldosterone (S)		Erect – 220–970 pmol/l
Ammonia (P) to lab without delay		4–50 μmol/l
Amylase (S or P)		70–300 U/l
α_1-Antitrypsin (S or P)		2.1–4.0 g/l
Aspartate aminotransferase (AST) (P)		6–42 U/l
Bicarbonate (P)		22–32 mmol/l
Bilirubin (total) (S or P)		3–17 μmol/l
Bilirubin (direct) (S or P)		2–9 μmol/l
Caeruloplasmin (S or P)		0.20–0.60 g/l
Calcium (S or P)		2.25–2.65 mmol/l
Carotene (S or P)		1.0–4.8 μmol/l
Chloride (S or P)		98–108 mmol/l
Cholesterol (S or P)		3.1–6.5 mmol/l
Copper (S or P)		11–23 μmol/l
Cortisol (S or P)	8–9 am	300–800 nmol/l
	4–5 pm	100–600 nmol/l
Creatinine (P)		50–120 μmol/l
Creatinine clearance		> F1.3 ml/s
Creatinine kinase (P)		20–130 U/l
Creatinine kinase isoenzymes		Qualitative
Digoxin (S)	toxic	> 2 μg/l
Effective thyroxine ratio (ETR) (S)		0.90–1.09
FSH (S) Male		3–19 U/l
Female Follicular		5–20 U/l
Mid-cycle		15–30 U/l
Luteal		5–15 U/l
Postmenopausal		50–100 U/l
Glucose (fasting) (fluoride) (P)		3.9–6.2 mmol/l
γ-Glutamyl-transferase (γ-GT) (P)	F	7–30 U/l
	M	10–50 U/l
Growth hormone (fasting, resting) (S)	M	<6 mU/l
	F	<16 mU/l
	Child	<10 mU/l
Insulin (fasting) (S)		3–28 mU/l
Iron (S or P) (1) Iron	M	14–31 μmol/l
8–10 am	F	11–29 μmol/l
(2) Iron binding capacity	M	41–70 μmol/l
	F	37–77 μmol/l

Continued

Lactate (special collection)		0.3–1.3 mmol/l
LDH (S or P)		< 80 U
Lead (HWB)		< 2 μmol/l
Lithium (S) not plasma		0.8–1.2 mmol/l (therapeutic range)
Magnesium (S or P)		0.7–1.1 mmol/l
Oestriol (pregnancy) (S)		Depends on gestation
Osmolality (S or P)		275–295 mosm/kg
Phosphatase		
A. Prostatic (S or P) (stabilise plasma with 5 mg/ml of $NaHSO_4$ or freeze)		0–4 U/l
B. Alkaline (S or P)		100–350 U/l
Phosphate (inorganic) (P)		0.8–1.4 mmol/l
Porphyrins (red cell) (HWB)		< 1.2 μmol/l
Potassium (P)		3.4–5.0 mmol/l
Prolactin (S) (resting)		25 μg/l
Proteins		
A. (1) Total (S)		63–78 g/l
(2) Albumin (S)		35–45 g/l
B. Electrophoresis (S) not plasma:		
Albumin		35–45 g/l
α_1-Globulin		2–4 g/l
α_2-Globulin		5–9 g/l
β-Globulin		6–10 g/l
γ-Globulin		8–16 g/l
Pyruvate (special collection)		30–80 μmol/l
Renin (special tubes – keep blood cold)		
100–180 mmol Na intake:		
Supine (6 hours)		<0.58 ng/s/l
Upright (4 hours)		0.28–1.25 ng/s/l
Sodium (P)		134–146 mmol/l
Thyroxine (S)		60–150 nmol/l
Transferrin (S or P)		2.1–3.5 g/l
Triglyceride (fasting) (P)		1.80 mmol/l
Tri-iodothyronine (S)		1.3–2.9 nmol/l
TSH (S)		1–11 mU/l
Urea (P)		3.0–8.0 mmol/l
Uric acid (P)	M	0.18–0.48 mmol/l
	F	0.12–0.42 mmol/l
Zinc (P)		12–20 μmol/l

II URINE

AA = 20 ml 50% acetate
d = 24-hour collection
Sp = spot urine

Aldosterone (d, AA)		14–55 nmol/d
ALA (delta amino laevulinic acid) (Sp or d, AA)	Sp:	< 50 μmol/l
	d:	10–50 μmol/d

Continued

Amylase (Sp or d, NO ACID)	Sp:	< 900 U/l
	d:	100–1000 U/d
Calcium (d, AA)		< 7.5 mmol/d
Catecholamines and derivatives (d, 20 ml 50% HCl):		
1. HMMA (VMA) Hydroxymethoxymandelic acid		< 35 μmol/d
2. Metadrenaline		< 5.6 μmol/d
3. Catecholamine		< 1.6 μmol/d
Copper (d, AA)		< 1.6 μmol/d
Coproporphyrin (collect 24-hour urine into 8 g sodium carbonate)		< 245 nmol/d
Creatinine (d, AA)		10–20 mmol/d
5-Hydroxyindole-acetic acid (5-HIAA) (d, AA)		5–37 μmol/d
Hydroxyproline (d, AA)		< 0.35 mmol/d (gelatin-free diet)
Indican (d, AA)		0.04–0.36 mmol/d
Lead (d, AA)		0.4 μmol/d
Magnesium (d, AA)		2.0–6.6 mmol/d
Melanin (fresh Sp)		Qualitative
Oestriol (in pregnancy) (d, AA)		50–160 μmol/d at 36 weeks' gestation
Osmolality (Sp)		300–1300 mosm/kg
Oxalate (d, AA)		< 300 μmol/d
Phosphorus (d, AA)		10–42 mmol/d
Porphobilinogen (fresh Sp)		Qualitative
Potassium (d or Sp, AA)		25–100 mmol/d
Protein (d or Sp, AA)		0.02–0.06 g/d
Sodium (d or Sp, AA)		40–210 mmol/d
Steroids (d, AA):		
1. 17-Oxosteroids	M	28–80 μmol/d
	F	14–60 μmol/d
2. 17-Hydroxy corticosteroids	M	14–70 μmol/d
	F	7–50 μmol/d
Urea (d or Sp, AA)		170–500 mmol/d
Uric acid (d, 8 g sodium carbonate)		< 3.6 mmol/d (purine-free diet)
Urobilinogen (fresh Sp)		Qualitative
Uroporphyrin (collect as for Coproporphyrin)		< 50 nmol/d
Xylose absorption:		
Xylose excretion in 5 hours		> 27 mmol
Plasma value at 2 hours		1.7–3.4 mmol/l

III FAECES

Fat (3-day collection)	< 5 g/l
Porphyrins (single stool)	
Coproporphyrins	< 30 nmol/g dry wt
Protoporphyrins	< 135 nmol/g dry wt

IV CSF

Protein	0.15–0.45 g/l
Glucose	2.7–4.2 mmol/l
IgG	< 0.05 g/l
IgG:Total protein ratio	5–14%

Appendix 2

Système International (SI) units

BASIC SI UNITS			PREFIXES					
Physical quantity	Name	Symbol	Factor	Name	Symbol	Factor	Name	Symbol
Length	Metre	m	10^{18}	Exa-	E	10^{-18}	Atto-	a
Mass	Kilogram	kg	10^{15}	Peta-	P	10^{-15}	Femto-	f
Time	Second*	s	10^{12}	Tera-	T	10^{-12}	Pico-	p
Electric current	Ampere	A	10^{9}	Giga-	G	10^{-9}	Nano-	n
Thermodynamic temperature	Kelvin	K	10^{6}	Mega-	M	10^{-6}	Micro-	μ
Luminous intensity	Candela	cd	10^{3}	Kilo-	k	10^{-3}	Milli-	m
Amount of substance	Mole	mol	10^{2}	Hecto-	h	10^{-2}	Centi-	c
			10^{1}	Deca-	da	10^{-1}	Deci-	d

*Minute (min), hour (h) and day (d) will remain in use although they are not official SI units.

DERIVED SI UNITS

Quantity	SI units	Symbol	Expression in terms of SI base units or derived units
Frequency	Hertz	Hz	1 Hz = 1 cycle/s ($1\ s^{-1}$)
Force	Newton	N	1 N = 1 $kg.m/s^2$
Work, energy, quantity of heat	Joule	J	1 J = 1 N.m ($1\ kg.m^2.s^{-2}$)
Power	Watt	W	1 W = 1 J/s ($1\ J.s^{-1}$)
Quantity of electricity	Coulomb	C	1 C = 1 A.s
Electric potential, potential difference, tension, electromotive force	Volt	V	1 V = W/A ($1\ W.A^{-1}$)
Electric capacitance	Farad	F	1 F = 1 A.s/V ($A.sV^{-1}$)
Electric resistance	Ohm	W	1 W = 1 V/A ($1\ V.A^{-1}$)
Flux of magnetic induction, magnetic flux	Weber	Wb	1 Wb = 1 V.s
Magnetic flux density, magnetic induction	Tesla	T	1 T = 1 Wb/m^2 ($1\ Wb.m^{-2}$)
Inductance	Henry	H	1 H = 1 V.s/A ($V.s.A^{-1}$)
Pressure	Pascal	Pa	1 Pa = 1 N/m^2 ($1\ N.m^{-2}$) = 1 $kg/m^2.s^2$ ($1\ kg.m^{21}.s^{-2}$)

The litre (l) ($10^{-3}\ m^3 = dm^3$), though not official, will remain in use as a unit of volume as also will the dyne (dyn) as a unit for force (1 dyn = 10^{-5} N).

PRESSURE MEASUREMENTS

SI unit	Old unit	Conversion factors	
		Old to SI (exact)	SI to old (approx.)
kPa	mmHg	0.133	7.5
kPa	1 standard atmosphere (approx. 1 Bar)	101.3	0.01
kPa	cmH_2O	0.0981	10
kPa	lbs/sq in	6.894	0.145

HAEMATOLOGY

Measurement	SI unit	Old unit	Conversion factors	
			Old to SI	SI to old
Haemoglobin (Hb)	g/dl	g/100 ml	Numerically	equivalent
Packed cell volume	No unit*	Per cent	0.01	100
Mean cell Hb concentration	g/dl	Per cent	Numerically	equivalent
Mean cell Hb	pg	uug	Numerically	equivalent
Red cell count	Cells/litre	Cells/mm^3	10^6	10^{-6}
White cell count	Cells/litre	Cells/mm^3	10^6	10^{-6}
Reticulocytes	Per cent	Per cent	Numerically	equivalent
Platelets	Cells/litre	Cells/mm^3	10^6	10^{-6}

*Expressed as decimal fraction.

pH	H1
pH	nmol/litre
6.80	158
6.90	126
7.00	100
7.10	79
7.20	63
7.25	56
7.30	50
7.35	45
7.40	40
7.45	36
7.50	32
7.55	28
7.60	25
7.70	20

Appendix 3

Respiratory physiology symbols and normal values

SYMBOLS

Primary

- C Concentration of gas in blood
- F Fractional concentration in dry gas
- F Frequency of respiration (breaths/min)
- P Pressure or partial pressure
- Q Volume of blood
- $\dot{Q}$ Volume of blood per unit time
- R Respiratory exchange ratio
- S Saturation of haemoglobin with O_2
- $\dot{V}$ Volume of gas per unit time

Secondary symbols for gas phase

- A Alveolar
- B Barometric
- D Dead space
- E Expired
- I Inspired
- L Lung
- T Tidal

Secondary symbols for blood phase

- a arterial
- c capillary
- ć end-capillary
- i ideal
- v venous
- $\bar{v}$ mixed venous
- – above any symbol denotes a mean value
- · above any symbol denotes a value per unit time

NORMAL VALUES

1. Blood

(a) ***Arterial***

pH	:	7.36–7.44	(H^+ = 44–36 nmol/l)
Pa_{O_2}	:	85–100 mmHg	(11.3–13.3 kPa)
Pa_{CO_2}	:	36–44 mmHg	(4.8–5.9 kPa)
O_2 content	:	20–21 vols%	(8.9–9.4 nmol/l)
CO_2 content	:	48–50 vols%	(21.6–22.5 nmol/l)

(b) ***Venous***

pH	:	7.34–7.42	(H^+ = 38–46 nmol/l)
P_{O_2}	:	37–42 mmHg	(5–5.6 kPa)
P_{CO_2}	:	42–50 mmHg	(5.6–6.7 kPa)
O_2 content	:	15–16 vols%	(6.7–7.2 mmol/l)
CO_2 content	:	52–54 vols%	(23.3–24.2 mmol/l)

2. Gases

(a) ***Inspired air***

O_2	:	20.93%	
PIO_2	:	149 mmHg	(19.9 kPa)
N_2	:	79.04%	
PIN_2	:	563 mmHg	(75 kPa)
CO_2	:	0.03%	

(b) ***Expired air***

O_2	:	16–17%	
PEO_2	:	113–121 mmHg	(15–16 kPa)
N_2	:	80%	
PEN_2	:	579 mmHg	(77 kPa)
CO_2	:	3–4%	
$PECO_2$	:	21–28 mmHg	(2.8–3.7 kPa)

3. Ventilation:perfusion

(a) ***Alveolar–arterial oxygen gradient:***

5–20 mmHg	(0.7–2.7 kPa) breathing air
25–65 mmHg	(3.3–8.6 kPa) breathing 100% oxygen

(b) ***Venous admixture*** **($\dot{Q}_S$:$\dot{Q}_T$): 5% of cardiac output**

(c) ***Right to left physiological shunt:*** **3% of cardiac output**

(d) ***Anatomical dead space:*** **2 ml/kg body weight**

(e) ***Dead space: tidal volume ratio*** **V_D:V_T): 0.25–0.4 or 33 + $\frac{\text{Age}}{3}$ per cent**

4. Lung volumes

Approximate values in adults are listed. Values are less in smaller subjects and in females.

Tidal volume	:	400 ml or 6 ml/kg
Inspiratory capacity	:	3.6 litres
Inspiratory reserve volume	:	3.1 litres
Expiratory reserve volume	:	1.2 litres
Functional residual capacity	:	2.4 litres
Residual volume	:	1.2 litres
Total lung capacity	:	6.0 litres
Vital capacity	:	4.8 litres

or 2.5 l/sq m body surface or 2.5 l/m height in males
2.0 l/sq m body surface or 2.0 l/m height in females

or 65–75 ml/kg

5. Lung mechanics

(a) *Peak expiratory flow rate*	:	450–700 l/min (males)	
	:	300–500 l/min (females)	
(b) *Forced expiratory volume in 1 sec* (FEV_1)	:	70–83% of vital capacity	
(c) *Compliance* (approximate values)	:		
(i) Lung compliance (CL)			
		Static	*Dynamic*
conscious (erect)	:	200 ml/cmH_2O	180 ml/cmH_2O
paralysed anaesthetised (supine)	:	160 ml/cmH_2O	80 ml/cmH_2O
(ii) Chest wall compliance (CCW)	:	200 ml/cmH_2O	
(iii) Total compliance (CT):			
conscious (erect)	:	150 ml/cmH_2O	100 ml/cmH_2O
*paralysed anaesthetised (supine)	:	74 ml/cmH_2O	56 ml/cmH_2O
(d) *Airways resistance*	:		
conscious	:	0.6–3.2 cmH_2O/l per second	

sedated, partially paralysed and ventilated (includes resistance of endotracheal tube and catheter mount): 5–10 H_2O/l per second

(e) *Work of breathing*: 0.3–0.5 kg m/min
or oxygen consumption of 0.5–1 ml/l ventilation

*Compliance values would be lower for the sedated, partially paralysed, ventilated patient in the intensive care unit, i.e. effective dynamic compliance = 40–50 ml/cmH_2O

6. Cardiovascular – pressures in kPa are given within brackets

(a) Cardiac index	:	2.5–3.6 l/min per m^2
(b) Stroke volume	:	42–52 ml/m^2
(c) Ejection fraction	:	0.55–0.75
(d) End diastolic volume	:	75 ± 15 ml/m^2
(e) End systolic volume	:	25 ± 8 ml/m^2
(f) Left ventricular stroke work index	:	30–110 g-m/m^2
(g) Left ventricular minute work index	:	1.8–6.6 kg-m/min per m^2
(h) Oxygen consumption index	:	110–150 ml/l
(i) Right atrial pressure	:	1–7 mmHg (0.13–0.93)
(j) Right ventricular systolic pressure	:	15–25 mmHg (2.0–3.3)
(k) Right ventricular diastolic pressure	:	0–8 (0–1)
(l) Pulmonary artery systolic pressure	:	15–25 mmHg (2.0–3.3)
(m) Pulmonary artery diastolic pressure	:	8–15 mmHg (1–2)
(n) Pulmonary artery mean pressure	:	10–20 mmHg (1.3–2.7)
(o) Pulmonary capillary wedge pressure	:	6–15 mmHg (0.8–2.0)
(p) Systemic vascular resistance	:	770–1500 dyne-s/cm^5
	:	77–150 kPa-s/l
(q) Pulmonary vascular resistance	:	20–120 dyne-s/cm^5
	:	2–12 kPa-s/l

Appendix 4

Physiological equations

RESPIRATORY EQUATIONS

(a) *Oxygen consumption* (250 ml/min)

Oxygen consumption = amount of oxygen in inspired gas minus amount in expired gas

i.e. $\dot{V}O_2 = (\dot{V}I \times FIO_2) - (\dot{V}E \times F\bar{E}O_2)$

(b) *Carbon dioxide production* (200 ml/min)

Volume CO_2 eliminated in expired gas = expired gas volume × CO_2 concentration in mixed expired gas

i.e. $\dot{V}CO_2 = \dot{V} \times F\bar{E}CO_2$

As expired volume is made up of alveolar and dead space gas,

$$\dot{V}CO_2 = (\dot{V}A \times FACO_2)\ (\dot{V}D \times FICO_2)$$

As $FiCO_2$ is negligible, especially if there is no rebreathing,

$$\dot{V}CO_2 = \dot{V}A \times FACO_2$$

or $$FACO_2 = \frac{\dot{V}CO_2}{\dot{V}A}$$

or $$PACO_2\ (\text{mmHg}) = \frac{\dot{V}CO_2(\text{ml/min STPD})}{\dot{V}A(\text{l/min BTPS})} \times 0.863$$

or $$PACO_2\ (\text{kPa}) = \frac{\dot{V}CO_2(\text{mmol/min})}{\dot{V}A(\text{l/min BTPS})} \times 2.561$$

STPD: Standard temperature (0°C) and pressure (760 mmHg or 101.35 kPa) dry gas

BTPS: Body temperature and ambient pressure, saturated with water vapour

(c) *Physiological dead space*

Bohr's equation, $$\frac{V_D}{V_T} = \frac{PACO_2 - P\bar{E}CO_2}{PACO_2}$$

or $$\frac{V_D}{V_T} = \frac{PaCO_2 - P\bar{E}CO_2}{PaCO_2}$$

(d) *Alveolar oxygenation*

$$PAO_2 = PIO_2 - \frac{PaCO_2}{R}$$ where R is the respiratory quotient (normally 0.8)

$$PAO_2 = PIO_2 - PaCO_2\frac{PIO_2 - P\bar{E}O_2}{P\bar{E}CO_2}$$

or $$PAO_2 = PIO_2 - PACO_2\left(FIO_2 + \frac{1 - FIO_2}{R}\right)$$

when $FIO_2 = 1.0$ (patient breathing 100% oxygen),
then PAO_2 = (PB – saturated water vapour pressure) $-PACO_2$
$= (PB - 47) - PaCO_2$

(e) *Venous admixture*

$$\frac{\dot{Q}_S}{\dot{Q}_T} = \frac{C\acute{c}O_2 - CaO_2}{C\acute{c}O_2 - C\bar{v}O_2}$$

$$= \frac{(PAO_2 - PaO_2) \times 0.0031}{CaO_2 + (PAO_2 - PaO_2) \times 0.0031 - C\bar{v}O_2}$$

$$= \frac{(PAO_2 - PaO_2) \times 0.0031}{(PAO_2 - PaO_2) \times 0.0031 + 5} \text{ (simplified)}$$

$$= C\acute{c}O_2 - C\bar{v}O_2$$

(f) *Fractional inspired oxygen concentration*

$$FiO_2 = \frac{O_2 \text{ flow in l/min} + (\text{Airflow in l/min} \times 0.21)}{\text{Total } O_2 + \text{Airflow in l/min}}$$

(g) *Henderson–Hasselbalch equation*

$$pH = pKA + \log \frac{(HCO_3^-)}{(CO_2)}$$

$$pH = 6.1 + \log \frac{(HCO_3^- \text{ in mmol/l})}{(PCO_2 \text{ in mmHg}) \times 0.03}$$

$$[H^+] \text{ nmol/l} = 24 \times \frac{(PCO_2 \text{ in mmHg})}{(HCO_3^- \text{ in mmol/l})}$$

$$[H^+] \text{ nmol/l} = 180 \times \frac{(PCO_2 \text{ in kPa})}{(HCO_3^- \text{ in mmol/l})}$$

CARDIOVASCULAR EQUATIONS

(a) *Mean blood pressure* (BP = DBP + 1/3 (SBP – DBP)

(b) *Rate pressure product* (RPP) = P × SBP

(c) *Body surface area* (BSA) in $m^2 = (Ht)^{0.725} \times (Wt)^{0.425} \times 71.84 \times 10^{-4}$

(d) **Cardiac Index* (CI) $= \dfrac{CO}{BSA}$ = ml/min per m^2

(e) *Stroke volume* (SV) $= \dfrac{CO}{P}$ = ml/beat

(f) **Stroke volume index* (SVI) $= \dfrac{SV}{BSA}$ = ml/beat per m^2

(g) **Left ventricular stroke work index* (LVSWI) = (BP – PCWP) (SVI) (0.0136) = g-m/m^2 per beat

(h) *Systemic vascular resistance* (SVR) $= \dfrac{BP - RAP}{CO}$ resistance units

(Multiply × 79.9 to convert to absolute resistance units, dynes sec cm^{-5})

(i) *Pulmonary vascular resistance* (PVR) $= \dfrac{PAP - PCWP}{CO}$ resistance units

(Multiply × 79.9 to convert to absolute resistance units, dynes sec cm^{-5})

(j) *Left ventricular pre-ejection period* (PEP) = QS_2 – LVET m sec

(k) *Other systolic time index ratios* may easily be calculated:

$$\frac{1}{PEP^2} \text{ and } \frac{PEP}{LVET}$$

*For interpatient comparisons and reference standards, the 'index' term, output normalised to body surface, may be used when

SBP = systolic blood pressure in mmHg
DBP = diastolic blood pressure in mmHg
P = heart rate in beats/min
Ht = height in cm
Wt = weight in kg
CO = cardiac output in ml/min
PCWP = pulmonary capillary wedge pressure in mmHg
RAP = right atrial pressure in mmHg
PAP = mean pulmonary artery pressure in mmHg
LVET = left ventricular ejection time in m sec
QS_2 = total electromechanical systole in m sec

RENAL EQUATIONS

(a) *Standard creatinine clearance* (ml/min/1.73 m^2)

$$= \frac{\text{urine creatinine(mmol/l)}}{\text{serum creatinine(mmol/l)}} \times \text{urine volume (ml/min)} \times \frac{1.73}{\text{body surface area}(m^2)}$$

(b) *Per cent filtered Na^+* excreted

$$= \frac{\text{urine } Na^+\text{(mmol/l)}}{\text{serum } Na^+\text{(mmol/l)}} \times \frac{\text{serum creatinine(mmol/l)}}{\text{urine creatinine(mmol/l)}} \times 100$$

(c) *Free water clearance* (ml/min)

$$= \text{urine vol (ml/min)} - \frac{\text{urine osmolality(mosm/kg)}}{\text{plasma osmolality(mosm/kg)}} \times \text{urine vol (ml/min)}$$

(d) *Additional calculated parameters*:

(i) $\frac{\text{urine}}{\text{plasma}}$ osmolality ratio

(ii) $\frac{\text{urine}}{\text{serum}}$ creatinine ratio

(iii) $\frac{\text{blood urea}}{\text{serum creatinine}}$ ratio

(iv) $\frac{\text{urine}}{\text{plasma}}$ urea ratio

(v) urinary Na^+ and K^+ excretion (mmol)

(vi) $\frac{\text{urinary } Na^+}{\text{urinary } K^+}$ ratio

Appendix 5

Plasma drug concentrations and American nomenclature

PLASMA DRUG LEVELS

Drug	Normal or therapeutic concentration mg/l	Toxic concentration mg/l	Lethal or potentially lethal concentration mg/l
Acetazolamide	10–15	–	–
Acetohexamide	21–56	–	–
Acetone	–	200–300	550
Aluminium	0.13	–	–
Aminophylline (Theophylline)	10–20	20	–
Amitriptyline	50–200 μg/l	400 μg/l	10–20
Ammonia	500–1700	–	–
Amfetamine	20–30 μg/l	–	2
Arsenic	0.0–20 μg/l	1.0	15
Barbiturates			
Short-acting	1	7	10
Intermediate-acting	1–5	10–30	30
Phenobarbital	15	40–70	80–150
Benzene	–	Any measurable	0.94
Beryllium	Tissue levels generally used (lung and lymph)	–	–
Boric acid	0.8	40	50
Bromide	50	0.5–1.5 g/l	2 g/l
Brompheniramine	8–15 μg/l	–	–
Cadmium	0.1–0.2 μg/l	50μg/l	–
Caffeine	–	–	100
Carbamazepine	6–12	12	–
Carbon monoxide	1% saturation of Hb	15–35% saturation of Hb	50% saturation of Hb
Carbon tetrachloride	–	20–50	–
Chloral hydrate	10	100	250
Chlordiazepoxide	1.0–2.0	6	20
Chloroform	–	70–250	390
Chlorpromazine	0.3	1–2	3–12
Chlorpropamide	30–140	–	–

Continued

Drug	Normal or therapeutic concentration mg/l	Toxic concentration mg/l	Lethal or potentially lethal concentration mg/l
Codeine	25 μg/l	–	–
Copper	1–1.5	5.4	–
Cyanide	0.15	–	5
DDT	13 μg/l	–	–
Desipramine	0.59–1.4	–	10–20
Dextropropoxyphene	50–200 μg/l	5–10	57
Diazepam	0.5–2.5	5–20	50
Dieldrin	1.5 μg/l	–	–
Digitoxin	20–35 μg/l	–	320 μg/l
Digoxin	1–2 μg/l	2–9 μg/l	–
Dinitro-o-cresol	–	30–40 μg/l	75
Diphenhydramine	5	10	–
Disopyramide	3–7	–	–
Ethosuximide	40–80	–	–
Ethyl chloride	–	–	400
Ethylene glycol	–	1.5 g/l	2–4 g/l
Fluoride	0.5	–	2
Gentamicin	5–8	10–12	–
Glutethimide	1–5	10–30	30–100
Gold (sodium aurothiomalate)	3–6	–	–
Hydrogen sulphide	–	–	0.92
Hydromorphone (Dihydromorphinone)	–	–	0.1–0.3
Imipramine	0.1–0.3	0.7	2
Iron	500 (erythrocytes)	6 (serum)	–
Lead	0.05–1.3	1.3	–
Lidocaine	2–4	6	–
Lithium	0.8–1.2 mmol/l	1.5 mmol/l	4 mmol/l
LSD (lysergic acid diethylamide)	–	1–4 μg/l	–
Magnesium	0.7–1.1 mmol/l	–	–
Manganese	0.15	4.6	–
Meprobamate	10	100	200
Mercury	60–120 μg/l	–	–
Mesuximide	2.5–7.5	–	–
Methadone	480–860 μg/l	2	4
Methanol	–	200	890
Methapyrilene	2 μg/l	30–50	50
Methaqualone	1–2	5–30	30
Methylamphetamine	–	5	40
Methyprylon	10	30–60	100
Mexiletine	0.6–2.5	–	–
Morphine	0.1	–	0.5–4
Nickel	0.41	–	–
Nicotine	–	10	5–52
Nitrofurantoin	1.8	–	–
Nortriptyline	50–200 μg/l	400 μg/l	10–20
Orphenadrine	–	2	4–8

Drug	Normal or therapeutic concentration mg/l	Toxic concentration mg/l	Lethal or potentially lethal concentration mg/l
Oxalate	2	–	10
Papaverine	1	–	–
Paracetamol	5–25	30	250 at 4 hours 50 at 12 hours
Paraldehyde	50	200–400	500
Paramethoxyamphetamine (PMA)	–	–	2–4
Pentazocine	0.1–1	2–5	10–20
Perphenazine	–	1	–
Pethidine	600–650 μg/l	5	30
Phenacetin	5–25	30	400
Phencyclidine	–	0.5	1
Phensuximide	10–19	–	–
Phenylbutazone	100	–	–
Phenytoin (Dilantin)	8–20	30	100
Phosphorus	Concentration in tissues usually used	–	–
Primidone	10	50–80	100
Probenecid	100–200	–	–
Procainamide	3–8	10	–
Prochlorperazine	–	1	–
Promazine	–	1	–
Propoxyphene	0.1–1	5–20	57
Propranolol	0.025–0.1	–	8–12
Propylhexedrine	–	–	2–3
Quinidine	3–6	10	30–50
Quinine	–	–	12
Salicylate (acetylsalicylic acid)	100–350	350–400	500
Strychnine	–	2	9–12
Sulfadiazine	80–150	–	–
Sulfaguanidine	30–50	–	–
Sulphafurazole	90–100	–	–
Sultiame	4–10	–	–
Theophylline	10–20	20	–
Thioridazine	1–1.5	10	20–80
Tin	0.12	–	–
Tobramycin	5–8	10–12	–
Tolbutamide	53–96	–	–
Toluene	–	–	10
Tribromoethanol	–	–	90
Tricyclics	50–200 μg/l	400 μg/l	10–20
Trimethobenzamide	1.0–2.0	–	–
Valproate	50–100	–	–
Warfarin	1.0–10	–	–
Zinc	0.68–1.36	–	–
Zoxazolamine	3–13	–	–

AMERICAN NOMENCLATURE

Adrenaline	Epinephrine
Cinchocaine	Dibucaine
Desferrioxamine	Deferoxamine
Dextropropoxyphene	Propoxyphene
Dihydromorphinone	Hydromorphone
Ergometrine	Ergonovine
Hyoscine	Scopolamine
Isoprenaline	Isoproterenol
Meclozine	Meclizine
Mepivacaine	Carbocaine
Methylamphetamine	Methamphetamine
Noradrenaline	Norepinephrine, Levarterenol
Orciprenaline	Metaproterenol
Oxybuprocaine	Benoxinate
Paracetamol	Acetaminophen
Pethidine	Meperidine
Salbutamol	Albuterol

REFERENCES

1. Koch-Weser J. Serum drug concentrations as therapeutic guides. *N Engl J Med* 1972; **287**: 227–31.
2. Winek CL. Tabulation of therapeutic, toxic and lethal concentrations of drugs and chemicals in blood. *Clin Chem* 1976; **22**: 832–6.
3. Richens A, Warrington S. When should plasma drug levels be monitored? *Curr Ther* 1979; **20**: 167–85.
4. Koch-Weser J. The serum level approach to individualization of drug dosage. *Eur J Clin Pharm* 1975; **9**: 1–8.
5. Davies DS, Prichard BNC. *Biological Effects of Drugs in Relation to their Plasma Concentrations.* London: Macmillan; 1973.

Appendix 6

Confirmation of intubation

This is a frequently performed procedure in anaesthesia, in the ICU and in a wide range of emergency situations with very variable availability of sophisticated equipment. It is also the cause of significant morbidity and mortality.

This is a simple check list which can be modified depending on the equipment available.

Always:

- Visualise the passage of the tip of the endotracheal tube through the vocal cords at intubation, where possible (most reliable but not perfect).
- Observe. Continuous observation of rise and fall of the chest on ventilation.
- Auscultate. Confirm air entry by auscultation in the axillae and also listen over the stomach. The axillae will confirm bilateral air entry (and indicate endobronchial intubation if air entry is unilateral). Auscultation over the stomach will allow differential breath sounds between axillae and stomach and may indicate oesophageal tube placement if the stomach sounds are louder.
- Observe the patient's colour – they should remain pink.

Equipment should be available that will also assist.

- Capnography. CO_2 in the exhaled air is a reliable indicator of correct tube placement. Capnography should always be available for anaesthesia and certainly for transfer of critically ill patients. Ideally, it should be easily available in any ICU.
- Oximetry helps confirm oxygenation.

Of these, visualisation and capnography are most reliable for intubation but all have a part to play and anyone intubating a patient must have a checklist to confirm correct placement.

'If in doubt, take it out.' Sometimes some of the four basic signs are unconvincing but if there is any doubt the tube should be replaced or mouth to mouth/mask ventilation should be used.

Appendix 7

Parameters monitored and measured by the PiCCO monitor

New non-invasive monitors have introduced some new 'measurements' into clinical practice.

Parameter normal value	Symbol
Pulse contour cardiac output/index CI 3.0–5.0 l/min per m^2 Pulse contour cardiac output is calibrated by means of a simple transcardiopulmonary thermodilution measurement	PCCO/PCCI
Global end diastolic volume/index 680–800 ml/m^2 (indexed) The total end-diastolic volume of all four chambers of the heart	GEDV/I
Intrathoracic blood volume/index 850–1000 ml/m^2 (indexed) The global end-diastolic volume plus the pulmonary blood volume	ITBV/I
Extravascular lung water/index 3.0–7.0 ml/kg (indexed) Quantifies lung status in terms of pulmonary permeability	EVLW/I
Cardiac function index 4.5–6.5 l/min (indexed) CO/GEDV = preload independent variable of heart function	CFI
Stroke volume/index 40–60 ml/m^2	SV/I
Stroke volume variation <10% Percentage difference of biggest to smallest stroke volumes over the last 30 seconds	SVV
Left ventricular contractility 1200–2000 mmHg/sec Maximum velocity of blood pressure curve corresponds to maximum power or contractility of the left heart	dP/dtmax
Systemic vascular resistance/index 1200–2000 dyn/s/cm^{-5} per m^2 (indexed)	SVR/SVRI

EVLW
There are two mechanisms by which the EVLW may be raised – increased intravascular filtration pressure (left heart failure, volume overload), and increased pulmonary vascular permeability as in endotoxic shock and sepsis.
There is a direct relationship between the mortality of intensive care patients with acute respiratory distress syndrome and high extravascular lung water.

SVV
Large variations in stroke volume are an indication of reduced intravascular volume (also atrial fibrillation, heart valve disease).

Appendix 8

Paediatric risk of mortality (PRISM) score. Mortality risk assessment.

Parameter	Age limit	Ranges	Points
Systolic blood pressure (mmHg)	Infants	130–160	2
		55–65	2
		>160	6
		40–54	6
		< 40	7
	Children	150–200	2
		65–75	2
		>200	6
		50–64	6
		< 50	7
Diastolic blood pressure (mmHg)	All ages	>110	6
Heart rate (beats/min)	Infants	>160	4
		<90	4
	Children	>150	4
		<80	4
Respiratory rate (breaths/min)	Infants	61–90	1
		>90	5
		Apnoea	5
	Children	51–70	1
		>70	5
		Apnoea	5
Pao_2/Fio_2	All ages	200–300	2
		<200	3
$Paco_2$ in torr (mmHg)	All ages	51–65	1
		>65	5
Glasgow coma score	All ages	<8	6
Pupillary reactions	All ages	Unequal or dilated	4
		Fixed and dilated	10
PT/PTT	All ages	1.5 times control	2
Total bilirubin mg/dl	>1 month	>3.5	6
Potassium in mEq/l	All ages	3.0–3.5	1
		6.5–7.5	1
		<3.0	5
		>7.5	5
Calcium in mg/dl	All ages	7.0–8.0	2
		12.0–15.0	2
		<7.0	6
		>15.0	6
Glucose in mg/dl	All ages	40–60	4
		250–400	4
		<40	8
		>400	8
Bicarbonate in mEq/l	All ages	<16	3
		>32	3

Infants: 0–1 year of age. PRISM score = (systolic blood pressure points) + (diastolic blood pressure points) + (heart rate points) + (respiratory rate points) + (oxygenation points) + (Glasgow coma score points) + (pupillary reaction points) + (coagulation points) + (bilirubin points) + (potassium points) + (calcium points) + (glucose points) + (bicarbonate points).

Sepsis-related organ failure assessment (SOFA) score. Easy to calculate, describes the sequence of complications in a critically ill patient rather than predicting outcome.

Organ system	Measure
Respiration	Pa_{O_2} to Fi_{O_2} ratio
Coagulation	Platelet count
Liver	Serum bilirubin
Cardiovascular	Hypotension
Central nervous system	Glasgow coma score
Renal	Serum creatinine or urine output

Measure	Finding	Points
Pa_{O_2} to Fi_{O_2} ratio	≥ 400 (mmHg)	0
	300–399 (mmHg)	1
	200–299 (mmHg)	2
	100–199 (mmHg)	3
	<100 (mmHg)	4
Platelet count	≥ 1500/μl	0
	1000–149 999/μl	1
	500–99 999/μl	2
	200–49 999/μl	3
	<200 per μl	4
Serum bilirubin	<1.2 mg/dl	0
	1.2–1.9 mg/dl	1
	2.0–5.9 mg/dl	2
	6.0–11.9 mg/dl	3
	≥ 12.0 mg/dl	4
Hypotension	Mean arterial pressure ≥ 70 (mmHg)	0
	Mean arterial pressure <70 then (no pressor agents used) (mmHg)	1
	Dobutamine any dose	2
	Dopamine ≤ 5 μg/kg per min	2
	Dopamine >5–15 μg/kg per min	3
	Dopamine >15 μg/kg per min	4
	Adrenaline ≤ 0.1 μg/kg per min	3
	Adrenaline >0.1 μg/kg per min	4
	Noradrenaline ≤ 0.1 μg/kg per min	3
	Noradrenaline >0.1 μg/kg per min	4
Glasgow coma score	15	0
	13–14	1
	10–12	2
	6–9	3
	3–5	4
Serum creatinine or urine output	Serum creatinine <1.2 mg/dl	0
	Serum creatinine 1.2–1.9 mg/dl	1
	Serum creatinine 2.0–3.4 mg/dl	2
	Serum creatinine 3.5–4.9 mg/dl	3
	Urine output 200–499 ml/day	3
	Serum creatinine >5.0 mg/dl	4
	Urine output <200 ml/day	4

Pa_{O_2} is in mmHg and Fi_{O_2} in per cent, from 0.21 to 1.00.
Adrenergic agents as administered for at least 1 hour with doses in μg/kg per min.
A score of 0 indicates normal and a score of 4 indicates most abnormal.
Data can be collected and the score calculated daily during the course of the admission.
Interpretation: minimum total score: 0; maximum total score: 24.
The higher the organ score, the greater the organ dysfunction.
The higher the total score, the greater the multiorgan dysfunction.

Mortality rate by SOFA score.[1]

Organ system	0	1	2	3	4
Respiratory	20%	27%	32%	46%	64%
Cardiovascular	22%	32%	55%	55%	55%
Coagulation	35%	35%	35%	64%	64%
CNS	32%	34%	50%	53%	56%
Renal	25%	40%	46%	56%	64%

LOGISTIC ORGAN DYSFUNCTION SYSTEM (LODS)

Assess patients for severity of critical organ dysfunction. To predict the probability of death for the patient.

Data collection	During the first 24 hours in the ICU
Data point	If not measured then it is assumed to be normal for scoring purposes
	If several measurements, use the most severe value

LOD score = (neurologic score) + (cardiovascular score) + (renal score) + (pulmonary score) + (haematological score) + (hepatic score).

Neurologic score.

Glasgow coma score	Points
14–15	0
9–13	1
6–8	3
< 6	5

Use lowest value. If sedated, estimate the score prior to sedation.

Cardiovascular score.

Heart rate (beats/min)		Systolic BP in (mmHg)	Points
30–139	*and*	90–239	0
≥ 140	*or*	240–269	1
		70–89	1
		≥270	3
		40–69	3
<30	*or*	<40	5

The most abnormal value for heart rate or systolic blood pressure either minimum or maximum.

Renal score.

Serum urea nitrogen mg/dl		Creatinine mg/dl		Urine output (l/d)	Points
<17	*and*	< 1.20	AND	0.75–9.99	0
17–27.99	*or*	1.2–1.59			1
28–55.99	*or*	≥1.60	OR	≥10	3
				0.5–0.74	3
≥56					5
				<0.5	5

Highest value for urea nitrogen and for creatinine.
If the urine output data are for less than a 24-hour period, adjust that value to 24 hours, assuming the same rate of excretion.
On haemodialysis, use the value of urine output prior to initiating haemodialysis

Pulmonary score.

On ventilation or CPAP?		Ratio (PaO_2 in mmHg)/(FiO_2)	Points
No			0
Yes	*and*	≥ 150	1
Yes	*and*	< 150	3

Respiratory support; use the lowest ratio of PaO_2 to FiO_2.

Haematological score.

White blood cell count 10^9/l		Platelet count 10^9/l	Points
2.5–4.9/μl	*and*	$\geq$ 50/μl	0
$\geq$ 50/μl			1
1–2.4/μl	*or*	< 50/μl	1
<1/μl			3

Note: Most abnormal value for the white cell count either minimum or maximum.
Minimum platelet count if several values are available.

Hepatic score.[2]

Bilirubin		Prothrombin time	Points
< 2.0 mg/dl (< 34.2 μmol/l)	*and*	$\leq$ 3 seconds above standard ($\geq$ 25% of standard)	0
$\geq$ 2.0 mg/dl ($\geq$ 34.2 μmol/l)	*or*	> 3 seconds above standard (< 25% of standard)	1

Highest value for bilirubin available. Highest value for prothrombin time in seconds.

MPM II, MORTALITY PROBABILITY MODELS.[3,4]

Excluded
- Age < 18 years
- Burn patients
- Coronary care patients
- Cardiac surgery patients

(The scoring is either present or not present)

Definitions

Coma or deep stupor at time of ICU admission
- Not due to drug overdosage
- If patient is on paralysing muscle relaxant, awakening from anaesthesia or heavily sedated, use best judgement of the level of consciousness prior to sedation
- *Coma*: no response to any stimulation; no twitching, no movements in extremities, no response to pain or command; Glasgow coma score 3
- *Deep stupor*: decorticate or decerebrate posturing; posturing is spontaneous or in response to stimulation or deep pain; posturing is not in response to commands; Glasgow coma score 4 or 5

Heart rate at ICU admission
- Heart rate $\geq$ 150 beats/min within 1 hour before or after ICU admission

Systolic blood pressure at ICU admission
- Systolic blood pressure $\leq$ 90 mmHg within 1 hour before or after ICU admission

Chronic renal compromise or insufficiency
- Elevation of serum creatinine > 2 mg/dl and documented as chronic in the medical record
- If there is the acute diagnosis on chronic renal failure then only record yes for acute renal failure

Cirrhosis
- History of heavy alcohol use with portal hypertension and varices
- Other causes of liver disease with evidence of portal hypertension and varices
- Biopsy confirmation of cirrhosis

Metastatic malignant neoplasm
- Stage IV carcinomas with distant metastases
- Do not include involvement only of regional lymph nodes
- Include if metastases are obvious by clinical assessment or confirmed by a pathology report
- Do not include if metastases not obvious, or if pathology report is not available at the time of ICU admission
- Acute haematological malignancies are included
- Chronic leukaemias are not included unless there are findings attributable to the disease or the patient is under active treatment for the leukaemia. Findings include sepsis, anaemia, stroke caused by clumping of white blood cells, tumour lysis syndrome with elevated uric acid following chemotherapy, pulmonary oedema or the lymphangiectatic form of acute respiratory distress syndrome

Acute renal failure
- Acute tubular necrosis or acute diagnosis on chronic renal failure
- Prerenal azotaemia is not included

Cardiac dysrhythmia
- Cardiac arrhythmia, paroxysmal tachycardia, fibrillation with rapid ventricular response, second- or third-degree heart block
- Do not include chronic and stable arrhythmias

Cerebrovascular incident
- Cerebral embolism, occlusion, cerebrovascular accident, stroke, brainstem infarction, cerebrovascular arteriovenous malformation (acute stroke or cerebrovascular haemorrhage, not chronic arteriovenous malformation)

Gastrointestinal bleeding
- Haematemesis, melaena
- A perforated ulcer does not necessarily indicate GI bleeding; may be identified by obvious 'coffee grounds' in nasogastric tube
- A drop of haemoglobin by itself is not sufficient evidence of acute GI bleeding

Intracranial mass effect
- Intracranial mass (abscess, tumour, haemorrhage, subdural) as identified by CT scan associated with any of the following: (1) midline shift; (2) obliteration or distortion of cerebral ventricles; (3) gross haemorrhage in cerebral ventricles or subarachnoid space; (4) visible mass > 4 cm; or (5) any mass that enhances with contrast media
- If the mass effect is known within 1 hour of ICU admission, it can be indicated as yes
- CT scanning is not mandated and is only indicated for patients with major neurological insult

Age in years
- Patient's age at last birthday

CPR within 24 hours prior to ICU admission
- CPR includes chest compression, defibrillation or cardiac massage
- Not affected by the location where the CPR was administered

Mechanical ventilation
- Patient is using a ventilator at the time of ICU admission or immediately thereafter

Medical or unscheduled surgery admission
- Do not include elective surgical patients (surgery scheduled at least 24 hours in advance) or preoperative Swan-Ganz catheter insertion in elective surgery patients

REFERENCES

1. Vincent JL, Moreno R, Takala J *et al.* The SOFA (Sepsis-related Organ Failure Assessment) score to describe organ dysfunction/failure. *Int Care Med* 1996; **22**: 707–10.
2. Le Gall J, Klar J, Lemeshow S *et al.* The logistic organ dysfunction system. *JAMA* 1996; **276**: 802–10.
3. Lemeshow S, Teres D, Klar J *et al.* Mortality Probability Models (MPM II) based on an international cohort of intensive care patients. *JAMA* 1993; **270**: 2478–86.
4. Lemeshow S, Le Gall J-R. Modeling the severity of illness of ICU patients. *JAMA* 1994; **272**: 1049–55.

Index

Notes: This index is presented in a letter-by-letter order, whereby hyphens and spaces between words are ignored. Cross-references in *italics* refer to general references (e.g. *see also specific drugs*).

B

E

H

I

J

K

L

M

N

P

Q

R

T

U

V

W

Y

Z